Clinical Pathways

Exemplars

Critical Care Nursing

Linda Bucher, DNSc, RN
Associate Professor of Nursing
University of Delaware
Newark, Delaware

Sheila Melander, DSN, RN, FCCM
Associate Professor of Nursing
University of Southern Indiana
Evansville, Indiana

W.B. SAUNDERS COMPANY
A Division of Harcourt Brace & Company
Philadelphia   London   Toronto   Montreal   Sydney   Tokyo

W.B. SAUNDERS COMPANY
A Division of Harcourt Brace & Company

The Curtis Center
Independence Square West
Philadelphia, Pennsylvania 19106

NOTICE

Nursing is an ever-changing field. Standard safety precautions must be followed, but as new research and clinical experience broaden our knowledge, changes in treatment and drug therapy become necessary or appropriate. Readers are advised to check the product information currently provided by the manufacturer of each drug to be administered to verify the recommended dose, the method and duration of administration, and the contraindications. It is the responsibility of the treating physician, relying on experience and knowledge of the patient, to determine dosages and the best treatment for the patient. Neither the publisher nor the editors assumes any responsibility for any injury and/or damage to persons or property.

THE PUBLISHER

Library of Congress Cataloging-in-Publication Data

Bucher, Linda.
Critical care nursing / Linda Bucher and Sheila Melander.—1st ed.

p.   cm.

ISBN 0–7216–6917–4

1. Intensive care nursing.   I. Melander, Sheila.   II. Title.
[DNLM: 1. Critical Illness—nursing.   2. Critical Care nurses'
instruction.   WY 154 M517c 1999]

RT120.I5B8 1999   610.73'61—dc21

DNLM/DLC   98–7040

CRITICAL CARE NURSING   ISBN 0–7216–6917–4

Printed in the United States of America.

Last digit is the print number: 9   8   7   6   5   4   3   2   1

The editors would like to dedicate this textbook to you—the critical care nursing student. We sincerely hope that the content and special features of this book will help prepare you to enter the critical care arena with confidence and enthusiasm. Every effort has been taken to provide the most current and relevant information needed by students to meet the challenges of the critical care environment in the 21st century. You have chosen to study one of the most rewarding specialties in nursing. Enjoy your journey.

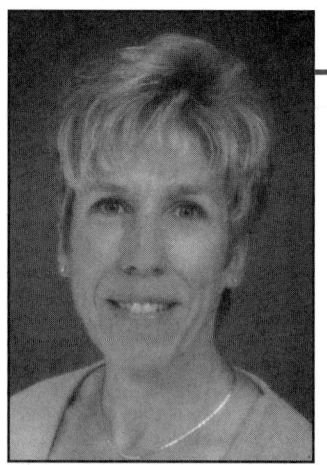

Linda Bucher, DNSc, RN, is an Associate Professor of Nursing in College of Health and Nursing Sciences at the University of Delaware. She teaches the graduate, undergraduate, and RN nursing students. In 1993, she implemented an elective honors program in critical care nursing which was developed in collaboration with a major health care center, for senior baccalaureate students. Students who complete the program have been consistently hired into a variety of critical care settings.

Dr. Bucher's experiences in nursing have covered a variety of settings and positions. Over the past 20 years, she worked as a staff nurse in medical-surgical, home care, and critical care nursing. She also served as a patient and staff development educator. Currently, Dr. Bucher also works as a per diem nurse in Critical Care/Emergency.

Dr. Bucher has been active in the American Association of Critical Care Nurses since 1987 and is a past president of the Southeastern Pennsylvania chapter of AACN.

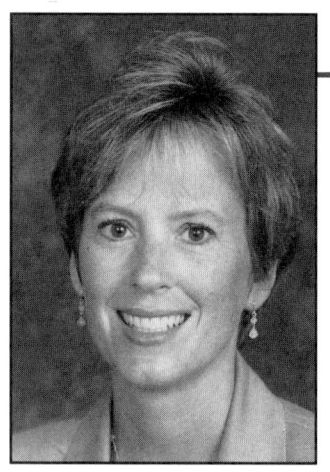

Sheila Melander, DSN, RN, is an Associate Professor of Nursing in the School of Nursing and Health Professions at the University of Southern Indiana. Dr. Melander is the course coordinator for the baccalaureate level critical care course and the graduate theory course. She received her BSN and MSN from the University of Evansville, Evansville, Indiana, and her DSN from the University of Alabama at Birmingham. Dr. Melander will earn her Acute Care Nurse Practitioners degree at Vanderbilt University in the summer of 1999. She has been a member of the American Association of Critical Care Nurses for many years and currently is serving as the chair of the Professional Development Think Tank. Dr. Melander has taught baccalaureate level critical care nursing students for 9 years and is the author of *Review of Critical Care Nursing: Case Studies and Applications* (W.B. Saunders Company).

Contributors

Rubi Agana-Defensor, RN, MS
Nurse Analyst
National Institutes of Health
Bethesda, Maryland

Marian S. Altman, MS, RN, ANP, CCRN
Adjunct Faculty
Medical College of Virginia School of Nursing
Richmond, Virginia
Adult Nurse Practitioner for GI/Renal Faculty
    Attending Service
Medical College of Virginia Hospital
Richmond, Virginia

Karen L. Baker, MSN
Clinical Nurse Specialist
National Institutes of Health
Clinical Center Nursing Department
Bethesda, Maryland

Deborah Becker, MSN, RN, CCRN
Lecturer
Adult Critical Care Nurse Practitioner Program
University of Pennsylvania School of Nursing
Philadelphia, Pennsylvania

Lisa Anne Bove, MSN, RN,C, CCRN
Project Manager
Shared Medical Systems
Malvern, Pennsylvania

Elisabeth G. Bradley, BSN, MS
Adjunct Instructor
Department of Nursing
University of Delaware
Newark, Delaware
Clinical Nurse Specialist—Critical Care
Christiana Care Health Services
Wilmington Hospital
Wilmington, Delaware

Jo Ann Brooks-Brunn, DNS, RN, FAAN
Assistant Professor
Pulmonary, Critical Care, and Occupational Medicine
Associate Scientist
Mary Margaret Walther Cancer Care Program
Indiana University School of Nursing
Indianapolis, Indiana
Past Member, Board of Directors
American Association of Critical-Care Nurses

Danni Brown, MS, RN
Manager, Hypothermia Project
University of Pittsburgh Medical Center
Pittsburgh, Pennsylvania

Linda Bucher, DNSc, RN
Associate Professor of Nursing
University of Delaware
Newark, Delaware

Karen K. Carlson, MN, RN, CCRN
Clinical Faculty
School of Nursing
Department of Biobehavioral Nursing
University of Washington
Seattle, Washington
Critical Care Nurse Specialist
Carlson Consulting Group
Bellevue, Washington

Belinda Childs, MN, RN, ARNP, CDE
Adjunct Faculty
Department of Nursing
Wichita State University
Diabetes Clinical Nurse Specialist
Clinic Coordination
Mid-America Diabetes Associates
Wichita, Kansas

Margaret H. Doherty, MSN, RN, CCRN
Instructor
Department of Nursing
Sonoma State University
Rohnert Park, California
Staff Nurse
Intensive Care Unit
Petaluma Valley Hospital
Petaluma, California

Catharine Dorozinsky, MSN, RN, CCTC, CRNT
Heart Transplant Coordinator
University of Pennsylvania Medical Center
Philadelphia, Pennsylvania

Sharon E. Douglass, MS
Associate Professor
Department of Health Professions and Physical
    Therapy
Director, HIV/AIDS Education Office
University of Central Florida
Orlando, Florida

Carolyn J. Driscoll, MSN, RN, FNP
Staff Nurse
Surgical Intensive Care Unit
University of Virginia Health System
Charlottesville, Virginia

Phyllis Dubendorf, MSN, RN, CCRN, CNRN
Faculty
Acute/Adult Tertiary Nurse Practitioner Program
University of Pennsylvania School of Nursing
Neurosurgical Nurse Practitioner
Thomas Jefferson University Hospital
Philadelphia, Pennsylvania

Carol Germain, EdD, RN, FAAN
Associate Professor
University of Pennsylvania School of Nursing
Philadelphia, Pennsylvania

Karen K. Giuliano, MSN, RN, CCRN, ANP
Clinical Nurse Specialist
Critical Care
Baystate Medical Center
Springfield, Massachusetts

Mary Linn Green, MSN, JD, RN
Nurse Attorney
Law Firm of Kostantacos, Traum, Rueterfors &
    McWilliams, P.C.
Rockford, Illinois

Elisabeth Greenfield, MSN, RN, CCRN
Colonel, Army Nurse Corps (Ret.)
Research Nurse
United States Army Institute of Surgical Research
Fort Sam Houston, Texas

Donna F. Hardwick, RN,C
Clinical Staff Nurse
Clinical Center Nursing Department
National Institutes of Health
Bethesda, Maryland

Debbie Hinnen, MN, RN, ARNP, CDE
Assistant Clinical Professor
University of Kansas School of Medicine
Adjunct Faculty
Department of Nursing
Wichita State University and
    Butler County Community College
Wichita, Kansas
Manager, Diabetes Services
Via Christi Regional Medical Center, St Joseph
    Campus
Wichita, Kansas

Julie A. Jamison, MN, RN, ARNP, CDE
Program Director
Diabetes Education
Wichita Clinic
Wichita, Kansas

Connie A. Jastremski, MS, MBA, RN, ANP
Assistant Professor
College of Nursing
SUNY Health Science Center
Syracuse, New York

Kimmith M. Jones, MS, RN, CCRN
Faculty Associate
University of Maryland School of Nursing
Baltimore, Maryland
Advanced Practice Nurse
Critical Care/Emergency Center
Sinai Hospital of Baltimore
Baltimore, Maryland

Carleen B. Kelley, MS, CCRN
Clinical Specialist, Surgical Nursing
Washington Hospital Center
Washington, D.C.

Joanne Konick-McMahan, MSN, RN, CCRN
Clinical Lecturer
Graduate Division
Adult Health and Illness
University of Pennsylvania
Clinical Nurse Specialist
Heart Failure Study
School of Nursing
University of Pennsylvania
Philadelphia, Pennsylvania

Catherine Nuss Kotecki, DNSc, RN, CNS,C
Assistant Professor
School of Nursing
University of Medicine and Dentistry of New Jersey
Stratford, New Jersey

Linda Laskowski-Jones, MS, RN, CS, CCRN, CEN
Trauma Program Coordinator/Clinical Nurse
   Specialist
Christiana Care Health Services
Newark, Delaware

Nancy Livingston, MSN, RN, FNP
Nurse Practitioner
Cardiomyopathy Center
University of California, Los Angeles
Los Angeles, California

Karen March, MN, RN
Clinical Faculty
Department of Biobehavioral Nursing
University of Washington
Seattle, Washington
Neuroscience Clinical Nurse Specialist
Harborview Medical Center
Seattle, Washington

Donna W. Markey, MSN, RN, ACNP
Clinician IV–General Surgery and Surgical Oncology
Acute Care Nurse Practitioner
University of Virginia Health Sciences Center
Charlottesville, Virginia

Kathy McCloy, MSN, RN, ACNP
Assistant Clinical Professor of Nursing
School of Nursing
University of California, Los Angeles
Acute Care Nurse Practitioner
Interventional Cardiology
UCLA Medical Center
Los Angeles, California

Debra Lynn-McHale, MSN, RN
Doctoral Candidate
University of Pennsylvania
Staff Nurse, Medical and Surgical Critical Care Units
Thomas Jefferson University Hospital
Philadelphia, Pennsylvania

Mary G. McKinley, MSN, RN, CCRN
President, American Association of Critical-Care
   Nurses, 1998–1999
Clinical Nurse Specialist, Critical Care
Ohio Valley Medical Center
Wheeling, West Virginia

Sheila Melander, DSN, RN
Associate Professor of Nursing
University of Southern Indiana
Evansville, Indiana

Paulette Morelli, MSN, RN, CNS, FNP, CCRN
Adjunct Instructor
Department of Nursing
University of Delaware
Newark, Delaware
Clinical Nurse Specialist/Nurse Practitioner
Christiana Care Health Services, Heart Center
Christiana, Delaware

Janet Flynn Mulroy, MSN, RN, CCRN
Staff Nurse Respiratory ICU
Baptist Memorial Hospital
Memphis, Tennessee

Susan A. Pfettscher, DNSc, RN
Associate Professor
Department of Nursing
California State University, Bakersfield
Bakersfield, California

Lisa Plowfield, PhD, RN
Assistant Professor
Department of Nursing
University of Delaware
Program Director
HEALTH Center
University of Delaware
Newark, Delaware

M. Lynn Rodgers, MSN, RN,C, CCRN, CNRN
Critical Care Clinical Nurse Specialist
Deaconess Hospital
Evansville, Indiana

Bonnie R. Sakallaris, MSN
Patient Care Director, CVICU
Inova Fairfax Hospital
Falls Church, Virginia

Susan S. Scott, BSN, RN, CCRN
Critical Care Educator
Baystate Medical Center
Springfield, Massachusetts

Diane Schwenker, MSN, RN, CCRN, CNRN
Staff
Neuroscience Consultant
University of Pennsylvania Health System
Philadelphia, Pennsylvania

Tess L. Sierzant, MS, RN, CNRN
Clinical Nurse Specialist, Neuroscience
Abbott Northwestern Hospital
Minneapolis, Minnesota

Rebecca S. Sloan, PhD, MSN
Assistant Professor of Nursing
Department of Family Health
Indiana University School of Nursing
Indianapolis, Indiana
Research Consultant and Advanced Nurse
   Practitioner
Kidney Disease Program
University of Louisville
Louisville, Kentucky

June Stark, BSN, MEd, RN
Critical Care Consultant
Director of Care Management and Utilization
St. Elizabeth Medical Center
Boston, Massachusetts

Jane Van Tatenhove, MSN, CCRN
Clinical Supervisor, Surgical Nursing
Washington Hospital Center
Washington, D.C.

Carla Ware, BSN, RN
Staff Nurse, Intensive Care Unit
California Pacific Medical Center
San Francisco, California

Claudia M. West, MS, RN
Associate Clinical Professor
Department of Physiological Nursing
University of California, San Francisco
San Francisco, California

Una Elizabeth Westfall, PhD, RN
Professor
Population-Based Nursing Department
Oregon Health Science University School of Nursing
Portland, Oregon

Anne W. Wojner, MSN, RN, CCRN
President-Elect, AACN
Assistant Professor of Clinical Nursing
The University of Texas at Houston Health Science
   Center
Houston, Texas
President
Health Outcomes Institute, Inc.
The Woodlands, Texas

Reviewers

Kathleen Andrews, MN, RN, CCRN
Missouri Western State College
St. Joseph, Missouri

Susan Appel, MN, RN, CCRN, CS
Carolinas College of Health Sciences
Charlotte, North Carolina

Maddy A. Biggs, BSN, RN
Johns Hopkins Hospital
Baltimore, Maryland

Wendy Blackburn, BScN, MA(Ed), RN, PG(MNI), CNN,C
Parkwood Hospital
London, Ontario

Betty Nash Blevins, MSN, RN, CCRN, CS
Bluefield State College
Bluefield, West Virginia

Mary Ann Boucher, MS, RN
Pikeville College
Pikeville, Kentucky

Jo Anne Brocksmith, MSN, RN, AAS
Vincennes University
Vincennes, Indiana

Luann M. Daggett, MSN, RN
The University of Southern Mississippi
College of Nursing
Meridian, Mississippi

Marla J. DeJong, MS, RN, CCRN, CEN
Captain Wilford Hall Medical Center
Lackland Air Force Base
Texas

Michele A. DeBiasse, MS, RD, CS, CNSD
Quincy Hospital
Quincy, Massachusetts

Mary Fabick, MSN, MEd, RN, CEN
Milligan College
Milligan College, Tennessee

Carol Goodyear-Bruch, MSN, RN, CCRN
Graceland College
Independence, Missouri

Marcia D. Gragert, PhD, RN
Montana State University–Bozeman
Great Falls, Montana

Joan S. Grant, RSN, RN, CS
University of Alabama at Birmingham
School of Nursing
Birmingham, Alabama

Debra Hagler, MS, RN, CS, CCRN
Arizona State University
College of Nursing
Tempe, Arizona

Karolyn R. Hanna, MSN, RN, PhD
Santa Barbara City College
Santa Barbara, California

Denise Haught
Oklahoma City Community College
Oklahoma City, Oklahoma

Patricia A. Kelly, PhDc, RN, CS, FNP, CCRN, CEN
Family Health Care of Albany and Muncie
Albany, Indiana/Muncie, Indiana

Ruth M. Kleinpell, PhD, RN, CCRN
Rush University
College of Nursing
Chicago, Illinois

Marilyn Leichty, PhD, RN
Iowa Wesleyan College
Mount Pleasant, Iowa

Maureen E. Leonardo, MN, RN
Duquesne University
Pittsburgh, Pennsylvania

Deborah Marantides, MSN, RN
Case Western Reserve University
Cleveland, Ohio

Lisa Mason, MS, RN, CS
Raritan Bay Medical Center
Perth Amboy, New Jersey

Lisa Massarweh, MSN, RN, CCRN
Kent State University
Ashtabula, Ohio

Diane Bateman McDougal, MNEd, RN
Youngstown State University
Youngstown, Ohio

Ronald Mitchell, PhD, RN
Idaho State University
Pocatello, Idaho

Kathryn Embrey Moss, RN, CCRN, CEN, ICP
Prince William Hospital
Manassas, Virginia

Sera Nicosia, BScN, MA(Ed), CNNc
Hamilton General Hospital
Hamilton, Ontario

Mary Jean Osborne, MSN, RN, CCRN
Lehigh Valley Hospital
Allentown, Pennsylvania

Phyllis G. Peterson, MN, RN, AOCN
Our Lady of Holy Cross College
New Orleans, Louisiana

Kimberly Quinn, MSN, RN, CCRN
Johns Hopkins Hospital
Baltimore, Maryland

Dolores A. Robertson, MSN, RN, CEN
Graceland College
Division of Nursing
Independence, Missouri

Nancy L. Sarpy, MS, RN, CCRN, CS
Loma Linda University
Loma Linda, California

Cynde C. Small, MSN, RN
Lake Michigan College
Benton Harbor, Michigan

Myra A. Smith, PhD, RN
University of Alabama at Birmingham
School of Nursing
Birmingham, Alabama

Janice M. Sylakowski, MS, RN
State University of New York at Buffalo
Buffalo, New York

Lyn A. Tepper, MS, RN
Northwest Community Hospital
Arlington Heights, Illinois
University of Illinois at Chicago
College of Nursing
Chicago, Illinois

Cynthia Lee Terry, MSN, RN, CCRN
Lehigh Carbon Community College
Schnecksville, Pennsylvania

Maureen Tess
Rush University
College of Nursing
Chicago, Illinois

Nancy Thornton, MSN
Canadian Association of Neuroscience Nurses
World Federation of Neuroscience Nurses
Vancouver, British Columbia

Pamela Becker Weiletz, MSN(R), RN, CS, ANP
Barnes-Jewish College Health System
Barnes-Jewish Hospital
St. Louis, Missouri

Pamela Wetter, BSN, MS, RN
St. Elizabeth School of Nursing
Lafayette, Indiana

Kathleen S. Whalen, MN, RN, CCRN
Community College of Denver
Denver, Colorado

Kathryn M. Wirtz, MSN, RN-CS, CCRN, CNRN
Veterans Administration
Chicago Health Care System
Chicago, Illinois

Preface

The next millennium will herald many exciting challenges for critical care nursing. This textbook, *Critical Care Nursing*, has been developed especially for nursing students who will be entering practice during that time. The primary purpose of this book is to provide students with the essential concepts that form the basis of critical care nursing. These concepts are built on a strong medical-surgical foundation and will be needed by students to adequately prepare them for practice in the present and future health care environment.

Today, patients are admitted to acute care facilities sicker than ever before and discharged from these facilities quicker than ever before. Critical care technology, such as cardiac monitoring, ventilators, and arterial pressure monitoring, is commonplace both inside and outside the traditional critical care unit. Tomorrow's hospitals are expected to become predominantly large critical care and intermediate care units. The nurse with critical care skills will find practice opportunities across the health care continuum as critically ill patients will increasingly be managed in outpatient centers (e.g., heart failure clinics), transitional care settings, and the home. To address these future trends, schools of nursing are designing curricula that require a course in critical care nursing. This type of visionary thinking will arm students with the essential critical care knowledge and skills needed to manage the acute care population of the next millennium.

In preparing *Critical Care Nursing*, contributors from 19 different states, representing state-of-the-art critical care nursing practice across the United States, were solicited. These nationally recognized nurse experts are engaged in a variety of roles: clinical educator, clinical nurse specialist, staff nurse, lawyer, nurse practitioner, nurse consultant, faculty member. Reviewers from both educational and clinical settings provided their suggestions to produce a timely and relevant textbook.

ORGANIZATION

Content of Units

The book is organized into eight units. Unit 1, **Introduction to Critical Care,** contains five chapters that provide the foundation for professional critical care nursing practice. In addition, information in these chapters is aimed at assisting the student to understand and manage the complex role of the critical care nurse. Chapter 1, *Critical Care Across the Health Care Continuum,* explores the current trends and future predictions for health care and their potential impact on the critical care nurse and environment. Chapter 2, *Legal and Ethical Issues in Critical Care Nursing,* presents information that will prepare the student to approach patient care within the boundaries of the law while addressing the ethical dilemmas that frequent the critical care environment. Chapter 3, *Professional Role of the Critical Care Nurse,* defines standards for critical care nursing practice and examines the evolving and complex role of the critical care nurse. In addition, there is emphasis on the importance of the professional organization and personal stress management for the critical care nurse. Chapter 4, *Impact of Critical Illness on the Patient and Family,* the longest chapter in Unit 1, reviews the stress response as it relates to critically ill adult patients and explores, in detail, the impact of critical illness on the adult patient and family. The needs of families (e.g., visitation, information, coping) are identified, and management strategies are presented from a collaborative perspective. Major needs that are common to most critically ill patients (e.g., relief from pain and anxiety, sleep, coping, communication, sexuality, spirituality) are fully explored by presenting the underlying theory (or theoretical definition), collaborative management strategies, and anticipated patient outcomes. Finally, this chapter also includes content on the unique physiological and psychosocial needs of the critically ill elderly patient. Unit 1 closes with a chapter on *Cultural Issues in Critical Care Nursing*. This chapter provides information on projected population demographics for the next millennium and their implications on critical care nursing practice. Critical care nurses need to be culturally self-aware and sensitive to the diversity of beliefs and values. Different cultural perspectives on responses to health crises, pain expression, grief, and death are presented.

Units 2 through 7 address various disorders commonly seen in critical care nursing practice. Units are organized according to body systems and include **Cardiovascular, Respiratory, Renal, Endocrine, Gastrointestinal, and Neurologic Disorders.** These units are organized in a similar fashion. The first chapter in each unit presents an overview of the anatomy and physiology of the body system. A review of the relevant history and physical assessment is provided in the second chapter. Both of these chapters provide sections that address the normal variations associated with aging. The third chapter in each unit presents detailed information on the laboratory and diagnostic testing specific to the body system. The remaining chapters in the unit discuss specific disorders that are commonly seen in adult critically ill patients (e.g., *Acute Myocardial Infarction, Acute Respiratory Failure, Acute Renal Failure, Diabetic Ketoacidosis and Hyperglycemic Hyperosmolar Nonketotic Coma, Acute Gastrointestinal Bleed, Acute Head Injury*).

Unit 8 presents information on common **Multisystem Disorders** seen in critical care nursing. Chapters on *HIV, Shock, Burns, Multiple Organ Dysfunction Syndrome*, and *Trauma* present inclusive information on managing the care of patients experiencing these problems.

Content of Disorder Chapters

Content in each disorder chapter in Units 2 through 8 is organized in a similar format to allow faculty and students to approach the content consistently from chapter to chapter. The *etiology and pathophysiology* of the disorder are presented first and provide the student with a foundation on which to relate the subsequent nursing care. Following the nursing process format, the *assessment* findings (history, physical, and diagnostic work-up) associated with the disorder are presented. Appropriate *nursing diagnoses* are discussed and delineated (Table) using the North American

Nursing Diagnosis Association's (NANDA) Taxonomy and include the problem statements and possible etiologic factors. A comprehensive section on the *collaborative management* of a patient with the disorder is presented. Interventions are fully discussed and a collaborative approach is emphasized. The roles and responsibilities of the various members of the multidisciplinary team (e.g., nurse, physician, respiratory therapist, dietitian, social worker, clergy, pharmacists, physical therapist, rehabilitation specialists) are discussed whenever appropriate. Finally, the anticipated *multidisciplinary outcomes* for patients presenting with the disorder are identified (Chart) and examined.

SPECIAL FEATURES

Features Found in Every Chapter

Objectives: Each chapter opens with a list of student objectives that were developed to reflect the higher level of complex information contained in the book. These are presented to help focus the student on the material that follows.

Key Concepts: Each chapter closes with a list of key concepts that provides the reader with a succinct review of the key information presented in the chapter.

References: Students are encouraged to explore the reference list provided at the end of each chapter. References are current (more recent than 1994 in most cases) and relevant (most references are primary references).

Features Found Throughout Chapters When Appropriate

Beyond the ICU: This unique feature gives insight into the nature of care that critically ill patients often require in nontraditional critical care settings and provides the student with opportunities to explore critical care nursing across the health care continuum (e.g., home care, rehabilitation, out-patient clinics).

Research Utilization: As described in Chapter 3, the knowledge-practice gap in critical care nursing practice must be eliminated. The Research Utilization chart has been designed with this challenge in mind and presents critical care research that was selected to enhance the content through an abstract, research critique, and nursing implications. In several instances the research was conducted by the chapter author.

Ethical Dilemma: The complex, interdependent relationship between critically ill patients and the critical care environment often produces ethical-legal dilemmas. Chapter 2 introduces a framework for resolving many of the common ethical-legal issues in critical care. This feature builds on this foundation by presenting hypothetical practice situations that deal with ethical dilemmas. Questions are posed in such a way as to generate sensitive, introspective discussions. As nurses are faced with increasingly complex patient care situations, scarcity of resources, and greater use of technology, ethical dilemmas will flourish. This teaching-learning strategy will encourage students to explore these scenarios in a safe environment as a way to prepare for future practice.

Clinical Pathway: Numerous and varied clinical pathways (critical paths, algorithms, etc.) are included throughout the disorder chapters. These pathways have been obtained directly from clinical agencies and represent practice guidelines across the United States and, in one case, Canada. It is anticipated that exposure to a variety of pathways will enable students to feel more comfortable with the differences across these forms.

Critical Thinking Exercise: This exercise is provided at the end of each disorder chapter. A clinical situation is presented followed by questions to stimulate critical thinking. This teaching-learning strategy provides opportunities for students to apply new knowledge to hypothetical situations. Answers to these questions can be found in the Instructor's Manual.

Additional Features

Exemplars: This truly unique feature of the book is found in the two-page unit openers. The clinical exemplar represents an example of caring and competent nursing practice which was written by critical care nurses who were nominees for the AACN Excellence in Caring Practice or Clinical Practice Awards. Five of these authors were, in fact, award recipients. These descriptive and compelling real-life narratives provide students with rare insights into the complexities of the role of the critical care nurse and the impact that excellent practice can make on patient and family outcomes.

Appendix: The most current 13 ACLS Guidelines are provided as the appendix. This allows students to refer to the individual algorithms when referenced in specific chapters.

Glossary: This feature is placed at the end of the book and provides easy access to the definitions of critical terms.

ANCILLARY PACKAGE

A complete package that fosters effective teaching and learning accompanies this text. The *Instructor's Manual* includes teaching strategies, clinical learning activities, critical thinking exercise worksheets, answer guidelines to critical thinking exercises in the text, practice ECG strips, suggested Internet and other resources, and transparency masters. A comprehensive *Test Manual* is available with over 500 multiple-choice questions in both printed and CD-ROM versions.

Pocket Companion to Critical Care Nursing by Sheila Melander and Linda Bucher provides quick access to important clinical information in any critical care setting. It includes selected tables, charts, and figures from the text in a pocket-sized format for portability and utility.

Feedback from Readers

Our goal is to provide the most current, clinically applicable content for the dynamic practice of critical care nursing. To that end we welcome comments from faculty and students as you use this book so that we may continue to achieve our goal in any future editions. Please feel free to write us in care of the Publisher.

Best wishes for a successful nursing career,

Linda Bucher

Sheila Melander

Acknowledgments

We would like to express our sincere appreciation to Barbara Nelson Cullen, former Senior Editor in Nursing Books at W. B. Saunders Company, who had the foresight to see a need for this textbook. To Robin Carter, Senior Editor, and Robin L. Richman, Senior Developmental Editor, both in Nursing Books, W. B. Saunders Company, and to Karen Gulliver of Karen Gulliver Productions, we offer a very special thank you; this project could never have come to fruition without your expertise, endless patience, and steady guidance.

We would also like to thank the following people at W. B. Saunders: Shelley Hampton, Production Manager; Agnes Byrne, Project Supervisor; Matt Andrews, artist; and Jonel Sofian, designer, whose combined efforts have produced a truly beautiful textbook.

Finally, we would like to express our deepest gratitude to each of the contributors and reviewers of this textbook. Their expertise and commitment to the profession of nursing are clearly reflected in their written words.

Linda Bucher
Sheila Melander

I would like to thank Dr. Kathleen McCauley for her confidence in my ability to undertake this endeavor. Her early support started this three-year journey. I would also like to express my gratitude to Dr. Betty Paulanka, Dean of the College of Health and Nursing Sciences, University of Delaware, for having the wisdom to suggest that this project might best be completed during a sabbatical leave. Her assistance in arranging for this time was pivotal in our ability to produce this book on schedule. To my family, a special thanks for always being there even when I was not. Finally, to my husband, Bill, my love and appreciation for your endless support—you continue to be my inspiration.

—LB

I would like to thank Dr. Nadine Coudret, Dean of the University of Southern Indiana School of Nursing and Health Professions, and Ann White, Director of the Baccalaureate Nursing Program. The resources, support, and encouragement given by Dean Coudret and Ann have made it possible for me to complete this endeavor. I also want to acknowledge Amy Shively for her friendship and unselfish gift of her time to this project. Most importantly, I would like to thank my husband, Chuck, and my two sons, Ryan and Matthew, for their constant patience and unconditional support.

—SM

Brief Contents

Contents

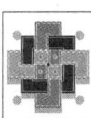

5 Cultural Issues in Critical Care Nursing   93

Carol Germain

6 Cardiovascular Anatomy and Physiology   109

Paulette Morelli

7 Cardiovascular Assessment   129

Elisabeth G. Bradley

8 Cardiovascular Laboratory and Diagnostic Tests   142

Kathy McCloy and Nancy Livingston

9 Coronary Artery Disease   201
Deborah Becker

10 Acute Myocardial Infarction   227
Linda Bucher

11 Heart Failure   258
Catherine Nuss Kotecki

12 Infectious Cardiac Disorders   286
Catherine Nuss Kotecki

13 Cardiac Surgery and Heart Transplantation   308
Debra Lynn-McHale and Catharine Dorozinsky

UNIT 3

Respiratory Disorders   351

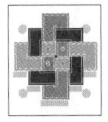

UNIT 4

Renal Disorders   509

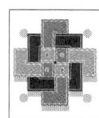

UNIT **5**

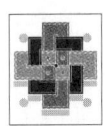

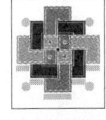

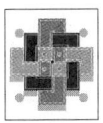

UNIT 8

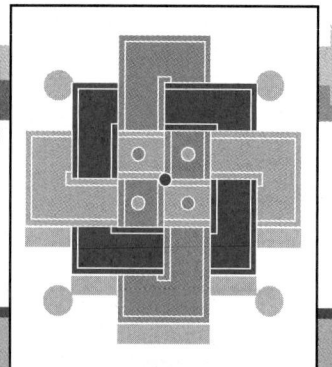

Introduction to Critical Care

The Power to Live and Die on One's Own Terms

Two years ago, I met an incredible woman and her daughter. On this day, Ms. X. was admitted to the intensive care unit (ICU) for respiratory management and possible ventilatory support. She was 88 years old and had recently been diagnosed with amyotrophic lateral sclerosis (ALS), also known as Lou Gehrig's disease. Her chief complaints were shortness of breath and dysphagia. Her daughter was also present.

After admitting Ms. X. to the ICU, I formally introduced myself and the concept of primary nursing. I began to collect nursing history and assessment data to generate a preliminary nursing plan of care.

I learned that Ms. X. had a living will, but at this time she was considering tracheostomy placement and whatever else was needed to make it possible for her to return home. She expressed concern for her quality of life. "I don't want to live if I can't bring any happiness to my family or if I become a burden. Do you think this would make me a burden?"

The question was a good one, but not for me to answer. I listened and encouraged Ms. X. to take time to consider and discuss the pros and cons of tracheostomy placement with her daughter. I contacted the clinical nurse specialist and the chaplain to provide additional support and resources. My interventions were incorporated in my care plan: decisional conflict.

I returned after the weekend and learned that Ms. X. had decided to have a tracheostomy as well as a gastrostomy and needed ventilatory support at night. My focus had changed.

The implications of tracheostomy placement were many. There was a clear knowledge deficit, and much teaching was needed to empower Ms. X. and her daughter to manage home care successfully, to handle the progressive nature of ALS, and to identify community resources.

I remember Ms. X.'s daughter saying to me, "This is what Mama wants, but I don't know that I can do this."

Ms. X. and her daughter lived in a rural area. In addition to caring for Ms. X., her daughter was caring for a son with muscular dystrophy. Family support systems were nonexistent.

I had serious doubts about their undertaking this endeavor—not only about logistics, but also about how Ms. X.'s daughter would be relieved in times of stress or illness or if she just wanted a little time to herself. I expressed my concerns to both Ms. X. and her daughter. However, both clearly stated that they did not want Ms. X. placed in a nursing home.

As health care providers, we sometimes become paternalistic and forget the golden rule: Do what the patient wants. Whenever I forget this, I whisper the American Association of Critical-Care Nurses' vision: a health care system driven by the needs of patients in which critical care nurses make their optimal contribution.

Thus began a 2½-week intensive teaching plan to prepare Ms. X. and her daughter for home transition. This experience was new to me. I had cared for patients on ventilatory support, but I had never prepared a patient for home ventilatory therapy. It was a challenge.

I moved Ms. X. to a private room and began to consult members of our interdisciplinary team. A colleague who specializes in pulmonary management of patients provided me with a detailed home ventilatory therapy teaching plan. I used this as the foundation for a highly individualized, interdisciplinary plan of care.

I sat down with Ms. X. and her daughter to develop a schedule of daily activities in an effort to help Ms. X.'s daughter organize her learning and day-to-day activities, both at the hospital and later at home. A schedule, posted in Ms. X.'s room, provided Ms. X. consistency and security.

Ms. X.'s daughter was highly involved. I could not do all this teaching myself. I communicated with my associates during change of shift report, by documentation, and with updated plans of care. Weekly, the interdisciplinary team reviewed Ms. X.'s plan and progress. Respiratory therapists followed up on suction technique and tracheostomy care. Nutritional support staff provided guidance on tube feedings and gastrostomy care. Nurses taught skin care, medications and their administration, and ways to enhance communication. Physical and occupational therapists addressed proper body mechanics as well as positioning and transfer techniques. Social services arranged for a home health team to assist in setting up a hospital bed, security supplies, the ventilator, and a backup electrical generator.

The day of discharge was filled with anxiety and joy. Had we done everything we could to ensure success? I pulled Ms. X.'s daughter aside and reviewed with her all the available resources should problems arise. We hugged and said our goodbyes.

During the next 2 years, Ms. X. was rehospitalized for everything from reinsertion of her gastrostomy to pneumonia. I sadly watched Ms. X.'s condition deteriorate.

During Ms. X.'s last admission, her daughter decided to act in her mother's interest by using her medical durable power of attorney to withdraw ventilatory support. Ms. X. had finally become unable to interact with those in her environment or her family. She could not participate in her own care.

Her daughter recognized that this was not what her mother had envisioned to be quality of life. Ironically, Ms. X. died in the same room from which she began her journey. I was fortunate to be present and to ensure that her death was peaceful. Her daughter was comforted by my presence because I understood her pain and grief, but also peace.

I used the hospital's standard of care for terminal weaning to guide team members in withdrawing ventilatory support. A member of the hospital's ethical review board and risk management team were consulted. A speech therapy consultation was obtained to evaluate whether we could establish a consistent method of communication with Ms. X. The doctor wanted to make sure that withdrawing ventilatory support was her wish.

The evaluation confirmed that Ms. X. was unable to communicate with others around her. I paged the chaplain, who was familiar with Ms. X. and her family. I turned off the monitor alarms, closed the doors, and allowed Ms. X.'s daughter to sit next to her and hold her hand. Ventilatory support was removed by the respiratory therapist, and supplemental oxygen was provided. Pain medication was administered by the doctor to provide comfort during this time.

I had empowered Ms. X. to go home on her own terms and to die on her own terms. What a precious gift it was, especially in this technology-filled environment of health care.

I have since spoken with Ms. X.'s daughter as part of a bereavement follow-up program in our unit. She said, "Thank you for taking what seemed impossible to me and putting it within my reach. Thank you for listening to our needs. Thank you for putting the humanity back in the hospital setting." My response: "No, thank you for allowing me to share in your journey and give you the best I could and that the system could provide."

Kathryn T. Parker, RN, BSN, MEd
Neuroscience ICU
Medical College of Virginia Hospitals
Disputanta, Virginia

1996 AACN-Siemens Excellence in Caring Practices Award Recipient
© 1997 by the American Association of Critical-Care Nurses.

1

Critical Care Across the Health Care Continuum

Linda Bucher and Sheila Melander

Objectives

After completing this chapter, the student will be able to:

1. Analyze the impact of the document, *Healthy People 2000*, on the acute care patient population and nurses practicing in critical care.
2. Evaluate the different types of provider services available for health care.
3. Differentiate consumer concerns regarding self-pay versus private insurance companies and government-funded services.
4. Discuss how the role of the patient as a "consumer of health care" has affected the health care industry.
5. Relate the history of critical care nursing to the predicted changes in critical care nursing in the next century.
6. Examine predictions for critical care technology in the next century.
7. Evaluate the nursing skills necessary for the next century.
8. Relate the significance of the expanding critical care environment to opportunities for nurses.

HEALTH CARE SYSTEM OF THE 21st CENTURY

As the 20th century draws to an end, there has never been more attention focused on any single industry than that focused on the health care system. Americans have long believed that the United States provides them with the best health care in the world. It is certainly the most expensive. Recently, the health care industry has witnessed a plethora of changes, changes in the delivery as well as the reimbursement of services and shifts in emphasis toward health promotion and greater consumer participation in health care decisions. Because these changes are expected to lead the way for the health of Americans in the next century, they also have many implications for our nursing profession.

The acuity level of critical care patients has kept pace with the complexity of the technology used to care for these patients. Concurrent with advances in technology is the need for the nurse to master the complex, psychomotor skills related to using the technology. Consequently, patients often require intense,

one-to-one, nurse–patient care, and, at times, two-to-one nurse-to-patient ratios are necessary to provide quality care. The needs of these patients must be kept in mind as we consider changes within our health care system to meet societal needs. It is vital that we focus on preventive care to decrease the need for acute care whenever possible. However, when complex, critical care is necessary for quality care, we must be prepared to deliver this level of care.

Nurses practicing in critical care can no longer focus only on the patient's acute illness event. Nurses must broaden their focus to include preventive care and risk factor modification education to decrease future patient admissions to acute care facilities. At the governmental level, initial efforts toward this goal have been focused on preventive care issues. These efforts have resulted in the identification of populations at risk of health crises. Further, by addressing population risk factors, decreases in the number of episodes of acute and chronic disease are being realized. This change has substantial monetary implications for our health care system. The original document that addresses these preventive care issues is *Healthy People 2000*.

Healthy People 2000

Healthy People 2000 is a document that contains plans for the significant improvement of the health of the United States. The document includes strategies for prevention of major chronic illnesses, infectious diseases, and injuries. The development of *Healthy People 2000* involved people all across the United States. Thousands of people, including all state health departments, more than 300 national organizations, 22 expert working groups, and the Institute of Medicine of the National Academy of Sciences, participated in the development of these goals. This document was begun in 1987, with the thought that the year 2000 could be a turning point characterized by decreases in preventable disabilities and deaths and enhanced quality of life.[1]

The major goals of the *Healthy People 2000* document include an increase in the healthy life span of Americans, a reduction of health disparities among Americans, and access to preventive services for all Americans. Each of these goals is discussed next in further detail.

Increase in the Span of Healthy Life for Americans

During this century, the average life span has risen from 47 years in 1900 to 75 years in 1987. This change is due to advances in the sciences that have decreased deaths from communicable diseases and have increased prevention and management of chronic diseases. Life expectancy at birth, death rates for people age 74 years and younger, infant mortality rates, years of healthy life as a proportion of life expectancy, and percentage of people experiencing limitations of major activity are the indicators used to measure overall progress in the goal of increasing the span of healthy life. During the measurement of these criteria, keep in mind that quality of life is the ultimate, defining characteristic. Years of healthy life in this study included both physical and psychological welfare. The ability of the individual to remain in his or her usual social role, whether as a housewife or in the outside work setting, was also considered.[1]

Reduction in Health Disparities Among Americans

This goal deals with the need to address the health care needs of vulnerable populations of Americans who are at greater risk of premature death, disease, and disability. Examples of vulnerable populations with complex needs are people with low income or disabilities and people in minority groups. These special populations experience areas of great risk.

For example, Native Americans, including Native Alaskans, appear to be a youthful group when looking at their age statistics. The median age for Native Americans living on a reservation is around 23 years, as compared with 32 years for the United States population as a whole. The reason is the large proportion of Native Americans who die before the age of 45 years. This death rate can be traced to six causes: unintentional injuries, cirrhosis, homicide, suicide, pneumonia, and complications of diabetes. Alcohol and obesity are specific risk factors that have been identified for the Native American. One estimate is that 95% of Native American families are affected either directly or indirectly by the use and abuse of alcohol.

Life expectancy at birth, infant mortality rates, and death rates for people aged 74 years and younger are measured for racial groups. Another possible measure could be potential years of lost life before age 65 years among the high-risk groups.[1]

Access to Preventive Services for All Americans

This goal addresses support for improvement and strengthening of all preventive care areas. This prevention strategy has three components: health promotion, health protection, and preventive services. Priorities are grouped under each of these areas. However, success depends on all three areas, not just one. One cannot assume that just because providers have conducted health promotion teaching, people will be persuaded to change their behaviors, nor can one assume making environmental changes will alone ensure increased health.

Particular attention is paid to those areas in which health professionals in both public and private sectors have the most responsibility. One of these areas is that of preventive services. Involvement at this level can help in the achievement of many of the prevention goals. For example, prenatal health care services are vital for the birth of a healthy infant. They also can be useful as resources and reinforcers of health promotion activities and can also serve as monitors for protective services by monitoring for exposure to toxic substances such as lead and radiation; by basic monitoring of child growth and development; by providing immunizations against childhood diseases and appropriate immunizations for vulnerable adults against pneumonia and influenza; by screening to detect hypertension, high blood cholesterol, and breast, cervical, oropharyngeal, and colorectal cancers; and by counseling on nutrition, smoking cessation, and injury prevention.[1] Other information collected includes the percentage of children immunized before school entry, the percentage of people who lack a source of primary care, and health insurance coverage for people age 64 years and younger and type of coverage (Table 1–1).

TABLE 1–1
Priorities for Health Promotion and Disease Prevention

Priority	Goals
Health Promotion	
Physical activity and fitness	Increase daily physical activity to at least 30% of the population (36% increase)
	Reduce a sedentary lifestyle to no more than 15% of population (38% decrease)
Nutrition	Reduce the overweight population to no more than 20% of the population (23% decrease)
	Reduce dietary fat intake to an average of 30% of calories (17% decrease)
Tobacco	Reduce cigarette smoking to no more than 15% of adults (48% decrease)
	Reduce initiation of smoking to no more than 15% of population by age 20 (50% decrease)
Alcohol and other drugs	Reduce-alcohol related vehicle crash deaths to no more than 8.5 per 100,000 people (12% decrease)
	Reduce alcohol use by school children ages 12–17 to less than 13%; marijuana use by ages 18–25 to less than 8%; cocaine use by ages 18–25 to less than 3% (50% decrease)
Family planning	Reduce teenage pregnancies to no more than 50 per 1000 girls ages 17 and younger (30% decrease)
	Reduce unintended pregnancies to no more than 30% of pregnancies (46% decrease)
Mental health and mental disorders	Reduce suicides to no more than 10.5 per 100,000 people (10% decrease)
	Reduce adverse effects of stress to less than 35% of population (18% decrease)
Violent and abusive behavior	Reduce homicides to no more than 7.2 per 100,000 people (15% decrease)
	Reduce assault injuries to no more than 10 per 1000 of population (10% decrease)
Educational and community-based programs	Provide quality K–12 school health education in at least 75% of schools; provide employee health-promotion activities in at least 85% of workplaces with 50 or more employees (31% increase)
Health Protection	
Unintentional injuries	Reduce unintentional injury deaths to no more than 29.3 per 100,000 people (15% decrease)
	Increase automobile safety restraint use to at least 85% of occupants (102% increase)
Occupational safety and health	Reduce work-related injury deaths to no more than 4 per 10,000 workers (33% decrease)
	Reduce work-related injuries to no more than 6 per 100 workers (22% decrease)
Environmental health	Eliminate blood lead levels above 25 μg/dL in children under age 5
	Increase protection from air pollutants so that at least 85% of population live in counties that meet EPA standards (71% increase)
	Increase protection from radon so that at least 40% of population live in homes tested by home owners and found to be/made safe (700% increase)
Food and drug safety	Reduce *Salmonella* infection outbreaks to fewer than 25 yearly (68% decrease)
Oral health	Reduce the prevalence of dental caries to no more than 35% of children by age 8 (34% decrease)
	Reduce edentulism to no more than 20% in population aged 65 and older (44% decrease)
Preventive Services	
Maternal and infant health	Reduce infant mortality to no more than 7 deaths per 1000 births (31% decrease)
	Reduce low birth weight to no more than 5% of live births (28% decrease)
	Increase first trimester prenatal care to at least 90% of live births (18% increase)
Heart disease and stroke	Reduce coronary heart disease deaths to no more than 100 per 100,000 people (26% decrease)
	Reduce stroke deaths to no more than 20 per 100,000 people (34% decrease)
	Increase control of high blood pressure to at least 50% of people diagnosed (108% increase)
	Reduce blood cholesterol to an average of no more than 200 mg/dL (6% decrease)
Cancer	Reverse the rise in cancer deaths to no more than 130 per 100,000 people
	Increase clinical breast examinations and mammography every 2 years to at least 60% of women aged 50 and older (140% increase)
	Increase Pap tests every 1–3 years to at least 85% of women aged 18 and older (13% increase)
	Increase fecal occult blood testing every 1–2 years to at least 50% of people aged 50 and older (85% increase)
Diabetes and chronic disabling conditions	Reduce disability from chronic conditions to no more than 8% of people (15% decrease)
	Reduce diabetes-related deaths to no more than 34 per 100,000 people (11% decrease)
HIV infection	Confine HIV infection to no more than 800 per 100,000 people
Sexually transmitted diseases	Reduce gonorrhea infections to no more than 225 per 100,000 people (25% decrease)
	Reduce syphilis infections to no more than 10 per 100,000 people (45% decrease)

Table continued on following page

TABLE 1–1
Priorities for Health Promotion and Disease Prevention Continued

Priority	Goals
Immunization and infectious diseases	Eliminate measles
	Reduce epidemic-related pneumonia and influenza deaths to no more than 7.3 per 100,000 people aged 65 and older (20% decrease)
	Increase childhood immunization levels to at least 90% of 2 year-olds (20% increase)
Clinical preventive services	Eliminate financial barriers to clinical preventive services
Surveillance and Data Systems*	
	Develop and implement common health status indicators for use by federal, state, and local health agencies

*The surveillance and data systems have not been specifically discussed. Data for the *Healthy People 2000* project need to be tracked and analyzed to determine its effectiveness.

An example of the impact of the *Healthy People 2000* project on the promotion of health and prevention of disease is obvious in the area of cardiovascular health. During the 1980s, the United States experienced major declines in the death rate associated with heart disease, stroke, and unintentional injuries. The more than 40% drop in heart disease mortality is due largely to early detection and control of hypertension, a decline in cigarette smoking, and an increased awareness of the impact of cholesterol and dietary fats.

Evaluation of Goals

The *Healthy People 2000: Midcourse Review* and 1995 revisions provide an overview of progress made in the years after the release of the *Healthy People 2000* document.[2] This document reflects the placement of an interstate network consisting of 41 states and 2 territories to translate the national objectives into state priorities. The document also states that 70% of local health departments are using *Healthy People 2000* as a framework to put prevention into action in their communities. This positive experience has served to exemplify that we can prevent disease and injury and promote both physical and mental health. Hundreds of community organizations have joined the *Healthy People 2000* consortium and are working through their memberships to make *Healthy People 2000* their standard (Table 1–2).

In the preface of *Healthy People 2000: Midcourse Review*, Donna Shalala, Secretary of Health and Human Services, states that this report documents that health care providers are partners at both federal and state levels with the private sector as well as with volunteer organizations to carry out the agenda of *Healthy People 2000* (Figure 1–1). This report demonstrates a positive trend toward the accomplishment of two-thirds of the national objectives. Trends are identified as declines in heart disease and stroke deaths, more women seeking prenatal care during the first trimester, infant mortality rates at an all time low, increases in childhood immunizations, declining tobacco use, more women over the age of 50 years receiving mammograms, increasing life expectancy rates, and changing dietary habits, with consumption of fewer fats and more fruits.

TABLE 1–2
Number of States with Healthy People 2000 Objectives by Priority Area

Priority Area	Number of States
Health Promotion	
Physical activity and fitness	33
Nutrition	41
Tobacco	43
Substance abuse: alcohol and other drugs	38
Family planning	37
Mental health and mental disorders	27
Violent and abusive behavior	42
Educational and community-based programs	28
Health Protection	
Unintentional injuries	44
Occupational safety and health	29
Environmental health	42
Food and drug safety	25
Oral health	36
Preventive Services	
Maternal and infant health	45
Heart disease and stroke	42
Cancer	44
Diabetes and chronic disabling conditions	40
HIV infection	45
Sexually transmitted diseases	42
Immunization and infectious diseases	44
Clinical preventive services	30
Surveillance and Data Systems	31

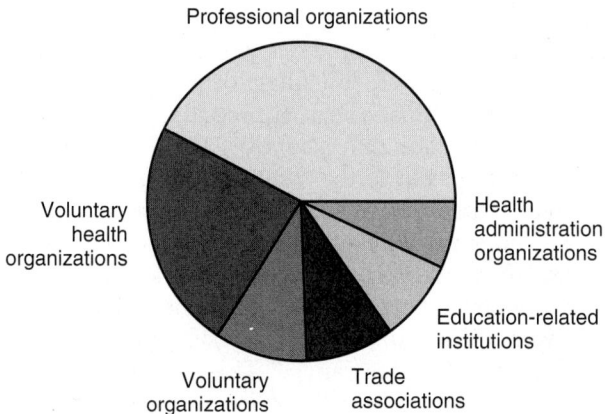

Figure 1–1

Participation of private and voluntary organizations in the *Healthy People 2000* agenda.

The progress of the *Healthy People 2000* plan can be evaluated by examining its three major goals.

Goal 1: Increase the Healthy Life Span of Americans. This goal relates to the estimates that reflect that Americans are living longer, but because of limitations that are a part of the aging process, the quality of life decreases. Based on information received from self-reported health status, activity limitation data found in the National Health Interview Survey, and statistics from Centers for Disease Control and Prevention and the National Center for Health Statistics, 64 years of life or 85% of life years are estimated as healthy. Years of unhealthy life or life with limitations of major life activities such as bathing, grooming, cooking, recreation, school, or work are estimated at 11.4 or 15% of life years. The challenge accompanying this goal is to minimize disability, to increase the independence as well as the health of our older adults, and to move from merely tracking mortality rates to looking at quality of life issues.[2]

Goal 2: Reduce Health Disparities Among Americans. This goal involves closing the gap between the health status of vulnerable populations and the general population and provides outcomes for racial and ethnic minorities that are similar to those experienced by the general population. At this point, the disparities between nonwhites and whites continue to

be substantial (Table 1–3). This study has discovered that a lack of data exists for subgroups of populations and populations in small geographic areas. As the United States become more diverse, the problems of identifying disparities as they emerge and of addressing differences in outcomes will increase. This goal calls for an improvement in the information available on health status and clinical preventive services used by populations at risk. These risk populations include racial and ethnic minorities and people with low incomes and disabilities.[2]

Goal 3: Achieve Access to Preventive Services for All Americans. This goal has varied results at this point. As a result of work from the US Preventative Services Task Force in 1996,[3] almost full consensus has emerged regarding which services should be made available to various groups at regular intervals. However, the number of Americans with health insurance coverage has declined. Before *Healthy People 2000*, 77% of people under age 65 years had private insurance. At this midpoint review, only 71.9% of this age group has private insurance. Among the Hispanic and black populations, the numbers of uninsured are increased. In 1993, the Census Bureau estimated that 39.7 million people or 15.3% were without health insurance. In another area, infant mortality rates show continued progress. However, the infant mortality rate per 100,000 live births for black babies is more than double that of white babies. Therefore, emphasis for reducing the incidence of low birth weight and for decreasing birth defects is still a major agenda item.[3]

Demographics have changed as a result of the *Healthy People 2000* initiative. For example, instead of coronary artery disease and stroke, adults now face cancer as the leading cause of death in the age group of 25 to 65 years. Slowing the rise of cancer and HIV deaths is now the obstacle for this age group for the year 2000. In addition, special population groups with special needs remain. By the year 2000, there will be 4 million more Americans over the age of 65 years than there were in 1990. This special population exists because the average age of the population is rising, and the number of those who live longer than 85 years is at a record level. This aging of America's population will challenge the system's ability to handle physical as well as mental illnesses. Primary providers will

TABLE 1–3
Years of Healthy Life and Life Expectancy by Race and Hispanic Origin*

	All Races	**White**	**Black**	**Hispanic**
Healthy years	64.0	65.0	56.0	64.8†
Life expectancy	75.4	76.1	69.1	Not available

*Data from 1990.
†Estimated from preliminary data.
From Centers for Disease Control and Prevention (CDC)/National Center for Health Statistics (NCHS).

need to identify risks to independence and health, so that patients can be counseled to remain physically healthy and active. Screenings for cancer, heart disease, and life-threatening illnesses as well as immunizations for pneumonia and influenza will be necessary. This population will offer great challenges for our current health care system. A data tracking set will also need to be established to follow developments as they occur from this special population.[3]

The midcourse review of the *Healthy People 2000* goals has demonstrated that great challenges are still related to the 22 priority areas (see Table 1–1). Americans who are from lower income families, members of minority groups, and who have disabilities still experience much poorer health outcomes than other Americans. To accomplish the goals of the document and to reach the vision of healthy people in healthy communities, these gaps must be closed. Data systems must be initiated and then maintained to provide information regarding the emergence of new diseases, the adequacy of child and adult immunizations, and the use of preventive services that are cost effective and provide life-saving information and services. In addition, payment systems need to reward providers and health plans that keep their constituents healthy. The midcourse review data confirm that even though goals are being reached, efforts need to continue toward focused activities that decrease illness and move toward health. The translation of this information into national health care policies that promote health and into information that the public can use to choose a healthy lifestyle is the challenge the United States and nursing faces for the next century.

FINANCIAL BASIS OF THE HEALTH CARE SYSTEM: QUALITY VERSUS COST

Health care costs have been rising faster than the inflation rate since 1960, and the United States spends more of its gross national product on health care than does any other country in the world. Even with this investment in health care, the United States trails many of the world's industrial nations on health indicators such as life expectancy and infant mortality.[3] As stated by Kovner,[4] all money for health services ultimately comes from the people. Because of an overwhelming economic burden from health care, the US Congress passed several pieces of legislation that facilitated the growth of managed care. Congress passed the Health Maintenance Organization (HMO) Act of 1974 that allowed for the expansion of HMOs as a cost containment effort without violating antitrust laws. In 1983, the Congressional Omnibus Reconciliation Act (COBRA) was passed. This legislation dramatically changed Medicare reimbursement to hospitals. Previously, the health care industry was based on "fee for

service," that is, the more services provided by hospitals, the higher the fees. The new legislation called for a system regulated by diagnostic-related groups (DRGs). Under this system, a predetermined amount was established for each diagnosis. The predetermined amount was payed to the institution regardless of the actual costs incurred. If hospitals could provide care at a cost under the allotted DRG fee, the hospital made money. If the cost of care was in excess of the designated DRG fee, the institution lost money. Many incentives were offered to providers to give care that stayed "within the DRG fee range." This practice has provided a situation in which quality of care could possibly be compromised in order to stay within a designated fee range. Because these initial efforts were effective in decreasing the costs of health care services, the government and other providers are continuing the search for other methods to contain costs.[5]

Other health care consumer concerns arise from proposed budget cuts from the federal government. According to Pera,[6] Medicare and Medicaid are major sources of federal expenditures, and they are also major targets for cost reductions. Restructuring proposals have been established that, if implemented, would cut funding for these programs by $450 billion dollars over the course of a 7-year period. To handle expected reductions in reimbursements, hospitals are looking for ways to reduce costs and to compete more effectively in the managed care market. Many health care professionals, as well as health care consumers, are fearful of the possible impact of these cuts on the consumer. The influence and growth of managed care have been tremendous. With such growth comes responsibility continually to monitor and evaluate the progress of managed care toward reducing health care costs without sacrificing quality and access. If data from California, which boasts heavy enrollments in HMOs, can be generalized across the country, further reductions in the use of services can be anticipated. In California, the average number of hospital admissions has decreased to 26% below the national average, and the average length of hospitalization has decreased to 31% below the national average. Research has shown that these decreases can be directly related to managed care models that put providers' incomes at risk through the use of capitation and salary-based plans.[7] Research on patient care outcomes related to these changes is inconclusive, and it is unclear whether this managed care environment in California has resulted in improvements in quality patient care outcomes.[8]

Under managed care, providers must balance conflicting interests, such as providing the highest quality of care possible while remaining financially solvent and even profitable. Under managed care, the more services provided, the less money made, and, in some cases, money is lost. At the same time, under managed care, hospitals are rewarded financially for decreasing a patient's length of stay. In a study by Rakich and colleagues,[9] even provider satisfaction can be negatively affected under managed care. These investigators found that HMO physicians' rates of job turnover are affected by the financial contingencies as well as the percentage of HMO patients in their caseload. The American Medical Association (AMA) also reported that physicians have reacted negatively to the decreased professional autonomy associated with managed care organizations. The AMA further reported that physicians believe that the extensive utilization review procedures interfere with their professional clinical decision making.[10] In terms of the physicians' perceptions of quality of care, a questionnaire was given to physicians before entering an HMO and, again, 2½ years after joining an HMO plan. The results revealed that 20 to 34% of the physicians believed that the quality of care they provided had diminished under the managed care system.[11] It appears that there are significant reasons for consumer concern that cost savings produced by managed care plans may be leading to physician and consumer dissatisfaction with access to care and quality of services when compared with fee-for-service plans.

EVOLUTION OF HEALTH CARE SERVICES

Today's health care delivery system may appear to the consumer as a complex maze of organizations and alliances. Physicians and physicians' groups are aligning with hospitals, corporations are negotiating with physicians and physicians' groups to provide selected services for their employees, and hospitals are competing with one another for patients as well as for procedures. Before the 1980s, the health care system functioned almost entirely as a fee-for-service entity. The third-party payers such as the federal government, insurance companies, or private insurers paid the services billed by the institution and the physician without questioning the cost of the services, necessity for the service, or cost effectiveness. As a result, institutions or physicians had no incentives to provide cost effective care. Quality of care became associated with quantity of diagnostic tests ordered or number of treatments performed. In 1983, the financial environment of the health care system changed. The federal government introduced the use of the prospective payment system for Medicare recipients. This payment system implemented the use of DRGs as basis for fee for services.[12] Once a medical diagnosis was made, the institution knew immediately how much money would be received from the federal government for that service. If the cost of care was less than the amount the federal government identified for that case, the hospital kept the remaining funds as profit; however, if the amount

was insufficient to cover expenses associated with that diagnosis, the institution lost money.[13]

The use of the prospective payment system for pay for Medicare services was considered a success because of its cost effectiveness and identified savings by the federal government. As a result of this success, other third-party payers began to implement similar systems. Along with this change came the realization from the public that cost of health care was exorbitant. Large corporations began to identify strategies to decrease the cost of health care coverage, and in doing so income decreased for health care institutions, primarily because of the decrease in hospital occupancy rates. Marketing campaigns were developed by hospitals to acquire new customers and to initiate new services. New strategies that provided health care services to employees of large corporations at reduced costs were developed. Managed care organizations, including HMOs and Preferred Provider Organizations (PPOs), were implemented. HMOs were developed to provide incentives to decrease the number of patients admitted to hospitals for care. People enrolled in an HMO select a package consistent with the level of care they require and pay a monthly fee for service. One advantage to the consumer of an HMO is easier access to services. HMOs typically provide full medical care, diagnostic testing, and pharmacy needs. A disadvantage of an HMO is that the consumer may be limited regarding the number of physicians involved in a specific HMO. If a patient sees a physician who is not a participant of the HMO, the monthly fee will not cover these costs. Advantages for physicians to participate in an HMO include the decrease workload regarding administrative responsibilities. The HMO provides clerical and assistive personnel to the provider group.[13]

PPOs, Exclusive Provider Associations (EPAs), and Independent Practice Associations (IPAs) are other types of managed care programs or plans A PPO typically provides more flexibility for the consumer by contracting with numerous hospitals and physicians to establish specific fees for services. These fees are usually discounted from the standard charges. Individuals may choose a preferred provider for care that will result in full payment of services by the PPO, or the consumer has the option to select a hospital or physician not part of the preferred organization. If this option is chosen, the consumer will be required to pay generally 15 to 20% of the total charges.[13]

Integrated delivery networks (IDNs) have been developed for the purpose of streamlining ambulatory care through care in the nursing home. This plan addresses health care needs across the life span. IDNs currently have integrated with many HMOs and PPOs.[14] No ideal model for health care delivery exists at this time. Selected models have been successful in certain areas because of the organization's ability to identify and to meet community health care needs.

Another component of managed care is the use of case management. Case management is the strategic management of cost and quality outcomes.[9] Kongstvedt[15] describes case management as a "system of health care delivery that tries to manage the cost of health care, the quality of health care, and access to health care." The case manager, typically working in some type of managed care organization, works with the patient, family, and health care professionals to plan and provide the best possible and most cost-effective services to the patient. Many times, case managers are used to manage complex cases when care requires the coordination of many health care providers or when complications arise that slow the recovery phase. Once again, the expertise of case managers is used to place the patient on the path that will provide the quality of care needed with cost effectiveness in mind.

The initiation of managed care into our health care systems has caused much reorganization in the delivery of health care services. The implementation of managed care has refocused the emphasis of care for many health care providers. Managed care has caused physicians and providers to place a much greater emphasis on promotion of health and on health-seeking behaviors for their clients. The tables have dramatically turned in our health care system. No longer are financial statements prospering because of increased hospital occupancy rates. Finances are stronger now for physicians when patients are kept out of the hospital and free from health problems and problems requiring referrals.

Capitation, the strict prepayment of services per patient per month, has also played a major role in the changes seen in our health care system. The organization paying for the health care negotiates this payment with the organization providing the care. As a result, the organization providing the care assumes greater risk. If actual costs to the health care facility are greater than the predicted costs, the health care facility stands to lose a great deal of money.[15] The implementation of capitated reimbursement has caused extensive reorganization within the health care world. Across the United States, physicians' groups commonly form alliances with nurse practitioners (NPs) or physician assistants (PAs) to act as midlevel providers of services.

ROLE OF THE CONSUMER IN THE HEALTH CARE SYSTEM

Managed care is dramatically influencing the delivery of health care services. Payer-driven health care forces the providers to limit the amount of care received while directing consumers to the least expensive treatments available. In some situations, this has led to physician and consumer dissatisfaction. Balancing costs of care with quality and access is an unending struggle. When managed care is used exclusively as a cost-containment strategy, quality and access of care can be jeopardized. All health care providers should function as advocates for better services for their clients under a managed care system. This advocacy helps others in society to become aware that cost-saving methods may come at a risk to consumers. From the consumer's end, people must stay abreast of health care legislation and must evaluate how it may affect their health care services. Consumers can no longer be complacent with their health care needs; they must have a voice.

Today's health care consumers must also be prevention oriented and must function as active participants in their health care. As discussed in *Healthy People 2000* and the *Healthy People 2000: Midcourse Review* and revisions, the goals established by these documents require an active role on behalf of the consumer. Without active consumer participation, these goals cannot be met. The challenge is how to entice the public into playing a more proactive role in their health care. As stated previously, managed care has provided the physicians with incentives to keep their patients healthy and out of hospitals. The 21st century presents exciting opportunities for the health care consumer to participate in the shift from the treatment of illness to the prevention of illness and the maintenance of health. The rewards are lifelong.

CRITICAL CARE ENVIRONMENT IN TRANSITION

Changes in the health care delivery system will necessarily affect the critical care environment. At the 21st century unfolds, critical care nurses will be at the forefront of these transitions. A brief overview of the history of critical care nursing can help to place the current and future directions for critical care nursing in perspective.

History of Critical Care Nursing

The history of critical care nursing in the United States is actually a study of the reorganization of patient care in acute care hospitals. From the early 1900s to the late 1950s, hospitals were organized into large units, usually consisting of 45 to 60 patient beds. Care was delivered to groups of 15 to 20 patients by a team of registered nurses (RNs; 1–2), nursing students (3–4), and licensed practical nurses (LPNs) or aides (1–2). If a patient became critically ill and if the family had adequate finances, a private duty nurse was often employed. Most times, however, the demand for private duty nurses exceeded the supply.[16]

In the 1930s, recovery rooms were introduced, and hospitals began to hire a core of RNs to work in this arena, replacing the nursing students assigned to this area and private duty nurses frequently hired by patients' families. This innovation represented a major shift in the organization and delivery of care to postoperative patients recovering from anesthesia. The benefits of the recovery room nurses' expertise were immediately seen in the reduction of postanesthesia complications. Unfortunately, it was many years before this concept found application to other groups of seriously ill patients.[16]

General patient care during this period was dynamic, and patients requiring a wide range of nursing skills could be found in any given unit at any given time. The main approach to care was similar to "putting out brush fires." Nurses often reported having difficulty in providing care to the sickest patients. This problem was portrayed by one nurse, who recalled: "I remember having a patient on an Aramine (metaraminol bitartrate) drip. He was just across from the nurses' station, supposedly so I could keep a close eye on him. But I also had 15 or 20 other patients with varying degrees of illness on my floor. I would run in to take a blood pressure; if it was all right, I would breathe a sigh of relief and go on to my other patients. When the drip needed titrating, I would speed it up or slow it down a bit (with a roller clamp) and hope for the best." Both nurses and physicians were frustrated by these hectic conditions, as well as by the unpredictable quality of patient care and patient care outcomes.[16]

Using lessons learned from wars and disasters, the concept of triage, combined with specialty nursing, was introduced to hospitals in the late 1950s and early 1960s. This combination allowed physicians and nurses to identify the most seriously ill patients who also had a chance of recovery. Once done, these patients were placed in a common area and were cared for by nurses around the clock. The origins of critical care nursing and intensive care units (ICUs) had begun. Technology at this time was limited and consisted of blood pressure cuffs, suction equipment, oxygen catheters, chest tubes, and intravenous fluids. What was different was that the technology, nurse, and critically ill patient were together, in one place.[16]

The early days of critical care nursing were marked by large numbers of seriously ill patients with complex needs, an inadequate number of physicians available to care for these patients, and an alarmingly high number of patient deaths. The emotional toll on critical care nurses was high. These circumstances fueled the desire of nurses to learn what the physician knew and to manage situations when the physician was not available. During this time, nurses and physicians joined forces to share knowledge. Physicians taught nurses how to interpret electrocardiograms (ECGs),

evaluate laboratory values, and apply principles of pathophysiology; nurses taught physicians how patients responded to different interventions and what patient behaviors could be anticipated over the course of an illness.[16]

Throughout the 1950s and 1960s, patient admissions to hospitals were at an all-time high. Cardiovascular disease had replaced infectious disease as the most common diagnosis and the diagnosis with the highest morbidity and mortality rates. In the 1960s, 30 to 40% of the patients experiencing a myocardial infarction died, most from lethal dysrhythmias. Technology and knowledge regarding the treatment of cardiac disease exploded during this time, and nurses were soon involved in diagnosing dysrhythmias, initiating drug therapies, and defibrillating patients. Consequently, in 1965, the first specialty ICU, the coronary care unit, was opened at Abington Hospital outside Philadelphia.[16]

Continued advances in diagnosing and treating critically ill patients, as well as in technology, led to the emergence of additional specialty ICUs that usually addressed a specific organ system, problem, or age group (e.g., neurologic ICU, respiratory ICU, surgical ICU, burn ICU, pediatric ICU, and neonatal ICU). Nurses working in these units were committed to the idea of continuing and advanced education and certification in their specialty. The creation of the American Association of Critical-Care Nurses (AACN), known initially as the American Association of Cardiovascular Nurses, in 1969 was a major force in providing the educational support and certification opportunities needed by these pioneer critical care nurses. Today, the AACN remains the largest professional, specialty nursing organization, with more than 70,000 members.

Throughout the 1970s and 1980s, hospitals continued to experience tremendous growth. The United States was proud of its health care system, and public and financial support for ICUs and for the nurses needed to staff ICUs was seemingly endless. Reimbursement systems, including Medicare, Medicaid, and Blue Cross and Blue Shield, were expanding. By the 1980s, hospitals across the United States were facing a serious nursing shortage. In ICUs, where the RN-to-patient ratio was usually 1:2, the impact of the shortage was particularly notable. The demand for critical care nurses now exceeded the supply. Many variables contributed to the nursing shortage of the 1980s: increased numbers of hospital beds, declining enrollments in schools of nursing, declining numbers of 18 to 22 year olds, and increases in career choices for women. Unfortunately, only one of these variables (hospital beds) changed in the 1990s. Most nurse leaders predict that by the year 2000, the number of critical care nurses needed will reach 450,000.[16]

The 1990s has seen a major shift in the emphasis of health care from treatment to prevention. In spite of serious downsizing efforts, the demand for critical care beds in the 1990s has increased and, with it, the demand for skilled critical care nurses. Some factors that account for this change include the acquired immunodeficiency syndrome (AIDS) pandemic, the widespread prevalence of trauma and substance abuse, and the continued, technologic advances in the diagnosis and treatment of cardiac, oncologic, and respiratory disorders. In addition, almost half the patients in ICUs are more than 65 years of age, enter the hospital more acutely ill, and leave the hospital sooner than ever before. Most hospitals will soon resemble large critical care units as more and more general care units are converted to intermediate care or telemetry units.[16] Although the history of critical care nursing may still be in its infancy by some standards, the achievements of critical care nurses have been powerful. The AACN's vision perhaps charts best the direction for critical care nursing in the next century: *A health care system driven by the needs of patients and their families in which critical care nurses make their optimal contribution.*

Predictions for Critical Care Technology in the Next Century

As the health care industry embarks on the 21st century, some of the greatest changes predicted will be those related to critical care nursing. In the United States, critical care units account for approximately 8% of all hospital beds, and roughly 20% of all patients will spend some portion of their stay in a critical care bed. The cost of delivering these critical care services accounts for almost 20% of all hospital expenditures.[17] As hospitals continue to downsize in an effort to contain these costs, the challenge for critical care nursing remains clear—the delivery of high-quality, holistic care that responds to the needs of patients and their families. Consequently, the critical care technology of the 21st century will be designed to function efficiently and invisibly to allow nurses to meet this challenge. Other factors, such as cost effectiveness and consumer demand, will also influence the development of critical care technology.[18]

Overall, the technology of the 21st century will allow nurses to detect physiologic changes earlier and to confront problems proactively. Noninvasive technology will become the standard for many of the new diagnostic and monitoring devices. Benefits of noninvasive technology include greater patient and nurse safety, reduced costs, and increased opportunities to use the devices on patients because sterile technique is not required for application. One example of advanced noninvasive technology is the Diasensor 1000, a glucometry device that replaces the fingerstick device. The device works by passing infrared light through the skin to the blood, where it is then reflected back to a computer sensor, analyzed, and converted into a blood glucose level. The procedure is painless and requires no supplies.[18]

Similarly, regional cerebral oxygen saturation and perfusion of the microcirculation of the adult brain can also be measured using harmless, near-infrared light. This monitoring device is applied to the patient's forehead using a simple adhesive. Unlike pulse oximetry, cerebral oximetry does not depend on pulsatile blood flow and, consequently, can function if a patient is hypotensive, on cardiopulmonary bypass, experiencing hypothermia, or in cardiac arrest.[18]

On-line analysis of ECG changes is an example of noninvasive technology that offers unique opportunities to monitor patients in several categories: patients with chest pain of unknown origin or unstable angina, patients undergoing percutaneous transluminal coronary angioplasty, and patients who have had a myocardial infarction. The Hewlett-Packard myocardial ischemic dynamic analysis (HP MIDA) system uses an eight-lead configuration to monitor cardiac activity fully. Real-time computer analysis of ischemic (ST depression or elevation) and myocardial (QRS variations) changes in these high-risk patients may provide critical information long before clinical symptoms develop. This information may promote proactive clinical decisions regarding therapeutic interventions, transfers, and discharges.[18]

Emerging invasive technologies include in-line and continuous intra-arterial blood gas (ABG) and pH monitoring. Marquette Medical System's On-line ABG is an example of an in-line, intra-arterial monitoring system that measures the partial pressures of oxygen and carbon dioxide (PaO_2 and $PaCO_2$), and pH in 60 seconds (Figure 1–2). Continuous intra-arterial monitoring, which uses a disposable, fiberoptic, intravascular sensor, provides real-time information and allows nurses and other health care providers to make clinical decisions arising from ABGs and pH based on trends rather than individual readings. Investigators anticipate that the ability to detect physiologic changes before the development of signs and symptoms and to make rapid therapeutic decisions will result in the selection of more appropriate interventions and may even reduce or avoid complications. Additional advantages of these types of systems include a decrease in iatrogenic blood loss and less exposure to blood by health care providers.[18]

Point-of-care testing refers to laboratory technology that can be operated by clinicians in nonlaboratory settings. This type of technology offers several advantages: simplicity, quick results (usually within 2 to 5 minutes), and minimal maintenance. The Diametrics IRMA SL is an example of a portable analyzer that performs blood gas and electrolyte analyses at the bedside (Figure 1–3). Unlike traditional laboratory collections,

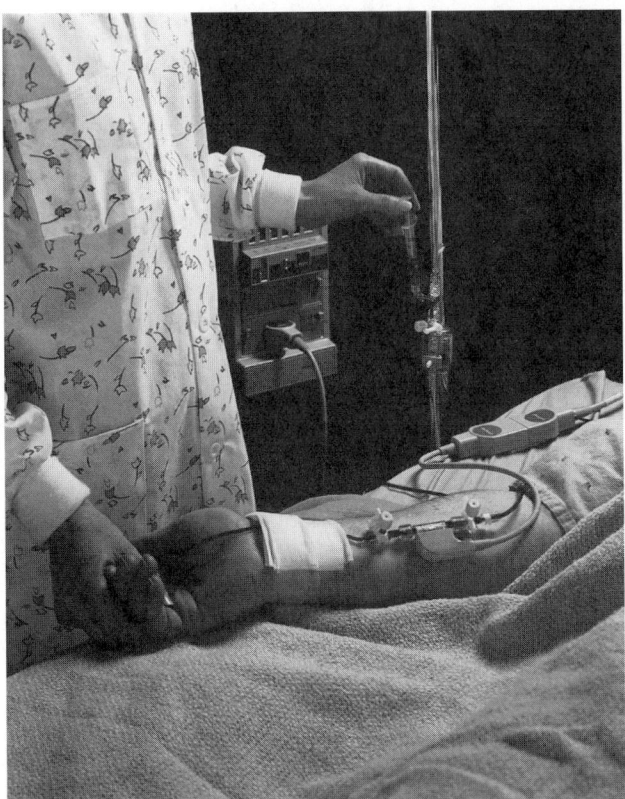

Figure 1–2

Marquette Medical System's on-line intra-arterial blood gas setup. (Courtesy of Marquette Medical System, Milwaukee, WI)

only two drops of whole blood are required for analysis. Investigators anticipate that this microsample technology will reduce phlebotomy-related blood loss, deliver cost-effective care, and provide rapid clinical information. For critically ill patients, such as those requiring emergency intubation or transcutaneous pacing, receiving complex pharmacotherapeutics, undergoing surgery, or experiencing cardiopulmonary arrest, the rapid identification of vital laboratory values can guide treatment decisions and, ultimately, can improve patient outcomes. It is predicted that future versions of point-of-care technology will be able to interface with wireless communication systems. In this way, patient data will be transmitted to health care providers from various settings, including the patient's home.[18]

Other emerging technologies will be designed to serve as bridges to either normal function or transplantation or as permanent implants. Within the field of respiratory care, pressure-regulated volume-controlled (PRVC) ventilation may become a primary mode of ventilation in the future. By combining the advantages of both volume-controlled and pressure-regulation ventilation, the "smart" ventilator can vary the inspiratory pressure control level according to the mechanical properties of the patient's lungs. The consequences of

this advance include lower inspiratory pressures with a controlled volume of ventilation, increased patient comfort, and decreased length of stay in the ICU.[18]

Initially, the left ventricular assist device (LVAD) was designed to serve as a bridge to heart transplantation. This continues to be a viable aim of the device. Since its development, the LVAD has become completely portable, and patients function with the device outside the hospital. These patients still require the constant presence of a trained companion to carry a manual pump should the device malfunction. Knowing that the demand for donor hearts will always exceed the supply and that some patients are not candidates for a heart transplant, the purpose of LVAD technology has been expanded to include an alternative to heart transplantation. Clinical trials are currently underway in England to evaluate the efficacy of using the LVAD for patients in end-stage heart failure who are not candidates for a heart transplant.[18]

One of the most eagerly anticipated devices is the implantable infusion pump for the delivery of insulin. By incorporating a closed-loop system, input from a glucose sensor is analyzed by a computer-controlled insulin infusion system. Once data are analyzed, the pump delivers a measured dose of insulin. This technology, once perfected, will likely be applied to other treatment modalities. For instance, many of the new, genetically engineered drugs are proteins and, like insulin, cannot be administered orally.[18]

As the technology explosion continues into the next century, research will be designed to determine

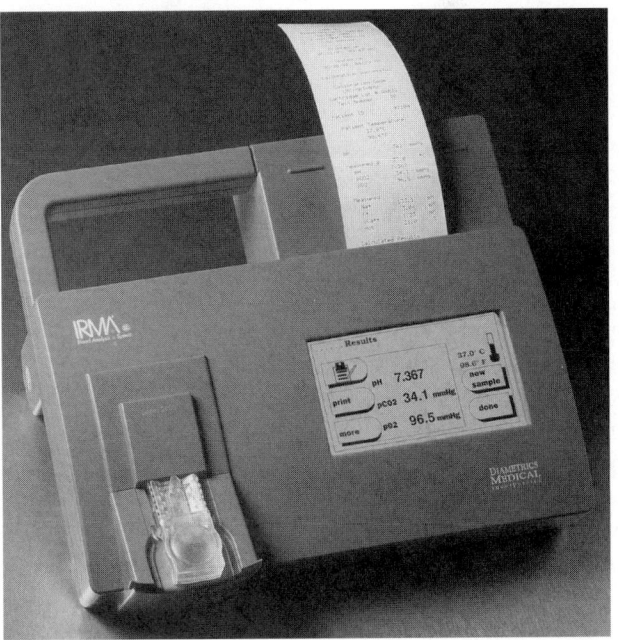

Figure 1–3

Diametrics IRMA SL blood analysis system. (Courtesy of Diametrics Medical, Inc., St. Paul, MN.)

whether the benefits justify the costs and whether patient care outcomes are improved. Nurses will need to be intimately involved in this process. In addition, the most effective nurses of the 21st century will be able to merge technology and patient care because patients and their families will see nurses as the vital link between them and the technology. The "high tech—high touch" metaphor will never have greater meaning. Nurses will be challenged to maintain the balance between the two and to keep the humanity in critical care nursing. To achieve this goal, nurses will need an open and inquisitive mind as well as the confidence to welcome change and to regard new technology as an opportunity to do something better for patients and their families.[18]

Skills Needed for the Next Century

Specific skills needed for the nurse of the next century include critical thinking, collaboration, delegation, and computer skills. These skills, once mastered, can be applied in the various settings of critical care nursing. Armed with the tools to meet the demands of the changing health care environment, nurses will be able to make their optimal contributions.

Critical Thinking Skills

In a single day, nurses are required to make seemingly endless and, many times, complex decisions regarding the care of patients and their families. Ideally, these decisions should be made using critical thinking skills. Critical thinking involves both an attitude and an approach to ideas or decisions. First, the proper attitude relates to a degree of willingness to give fair and equal consideration to all possible ideas or decisions. Second, the approach involves accepting an idea or decision only after carefully reflecting on it.[19] For many nurses, decisions regarding patient care are guided by the nursing process. The incorporation of reflective analysis in this process defines the essence of critical thinking and is key to improving patient outcomes (Figure 1–4). When providing care, nurses are encouraged to pose questions such as: "What did I learn from this patient situation that would allow me to care for similar patients more effectively?" "Did I rely solely on previous knowledge to manage this patient's clinical problems?" "Should I consider creative alternatives to arrive at superior patient outcomes?"

The development of critical thinking skills takes time. As clinical experiences are accumulated and expert knowledge amassed, critical thinking skills guide clinical decisions, and the application of the nursing process to patient care issues becomes a highly dynamic process (Table 1–4).[20]

Collaborative Skills

The care of patients and their families involves various disciplines: nursing; medicine; respiratory, occupational, and physical therapy; dietetics; rehabilitation; ministry; social services; pharmacy; and other ancillary services and workers such as patient transport, unlicensed assistive personnel (UAP), and even volunteers. It is most often the nurse's responsibility to coordinate patient care activities, and this is best achieved if a collaborative approach is taken. Collaboration, by definition, implies shared attention to a problem in which the unique talents and contributions of all concerned parties are considered. In a collaborative environment, the focus is on finding the best solutions to patient care issues. Individual interests are set aside, and the patient's interests become the primary concern of the multidisciplinary team.[21]

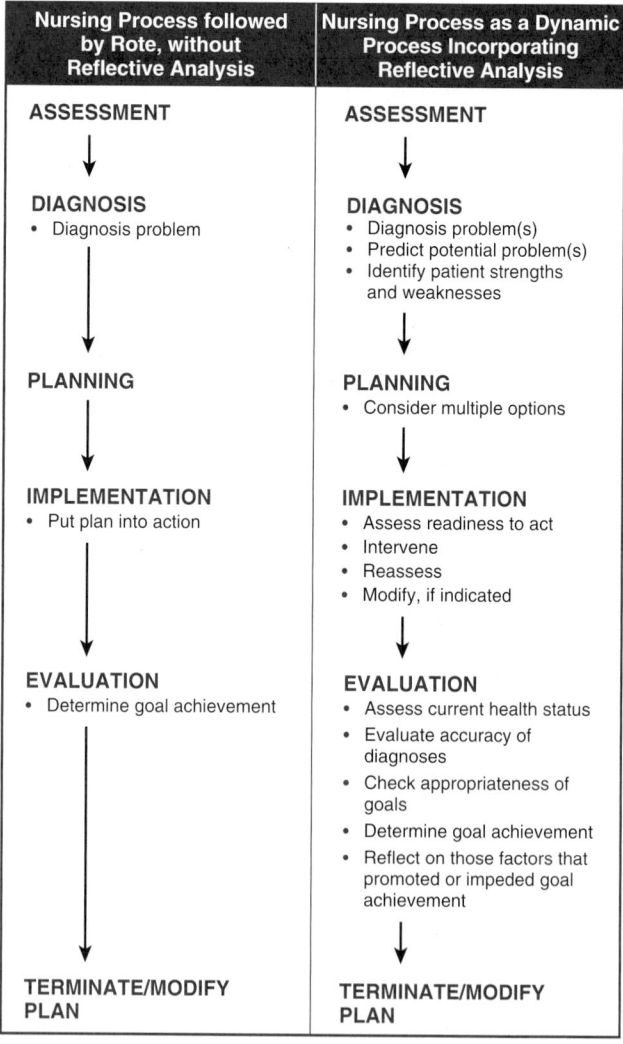

Figure 1–4

Comparison of the use of the nursing process with and without reflective analysis. (Modified from Alfaro-LeFevre R: Critical Thinking in Nursing: A Practical Approach. Philadelphia, W.B. Saunders, 1995, p. 45.)

TABLE 1–4
Novice Nurse Thinking Compared With Expert Nurse Thinking*

Novice Nurses	Expert Nurses
Knowledge is organized as separate facts; must rely heavily on resources (texts, policies, preceptors); lack knowledge gained from actually *doing* (e.g., listening to breath sounds)	Knowledge is highly organized and structured, making recall of information easier; have a large storehouse of experiential knowledge (e.g., what abnormal breath sounds sound like, what associated but subtle changes look like)
Focus so much attention on *actions*, they tend to forget to *assess* before acting	*Assess* and think things through before *acting*
Need clear-cut rules	Know when to bend the rules
Are often hampered by unawareness of resources	Are aware of resources and how to use them
Are often hindered by anxiety and lack of self-confidence	Are usually more self-confident, less anxious, and more focused
Must be able to rely on step-by-step procedures; tend to focus more on *procedures* than patient response to the *procedure*	Know when it is safe to skip steps or to do two steps together; are able to focus on both the parts (the procedure) and the whole (the patient response)
Become uncomfortable if patient needs preclude performing procedures exactly as learned.	Are comfortable with rethinking procedure if patient needs require modification of the procedure
Have limited knowledge of suspected problems; therefore, question and collect data more superficially	Have an intuitive sense of suspected problems that allows them to question more deeply and to collect more relevant and in-depth data
Tend to follow standards and policies by rote	Analyze standards and policies, looking for ways to improve them
Learn more readily when matched with a supportive, knowledgeable preceptor or mentor	Are challenged by novices' questions, clarifying their own thinking when teaching novice nurses

*The depth and breadth of expert knowledge, largely gained from opportunities to apply theory in *real situations*, greatly enhance the development of critical thinking skills.
Adapted from Alfaro-LeFevre R: Critical Thinking in Nursing: A Practical Approach. Philadelphia, W.B. Saunders, 1995, p 43.

In a recent study,[22] physicians and nurses identified being available (being in the right place, at the right time, and with the right information) and being receptive (being interested in collaboration and having trust and respect in each other) as the prerequisite conditions for effective collaboration. They also reported that collaboration resulted in improved patient care and job satisfaction and controlled costs.[22] Open and effective communication and mutual trust and respect among members of all involved disciplines are integral to the success of a collaborative, team approach to patient care (see Chapter 3).

Delegation Skills

Nurses have traditionally represented the largest portion of patient care providers. In the struggle to downsize and redesign acute care delivery systems, hospitals have frequently opted to use less expensive nursing personnel (e.g., nurse extenders, critical care technicians, assistive personnel). It has been reported that approximately 97% of hospitals employ some type of UAP.[23] The incorporation of UAP has magnified the need for the nurse of the future to have the ability to delegate effectively.

UAP have been incorporated into patient care delivery systems in various ways. Clinical models refer to delivery systems that use UAP to provide direct patient care tasks. The range of patient care tasks provided by UAP varies from institution to institution and can include obtaining vital signs, measuring intake and output, obtaining a 12-lead ECG, discontinuing peripheral intravenous lines, and endotracheal suctioning. The clinical model can be further divided into partnered and nonpartnered designs. In partnered models, the RN and designated UAP work the same schedule and care for the same patients. In nonpartnered models, the UAP are assigned to work with RNs as needed.[23]

Nonclinical models incorporate UAP to perform various nonnursing tasks that do not typically involve direct patient contact. These tasks include making unoccupied beds, assisting with patient transports, delivering laboratory specimens, answering call lights, and restocking supplies. Integrated models incorporate multiple levels and types of UAP. Research to date has been inconclusive regarding the ability of UAP to reduce hospital costs while maintaining or improving patient outcomes. One major concern regarding the use of UAP identified in the literature was the need for RNs to have expertise in both delegation and supervision.[23]

Certain institutional requirements should be established before UAP are incorporated into the nursing

CHART 1–1

Thomas Jefferson University Hospital Department of Nursing: Position Description

Title: Critical care technician

Source of Supervision: Nursing care coordinator

Employees Supervised: None

General Description: A technician who under the direct supervision of a registered nurse participates in the delivery of patient care within the critical care environment.

Requirements:
1. High school graduate.
2. Successful completion of a state-approved emergency medical technician training program.
3. Emergency medical technician certification required.
4. Minimum of 1 year experience in an emergency room, critical care environment, or related area preferred.
5. Certified in cardiopulmonary resuscitation.

General Responsibilities:
1. Demonstrates an awareness of individual liability for actions.
2. Functions within the established policies and procedures of the Nursing Department of Thomas Jefferson University Hospital.
3. Provides for patient rights.
4. Maintains confidentiality of patient information and records.
5. Demonstrates knowledge of fire regulations, disaster plans, and code blue procedures.
6. Takes necessary electrical, radiation, and oxygen precautions.
7. Follows approved and established techniques and procedures, asepsis, infection control, and safety.
8. Exhibits responsibility through collaboration with others and for efficient, cost-effective use of time and equipment.
9. Establishes priorities based on patient's care requirements in collaboration with the professional nurse based on a basic understanding of a patient's health problems, psychosocial needs, age, and functional status.
10. Identifies self-limitations and appropriately seeks assistance for the provision of safe patient care.

11. Initiates and follows through with appropriate nursing action identified in the patient's plan of care under the direction of the professional nurse.
12. Maintains open channels of communication with nursing staff and other health care providers.
13. Contributes to the maintenance of adequate unit staffing based on patient care needs as identified by the nursing care coordinator.
14. Participates in committees, staff meetings, and activities as assigned or required.
15. Attends all required inservices.

Specific Responsibilities and Functions:
   Under the directions and supervision of a registered nurse:

1. Assists in providing optimal patient care to critically ill patients.
2. Cleans up after procedures including making up stretchers and beds and restocking of area.
3. Stocks unit before the end of each shift according to established guidelines and reports items needed to charge nurse.
4. Initiates and maintains cardiopulmonary resuscitation.
5. Applies electrodes for cardiac monitoring and assists with dysrhythmia monitoring.
6. Applies electrodes for electrocardiography and performs 12-lead ECGs.
7. Performs oral suctioning as needed; assists with endotracheal suctioning as needed.
8. Performs tracheostomy care, ear, nose, and throat care, mouth care as needed.
9. Performs respiratory care such as chest physiotherapy and turn-cough-deep breathe protocols as directed.
10. Assists in admitting and transferring of patients.
11. Obtains vital signs, temperature, pulse, respiration, and blood pressure and records on patient chart.
12. Performs neurologic checks and records data: a) level of consciousness; b) motor ability; c) pupil size, equality, and reactivity.
13. Monitors intake and output.
14. Provides bed pans and urinals and assists patients with toileting activities as needed.
15. Performs Hematest.

CHART 1–1—Continued

16. Applies hot or cold packs as directed.
17. Assists in collecting specimens, properly labeling and transporting to laboratory: a) urine by way of catheter and clean catch; b) sputum; c) throat culture; d) wound culture; e) blood (labeling and transporting only).
18. Assists in positioning patients as directed for coma, shock, seizures, dyspnea, and combativeness.
19. Assists in maintaining patient's hygiene and functional needs.
20. Lifts and moves patients by means of proper body mechanics.

21. Utilizes protective devices (restraints) as directed in the safest and most effective manner.
22. Maintains appropriate documentation on all assigned patients.
23. Sets up for diagnostic procedures such as: a) chest and other portable radiographs; b) line insertion; c) lumbar puncture; d) thoracentesis and paracentesis; e) chest tube insertion.
24. Applies dressings as directed: a) surgical; b) compression for control of bleeding; c) sterile.
25. Other duties as assigned.

Courtesy of Thomas Jefferson University Hospital Department of Nursing, Philadelphia, PA., 1994.

care delivery system. These include a written job description that complies with the state nurse practice act and board of nursing rules and regulations (Chart 1–1), training requirements for UAP, baseline and intermittent documentation of competency to perform tasks, and the assignment and supervision of UAP by RNs only.[24] When delegating direct patient care activities to UAP, responsibility and accountability for the patient's care invariably remain with the RN (Chart 1–2).[25] At all times, the RN delegates patient tasks after conducting a thorough patient assessment and determining an individualized plan of care. The AACN recommends that the RN assess five factors before deciding to delegate patient care tasks. Table 1–5 provides a guide based on these factors to assist nurses in making appropriate decisions relative to delegating to UAP.[24]

Computer Skills

Computers will continue to fill an important role in health care in the next century. Currently, nurses find computer applications in most every health care delivery setting. Computers are used to document patient care, to monitor physiologic data, and to manage patient information. Most critical care technology relies on computer technology (e.g., dysrhythmia detection systems, portable analyzers, infusion pumps, and pulse oximetry). Nurses will need to update and

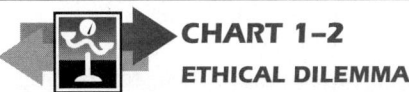

CHART 1–2

ETHICAL DILEMMA

You a are nurse working in a 36-bed, fully monitored, intermediate care unit. Patients in this unit may have any of the following diagnoses: acute myocardial infarction, recent open heart surgery, congestive heart failure, cardiac dysrhythmias, recent pacemaker implant, or coronary artery disease. The unit is filled to capacity, and you are assigned 6 patients. A critical care technician (CCT) from the intensive care unit has been floated to your unit to fill a vacancy due to a call-out by the unit's full-time technician. When the CCT provides you with the vital signs for your patients, you note that all the blood pressures are in the 120s/80s, the pulses are all in the 70s, and the respirations are all 18. Knowing that your patients represent various clinical diagnoses and have varying levels of physiologic stability (based on information from report), you question the accuracy of this information.

1. How would you proceed at this point? Explore the potential consequences of all choices.
2. What are the potential ethical implications in this situation?
3. What are the potential legal ramifications in this situation?
4. What resources are immediately available to assist you in this dilemma?

TABLE 1–5
Decision Grid for Delegation: Five Factors Affecting the Decision to Delegate*

Task and Specific Patient Combination	Potential for Harm	Complexity of Task	Problem Solving and Innovation Necessary	Unpredictability of Outcome	Level of Patient Interaction	Total
Suctioning: Patient has closed head injury and increased intracranial pressure	3	2	3	3	2	13
Suctioning: Patient is comatose with stable vital signs	1	2	1	1	2	7

*This grid can be used as a guide to evaluate patient care tasks being considered for delegation to an unlicensed person. For each task, consider both the individual patient and the task. Score each factor for each patient (0, none; 1, low; 2, moderate; 3, high). The higher the score, the less likely the nurse would delegate the task. As can be seen in the above example, the scores for the same activity—suctioning—are different for two different patients. The range of scores considered acceptable for delegation needs to be determined by each institution.

From Biel M (ed): Delegation: A Tool for Success in the Changing Workplace. Aliso Viejo, CA, American Association of Critical Care Nurses, 1995, p 6.

expand their computer literacy skills to effectively function in the next century. For example, wireless communication systems will transport patient data (e.g., ECGs, physiologic waveforms, laboratory data, and vital signs) to health care providers off site, thus allowing for more rapid decision making. Voice-activated computer charting will replace the traditional keyboard for data entry. On-line access to the Internet will increase the capacity for rapidly acquiring information on new and best practices. It may also play a role in communicating with families, by keeping them up to date on a patient's status.[26] Virtual reality will become a reality, by allowing health care providers to learn new skills and to practice with new equipment without actually involving a real patient. Expert systems will process complex patient information, will reason, and will even provide clinical decisions. Nurses must be comfortable with the expansion in computer technology to collaborate with system developers effectively in the creation of systems that will support critical care nursing practice.[17,18,21]

EXPANDING THE BOUNDARIES OF CRITICAL CARE NURSING

Once thought to only exist in traditional ICUs, critical care nursing in an acute care setting can be found in intermediate care (telemetry or step-down) units and, with the advance of flexible monitoring systems, in medical–surgical units. Patients in intermediate care units can be monitored for heart rhythm, blood pressure through an arterial line, oxygen saturation, and end-tidal CO_2. Most units are also able to manage patients on various medicated drips (e.g., nitroglycerin, dopamine, and dobutamine) and to wean patients from ventilators. Patients undergoing coronary artery stent placement and percutaneous transluminal coronary angioplasty, as well as those awaiting a heart transplant, are often cared for in intermediate care units.[26]

In an effort to monitor patients who do not need the full services of an ICU or intermediate care unit, flexible and portable monitoring systems can be brought to the patient in a general (or medical-surgical) unit. Versions of this system range from monitoring oxygen saturation and noninvasive blood pressure to vital signs, including heart rate, invasive blood pressure, cardiac rhythm, respiration and apnea, temperature, and end-tidal CO_2. Using this system, the nurse can quickly and easily convert any bed in the hospital to a monitored bed.[27]

As more and more procedures are moved to less costly, alternative sites (e.g., outpatient surgical and diagnostic centers), it is believed that hospitals will evolve into giant ICUs that will only treat the sickest patients. In an effort to remain financially solvent, many hospitals have redesigned and formed integrated delivery systems that provide services to support patients across the care continuum: health maintenance organizations, home health care agencies, outpatient surgical centers, clinics, and transitional care facilities. Patients entering hospitals today are older and sicker and are discharged sooner. Patients often require some degree of transitional care after discharge from an acute care setting and before going home. Transitional care is a broad term that refers to various health care settings including subacute, skilled, rehabilitative, and long-term care.[28] Patient acuity across the various levels differs, and many patients require critical care nursing skills.

Subacute care is in its infancy but is expected to develop quickly over the next decade. Patients admitted to this level of transitional care are usually severely impaired but medically stable (e.g., ventilator-dependent patients, comatose patients, and patients with stage III or greater decubitus ulcers). At this level, patients require continuous monitoring and therapy, close supervision by a skilled, multidisciplinary team, or highly technical medical equipment. The goal of care at this level is focused on stabilization.[28]

Skilled care units are designed to address the needs of recently hospitalized patients who have multiple, complex needs. Patients requiring complex wound care, total parenteral nutrition, intravenous therapy, gait training, or intermittent catheterization are often referred to these units for continued care by nurses and physical, occupational, and respiratory therapists. The goal of care at this level is restoration of function.[28]

Acute rehabilitative units provide an intensive program for patients usually recovering from traumatic, neurologic, or orthopedic injuries. The goal of care at this level is focused on adaptation. Patients are taught to identify and to maximize their strengths and to adapt to limitations in activities of daily living. Aggressive physical therapy, often in conjunction with adaptive equipment (e.g., prostheses and wheelchairs), is conducted under the supervision of skilled providers. Frequently, skilled care is combined with acute rehabilitation (skilled rehabilitation), and the goal becomes both restorative and adaptive. Subacute care units, skilled care units, and rehabilitation units can be found in hospitals and long-term care facilities, or they may be freestanding.[28]

Long-term or extended care focuses on support and provides services to patients requiring assistance with living with chronic illnesses such as Alzheimer's disease, multiple sclerosis, or emphysema. In long-term care facilities, patients reside in a homelike environment, and socialization is encouraged. For example, group dining is the norm.[28] Table 1–6 provides a summary of the various levels of transitional care.

Many patients discharged from acute care settings require home health nursing rather than transfer to a transitional care unit. For example, the goal for patients undergoing the minimally invasive direct coronary artery bypass procedure is discharge on postoperative day 2.[26] Patients currently receive chemotherapy, dialysis, blood products, intrathecal infusions, and enteral and parenteral nutrition in the home setting. Portable technology, such as the LVAD and home ventilators, has made it possible for more patients to live outside the acute care setting and in the comfort of their homes. Advances in the treatment of heart failure have led to the successful management of these patients in nurse-controlled, outpatient clinics. Similarly, patients are being treated in outpatient surgical centers in greater numbers than ever before. All these patients are prime candidates for and benefit from follow-up by a home health nurse. In Denmark, open heart surgery is performed in mobile units, after which the patients are transported to their homes with a critical care nurse assigned to them around-the-clock.[29]

The acuity of patients discharged from acute care settings will continue to be higher than ever before. Shorter hospital stays, alternate treatment settings, and "high-tech" home care will become the standard rather than the exception in the next century.[26, 29] As critical care nursing prepares for a "boundless health care system," telemedicine will most likely provide the information link between patients and providers. Through the use of the telephone, interactive television, and computer, both audio and video information can be delivered between two or more distant sites. For example, a home health nurse visiting a patient receiving dobutamine therapy for heart failure can obtain and transmit an ECG and even lung sounds,

TABLE 1–6
Levels of Transitional Care

Transitional Care Level	Approximate Patient-to-RN Ratio	Average Length of Stay	Focus of Care
Subacute	6:1 (hospital) 8:1 (freestanding)	1–3 months	Stabilization
Skilled	8:1 (hospital) 10:1 (freestanding)	2–4 weeks	Restoration
Acute rehabilitation	10:1 (hospital) 14:1 (freestanding)	2–4 weeks	Adaptation
Long term or extended	12:1 (daytime) 16:1 (night/weekend)	3 months+	Support

Adapted from Jones AM, Foster N: Transitional care: bridging the gap. Med Surg Nurs 6:33, 1997.

using a telestethoscope, back to the primary care provider. In this way, health care comes to the patient, even the patient living hundreds of miles from a health care facility.[18, 30]

EXPANDING OPPORTUNITIES FOR THE CRITICAL CARE NURSE

"I think we need to get out of the whole mind-set of *'bedside'* and think of things in terms of *'patient-side,'* because wherever the patient is, we're going to be by their side." These words by Joan Vitello,[26] past president of the AACN, describe the essence of the expanding boundaries of critical care nursing and, ultimately the opportunities. In the next century, critical care nurses will be caring for patients across the entire continuum of care, including preventive services, traditional ICU care, care in intermediate, medical–surgical, and transitional care units, and care in clinics and the home. To maximize their marketability, nurses will need to develop clinical skills that cross over several different settings. The home care environment will perhaps hold the greatest opportunities for nurses. Given the shorter length of stays and the movement of high-technology equipment into the home coupled with the burden of patient care on the families, nurses will provide the essential information and support needed by the family to care for their loved one properly. According to Joan Vitello,[26] the greatest challenge in these exciting times will be to remember to treat the patient and the family holistically, regardless of the setting.

Flexibility and an openness to change will keep nurses in the forefront of health care in the next century. A commitment to being an active participant in the change process will further open doors to new and inspiring opportunities in the field of critical care nursing.

Key Concepts

➠ The 21st century, guided by the *Healthy People 2000* plan, will emphasize health promotion, illness prevention, and health maintenance.

➠ The major goals for the United States from the *Healthy People 2000* document include the increase in the span of healthy lives for Americans, the decrease in health disparities among Americans, and the increase in access to preventive services for all Americans.

➠ The *Healthy People 2000: Midcourse Review* and 1995 revisions demonstrated a positive trend towards achieving many of the national health objectives but work remains to be done.

➠ Several acts of legislation, including the HMO Act of 1974 and the COBRA Act, served to change the

reimbursement of health care services dramatically. Emphasis shifted from fee for service to fees based on DRGs.

➠ The development of HMOs has led the way in the attempts to reduce the costs of health care services further.

➠ Cost-containment efforts must be balanced with quality patient outcomes. Providers and consumers must remain the gate-keepers as changes in health care delivery systems continue to evolve.

➠ The role of the health care consumer in the 21st century will be that of an active participant in all decisions related to health.

➠ The history of critical care nursing is a study of the reorganization of patient care in hospitals. Recovery rooms and experiences with triage led the way in the development of specialty ICUs.

➠ Although hospitals are downsizing, the number of critical care beds is increasing. The demand for critical care nurses in the year 2000 is likely to exceed the supply.

➠ Critical care nursing can be found across the health care continuum—ICUs and intermediate care units, transitional care units, outpatient surgical centers and clinics, and home health care.

➠ Advances in critical care technology will continue well into the next century, with the emphasis on noninvasive technology, including point-of-care testing.

➠ Merging "high tech" with "high touch" will be the greatest challenge for critical care nurses in the future.

➠ Nurses preparing for the 21st century will need to develop critical thinking, collaboration, delegation, and computer skills.

➠ Flexible and portable monitoring systems and advances in telemedicine will bring the health care provider to patients, as the boundaries of critical care become "seamless" in the next century.

➠ Opportunities for critical care nurses will exist in various settings. Flexibility and an openness to change will keep nurses marketable.

References

1. Healthy People 2000: DHHS Publication No. (PHS) 91-50213. Washington, DC, US Department of Health and Human Services, 1990.
2. Healthy People 2000 Midcourse Review: US Department of Health and Human Services. Boston, Jones & Bartlett, 1996.
3. US Preventative Services Task Force: In: Healthy People 2000 Midcourse Review: US Department of Health and Human Services. Boston, Jones & Bartlett, 1996.
4. Kovner A: Health Care Delivery in the United States. New York, Springer, 1995.
5. Mackelprang R, Johnson P: Managed care: Balancing costs, quality and access. SC Psych Proc 8:175–178, 1995.
6. Pera M: Medicare/Medicaid cuts to hit nurses too. N M Nurse 40(4): 7–8, 1995.

7. Feldstein M.: Health plan's financing gap. Society 32:64–66, 1994.

8. Luft H: (1997). Modifying managed competition to address cost and quality. In: Lee PR, Estes CL (eds): The Nation's Health, 5th ed. Boston, Jones & Bartlett, 1997, pp 334–348.

9. Rakich J, Longest B, Darr K: Managing Health Services Organizations. Baltimore, Health Professions Press, 1997.

10. Kerstein J: Primary care physician turnover in health maintenance organization. Health Serv Res 29:17–38, 1994.

11. Schulz R, Girard C, Scheckler WE: Physician satisfaction in managed care environment. Fam Pract 34(3):298–305, 1992.

12. Enthoven A, Kronick R: Managed care, mergers, and role of corporations. In: Lee PR, Estes CL (eds): The Nation's Health, 5th ed. Boston, Jones & Bartlett, 1997.

13. Cleverly WO: Essentials of Health Care Finance, 3rd ed. Gaithersburg, MD, Aspen, 1997.

14. Ummel S: Pursuing the elusive integrated delivery network. Health Care Forum J 40(2): 13–19, 1997.

15. Kongstvedt P: Essentials of Managed Health Care, 2nd ed. Gaithersburg, MD, Aspen, 1997.

16. Lynaugh JE, Fairman J: Critical care nursing: a history. Philadelphia, University of Pennsylvania Press, 1998.

17. Henry SB, Dolter KJ, Reilly CA: Critical care information systems. Crit Care Clin North Am 7:191–202, 1995.

18. McConnell EA: The future of technology in critical care. Crit Care Nurse 16(Suppl 1):3–16, 1996.

19. Tappen RM: Nursing Leadership and Management: Concepts and Practice, 3rd ed. Philadelphia, F.A. Davis, 1995.

20. Alfaro-LeFevre R: Critical Thinking in Nursing: A Practical Approach. Philadelphia, W.B. Saunders, 1995.

21. Sullivan EJ, Decker PJ: Effective Leadership and Management in Nursing, 4th ed. Menlo Park, CA, Addison Wesley Longman, 1997.

22. Baggs JG, Schmitt MH: Nurses' and resident physicians' perceptions of the process of collaboration in an MICU. Res Nurs Health, 20:71–80, 1997.

23. Krapohl GL, Larson E: The impact of unlicensed assistive personnel on nursing care delivery. Nurs Econ 14:99–110, 1996.

24. Biel M (ed): Delegation: A Tool for Success in the Changing Workplace. Aliso Viejo, CA, American Association of Critical Care Nurses, 1995.

25. National Council of State Boards of Nursing: Statement on the Nursing Activities of Unlicensed Persons [Position statement]. Chicago, National Council of State Boards of Nursing, 1990.

26. Macready N: Beyond the boundaries: a continuum of cardiac care. Crit Care Nurse 17(Suppl 1):3–16, 1997.

27. Macready N: Flexible monitoring: mobilizing critical care. Am J Crit Care Nurs 6(Suppl 1):3–15, 1997.

28. Jones AM, Foster N: Transitional care: Bridging the gap. Medsurg Nurs 6:32–38, 1997.

29. Paladichuk A: Breaking down the walls: critical care at home and on the road. Crit Care Nurse 17:94–99, 1997.

30. Villaire M: Telemedicine: tuning in critical care's future? Crit Care Nurse 16:102–107, 1996.

2

Legal and Ethical Issues in Critical Care Nursing

Mary Linn Green

Objectives

After completing this chapter, the student will be able to:

1. Describe the ethical foundations of nursing practice.
2. Identify the legal foundations of nursing practice.
3. Summarize the elements of ethical decision making in critical care.
4. Analyze the key legal and ethical issues that are relevant to critical care nursing.

Over the past few decades, the innovations and technologic advances in health care have progressed at a staggering rate. Nowhere in nursing is this more evident than in the area of critical care, in which increasingly complex technology is used to care for increasingly critically ill patients. Such technologic devices as ventilators, cardiac monitors, arterial lines, central venous catheters, and intravenous drip regulators are common tools used by critical care nurses for their patients. The health care team now has complex technologic interventions at its fingertips that were virtually unheard of some 25 years ago. Because of these capabilities, there may be a tendency to focus on the technology, rather than on the actual patient. Often, the health care team responds to the patient's illness with increasing levels of technology without completely assessing whether these interventions will contribute to that patient's overall well-being. Simply because a technique is available should not be the reason to use it for a particular patient. Critical care nurses must keep in mind that their primary role is to hold foremost the overall well-being of the patient and to advocate for their patients and not for technology.[1]

The fields of ethics and law have had difficulty in keeping pace with the breakneck speed of health care technology. Within the past decade, health care institutions have developed ethics committees to review and discuss various patient care situations. Consultations with ethicists are becoming more readily available to the health care team. In the legal arena, an increasing number of courts have dealt with such issues as a patient's right to refuse treatment and the withdrawal of life-sustaining treatment. State legislatures have passed laws concerning such issues as surrogate decision making for incompetent patients. Although great progress has been made, many questions are still left unanswered when the fields of health care, ethics, and law are drawn together into a complex patient care situation.

This chapter reviews the ethical and legal foundations of nursing practice and thus allows the critical care nurse to reflect on the importance of these areas in his or her own practice. The elements of ethical decision making are presented, and the critical care nurse is encouraged to incorporate this process into practice. Finally, the key legal and ethical issues in critical care are analyzed to enable the critical care nurse to be better equipped to deal with these complex issues in practice.

ETHICAL FOUNDATIONS OF NURSING PRACTICE

To have a clear concept of his or her role as a nursing professional, the critical care nurse must be able to understand the ethical foundations of nursing practice. These foundations include underlying ethical principles and theories and the nursing profession's code of ethics.

Ethical Principles

Several important concepts or principles of ethics are considered to represent the common morality shared by members of society.[2] Because these principles often underlie many ethical dilemmas, it is important for the nurse to be able to recognize them.

Veracity

Veracity is the principle of truthfulness. This requires that the nurse tell the truth to patients and not intentionally deceive or mislead them. Although the nurse may feel uncomfortable about discussing bad news with patients, this is not a good enough reason to avoid telling the truth to patients about their diagnosis, treatments, or prognosis. However, the principle of veracity has a limit. This occurs when telling patients the truth may seriously harm their ability to recover or may produce greater illness.[3]

Nonmaleficence

Nonmaleficence is the principle that the nurse do no harm to patients. This requires one to consider whether the pain and discomfort caused by medical interventions are outweighed by the benefits that patients receive.[4] This principle also requires that the nurse protect those from harm who are unable to protect themselves. This group includes such patients as children, the unconscious, the mentally incompetent, and the extremely debilitated.[5]

Fidelity

Fidelity is the principle of faithfulness to commitments made to oneself and to others. This requires the nurse to be faithful and loyal to the responsibilities he or she has accepted as part of the practice of the profession. The nurse must be responsible and accountable both to patients and to the nursing profession.[5]

Beneficence

Beneficence is the principle of doing good. This requires nurses to promote the health, welfare, and safety of patients. Inherent in this principle is a consideration of the consequences of nursing actions. The nurse must assess whether the overall result of various interventions will benefit patients.[4]

Autonomy

Autonomy is the principle of independence and self-determination. This requires the nurse to respect patients' rights to make decisions for themselves, even if the nurse disagrees with these decisions. The principle of autonomy has limitations. This situation occurs when one patient's autonomy interferes with another patient's health and well-being, as in the case of forced isolation to prevent the spread of disease.[6]

Justice

Justice is the principle of fairness and equality for all persons. This requires the nurse to treat similar patients equally and to avoid discriminating against patients based on cultural or ethnic background, religion, age, sex, social status, or diagnosis. Justice also refers to the distribution of limited resources. In the context of health care, this involves equal access to health care by patients with similar problems. In cases of limited health care resources, ethical problems concerning rationing of these resources may arise.[4]

These ethical principles do not exist in a vacuum. There is continual interplay, and at times tension, among these principles for all persons in their daily lives. The critical care nurse encounters these same principles routinely in practice. It is important for the nurse to be able to recognize such principles as beneficence versus nonmaleficence as they relate to a patient care situation. The process of ethical decision making, based on these principles, is discussed later in this chapter.

Nursing Code of Ethics

In addition to ethical principles, another ethical foundation of nursing practice is the Nursing Code of Ethics. In an attempt to define and apply the basic ethical principles to the profession of nursing more fully, the American Nurses Association published the Code for Nurses with Interpretative Statements.[7] This code, through its interpretations, provides guidance to nursing for conduct and relationships in carrying out responsibilities that are consistent with the ethical obligations of the profession and high quality in nursing care.[8] Every nurse has a personal and professional responsibility to uphold and adhere to the code and to ensure that their nursing colleagues do so as well.[9]

Provides Services with Respect

"The nurse provides services with respect for human dignity and the uniqueness of the client, unrestricted by considerations of social or economic status, personal attributes, or the nature of health problems."[10] The most fundamental basis of nursing practice is respect for the worth and dignity of every patient. Nurses must work to protect and preserve human life if there is hope of recovery or reasonable hope of benefit from treatment that prolongs life.[10] Patients should have the right to determine what will be done with their person. They should be provided with accurate information and should be allowed to accept, refuse, or terminate treatment. Nurses are obliged to understand the moral and legal rights of all patients and to protect and support those rights.[10]

Nurses should consider patients' individuality, lifestyles, and value systems in planning and tailoring care to meet these specific needs. Nurses' respect for patients' worth and dignity should not be influenced by the nature of their patients' health problems. Nurses do not act deliberately to terminate the life of anyone.[11] Nurses should not limit the provision of nursing care by their attitudes or beliefs. If a nurse is ethically opposed to the care expected for a specific patient, the nurse is justified in refusing to participate in that care.[11] This refusal must be made in a timely fashion, to provide opportunity for other arrangements to be made for the patient's care. However, if the patient's life is in jeopardy, the nurse must not abandon the patient and may only withdraw from care when alternative sources of nursing care become available.[12] Nurses should respect patients and render or obtain needed services for them irrespective of the setting.[12]

Safeguards Right to Privacy

"The nurse safeguards the client's right to privacy by judiciously protecting information of a confidential nature."[12] The right to privacy is inalienable, and the patient trusts the nurse to hold all information in confidence.[12] Only information that is pertinent to the patient's welfare and treatment should be disclosed, and then only to those involved in the patient's care. Information required for quality of care review should be disclosed pursuant to defined protocols.[13] Even though the patient's records belong to the agency in which the information is collected, the patient maintains the right of control over the information within the records. For a nurse to use a patient's record for research or other purpose in which anonymity cannot be guaranteed, the patient's consent must first be obtained.[13]

Incompetent, Unethical, or Illegal Practice

"The nurse acts to safeguard the client and the public when health care and safety are affected by incompetent, unethical or illegal practice by any person."[14] Because the nurse is committed to the health and safety of the patient, the nurse must be vigilant and take action if the rights or best interests of the patient are threatened by incompetent, unethical, or illegal practice by any member of the health care team or health care system.[14] If the nurse becomes aware of inappropriate practice in the provision of care, concern

should be expressed to that individual about the patient's welfare. If factors in the health care system threaten the patient's welfare, the nurse should express concern to the appropriate administrative person. If necessary, the inappropriate practice should be reported to the appropriate authority within the larger system.[14] The nurse should participate in organized review mechanisms that serve to safeguard patients.[15]

Assumes Accountability and Responsibility

"The nurse assumes responsibility and accountability for individual nursing judgments and actions."[15] Individual professional nurses must bear the primary responsibility for the nursing care that patients receive, and nurses must be accountable for their own practice.[16] The nurse is responsible for nursing judgment and action. A collaborative relationship between the nurse and the patient must be attained through the use of the nursing process.[16] The nurse is held accountable for judgments and actions undertaken in the course of nursing practice. The accountability of the nurse for actions taken and judgments made is not relieved by physicians' orders or agency policies.[17]

Maintains Competence

"The nurse maintains competence in nursing."[17] It is the personal responsibility of every nurse to maintain competency in practice.[17] Nurses should acquire knowledge of new developments and techniques in their field of practice, both for the nurses' own professional development and for the well-being of their patients.[17] Nurses should engage in ongoing self-evaluation of their competency, as well as have their practice reviewed and evaluated by their peers.[17] Nurses should consult with and refer patients to other nurses with expertise in various areas of practice.[18]

Exercises Informed Judgment and Uses Individual Competence

"The nurse exercises informed judgment and uses individual competency and qualifications as criteria in seeking consultation, accepting responsibilities, and delegating nursing activities."[18] Because of the changing scope of nursing practice, the nurse must exercise judgment in accepting responsibilities, requesting consultation, and assigning responsibilities to others.[18] The nurse must not engage in practices that are prohibited by law, nor should the nurse delegate activities to others that are also prohibited. If the nurse determines that he or she lacks the knowledge or competence to perform certain care, the nurse should refuse to do so and should seek alternative sources of care based on concern for the patient's welfare.[19] If the needs of the patient are beyond the competency and qualifications of the nurse, consultation and collaboration must be sought with qualified nurses or other health professionals.[19] The nurse is accountable for delegation of nursing care activities to other health workers. The nurse must assess the competency of these other workers and must not delegate functions to them for which they are not prepared or qualified. Institutional policies do not relieve the nurse of the accountability for judgments about delegation of nursing care.[19]

Every nurse has the responsibility to familiarize himself or herself with this nursing code of ethics in its entirety and to incorporate its principles into the practice of nursing.

Nurse as Patient Advocate

One of the fundamental roles of the profession of nursing has long been that of patient advocacy. As primary caregivers who have traditionally spent the most time caring for a patient, nurses are in a unique position to serve as patient advocates. Perhaps the most accurate definition of advocacy, as it pertains to nursing, is "acting to safeguard and advance the interests of another."[20] This means that nurses act to safeguard and advance the interests of the patient for whom they care. The role of advocacy for nurses is multifaceted and includes advising, acting as liaison, sharing information, making recommendations, and assisting patients to make informed choices.[21] Not only do nurses assist patients or their designated surrogate to make informed decisions that are in the patient's best interests, but also, as advocates, nurses must support and respect these decisions.

In yet another advocacy role, nurses serve as liaisons between the patient and other members of the health care team. In this capacity, nurses represent and define the patient's decisions to other health team members involved in the patient's care. If a treatment decision is made that is not in the patient's best interest, nurses should intervene to question that decision.

Patient advocacy is an ongoing process for nurses during the entire course of the patient's care. This process has been described as "facilitating, educating, advocating, communicating, and understanding the values, preferences and goals of others."[21] To be effective advocates, nurses need to understand and respect the values, culture, religion, and beliefs unique to each patient. To facilitate patient advocacy within the health care system, nurses must understand the values and hierarchy of the institution in which they work, and they must learn how to work within that system.[22]

Risks of Advocacy

The role of patient advocate, particularly for critical care nurses, is one that inherently involves some risks. These risks of advocacy have been well described by Rushton in four basic areas.[22] The first area of risk can be conflict between nurses and others involved in a particular patient's situation. This could include conflict with the patient, the patient's family or surrogate, the physicians, other members of the health care team, or the institution. Often, this conflict is based on varying interpretations of what is in the best interests of the patient.[22]

The second area of risk can be more personal and can be directed at nurses' professional positions. Nurses have been found to be insubordinate or have sustained damage to their reputations, or even friendships, because of their advocacy for their patients. These risks are uniquely influenced by the values and directives of the health system in which the nurses work, and some systems encourage advocacy by nurses more than others.[22]

The third area of risk can be to the personal integrity of nurses. This can occur when nurses experience a dilemma between what they perceive to be their professional nursing duties to a patient and their own personal convictions. This tug-of-war between their perception of duty and their personal convictions can lead to stress and, ultimately, a loss of integrity and self-esteem.[22]

The fourth area of risk can be the potential for personal suffering that nurses experience through their care of patients. Nurses are in a unique position to recognize and respond to their patients' suffering. However, if they are unable to relieve patients' suffering, or if they believe that their advocacy for the patient is inadequate, nurses themselves can also personally suffer.[23] Although critical care nurses learn that patient advocacy carries risks, they also realize that the personal and professional satisfaction in effectively advocating for a patient are well worth these risks.

Nurse's Obligation to Self

In reviewing the ethical foundations of nursing practice, nurses should give consideration and thought to their obligations or duties to self. Often, nurses concentrate so intently on their duties to their patients and to others that they do not take the time to reflect on their duties to themselves. However, when nurses fulfill their duties to themselves, they become more effective in fulfilling their duties to others, including patients. Jameton has identified three aspects of duties to self that are expressed in ethical concerns involving critical care nurses: identity, self-regarding duties, and integrity.[24]

Identity encompasses both professional and personal identities for nurses. The goal in this area is to integrate nurses' professional identities with their personal identities. This duty enables critical care nurses to express their opinions, based on their own moral viewpoints, when discussing the appropriateness of a patient's care with other staff members.[25] Maintenance of a personal identity is not something that is isolated and uninvolved with the practice of nursing. Rather, this duty to self requires active participation in ethical judgment by nurses, both in the work setting and in their personal lives.[26]

Self-regarding duties are those that primarily apply to or affect oneself. In nursing, professional competence is a major self-regarding duty. Competence is maintained by an honest assessment of the nurses' own capacities and an adequate level of self-care.[27] Competence is primarily a self-attribute that is developed by nurses and secondarily has a positive effect on patient care.

Integrity is viewed as wholeness of character, which is an individual concern and therefore a duty to oneself. Integrity is threatened when nurses face conflicting duties to self because they are divided by personal and professional concerns. This is particularly true when their professional activities require a level of dedication that threatens the welfare of their personal lives.[28] Nurses may struggle between these two significant commitments, while they attempt to strike a balance between them.[29] Reaching an acceptable balance is unique to each individual nurse and contributes to his or her wholeness of character.

Being able to recognize their obligations and duties to self contributes greatly to the ethical foundation in nurses' personal and professional lives. When viewed in the context of ethical principles, duties to self are not based on selfishness, but rather on the importance of including oneself in ethical considerations. By developing this sense of self-respect and dignity, nurses will be better equipped to respect the dignity and needs of their patients.

LEGAL FOUNDATIONS OF NURSING PRACTICE

In addition to understanding the ethical foundations of nursing practice, an understanding of the legal foundations of nursing practice is also of vital importance to the critical care nurse. Never before have legal issues affected the practice of nursing as they do currently, and on a seemingly daily basis. Both general and specific legal principles have an impact on nurses' professional and personal lives. General legal principles include consent, various types of torts, negligence, and liability. More specific legal issues such as informed consent and advance directives are discussed later in this chapter.

Consent

Consent is the legal doctrine that provides an individual the right to determine what will or will not be done to himself or herself. Consent is legally defined as a "willingness in fact that an act or an invasion of an interest shall take place."[30] The doctrine of consent in patient care was established in the case of *Schloendorff v. Society of New York Hospitals*,[31] in which Justice Cardozo wrote:

> *Every human being of adult years and sound mind has a right to determine what will be done with his own body; and a surgeon who performs an operation without his patient's consent commits an assault, for which he is liable in damages. This is true except in cases of emergency where the patient is unconscious, and where it is necessary to operate before consent can be obtained.[32]*

Thus, the patient's right of self-determination and the importance of consent to treatment were firmly established.

Types of Consent

There are basically two types of consent: express and implied. Express consent is directly given, either verbally or in writing. In health care, the most common type of express consent is a written consent form that is signed by the patient.[33] These forms include such documents as general consent for treatment, consent for a specific procedure, or consent for administration of blood.

Implied consent is given by a person's actions or inactions, rather than verbally or in writing. A common example of implied consent is when a patient rolls to one side to receive an injection in the hip. The courts have also found implied consent by a patient to exist in other selected circumstances. One is when an emergency exists and the patient is unable to give express consent. Another is during a surgical procedure, when more extensive surgery is needed that is substantially similar to that to which the patient gave express consent. Yet another circumstance is when the patient continues to take treatments without objecting to them.[33]

Elements of Consent

For a patient to give valid consent, four elements must be met. The first is that the patient must have decision-making capacity. This means that the patient has the "ability to appreciate the nature, extent, or probable consequences of the (health care provider's) conduct to which consent is given."[33] There is a general presumption of decision-making capacity for adults. When a patient's decision-making capacity is called into question, the patient should be evaluated for the potential need for an appointed guardian or determination of an appropriate surrogate decision maker for the patient.[34] The second element required for valid consent is that it must be given voluntarily by the patient. This means that it is given freely and not as a result of duress, coercion, or undue influence.[34] The third element required is that the patient's consent is not obtained in any fraudulent manner.[34] The final element for valid consent is that the patient knows and understands what treatment he or she will receive.[35] This final element of knowledge and understanding by the patient becomes the substance of the doctrine of informed consent. The issue of informed consent is addressed more specifically later in this chapter.

Types of Torts

Tort law is an area of civil law, as opposed to criminal law. A tort is best defined as "a private or civil wrong, or injury, other than a breach of contract, for which the court will provide a remedy in the form of an action for damages."[36] The civil action for a tort is brought by an injured person (the plaintiff) in order to be compensated for damage he or she suffered by a wrongdoer (the defendant). Various torts have been categorized as intentional or quasi-intentional, depending on the requirement of intent by the defendant. Other critical areas of tort law, particularly to nurses, are those of negligence and liability. Each of these areas of tort law is considered as it relates to health care, and to nurses in particular.

Intentional Torts

Intentional torts are classified as such because they are based on the concept of intent by the person who commits a tort. The concept of intent is composed of three basic elements: "(1) it is a state of mind, (2) about consequences of an act and not about the act itself, (3) it extends not only to having in mind a purpose to bring about given consequences but also to having in mind a belief that given consequences are substantially certain to result from the act."[37] This intent, which is particular to tort liability, does not need to be a hostile intent, or even a desire to do any harm. It is simply an intent to invade the interests of another in an unlawful way.[37] The intentional torts that are encountered in health care are assault, battery, false imprisonment, and intentional infliction of emotional distress.

Assault

The tort of assault relates to a person's interest in freedom from apprehension of a harmful or offensive contact.[38] No actual physical contact is necessary, but rather only the fear or apprehension that the contact will occur. Assault is considered to be a mental, rather than a physical, invasion.[38] If a person is unaware of the threat, no assault has occurred. The important element of this tort is the threat perceived by the victim. This tort can be applicable to patient care. If a nurse threatens to give a patient an injection against his or her will, and approaches the patient with a syringe in hand, the patient may well have an action against the nurse for assault. Most often, the tort of assault is combined with that of battery.

Battery

The tort of battery is a harmful or offensive contact with a person or apprehension that such a contact is imminent.[39] This contact extends to anything that may be attached to or extending from a person, including such things as clothing, or even assistive devices such as canes. Unlike in assault, the person need not be conscious of the contact at the time it occurs.[40] Battery is most often encountered in patient care when no consent is given for treatment, such as surgery performed without the patient's consent. If a nurse gives the patient an injection or inserts an IV line over the patient's objection, the nurse may be liable for battery.

False Imprisonment

The tort of false imprisonment protects a person's freedom from restraint of movement.[41] There must be some direct restraint of movement against the person's will and no means for the person to escape from the confinement. The restraint of movement may be even for a brief period, and the person must be aware of the confinement. In patient care, false imprisonment is most often alleged when a patient is admitted to the hospital against his or her will.

Intentional Infliction of Emotional Distress

The tort of intentional infliction of emotional distress protects a person's peace of mind.[42] The conduct of the defendant must be extreme and outrageous, exceeding the bounds tolerated by decency, and must cause severe emotional distress.[43] In patient care, the intentional infliction of emotional distress may be alleged not only by the patient, but the patient's family as well. A wife who is subjected to observing her husband being futilely resuscitated and die may well have a valid cause for action against the health care providers for the infliction of emotional distress.

Quasi-Intentional Torts

Quasi-intentional torts are different from intentional torts because the intent may not be as clear. However, these torts do involve a voluntary act by the defendant and a subsequent interference with an interest of the plaintiff.[44] The quasi-intentional torts that are encountered in health care are defamation and invasion of privacy.

Defamation

Defamation is an invasion of a person's interest in reputation and good name. It is made up of the twin torts of libel and slander, one being written and the other oral.[45] Defamation requires a communication about a person to a third party. This communication is one that tends to injure the plaintiff's reputation and to diminish the esteem, respect, or confidence in which the plaintiff is held.[46] Generally, only a living person may be defamed, and defamation aimed at a general group or class of people is not actionable.[47] The statements must be understood by others to be defamatory. There are differing standards of proof for defamation if it involves a public figure as opposed to a private person.

Libel is defamation that is written. However, this meaning has been extended to include such things as pictures, signs, movies, and television.

Slander is defamation that is spoken. Slander per se occurs, and the plaintiff's damages are presumed, if the oral defamatory communication imputes the following: the plaintiff is guilty of a crime involving moral turpitude, the plaintiff is suffering from a loathsome disease, unchastity in a female plaintiff, and statements relating to the plaintiff's business, trade, or profession.[48] It is easy to recognize that certain situations in health care may lend themselves to actions based on defamation. Nurses can be held liable for such things as making false statements about a patient's condition or derogatory comments about physician's reputations.

Invasion of Privacy

Invasion of privacy is the interference with a person's right to be left alone and is composed of four separate causes of action.[49] The first is the appropriation of the plaintiff's name or likeness for the benefit of the defendant. This occurs when the plaintiff's name, picture, or other likeness is used without the plaintiff's consent to further a business purpose of someone else.[49]

The second is the unreasonable intrusion on the plaintiff's seclusion or private affairs. This includes intrusion on the plaintiff's physical solitude.[50] The intrusion must be one that would be offensive or objection-able to a reasonable person. This cause of action has particular importance in the health care setting. Nurses can be held liable for allowing a patient's care to be observed by others without the patient's consent.

The third is the public disclosure of private facts about the plaintiff. This requires that the disclosure must be public, the facts disclosed must be private, and the matter made public must be highly offensive and objectionable to a reasonable person.[51] This cause of action also has relevance to the health care setting. Nurses can be held liable for releasing information about the patient's diagnosis and treatment to the public.

The fourth cause of action for invasion of privacy is placing a person in a false light in the public eye. The false light must be something that would be objection-able to a reasonable person.[52]

Negligence

Negligence is the area of tort law that is perhaps the most commonly identified by nurses. Causes of action based on the theory of negligence are those most frequently filed against nurses. Therefore, it is important to understand the concept of negligence in general and professional negligence in particular.

Unlike intentional and quasi-intentional torts, discussed previously, in negligence, the defendant does not intend or desire to bring about the consequences that occur. However, the risk of these consequences would be great enough that a reasonable person would anticipate and would take steps to guard against them.[53] Negligence has been defined as "conduct which falls below the standard established by law for the protection of others against unreasonable risk of harm."[53] The elements that must be proven in a cause of action in negligence are 1) a duty owed by the defendant to the plaintiff; 2) a breach of this duty; 3) the breach of duty as the legal or proximate cause of the plaintiff's injuries; and 4) experience by the plaintiff of damage or loss.[54]

In negligence actions, the conduct of the defendant is scrutinized and is compared with the conduct of a reasonably prudent person. In the trial of a negligence case, this comparison of conduct is defined for the jury. In Illinois, for example, the jury receives the following definition of negligence: "the failure to do something which a reasonably careful person would do, or the doing of something which a reasonably careful person would not do, under circumstances similar to those shown by the evidence."[55] Thus the jury compares the conduct of the defendant to the standard of the reasonably prudent or careful person and decides whether or not the defendant was negligent. Most general negligence cases have to do with property damage and personal injury such as slips and falls and car accidents. However, general negligence cases have been filed against hospitals for such things as falls by patients and visitors, injuries caused when patients step on needles embedded in the carpet of their rooms, and accosting of visitors in the parking lot.

Professional Negligence

Negligence cases that are filed against nurses are known as professional negligence or professional malpractice cases. In a professional negligence case, the plaintiff, most commonly the patient, must prove the same four elements against the nurse as in a general negligence case. By way of example, consider these elements in the context of a situation in critical care. An ICU nurse is assigned to a patient on a busy shift. The physician orders an IV medication, and the nurse mistakenly gives the patient triple the amount that is ordered. The patient immediately goes into cardiopulmonary arrest and dies. In the subsequent lawsuit, the patient's wife (plaintiff) must prove the four elements of negligence against the nurse. The first element is a duty owed by the nurse to the patient. The nurse was assigned to care for the patient, and thus a duty of due care immediately attached and was owed by the nurse to the patient. The second element is a breach of this duty. By the nurse's inattention to the appropriate dose of medication and by the injection of triple the ordered amount, the nurse breached her duty to the patient. The third element is that the nurse's breach of duty must be the legal or proximate cause of the patient's injuries. The patient's cause of death was determined to be an overdose of the medication given by the nurse. Therefore, there is a direct causal connection between the nurse's breach of duty and the patient's injuries. The fourth element is that the patient must have experienced damages. Not only did the patient die, but also his wife suffered the loss of her spouse. Thus, the plaintiff would be able to prove negligence on the part of the nurse and could recover monetary damages.

In a professional negligence case against a nurse, his or her conduct is judged according to the standard of conduct for professional nurses. In a general negligence case, the defendant's conduct is compared with that of a reasonably prudent person. However, in a professional negligence case against a nurse, his or her conduct is compared with that of a reasonably well-qualified nurse. This is known as the professional standard of care. In Illinois, for example, the jury receives the following definition of professional negligence: "in providing professional services to the patient, a registered professional nurse must possess and apply the knowledge and use the skill and care ordinarily used by a reasonably well-qualified registered professional nurse under the circumstances similar to those shown by the evidence. A failure to do so is professional negligence."[56] To prove whether or not the defendant nurse met this standard of care, expert testimony is re-

quired. Therefore, both the defendant and the plaintiff must present a nurse expert witness to testify that the defendant nurse did or did not act as a reasonably well-qualified nurse would act in a similar situation. A nurse will be found guilty of professional negligence if he or she breached the standard of care and if that breach caused damages to the patient.

Many standards govern the practice of critical care nursing. Standards of nursing care are established measures of the quality and quantity of care and agreed-on levels of performance for nurses. These standards are established by many sources: policies and procedures, standards of practice, standards of care, and performance criteria. On a national level, there are the American Nurses Association (ANA) Standards of Nursing Care, both in general and specialized areas. Of particular importance to the critical care nurse are the American Association of Critical-Care Nurses (AACN) Standards of Care for the Critically Ill. The critical care nurse should become familiar with these standards of care and should adhere to them in his or her own practice. These standards serve two important purposes. The first is to ensure safe, competent, and effective care for patients. The second is to provide the nurse with some measure of professional protection if the nurse's care of a patient should be called into question. Evidence that the nurse adhered to these professional standards in his or her care of the patient is extremely useful in proving that the nurse met the standard of care.

Types of Liability

Liability has been generally defined as "the responsibility for a possible or actual loss, penalty, evil, expense or burden for which law or justice requires the individual to do something for, pay, or otherwise compensate the victim."[57] Two basic types of liability apply to nurses: personal and vicarious.

Personal Liability

It has long been an accepted principle that everyone is responsible for his or her own behavior. Nurses are certainly no exception to this rule, and they are held accountable for their behavior, whether negligent or not. Nurses are individually held accountable for the care they render to patients. Along with this personal accountability comes personal liability if the care they render is negligent. The development of the profession of nursing as separate and distinct from the profession of medicine has not been overlooked in the eyes of the law. Patients are filing professional negligence lawsuits that name the nurse, as well as the physician, individually as defendants. Although traditionally, the nurse's employer (such as a hospital) has been sued for the actions of the nurse, increasingly both the individual nurse and the nurse's employer are named as defendants. Critical care nurses are in a unique situation that serves to increase their individual liability. Not only does the critical care nurse serve as the patient's primary nurse (particularly in a 1:1 situation), but also the patient's illness is usually severe and fraught with complications.

Vicarious Liability

The second type of liability that applies to nurses is vicarious liability. Vicarious liability is also called "imputed liability and refers to the responsibility one is found to have for the actions of other individuals because a special relationship exists between those individuals."[58] This refers to the special relationship between an employer (such as a hospital) and an employee (the nurse). The term "respondeat superior" is based on vicarious liability and means "let the master speak."[57] This requires the employer to be vicariously liable for the negligent acts of its employees. However, for the employer to be held liable, the act must have occurred when the person was working and must also have been part of the employee's job responsibilities.[59] Thus, if a critical care nurse is employed by a hospital and is acting within his or her job description when an injury to a patient occurs, the hospital can be held vicariously liable for the nurse's negligence by the patient.

ETHICAL DECISION MAKING IN CRITICAL CARE

To incorporate the process of ethical decision making into his or her own practice, the critical care nurse must possess an understanding of the elements of ethical decision making. Earlier, the basic ethical principles and nursing code of ethics were delineated. Additionally, the nurse's role as patient advocate, the risks of this advocacy, and the nurse's obligation to self were all discussed in the context of the ethical foundations of critical care nursing practice. In building on this foundation, we now consider the process of ethical decision making as it relates to critical care.

Decision making in critical care is a process that usually is neither neat nor uncomplicated. Frequently, this decision-making process is "marked by soul-searching discussions, agonizing dialogue among health care professionals, and sometimes even battles over the appropriate course of action."[60] Decisions are individual, personal determinations based on one's values. People possess certain personal, cultural, and religious values that are important to them, and they make choices in their lives based on these values. Other factors that influence a person's decisions are age, gender, religion, and culture.[60] Each person possesses a set of values and factors in his or her life that

combines to form a basis for decision making unique to that individual. When a person becomes a patient in a critical care unit, these personal values are not left at home, but rather they accompany the patient and serve as a basis for the decisions the patient makes concerning his or her care. Critical care nurses, in helping to facilitate ethical decision making, must not lose sight of this issue.

The critical care setting is the area of health care in which ethical dilemmas occur the most frequently. According to Genesen,[61] the critical care unit lends itself to ethical concerns for two reasons. The first is that critical care units contain the most sophisticated medical technology currently available, which presents issues concerning its proper application.[61] The second is that patients in critical care units are often unable to make decisions about their care, either because their illness has caused them to lose their decision-making capacity or because the extent and prognosis of their illness are not clear.[61]

The foundation of ethical decision making should be a self-assessment by each critical care nurse of his or her own values concerning illness, life, and death. This self-assessment is accomplished by the nurse's considering difficult questions. What is most important in my life? If I knew I was dying, what would be most important? How would I feel about life-sustaining procedures if I were dying? What is my religion? How does my religion affect my beliefs about death and illness? Who would I want to make decisions for me if I could not make them for myself?[62] The answers to these questions vary with each individual and enable the nurse to identify and consider his or her own values. Armed with this knowledge of self, the nurse can then approach ethical decision making in patient care. The nurse should then separate his or her own personal values from those of the patient, the patient's family, and other health care providers.[62]

The process of clinical and ethical decision making has been well delineated by Jonsen and colleagues in their decision-making model.[63] According to this model, four areas of information must be taken into consideration in ethical decision making. These are medical indications, preferences of patients, quality of life, and contextual (external) issues.[64] When deliberation concerning the ethical appropriateness of a patient's plan of care occurs, the decision must include a consideration of each of these areas.[65] Each of these four areas is considered individually.

Medical Indications

Medical indications consist of objective information. This includes the patient's medical history, an accurate diagnosis, and an accurate prognosis. Dependent on these indications, all treatment options are identified for the patient.[64]

Preferences of Patients

The area of preferences of the patient consists of subjective information that is unique to each patient. This includes the patient's personal history and religious and personal values. Also included are any preferences that the patient has expressed. Any advance directives executed by the patient are considered, as is any self-assessment about the quality of life that may be made by the patient. Finally, the patient's ability to make and communicate decisions is also taken into account.[64]

Quality of Life

The area of quality of life also consists of subjective information. This includes an external assessment of the benefits and burdens of the treatment on the patient. If the patient cannot decide for himself or herself about the desired quality of life, someone must be identified to do so for the patient. Preferences of the patient's family members and the potential burdens on the patient's caregiver are also issues to be considered.[64]

External Issues

The area of external or contextual issues consists of objective information. This includes economic factors such as insurance availability and cost of care. Legal issues and any constraints that are particular to the health care institution are also included in this area.[64]

The areas of medical indications and preferences of patients are the two most important areas to be considered in shared decision making and are of a higher priority than the quality of life and external issues. This is because a patient or surrogate decision maker who is thoroughly informed about the patient's medical indications has the right to consent to or refuse the care that is recommended.[65] Quality-of-life issues are subjective and are difficult to evaluate. However, due consideration should be given to these issues as the patient or surrogate decision maker weighs the benefits and burdens of treatment. Although external issues deserve some consideration in the decision-making process, they are often general and are not necessarily focused on the individual patient.[65] To facilitate the process of ethical decision making, communication is essential. The entire health care team must discuss the patient's situation with one another and, in turn, must discuss this with the patient, family, and surrogate. There is no magic formula that enables critical care nurses to arrive at ethical decisions for all patients automatically. Rather, this decision-making process is based on respect for self, patients, and families, thoughtful consideration of the areas described previously, and a recognition that each patient's situation is unique. See Chart 2–1 for an example of an ethical dilemma.

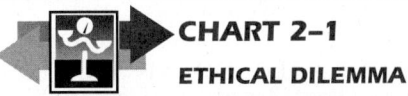

CHART 2–1

ETHICAL DILEMMA

Timmy C. is a "street person" in his late 60s who was found unresponsive on the sidewalk outside a bar. He had no heart rate or respirations, and no one could determine how long he had been unconscious. Paramedics resuscitated him at the scene, and his heart rate returned, his pupils reacted sluggishly and he exhibited decerebrate posturing. In the emergency room, he was in normal sinus rhythm, he had an arterial line and a Swan-Ganz catheter inserted, and was placed on a ventilator. He was sent to the ICU during the night shift.

At 7:00 AM, you are assigned to be the primary nurse for Timmy on the day shift. As you are receiving report, he goes into asystole, and a full code is called. His heart rate is reestablished at 50 to 60 beats per minute, but he has no blood pressure. He exhibits no pupillary response, nor does he have any gag reflex when suctioned. To maintain his systolic blood pressure in the range of 80 to 90 mm Hg, the physician has ordered Levophed (norepinephrine bitartrate), an expensive medication. If the IV Levophed is decreased to anything less than the maximum dose, Timmy loses his blood pressure.

Timmy has no living relatives or friends. He has not left any living will or advance directive of any kind. He has no family doctor.

- If you, as Timmy's primary nurse, decide that it is contrary to your personal ethics and beliefs to continue to treat him with the IV Levophed, what would be your course of action?
- What, if any, bearing does the fact that Timmy is a "street person" with no known relatives or family have on what his course of treatment should be?
- Should costly medication, such as Timmy is receiving, be withheld if it will not result in his recovery?
- Whose responsibility is it to determine that the medication should be discontinued and that Timmy should be allowed to die?

LEGAL AND ETHICAL ISSUES IN CRITICAL CARE

As new advances in health care technology continue to be made at a rapid rate, these same advances have contributed to increasingly complicated legal and ethical issues in patient care. Nowhere in health care is this more obvious than in the area of critical care. It is imperative that critical care nurses be familiar with these legal and ethical patient care issues, which are encountered daily in their practice of nursing. The key issues relevant to critical care are advance directives and end-of-life decisions, resuscitation, informed consent, brain death and organ donation, and allocation of resources.

Advance Directives and End-of-Life Decisions

Advance directives are legal documents that allow individuals to give instructions about their future health care if they should become incapable of making their own decisions. There are two types of advance directives: an instruction directive (living will) and a proxy directive (durable power of attorney). A living will is a written instruction of a person's treatment wishes. Most states have statutes that govern the format and the use of a living will, so it is best for the nurse to be familiar with the law in his or her own state. In general, a living will contains instructions concerning the use or withdrawal of life support in end-of-life situations. A patient must have a terminal illness or permanent unconsciousness for a living will to take effect. The patient's condition and the anticipation that it is not expected to improve must be certified in the medical record by at least one, and sometimes two, physicians.[66]

A durable power of attorney is a proxy advance directive, in which another individual (agent) is designated to make health care and treatment decisions for a person if he or she becomes unable to do so. This document is a much broader directive than the living will because it allows the agent to step in and actually make the decisions for the patient. The durable power of attorney does not take effect until the patient is incapable of making a decision. As with the living will, most states have statutes that govern the durable power of attorney. In general, most of the statutes require that the agent make health care decisions according to the patient's wishes. The agent also has the authority to make all health care decisions for the patient and is not simply limited to end-of-life decisions. Some states have restrictions on who can serve as agent, and they specifically prohibit health care workers from doing so.[67] As a critical care nurse, there are a few guidelines to keep in mind concerning advance directives. If a patient has an advance directive, a copy should be placed in the medical record. If the patient has a designated agent pursuant to a durable power of attorney, that agent should be identified in the record. If the nurse suspects that the patient may be incapable of making his or her own decisions, this possibility should be brought to the physician's attention. The nurse should be familiar with the protocols of the institution regarding the appropriate procedure to be followed with advance directives. Finally, the nurse should become familiar with the applicable state law governing advance directives.

Patient Self-Determination Act

The Patient Self-Determination Act was passed by the United States government in 1990, and it concerns the issue of end-of-life decisions. The act was designed to encourage communication among patients, health care workers, physicians, and family members about advance directives and patients' rights. The act requires health care facilities to 1) provide written information to each patient admitted explaining the patient's right to make decisions concerning health care and to formulate advance directives, as well as the institution's policies that address these rights; 2) document in the medical record whether or not the patient has an advance directive; 3) refrain from discrimination against the patient if he or she has no advance directive; 4) ensure compliance with state law concerning advance directives; and 5) educate staff members and the community about advance directives.[68] The basic effect of this act is to raise the patient's awareness of the right to make end-of-life decisions. The critical care nurse should be familiar with his or her institution's policies pursuant to this act.

Surrogate or Family Decision-Making Statutes

For those patients who do not have any advance directives and who have become incapable of decision making, yet another type of state statute may provide assistance. These laws are known as surrogate or family decision-making statutes and have been passed in about half of the states. In general, these surrogate statutes provide a list of individuals (such as spouse, parent, and adult child) who are authorized to make decisions on behalf of an incompetent patient with no advance directives. The surrogate is required to consider the patient's values, beliefs, and personal preferences when making decisions on the patient's behalf. The surrogate statutes provide for decision making concerning end-of-life decisions to return to the incompetent patient's family and close friends, who have traditionally made these decisions.[69] The critical care nurse should be familiar with applicable state surrogate or family decision-making statutes. If such a statute is in effect in his or her state, the nurse should be familiar with the institution's policies pursuant to this statute. Finally, the nurse will be in a unique position to identify, communicate with, and support the patient's surrogate while caring for the critically ill patient.

Various avenues are now available to enable patients to make end-of-life decisions. If a patient is competent to make his or her own decision to withdraw or withhold life-sustaining treatment, then he or she may do so (Chart 2–2: Beyond the ICU). When a patient is not competent to make his or her own decision about

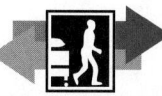

CHART 2–2

BEYOND THE ICU: THE RIGHT TO DIE

Kenneth, a 10-year-old boy, is admitted to the ICU after a diving accident. He is diagnosed with a high cervical fracture that has rendered him quadriplegic and is placed in cervical skeletal traction. He is intubated and is placed on a ventilator, and his parents are understandably distraught. Over the next week, his condition stabilizes to a point where a cervical fusion is successfully performed. However, he does not regain any spontaneous respiration; it is determined that he will remain ventilator dependent, and a tracheostomy is performed. All the technology at the disposal of the critical care unit staff has been brought into use successfully to save Kenneth's life. The nursing staff has spent a considerable amount of time with him and his parents in trying to support them through this devastating event. The social services staff has worked with the nursing staff and with Kenneth's doctor to arrange for an appropriate transfer. With support and good wishes from the ICU staff, Kenneth, stable but still ventilator dependent, is transferred to a rehabilitation facility.

Twenty-one years later, Kenneth was living in his parents' home. He was able to read, watch television, and orally operate a computer; he was wheelchair bound and ventilator dependent. Over the years, his parents had cared for him at home with only occasional outside help. His mother died when Kenneth was 20 years old, and his father continued to care for him alone. When Kenneth was 31 years old, his father was diagnosed with a terminal illness. Faced with what appeared to be the imminent death of his ill father, Kenneth decided that he wanted to be released from a life of paralysis held intact by the life-sustaining properties of a ventilator. He despaired over the prospect of life without the attentive care, companionship, and love of his father. His quality of life would never be the same.

Kenneth was evaluated by a neurosurgeon, who determined that his quadriplegia was irreversible. He was next evaluated by a psychiatrist, who found him to be competent and able to understand the nature and consequences of his decision. Kenneth arrived at his decision to be removed from the venti-

lator after substantial deliberation. His father understood the basis for his son's decision and reluctantly approved. Although Kenneth's quadriplegia was irreversible, it was not a terminal condition as long as he was on the ventilator.

Kenneth petitioned the district court as a non–terminally ill, competent, adult quadriplegic for an order permitting the removal of his ventilator by someone who could administer a sedative and thereby relieve the pain that would precede his death. He also sought an order of immunity from civil or criminal liability for anyone providing the requested assistance. Finally, he petitioned the court for a declaration absolving him of suicide in the removal of his life-support system.

The district court determined that Kenneth was a mentally competent adult fully capable of deciding to forego continued life connected to a ventilator. The court also found that he understood that the removal of his life support system would shortly prove fatal. Finally, the district court concluded that Kenneth had a constitutional privacy right to discontinue further medical treatment and that Kenneth was entitled to the relief he sought.

The Attorney General of the state in which Kenneth resided appealed the issue to the state Supreme Court. Before the Supreme Court could hear this case, Kenneth died. Within a few days after Kenneth's death, his father also died. The state Supreme Court decided Kenneth's case, even though he had died, because it concluded that the issues presented were of great importance to the citizens of that state. The Supreme Court held that Kenneth's right to withdraw the ventilator outweighed the interests of the state. (This is based on the actual case of McKay v. Bergstedt, 180 P.2d 617, Nevada, 1990.)

Despite the best efforts of critical care nurses to support and maintain a patient's life, they must never lose sight of the fact that the patient ultimately evaluates the quality of his or her life and decides whether life-sustaining measures should be withdrawn.

this treatment, the issue becomes problematic. However, with such tools as advance directives and surrogate or family decision-making statutes, even a patient who is not competent is allowed to make this decision through alternate channels.

Resuscitation

Cardiopulmonary resuscitation (CPR) is another key legal and ethical issue in critical care. CPR is the provision of temporary ventilation and circulation through artificial means and is meant to restore health, to eliminate suffering, and to preserve life.[70] Based on the doctrine of implied consent, it is commonly presumed that all hospitalized patients would want CPR. Unless there is a written "Do Not Resuscitate" (DNR) or "No Code" order for a patient, CPR is provided for all patients. The decision not to resuscitate is one that must be made by the patient or surrogate after a full discussion with the patient's physician. This decision is difficult at best and is based on the patient's unique values, beliefs, and medical condition. The physician must document in the patient's medical record that the issue of resuscitation was fully discussed with the patient or surrogate and that the decision not to resuscitate was made. The physician must also write a DNR order in the patient's medical record. The decision to forgo resuscitation must be constantly reevaluated, because the patient's condition may change.

Often, patients are transferred to the critical care unit because they have been resuscitated on other nursing units. The status of each patient should be reviewed on admission to the critical care unit, and the issue of continued resuscitation versus no further resuscitation must be addressed if necessary. Not all patients benefit from CPR. This is particularly true of patients who have an end-stage terminal condition or multiple-system organ failure, for whom further aggressive care would be considered futile.[71] Each patient's case must be reviewed on an individual basis to determine whether resuscitation would meet a clinical goal for that patient. If no clinical goal is to be met by resuscitation, then the decision by the patient or surrogate to withhold it is appropriate.

Critical care nurses are in a unique position to assist in facilitating the discussion between the patient or surrogate and the patient's physician concerning the patient's resuscitation status. Often, it is the nurse who raises the issue to the physician for discussion with the patient. The nurse may also be the person to whom the patient or surrogate may communicate their desire to forgo resuscitation. The role of the critical care nurse is to ensure that the patient or surrogate be given the opportunity to decide on the appropriate resuscitation status for the patient and that the patient's decision be adhered to in the event of cardiopulmonary arrest.

Informed Consent

The concept of consent in general is reviewed earlier in the chapter. One of the elements necessary for a patient to give valid consent is that the patient knows and understands what treatment he or she will receive. This requirement of patient knowledge and understanding forms the basis of the doctrine of "informed" consent. The issue of informed consent is a basic and fundamental legal and ethical issue in critical care. It is only through the process of informed consent that a patient can determine in a knowledgeable manner exactly which health care interventions he or she requires and should receive. The responsibility for obtaining a patient's informed consent rests with the patient's physician, and not with the nursing staff. Obtaining informed consent from a patient is a process of sharing information and involves much more than simply having the patient sign a consent form.

The doctrine of informed consent requires that the physician provide the patient with the following information: (1) the patient's diagnosis and the name of the proposed treatment; (2) an explanation of the treatment and its intended purpose; (3) the anticipated benefits of the treatment; (4) the material risks of the treatment; (5) any alternative treatments; and (6) the prognosis if the treatment is refused.[35] The physician must first provide the patient with sufficient information about the proposed treatment and available alternatives. Next, the physician must help the patient to understand the information so that the patient can make a decision that is consistent with his or her personal beliefs and values. Finally, the physician must be certain that the patient's decision to accept or reject the treatment is voluntary.[72] Informed consent is based on patient autonomy and a collaborative decision-making process with the physician.

There are, however, some exceptions to the informed consent doctrine. In the case of an emergency, in which the life of the patient is threatened and informed consent cannot be obtained, the health care provider may render the necessary treatment, and the patient's consent will be implied. Another exception is a patient waiver. This occurs when the patient does not want to be given information about the proposed treatment. If a patient insists that he or she not be given the information, the request should be honored, and this should be noted in the patient's record by the physician.[73]

If a patient lacks the capacity to make a decision about his or her care, other methods must be used to obtain informed consent. The physician must discuss all of the same information with the patient's agent under a health care power of attorney, or the patient's surrogate pursuant to state law, as the physician would have discussed with the patient. It is then the patient's agent or surrogate's responsibility to give the necessary informed consent for the patient's care.

The substance of the discussion between the physician and the patient (or agent or surrogate) in which informed consent is obtained must be documented in the patient's medical record. Although the nurse is not directly responsible for obtaining a patient's informed consent, he or she is usually involved in the process in some way. If the nurse learns that the patient or surrogate does not have a clear understanding of the proposed treatment, this should be brought to the physician's attention. If the nurse has reason to question the patient's ability to make an informed decision, this should also be reported. Finally, the nurse can be instrumental in clarifying information for the patient or surrogate.

Brain Death and Organ Donation

The issues of brain death and organ donation are frequently encountered in critical care and often pose some difficult legal and ethical issues for the critical care nurse.

Brain Death

Death was once defined as the cessation of cardiopulmonary function. However, with the life-support systems that are currently available, this definition has become obsolete. The definition of death has now become focused on the cessation of brain activity alone. The most frequently used criterion for determining death is whole-brain death. Whole-brain death is defined as "the permanent, irreversible cessation of the functioning of all areas of the brain."[74] The determination of death by whole-brain criteria requires (1) the demonstration of coma (indicating loss of cerebral hemispheric function) and (2) the documentation of absent corneal, oculovestibular, oropharyngeal, and ventilatory reflexes (indicating loss of function of the brain stem).[75]

The formal determination of brain death is generally performed in two groups of patients in critical care units. The first group is composed of patients who appear to be dead and from whom life-sustaining treatment will be removed. The second group is composed of patients who appear to be dead and whose organs will be transplanted.[75] The role of the critical care nurse, in addition to caring for the patient, is to serve in a supportive role to the patient's family.

Organ Donation

Organ donation is another legal and ethical issue frequently encountered in critical care nursing. This situation includes patients who are critically ill and are waiting for an organ donation and patients who are brain dead and whose organs will be transplanted.

Both these groups of patients and their families have different needs that require the skill and support of the critical care nurse. Organ and tissue donation has become accepted, and commonplace, in our society. Transplants of the heart, lungs, kidneys, liver, pancreas, corneas, bone, and even skin are possible. Although science has achieved success with organ transplantation and the technical ability to manage donor patients, there remains a distinct shortage of organ donation. In the United States, more than 40,000 patients are on organ transplantation waiting lists, and approximately six patients die every day while waiting for an organ transplant.[76] The most organs for transplant are procured from patients in the critical care setting. However, many families are reluctant to donate the patient's organs when asked, and many health care workers are reluctant to discuss the issue of organ donation with families. In an attempt to increase organ donation, most states have passed legislation that requires hospitals to have administrative or nursing staff approach the families of eligible donors to give them the opportunity to donate patients' organs.[77]

The medical criteria for organ donation vary among regions of the United States. Within each region, at least one organization deals with organ procurement. It is recommended that the critical care nurse become familiar with the organization in the area in which they practice. Generally, organs can be procured from patients up to 75 years of age, although this criterion may vary from region to region. Patients with active systemic infections are not permitted to be donors, nor are patients with active systemic cancers.[78] The final determination regarding patients' eligibility to donate organs is made by the procurement agencies.

The Uniform Anatomical Gift Act is a uniform law that has been passed in all states and governs the donation of organs and tissues. The act allows a competent adult to donate all or part of his or her body as a gift, in writing, before his or her death, and is effective at the time of death. If a person has not agreed to organ donation before his or her death, the act specifies a list of individuals who can consent for donation at the time of the person's death.[79]

In addition to cadaver donation, another major source of organs is from living donors who are related to the patients in need of transplant. An adult with decision-making capacity is competent to volunteer to donate an organ to a relative. However, in some cases, ethical problems could arise if the donor has been coerced to donate by other family members. An even greater ethical and legal problem arises if the proposed donor is a minor or is mentally incompetent. The issue of organ donation by a minor is controversial and may involve conflicting interests for the parents. In cases of proposed organ donation by a minor or a person who is mentally incompetent, a review by a court with a resulting court order is required.[80]

The critical care nurse may be personally faced with an emotional and psychological challenge in caring for patients who are either the donor or the recipient of organ transplantation. The care of a patient who is a potential organ recipient includes sophisticated physical interventions aimed at support of the patient's particular organ system failure. Psychological and emotional support of both the patient and the family is critical during the harrowing vigil of waiting for a donor organ in time to save the patient's life. The critical care nurse is also faced with a patient care challenge in the opposite situation. The care of a patient who has been declared brain dead involves supportive care for the patient and emotional support for the family. The critical care nurse can be a key facilitator in the discussion with the family about potential organ donation. Finally, the critical care nurse is instrumental in assisting the family in processing their feelings about consent to organ donation.

Allocation of Resources

The final key legal and ethical issue that is relevant to critical care is the allocation of resources. One of the most far-reaching issues for our society in general is the allocation of financial resources for health care. In the past, health care services were reimbursed retrospectively, and the cost of health care was not commonly questioned. Today, with an increased emphasis on prospective reimbursement and managed care, health care institutions have had to become increasingly cost conscious. The cost of critical care is extraordinarily high and is not always fully reimbursed by third-party payers. Acute care facilities face decreasing payments for patient care by public funding sources. In an increasingly competitive environment, these acute care facilities are called on to provide higher levels of technology with decreasing funds at their disposal.

A related issue, and one that is relevant to critical care nurses, is the deliberate decrease in the number of professional nursing staff by health care institutions. In an effort to contain costs, many acute care facilities have made cuts in the number of their professional staff. Nurses with seniority are offered early retirement packages, and vacancies in staff are not always filled. Critical care nurses are especially sensitive to these issues, because of the high nurse-to-patient ratio that is required by critically ill patients.

Health care rationing is a controversial issue. The rationing of limited health care resources has been debated by philosophers and practitioners alike. The concept of rationing health care on the basis of such patient characteristics as age, mental competency, or illness is at odds with the long-accepted principle that health care should be available and equitable for all persons in our society. Ethical and legal debates concerning the allocation of health care resources will continue to increase in the foreseeable future.

The ethical and legal principles that are relevant to critical care nursing are not always easy to grasp. Most of these issues will be confronted by the critical care nurse at some point in his or her career. The fields of nursing, ethics, and law are inextricably entwined. In recognizing and dealing with the issues presented, the end result will be quality professional nursing care for critically ill patients.

Critical Thinking Exercise

Stephanie S. is an 88-year-old woman who has sustained a massive cerebrovascular accident, which has rendered her completely unresponsive. She was admitted to the ICU and is being maintained on a ventilator and artificial nutrition and hydration. Stephanie is a widow and has three adult children, one son and two daughters. Her son and older daughter live nearby and see or speak to her on a daily basis. Her younger daughter lives across the country, speaks with her once a month, and comes to visit her every few years. Stephanie does not have a living will or a power of attorney for health care. However, she lives in Illinois, which has a health care surrogate statute in effect.

The physicians have thoroughly evaluated Stephanie's condition and have determined that it is irreversible. According to the health care surrogate statute, a person without an advance directive (living will or health care power of attorney) may have life-sustaining treatment withdrawn based on the decision to do so by the person's surrogate.

The person must have a qualifying condition, which is certified in writing in the patient's medical record by her attending physician and at least one other qualified physician. "Permanent unconsciousness" is considered a qualifying condition. Stephanie's family physician and the consulting neurologist have both documented in her medical record that she has this qualifying condition.

The law provides that Stephanie's adult children can be named as appropriate surrogates to decide whether her life-sustaining treatment should be withdrawn and she should be allowed to die. Because Stephanie has three adult children available to act as her surrogates, all three are allowed to participate equally in this decision. Her younger daughter has flown in to be available to participate, and all three children have agreed to act as Stephanie's surrogates.

The law further provides that the patient's surrogates must carefully weigh the benefits and burdens of the life-sustaining treatment to the patient. The surrogates must then come to a decision about the life-sustaining treatment that the patient would have made for herself. Stephanie's children have thoroughly discussed the benefits and the burdens that the life-sustaining treatment would have on her. Her son and older daughter firmly believe that Stephanie would not wish to be kept alive in a completely unresponsive state. Her younger daughter disagrees with her siblings and firmly believes that Stephanie would want to be maintained on life supports. The law provides that if multiple surrogates are making the decision, and if there is a conflict regarding what should be done, the majority decision rules.

You have been assigned as Stephanie's primary nurse.

1. Stephanie's three children come to you about the conflict they are having in the decision to withdraw her life-sustaining treatment. What do you do?
2. Can the daughter who objects to the withdrawal of life-sustaining treatment do anything to prevent this?
3. What, if anything, would be the role of the hospital ethics committee in this case?
4. Assume that the decision is made by all the children that Stephanie's life-sustaining treatment should be withdrawn. The physician orders that this treatment should be discontinued. You are still Stephanie's primary nurse. However, because of your own convictions and beliefs, you do not believe that you can personally withdraw these supports. What options are available to you?

Key Concepts

→ The ethical principles that are basic to critical care nursing include veracity, nonmaleficence, fidelity, beneficence, autonomy, and justice. The recognition and identification of these ethical principles form a basis for ethical decision making in patient care situations.

→ The Nursing Code of Ethics with interpretive statements was developed by the American Nurses Association and provides guidance to nurses that is consistent with the ethical obligations of the profession.

→ Patient advocacy is a fundamental role of the profession of nursing and includes advising, acting as liaison, sharing information, making recommendations, and assisting patients to make informed choices. The role of patient advocacy for critical care nurses inherently involves both personal and professional risks.

→ Nurses should identify and should give thoughtful consideration to their own obligations and duties to self, which contribute greatly to the ethical foundation in nurses' personal and professional lives.

→ There are two types of consent: express and implied. Express consent is directly given, either verbally or in writing. Implied consent is given by a person's actions or inactions.

→ The elements of valid consent are as follows: 1) the patient must have decision-making capacity; 2) consent must be given voluntarily; 3) consent is not obtained in any fraudulent manner; and 4) the patient knows and understands the treatment that will be received.

→ Tort law is an area of civil law, as opposed to criminal law. The major areas of tort law are intentional torts, quasi-intentional torts, and negligence.

→ The intentional torts that are encountered in health care are assault, battery, false imprisonment, and intentional infliction of emotional distress. The quasi-intentional torts encountered in health care are defamation and invasion of privacy.

→ The elements in a cause of action for negligence are 1) a duty, 2) a breach of this duty, 3) injury caused by the breach of duty, and 4) actual damages or loss.

→ The two types of liability are personal liability and vicarious liability. Personal liability is responsibility for one's own behavior. Vicarious liability is imputed and involves responsibility for the actions of others.

→ Areas of information that must be taken into consideration in ethical decision making include medical indications, preferences of patients, quality of life, and external issues.

→ Advance directives are legal documents that allow individuals to give instructions about their future health care if they should become incapable of making their own decisions. The two types of advance directives are instruction directives (living wills) and proxy directives (durable powers of attorney).

→ Surrogate and family decision-making statutes are state laws that identify individuals (such as spouses or parents) who are authorized to make decisions on behalf of incompetent patients with no advance directives.

→ The decision not to resuscitate a patient is one that must be made by the patient or patient's surrogate after a full discussion of the benefits and burdens with the patient's physician.

→ The doctrine of informed consent requires that the physician provide the patient with the following information: 1) diagnosis and proposed treatment; 2) explanation of treatment and its intended purpose; 3) anticipated benefits of treatment; 4) material risks of treatment; 5) alternative treatments; and 6) prognosis if treatment is refused.

→ The most frequently used criterion for determining death is whole-brain death, which is defined as the permanent, irreversible cessation of the function of all areas of the brain.

→ The medical criteria for organ donation vary among regions of the United States. Within each region, at least one organization sets the criteria and deals with organ procurement.

→ The allocation of resources in health care includes the cost of health care, decreases in professional staff, and rationing of health care resources.

References

1. Drought T: Ethical practice in a technological age. Crit Care Nurs Clin North Am 7:297–304, 1995.
2. Jecker N: Principles and methods of ethical decision making in critical care nursing. Crit Care Nurs Clin North Am 9:29–33, 1997.
3. Catalano J: Ethical decision making in the critical care patient. Crit Care Nurs Clin North Am 9:45–52, 1997.
4. Jecker, op. cit., p 30.
5. Catalano, op. cit., p 46.
6. Catalano, op. cit., p 45.
7. American Nurses Association: Code for Nurses With Interpretative Statements. Washington, DC, American Nurses Publishing, 1985.
8. Ibid., p i.
9. Ibid., p iv.
10. Ibid., p 2.
11. Ibid., p 3.
12. Ibid., p 4.
13. Ibid., p 5.
14. Ibid., p 6.
15. Ibid., p 7.
16. Ibid., p 8.
17. Ibid., p 9.
18. Ibid., p 10.
19. Ibid., p 11.
20. Rushton C: Creating an ethical practice environment: a focus on advocacy. Crit Care Nurs Clin North Am 7:387, 1995.
21. Ibid., p 388.
22. Ibid., p 389.
23. Ibid., p 390.
24. Jameton A: Duties to self: professional nursing in the critical care unit. In: Ethics at the Bedside: A Source Book for Critical Care Nurses, Philadelphia, J. B. Lippincott, 1987, p 115.
25. Ibid., p 120.
26. Ibid., p 123.
27. Ibid., p 125.
28. Ibid., p 127.
29. Ibid., p 128.
30. Restatement of the Law (Second) Torts, Section 10A (1965).
31. Schloedorff v Society of New York Hospitals, 105 N.E. 92, 93 (NY 1914).
32. Ibid., p 93.
33. Brent N: Nurses and the Law: A Guide to Principles and Applications. Philadelphia, W. B. Saunders, 1997, p 240.
34. Ibid., p 241.
35. Ibid., p 242.
36. Black H: Black's Law Dictionary, 5th ed. St. Paul, West, 1983, p 774.
37. Keeton W (ed): Prosser and Keeton on the Law of Torts, 5th ed. St. Paul, West, 1984, p 34.
38. Ibid., p 43.
39. Ibid., p 39.
40. Ibid., p 40.
41. Ibid., p 49.
42. Ibid., p 56.
43. Ibid., p 60.
44. Brent, op. cit., p 111.
45. Keeton, op. cit., p 771.
46. Ibid., p 773.
47. Brent, op. cit., p 114.
48. Ibid., p 115.
49. Keeton, op. cit., p 851.
50. Ibid., p 854.
51. Ibid., p 856.
52. Ibid., p 863.
53. Ibid., p 169.
54. Ibid., p 164.
55. Illinois Pattern Jury Instructions: Civil, 3rd ed. St. Paul, West, 1994, sect 10.01.
56. Ibid., sect 105.01.
57. Brent, op. cit., p 43.
58. Ibid., p 566.
59. Ibid., p 44.
60. Pierce P: What is an ethical decision? Crit Care Nurs Clin North Am 9:2, 1997.
61. Genesen L: Ethical decision making in the critical care unit. Crit Care Nurs Clin North Am 9:116, 1997.
62. Hall JK: Nursing Ethics and Law. Philadelphia, W. B. Saunders, 1996, p 64.
63. Jonsen AR, et al.: Clinical Ethics. New York, McGraw-Hill, 1992.
64. Genesen, op. cit., p 118, citing Jonsen.
65. Ibid., p 117.
66. Fade A: Advance directives: an overview of changing right-to-die laws. J Nurs Law 2:28, 1996.
67. Ibid., p 29.
68. Grafius L: Ethics for Everyone. Chicago, American Hospital Association, 1995, p 36.
69. Fade, op. cit., p 30.
70. Grafius, op. cit., p 46.
71. Luce J: Ethical principles in critical care. JAMA 263:697, 1990.
72. Grafius, op. cit., p 33.
73. Brent, op. cit., p 243.
74. Grafius, op. cit., p 42.
75. Luce, op. cit., p 698.
76. Siminoff L: Withdrawal of treatment and organ donation. Crit Care Nurs Clin North Am 9:85, 1977.
77. Ibid., p 86.
78. Ibid., p 87.
79. Brent, op. cit., p 259.
80. Siminoff, op. cit., p 88.

3

Professional Role of the Critical Care Nurse

Mary G. McKinley

Objectives

After completing this chapter, the student will be able to:

1. Define critical care nursing practice.
2. Differentiate the various professional roles that a nurse working in critical care may assume.
3. Defend the benefits of belonging to a professional organization.
4. Analyze the stressors present in the work setting of the critical care nurse.
5. Implement methods to reduce the stress of working in critical care.
6. Incorporate the research process and research utilization in critical care nursing practice.

DEFINING CRITICAL CARE NURSING PRACTICE

Critical care nursing is a specialty area of nursing that involves caring for patients and families who are undergoing life-threatening illness or injury or potentially life-threatening illness or injury.[1] The specialty of critical care nursing does not exist separately from the profession of nursing as a whole. The difference is in dealing with life-threatening problems. Nurses working in critical care are committed to protecting, maintaining, and restoring the health of those entrusted to their care. In caring for critically ill patients, critical care nurses continuously monitor and observe patients for alterations in their physiologic status, plan and implement interventions that assist the patient who has alterations in function, and evaluate responses to these interventions and outcomes of care. Critically ill patients are in a highly complex and technologic environment and require critical care nurses who have a broad knowledge base, high-level decision-making skills, and a high regard for the patients in their care. The challenge of the critical care nurse is to create safe passage for the patients and families who are in vulnerable circumstances.

The roots of critical care nursing come from the need of patients for specialized care. Patients who require critical care are those who are physiologically unstable and at risk of dying but who are more likely to survive if they are given specialized care. Florence

Nightingale established the first "intensive care unit" (ICU) during the Crimean War when she placed the sickest patients in close proximity to the nurses. In the polio epidemics of the 1950s, patients with respiratory failure were treated with iron lungs and required specialized care in large common areas or wards that were a predecessor of the current critical care area.[2] Critical care units were invented because of problems arising from patients who were desperately ill and needed one nurse.[3] In the 1960s, specialized care was required for patients in postanesthesia care units or recovery rooms. These patients required expertise to prevent postoperative complications and catastrophes. Nurses who were provided with special training and education could provide this care. It was recognized that specialized nursing care could make a difference in patient outcomes, and ICUs were formed. From this beginning, critical care nursing has expanded beyond the boundaries of the traditional ICU. Today, specialized units are designed to care for cardiovascular or neurologic surgical, trauma, pediatric, or neonatal patients, to name just a few. Critical care can also be found in subacute areas, in home care, and in the community.

The basic premise of critical care is to provide high-level care to patients who are desperately ill. Because of the delicate balance needed by these patients, the care delivered must include collaboration of all the disciplines involved in the care and a consistent approach based in knowledge and science.

Collaboration in Critical Care

Critically ill patients require care that is comprehensive as well as specialized. A collaborative practice model that facilitates multidisciplinary problem solving and decision making is essential. Collaboration means working together. The National Joint Practice Commission defined collaborative practice as the "jointly determined relationship between the nurses and physicians, in the hospital setting, for the purpose of integrating their care regimens into a single comprehensive approach to their patients' needs."[4] Norsen and colleagues[5] defined collaborative practice in health care as "working together in a joint effort toward a mission of excellent patient care." Other definitions can be found in the health care literature, but whatever the definitions may say, one thing is clear: collaboration is a key factor in the delivery of quality care for patients in critical care.

A study done by Knaus and colleagues[6] identified the difference between actual and predicted death rates in 13 ICUs. These investigators found that the difference was not attributed to the technology or the physiologic status of the patients but rather to the interaction and communication between the nurses and physicians.[6] This landmark study identified the importance of establishing a collaborative practice model in caring for patients in critical care. Successful collaboration requires cooperative decision making, open communication, trust, and sharing of knowledge and goals among care givers. The result of successful collaboration can be seen in positive patient outcomes. Collaboration extends not only to the physician but also to others who assist in the care of patients in critical care. Respiratory, occupational, physical, dietary, and pharmacy therapists, for example, have a role to play in the care of the critically ill. Nurses have the greatest opportunity to interact with all the health care professionals caring for the patients. Because of this contact, nurses have the role of coordination and integration of services within the plan of care.

Standards

Standards serve as guides for the provision of care and as criteria for evaluating care. Standards must be clearly defined and are validated by knowledge, science, or some body of authority. The three forms of standards are structure, process, and outcome.

Structure Standards

Structure standards are the rules of the system. These include the mission, philosophy, and administrative policies that exist within a system. Structure standards that are present in nursing include the American

---

CHART 3–1

American Nurses Association Standards of Nursing Practice

Assessment
   The nurse collects patient health data.
Diagnoses
   The nurse analyzes the assessment data in determining diagnoses.
   The nurse identifies expected outcomes individualized to the patient.
Planning
   The nurse develops a plan of care that prescribes interventions to attain expected outcomes.
Implementation
   The nurse implements the interventions identified in the plan of care.
Evaluation
   The nurse evaluates the patient's progress toward attainment of outcomes.

From Standards of Clinical Nursing Practice. Washington, DC, ANA Publishing, 1991, p. 2.

Nurses Association (ANA) standards of practice (Chart 3–1)[7]. An institution may have structure standards, such as policies, that clearly state what a nurse should or should not do within the role or in a given situation. For example, the nurses' job description outlines specific roles and responsibilities for a nurse in a given setting.

Process Standards

Process standards are the working standards. There are many examples of process standards in nursing. Procedure books are one example. These types of standards describe what and how something is to be done. Other examples of process standards include the nursing care plan, practice guidelines, clinical pathways, and protocols. All these standards are tools to help the nurse in providing quality care.

Outcome Standards

The outcome standards are how quality can be measured. These standards do not stand alone but are built on all the other standards and are the overall standard that nursing is trying to achieve. A standard of care, which identifies actual patient outcomes, is an example of an outcome standard. Outcomes that may be evaluated include patient satisfaction with care, functional health status, quality of life scales, readmission rates, and length of stay. Outcome measures may also be physiologic, such as resting heart rate, minute volumes, blood pressure, and comfort levels. The American Association of Critical-Care Nurses (AACN) established outcome standards for critical care patients. These outcomes use nursing diagnosis as a framework and include outcome criteria, defining characteristics, causes or related factor interventions, monitoring, and related medical diagnoses. The AACN standards were published as *Outcome Standards for Nursing Care of the Critically Ill* in 1990.[8]

The use of standards is important to the practice of nursing. Standards help to identify high-quality care for patients, they give nurses the knowledge of what is necessary for continuous and consistent high-quality care, and they can help to determine that care meets the acceptable level. This final criterion is important for administrators and regulatory agencies because it allows them to identify whether appropriate care is given according to acceptable standards.

Critical care nursing is a dynamic and evolving specialty. Changes in society, technology, the nursing profession, and the health care environment will affect the future both of this specialty and of the profession. These changes can sometimes be difficult to face and may require an examination of the various roles of the nurse. By keeping the needs of the patient as the primary driving force for their actions, critical care nurses will meet the challenges of the future.

CHANGING ROLE OF THE CRITICAL CARE NURSE

Changes within the health care environment have resulted in role changes for nurses working in critical care. These role changes can be seen at both staff and advanced practice levels.

Staff Nurse Role

As noted, the traditional boundaries of the ICU are gone. Critical care knowledge and skills are needed in areas outside the four walls of the ICU. This expansion has served to broaden the role of the staff nurse in critical care. Critical care skills are portable and useful in various settings. For example, some units are available for chronically ventilator-dependent patients, or these patients may be found in a home care setting. Other examples are in the areas of heart failure, renal failure, and other chronic diseases during which staff nurses follow the patient throughout the continuum of care. Nurses with critical care skills are needed to assist in the care of these patients regardless of the setting.

The tumultuous health care environment has also prompted an examination of the role of the nurse in the critical care setting. Complexity of care is increasing, and this serves to challenge the traditional role of the nurse. Caring for individuals with multisystem dysfunction who require advanced technology is part of this challenge. The staff nurse in critical care is called on to use the nursing process to its fullest capacity in assessing, diagnosing, planning, implementing, and evaluating the care of these complex critically ill patients.

As complexity increases, ethical issues also increase. Dealing with issues such as end-of-life care, organ transplantation, and allocation of resources can be difficult, but these issues are part of the daily work of the critical care nurse. As complexity increases, so does expense, and the nurse in critical care is challenged to reduce costs and length of stay. Sicker and more acutely ill patients are transferred from the critical care unit and are discharged from the hospital earlier. Critical care nurses are challenged to provide high-quality care for patients in this ever-changing environment.

Advanced Practice Roles

The current health care environment calls for nurses to have advanced knowledge and skills to deliver the highest level of care to their patients. This need for ever-increasing knowledge and skill has provided a niche for advanced practice nurses within the acute and critical care setting. Studies show that between 60 and 80% of basic health care required by patients can be delivered by advanced practice nurses. Investigators have also documented that advanced practice nurses provide effective, quality health care at an affordable cost.[9] As critical care has expanded beyond the walls of the critical care units, these advanced practitioners have demonstrated that advanced knowledge and expertise are needed throughout the continuum of care.

Advanced practice roles require additional education and clinical requirements beyond basic education. A minimum of a graduate degree with a major in nursing is required. The ANA definition of advanced clinical practice can be found in Chart 3–2.[10] The main advanced practice roles within critical care include acute care nurse practitioner (ACNP) and critical care clinical nurse specialist (CNS). These two roles sometimes overlap. The CNS has traditionally practiced in the acute care setting, and the ACNP has a primary care focus. That traditional view is being challenged as those boundaries are crossed and a newer generation of advanced clinical practice roles is emerging.[11] Some other advanced practice roles that are evolving include those involving case and outcomes management. These newer roles also show a shifting of perspectives.

CHART 3-2

American Nurses Association Definition of Advanced Practice

Advanced practice registered nurses manifest a high level of expertise in the assessment, diagnosis, and treatment of the complex responses of individuals, families, or communities to actual or potential health problems, prevention of illness and injury, maintenance of wellness, and provision of comfort. The advanced practice registered nurse has a master's or doctoral education concentrating in a specific area of advanced nursing practice, has supervised practice during graduate education, and has ongoing clinical experiences. Advanced practice registered nurses continue to perform many of the same interventions used in basic nursing practice. The difference in this practice relates to a greater depth and breadth of knowledge, a greater degree of synthesis of data, and greater complexity of skills and interventions.

From Scope and Standards of Advanced Practice Registered Nursing. Washington, DC, ANA Publishing, 1996, p. 2.

Case and outcome managers are involved in the care of the patient across the continuum and beyond the boundaries of the critical care unit. Whatever the title or role, the need exists for nurses with advanced practice skills in critical care. The need for advanced practice nurses will increase in the future.[12]

Clinical Nurse Specialist

The CNS represents the largest group of advanced practice nurses, with more than 58,000 nurses.[12] The CNS functions as an advanced practitioner by completing the roles of educator, consultant, researcher, and manager.[13] For example, nurses in the unit may consult the CNS if they have a particularly challenging patient or family. The CNS may use the role of researcher if a problem is identified in the unit. By completing a review of the literature and researching information, the CNS may be able to analyze corrective measures and thereby to solve problems. Nurses working in CNS positions function autonomously and in collaboration with health care providers. The CNS may function in a specialty area or may specialize in the management of a particular type of condition, such as cardiovascular disease or trauma. The primary aim of the CNS in critical care is to create a practice environment that provides optimal patient outcomes. In

some areas, the CNS role includes case management or outcomes management functions. These additions to the role are relatively new and are seen in some areas as a way to advance and secure the role.

Acute Care Nurse Practitioner

The ACNP is a newer role and includes the functions of researcher and practitioner. The purpose of the ACNP is to provide advanced nursing care across the continuum of acute care services to patients who are acutely and critically ill. These nurses may function in various settings. The ACNP practices in any setting in which patient care requirements include complex monitoring and therapies, high-intensity nursing intervention, or continuous nursing vigilance within the full range of high-acuity care. For example, the ACNP, in some settings, conducts patient rounds with the staff, assesses the needs of the patient, and implements the plan of care for the patient, a plan that may include insertion of central venous lines or removal of chest tubes. The ACNP acts autonomously to manage patient care. The care that these nurses give is based in their knowledge of the full spectrum of high-acuity patient care needs.[14] These nurses are working within the acute care practice setting in advanced roles. The knowledge and skills required for this position require master's level preparation and certification in acute care. This specialty has seen an increase in recent years as managed care has increased its impact on the health care environment.[15]

The roles of both CNSs and ACNPs are valuable within the context of the health care environment. The competencies for each role are different. The key to success in these roles is matching the competencies with the demands of patients and the system. Because these roles are evolving, they may change to meet the needs of the patient and families.

Other Roles

Case managers and outcomes managers are newer positions in advanced practice. These practitioners use case or outcomes management models to effect changes within the acute care environment. Case management became a focus of health care in the early 1980s. Usually, case managers use a pathway to assist in outlining the care needs of the patient. The nurse case manager facilitates the patient's movement through the system by using resources effectively and by implementing cost-control measures. Outcomes management focus began in the late 1980s. In outcomes management, the focus is on the measurement of health outcomes among populations receiving medical care.[16] Outcomes managers can facilitate an exploration of possible contributors to untoward outcomes and can assist with the examination of new approaches to practice. Because of nursing's unique contribution to patient care and the educational preparation of nurses in advanced practice, nurses are ideally suited for the positions of case or outcomes managers. In today's highly volatile health care environment, roles such as CNS, ACNP, and case and outcomes managers are key to increasing the visibility and viability of the nursing profession.

ROLE OF THE PROFESSIONAL ORGANIZATION

Associations consist of groups of people who come together because of a common interest. Professional organizations allow professional colleagues to come together and to perform functions that they cannot perform as individuals. Nursing organizations have had a tremendous impact on the profession. State rules and regulations exert legal control over nursing licensure, but professional associations exert voluntary control. This voluntary interest can assist in assuring the public of the quality and availability of services from the profession. Nursing organizations have provided a mechanism for effective changes in the profession. They have served as a forum for the exchange of ideas and collective action with regard to issues facing nursing and the profession as a whole.

Some of the major nursing organizations (e.g., the ANA and the National League for Nursing [NLN]) began at about the turn of the century and did assist in ensuring the interests of the public in professional nursing. At the beginning, these organizations had two concerns: 1) laws to protect the public from poorly prepared nurses; and 2) lack of standardization in preparation of nurses. Because of the efforts of these associations, these two concerns were addressed. Nursing lobbied successfully for state licensure laws, and the promotion of accreditation for schools of nursing was accomplished.[17]

Nursing associations have the public, the nursing profession, and individual nurses as their constituents. Associations serve these three constituents in different ways. The code of ethics and standards of practice are ways in which nursing associations have served the public and nursing as a whole. Individual practitioners of nursing are served by associations through continuing education offerings, identifying credentialing, and providing a method for communication of the concerns of the profession. Therefore, nursing associations strive to meet the needs of the nurses who are their members.

As nursing has grown and as the health care needs of patients have changed, many nurses began working in specialty practice. These nurses found that their needs were specific to the area of clinical practice in which they worked. One organization that has critical care as its specialty practice focus is the AACN.

American Association of Critical-Care Nurses

The AACN was established in 1969. The organization is the world's largest nurse's specialty organization, with more than 70,000 members and more than 270 local chapters. The mission of the organization is to inspire and provide leadership to establish work and care environments for critical care nurses and their patients that are respectful, healing, and humane. The vision of the organization is to create a health care system driven by the needs of patients and families in which critical care nurses make their optimal contribution. The values of accountability, advocacy, integrity, collaboration, leadership, stewardship, lifelong learning, commitment to quality, innovation, and passion form an integral part of the organization. The mission, vision, and values are framed within an ethic of care and the basic ethical principles of respect for persons, beneficence, and justice. Essential to the ethic of care are compassion, collaboration, accountability, and trust. The relationship of the mission, vision and values, and an ethic of care are depicted in Figure 3–1. The AACN strives to meet the needs of nurses working in critical care. Through this responsive organization, critical care nurses have gained collective strength in their knowledge and abilities in caring for patients.

Benefits to Belonging

Every association offers various benefits to its members. The AACN offers excellent educational opportunities such as the annual National Teaching Institute and Critical Care Exposition, in which as many as 4000 to 5000 critical care nurses meet to explore the cutting edge information in critical care and see the latest in technological advances. Included in the National Teaching Institute is the Advanced Practice Institute, where nurses in advanced practice roles in critical care have the opportunity to present and discuss practice issues and concerns. The Leadership Connections program, an annual offering, provides nurses in critical care with helpful topics in developing leadership skills. This program is for the bedside nurse as well as for nurses in management and education positions. The AACN offers these programs at a discount to members.

The AACN has excellent publications and journals as a benefit to assist members in their educational development. *Critical Care Nurse* and the *American Journal of Critical Care* are the two main publications. A monthly newsletter with association-related information, *AACN News*, is another publication that is a member benefit. In addition, many foundational resources are available to the members of AACN; these

AN ETHIC OF CARE

AACN's mission, vision, and values are framed within an ethic of care and ethical principles. An ethic of care is a moral orientation, which acknowledges the interrelatedness and interdependence of individuals, systems, and society. An ethic of care respects individual uniqueness, personal relationships, and the dynamic nature of life. Essential to an ethic of care are compassion, collaboration, accountability, and trust. Within the context of interrelationships of individuals and circumstances, traditional ethical principles provide a basis for deliberation and decision making. These ethical principle include:

• **Respect for Persons:** a moral obligation to honor the intrinsic worth and uniqueness of each person; to respect self-determination, diversity, and privacy.

• **Beneficence:** a moral obligation to promote good and prevent or remove harm; to promote the welfare, health, and safety of society and individuals in accordance with beliefs, values, preferences, and goals.

• **Justice:** a moral obligation to promote good and to prevent or remove harm; to be fair and promote equity, nondiscrimination, and the distribution of benefits and burdens based on needs and resources available; to advocate on another's behalf when necessary.

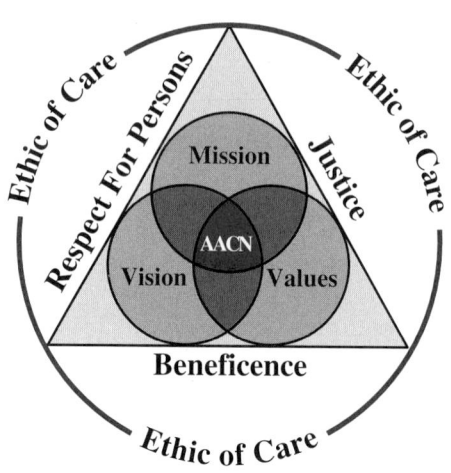

Figure 3–1

Model of American Association of Critical-Care Nurses (AACN) Ethic of Care. (With permission from Mission, Vision, and Values, AACN Board of Directors, Aliso Viejo, CA, 1997.)

are offered at a discount or are free of charge in some cases. These resources include, for example, the *Core Curriculum for Critical Care Nursing, Orientation to the Care of the Acute and Critically Ill Patient,* and the *AACN Procedure Manual for Critical Care.* The AACN is also committed to making information accessible to their members by electronic format. The AACN has a strong on-line presence in its web site, which has a members-only area. This web site provides members with up-to-the-minute organization information and a direct link to the national office. The members-only area includes resource databases and information. Within the area are access to CINAHL (Cumulative Index for Nursing and Allied Health Literature) for literature searches, access to the PRN (Practice Resource Network) line (a clinical reference resource and information link to an on-line bulletin board), and access to AACN journals.

Another major benefit of belonging to the AACN is the opportunity offered for developing leadership skills. The AACN believes strongly in its members and has actively sought ways to involve them. Most recently, the AACN has offered the 50 Plus Ways to Volunteer. Opportunities are varied and can include working in task forces, work groups, and think tanks, serving as chapter leaders, serving in elected positions such as the Board of Directors, completing surveys for the Volunteers in Participation program, and being on conference calls with the Board as an Advisory Team

member. The purpose of these activities is to strengthen members' leadership skills to assist in dealing with today's health care environment. Volunteer activities with the AACN also offer outstanding opportunities to network with other critical care professionals who are dealing with the same challenging health care environment. This networking can be key to dealing with problems or concerns in the demanding area of critical care. The AACN is also focused on networking within the public policy arena in the development of Public Policy Advisory Teams. These volunteers help to assess and provide information on changes or potential changes in public policy on a state or regional level. The AACN also provides a collective voice for specialty nursing as a liaison to other organizations. This leadership is essential in the current changing health care environment.

The AACN has a foundation that strives to meet the cause-driven portion of its vision. This foundation offers members assistance in increasing the public's awareness of critical care, in meeting the needs of families in critical care, and in working to educate consumers about the importance of advance directives as well as how to complete these important documents.

The AACN offers research grants and scholarships in many different areas as another member benefit. More than $80,000 in research grants and $100,000 in scholarships are offered per year. The grants can assist in resolving practice issues and concerns within the critical care area. The scholarships can be for basic or graduate education.

Certification in nursing is awarded to a nurse who has mastered a body of knowledge and has acquired skills in a defined area of practice. The AACN Certification Corporation regulates certification in critical care. The certification granted is known as the CCRN. In some areas, certified nurses have greater earning potential, increased employment opportunities, and greater status, and in some states, they are eligible for insurance reimbursement. Requirements for the CCRN credential include caring for the critically ill patient within the environment and completion of a computerized test. The certification is available for adult, pediatric, and neonatal patient populations. Certification in critical care is offered at a discount rate to members of AACN. More than 50,000 nurses currently hold the CCRN credential in their area of practice.

The AACN is an outstanding organization that has critical care nursing as its focus. It has been a strong force for assisting nurses in critical care with the specialized needs presented by this demanding area of clinical practice. From education to research to practice, the AACN strives to assist nurses working in critical care to make their optimal contribution in caring for patients with life-threatening problems.

Other Specialty Organizations

As noted, other nursing specialty organizations may be helpful to the nurse in critical care. If the focus of practice is spinal injuries, there is the American Association of Spinal Cord Injury Nurses. Other organizations have emergency, nephrology, or neuroscience nursing as their focus—the Emergency Nurses Association, the American Nephrology Nurse Association, and the American Association of Neuroscience Nurses. Each of these organizations has its own focus and offers benefits of belonging. Nurses also belong to other professional organizations such as the Society for Critical Care Medicine. This organization includes nursing as a part of the interdisciplinary care team that is needed in the critical care area.

STRESS IN CRITICAL CARE

The critical care area provides nurses with a double-edged sword. It is an exciting, challenging, and rewarding place to work. It is also a tension-filled and stressful place to work. Early discussions of stress in the ICU likened the unit to a war bunker. The fast-paced situations, the continual stress of rapid-fire decision making, the never-ending noise from alarms beeping and phones ringing, and the emotional roller coaster of facing life-and-death decisions place enormous stress on the nurses who choose to work in these areas. Stresses in critical care practice can be broken down into several areas: Workload, environment, psychological factors, and interpersonal factors.

Sources of Stress

Workload

The first area that can be a source of stress is the workload in critical care. Working in critical care brings with it the physical stress and strain of lifting and moving heavy patients and equipment. Depending on the design of the unit, the nurse most likely spends much of the shift standing and walking. The actual physical labor is difficult in these units. There are also the demands of shift rotation and of working holidays, weekends, and long hours. Changes in scheduling in the 1980s allowed for more flexible staffing schedules and even self-scheduling. However, with the flexibility came shifts that can include 12-hour, 8-hour, and 4-hour shifts all in one week. The demands of this type of scheduling bring its own stress on the nurse as a person with a personal and family life.

All this makes the critical care area a demanding place to work in a physical sense. Nurses working in critical care can become exhausted from these physical demands. It can also be exhausting to keep up with the rapidly changing technology within the unit. Technology has a powerful impact on critical care units. Most of that impact has been positive by decreasing the time nurses spend on tasks and thus increasing the time nurses spend with patients. Technology does have its down side, however, and staff members often struggle to keep up with the many changes and challenges that technology brings.

Overall changes in the health care environment, such as managed care and capitation, have added another stress for the critical care nurse (Chart 3–3). "Doing more with less" has become a familiar phrase in health care today, and the critical care unit is no exception. Nurses may be faced with shortages of staff, equipment, and resources. Frequently, nurses are asked to "float" to other units. The critical care nurses who pride themselves on knowing their patients can be overwhelmed by a multiple-bed patient assignment in an unfamiliar unit. The experience of "floating" can be extremely stressful. Having nurses "float" to the unit can also be a stress for the critical care staff member. Dealing with a nurse who is inexperienced and uncertain of the equipment and routine of the unit can add stress to the critical care nurse's already busy day. Another workload stress is the decreasing length of stay of patients in critical care. The rapid turnover of patients within units can lead to stress, and the

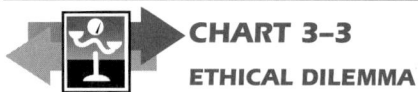

CHART 3-3

ETHICAL DILEMMA

You are the staff nurse in a rural community hospital. This hospital is the major health care facility for this area. You have just received an interdepartmental memo from the administration stating that there will not be a raise or any additional benefits this year. This is the third year in a row that this has happened. Many of the coworkers in your unit are beginning to talk about a strike or a walkout. Several nurses have talked with the director of nursing, who says that her hands are tied. A meeting has been scheduled, off hospital property, for employees to discuss a strike or walkout.

1. Would you attend this meeting, and why or why not?
2. Do you think it is ethical for nurses to strike? Why or why not? Is there a good reason to strike?
3. Do you believe in unions for professional groups? Why or why not?

Adapted from Uustal D: Values and Ethics in Nursing: From Theory to Practice. East Greenwich, RI, Educational Resources in Nursing and Wholistic Health, 1992.

concern of patients' being discharged too soon can bring stress on the nurse (Chart 3–4).

Environment

The stressors that come from the critical care environment are what could be termed hidden stressors. These entities that are present in the environment are so common and so prevalent that they can easily become ignored as a focus of stress. Because of their constant presence, these concerns add to the already stressful working conditions for the nurse in critical care. Some of these stressors include noise, lighting, and occupational hazards.

The continual noise inherent in the critical care unit is a source of stress for the nurse working in the unit. There is the constant noise from the equipment needed for patients in critical care. Ventilators, monitors, intravenous pumps, and specialized beds all have their own sounds, and all have their own alarms. Something always seems to be buzzing, beeping, or ringing. Add to these noises the constant hum of people working. Even though sincere attempts are made to keep voices to a minimum, noise is always made when caring for patients.

Along with the noise as a stress are the lights in the unit. Rarely are units designed to allow for natural lighting. A nurse who works in the unit may not know

what the weather or the time of day is because of this lack of exposure to natural light. Most units are harshly lit. Many times, monitors and alarms are not only beeping but also flashing. This abnormal lighting can compound the environmental stress a nurse may experience.

The nurse may be exposed to multiple occupational hazards, including chemicals, infectious disease, and radiation. These occupational concerns are present in the everyday work of the nurse in critical care, and fear of physical illness or injury related to these factors can be a source of stress for the nurse.

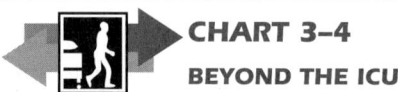

CHART 3-4

BEYOND THE ICU

The current health care environment has caused some major changes in hospitals. These changes have led to the utilization of critical care nurses in many settings other than the traditional ICU. Critical care technology and skills have become useful in many different areas. From using monitors in medical–surgical areas to having patients on ventilators at home, critical care technology is improving care for patients outside the boundaries of the ICU. The critical care nurse's skill and knowledge of the technology and its application to the care of patients are needed in these different settings.

The critical care nurse may require cross-training to care for patients in untraditional critical care settings. For example, a need may exist for critical care skills and technology in obstetrics. The critical care nurse may be comfortable with the cardiac monitor and the intravenous pumps but not so comfortable with the fetal monitor and the oxytocin drip. The critical care nurse in such a setting may require review and training in the unfamiliar areas. It is helpful to have experienced nurses or preceptors in these areas to assist less-experienced nurses. A preceptor can be helpful with skills, techniques, and overall guidance in areas unfamiliar to the less-experienced nurse. Cross-training is a part of nearly every hospital's operation. Nurses are "floating" and being "pulled" to assist in caring for patients in many settings. Nurses in other settings are also being "pulled" to assist in the ICU. Nurses are concerned about "pulling" and maintaining a standard of care for patients. These concerns have not been resolved in our profession. It is beneficial to the nurse to become familiar with working in various settings to improve care for patients.

Psychological Factors

Another general source of stress in critical care is psychological. These issues can be a most subtle source of stress for the nurse working in the unit, and because they are subtle, these stressors can be the most dangerous. The critical care unit is a unit in continual crisis. There are the fears of facing physiologic crises, never knowing when a patient may suffer a cardiac arrest, to the psychological stresses of dealing with pain, suffering, death, and dying. There are the fears of not being able to deal with these crises and of making mistakes.

The constant interruptions in the day of the nurse working in critical care can lead to disorganization and increasing stress. Although many nurses choose to work in these units because of the constant challenges and changes, these factors can be a source of stress. Nurses who work in critical care often have high expectations for themselves and are fearful of not meeting those expectations.

The ethical dilemmas that the critical care nurse faces are a part of the psychological stress. So many situations can present themselves in critical care that it is difficult for the nurse to keep up with them, from families who want everything done when no hope exists for survival to patients who are depressed and are willing to give up too soon. Ethical dilemmas increase the stress that nurses face in critical care.

Another psychological stress that is common in critical care is the lack of direct reward. It seems that patients often do not remember their time in the unit or the nurses who cared for them in their time of crisis. It can be frustrating for nurses who have done their best and have given their all to have patients not acknowledge that work. In addition, nurses working in critical care rarely see the final results of the efforts made.

Patients who improve transfer to another unit, where they recover, and they may be discharged, never knowing or recognizing the nurses who dealt with them in their most fragile state. This lack of continuity can result in stress for the nurse who went into critical care to help people and to make a difference in people's lives. The lack of recognition and support can extend to fellow staff members. Staff members in critical care are often too busy or too stressed themselves to give each other the assistance and recognition of work well done that can help to ease the strain of a busy day.

Interpersonal Factors

Interpersonal relationships can be a source of stress for the nurse working in critical care. Dealing with difficult patients, families, and other health team members can result in stress for the nurse. Conflict with administration and management can be another interpersonal stress. Nurses also have a life outside work. That personal life may have areas of interpersonal conflict such as family crises or problems with children or a spouse that can increase stress.

Reducing Stress in Critical Care

Nurses can deal with the stress of working in critical care in many positive ways. The first important step is to recognize the presence of stress within the work setting. The acknowledgment of the existence of stress is vital to reducing the problems that can occur secondary to stress and stress overload. With that recognition are two other important points: maintaining a sense of humor and limiting exaggeration. Even in the tension-filled critical care unit, the nurse must maintain a sense of humor. The ability to laugh at oneself, not at the expense of patients or families, is essential in keeping a balance in life. Exaggeration is a human tendency. Unfortunately, exaggeration allows stress to get out of control. Any time an upsetting incident happens, the nurse should take a deep breath and should consider the overall implications of the incident and not exaggerate it out of proportion. The larger a concern becomes, the more stress it creates.

The second step in dealing with the stress of working in critical care is to take care of you. This may include health maintenance activities such as proper nutrition, adequate sleep, and exercise. Using stress reduction techniques is also important. Taking time away from the unit—breaks and vacations—is one technique that can increase tolerance to stress. Identifying diversional activities can be another way of caring for you. It can be as simple as taking a hot bath, reading an enjoyable book, or going to a museum or a football game. Whatever activities you may find relaxing and rejuvenating can help to increase tolerance of stress.

Establishing good time-management skills can assist in reducing stress. Time management is particularly important for dealing with the constant changes that occur in critical care. Patient admissions and conditions can change suddenly, and the nurse who has the best time-management skills can adapt and adjust to the alterations in workload.

One of the most effective ways of dealing with stress is discussing the problem with others. This approach is most effective when the discussion occurs with people who are in a similar situation. Some units have established discussion groups that meet to review any crisis situations that have occurred. Other units use outside sources, such as a psychologist or psychiatric CNS, to review and discuss upsetting or traumatic occurrences. Whatever the method, critical care nurses need to have an outlet to assist in dealing with the multiple stressors of the work environment.

Learning to use relaxation techniques can also be a tool to assist in the management of stress. Relaxation techniques can include simple 10-second skills, such as closing your eyes and taking a deep breath, to more advanced tools such as progressive muscle relaxation and yoga.

A word of caution in dealing with stress: Do not accept substitutes. Substitutes for good stress-management skills can include using drugs and alcohol, smoking, overeating, and drinking excessive caffeine. These substitutions serve to increase the stress response. There are no substitutes for good stress management skills.

RESEARCH AND RESEARCH UTILIZATION IN CRITICAL CARE

In the 1960s, nursing scholars realized that nursing could achieve its potential and desired professional status only by developing a scientifically derived body of knowledge unique to nursing. With this realization, nurse researchers set about developing science-based knowledge, and theorists began to formulate nursing theories. Two other developments were the growth and maturing of critical care nursing and the realization that patient care practices needed to be examined within the context of nursing science.[17] It was clear that using traditional methods to deal with patient problems was no longer acceptable. To move critical care nursing and patient care forward, a solid scientific basis was necessary. Critical care nursing, therefore, has always had a focus on research and the use of research in practice.

Some nurses and students of nursing do not always value nursing research. One of the reasons frequently cited is that research is too theoretically oriented. Therefore, one should consider the value of research in relation to the care of patients. By applying research to everyday practice, nurses can truly see value in research. To examine questions that nurses and patients deal with on a daily basis and to attempt to find answers that make health care efficient and more effective can only make research more relevant and valuable.

Since the early evolution of nursing research, concern has been expressed about the utilization of research in practice.[18] This issue remains a concern today because articles continue to be published on the knowledge–practice gap. The expanding knowledge base must be used to enhance nursing practice for it to have relativity and applicability. Research and research utilization are not separate, independent activities but are interdependent.

Research Process

The research process is highlighted in Chart 3–5. The process begins by identifying a problem. In critical

CHART 3–5

Steps of the Research Process

1. Identification of research problems
2. Review of the literature
3. Formulation of the research question or hypothesis
4. Design of the study
5. Obtaining consent
6. Implementation
7. Drawing conclusions based on findings
8. Discussion of implications
9. Dissemination of findings

care, patients and nurses can have many problems. Once a specific problem is identified, there needs to be a thorough review of the literature. Before the 1970s, no large database for critical care research existed, but now there is an abundance of literature. Computerization has been a tremendous aid to this step in the process. Once literature has been identified about the problem, the next step is to formulate a question or hypothesis. A frequent focus of critical care literature concerns the needs of families in critical care, so a possible hypothesis could be to test an intervention to meet the needs of families (e.g., issuing beepers to families to maintain contact and to provide timely information). The next step in the research process is to design a study. This could be experimental or nonexperimental. In looking at the example of family needs, this could involve distributing beepers to families of patients in one ICU (intervention) and comparing satisfaction levels of these families (experimental group) with families of patients in another ICU who did not receive beepers (control group). Next is to consider how data for the study are to be collected and analyzed. This step can be complex, involving protocols, subject selection, and informed consent. Implementation of the research study includes actual data collection and analysis of the data with implications. Then the research must be disseminated. Often, this is the point at which the standard nursing text ends its discussion of nursing research. However, an important part of research is the utilization of the information.

Research Utilization

Data are just data unless they are applied and used in the clinical setting. Nurses must make an effort to incorporate research to improve practice. For too long, research and practice have existed in two separate worlds. In critical care, with the rapidly changing pace and increasing technology, opportunities to put research into practice are abundant. Research has been done that is applicable to the nurse in critical care and to everyday practice in that setting. For example, research has demonstrated that the use of saline solution in endotracheal tubes is ineffective and actually may be detrimental to patients. Yet this practice continues in some ICUs. How can the application of research become more a part of everyday practice? Barriers to using research must be eliminate or minimized, and nurses must facilitate research use in practice.

Barriers to Research Utilization

Barriers to research utilization have been studied. Some of the barriers to consider are lack of awareness, unwillingness to change, failure to see the value of research, and lack of understanding. These barriers can be overcome with work on the part of the researcher and the nurse in the clinical setting. Increasing awareness by reviewing journals and staying current with information are important. Being open to change and new ideas can be difficult, but in the current environment, change is a constant. Researchers need to make their research clear and understandable. Research must be applicable to the clinical setting. With efforts from both researchers and nurses, we can improve the utilization of research in practice.

Facilitators of Research Utilization

One way to facilitate the use of research is to create an environment in which nurses can question and evaluate their practice. Administrators and health care institutions can be major players in this area. This can include the development of journal clubs and research committees in which nurses can collaborate and discuss research concerns. Collaboration with colleagues in area teaching institutions as well as health care facilities can be a facilitator to the use of research. Educational efforts must be part of the facilitation of the use of research in practice. Researchers can increase this use by making their studies more user friendly. By decreasing the use of research jargon, writing more clearly, and increasing the emphasis on the application of research to the clinical setting, the researcher can assist in the facilitation of research utilization.[19,20]

Improving practice requires a commitment by nurses to read and use research findings. The gap between the research and the use of research must be eliminated to improve the outcomes of our care.

Key Concepts

➧ Critical care nursing is a nursing specialty that deals with patients and their families who are ex-

periencing life-threatening illness or injury or potentially life-threatening illness or injury.

➧ Collaboration in critical care requires that all members of the health team (nurses, physicians, respiratory therapists, social workers, etc.) work together to develop and implement an *integrated* plan of care.

➧ Advanced practice roles in critical care nursing have recently expanded in response to the changes in health care and include the roles of CNS, ACNP, case manager and outcomes manager.

➧ Critical care nursing is no longer restricted to the boundaries of the ICU and can be found in outpatient clinics, transitional care settings, and home care. Nurses are encouraged to expand their skills to increase their marketability.

➧ Professional nursing organizations (e.g., ANA) serve to maintain quality nursing care by delineating standards for practice. These standards are used to guide and evaluate nursing care and include structure, process, and outcome standards.

➧ The specialty organization for critical care nurses is the AACN. This organization works to provide education, research, and leadership opportunities to its members.

➧ AACN's vision for health care is a system driven by the needs of patients and families in which critical care nurses make their optimal contribution.

➧ Numerous stressors exist in critical care nursing. These stressors can be generated by workload (e.g., long hours), environment (e.g., occupational hazards), psychological factors (e.g., dealing with patients' pain), and interpersonal factors (e.g., family responsibilities).

➧ Critical care nurses must recognize stress in the work setting and develop strategies to minimize the effects of stress (e.g., scheduled time off, exercise, adequate sleep).

➧ Research is a critical component of nursing practice. Critical care nurses must be committed to reducing the research–practice gap by participating in research studies and applying appropriate research findings to their practice.

References

1. American Association of Critical Care Nurses (AACN): Scope of Practice for the Nursing Care of the Critically Ill Patient and Family. Aliso Viejo, CA, AACN, 1997.
2. Rudy E, Grenvik A: Future of critical care. Am J Crit Care 1:33–37, 1992.
3. Lynaugh J, Fairman J: New nurses, new space: a preview of the AACN history study. Am J Crit Care 1:19–24, 1992.
4. National Joint Practice Commission: Guidelines for establishing joint collaborative practice in hospitals. Chicago, National Joint Practice Commission, 1981.
5. Norsen L, Opalden J, Quinn J: A practice model: collaborative practice. Crit Care Nurs Clin North Am 7:43–52, 1995.

6. Knaus W, et al: APACHE II: a severity of disease classification system. Crit Care Med 13:818–829, 1985.

7. American Nurses Association (ANA): Standards of Clinical Nursing Practice. Washington, DC, ANA Publishing, p. 2, 1991.

8. American Association of Critical-Care Nurses (AACN): Outcome Standards for Nursing Care of the Critically Ill. Aliso Viejo, CA, AACN, 1990.

9. Brown S, Grimes D: Nurse Practitioners and Certified Midwives: a Metaanalysis of Studies on Nurses in Primary Care Roles. Washington, DC, ANA Publishing, 1993.

10. American Nurses Association (ANA): Scope and Standards of Advanced Practice Registered Nursing. Washington, DC, ANA Publishing, p. 2, 1996.

11. Mirr M: Advance clinical practice: a reconceptualized role. AACN Clin Issues 4:599–602, 1993.

12. American Association of Critical Care Nurses (AACN): Advanced Practice Key Messages and Action Strategies. Aliso Viejo, CA, AACN, 1995.

13. Gawlinski A, Kerns L: Clinical Nurse Specialist in Critical Care. Philadelphia, W.B. Saunders, 1994.

14. Keane A, Richmond T, Kaiser L: Critical care nurse practitioners: evolution of the advanced practice nursing role. Am J Crit Care 3:232–237, 1994.

15. Dracup K: Advanced practice nurses in critical care: yes or no? Am J Crit Care 3:163–164, 1994.

16. Wojner A: Outcomes management: an interdisciplinary search for best practice. AACN Clin Issues, 7:133–145, 1996.

17. Chitty K: Professional Nursing: Concepts and Challenges. Philadelphia, W.B. Saunders, 1997.

18. Lindeman C: Priorities in clinical nursing research. Nurs Outlook 23:693–698, 1975.

19. Dracup K: The three Rs: reading, writing, and research. Am J Crit Care 3:328–330, 1996.

20. Funk S, Tornquiest E, Champagne M: Barriers and facilitators of research utilization. Nurs Clin North Am 30:395–407, 1995.

4

Impact of Critical Illness on the Patient and Family

Margaret H. Doherty, Lisa Plowfield, Carla Ware, and Claudia M. West

Objectives

After completing this chapter, the student will be able to:

1. Describe the physiologic effects of stress on the patient and family.
2. Compare the effects of specific physiologic, psychological, and environmental stressors on the critically ill patient.
3. Apply family and crisis theories to the care of the critically ill patient and family.
4. Use a systematic approach for the psychosocial assessment of the critically ill patient and family.
5. Develop specific nursing diagnoses that pertain to selected physiologic and psychosocial needs of the critically ill patient and family.
6. Plan appropriate nursing interventions that address selected physiologic and psychosocial needs of the critically ill patient and family.
7. Identify favorable outcomes for selected physiologic and psychosocial needs of the critically ill patient.
8. Relate the impact of the increase in the number of elderly patients requiring critical care nursing to changes in the health care delivery system.
9. Discuss the nursing implications of the physiologic and psychological age-related changes in patients who are critically ill.

The impact of critical illness on the patient and family is enormous. Initially, the stress response is activated, directly affecting the course of the patient's illness and ultimate recovery. At the same time, the family is anxious about the patient's condition and has specific informational needs that need to be met. Families are in crisis, and the nurse is in a key position to help the patient and family to cope effectively.

To do this, the nurse must assess the patient's physiologic and psychological status on an ongoing basis. The nurse must also assess the family in terms of their ability to cope with this situation and their ability to help the patient recover. Family theory is used to optimize care of these patients. The family's input is essential to individualize the care of the patient. The nurse frequently needs to interview the family to obtain the patient's medical and social history, as well as usual patterns of coping. Once the family is involved in the care, they have less anxiety about the welfare of their relative, they have their informational needs met, and

they feel a part of the total management of the patient. With elderly critically ill patients, the nurse must be cognizant of the physiologic and psychosocial changes associated with aging that may affect these patients. Knowledge of these important areas of nursing must be part of every nurse's education.

To achieve the desired patient outcomes of comfort, safety, dignity, and recovery, the nurse must provide many essential interventions. Effective pain management is necessary for the patient's comfort and recovery. Pharmacologic and nonpharmacologic measures that are specific to each patient should be considered. Health team members including nurses, physicians, pharmacists, discharge planners, and respiratory therapists must work collaboratively to provide comprehensive care to patients. Noise in the unit must be reduced to facilitate the patient's rest and to decrease anxiety. Frequent explanations of procedures and frequent orientation of the patient must occur. Spiritual needs and sexual needs of the patient must also be addressed as soon as possible, and the patient's sense of control must be maximized to meet the patient's psychological needs.

Competent and caring nurses must be eager to improve the care they currently provide to critically ill patients and their families. Nurses must use their creativity, knowledge, and technical expertise to provide comprehensive care. Making the critical care unit a warm, caring environment maximizes patient outcomes, increases staff satisfaction, and provides an excellent standard of professional practice.

OVERVIEW OF THE STRESS RESPONSE

Stress is a phenomenon that is relevant to critically ill patients and critical care nurses. Selye[1] defined stress as "a nonspecific response of the body to any kind of demand made upon it," manifested by specific physiologic events. Stress is a sociopsychophysiologic process that consists of behavioral, humoral, metabolic, intellectual, immune, and other physiologic responses to stressors.[2] Stressors are the actual stimuli that elicit the stress response. Stressors are physical, psychological, and environmental. They may be an actual threat or some afferent input signaling injury, illness, or other conditions such as pain.[2] Stimuli that can be perceived as stressors include physiologic stressors, such as trauma, thermal injuries, physical injury, drugs, hormonal changes, microorganisms, dietary deficiencies, and hypoxia. Psychological stressors include emotional demands, vocational pressures, sense of isolation, social pressures, and cultural factors.[3] Finally, environmental stressors include sensory overload, sleep deprivation, excessive lighting, and excessive noise.[3]

The patient's perception of the stress and his or her reaction to it, as well as the stress itself, define the stimuli as stressful or not. Consider the following two situations. A patient scheduled for emergency coronary artery bypass surgery may view the event as extremely stressful. This view is appropriate given the complex physiologic and psychological events associated with this type of surgery and subsequent recovery. For another patient having elective bypass surgery, the situation may be viewed differently. This patient is generally healthier and may see the operation as a means to improve his or her quality of life. This patient's stress may be far less severe.

Physiologic Responses to Stress

A person's response to stress or stressors is complex. After stimulation of the central nervous system by the afferent stimuli of the stressor, a neuroendocrine response occurs that involves many organs and tissues.

This complex response is viewed as protective because the activation of the neurologic and endocrine systems maintains homeostasis. It is also adaptive, such as the tachycardia that results to meet increased metabolic needs of the tissues and organs (Figure 4–1). The response to the stressors is graded, in that the extent of the response depends on the intensity and duration of the stressors or afferent stimuli.[2] The sum of these physiologic changes in response to stress is called the general adaptation syndrome.[1] This syndrome consists of three stages: the alarm reaction, the stage of resistance, and the stage of exhaustion. The alarm reaction and the stage of resistance attempt to maintain resistance against stress, to stabilize the body's reaction to stressors, and to maintain homeostasis. Death often results in the stage of exhaustion, when the magnitude of the stressors is too great for the patient's physiologic and psychological reserves.[1]

Although the stress response is usually protective, it can lead to pathologic conditions because of the complex physiologic events that occur with its activation. For example, tachycardia is part of the normal stress response to pain. In the patient with an acute myocardial infarction (AMI), this response can actually precipitate additional angina, can decrease cardiac output, and can even cause life-threatening dysrhythmias. With repeated episodes of stress or an excessive number of stressors, diseases can occur, such as hypertension, heart disease, renal disease, infections, neurologic diseases, digestive diseases, and some metabolic diseases.[3] These stress-related diseases can lead to or can complicate a critical illness. Nurses caring for critically ill patients must be knowledgeable of the stress response and the potential consequences of the stress response in individual patients. Ultimately, nursing care must focus on minimizing the stress response in all critically ill patients.

Stressors Specific to Critical Illness and Critical Care Environment

Specific physical, psychological, social, emotional, and environmental stressors have been identified in the critical care unit. Examples of physical stressors include pain, immobility, confusion, sore throat from intubation, sleeplessness, chest tube removal, and suctioning.[4] Psychological and social stressors include a sense of isolation, powerlessness, anxiety, depression, communication problems, emotional distress, hostility, fear of the unknown, and fear of death.[5] Finally, environmental stressors include equipment, alarms, loud noises, staff conversations, and lights.[6] Specifically, cardiac surgical patients have reported that the endotracheal tube, pain, and the inability to talk were the most stressful aspects of their critical care stay.[5]

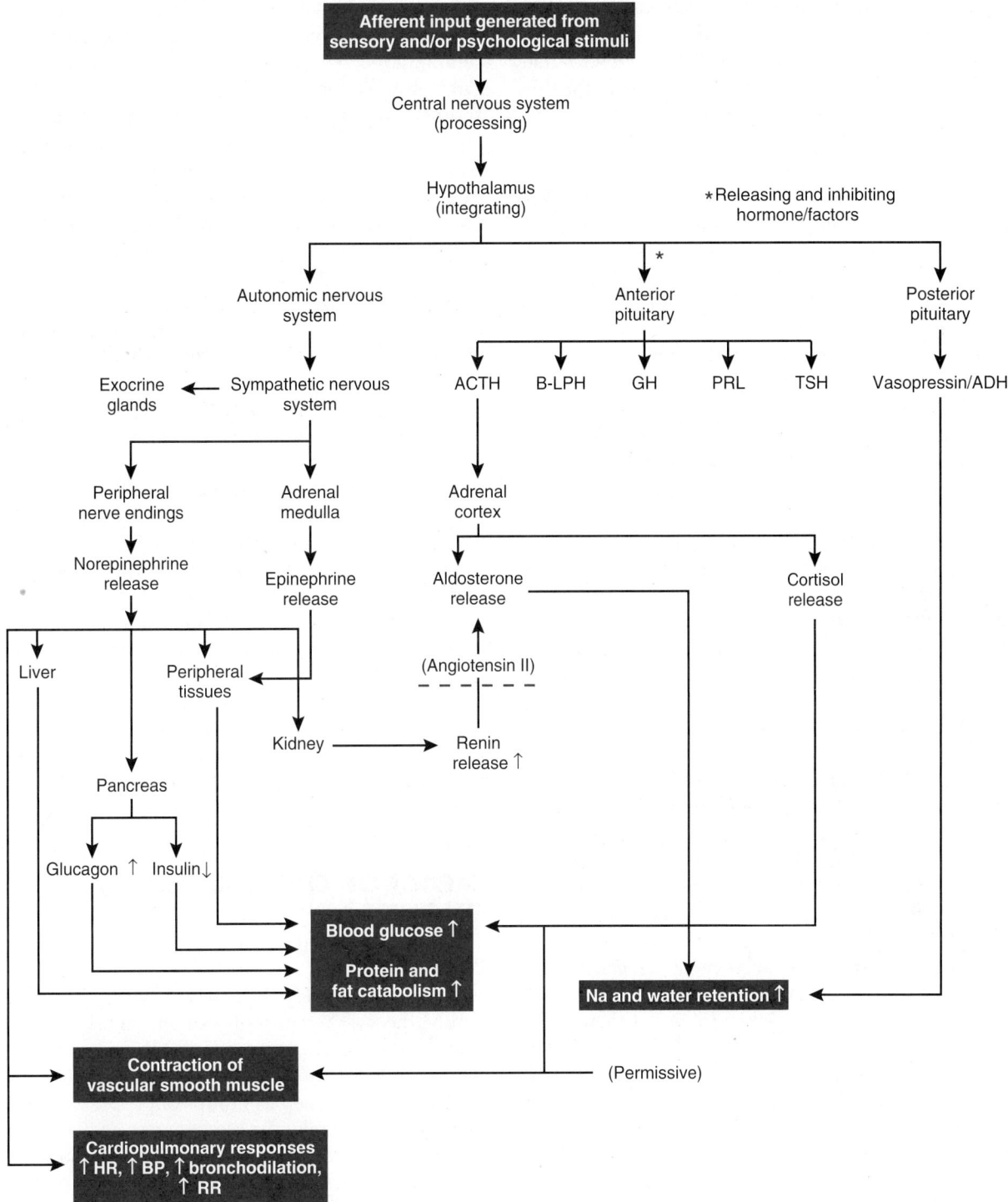

Figure 4–1

Systems participating in the stress response. ADH, antidiuretic hormone; ACTH, adrenocorticotropic hormone; B-LPH, beta-lipoprotein hormone; BP, blood pressure; GH, growth hormone; HR, heart rate; PRL, prolactin; RR, respiratory rate; TSH, thyroid-stimulating hormone. (Adapted from Carri-eri-Kohlman V, Lindsey AM, West CM: Pathophysiological Phenomena in Nursing, 2nd ed. Philadelphia, W.B. Saunders, 1993, p 401.)

Critically ill patients are especially vulnerable to both the initial stressors of their illness and the activation of the stress response itself. This vulnerability is depicted in the following situations. A 19-year-old His-panic man is admitted to the intensive care unit (ICU) after sustaining head and abdominal injuries from a motorcycle accident. He has a decreased level of consciousness and responds to repositioning with moaning. His multiple physiologic stressors include pain, tissue injury, alterations in cerebral perfusion, and increased intracranial pressure. His psychological stressors include isolation, fear, and anxiety because neither he nor his family speaks English. The nurse must address each of these stressors in caring for this patient. Aggressive interventions to decrease increased intracranial pressure and to maintain neurologic function are provided, in collaboration with physicians, respiratory therapists, and other members of the health team. Effective pain management is implemented for comfort and to limit activation of the stress response. Caring and competent nursing care is provided to decrease the patient's and the family's anxiety and fear of the unknown.[7] The patient's and the family's stress are reduced further by obtaining an interpreter. A collaborative and comprehensive approach facilitates recovery of this patient.

Another example of the effects of stress on critically ill patients is a 66-year-old male patient who is recovering from the surgical repair of a ruptured abdominal aortic aneurysm and who is experiencing hemodynamic instability postoperatively. His hypovolemic state requires aggressive fluid resuscitation and inotropic support with intravenous dopamine (Intropin). He has to recover not only from the psychological stress of the emergency surgery but also from the physiologic stressors of the surgery. The surgical stress response includes neuroendocrine, metabolic, and inflammatory responses to the acute injury (see Figure 4–1). This injury stimulates the release of cortisol within a few hours after surgery.[2] This increased blood cortisol stimulates an increase in blood glucose by potentiating the effects of glucagon and catecholamines on hepatic glucose production. Cortisol also affects the vascular smooth muscle response to catecholamines to sustain the vascular changes associated with stress.[2] These complex physiologic consequences of the stress response must be considered when caring for this unstable postoperative patient.

Psychosocial stress may extend beyond the critical phase of a patient's illness. In one study of patients recovering from an AMI, at least 25% had significant long-term difficulties in psychosocial adaptation that was independent of their physical recovery. Many failed to return to their previous work, leisure, and sexual activities even when they were physically able to do so.[4] When patients adapt poorly psychosocially, they often feel isolated, have low compliance with medical and exercise regimens, and have negative feelings about their health in general.[4] Considering these findings, the nurse must provide interventions that foster the patient's psychosocial and physical recovery early in the critical care experience.

Environmental stressors in critical care units include excessive noise, sophisticated equipment, excessive lighting, and offensive odors resulting in alterations in the patient's sleep patterns and sensory stimulation. Sensory overload or excess develops from extraneous staff conversations at the bedside, paging systems, and equipment alarms. These stimuli are compounded by continuous lighting and unfamiliar sights in the critical care setting. The lack of privacy is another stressor in the ICU that may increase the patient's discomfort and may increase the level of stress. Many environmental stressors can be controlled. The nurse should minimize extraneous noises at the bedside and should turn the lights down whenever possible, especially at night. Staff conversations should be limited at the bedside to conversations that include the patient. Ventilator alarms can be suspended for 3 minutes during suctioning. The patient's privacy should be respected and provided for whenever possible.

In summary, a critically ill patient's response to stress varies. If the stressor is great, the stress response requires tremendous energy and taps the patient's metabolic reserves. If adaptive mechanisms fail, death can occur. Even though the stress response is protective, pathologic consequences occur when the magnitude of the stressor overtaxes the homeostatic mechanisms.[2] Many critically ill patients face this situation because the stressors are too great for physiologic or psychological adaptation. Environmental stressors compound the stress response by interfering with rest and by increasing discomfort and anxiety. Consequently, the health of the patient is further threatened. Nurses must assess patients thoroughly to protect them from unnecessary stressors and to maximize their defenses against the consequences of stress.

IMPACT OF CRITICAL ILLNESS ON THE FAMILY

When considering the impact of critical illness on the patient and family, the nurse should incorporate family theory. A thorough patient assessment must include the family because no one lives without a family.[8] Whether orphaned or homeless, all persons have families, defined as groups of people with whom they share intimate details of everyday life. Most persons, however, have either blood or marital ties that create their families. Whatever the origin of one's family, family members are persons who are concerned when someone is critically ill or injured. Each nurse and each patient live within the context of a family system and bring their own values, beliefs, and culture with them.

The nurse has a well-defined opportunity to deliver nursing care within the context of a family. Many critically ill patients are intubated or have an altered level of consciousness. Effective communication with the patient may be hindered or impossible. It is the family who can best interpret the patient's behavioral cues and responses and can provide the health team with important assessment data. It is the family who can also best describe the impact of the illness on the patient and the family.

Definition of Family

The family has been defined by the United States Census Bureau as a group of two or more persons related by blood, marriage, or adoption. For many years, nurses used this same definition, but as lifestyles have become more relaxed and openly disclosed, family definitions have become broader. For the purposes of this text, family is defined as two or more persons who depend on one another for emotional, physical, or economic support; the members of one's family are self-defined.[9]

The definition of family in the critical care setting often becomes important from the legal standpoint. Many times, critically ill patients are unable to speak for themselves, at least temporarily. Identifying who can legally make decisions for these patients is essential. For example, a motorcycle accident victim may be his parents' adult son, but he may also have lived with his girlfriend for 3 years. Other situations include the absence or unavailability of blood relatives or marriage-related persons for decision-making purposes or advance directives with a designated health

care power of attorney who is not a family member. All these situations require the health care team to redefine family on a patient-by-patient basis.

Family System Perspectives

Because the family consists of more than one person, a systems approach to family nursing may be used. A family system is "an open, ongoing, goal-seeking, self-regulating, social system."[10] Patients live within the context of a family, and because it is within this context that they will return, critical care nursing requires that nurses look beyond the patient to the family members who anxiously wait for information. As a system, each person's actions within the family can affect every other family member. See Table 4–1 for the major theoretical concepts of family systems theory.[11] For example, when a parent of toddlers becomes ill, the remaining well parent takes on the full responsibility of the children as well as maintaining the household. The effects of a parent's illness on young children can be demonstrated by greater acting-out behaviors and increased clinging to the well parent.

When the family enters the critical care setting, the physical unit and the team of care providers become part of the family's system. The wife of an ill patient may look to the nurses for psychological support, reas-

TABLE 4–1
Major Theoretical Concepts of Family Systems Theory

Theoretical Concept	Expanded Meaning
A family system is part of a larger suprasystem and is composed of many subsystems.	This concept identifies the family as a part of the larger society and also identifies smaller subsets of the family. Common family subsystems include the marital subsystem, the parental subsystem, the child subsystem, and the same-gender subsystems.
The family as a whole is greater than the sum of its parts.	Knowing each member of a family does not equate with knowing the whole family as an interacting groups of persons. The behavioral patterns, values and norms, and cultural mores of the family may not be fully understood by simply assessing individual members of the family.
A change in one family member affects all family members.	Any alteration in one member's roles or responsibilities will create change for all members. Not all family members change in the same way or to the same extent.
The family is able to create a balance between change and stability.	Change is normal for all families, and they work to maintain a balance that supports their own belief system and behavioral patterns. Change, however, can be distressful, particularly a change that is sudden and unexpected and may alter the family composition. Family members work together to restore some stability to their lives; this work is part of the self-regulating function of the family system. It is often when families have difficulty in regaining some sense of stability that crisis may result.
Behaviors of family members are best described as circular, as compared with linear.	Linear patterns of behavior are cause-and-effect relationships. Circular behaviors are patterns that can be noted within families and depicted as interdependent. The behaviors and actions of one member affect other members, and the responses to another's behavior, in turn, can affect the first member's behaviors. This pattern of circularity continues over time and reflects the dynamic nature of families.

TABLE 4–2
Family Assessment

Category	Areas to Assess
Initial patient assessment	Usual family roles; anticipated changes
	Family concerns
	Desire for family involvement in care
	Decision making (who should be involved)
	Supportive family members
Initial family assessment	Family structure
	Family constellation
	Family availability
	Family roles
	Role of patient in family
	Family decision maker
	Family spokesperson
	Family perceptions and understanding
	Knowledge of patient's condition
	Experience with critical illness
	Immediate need for information
	Expectations regarding care and patient outcomes
	Immediate logistical needs
	Transportation
	Lodging
	Family coping
	Past responses to crises
	Perceived effective and ineffective coping strategies

From Dunbar S, McLain RM: Family care. In: Kinney MR, Packa DL, Dunbar SR (eds): AACN's Clinical Reference for Critical Care Nursing. Philadelphia, C. V. Mosby, 1993, pp 411–425.

surance, hope, and empathy. She may look to the physicians, social workers, and discharge planners for information and guidance on decision making. The daily needs of the wife may have been previously met within the system of her family and her neighbors, but with the stress of a critical illness, she has more urgent needs that can only be met by the health care team. A systems perspective of families of the critically ill patient can assist the nurse in understanding the patient and the context within which he or she lives. The nurse can also assess the family in terms of their structure and coping skills. This initial assessment includes collecting pertinent information about the patient and family that will help to plan the patient's care (Table 4–2).[8]

Family Stress and Crisis Theories

Whenever a patient is hospitalized in a critical care unit, the threat of death exists. Not only do the illness and hospitalization affect the family and its function, but also the threat of death brings a host of additional alterations on the family. The rapid changes in physiologic function and the threat of loss of life can precipitate crises for many families of critically ill patients.

Families respond with a wide range of behaviors characterized by stress and coping responses. The origin of family stress and crisis theories began with Hill's ABCX model of family crisis.[12] In helping families to adjust and adapt to both normative and nonnormative crises, Hill proposed that several interacting factors could be identified that led to either crisis or noncrisis (Figure 4–2). The interaction of the stressor

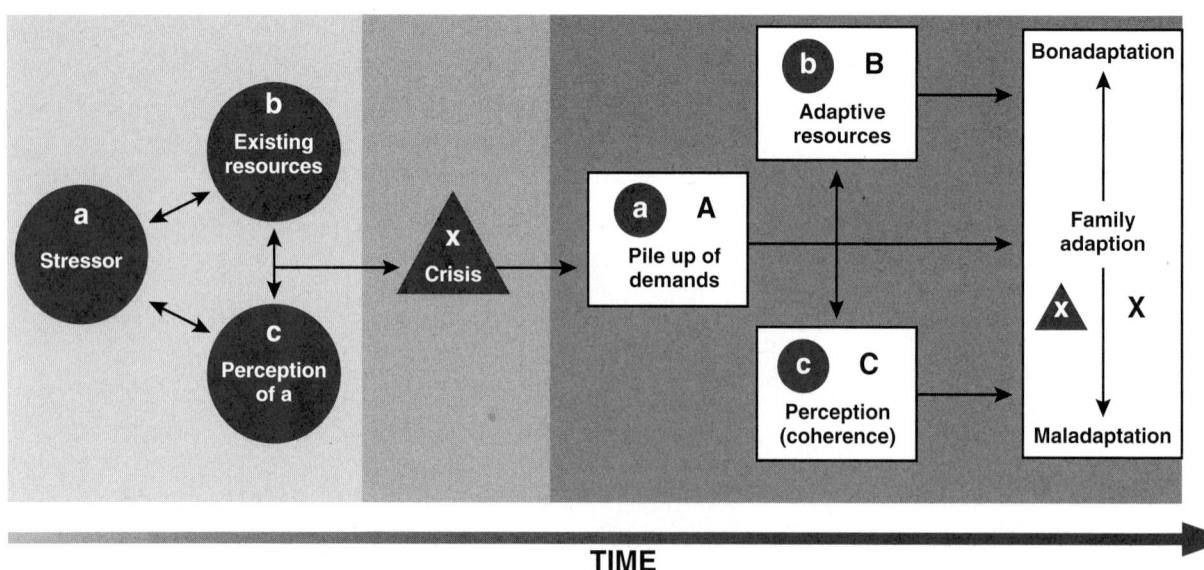

TIME

Precrisis   Postcrisis

Figure 4–2
The ABCX model and double ABCX model. (Adapted from McCubbin HI, Patterson J: The family stress process: the double ABCX model of adjustment and adaptation. In: McCubbin HI, Sussman MB, Patterson JM (eds): Social Stress and the Family. New York, Haworth, 1983, p 12.)

TABLE 4–3
Phases of Crisis

Phase	Characteristics
I	Stressful event has occurred
	Family's anxiety level is raised
	Family relies on usual patterns of coping
II	Usual coping strategies do not alleviate the stressor
	Family's anxiety increases further
III	Heightened anxiety is painful
	Family uses every resource known to cope with the stressful situation (some of the resources may be new to the family because the members are willing to do almost anything to alleviate some of the tension)
IV	State of active crisis exists
	Family is unable to alleviate anxiety

event, the family's existing resources, and the meaning of the stressor event for the family may interact together to cause a crisis. The family uses its existing resources to cope with the current critical care illness. These include those patterns of responding to stressful events that have been successful in former situations. The family also assigns meaning to the critical care experience. If the severity of the illness and the changes the illness produces can be met with the family's current resources, crisis will be avoided. If the illness presents the family with an overwhelming severity that cannot be met by the available resources, crisis may occur.[12] Families in crisis are unable to solve problems in their usual way and are emotionally upset by their concern for the patient.[13]

Four phases of a crisis have been identified (Table 4–3).[14] The first phase occurs when a stressful event has occurred and the family's anxiety is raised. A person's usual patterns of coping are relied on to alleviate the anxiety. During the second phase, the usual coping strategies do not alleviate the stressor, and the family's anxiety increases further. In the third phase, the heightened anxiety is so painful that the family uses every known resource to cope with the stressful situation. Some of the resources may be new to the family because the members are desperate to alleviate some of the tension. The fourth phase is a state of active crisis. It results when the family lacks internal strength and social support, when the stressor remains unresolved, and when the anxiety is unbearable.[13] Crisis occurs when the family system's resources are unable to meet the demands of the crisis-provoking event, such as a critical illness.[14] At this point, the stressor event is also perceived as a threat and not as a challenge.

Based on various frameworks, Hoff's crisis paradigm can be applied to both individuals and families experiencing crises (Figure 4–3).[13] The crisis paradigm

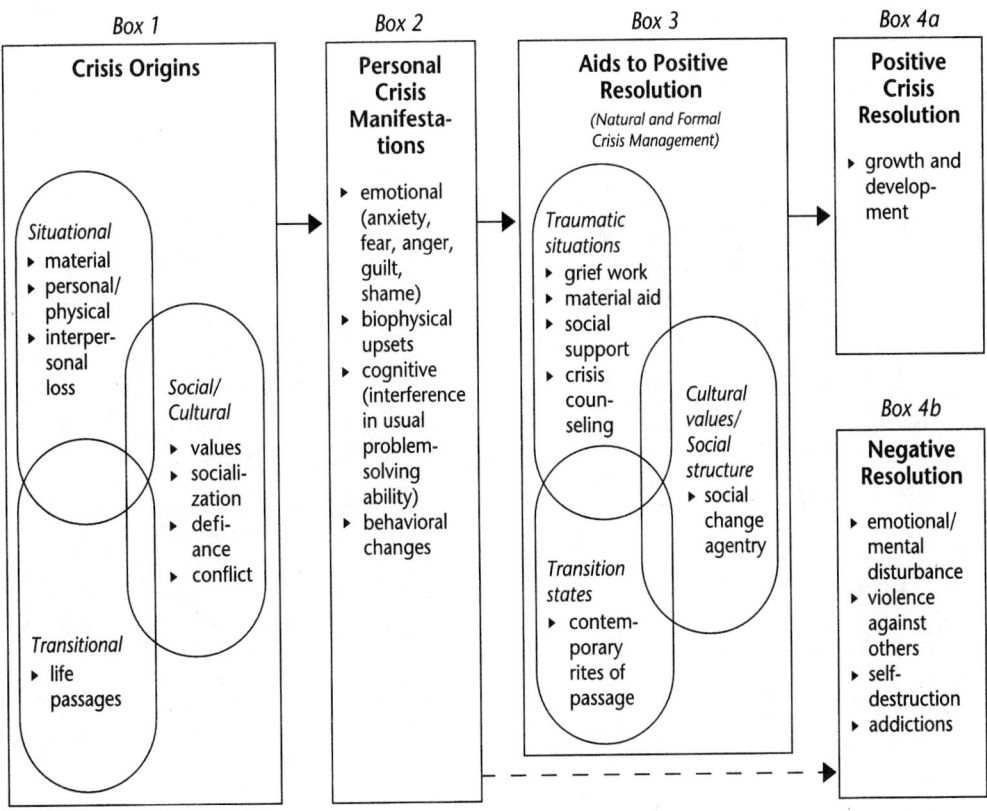

Figure 4–3

Hoff's crisis paradigm. (From Hoff LA: People in Crisis: Understanding and Helping, 4th ed. San Francisco, Jossey-Bass, 1996.)

depicts four phases of crisis intervention. Unique to Hoff's model is the inclusion of sociocultural factors. Using this crisis paradigm encourages health care providers to examine situational factors, transitional stages of families, and the sociocultural structure that may influence the outcomes of crisis. Examination of these factors may also identify appropriate areas of intervention for nurses, so bonadaptation may result. Bonadaptation is the successful, growth-producing result of crisis. Because families develop a norm of behavior before crisis events, families may alter their level of functioning with the use of their resources, interventions, and the passage of time. It is a basic goal of the health care team to return families to their former level of functioning after crisis events, but optimally, the goal is to develop a higher level of functioning.[15]

Another important model of family adjustment to stressors is the double ABCX model of family adjustment and adaptation to stress (see Figure 4–2). The double ABCX model added the postcrisis period and an interaction of postcrisis factors.[16] These factors eventually determine whether a family's adaptation was positive or negative. Once crisis has occurred and a family's usual coping resources have been unable to meet the demands of the stressful event, families will have additional needs. In the postcrisis phase, families can adapt well or poorly to the situation.[17]

During the critical illness, family members continue to face the tasks of everyday life (e.g. laundry, eating meals, getting children to school). This pileup of demands requires families to use additional resources. If these resources are not readily available, even greater stressors can develop for the family. In addition, when the family's usual methods of coping are unable to meet the severity of the stressful event, other unknown resources must be identified and used to cope with the critical illness. When additional resources are available to meet the crisis needs and the pileup of demands, families may develop greater coping resources and may perceive the crisis as a challenge. When families are unable to cope with the crisis and feel threatened, poor adjustment and a lower level of family functioning can result.

In all the family stress and crisis theories, families are viewed as dynamic systems with members who interact to restore a sense of balance to their world. Family perceptions and the personal meaning of the crisis situation need to be explored if the health care team is to assist families in crisis as a result of critical illness or injury. Only when the health care providers fully understand the impact of the illness on the family will they be able to intervene to promote bonadaptation (Chart 4–1).

An example of the importance of family theory with critically ill patients is demonstrated by the following case. Mr. J., a 32-year-old husband and expectant father, is admitted to the critical care unit after a right frontoparietal craniotomy for an arteriovenous malformation that had caused severe headaches and photophobia. After the operation, he is alert, oriented, and moving all extremities well. He has reported some photophobia. Within 6 hours of surgery, Mr. J. develops slurred speech and left-side hemiparesis. His neurologic function declines rapidly. A computed tomog-

CHART 4–1

Nursing Diagnosis: Ineffective Family Coping

Etiologic Factors: Catastrophic illness of a family member, inadequate coping skills, inadequate support systems.

Manifestations: Verbalizations of an inability to cope, inability of family members to make decisions, requests for help.

Expected Patient Outcomes:
1. Family members will identify usual patterns of coping and ineffective coping strategies.
2. Family members will demonstrate ability to assess, to solve problems, and to make decisions.
3. Family members will express realistic expectations of each other.

Interventions:
1. Establish trusting relationship with family members.
2. Observe family dynamics.
3. Assess the family's coping strategies and suggest new ones, as appropriate.
4. Support the family's effective coping strategies.
5. Consult psychiatric liaison nurse, clergy, or social services to facilitate effective family coping, as appropriate.
6. Consider team conferences to discuss how to best help the family effectively cope with the patient's critical illness.
7. Evaluate and document the family's response to interventions.

raphy scan documents bleeding at the surgical site and cerebral edema. Mrs. J. is notified immediately. Her response is to arrive at the unit with her own mother by her side.

The nurse needs to examine the support system of Mrs. J. and her response to this life-threatening situation. Mrs. J.'s definition of the situation, as well as her coping resources, will help to define whether or not this family will experience a crisis. Her pregnancy may be viewed either as an additional stressor that may increase the likelihood of crisis or as a resource (or comfort) that may help to decrease the risk of crisis. The nurse can gain greater insight into the meaning of neurologic illness to this family if he or she assesses the family as a whole and understands the roles and responsibilities of each family member, as well as the cultural norms that influence the family's definitions of the stressor event.

Collaborative Management of Specific Family Needs

The needs of families of critically ill patients have been well documented in the nursing literature. Two of the greatest priorities of families are the need for information and the need to visit the patient.[18–20] In a review of family needs literature, three major categories of needs were identified: informational needs, reassurance needs, and convenience needs (Chart 4–2). Whether patients were hospitalized in a critical care setting for days or weeks, the family's needs remained the same.[20] However, the needs of families of elderly patients had slightly altered priorities, with an increased need for reassurance that the best care is being given, a need to visit at any time, and a need to have the clergy visit. Additionally, these families indicated a need to talk with the physician daily, to have a place to be alone, to have flexible visiting hours, to have someone help with financial services, and to provide some physical care to the patient.[21] These important needs of families must be addressed by the health care team.

Collaboration among health care professionals is required for the comprehensive management of the critically ill patient and family. Nurses at the bedside must collaborate with physicians, respiratory therapists, discharge planners, dietitians, chaplains, and social workers who are involved in the care of the patient. Each discipline contributes specific knowledge and expertise about various aspects of patient care. The nurse must coordinate this collaborative approach, so that the patient receives the most comprehensive care and family needs can be met.

An example of family needs is demonstrated by the following case. Mr. S. is a 53-year-old man, admitted to the medical ICU with a diagnosis of acute gastrointestinal bleeding secondary to chronic alcohol abuse. He is awake, restless, hemodynamically unstable, and receiving multiple blood products. He also has a family history of cerebral aneurysm. His wife is a school teacher, and she is anxious and unclear about his prognosis. Clearly, the patient's physiologic and psychological needs must be met. In addition, his wife needs open and effective communication with the physician and nursing staff to decrease her anxiety and to assist her to cope with her husband's illness and subsequent management regimen. This patient and his wife illustrate the interrelatedness of the complex physiologic and psychological needs of the patient and the psychosocial needs of the family.

The nurse addresses these multiple needs of the family by first conducting a family assessment that explores the family's knowledge of the patient's illness and required care (see Table 4–2). Appropriate information is then presented to the family in both verbal and written formats. This should include information about the unit's visiting hours, telephone number, usual routines, physical setting, and patient equipment. Family members should be prepared as much as possible before visiting their relative to decrease their own stress and anxiety. Finally, allowing time at the

---

CHART 4–2

Needs of Families Dealing With a Critical Illness

Informational Needs
To have questions answered honestly.
To know the patient's prognosis.
To know specific facts about the patient's progress.
To know how the patient is being treated medically.
To have understandable explanations.
To be called about changes in the patient's condition.

Reassurance Needs
To be assured that the best care possible is being given to the patient.
To feel that there is hope.
To believe that hospital personnel care about the patient.
To know exactly what is being done for the patient and why.

Convenience Needs
To have access to a telephone and restroom.
To visit at any time.

patient's bedside is comforting to family members and helps to meet some of their needs.

The most advanced technology in health care is found in the critical care setting. Patients in this setting are the most physiologically unstable or have the potential to become unstable. An important part of this technologically advanced care is the family.[22] Nursing practice with families in the critical care setting was researched using narrative accounts from clinical practice. It was found that "some nurses approach care as a set of curative tasks. For these nurses, the challenge of the situation was the complex physiologic care that patients require and the medical and technologic procedures that can be employed. Nurses who practice in this way often viewed the family as an obstacle or impediment" (p. 200).[22] Instead of excluding families, they should be incorporated into specific aspects of care. Family members can hold the patient's hand, thus permitting the patient's extremity to be unrestrained during that time. The family should be encouraged to talk to the patient and to discuss family activities or current events. The family can also provide basic nursing care such as washing the patient's hands, applying lotion to the patient's feet, or assisting with mouth care. These activities increase the patient's comfort and allow the family to participate in patient care activities. This provides family members with a sense of control over the situation and acceptance as a member of the health team.[4] Conversely, the nurse must not simply thrust responsibilities onto families but should include them as much as they desire. Nursing standards of care, such as those established by the American Association of Critical Care Nursing (AACN),[23] clearly state that patients and their families are the appropriate focus of nursing care. Consequently, nurses must be knowledgeable about the application of family theory in the critical care setting and must incorporate it in their bedside practice.

Visitation Issues in Critical Care

Sometimes, nurses are uncomfortable with the family's presence in the critical care unit, and this discomfort may create a barrier to family involvement. A study by Chesla and Stannard[24] explored the critical care nursing activities that specifically restricted family involvement. The nursing activities identified included keeping the families physically away from the patient, avoiding the patient when family members were present, and considering the family's perspective to be a problem. Even though critically ill patients are unstable and require extensive nursing time, the nurse should allow the family to be part of the patient's care. At the same time, the nurse may believe that opportunities to talk with the family are limited when patient care activities are so demanding and

time consuming. This can be a realistic concern when the nurse is titrating multiple infusions, managing invasive equipment, and monitoring hemodynamic stability. During these times, another nurse or member of the health team should be asked to communicate with the family. Alternately, the nurse may inform the family that he or she will have a few minutes in an hour and will be able to speak with them at that time.

Unfortunately, some nurses continue to limit family involvement in critical care by restricting visiting hours (Chart 4–3).[25] However, research has validated the finding that families have a strong need to visit their critically ill family member in the critical care setting. The physiologic effects of visitation on patients has been and continues to be a controversial issue and may, in part, account for nurses' concerns regarding family involvement. Kleman and colleagues[26] examined the physiologic effects of visiting on 48 patients with AMIs and found no significant changes in any cardiovascular variables over time. However, a large individual variability in cardiovascular parameters was noted. Patients with the greatest heart rate change from baseline to 15 minutes after the visit had ejection fractions of less than 40%. In addition, 89% of these pa-

---

CHART 4–3

Comparison of Restrictive and Flexible Visitation Policies

Restrictive Policy

Visitors are limited to the immediate family.

Visits are limited to 10 to 20 minutes per hour, as determined by the nursing staff.

Visiting hours are from 11:00 AM to 8:00 PM.

A sign on the door instructs visitors to use the intercom to announce their arrival and to state their relationship with the patient, and then the nurse decides whether the visitor gains access.

Flexible Policy

Visiting hours are from 8:00 AM to 8:00 PM for all visitors; family members or significant others have 24-hour visiting privileges.

The patient may restrict visitors or may designate who may visit.

The nursing staff may restrict visitors during procedures or as the patient's condition changes, using patient assessment and professional judgment.

The family has a designated spokesperson who updates visitors on the patient's condition and whom the physician can contact.

tients with large changes had smoked for 25 years or more. Even though some patients experienced some physiologic changes during the visits, they stated that they believed that family visits were positive.[26] Although this study determined that visits were not harmful to patients, the researchers stressed the importance of closely monitoring critically ill patients' physiologic parameters during visits.

Although the literature supports flexible visitation policies in critical care settings, many individual patient variables must be considered when determining visitation needs. These include the patient's need for rest, the nurse's workload, environmental noise and activity, and the effects on the patient and family members. Research has shown that open visitation actually decreases patients' anxiety, and any restrictions that may be made on visitation should depend on the nurse's judgment, the patient's comfort, and the patient's physiologic status.[27]

An important part of a flexible visitation policy is the development of a contract with the patient and family. With a contract, the patient can determine who will visit and when, thus allowing the patient some control over the situation. Contract questions for the patient could include the following: Who would you like to visit you? When would you like to have visitors? For the family, an important question would be: Who will be the spokesperson for the patient? [28] A statement should be included in the contract that states the need to limit visitors, based on the clinical status of the patient and the general activity of the unit. This contract should be in written form and verbally discussed with the patient and family.

In one study, alert and hemodynamically stable patients with AMIs were encouraged to indicate their desire for visitors by activating a green or red light.[29] Physiologic variables measured included heart rate, blood pressure, temperature, salivary cortisol levels, and the presence of premature ventricular beats. Psychological variables measured included the level of visit stress, perceived control of visits, and perceived rest between visits. By using a light that registered red or green, patients were able to indicate their preference for visits. The researchers found that patients with the control mechanism ($N = 30$) believed they had more control of their environment and were able to obtain more rest than patients without the mechanism ($N = 30$). In addition, heart rate and diastolic blood pressure decreased in patients with the control mechanism.[29] Many critically ill patients are not alert or hemodynamically stable, and, consequently, this type of mechanism would not be indicated. However, this research supports the positive impact of patient control in the critical care environment. The application of this type of device or of other similar measures is an important adjunct in the comprehensive care of patients and families.

Finally, in some critical care settings, visitation has been expanded to include pets. Pet visitation or animal-assisted therapy has been shown to be beneficial to patients in acute care settings. The positive effects of animal-assisted therapy on patients include decreases in blood pressure and anxiety. Survival has even been correlated with pet ownership.[30] Pets must have current immunizations and should be brought to the ICU in a carrier or on a leash. Once in the unit, the pets should be placed on or next to the patients' beds. Many patients have developed strong bonds with their pets. Many elderly patients are concerned about their pets' welfare during the hospitalization. The benefits of animal-assisted therapy far outweigh the potential risks (such as the transmission of an infection from pet to owner) and should be considered part of the critical care unit's visitation policy.

Financial Issues Related to Critical Illness

When a patient is critically ill, the illness frequently has many financial consequences on the family. The economic impact on the family both during hospitalization and after recovery has been studied. Covinsky and associates[31] found that 33% of the patients studied required ongoing care from a family member after hospital discharge. Twenty percent of the patients' family members had to quit their jobs to care for the patient at home. Thirty-one percent of families lost the family savings, and 29% reportedly lost the major source of income. These burdens occurred even though 96% of the patients had hospitalization insurance. The survey also suggested that a large part of home care expenses was not reimbursed by either private or public insurance.[31] Nurses need to be attentive to the cost of critical care when caring for these patients. For example, nurses should know the cost of items and should use expensive supplies cautiously. Daily arterial blood gas determinations may not be necessary if the patient is stable on the ventilator and continuous pulse oximetry is used. Social workers or case managers have the expertise to guide the family through these financial challenges and should be consulted as needed. Interventions such as these are indicated whenever possible to minimize the financial impact of the critical illness on the family.

Outcomes

Collaborative management of families in the critical care setting requires that health care professionals work together to assess the needs of the family, to plan and implement the best care, and to evaluate outcomes for each family. Family members need to be kept informed of the patient's condition and the care the patient is receiving. Family members also need to be allowed to visit the patient and to participate in the care whenever possible. The incorporation of flexible visitation policies, including policies that permit pet visitation, has many positive psychological outcomes on the patient and family. Flexible visitation also affords families the opportunity to meet their two greatest needs: the need to see their family member and the need for information. Finally, the financial impact of the critical illness on the family can be devastating. Early involvement with social service workers or a case manager is essential to achieving optimal outcomes related to the family's financial stability.

IMPACT OF CRITICAL ILLNESS ON THE PATIENT

To explore the impact of a critical illness on the patient, the nurse must first perform a thorough psychosocial assessment (see Table 4–2). During this assessment, the nurse applies knowledge from family, crisis, and normal growth and development theories. Erickson's model of the developmental stages of psychosocial growth describes psychosocial development as a continuum beginning at birth and extending to death. This continuum includes four major life-cycle phases: childhood, adolescence, adulthood, and old age. These phases are further subdivided into eight psychosocial stages, with specific developmental tasks for each stage (Table 4–4).[32] With the stress of critical illness, a patient may not progress from one developmental stage to the next stage or may digress to a lower developmental stage.[32] The patient's self concept, physiologic and psychological stressors, emotional health, and developmental stage are key parts of psychosocial assessment.

Patients experience the stress of critical illness differently, depending, in part, on their stage of psychosocial development. Although general definitions exist for each stage, the specific psychosocial needs of each patient may vary. For example, a 65-year-old woman, diagnosed with breast cancer, has different psychosocial needs from those of a 40-year-old woman with the same diagnosis. The developmental task for the 65-year-old woman is concerned with the maintenance of life goals, whereas the developmental task for the 40-year-old woman is concerned with developing intimate relationships.

TABLE 4–4
Erickson's Psychosocial Stages of Development

Stage	Phase	Ego Strength	Unresolved	Task
Early infancy: birth–1 yr	Trust versus mistrust	Hope	Mistrust, dependency	Development of trust, establish separation from mother
Later infancy: 1–3 yr	Autonomy versus shame and doubt	Will	Shame and doubt, poor self-control	Feelings of security, acceptance
Early childhood: 4–5 yr	Initiative versus guilt	Purpose	Guilt, feelings of of inadequacy	Development of initiative
Middle childhood: 6–11 yr	Industry versus inferiority	Competence	Self-concept disturbances	Identification with significant elders, peer acceptance
Puberty and adolescence: 12–20 yr	Ego identity versus role confusion	Belonging	Role confusion, sexual confusion, self-consciousness	Development of sexual identity, development of own perceptions of the world
Early adulthood: 20–40 yr	Intimacy versus isolation	Love	Isolation, lack of responsibility	Ability to develop intimate relationships, appropriate channeling of emotions
Middle adulthood: 40–60 yr	Generativity versus stagnation	Care	Stagnation, poor motivation	Maintenance of life goals
Late adulthood: 60 yr and older	Ego integrity versus despair	Wisdom	Despair, loss of hope	Ability to resolve loss, acceptance of uncertain future

Another important aspect of psychosocial assessment is the patient's self-concept. "Self-concept refers to ideas, feelings, and attitudes that compose a person's identity, worth, capabilities, and limitations. The values and opinions of others, especially those provided during early childhood years, play an important role in self-concept development."[33] A critical illness activates patient coping behaviors that are directly associated with self-concept. A critically ill patient, such as a patient with a spinal cord injury, needs to grieve the loss of high-level wellness. The critical illness involves the loss of the familiar self-image and its replacement with a new one. These losses result in a temporary or permanent phase of lowered self-esteem.

Critically ill patients appropriately fear for their lives and, at the same time, feel isolated because they are removed from their familiar environments. Further, a sense of inadequacy or inferiority may develop if the patient does not understand the disease process and necessary treatment plan. The nurse must be aware of the psychosocial alterations that result from the critical illness and must identify how these changes affect the patient's ability to cope with the critical illness. It is a challenge for nurses to incorporate the psychosocial assessment into the plan of care, to help patients maintain their self-image and developmental stage.[31]

Management of Psychosocial Needs

The assessment and effective management of the patient's psychosocial needs require a multidisciplinary approach. Members of the health care team should confer to develop a plan of care to maximize the patient's coping abilities. Family members can be involved by providing information about prior coping strategies and family support systems. Clergy can provide emotional support to the patient, family, and staff caring for a critically ill patient. Social services can provide important information to the patient and families regarding discharge planning and financial resources. Psychologists and psychiatric nurse liaisons can work together to help the patient, family, and staff cope with the complex implications of the critical illness.

An example of the importance of a psychosocial assessment and management plan is demonstrated by the following case. Mr. W. is a 59-year-old white man who is admitted to the ICU with end-stage congestive heart failure. Both Mr. W.'s father and his only sibling died of heart attacks in their late forties. Currently, Mr. W. is divorced and has two adult sons. However, Mr. W.'s sons have limited contact with him and are not aware of this hospitalization. Mr. W. is alert and on mechanical ventilation. He is hemodynamically unstable and has an ejection fraction of 19%. Mr. W. has a history of six coronary artery bypass grafts and has been on the heart transplant list for 8 months. Although he is unable to communicate verbally, he shows signs of emotional distress through facial expressions, restlessness, and intermittent episodes of crying.

Using Erickson's model of psychosocial development, the nurse can identify Mr. W.'s expected developmental stage and can anticipate the associated developmental tasks (see Table 4–4). In fact, the nurse may find that Mr. W. may be experiencing a crisis in more than one psychosocial stage. For example, the phase of intimacy versus isolation may apply because Mr. W. is unable to speak, reinforcing feelings of isolation and inhibiting the appropriate channeling of emotions. In addition, his sons are not aware of this current hospitalization, a situation that further contributes to his sense of isolation. The phase of generativity versus stagnation is applicable not only chronologically but also because Mr. W.'s health is severely threatened by the illness and poor prognosis. He may also be experiencing a lack of motivation to live and disinterest in the future, related to the lack of family support and frustration with the unavailability of a heart for transplant. In fact, Mr. W. may also be dealing with the developmental tasks related to the phase of ego integrity versus despair. The nurse may sense a loss of hope and fear of death in Mr. W. As can be seen by this example, Mr. W. has many complex physiologic and psychosocial stressors that need to be identified and managed.

Nursing interventions for this patient should first include establishing a method of effective communication. Communication strategies could include using a clipboard and pencil, as well as nonverbal communication strategies such as the use of touch and eye contact. All members of the health care team (physician, respiratory therapist, clergy) should be encouraged to use these strategies. Social services should be consulted to contact family members if Mr. W. agrees. Ongoing emotional support should be provided, but the nurse must also avoid offering Mr. W. false hope. The nurse needs to assess Mr. W. continually for signs and symptoms of emotional distress. These signs could include expressions of anger, denial, irritability, withdrawal, inability to trust, crying, and noncompliance with treatments. Physiologic symptoms may include decreased appetite, activation of the stress response, sleeplessness, and restlessness.[3]

A critical illness has numerous and complex effects on patients including pain, anxiety, sleep alterations, communication needs, coping needs, and sense of powerlessness, as well as sexuality, spirituality, and patient education needs. Each of these is discussed in terms of theoretical definition, collaborative management, and anticipated outcomes.

Pain

Pain is common among patients in the critical care unit. Pain is defined as an unpleasant sensory and emotional experience associated with tissue damage that is described by the person experiencing the pain.[34] The gate control theory of pain explains the transmission of pain within the central nervous system. A gating mechanism in the substantia gelatinosa of the central nervous system balances impulses between large-diameter, nonpain fibers and smaller-diameter pain fibers. This mechanism can block or modulate the pain sensation from the periphery to the central nervous system. It can also modify the cerebral processes in the thalamus and cerebral cortex and can decrease the noxious stimuli at the level of the spinal cord.[35] This theory is applicable to many pain-management interventions for the critically ill patient.

Many critically ill patients have complex pathologic conditions that cause pain or require treatments that cause pain, such as chest tube insertion or removal, endotracheal suctioning, and central line insertion.[36] The most common reason for unrelieved pain among hospitalized patients in the United States is the failure of hospital staff to assess pain routinely and to provide adequate pain relief.[22] To provide comprehensive care with optimal outcomes, the nurse must accurately assess the patient's pain, provide the most appropriate interventions, and reassess the effectiveness of these interventions.

Collaborative Management

Collaborative and comprehensive management of pain is necessary to achieve patient comfort. Standards for the treatment of acute pain have been established by the Agency for Healthcare Policy and Research (AHCPR).[34] The major goals of these guidelines are to reduce the incidence and severity of patients' acute postoperative pain, to educate patients about the need to communicate unrelieved pain so they can receive prompt evaluation and effective treatment, to enhance patient comfort and satisfaction, and to contribute to fewer postoperative complications.[34]

A comprehensive pain assessment is the first step in effective pain management. Because pain involves physiologic tissue alterations, subjective interpretation, cultural influences, and historical perspective, it is challenging to assess accurately (Figure 4–4). Patient self-report is considered to be the most valid assessment strategy.[34] With the use of standardized pain scales, the patient can report ongoing pain using numbers, word descriptors, or FACES (Figure 4–5). These tools can be adapted to meet the needs of intubated patients and of non–English-speaking patients as well.

If patients cannot report their pain, nurses must use nonverbal indicators to assess and manage a patient's pain. These include patient behaviors, such as facial grimacing, grabbing at the pain site, crying, guarded movement, and restlessness.[37] Nurses also assess a patient's pain using physiologic indicators such as changes in blood pressure, heart and respiratory rate, electrocardiogram (ECG), and mixed venous oxygen saturation (SvO_2).[37] These physiologic indicators reflect the activation of the sympathetic nervous system as part of the stress response (Chart 4–4).

The nurse must provide the most effective intervention for the management of a patient's pain. Patients and their families should be questioned to explore fully their fears and concerns related to the use of pain medications, the cultural influences on the management of pain, and the level of knowledge regarding pain management. The assessment and documentation of a patient's pain must be ongoing and must include the patient's self-report whenever possible as well as the presence of any physiologic or behavioral indicators.

Pharmacologic Management. Effective pain management involves appropriate medication orders, pharmacy consultation, and safe and timely medication administration by the nurse. Pharmacologic intervention is a complex nursing responsibility that involves pain assessment, consideration of drug timing and dosing, drug interactions, and the possibility of adverse effects. Morphine sulfate (MSO_4) is considered the standard of narcotics and is used for equianalgesic comparison with other narcotics.[34] For example, a 55-year-old woman is admitted to the critical care unit after surgical repair of an abdominal aortic aneurysm. On postoperative day 2, she is hemodynamically stable and reports a pain level of 7/10. She is medicated with MSO_4, 5 mg intravenously, with good relief reported after 20 minutes (pain rated as 2/10). She is also premedicated before being moving out of bed to a chair. When pain is managed effectively, patient cooperation is also enhanced, and the risk of developing atelectasis, deep vein thrombosis, or pneumonia from immobility is decreased. However, if this patient were hypovolemic, she would be at risk of developing symptomatic hypotension from the vasodilatory effect of the narcotic.[38]

When managing a patient's pain, the nurse must consider the drug's pharmacologic effects and the patient's physiologic variables. To achieve this goal, a collaborative approach involving physicians and pharmacists is recommended. Many nurses are reluctant to medicate patients with narcotics because of the fear of complications.[39] However, according to the AHCPR, the incidence of narcotic-related complications (respiratory depression, tolerance, physical dependence, and addiction) is low, and treatment for these adverse effects is available.[34]

Initial Pain Assessment Tool

Date_____

Patient's name _____Age _____Room_____

Diagnosis_____Physician_____

Nurse_____

I. Location: Patient or nurse marks drawing.

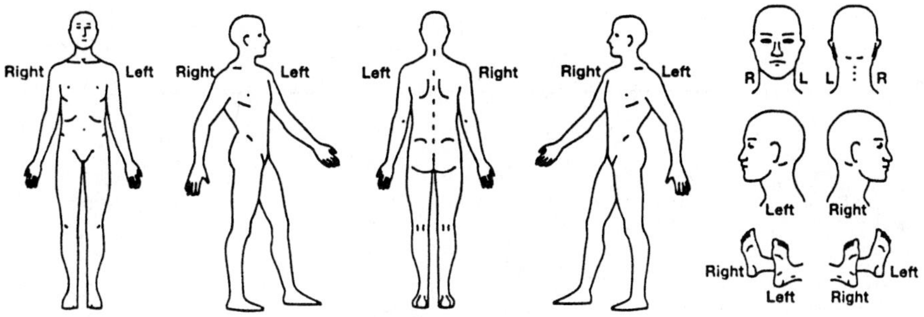

II. Intensity: Patient rates the pain. Scale used_____

    Present:_____

    Worst pain gets:_____

    Best pain gets:_____

    Acceptable level of pain:_____

III. Quality: (Use patient's own words, e.g., prick, ache, burn, throb, pull, sharp)

_____

IV. Onset, duration, variations, rhythms:_____

_____

V. Manner of expressing pain:_____

VI. What relieves the pain?_____

VII. What causes or increases the pain?_____

VIII. Effects of pain: (Note decreased function, decreased quality of life.)

    Accompanying symptoms (e.g., nausea) _____

    Sleep_____

    Appetite_____

    Physical activity_____

    Relationship with others (e.g., irritability)_____

    Emotions (e.g., anger, suicidal, crying)_____

    Concentration_____

    Other_____

IX. Other comments:_____

_____

X. Plan:_____

_____

Figure 4–4

Initial pain assessment tool. (From McCaffery M, Beebe A: Clinical manual for nursing practice. St. Louis, C.V. Mosby, 1989.)

Research has shown that the incidence of narcotic-induced ventilatory depression is less than 1%.[39] However, the nurse must still closely monitor the patient's response to narcotics, especially the first dose. The response to narcotics is individualized and depends on many physiologic factors such as the patient's hemodynamic status, age, and respiratory status.

Tolerance, on the other hand, is a physiologic response to narcotic analgesia after repeated administra-

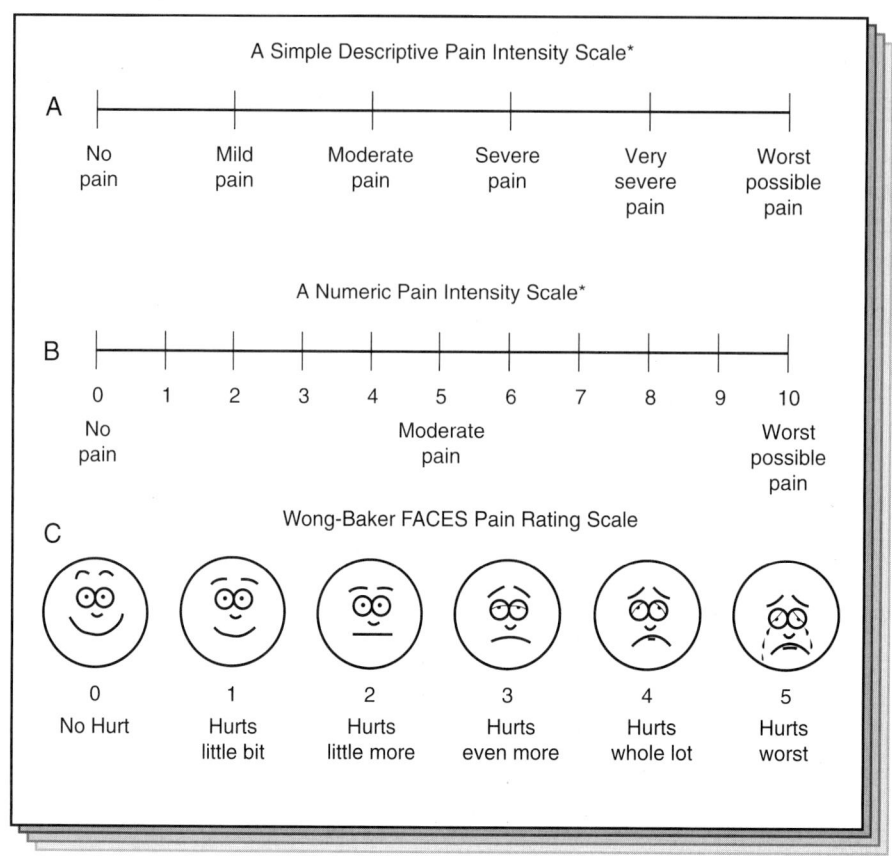

Figure 4–5

Pain scales. *A, Simple descriptive pain intensity scale. B, 0 to 10 Numeric pain intensity scale. C, Wong–Baker FACES pain rating scale.* (*A* and *B*, from Acute Pain Management: Operative or Medical Procedures and Trauma. Clinical Practice Guidelines. Publication No. 92-0032.35. Rockville, MD, Agency for Health Care Policy and Research, Public Health Service, US Department of Health and Human Services, 1992. *C*, from Wong D: Whaley and Wong's Essentials of Pediatric Nursing, 5th ed. Chicago, Mosby-Year Book, 1997, p 1215. Copyrighted by Mosby-Year Book, reprinted by permission.)

tion of the medication and can develop in the critically ill patient who requires extensive use of narcotics for pain control.[40] Because the narcotic binds to opioid receptors in the central and peripheral nervous system, the opioid receptors downregulate in number or change their shape.[41] Consequently, it takes more drug to cause the same level of analgesia, so the patient requires more drug for the same effect. With acute pain, the chance of developing tolerance is less, but if it does exist, the narcotic dose can be decreased by 10% daily over a 10-day period to prevent physiologic symptoms of withdrawal.[39]

Physical dependence is defined as the physiologic adaptation of the body to the presence of a narcotic, and this narcotic is required to maintain the same level of analgesia.[40] Tolerance and physical dependence can be anticipated with long-term use of narcotics for chronic pain. These complications should not be confused with psychological dependence or addiction. Addiction is defined as a pattern of compulsive drug use characterized by a continuous craving for a nar-

cotic and the need to use the narcotic for effects other than pain relief.[40] Research studies have shown that the incidence of addiction with the use of narcotics for pain relief is less than 1%.[39] Ongoing collaboration with other health care team members and appropriate documentation of the patient's response to narcotics can assist nurses to provide safe narcotic administration to patients in pain.

Nonpharmacologic Management. Many effective nonpharmacologic interventions complement pharmacologic approaches to pain management, such as relaxation techniques, family involvement in care, and calm reassurance. Currently, music therapy has gained in popularity as a nonpharmacologic adjunct to pain management. Music is defined as the combination of rhythm, harmony, and melodic sounds that promote pleasure and may have medicinal purposes.[35] Specifically, music with a simple, repetitive rhythm, slow tempo, string composition, and recognized instrumental and vocal timbre has been shown to reduce anxiety.[42] Music is also soothing to hear, provides di-

CHART 4–4

Physiologic and Behavioral Indicators of Acute Pain

Sympathetic-Adrenergic Responses
Increased heart rate
Increased respiratory rate
Increased blood pressure
Increased oxygen consumption rates
Increased muscle tension and motility
Increased pupillary dilatation
Increased palmar and plantar sweating
Increased anxiety
Decreased gastrointestinal motility

Behavioral Indicators
Increased movement: restlessness
Decreased movement: rigid posture, splinting
Facial grimacing
Crying

CHART 4–5

How to Start a Music Therapy Program in Your Unit

Select patients experiencing pain or anxiety.
Obtain tape players that are small, portable, and contain headphones.
Collect music tapes that have been shown to reduce anxiety, such as Bach, Beethoven, Brahms' lullaby, guitar music, and sound tracks from Born Free and The Sound of Music.
Help patients to identify the type of music they prefer.
Combine music therapy with other comfort measures, including analgesics, for best results.
Schedule specific times for music therapy, 25 to 90 minutes per day, uninterrupted whenever possible.
Evaluate outcomes: monitor heart rate, blood pressure, and self-reports of changes in pain and anxiety levels.
Include the family as much as possible.

version for the patient, and decreases pain.[35] Music therapy has also been used to decrease cough during bronchoscopy and to decrease heart rate and blood pressure in patients undergoing cardiac surgery.[35, 43] Music therapy, as a means to reduce anxiety and pain, is appropriate in the critical care setting. Critically ill patients should be able to consider complementary approaches to pain management such as music therapy. Chart 4–5 describes the steps that can be taken to initiate a music therapy program in a critical care unit.[35]

Outcomes

Effective pain control is an expected outcome for the critically ill patient. Chart 4–6 provides information for effective pain management. Pain management involves accurate assessment of the patient's pain, collaboration among health care team members, individualized interventions, and ongoing evaluation of the effectiveness of the interventions. Patient comfort increases and fewer physiologic complications develop when pain is comprehensively managed in the critical care setting.

Anxiety

Anxiety plays a significant role in the general adaptation syndrome that is part of the critically ill patient's experience. Anxiety is defined in terms of a generalized anxiety disorder that includes the following crite-

ria: excessive worry, difficulty in controlling the worry, restlessness, irritability, decreased ability to concentrate, and disturbed sleep.[44] The stressor that precipitates anxiety is whatever the patient perceives as a threat, loss, or danger. Consequently, anxiety is an alerting response that results from a real or perceived threat to a patient's biologic, psychological, or social integrity.[45] The greater the threat to the patient, the greater level of anxiety that will develop in the patient.

Collaborative Management

Once the nurse assesses the presence of anxiety in the patient, a collaborative plan can be established to reduce the anxiety. The nurse can decrease the patient's anxiety by helping him or her to identify and build on previously successful coping mechanisms as well as to develop new mechanisms.[45] When providing care, the nurse should convey calm attentiveness and interest. Whenever possible, the nurse should maintain eye contact with the patient, listen carefully when the patient verbalizes fears or anxiety, and allow time for the patient to initiate appropriate coping mechanisms or to develop new ones.[45]

The presence of a support system, such as family, friends, and clergy, can also help to reduce the patient's anxiety. The nurse should also promote the

CHART 4–6

Nursing Diagnosis: Pain

Etiologic Factors: Trauma, disease, or treatments and procedures.

Manifestations: Patient self-reports; physiologic or behavioral indicators such as crying, grimacing, tachycardia, restlessness, rigid posture, and splinting.

Expected Patient Outcomes:
1. The patient will communicate the pain level to the nurse.
2. The patient will express an acceptable level of pain relief.

Interventions:
1. Obtain a comprehensive baseline pain assessment from the patient or family.
2. Assess the patient's pain regularly and before and after interventions, using appropriate rating scales.
3. Evaluate the efficacy of current pain medication and consult with the physician or pharmacist to adjust the dose accordingly.
4. Premedicate the patient before painful activities or procedures, such as turning, suctioning, chest tube removal, and central line insertion.
5. Observe for potential side effects of narcotics (sedation, constipation, respiratory depression, or tolerance).
6. Provide nonpharmacologic interventions for pain management, such as music therapy when available.
7. Document effectiveness of pain management strategies.
8. Teach the patient and family about effective pain-management strategies, such as requesting pain medication before pain becomes severe.
9. Arrange team conferences to plan and evaluate pain management strategies, as necessary.

---

patient's sense of control when possible, such as allowing the patient to select the timing of procedures and routine activities. Relaxation techniques may be helpful with alert patients who are interested in using them. When a patient has severe anxiety, anxiolytic drugs, such as benzodiazepines, may be appropriate.[45] Additionally, consultations with psychiatric nurse liaisons, psychologists, or psychiatrists should also be considered.

Anxiety may also be manifested as a part of the syndrome called ICU psychosis. This term refers to acute delirium or a disturbance of consciousness.[46] This acute confusional state or delirium can be manifested by restlessness, agitation, combativeness, disorientation, or communication impairment.[45] Criteria for delirium include the following: disturbance in consciousness, change in cognition, and rapid development over a short period.[44] The etiologies of delirium include physiologic disorders, such as hypoxia, cerebral hypoperfusion, metabolic abnormalities, and medication toxicities, as well as environmental factors such as sleep deprivation and sensory overload (Chart 4–7).[47]

Nurses must identify patients at risk for developing anxiety or delirium. They must minimize the risk factors contributing to the development of these conditions, ensure patient safety with physical and pharmacologic restraints, and correct the cause as soon as possible. Once the underlying cause is identified and

CHART 4–7

Causes of Delirium

Physiologic Causes
Trauma: head injuries, hypovolemic shock
Medication withdrawal or intoxication: antibiotics, anticonvulsants, cardiac drugs, diuretics, histamine blockers, sedative-hypnotics, alcohol, opiates
Metabolic disorders: hepatic failure, uremia, acid–base imbalance, electrolyte imbalance
Nutritional disorders: hypoglycemia, hyperglycemia
Organ dysfunction: neurologic, pulmonary, cardiac, gastrointestinal, renal
Infections: sepsis, pneumonia, fever
Pain

Environmental Causes
Immobility
Sleep deprivation
Excessive noise

corrected, recovery from both anxiety and delirium is more likely to be complete.[46]

Outcomes

Effective management of anxiety and delirium is an expected outcome for the critically ill patient. This involves a collaborative effort that includes nurses for accurate patient assessment and evaluation, pharmacists for guidance regarding appropriate anxiolytic medications, physicians for overall management, and clergy for spiritual support. Family involvement in the plan of care is also important when dealing with an anxious patient. An individualized plan of care and ongoing evaluation of the effectiveness of the plan are essential to the patient's recovery and sense of well-being (Charts 4–8 and 4–9).

Sleep Alterations

Sleep pattern disturbances are common in critically ill patients. Sleep pattern disturbances consist of impaired sleep, resulting in altered daytime functioning and altered sleep architecture.[48] Normal sleep consists of two states. The first sleep state is characterized by the sleeping posture, with eyes closed. This state, called non–rapid eye movement sleep, has four stages and lasts 70 to 80% of total sleep time. The second sleep state consists of rapid eye movement sleep and is character-

ized by increased cortical activity. This state comprises 20 to 25% of total sleep time or 50 to 60 minutes.[48]

More than 50% of all patients in the critical care setting experience some degree of sleep deprivation.[49] These altered sleep patterns result from environmental, physiologic, and psychological stressors. Environmental stressors include equipment alarms, staff conversations, lighting, and extraneous noises. Physiologic stressors include the pathophysiologic condition, coughing, nursing and medical interventions, difficulty achieving comfort, medications, and inadequate pain control.[50] Psychological stressors that contribute to sleep deprivation include fear, pain, loss of control, severity of illness, and anxiety.[51] Sleep deprivation is particularly harmful to the critically ill patient because of the numerous physiologic effects (Chart 4–10).[52] The competent and caring nurse must allow for adequate sleep to minimize further physiologic complications.

Collaborative Management

The therapeutic goal for a patient with sleep alteration is to restore the patient's normal sleep–wake cycle and facilitate rest and recovery.[48] Many of the causes of sleep deprivation can be corrected with appropriate nursing interventions. Successful interventions include promoting at least 90-minute rest–sleep cycles, decreasing extraneous noises, effectively treating pain, reducing fear, considering anxiolytics, providing reassurance, and encouraging family participation (Chart 4–11).

CHART 4–8

Nursing Diagnosis: Anxiety

Etiologic Factors: Trauma, sudden critical illness or hospitalization, medical or nursing procedures or treatments, unknown prognosis.

Manifestations: Verbalizations of anxiety, fear of death; activation of stress response (restlessness, noncompliance with mechanical ventilation, changes in vital signs).

Expected Patient Outcomes:
1. The patient will demonstrate a decrease in restless behavior.
2. The patient will decrease verbalizations of fear of death and anxiety.
3. The patient's vital signs will stabilize.
4. The patient will activate appropriate and effective coping strategies to manage stressors related to critical illness.

Interventions:
1. Establish a trusting relationship with the patient and family.
2. Allow the family to visit and to participate in care as much as possible and as the patient's condition permits.
3. Allow the patient to control the environment whenever possible.
4. Provide adequate periods of rest or sleep by planning care to allow 90-minute uninterrupted periods of rest.
5. Provide information to the patient and family about therapies and prognosis using simple explanations.
6. Consider anxiolysis with benzodiazepines.
7. Consult with the pharmacist, physician, clergy, for example, regarding additional strategies.
8. Evaluate and document the patient's response to interventions.

CHART 4–9

Nursing Diagnosis: Altered Thought Processes (Delirium)

Etiologic Factors: Physiologic disorders (hypoxia, metabolic abnormalities, drug toxicity); environmental factors (sleep deprivation, sensory overload or deprivation).

Manifestations: Acute onset of disorientation, impaired cognition, combativeness, agitation, or hallucinations.

Expected Patient Outcomes:
1. The patient will regain the usual level of orientation and cognitive abilities.
2. The patient will be free of injury.
3. The patient will respond to environmental stimuli appropriately.

Interventions:
1. Identify the cause and correct as appropriate (e.g., for hypoxia, increase oxygen).
2. Reorient the patient frequently to person, place, and time, using verbal cues, calendars, and clocks.
3. Provide appropriate periods of uninterrupted rest to facilitate 90-minute sleep cycles.
4. Provide adequate sedation to ensure the patient's safety and to limit adverse side effects.
5. Include the patient's family in care to provide emotional support and reassurance to the patient.
6. Reduce the demand for cognitive functioning until the delirium resolves.
7. Promote communication that increases the patient's sense of integrity.
8. Evaluate and document the effectiveness of strategies.

Outcomes

The outcomes of these interventions are best demonstrated by the following case. Mr. B. is an 87-year-old man admitted to the critical care unit with a diagnosis of an exacerbation of chronic obstructive pulmonary disease (COPD) complicated by a left lower lobe pneumonia. He requires intubation and mechanical ventilation to support his respiratory status. He is awake and alert most of the time, appears anxious, and becomes agitated during pulmonary hygiene activities, including suctioning. His nurse, physician, pharmacist, and respiratory therapist recognize the patient's need for sleep and have instituted the following interventions. His wife is permitted to stay at the bedside for most of the day but is encouraged to go home at night to rest. All procedures are explained to Mr. B. before they are instituted, to reduce his fear of the unknown. Low-dose anxiolytic agents are used on a routine basis to decrease Mr. B.'s anxiety and to increase compliance with necessary pulmonary interventions. Nursing care is done in a scheduled manner to allow for 90-minute rest–sleep periods twice during the day and several times during the night. In-line arterial blood gas measurements, daily chest radiographs, and continuous pulse oximetry are used to monitor Mr. B.'s pulmonary status by being as minimally invasive as possible. The nurses consistently demonstrate a caring and competent attitude when providing care for Mr. B. and his wife. With these interventions, the stressors that interfere with Mr. B.'s sleep will be minimized, and his chances for recovery will be maximized. Nurses who realize the importance of sleep will allow patients to rest, thereby promoting recovery from the critical illness.

CHART 4–10

Consequences of Sleep Deprivation

The following are increased with sleep deprivation:

Hemodilution
Cortisol
Serum levels of triiodothyronine, thyroxine
Insulin levels
Blood glucose
Agitation

The following are decreased with sleep deprivation:

Red blood cell count
Hematocrit
Oxygen consumption
pH
Motivation

CHART 4–11

Nursing Diagnosis: Sleep Pattern Disturbance

Etiologic Factors: Sleep deprivation secondary to excessive noise, pain, anxiety, immobility, fear of death, or isolation.

Manifestations: Self-report of inadequate rest or sleep or sense of exhaustion, physiologic and behavioral indicators (e.g., agitation, noncompliance with therapy, lack of motivation).

Expected Patient Outcomes:
1. The patient will sleep for at least 90-minute segments without interruptions, especially at night.
2. The patient will verbalize a sense of feeling adequately rested.
3. The patient will demonstrate physiologic and behavioral signs of adequate rest or sleep.

Interventions:
1. Assess the patient for signs of inadequate rest or sleep.
2. Eliminate extraneous stimuli such as lights, unnecessary activities, noise, and verbal exchanges between staff members at the patient's bedside.
3. Communicate with all members of the health team to allow 90-minute rest or sleep periods between interventions.
4. Consider incorporating music therapy to facilitate rest or sleep, if available.
5. Position the patient for maximum comfort.
6. Medicate the patient for pain, if necessary.
7. Consult with the physician or pharmacist regarding the use of medications to facilitate sleep.
8. Evaluate and document the patient's response to interventions.

Communication Needs

Effective therapeutic communication between nurses and patients is essential for the patient's psychological integrity.[51] This type of communication is defined as interactive verbal and nonverbal strategies that focus on the needs of the patient and facilitate a goal-directed communication process.[44]

Collaborative Management

Unfortunately, many critically ill patients are intubated or may be experiencing changes in mental status that leave them unable to communicate their needs and fears to the staff effectively. This problem can be frustrating both to the patient who tries to make his or her needs known to the nurse and to the nurse who attempts to understand or interpret them. In these situations, the nurse must always explain what will happen to the patient before initiating patient care activities. With intubated, alert patients, various devices can improve communication with the patient. For example, a letter board that has large letters or short words to which the patient can point is often helpful. Picture boards are also effective, especially with non–English-speaking patients. In addition, computers can be used to help with communication. One patient, a 28-year-old man with a traumatic brain injury, was unable to communicate verbally because of a tracheostomy. However, he was alert and could use one hand to work a keyboard to communicate his needs. Nurses must be creative to maximize communication with patients.

Nonverbal communication is also important in the critical care setting. Nurses must have a caring, warm approach to their patients and must offer reassurances whenever possible. Nurses can enhance a trusting relationship with patients by decreasing the depersonalization that often accompanies hospitalization. Use of eye contact, a warm smile, and touch are positive nonverbal communication techniques for both conscious and unconscious patients. Nurses should always introduce themselves to the patient and family and include pertinent information from the family in the plan of care. Effective nonverbal communication can decrease stress on both patient and family during this critical time.

Outcomes

Communication is an essential part of critical care nursing. Verbal and nonverbal communication with the patient will decrease anxiety, facilitate cooperation with treatments, and maximize optimal recovery from the critical illness. An interdisciplinary approach facilitates effective communication with critically ill patients. Hospital administrators may financially support the use of bedside computers for intubated patients. Social services may be able to locate an interpreter for non–English-speaking patients. Team conferences that address the communication needs of the patient also reinforce the effective management of these needs (Chart 4–12).

CHART 4–12

Nursing Diagnosis: Impaired Communication

Etiologic Factors: Intubation, decreased level of consciousness, language differences, side effects of medications.

Manifestations: Inability to speak or to communicate needs effectively.

Expected Patient Outcome:
1. Patient will be able to communicate needs effectively.

Interventions:
1. Assess the patient's level of consciousness and level of comprehension.
2. Provide tools for alternate means of communication: paper and pencil, pointer, or picture board.
3. Use nonverbal communication techniques to provide additional emotional support (touch, eye contact).
4. Try to lip read if the patient attempts to mouth words.
5. Include the family in developing and using communication strategies.
6. Speak slowly and succinctly for maximal patient comprehension.
7. Consult with a speech therapist to plan communication strategies.
8. Explain communication strategies to all health team members to ensure consistency.
9. Contact social services for an interpreter if patient does not speak English.

Facilitating Coping

Facilitating coping is an important role of the critical care nurse. Coping is defined as "constantly changing cognitive and behavioral efforts to manage specific external and/or internal demands that are appraised as taxing or exceeding the resources of the person."[53] The critically ill patient and the family use familiar coping strategies when their own instinctive defense mechanisms have not been able to meet the demands of the stressful situation, such as a critical illness. Available coping strategies are often patterns of responses that have developed from earlier life experiences or similar situations. The strategies are directed toward lessening the current stressful situation so that successful adaptation can result.[53]

Stress is the result of an interaction between the patient and the environment and is regulated by cognitive appraisal and coping activities. Cognitive appraisal, which occurs at all levels of consciousness, is an assessment activity that evaluates the stressfulness of the stressor.[53]

Collaborative Management

A patient's ability to cope with a stressful and threatening event depends on many factors, including individual coping skills (Figure 4–6; see Figure 4–2). However, the critically ill patient may be unable to use previous coping mechanisms to minimize stress, usually because of many physiologic and psychosocial factors, including physiologic instability, pain, lack of control, loss of privacy, and social isolation from family and friends (Chart 4–13).[32] Consequently, the critically ill patient may need to develop new coping skills. Listening, communicating, advocating, and educating are strategies the nurse can use to help the patient and family cope with the critical illness. Active listening to the patient and family provides time for a verbal account of the patient's and family's definitions

---

CHART 4–13

Coping Challenges Related to Critical Illness

Illness-Related Coping Challenges
Coping with pain and helplessness
Coping with the hospital and intensive care environment
Coping with medical and nursing procedures
Coping with many different team members
Coping with an unknown future

General Coping Challenges
Maintaining an emotional balance
Maintaining self-esteem
Maintaining meaningful relationships with family and friends
Maintaining a sense of productivity

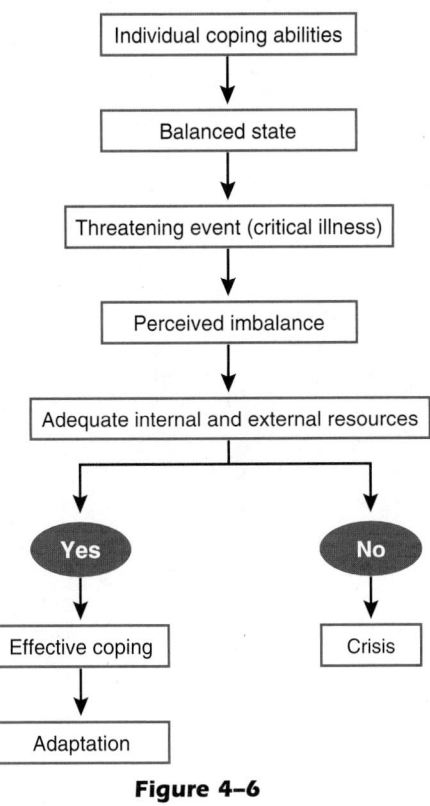

Figure 4–6

Coping response.

of the stressful illness, clarification of misinformation, and knowledge acquisition. In addition, patients gain a sense of personal worth in relation to the stressful event. Creativity with coping implies helping the patient to redefine the situation. For example, if a patient views the illness as a death threat from God, he or she may use energy in this area instead of using energy to adapt. If the nurse can help the patient to redefine the situation, the patient may be able to develop a more positive view of the illness event.[15] For some patients, it may be appropriate to teach relaxation techniques to deal with both physiologic and psychological stressors.

Collaboration with the health care team, the patient, and the family will help the patient to cope with the critical illness. The nurse should assess and support the coping abilities of the patient and family. If the coping abilities are inadequate to meet the demands of the illness, then crisis and ineffective coping may result (see Figure 4–3). Specific symptoms of ineffective coping include moderate to high levels of anxiety, depression, noncompliance with therapies, and avoidance of friends and family.[52]

Social services, clergy, and psychiatric nurse liaisons can provide helpful information for the patient and family to increase their ability to cope with the critical illness. A team conference that includes the patient and family can be an effective mechanism through which the patient's illness can be discussed.

Expectations of the whole team, including the family, can be discussed, and realistic goals can be developed.

Outcomes

Crisis can be minimized with critically ill patients through effective coping. Patients and families can adapt if resources are provided. Using collaborative management, the impact of the illness and the resources needed for the patient and family to cope can be identified and enhanced when needed (Chart 4–14).

Powerlessness

A sense of powerlessness is common in critically ill patients. Powerlessness develops from a lack of warning about the critical illness and causes the patient to have a limited influence on the event.[32] Powerlessness also occurs with other unpredictable events, such as acts of war, natural disasters, and accidents. In each of these situations, the person does not have time to adapt and feels completely overwhelmed. These events can lead to ineffective coping, as just described.

In this unbalanced psychological state, the patient goes through a process of psychological adaptation and coping in an attempt to regain a sense of equilibrium in his or her life.[32] The nurse must assess critically ill patients for this sense of powerlessness and must provide the most appropriate interventions. Knowing that powerlessness is a natural reaction to critical illness, the nurse can be prepared to help the patient to cope more effectively.

Collaborative Management

An interdisciplinary plan of care is indicated for the diagnosis of powerlessness. Psychiatric liaison nurses, psychologists, social workers, clergy, nurses, and physicians can develop a plan of care that includes interventions to help the patient to cope effectively. Patients can have some control of their situation by participating in decisions about their care. For example, a patient with an AMI can decide when to have his or her bath and who can visit. Family members should be involved in patient care as much as possible and according to the patient's wishes and physiologic status.

Outcomes

Powerlessness is a significant reaction to the stress of critical illness. By acknowledging its existence, the health care team can help patients to cope with the critical illness and to regain control of the situation. By helping the patient to restore a sense of power, the nurse facilitates both physiologic and psychological recovery (Chart 4–15).

CHART 4–14

Nursing Diagnosis: Ineffective Individual Coping

Etiologic Factors: Catastrophic illness, inadequate coping skills, inadequate support systems.

Manifestations: Fatigue, insomnia, frequent crying, inability to make decisions, verbalizations of inability to cope, requests for help.

Expected Patient Outcomes:
1. The patient will identify ineffective coping strategies (e.g., defense mechanisms).
2. The patient will demonstrate an ability to assess, to solve problems, and to make decisions.
3. The patient will express realistic expectations of self.
4. The patient will learn and use new and effective coping skills.

Interventions:
1. Establish a trusting relationship with the patient.
2. Assess the patient's usual coping strategies and suggest new ones, if appropriate.
3. Provide emotional support to the patient to maximize effective coping.
4. Involve the family in the plan.
5. Consult with the psychiatric nurse liaison to facilitate development of new coping skills.
6. Consult with clergy to provide spiritual support to the patient, if desired.
7. Arrange a team conference to discuss how to help patient effectively cope with the illness.
8. Evaluate and document the patient's response to interventions.

Sexuality Needs

Intimacy and sexuality are important aspects of a patient's psychosocial needs in the critical care setting because a patient's sexual functioning is often affected by a serious illness.[32] Altered sexuality patterns are defined as the state in which an individual expresses concern regarding his or her sexuality. The patient's fears, myths, and comfort level related to sexual function should be addressed with all patients who express a concern regarding an alteration in sexuality. The psychological effects of a critical illness can have a far greater impact on sexual function than the physiologic effects.[54] A person's beliefs, attitudes, and knowledge of sexuality can affect the achievement of sexual integrity. These factors become particularly important after a life-threatening illness.[54]

CHART 4–15

Nursing Diagnosis: Powerlessness

Etiologic Factors: Sudden critical illness, trauma, dependence on health team for all needs.

Manifestations: Inability to communicate related to intubation, fear demonstrated through facial expressions or verbalizations, withdrawal, anger, frustration.

Expected Patient Outcomes:
1. The patient will identify feelings of helplessness.
2. The patient will participate in decision making, as appropriate.
3. The patient will report a restored sense of control.

Interventions:
1. Encourage the patient to express feelings regarding the hospitalization and illness.
2. Provide emotional support, including acknowledgment of normality of the patient's feelings of helplessness and the use of nonverbal communication techniques.
3. Incorporate all members of the health team, including the family, in strategies to restore the patient's sense of control.
4. Facilitate effective verbal and nonverbal communication.
5. Allow the patient to make care decisions whenever possible.
6. Provide positive feedback for the patient's participation in care decisions.

Collaborative Management

Sexual function is a topic that is often avoided by nurses caring for critically ill patients. This neglect could stem from the discomfort level of the nurse or the discomfort level of the patient. Nurse discomfort is often associated with personal attitudes and values toward sexuality as well as the nurse's belief that it is not a part of his or her role.[55] In addition, the critically ill patient may be too ill to discuss sex, or the discussion of sexuality may cause anxiety. For example, a study of the sexual counseling of patients with AMIs showed that the lack of information regarding sexuality was frustrating to these patients, and vague references to sexuality led to insecurity, confusion, and depression.[56]

Before discussing sexual function with a patient, nurses should take a personal inventory regarding their own sexual beliefs and attitudes (Chart 4–16).[56] Nurses need to assess their own comfort level surrounding the sexual counseling of patients and to address any concerns. Nurses should also recognize the importance of discussing patients' concerns about sexuality and sexual function. These discussions can only take place when nurses take the responsibility for acquiring the knowledge and skill needed to provide sexual counseling effectively to their patients.

The nurse must assess sexuality needs and not make assumptions about a patient's sexual activity. Assessment and teaching should begin early in the nursing care of the patient and as the patient's physiologic status allows. The nurse should reassure the patient that it is normal to have questions regarding sexual activity and function after the illness. By using a general statement, the nurse can initiate a discussion in a nonthreatening manner. For example, the nurse could have the following conversation with an alert patient. "Many patients have concerns about resuming sexual activity. What concerns do you have?"[56] To be touched and held is vital to the healing process and to feeling "normal" again. Nurses can help patients by teaching that kissing and intimate touch are good places to begin resuming their previous level of sexual function.[56]

Sexual counseling and suggested interventions should be approached in a sensitive, straightforward manner. It may be appropriate to include the patient's partner in these discussions. As the patient improves physiologically, the nurse should provide specific guidelines that will aid the patient in resuming sexual activity after hospitalization.[56] The nurse should also consider consulting with other members of the health care team (physician, physical therapist, counselor) when identifying these guidelines.

Outcomes

Sexual concerns can adversely affect the recovery of the critically ill patient. By addressing these concerns, the nurse can develop a plan of care that includes information on sexual function and allows the patient the opportunity to discuss these issues. A team approach should be considered when helping patients and partners deal with these concerns. The outcome will be less anxiety, a return to normal sexual function, and a positive quality of life for the patient and partner (Chart 4–17).

Spirituality Needs

Spiritual well-being is defined as the belief or value system that provides strength, hope, and meaning to life. Spiritual well-being can be the center of a healthy lifestyle allowing holistic integration of a person's inner resources. Spirituality is a source of inner strength and peace and helps us to express our views and behaviors, in the search for hope and meaning in our lives.[57] Even in Plato's era, health care providers were encouraged to care for the whole person: "As you ought not to attempt to cure the eyes without the head, or the head without the body, so neither ought you to attempt to cure the body without the soul." The "part," Plato added, "can never be well unless the whole is well."[58]

Collaborative Management

Spiritual needs are an important component of the human existence, and care of the spiritual and psychosocial needs of patients has an impact on health

---

CHART 4–16

Exploring Attitudes Toward Sexual Counseling

1. In general, what are your attitudes towards sexuality?
2. How comfortable are you discussing sex?
3. Would you be uncomfortable asking a peer for help discussing sexual issues with a patient or family?
4. Would you be willing to chart your discussion about sexual function with the patient?
5. Do you believe you possess enough knowledge about changes in sexual function to counsel a patient?
6. Do you think it is part of a nurse's role to address issues about sexual function?

CHART 4–17

Nursing Diagnosis: Altered Sexuality Patterns

Etiologic Factors: Side effects of medications, sudden illness, change in body image.

Manifestations: Expressed fear of resuming sexual activity secondary to exertional effects, self-report of sexual concerns.

Expected Patient Outcomes:
1. The patient will verbalize concerns regarding sexual function.
2. The patient will identify stressors in his or her life that may interfere with sexual functioning.
3. The patient will resume previous sexual activity when physiologically able to do so.

Interventions:
1. Conduct a personal inventory of your own attitudes toward sexuality and discussing sexual issues with patients and families.
2. Obtain a sexual history from the patient.
3. With the patient's permission, include the patient's partner in discussions about sexuality when the patient's physical status permits.
4. Encourage the patient to ask questions and to discuss sexuality as related to the diagnosis and future sexual activity.
5. With stressors that negatively affect sexual activity, assist the patient to
   a. Modify lifestyle to reduce stress.
   b. Participate in rehabilitation or an exercise program to increase physical endurance after discharge and if indicated.
   c. Identify stressors that can be controlled by the patient and help the patient to identify methods of reducing or eliminating them.
6. Involve additional members of the health team, as appropriate.
7. Provide information on additional community resources, as appropriate.

---

and survival.[59] Because spirituality is associated with hope, meaning, and connectedness, the nurse needs to help the patient to maintain spiritual well-being. Although this is a difficult task, patient well-being is enhanced by attending to the spiritual and psychosocial crises that are often associated with a life-threatening illness.[57]

Some nurses may not address the spiritual concerns of patients because they do not recognize the signs and symptoms of spiritual distress. These signs include the patient's asking "Why me?" and "What did I do to deserve this?", crying, expressing a sense of hopelessness, and requesting to see a priest or rabbi. The nurse should also observe patient's interactions with family members and health care team members and the patient's nonverbal communication. Cues, such as body language, facial expressions, and restlessness, can often point toward spiritual distress.[59] Even though nurses tend to place a greater emphasis on the physiologic needs than on the psychosocial needs of the critically ill patient, the spiritual needs must be addressed as well.[59]

A thorough psychosocial assessment is essential for identifying and effectively managing spiritual distress. After the nurse has assessed the patient and the patient is found to be experiencing spiritual distress, appropriate action can be taken to maximize recovery. Spiritual well-being is enhanced by allowing open discussion of spiritual feelings, showing respect for individual beliefs, giving patients privacy for prayer, and making referrals to the clergy, if requested.[57] Another effective intervention is including the patient's family in the plan. This approach supports the patient's spirituality by providing a familiar support system and provides comfort for both the patient and family. The nurse should ask the family for information about the patient's spiritual needs and find out how these needs are normally addressed. The nurse should show acceptance of the patient's spiritual beliefs and support them whenever possible. For example, if a patient is Jewish, the nurse can ask the patient and family if they would like a rabbi to visit. If the patient has no formal religion, the nurse can offer the services of the hospital chaplain. The following questions are helpful in obtaining useful information for assisting patients and families: In what or in whom do you find a source of strength in this time of crisis? Is there someone I could call for you, such as a rabbi or priest? How can I support you in your spiritual beliefs? Are specific practices important for your spiritual well-being?

Outcomes

It is challenging for the nurse to help patients find hope and meaning in life during a time of physical and emotional crisis.[57] Because every patient is unique, with different coping techniques, nurses should use spiritually related nursing interventions when deter-

CHART 4–18

Nursing Diagnosis: Spiritual Distress

Etiologic Factors: Sudden illness, uncertain prognosis or future, multiple treatments and invasive procedures.

Manifestations: Emotional detachment, expressed feelings of isolation or abandonment, questioning of belief system.

Expected Patient Outcomes:
1. The patient will express decreased feelings of anxiety, fear, isolation, and abandonment.
2. The patient will continue spiritual practices.
3. The patient will express satisfaction with his or her spiritual belief system.

Interventions:
1. Ask the patient about past spiritual beliefs and experiences that were comforting during crises.
2. Express a willingness to help the patient meet his or her spiritual needs.
3. Provide nonjudgmental care and support of the patient's spiritual needs and traditions.
4. Provide spiritual support by contacting local religious leader of the patient's choice or the hospital chaplain.
5. Actively listen when the patient expresses feelings of doubt, fear, or abandonment.
6. Evaluate and document the effectiveness of interventions.

---

mined to be appropriate for a patient. The spiritual well-being of the critically ill patient has a profound impact on the outcome of the critical illness. The nurse must address the spiritual needs of patients and must provide spiritual support when possible to maximize recovery from the critical illness (Chart 4–18).

Patient Education Needs

Patient education is an important part of critical care nursing. Principles of adult education that apply in this setting include individualized content, impact of past experience on learning, trust as a basis for learning, maximal use of senses, progression from simple to complex content, and familiarity of concepts.[3] Critically ill patients have many barriers to learning, including the pathologic processes they are enduring. The nurse must adapt the principles of adult learning to each patient in an individualized manner (Chart 4–19).

Collaborative Management

Patients' perceptions about their disease play an important part in the education required in the critical care setting and in the patients' long-term recovery. For example, in one study of ICU patients with cardiovascular disease, 64% knew that smoking was a risk factor, but only 15% recognized hypertension as a contributor to the development of the disease. Seventy-five percent of the patients studied were knowledgeable about diet as a risk factor, but 19% of patients with AMIs and 40% of patients undergoing angioplasty indicated that they were unsure of what caused their cardiovascular disease.[60] These identified educational needs are important to address, to prevent progression of the patient's disease once discharged.

In another example, a patient who is intubated and is receiving mechanical ventilation may have varying levels of consciousness. The nurse should provide simple explanations relevant to the patient during periods of improved cognition. The education can be reinforced by the respiratory therapist when it pertains to compliance with the ventilator or suctioning. Addi-

---

CHART 4–19

Principles of Adult Learning and Education

1. Assess the patient's willingness to learn as well as his or her personal goals.
2. Assess the patient's physical and mental readiness to learn before starting the teaching.
3. Maximize comfort with adequate pain relief and repositioning before teaching.
4. Include the family as appropriate.
5. Assess factors that influence patient's ability to learn, such as level of consciousness, education, and cultural background.
6. Use visual aids whenever possible, such as written materials, videos, and posters.
7. Use simple terms and explanations to present complex information.
8. Provide written material to reinforce verbal information whenever possible.

tional educational content should include pertinent information about the patient's necessary therapies, such as weaning from the ventilator and adequate pain control.

Preoperative patient education can decrease anxiety and can increase the sense of control of both patients and family members. A tour of the critical care unit before a patient undergoes cardiac surgery provides information about the critical care setting and education about the postoperative period, and it reduces the patient's and family's anxiety about the hospitalization.[61] Other means of education can include the use of videotapes for patient and family education. A videocassette recorder can be used for viewing educational videotapes in the patient's room or the waiting room. It may even be possible to lend these videotapes to families for overnight viewing. Patient and family education can also be enhanced with the use of educational pamphlets from the AHCPR such as *Pain Control After Surgery: A Patient's Guide from the AHCPR*.[34] Similar patient guides are also available for angina, cancer pain, early HIV management, heart failure, poststroke rehabilitation, cardiac rehabilitation, and other common clinical disorders.

Outcomes

Patient and family education can help the patient and family to cope with the critical illness and can maximize recovery. For this to occur, nurses must provide ongoing education related to the patient's treatment plan as well as essential information needed for the patient to return home safely (Chart 4–20).

IMPACT OF CRITICAL ILLNESS ON THE ELDERLY

Elderly patients, defined as those 65 years old or older, represent a specialized population in the critical care setting because of their unique problems and responses to critical illness. In addition, they are the fastest growing segment of the population of the United States.[62] Because of increased life expectancy, the numbers of elderly are estimated to increase from 31.4 million to 52 million by the year 2025.[63] The segment of the population that is older than 85 years will increase even more rapidly, from 3.5 million in 1994 to 7 million by 2020 and to 14 million in 2040.[62] A survey of adult critical care units in the United States found that the elderly accounted for 58% of all occupied beds.[64]

Spiraling health care costs and scarce resources raise the question of whether age should be used as a criterion for rationing critical care to the elderly.[65] Many argue that the elderly, with their diminished physiologic reserve and chronic illnesses, are less likely to benefit, and needed resources should be directed toward the young, who have a greater potential to recover and contribute to society.[66, 67] Studies of the outcomes of critical illness and trauma have shown consistently that increasing age is associated with increased morbidity and mortality. Yet, when the severity of illness and the presence of chronic illness are controlled for, age becomes a weak predictor of outcome or has no predictive value.[65, 66, 68–71] In addition to the severity of illness and preexisting chronic illnesses, other factors that predict outcome in the elderly are decreased functional status at the time of

---

CHART 4–20

Nursing Diagnosis: Knowledge Deficit (Learning Need)

Etiologic Factors: Lack of experience with the illness or disease process, misinterpretation of information, lack of experience with treatments and procedures.

Manifestations: Requests for information regarding the condition, prognosis, discharge needs; expressions of confusion regarding the illness or disease process and treatments and procedures.

Expected Patient Outcomes:
1. The patient will explain the disease process, purpose of treatments, and prognosis.
2. The patient will restate pertinent information related to discharge.

Interventions:
1. Assess the patient's knowledge regarding illness, treatments, prognosis.
2. Include the family in all teaching whenever possible.
3. Provide written information whenever possible.
4. Allow the patient and family ample opportunity to ask questions.
5. Repeat information as often as needed.
6. Evaluate learning of one topic before proceeding to a new topic.
7. Convey a positive, supportive attitude toward the patient and family during teaching sessions.

admission, domicile at the time of admission (i.e., own home or institutional setting), the presence of a closed head injury, and intercurrent events such as sustained periods of hypotension, cardiac arrest, prolonged mechanical ventilation, and placement of a pulmonary artery catheter.[67, 71]

The question also arises whether cardiopulmonary resuscitation (CPR) is beneficial in the elderly. Age is not a good predictor of CPR outcome. The outcome is most often associated with the severity of illness and the presence of coexisting diseases. A large clinical trial found no difference between those over 65 years and those under 65 years in the frequency of good neurologic and functional status recovery 6 months after successful CPR.[72] The factors that predicted good neurologic recovery in this large clinical trial were no history of diabetes mellitus, a cardiac cause of the arrest, short arrest time, and short CPR time.

Most elderly patients who survive hospitalization are able to return to their homes at discharge or after varying periods in a transitional setting. Quality of life has been measured by functional status, cognitive function, sensory function, pain, mood, and perception of health. These measures improve to baseline or near-baseline levels for most patients over the months after discharge.[65, 66, 69, 71] More research is needed to determine long-term outcomes beyond the first 12 to 18 months after discharge.

Physiologic Changes Related to Aging

Scientists are becoming aware that aging and disease are separate processes. What is diagnosed as disease is not "normal" aging. For example, it has been accepted for many years that aging inevitably results in coronary artery disease. Yet, data have shown that some populations, such as traditional Japanese and Eskimos, live to an extremely old age without evidence of this chronic disease.[73] Many diseases and disabilities are the result of years of exposure to injurious environmental and lifestyle factors.[74] Because of these factors, people age at different rates and in different ways, making it difficult to predict the occurrence of disease and individual responses to it. This variability accounts for the great heterogeneity seen in the elderly and the finding that chronologic age often does not correlate with biologic age in older adults.[74] For example, Mrs. S. is a 72-year-old woman with well-controlled hypertension and mild osteoporosis of the thoracic spine. She works in her garden, volunteers at a local nursing home 1 day a week, and walks 2 miles 2 or 3 days a week. In contrast, Mrs. W., a 67-year-old woman with a history of long-standing type 2 diabetes mellitus and two myocardial infarctions, is able to tolerate only light housework and cooking before her angina forces her to rest. She must rely on her neighbors to do her grocery shopping and yard work. The presence of a chronic disease and of its complications has resulted in a greater loss of function and physiologic reserve for Mrs. W. than for Mrs. S., although Mrs. S. is the elder by 5 years.

Despite the failure of research to differentiate the changes associated with "normal" aging from those of disease, a decrease in function of most organ systems begins in the early adult years.[74] This loss of function occurs at different degrees and rates in different organ systems. Humans are born with a tremendous built-in reserve, an organ system "redundancy," so that many of these losses do not become evident until late in life or when the limited reserve is stressed by disease or other conditions.[74] However, because of these age-related changes, the elderly are at high risk of disease, and their response to disease can be different from that in younger patients. For example, Mr. L. is a 74-year-old man in the ICU who has undergone bowel resection 2 days earlier. He has been progressively well in regard to hemodynamic values and activity. On the third day, as the nurse prepares to transfer him to an intermediate care unit, he appears lethargic and says, "I'm just so tired." Mr. L. also complains of shortness of breath. He has no history of heart disease or angina. When his fatigue and shortness of breath worsen during the day, an ECG is performed and reveals ST elevations of more than 1 mm in leads V_1, V_2, and V_3. Serum creatine phosphokinase and isoenzymes are elevated, diagnostic of an AMI. This patient's AMI presented atypically, with fatigue and shortness of breath. The diminished perception of painful stimuli (angina) may account for his failure to feel chest pain. In addition, with decreased physiologic reserves diminished further by recent surgery, even a relatively small impairment in myocardial function could result in fatigue and shortness of breath.

It is against the background of age-related changes that chronic disease is overlaid, serving to confound the responses to acute illness further. Table 4–5 presents a list of selected aging-related changes in each organ system and their functional consequences.[75] These changes have implications for the critically ill elderly patient and for appropriate nursing management. The following is a discussion of those changes as they relate to the stress response, the immune system, the neurologic system, nutritional status, and response to medications.

Stress Response

The major age-related changes in the stress response are an elevation of the pituitary and adrenal hormones at baseline and in response to a stressor and a decreased responsiveness of the target tissues to the stress hormones.[76] A study of otherwise healthy elderly patients undergoing intra-abdominal surgery found that they had higher serum levels of epinephrine, norepinephrine, cortisol, and antidiuretic

TABLE 4–5
Selected Age-Related Changes and Their Consequences

Organ or System	Age-Related Physiologic Change	Consequences of Age-Related Physiologic Change
General	↑ Body fat ↓ Total body water	↑ Volume of distribution for fat-soluble drugs ↓ Volume of distribution for water-soluble drugs
Eyes and ears	Presbyopia Lens opacification ↓ High-frequency acuity	↓ Accommodation ↑ Susceptibility to glare Difficulty in discriminating words if background noise is present
Endocrine	Impaired glucose tolerance ↓ Thyroxine clearance (and production) ↑ Antidiuretic hormone, ↓ renin, and ↓ aldosterone	↑ Glucose level in response to acute illness ↓ Thyroxine dose required in hypothyroidism
Respiratory	↓ Lung elasticity and ↑ chest wall stiffness	Ventilation–perfusion mismatch and ↓ PaO_2
Cardiovascular	↓ Arterial compliance and ↑ systolic blood pressure left ventricular hypertrophy ↓ Beta-adrenergic responsiveness ↓ Baroreceptor sensitivity and ↓ sinoatrial note automaticity	Hypotensive response to ↑ heart rate, volume depletion, or loss of atrial contraction ↓ Cardiac output and heart rate response to stress, standing, volume depletion Impaired blood pressure response to standing, volume depletion
Gastrointestinal	↓ Hepatic function ↓ Gastric acidity ↓ Colonic motility ↓ Anorectal function	Delayed metabolism of some drugs ↓ Calcium absorption on empty stomach Constipation
Hematologic and immune systems	↓ Bone marrow reserve (possible) ↓ T-cell function ↓ Autoantibodies	 False-negative purified protein derivative (PPD) response False-positive rheumatoid factor, antinuclear antibody
Renal	↓ Glomerular filtration rate ↓ Urine concentration-dilution (see also Endocrine, above)	Impaired excretion of some drugs Delayed response to salt or fluid restriction or overload; nocturia
Genitourinary	Vaginal or urethral mucosal atrophy Prostate enlargement	Dyspareunia, bacteriuria ↑ Residual urine volume
Musculoskeletal	↓ Lean body mass, muscle ↓ Bone density	 Osteopenia
Nervous system	Brain atrophy ↓ Brain catechol synthesis ↓ Brain dopaminergic synthesis ↓ Righting reflexes ↓ Stage 4 sleep	Benign senescent forgetfulness Stiffer gait ↑ Body sway Early awakening, insomnia

↑, increase; ↓, decrease; →, leading to.
From Resnick NM: Geriatric medicine. In: Fauci AS, Braunwald E, Isselbacher KJ, et al (eds): Harrison's Principles of Internal Medicine, 14th ed. New York, McGraw-Hill, 1998, p. 38.

hormone at baseline and in response to the stress of the surgery when compared with the findings of other studies of patients less than 65 years of age. Nevertheless, despite these elevations, blood pressure and heart rate did not increase in the older patients. Because of these diminished responses to circulating catecholamines, hemodynamic changes cannot be used reliably to evaluate the response of an elderly patient to a stressor such as pain or dehydration. In addition, because of the decreased physiologic reserve of elderly patients, they may not be able to sustain a prolonged response to a major stressor, such as sepsis or trauma.

Immune System

An overall decrease of immune function occurs as a person grows older. This change is probably the single most important functional loss in the elderly because it puts them at risk of many diseases.[77] Major sequelae of this loss are decreased helper and killer T-cell function, decreased migration of leukocytes and phagocytosis, decreased inflammatory response, reduced hypersensitivity reaction to antigens, and decreased production of autoantibodies. The elderly are susceptible to infections, sepsis, cancer, delayed wound healing, and autoimmune disorders.[77, 78] Because of the impaired immune responses in these patients, signs of infection, such as fever or purulent drainage, are often muted or absent.[78] Frequently, an acute change in mental status or incontinence is the only sign of infection.

Infections carry a high mortality rate because of the severe strain they place on the elderly patient's physiologic reserve. Infections also carry a high mortality rate because of the aggressive antibiotic and fluid management the patient receives.[74, 78] Prevention of infection must be directed at frequent hand washing of all health care workers in contact with the patient and meticulous care of the skin, invasive lines, and urinary catheters. The skin is the largest organ of the immune system and is the primary barrier to invasive organisms, but it becomes colonized by many pathogenic organisms soon after admission to an ICU.[78] Decubitus ulcers, urine, feces, and wet dressings all interrupt the integrity of the skin and allow access of this abnormal skin flora to the blood, thereby increasing the risk of sepsis. Sepsis is known to be a poor prognostic sign in critically ill elderly patients.

Most bladder infections in critically ill patients are due to *Escherichia coli*. The nurse should recommend routine urine cultures every 72 hours in elderly patients. This approach provides earlier detection in the elderly who do not manifest fever, leukocytosis, or cloudy urine.[78] Chart 4–21 summarizes the management of a patient at risk of infection.

CHART 4–21

Nursing Diagnosis: Risk of Infection

Etiologic Factors: Age-related changes that depress immune function; chronic illness, invasive lines and procedures, colonization with ambient organisms, skin breakdown, immobility, medications.

Manifestations: +/− altered mental status, +/− fever, +/− cough, +/− leukocytosis, +/− urinary incontinence, +/− purulent drainage, +/− heat or redness.

Expected Patient Outcomes:
1. The patient will achieve or maintain baseline mentation.
2. The patient will achieve or maintain normalization of temperature, white blood cell count, and urinary patterns.
3. The patient will achieve or maintain skin integrity.

Interventions:
1. Use meticulous hand washing and aseptic technique with all lines and all procedures.
2. Assess the patient for silent urinary tract infection with a urine culture every 72 hours.
3. Assess the lungs for retained secretions and diminished breath sounds.
4. Minimize the patient's exposure to other patients or visitors with active infections.
5. Provide adequate caloric and nitrogen nutrition to meet metabolic needs.
6. Keep the skin clean and dry; apply lotion as needed.
7. Consult with the physician or pharmacist to assess for the effectiveness of antibiotics.
8. Consult with the enterostomal therapist or wound care team as needed for additional recommendations.
9. Perform skin assessment at least once a week and document findings.
10. Evaluate and document the effectiveness of interventions.

Neurologic System

Changes in sensory input may occur in the elderly. When these changes are accompanied by critical illness and a strange environment, anxiety and altered mental status may result. The nursing history should determine the use of eyeglasses and hearing aids, and these aids should be made available to the patient when possible. Changes in vision result in a decreased ability to distinguish objects, to differentiate colors (except for bright colors), and to see in the dark.[77] There also is an increased susceptibility to glare, which, when considering that much of the equipment in an ICU is shiny or glossy, can cause significant eye discomfort and decreased visual acuity.[79] Changes in hearing make it difficult for the elderly person to filter background noise from meaningful sounds, such as the nurse's voice. Additionally, the elderly patient is less perceptive to pitches in the higher range, which is the range of many women's voices.[79] The nurse must be aware of the interference of background noise and must gauge the pitch of his or her own voice when speaking to the patient.

With aging, brain size is reduced by loss of the number and size of neurons. This change results in a decreased capacity of the brain to adapt to acute and sudden changes in its chemical environment, often resulting in changes of mental status known as delirium. St. Pierre[80] defines delirium as "an acute confusional state characterized by an abrupt onset that can develop over hours, a fluctuating mental status, and an inability to maintain attention." Delirium may be the first and only sign of an acute problem. For example, Mrs. C. is 85 years old and presents to the emergency department with her daughter. Her daughter reports that her mother has experienced fluctuating confusion and occasional urinary incontinence for the last 2 days. The daughter is concerned because her mother has had no history of these behaviors. On questioning, Mrs. C. can describe no additional symptoms. Her vital signs are normal, her temperature is 97.7°F, few bibasilar crackles are heard, but otherwise her physical examination is unremarkable. A pulse oximeter reading of 85% prompts a chest radiograph to be taken, which reveals a right middle lobe consolidation. She is diagnosed with pneumonia, and deteriorating blood gases over the next few hours necessitate intubation and mechanical ventilation. This presentation of pneumonia is atypical because the patient has no history of cough, fever, or shortness of breath. The acute hypoxemia was sufficient to cause delirium, and the incontinence was probably secondarily related to the patient's altered mental status.

Delirium can be subtle, characterized by lethargy, and can go undetected, or it can be a severe agitation with attempts by the patient to remove noxious stimuli such as intravenous lines, catheters, or endotracheal tubes. Because this change often indicates an acute physiologic problem, it occurs frequently, in approximately half the elderly admissions to critical care units. Failure to recognize this condition and to treat its cause can result in serious morbidity or death. Therefore, delirium should be considered a medical emergency that needs rapid detection and treatment.[80]

Detection and diagnosis of delirium can be difficult when it is superimposed on preexisting dementia. Table 4–6 lists the major differences between delirium and dementia. The main characteristic of delirium is an impaired awareness and change in the level of alertness that is usually reversible if treated quickly (see Chart 4–9). Delirious persons have fluctuating periods of agitation or lethargy, disturbed sleep patterns, occasional visual hallucinations, and bizarre thought patterns. Dementia, on the other hand, is gradual in onset, occurring over months or years, and is not reversible. It is usually stable, without frequent fluctuations in behavior patterns. Attention and ability to focus on a task or a simple command are usually intact until the advanced stage. Thought processes are simple and usually impoverished, and perceptual disturbances and hallucinations are unusual.[80]

The nurse must thoroughly assess the elderly patient to determine the presence of delirium or dementia. Assessment of mental status is done at admission and should be repeated once or twice a day or with any change in the patient's status. Knowledge of the patient's usual cognitive status and behavior is important and should be obtained from family or friends when possible. Systematic assessments of mental status can be done using the Folstein mini-mental state examination (MMSE) (Figure 4–7),[81] which tests the patient's orientation, registration (naming objects), attention and calculation, recall, and language. This test is frequently used in acutely ill adults. The disadvantages to its use in the critical care area are that the patient must be able to speak and to write, requirements that preclude its use in intubated patients or in those who cannot hold a pencil or write.

An alternative tool for assessment of mental status is the Clinical Assessment of Confusion-A (CAC-A).[82] This instrument is currently being tested and may have wider application in the critical care setting than the MMSE (Figure 4–8). The CAC-A is a list of 25 behaviors denoting confusion. The dimensions of the behaviors are cognition, general behavior, motor activity, orientation, and psychotic/neurotic behaviors.[82] The nurse completes the assessment by observing the patient and circling the behaviors exhibited by the patient. Each behavior is assigned a weighted score, and the scores are summed. A score higher than 0 indicates confusion. The severity of the confusion is associated with the magnitude of the score. The CAC-A was tested in a group of critically ill patients and was compared with the MMSE.[83] A high degree of agreement was seen

TABLE 4–6

Comparison of Delirium and Dementia

	Delirium	Dementia
Onset	Abrupt: hours to days	Gradual: months to years
Duration	Hours to days; usually less than 1 week	Ongoing, irreversible
Course	Fluctuates	Essentially stable; may be progressive over time
Attention	Attention deficit; unable to focus or shift attention, easily distracted	Normal, except in advanced dementia; may fixate on one thing for long periods
Consciousness	Fluctuates; may be hyperalert or difficult to arouse	Normal
Orientation	Usually disoriented, but fluctuates	Often disoriented, especially in unfamiliar surroundings
Thought	Disordered, fragmented; may be delusional or bizarre, slowed or accelerated; lucid intervals; fund of knowledge intact	Usually ordered; content impoverished; abstraction poor; may confabulate; loss of common knowledge; attempts to conceal
Perception	Illusions, hallucinations (usually visual), or delusions common	Perception usually normal; occasionally paranoid
Insight	May be present in lucid intervals	Absent
Behavior	Hyperactivity or hypoactivity, may be mixed	May be agitated or apathetic; may pace or have other ritualistic behaviors
Sleep–wake cycle	Always disturbed, often reversed	Fragmented, "sundowning" common
Speech	Disorganized, often incoherent; slow or rapid	Ordered, except in advanced dementia; may have word-finding difficulty, may perseverate

From St. Pierre J: Delirium in hospitalized elderly patients: off-track. Crit Care Nurs Clin North Am 8:53–60, 1996.

between the two instruments, with the CAC-A having the advantage of not requiring the patient to be able to speak or write.

The nurse must examine many factors that can cause acute changes in mental status of the critically ill patient because some causes may require immediate rapid treatment or drug reversal. For example, some medications that can cause confusion include sedatives, narcotics, and drugs with anticholinergic activity, such as diphenhydramine (Benadryl), haloperidol (Haldol), amitriptyline (Elavil), promethazine (Phenergan), metoclopramide (Reglan), diphenoxylate (Lomotil), and disopyramide (Norpace). Other treatable causes include infection, hypoxemia, hypoglycemia or hyperglycemia, acid–base or electrolyte imbalances, volume depletion, or other causes of decreased cerebral perfusion.[80]

Once the cause of the delirium is found, appropriate treatment must be instituted immediately, and supportive measures must be implemented to prevent complications. Complications, such as falls, self-injury, or removing endotracheal tubes or arterial catheters, can cause serious problems. The use of chemical and physical restraints may increase the agitation, may precipitate further mental status changes, or may cause injury. Therefore, these measures should be used only when the risk of self-injury is high and when all other attempts to reduce environmental stimulants (e.g., noise, large number of contacts with the patient) have been determined to be ineffective. When the use of restraints is deemed necessary, the least restrictive restraint should be used for the shortest time possi-

ble.[84] This approach requires frequent assessment of mental status.

Sometimes, asking a close family member or friend to remain at the patient's bedside during delirious periods can be effective. An example is Mr. R., a 77-year-old man, who was admitted to the ICU with severe hypoxemia secondary to pneumonia. In his agitation, he repeatedly removed his pulse oximeter and was restrained with a Posey belt when he attempted to climb out of bed. His agitation increased, resulting in serious oxygen desaturation and the need for higher inspired oxygen concentration. The nurse realized that sedating Mr. R. could depress his respirations and lead to intubation. Thinking that having his wife beside him might calm him, the nurse asked Mrs. R. to remain at the patient's bedside and to talk to him. When his agitation quieted, the nurse moved a bed into the room for her to spend the night. The patient successfully avoided chemical and physical restraint, and with a good response to antibiotics, he did not have to be intubated.

Nutritional Status

The elderly are at risk of malnutrition because of many psychosocial and physical problems common to the aged. The many losses sustained by the elderly (see the section later on psychosocial issues) may lead to depression and social isolation, which can cause anorexia and poor food intake. Diminished taste perception, which often accompanies aging, chronic illness, polypharmacy, and unpalatable special diets,

Maximum Score	Score	
		Patient _____ Examiner _____ Date _____
		Orientation
5	( )	What is the (year) (season) (date) (day) (month)?
5	( )	Where are we: (state) (county) (town) (hospital) (floor)
		Registration
3	( )	Name three objects: 1 second to say each. Then ask the patient all three after you have said them. Give 1 point for each correct answer. Then repeat them until he or she learns all three. Count trials and record. Trials _____
		Attention and Calculation
5	( )	Serial 7's. 1 point for each correct. Stop after five answers. Alternatively spell "world" backwards.
		Recall
3	( )	Ask for the three objects repeated above. Give 1 point for each correct.
		Language
9	( )	Name a pencil, and watch (2 points)
		Repeat the following "No ifs, ands, or buts." (1 point)
		Follow a three-stage command:
		"Take a paper in your right hand, fold it in half, and put it on the floor." (3 points)
		Read and obey the following:
		Close Your Eyes (1 point)
		Write a sentence (1 point)
		Copy design (1 point)
_____		*Total Score*
		ASSESS level of consciousness along a continuum _____
		Alert Drowsy Stupor Coma

Instructions for Administration of Mini-Mental State Examination

Orientation

(1) Ask for the date. Then ask specifically for parts omitted, e.g., "Can you also tell me what season it is?" One point for each correct.
(2) Ask in turn "Can you tell me the name of this hospital?" (town, country, etc.). One point for each correct.

Registration

Ask the patient if you may test his or her memory. Then say the names of three unrelated objects, clearly and slowly, about 1 second for each. After you have said all three, ask him or her to repeat them. This first repetition determines his or her score (0–3), but keep saying them until he or she can repeat all three, up to six trials. If he or she does not eventually learn all three, recall cannot be meaningfully tested.

Attention and Calculation

Ask the patient to begin with 100 and count backwards by 7. Stop after five subtractions (93, 86, 79, 72, 65). Score the total number of correct answers.
If the patient cannot or will not perform this task, ask him or her to spell the word "world" backwards. The score is the number of letters in correct order, e.g., dlrow = 5, dlorw = 3.

Recall

Ask the patient if he or she can recall the three words you previously asked him or her to remember. Score 0–3.

Language

Naming: Show the patient a wrist watch and ask him or her what it is. Repeat for pencil. Score 0–2.
Repetition: Ask the patient to repeat the sentence after you. Allow only one trial. Score 0 or 1.
Three-stage command: Give the patient a piece of plain blank paper and repeat the command. Score 1 point for each part correctly executed.
Reading: On a blank piece of paper print the sentence "Close your eyes," in letters large enough for the patient to see clearly. Ask him or her to read it and do what it says. Score 1 point only if he or she actually closes his eyes.
Writing: Give the patient a blank piece of paper and ask him or her to write a sentence for you. Do not dictate a sentence, it is to be written spontaneously. It must contain a subject and verb and be sensible. Correct grammar and punctuation are not necessary.
Copying: On a clean piece of paper, draw intersecting pentagons, each side about 1 inch, and ask him or her to copy it exactly as it is. All 10 angles must be present, and 2 must intersect to score 1 point. Tremor and rotation are ignored.
Estimate the patient's level of sensorium along a continuum, from alert on the left to coma on the right.

Figure 4–7

Mini-mental state examination. (From Folstein MD, Folstein SE, McHugh PR: Mini-mental state: a practical method for grading the cognitive state of patients for the clinician. J Psychiatr Res 12:189–198, 1975.)

Patient _____

Nurse _____

Date _____ Time _____

Directions: Under each category circle the number for each behavior the patient has exhibited. Next, sum the numbers for each category and for the total scale.

Cognition
  1. Extreme forgetfulness 4
  2. Forgetful 3
  3. Decreased ability to concentrate 3
  4. Altered conceptualization 3

  (Maximum = 13) Sum _____

General behavior
  5. Noisy 3
  6. Not recognizing limitations of illness 3
  7. Restlessness 3
  8. Difficulty relating to others 3
  9. Antagonistic 3
  10. Withdrawn 2
  11. Irritability 2
  12. Demanding 2
  13. Apathy 2

  (Maximum = 23) Sum _____

Motor activity
  14. Speech slurred 3
  15. Altered voluntary motor response 3
  16. Absence of any meaningful response 3
  17. Altered involuntary motor response 2
  18. Little body movement 2

  (Maximum = 13) Sum _____

Orientation
  19. No idea of place 4
  20. Calling people from past 4
  21. Calls someone known to him/her by another name 4

  (Maximum = 12) Sum _____

Psychotic/neurotic behaviors
  22. Delusional 4
  23. Paranoid ideation 4
  24. Talking to people not actually present 4
  25. Behavior regressed, repulsive, and/or repetitive 4

  (Maximum = 16) Sum _____
  (Maximum = 77) Total score _____

Additional behaviors:

Directions: On the line place a "/" indicating your overall assessment of the patient's level of confusion.

_____
         No confusion   Severe confusion

Figure 4–8

Clinical assessment of confusion. (From Vermeersch PEH: The clinical assessment of confusion-A. Appl Nurs Res 3:128–133, 1990. Originally adapted from Nagley SS: Prevention of confusion in hospitalized elderly persons. University Microfilms No. 8420848. Dissertation Abstracts Int 45:1732, 1990.)

adds to disinterest in food. Compounding the problem may be difficulties related to ill-fitting dentures, poor oral health, and impaired swallowing.

For these reasons, the elderly patient may be undernourished on admission to the ICU. All too often, because of the immediate need to treat life-threatening problems, nutrition may be ignored for several days. Research has shown that malnutrition results in increased infections, delayed wound healing, prolonged weaning from mechanical ventilation, longer hospital stays, and increased mortality. The nurse must assess nutritional status and must advocate for early nutritional support. A simple assessment can identify a recent history of weight loss and poor dietary intake and evidence on physical examination of muscular wasting and loss of subcutaneous tissue. The presence of these indicators reliably points to malnutrition. If, in addition, the serum albumin level is below normal, the nurse has strong evidence that a more thorough nutritional assessment and prompt institution of nutritional support are needed.[85]

The maxim of nutritional support is "If the gut works, use it!" Studies have shown that the direct supply of nutrients to the gastrointestinal tract, which is provided by oral intake and enteral tube feedings, maintains the health and integrity of the intestinal mucosa. A healthy mucosa is a barrier between the intestinal flora and the blood. Breakdown of this barrier during periods without enteral nutrition (as with total parenteral nutrition) has been implicated in the migration of enteric bacteria into the blood, sepsis, and multiorgan system failure.[86]

An adequate oral diet is frequently not feasible in the critically ill elderly patient, and such attempts may result in inadequate caloric and nitrogen intake. Use of nasoenteric tube feedings is economical, convenient, and usually capable of delivering sufficient nutrients, but diarrhea can be a major complication with this mode of nutritional support. Diarrhea can be due to too rapid administration or use of a hypertonic formula, but it can also be due to many medications (e.g., antibiotics) or bacterial contamination of the feeding. Sometimes, changing medications may be all that is needed to eliminate the diarrhea. The other alternative is to provide total parenteral nutrition through a central intravenous line. This method can provide complete nutritional support when the gastrointestinal tract cannot be used (e.g., short-bowel syndrome) or when the patient's nutrient requirements are too great to be provided by the other routes. However, the risks of infection and hyperosmolar hyperglycemic nonketotic coma are serious complications of total parenteral nutrition, and require meticulous attention to site care and blood glucose monitoring.[86]

Pharmacology

Polypharmacy is a common situation in elderly persons because they are frequently treated for several medical problems simultaneously. Age-related changes can compound the problems of side effects and toxicity. Body fat increases and thus allows for greater distribution of fat-soluble drugs, with a resulting longer drug half-life and a greater risk of drug toxicity. When this change is considered in addition to the decreased renal or hepatic clearance of drugs that occurs in many elderly patients, the chance of serious toxicities can be great. In addition, these patients have decreased hepatic synthesis of protein and a resultant lowering of serum albumin levels. Malnutrition and fluid volume excess also may lower albumin levels. Albumin binds with many drugs to transport them through the blood. A lowered serum albumin decreases drug binding capacity and allows elevated plasma levels of free drug to circulate. Thus, drug side effects and the risk of toxicity increase, even at usually safe doses. Examples of drugs that are highly protein bound include antipsychotics, benzodiazepines, hydralazine (Apresoline), propranolol (Inderal), furosemide (Lasix), phenytoin (Dilantin), quinidine (Duraquin), and warfarin (Coumadin).[87]

Table 4–7 provides a list of commonly administered drugs in the critically ill, their routes of elimination, and implications for care of the elderly.[77] The nurse must titrate medications and must evaluate the patient's response to them carefully. One or more medications may require less frequent dosing or a lower dose to achieve the therapeutic effects.[87]

Psychosocial Issues Related to the Elderly

Many psychosocial risk factors in elderly patients have implications for their recovery and rehabilitation from a critical illness. The elderly often experience multiple losses: loss of independence, retirement and loss of a social role, lowered income level, lowered health status, decreased functional ability, loss of a home, and loss of loved ones. The individual's response to these stressors depends on the meaning of these losses, the ability to find meaningful substitutes for them, and the presence of an effective support system. For example, many elderly persons acquire new hobbies or volunteer their time to help others, thus developing new skills and social roles. Some elderly persons are not able to cope effectively with these losses and become depressed, socially isolated, and at risk of further illness.

Elder Abuse

Elder abuse has become an increasing problem as many more elderly patients, often with severe behavioral problems and multiple physical care needs, are cared for at home. Abuse can result from physical violence against the elder, from neglect, and from financial exploitation.[88] Investigators estimate that 2.5 million elderly persons are abused and neglected in the United States.[79] The profile of the typical, abused elder is that of a woman, more than 70 years old, with physical and mental problems, who depends on a family member for care, usually an adult child or spouse, and who is socially isolated. Often, the abused elder has limited financial resources, no options for alternate living arrangements, and is frail and smaller than the abuser.[79, 88] The abuser most often is an adult child who is the primary care giver. This care giver may be responding to years of stress caused by caring for the elder without respite, perhaps unable to cope with the reversal in roles (e.g., from being the child of the parent to being the "parent" of the parent), or the care giver may have been abused at one time. Alcohol or drug abuse may also be a factor.[88]

The nurse must be aware of signs of possible abuse. These signs include a history of repeated emergency room visits for injuries, malnutrition, dehydration,

TABLE 4–7
Pharmacologic Considerations in the Elderly

Drug	Route of Elimination	Clinical Implications
Analgesics		
Acetaminophen	Hepatic	No substantial age-related change in kinetics
Aspirin	Renal	Highly protein bound; half-life may be prolonged
Narcotics	Hepatic	Blood levels higher; pain relief longer
		Lower doses are usually effective
		Constipation is major side effect in elderly patients
Antimicrobials		
Aminoglycosides	Renal	Prolonged half-life may require increased dosage intervals (e.g., q12h, q24h)
		Nephrotoxicity and ototoxicity are major problems; monitor blood levels, serum creatinine, creatinine clearance
		Formula for calculating age-referenced, creatinine clearance interval in men: [140 − age × kg body wt/72 × serum creatinine] woman: 85% of this calculated value
Cephalosporins	Renal	Half-life prolonged
Penicillins	Renal	Half-life prolonged
	Hepatic	Some highly protein bound
Tetracycline	Renal	Half-life prolonged
Amphotericin	Renal	Nephrotoxicity a major problem in elderly patients with underlying renal dysfunction
Cardiovascular Drugs		
Beta-adrenergic agents	Renal	Elderly patients may require increased dosage to achieve therapeutic effect
Digoxin	Renal (15–40% nonrenal)	Decreased clearance; half-life prolonged
Lidocaine	Hepatic	Volume of distribution increased; half-life prolonged; clearance unchanged
Procainamide	Renal	Clearance decreased; highly protein bound
		Half-life prolonged; steady-state levels higher
Quinidine	Hepatic	Highly protein bound; clearance decreased
		Half-life prolonged
Verapamil	Hepatic	Clearance decreased
		Effects more pronounced and prolonged
Antihypertensives		
Diltiazem	Hepatic	Clearance decreased; use cautiously in sinus node dysfunction
Hydralazine	Hepatic	Highly protein bound
Propranolol	Hepatic	Highly protein bound
		Half-life prolonged; clearance decreased; blood levels higher
		Sensitivity to effects decreased
Diuretics		
Furosemide	Renal	Highly protein bound
		Elderly patients at high risk of dehydration and electrolyte imbalance

From Rauen CA, Britt TL: Elderly patients. In: Clochesy JM, Bren C, Carding S, et al (eds): Critical Care Nursing, 2nd ed. Philadelphia, W.B: Saunders, 1996, p 1507. Adapted from Kane R, Ouslander J, Abrass I: Essentials of Geriatrics, 3rd ed. New York, McGraw-Hill, 1994, pp 356–357.

overmedication or undermedication, poor hygiene, excessive drowsiness, ecchymosis of the wrists and ankles where the elder may have been restrained, old scars, old and new contusions especially on the upper arms where these patients may have been held and shaken, and cigarette burns in unusual locations. The presence of such signs warrants questioning of the care giver and being alert to inconsistencies in the explanations.[79, 88] The United States government has mandated that all suspected cases of neglect or abuse be reported to appropriate state agencies, and persons who report such cases are protected from liability. Placement in protective services, reassignment of legal guardianship to someone other than the primary care giver, and family counseling are the types of interventions implemented.[79, 88] The nurse plays an important role in the early identification of those at risk of abusing or of being abused, so that interventions can be initiated before abuse occurs.

Collaborative Management

In this era of managed care and shorter hospital stays, patients are being discharged to the community with greater health care needs. In the case of the elderly, many have fewer resources to assist them, such as family to care for them at home. ICU length of stay is also becoming shorter as health insurers put stringent limits on what types of care will be reimbursed, and the nurse no longer has the luxury of waiting until transfer to the general nursing unit to begin discharge planning. Additionally, direct discharge to the community is becoming more frequent.[89]

With these constraints superimposed on the complex health care requirements of the elderly, discharge planning must occur on admission to the critical care unit and must incorporate the expertise of a multi-disciplinary team including the nurse, physician, social worker, and others as appropriate. In fact, the Health Care Financing Administration (HCFA) mandates a multidisciplinary approach to discharge planning that is clearly documented in the medical record.[89] For complex patients, such as the critically ill elderly, a case management model is strongly recommended to coordinate the many services and levels of care that will be required and to facilitate a smooth transfer from the ICU, to a general unit, to the community.

Discharge planning should consist of assessment of the patient's functional, cognitive, and emotional status and limitations, social support system, living situation, level of nursing care required, and medications and treatments.[89] Options to consider, if further care is needed, include the patient's home, a transitional care facility, or other living arrangements. Before a patient can be discharged to the home, an assessment must be made of the living situation, that is, the presence of someone who can assume the patient's care such as a spouse, the ability of that individual to adopt this role in terms of her or his own health and willingness to provide the care, the potential of the home to accommodate special aids and medical equipment, and safety hazards.

Discharge to a transitional care facility may be short or long term, depending on the potential for rehabilitation and return to functional independence. The inability to return to their own home is a difficult situation for most elderly people to accept. They may feel abandoned and as if their lives are over. The nurse is challenged to assist in this transition and can help patients to find out more about the facility to which they are being transferred, such as whether they can have some of their personal belongings with them. The nurse can encourage family and friends to visit as much as possible and to bring favorite foods if these are not contraindicated. Sometimes, all the nurse is able to do is to listen to the elderly patient, to correct misinformation, and help her or him to achieve a realistic and optimistic view of the future.

Other members of the health care team can facilitate recovery of the elderly critically ill patient. Clergy may provide spiritual support to the patient and family. Pharmacists are closely involved in the assessment of medications and their effectiveness. Social services and discharge planning can facilitate appropriate discharge when the patient is able to leave the hospital.

Outcomes

The elderly patient in the critical care setting has specific needs that must be addressed. Physiologic changes must be supported to encourage recovery. Alterations in consciousness can be minimized if the patient is assessed frequently and accurately. Competent and safe nursing care of the elderly must include the following: awareness that elderly patients comprise a heterogeneous group that demonstrates varying degrees of health and illness; knowledge of the normal changes associated with aging, which can result in the atypical presentation of acute illness and response to therapies; and knowledge of the psychosocial risk factors that can limit their recovery from critical illness. With this awareness, the chance for optimal recovery is enhanced.

Critical Thinking Exercise

Mr. L. is a 74-year-old man admitted to the ICU in acute respiratory failure. He had been experiencing flulike symptoms for several days before this admission.

Past Medical History: Emphysema, coronary artery disease with four bypass grafts, atrial fibrillation, and benign prostatic hypertrophy.

Current Medications: Digoxin, warfarin (Coumadin), theophylline (Theo-dur), furosemide (Lasix), and potassium supplement (Slow-K).

Allergies: Penicillin.

Social History: Cigarettes (1–2 packs per day for 40 years), stopped 20 years ago; three to four glasses of wine per week; no recent travel outside of the United States.

Family History: Father died of lung cancer at age 66 years; mother is alive, severely debilitated from a stroke, and lives with the patient; two grown children, ages 44 and 46 years; wife cares for patient's mother.

Physical Examination:

Respiratory: Coarse breath sounds with expiratory wheezes throughout lung fields, respirations at 8 per minute with peripheral cyanosis. Initial arterial blood gases (ABGs) on 100% nonrebreather mask: pH, 7.24; $PaCO_2$, 76 mm Hg;

Pa_{O_2}, 48 mm Hg; HCO_3, 32 mEq/L; Sa_{O_2}, 84%. *The patient underwent emergency intubation and mechanical ventilation. Initial ventilator settings:* Fi_{O_2}, 100%; V_T, 1000 mL; *intermittent mandatory ventilation (IMV), 12 breaths per minute; pressure support, 10 cm; positive end-expiratory pressure, 10 (patient's admission weight, 92.4 kg).*

Cardiovascular: *Atrial fibrillation with a rapid ventricular response; heart rate, 135 beats per minute and irregular; blood pressure, 182/100 mm Hg, temperature, 100.9°F. Skin is clammy with poor capillary refill; no peripheral edema noted; pedal pulses by Doppler.*

Neurologic: *Patient has decreased level of consciousness and responds to tactile and painful stimuli only.*

Gastrointestinal: *Hypoactive bowel sounds in all quadrants.*

Genitourinary: *Patient was incontinent of urine on admission. Foley catheter inserted; urine output, 50 mL over past hour, dark amber in color.*

Additional Laboratory Values: *Complete blood count: white blood cells, 13.5 (normal, 5–10); hemoglobin/hematocrit 13.1/40.8 (normal, 11–16/36–47); neutrophils, 8.4 (normal, 2–6.9); glucose, 412 mg/dL (normal 65–105); sodium, 138 mEq/L (normal, 135–145); potassium, 4.2 mEq/L (normal, 3.6–5.0); chloride, 106 mEq/L (normal, 98–107); digoxin level, 0.3 ng/mL (normal, 0.5–2.0); theophylline level, 8 μg/mL (normal, 10–20).*

After 2 hours, the patient's vital signs are as follows: blood pressure, 146/84 mm Hg; heart rate, 108 beats per minute (atrial fibrillation); respirations, 14 (IMV, 12; spontaneous respirations, 2). The patient is responsive to verbal stimuli but somnolent; color is improved. ABGs: pH, 7.34; Pa_{CO_2}, 54 mm Hg; Pa_{O_2}, 88 mm Hg; HCO_3, 31 mEq/L; Sa_{O_2}, 94%.

Psychosocial Status: *Mr. L.'s wife is at the bedside, holding his hand. His other hand is loosely restrained to prevent accidental extubation. Mrs. L. has many questions about what happened to her husband and why. She also asks when he will be able to breathe on his own. The patient's children arrive shortly and provide emotional support to their mother. Mrs. L. is concerned not only with her husband but also with her mother-in-law. Mrs. L. has had to ask a neighbor to watch her.*

Management: *Mr. L. remains on the ventilator for 3 more days, and his respiratory status gradually improves. As he becomes more alert, he is visibly anxious and frustrated with the breathing tube and the suctioning procedures. He has difficulty using paper and pen to communicate his needs, although his wife is able to read his lips well. His respiratory infection is treated with intravenous antibiotics, his heart rate decreases with intravenous doses of digoxin, and he is receiving intravenous aminophylline. Mr. L.'s family is permitted to stay at his bedside, except during change of shift. The family members are encouraged to return home at night to sleep.*

1. What psychosocial needs do the patient and family have that can be met during this crisis?

2. What multidisciplinary resources should be used to assist the patient and family to meet these needs?

3. What interventions can be used to decrease Mr. L.'s anxiety and sense of powerlessness while he is intubated and physically restrained? Provide rationales for your suggestions.

4. How would you assess Mr. L.'s level of pain? If he were experiencing pain, what interventions would be appropriate to consider and why?

5. What education does the patient and family need at this time? After extubation? At discharge? Provide rationales.

6. What community resources would you suggest to meet this family's needs after discharge?

7. What specific considerations are indicated for Mr. L. and his wife related to their ages?

8. What age-related complications is Mr. L. at risk of developing during this hospitalization and why?

Key Concepts

➡ A critical illness activates the body's stress response.

➡ Patients live within the context of a family, and because it is within this context that they will return, nurses must look beyond the patient to the family members.

➡ Families of critically ill patients are in crisis. This crisis occurs when the family's resources are unable to meet the demands of the crisis-provoking event.

➡ A crisis can be perceived as either a challenge or a threat.

➡ Ongoing assessment of the patient's physiologic and psychological status is necessary to provide comprehensive care.

➡ Nurses need to collect a complete psychosocial history to identify the patient's and family's normal coping strategies and to recognize when these strategies are ineffective.

➡ Family involvement in the patient's care is critical to the patient's recovery.

➡ Effective pain management is necessary for optimal recovery and includes both pharmacologic and nonpharmacologic interventions.

➡ Pain assessment should be made by the patient's self-report as well as nurses' observations of physiologic and behavioral indicators. In addition, nurses must be aware of pain that accompanies treatments and procedures and must premedicate the patient appropriately.

➡ Anxiety and powerlessness are present to some degree in all critically ill patients.

➡ Delirium is a potential development in critically ill patients. When present, the physiologic or environmental causes should be identified and corrected as quickly as possible.

➠ Nurses can enhance coping with active listening, effective communication, appropriate patient and family education, and creative problem solving.

➠ The number of elderly persons is growing rapidly, with the group over 85 years the fastest growing segment of the population.

➠ The cost of health care and the scarcity of resources raise the question of rationing critical care to the elderly.

➠ Age should not be used as a predictor of the outcomes of critical illness and injury. Other factors such as severity of illness, functional status at baseline, and preexisting chronic health conditions are better predictors of poor outcomes than is age.

➠ The elderly are a heterogeneous population group. Chronologic age and biologic age may be different in some people, and this difference makes it difficult to predict disease or response to treatment.

➠ Distinguishing the effects of aging from those of disease is difficult, but several things once thought inevitable with aging can be prevented with diet and lifestyle modification.

➠ Many age-related physiologic changes that occur in every organ system lower physiologic reserve, but they do not pose a problem unless an acute stressor or chronic condition is superimposed on them.

➠ Age-related changes alter the presentation of disease from that seen in younger patients, so nurses require a high index of suspicion and careful assessment. Often, the first clue to an acute problem is an alteration in the patient's mental status because of the brain's limited capacity to adjust to a sudden change in its chemical environment.

➠ Changes in immune function are the most functionally important changes in the elderly and put them at high risk of infection, cancer, and autoimmune disorders.

➠ Delirium should be considered a medical emergency because of its high mortality rate. Every effort to diagnose and treat it should be made.

➠ Many functional and psychosocial risk factors that are prevalent in the elderly can lead to malnutrition.

➠ The elderly sustain many losses, which can impede their recovery from critical illness.

➠ Elder abuse is a rising problem, and the nurse can play a key role in identifying the abused and abusing individuals and those at risk of either role.

➠ Discharge planning requires a multidisciplinary approach, which should begin at the point of admission.

References

1. Selye H: The Stress of Life. New York, McGraw-Hill, 1956.
2. Lindsey AM, Carrieri-Kohlman V, Page GG: Stress response. In: Carreri-Kohlman V, Lindsey AM, West CM (eds): Pathophysiological Phenomena in Nursing, 2nd ed. Philadelphia, W.B. Saunders, 1993, pp 397–419.
3. Ignatavicius DD, Workman ML, Mishler MA: Medical-Surgical Nursing: A Nursing Process Approach, 2nd ed. Philadelphia, W.B. Saunders, 1995.
4. Moser DK, Dracup K: Psychosocial recovery from a cardiac event: the influence of perceived control. Heart Lung 24:273–280, 1995.
5. Pennock BE, Crawshaw L, Maher T, et al: Distressful events in the ICU as perceived by patients recovering from coronary artery bypass surgery. Heart Lung 23:323–327, 1994.
6. Soehren P: Stressors perceived by cardiac surgical patients in the intensive care unit. Am J Crit Care 4:71–76, 1995.
7. Holland C, Cason CL, Prater LR: Patients' recollections of critical care. Dimensions Crit Care Nurs 16:132–140, 1997.
8. Dunbar S, McLain RM: Family care. In: Kinney MR, Packa DL, Dunbar SR (eds): AACN's Clinical Reference for Critical Care Nursing. Philadelphia, C.V. Mosby, 1993, pp 411–425.
9. Hanson SMH, Boyd ST: Family Health Care Nursing: Theory, Practice, and Research. Philadelphia, F.A. Davis, 1996.
10. Broderick CB: Understanding Family Process: Basics of Family Systems Theory. Newbury Park, CA, Sage, 1993.
11. Wright L, Leahey M: Nurses and Families: A Guide to Family Assessment and Intervention, 2nd ed. Philadelphia, F.A. Davis, 1994.
12. Hill R: Generic features of families under stress. In: Parad HJ (ed): Crisis Intervention: Selected Readings. New York, Family Service Association of America, 1965, pp 32–52.
13. Hoff LA: People in Crisis: Understanding and Helping, 4th ed. San Francisco, Jossey-Bass, 1996.
14. Caplan G: Principles of Preventive Psychiatry. New York, Basic Books, 1964.
15. Burr WR, Klein SR: Reexamining Family Stress. Thousand Oaks, CA, Sage, 1994.
16. McCubbin MA, McCubbin HI: Families coping with illness: the resiliency model of family stress, adjustment, and adaptation. In: Danielson CB, Hamel-Bissell B, Winstead-Fry P (eds): Families, Health, and Illness: Perspectives on Coping and Intervention. Philadelphia, C.V. Mosby, 1993, pp 21–63.
17. McCubbin MA: Family stress theory and the development of nursing knowledge about family adaptation. In: Meetham SL, Meister SB, Bell JM, et al (eds): The Nursing of Families. Newbury Park, CA, Sage, 1993.
18. Molter NC: Needs of relatives of critically ill patients: a descriptive study. Heart Lung 8:332–339, 1979.
19. Price DM, Forrester A, Murphy PA, et al: Critical care family needs in an urban teaching medical center. Heart Lung 20:183–188, 1991.
20. Davis-Martin S: Perceived needs of families of long-term critical care patients: a brief report. Heart Lung 23:515–518, 1994.
21. Peirce AG, Wright F, Fulmer TT: Needs of the family during critical illness of elderly patients. Crit Care Nurs Clin North Am 4:597–606, 1992.
22. Chesla CA: Reconciling technologic and family care in critical-care nursing. IMAGE 28:199–203, 1996.
23. American Association of Critical-Care Nurses (AACN): AACN Standards for Nursing Care of the Critically Ill, 2nd ed. Norwalk, CT, Appleton & Lange, 1989.
24. Chesla CA, Stannard D: Breakdown in the nursing care of families in the ICU. Am J Crit Care 6:64–71, 1997.
25. Simpson T, Wilson D, Mucken N, et al: Implementation and evaluation of a liberalized visiting policy. Am J Crit Care 5:420–426, 1996.
26. Kleman M, Bickert A, Karpinski A, et al: Physiologic responses of coronary care patients to visiting. J Cardiovasc Nurs 7:52–62, 1993.
27. Simon SK, Phillips K, Badalamenti S, et al: Current practices regarding visitation policies in critical care units. Am J Crit Care 6:210–217, 1997.
28. Marfell JA, Garcia JS: Contracted visiting hours in the coronary care unit. Nurs Clin North Am 30:87–95, 1995.

29. Lazure LL, Baun MM: Increasing patient control of family visiting in the coronary care unit. Am J Crit Care 4:157–164, 1995.

30. Cole KM, Gawlinski A: Animal-assisted therapy in the intensive care unit. Nurs Clin North Am 30:529–537, 1995.

31. Covinsky K, Goldman L, Cook EF, et al: The impact of serious illness on patients' families. JAMA 272:1839–1844, 1994.

32. Barry PD: Psychosocial Nursing: Care of the Physically Ill Patients and Their Families. Philadelphia, Lippincott-Raven, 1996.

33. Morton PG: Health Assessment in Nursing. Philadelphia, F.A. Davis, 1993.

34. Acute Pain Management Guideline Panel, Health Care Agency for Policy and Research: Acute Pain Management: Operative or Medical Procedures and Trauma. Clinical Practice Guidelines. Publication No. 92-0032.35. Rockville, MD, US Department of Health and Human Services, 1992.

35. Henry LL: Music therapy: a nursing intervention for the control of pain and anxiety in the ICU. A review of the research literature. Dimensions Crit Care Nurs 14:295–304, 1995.

36. Puntillo KA: Effects of interpleural bupivacaine on pleural chest tube removal pain: a randomized controlled trial. Am J Crit Care 5:102–108, 1996.

37. Puntillo K, Miaskowski C, Kehrle K, et al: Relationship between behavioral and physiological indicators of pain, critical care patients' self-reports of pain, and opioid administration. Crit Care Med 25:1159–1166, 1997.

38. Guyton-Simmons J, Ehrmin JT: Problem solving in pain management by expert intensive care nurses. Crit Care Nurse 14:37–44, 1994.

39. Gujol MC: A survey of pain assessment and management practices among critical care nurses. Am J Crit Care 3:123–129, 1994.

40. Agency for Health Care Policy and Research: Management of Cancer Pain Guideline Panel. Publication No. 94-0592. Rockville, MD, US Department of Health and Human Services, 1994.

41. Puntillo K, Casella V, Reid M: Opioid and benzodiazepine tolerance and dependence: Application of theory to critical care practice. Heart Lung 26:317–324, 1997.

42. Watkins GR: Music therapy: proposed physiologic mechanisms and clinical implications. Clin Nurse Specialist 11:43–50, 1997.

43. Byers JF, Smyth KA: Effect of a music intervention on noise annoyance, heart rate, and blood pressure in cardiac surgery patients. Am J Crit Care 6:183–191, 1997.

44. Keltner NL, Schwecke LH, Bostrom CE: Psychiatric Nursing, 2nd ed. St. Louis, C.V. Mosby, 1995.

45. Barry PD (ed): Psychosocial Nursing, 3rd ed. Philadelphia, Lippincott-Raven, 1996, pp 323–339.

46. Diagnostic and Statistical Manual of Mental Disorders, 4th ed. Washington, DC, American Psychiatric Press, 1994.

47. Haskell RM, Frankell HL, Rotondo MF: Agitation. AACN Clin Issues 8:335–350, 1997.

48. Robinson CR: Impaired sleep. In: Carrieri-Kohlman V, Lindsey A, West CM (eds): Pathophysiological Phenomena in Nursing, 2nd ed. Philadelphia, W.B. Saunders, 1993.

49. Simpson T, Lee ER: Individual factors that influence sleep after cardiac surgery. Am J Crit Care 5:182–189, 1996.

50. Simpson T, Lee ER, Cameron C: Patients' perceptions of environmental factors that disturb sleep after cardiac surgery. Am J Crit Care 5:173–181, 1996.

51. Chulay M, Guzzetta C, Dossey B: AACN Handbook of Critical Care Nursing. Stamford, CT, Appleton & Lange, 1997.

52. Guyton AC: Textbook of Medical Physiology, 8th ed. Philadelphia, W.B. Saunders, 1991.

53. Lazarus RS, Folkman S: Stress, Appraisal, and Coping. New York, Springer, 1984.

54. Steinke EE, Patterson P: Sexual counseling of MI patients by cardiac nurses. J Cardiovasc Nurs 10:81–87, 1995.

55. Steinke EE, Patterson-Midgley P: Sexual counseling of MI patients: nurses comfort, responsibility, and practice. Dimensions Crit Care Nurs 15:216–223, 1996.

56. Steinke EE, Patterson-Midgley P: Sexual counseling following acute myocardial infarction. Clin Nurs Res 5:462–472, 1996.

57. Clark C, Heidenreich T: Spiritual care for the critically ill. Am J Crit Care 4:77–81, 1995.

58. Leetun MC: Wellness spirituality in the older adult: assessment and intervention protocol. Nurse Pract 21:60–70, 1996.

59. Twibell RS, Wieseke AW, Marine M, et al: Spiritual coping needs of critically ill patients: validation of nursing diagnoses. Dimensions Crit Care Nurs 15:245–253, 1996.

60. Zerwic JJ, King KB, Wlasowicz GS: Perceptions of patients with cardiovascular disease about the causes of coronary artery disease. Heart Lung 26:92–94, 1997.

61. Lynn-McHale DJ, Corsetti A, Brady-Avis E, et al: Perioperative ICU tours: are they helpful? Am J Crit Care 6:106–115, 1997.

62. Waite LJ: The demographic face of America's elderly. Inquiry 33:220–224, 1996.

63. Schneider EL, Guralnik JM: The aging of America: impact on health care costs. JAMA 263:2335–2340, 1990.

64. Groeger JS, Guntupalli KK, Strosberg M, et al: Descriptive analysis of critical care units in the United States: patient characteristics and intensive care unit utilization. Crit Care Med 21:279–291, 1993.

65. Chellurie L, Grenvik A, Silverman M: Intensive care for critically ill elderly: mortality, costs, and quality of life. Arch Intern Med 155:1013–1022, 1995.

66. Layon AJ, George BE, Hamby B, et al: Do elderly patients overutilize health care resources and benefit less from them than younger patients? A study of patients who underwent craniotomy for treatment of neoplasm. Crit Care Med 23:829–834, 1995.

67. Wu AW, Rubin HR, Rosen MJ: Are elderly people less responsive to intensive care? J Am Geriatr Soc 38:621–627, 1990.

68. Johnson CL, Margulies DR, Keraney TJ, et al: Trauma in the elderly: an analysis of outcomes based on age. Am Surg 60:899–902, 1994.

69. Konopad E, Noseworthy TW, Johnston R, et al: Quality of life measures before and one year after an admission to an intensive care unit. Crit Care Med 23:1653–1659, 1995.

70. Swinburne AJ, Fedullo AJ, Bixby K, et al: Respiratory failure in the elderly: analysis of outcome after treatment with mechanical ventilation. Arch Intern Med 153:1657–1662, 1993.

71. Zeitlow SP, Capizzi PJ, Bannon MP, et al: Multisystem geriatric trauma. J Trauma 37:985–988, 1994.

72. Rogove HJ, Safar P, Sutton-Tyrell K, et al: Old age does not negate good cerebral outcome after cardiopulmonary resuscitation: analyses from the brain resuscitation trials. Crit Care Med 23:18–25, 1995.

73. Stone NJ: Diet, lipids, and coronary artery disease. Endocrinol Metab Clin North Am 19:321–344, 1990.

74. Kane RL, Ouslander JG, Abrass I: Essentials of Clinical Geriatrics, 3rd ed. New York, McGraw-Hill, 1994.

75. Resnik NM: Geriatric medicine. In: Isselbacher K, Braunwald E, Wilson J, et al (eds): Harrison's Principles of Internal Medicine, 13th ed. New York, McGraw-Hill, 1994, pp 30–33.

76. Furuya K, Shimizu R, Hirabayashi Y, et al: Stress hormone responses to major intra-abdominal surgery during and immediately after sevoflurane-nitrous oxide anaesthesia in elderly patients. Can J Anaesth 40:435–439, 1993.

77. Rauen CA, Britt TL: Elderly patients. In: Clochesy JM, Breu C, Cardin S, et al (eds): Critical Care Nursing, 2nd ed. Philadelphia, W.B. Saunders, 1996, pp 1493–1509.

78. Stanley M: Sepsis in the elderly. Crit Care Nurs Clin North Am 8:1–6, 1996.

79. Matteson MA: Psychosocial aging changes. In: Matteson MA, McConnell ES, Linton AD (eds): Gerontological Nursing, 2nd ed. Philadelphia, W.B. Saunders, 1997, pp 555–601.

80. St. Pierre J: Delirium in hospitalized elderly patients: off track. Crit Care Nurs Clin North Am 8:53–60, 1996.

81. Folstein MF, Folstein SE, McHugh PR: Minimental state: a practical method for grading the cognitive state of patients for the clinician. J Psychiatr Res 12:189–198, 1975.

82. Vermeersch PEH: The clinical assessment of confusion-A. Appl Nurs Res 3:128–133, 1990.

83. Scherubel JC, Tess MM: Measuring clinical confusion in critically ill patients. J Neurosc Nurs 26:146–150, 1994.

84. Fletcher K: Use of restraints in the elderly. AACN Clin Issues Crit Care 7:611–620, 1996.

85. Dempsey DT, Mullen JL, Busby GP: The link between nutritional status and clinical outcome: can nutritional intervention modify it? Am J Clin Nutr 47:352–356, 1988.

86. Alexander JW: Nutrition and translocation. JPEN J Parenter Enteral Nutr 14:170S–174S, 1990.

87. Planchock NY, Slay LE: Pharmacokinetics and pharmacodynamic monitoring of the elderly in critical care. Crit Care Nurs Clin North Am 8:79–89, 1996.

88. Lay T: The flourishing problem of elder abuse in our society. AACN Clin Issues Crit Care Nurs 5:507–515, 1994.

89. Girard NJ: Gerontological nursing in acute care settings. In: Matteson MA, McConnell ES, Linton AD (eds): Gerontological Nursing: Concepts and Practice, 2nd ed. Philadelphia, W.B. Saunders, 1997, pp 854–895.

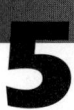

5

Cultural Issues in Critical Care Nursing

Carol Germain

Objectives

After completing this chapter, the student will be able to:

1. State the projected demographic and other societal changes likely to affect critical care nursing in the 21st century.
2. Increase self-awareness of his or her own cultural beliefs and values, to become more sensitive to the diversity of beliefs and values of those from other cultures and subcultures.
3. Value nursing models and theories as guides to culture-specific care.
4. Increase potential for delivering culturally competent critical care nursing in multiple settings.
5. Use culture-specific knowledge as a general base for individual assessment for the planning and delivery of care.
6. Articulate the population projections for the United States in the 21st century as these relate to critical care nursing.
7. Use cultural concepts such as ethnocentrism, world view, cultural diversity, and cultural relativism to understand and analyze patient or family and staff behaviors in critical care settings.
8. Distinguish among concepts of health, sickness, disease, and illness from a cultural perspective to understand differing patient and provider explanatory models (perceptions of an illness event).
9. Apply knowledge of differing cultural perspectives on responses to health crises, pain expression, grief and grieving, and dying and death when planning and delivering nursing care.
10. Use quality resources for continuing acquisition of cultural knowledge and understanding, attitudes, and skills.

This chapter provides an introduction to knowledge of culture, its characteristics, its pervasive influence on health, and its crucial importance in critical care nursing. Because people respond as whole persons, not just physiologically, to sickness, disease, or injury of a body part or the mind, skill in applying cultural knowledge influences the outcomes of care.

CULTURE

Culture is defined in numerous ways. A simple definition is that culture is the way of life of a particular, unified group of people. An ideational or cognitive definition emphasizes what people *think,* for example, their world view or the lens through which they perceive and understand the world they inhabit, as well as their ideas, language, communications, systems of concepts, and meanings. A materialist definition emphasizes *behavior,* that is, the manifest patterned ways of group living. Material culture includes, but is not limited to, technology, artifacts, clothing, housing, dietary practices, musical instruments, and systems of law, education, and health care. An holistic approach to culture necessitates both ideational and materialist perspectives.[1]

Culture also provides for the transmission of guidelines for living to current and future generations in the form of norms (rules), both prescriptive and proscriptive, and the sanctions for ignoring or violating the norms. In many cultures, religion is an essential and intertwined component and provides a source of beliefs and values by means of symbols, language, and rituals. Thus, culture is the integrating core of human groups that provides the structure and context for daily life experiences as well as defining that which is passed from generation to generation, largely in families. The definition of family, however, varies widely among cultures and subcultures, from the small nuclear group of parents and children to widely extended family groups whose members may not all be blood-related kin, and to other groupings, neither genetically nor legally related, such as lesbian or gay male domestic partners.[2] In many of the more than 500 Native American subcultures, the tribe, not the individual or family, is the major cultural unit.

The insider's knowledge or view of a culture is termed *emic,* whereas the outsider's view, which may be obtained partially through travel, films, literature, textbooks, friendships, work experiences, or study, or may be learned from patients from other cultures, is termed *etic.* Sharing emic and etic perspectives leads to the widening of each party's cultural horizon. Cultures are dynamic, not static, and they have historical, economic, social, political, and geographic elements.[3]

Subcultures

Smaller groups of a society or a culture, not necessarily associated with racial or ethnic heritage or identity, but definitely with shared beliefs, values, and norms, are called subcultures. They have distinctive unifying characteristics that set them apart from the cultural mainstream and include adolescent groups of different types, street gangs, musicians of widely varying tastes, migrant farm workers, religious communities, homeless people, gay male and lesbian subcultures, and professional groups of scientists. Nursing and medicine are separate professional subcultures with distinct world views.

Clinical units in hospitals, such as critical care, intermediate care, and trauma units, can also be considered subcultures. These units have their own norms, beliefs, values, mode of dress, rituals, expected staff role behaviors, priorities, and practices that make them distinct from other hospital units. These cultural characteristics are passed down from existing staff to new staff. A nursing cultural perspective in critical care always includes the culture of the patient and family, the cultures of the nurse and other care providers, and the sociocultural context in which care takes place, which could be the acute care hospital setting, a skilled nursing facility, or the home. The nurse is influenced by culture from at least four sources: family heritage (or family of orientation); childhood socialization (enculturation); socialization to the discipline and profession of nursing through formal education; and, later, socialization to the culture of nursing within various work settings.

Cultural Diversity, Prejudice, Discrimination, and Racism

In the United States, the biomedical model and culture have been dominant in critical care, and the biotechnologic emphasis of our society is clearly evident. To such units, which are primarily staffed by white, middle- and upper-class nurses, physicians, and other health team members, comes a steady stream of society's sickest persons from a multitude of cultures and subcultures. Some patients may attribute their sickness (perhaps silently) to nonbiologic causes such as spirit possession, loss of soul, or fate, which the biomedical system does not address. Only professional care that is culturally competent can help to bridge this patient–provider cultural gap. Such care is not a luxury. It is a right, and for nursing, an ethical mandate.[4]

The United States is a relatively young country with citizens of many racial and ethnic heritages. At one time, the mass of native and immigrant cultures in the United States was referred to as the "melting pot," but this notion of a congealed, homogeneous mass has been replaced by new metaphors such as "alphabet soup" or "salad bowl." These metaphors imply that the distinct ingredients and flavors are identifiable, although mixed together. Other metaphors used include a mosaic of different parts, or a fine tapestry woven of many distinct threads that make up a unique whole society. Although valuing cultural diversity is an important goal, there are societal obstacles to its accomplishment. One is the notion of ethnocentrism that posits "my way is the best way and only way." Ethnocentrism is the inability of members of the dominant culture to see any culture apart from its own as having value or the consistent measuring of the worth of others' cultures using only its own as the norm or point of reference. The nondominant or minority individuals or groups who do not meet the dominant cultural norms, whether through inherited physical racial characteristics such as skin color or through socioeconomic, educational, or religious status, suffer from negative stereotyping and prejudicial attitudes. If unchecked, these attitudes can lead to acts of discrimination in access to health care or in actual health care situations.

The belief that membership in one race makes one superior to those of other races is racism. Prejudiced attitudes or overt discriminatory acts also occur in response to older age, gender, disabilities, sexual orientation, or nationality. Having minority status in this society refers more to unequal power status in social systems rather than to numeric representation in the total population. Racial and ethnic minority groups, for example, do have middle and upper socioeconomic classes, but they may lack the power and privileges of the dominant white majority. Racism and other prejudiced attitudes or ethnocentric biases operate at an institutional as well as an individual level. Institutional racism, according to Giachello, refers to the "established, customary, and respected ways in which society operates to keep the minority in a subordinate position."[5] Racism may be conscious and deliberate, but it also may be unconscious and unintentional. One dimension of professional nursing practice includes assessment of the practice unit as it relates to the larger sociocultural system.[6] Instances of institutional racism or other prejudiced or ethnocentric attitudes that lead to discriminatory practices require collective action for change to take place.

Immigration, Ethnicity, and Marginalization

Serious sickness is a cultural leveler because it can be experienced by anyone. In the crisis-oriented, fast-paced, high-powered, biomedical, technologic environment of critical care, all patients become disempowered and at least temporarily marginalized to some degree by their status in the social system of the institution. Meleis noted that "When people are marginalized they are stripped of their voice, their power, and their rights to resources. . . . The definition of marginalization highlights the effects of disenfranchisement based on race, sexual orientation, socioeconomic circumstances, and national origin."[7] The most marginalized people in health care institutions are those who live their daily lives as marginalized people. These include the poor, the homeless, the battered women, and others who do not have the resources to enter the health care system until they are critically sick. For many reasons, the poor from all racial and ethnic groups often lack access to health care resources, and this partially explains their higher rates of hypertension, heart disease, stroke, AIDS, and other diseases.

Ethnicity refers to the identification (by self, other insiders, and outsiders) with a cultural group, irrespective of color, that has shared ancestry, geography, history, language, religion, politics, and social interaction patterns and, more extensively, literature, art, music, and artifacts. Thus, racial groups such as American Indians or Alaskan tribes, whites of European, South African, Near Eastern, and Lebanese origin, blacks who are recent immigrants from African countries, the West Indies, or the Carribean islands, Asians from the Phillipines, Thailand, Korea, Japan, or Taiwan, and South Asian Indians exhibit considerable ethnic variations between and within their own racial groups. Persons of Hispanic origin may be of any race, including white, which they self-identify. Their ethnicity varies because they or their ancestors come from many countries with considerable cultural or ethnic

variation such as Mexico, Puerto Rico, Cuba, Spain, or other countries in Latin and South America.

As persons emigrate from their homeland where they were enculturated and become immigrants in another country, or as people migrate within the boundaries of their country such as the United States, they become gradually more or less acculturated to the dominant national, regional, or local cultures for political, economic, social, or other reasons. Some immigrants and migrants experience a period of grief over the losses that often accompany such moves. Many new immigrant families live their lives biculturally, adhering to the culture of the workplace while at work, but maintaining their traditional cultural beliefs and practices while in the privacy of their homes. Later generations of immigrant families may become selectively traditional based on the degree of assimilation into American society. Intermarriage between persons of different racial or ethnic heritages adds another dimension to the culture of individuals and families. So does the resultant mixed racial or ethnic heritage of the next generation and the children of interracial and international adoptions.

NATIONAL POPULATION PREDICTIONS FOR THE 21ST CENTURY

As the 21st century approaches, the United States continues to open its doors to immigrants who leave their native lands for further economic or educational opportunities for themselves and their families, to seek refuge from wars or political oppression, or to flee severe environmental hazards. However, immigrant groups in the late 1990s and 21st century will differ in racial and ethnic identities and proportions compared with the white European groups that dominated immigration at the turn of the 20th century. In addition to immigration, other changes that are considered in projecting demographics for the first half of the 21st century are fertility and births of the population as a whole, extended life expectancy, and mortality in older age groups.

In 1995, approximately 83% of the US population was white, although 74% were non–Hispanic white. By 2050, it is projected that the white population will comprise 75% of the population, but the non–Hispanic white population will decline to 53%, almost equal to the sum of the remaining census categories. This decline in the white population is in contrast to projected surges in the populations of Hispanic origin and Asian and Pacific Islanders. Every year from 1995 to 2050, the Hispanic-origin population will add the largest number of people to the US population and will increase to 25% of the population by 2050. Puerto Ricans hold US citizenship but those who reside in the commonwealth of Puerto Rico rather than the United States are not included in the US census figures; only persons in the 50 states and the District of Columbia are included. After 2016, more blacks than non–Hispanic whites will be added to the population each year, and by 2050, the black population will nearly double its 1995 size to 61 million or 15% of the population from 13% in 1995. In 2050, 9% of the population will be Asian and Pacific Islander, compared with 4% in 1995. The American Indian, Eskimo, and Aleut population, although the smallest racial constituent, is predicted to grow by natural increase from 0.9% in 1995 to 1.1% by 2050 (Table 5–1).[8] These projected population shifts have given rise to the current notion of the "browning" of the United States. Over time, because of intermarriage or interracial relationships, the number of mixed racial children will add to the nation's multiracial diversity.

Another important projection for critical care nursing is that, if current demographic trends continue, the fastest-growing group in the United States over the next five to six decades will be the elderly, especially the oldest component. In 1995, there were 4 million people aged 85 years. That number will double by the year 2030 and will more than double again to 18.2 million by 2050. A large number of these elderly people will be post–1970 immigrants.[8]

CHANGES IN THE US HEALTH CARE SYSTEM

Two alarming trends in the 1990s have been the early discharge of extremely sick patients from hospitals to their homes and the decline in the total number of minority students graduating from RN preparation programs. Even though admissions of minority students have increased, there has been a decline in graduations for both African-Americans and Hispanics, but a slight increase among Asian and American Indians.[9]

Nursing has a history of more than a century of caring for vulnerable populations in their homes, many of these patients immigrants. As we near the turn of the century, the intensive, high-technology care that marked the early hospital critical care units of the 1960s is, and will continue to be, delivered in patients' homes under nursing supervision and in collaboration with off-site physicians and on-site families or other support systems. Although patients most likely would prefer nurses who share their racial or ethnic heritage as providers of care in their homes, RN graduation trends indicate that this goal is not a possibility. Increasing minority recruitment and graduations will help, but given the realities, all nurses must be prepared to deliver culturally competent critical care in patients' homes. For care to be culturally competent, the nurse must have a high degree of cultural self-awareness and the ability to take into account patients' and families' racial and ethnic identities, health beliefs, values, lifestyles, lan-

guage, usual coping patterns, socioeconomic status, sociopolitical societal context, and a host of other considerations grouped broadly under the umbrella term of culture. Regardless of the setting for care, sometimes it is necessary to use a more culturally knowledgeable and skilled nurse or other specialist. These persons, called "culture brokers," can negotiate situations in which quality care is impeded by a cultural "disconnect" between patient or family and provider.

CULTURALLY COMPETENT NURSING CARE

As critical care moves out of hospital system boundaries to patients' homes, nurses themselves may experience the culture shock that patients feel when they enter the foreign territory of the hospital. A critically ill patient is a stranger to the culture of the institutional critical care unit. Try to imagine how you would feel if one of your family members or friends, while traveling in a foreign country, had to be hospitalized in a critical care unit. From your experienced (and, possibly, ethnocentric) point of view, the technology is primitive, the ward ancient, the medical and nursing care far from your accustomed standards, and the language completely foreign to you. In addition to the anxiety over the sickness of your companion, you (or another in your group) may be experiencing culture shock, from being a stranger not just to the culture of the country but to the institutional culture as well. Culture shock is a type of crisis manifested by frustration and irritation at one's inability to understand or control a new situation. It also includes the frustration that accompanies the loss of the usual methods, symbols, and supports of social interaction. For example, culture shock can be experienced by a graduate nurse new to the staff of a critical care unit or by an experienced nurse who encounters a patient or family situation that is radically culturally different from his or her prior experiences. Culture shock is a reaction to stress and subsides as one acquires the necessary skills appropriate to the new environment or new situation. An exercise, such as imagining oneself as the stranger to a culture and trying to understand what critically ill patients are going through, can promote cultural sensitivity, particularly if it is discussed in a group session with a knowledgeable leader. However, cultural sensitivity, although important, is not sufficient for a professional nurse. For culturally competent care, sensitivity must be combined with specific cultural knowledge of each patient's racial, ethnic, and religious or spiritual needs. An attitude of openness to change is necessary, so that understanding of the patient's cultural needs and the skills needed to meet those needs can be integrated with the requisite physiologic or technologic critical care knowledge and skills.

TABLE 5-1

Percentage Distribution of the Population by Race and Hispanic Origin: 1995 to 2050

| Year | Race | | | | | Not of Hispanic Origin | | | |
	Total	White	Black	American Indian*	Asian[†]	Hispanic Origin[‡]	White	Black	American Indian*	Asian[†]
Projections										
Middle Series										
1995	100.0	83.0	12.6	0.9	3.6	10.2	73.6	12.0	0.7	3.3
2000	100.0	82.1	12.9	0.9	4.1	11.4	71.8	12.2	0.7	3.9
2030	100.0	77.6	14.4	1.0	7.0	18.9	60.5	13.1	0.8	6.6
2050	100.0	74.8	15.4	1.1	8.7	24.5	52.8	13.6	0.9	8.2

*American Indian represents American Indian, Eskimo, and Aleut.
[†]Asian represents Asian and Pacific Islander
[‡]Persons of Hispanic origin may be of any race. The information on the total and Hispanic population shown in this report was collected in the 50 states and the District of Columbia and therefore does not include residents of Puerto Rico.
  From the United States Department of Commerce: Population Projections of the United States by Age, Sex, Race, and Hispanic Origin. Washington, D.C.: Bureau of the Census Publication P25-1130, middle series, 1996.

Although this chapter and this text emphasize scientific knowledge, including knowledge of culture, culturally competent care requires other types of knowing. Carper's typology of empirics (the science of nursing), personal knowledge or knowledge of self and the other, esthetics (the art of nursing), and ethical knowledge provide a more sufficient framework for advancing in cultural competence than science and technologic knowledge alone.[10] This effort can be aided by analysis of case studies in critical care such as those provided by Galanti.[11] Discussion of Beauchamp's case study of nursing a dying gay man who opted to terminate hospital care and to receive nursing care while dying at home could be helpful in preparing for such experiences.[12] Clinical conferences or debriefing sessions after culturally complex clinical experiences can aid staff in growth in cultural competence through analysis of stories involving individual or group attitudes, values conflicts, cultural missteps or successes, or instances of institutionalized prejudice or discrimination.

A further clarification of culturally competent care according to the American Academy of Nursing is "care that takes into account issues related to diversity, marginalization and vulnerability due to culture, race, gender and sexual orientation. This care is guided by nursing theories, models, and/or research principles. . . . It is also care that is provided within the historical and 'dailiness' context of clients."[13]

Nursing Conceptualizations and Culturally Competent Care

Several conceptual models of nursing specifically address the cultural component of care. For example, in the Neuman Systems Model, the sociocultural variable is one of the five variable areas that make up the client–client system.[14] In Orem's Self-Care Framework, culture is one of the basic conditioning factors that the nurse must address in an assessment of the patient.[15] Orem's framework may require more cautious application in cultures in which family structure is more hierarchical and the norms for the care of the sick and elderly do not have self-care as a goal.

Theory of Cultural Diversity and Universality

Leininger, a nurse anthropologist, developed a theoretic model that has culturally specific and congruent care as major foci. Components are graphically depicted in Leininger's Sunrise Model, a conceptual guide encompassing cultural and social structure dimensions (Figure 5–1). The major cultural components of the theoretic model are technologic, religious and philosophic, kinship and social factors, cultural values and lifeways, political and legal factors, and economic and educational factors. These components are interactive with environmental context, language, and ethnohistory. Leininger has developed culturalogic assessment guides, both long and short forms, for practice and research called enablers that are consistent with the theoretical model. These enablers assist the nurse to obtain the patient's cultural views and to examine the nurse's own behaviors in relation to those of the patient.[16]

Leininger has criticized the value orientation and descriptors of the North American Nursing Diagnosis Association (NANDA) taxonomy as ethnocentric and Anglo-American Western culture-bound, with little focus on cultural care nursing phenomena. In her conceptualization of the nursing process, Leininger does not use the term "nursing diagnosis." After assessment, the terms "nursing judgments" or "decisions" are used. "Nursing actions" is the term used instead of "interventions," which is also considered a Western culture-bound term. Nursing assessments, decisions, and actions are aimed at cultural care preservation or maintenance, cultural care accommodation or negotiation, or cultural care repatterning or restructuring. For example, the nurse is preserving or maintaining a patient's cultural beliefs, values, and expressions when he or she obtains and respects a family patriarch's view regarding who will be the major decision maker in his health crisis. Of course, legal considerations have to be taken into account as well. Accommodation and negotiation come into play when a nurse helps a patient to use traditional healing rituals to complement biomedical practices. Repatterning and restructuring may consist of educational and persuasive actions on the part of the home care nurse to help the patient and family adjust to new technology, to promote sterility of supplies, and to understand how to avoid practices that pose a risk of infection to patient or family members.[16]

Acquiring Knowledge of Specific Cultural Groups

Other textbooks that provide general guidelines for culture-specific care of major groups have been provided by Spector[17] and Giger and Davidhizar.[18] These latter authors use the concepts of space, communication, social organization, time, environmental control, and biologic variations to organize material related to the assessment and care of persons from 16 specific cultural groups. In presenting the evolving Purnell's Model for Cultural Competence, Purnell and Paulanka provide a framework of 12 domains and their concepts deemed essential for assessing the ethnocultural attributes of an individual, family, or group. These include inhabited localities and

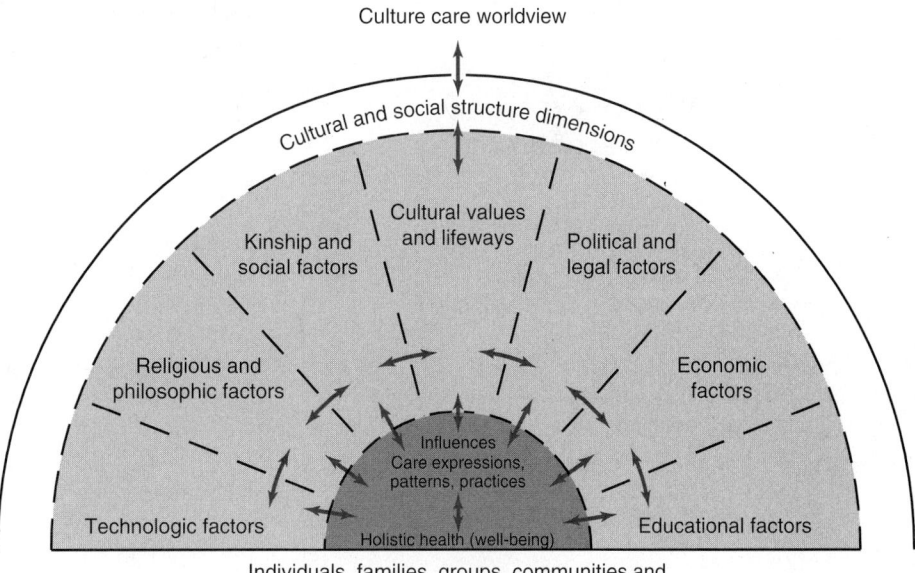

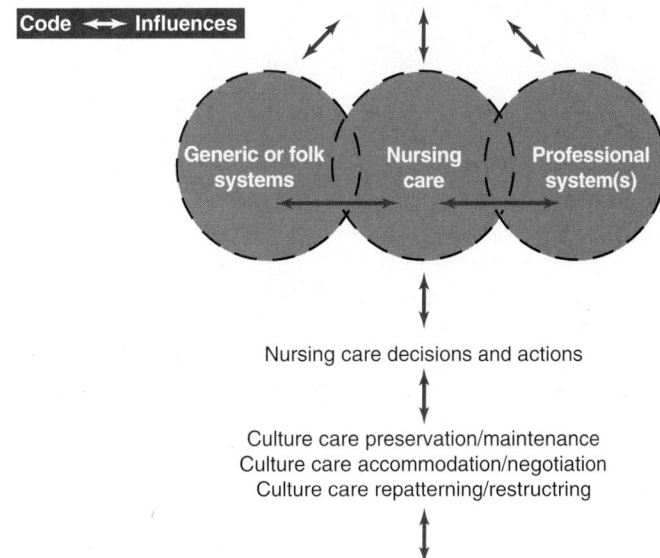

Figure 5–1

Leininger's sunrise model depicts the theory of cultural care diversity and universality. (From Leininger M: Culture Care Diversity and Universality: A Theory for Nursing. New York, National League for Nursing, 1991.)

topography, communication, family roles and organization, workforce issues, biocultural ecology, high-risk health behaviors, nutrition, pregnancy and childbearing practices, death rituals, spirituality, health care practices, and health care practitioners.[19] Lipson, Dibble, and Minarik, in their profiles of 24 cultural groups in US society, specifically address areas that have high utility for critical care including communication, serious or terminal illness, death rituals, family relationships, and spiritual or religious orientation. These authors also provide a guide for a minimal cultural assessment that can be more specifically tailored for use in critical care nursing[20] (Chart 5–1).

Textbooks such as these do not promote the racial or ethnic stereotyping of members of a specific culture; rather, they present general characteristics that provide guidelines for individualized assessments. Intracultural diversity, even differences between patient and family,

can be more varied than differences among members of different cultures. In addition, the areas of socioeconomic level, education, occupation, gender, sexual identity, daily living environment, language, and social roles (e.g., parent, coach, political leader, prisoner) are part of the sociocultural makeup of an individual regardless of race or ethnicity. Assessment of these variables is essential to a full cultural nursing history of the patient as soon as the patient's condition is stabilized. The patient, or a family member if the patient cannot be directly questioned, is the one who self-identifies racial or ethnic identity. Inferring a patient's or staff member's or any person's racial or ethnic identity, education, or socioeconomic level, and assuming needs on the basis of appearance, physical characteristics, first name or surname, accent or dialect is culturally insensitive.

CHART 5-1

Minimum List of Questions for a Cultural Assessment

- Where was the patient born? If an immigrant, how long has the patient lived in this country?
- What is the patient's ethnic affiliation, and how strong is the patient's ethnic identity?
- Who are the patient's major support people: family members, friends? Does the patient live an ethnic community?
- What are the primary and secondary languages, speaking ability, and reading ability?
- How would you characterize the nonverbal communication style?
- What is the patient's religion, its importance in daily life, and current practices?
- What are the patient's food preferences and prohibitions?
- What is the patient's economic situation, and is the income adequate to meet the needs of the patient and family?
- What are the health and illness beliefs and practices?
- What are the customs and beliefs around such transitions as birth, illness, and death?

Lipson, J. Dibble, S. & Minarik, P. (Eds). (1996). *Culture and nursing care: A pocket guide.* San Francisco, UCSF Nursing Press. p. 3.

Providing an interpreter for a non–English-speaking patient or family is sometimes essential to obtain an accurate and complete assessment including a cultural history, as well as for aiding accurate nursing diagnoses, interventions, and evaluation of nursing outcomes. The interpreter should be a neutral or noninvolved but reliable person of the same sex, to avoid conflicts in translation or reporting related to personal or sexual matters.

Although it may be interesting to read about world cultures, the nurse's responsibility is to learn the common cultural characteristics of those groups who make up the usual patient population of the unit as a starting point for an individual assessment. The cultural language or professional jargon of a critical care unit is a foreign language for most English-speaking patients and needs interpretation for safe and effective care. Basic textbooks cannot address all cultures. When a patient is a traveler or an international student or business person from a culture that is not known to the staff, guidelines for culturally congruent care can be systematically developed by using categories from the aforementioned texts.

CULTURAL DIMENSIONS OF COMMON RESPONSES IN CRITICAL CARE

Nurses, regardless of setting, deal with the results of common events that affect human beings. Childbirth complications, trauma, war, major infections, environmental disasters, diseases, drug overdoses, and criminal attacks are types of events that provoke crises for individuals and families throughout the world, but responses to these events are variously expressed within and among cultures. Four interrelated responses are briefly discussed. They are sickness as crisis, pain, dying and death, and grief.

Sickness as Crisis

People of all cultures experience sickness, or the threat of it, in the course of their lives. The term "sickness" encompasses the symptoms and distress associated with the wide variety of human events that people describe when they say, "I'm sick." These events range from sea sickness, a bout with the flu, a life-threatening myocardial infarction, the multiple-systems response to trauma, the experience of grief after the death of a loved one, or a curse or spirit possession imposed on a person for breach of a cultural taboo.[21]

Explanatory Models of Sickness and Illness

A conceptual distinction between sickness as disease and sickness as illness is helpful in understanding sickness from a cultural context. Pathologic processes of the body organ or injured body part, or the disordered mind, that biomedicine diagnoses and treats, are considered disease. Patients have symptoms and feel sick, but patients also interpret sickness. This interpretation is not just in relation to the disease or disordered mind, but as illness, which is the whole experience of the disease with its meaning and significance. Explanatory models vary because of cultural influences. Thus, all other things being equal, two people can have the same medical diagnosis and the same treatment (e.g., coronary artery bypass surgery), but have entirely different illness experiences. One person will recover medically and will achieve maximal functional status as predicted, and the other will recover medically but will remain ill and will fail to achieve maximal functional status. Again, all other things being equal, the meaning and significance of the illness to the person will vary. For example, the illness may mean a welcomed retirement opportunity, a remaining curse, or punishment for transgressions. These meanings will influence whether illness persists when the injury or disease has been treated and "cured." This situation indicates that a patient may have a different explanatory model (perspective) of the sickness than the biomedically oriented provider. For care to be culturally competent, the patient's and the provider's explanatory models must be shared, so that each understands the perceptions of the other, and negotiation can ensue. This is necessary to achieve the most successful outcome for the patient. Eliciting the patient's explanatory model guards against cultural imposition, the practice of imposing one's own world view without identifying an individual's critical beliefs and values[21,22].

Health deviations sometimes reach a crisis level when the underserved poor and deprived minorities of this country, as well as new immigrants and refugees faced with major transitional crises and few personal resources, turn to popular (herbal remedies, over-the-counter drugs) or folk remedies (provided by a cultural healer). Often, these remedies take priority in the person's hierarchy of resort before relief from the professional health care system is sought. Some popular or folk remedies are not successful, and professional care is delayed until emergency room or other critical care becomes the last option. Even people who are not economically deprived but who have strong cultural roots tend to use their popular or folk remedies as first-line treatments for common sicknesses. It is important that the history of the use of these remedies be obtained as part of the nursing assessment when the person seeks professional care, particularly in emergency departments or urgicenters. However, this history should be obtained in a nonjudgmental manner, so that the patient or family is not demeaned by reference to their health decisions. Blaming may result in the withholding of vital information and future delays in seeking professional care.[23]

Persons and their families in health crises may find comfort in basic religious and cultural beliefs and practices, although they may ignore these beliefs when they are well. Some cultural practices or rituals may initially seem strange to the nurse, but they may become less so when the nurse makes the effort to understand the patient's world view and the meaning of symbols, such as medals or oils, and religious rituals of the cultural group.

Culture and Pain

The meaning of pain, how pain is expressed, and what pain relief measures are requested or given are culturally influenced. Like other cultural patterns, cultural expectations and responses to pain are passed down to children early in their development. The cultural value of pain relief in the larger US society is evident in the widespread advertising of nonprescription analgesics on television and in other media and their ready availability in drug stores and food markets. However, in some cultures, the expectation is that pain is something to be endured. One cannot assume that people of the same heritage but somewhat different culture share the same views on pain. For example, Lipson, Dibble, and Minarik noted the difference between two Hispanic (Latino) cultures and the cultural responses to pain. Mexican-Americans were described as valuing inner control and self-endurance. Men may interpret expression of pain as showing weakness and possible loss of respect. The social expression of pain is more acceptable in Mexican-American women. However, stoicism is common, and patients tend not to complain of pain. The nurse would need to assess pain by nonverbal cues. In contrast, the pain response of Puerto Rican Hispanics (Latinos) is described as loud and outspoken, with verbal moaning and crying out of "dolor" (pain). Their preference is for oral or intravenous medications rather than intramuscular or rectal medications. Herbal teas, heat, and prayer are also used to manage pain.[20] Use of a scale or diagram that permits patients to indicate the degree of their pain can be helpful in the initial assessment and the continual monitoring of pain-relief mechanisms, particularly for non–English-speaking patients.

In her ethnographic research of cultural meanings, expressions, and self-care and dependent-care actions associated with experiences of pain in Mexican-Americans, Villaruel identified four themes providing a cultural context within which the pain experience of Mexican-Americans may be understood. These are as follows: 1) pain is an encompassing experience of suffering; 2) pain is an accepted obligation of life and of one's role within the family, a burden one must bear so as not to inflict pain on others; 3) to endure pain stoically is expected and esteemed; and 4) the primacy of caring for others is the essence of the family. The nursing implications of the study include that nurses caring for Mexican-Americans must not equate the absence of pain behaviors or the absence of verbal expressions of pain with the absence of pain. Suggestions are made regarding how the nurse can involve the patient in accepting pain-relief measures while helping her or him maintain personal integrity.[24] Further study of pain in critical care situations with specific populations such as Mexican-American patients is needed.

In the critical care unit, pain related to disease, surgery, or injury or its treatment, although acute, may be superimposed on a patient's chronic pain due to prior injuries or bone and joint diseases such as arthritis. Patients have a right to adequate pain control. Patients in chronic pain may have learned to manage it using nonmedical alternatives or complementary approaches. Nurses should try to make it possible for patients to continue their pain-management strategies whenever possible. This may include arranging to continue such therapies as massage or meditation whenever such therapies are not medically contraindicated. Nurses are in the position to make decisions about pain relief for patients, but nurses' inferences about patients' pain are influenced by their own cultural and religious backgrounds, as well as by the culture of the unit and the larger sociocultural context. This is another reason that self-awareness of the nurse's and nursing staff's biases and belief systems can contribute to culturally competent care. The management of pain, both acute and chronic, in specific subcultures of patients such as those who use and abuse illegal drugs, would benefit from consultation with an advanced practice nurse specialist in pain control.

Cultural Perspectives on Dying and Death

Customs surrounding dying and death vary widely between and among cultures. Among the more than 500 American Indian tribes, for example, some avoid contact with the dying; in others, tribal members remain near their dying members. In some tribes, it is preferred to die at home, whereas in others, the dying person is brought to the hospital to die because a death in the home would necessitate abandonment of the family dwelling place.

Religion is a major, essential, and intertwined component of many cultures. For the Navajo and other American Indians, religion and health are so closely related that they are said to be two sides of the same coin. The nurse should consult with the native healer, clergy, hospital chaplain, or other religious practitioner regarding what may be helpful in the spiritual care of the dying. Rituals such as the Sacrament of the Sick for Roman Catholics, chants by a native healer, and formal prayers for the dying may be conducted at the bedside, and space and time may need to be made available for these traditions. Because some of these events are considered private, it should be determined whether privacy requirements would exclude the nurse from the ceremony. However, the nurse needs to apprise the visitors of certain restrictions, such as not having lighted candles near oxygen equipment.

In Islamic cultures and with some Orthodox Jews, the possibility of death is not discussed with the patient or among family members. Such discussion could be viewed as increasing the individual's chance of dying, destroying hope, or taking away some of the will to live. For some patients, knowledge of a dreaded diagnosis such as advanced cancer can even prompt suicide so as not to burden one's family. The nurse who values the patient's right to know must respect the patient's cultural practices while developing an advocacy role in each particular situation. People from cultures who proscribe discussion of the possibility of death would be expected to be reluctant to discuss advance directives or do not resuscitate (DNR) options. Organ donation and autopsy consent also vary with culture. The belief of some cultures is that the body needs to be intact for resurrection or the afterlife. If the patient is prohibited from or is unable to participate in discussions of such issues, the family spokesperson (e.g., spouse, eldest in authority, eldest son) should be consulted. Family meetings, with staff support and legal and spiritual advice, may help to promote family communication with the dying member and gradual acceptance of the reality of death by distressed family members. In the hospital, a private room or area for the visitors of the dying patient to grieve is important, as is a place for overnight rest for those designated to be readily available to the dying person.

In some cultures, a constant vigil by one or two individuals at the bedside of the dying is an expectation, and families should be assisted to accomplish this goal. In Gypsy and other cultures, numerous family members may expect to surround the critically ill patient as a sign of love and respect, but limits may need to be set for efficient and effective nursing of all patients to take place. The nurse should approach the patient's spokesperson, or the leader of the visiting group, to develop a visitation plan that accommodates needs of patient, family, and staff.

Other variations from the norms of the unit may be helpful. For example, some Muslims may request support for the ritual of turning the bed of the dying toward the direction of the Holy City of Mecca. In other belief systems, relatives may request that a nearby window be kept open to allow the spirit of the person to leave when death occurs. A self-aware staff views visitors as helpful to dying patients in most situations, and staff members are comfortable in asking visitors about their customs with the dying.

Care of the body immediately after death and funeral and burial customs also vary among ethnic and religious groups. When a final bathing of the deceased is part of a religious or cultural ritual (e.g., among religious Jews or Muslims), the family or designated group should be permitted to provide this aspect of postmortem care on the unit whenever feasible. Local guides for such customs should be part of each unit's literature.

Cultural Influences on the Grieving Process

Grief is always preceded by loss, thus change. The most frequent cause of acute grief is loss of a loved one. Other losses provoking grief include loss of one's previous state of wellness, loss of physical function after a stroke or other catastrophe, loss of independence or mobility including driving privileges, loss of social roles, and loss of one's home or job or a valued object.

An analysis of the concept of grief by Cowles and Rodgers resulted in a definition of grief as a "dynamic, pervasive, highly individualized process, with a strong normative component."[25] The term "dynamic" refers to a constantly changing state; "pervasive" means having the potential to affect every aspect of the griever's existence. Grief is highly individualized in that the combination of objective and subjective experiences associated with grief (e.g., crying, anxiety, anger at the staff, physical or somatic symptoms, loss of ability to concentrate) are influenced by many factors. These include the relationship between the grieving person and the lost being or object, whether the loss is sudden or anticipated, the support systems available, the grieving individual's prior experiences with loss or grief, and the person's culture and religious beliefs. A normative component to grief implies that people learn how to grieve, or learn the norms of grief expression, through the process of enculturation. Different cultures have "limits beyond which grief becomes unacceptable or inappropriate."[25]

The process of grieving does not happen as a discrete set of steps over a set period. There is an emerging consensus on the enduring nature of grief, that is, that grief has no assigned time limit such as 6 months or 2 years. Rather, how an individual adjusts to the changes provoked by prior losses, or to new situations with reminders of prior losses, or other reminders such as anniversaries, for example, may revive aspects of grief for unlimited periods. Given culturally approved constraints against prolonged public grief expression, the bereaved individual may continue to grieve privately. Cowles and Rodgers also pointed out that the popularized staging theory of Elizabeth Kubler-Ross is a theory of dying, not a theory of grief.[25]

The nurse, regardless of practice setting, can expect a variety of expressions of grief in response to the anticipation or actuality of a patient's death. Loud wailing or deep sobbing may be culturally appropriate. A private place where relatives of the deceased can assemble to support each other and to receive support from staff should be part of every unit. Nurses and other staff members may also have formed attachments with patients and grieve their loss. The nursing ritual of postmortem care, attentively given by the nursing staff, helps to bring the patient–nurse relationship to closure and the nurses to composure, so that care can be rendered competently to other patients in the setting.

PATIENT AND NURSE ADVOCACY

The American Association of Critical-Care Nurses (AACN) clearly positions the nurse as patient advocate and the health care institution as instrumental in providing an environment with the expectation and support for the nurses's advocacy role.[26] The nurse also has the right to self-advocacy based on self-awareness. Conflicts between the nurse's personal and professional values and the cultural practices of patients and families need to be examined by the nurse, so that neither the nurse's values are imposed on vulnerable persons nor the nurse's own professional integrity is diminished. This examination involves continuous introspection, dialogue with colleagues, and acquisition of cultural knowledge to achieve greater self-awareness. Without such examination and awareness, attitudes of the nurse can be conveyed to patients and family and may thus indicate a less than acceptable level of cultural competence. While the patient is under the nurse's accountability, the basic principle is to support the patient's cultural practices if these are not harmful to the patient or to others in the environment, including other patients, families, and staff, or the environment itself. If the nurse cannot resolve a conflict between his or her own personal and professional values and those of the patient or family, or the demands of other staff, he or she has the responsibility and the right to activate a process for transfer of the care of a patient to another qualified nurse. The self-aware nurse can also more confidently and competently deal with the occasional offensive racist or sexist (male or female) remarks, sexual overtures, or other demeaning behaviors of patients or visitors whose enculturation has not prepared them to regard the nurse as a professional.

CULTURAL DIVERSITY AND CULTURAL RELATIVISM

The principle of cultural relativism refers to the perspective that the behaviors of individuals should be judged from the context of their own cultural systems. This principle supports the notion of respecting and supporting cultural diversity. However, this does not mean that "anything goes."[27] Cultures of origin have norms, laws, taboos, and sanctions for violators. However, when immigrants come to the United States, whether as refugees or voluntarily, certain of their practices may be viewed as violations of human rights. An example of this is female circumcision with its variety of forms (e.g., female genital mutilation, clitoridectomy, infibulation).[28] Each procedure involves ritual surgery on the female genitalia, justifiable to both men and women in many African countries and some countries of Islamic tradition. Female circumcision can become an issue for critical care nursing because hemorrhage, infection, and even death can follow such primitive ritual surgeries. In Western countries, such as the United States and France, nurses and physicians may be requested to perform or to participate in such practices for refugee groups such as Somalians. However, such ritual practices are perceived in Western societies as abhorrent abuse of children and women. Further, these practices are considered unethical, if not illegal, and requests are usually denied.[27, 28] Cultural accommodation could take the form of a symbolic substitute for the procedure. That type of cultural change, however, would take time and education to become acceptable.

THE NURSE AS CULTURE LEARNER

Because of the wide variations in cultural beliefs, attitudes, and practices of patients, families, and staff in this heterogeneous, multicultural society, the nurse's attitude should be one of eagerness to learn rather than presuming to know. Puzzling patient behaviors or unusual symbols (often on the skin) should prompt the nurse to ask what such behaviors or symbols mean to the patient or family and how the staff can help. For example, a Chinese-American or Puerto Rican patient who refuses certain foods or who leaves certain beverages on the meal tray, especially when requested to force fluids, may be reflecting a belief in the humoral theory of disease. This theory aims at maintaining or reestablishing harmony in the body by balancing certain humors. Heat and cold are opposites. Cold remedies are used for hot conditions such as kidney disease or arthritis. Hot and cold have less to do with actual temperature and more to do with the symbolic power of a substance. The classification of hot and cold conditions and remedies is complex and is passed on by word of mouth. Thus, classifications vary widely within and among cultures. The patient should be encouraged to share her or his emic perspective or explanatory model that explains the illness and guides the patient's choice of hot or cold remedies.

Affirmative nodding of the head to the nurse's comments or smiling responses to questions posed by staff to a non–English-speaking patient may indicate attempts to please, embarrassment over not understanding the English language, or deference to authority. This can be dangerous. Every effort must be taken to ascertain the patient's understanding. Avoidance of eye contact by a Filipino patient is likely to indicate respect, not evasion or aversion. Such situations require further investigation and represent cultural challenges. The patient cannot be left out of the interpretation of what her or his behavior means.

Sometimes cultural missteps are made, many of them through miscommunication or unrefined communication skills. Patients can usually tolerate missteps if they feel respected by committed staff members who consistently remember the common needs of extremely sick people (Chart 5–2).

The challenges of promoting cultural diversity in critical care nursing provide opportunities for the nurse to gain experiential knowledge of culture. When such experiences are thoughtfully reflected on, the nurse can be personally satisfied that continued growth in cultural competence is obtained.

CHART 5–2

Basic Cultural Needs of the Critically Ill

- To be addressed respectfully as the patient wishes to be addressed
- To be spoken to so as to be able to understand
- To know the names and the professional identities of the staff who care for them
- To have modesty protected and privacy preserved
- To be touched gently
- To have cultural gender roles taken into consideration when intimate body care is required
- To be cared for by those with expert knowledge and technologic skills assisted with state-of-the-art technology
- To have access to appropriate cultural supports
- To have their cultural explanations heard and incorporated into the plan of care

Key Concepts

➡ Culture provides for the transmission of guidelines for living to current and future generations. Included in these guidelines are norms (rules), both prescriptive or proscriptive. In addition, cultures provide sanctions for ignoring or violating the norms.

➡ Adolescents, migrant farm workers, musicians, homeless people, and scientists are examples of groups who form subcultures within a larger culture or society.

➡ Currently, one metaphor for the cultural diversity found in the United States is a fine tapestry woven of many distinct threads that make up a unique whole society.

➡ Racism may be conscious and deliberate, but it may also be unconscious and unintentional. When institutional racism leads to discriminatory practices, collective action is required for changes to occur.

➡ Many immigrant families live their lives biculturally, that is, they adhere to the culture of the workplace while at work, but maintain traditional cultural beliefs and practices while at home.

➡ Intermarriage between persons of different racial or ethnic heritages adds another dimension to the culture of individuals and families.

➡ Significant increases in the Hispanic and black populations and a decrease in the non–Hispanic white population are predicted for the first half of the 21st century.

➡ Predicted changes in health care include the continued early discharge of extremely sick patients and the delivery of high-technology care in the patient's home.

➡ For a nurse to deliver culturally competent care, he or she must first have a high degree of cultural self-awareness.

➡ Culture shock refers to a type of crisis that occurs when one is unable to understand or control a new situation and one's usual coping methods, symbols, and social supports are not available.

➡ Leininger, a nurse anthropologist, has developed a theoretic model that has culture-specific and congruent care as major foci.

➡ Nurses are expected to study culture-specific care, emphasizing knowledge of those groups who make up the usual patient population in their work setting.

➡ Patients interpret sickness not just in relation to the pathology of the disease, but as illness, the whole experience of the disease with its personal meaning and significance.

➡ The meaning of pain, how pain is expressed, and what pain relief measures are used are all strongly influenced by one's culture.

➡ Cultural practices related to dying and death need to be explored with families and accommodations should be made to facilitate these practices whenever possible.

➡ In critical care, the nurse should be prepared to witness a wide range of visitors' grief-related behaviors. In addition, the nurse may experience personal grief over the death of a patient.

➡ When a conflict between the cultural values of a patient and a nurse cannot be resolved, the nurse should activate a process for transferring the care of the patient to another qualified nurse.

➡ Respecting and supporting cultural diversity does not mean that "anything goes." Some cultural practices may be morally or legally unacceptable in a different context.

➡ A nurse may make a cultural error but patients are usually tolerant if they are generally treated with respect and their other needs for care are met. Reflection on cultural care experiences can help the nurse progress toward cultural competency.

References

1. Germain C: Ethnography: the method. In: Munhall P, Oiler Boyd C (eds): Nursing Research: A Qualitative Perspective, 2nd ed. New York, National League for Nursing Press, 1993, pp 237–268.
2. Eliason M: Caring for the lesbian gay, or bisexual patient. Crit Care Nurs Q 19:65–72, 1996.
3. Helman C: Culture, Health and Illness, 3rd ed. London, Butterworth-Heinemann, 1994.
4. Eliason M: Ethics and transcultural nursing care. Nurs Outlook, 41:225–228, 1993.
5. Giachello A: Cultural diversity and institutional inequality. In: Adams D (ed): Health Issues for Women of Color: A Cultural Diversity Perspective. Thousand Oaks, CA, Sage, 1995, pp 5–25.
6. Germain C: Cultural concepts in critical care. Crit Care Q 82:61–78, 1982.
7. Meleis A: Culturally competent scholarship: substance and rigor. Adv Nurs Sci 19:1–16, 1997.
8. United States Department of Commerce: Population Projections of the United States by Age, Sex, Race, and Hispanic Origin. Washington, DC, Bureau of the Census publication P25-1130, middle series, 1996.
9. National League for Nursing: Nursing DataSource 1994, vol. 1. New York, National League for Nursing Press, 1994.
10. Carper BA: Fundamental patterns of knowing in nursing. In: Nicoll LH (ed): Perspectives on Nursing Theory, 3rd ed. Philadelphia, J.B. Lippincott, 1997, pp 247–255. (Reprinted from Adv Nurs Sci 1:13–23, 1978.)
11. Galanti G-A: Caring for Patients From Different Cultures: Case Studies From American Hospitals. Philadelphia, University of Pennsylvania Press, 1991.
12. Beauchamp C: The centrality of caring: a case study. In: Munhall P, Oiler Boyd C (eds): Nursing Research: A Qualitative Perspective, 2nd ed. New York, National League for Nursing Press, 1993, pp 338–358.
13. Meleis A, Isenberg M, Koerner J, et al: Diversity, Marginalization and Culturally Competent Health Care: Issues in Knowledge Development. Washington, DC, American Academy of Nursing Press, 1995, p 4.
14. Neuman B: The Neuman Systems Model, 3rd ed. East Norwalk, CT, Appleton & Lange, 1995.
15. Orem D: Nursing: Concepts of Practice, 5th ed. St. Louis, Mosby-Year Book, 1995.
16. Leininger M: Transcultural Nursing: Concepts, Theories, Research, and Practices. New York, McGraw-Hill, 1995.
17. Spector R: Cultural Diversity in Health and Illness, 4th ed. Stamford, CT, Appleton & Lange, 1996.
18. Giger J, Davidhizar R (eds): Transcultural Nursing: Assessment and Intervention, 2nd ed. St. Louis, Mosby-Year Book, 1995.
19. Purnell L, Paulanka B: Transcultural Health Care: A Culturally Competent Approach. Philadelphia, F.A. Davis, 1998.
20. Lipson J, Dibble S, Minarik P (eds): Culture and Nursing Care: A Pocket Guide. San Francisco, UCSF Nursing Press, 1996.
21. Germain C: (1992). Cultural care: a bridge between sickness, illness, and disease. Holistic Nurs Prac 6:1–9, 1992.
22. McSweeney J, Allan J, Mayo K: Exploring the use of explanatory models in nursing research and practice. Image: J Nurs Scholarship 29:243–248, 1997.
23. Germain C: Cultural concepts and office practice. Office Nurse 6:29–32, 1991.
24. Villaruel A: Mexican-American cultural meanings, expressions, self-care and dependent care actions associated with experiences of pain. Res Nurs Health 18:427–436, 1995.
25. Cowles K, Rodgers B: The concept of grief: an evolutionary perspective. In: Rodgers B, Knafl K (eds): Concept Development in Nursing. Philadelphia, W.B. Saunders, 1993, pp 93–106.
26. American Association of Critical-Care Nurses: Position Statement: Role of the Critical Care Nurse as Patient Advocate. Aliso Viejo, CA, American Association of Critical-Care Nurses, 1989.
27. Baker C: (1997). Cultural relativism and cultural diversity: implications for nursing practice. Adv Nurs Sci 20:3–11, 1997.
28. Morris R: (1996). The culture of female circumcision. Adv Nurs Sci 19:43–53, 1996.

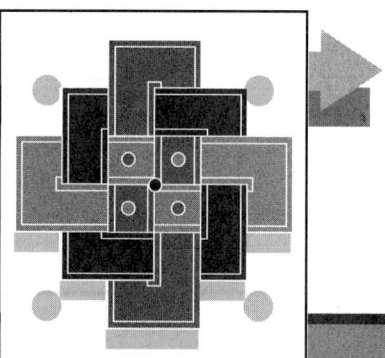

Cardiovascular Disorders

Helping Someone See Past Regret and Toward a Second Chance at Life

R. is a gentleman in his early fifties who had a heart transplant 8 years earlier. He was admitted to the thoracic transplant intensive care unit (ICU) after experiencing shortness of breath at home. A cardiac catheterization revealed advanced coronary artery disease for which bypass surgery was his only option. Although R. was medically stable for the time being after medication changes, emotionally he required astute critical care nursing skills to help him adapt to psychosocial issues.

R. had guilty feelings related to his present physical state. After his heart transplant, he had felt so much better that he quickly reverted to his previous lifestyle. He resumed smoking one and a half packs of cigarettes per day only 4 months after receiving the heart transplant. Additionally, he did not follow the no-added-salt, low-fat, low-cholesterol diet that had been prescribed for him. Despite this, he was compliant with his medication regimen and had only experienced one bout of mild graft rejection.

After taking care of R. a couple of times, I had developed a good, trusting relationship with him. He opened up to me while maintaining a quiet, reserved attitude with most of the other staff members. I tried to let R. know that not only was I interested in a positive outcome in his health, but also I was genuinely interested in who he was as a person. I was his primary nurse and a firm believer in continuity of care. Whenever I was working, I arranged to be assigned to deliver his care.

When beginning our conversations, I tried to provide an environment conducive to therapeutic communication, not always an easy task in an ICU. I ensured that we had a private room to talk in and comfortable furniture, as well as adequate lighting and temperature. We turned off the television, and R. often would have his much loved classical music lulling softly in the background. During each of these conversations, R. relaxed more and more.

I wanted R. to open up and verbalize his thoughts and feelings about his current situation. I knew from observing others and their interactions with R. that if he felt pressured, he became quiet and withdrawn. I always began our conversations with small talk about the weather or some trivial thing that had happened to me that day. This helped R. to see that I was a person, too, and not just a nurse doing physical and technical tasks to get her job done.

Slowly, I introduced subjects that were deeper in context and emotion. I gave R. the time to express himself without interruption. I asked a lot of open-ended questions so R. could answer in his own words and tell me how he really felt. I knew from previous conversations with R. that he believed that many of the nurses blamed him for his declining health, primarily because of his poor compliance. I made it a point to ask questions in a nonjudgmental way, while assuring him that we were all here for him.

Once I had R.'s trust and he felt comfortable with me, he began to discuss his interpretation of his life. This was important because the way that he saw the situation before him could be very different from the way we "medical people" viewed the very same information. Also, by knowing how he felt, we could all collaborate and include his wishes in his plan of care.

He began expressing feelings of guilt and loss of self-respect secondary to his choice of returning to poor lifestyle habits. I pointed out to R. that although those habits certainly did play a part in his current physical state, his immunosuppressive medication also had a role by accelerating the atherosclerotic process. I pointed out that all actions, positive or negative, from that day on would be decided by himself. He could continue on the same path at the time of discharge, or he could again conform to the recommended lifestyle. We worked through these feelings and redirected them to positive outlets, including early verbalization of any concerns. He related that he was feeling emotionally better after realizing that all was not lost; he had already quit smoking and intended to stay that way. He also verbalized an increased satisfaction with the no-added-salt, low-fat, low-cholesterol diet. I invited his wife (with R.'s permission) into our conversations often because she did the meal planning and preparation. She thoroughly supported him in his new choices and even presented him with a gift of an American Heart Association cookbook that was recommended by the hospital dietary staff. I had consulted with the dietitian to meet with R. and his wife for additional instruction, to answer questions and to provide reinforcement of his positive dietary choices. He was given support and praise for his compliance with medications and his exercise regimen. R. had expressed feeling depressed because he could not participate in his normal exercise routine. Before admission, he was involved in cardiac rehabilitation three times a week and routinely took an evening walk with his wife. Cardiac rehabilitation was resumed on hospital admission, but because of his heart failure, it was necessary to drop to a lower metabolic equivalent level.

R. had not been outside during the 2 weeks he had been hospitalized. I thought that a trip outside would be significant to further R.'s emotional healing. I felt that something as simple as fresh air and a change of environment, especially from the confinement he perceived in the ICU, could help to elevate his spirits. I passed the request to his day shift nurse, who presented the idea to his physician the next morning. The order was obtained from the primary physician, and when R.'s wife was visiting the next night, we surprised her and had R. hooked up to a portable monitoring system with defibrillatory capabilities, and outside we went.

It was refreshing and enlightening to see R. light up, walking hand in hand with his wife. Our conversation suddenly had begun to focus on the future instead of regrets from the past. Despite still being on hospital grounds and accompanied by myself, just stepping outside the sterile environment of the ICU allowed R. to rediscover a sense of freedom both emotionally and physically. He expressed to his wife all his fears about not living through his upcoming coronary artery bypass graft (CABG) surgery and possibly having a short time of independent life after recovery. I allowed them the time to deal with these issues in as much privacy as could be afforded. She held him closely for a long time, they looked into each other's tearful yet twinkling eyes, kissed, and asked me to join them in prayer, not just for a speedy recovery, but also for acceptance of the future, whatever it would be. After this solemn time, they told me of their life together, the good times and the bad. Their stories included R.'s suffering a massive myocardial infarct with resulting cardiomyopathy at the young age of 38. The illness

forced him to retire from a job that he loved. They also shared joyous moments, such as the time when they could not make it to the hospital in time, and R. had to help his wife deliver their third child in the front seat of a Volkswagen Bug. I felt that, because R. and his wife had told me these personal stories, I had succeeded in having them see me not only as a nurse, but also as *their* nurse and their friend.

Unfortunately, R. had many questions that could only be answered with time. He had so many things that he wanted to say to his wife that he felt he could not say in the impersonal, busy confines of the ICU. Simply taking the time to allow him the freedom to express himself outside an area that represented his regrets and fears helped R. to overcome or at least face his fears with the support of his wife.

The day before surgery, R.'s wife asked whether she could spend the night at R.'s bedside. Although this request was not a standard or accepted norm in the unit, I realized that it meant so much to him. After assessing the situation and feeling that it would not interfere with either the care or the privacy of the other patients in the unit, I passed the request on to my supervisor, who granted permission. We felt that, if nothing else, the closeness of a loving partner would aid in a more restful night with less anxiety. This solitary act probably did more to heal both their hearts than we can ever appreciate.

The next morning, R. underwent his CABG surgery and recovered without complications. He was discharged from the hospital, but not from the lives of the many hospital employees, to whom he always offered a kind word and an innocent, cheerful smile. As nurses, we can teach our patients so much—what to do, what not to do—but we also need to keep our ears open and our lips closed at times to learn about the people whom we call "patients." We must remember that we provide care to individuals and not to machines; all areas of nursing may not be cardiac centered, but we should strive to have all interactions centered on "heart care."

Maureen M. Popke, RN, BS, CCRN
Emergency Services
Celebration Health, Florida Hospital
Orlando, Florida

1997 AACN-3M Health Care Excellence in Clinical Practice Nominee

6

Cardiovascular Anatomy and Physiology

Paulette Morelli

Objectives

After completing this chapter, the student will be able to:

1. Describe the major structures of the heart and their functions.
2. Outline the normal physiologic changes in the cardiovascular system that occur with aging.
3. Explain the different components of hemodynamic monitoring.
4. Discuss the value and limitations of hemodynamic monitoring.
5. Relate the potential complications of hemodynamic monitoring with early detection assessment findings.
6. Analyze determinants of cardiac output.
7. Formulate nursing interventions to improve the balance between oxygen supply and demand.

The significance of this chapter is to lay the foundation of knowledge of the cardiovascular system needed by the nurse to make accurate assessments and to investigate patients' problems thoroughly. It is important to review normal anatomy and physiology before attempting to understand pathophysiology. Knowledge of cardiovascular anatomy and physiology will help the nurse to analyze and respond to consequences of abnormalities in this system.

ANATOMY

Heart

The heart is a hollow, muscular organ located in the mediastinal space of the chest, between the lungs and thoracic cavity (Figure 6–1). The average, healthy heart is approximately the size of the owner's clenched fist, about 12 cm long and 9 cm wide, weighing approximately 250 to 400 g, according to body size. The top of the heart is the base and the bottom is the apex. The apex of the heart is approximately two-thirds of its mass and it is located to the left of the midsternal line. The anterior view of the heart primarily consists of the right ventricle. The left atrium is the most posterior chamber. The apex or lateral surface is mostly composed of the left ventricle.

There are four distinct layers of the heart (Figure 6–2). The pericardium is a thin fibroserous sac that encases the heart. The space between the surface of the heart and the pericardium contains approximately 10 to 15 mL of fluid. This fluid serves as a lubricant to reduce friction during muscle contraction. It also serves as a protective barrier against infection and neoplasm.

The other three layers of the heart muscle are the endocardium (internal layer), the myocardium (middle layer), and the epicardium (external layer). The endocardium is a smooth layer of tissue forming the innermost lining of the heart and valves. The myocardium (heart muscle) is the thickest layer of the heart, located between the epicardium and the endocardium. It consists of fibrous skeletal tissue, cardiac muscle tissue, conduction tissues, and arteries and veins. The fibrous skeletal framework provides support for the atrial and ventricular musculature as well as the valvular tissue. The cells in this layer of the heart have the property of automaticity; they are responsible for the ability of the heart to contract. The myocardium uses high amounts of oxygen and does not fatigue easily. The epicardium (visceral pericardium) is the outermost layer of the

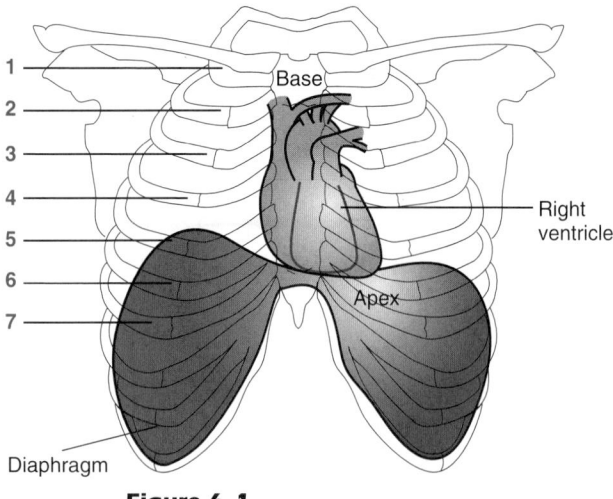

Figure 6–1

Location of the heart in the thoracic cavity.

heart. The coronary arteries cross this layer before entering the myocardium.

Chambers of the Heart

The heart can be divided into two anatomically distinct sides, the right side and the left side. Each side is further subdivided into an upper and lower chamber (Figure 6–3). The upper chambers, the atria, are separated by the interatrial septum. The atria receive blood from various parts of the body. The lower chambers, the ventricles, are separated by the interventricular septum. The ventricles pump blood to various parts of the body.

The right atrium is a thin-walled chamber that receives deoxygenated blood from the inferior vena cava, the superior vena cava, and the coronary sinus. Blood returns to the right side of the heart from all parts of the body through the vena cava. The inferior vena cava receives deoxygenated blood from the lower half of the body, and the superior vena cava drains deoxygenated blood from the upper portion of the body. Blood from the coronary veins drains into the right atrium through the coronary sinus. Blood flows from the right atrium into the right ventricle and is ejected through the pulmonary artery into the pulmonary circuit.

The ventricles serve as the pumps of the heart. The right ventricle is a thin-walled chamber, approximately 2 to 4 mm thick, that composes the inferior portion of the heart's apex. Blood leaves the right ventricle through the pulmonary artery and is pumped to the lungs, where it is reoxygenated.

The left atrium is slightly thicker than the right atrium. It receives oxygenated blood from the lungs through four pulmonary veins and empties into the left ventricle.

The left ventricle is three to five times thicker than the right ventricle, approximately 8 to 12 mm thick. This increase in musculature is necessary for the left

ventricle to be able to pump blood against the resistance of the entire circulation. For all intents and purposes, the left ventricle is the major pump of the heart. The heart propels blood from the left side of the heart across the aortic valve through the aorta into the arterial system.

Valves

There are two types of cardiac valves in the heart, the atrioventricular (AV) valves (tricuspid and mitral) and the semilunar valves (pulmonic and aortic). Together, these valves open to facilitate the forward flow of blood and close to seal the orifice, thus preventing regurgitation from one chamber to another (see Figure 6–3). The valves open and close in response to pressure gradients. The AV valves are inflow valves, situated between the atria and the ventricles. The semilunar valves sit in the outflow tracts of the ventricles. Each valve is composed of flexible fibrous tissue and a fibrous supporting ring (annulus). The AV valves have leaflets (cusps) attached by the chordae tendineae to papillary muscles (Figure 6–4). Contraction of the papillary muscles tenses the chordae tendineae, thus preventing the valves from everting into the atria during systole (contraction). The tricuspid valve, which is composed of three cusps, separates the right atrium and the right ventricle. The mitral valve, which separates the left atrium and the left ventricle, is made up

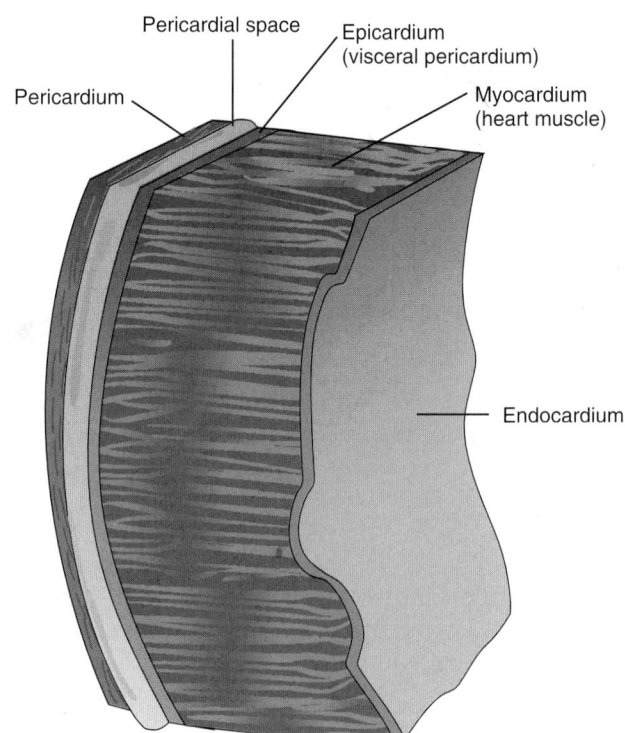

Figure 6–2

The heart has four distinct layers. The pericardium is a thin, fibroserous sac that encases the heart muscle (myocardium), the endocardium (internal layer), and the epicardium (external layer).

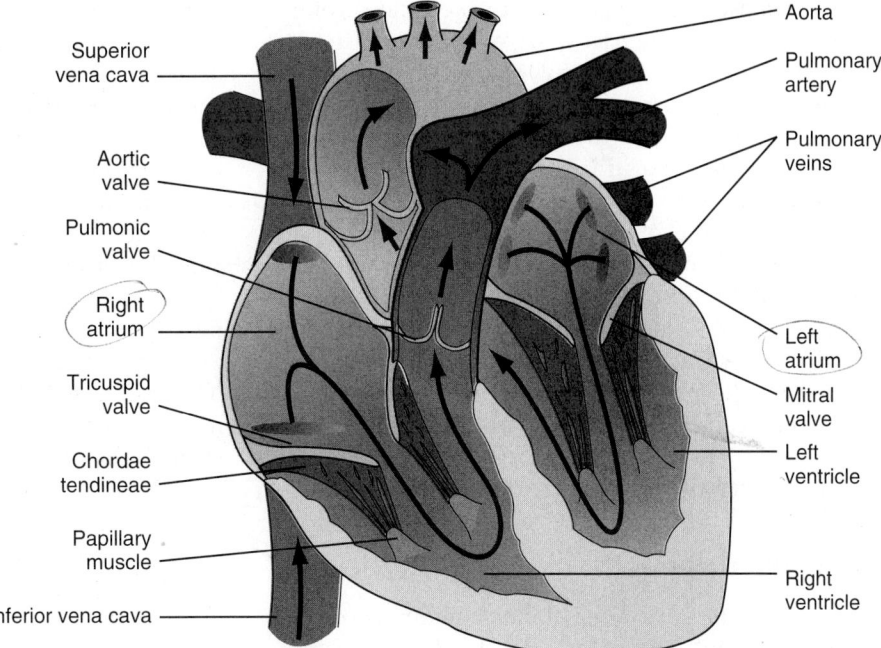

Figure 6–3

Normal heart cross section, illustrating the four chambers, the valves, and the major blood vessels. Arrows illustrate the flow of blood.

Superior vena cava

Aortic valve

Pulmonic valve

Right atrium

Tricuspid valve

Chordae tendineae

Papillary muscle

Inferior vena cava

Aorta

Pulmonary artery

Pulmonary veins

Left atrium

Mitral valve

Left ventricle

Right ventricle

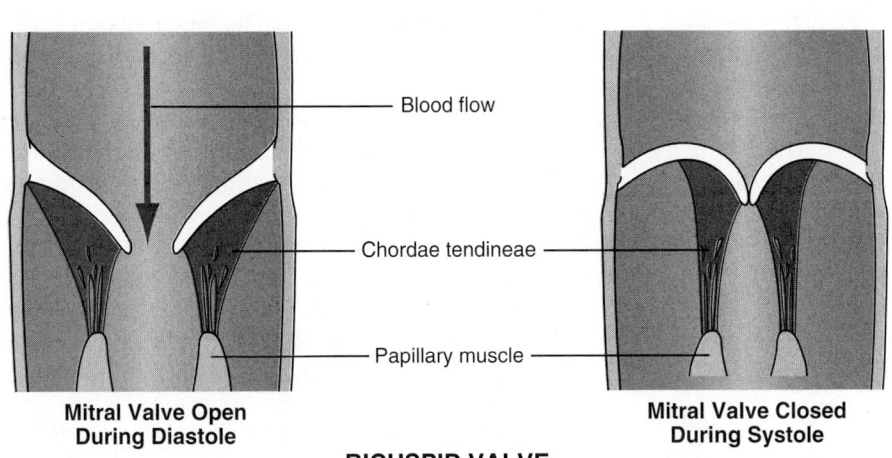

Blood flow

Chordae tendineae

Papillary muscle

Mitral Valve Open During Diastole

Mitral Valve Closed During Systole

BICUSPID VALVE

Figure 6–4

Close-up visualization of the bicuspid (mitral) and semilunar (aortic) valves.

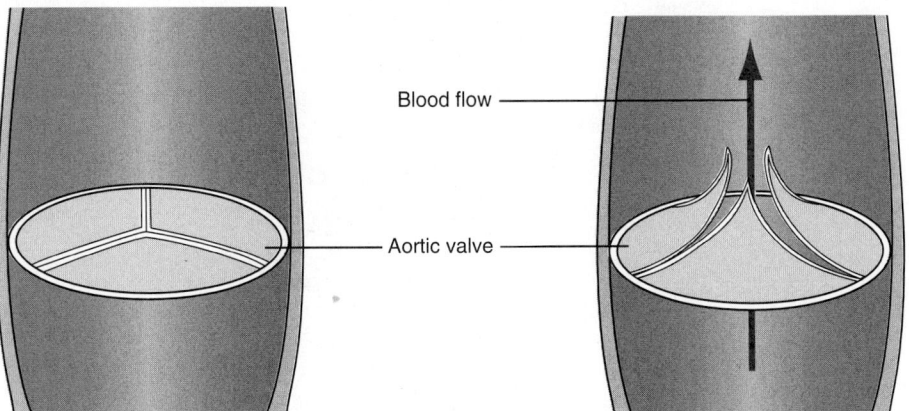

Blood flow

Aortic valve

Aortic Valve Closed During Diastole

Aortic Valve Open During Systole

SEMILUNAR VALVE

of two cusps. These cusps are thicker and stronger than the cusps of the tricuspid valve because the left ventricle is a more powerful pump. The semilunar valves consist of the pulmonic valve, situated in the summit of the outflow tract of the right ventricle, and the aortic valve, situated in the outflow tract of the left ventricle (see Figure 6–3). Structurally, these valves are not similar to the AV valves. The semilunar valves, which consists of three cusps of equal size, are composed of tough fibrous tissue to withstand the higher pressures in the ventricles (see Figure 6–4). During ventricular contraction, the free edges of the valves are opened by the pressure of the blood being expelled from the ventricles. During diastole (ventricular filling), the cusps fill with blood, closing the communication between the ventricles and the outflow vessels.

Coronary Arteries

The coronary arteries supply blood containing oxygen and essential nutrients to the heart. The two main coronary arteries, the left and right coronary arteries, originate from the coronary ostia in the aorta (Figure 6–5). The normal anatomy of coronary arteries has numerous variations. The left main coronary artery is short and bifurcates, shortly after its origin, into the left anterior descending artery and the circumflex artery. The left anterior descending artery supplies blood to the anterior portion of the left ventricle, a portion of the interventricular septum, and usually some portion the right ventricle. It usually supplies the anterior wall of the heart, as well as portions of the posterior and inferior portion of the apex. The circumflex branch curves at a 90° angle to the lateral left ventricle and apex. Branches of the circumflex artery supply blood to the left atrium and the posterior and lateral walls of the left ventricle,

and they usually terminate before reaching the posterior portion of the left AV groove. Should the circumflex artery continue in the AV groove, the coronary circulation is said to be left dominant.

The right coronary artery extends along the groove of the right atrium and right ventricle and along the posterior aspect of the interventricular septum. It supplies blood to the right atrium and right ventricle. Branches from the right coronary artery supply blood to the inferior surface of the left ventricle, where it terminates. When this artery supplies the posterior aspect of the heart, the coronary circulation is said to be dominant right. It also supplies blood to the sinoatrial (SA) node, the AV node, and the posterior papillary muscle in the right ventricle.

Collateral circulation consists of minute anastomoses or connections that exist between the smaller coronary arteries. These connections dilate during times of acute coronary occlusion. They increase in number in response to demand imposed by atherosclerotic heart disease, chronic anemia, or hypoxia.

Vascular System

Central Vascular System. The major vessels transporting blood to the heart include the inferior and superior vena cava and the pulmonary veins. The superior vena cava and the inferior vena cava empty deoxygenated blood into the right side of the heart, and this blood flows across the tricuspid valve into the right ventricle. Blood then travels past the pulmonic valve and into the pulmonary artery, to the lung capillaries, the pulmonary veins, and the left atrium. The oxygenated blood received from the lungs returns to the left atrium and moves through the mitral valve to the left ventricle, through the aortic valve to the aorta,

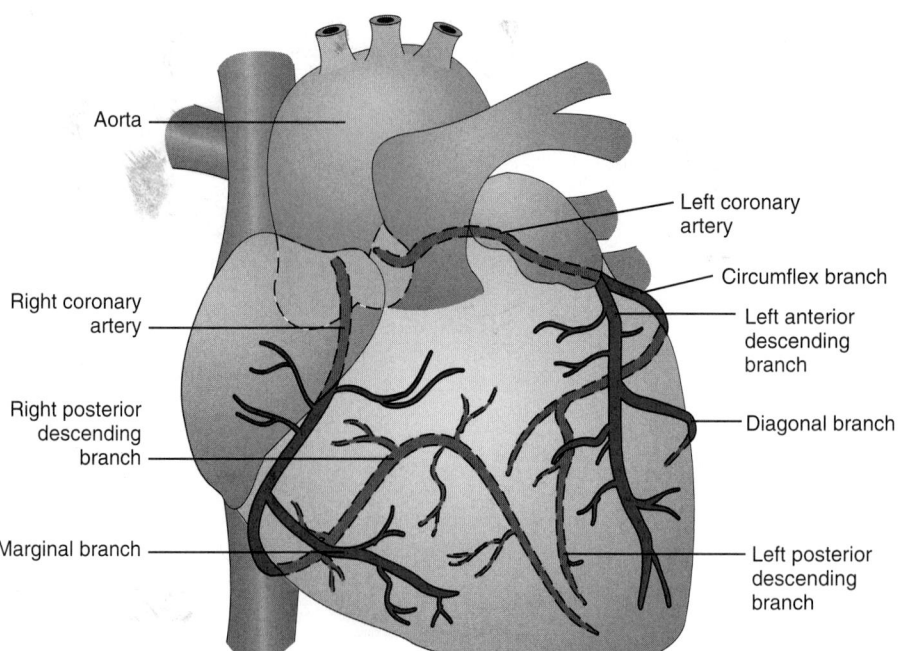

Figure 6–5

Normal heart, illustrating the origin and route of the major coronary arteries.

and out to the rest of the body (e.g., muscles, kidneys, brain). The aorta is the major vessel transporting oxygenated blood away from the heart for distribution to peripheral tissues.

Peripheral Vascular System. The peripheral system is a complex network of blood vessels composed of communicating systems within a larger system. Arteries have thick elastic walls that expand in response to the stroke volume or the volume of blood pumped out of the left ventricle with each contraction. The propagation of this pulse wave constitutes the pulse felt during an assessment.

Arteries divide and subdivide to arterioles, the smallest of these vessels. Arterioles are primarily composed of smooth muscle, which has the ability to constrict or dilate, thus controlling blood flow to different areas. These vessels receive their stimulation from the autonomic nervous system, which regulates the degree of vasoconstriction or vasodilation. Resistance to blood flow offered by the arterioles is called peripheral or systemic vascular resistance.

Capillaries are numerous vessels, one cell layer thick, that bring blood to the cellular level for the exchange of oxygen and carbon dioxide, the delivery of nutrients, and the removal of waste products. These exchanges occur by diffusion, osmosis, and hydrostatic pressure gradients among the blood, the capillary wall, and the cells. After the exchanges are complete, blood leaves the capillaries and is returned to the heart through the venules. Venules carry blood to larger vessels called veins.

Veins are thin-walled vessels composed of smooth muscle. They can expand and act as a reservoir for blood. Venous return to the heart is facilitated by the pumping action of the leg muscles and the one-way valves located in the leg veins.

Conduction System

The electrical activity (stimulation) of the heart is coupled with the mechanical activity (contraction) of the heart. The electrical activity occurs spontaneously before a contraction. This inherent property of cardiac muscle is known as automaticity. The conduction system of the heart is composed of the SA node, the AV node, the AV bundle (bundle of His), and the Purkinje fibers (Figure 6–6). These structures consist of highly specialized cardiac cells that permit either the generation or rapid conduction of an action potential (nerve impulse) throughout the heart.

The SA node is located in the wall of the right atrium, near the opening of the superior vena cava. The AV node sits in the interatrial septum, just above the opening of the coronary sinus. The AV bundle (bundle of His) stems from the AV node and divides into the right and left bundle branches on either side of the muscular part of the septum. The right bundle branch travels down the septum to the anterior wall of the right ventricle, further branching into a plexus of Purkinje fibers. The left bundle branch also travels down the septum to the anterior wall of the left ventricle, further branching into a plexus of Purkinje fibers.

The electrical stimulation required for muscle contraction and determination of the heart rate normally arises in the SA node, the "pacemaker" of the heart. This component of the conduction system has the fastest rate of automaticity, although each component of the conduction system can potentially become the "pacemaker" of the heart, with its own inherent rate. Normally, the electrical impulse is generated at the SA node and travels down to the AV node, to the AV bundle (bundle of His), which then quickly divides into the right bundle branch and the left bundle branch.

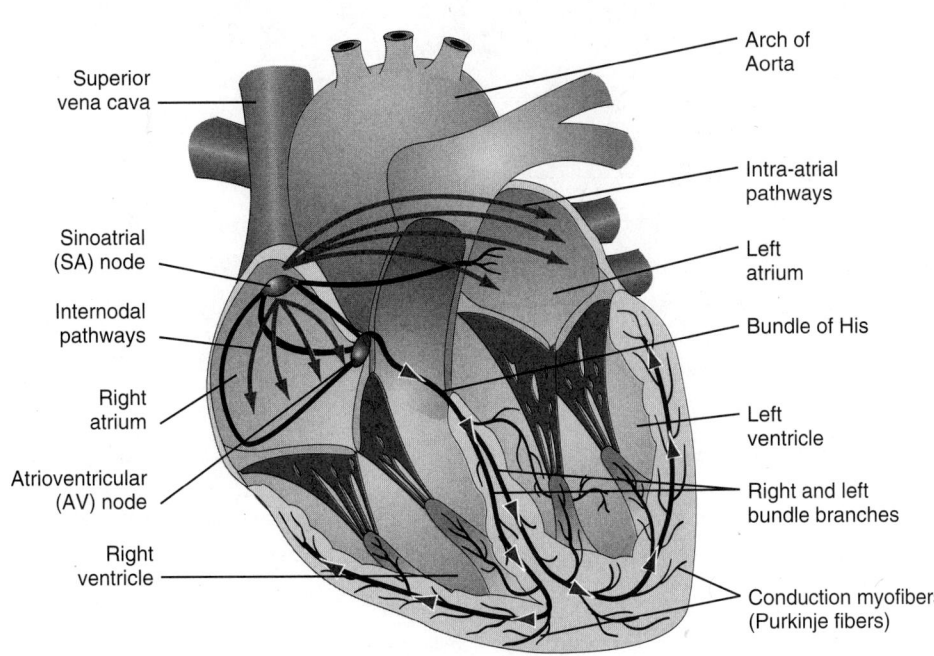

Superior vena cava

Sinoatrial (SA) node

Internodal pathways

Right atrium

Atrioventricular (AV) node

Right ventricle

Arch of Aorta

Intra-atrial pathways

Left atrium

Bundle of His

Left ventricle

Right and left bundle branches

Conduction myofibers (Purkinje fibers)

Figure 6–6

The conduction system. The arrows indicate the path the electrical impulse normally travels, beginning at the sinoatrial node.

Impulse excitation is then spread throughout the ventricles through a network of conduction myofibers called Purkinje fibers. The conduction of the impulse throughout the ventricle results in the depolarization of the myocardium and subsequent contraction.

PHYSIOLOGY

Heart

The healthy average heart beats 60 to 100 times a minute, ejecting approximately 60 to 80 mL blood (or stroke volume) from each ventricle with each contraction. The total cardiac output is approximately 5 L blood per minute and is calculated by multiplying the heart rate times the stroke volume. For example, if a person's heart rate is 70 beats per minute and the stroke volume is 70 mL, then this person's total cardiac output is 4900 mL per minute. Consider that an average person's heart rate is 80 beats per minute, beating 24 hours a day, for a life span of 80 years. This person's heart will beat a total of 33,638,400,000 times in a lifetime, without taking a rest.

Cardiac Cycle

The heart pumps blood throughout the body, thus supplying oxygen and essential nutrients to tissues and removing metabolic end products and gases from these same tissues. This process is accomplished through the cardiac cycle. The mechanical events of the cardiac cycle begin with relaxation of the ventricles during diastole and end with the closure of the semilunar valves at the conclusion of systole (contraction) (Figure 6–7). Both atria and ventricles contract and relax in unison to propel blood efficiently through the heart.

Diastole. Diastole comprises 60% of the cardiac cycle. This phase of the cardiac cycle has four components: isovolumetric relaxation of the ventricles, rapid filling of the ventricles, slow filling of the ventricles, and atrial contraction. During the isovolumetric relaxation of the ventricles, all the valves in the heart are closed, and the volume of blood in the ventricles remains constant. The tricuspid and mitral valves open when the pressures in the ventricles fall below the pressures in the atria. During this period, the atria and ventricles are essentially one chamber with equal pressure. Then rapid filling of the ventricles begins as

Figure 6–7

The cardiac cycle. The graphs demonstrate the relationships of the cardiac cycle, the generation of pressures within the heart, and the electrical activity of the heart. ECG, electrocardiogram.

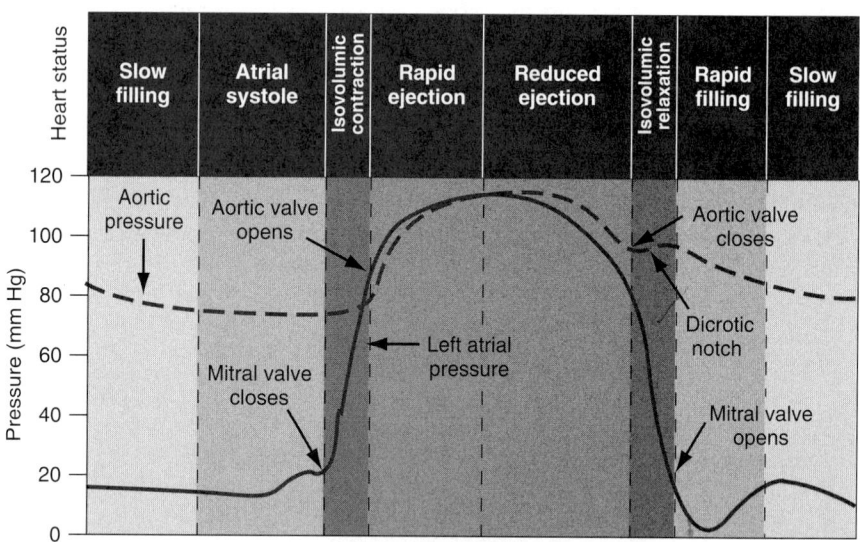
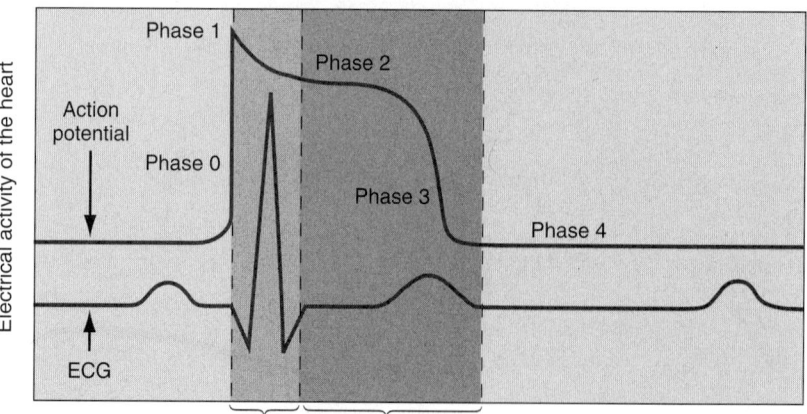

a result of the change in the pressure gradients and gravity. As the pressure gradient becomes less, the ventricles fill at a slower pace. Toward the end of diastole, the atria contract ("atrial kick"), raising the pressure within the atria and forcing blood into the ventricles. This additional blood volume can contribute an additional 30% to the cardiac output. At this point, the large volumes of blood in the ventricles create pressures that exceed those of the atria, thereby causing closure of the mitral and tricuspid valves. Closure of the mitral valve occurs slightly before closure of the tricuspid valve because left-sided pressures are greater and are created more quickly than right-sided pressures. During this relaxation phase of the cardiac cycle or diastole, blood flows through the coronary arteries. Closure of the AV valves heralds the onset of systole.

Systole. Systole constitutes 40% of the cardiac cycle. This phase of the cardiac cycle also has four components: isovolumetric contraction of the ventricles, rapid ventricular ejection, reduced ventricular ejection, and protodiastole. At the point at which all the valves are closed and the volume in the ventricles is constant, the ventricles begin to contract. When the pressures in the ventricles exceed the pressure in the outflow tract, the aortic and pulmonic valves open. During the rapid ventricular ejection, the ventricles propel blood into the aorta and pulmonary artery at a rapid rate. As the volume of blood remaining in the ventricles diminishes, there is less of a pressure gradient between the ventricles and their respective outflow tract, resulting in a slower rate of propulsion. During protodiastole, the ventricular pressures actually fall below the pressure of the aorta and pulmonary artery, thus causing the aortic and pulmonary valves to close. The amount of volume propelled out of the left ventricle, which is usually more than half, in proportion to the blood volume remaining in the left ventricle at the end of systole is called the ejection fraction. The normal ejection fraction is greater than 50%. The AV valves open, and ventricular filling begins, hence marking the beginning of another diastole.

Conduction System

The cycle of cellular activity that triggers the heartbeat (contraction) is known as the action potential. The difference in electrical charge on either side of the myocardial cell membrane is referred to as the membrane (resting) potential. At this stage, the membrane is said to be polarized. When an electrical stimulus is initiated, an exchange of ions inside and outside the cell establishes an action potential.

Phases of the Action Potential. There are five phases of an action potential (see Figure 6–7) involving four major electrolytes: sodium (Na^+), potassium (K^+), calcium (Ca^{++}), and chloride (Cl^-). Phase 0 of the action potential begins with a depolarizing stimulus, during which time the fast Na^+ channels open and the cross membrane potential of the cell switches from a negatively charged cell to a positively charged cell. This phase corresponds with ventricular depolarization (contraction). Phase 1 is equated with early repolarization, a brief period when the cells are less permeable to Na^+ and Cl^- flows into the cell. Phase 2 is known as the plateau phase of repolarization. Cells are less permeable to Na^+, and the slow inward flow of Ca^{++} maintains the plateau. Late repolarization, phase 3, results from the slow channels allowing equally charged ions through the cell membrane. The slow Ca^{++} channel becomes inactivated, and K^+ leaves the cell. The cell returns to its resting state. Phase 4 is known as complete repolarization and occurs synchronously with diastole. This phase is a refractory period and needs to occur so that the membrane can fully recover before accepting another stimulus.

After depolarization of the heart, the discharge of an electrical impulse through the myocardium results in a ventricular contraction. This type of action potential is found in the pacemaker cells of the heart, which propagate to adjacent cells, spontaneously depolarizing, without an outside stimulus. This property is referred to as automaticity and is an inherent property of the cardiac cells.

Cardiac Output

Cardiac output is the measurement of the heart's overall performance and a measure of blood flow to the periphery. It can be defined as the volume of blood that is pumped out of the heart per minute. It is best understood by the following equation:

$$CO = HR \times SV$$

where cardiac output (CO) is the product of heart rate (HR) and stroke volume (SV).

Cardiac output can be adjusted to meet the body's needs. During restful periods, metabolic requirements are low, and cardiac output may only be 2 to 3 L per minute. However, during periods of increased body needs (e.g., exercise), cardiac output increases by increasing the parameters that determine cardiac output. For example, the heart rate can increase to meet metabolic demands of the body.

Stroke volume is the amount of blood ejected from the ventricle with each heart beat. The normal range for stroke volume is 60 to 80 mL per beat, but it can also increase to meet the metabolic demands of the body. It can increase in conjunction with the heart rate or in response to a lower heart rate in an attempt to maintain a normal cardiac output. The three determinants of stroke volume are preload, afterload, and contractility. Table 6–1 summarizes the parameters for cardiac output and includes important formulas and normal ranges for additional hemodynamic parameters as well as causes of deviations in these parameters.

TABLE 6-1

Hemodynamic Parameters

Parameter	Normal	Formula	Causes of High Values	Causes of Low Values
Cardiac index (CI)	2.5–4 L/min/m^2	CO/BSA	Sepsis (due to peripheral vasodilation)	Abnormal heart rate ↓Contractility ↓Preload ↑Afterload
Cardiac output (CO)	4–8 L/min	HR × SV	Sepsis (due to peripheral vasodilation)	Abnormal heart rate ↓Contractility ↓Preload ↑Afterload
Central venous pressure/right atrial pressure (CVP/RAP)	2–6 cm H$_2$O 2–8 mm Hg		Fluid overload, venous constriction, pulmonary hypertension	Dehydration, diuretics, hemorrhage venodilation, third spacing, dysrhythmias
Left ventricular stroke work index (LVSWI)	40–70 g/m^2/beat	SVI(MAP − PAOP) × .0136	Response to catecholamines (β stimulants, milrinone), normal electrolyte levels, aerobic metabolism, <40% loss of functional myocardium, increased preload	Myocardial infarction, drugs (β blockers, calcium channel blockers), hyponatremia, hyperkalemia, anaerobic metabolism, >40% loss of functional myocardium, decreased preload, myocardial depressant factor
Mean arterial pressure (MAP)	70–105 mm Hg	$\dfrac{SBP + (2 \times DBP)}{3}$	Vasoconstriction, inotropic agents, polycythemia, shock (cardiogenic, hypovolemic), atherosclerosis	Vasodilation, modest hypoxemia, anemic states, drugs (nitrates, milrinone, β and calcium channel blockers), shock (septic, anaphylactic, neurogenic)
Mixed venous oxygen saturation (SVO$_2$)	60–80%		↑O$_2$ supply: ↑SaO$_2$ 　　　　　↑Hgb ↓O$_2$ demand: ↓VO$_2$ 　　　　　VO$_2$, O$_2$ ↓Utilization of O$_2$ by tissues	↓O$_2$ supply: ↓CO 　　　　　↓SaO$_2$ 　　　　　↓Hgb ↑O$_2$ demand: ↑VO$_2$ 　　　　　↑CO

Parameter	Normal value	Formula	Increased by	Decreased by
Pulmonary artery occlusive pressure (PAOP) or wedge	8–15 mm Hg		Hypertension, fluid overload, pulmonary hypertension	Dehydration, diuretics, vasodilation
Pulmonary artery pressures (PAP)	15–30 mm Hg (systolic), 8–15 mm Hg (diastolic), 10–20 mm Hg (mean)		Hypertension, vasoconstriction, pulmonary edema, pulmonary hypertension	Dehydration, diuretics, β and calcium channel blockers
Pulmonary vascular resistance index (PVRI)	180–285 dynes/s/cm^{-5}-m^2	$\dfrac{PAM - PAOP}{CI} \times 80$	Hypoxia, hypercapnia, vasoconstriction, pulmonary edema, pulmonary embolus, COPD, mitral stenosis, shock (cardiogenic, hypovolemic)	Vasodilation, drugs (nitrates, milrinone, β and calcium channel blockers) shock (septic, anaphylactic, neurogenic)
Right ventricular pressures (RVP)	15–30 mm Hg (systolic), 2–8 mm Hg (diastolic)		Fluid overload, venous constriction, pulmonary hypertension	Dehydration, diuretics, hemorrhage venodilation, third spacing, dysrhythmias
Right ventricular stroke work index (RVSWI)	7–12 g/m^2/beat	$SVI(PAM - CVP) \times .0136$	Response to catecholamines (β stimulants, milrinone), normal electrolyte levels, aerobic metabolism, <40% loss of functional myocardium, increased preload	Myocardial infarction, myocardial depressant factor, drugs (β blockers, calcium channel blockers), hyponatremia, hyperkalemia, anaerobic metabolism, >40% loss of functional myocardium, decreased preload
Stroke volume (SV)	60–80 mL/beat	CO/HR	Exercise, bradycardia, positive inotropic agents	Tachydysrhythmias, extreme vasodilation, cardiac tamponade
Systemic vascular resistance index (SVRI)	1970–2390 dynes/s/cm^{-5}-m^2	$\dfrac{MAP - CVP}{CI} \times 80$	Vasoconstriction, inotropic agents, polycythemia, shock (cardiogenic, hypovolemic), atherosclerosis	Vasodilation, modest hypoxemia, anemic states, drugs (nitrates, milrinone, β and calcium channel blockers), shock (septic, anaphylactic, neurogenic)

BSA, body surface area; DBP and SBP, diastolic and systolic blood pressure; HR, heart rate; PAM, pulmonary artery mean pressure; SaO$_2$, arterial oxygen saturation

Preload is the volume and pressure generated within the ventricle at the end of diastole; it is a measurement of ventricular end-diastolic volume. Preload is reduced with rapid heart rates, hemorrhage, and dehydration, to name a few examples. It is increased when the heart's pumping abilities are reduced, as in congestive heart failure and cardiogenic shock. This volume determines the degree of stretch or pressure in the ventricle at the end of diastole. It is best explained using Starling's law, which states that the more a myocardial fiber is stretched further during diastole, the more it shortens in systole and the greater the force of contraction. Increased force and shortening are required to convert increased venous return into increased stroke volume.

Essentially, Starling's law explains the heart's ability to adjust its output according to venous return. Several direct hemodynamic measurements measure preload. Right atrial pressure (RAP) or central venous pressure (CVP) reflects preload in the right side of the heart, and pulmonary artery occlusive pressure (PAOP) is a measurement of preload in the left side of the heart.

The force of resistance against which the heart has to pump to eject blood during systole is afterload. The greater the resistance, the greater is the tension within the ventricles. High afterload values result in a decreased stroke volume, and low afterload values result in an increased stroke volume. Afterload values are determined through derived parameters. The pulmonary vascular resistance (PVR) pressure reflects right ventricular afterload, and the systemic vascular resistance (SVR) pressure reflects left ventricular afterload.

Contractility, also called inotropy, is the force generated by the contracting myocardium. It is an inherent property of the heart, but it can be altered. Contractility can be increased by elevated levels of circulating catecholamines, by sympathetic neuronal activity, and by certain drugs. A classic example is digoxin, a positive inotrope, which is usually given to increase the force of contraction. Beta blockers typically have a negative inotropic effect on the heart and depress the force of contraction.

NORMAL STRUCTURE AND FUNCTIONAL CHANGES ASSOCIATED WITH AGING

It is reported that 83% of people who die of heart attacks are 65 years or older, but whether age-related changes or cardiac disease places the elderly at a higher risk is unclear. The common belief that "all old people are alike" is so much in error. The truth is that age-related cardiac changes vary in this population. However, the challenge of distinguishing changes associated with aging from those caused by disease remains. Table 6–2 summarizes the key physiologic changes and associated consequences in the cardiac system that occur with aging.

The heart, as it ages, remains the same or becomes slightly smaller. The heart rate, stroke volume, and cardiac output decrease.[1, 2] At ages 20 through 80 years, there is a linear regression in cardiac indices, although this change is more evident at ages 60 through 70 years and also is more pronounced at the upper

TABLE 6–2
Cardiac Changes Associated With Aging

Anatomic or Physiologic Change	Potential Consequences
Cardiac Changes	
LV hypertrophy	Decreased LV reserve
	Decreased cardiac output
Thickening and calcification of cardiac valves	Increased heart pressures
Conduction Changes	
Fibrosis of SA node	Decreased heart rate
	Sick sinus syndrome
Altered baroreceptor reflex	Decreased heart rate
	Orthostatic hypotension
Vascular Changes	
Elongation and stiffness of aorta	Decreased cardiac output
	Slightly increased BP
Arterial stiffening and thickening	Slightly increased BP

BP, blood pressure; LV, left ventricle; SA, sinoatrial

limits with maximal exercise.[3] The overall decrease in the number of pacemaker cells and the fibrosis of the SA node contribute to the decrease in heart rate. These factors often result in decreased efficiency of the conduction system and can lead to cardiac dysrhythmias. In addition, the heart becomes less responsive to the impulses of the sympathetic nervous system and more prone to irritability.

The blood vessels, particularly the aorta and its major branches, become stiffer, leading to an increase in peripheral resistance in the elderly. As people age, the walls of their blood vessels have less elastin and less smooth muscle fiber. This change, in conjunction with an increase in collagen, calcium, and lipid deposition and decreases in connective tissue and in elasticity, results in vascular rigidity and increased vascular resistance to blood flow. These changes all contribute to increased impedance against which the ventricle has to pump. The resultant elevated blood pressure is considered to be a result of advancing age.[3,4]

The dilation of the aorta and elevation of the systolic blood pressure result in hypertrophy of the left ventricular wall.[3] This hypertrophy is also a consequence of a degenerative process in the connective tissue and results in increased ventricular wall thickness with or without chamber dilation. Although advancing age alone is a risk factor for the development of left ventricular hypertrophy, coexisting hypertension and obesity increase the prevalence and severity of this condition.

A higher prevalence of systolic ejection murmurs is encountered in the elderly population. With aging, an increase in fibrosis and calcification of the aortic valve cusps causes these cusps to become more rigid. This substantial thickening, together with the dilation of the aorta, produces the systolic murmurs often heard in this population.

A diminished baroreceptor reflex and thus a reduction in vasomotor responsiveness are associated with advanced age and do make the elderly more prone to orthostatic hypotension.[2] The baroreceptors in the large arteries lose their effectiveness in controlling blood pressure, especially during postural changes.

Atherosclerosis, which involves a buildup of fatty substances in and fibrosis of the inner layer of arteries, is common in the elderly population. Autopsy studies have demonstrated evidence of atherosclerosis in 70% of persons past the seventh decade of life.[5] In actuality, atherosclerosis begins at a young age and takes many years to progress to the symptomatic stage.

Many cardiac changes occur as a part of the aging process, and these complex phenomena often obscure the cause of acute cardiac problems in the elderly. More research in this area is needed, to understand better the fine line that separates "normal" physiologic processes from pathologic cardiac changes in this population.

BASIC CONCEPTS OF HEMODYNAMICS

Hemodynamic Monitoring

Hemodynamic monitoring is a common and vital practice in intensive care and step-down units. It provides for immediately accessible information regarding the cardiovascular functioning of the patient, so that rapid response to and treatment of actual or potential problems can occur. The purpose of hemodynamic monitoring is to assess, diagnose, and evaluate treatment modalities for the acutely ill patient. This goal can be accomplished by inserting an intra-arterial catheter (A-line) or a flow-directed, balloon-flotation pulmonary artery catheter. Either catheter, attached to an oscilloscope (Figure 6–8), can provide invaluable data. It is important to understand general concepts related to direct monitoring. The pressure transducer converts pressure within a vessel into electrical impulses that are then displayed on an oscilloscope by way of a pressure curve. The oscilloscope also displays pressure values sensed by the transducer.

Arterial Catheter

Insertion of an arterial catheter provides continuous readouts of direct blood pressure measurements. Candidates for A-lines include the following: 1) patients experiencing sustained hypotension or hypovolemia; 2) patients receiving vasoactive drugs that require continuous blood pressure monitoring; 3) patients needing continuous or intermittent blood pressure monitoring because of difficulties in obtaining blood pressure by the cuff method; and 4) patients requiring access for frequent blood sampling.

An A-line can be inserted into a radial, brachial, axillary, femoral, or dorsalis pedis artery. The radial artery is the most common site for the insertion of an A-line. This is because of the ease in accessing this artery and the collateral circulation available through the radial and ulnar arcade. Adequate collateral circulation is verified by performing an Allen test before insertion of the catheter (Figure 6–9). The femoral artery is probably the second most popular site for A-line insertion. It is frequently targeted in emergency situations because insertion through this larger artery can be accomplished quickly. However, this site carries a higher risk of infection because of its proximity to the perineum.

Arterial blood pressure is generated by two forces, one created by the volume of blood in the arteries and the other by the vessels imposing resistance against which the heart has to pump. Cardiac output, the amount of blood ejected by the ventricle, and the SVR are two important factors that determine arterial blood pressure. The normal blood pressure is 100 to 140 mm Hg systolic and 60 to 90 mm Hg diastolic. The normal mean arterial pressure (MAP) is 70 to 100 mm Hg. MAP

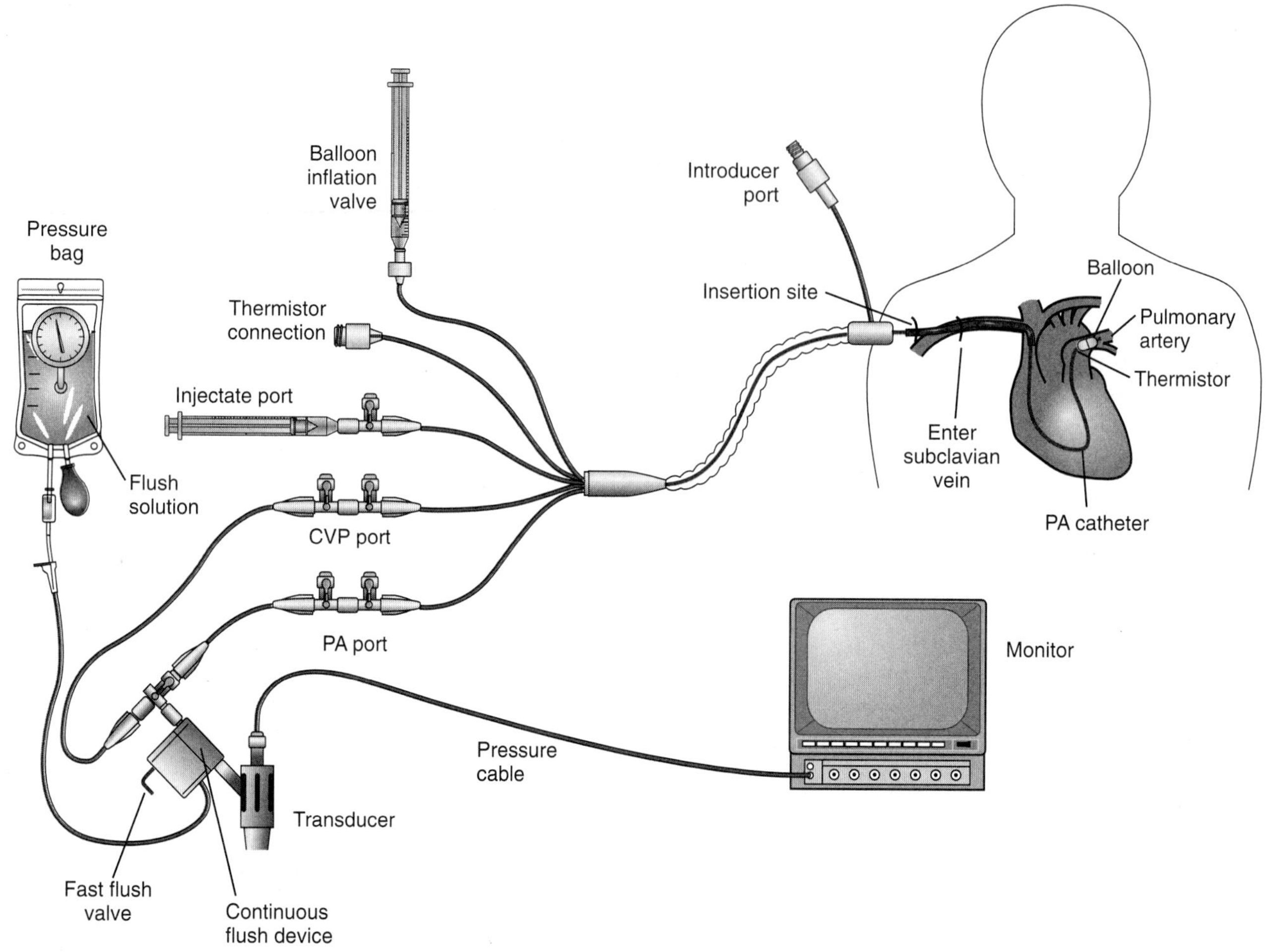

Balloon
inflation
valve

Pressure
bag

Thermistor
connection

Injectate port

Flush
solution

CVP port

PA port

Fast flush
valve

Continuous
flush device

Transducer

Introducer
port

Insertion site

Balloon

Pulmonary
artery

Thermistor

Enter
subclavian
vein

PA catheter

Monitor

Pressure
cable

Figure 6–8

Basic setup for hemodynamic monitoring. CVP, central venous pressure; PA, pulmonary artery.

is the most frequently used parameter to assess perfusion pressure throughout the cardiac cycle. A minimum MAP of 60 mm Hg is needed to perfuse the vital organs. MAP can be calculated from blood pressure (BP):

$$MAP = systolic\ BP + (2 \times diastolic\ BP)/3$$

Systole consists of one-third of the cardiac cycle, and diastole consists of two-thirds of the cardiac cycle.

The normal waveform for an invasive blood measurement pressure begins with an initial sharp rise, indicating the ejection of blood from the left ventricle and an increase in pressure in the arterial system

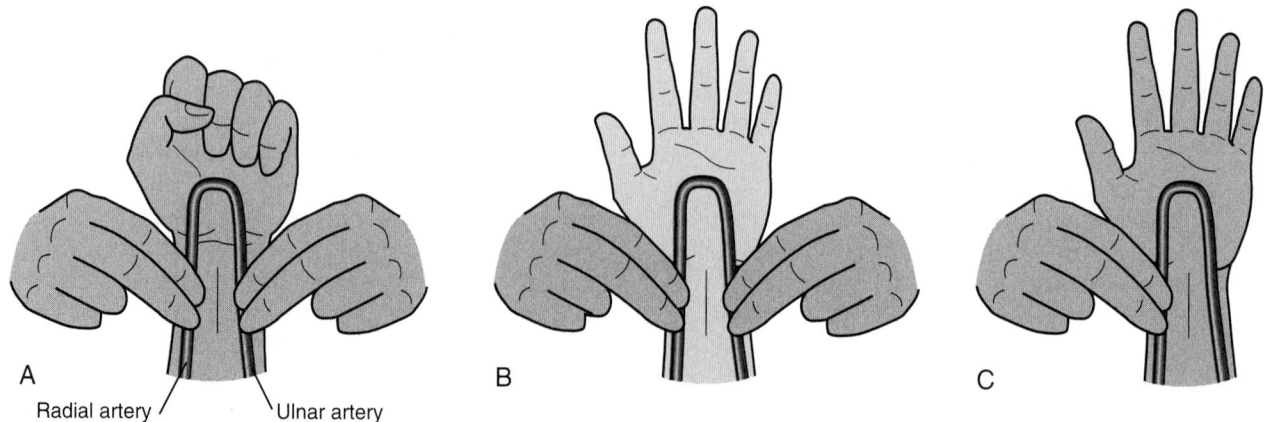

A

Radial artery   Ulnar artery

B

C

Figure 6–9

The Allen test. A, The patient is instructed to clench the fist and elevate the hand. The radial and ulnar arteries are simultaneously occluded by the nurse. B, The patient's hand should be observed for blanching. C, The hand is then lowered and opened, and only the pressure on the ulnar artery is released. Color should return to the hand within 6 seconds, thus indicating adequate collateral blood flow to the hand by the ulnar artery.

(Figure 6–10). The rounded top represents the peak systolic pressure. After the peak systolic pressure, force of contraction diminishes, and the pressure drops. The slight upswing of the waveform is called the dicrotic notch and represents the closure of the aortic valve. Tapering off after the dicrotic notch is the lowest point in diastole. The arterial pressure waveform always occurs just after the depolarization of the ventricles (QRS complex on the ECG).

Abnormal waveforms can result in erroneous measurements, and treatment based on this determination could result in detrimental outcomes. Some causes of abnormal waveforms include dampening, respiratory artifact, catheter fling, dysrhythmias, aortic stenosis, and aortic regurgitation.

Nursing management of an A-line is as critical as the management of the critically ill patient. An A-line is in an artery, and if it should become disconnected, the patient could exsanguinate within minutes. Consequently, all connections should be secured tightly on setup and checked frequently. In addition, the patient needs to be assessed for adequate circulation to the cannulated limb. This assessment includes inspection of skin color, palpation of skin temperature, and assessment of capillary refill and distal pulses, if appropriate. Motor function and sensation of the cannulated limb also need to be assessed. This direct method of obtaining arterial blood pressure measurements needs to correlated with an indirect method routinely or when the obtained value is in question. Keep in mind that the direct method of obtaining a blood pressure results from a pulse of pressure generated from ventricular contraction. The indirect method (cuff) of ob-

taining a blood pressure measures blood flow, not a pulse of pressure. Usually, the higher blood pressure value is used to direct interventions. Observation of the patient, management of equipment, and close analysis of the trends of direct blood pressure measurements prove invaluable in the management of the critically ill patient.

As with any invasive line, complications can occur. These complications include hemorrhage, infection, thrombosis, vasospasm, compromised circulation, and nerve injury. It is imperative that the institution's guidelines for management of an invasive line be strictly adhered to, to avoid potential problems.

Balloon-Flotation Pulmonary Artery Catheter

Placement of a flow-directed, balloon-flotation pulmonary artery catheter is a more complex procedure. Reasons for selecting this invasive method of hemodynamic monitoring include the following: (1) measuring intracardiac pressures; (2) determining cardiac output; and (3) obtaining intracardiac and mixed venous blood samples. The catheter used for insertion is usually 110 cm long and has four to five ports (Figure 6–11). A proximal port opens to the right atrium. This port is used to instill injectate for cardiac output determinations. The ventricular port terminates in the right ventricle and is approximately 19 cm from the tip of the catheter. This port offers an extra line for infusion of fluids or drugs. The distal port terminates at the end of the pulmonary artery catheter and is attached to the flush system. The balloon-inflation port terminates 1 cm from the tip of the catheter and terminates in the pulmonary artery. By inflating the balloon, the catheter floats forward in the pulmonary artery until it is in a wedged position. Finally, the fifth port is the thermistor, which is located 3.7 cm from the tip of the catheter and is used for measuring core temperature and for calculating cardiac output.

For insertion, the pulmonary artery catheter is passed through a central vein (subclavian, brachial, internal jugular, or femoral) to the right atrium, right ventricle, and then into the pulmonary artery. The right atrium is a low-pressure chamber and generates its own waveform. Mean right atrial pressures range from 0 to 8 mm Hg. From the right atrium, the catheter is then passed to the right ventricle, where the chamber pressure is greater because of the dynamic pumping action of the heart. In this chamber, diastolic pressure is about the same as in the right atrium (during diastole, the tricuspid valve is open and the right side is essentially one chamber), but systolic pressure is much higher. As the catheter is advanced into the pulmonary artery, again the pressure changes, reflecting the even higher pressure in the pulmonary artery. The last waveform is produced by floating the

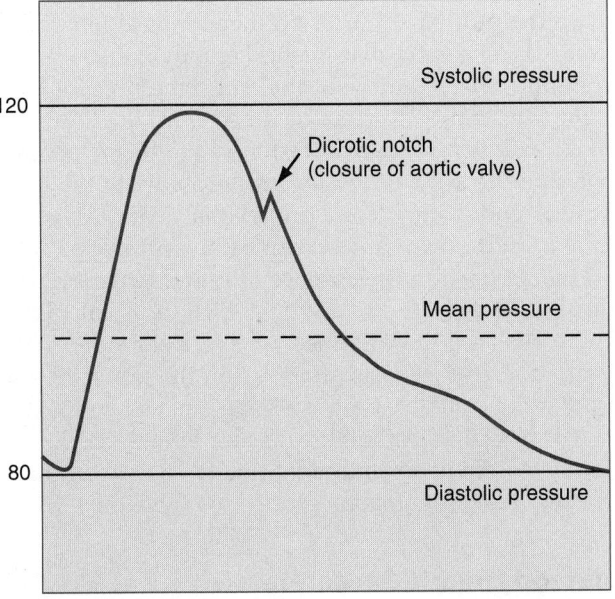

Figure 6–10

Normal arterial waveform. The sharp rise signifies left ventricular systole, the rounded slope represents the peak systolic pressure, the dicrotic notch occurs with closure of the aortic valve, and the descending slope signifies the beginning of diastole.

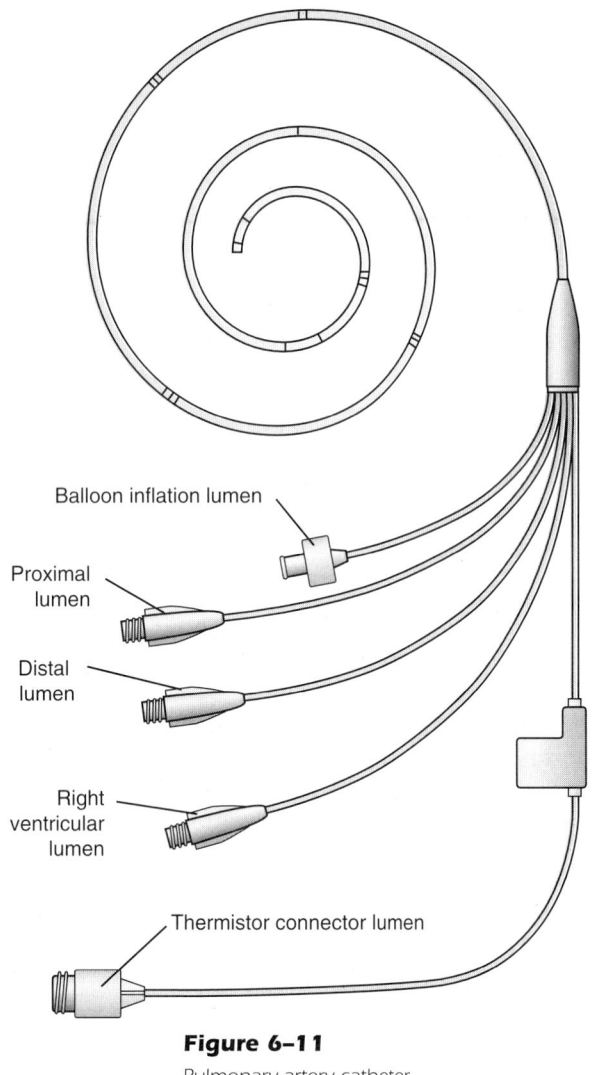

Balloon inflation lumen

Proximal lumen

Distal lumen

Right ventricular lumen

Thermistor connector lumen

Figure 6–11

Pulmonary artery catheter.

balloon-filled catheter into a branch of the pulmonary artery. This pressure is the PAOP, formerly known as pulmonary capillary wedge pressure. When the balloon is inflated, forward blood flow is occluded, and pressures can be measured beyond the tip of the catheter. This measurement reflects performance of the left side of the heart, specifically the left ventricular end-diastolic pressure (LVEDP) or left ventricular end-diastolic volume (LVEDV), or left ventricular preload. The PAOP waveform is similar to the right atrial waveform, although the PAOP reading is usually slightly higher. The various pressure tracings are depicted in Figure 6–12.

To obtain periodic PAOP readings, the balloon should be inflated slowly up to the amount recommended by the manufacturer, which is clearly marked on the catheter, or until the waveform dampens. As the waveform dampens from the pulmonary artery waveform to the PAOP waveform, the nurse should obtain the reading at the end of expiration for greatest accuracy and consistency. During the respiratory cycle, and

especially during inspiration, changes in the intrathoracic pressure exert significant changes in the intracardiac pressure. Positive-pressure ventilation also affects intracardiac pressure, and this is reflected by an increase in the PAOP. For patients on ventilators, it may serve better to obtain readings on and off the ventilator. This information provides for the actual effects of the positive-pressure ventilation on PAOP. Regardless of the steps taken to obtain PAOP readings, a consistent pattern must be followed so that trends are accurately interpreted.

A few tips to remember when taking a PAOP reading are as follows. Keep the balloon inflated for only 5 to 10 seconds, do not overinflate, and limit the frequency and duration of the inflation. The balloon should always be allowed to deflate passively: do not pull back on the syringe. If the balloon has ruptured, tape the port closed, tag a sign to this port, and communicate the problem. In this event, the pulmonary artery diastolic pressure can be used to estimate the PAOP. The PAOP is usually 1 to 4 mm Hg lower than the pulmonary artery diastolic pressure, except in patients with lung disease or severe mitral valve dysfunction. In these patients, the PAOP may be 5 mm Hg or more than the pulmonary artery diastolic pressure.

Understanding and recognizing waveforms and respective pressures provide invaluable information regarding the critically ill patient's cardiovascular status. Monitoring trends in these parameters aids the health team to detect and treat imminent problems and to evaluate the efficacy of different therapeutic modalities.

Hemodynamic Pressures

Once the pulmonary artery catheter is inserted and is verified for correct placement, hemodynamics can be continuously monitored. Preload pressures on the right side of the heart are obtained from the CVP and RAP readings. These values reflect the blood volume entering the right ventricle and the ability of the right atrium and ventricle to propel that volume to the lungs. On the left, preload can be measured by PAOP measurements. In the absence of mitral valve disease, the PAOP reflects the LVEDV. PVR is a calculated value that reflects afterload on the right side of the heart, and SVR reflects afterload on the left. PVR and SVR can be indexed by dividing the values by the body surface area (BSA). Indexing allows the health team to account for individual body size when interpreting hemodynamic pressures (see Table 6–1).

Hemodynamic Parameters

Table 6–1 provides a summary of normal hemodynamic parameters as well as situations that can cause values to be elevated or decreased. The pressures that

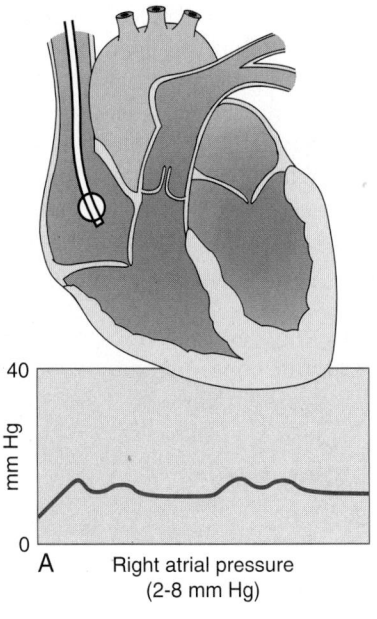

40

mm Hg

0

A   Right atrial pressure
(2-8 mm Hg)

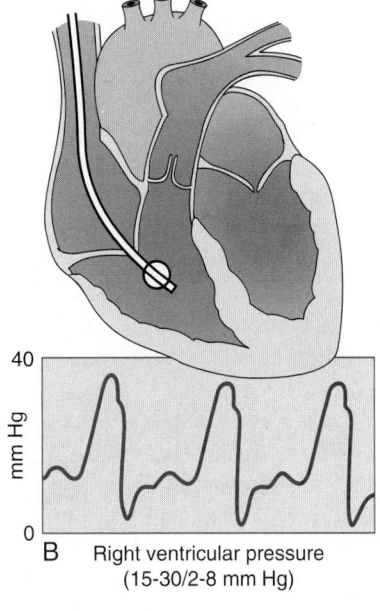

40

mm Hg

0

B   Right ventricular pressure
(15-30/2-8 mm Hg)

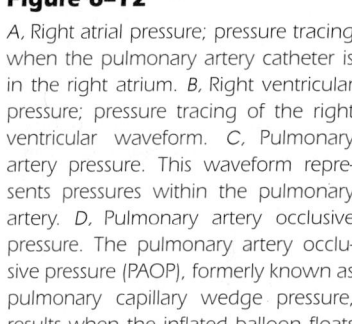

Figure 6–12

A, Right atrial pressure; pressure tracing when the pulmonary artery catheter is in the right atrium. *B*, Right ventricular pressure; pressure tracing of the right ventricular waveform. *C*, Pulmonary artery pressure. This waveform represents pressures within the pulmonary artery. *D*, Pulmonary artery occlusive pressure. The pulmonary artery occlusive pressure (PAOP), formerly known as pulmonary capillary wedge pressure, results when the inflated balloon floats into a branch of the pulmonary artery.

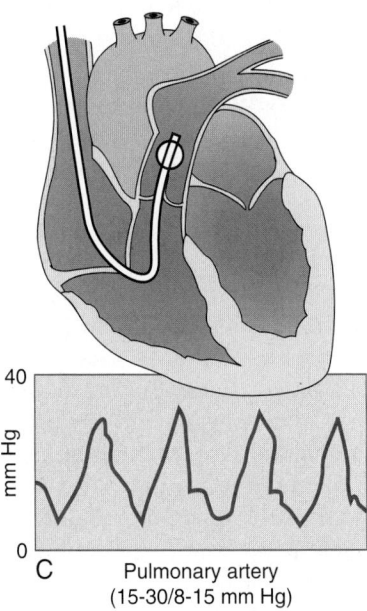

40

mm Hg

0

C   Pulmonary artery
(15-30/8-15 mm Hg)

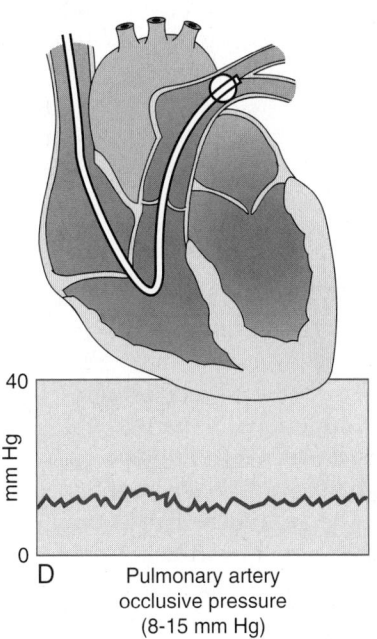

40

mm Hg

0

D   Pulmonary artery
occlusive pressure
(8-15 mm Hg)

can be measured directly include the right atrial, right ventricular, pulmonary artery, and PAOP pressures and the cardiac output. These direct measurements can be obtained using a flow-directed balloon-tipped pulmonary artery catheter and are incorporated into formulas to calculate parameters reflective of pressures on the left side of the heart. A single abnormal value is not a reason to initiate or change a therapy. Hemodynamic values must be trended and correlated with clinical findings.

Cardiac Output. Measurements for cardiac output determinations can be obtained by continuous readings or by intermittent readings. In a comparison study between continuous cardiac outputs and intermittent thermodilution cardiac outputs, results showed that these methods were clinically comparable.[6] The intermittent method consists of a minimum of three injections of 10 mL normal saline at room temperature pushed quickly (up to 4 seconds) and evenly through the proximal port of the pulmonary artery catheter at the end of expiration. Measurements are determined by the temperature change sensed by the thermistor at the distal end of the pulmonary artery catheter. Cardiac output measurements generate a waveform on the monitor determined by the integration of the area under the curve. At least three measurements within 10% of the median value are averaged to provide the mean cardiac output. Continuous cardiac output determinations are calculated in a similar manner. However, the continuous cardiac output method employs heat rather than cold. The heater and thermister probe of the pulmonary artery catheter are connected to the continuous cardiac output monitor for continuous measurements displayed on the monitor.[6]

Newer technology has afforded cardiac output to be monitored nonivasively and also continuously by a method called thoracic electrical bioimpedence (TEB), using the electrocardiogram tracing and changes in impedence. This technique measures pulsatile changes in the electrical conductivity of tissue as it passes through the chest. TEB measurements can be accomplished with the use of gelled electrode pads placed on the patient's anterior chest and lateral sides of the neck and attached to the cardiac monitor. One study cited clinically unacceptable errors with TEB measurements in earlier research studies, as well as the researcher's own current work, which revealed errors in evaluating cardiac performance in patients with heart disease.[7] Although much research has been conducted on the accuracy of TEB measurements, posing limitations on use in certain patient populations, research continues to aid in refining this easy, convenient, noninvasive, and continuous alternative for assessing and monitoring cardiovascular parameters.

Mixed Venous Oxygen Saturation Monitoring

Mixed venous oxygen saturation (SVO_2) monitoring is a significant and more sophisticated addition to hemodynamic monitoring. It provides accurate and continuous measurement of SVO_2 by the use of a fiberoptic, flow-directed, thermodilution pulmonary artery catheter. Readings from this catheter reflect the percentage of hemoglobin that is bound with oxygen in venous blood and is monitored as an indicator of circulatory adequacy. SVO_2 represents how much oxygen is attached to hemoglobin (Hgb) in venous blood (the amount of oxygen "left over"). It is determined by Fick's principle:

$$CO\ (1.34 \times Hgb \times SaO_2) \times 10$$

SVO_2 values reflect the relationship between the oxygen supply and oxygen reserve, the body's ability to provide adequate oxygen to satisfy tissue demands. Oxygen demand is the amount of oxygen the tissues require to meet the metabolic needs and is influenced by cellular metabolic rate, body temperature, and exercise. When tissues require more oxygen, or if the available oxygen diminishes, tissues extract more oxygen than usual from capillary blood. The result is that less oxygenated blood returns to the heart. SVO_2 measurements between 60 and 80% suggest adequate tissue oxygen delivery and utilization. Measurement trends that fall outside this range require reevaluation of the patient as well as the current therapies. A low value indicates decreased oxygen availability or increased use of oxygen. This information is of utmost value when planning nursing care. A summary of causes of high and low SVO_2 values is available in Table 6–1. If a patient has a low SVO_2, then the nurse must consider the physiologic effects of certain nursing care activities. Repositioning, suctioning, and bathing, for example, could further deplete oxygen reserves by increasing the metabolic demands associated with these activities. "Routine" nursing care activities, in this case, would not have a routine consequence.

Complications of Pulmonary Artery Monitoring

The benefits of pulmonary artery monitoring have been presented, but this intervention is not without hazard. Awareness of the potential risks of inserting, maintaining, and removing the catheter can alert the nurse to prevent or quickly respond to actual or potential complications.

Infarction. Pulmonary artery infarction is an uncommon, but potentially lethal, emergency that can occur from overinflating the pulmonary artery balloon or from prolonged or frequent wedging. This unfortunate complication can also result from distal migration of the pulmonary artery catheter tip. Signs and symptoms of a pulmonary artery infarction include a sudden rise in the pulmonary artery pressure, followed by hemoptysis, hemodynamic instability, or change in respiratory status. Depending on the size of the infarct, the patient may present with chest pain, dyspnea, tachycardia, tachypnea, hypotension, changes in level of conciousness, or a pleural friction rub. The pulmonary artery waveform must be continuously displayed, so that any spontaneous wedging is immediately detected, evaluated, and corrected.

Premature Beats and Tachycardia. Atrial and ventricular premature beats and ventricular tachycardia are some of the common dysrhythmias that can occur from irritation of the catheter as it comes in contact with the endocardium. Dysrhythmias can also occur during insertion if the catheter is not fully inflated to the manufacturer's recommended volume, so that the balloon surrounds the tip of the catheter as it is advanced, thus preventing the tip of the catheter from irritating the wall of the myocardium. Dysrhythmias are detected on the oscilloscope and should be constantly monitored. An increase in frequency of dysrhythmias or sustained dysrhythmias can lead to hypotension, decreased level of consciousness, and death.

Infection. Infection is a complication that can occur with any invasive line. In fact, it is the most frequent life-threatening, catheter-related complication associated with use of a pulmonary artery catheter.[8] For this reason alone, special attention to aseptic technique is of utmost importance. Other predisposing risks for infection include the site of cannulation, the length of time the catheter is in place, frequent positioning of the catheter, fluid contamination, and poor or inadequate dressing technique. As a result of an extensive literature review regarding the infectious complications of pulmonary artery catheters, Mermel and Maki recommended that the clinician inserting the catheter be knowledgeable and experienced in the insertion procedure, maintenance, and use of these catheters.[8] Further, the site of choice should be subclavian, peripheral arm vein, or internal jugular vein. Other recommendations to reduce the risk of infectious complications include use of personal protective equipment during insertion and any manipulation of the catheter thereafter, site preparation using 1 or 2% tincture of iodine, and selection of a heparin-bonded catheter. These authors also found that the risk for infection rose sharply once the catheter had been in place for 4 days.

Thrombophlebitis. Thrombophlebitis, a compromise to venous circulation, can occur by entry of cutaneous microorganisms, improper skin preparation, or long-term catheter movement at the site of entry. This problem is evidenced by tenderness, pain, edema, redness, and increased skin temperature at the area of the insertion site. Merkel and Maki further reported that the use of heparin-bonded pulmonary artery catheters reduced the risk of thrombosis.[8]

Air Embolism. Air emboli occur primarily by failing to eliminate air during the catheter insertion procedure. This complication can be avoided by backfilling the introducer with blood or by flushing all the ports to the invasive line before insertion. Air emboli can also result from loose connection. Depending on the severity, the patient may exhibit hypotension, cyanosis, tachycardia, or loss of consciousness to death. Should the nurse suspect an air embolism, the patient should be placed in Trendelenburg's position and on the left side.

Pneumothorax. The risk of pneumothorax is greatest during insertion of the pulmonary artery line, but this complication can occur after the procedure, especially if the patient is restless. Consequently, the internal jugular vein has become the preferred site for catheter insertion because of the decreased risk of puncturing the apex of the lung. Most commonly, the patient with a pneumothorax presents with dyspnea, pleuritic pain, tachycardia, diminished chest excursions, and decreased breath sounds on the left side. To avoid this complication, special attention to proper positioning of the patient during the procedure is emphasized. Position the patient's head to the contralateral side and place a rolled towel between the scapulae for a subclavian approach. In addition, placement of the patient in Trendelenburg's position helps to distend and visualize the vessels (internal jugular). Sedation may be indicated for the restless patient. A chest radiograph confirms proper placement of the catheter and rules out complications such as pneumothorax.

Other Risks. Excessive catheter length or insertion and advancement of the catheter with the balloon deflated increases the risk of knotting in the catheter. This problem is evident on a chest radiograph or is apparent during the withdrawal of the catheter when resistance is met.

Myocardial perforation with tamponade and valvular disruption can occur by advancing the catheter with a partially inflated balloon. The incidence of tamponade is higher in patients with a noncompliant ventricle. Tamponade may initially be suspected in patients with equalization of intracardiac pressures, muffled heart tones, increased heart rate, distention of the jugular veins, and paradoxic pulse.

Valvular damage can result from withdrawing the catheter with the balloon inflated, thereby causing damage to the pulmonic valve or tricuspid valve. Symptoms of valvular damage can be manifested by a new murmur, heart failure (right sided), edema, and elevated RAP.

It is imperative that the nurse be knowledgeable about the potential risks associated with invasive hemodynamic monitoring. Some risks can be minimized by astute nursing care, whereas other risks should be detected early enough to avoid or limit a detrimental outcome.

General Nursing Guidelines for Insertion of Hemodynamic Monitoring

Care of the patient who undergoes hemodynamic monitoring requires knowledge and understanding of cardiac anatomy and physiology, monitored parameters, and management of equipment. Equipment preparation and maintenance need special attention, so that the readings are accurate from the moment the invasive line is placed.

Obtain a 500-mL bag of normal saline solution (some centers use 5% dextrose in water), add heparin (if a part of the hospital's protocol), and flush the system free of air and air bubbles. Apply pressure to the IV bag and inflate to 300 mm Hg to activate the intraflow device. This device automatically delivers 3 mL flush solution per hour through the distal port of the catheter and limits the risk of catheter occlusion.

Turn on the monitor and allow the transducer to warm up for 20 minutes before zeroing and obtaining the first set of readings.[9] Level the transducer with the patient's right atrium, which is located at the fourth intercostal space, midaxillary line (phlebostatic axis)

Figure 6–13

The phlebostatic axis is a baseline reference point on the chest used for consistent transducer height placement. It is located at the fourth intercostal space at the midaxillary line. This point is an approximation of the level of the right atrium.

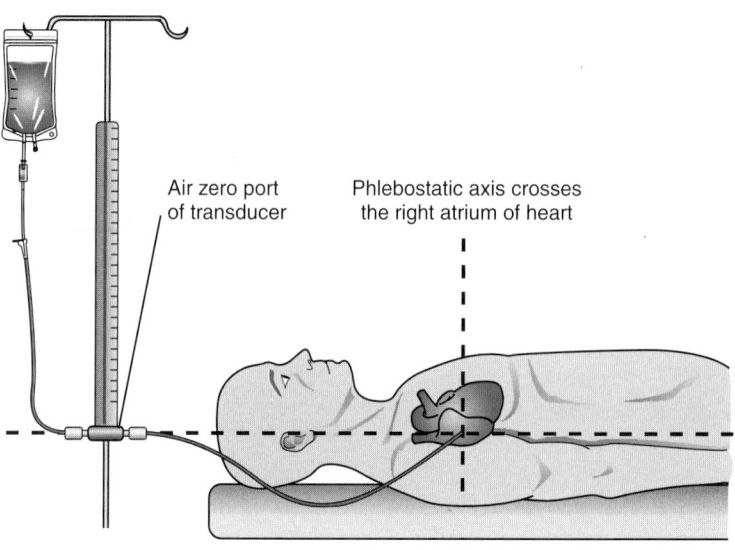

Air zero port of transducer

Phlebostatic axis crosses the right atrium of heart

(Figure 6–13), and calibrate the equipment according to manufacturer's guidelines. For patients with thoracic changes, such as the "barrel chest" associated with emphysema, the level of the right atrium should be approximated at halfway between the anterior and posterior axillary lines at the fourth intercostal space. Leveling the transducer should be done every time the patient or the transducer is moved.[9] To zero the transducer to atmospheric pressure, the transducer is exposed to atmospheric pressure by opening the proximal stopcock to air and creating an air–fluid interface. The zero button on the pressure module is activated and the monitor displays a message indicating that that the system is zeroed. Last, calibrating the system to a known value allows for an upper scale limit to be calibrated while the system stays open to air. A reference value of 200 should appear on the pressure module. Recap the stopcock, and turn the stopcock off to air and back on to the patient. The A-line or pulmonary artery line has been zeroed and the system has been calibrated. Pull the pigtail to fast flush the line. Transducers should be calibrated on initial setup and on disconnection of the transducer from the amplifier or in accordance with the institution's protocols.[9] Frequent patient transfers or position changes necessitate more frequent leveling. Finally, the nurse should check the module to ensure that it is set for the type of waveform being monitored.

The patient must be prepared for the procedure by receiving appropriate patient education. During the procedure, patients need emotional support. In addition, the nurse also assists the physician. On completion of the procedure, it is imperative that the equipment be checked again. The system needs to be fast flushed because there may be blood in the catheter that may interfere with obtaining accurate readings. Clean the insertion site, cover it with a dressing that is dated and initialed, and then anchor the tubing. Reassess the

patient's circulation, motor function, and sensation of the affected limbs, as appropriate.

Remember, individual hemodynamic values are rarely significant. It is important to look at the whole picture and to correlate the hemodynamic values with clinical findings when caring for the critically ill patient.

Key Concepts

➡ The heart muscle is located in the mediastinal space in the chest.

➡ The four layers of the heart are the pericardium, the endocardium (internal layer), the myocardium (middle layer), and the epicardium (external layer).

➡ The heart pumps blood throughout the body, thus supplying oxygen and essential nutrients to the tissues and removing metabolic end products and gases from these same tissues.

➡ The right atrium receives deoxygenated blood from all areas in the body through the inferior vena cava, superior vena cava, and coronary sinus. The deoxygenated blood flows from the right atrium through the tricuspid valve to the right ventricle. It then is ejected into the pulmonary artery to the lungs, where it is reoxygenated.

➡ The left atrium receives oxygenated blood from the lungs and empties it into the left ventricle. This blood is then ejected through the aorta away from the heart for distribution to the peripheral tissues.

➡ Cardiac valves open to facilitate forward flow of blood and close to seal the orifice, thereby preventing regurgitation from one chamber to another.

➡ The two main coronary arteries, left and right, originate from the coronary ostia in the aorta.

➡ Normally, the electrical impulse is generated at the sinoatrial (SA) node and travels down to the atrioventricular (AV) node, to the AV bundle (bundle of His), which quickly divides into the right bundle branch and the left bundle branch. Impulse excitation is then spread throughout the ventricles by a network of conduction myofibers called Purkinje fibers.

⇒ The conduction of the impulse throughout the ventricle results in the depolarization of the myocardium and subsequent contraction.

⇒ There are four phases of an action potential involving four major electrolytes: sodium (Na^+), potassium (K^+), calcium (Ca^{++}), and chloride (Cl^-).

⇒ The five phases of a cardiac cell action potential are as follows: phase 0 corresponds with ventricular depolarization (contraction); phase 1 corresponds with early repolarization; phase 2 is the plateau phase; phase 3 corresponds with late repolarization; and phase 4 corresponds with complete repolarization.

⇒ Diastole comprises 60% of the cardiac cycle. This phase of the cardiac cycle has four components: isovolumetric relaxation of the ventricles, rapid filling of the ventricles, slow filling of the ventricles, and atrial contraction.

⇒ Systole constitutes 40% of the cardiac cycle. This phase of the cardiac cycle also has four components: isovolumetric contraction of the ventricles, rapid ventricular ejection, reduced ventricular ejection, and protodiastole.

⇒ Cardiac output (CO) is the measurement of the heart's overall performance and a measure of blood flow to the periphery. Cardiac output is the product of heart rate (HR) and stroke volume (SV).

⇒ There are three determinants of SV: preload, afterload, and contractility.

⇒ Several direct hemodynamic measurements measure preload: right atrial pressure (RAP) or central venous pressure (CVP) reflects preload in the right side of the heart, and pulmonary artery occlusive pressure (PAOP) is a measurement of preload in the left side of the heart.

⇒ Afterload of the heart cannot be directly measured and therefore is derived from formulas obtained using direct measurements. The pulmonary vascular resistance (PVR) pressure, which reflects right ventricular afterload, and the systemic vascular resistance (SVR) pressure, which reflects left ventricular afterload, are derived measurements.

⇒ Contractility is another derived hemodynamic parameter and is reflected in the stroke volume index (SVI): the right ventricular stroke work index (RVSWI) reflects contractility of the right ventricle, and the left ventricular stroke work index (LVSWI) reflects contractility of the left ventricle.

⇒ Cardiovascular changes resulting from aging are apparent in the cardiac structure, cardiac conduction system, and cardiovascular system.

⇒ Hemodynamic monitoring is accomplished by inserting an intra-arterial catheter (A-line) or a flow-directed, balloon-flotation pulmonary artery catheter.

⇒ Indications for an A-line include the following: (1) patients experiencing sustained hypotension or hypovolemia; (2) patients receiving vasoactive drugs that require continuous blood pressure monitoring; (3) patients needing continuous or intermittent blood pressure monitoring because of difficulties in obtaining blood pressure through the cuff method; and (4) patients requiring access for frequent blood sampling.

⇒ An A-line can be inserted into a radial (most common), brachial, axillary, femoral, or dorsalis pedis artery.

⇒ Abnormal waveforms and erroneous measurements result from dampening, respiratory artifact, catheter fling, dysrhythmias, aortic stenosis, and aortic regurgitation.

⇒ Nursing responsibilities for management of a patient with hemodynamic lines include checking all connections to ensure that they are tight on setup and thereafter. In addition, the patient needs to be assessed for adequate circulation to the cannulated limb. This assessment includes inspection of skin color, palpation of skin temperature, and assessment of capillary refill and distal pulses, if appropriate. Motor function and sensation of the cannulated limb also need to be assessed.

⇒ Formulation of nursing interventions to improve the balance between oxygen supply and demand can be accomplished through monitoring of mixed venous oxygenation (SVO_2).

⇒ SVO_2 values reflect the percentage of hemoglobin that is bound with oxygen in venous blood and is monitored as an indicator of circulatory adequacy. It represents how much oxygen is attached to hemoglobin in venous blood (the amount of oxygen "left over").

⇒ The potential risks of inserting, maintaining, and removing a pulmonary artery catheter can alert the nurse to the following actual or potential complications: pulmonary artery infarction, dysrhythmias, infection, thrombophlebitis, air emboli, pneumothorax, catheter knotting, myocardial perforation, and valvular damage.

References

1. Kopec C: Care of the aging adult. In: Millonig V (ed): Adult Nurse Practitioner Certification Review Guide. Potomac, MD, Health Leadership Associates, 1994, pp 573–613.
2. Smith-Rossi M: The octogenarian cardiac surgery patient. J Cardiovasc Nurs 9:75–95, 1995.
3. Lakatta E, Gerstenblith M, Weisfeldt ML: The aging heart: structure, function, and disease. In: Braunwald E (ed): Heart Disease, 5th ed. Philadelphia, WB Saunders, 1997, pp 1687–1700.

4. Lavie D, Milani R, Messerli F: Prevention and reduction of ventricular hypertrophy in the elderly. Clin Geriatr Med 12:57–65, 1996.

5. Aronow W, Tresch D: Coronary artery disease in the elderly. Clin Geriatr Med 12:89–99, 1996.

6. Ditmyer C, Shively M, Burns D, et al: Comparison of continuous with intermittent bolus thermodilution cardiac output measurements. Am J Crit Care 4:460–465, 1995.

7. Yakimets J, Jensen L: Evaluation of impedence cardiography: comparison of NCCOM3-R7 with Fick and thermodilution methods. Heart Lung 24:194–206, 1995.

8. Mermel L, Maki D: Infectious complications of Swan-Ganz pulmonary artery catheters. Am J Respir Crit Care Med 109:1020–1036, 1994.

9. Ahrens T, Penick J, Tucker M: Frequency requirements for zeroing transducers in hemodyanmic monitoring. Am J Crit Care 4:466–471, 1995.

7

Cardiovascular Assessment

Elisabeth G. Bradley

Objectives

After completing this chapter, the student will be able to:

1. Perform a comprehensive assessment of a patient for cardiovascular risk factors.
2. Locate the anatomic landmarks for cardiac auscultation.
3. Describe the timing and grading of systolic and diastolic murmurs within the cardiac cycle.
4. Describe the four-point scale used to characterize pulse amplitude.
5. Recognize the importance of a comprehensive history for the elderly patient.

Experienced nurses are recognized by their ability to assess a patient's condition accurately and quickly. What may appear to be a "sixth sense" or "gut feeling" is, in actuality, the result of finely tuned assessment skills. Cardiovascular assessment includes cardiac auscultation, and this demands a high level of proficiency. This skill only comes with practice in the clinical setting. Despite all the advances in modern technology, cardiac auscultation remains a cost-effective diagnostic tool.[1] In addition to identifying critical assessment findings, the ability to identify abnormal heart sounds and murmurs accurately is personally rewarding for the nurse.

HEALTH HISTORY

The health history is an interview. In a controlled situation, the standard history is performed in a logical sequence beginning with the chief complaint, followed by the history of present illness, past medical history, family history, social history, and medication history. With the critically ill patient, several factors come into play that require modification of this process. With the hemodynamically unstable patient, initial management is focused on critical actions such as establishing an airway; the history is then deferred until later. A patient who may be unconscious, sedated, paralyzed with neuromuscular blockers, combative, or in severe pain is unable to provide a history. None of this negates the importance of obtaining pertinent information for the health history. When the patient is

unable to give a history, valuable information is obtained from the family or significant other, friends, paramedics or emergency medical technicians present in the field, the primary care physician, and old medical records.

The process of obtaining the health history begins with the patient's arrival to the emergency department. If arrival is by ambulance or helicopter, a verbal report provides a baseline for future assessments. Every effort is made to streamline the history-taking process so as not to overburden the patient and family with repetitive questions regarding medications and past medical history. A discussion of advance directives is initiated early in the admission process to establish resuscitation status. For the patient who is unable to give informed consent, the legal guardian should be identified.

Risk Factors Associated With Cardiovascular Disease

Integral to the cardiovascular history is an assessment of risk factors for coronary heart disease. The terms primary and secondary prevention are used in relation to risk factor modification, but the use of the terms in the medical literature is inconsistent. Primary prevention refers to risk factor modification in healthy individuals with no clinical evidence of disease. Secondary prevention describes risk factor modification in individuals with known cardiac disease such as angina pectoris or a history of myocardial infarction.[2]

129

TABLE 7–1

Cardiovascular Risk Factors

Modifiable	Nonmodifiable
Cigarette smoking	Age
Hypertension	Gender (male sex)
High LDL-C	Heredity (family history)
Low HDL-C	Race (African-American)
Diabetes mellitus	
Sedentary lifestyle	
Obesity	
Lack of reproductive hormones	
Psychosocial factors:	
Type A behavior pattern	
Psychological stress	
Low socioeconomic status	

LDL-C, low-density lipoprotein cholesterol; HDL-C, high-density lipoprotein cholesterol

Modifiable and Nonmodifiable Risk Factors

Cardiovascular risk factors may be classified as modifiable or nonmodifiable (Table 7–1). The risk of coronary heart disease increases as the total number of risk factors increases, illustrating the necessity of a comprehensive risk factor assessment.[3] All members of the health care team have a role in risk factor management. Cardiac rehabilitation is initiated while patients are in the coronary or intensive care units, thus placing the critical care nurse in a prime location to identify high-risk patients. A sample health assessment form demonstrates an initial risk appraisal typically performed by cardiac rehabilitation professionals (Figure 7–1). The modifiable risk factors identified become the focus of patient teaching efforts for the entire team. Incorporated into the cardiac risk factor review is an assessment of the patient's physiologic status (Table 7–2). This assessment guides cardiac rehabilitation professionals in determining the need for monitoring during the patient's exercise routine. For example, a patient classified as a high risk for developing complications during exercise would require continuous ECG monitoring, whereas a patient classified as a low risk would be supervised using pulse checks.

Many risk factors associated with an increased risk for cardiovascular disease have been identified, and the public's awareness of the benefits of "heart-healthy" living has been elevated. Despite this fact, risk factor modification in high-risk patients (secondary prevention) is not consistently initiated.[4] A Guide to Comprehensive Risk Reduction for Patients with Coronary and Other Vascular Disease, endorsed by the American College of Cardiology, provides an example of recommendations for the management of the major modifiable risk factors (Table 7–3).

Recommendations from national experts in the form of practice guidelines and consensus statements

TABLE 7–2

Risk Stratification Parameters for Monitoring Guidelines During Exercise

Risk Level	Characteristics
Low	Uncomplicated clinical course
	No evidence of myocardial ischemia
	Function capacity >7 METs
	Normal LV function (EF >50%)
	Absence of significant ventricular ectopy
Intermediate	ST depression >0.2 mm, flat, or downsloping
	Reversible thallium deficit
	Moderate to good LV function (EF 35–49%)
	Changing or new pattern of angina pectoris
	Failure to comply with exercise intensity prescription
High	Prior MI or infarct involving >35% of LV
	EF <35% at rest
	Fall in exercise systolic BP or failure to rise more than 10 mm Hg on exercise tolerance test
	Functional capacity <5 METs with hypotensive blood pressure response or >1 mm ST segment depression
	Congestive heart failure syndrome in hospital
	High-grade ventricular ectopy
	Previous cardiac arrest

EF, ejection fraction; LV, left ventricular; MET, metabolic equivalent; MI, myocardial infarction.
Courtesy of Department of Cardiac Rehabilitation, Christiana Care Health Services, Wilmington, DE.

<u>CHRISTIANA CARE HEALTH SERVICES - DEPARTMENT OF CARDIAC REHABILITATION</u>
<u>HISTORY AND PHYSICAL - PAGE 3</u>

<u>CARDIAC RISK FACTOR INQUIRY</u>

Name:_____

MR #:_____

NON-MODIFIABLE RISK FACTORS:

    <u>Family History:</u> ___MI   ___CVA   <u>Gender:</u>   ___Female after menopause _____Age at onset
                 ___Surgery ___HTN   ___Female not receiving estrogen placement
                                            ___Male ___Male after age 65

MODIFIABLE RISK FACTORS:

    <u>Hypertension:</u>   How long:_____Treatment:_____

    <u>Diabetes:</u>   Type:_____Age at Onset:_____Treatment:_____
                       Glucose Monitoring: Blood_____Urine_____Frequency_____HgbA$_1$C_____
                       Patient will bring glucometer to exercise session_____

    <u>Tobacco Abuse:</u> Present_____Past_____
                       Type_____Amount_____
                       Cessation Date_____Method used_____
                       Reason for cessation_____
                       Interested in a smoking cessation program_____

    <u>Hyperlipidemia:</u>
                       Patient is unaware of current cholesterol levels_____
                       Current levels: Date:_____Total_____HDL_____LDL_____Trig_____
                       Diet: AHA/NCEP 1_____NCEP 2_____Ornish_____Other_____
                               ADA_____Calories_____
                               Alcohol intake_____Caffeine intake_____
                       Would the patient like to meet with the nutritionist while in the program?_____

    <u>Obesity:</u>   More than 15 lbs. overweight
                       Current weight_____Height_____
                       Patient's desired weight_____Desired weight loss_____

    <u>Stress:</u>   Do you currently have any stress that might effect your health?_____
                       Type A Personality_____
                       Stressors:_____
                       _____
                       Are you interested in learning more about stress management?_____

    <u>Sedentary Lifestyle:</u>
                       Currently compliant with discharge program_____Able to check pulse_____
                       Able to resume normal sexual functioning_____
                       Home exercise equipment or health facility_____
                       _____

Signature:_____   Date:_____   history.doc(01/23/97)emm

Figure 7–1

Cardiac risk factor inquiry. (Courtesy of the Department of Cardiac Rehabilitation, Christiana Care Health Services, Wilmington, DE.)

may facilitate a more consistent approach to risk factor management in high-risk patients. The National Cholesterol Education Program (NCEP) provides such guidelines for the detection and management of hypercholesterolemia. For adults 20 years of age and older who have no evidence of cardiovascular disease, the panel recommends measurement of total and high-density lipoprotein (HDL) cholesterol levels every 5 years, provided the total cholesterol level is less than 200 mg/dL at the first measurement.[5] The Joint Na-

TABLE 7–3
Guide to Comprehensive Risk Reduction
for Patients With Coronary and Other Vascular Disease

Risk Intervention	Recommendations
Smoking: <u>Goal</u> complete cessation	Strongly encourage patient and family to stop smoking. Provide counseling, nicotine replacement, and formal cessation programs as appropriate.

Lipid management:
  <u>Primary goal</u>
  LDL<100 mg/dL
  <u>Secondary goals</u>
  HDL>35 mg/dL;
  TG<200 mg/dL
	Start AHA Step II Diet in all patients: ≤30% fat, <7% saturated fat, <200 mg/d cholesterol.
	
	Assess fasting lipid profile. In post-MI patients, lipid profile may take 4 to 6 weeks to stabilize. Add drug therapy according to the following guide:

LDL<100 mg/dL	LDL 100 to 130 mg/dL		LDL>130 mg/dL	HDL<35 mg/dL
No drug therapy	Consider adding drug therapy to diet, as follows:		Add drug therapy to diet, as follows:	Emphasize weight management and physical activity. Advise smoking cessation. If needed to achieve LDL goals, consider niacin, statin, fibrate.
	↘	Suggested drug therapy	↙	
	TG <200 mg/dL	TG 200 to 400 mg/dL	TG >400 mg/dL	
	Statin Resin Niacin	Statin Niacin	Consider combined drug therapy (niacin, fibrate, statin)	
	If LDL goal not achieved, consider combination therapy.			

Risk Intervention	Recommendations

Physical activity:
  <u>Minimum goal</u>
  30 minutes 3 to 4
  times per week
	Assess risk, preferably with exercise test, to guide prescription.
	Encourage minimum of 30 to 60 minutes of moderate-intensity activity 3 or 4 times weekly (walking, jogging, cycling, or other aerobic activity) supplemented by an increase in daily lifestyle activities (eg, walking breaks at work, using stairs, gardening, household work). Maximum benefit 5 to 6 hours a week.
	Advise medically supervised programs for moderate- to high-risk patients.

Weight management:	Start intensive diet and appropriate physical activity intervention, as outlined above, in patients >120% of ideal weight for height. Particularly emphasize need for weight loss in patients with hypertension, elevated triglycerides, or elevated glucose levels.
Antiplatelet agents/anticoagulants:	Start aspirin 80 to 325 mg/d if not contraindicated. Manage warfarin to international normalized ratio=2 to 3.5 for post-MI patients not able to take aspirin.
ACE inhibitors post-MI:	Start early post-MI in stable high-risk patients (anterior MI, previous MI, Killip class II [S_3 gallop, rales, radiographic CHF]). Continue indefinitely for all with LV dysfunction (ejection fraction≤40%) or symptoms of failure. Use as needed to manage blood pressure or symptoms in all other patients.
Beta-blockers:	Start in high-risk post-MI patients (arrhythmia, LV dysfunction, inducible ischemia) at 5 to 28 days. Continue 6 months minimum. Observe usual contraindications. Use as needed to manage angina rhythm or blood pressure in all other patients.
Estrogens:	Consider estrogen replacement in all postmenopausal women. Individualize recommendation consistent with other health risks.
Blood pressure control: <u>Goal</u> ≤140/90 mm Hg	Initiate lifestyle modification—weight control, physical activity, alcohol moderation, and moderate sodium restriction—in all patients with blood pressure >140 mm Hg systolic or 90 mm Hg diastolic. Add blood pressure medication, individualized to other patient requirements and characteristics (ie, age, race, need for drugs with specific benefits) if blood pressure is not less than 140 mm Hg systolic or 90 mm Hg diastolic in 3 months or if *initial* blood pressure is >160 mm Hg systolic or 100 mm Hg diastolic.

ACE indicates angiotensin-converting enzyme; MI, myocardial infarction; TG, triglycerides; and LV, left ventricular.
From Smith, S.C., et al. *Preventing heart attack and death in patients with coronary disease. Circulation 92:3, 1995.* With permission of the American Heart Association.

tional Committee on Detection, Evaluation, and Treatment of High Blood Pressure publishes reports to guide health professionals in the management of hypertensive patients. Techniques for accurate blood pressure measurement are outlined, and blood pressure readings for adults 18 years of age and older are categorized as normal, high normal, or hypertensive. Normal blood pressure is defined as a systolic reading of less than 130 mm Hg and a diastolic reading of less than 85 mm Hg.[6] Practice guidelines provide the nurse and other health team members with accurate research- based information to guide their practice and to teach patients and families.

A common misconception is that cardiovascular disease only affects men. In reality, this disease is the number one cause of death in women in the United States.[7] Women are affected by the same risk factors as men; however, the disease manifests itself approximately 10 to 20 years later in women. Endogenous estrogen may have a cardioprotective effect that is lost as a woman reaches menopause. The Post Menopausal Estrogen/Progestin Interventions (PEPI) trial has established that hormone replacement therapy is effective in the primary prevention of coronary artery disease.[8] The American College of Cardiology recommends consideration of estrogen therapy in all postmenopausal women.[9]

The use of oral contraceptives has been associated with an increased risk of cardiovascular disease. The older high-dose oral contraceptives tended to increase blood pressure, increase some clotting factors, increase levels of low-density lipoprotein (LDL) cholesterol, and decrease levels of HDL cholesterol.[7] Newer lower-dose oral contraceptives have been found to pose a much lower risk for women.[10] General recommendations from the American Heart Association include avoiding the use of oral contraceptives by women who smoke and considering other forms of birth control for women over the age of 35 years. Cigarette smoking, in combination with the use of oral contraceptives, results in 10 times the risk for death from coronary artery disease.[11]

Congenital Defects. Information is gathered to determine the presence of a family history of congenital heart defects. Although this field was once considered a pediatric specialty, more children with congenital heart defects are surviving to adulthood.[12] Approximately 960,000 persons in the United States with congenital heart defects are alive today.[13] Most corrective operations are performed during infancy or childhood, but not all adults have had surgical intervention. A key component for this area of assessment is the patient's understanding of the cardiac procedure and the follow-up required.

Rheumatic Disease. An estimated 1,360,000 persons in the Unted States have rheumatic heart disease.[13] A history of rheumatic fever should alert the

TABLE 7–4

Signs and Symptoms of Cardiovascular Disease

Signs and Symptoms	Possible Cardiac Cause
Dyspnea	Left ventricular failure
	Mitral stenosis
Syncope	Dysrhythmias, especially heart rates >180 and <30
	Aortic stenosis and hypertrophic cardiomyopathy
	Postural hypotension
	Vasovagal reflex
Chest pain or discomfort	Coronary heart disease
	Dissecting aortic aneurysm
	Aortic valve disease
Cyanosis	Congenital heart disease
	Low cardiac output
Dependent edema	Congestive heart failure
Fatigue	Congestive heart failure
	Mitral valve disease
Hemoptysis	Mitral stenosis
Palpitations	Tachydysrhythmias: PSVT, atrial flutter, atrial fibrillation, MAT, VT
	Bradydysrhythmias: heart block, sinus arrest
	Premature beats

PSVT, paroxysmal supraventricular tachycardia; MAT, multifocal atrial tachycardia; VT, ventricular tachycardia

critical care nurse to the possibility of valvular disease, because acute rheumatic fever may result in fibrosis of the heart valves.[14] More than 66,000 operations are performed annually on patients with defective heart valves, many of which were acquired secondary to rheumatic heart disease.[13]

Signs and Symptoms Associated With Cardiovascular Illness

Common signs and symptoms of cardiac disease are listed in Table 7–4. Each symptom, although frequently related to cardiac disease, may have other causes (e.g., pulmonary or neurologic). When obtaining information from patients regarding the various symptoms, details such as onset, duration, precipitating factors, and alleviating factors should be recorded.

PHYSICAL EXAMINATION

The health history and physical examination are described as separate entities. In reality, both typically occur simultaneously. The experienced critical care nurse obtains much of the health history during the physical examination. A head-to-toe, systematic approach is recommended.

General Appearance

Observation of a patient's general appearance begins with the initial contact and continues throughout the physical examination. Note the patient's facial expression, level of consciousness, body posture, and mobility. Height and weight are obtained as early as possible for calculation of drug dosages, as well as for accurate evaluation of daily fluid status.

Vital Signs

Assessment of vital signs includes measurement of temperature, heart rate, respiratory rate, and blood pressure. For patients with an irregular heart rate, auscultate the apical rate of the heart at the apex for 1 full minute while simultaneously palpating the radial pulse. Dysrhythmias such as premature ventricular contractions and atrial fibrillation may result in weak contractions of the heart that are not perfused to the periphery. In this case, the radial pulse rate will be less than the apical heart rate, and this difference is described as a pulse deficit.

Assess bilateral blood pressures (both arms) on admission. A difference of 5 to 10 mm Hg is acceptable, and when different values are obtained, the higher pressure is used. A difference of 10 to 15 mm Hg may indicate arterial compression or obstruction (e.g., atherosclerosis) on the side with lower pressures, because blood flow would be inhibited. A significant difference in blood pressure between the two arms is often an assessment found in patients with aortic dissection. A Doppler device may be used to measure systolic blood pressure when Korotkoff sounds are not readily audible. Systolic blood pressure measurements obtained with a Doppler device over the radial artery have been shown to correlate well with intra-arterial pressure in the radial artery.[15]

Orthostatic (postural) hypotension is a drop in systolic pressure of 20 mm Hg or more and an increase in heart rate associated with postural changes (rising from a supine position to a sitting or standing position). The patient may present with symptoms of vertigo or syncope associated with changing positions. Predisposing factors include hypovolemia, prolonged bed rest, and use of antihypertensives, vasodilators, and narcotics. To assess a patient for orthostatic hypotension, blood pressure measurements are taken with the patient supine, sitting, and standing (if tolerated). Start with the patient supine and wait 1 to 3 minutes after each position change before measuring the blood pressure.

Head and Neck

Carotid Arteries

Inspection. The neck is inspected for signs of visible arterial pulsations. A pulsating bulge may be seen unilaterally with a tortuous or kinked carotid artery.[16]

Auscultation. Auscultation of the carotid arteries is performed in patients with suspected cerebrovascular disease and in middle-aged and older adults. Auscultation of a carotid bruit may indicate arterial narrowing. A bruit, if heard, sounds similiar to a heart murmur, but it is vascular in origin.

Palpation. The carotid arteries are palpated in the lower third of the neck to avoid pressure on the carotid sinus, because stimulation of the baroreceptors may cause a decrease in heart rate.[17] Standing on the same side that is being palpated, locate the carotid artery by placing the index and third fingers on the patient's thyroid cartilage and sliding them toward you between the trachea and the sternocleidomastoid muscle. The carotid arteries are never palpated simultaneously, because this could compromise blood flow to the brain. A thrill feels much like the vibration produced by a purring cat and may be detected on palpation. The presence of a thrill may indicate arterial narrowing.

Jugular Veins

Inspection. Inspect the internal and external jugular veins for distention and abnormal pulsations. The neck veins are normally flat when the patient is sitting erect and only become visible when the patient is supine. Jugular venous distention is abnormal and occurs when central venous pressure is elevated.

To assess for jugular venous distention, position the patient supine, with the head of the bed elevated 30 to 45°. Keep the patient's neck in a relaxed position, not flexed, and turn the patient's head slightly to the left. Standing on the right side of the patient, identify the internal and external jugular veins. The internal jugular vein lies anterior to the external jugular vein and parallel to the carotid artery and trachea (Figure 7–2). Measure the vertical distance between the angle of Louis (sternal angle) and the highest level of jugular pulsation in the internal jugular vein in centimeters. To visualize the internal jugular vein, it is helpful to shine a flashlight tangentially across the patient's neck. The external jugular vein lies superficially and is typically easier to visualize; however, the internal jugular vein is the preferred vein to assess. Measurements greater than 3 to 4 cm above the sternum at the angle of Louis and with the head of the bed elevated 30° indicate an elevation in central venous pressure. Assessment of jugular venous distention provides an estimation of

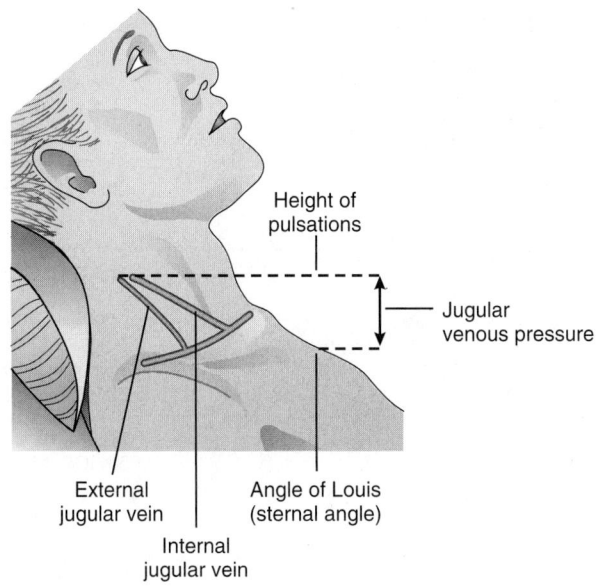

Figure 7–2

Assessment of jugular venous distention.

central venous pressure without the use of an invasive line.

Skin

Color

Color of the skin and mucous membranes is assessed to note the presence of cyanosis, jaundice, pallor, and redness. Cyanosis, seen as a bluish discoloration, is further differentiated as peripheral or central, based on arterial oxygen saturation. Peripheral cyanosis is related to decreased perfusion and is seen in the extremities, nail beds, and nose (cool, exposed areas). Clinical causes include heart failure and shock, but this condition can also be triggered by anxiety or exposure to cold. Arterial oxygen saturation is typically normal. Central cyanosis, also a bluish discoloration, is seen in the mucous membranes, lips, and conjunctivae (warm, well-perfused areas). Clinical causes include congenital right-to-left shunts and pulmonary disease (e.g., pneumonia). Arterial oxygen saturation is typically low. To assess patients with darker skin color, inspect the conjunctivae, sclerae, buccal mucosa, tongue, lips, nail beds, palms, and soles.

Temperature and Moisture

Skin temperature is evaluated as cold, cool, normal, warm, or hot. The presence of diaphoresis is also noted. Bilateral assessment of the upper and lower extremities is performed simultaneously, to note any differences in temperature and moisture.

Capillary Refill

To evaluate arterial circulation, the nail bed is compressed (causing blanching), and then pressure is released. Normal capillary refill is rapid and occurs in less than 2 seconds.

Heart

Inspection and palpation are performed with the patient supine and with the nurse preferably standing on the right side of the patient. For patients in stable condition, auscultation is performed with the patient in two additional positions: sitting while leaning forward and lying in a left lateral position. Changing positions brings various parts of the heart closer to the chest wall and accentuates heart sounds.

Inspection. Inspect the patient's precordium for pulsations and attempt to visualize the apical impulse or "point of maximal impulse" (PMI). Tangential lighting is helpful in sighting impulses. The apical impulse, seen with each contraction or thrust of the left ventricle, is a visible pulsation in the fifth intercostal space at the midclavicular line. It is visible in approximately one-half of the population. Located close to the cardiac apex, the PMI provides an estimation of cardiac size. The PMI may be displaced laterally or may appear more forceful in patients with left ventricular hypertrophy. Identify any abnormal pulsations, remembering the PMI is the only "normal" visible pulsation on the precordium.

Outward motion of the heart or great vessels against the chest wall can be described as a lift or a heave. A heave is a more excessive thrust than a lift. Describe the location of the pulsation using anatomic reference lines and intercostal spaces. Location provides insight into the possible cause of the abnormality. For example, a heave or lift visualized along the left sternal border indicates right ventricular hypertrophy.

Palpation. Palpate the patient's precordium for pulsations and thrills, using your fingertips and the palmar surface of the hand. In a systematic fashion, palpate the key areas illustrated in Figure 7–3. The process begins at the apex of the heart with palpation of the PMI. This normal pulsation is usually felt as a quick tap, approximately 2 cm in diameter. As mentioned earlier, the location of the apical impulse provides the critical care nurse with clues to the patient's underlying clinical condition. Detection laterally may occur with upward displacement of the diaphragm (due to pregnancy, ascites, or tumor), right-to-left mediastinal shift, and left ventricular dilatation. A medial location of the PMI may occur with downward displacement of the diaphragm (due to chronic obstructive pulmonary disease) and left-to-right mediastinal shift. Dextrocardia is a rare condition in which the po-

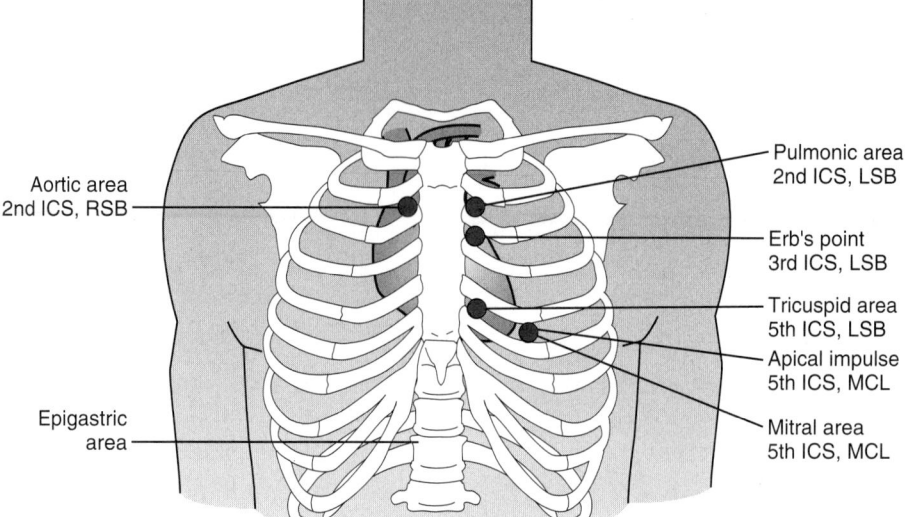

Figure 7–3

Cardiac palpation and auscultation points. ICS, intercostal space; LSB and RSB, left and right sternal border; MCL, midclavicular line.

In the figure:
- Aortic area 2nd ICS, RSB
- Pulmonic area 2nd ICS, LSB
- Erb's point 3rd ICS, LSB
- Tricuspid area 5th ICS, LSB
- Apical impulse 5th ICS, MCL
- Mitral area 5th ICS, MCL
- Epigastric area

sition of the heart is reversed. The apex, and therefore the PMI, is located on the right side of the chest. From the apex, move upward to the right and left sternal borders and finally to the base of the patient's heart, located at the second intercostal space and right and left sternal borders. Finally, palpate the patient's epigastric area. Describe both the location and the sensation felt. A thrill describes a vibration, much like the vibration of a purring cat. Turbulent blood flow associated with heart murmurs may produce a palpable thrill. Pulsations are felt as tapping sensations.

Auscultation. When assessing the heart, it is tempting to begin at once with auscultation. Valuable information is obtained by performing inspection and palpation, and then using auscultation to confirm earlier findings. The bell and diaphragm of the stethoscope are used to assess heart sounds. The diaphragm detects high-pitched sounds (S_1, S_2, murmurs due to stenosis) and is pressed firmly against the patient's chest wall. The bell detects low-pitched sounds (S_3, S_4, diastolic murmurs due to ventricular filling) and is placed lightly on the chest wall. Pressing the bell firmly against the chest wall causes the skin to function as a diaphragm and results in loss of the low-pitched sounds.

Auscultation is performed at five areas on the precordium: aortic area, pulmonic area, Erb's point, tricuspid area, and mitral area (see Figure 7–3). The focus must first be on heart sounds, then murmurs. Attention is given to each sound individually, S_1, S_2, and finally to the normally quiet time between the two sounds. Variations in heart sounds, including changes in the loudness of the sound, provide additional clues to the patient's clinical condition. For example, detection of an S_3, the third heart sound, may be an early warning sign of heart failure.

FIRST HEART SOUND. S_1, the first heart sound, is produced when the mitral and tricuspid valves close. S_1 marks the end of diastole and the start of ventricular systole. The sound of S_1 is described as "lub" and is high pitched. S_1 is louder than S_2 at the apex because of the close proximity of the mitral and tricuspid valves and is synchronous with the upstroke of the carotid pulse. Normally, the mitral valve closes slightly before the tricuspid valve because of the higher pressure gradients on the left side of the heart. The two components of S_1 are identified as M_1 (mitral valve closure) and T_1 (tricuspid valve closure) and are usually heard as one sound.

SECOND HEART SOUND. S_2, the second heart sound, is produced when the aortic and pulmonic valves close. S_2 marks the end of systole and start of diastole. The sound of S_2 is described as "dub" and is higher in pitch and shorter in duration than S_1. S_2 is louder than S_1 at the base of the heart because of the close proximity of the aortic and pulmonic valves.

A split S_2 occurs when the aortic valve closes before the pulmonic valve. The two components are identified as A_2 and P_2. Normal, physiologic splitting of S_2 may occur on inspiration because of increased venous return to the heart. Pathologic splitting of S_2 is suspected when the split persists throughout the respiratory cycle or appears on expiration and disappears on inspiration.[16]

THIRD HEART SOUND. S_3, the third heart sound, is produced during rapid ventricular filling in early diastole and occurs after S_2. It is described as "Ken-tuc-ky" (S_1–S_2–S_3). This finding may be normal in children and young adults. A pathologic S_3 is caused by decreased ventricular compliance or increased volume that results in vibration of the ventricle during diastole. A pathologic S_3, referred to as a ventricular gallop, often indicates left ventricular failure.

FOURTH HEART SOUND. S_4, the fourth heart sound, is produced during atrial contraction and represents the "atrial kick" at the end of diastole. The sound occurs just before S_1 and is caused by decreased ventricular compliance, which creates resistance to ventricular filling. It is described as "Ten-nes-see" (S_4–S_1–S_2). When an S_4 is heard, it is often referred to as an atrial gallop.

Conditions that affect left ventricular compliance include hypertension, coronary artery disease, aortic stenosis, and cardiomyopathy. Conditions that affect right ventricular compliance include pulmonary hypertension and pulmonic stenosis.[16]

The term "summation gallop" describes the occurrence of both S_3 and S_4 together.

MURMURS. Murmurs are sounds created by turbulent blood flow. The presence of a murmur is not an automatic indication of cardiac disease,[18] nor does the loudness of a murmur necessarily correlate with the severity of heart disease. Valvular problems may result in production of a heart murmur. Sounds are produced by forward blood flow through a stenotic (narrowed) valve or backward blood flow (regurgitation) through an incompetent valve. Additional causes of murmurs are blood flow through an abnormal opening (e.g., ventricular septal defect) or simply increased blood flow across normal structures.

To assess murmurs accurately, it is essential first to identify timing of the murmur within the cardiac cycle and to consider valve positions at that time (Figure 7–4). Murmurs are classified as systolic, diastolic, or continuous. Systolic murmurs are described further as midsystolic murmurs that begin after S_1 and end before S_2 and pansystolic (holosystolic) murmurs that start with S_1 and end at S_2. Late systolic murmurs begin in midsystole to late systole and end at S_2. Diastolic murmurs are described as early, middiastolic, or late (presystolic). Assessment of where the sound is heard the loudest and where the sound may radiate is helpful in identifying the valve involved.

In addition to timing, the following characteristics of murmurs are assessed: intensity, pattern, pitch, quality, and radiation. The intensity of a murmur is graded based on the loudness of the sound (Table 7–5). The shape or pattern of a murmur further describes the intensity. The following terms are used to describe the pattern of a murmur: crescendo: quiet to loud; de-

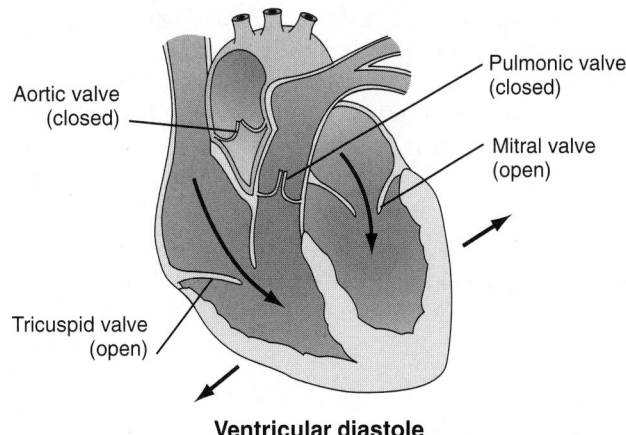

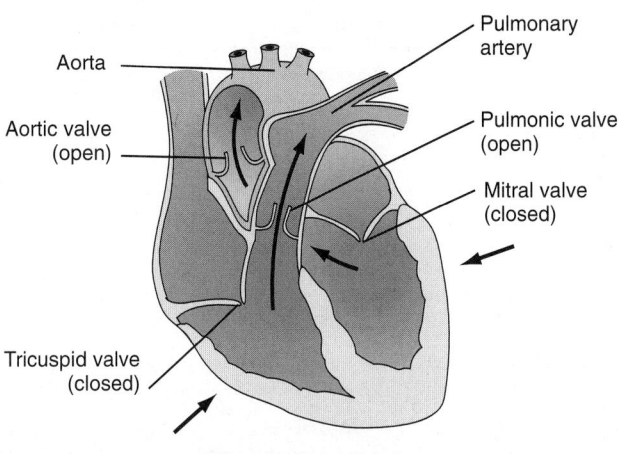

Figure 7–4

Valve positions during ventricular diastole and systole.

crescendo: loud to quiet; crescendo-decrescendo: quiet to loud to quiet; or plateau: same intensity throughout. Pitch is described as low, medium, or high. High blood flow generally results in a high-pitched murmur, whereas slower rates of blood flow produce a low pitch. The quality of a murmur is described as harsh, musical, rumbling, or blowing. Finally, radiation of the sound is noted. Radiation is affected by the direction of blood flow, the intensity of the murmur, and the sound transmission through the tissues.

Grading of murmurs is an advanced skill that develops with practice in the clinical setting. An important role of the critical care nurse is the assessment and monitoring of the physiologic consequences associated with heart murmurs. For example, acute mitral regurgitation, a potential complication of myocardial infarction, is associated with development of a new, loud holosystolic murmur over the apex. Specific types of systolic and diastolic murmurs, with their characteristic findings, are summarized in Tables 7–6 and 7–7.[16]

PERICARDIAL FRICTION RUBS. Inflammation of the pericardial sac may result in a pericardial friction rub. The

TABLE 7–5
Grading of Heart Murmurs

Grade	Description
Grade 1 (1/6)	Faint
Grade 2 (2/6)	Quiet
Grade 3 (3/6)	Moderately loud
Grade 4 (4/6)	Loud
Grade 5 (5/6)	Very loud
Grade 6 (6/6)	Heard with stethoscope entirely off chest

parietal and visceral surfaces rub together, producing harsh, grating sounds classically described as "leather rubbing together, sandpaper, or scratching." Heard best in the third intercostal space and left sternal border, a pericardial rub becomes more intense when patients lean forward and exhale.[16] In the alert patient, differentiation of a pericardial rub from a pleural rub is made by asking the patient to hold his or her breath momentarily. A pericardial friction rub will continue to be auscultated, whereas a pleural rub will stop. Pleural rubs are typically confined to one area of the chest; pericardial rubs can be heard anywhere on the precordium.

EXTRA HEART SOUNDS. Normally, heart valves open silently. Extra heart sounds may be produced with valvular disease. An "opening snap" of the mitral valve is a snap or click produced by opening of the mitral valve, heard in early diastole. An "ejection click" of the semilunar valves is produced by aortic or pulmonic stenosis. A click is heard in early systole as

TABLE 7–6
Systolic Murmurs*

Type	Condition/ Cause	Location	Intensity/ Pitch	Pattern/ Quality	Radiation
Ejection murmur (midsystolic)	**Aortic stenosis** Forward blood flow through stenotic valve	Second intercostal space, right sternal border	Often loud with a thrill Medium to high	Crescendo to decrescendo "diamond shaped" S_1 ⎰ S_2 Often harsh, musical at apex	Neck → left sternal border → apex
Ejection murmur (midsystolic)	**Pulmonic stenosis** Forward blood flow through stenotic valve	Second intercostal space, left sternal border	Soft to loud Medium	Crescendo to decrescendo "diamond shaped" S_1 ⎰ S_2 Often harsh	Left shoulder and neck
Ejection murmur (holosystolic)	**Ventricular septal defect** Blood flow from left to right ventricle	Left sternal border	Often very loud with a thrill High	Plateau S_1 ▮ S_2 Often harsh	Wide
Regurgitant murmur (holosystolic)	**Mitral regurgitation** Backflow of blood into left atrium	Apex	Soft to loud Medium to high	Plateau S_1 ▮ S_2 Blowing	Left axilla
Regurgitant murmur (holosystolic)	**Tricuspid regurgitation** Backflow of blood into right atrium	Left lower sternal border	Variable Medium	Plateau S_1 ▮ S_2 Blowing	Right of sternum and xiphoid area

*Systolic murmurs occur between S_1 and S_2; valve positions: aortic/pulmonic → open; mitral/tricuspid → closed.

TABLE 7–7
Diastolic Murmurs*

Type	Condition/ Cause	Location	Intensity/ Pitch	Pattern/ Quality	Radiation
Ejection Murmur	**Mitral stenosis** Forward blood flow through stenotic valve	Apex	Grade 1–4 Low	Decrescendo to crescendo S_2 S_1 Rumbling	Little to none
Regurgitant murmur	**Aortic regurgitation** Backflow of blood into ventricle	Second to fourth left intercostal space	Grade 1–3 High	Early decrescendo S_2 S_1 Blowing	Apex

*Common diastolic murmurs occur between S_2 and S_1; valve positions: aortic/pulmonic → closed; mitral/tricuspid → open.

the semilunar valves open. Mechanical prosthetic valves also produce loud clicks as they open and close.[19]

Extremities

Pulses

The common sites for palpation include the carotid, brachial, radial, popliteal, dorsalis pedis, and posterior tibial arteries. The dorsalis pedis and posterior tibial arterial pulses may be absent in normal, healthy patients. The peripheral pulses are palpated to assess rate, rhythm, amplitude (strength), and equality bilaterally. Contour of the pulse is best assessed using the carotid artery or brachial artery. The contour (shape) normally has a smooth, rapid upstroke after S_1.[16] Corresponding pulses are palpated simultaneously (Figure 7–5), with the exception of the carotid pulse. Assessment of pulse amplitude is based on a four-point scale (Chart 7–1).[17] Documentation of pulse

strength must include reference to the scale because both three-point and four-point scales are used in practice.

Edema

Assessment of edema is performed on the dorsum of each foot, behind the medial malleolus, and the pretibial areas. Firm pressure is applied for at least 5 seconds and then is released.[16] The sacral area is assessed in patients on bed rest. A four-point scale is used to describe and document edema, with slight edema (1+) the

---

CHART 7–1

Pulse Amplitude

0 = Absent
1 = Diminished
2 = Normal
3 = Increased
4 = Bounding

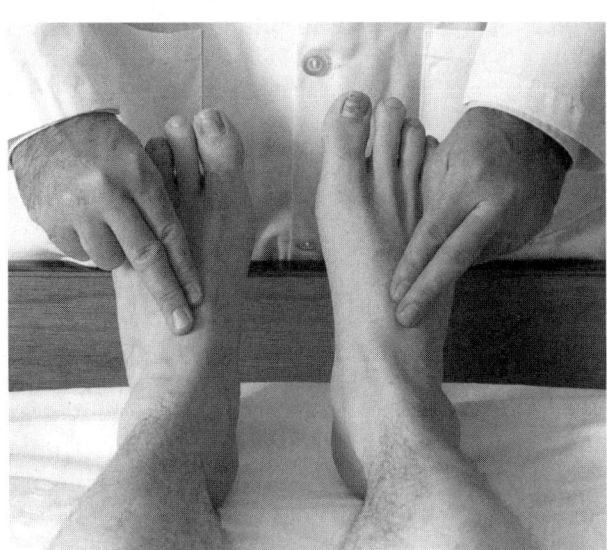

Figure 7–5
Simultaneous palpation of dorsalis pedis pulses. (From Swartz MH: Textbook of Physical Diagnosis: History and Examination, 3rd ed. Philadelphia, W.B. Saunders, 1998, p 330.)

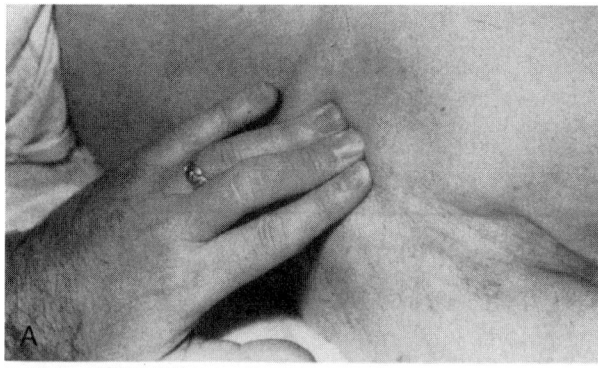

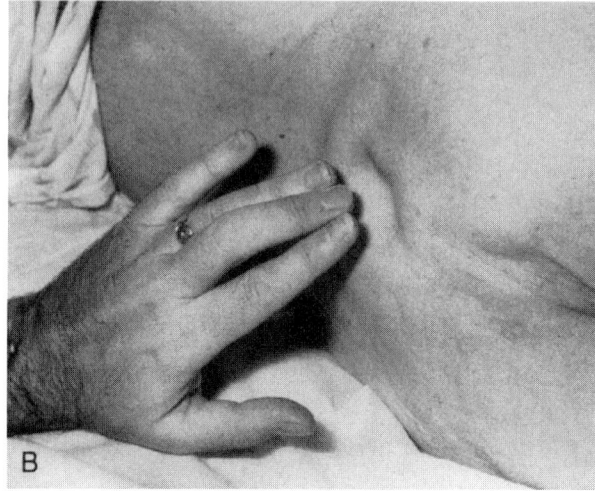

Figure 7–6

A and B, Pitting edema of the sacrum. (From Swartz MH: Textbook of Physical Diagnosis: History and Examination, 3rd ed. Philadelphia, W.B. Saunders, 1998, p 311.)

mildest and marked edema (4+) the most severe.[16] An indentation that remains when pressure is released is described as pitting. Slight pitting disappears rapidly, whereas marked or severe pitting may take 2 to 5 minutes to return to baseline. Figure 7–6 illustrates 4+ pitting edema.

NORMAL VARIATIONS ASSOCIATED WITH AGING

Assessment of elderly patients (age 65 years and older) requires the same systematic approach outlined for younger adults. Meticulous attention to identification of risk factors is an integral component of the health history because cardiovascular disease accounts for more than 50% of all deaths in the elderly population.[20] Hypertension is increasingly prevalent in older adults, with more than 50% requiring medical attention for hypertension. Isolated systolic hypertension is the most common form seen.[20] Despite these statistics, risk factor management is not consistently initiated.[21] The history must also include a detailed medication assessment.

Older adults are often treated with multiple medications that place them at increased risk of adverse drug effects and drug interactions.[22] Frequently, one drug affects the absorption of another. Slower intestinal motility may delay absorption of medications and may extend their duration of action. Declining liver and renal function delays metabolism and excretion of drugs.[23] After absorption, many drugs (e.g., digoxin) bind to protein. The protein-bound portion of the drug is pharmacologically inactive, whereas the unbound, free fraction of the drug exerts the therapeutic and toxic effects. In older adults, low serum albumin levels may result in more free, unbound drug in circulation, thereby increasing the risk of adverse effects and toxicity.[24] Knowledge of these age-related physiologic changes is integral to performing a thorough medication assessment and effective patient teaching.

Aging affects the body's ability to respond to physiologic stress. Changes specific to the cardiovascular system include decreased heart rate response to stress, decreased cardiac output, and decreased compliance of peripheral blood vessels.[22] Dysrhythmias and postural hypotension may cause syncope.[16] Early systolic murmurs are common and are usually benign. Because of decreased compliance of the heart, an S_4 may be auscultated. The PMI may be displaced secondary to kyphosis or scoliosis and does not necessarily indicate cardiac enlargement.[18]

Key Concepts

⇒ Primary prevention is risk factor modification before the onset of disease. Secondary prevention is risk factor modification in individuals with known cardiac disease.

⇒ The risk of coronary heart disease increases as the total number of risk factors (modifiable and nonmodifiable) increases.

⇒ Risk factor modification in high-risk patients and the elderly is not consistently initiated, making this area a priority for nurses.

⇒ The apical impulse, or "point of maximal impulse" (PMI), is palpated in the fifth intercostal space left midclavicular line. The PMI provides an estimate of cardiac size.

⇒ The first heart sound (S_1) is produced when the mitral and tricuspid valves close. This sound marks the start of ventricular systole. S_1 is louder than S_2 at the apex.

⇒ The second heart sound (S_2) is produced when the aortic and pulmonic valves close. This sound marks the start of ventricular diastole. S_2 is louder than S_1 at the base of the heart.

⇒ A splitting of S_2 occurs when the aortic valve closes before the pulmonic valve. This condition may be physiologic or pathologic.

➡ The third heart sound (S₃) is often indicative of left ventricular failure.

➡ The fourth heart sound (S₄) is related to decreased ventricular compliance.

➡ Presence of a murmur is not an automatic indication of cardiac disease.

➡ Murmurs are frequently produced by forward flow of blood through a stenotic valve or backward flow of blood through a regurgitant valve.

➡ Murmurs are classified as systolic, diastolic, or continuous based on their timing in the cardiac cycle. Diastolic murmurs are usually pathologic.

➡ Inflammation of the pericardial sac may result in a pericardial friction rub. Inflamed parietal and visceral surfaces of the heart rub together to generate a harsh, grating sound.

➡ Arterial pulses are assessed for pulse strength (amplitude) using a four-point scale.

➡ Normal capillary refill occurs in less than 2 seconds.

➡ A four-point scale is used to describe and to document edema of the lower extremities; the sacral area is assessed, in addition to the extremities, for patients on bed rest.

➡ The normal physiologic changes associated with aging affect the absorption, metabolism, and excretion of medications. This feature of aging, combined with polypharmacy, places the older adult at an increased risk of adverse drug effects and drug interactions. A thorough medication assessment is essential.

➡ Dysrhythmias and postural hypotension often cause syncope in the elderly.

References

1. Mangione S, Nieman LZ, Gracely E, et al: The teaching and practice of cardiac auscultation during internal medicine and cardiology training. Ann Intern Med 119:47–54, 1993.
2. Swan HJC, Gersh BJ, Graboys TB, et al: 27th Bethesda Conference: matching the intensity of risk factor management with the hazard for coronary disease events. Task force 7. Evaluation and management of risk factors for the individual patient (case management). J Am Coll Cardiol 27:1030–1039, 1996.
3. Blackburn H: The concept of risk. In: Pearson TA, Criqui MH, Luepker RV, et al (eds): Primer in Preventive Cardiology. Dallas, American Heart Association, 1994.
4. Pearson TA, Fuster V: 27th Bethesda Conference: matching the intensity of risk factor management with the hazard for coronary disease events. Executive summary. J Am Coll Cardiol 27:961–963, 1996.
5. US Department of Health and Human Services: Second Report of the Expert Panel on Detection and Treatment of High Blood Cholesterol in Adults. NIH publication no. 93-3096. Rockville, MD, National Cholesterol Education Program, 1993.
6. Joint National Committee on Detection, Evaluation, and Treatment of High Blood Pressure. The fifth report of the joint national committee on detection, evaluation, and treatment of high blood pressure. Arch Int Med 153:154–183, 1993.
7. Barrett-Connor E: Estrogen and coronary heart disease. In: Pearson TA, Criqui MH, Luepker RV, et al (eds): Primer in Preventive Cardiology. Dallas, American Heart Association, 1994.
8. Writing Group for the PEPI Trial: Effects of estrogen or estrogen/progestin regimens on heart disease risk factors in postmenopausal women. JAMA 273:199–208, 1995.
9. Smith SC, Blair SN, Criqui MH, et al: Preventing heart attack and death in patients with coronary disease. Circulation 92:2–4, 1995.
10. Froelicher ES, Berra K, Stepp C, et al: Risk profile screening. J Cardiovasc Nurs 10:30–50, 1995.
11. Miller M, Vogel RA: The Practice of Coronary Disease Prevention. Baltimore, Williams & Wilkins, 1996.
12. Sparacino PSA: Adult congenital heart disease, an emerging population. Nurs Clin North Am 29:213–219, 1994.
13. American Heart Association: Heart and Stroke Facts: 1996 Statistical Supplement. Dallas, American Heart Association, 1995.
14. Dajani AS: Rheumatic fever. In: Braunwald E. (ed): Heart Disease, 5th ed. Philadelphia, W.B. Saunders, 1997.
15. Cummins, RO (Ed.): Textbook of advanced cardiac life support (AHA Pub. No. 70–1050). Dallas, TX, AHA (1994).
16. Bates B, Bickley LS, Hoekelman RA: A Guide to Physical Examination and History Taking, 6th ed. Philadelphia, J.B. Lippincott, 1995.
17. Swartz MH: Textbook of Physical Diagnosis, History and Examination, 2nd ed. Philadelphia, W.B. Saunders, 1994.
18. McGovern M, Kuhn JK: Cardiac assessment of the elderly client. J Gerontol Nurs 18:40–44, 1992.
19. Fabius DB, Stunkard J: Uncovering the secrets of snaps, rubs, and clicks. Nursing 94 24:45–50, 1994.
20. Kannel WB, Vokonas PS: Preventive cardiology in the elderly: the Framingham study. In: Pearson TA, Criqui MH, Luepker RV, et al (eds): Primer in Preventive Cardiology. Dallas, American Heart Association, 1994.
21. Williams MA: Cardiovascular risk-factor reduction in elderly patients with cardiac disease. Phys Ther 76:469–480, 1996.
22. Kane RL, Ouslander JG, Abrass IB: Essentials of Clinical Geriatrics, 3rd ed. New York, McGraw-Hill, 1994.
23. Redeker NS, Sadowski AV: Update on cardiovascular drugs and elders. Am J Nurs 95:34–41, 1995.
24. Lee M: Drugs and the elderly: do you know the risks? Am J Nurs 96:25–32, 1996.

8

Cardiovascular Laboratory and Diagnostic Tests

Cathy McCoy and Nancy Livingston

Objectives

After completing this chapter, the student will be able to:

1. Identify pertinent laboratory tests used in the assessment and management of patients with cardiovascular disease.
2. Identify noninvasive cardiac diagnostic tests, including their indications and pertinent associated nursing care.
3. Identify invasive cardiac diagnostic tests, including their indications and pertinent associated nursing care.
4. Formulate a systematic approach to basic electrocardiographic (-gram) (ECG) interpretation.
5. Identify basic and life-threatening dysrhythmias and the appropriate interventions.
6. Identify the appropriate lead placement for bedside ECG monitoring.
7. Recognize ECG changes associated with acute myocardial infarction (AMI).
8. Identify the basic principles of pacemaker therapy and ECG signs of pacemaker malfunction.

The diagnosis of cardiovascular disease presents a challenge to the nurse and the multidisciplinary team. Advances in technology now provide the health care team with detailed information for cardiovascular assessment. This chapter addresses various noninvasive and invasive diagnostic tests used in the evaluation of cardiac patients ranging from simple serum laboratory tests to nuclear imaging modalities and invasive catheterization. A basic foundation for ECG interpretation is also presented. Knowledge of various cardiovascular laboratory and diagnostic tests provides the nurse with the information necessary to deliver safe and comprehensive care to the critically ill cardiac patient.

LABORATORY TESTS

Blood Assessment

Laboratory diagnostic tests are of critical importance in the assessment of the cardiac patient. The results of serum laboratory diagnostic tests often form the basis for diagnosis, intervention, and evaluation of treatment measures. It is important to collect blood speci-

mens properly to ensure the accuracy of test results. Familiarity with the types of serum laboratory tests, normal values, and physiologic rationale for each test guides the critical care nurse in decision making.

Serum Electrolytes

Electrolytes serve many functions in the body. Water provides volume for the body fluid, and the electrolytes contribute to the function of these fluids. Electrolytes assist in regulating acid–base and water balance, and they contribute to enzyme reactions and to cardiac and neuromuscular activity. Sodium, potassium, calcium, and magnesium are the key ions in the depolarization and repolarization process, which is vital to cardiac function. Table 8–1 lists normal laboratory values for serum electrolytes, blood urea nitrogen (BUN), and creatinine.

Serum Sodium

Sodium (135–145 mEq/L) is the most abundant cation in the body. Sodium is essential for maintaining the osmolality of extracellular fluids, acid–base balance, transmis-

TABLE 8-1
Normal Serum Electrolyte, Blood Urea Nitrogen, and Creatinine Values

Component	Normal Range
Sodium	135–145 mEq/L
Potassium	3.5–5.0 mEq/L
Calcium, total	8.5–10.5 mg/dL
Calcium, ionized	4.5–5.1 mg/dL
Magnesium	1.5–2.5 mg/dL
Blood urea nitrogen	6–20 mg/dL
Creatinine	0.8–1.2 mg/dL
Blood urea nitrogen:creatinine ratio	10:1

sion of nerve impulses, and vital chemical reactions.[1] The body loses sodium through the kidneys, skin, and gastrointestinal tract. An important physiologic principle to remember in fluid and electrolyte balance is that where sodium goes, water follows. If the kidneys retain sodium, then water is also retained. Conversely, if the kidneys excrete sodium, water is also excreted. An increase in sodium intake results in water retention and increased blood volume. Therefore, when large amounts of sodium are excreted, less water is retained, and hypovolemia may occur. This situation can happen when a patient is aggressively treated with diuretics.

Sodium concentration is primarily regulated by the kidneys. A decrease in renal blood flow secondary to hypovolemia, decreased cardiac output, and medications may cause sodium retention by means of the renin–angiotensin–aldosterone mechanism (see Chapter 20). This mechanism stimulates the adrenal cortex to produce the hormone aldosterone. Aldosterone increases sodium reabsorption by the kidneys and also leads to water reabsorption, to increase blood volume and subsequent increased blood flow to the kidneys.

Skin losses of sodium are usually small, but sweat losses can be extensive during exercise and during periods of exposure to a hot environment. Loss of skin surface, which can occur with extensive burns, also leads to excessive losses of sodium. Sodium moves freely between the extracellular fluid and the contents of the gastrointestinal tract. Sodium losses also occur with vomiting, diarrhea, fistula drainage, and gastrointestinal suction.

Hyponatremia is defined as a serum sodium concentration of less than 135 mEq/L. Sodium deficit may occur from an actual loss of sodium from the body (depletional hyponatremia), or it may occur from retention of excess water causing sodium dilution (dilutional hyponatremia). With respect to the cardiac patient, hyponatremia is most likely in patients with untreated heart failure who are taking diuretics that waste sodium. Hyponatremia may also occur from salt and water loss from diarrhea, vomiting, excessive sweating, and diabetic acidosis.[2]

The signs and symptoms of hyponatremia depend on the rapidity of onset and the severity of the sodium deficiency. If the low serum level occurs slowly, the signs and symptoms are usually not apparent until the levels approach 125 mEq/L. Seizures may occur at levels less than 125 mEq/L. Patients who have water excess intoxication (dilutional hyponatremia) and sodium loss may have physical findings that include headache, lethargy, confusion, weight gain, edema, and ascites. Laboratory values include a low serum osmolality; decreased hematocrit, chloride, and BUN; and decreased urinary sodium. If the patient has lost sodium in excess of water, signs and symptoms may include weakness, headache, poor skin turgor, nausea, vomiting and diarrhea, abdominal pains, confusion, lethargy, and coma.

Treatment of hyponatremia varies, depending on the cause. For water intoxication, fluid restriction, diuretic therapy, and demeclocyline (Declomycin) may be effective. Treatment of water and sodium loss is intravenous replacement with normal or hypertonic saline and liberalization of dietary sodium.

Hypernatremia is a serum sodium concentration in excess of 145 mEq/L. This disorder occurs when the ratio of sodium ions to water molecules is increased, leading to intracellular dehydration. In the cardiac patient, this situation is most likely to occur when the patient becomes dehydrated from excessive diuresis. Dehydration may also occur in persons who are unable to express their thirst or obtain water to drink. The unconscious person is at risk of developing hypernatremia. Patients with diabetes insipidus and uncontrolled diabetes mellitus with osmotic diuresis may experience dehydration that can lead to hypernatremia.

The signs and symptoms of hypernatremia vary, depending on the mechanism of hypernatremia. In both types, patients have central nervous system (CNS) irritability including lethargy, confusion, seizures, and coma. In water deficit, signs and symptoms of dehydration are usually present, and hypotension with postural changes and compensatory tachycardia may occur. The patient may complain of thirst, muscle cramps, and weakness. In sodium excess, signs and symptoms of fluid overload are observed. Laboratory values for both causes include increased hematocrit, BUN, and serum and urine osmolality. Seizures, coma, and symptoms of volume depletion may occur with serum sodium levels higher than 160 mEq/L.

Treatment of hypernatremia is to normalize the ratio of sodium to water by replacing water. In a patient with congestive heart failure, fluid replacement should be done slowly, to prevent volume overload and to avoid exacerbating heart failure. Daily weights and intake and output should be monitored closely. Dietary sodium should be restricted. Diuretics may be used to lower sodium levels if the cause is sodium excess.

Serum Potassium

Potassium (3.5–5.0 mEq/L) is the major cation in intracellular fluid. Ninety percent of potassium is concentrated within the cell; only small amounts are contained in blood and bone. Damaged cells release potassium into the blood. The functions of potassium include maintenance of intracellular osmolality, which is necessary for neuromuscular control and the regulation of skeletal, cardiac, and smooth muscle activity, regulation of acid–base balance, and participation in many intracellular enzyme reactions. Potassium, along with calcium and magnesium, affects the rate and force of contraction of the heart. Potassium contributes to the intricate chemical reactions that convert carbohydrates into energy, change glucose into glycogen, and convert amino acids to proteins.[1] The kidneys play the primary role in potassium excretion. If kidney function is impaired, serum potassium concentrations may reach toxic levels. Abnormally high or low serum potassium levels can have serious and often life-threatening consequences that include ventricular dysrhythmias.

The most common cause of *hypokalemia* in the cardiac patient occurs with the use of potassium-wasting diuretics. Loss of intestinal secretions, liver disease, aldosterone excess, metabolic alkalosis, inadequate dietary intake, and intracellular shifts can also decrease serum potassium levels.

Patients with decreased potassium levels may complain of nausea and vomiting, anorexia, constipation, muscle cramps, and muscle weakness. Diaphragm weakness can occur, leading to decreased ventilation and respiratory arrest. Changes in the ECG may occur with low potassium levels. The ECG may display flattened T waves, prominent U waves, and a prolonged PR interval. The prolonged repolarization period increases the risk of ventricular tachydysrhythmias.[3]

Hypokalemia is treated by replacing potassium. Oral potassium is given initially. Patients who chronically have low potassium levels should be encouraged to eats foods high in potassium (i.e., bananas and oranges) or to take a potassium supplement prescribed by their physician. If the potassium level is dangerously low (<3.0 mEq/L), a slow intravenous (IV) infusion of potassium (10 mEq per hour) should be administered. Undiluted potassium is *never* given intravenously. A rapid infusion of a concentrated potassium solution has been known to cause death due to cardiac arrest. Serum potassium levels and the ECG should be monitored closely while the level is low. If the patient is taking digitalis, serum potassium levels must be closely monitored because hypokalemia enhances the action of digitalis and potentiates digitalis toxicity.

The most common cause of *hyperkalemia* is renal failure or renal insufficiency in which potassium secretion is diminished. Patients in heart failure frequently experience hyperkalemia. They often are taking angiotensin-converting enzyme (ACE) inhibitors, which can cause retention of potassium. Patients who take diuretics with potassium supplementation and who experience renal insufficiency or worsening heart failure may not excrete the excess potassium. Hyperkalemia may also occur in patients who have experienced trauma, in which potassium from the damaged cells is released into the blood.

Hyperkalemia alters the electrophysiology of myocardial cells and can produce marked cardiac conduction delays. The increase in intracellular potassium reduces the resting membrane potential. As a result, phase 0 of the action potential is reduced, with resulting slowing of conduction. Phase 3 of the action potential is accelerated, resulting in a faster repolarization. This situation can cause bradycardia, heart block, escape rhythms, sinus arrest, ventricular fibrillation, and cardiac arrest. These ECG rhythms are discussed in further detail later in this chapter.

The clinical presentation of hyperkalemia (>5.5 mEq/L) includes complaints of nausea, vomiting, diarrhea, abdominal cramping, drowsiness, irritability, tetany, and mental confusion. Neuromuscular changes such as fatigue, muscle weakness, paresthesia, and muscle pain may occur. ECG changes that may occur include elevated (peaked) T wave, flattened P wave, decreased R-wave amplitude, widened QRS complex, and depressed ST segment.

Treatment of hyperkalemia is aimed at moving potassium out of the extracellular fluid. IV glucose and insulin can be given to help drive potassium into the cells. Oral or rectal sodium polystyrene sulfonate (Kayexalate) and sorbitol can also help further to mobilize potassium out of the body. Kayexalate exchanges sodium for potassium at a 1.5:1 ratio in the bowel, and sorbitol causes osmotic diarrhea to eliminate the potassium.[4] If the foregoing treatments are unsuccessful, hemodialysis may be necessary. An infusion of calcium may be given that does not reduce the serum potassium concentration but immediately antagonizes the cardiac conduction abnormalities. Calcium (2.25–14 mEq) should be given over a 2-minute period and may be repeated after 5 minutes if no benefit had occurred. Close continuous monitoring of the ECG and frequent serum potassium levels are necessary until the level returns to normal.

Serum Calcium

Calcium is an important cation necessary for cellular excitability, smooth muscle contractility, transmission of nerve impulses, blood clotting, bone and tooth formation, and intracellular energy formation. Most of the body's calcium (98–99%) is stored in the skeleton and teeth. The rest of the calcium can be found ionized in the serum (50%) and bound to protein (50%). The ionized form of calcium is the biologically active form responsible for cardiac and neuromuscular excitability and for blood clotting. Total serum calcium (8.5–10.5 mg/dL) is influenced by vitamin D, parathyroid hormone, and calcitonin. Calcium regulation is essential for cardiac function. It is responsible for prolonging the action potential and for decreasing the threshold potential of the cardiac electrical cells. It is also necessary for the actin–myosin interaction that causes muscle fiber contraction.

The most common causes of *hypocalcemia* in the cardiac patient are dietary deficiencies and malabsorption of vitamin D or calcium. Chronically ill cardiac patients with reduced albumin levels have less protein available on which calcium can bind, leading to hypocalcemia. Patients in heart failure may have decreased calcium levels because of diuretic use, volume overload, and hypoparathyroidism or hyperphosphatemia, which prevent calcium from being absorbed in the intestines.[4]

Hypocalcemia prolongs the action potential and increases the threshold potential in myocardial cells. This change can increase the risk of ventricular tachydysrhythmias and may enhance the toxic effects of digitalis.[3] ECG changes include prolonged ST and QT intervals, and the disorder may decrease cardiac contractility.

Clinical findings in hypocalcemia include muscle cramping, paresthesia, and tetany. Tetany is a continuous muscle contraction similar to a muscle spasm. In addition, calcium affects the excitability of the cardiac muscle and, if uncorrected, can result in heart failure. Other signs include laryngeal spasm, convulsions, decreased prothrombin time (PT), and positive Chvostek's and Trousseau's signs (see Chapter 26).

Treatment of hypocalcemia is aimed at increasing the serum calcium level. Calcium supplementation can be given by the IV or oral route. If the cause of the deficiency is vitamin D deficiency, then vitamin D supplementation should be provided. The patient should be monitored for ECG and neuromuscular changes throughout treatment.

The most common cause of *hypercalcemia* is excessive bone reabsorption with release of calcium. This is due to hyperparathyroidism, metastatic carcinoma, hyperplasia of the parathyroid glands, hypophosphatemia, and prolonged immobility. Increased intake of vitamin D can lead to increased absorption of calcium. Long-term use of thiazide diuretics can raise total serum calcium levels by 0.5 to 1.0 mg/dL. This drug use is the most likely cause of hypercalcemia in the cardiac patient.

Signs and symptoms associated with hypercalcemia include diminished neuromuscular excitability resulting in fatigue, muscle pain and weakness, personality changes, and gastrointestinal symptoms. Hypercalcemia reduces the action potential and the threshold potential, making the cardiac cells more receptive to dysrhythmias. The ECG shows shortening of the ST and QT segments, indicating shortened ventricular systole. Decreased impulse formation and conduction may appear as bradycardia or heart blocks. Hypercalcemia potentiates digitalis, so dysrhythmias associated with digitalis toxicity may occur. Renal calculi and flank pain may occur. Heart failure may occur or may be exacerbated by the increased force of contractions that causes an additional workload on the heart.

Treatment of hypercalcemia is directed toward correcting or controlling the condition causing the disorder. For chronic hypercalcemia, a low-calcium diet should be maintained. Plicamycin (Mithracin) can be given if the cause is bone reabsorption. Loop diuretics are given to promote excretion of calcium in the urine. The patient should be observed for signs and symptoms of heart failure, dysrhythmias, and neurologic changes throughout treatment.

Serum Magnesium

Magnesium (1.5–2.5 mg/dL) is the second most abundant intracellular cation. Fifty percent of total magnesium is stored in bone, and 50% is contained in the body cells. Magnesium is required for the use of adenosine triphosphate as a source of energy. Magnesium plays a role in many enzymatic activities, such as carbohydrate metabolism, protein synthesis, nucleic acid synthesis, and muscular contraction.[1] Magnesium also plays a vital role in neuromuscular activity, in blood clotting, and in the cessation or generation of dysrhythmias.[3]

Hypomagnesemia usually results from impaired intestinal absorption, alkalosis, alcoholism, and excessive adrenal corticoid secretion. The most common cause in the cardiac patient is diuretic use and renal loss of magnesium. Magnesium also plays a role in maintaining serum potassium levels; therefore, laboratory values should be closely monitored in patients receiving diuretic therapy.

Clinical manifestations associated with hypomagnesemia are hyperactive deep tendon reflexes, tremors, confusion, and disorientation. The patient may also have nausea, vomiting, and mental status changes from mild lethargy to coma, seizures, and a positive Chvostek's or Trousseau's sign. ECG changes include flat or inverted T waves, ST-segment depression, and a prolonged QT interval. These changes put the patient at risk for ventricular dysrhythmias, especially torsades de pointes, which have been associated with magnesium deficiency after myocardial infarction (MI).

The degree of hypomagnesemia guides the type of therapy needed. Oral magnesium tablets may be given for mild magnesium deficiency. More severe hypomagnesemia is treated with an IV infusion of magnesium sulfate. Hypokalemia often occurs concurrently with magnesium deficiency and should also be corrected. ECG and neuromuscular monitoring is necessary throughout treatment.

Hypermagnesemia has three primary causes. It may be caused by renal failure, hyperparathyroidism, and excessive intake of parenteral magnesium commonly found in laxatives. The clinical presentation of hypermagnesemia includes neuromuscular sedation such as muscle weakness, confusion, and respiratory paralysis. Levels more than 6.0 mEq/L can cause respiratory depression and apnea, as well as bradycardia leading to asystole.[2, 3] Blood pressure may be decreased, and the ECG may show an increase in the PR interval, a widened QRS complex, and elevation of the T wave.

The treatment of hypermagnesemia is to discontinue the administration of magnesium-containing drugs and to remove magnesium by using diuretics or by dialysis. IV administration of calcium gluconate is often used to remove excess magnesium from the body. As with hypomagnesemia, ECG and neuromuscular monitoring is recommended throughout treatment.

Renal Function Assessment

BUN (6–20 mg/dL) and creatinine (0.8–1.2 mg/dL) reflect renal function and overall hydration. Elevations of both BUN and creatinine indicate that renal function is impaired because of decreased renal perfusion (low cardiac output or renal artery stenosis) or chemotoxic effects of medications. Certain cardiac medications, such as ACE inhibitors and diuretics, can cause elevations in BUN and creatinine that indicate impaired renal function. An elevated creatinine level is a more specific and sensitive indicator of kidney disease and impaired renal function than an elevated BUN level. In terms of hydration, an elevated BUN level and a normal creatinine level may indicate dehydration. A decreased BUN level and a normal creatinine level may indicate that the patient is overhydrated.

A normal BUN-to-creatinine ratio is 10:1. A ratio greater than 10:1 may indicate volume depletion, excessive protein intake, or catabolic state. A decreased ratio, less than 10:1, may indicate liver disease, excessive fluid intake, or decreased protein intake. A ratio of 10:1, along with an elevated BUN and creatinine level, suggests acute renal failure, chronic renal failure, or renal toxicity related to medications.

Glucose Levels

Serum glucose levels (80–120 mg/dL) should be assessed in the cardiac patient. An elevated fasting glucose level may indicate diabetes mellitus. Because diabetes is a risk factor for heart disease, it is important that it be well controlled. The peripheral vascular effects of diabetes mellitus and possible end-organ damage can affect the cardiovascular system over time.

Hematologic Studies

The complete blood count is a determination of the number of red and white cells per cubic millimeter of blood. The main function of the red blood cell (erythrocyte) is to carry oxygen to the cells from the lungs and carbon dioxide from the cells to the lungs. This process is achieved by hemoglobin, a component of the red blood cells. Hemoglobin combines with oxygen and carbon dioxide and gives the arterial blood its bright red color. The oxygen-carrying capacity of the blood is directly proportional to the hemoglobin concentration, rather than to the number of red blood cells. For this reason, hemoglobin levels are important in evaluating anemia.

Another component of the complete blood count is the hematocrit. This test looks at the red blood cell mass. It quantifies the percentage of packed red blood cells in a volume of whole blood. It is an important measurement in the determination of anemia. The normal values for hemoglobin and hematocrit vary with age, sex, and race (Table 8–2).

Anemia is a condition that occurs with an abnormally low number of circulating red blood cells or abnormally low hemoglobin, or both. Anemia can have a significant effect on the cardiovascular patient. The body compensates for acute blood loss in the presence of anemia by vasoconstriction, increased heart rate, and increased cardiac output. The body attempts to maintain blood volume and perfusion of oxygen to the vital organs. The initial compensatory mechanism is not effective on a long-term basis. The increased heart rate causes an increase in myocardial oxygen demand because of the greater workload. This increased workload can cause palpitations, shortness of breath, congestive heart failure (CHF), and angina in the patient with coronary artery disease (CAD) and should be corrected (see Chapter 9 and 11).

TABLE 8–2
Normal Serum Hemoglobin and Hematocrit Values*

	Hemoglobin (g/dL)	Hematocrit (%)
Adult male	14.0–17.4	42–52
Adult female	12.0–16.0	36–48

*Values vary with age and race.

Thyroid Function Assessment

Thyroid function tests include thyroid-stimulating hormone (TSH), total thyroxine (T_4), and total triiodothyronine (T_3). Hyperthyroidism and hypothyroidism can affect cardiac conduction; therefore, it is important to assess these laboratory tests in cardiac patients. Hyperthyroidism can cause atrial fibrillation and subsequent heart failure. Hypothyroidism can cause heart failure and possible cardiac enlargement. It can also lead to bradycardia, a prolonged PR interval, a depressed P wave, and a flat or inverted T wave.

Lipid Profile

Elevated lipid levels have shown to be a risk factor for the development of CAD. The lipid profile measures the total cholesterol, triglycerides, and lipoprotein in the blood. An elevated lipid panel can be related to familial hyperlipidemia and hypercholesterolemia.

Cholesterol

Cholesterol is a fat-soluble steroid found in animal fats and oils. It is found in high concentrations in the brain and nervous system. Elevated cholesterol levels (>200 mg/dL) are associated with an increased risk of CAD.[5] In the Framingham study, women and men with serum cholesterol concentrations more than 295 mg/dL had higher than three times the risk of MI and CAD than those with cholesterol concentrations less than 240 mg/dL. The higher the level, the greater the risk. The desired total cholesterol level is less than 200 mg/dL in all patients with and without coronary risk factors[5] (Table 8–3).

Low-Density Lipoproteins

Low-density lipoproteins (LDLs) are the major carriers of plasma cholesterol; therefore, their measurement provides a good estimate of total blood cholesterol. The desirable goal for LDL levels is less than 130 mg/dL, and

TABLE 8–3
Goals for Blood Cholesterol and Lipid Levels*

Parameter	Goal (mg/dL)
Total cholesterol	<200
Low-density lipoprotein	<130
High-density lipoprotein	>35
Triglycerides	<200
Ratio of cholesterol to high-density lipoprotein	<4

*Although the reference range for values of cholesterol and lipids vary according to sex and age, the recommended target goals (for adults) are the same, regardless of age, race, or sex.

the LDL value is directly related to the risk of CAD (see Table 8–3). The higher the LDL level, the greater the risk of developing CAD. In a study by Marcus,[6] patients with LDL levels less than 100 mg/dL had a reduction in coronary artery–related events and a reduction in cardiac morbidity and mortality. LDL carries cholesterol into the cell, with resulting deposition of cholesterol throughout the body including the arterial vessel walls. LDL is catabolized mainly in the liver. High dietary intake of saturated fats and cholesterol results in elevated LDLs. Factors that lower LDL cholesterol include weight loss and a low dietary intake of fat and cholesterol.

High-Density Lipoproteins

High-density lipoproteins (HDLs) have a protective effect against CAD by removing cholesterol from vessel walls and transporting it to the liver, where it is removed from the body. HDL is composed mostly of protein. The desired HDL level is more than 35 mg/dL. An inverse relationship exists between HDL and CAD. The higher the HDL, the lower the risk of CAD. High HDL levels are associated with regular exercise and consumption of a moderate amount of alcohol (e.g., red wine). Smoking, diabetes, obesity, and a sedentary lifestyle are associated with high levels of LDL and low levels of HDL.

Triglycerides

The normal range for triglycerides is 40 to 200 mg/dL. Triglycerides account for more than 90% of dietary intake and comprise 95% of fat stored in tissues. They are stored in adipose tissue as glycerol, fatty acids, and monoglycerides, and the liver converts these to triglycerides. Elevated triglyceride levels (>200 mg/dL) can contribute to the development of atherosclerosis, which leads to CAD.[5] Serum blood levels should be obtained in the fasting state. Serum levels will be falsely elevated if blood is drawn with the patient in the nonfasting state (see Table 8–3).

Ratio of Cholesterol to High-Density Lipoproteins

The ratio of cholesterol to HDL is another value to assess when evaluating the lipid profile. It gives more information than the other values alone. The higher the cholesterol-to-HDL ratio, the greater the risk for developing atherosclerosis. The desired range is less than 4 mg/dL (see Table 8–3).

Assessment of Cardiac Enzymes

The diagnosis of AMI is usually confirmed by the patient's history, ECG changes, and elevation of serum enzymes released from the heart muscle after myocardial injury. The three major enzymes released into the blood that occur in abnormal levels after myocardial injury are creatinine phosphokinase (CPK), lactate dehydrogenase (LDH), and troponin I.

Creatine Phosphokinase

Creatine kinase (CK) is an enzyme found in the heart, skeletal muscle, and brain. CK can be divided into three isoenzymes: MM is found in the skeletal muscle; BB is found in the brain; and MB is found in cardiac muscle. The isoenzymes are used to differentiate the source of the injury. The MB isoenzyme is specific to cardiac muscle, and elevations higher than 3% are definitive in the diagnosis of MI.

CK elevations begin to appear within 4 to 6 hours after the onset of AMI. Serum levels of the enzyme usually begin to peak 12 to 24 hours after the onset of the infarction and return to normal within 3 to 4 days. The elevation of CK is nonspecific to cardiac injury. If a patient receives an intramuscular injection or physical trauma, an elevation in the CK level will occur secondary to skeletal muscle injury.

The use of CK-MB isoenzyme provides a means of quickly determining myocardial damage. In assessing MI using the CK-MB isoenzyme, it is important to obtain blood on admission and every 8 hours over a 24-hour period, because the serum isoenzyme begins to rise within 4 to 6 hours and peaks within 12 to 24 hours after injury. CK-MB isoenzyme is most useful in the early diagnosis of MI. If the patient is admitted more than 36 hours after the onset of symptoms, CK-MB isoenzymes may not provide an accurate assessment of the situation.

A disadvantage of the CK-MB isoenzyme is that it is not sensitive to microinfarctions, which can be associated with unstable angina. Another disadvantage is that early detection of infarction is not possible because no rise in CK-MB occurs until 4 to 6 hours after injury. Further, it often takes 1 to 2 hours for the laboratory to measure the isoenzyme. All these factors contribute to delays in diagnosis.

Lactate Dehydrogenase

Another enzyme released after MI is lactate dehydrogenase (LDH). LDH appears in abnormal levels in the blood 12 to 24 hours after the onset of MI. Peak levels occur in 3 to 6 days and return to normal 7 to 10 days after infarction. LDH is found in almost all tissues including the heart, lungs, kidneys, skeletal muscle, liver, and red blood cells. Damage to tissues causes the release of LDH into the circulation. LDH can be separated into five different isoenzymes. Cardiac muscle is rich in the isoenzyme LDH_1; therefore, after MI, the predominant isoenzyme is LDH_1. Serum levels of LDH_1 and LDH_2 normally have a ratio of 1:2. In AMI, the ratio is reversed. This pattern is known as the "flipped" LDH pattern and is seen after AMI.[7]

Troponin

Cardiac troponin I is another laboratory value currently used in some institutions to assess AMI. The absence of ST-segment elevations makes it difficult to determine whether a patient has an AMI or unstable angina. Patients who present within the first few hours of an AMI rarely have measurable elevations in CK isoenzyme. Troponin I is a sensitive and specific marker for myocardial necrosis and is detected in blood only if myocardial ischemia has occurred.[8] Troponin assay rises a couple of hours earlier than CK-MB in patients with AMI and has greater specificity and sensitivity in the diagnosis and exclusion of myocardial injury.[9, 10] Troponin assay allows early identification of patients with chest pain suggestive of ischemia or infarction and allows identification of patients with MI who present 48 hours to 6 days after infarction. In patients with unstable angina, troponin I appears to be a more sensitive indicator of myocardial cell injury than CK-MB.[10, 11]

Skeletal muscle injury can result in elevation in the CK total and in CK-MB. Troponin has helped to identify patients with false-positive CK-MBs under these circumstances. In a study of 215 patients, who presented without evidence of cardiac disease (no ECG changes), 59% of patients with skeletal muscle injury and 3.8% with renal failure had elevated CK-MB levels, but none of these patients had increased troponin I levels.[9] Table 8–4 outlines patterns of enzyme release commonly occur seen during AMI.

Coagulation Studies

Drug-induced anticoagulation is a routine procedure for many patients and requires close monitoring of blood coagulation levels by the nurse. Patients receive anticoagulants for treatment and prophylaxis of venous thrombosis, pulmonary embolism, and systemic embolism associated with tissue and mechanical heart valves, atrial fibrillation, and MI. Anticoagulation is also indicated for AMI, in conjunction with thrombolytic therapy, for unstable angina, and during cardiac surgery.

Partial Thromboplastin Time

Partial thromboplastin time (PTT) measures the intrinsic coagulation system and is used to assess patients receiving heparin therapy. The normal range is 30 to 45 seconds. A modified version of the PTT is the activated PTT (aPTT), which has a normal value of 21 to 35 seconds. The therapeutic range of PTT and aPTT should be maintained at 1.5 to 2.5 times the control. It is important to monitor PTT levels closely in patients receiving IV heparin (see Chapter 10). Blood levels should be checked 6 hours after making a dose adjustment, and

TABLE 8–4
Patterns of Cardiac Enzymes in Acute Myocardial Infarction

Enzyme	Earliest Rise	Peak	Normalization
CK	4–6 hours	12–24 hours	3–4 days
CK-MB	4–6 hours	12–24 hours	2–3 days
LDH	12–24 hours	3–6 days	7–10 days
Troponin I	3–7 hours	14–18 hours	5–7 days

CK, creatine kinase; CK-MB, creatine kinase–myocardial bands; LDH, lactate dehydrogenase.

they should be checked daily in those patients receiving a stable dose. Causes of prolonged PTT are vitamin K deficiency, liver disease, disseminated intravascular coagulopathy (DIC), and anticoagulant therapy.

Prothrombin Time

PT is used to monitor patients receiving oral anticoagulants such as warfarin (Coumadin), which alters the extrinsic coagulation pathway and interferes with the formation of vitamin K. Vitamin K causes blood to clot. Many patients with cardiovascular disease require anticoagulation therapy that prolongs the blood's ability to clot. Oral anticoagulants are used in the long-term treatment of patients with atrial fibrillation, prosthetic heart valves, pulmonary embolism, deep vein thrombosis, and ventricular or atrial thrombus. The normal range for the PT is 11 to 13 seconds, and the recommended therapeutic level is 1.5 to 2 times the control.

International Normalized Ratio

The international normalized ratio (INR) is a mathematical "correction" of the results of the one-stage PT. It is a common scale that standardizes reporting of PT determinations worldwide. The INR was developed because thromboplastin reagents used in the measurement of the PT varied significantly in their response to the effects of oral anticoagulants. Now all laboratories use the same calculation to compute the INR. The INR is considered the most accurate method of assessing anticoagulation therapy.[12] Normal range for the INR is 1.3 to 1.6. Recommended therapeutic ranges are listed in Table 8–5. Patients should have their INR levels checked every month even if they have been on the same dose of warfarin for several months.

RADIOGRAPHIC AND IMAGING STUDIES

Chest Radiograph

The chest radiograph is used to determine cardiac abnormalities, heart size and configuration, and changes in individual chambers, as well as pulmonary diseases

and disorders of the mediastinum and bony thorax. The chest radiograph can be obtained in the radiology department or at the patient's bedside with a portable machine. The chest radiograph can provide a record of sequential development or progression of a disease. Chest radiographs should be obtained after insertion of invasive lines (chest tubes, endotracheal tubes, intra-aortic balloon pump, Swan-Ganz catheter, and central lines) to determine whether these lines are in the correct anatomic position and to determine whether a pneumothorax related to the insertion has occurred. In the cardiac patient, the posteroanterior chest radiograph is useful in diagnosing heart failure and cardiomegaly by revealing pleural effusions and cardiac size (Figure 8–1).

Computed Tomography

Computed tomography (CT) uses x-rays to produce a planar image of the heart. CT has not been widely used in cardiovascular studies because of its slow image acquisition, which causes blurring of the moving heart and lungs. CT scans have limited use for cardiovascular assessment because the images gener-

TABLE 8–5
Recommended Therapeutic Range for Oral Anticoagulation

Indication	International Normalized Ratio (INR)
Primary and secondary prevention of venous thrombosis	
Treatment of pulmonary embolism	
Prevention of systemic embolism:	2.0–3.0
Tissue heart valves	
After myocardial infarction	
Valvular heart disease	
Atrial fibrillation	
Mechanical prosthetic valves	2.5–3.5

Adapted from Hirsch J, Dalen J, Deylein D, et al: Oral anticoagulants: mechanism of action, clinical effectiveness and optimal therapeutic range. Chest, 108:231S, 1995.

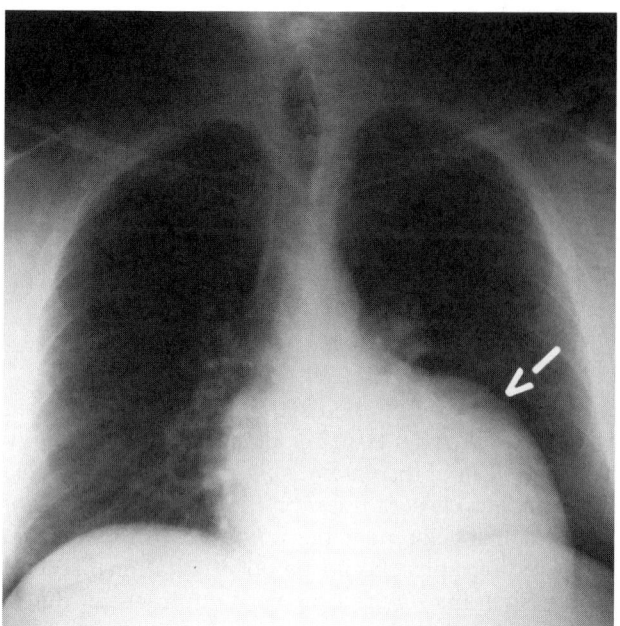

Figure 8–1

Posteroanterior chest radiograph depicting an enlarged cardiac silhouette (arrow) in a patient with end-stage cardiomyopathy.

ated appear to be distorted and have poor resolution. Studies have been limited to assess nonmoving structures such as the aorta, pericardium, and vena cava. Multiple cross-sectional images, or slices, are taken through a certain plane of the body. The test can be done with or without a contrast agent. If contrast is used, an IV bolus of contrast dye is injected, and then images are taken of illuminated areas.

Ultrafast Computed Tomography

Advances in imaging technology have improved the cardiologist's ability to detect and to quantify coronary artery calcification. The newer generation of CT scanners scan much more rapidly than before and allow for clear images of the moving heart and lungs. Magnetic fields are used to direct the x-ray beams in a rapid scan of the patient's body after contrast is injected. Ultrafast CT has shown high accuracy in delineating the inner and outer surfaces of cardiac walls, thus making it possible for more accurate calculations of chamber volumes, ventricular mass (thrombi), wall thickness, and stroke volume. Although ultrafast CT is expensive technology, it is considered superior in measuring cardiac function. Few other studies offer as many measurements in such a short time. Further developments in three-dimensional CT imaging are expected.

Patient Considerations

Before the test, the nurse should explain the rationale for the test and what the patient may experience

during the test. The patient undergoing a CT scan should take nothing by mouth for 4 hours before the procedure. The administration of the contrast agent is similar in both tests and requires an IV line. During the administration of the contrast, the patient may experience flushing, headache, nausea, or tingling for a few minutes or seconds. The patient should be instructed to report symptoms such as chest pain, shortness of breath, or severe itching. For conventional CT, the patient is expected to lie in the scanning tube for 30 to 90 minutes. The patient may be instructed to hold his or her breath for 30 to 45 seconds at a time. The ultrafast CT is a much shorter test requiring the patient to lie still in the scanning tube for approximately 30 minutes.

Magnetic Resonance Imaging

This diagnostic tool uses a powerful magnetic field and pulses of radiofrequency to obtain images of internal structures. It is a noninvasive technique that produces cross-sectional images of human anatomy through exposure to magnetic energy, but without using radiation. It provides further information on structural cardiovascular abnormalities when the results from tests such as the echocardiogram are inconclusive. Magnetic resonance imaging (MRI) provides detailed images of soft tissue structures and can be used to image various cardiac abnormalities because vessels and heart chambers are clearly outlined. Cardiac conditions that can be imaged with MRI include structural abnormalities (congenital heart defects, valvular disease, aortic disease, chamber size, and pericarditis), regions of myocardial infarction, cardiac masses (thrombi or tumors), and unusual blood flow (graft patency). Because of its high cost, it is rarely the test of choice in cardiac diagnosis.

Patient Considerations

Before the test, the nurse should explain why the test is indicated and what the patient may experience during the test. The patient should void before leaving the unit for the test. The patient only needs to take nothing by mouth (NPO) for 4 hours before the scan if contrast is used. The nurse should determine whether the patient has any contraindications to the test (Chart 8–1). The nurse should explain to the patient the need to lie flat for 60 to 90 minutes in a small tube. The nurse should explore with the patient any history or inclination toward claustrophobia. Premedication may be given to help the anxious or claustrophobic patient to relax if the situation warrants it. The patient cannot be attached to any machines, such as an infusion pump, cardiac monitor, or respirator (unless it is a magnet-safe ventilator), or have any metal implants, such as a pacemaker,

CHART 8–1

Contraindications to Magnetic Resonance Imaging

Absolute:

- Implanted cardiac pacemakers and implanted cardiac defibrillators; MRI may cause device to shut down, fire, or function inappropriately because of the strong magnetic field
- Epicardial pacemaker wires
- Implanted drug infusion pumps
- Cochlear (inner ear) implants
- Metal vascular or aneurysm clips, especially cerebral
- Metal artificial heart valve
- Certain intrauterine devices

Potential (should be assessed by a radiologist):

- Artificial joint replacements
- Dental braces and bridges
- Surgical wires and clips from healed surgical procedures
- Metal mesh and plates
- Other foreign objects in the body
- Pregnancy

because of the strong magnetic field. In most cases, the patient must be medically stable to have an MRI.

Echocardiography

Echocardiography is a noninvasive ultrasound imaging test that records the movement of the structures of the heart. It plays an important role in the diagnosis and serial evaluation of numerous cardiac disorders. Echocardiography has been a standard diagnostic tool since the mid–1950s.[13] Since then, echocardiography has become a widely used, safe, and inexpensive diagnostic tool in cardiology. It provides a noninvasive means to accurately assess left ventricular function (ejection fraction), cardiac chamber size, structure and function of the valves, wall motion and thickness, and size of pericardial effusion and to detect the presence of intracardiac thrombi.

The procedure involves the transmission of ultrasonic high-frequency sound waves with a piezoelectric transducer. The transducer sends out sound waves to the heart and receives "echoes" that are reflected back from the various structures within the heart. The pictures formed by the echoes are recorded on a video tape along with the ECG. In this way, the pictures can be referenced to the cardiac cycle and can be easily stored. Structures can be viewed from various angles by changing the position of the transducer.

The three basic types of echocardiographic studies are M-mode, two-dimensional, and Doppler.

M-Mode Echocardiography

The M-mode was the first mode used for cardiac diagnosis. This mode is currently rarely used alone because it uses a single ultrasonic beam and provides a one-dimensional image of the cardiac structures. The M-mode does remain useful for evaluation of wall thickness, heart chamber dimensions, and valve motion.

Two-Dimensional Echocardiography

Two-dimensional echocardiography allows for even greater analysis of the cardiac structures by transmitting multiple ultrasonic beams through a wide arch instead of a unidimensional time–motion display. Two-dimensional echocardiograms depict anatomic relationships and define the movement of cardiac structures relative to one another. This wider field of view allows for better determinations of anatomic structures, wall motion, abnormal communications, mitral valve orifice size, valvular vegetations, mitral valve prolapse, pericardial effusions, and thrombi[14] (Figure 8–2).

Doppler Echocardiography

Doppler echocardiography evaluates the direction of blood flow, turbulence, and velocity and allows for the estimation of gradients within the heart and great vessels. This technique is an important complement to echocardiographic imaging by allowing evaluation of normal and abnormal blood flow. This test uses the same hand-held transducer, which is placed on the patient's chest using conductive jelly, and is a valuable adjunct to conventional echocardiography for a more complete noninvasive evaluation of cardiac function. These sound waves can be heard through the stethoscope attached to the transducer. The transducer emits sound waves that bounce off moving red blood cells. Flow sounds are heard during systole and diastole. If

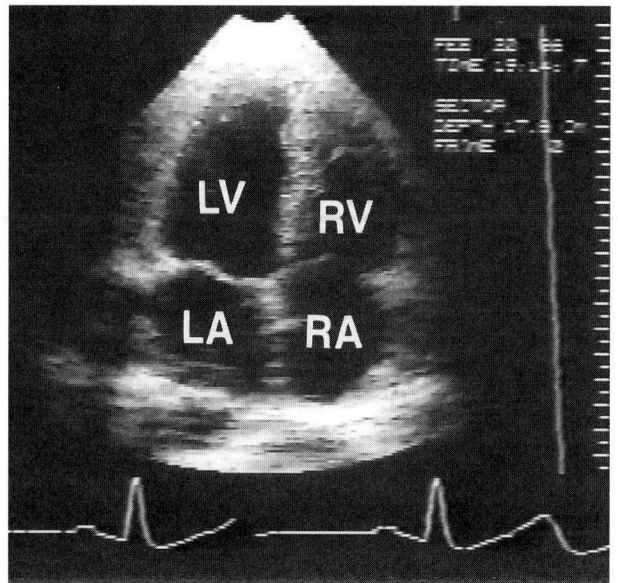

Figure 8–2

Two-dimensional apical four-chamber view echocardiogram. LA, left atrium; LV, left ventricle; RA, right atrium; RV, right ventricle.

blood flow in the area is decreased, the sounds will be decreased. If partial obstruction is present, one will hear a high-pitched sound at the obstruction and a weaker sound distal to it. If a complete obstruction is present, the sound may be almost absent. Doppler studies can record the location, timing, direction, and magnitude of blood flow.

Because Doppler echocardiography focuses on blood flow, it is a valuable diagnostic tool in determining the origin of heart murmurs, in locating intracardiac and extracardiac shunts, in assessing the presence of valvular regurgitation and stenosis and ejection fraction, and in evaluating the patency of coronary bypass grafts.[15] Doppler techniques are now a standard part of the routine echocardiogram in most institutions.

Doppler Color Flow Imaging

Doppler color flow imaging allows for visualization of blood flowing through the heart. It is an added feature that can easily be incorporated into the routine echocardiogram examination. Blood flow is analyzed at multiple points along the Doppler beam simultaneously. The different directions and velocities of blood flow are displayed on the monitor as different colors relative to the transducer position. The velocity of the blood flow is indicated by the intensity of the color. The result is a "noninvasive angiogram" that is a two-dimensional image of cardiac anatomy with a color representation of blood as it flows through the anatomic structures.

Doppler color flow imaging allows for the immediate visualization of the extent and direction of regurgi-

tant blood flow. When abnormal flows such as shunts or regurgitant or stenotic jets are detected, their directions are displayed on the monitor. The severity of the valvular regurgitant can be determined, based on the length and width of the regurgitant jet flow.

Ejection fraction can also be determined using color Doppler techniques. This is done during a two-dimensional echocardiogram by placing the color sector over the left ventricle. This technique is especially useful because the blood pool can be distinguished from the borders of the left ventricle.[16] Color flow Doppler allows for more accuracy in detecting flow abnormalities.

Patient Considerations

There is no special pretest patient preparation for an echocardiogram. The test can be done at the patient's bedside and repeated many times. At the beginning of the procedure, the patient is instructed to lie on the left side, with the head elevated slightly to enhance viewing of the heart. ECG leads are placed on the patient, and the tracing is displayed on the monitor. The transducer is placed on the chest after a generous amount of conductive gel is applied to the chest wall. The conductive gel allows for air-free contact between the transducer and the skin and allows the transducer to slide more easily across the chest (Figure 8–3). No risks are associated with the procedure, and it usually lasts 30 minutes to 1 hour, depending on the study ordered. The only discomfort the patient may experience is due to the pressure of the transducer on the chest wall.

Transesophageal Echocardiography

Transesophageal echocardiography (TEE) is an echocardiogram combined with endoscopy to give a better

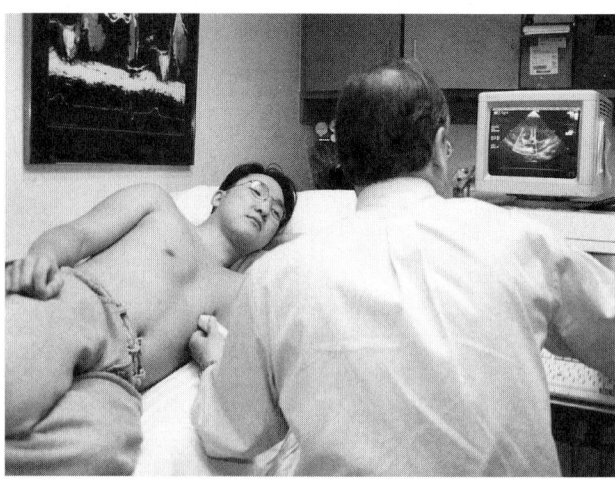

Figure 8–3

Echocardiogram being performed demonstrating standard patient and clinician positions.

view of the heart's structures. TEE uses a miniature transducer mounted on the end of a modified endoscope to transmit and receive ultrasound waves from within the esophagus, thus producing high-quality, high-frequency images of the nearby cardiac structures. It is especially useful in patients who have increased ultrasound attenuation in transthoracic echocardiograms, such as patients with chronic obstructive pulmonary disease (COPD) and obesity. TEE is used to visualize and evaluate heart valves and the functioning of prosthetic valves and to examine the heart for endocarditis, congenital heart disease, intracardiac thrombi, and tumors. It is also used to assess thoracic and aortic disorders, such as dissection and aneurysm. Surgeons have used TEE intraoperatively to assist in removing air from the heart before closing the chest and to help evaluate the success of surgical repair of congenital and valvular defects.[17,18] In addition, TEE is used widely intraoperatively to monitor left ventricular wall motion.[16] This procedure can be done on an inpatient or outpatient basis or while patients are under general anesthesia and are intubated.

The endoscope used in TEE has a flexible tip that can be manipulated 90° forward and 30° laterally to direct ultrasound. The scope is lubricated and is inserted into the patient's open mouth. A bite block with a hollow center is used to allow for easy passage of the tube and to prevent the patient from biting the endoscope. The scope is then advanced approximately 30 to 35 cm, which places the transducer behind the left atrium. Ultrasound images are then obtained and are recorded for review. Left ventricular inferior images may also be obtained by advancing the scope to 40 to 45 cm into the stomach and angling upward. See Chart 8–2 for nursing care of the patient undergoing TEE.

Myocardial Perfusion Scans

Thallium-201 and Technetium 99m Sestamibi

Thallium-201 (Tl-201) and technetium 99m (Tc 99m) sestamibi (Cardiolyte) are radioactive imaging agents used with treadmill stress ECG testing to diagnosis

---

CHART 8–2

Nursing Care of the Patient Undergoing Transesophageal Echocardiography

Before the procedure:

- Assessment for contraindications: history of esophageal dysfunction, cancer, strictures, or surgery
- History of adverse reactions to anesthetics or sedatives
- Explanation of the procedure to the patient
- Obtaining of signed informed consent
- Patient to have nothing by mouth for at least 4 to 6 hours before the procedure
- Insertion of intravenous line or heparin lock
- Removal of dentures or oral prosthesis
- Patient asked to void before the procedure
- Suction setup in place and functioning
- Resuscitation equipment available
- Patient placed on the cardiac monitor and pulse oximetry

During the procedure:

- Patient's throat may be sprayed with topical anesthetic that causes a bitter taste and the sensation of a swollen tongue
- Position the patient on the left side with the head flat or slightly elevated

- "Chin to chest" position, to allow for better passage of the endoscope through the oropharynx
- Continuous, conscious sedation
- Suction, as needed
- Informing the patient of progress and providing reassurance
- Continuous monitoring of blood pressure, heart rate, and oxygenation

After the procedure:

- Patient sitting up or positioned on one side
- Patient encouraged to cough
- Nothing by mouth till the gag reflex enables the patient to protect the airway (30 minutes to several hours)
- Provision of lozenges; a sore throat possible for a couple of days
- If done as an outpatient, patient instructed not to drive for the next 12 hours if sedation was given during the procedure; best to have someone drive the patient home
- Patient instructed to call the physician in the event of hemoptysis, pain, or dyspnea

ischemic heart disease and myocardial perfusion. These tests reveal wall motion and ventricular function during increased oxygen demand (exercise). Tl-201 and Tc 99m sestamibi are similar in that they collect more readily in healthy cells than in damaged ones. Regions of ischemia and infarction cannot take up this substance and therefore appear as "cold spots" when imaged. They both are distributed to myocardial cells in proportion to the blood supply, and thus they measure myocardial perfusion.

Tl-201 is a potassium analog normally taken up by myocardial cells. The most widely used clinical application for myocardial perfusion imaging is stress testing with Tl-201. It is injected IV at maximal exercise, when it is rapidly taken up from the blood by living myocardial cells, and an image of the heart is obtained. Images are taken at peak exercise and are repeated at rest 4 to 6 hours later. The images reveal absent, poor, or good uptake of the isotope. If regions of decreased thallium uptake (cold spots) are detected on the exercise study but are not seen after the resting images, a diagnosis of myocardial ischemia is made. If regions of limited or no thallium uptake are observed on the exercise scan and the rest scan, a diagnosis of prior MI can be made. The sensitivity of Tl-201 stress testing is more than 85%. In contrast, the sensitivity of standard ECG stress testing is about 50 to 70%. Resting thallium scans are used when patients have anginal symptoms at rest, and these scans demonstrate the presence of transient myocardial hypoperfusion and viable myocardium.[19]

Tc 99m sestamibi is used in a similar way as Tl-201. The patient exercises to an acceptable heart rate, the isotope is injected IV, and scanning images are taken of the heart. If a defect is seen in the myocardium, indicative of regional hypoperfusion resulting from coronary narrowing, then the patient must return in 24 hours for a reinjection and repeat imaging. If on the repeat scan, the defect remains, this indicates myocardial scar or old infarction. However, if on repeat injection, the defect is no longer present, this indicates that the patient has ischemia and probably a high-grade stenosis in the coronary artery supplying that segment of the myocardium. Tc 99m sestamibi not only helps in the diagnosis of ischemic abnormalities, but also aids in the assessment of wall motion abnormalities.

Technetium Pyrophosphate Scan

Tc 99m pyrophosphate (Tc-PYP) is an infarct-avid agent (hot spot imaging) and has been shown to be a sensitive method of detecting MI from 24 hours to 5 days after onset of chest pain. A Tc-PYP scan is not performed often and is only indicated when standard methods of imaging used to diagnose myocardial infarction are unreliable. Examples include 1) the period after cardiac surgery when high levels of creatine

kinase are present, 2) atypical chest pain with equivocal ECG or enzyme changes, 3) chest pain and ECG that do not allow assessment of transmural injury (i.e., left bundle branch block), 4) preexisting infarcts and evidence of infarct extension, and 5) myocardial contusion. This technique is normally used in bone imaging to assess activity in the ribs, sternum, and vertebral column. A normal pyrophosphate scan image shows no activity in the regions of the heart. It localizes infarct tissue at approximately 12 hours to 1 week after the acute event. The optimal imaging time is 24 to 72 hours, because during this time collateral blood flow develops to the infarcted area, and the level of calcium accumulation within necrotic cells is increased. Tc-PYP does not stay in infarcted tissue past 7 to 10 days; therefore, is useful only in the acute phase and for a short time thereafter.

It is not necessary to withhold food or medications from the patient before the scan. A single scan is required, lasting about 30 minutes. There is no special aftercare of the patient other than determining the patient's tolerance of the procedure.

Technetium 99m Teboroxime

Another technetium agent, Tc 99m teboroxime (Cardiotec), is an attractive testing agent because of its high myocardial extraction and washout. Currently, however, it is not commonly used. Because of the rapid washout, the patient must be imaged within 2 minutes of exercise, and image acquisition must be completed within 10 minutes, which allows for a more expeditious examination. Use of Tc 99m teboroxime may become more widespread when faster scanning equipment can be developed.

Pharmacologic Thallium Imaging: Dipyridamole (Persantine) and Adenosine (Adenocard)

In the past, myocardial perfusion imaging was limited to patients who could perform some form of exercise. However, many patients cannot exercise because of physical disabilities from chronic illness and aging. To broaden the clinical availability of perfusion scintigraphy, several nonexercise pharmacologic stressor agents have been used. The most commonly used coronary vasodilator agents are intravenous dipyridamole and adenosine. Both agents cause vasodilation in normal vessels as occurs in exercise, whereas less vasodilation is seen in stenotic vessels. In patients without CAD, dipyridamole causes vasodilation and increased coronary artery blood flow. In patients with CAD, dipyridamole does not cause vasodilation in the diseased artery, but vasodilation in the vessels distal to the stenotic areas is significant.[19] In addition, by causing the exercise effect, ischemia that normally would occur during exercise is induced with dipyridamole. Less significant coronary blockages are associated with transient thallium defects, whereas mild, persistent defects are consistent with severe coronary artery stenosis.

Dipyridamole is given IV, and the patient waits a few minutes until the drug takes effect, when the thallium is injected IV. The patient then goes to the nuclear medicine department to have images of the heart taken by a scanning machine. The patient goes back to his or her room to rest and returns to the nuclear medicine department in several hours to have more images of the heart taken. Before and during the test, the patient's blood pressure, heart rate, and ECG are monitored frequently.

In a comparison of dobutamine and dipyridamole in a dog model, dobutamine was the better agent for inducing wall motion abnormalities during ischemia, whereas dipyridamole resulted in greater flow heterogeneity.[20] These findings suggest that dipyridamole may be a better pharmacologic agent for perfusion imaging, and dobutamine may be better for use with an imaging modality that assesses wall motion during stress testing.

Positron Emission Tomography

Positron emission tomography (PET) scanning is useful in the detection of CAD and in the assessment of myocardial viability in patients with CAD and left ventricular dysfunction. The test allows for the noninvasive evaluation of regional cardiac metabolism through direct measurement of oxygen uptake and use. What distinguishes PET imaging from conventional imaging techniques is its ability to provide quantitative evaluation of tissue function. This means that PET scanning can identify metabolically active tissue. Identification of active tissue may allow for methods of reperfusion to be used and may permit preservation of myocardium and reduction of infarct size. PET imaging assists in determining which regions of the myocardium have viable tissue that could benefit from revascularization and which areas have suffered complete infarction. PET scans can localize and facilitate understanding of ischemia in discrete areas of myocardium resulting from an imbalance of oxygen supply and demand. The combined use of tracers provides a unique tool to identify myocardium with reduced blood flow and to determine the metabolic state (viability) of such compromised tissue. To determine the presence or absence of viable myocardium, a comparison of images is made using fluorodeoxyglucose-18 (^{18}FDG), and rubidum-82 or N-13 ammonia (^{13}NH$_3$) (Figure 8–4A).

If ^{13}NH$_3$ uptake is decreased or absent (indicating decreased coronary flow) and ^{18}FDG uptake is high (indicating intact metabolism), a mismatch is said to occur (Figure 8–4B). A mismatch means that there is little or no blood flow, but potentially salvageable ischemic myocardium. Matched images demonstrate that uptake of ^{18}FDG and ^{13}NH$_3$ is absent, a finding that indicates no blood flow and nonviable, necrotic myocardium. Limited widespread availability and high cost have prevented the general use of PET scanning for cardiac imaging.

Patient Considerations

The patient is NPO for 3 to 4 hours before the test. Often, patients are allowed a light breakfast if the test is later in the day, but they are restricted from caffeinated beverages for 24 hours before the test. Many scans require two sessions, and the restrictions should be continued until the second scan has been completed. The nurse must explain to the patient what occurs during the test. The nurse should tell the patient that radioactive isotopes will be injected into the body to assess the function of the heart. The nurse should also explain that the isotopes are not harmful and are rapidly removed from the body because of their short half-life. The patient will be placed in a doughnut-shaped scanning device (Figure 8–5). The patient's arms will be restrained at his or her sides to prevent movement during the scan. The isotopes will be injected IV. The patient will be able to communicate with the technician during the procedure by intercom from the adjoining room. The length of the scanning procedure ranges from 1 to 4 hours. There are no special patient care needs after these scans.

Radionuclide Ventriculography

The two types of radionuclide ventriculograms are the first-pass study and the multigated acquisition (MUGA) scan (blood pool study). These studies evaluate regional and global ventricular performance and ventricular volume. A stress MUGA scan (with exercise) may be performed to detect changes in ejection fraction and cardiac function during exercise. A MUGA scan may also complement other studies in assessing valve disease, cardiomyopathy, and transplant rejection, and it may be used as a screening test for CAD. These studies are helpful in noninvasive diagnosis, prognosis, and evaluation of therapy.

First-pass studies involve the IV injection of Tc 99m, which mixes with the blood, so that changes in count rate and isotope uptake correspond directly to changes in ventricular volumes. After injection, a scintillation camera records separate images of the isotope in its

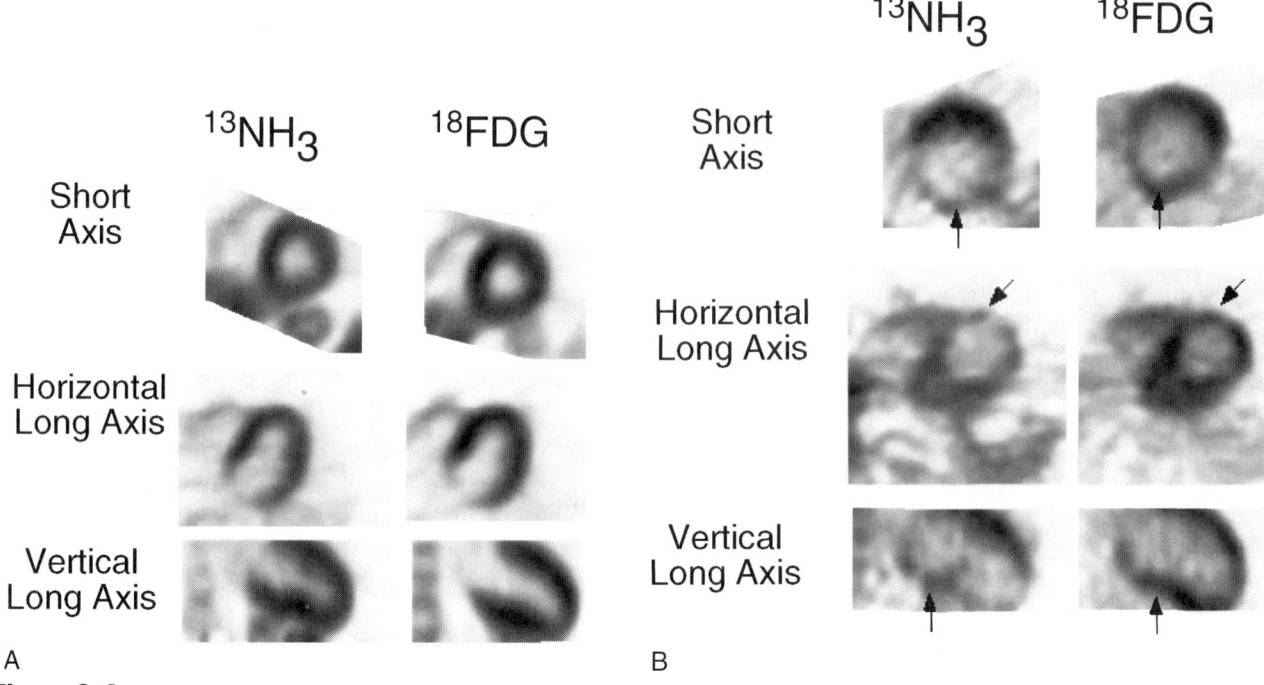

Figure 8–4

A, Normal positron emission tomography (PET) scan with N-13 ammonia ($^{13}NH_3$) perfusion images and fluorodeoxyglucose 18 (^{18}FDG) metabolic images obtained in a healthy person. Note the homogeneous tracer distribution throughout the entire left ventricular myocardium. B, PET scan image showing perfusion ($^{13}NH_3$) and metabolic (^{18}FDG) images obtained in a patient with ischemic cardiomyopathy who is referred for cardiac transplant evaluation. The short axis images of $^{13}NH_3$ perfusion shows a defect in the inferior wall. In contrast, glucose metabolic activity is preserved that is consistent with a blood flow metabolism mismatch, that is, viable myocardium. The vertical long axis images confirm this mismatch. An additional perfusion-metabolism mismatch is noted in the distal anterior wall and apex, as indicated by the arrows on the horizontal long axis cuts. Blood flow metabolism mismatches are the hallmark of myocardial viability. Viable segments are likely to improve contractile function after revascularization (coronary artery bypass).

initial pass through the left ventricle. This is called first-pass imaging. Counts are higher during diastole because there is more blood and, therefore, more radioactivity in the ventricular chamber. When the blood is ejected during systole, the counts fall. The procedure requires about 25 to 30 seconds of imaging. An advantage of first-pass imaging is its ability to assess the

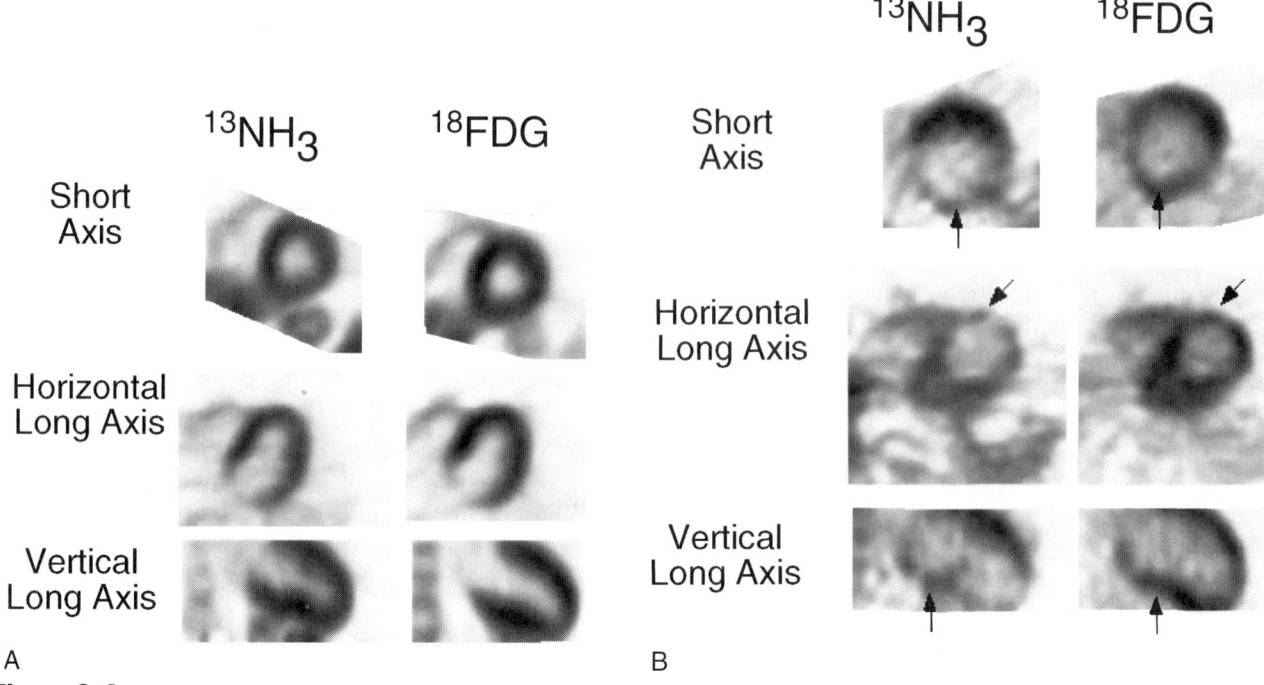

Figure 8–5

Position emission tomography scanner. The patient lies on the table and is positioned within the doughnut-shaped scanning machine during the test.

heart within a few seconds. During exercise studies, this procedure can be used to study the heart at various levels of exercise without having the patient maintain a steady, prolonged period of exercise.

The MUGA study differs from the first-pass technique in that data are collected continuously over hundreds of cardiac cycles. Once the Tc 99m is injected, images are obtained. The patient is attached to an ECG machine, which is essential for ECG gating of the acquired image. The R wave on the ECG signal is used to initiate the data collection. A certain number of images are taken with each heartbeat (16–64 frames per cardiac cycle). The portion of isotope ejected with each heartbeat can then be calculated by the images to determine the ejection fraction. In addition, the presence and size of intracardiac shunts can be determined.

Patient Considerations

There are no special preparations for patients undergoing radionuclide tests. Meals do not need to be withheld, but patients should not eat a heavy meal before the test. The patient should void before the procedure. He or she is attached to an ECG and has an IV line placed. Comfortable clothing should be worn if the patient is undergoing an exercise test. Although adverse effects are rare, patients should be assessed for any side effects from the radionuclide tracer. Patients who receive sestamibi often report a metallic taste in their mouth for several hours after injection. The tests last approximately 30 to 45 minutes.

STRESS TESTING

Exercise Stress Testing

Treadmill exercise stress testing is the most commonly used noninvasive test to detect CAD. Both physical and emotional stresses usually precipitate myocardial ischemia in patients with coronary artery stenosis. Exercise increases myocardial oxygen demand, and, once the available oxygen supply is depleted, angina develops. The exercise stress test attempts to induce ischemia and to document ECG changes that correlate with the patient's symptoms.

Exercise stress testing can be done using a treadmill or bicycle (Figure 8–6). Before starting the test, a baseline ECG, blood pressure, and heart rate are obtained

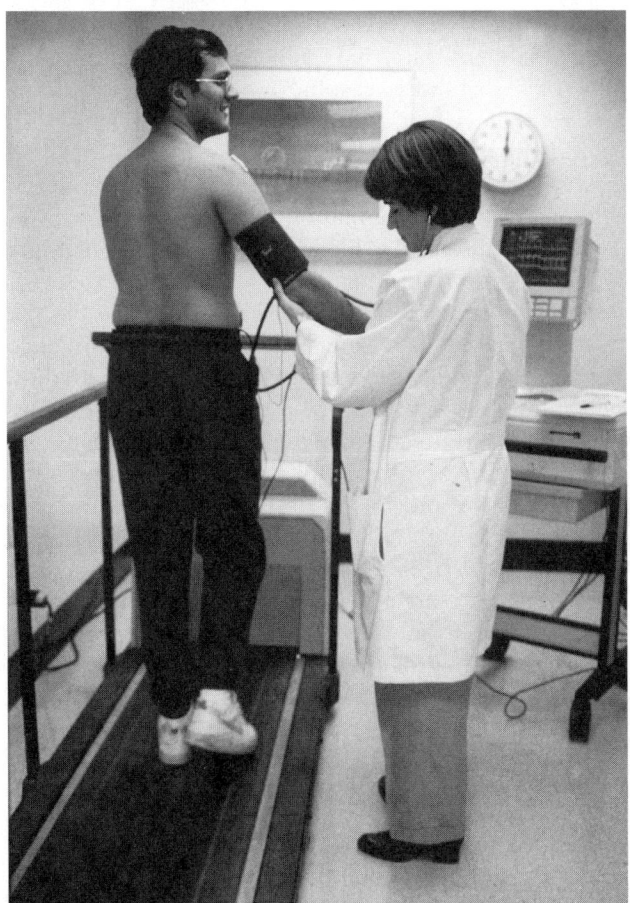

Figure 8–6

Exercise treadmill test. Patient undergoing testing with continuous 12-lead electrocardiographic monitoring and intermittent blood pressure monitoring by the clinician.

and are then monitored during exercise. The rate and the incline at which the patient exercises are progressively increased until the patient reaches 85 to 90% of age-predicted heart rate response. The exercise test is terminated before reaching the age-predicted maximum if the patient experiences runs of ventricular dysrhythmias, hypotension, chest pain, dyspnea, or ST-segment elevation greater than 1 mm or depression greater than 2 mm. The test may also be terminated because of leg fatigue or cramps, or if the patient is too tired to continue. Otherwise, the test can be stopped once 85% of the predicted maximal heart rate is reached.

A positive exercise test is defined as a downsloping of the ST segment of more than 1 mm or an upsloping of the ST segment of more than 2 mm occurring more than 0.08 seconds from the J point. The more marked the ST-segment deviation and the less the patient is able to exercise, the more severe the CAD is likely to be. Other criteria that indicate a positive test include the development of hypotension, inverted T waves, and angina.

Exercise stress testing is not always conclusive. Because the standard exercise stress test relies on ischemic related changes on the ECG, the test is less useful in patients with baseline abnormal ST segments, such as those with left bundle branch block or left ventricular hypertrophy. False-positive results are common among populations where the prevalence of CAD is low, and a "normal" test does not exclude the possibility of CAD.

Exercise Stress Echocardiography

Exercise stress echocardiography is a relatively new but widely used diagnostic test that is helpful in identifying the extent and location of CAD. When two-dimensional echocardiography is combined with standard exercise testing, it allows for more accurate evaluation of myocardial wall motion. Because of its high degree of sensitivity and specificity, stress echocardiogram can be used accurately to predict the number and location of significant (>50%) stenotic coronary lesions.[20] A normal response to exercise is hypercontractility throughout the myocardium. If decreased contractility is noted with exercise, CAD can be considered a likely cause.

The two types of stress echocardiograms are the bicycle test and the treadmill test. The most common is the treadmill echocardiogram. This combines the standard two-dimensional echocardiography with a treadmill stress test. At the beginning of a test, a baseline ECG, heart rate, blood pressure, and resting two-dimensional echocardiogram are obtained. The patient begins to walk or run on the treadmill while the ECG, heart rate, and blood pressure are continuously monitored. When the patient reaches peak exercise, determined by the patient or the physician, the exercise is stopped, and an echocardiogram is obtained. After the patient's heart rate and blood pressure have returned to normal, a posttest echocardiogram is obtained. Comparisons are then made among the three echocardiograms. The test is relatively inexpensive and can be performed in a physician's office.

Pharmacologic Stress Testing

Exercise stress testing, with or without nuclear or echocardiography imaging, is the noninvasive method of choice used for the detection of CAD and the functional assessment of the patient's heart. However, many patients are unable to perform adequate leg exercises because of neurologic, vascular, respiratory, or orthopedic limitations. For these patients, pharmacologic methods of evaluating coronary artery blood flow and myocardial function have been developed and do not require standard exercise. IV dobutamine (Dobutrex) is the medication commonly used. During exercise stress testing, ischemia occurs in most patients when myocardial oxygen demand exceeds coronary artery blood flow. Dobutamine increases myocardial oxygen demand by increasing myocardial contractility, heart rate, and blood pressure, similar to a standard exercise test, and thereby induces ischemia in most patients with severe coronary artery lesions. These medications, when used in combination with echocardiography, can provide valuable information about coronary artery stenosis.

The dobutamine echocardiogram is similar to the treadmill test in that frequent ECG monitoring, blood pressure, and heart rate measurements are taken. A two-dimensional echocardiogram is taken at baseline and with each dose increase. A dobutamine infusion is started at a low dose and is gradually increased by 5 μg/kg per minute every 3 minutes until the peak dose is reached. A high dose of dobutamine is necessary to increase myocardial oxygen demand to a level beyond the available supply.[20] The results of the test are based on a comparison of the echocardiogram at rest, at peak exercise (peak dose), and after exercise (after infusion). An abnormal test result shows regions of abnormal wall motion or contractility (hypokinesis) with drug-induced exercise.

Patient Considerations

Patients who are undergoing an exercise ECG test should be instructed to abstain from eating or drinking for 2 hours before the test and to avoid consuming caffeinated beverages for several hours before the test. The patient's clinical situation and the indication for the test will determine whether certain medications (e.g., beta blockers) should be withheld before the test. Patients should wear comfortable shoes and loose-fitting clothes for exercise. Patients undergoing exercise stress echocardiograms should be told that an echocardiogram will be taken before and after exercise. The procedure is the same as other echocardiogram tests, except exercise is added. Patients will be asked to walk on a treadmill or bicycle, and the speed or grade will gradually be increased. During both exercise echocardiography and standard stress testing, patients will be encouraged to continue exercising until they feel they can no longer exercise or develop symptoms that would require termination of the test, as previously described in each section. The entire test takes less than 1 hour. Patients undergoing pharmacologic stress testing should be assessed for side effects from the medications, including flushing, headache, and nausea.

Cardiopulmonary Exercise Testing

Cardiopulmonary exercise testing involves submaximal and maximal treadmill or bicycle exercise with continuous ECG monitoring, breath determination of oxygen uptake and carbon dioxide, and spirometry. This technique allows determination of exercise capacity, peak heart rate, maximal oxygen consumption, anaerobic threshold, respiratory gas exchange ratio, and ventilatory equivalent for oxygen. The test is indicated to evaluate patients with CHF, previous MI, and dyspnea, and those who are undergoing or have undergone heart transplantation.

Patients are asked to bicycle or walk with a breathing mouthpiece that is similar to a snorkel. Two different tests are performed. During the first test, the bike or treadmill stays at the same low speed for 8 minutes to test patients' abilities to perform normal daily activities. The second test evaluates how much they can do, and the difficulty of the test increases gradually. Patients are encouraged to continue until they can no longer exercise. ECG, heart rate, blood pressure, and breathing are monitored throughout the test. The total exercise time is approximately 20 minutes, and the whole test takes 1 hour. Maximal oxygen consumption is measured; this is the best indicator of maximal cardiac reserve and provides important prognostic information to guide the assessment and therapy of patients with heart failure as well as other cardiac conditions.

Patient Considerations

Patients should be told not to eat or drink 2 hours before testing. They should wear comfortable pants or shorts and tennis shoes to protect their feet. The nurse should explain to the patients that they will be asked to exercise until they no longer can. There are no special precautions after the test, except that patients may be tired, so they should not plan strenuous activity for the remainder of the day.

Electrophysiologic Studies

Electrophysiologic studies are performed to evaluate the electrical conduction system of the heart. This technique includes both diagnostic testing and interventional treatment procedures. Candidates for this procedure include those with refractory or life-threatening supraventricular or ventricular dysrhythmias (e.g., paroxsysmal supraventricular tachycardia or ventricular tachycardia), survivors of sudden cardiac arrest, and patients with unexplained syncope and atrioventricular (AV) accessory pathways. The procedure enables one to identify the origin of a dysrhythmia and to evaluate the effect of antidysrhythmic therapies such as medications, pacing, and surgical interventions. The electrophysiologic study is similar to cardiac catheterization. An electrode catheter is inserted into the femoral vein and is threaded through the inferior vena cava. It is advanced into the right atrium, through the tricuspid valve, and into the apex of the right ventricle. The patient is monitored continuously with intracardiac and external ECG leads to record the cardiac response.

With pacing of the atria and ventricle and introduction of premature extra stimuli, ventricular and supraventricular tachycardias can be induced in most patients who have significant dysrhythmias. Programmed electrical stimulation (PES) is used to examine the tachydysrhythmia by reproducing it through intracardiac catheters. PES is administered at different rates and at different timing intervals during the depolarization-repolarization cycle. It is designed to reproduce dysrhythmias so that the origin of conduction can be located. By moving the catheter, the area can be located and treated with radiofrequency ablation. Catheter ablation involves destroying localized areas of tissue with energy delivered by means of a temperature-monitoring intracardiac catheter. The radiofrequency energy is rarely felt by patients, although some have reported feeling mild chest discomfort during ablation using high energy. Ablation is not always successful, and if the patient does not respond to antidysrhythmic drug therapy, an implantable cardiodefibrillator (ICD) should be inserted (see Chapter 10). Although many dysrhythmias are treated successfully with ablation techniques, ventricular dysrhythmias have only a 30 to 40% success rate. For patients with these life-threatening dysrhythmias, ICDs are the treatment of choice.

Patient Considerations

Patients undergoing electrophysiologic studies should be NPO for 6 to 8 hours before the procedure. In some cases, antidysrhythmic agents are withheld for up to 3 days before the test, to assess dysrhythmias without the influence of the medication. The patient's groin is shaved in preparation for catheter insertion. If the patient receives anticoagulation during the procedure or afterward, a pressure dressing may be applied after the test for several hours to prevent bleeding from the groin puncture site. The procedure can vary from 1 to 4 hours, depending on the difficulty in reproducing the dysrhythmia and in locating the appropriate area to perform ablation.

CARDIAC CATHETERIZATION

Cardiac catheterization dates back to 1929, when Werner Forssmann performed the first cardiac catheterization on *himself*. Nearly a century later, cardiac catheterization has evolved into the most definitive means of diagnosing and, in some cases, treating various cardiovascular disorders. Cardiac catheterization is a combined hemodynamic and angiographic invasive procedure performed to confirm the presence of a clinically suspected heart condition, to define its anatomy and physiology, and, in appropriate cases, to perform therapeutic procedures. Intravascular catheters are used to measure pressures in blood vessels and heart chambers, to determine cardiac output, to measure oxygen saturation, and to inject radiopaque material to examine cardiovascular structures and blood flow. Depending on the clinical situation, many different diagnostic procedures or combinations of procedures may be used in cardiac catheterization. These diagnostic procedures include (but are not limited to) right and left heart catheterization, coronary angiography, ventriculography, aortography, and cardiac biopsy. Common indications for cardiac catheterization are listed in Chart 8–3.

Right and Left Heart Catheterization

The purpose of right and left heart catheterization is to measure intracardiac pressures, specifically in the right atrium, right ventricle, pulmonary artery, left atrium, and left ventricle. Determinations of valve function can also be made with right heart catheterization and left heart catheterization. Right heart catheterization involves directing a balloon-tipped, flow-directed catheter (pulmonary artery catheter or Swan-Ganz catheter) under fluoroscopy through an access vein. The veins commonly used for this include the internal jugular, femoral, and brachial vein. The catheter is advanced through the inferior or superior vena cava into the right atrium, where an initial measurement is obtained. The catheter is next guided across the tricuspid valve into the right ventricle and finally from the right

CHART 8–3

Indications for Cardiac Catheterization

1. Suspected or known coronary artery disease
   a. New-onset angina
   b. Unstable angina
   c. Evaluation before a major surgical procedure
   d. Silent ischemia
   e. Positive exercise treadmill test
   f. Atypical chest pain or coronary spasm
2. Acute myocardial infarction (AMI)
   a. Unstable angina after infarction
   b. Failed thrombolytic therapy
   c. Cardiogenic shock secondary to AMI
   d. Mechanical complications secondary to AMI (e.g., ventricular septal defect, rupture of ventricular wall, papillary muscle)
3. Sudden cardiovascular death
4. Valvular heart disease
5. Congenital heart disease (before anticipated corrective surgery)
6. Aortic dissection
7. Pericardial constriction or tamponade
8. Cardiomyopathy
9. Initial and follow-up assessment for heart transplant

From Kern MJ (ed): The Cardiac Catheterization Handbook, 2nd ed. St. Louis, Mosby–Year Book, 1994, p 3.

ventricle across the pulmonic valve and into the pulmonary artery. Normal pressure readings for these chambers are listed in Table 8–6. In addition, cardiac output, the amount of blood ejected from the heart per minute, may be obtained by the thermodilution method during right heart catheterization (see Table 8–6). The catheter may be withdrawn in the catheterization laboratory or left in place for continuous monitoring of hemodynamic status in the intensive care unit. For detailed information regarding hemodynamic monitoring and cardiac output measurement, refer to Chapter 6.

Left heart catheterization involves directing a catheter to the left heart under fluoroscopic guidance from an access artery, usually the femoral or brachial artery. The catheter is advanced through the aorta and ultimately across the aortic valve into the left ventricle, where a pressure reading is obtained (see Table 8–6). Once pressure recordings are obtained, the catheter is removed.

Coronary Angiography

Coronary angiography is a technique that uses radiopaque contrast dye to visualize the cardiac structures and the coronary arteries. A catheter is introduced into an artery, usually the brachial or femoral artery, and is directed toward the heart under fluoroscopic guidance. The catheter is guided through the aorta to the left and right coronary arteries. Once the catheter is in the appropriate position, a contrast agent or dye is injected, allowing visualization of the artery under examination. Individual coronary arteries and

their branches are injected separately and are viewed from different angles so that the entire coronary circulation may be visualized.[21] Several injections of the contrast agent are necessary to visualize thoroughly the anatomy and patency of the coronary arterial bed. A single exposure produces a single large film image, and a series of x-ray exposures is used to produce an x-ray motion picture or *cineangiography*. Figure 8–7 depicts angiographic visualization of the right and left coronary arteries.

TABLE 8–6

Normal Hemodynamic Parameters Obtained from Cardiac Catheterization

Chamber or Vessel	Pressure Reading (mm Hg)
Right atrium	2–8 (mean)
Right ventricle	15–30 (systolic)
	2–8 (diastolic)
Pulmonary artery	15–30 (systolic)
	4–12 (diastolic)
Pulmonary artery occlusive pressure	4–12 (mean)
Left atrium	4–12 (mean)
Left ventricle	100–140 (systolic)
	4–12 (diastolic)
Aorta	100–140 (systolic)
	60–90 (diastolic)
	70–90 (mean)
Cardiac output	4–8 L/minute
Cardiac index	2.5–4 L/minute

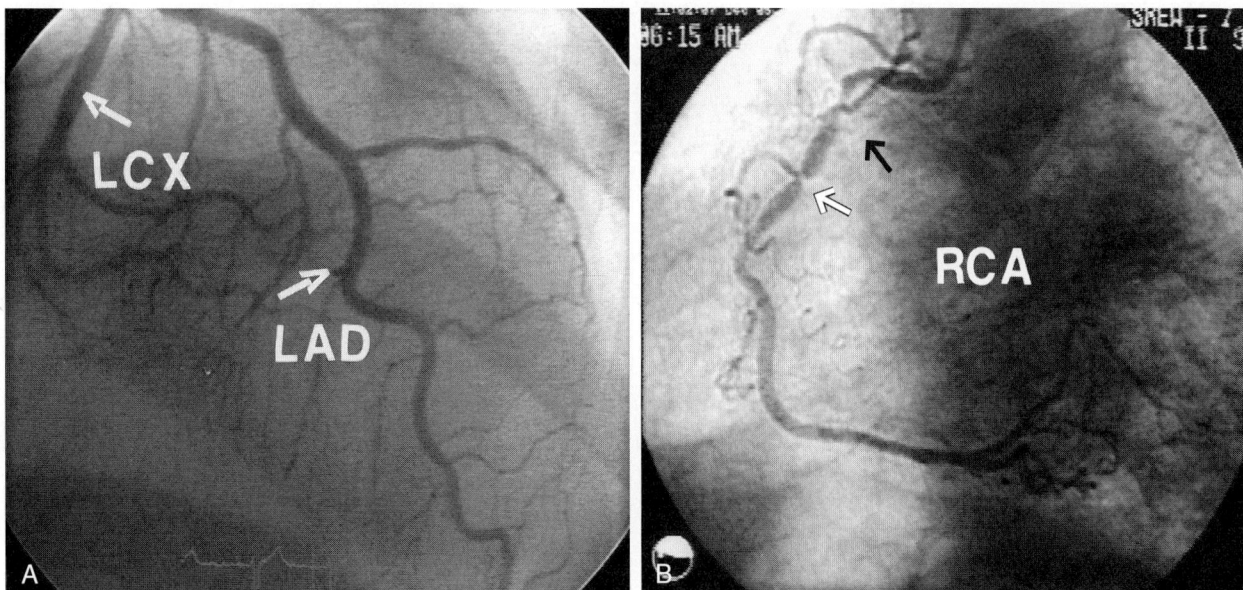

Figure 8–7

*A, Angiographic view of normal left anterior descending (LAD) and left circumflex (LCX) coronary arteries (left anterior oblique view). B, Angiographic view of the right coronary artery (RCA) (left anterior oblique view). The **black arrow** denotes an 80% proximal stenosis, followed by a 90% stenosis (white arrow).*

Ventriculography

Ventriculography refers to the selective injection of contrast dye into a chamber of the heart. Usually, ventriculography is used to evaluate the left ventricle; however, right ventriculography may be performed in patients with congenital heart disease.[22] As previously stated, the contrast agent is injected directly into the left ventricular chamber (Figure 8–8). As the ventricle contracts and

relaxes, ventricular wall motion can be analyzed by visualizing the silhouette of the ventricle during systole and diastole. Ventricular wall motion is observed for areas of decreased, abnormal, or absent movement. The determination of left ventricular ejection fraction (LVEF) is an important measurement obtained with ventriculography. In addition to evaluation of left ventricular function, ventriculography is also indicated to identify aortic and mitral valve competence, abnormal wall thickness, intracardiac shunts, thrombus, and congenital malformation and to determine the presence and location of ventricular aneurysms and septal defects.[22]

Aortography

Aortography is the injection of radiopaque contrast medium to visualize the aorta, the aortic valve leaflets, and the major branches of the aorta. Aortography is used to determine the presence of aortic valve insufficiency, aneurysms or dissections of the ascending aorta, coarctation of the aorta, and injuries to the aorta or its major branches.

Endomyocardial Biopsy

Endomyocardial biopsy is performed to remove a piece of tissue from the heart as a means of diagnosing and evaluating primary myocardial disease, myocarditis, and heart transplant rejection. Endomyocardial biopsy has become a safe procedure with the development of transvascular biotomes. The biotome is a

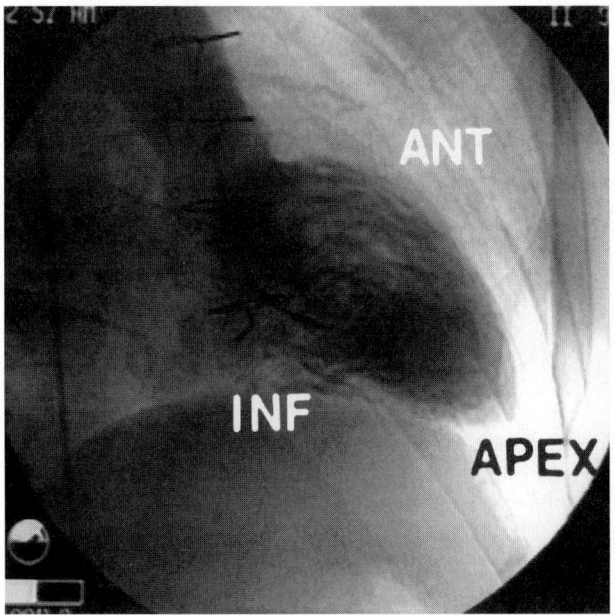

Figure 8–8

Angiographic right anterior oblique view of the end-diastolic frame of a left ventriculogram. ANT, anterior; INF, inferior.

special catheter with a scissor-like handle that controls a collection device at the opposite end. The biotome is introduced into a vascular sheath for placement through the brachial, internal jugular, or femoral vein. This technique allows the physician to scrape a small amount of tissue from the endomyocardial surface of the heart, most commonly the right ventricle. A series of specimens, three or four samples, is obtained, and then the tissues are microscopically examined. Left ventricular biopsy, when necessary, is approached from the brachial or femoral artery. Figure 8–9 depicts tissue samples obtained from the endomyocardial biopsy of the right ventricle in a cardiac transplant recipient for the purpose of rejection surveillance.

Risks of Cardiac Catheterization

Cardiac catheterization is the most widely performed invasive cardiac procedure in the United States.[23] Cardiac catheterization is generally accepted as the most definitive procedure for the evaluation and diagnosis of CAD. The procedure has relatively few contraindications (Chart 8–4).[24] Although cardiac catheterization is an invasive procedure that involves the heart and vascular system, the overall risk of serious complications associated with cardiac catheterization is less than 1%.[23] Major risks of cardiac catheterization are listed in Chart 8–5.[24]

Patient Considerations

Although this procedure is routinely performed, the prospect of undergoing cardiac catheterization can cause the patient and family anxiety. Patient and family education before the procedure should include written education materials and ample opportunity to discuss the procedure, including indications, risks, and alternatives with the physician and appropriate members of the health care team. Ideally, patient education should begin as soon as cardiac catheterization is discussed. The use of written materials along with audiovisual aids is useful when providing information about the purpose of the catheterization and the various aspects of the procedure, including what to expect during and after the procedure (Chart 8–6). Informed consent is necessary before cardiac catheterization, and it should be obtained by the appropriate personnel.

Preprocedure Considerations

Patients should be NPO at least 6 hours before cardiac catheterization to avoid nausea or vomiting during the procedure that may be induced by contrast agents or vagal reaction. The appropriate preprocedure laboratory studies, specifically, complete blood count, electrolytes, BUN, creatinine, and coagulation studies, should be performed and documented in the patient's chart. Patients receiving anticoagulants, such as warfarin (Coumadin), may be instructed to discontinue these medications 1 to 3 days before the procedure. The practice of discontinuing anticoagulants before cardiac catheterization varies among physicians and institutions. Patients are usually premedicated about 1 hour before the procedure with an antihistamine, such as diphenhydramine (Benadryl), and a benzodiazepine, such as diazepam (Valium), to minimize any reaction to the dye and to induce light sedation, respectively.

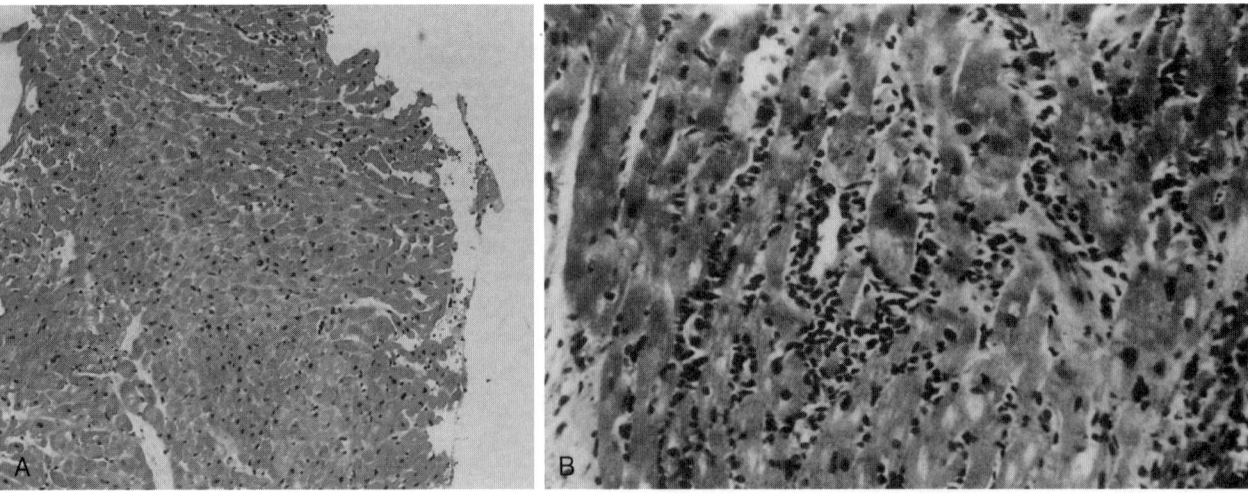

Figure 8–9

A, Endomyocardial biopsy of a patient who underwent orthotopic heart transplantation. Routine biopsy under a low-power field shows no significant rejection. *B,* Endomyocardial biopsy from a patient who underwent orthotopic heart transplantation who presented with congestive heart failure. Biopsy under a high-power field reveals mild diffuse mononuclear infiltrates consistent with mild diffuse rejection (International Society of Heart and Lung Transplantation category 1B).

CHART 8–4

Contraindications to Cardiac Catheterization

Absolute:

- Inadequate equipment, personnel, or catheterization facility

Relative:

- Uncontrolled congestive heart failure, hypertension, dysrhythmias
- Recent cerebral vascular accident (<1 month)
- Infection or fever

- Electrolyte imbalance
- Acute gastrointestinal bleeding or anemia
- Pregnancy
- Anticoagulation (or known, uncontrolled bleeding diathesis)
- Uncooperative patient
- Medication intoxication (e.g., digoxin)
- Renal failure

From Kern MJ, (ed): The Cardiac Catheterization Handbook, 2nd ed. St. Louis, Mosby–Year Book, 1994, p 4.

Postprocedure Considerations

After the procedure, the catheters are removed from the access site. Pressure may be held manually or with a compression device for 20 to 30 minutes to prevent bleeding from the access site. Some physicians may chose to use a synthetic collagen material or other type of vascular seal to achieve hemostasis at the arterial access site. These seals do not require prolonged manual compression or a pressure dressing after insertion. Once hemostasis is achieved at the access site, the patient is instructed not to bend or flex the affected extremity for 4 to 6 hours after catheter removal to promote complete arterial repair.[21] Practices related to femoral artery access site care vary from institution to institution. Oral and IV fluids are given to promote renal elimination of the contrast dye and to prevent renal damage. Assessment of vital signs, peripheral circulation distal to the access site, and the arterial access site must occur frequently and at regular intervals during the postcatheterization period to ensure that associated complications do not occur. Diminished or absent distal pulses, increased heart rate, increased or decreased blood pressure, or bleeding at the insertion site may indicate inadequate hemostasis, retroperitoneal bleeding, pseudoaneurysm, or femoral artery dissection.[21, 23] These conditions require prompt assessment and intervention by the nurse and physician.

CHART 8–5

Complications of Cardiac Catheterization

Death (<0.2%)

Myocardial infarction (<0.5%)

Cerebral vascular accident (<0.5%)

Serious dysrhythmia (<1.0%):
- Ventricular tachycardia
- Ventricular fibrillation
- Atrial fibrillation
- Supraventricular tachydysrhythmia
- Heart block asystole

Vascular injury (<1.0%):
- Hemorrhage (local, retroperitoneal, pelvic)
- Pseudoaneurysm

- Thrombosis, embolus, or air embolus
- Aortic dissection

Cardiac perforation, tamponade

Contrast reaction, anaphylaxis, or nephrotoxicity

Protamine reaction

Infection

Congestive heart failure

Vasovagal reaction

From Kern MJ (ed): The Cardiac Catheterization Handbook, 2nd ed. St. Louis, Mosby–Year Book, 1994, p 4.

CHART 8–6

Information for Patients Undergoing Cardiac Catheterization

The purpose of cardiac catheterization is to evaluate the function of your heart and its blood flow. Before the procedure:

- Do not eat or drink anything 6 hours before the test.
- If you are allergic to any medications or x-ray dye, inform your doctor prior to the test.
- Inform your doctor of all medications you are currently taking. If you are taking a medicine called warfarin (Coumadin), a blood-thinner, your doctor will instruct you when to stop taking this medicine before the test.

During the procedure:

- You will be placed on a narrow table.
- Cardiac catheterization should not be painful. Let your doctor or nurse know if you are uncomfortable during the procedure.
- One side of your groin (or one arm) will be shaved, and sterile drapes will be placed to keep the area as clean as possible. Do not touch these drapes.
- After giving you a local numbing medicine in your groin, your doctor will then place a catheter (similar to an intravenous line) into your groin.
- It will be important for you to cough and to hold your breath when you are asked to do so.

- Inform the staff if you have any chest pain or discomfort.
- A large camera will rotate around you and will take pictures of your heart as the doctor injects dye into your coronary arteries and heart. The dye will make you feel hot for a few seconds, and you may experience some chest pain.

After the procedure:

- Your doctor will be able to tell you the results of your test shortly after the catheterization. Together, you will be able to plan what to do if you are found to have heart disease.
- After the procedure, the catheter will be removed from your groin, and pressure will be held on your groin for about 30 minutes, to prevent bleeding. You must lie flat for 4 to 8 hours, as directed.
- During the recovery period, your vital signs, the groin dressing, and the pulses in your feet will be checked frequently. It is important to maintain bed rest as you are instructed.
- After the catheterization, you will be encouraged to drink as many fluids as possible to help flush the dye out of your body through the kidneys.

Adapted from Ricciuti CG: Cardiac Diagnostic Tests: A Guide for Nurses. Philadelphia, W.B. Saunders, 1997, p 289.

In the absence of complications, the patient may ambulate once hemostasis has been demonstrated for the allotted period. Discharge instructions should include activity restrictions for approximately 24 hours (e.g., no driving, minimal flexing of the affected extremity), access site care, and follow-up instructions with the cardiologist. After the procedure, when the patient is alert, the findings of the catheterization should be discussed with the patient and family. Any further interventions and changes to the treatment regimen may also be discussed with the patient at this time.

ELECTROCARDIOGRAPHY

The purpose of this section is to provide the nurse with a basic foundation on which to approach and interpret ECG testing. The ECG provides the clinician with im-

portant diagnostic information about the heart's conduction system and clues to various cardiac and extracardiac pathologic processes. ECG is an art that challenges the most experienced practitioner. A detailed explanation of the ECG is beyond the scope of this chapter. This section focuses on basic concepts that provide a foundation for normal ECG and dysrhythmia interpretation and thus establishes the groundwork on which to add more advanced concepts.

The ECG is a widely used diagnostic tool in the care of the patient with cardiovascular disease. The ECG is simple, inexpensive, and noninvasive. The ECG is used as a screening tool, as a guide to therapeutic intervention, and as an invaluable diagnostic tool for many cardiovascular diseases and conditions. The ECG allows us to record electrical activity of the cells of the heart externally through the skin that reflects the cardiac cycle. The concept of measuring electrical forces and the points on the body where they are best detected is founded on the work of Willem Einthoven, a Dutch scientist recognized as the father of the ECG.

Conduction System

A specialized system of cells located strategically throughout the heart provides for either spontaneous formation or rapid conduction of an electrical impulse in the myocardium (see Figure 6–6). These cells constitute the conduction system of the heart, specifically, specialized pacemaker cells in the sinoatrial (SA) node and the conduction cells of the AV node, bundle of His, and Purkinje fibers. These cells control the timing and synchronization of electrical impulses necessary for myocardial contraction. Impulses generated within this specialized system create a rhythmic repetition of events termed *cardiac cycles*.[25] Each cycle consists of electrical activation, or depolarization, followed by mechanical contraction. The ECG records electrical changes in the heart muscle, but it does not record the mechanical activity. For a more detailed explanation of the cardiac cycle, see Chapter 6.

Stimulation of the electrical activity of the heart originates in the sympathetic and parasympathetic branches of the autonomic nervous system. Each cardiac cycle is initiated by the generation of an action potential that begins at the SA node, a group of cells that initiates electrical impulses. The SA node, located in the posterior wall of the right atrium near the orifice of the superior vena cava, is the predominant pacemaker of the heart. The SA node generates a wave of impulses that travels through the atria, stimulating the right and left atrium, respectively. The normal rate of impulse formation in the SA node is 60 to 100 beats per minute. The activity of the SA node is regulated by the autonomic nervous system, which allows the heart to alter its intrinsic rate to meet the dynamic needs of the body.

Impulses generated from the SA node travel to the AV node after radiating through the atria. The AV node, located near the intra-atrial septum in the inferior wall of the right atrium, serves as a conduit for the wave of electrical stimulation as it travels from the SA node to the ventricles. The primary function of the AV node is to slow electrical conduction sufficiently to synchronize atrial and ventricular activity.[25] Slowing of the impulse at the AV node allows the ventricles to fill, during diastole, with blood from the atria. The AV node has an intrinsic rate of 40 to 60 beats per minute and can pace the heart in the event of SA node failure.

From the AV node, the electrical impulse spreads to the ventricles. The wave of electrical stimulation travels to the bundle of His. The bundle of His begins at the top of the intraventricular septum and descends along the interventricular septum before dividing into the left and right bundle branches. These branches provide a pathway for impulses to travel throughout the ventricle to their point of termination in the Purkinje fibers. The Purkinje fibers transmit the electrical impulse to the myocardial cells and cause simultaneous contraction of the ventricles. The intrinsic rate of the specialized cardiac cells in the ventricle, should the SA and AV node fail, is 20 to 40 beats per minute.

Electrical Activity of the Heart

During their resting phase, the cells of the myocardium are polarized, that is, they have positive charges on the outside of each cell and an equal number of negative charges on the inside of the cell. Electrical stimulation makes the cell membrane permeable to the flow of ions, which is responsible for the flow of electrical current throughout the myocardium.

Sodium and potassium ions are the predominant ions in this electrical milieu. In the resting cell, the potassium ion concentration is 50 times greater inside the cell than outside the cell. On depolarization, the first current flow consists of sodium ions moving from outside to inside the cell until the outer surface of the cell becomes negatively charged and the membrane is fully depolarized. The flow of potassium ions from inside the cell to outside begins shortly after the sodium ions start to move into the cell. When the potassium ion flow exceeds that of sodium ions, repolarization of the membrane begins, and the outer surface of the membrane again becomes positively charged. Simply stated, myocardial cells are charged or polarized in the resting state, but when electrically stimulated, they depolarize and contract. Thus, a progressive wave of depolarization passes through the heart and causes contraction of the myocardium that can be recorded on the surface ECG. Figure 6–7 represents the sequence of electrical changes that occurs in the cell membrane, known as the ventricular *action potential.*

During phases 0, 1, and 2, the myocardial cell is *absolutely refractory,* that is, it cannot accept another stimulus and is unable to depolarize. The cell is considered to be in a *relative refractory* period during phase 3 of the action potential, in which the cell can be stimulated but requires a stronger stimulus for depolarization to occur. At the end of phase 3 is a supernormal period during which a small stimulus may elicit an action potential.[26]

ECG Wave Identification

The electrical activity of the heart is recorded on the ECG as waves. These waves are arbitrarily labeled *P, QRS, T,* and *U* (Figure 8–10).

The initial wave of the cardiac cycle is the P wave. The P wave represents electrical activity of the contraction, or depolarization, of both atria.

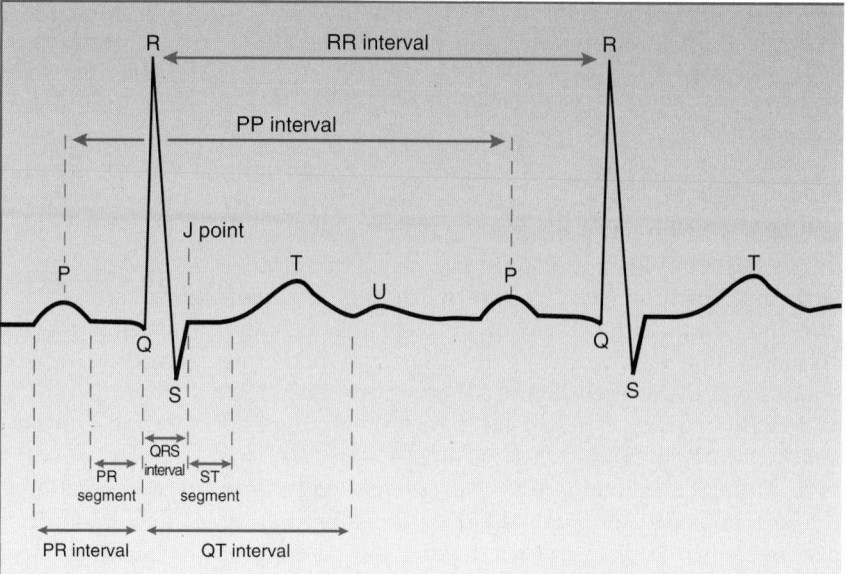

Figure 8–10

Various electrocardiographic waves and intervals of the normal cardiac cycle (lead II).

The QRS complex reflects the activation or depolarization of the ventricles. The QRS complex represents the electrical impulse as it travels from the AV node to the Purkinje fibers (ventricular conduction system) and into the myocardial cells. The Q wave is the first downward deflection of the QRS complex and it is normally followed by an upward R wave. The R wave is the first upward deflection of the QRS complex, whether or not it is preceded by a Q wave. The negative deflection after the R wave is called an S wave. Thus, the entire QRS complex represents the electrical activity of ventricular contraction or depolarization.

The ST segment follows the QRS complex. The normal ST segment is represented by an isoelectric pause after the QRS complex. The ST segment starts at the point at which the QRS complex returns to baseline, referred to as the *J point* or *junction point*. The ST segment terminates with a gradual sloping into the T wave. Variations in the quality of the ST segment, such as contour and position in relation to baseline, are discussed later in this section.

The T wave reflects the repolarization or recovery of the ventricles. The deflection of the T wave should be similar to that of the R wave. The mass of the ventricles is much greater than the atria and is reflected in the larger size of the QRS complex and T wave as compared with the P wave. The atria also have a repolarization wave; however, repolarization of the atria is not usually visualized because the corresponding wave is small and is obscured by the QRS deflection.

Finally, in some patients, a U wave may be present after the T wave. The source of the U wave is uncertain; however, its appearance may represent late ventricular repolarization or a pathologic state such as deficient potassium levels. On the ECG, one cardiac cycle is represented by the P wave, the QRS complex, and the T wave.

Lead System

The ECG measures the electrical activity of the heart along pathways called *leads*. Each lead is made up of two electrodes, one designated positive and the other negative, or with one electrode designated positive and the other designated a reference point. Current always flows toward the positive electrode. When the electrical current travels between the positive and negative poles, the lead records the current on the ECG. When electrodes are placed at certain locations on the body, the electrical activity of the heart can be viewed from different perspectives, depending on the position of the *positive* electrode.

The two types of ECG recording electrodes or leads are unipolar and bipolar. A bipolar lead is made up of two electrodes, one designated positive and one designated negative. A unipolar lead consists of one positive electrode and the other designated a zero electrical reference point at the center of the electrical field of the heart. When the electrical current in the heart flows toward the positive electrode or pole, the deflections on the ECG are upright (positive). When the electrical current in the heart flows away from the positive electrode, the deflections recorded on the ECG are inverted or negative. A biphasic complex occurs when depolarization moves perpendicular to the positive electrode.

Twelve-Lead ECG

The standard ECG consists of 12 separate leads, each viewing the pattern of the heart's electrical activity from a different perspective. The standard 12-lead ECG consists of six *limb* leads (three *standard* and three *augmented* leads) and six *chest* or *precordial* leads. The

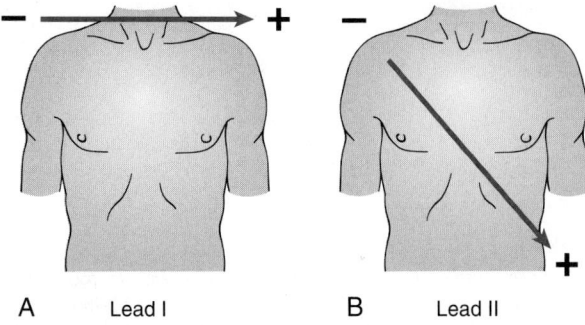
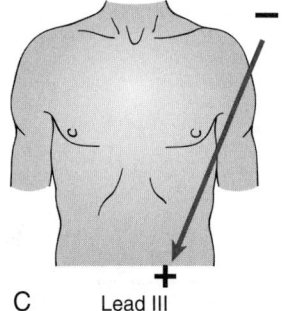

A   Lead I   B   Lead II   C   Lead III

Figure 8–11

Positions of the standard (bipolar) limb leads. *A*, Lead I. *B*, Lead II. *C*, Lead III.

standard limb leads, referred to as leads I, II, and III, are bipolar leads that record the electrical forces of the heart recorded between two electrodes placed on the arms and the legs. The limb leads record electrical activity of the heart in the frontal plane of the body. Lead I records electrical activity between the right arm and the left arm; lead II records activity between the right arm and the left leg; and lead III records electrical activity between the left leg and the left arm. The right arm is always considered the negative pole, whereas the left leg is always considered the positive pole. The left arm can be either positive or negative, depending on the lead. Figure 8–11 shows the standard position of the limb leads. The position of the three standard limb leads can be transposed into an equilateral triangle, termed *Einthoven's* triangle, with each side of the triangle formed by the three electrodes. Einthoven's triangle represents the relationship of the standard limb leads as they intersect in the center of the frontal plane at 60° angles. This is called a triaxial reference system for viewing cardiac electrical activity (Figure 8–12).[25]

The three augmented limb leads are unipolar and record electrical activity of the frontal plane of the body using the same electrodes as the standard limb leads. These unipolar leads consist of a positive electrode and a zero electrical reference point at the center of the electrical field of the heart. The amplitude of the unipolar leads is small, yet, by eliminating the negative electrode, the amplitude of the deflections is augmented or enhanced by 50%.[27] Such an augmented

limb lead is labeled *aV*, with the position of the positive electrode labeled according to the extremity on which it is located. The augmented limb leads are identified *aVR* (augmented right arm), *aVL* (augmented left arm), and *aVF* (augmented left foot). Figure 8–13 demonstrates the position of the augmented leads. When transposed on the triaxial reference system, a hexaxial reference system is produced for viewing cardiac electrical activity in the frontal plane, with the six leads now separated by 30° angles (Figure 8–14).

The remaining six leads of the 12-lead system are the unipolar precordial leads or chest leads. They are designated by the letter V and by a number, 1 to 6, which represents the position of the positive electrode on the chest wall or precordium. The positions of the precordial leads are depicted in Figure 8–15. Essentially, the chest leads encircle the heart in a horizontal plane. The position of the precordial leads reflects the electrical activity of the ventricles. V_1 and V_2 reflect the electrical activity of the right ventricle (and also right atrium), whereas V_3 through V_6 reflect the electrical activity of the larger left ventricle. These 6 leads demonstrate an increase in the amplitude of the R wave and a decrease in the amplitude of the S wave from V_1 to V_6, respectively, in the normal 12-lead ECG. This feature is commonly referred to as *R-wave progression*. Thus, the QRS complex, or R wave, in lead V_1 is mainly negative, whereas the R wave in lead V_6 is positive in the healthy myocardium. Figure 8–16 shows normal ECG tracings of each of the 12 leads and normal R-wave progression in the precordial leads.

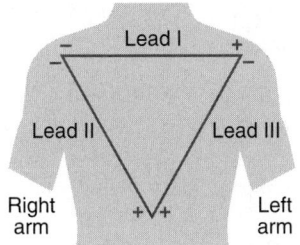

Figure 8–12

Standard limb leads form Einthoven's triangle. The triaxial reference system depicts cardiac electrical activity in the frontal plane of the body. (From Hansen M: Pathophysiology. Philadelphia, W.B. Saunders, 1998, p 411.)

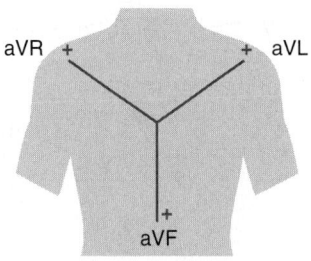

Figure 8–13

Position of the augmented (unipolar) limb leads. (From Hansen M: Pathophysiology. Philadelphia, W.B. Saunders, 1998, p 411.)

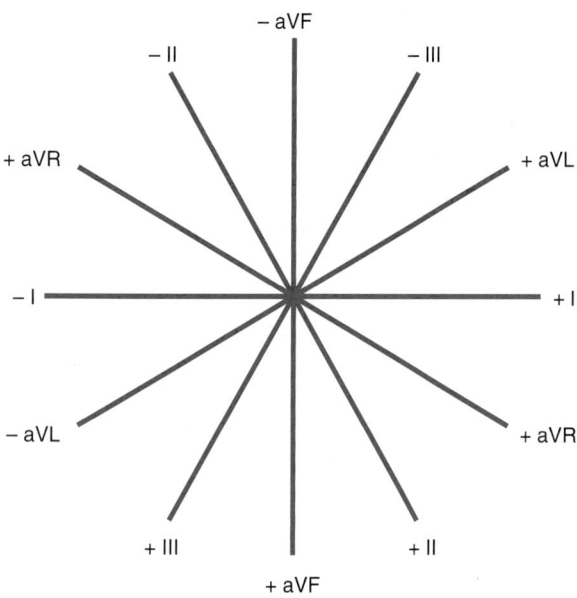

Figure 8–14

Hexaxial reference system depicts cardiac electrical activity in the frontal plane of the body. (From Hansen M: Pathophysiology. Philadelphia, W.B. Saunders, 1998, p 411.)

Figure 8–15

Position of the precordial (chest) leads as they encircle the heart in the horizontal plane. V_1, fourth intercostal space (ICS), right sternal border; V_2, fourth ICS, left sternal border; V_3, midway between V_2 and V_4; V_4, fifth ICS, left midclavicular line; V_5, fifth ICS, left anterior axillary line; V_6, fifth ICS, left midaxillary line. (From Hansen M: Pathophysiology. Philadelphia, W.B. Saunders, 1998, p 412.)

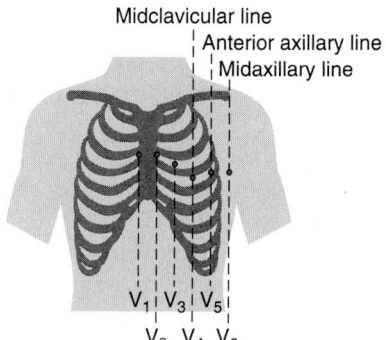

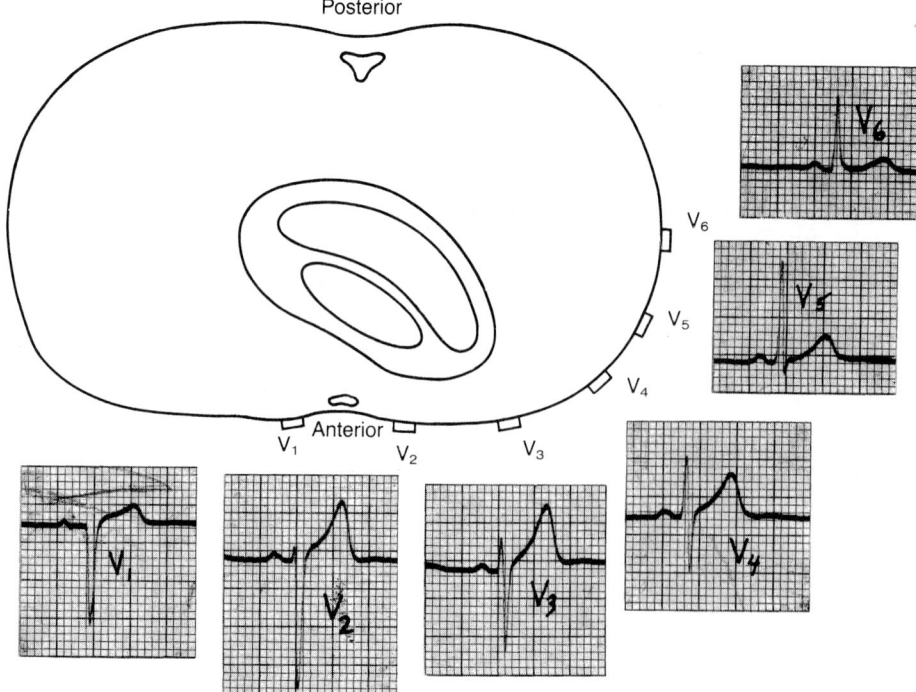

Figure 8–16

Normal R-wave progression of the precordial leads. Note the progressively larger R wave from lead V_1 to V_6. (From Phillips R, Feeney M: The Cardiac Rhythms, 3rd ed. Philadelphia, W.B. Saunders, 1990.)

Bedside ECG Monitoring

Continuous bedside ECG monitoring has undergone many transitions since its inception with the advent of cardiac care units in the 1960s. Continuous bedside cardiac monitoring has evolved into a routine yet essential component in the evaluation of critically ill patients in various settings. Thus, the goals of bedside cardiac monitoring have evolved from simple heart rate monitoring to the sophisticated detection of cardiac dysrhythmias. Many current bedside cardiac monitors have additional capabilities such as five-cable systems that allow monitoring of specific precordial leads, 12-lead ECG capability, and detection of ST-segment changes.

Many types of cardiac monitoring systems are available and are in use today. The general components of these systems include a monitor screen (cathode ray oscilloscope) on which the ECG is displayed and a printout system that directly transcribes the cardiac rhythm onto paper.[28] A rate meter triggered by the QRS complex is usually part of the system. If the heart rate falls below a preset low rate limit (usually 50 beats/minute) or exceeds a preset high rate limit (usually 120 beats per minute), the monitor will sound an alarm and will automatically print out a 6-second strip of the event. In addition, the monitor is preset to recognize certain dysrhythmias and to sound an alarm when they occur. Similar to rate limits, the monitor automatically prints out a 6-second strip recording the dysrhythmia. Rhythm strips of longer duration can usually be obtained manually. In addition to these alarms, most monitors provide some form of dysrhythmia storage in which the nurse can recall and print out various rhythms that have triggered the alarms over a period of time.

Bedside cardiac monitoring requires a minimum of three electrodes: positive, negative, and ground electrodes. Historically, bedside cardiac monitoring used the 3-lead system to monitor the bipolar limb leads: I, II, and III. The use of lead II has been preferred for bedside monitoring because of the easy visibility of P waves and an upright R wave, and it continues to be the lead of choice in a recent study of critical care nurses' monitoring preferences for a single lead.[29] Lead II can be obtained by placing the positive electrode in the lower left torso area, the negative electrode in the right shoulder area, and the ground electrode (usually placed) in the left shoulder area. Despite its appeal, the use of lead II has limited value in detecting bundle branch blocks and in diagnosing wide QRS complex tachycardias. Whenever possible, lead V_1 or V_6 should be selected to monitor critically ill patients.[30]

The *MCL,* or modified chest leads, are bipolar substitutes for the unipolar V_1 and V_6 leads. MCL_1 and MCL_6 can be obtained using a three-electrode system. Monitoring of the MCL leads, especially MCL_1, has become routine practice because the QRS morphologies in these leads have been noted to approximate V_1 and V_6.[31] MCL_1 can be obtained by placing the positive electrode in the fourth intercostal space at the right sternal border and the negative electrode in the left shoulder area; the ground electrode may be placed anywhere. To view MCL_6, the positive electrode is placed at the fifth intercostal space in the midaxillary line while the negative electrode is placed in the left shoulder area. Figure 8–17 depicts appropriate lead placement for leads MCL_1 and MCL_6. MCL_1 and MCL_6 are useful in detecting bundle branch blocks and in differentiating ventricular beats from aberrantly conducted beats, rendering them more valuable than monitoring in lead II.[27,31,32]

Many bedside cardiac monitors now use a five-cable system that allows monitoring of the unipolar precordial leads V_1 and V_6. One lead is placed on each limb, and the fifth lead is positioned on the appropriate precordial site. Drew and Scheinman[30] demonstrated that, when applying the morphologic criteria for diagnosing ventricular tachycardia, it is more accurate to observe the criteria in V_1 rather than the MCL_1 tracing. Thus, monitoring with MCL_1 is *not* recommended when it is possible to monitor V_1 (see Figure 8–17).

A few leads are available for continuous cardiac bedside monitoring. Choice of a monitoring lead depends on the capabilities of the monitoring system in use (i.e., three-cable system versus five-cable system) and the patient's clinical problem. Chart 8–7 outlines a research-based approach to lead placement recommended for bedside cardiac monitoring.

ECG Tracing

As previously stated, the ECG provides a recording of the electrical activity of the heart. The ECG is recorded on ruled paper. The smallest divisions are 1 mm by 1 mm squares (Figure 8–18). There are five small (1 mm $\times$ 1 mm) squares between the heavy lines, which represent one large square. The horizontal axis of the lines represents time, whereas the vertical axis represents voltage. The amount of time represented by the distance between the heavy lines, or one large square, is 0.2 seconds. Each small division or square, when measured horizontally, represents 0.04 seconds. By measuring along the horizontal axis, the duration of any part of the cardiac cycle or wave can be determined.

The height of one small square is equal to 1 mm, or 0.1 mV (voltage). By measuring along the vertical axis, the voltage of any part of the cardiac cycle can be determined.

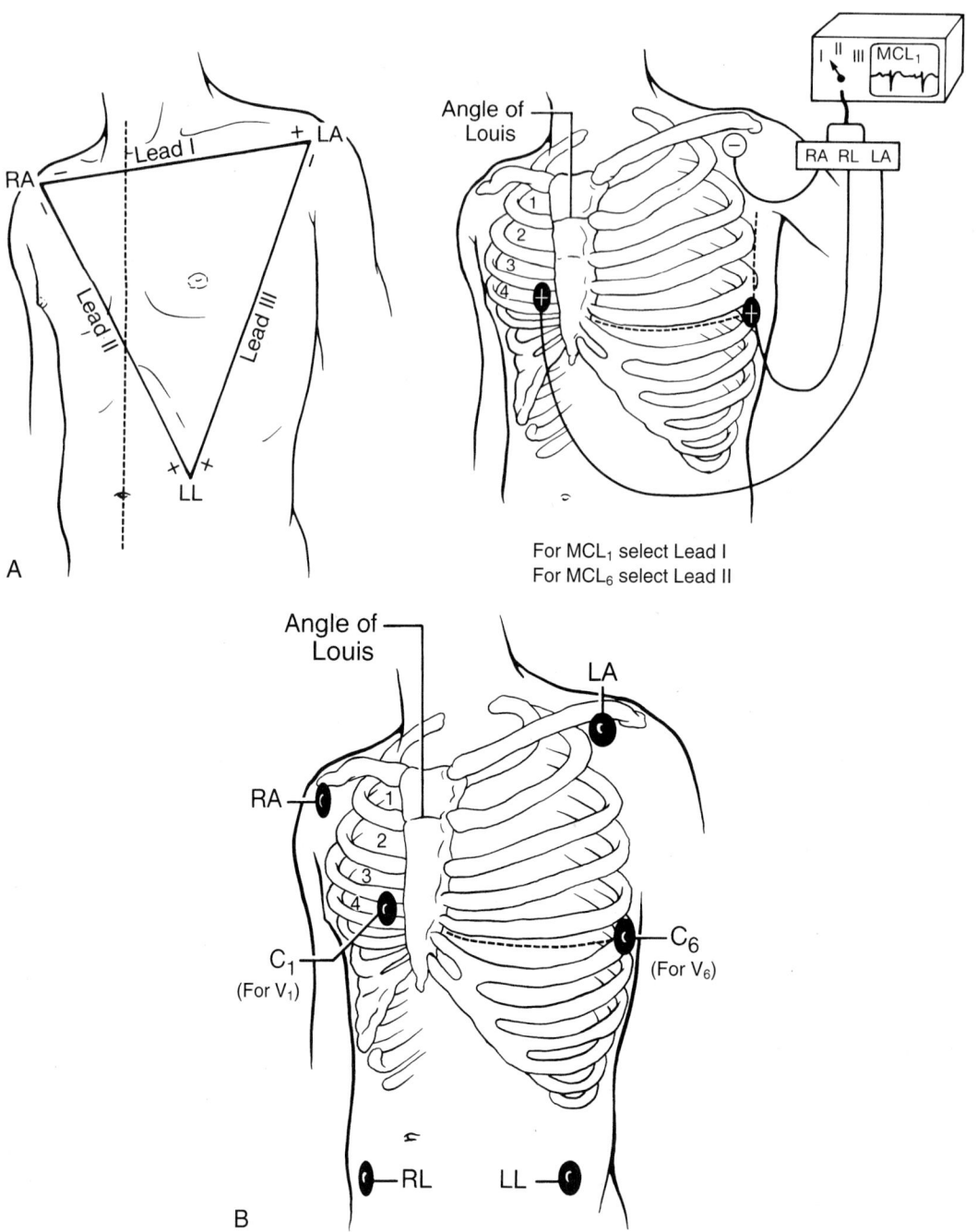

Figure 8-17

A, Proper lead position for leads MCL₁ or MCL₆ with the three-lead bedside monitor. *B*, Proper lead position for V₁ or V₆ with the five-lead bedside monitor. *C*, chest; *LA*, left arm; *LL*, left leg; *MCL*, modified chest lead; *RA*, right arm; *RL*, right leg. (From Drew BJ: Bedside electrocardiogram monitoring. AACN Clin Issues Crit Care Nurs 4:26, 28, 1993.)

ECG Interpretation

For the novice as well as the expert nurse, accurate ECG interpretation depends on developing a systematic routine when approaching the ECG. Systematic evaluation of the ECG enables the nurse to avoid the pitfalls associated with omission of important or subtle components of the ECG when diagnosing and treating cardiac dysrhythmias.

For every ECG, certain features should be examined systematically. These include, in the order of examination, heart rate, evaluation of specific waves and intervals, rhythm identification, and evaluation of the ST–T-wave segment. Once basic skills in ECG interpretation are perfected, more complex findings may be added to this systematic approach.

CHART 8–7

Recommended Leads for Cardiac Monitoring

For monitors with five-lead patient cables

First choice:
   Single-lead monitoring: V_1
   Dual-lead monitoring: V_1 plus the limb lead appropriate for clinical situation*
Second choice:
   Substitute V_6 for V_1 when patient cannot have electrode at sternal border
   or
   When QRS amplitude is not adequate for optimized computerized dysrhythmia monitoring

For monitors with three-lead patient cables

First choice:
   MCL_1
Second choice:
   MCL_6

Tips for selecting a limb lead appropriate for the patient's clinical situation:

1. Atrial flutter: II, III, or aVF
2. Inferior MI: II, III, or aVF (pick lead with maximum ST elevation on 12-lead ECG)
3. Anterior MI: pick lead with maximum ST elevation on 12-lead ECG
4. After angioplasty: III or aVF (whichever has the tallest R wave)
5. If three channels are available for ECG monitoring, the combination of V_1 + I + aVF has the following advantages:
   a. Best dysrhythmia lead—V_1
   b. Atrial flutter—aVF
   c. Inferior MI or postangioplasty—aVF
   d. Axis determination—I and aVF

Adapted from Drew BJ: Bedside electrocardiogram monitoring. AACN Clin Issues Crit Care Nurs 4:25–33, 1993; Drew BJ: Bedside electrocardiographic monitoring: state of the art for the 1990's. Heart Lung 20:610–623, 1991; Drew BJ; Tisdale LA: ST segment monitoring for coronary artery reocclusion following thrombolytic therapy and coronary angioplasty: identification of optimal bedside monitoring leads. Am J Crit Care 2:280–292, 1993.

Rate

The first factor to consider when interpreting the ECG is the heart rate. The rate is reported as cycles or beats per minute. Normally, there are the same number of P waves and QRS complexes, and either may be used to determine cardiac rate. The ventricular rate versus the atrial rate, however, is of primary importance in the critical care setting. The ventricular rate usually dictates how well the patient tolerates the rhythm; thus, heart rate is usually calculated in terms of the ventricular rate. In the presence of certain cardiac rhythm abnormalities (discussed later), the number of P waves and QRS complexes may not be the same, necessitating the determination of both the atrial and ventricular rates separately.

To calculate the approximate heart rate, a simple formula may be used. The cardiac rate per minute can be determined by counting the number of large squares on the ECG paper between cardiac cycles. Because there are 300 fifths of a second in 1 minute ($1/5 \times 300 = 60$), it is necessary only to determine the number of large squares (fifths of a second) between consecutive cycles and to divide this number into 300. By applying this formula, the nurse can easily determine the heart rate by glancing at the tracing of a relatively regular cardiac rhythm. Find a specific R wave that falls on a heavy black line. From that R wave, count down each successive heavy black line as "300, 150, 100, 75, 60, 50. . . ." The location of the next R wave determines the heart rate. If the next R wave falls on a heavy black line, use the countdown method to determine the exact rate. If the next R wave falls

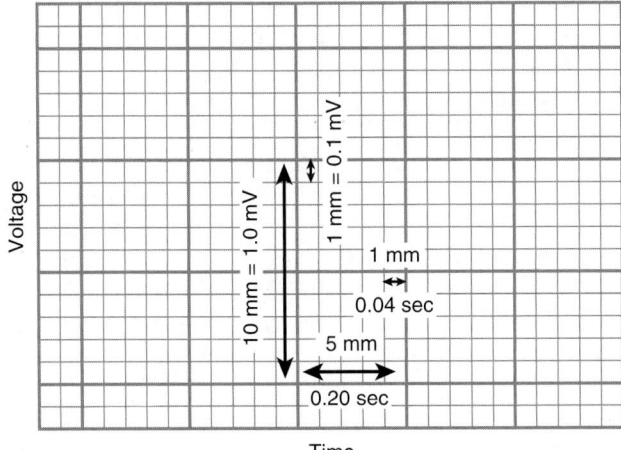

Figure 8–18

Standard electrocardiographic (ECG) paper. At the normal speed of 25 msec per second, each small square represents a 40-msec time interval, and each large square represents 200 msec. Height and depth of the ECG waveform are measured in millivolts (mV). Each small square is 1 mm high (10 = 1 mV). Routine ECGs are recorded with a 1 mV standard amplitude scale. (From Phillips R, Feeney M: The Cardiac Rhythms, 3rd ed. Philadelphia, W.B. Saunders, 1990).

between two heavy black lines, approximate the rate between the two values (Figure 8–19).

Heart rate may also be calculated by dividing the number of small boxes between QRS complexes into 1500. This method is generally used for tachycardias, in which the heart rate exceeds 100 beats per minute, for more precise measurement.

If the rhythm is irregular, the number of cardiac cycles over a particular interval of time should be counted to determine the average cardiac rate. A simple and quick method for estimating heart rate is to count the number of cardiac cycles in 6 seconds and to multiply by 10. Most ECG paper provides markings at 3-second intervals (Figure 8–19).

The next step in ECG interpretation is identification of the specific cardiac rhythm or pattern. This step in evaluation of the cardiac rhythm involves the consideration of many features of the ECG, including the regularity or irregularity of the rhythm and the characteristics of the individual waves and intervals that comprise the cardiac cycle.

Although the sinus node regulates cardiac rhythm with amazing precision, the cardiac rhythm is not always exactly regular.[25] Cardiac rhythm is greatly affected by innervation from the autonomic nervous system resulting in variations in cardiac rate, particularly with variations related to the respiratory cycle when an individual is at rest. This normal variation in heart rate is also referred to as *heart rate variability.* The regularity of the rhythm can be determined by measuring the distance between consecutive R waves. The distance between R waves should be equal or within 10% of each other to be considered regular.

Evaluation of Waves and Intervals

The P-wave contour is normally small, rounded, and smooth. The P wave should be clearly visible and should precede each QRS complex (see Figure 8–10). The P wave is normally upright in leads aVL, I, II, and V_4 through V_6. The P-wave duration is normally less than 0.12 seconds, and its amplitude is normally less than 0.25 mV in all leads. When evaluating P waves, the nurse should always determine whether each P wave is associated with a QRS complex.

The PR interval represents the time from the beginning of atrial depolarization to the beginning of ven-

tricular depolarization. It is measured from the beginning of the P wave to the beginning of the QRS complex. The PR segment is normally isoelectric. The normal duration of the PR interval ranges from 0.12 to 0.20 seconds. Normal variations may occur in the PR interval because of variation in heart rate. The PR interval is shorter at faster heart rates and longer at slower heart rates. The PR interval should be the same length with each cardiac cycle.

The QRS complexes are inspected to ascertain that each QRS complex is the same shape and width. The QRS interval represents the duration of the QRS complex denoting the time from the beginning of ventricular depolarization to the end of ventricular depolarization. It is measured from the beginning of the first appearing Q or R wave to the end of the last appearing R or S wave (see Figure 8–10). The normal duration of the QRS complex ranges from 0.04 to 0.12 seconds.

The QT interval represents ventricular depolarization and repolarization. It is measured from the beginning of the QRS complex to the end of the T wave (see Figure 8–10). The duration of the QT interval should be less than half of the previous RR interval. The QT interval varies with age, sex, and heart rate.

The ST–T-wave segment should also be evaluated and is discussed later, in the section on ECG changes associated with myocardial infarction.

Rhythm Interpretation

Knowledge of the characteristics of the normal ECG sets the foundation for determining variations and abnormalities of the cardiac rhythm. The term *dysrhythmia* refers to all rhythms other than normal sinus rhythm. Dysrhythmias can be classified in various ways. When classified according to rate, the term *bradydysrhythmia* is used to identify any rhythm with a rate less than 60 beats per minute. The term *tachydysrhythmia* is used to identify any rhythm with a rate more than 100 beats per minute. Cardiac rhythms may also be classified according to their site of origin. For example, dysrhythmias originating in the atrium or AV node are termed supraventricular dysrhythmias, whereas rhythms originating below the AV node are termed ventricular dysrhythmias. When a beat is conducted along pathways other than the normal conduc-

Figure 8–19

Simple methods for calculating heart (ventricular) rate. Counting the heavy lines between QRS complexes approximates the ventricular rate at 85 beats per minute. If using the 6-second method, the ventricular rate is 90; 9 QRS complexes are counted in 6 seconds, so 9 × 10 (6-second intervals in 1 minute) equals 90 beats per minute.

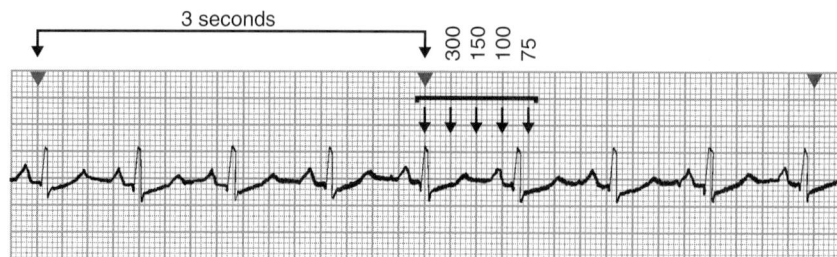

tion pathway, the complex is said to be *aberrantly* conducted. Aberrant ventricular beats are usually wide (longer than 0.12 seconds) because of prolonged conduction time through the ventricles.

Cardiac dysrhythmias result from either a disturbance in *automaticity* or an alteration in *conduction*. Problems of impulse formation or automaticity can originate in any cells of the pacemaking (SA node) or conducting system (AV node, bundle of His, right and left bundle branches, or Purkinje fibers). The SA node usually controls the cardiac rate and rhythm because of its inherent automaticity. Rhythms that originate from sites other than the sinus node are termed *ectopic*. Disturbances in automaticity may be related to ectopic foci, which usurp the control of the SA node by accelerating their own automaticity, or by a change in the automaticity (increased or decreased) of the sinus node itself. *Accelerated automaticity* results in cardiac rhythms with rates higher than 100 beats per minute and is limited by the maximal rate of impulse formation in the pacemaker cells.

Disturbances in conduction may occur in any area of the myocardium. When conduction is slowed or fails to occur at all, the term *block* is used. Cardiac impulses can be partially blocked, causing conduction delays, or totally blocked, causing conduction failure.[25] Partial or total block may occur within the pacemaking and conducting systems. Uneven, or heterogeneous, conduction can occur in any part of the myocardium, with resulting *reentry* of the impulse into an area that has just previously been depolarized and repolarized. Reentry produces a circular movement of the impulse that continues as long as the impulse encounters receptive cells. The result can be an isolated premature (or early) beat, multiple premature beats, nonsustained tachydysrhythmias, or sustained tachydysrhythmias. *Triggered activation* also implies an abnormality in electrical conduction. *Afterpotentials* exist immediately after repolarization and may *trigger* another action potential or depolarization, possibly resulting in tachydysrhythmias.

The identification of the cardiac rhythm involves incorporating the previous ECG characteristics including the heart rate, the regularity or irregularity of the rhythm, and the characteristics of the individual waves and intervals that comprise the cardiac cycle. The following discussion presents the ECG characteristics of specific cardiac rhythms and dysrhythmias.

Normal Sinus Rhythm. Recognition of normal sinus rhythm provides the nurse with a foundation on

CHART 8–8

Normal Sinus Rhythm

ECG criteria:

- Rate: 60 to 100 beats/minute
- Rhythm: regular; RR and PP intervals are constant
- P wave: normal and upright in lead II; P wave precedes each QRS complex
- PR interval: 0.12 to 0.20 seconds and constant
- QRS complex: 0.04 to 0.12 seconds

which to identify cardiac dysrhythmias (Chart 8–8). Normal sinus rhythm is recognized as having a normal P wave, followed by a normal QRS complex and T wave, with a physiologically appropriate heart rate of 60 to 100 beats per minute (Figure 8–20). The electrical impulse originates in the sinus node and travels along the normal conduction pathway. The sinus rate is higher in infants and young children and tends to decrease with aging.

Sinus Bradycardia. This term is used for a sinus rate of less than 60 beats per minute in the normal adult population (Figure 8–21). Sinus bradycardia may result from excessive parasympathetic activity and is considered normal in the trained athlete and during sleep. When the heart rate falls below 40 beats per minute, it may be considered abnormal when associated with signs and symptoms of low cardiac output and hemodynamic compromise, such as angina, dyspnea, hypotension, syncope, anxiety, and changes in level of consciousness (LOC) (Chart 8–9).

Sinus Tachycardia. This term refers to a normal sinus rhythm in which the heart rate exceeds 100 beats per minute, yet rarely exceeds 160 beats per minute (Figure 8–22). The mechanism of sinus tachycardia is physiologically enhanced automaticity[27] (Chart 8–10).

Sinus Dysrhythmia. This term refers to a sinus rhythm with physiologic variations in sinus rates (Figure 8–23). Sinus dysrhythmia occurs when an impulse is discharged from the sinus node at a normal rate but at an irregular interval.[33] The variation in sinus rates may be synchronized with the respiratory

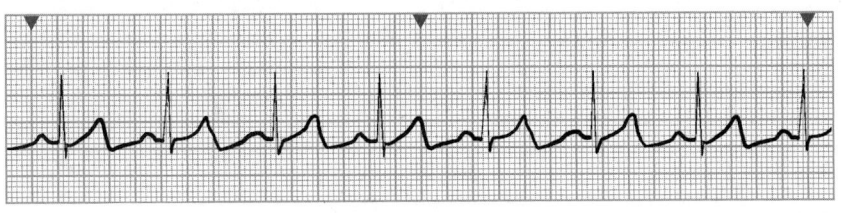

Figure 8–20
Normal sinus rhythm, lead II.

CHART 8–9

Sinus Bradycardia

ECG criteria:

- Rate: 40 to 60 beats/minute
- Rhythm: regular to slightly irregular
- P wave: normal and upright in lead II; one P wave precedes each QRS complex
- PR interval: 0.12 to 0.20 seconds and constant
- QRS complex: 0.04 to 0.12 seconds

Cause:

- Increased vagal stimulation
- Medical conditions: atherosclerotic heart disease, myocardial infarction, hypothermia, increased intracranial pressure, hypoendocrine states (e.g., Addison's disease, myxedema coma)
- Medications: digoxin, calcium channel blockers, beta blockers, central nervous system depressants (e.g., morphine, sedatives)

Treatment:

Usually no treatment is indicated. Patients who do demonstrate signs and symptoms of low cardiac output and hemodynamic compromise (e.g., hypotension, changes in level of consciousness, angina, syncope) may require one or more of the following:

- Identification and treatment of the underlying cause of the bradycardia
- Atropine
- Isoproterenol (Isuprel)
- Pacemaker: transcutaneous, temporary, or permanent
- See Appendix: ACLS: Bradycardia Algorithm

cycle, that is, slowing of the rate with expiration and acceleration of the rate with inspiration. Sinus dysrhythmia is marked in the young and becomes less frequent with the normal growth process (Chart 8–11).

Sinus Arrest. Sinus arrest or sinus pause (Figure 8–24) is failure of impulse formation in the sinus node. At times, alternate pacemaker cells may take over during the pause. Sinus arrest is often difficult to de-

termine on the resting ECG; however, it may be recognized by long pauses, in which beats are missing or "dropped" (Chart 8–12).

Dysrhythmias Originating in the Atria. The atrial dysrhythmias presented include premature atrial complexes (PACs), atrial tachycardia, atrial flutter, and atrial fibrillation. These disturbances in cardiac rhythm can be grouped under the broad desig-

CHART 8–10

Sinus Tachycardia

ECG criteria:

- Rate: 100 to 160 beats/minute
- Rhythm: regular to slightly irregular
- P wave: normal and upright in lead II; one P wave precedes each QRS complex; P waves are sometimes not visible at higher heart rates, but can usually be found on 12-lead ECG
- PR interval: 0.12 to 0.20 seconds and constant
- QRS complex: 0.04 to 0.12 seconds

Cause:

- Enhanced automaticity
- Caffeine-containing products: coffee, tea, chocolate

- Medical conditions: anxiety, pain, fever, hypotension, anemia, myocardial infarction, shock, congestive heart failure
- Medications: dopamine (Intropin), aminophylline, epinephrine (Adrenalin)

Treatment:

- Determining and treating the underlying cause (e.g., fever, pain, hypovolemia).
- Cardiac medications: beta blockers, calcium channel blockers
- CNS depressants: antianxiety agents, tranquilizers, pain medication
- See Appendix: ACLS: Tachycardia Algorithm

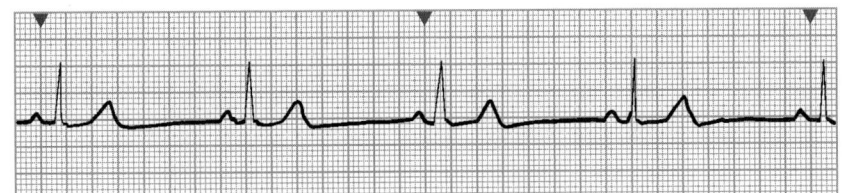

Figure 8–21
Sinus bradycardia.

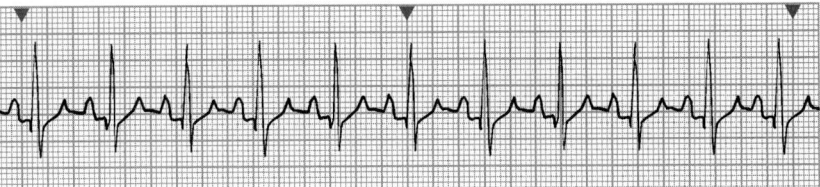

Figure 8–22
Sinus tachycardia.

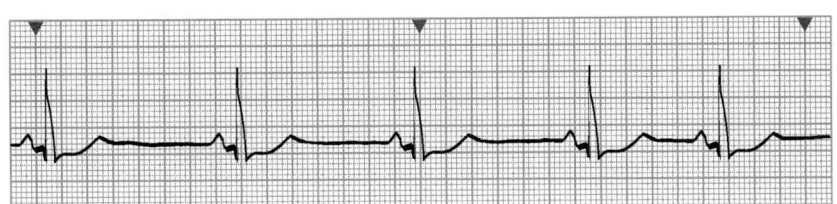

Figure 8–23
Sinus dysrhythmia.

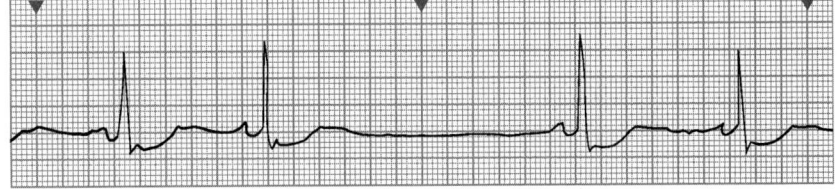

Figure 8–24
Sinus arrest.

CHART 8–11

Sinus Dysrhythmia

ECG criteria:

- Rate: 40 to 100 beats/minutes; periods of slower and faster heart rates may alternate
- Rhythm: irregular RR intervals with corresponding changes in the rate
- P wave: normal and upright in lead II; one P wave precedes each QRS complex
- PR interval: 0.12 to 0.20 seconds and may vary slightly
- QRS complex: 0.04 to 0.12 seconds

Cause:

- Respiratory variation most common

Treatment:

- None required

---

nation of supraventricular dysrhythmias. Conover[27] defined the term supraventricular as the area above the branching portion of the bundle of His.

PREMATURE ATRIAL CONTRACTIONS. Whenever the atrial impulse originates from a focus other than the sinus node, the result is an ectopic P wave. PACs occur when an ectopic atrial pacemaker generates an impulse before the next sinus beat is due (Figure 8–25). The P wave of the PAC usually differs in contour from the P wave of the sinus beat, depending on the origin of the impulse of the impulse in the atria. A PAC may or may not be conducted to the ventricles. In addition, PACs may occur randomly or in a pattern, such as bigeminal (every other beat), trigeminal (every third beat), or clustered. PACs generally depolarize and reset the sinus node, so that the next sinus beat occurs sooner than the expected sinus P wave. This process is known as an *incomplete compensatory pause* (Chart 8–13).

PAROXYSMAL ATRIAL TACHYCARDIA.. This dysrhythmia is caused by an ectopic focus in the atria that takes control from the SA node resulting in a (usually) regular and rapid rhythm originating from any location in the atria (Chart 8–14). Most often, it occurs spontaneously (thus

CHART 8–12

Sinus Arrest

ECG criteria:

- Rate: 60 to 100 beats/minute; often <60 beats/minute because of missed beats
- Rhythm: irregular RR intervals; rhythm is characterized by missed or "dropped" beats; rhythm remains regular before and after missed beats
- P wave: one P wave precedes each QRS complex; absent during missed beat
- PR interval: normal
- QRS complex: normal

Cause:

- Cardiac origin: cardiomyopathy, rheumatic heart disease, myocardial infarction
- See Sinus Bradycardia (Chart 8–9)

Treatment:

- No treatment necessary in asymptomatic patients
- Reduction or elimination of any medications that may be contributing to the cause
- Temporary pacing necessary in some symptomatic patients
- If sinoatrial node unable to restore normal pacing, permanent pacemaker may be indicated
- See Appendix: ACLS: Bradycardia Algorithm

---

the term, paroxysmal) and is precipitated by a PAC. Caused by sudden rapid firing from an ectopic atrial focus, paroxysmal atrial tachycardia often achieves rates of 150 to 250 per minute and usually starts suddenly and ends abruptly (Figure 8–26).

ATRIAL FLUTTER. This rapid and regular atrial rhythm has an atrial rate of approximately 300 beats per minute (Chart 8–15). Atrial flutter is thought to be due to a single reentry circuit located in the right atrium.[27] Atrial flutter is recognized on the ECG by undulating

---

CHART 8–13

Premature Atrial Contractions (PACs)

ECG criteria:

- Rate: variable; usually 60 to 100 beats per minute
- Rhythm: irregular; when PACs occur, the pause after the PAC is not usually compensatory; the sinus beat after the PAC does not occur at normal time because the SA node timing is interrupted
- P waves: premature P wave with possible abnormal configuration (flat, slurred, notched, inverted, diphasic, or wide) or lost in T wave or QRS complex of sinus beat; P wave of sinus beat normal
- PR interval: sinus beat; normal; PAC varies depending on site of ectopic pacemaker
- QRS complex: usually normal

Cause:

- Stimulants: catecholamines, caffeine, nicotine, excessive alcohol consumption
- Cardiac disease: myocardial infarction, congestive heart failure (CHF)
- Electrolyte disturbances: hypokalemia, hypermetabolic states
- Medical conditions: hypoxemia, chronic obstructive pulmonary disease
- Emotions: anxiety, fear
- Medications: central nervous system stimulants, digoxin, over-the-counter medications containing stimulants

Treatment:

- Usually no treatment needed; continued monitoring
- Treatment of underlying cause (e.g., decreased consumption of caffeine, correction of hypoxemia)
- Consideration of electrolyte imbalance, digoxin toxicity, early warning of CHF

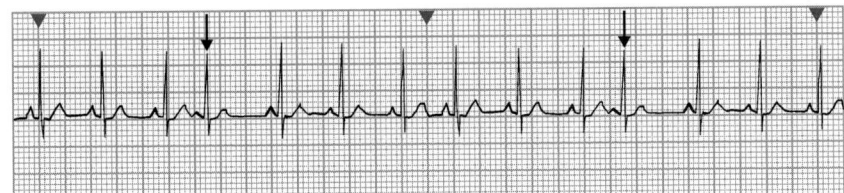

Figure 8-25

Premature atrial contraction (*arrow*).

Figure 8-26

Paroxysmal atrial tachycardia (PAT). Arrows indicate beginning and ending of PAT.

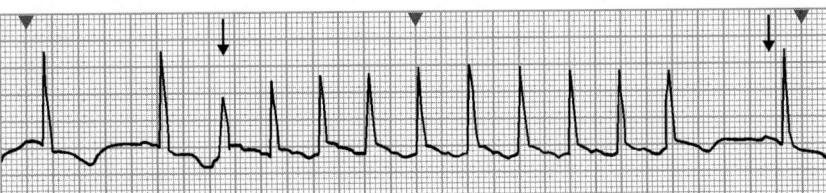

waves called F waves or flutter waves (Figure 8–27). F waves, which represent atrial activity, are often referred to as having a "saw-tooth" pattern. Many of the impulses generated with atrial flutter fail to pass through to the ventricles and result in variation in atrial and ventricular rates, that is, 300 atrial, 75 ventricular, for a ratio of 4:1. Conduction ratios usually occur in even intervals: 2:1, 4:1, 6:1. With a normal AV node, there is usually 2:1 conduction; however, conduction ratios vary with AV node disease, with increased vagal tone, or with use of medications that cause AV block. When ventricular rates are less than 100 beats per minute, the dysrhythmia is described as atrial flutter with a controlled ventricular response. Conversely, when ventricular rates are more than 100 beats per minute, the atrial flutter is said to have an uncontrolled ventricular response.

ATRIAL FIBRILLATION. Disorganized, ineffective contractions of the atria due to multiple irritable foci in the atria characterize atrial fibrillation (Figure 8–28). The dysrhythmia is distinguished by the absence of P waves and an irregular ventricular response (Chart 8–16). The atrial rhythm is chaotic, with atrial rates of 350 to 600 beats per minute, in which organized atrial activity cannot be detected. Essentially, the atria are fibrillating. The inherent capacity of the AV node to transmit impulses to the ventricle is exceeded by the rapid, chaotic atrial impulses. This usually results in a ventricular rate ranging from 100 to 180 beats per minute. As with atrial flutter, the ventricular response depends on the condition of the AV node, vagal tone, and the presence or absence of cardioactive drugs. Further, the term atrial fibrillation with an uncontrolled ventricular response is used to describe this

CHART 8-14

Paroxysmal Atrial Tachycardia

ECG criteria:

- Rate: atrial rate between 150 and 250 beats per minute; onset is usually sudden and often initiated by a premature atrial contraction
- Rhythm: regular or slightly irregular
- P waves: ectopic P waves with possibly abnormal contour or difficult to see in any of the 12 leads
- PR interval: <0.12 second; may be difficult to see or measure
- QRS complex: usually normal

Cause:

- See Premature Atrial Contractions (Chart 8–13)

Treatment:

- Often self-limiting
- Treatment aimed at correcting underlying cause
- Vagal nerve stimulation (e.g., carotid sinus massage, Valsalva maneuvers) may possibly slow rate
- Consideration of adenosine, beta blockers, calcium channel blockers, digoxin to slow rate
- Consideration of cardioversion if hemodynamically unstable (e.g. angina, hypotension, changes in level of consciousness)
- See Appendix: ACLS: Tachycardia Algorithm, Electrical Cardioversion Algorithm

CHART 8–15

Atrial Flutter

ECG criteria:

- Rate: atrial rate, between 250 and 350 beats/minute; ventricular rate, depends on degree of atrioventricular (AV) block; varying degrees of AV conduction or block may be present in ratios of 2:1, 3:1, 4:1
- Rhythm: atrial, usually regular (PP intervals constant), but can be irregular because of varying conduction ratios; ventricular, usually regular (RR intervals constant), but can be irregular because of varying conduction ratios
- AV conduction: depends on rate and degree of AV block
- P waves: "saw-tooth," flutter waves; usually peaked, uniform in width
- PR Interval: not usually measurable
- QRS complex: usually narrow

Cause:

- Rare in the absence of organic heart disease: coronary artery disease, cardiomyopathy, congestive heart failure, valvular heart disease
- Medical conditions: pulmonary disease, chronic obstructive pulmonary disease, pulmonary embolism

Treatment:

- Treatment aimed at the restoration of normal sinus rhythm
- Consideration of digoxin, propranolol, quinidine, diltiazem, verapamil to slow ventricular rate
- Consideration of cardioversion if hemodyamically unstable (e.g., angina, hypotension, changes in level of consciousness)
- See Appendix: ACLS: Tachycardia Algorithm, Electrical Cardioversion Algorithm

CHART 8–16

Atrial Fibrillation

ECG criteria:

- Rate: atrial, between 350 and 600 beats/minute; ventricular, range from 100 to 180 beats per minute, depending on atrioventricular (AV) conduction
- Rhythm: ventricular, irregular and usually rapid, depending on degree of AV block
- AV conduction: ventricles respond irregularly to excessive impulses from atria
- P waves: no visible P waves; fibrillating, wave-like, erratic baseline of varying shapes and sizes
- PR interval not visible or measurable
- QRS complex: usually narrow unless conduction delayed through the ventricles

Cause:

- Associated with underlying cardiac disease (e.g., coronary artery disease, valvular heart disease)
- and extracardiac disease (e.g., chronic obstructive pulmonary disease, pulmonary embolism, thyroid disorders)
- See also Premature Atrial Contractions (Chart 8–13)

Treatment:

- Treatment aimed at controlling the ventricular response and the restoration of sinus rhythm
- Consideration of digoxin, quinidine, beta blockers, calcium channel blockers to slow ventricular rate or to convert to normal sinus rhythm
- Cardioversion if patient hemodynamically unstable (e.g., angina, hypotension, changes in level of consciousness)
- See Appendix: ACLS: Tachycardia Algorithm, Electrical Cardioversion Algorithm

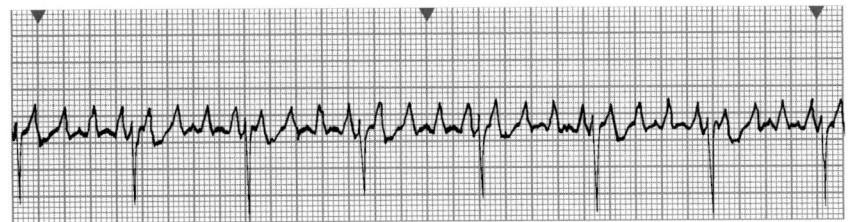

Figure 8–27
Atrial flutter with 4:1 conduction (four flutter waves to each QRS complex).

Figure 8–28
Atrial fibrillation. Note the irregular RR intervals.

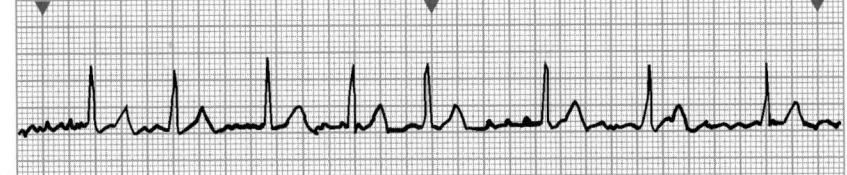

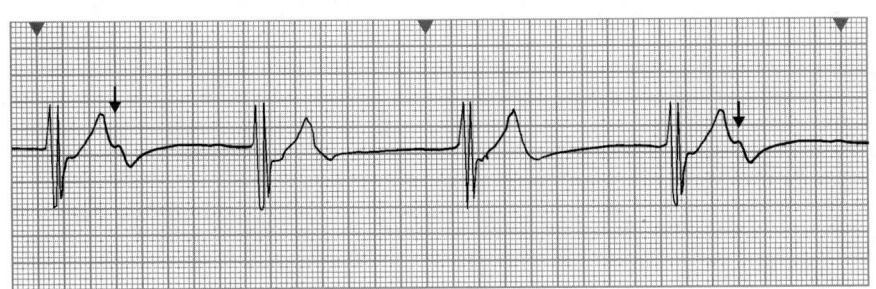

Figure 8–29
Junctional rhythm with ventricular rate of 40 beats per minute. Note the retrograde conduction of P waves (*arrows*).

Figure 8–30
Accelerated junctional rhythm.

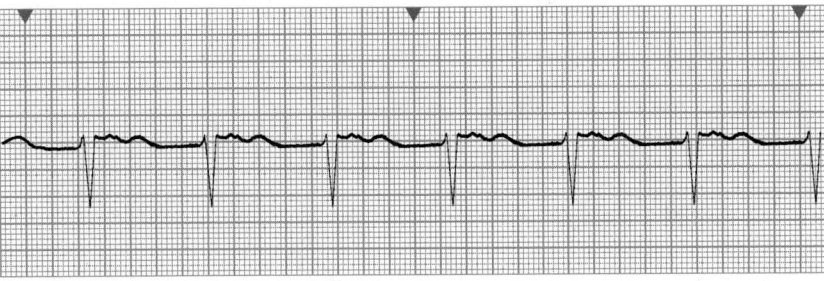

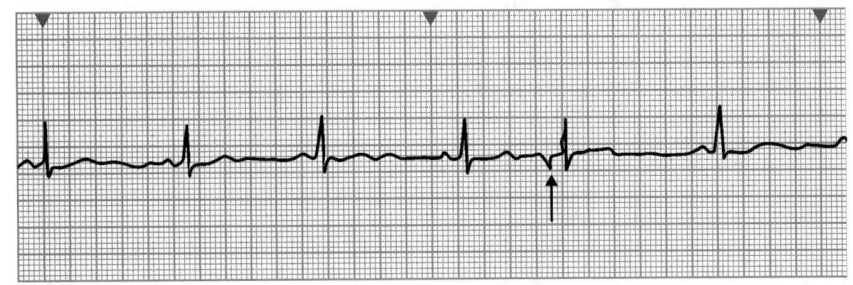

Figure 8–31
Premature junctional complex with retrograde conduction (lead II). Note the inverted P wave of the premature junctional complex (*arrow*).

Figure 8–32
First-degree atrioventricular block with a PR interval of 0.40 seconds (*arrows*).

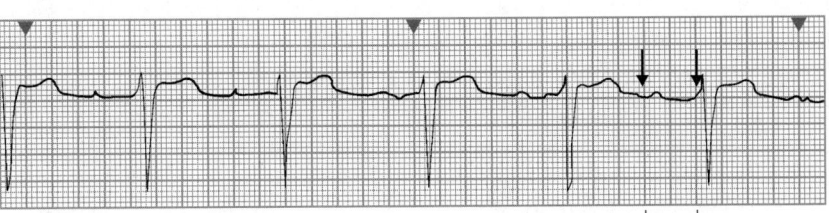

PR interval
.40 sec

dysrhythmia when ventricular rates exceed 100 beats per minute.

Junctional Dysrhythmias. When the AV node assumes the role of the pacemaker of the heart, junctional dysrhythmias result. Junctional dysrhythmias generally occur with organic heart disease, atrial ischemia, and myocardial infarction, and in response to certain medications, such as in digitalis toxicity.

JUNCTIONAL RHYTHMS. A junctional rhythm occurs when the AV node takes over the function of the SA node when the SA node has failed to fire or is blocked.[33] The inherent rate of the AV node (junctional rate) is 40 to 60 beats per minute and represents a slow or junctional *escape* rhythm (Figure 8–29 and Chart 8–17). The P waves of the junctional beats are usually upright in lead I and inverted in leads II and III. They may come before, during, or after the QRS complex, depending on the priority of atrial and ventricular depolarization. If the P wave precedes the QRS complex, the atria have been depolarized first, and the PR interval is usually short (less than 0.11 seconds). *Retrograde conduction* occurs with when the impulse originating in the AV node travels first to the ventricles, then rebounds to stimulate the atria; hence the P wave follows the QRS complex. If the junctional impulse stimulates both atrial and ventricular depolarization at the same time, then the P wave will be *hidden* in the QRS complex. If the atria are not depolarized, a P wave will not be present. The width of the QRS complex is usually normal because the ventricles are usually stimulated along the normal ventricular conduction pathway. Junctional rhythms that occur at a rate between 60 and 100 beats per minute are termed *accelerated junctional* rhythms (Figure 8–30). Junctional rhythms that occur

---

CHART 8–17

Junctional Rhythm

ECG criteria:

- Rate: 40 to 60 beats/minute
- Rhythm: usually regular, may be slightly irregular
- P waves: P wave may precede QRS complex; may be lost in QRS complex and not visible; may follow the QRS complex (retrograde conduction); may be upright in leads I, aVR, and aVL and inverted in leads II, III, aVF
- PR interval: if P wave precedes QRS complex, PR interval is usually short (<0.12 seconds)
- QRS complex: usually normal

Cause:

- Coronary artery disease, congestive heart failure, cardiomyopathy, rheumatic heart disease, myocardial infarction, electrolyte imbalances
- Sinus dysrhythmias: sinus bradycardia, sinus arrest
- Medications: beta blockers, calcium channel blockers, digoxin, central nervous system depressants

Treatment:

- Treatment aimed at eliminating underlying cause
- Treatment required similar to treatment for symptomatic sinus bradycardia: may require atropine, isoproterenol to increase ventricular rate; may require temporary or permanent pacemaker when patient is symptomatic (e.g., hypotensive)
- See Appendix: ACLS: Bradycardia Algorithm

CHART 8–18

Junctional Tachycardia

ECG criteria:

- Rate: accelerated, 60 to 100 beats/minute; junctional tachycardia, 100 to 180 beats/minute; paroxysmal junctional tachycardia, 180 to 250 beats/minute
- Rhythm: usually regular, may be slightly irregular
- P waves: P wave possibly preceding QRS complex, hidden in the QRS complex, or after the QRS complex (retrograde conduction); upright in leads I, aVR, and aVL and inverted in leads II, III, aVF
- PR interval: if P wave precedes QRS complex, PR interval is usually short (<0.12 seconds)
- QRS complex: usually normal

Cause:

- See Junctional Rhythm (Chart 8–17)

Treatment:

- Identification and treatment of underlying cause (e.g., digitalis toxicity, acute myocardial infarction, electrolyte disturbances)
- Consideration of vagal maneuvers (carotid sinus massage, Valsalva maneuvers)
- Consideration of medications useful to treat atrial tachycardias (e.g., calcium channel blockers, digoxin, central nervous system depressants)
- See Appendix: ACLS: Tachycardia Algorithm

at a rate higher than 100 beats per minute are termed *junctional tachycardias* (Chart 8–18).

PREMATURE JUNCTIONAL COMPLEX. Premature junctional complexes (PJCs) occur when the AV node or bundle of His takes over as the dominant pacemaker of the heart for only one beat or for isolated beats (Figure 8–31). The PJC occurs before the next sinus beat, interrupting the heart's regular rhythm, and may be followed by a complete or incomplete compensatory pause. These rhythms are rare and are not considered dangerous (Chart 8–19).

Atrioventricular Blocks. Atrioventricular block refers to a delay or interruption in electrical conduction between the atria and the ventricles. The severity of the block is denoted by the term *degree* (e.g., first-degree, second-degree, third-degree). Each degree of block may occur at the level of the AV node or below it.

FIRST-DEGREE AV BLOCK. First degree AV block (1° AVB) refers to prolongation of AV conduction because of an increased relative refractory period at the level of the AV node. It is characterized by a prolonged PR interval (>0.20 seconds) (Figure 8–32). Impulses are transmit-

ted normally from the SA node, but they are delayed at the AV node (Chart 8–20).

SECOND-DEGREE AV BLOCK. Second-degree AV block (2° AVB) is present when one or more, but not all, atrial impulses fail to reach the ventricles because of impaired conduction. With second-degree AV block, impulses from the atria never reach the ventricles, and QRS complexes are missed or *dropped*. Second-degree AV block usually occurs at the level of the AV node and is associated with reversible conditions such as inferior MI, rheumatic fever, and pharmacologic therapies such as the use of beta blockers and calcium channel blockers.

There are two types of second-degree AV block. Second-degree AV block type I (also known as Wenckebach or Mobitz type I) occurs when the PR interval of each successively conducted beat lengthens progressively until a P wave presents but is not followed by a QRS complex (Figure 8–33). This situation occurs when the signal from the SA node is blocked at the AV node. Usually, only a single impulse is completely blocked, and then the pattern begins again, producing group beating. When the AV conduction ratios remain constant, the cardiac rhythm can be considered *regularly irregular*. Wenckebach or Mobitz type I block usually results from progressive prolongation

CHART 8–19

Premature Junctional Complex (PJC)

ECG criteria:

- Rate: usually normal, dependent on rate of underlying rhythm
- Rhythm: usually irregular because of premature beat
- P waves: P wave of the PJC may come before, during, or after the QRS complex; usually upright in leads I, aVR and aVL; inverted in leads II, III, aVF
- PR interval: if P wave of the PJC precedes the QRS complex, the PR interval is usually short (<0.12 seconds)
- QRS complex: usually normal

Cause:

- Can occur in healthy individuals without a history of heart disease
- Coronary artery disease, congestive heart failure, cardiomyopathy, rheumatic heart disease, myocardial infarction
- Excessive caffeine, alcohol, tobacco consumption

Treatment:

- Treatment aimed at eliminating underlying cause

CHART 8–20

First-Degree Atrioventricular (AV) Block

ECG criteria:

- Rate: 60 to 100 beats/minute
- Rhythm: regular, RR intervals are constant
- AV conduction: prolonged
- P wave: normal and upright in lead II; one P wave precedes each QRS complex
- PR interval: >0.20 seconds and constant
- QRS complex: 0.04 to 0.12 seconds

Cause:

- Possibly a normal variant
- Associated with initial degenerative disease of the conduction system
- Coronary artery disease, myocarditis, myocardial infarction
- Medications: beta blockers, calcium channel blockers, digitalis toxicity

Treatment:

- Usually none; continue to monitor
- Consider modifying or eliminating causative medication, if appropriate

Figure 8–33

Second-degree atrioventricular block, Mobitz type I (Wenckebach). Note the progressive lengthening of the PR interval until a QRS complex is blocked.

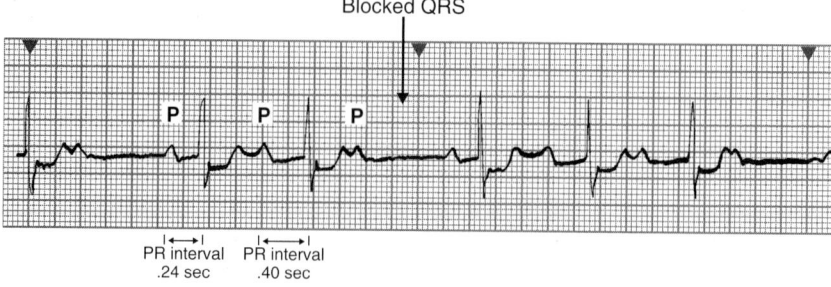

Blocked QRS

PR interval .24 sec   PR interval .40 sec

of the relative refractory period in the AV junction. It may be benign in patients without organic heart disease, but it is abnormal when associated with certain medications (e.g., beta blockers, calcium channel blockers), digitalis toxicity, MI, or cardiac surgery. In the setting of inferior MI, the diagnosis of second-degree AV block type I is usually transient; however, close observation is necessary because high-grade or complete AV block may develop (Chart 8–21).

Second-degree AV block type II (Mobitz type II) is characterized by the occurrence of blocked beats (QRS complexes), yet the PR interval remains constant and is usually normal. With Mobitz type II block, more than one nonconducted beat may occur in succession. When every other atrial impulse is blocked, 2:1 conduction occurs. This form of second-degree AV block usually occurs below the level of the AV node either at the bundle of His or the bundle branches, thus providing for the normal PR interval. A wide QRS complex is apparent when the level of the block is at the bundle branches because of prolonged ventricular conduction through the ventricles. When the block occurs at the level of the bundle of His, the QRS complex is normal in duration. When AV nodal disease is also present, the PR interval is prolonged. Mobitz type II block is usually associated with organic disease of the conduction system. In the setting of acute anteroseptal MI, the appearance of Mobitz type II block indicates a high-risk patient and may be a precursor to complete heart block (Chart 8–22).

Advanced or high-grade AV block is diagnosed when a blocked P wave occurs at more than a 2:1 AV conduction ratio, that is, two or more atrial beats fail to be conducted. Conduction ratios of 3:1, 4:1, 5:1, and 6:1 constitute high-degree AV block (Figure 8–34). Junctional escape beats may appear as a physiologic mechanism to provide a supplemental pacemaker.

THIRD-DEGREE AV BLOCK OR COMPLETE HEART BLOCK. The presence of third-degree AV block (3° AVB) indicates that none of the atrial impulses are conducted to the ventricles. In this situation, the atria and ventricles function independent of each other, leading to complete *AV dissociation*. Mapping out the P waves and R waves reveals independent pacemakers (Figure 8–35). The atrial rate is always faster than or equal to the ventricular rate. Depending on the level of the block, an

CHART 8–21

Second-Degree Atrioventricular (AV) Block, Mobitz Type I (Wenckebach)

ECG criteria:

- Rate: atrial, 60 to 100 beats/minute; ventricular, slower than atrial rate; depends on ratio of P waves to QRS complexes
- Rhythm: atrial, regular; ventricular, irregular, RR interval becomes progressively shorter; group beating usually occurs leading to a regularly irregular rhythm
- AV conduction: some impulses from the sinoatrial node do not conduct through to the ventricles; AV conduction ratios are usually constant
- PR interval: becoming progressively longer with each cycle until a "dropped" beat occurs (P wave present but lacks a succeeding QRS)
- QRS complex: usually normal

Cause:

- Almost always associated with some type of heart disease (e.g., myocardial infarction, coronary artery disease)
- See First-Degree AV Block (Chart 8–20)

Treatment:

- Often no treatment necessary; observation; continued monitoring
- Identification and treatment of underlying cause (e.g., drug toxicity, myocardial infarction)
- Consideration of atropine, temporary pacemaker if patient is symptomatic (e.g., angina, hypotension, changes in level of consciousness)
- See Appendix: ACLS: Bradycardia Algorithm

CHART 8–22

Second-Degree Atrioventricular (AV) Block, Mobitz Type II

ECG criteria:

- Rate: see Mobitz type I
- Rhythm: atrial, regular; ventricular, regular or irregular, depending on the block
- AV conduction: some impulses do not conduct through to the ventricles; AV conduction ratios are usually constant
- P wave: more P waves than QRS complexes
- PR interval: constant; may be prolonged >0.20 seconds
- QRS complex: periodically "dropped" after a P wave; normal duration if block is at level of bundle of His, >0.12 seconds if bundle branch block present

Cause:

- See First-Degree AV Block (Chart 8–20)
- Usually associated with cardiac disease

Treatment:

- Treatment aimed at preventing progression to third-degree AV block
- Identify underlying cause and treat (e.g., drug toxicity, myocardial infarction)
- Consideration of atropine, isoproterenol to increase ventricular rate
- Consideration of dopamine in the setting of hypotension
- Temporary transvenous pacemaker if patient is symptomatic (e.g., hypotension, angina, changes in level of consciousness)
- See Appendix: ACLS: Bradycardia Algorithm

escape rhythm may evolve, originating either from the AV junction or from the ventricles. A junctional escape rhythm is usually present when the block is at the level of the AV node. The ventricular rate is usually 40 to 60 beats per minute, and the QRS complex is of normal duration when ventricular conduction proceeds along its normal conduction pathway (Chart 8–23). If the level of the block is below the level of the AV junction, an *idioventricular* escape rhythm will ensue, with a ventricular rate often less than 40 beats per minute. The QRS complex is wide because of depolarization originating in the ventricle. This form of third-degree heart block carries a more ominous prognosis and usually requires emergency therapy.

Ventricular Dysrhythmias. Ventricular dysrhythmias can be the most serious and potentially lethal of all abnormal heart rhythms. Prompt recognition and immediate treatment may be necessary to prevent subsequent loss of cardiac output and pump failure often associated with these rapid and malignant rhythms.

PREMATURE VENTRICULAR COMPLEX. A premature ventricular complex (PVC) is a single beat that occurs before the expected sinus-conducted QRS complex as a result of firing from an irritable focus in one of the ventricles (Chart 8–24). A PVC is usually easily recognized because it is broad (longer than 0.12 seconds) and premature, has an increased amplitude, and has a T wave of opposite polarity to the sinus QRS complex (Figure 8–36). Usually, there is no related P wave, although retrograde conduction may occur with a P wave following the QRS complex. A PVC usually exhibits a full compensatory pause.

PVCs have many types and various presentation patterns. PVCs that are identical in form originate from the same ectopic focus in the ventricle and are referred to as *unifocal. Multifocal* PVCs originate from different foci and exhibit different shapes. *Ventricular bigeminy* occurs when every other beat is a PVC. A *trigeminal* rhythm is made up of groups of three, that is, every third beat is a PVC. When two PVCs occur in

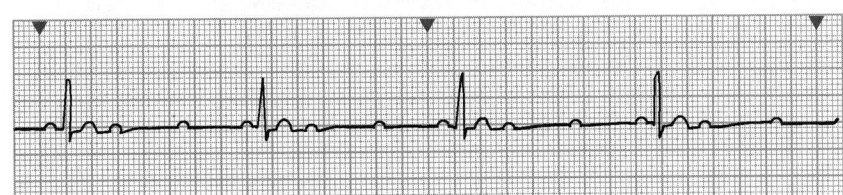

Figure 8–34

Second-degree atrioventricular block, Mobitz type II with 3:1 conduction.

Figure 8–35

Third-degree atrioventricular block (complete heart block). Note the complete dissociation between the P waves and the QRS complexes.

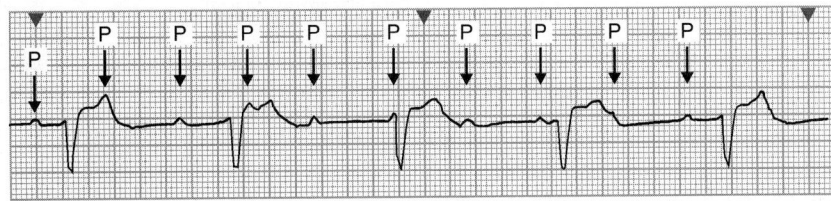

CHART 8-23

Third-Degree Atrioventricular (AV) Block

ECG criteria:

- Rate: atrial, 60 to 100 beats/minute; ventricular, 20 to 60 beats/minute
- Rhythm: atrial and ventricular rates regular but independent of each other
- AV conduction: no atrial impulses conducted to the ventricles; ventricular conduction is ectopic
- P waves: normal but not related to QRS complexes, and some hidden in QRS complexes
- PR interval: varies
- QRS complex: normal if impulse originated in AV junction; wide (>0.12 seconds) if originating in ventricles

Cause:

- Coronary artery disease, congestive heart failure, myocardial infarction
- Medications: beta blockers, calcium channel blockers, digitalis toxicity

Treatment:

- Identification of underlying cause; most patients are symptomatic (e.g., dizziness, hypotension, angina, changes in level of consciousness) and require urgent treatment
- Atropine, isoproterenol, dopamine
- Temporary or permanent transvenous pacing may be necessary
- See Appendix: ACLS: Bradycardia Algorithm

CHART 8-24

Premature Ventricular Complexes (PVCs)

ECG criteria:

- Rate and rhythm: determined by underlying rhythm
- P wave: P waves usually not visible in the PVC; if present, they may occur before, during (hidden in), or after the ectopic beat
- PR interval: determined by the underlying rhythm
- QRS complex: PVC, wide (>0.12 seconds), bizarre, distorted; T wave of PVC deflects in opposite direction (polarity) of QRS complex, may be unifocal or multifocal; compensatory pause usually follows PVC

Cause:

- Coronary artery disease, myocardial infarction, congestive heart failure, conduction system disease
- Electrolyte imbalances: hypokalemia, hypermetabolic states
- Anxiety, fear, stress
- Caffeine, excessive use of alcohol or nicotine
- Medications: epinephrine, dopamine, aminophylline
- May occur in individuals without a history of heart disease

Treatment:

- Consideration of treatment with frequent PVCs (>5–6/minute), bigeminy, trigeminy, multifocal PVCs
- Treatment aimed at determining and managing the underlying cause (e.g., electrolyte imbalance, myocardial infarction, congestive heart failure)
- Administration of lidocaine (LidoPen), procainamide (Pronestyl), bretylium (Bretylol), as needed

Figure 8-36

Premature ventricular complex (PVC). The arrows indicate every third beat is a PVC, also called ventricular trigeminy (lead V$_1$).

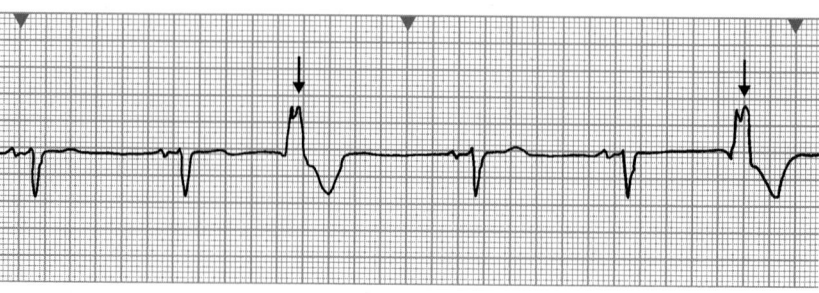

succession, they are described as a couplet, paired, or back to back. If three or more PVCs occur in succession, the rhythm is termed *ventricular tachycardia*.

VENTRICULAR TACHYCARDIA. This dysrhythmia is defined as three or more beats of ventricular origin in succession at a rate higher than 100 beats per minute (Figure 8–37 and Chart 8–25). The ventricular complexes are wide and bizarre. Ventricular tachycardia is usually a regular rhythm or is slightly irregular. AV dissociation is usually present as the SA node is depolarizing the atria in a normal manner at a rate either equal to or slower than the ventricular rate. A sinus P wave can sometimes be recognized between QRS complexes, but it does *not* have a fixed relation to the QRS complex. *Nonsustained* ventricular tachycardia is defined as lasting less than 30 seconds and does not lead to hemodynamic compromise. *Sustained* ventricular tachycardia, however, does last longer than 30 seconds and may lead to hemodynamic collapse. *Monomorphic* ventricular tachycardia has a uniform beat-to-beat QRS

morphology, whereas the *polymorphic* form has a constantly changing, sometimes subtle, beat-to-beat QRS configuration. *Torsades de pointes*, a form of polymorphic ventricular tachycardia, is identified by an undulating pattern associated with delayed ventricular repolarization, manifested on the ECG as a prolonged QT interval. Torsades de pointes means *twisting of the points*, derived from the finding that electrical activity appears to be twisted into a helix (Figure 8–38). Most cases of torsades de pointes are related to drugs that prolong myocardial repolarization and the QT interval such as procainamide or quinidine (Quinaglute). Other causes include hypokalemia, hypomagnesemia, hypocalcemia, high-grade AV block, and sinus bradycardia.[27]

Ventricular tachycardia may be well tolerated, or it may be associated with life-threatening hemodynamic compromise. In the setting of an MI, the mechanism contributing to this rhythm is commonly reentry. However, triggered activity may also contribute to the

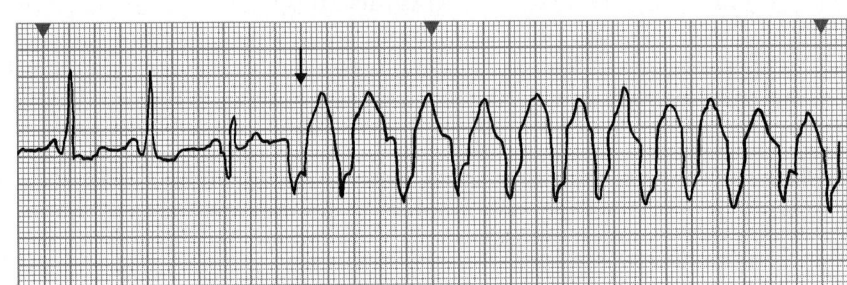

Figure 8–37
Sustained ventricular tachycardia. The arrow indicates the onset of ventricular tachycardia from sinus rhythm.

Figure 8–38
Torsades de pointes.

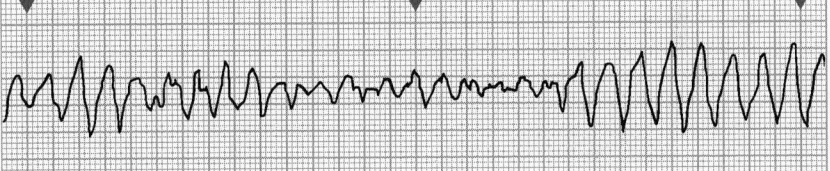

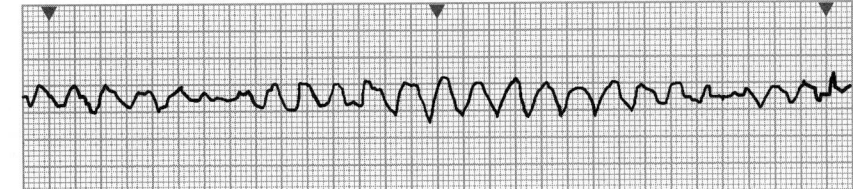

Figure 8–39
Ventricular fibrillation.

Figure 8–40
Asystole *(arrow)*.

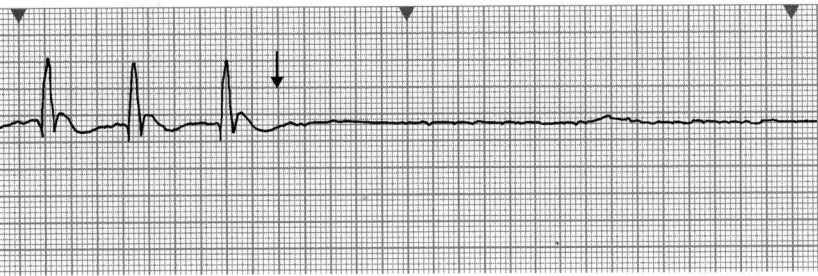

CHART 8–25

Ventricular Tachycardia

ECG criteria:

- Rate: ventricular: 150 to 250 beats/minute
- Rhythm: ventricular: regular or slightly irregular
- Conduction: originating in ventricles
- P waves: usually hidden in QRS complex
- PR interval: not visible and not measurable
- QRS complex: wide and bizarre; similar to PVCs

Cause:

- See Premature Ventricular Complexes (Chart 8–24)
- Coronary artery disease, congestive heart failure, myocardial infarction, cardiomyopathy
- Electrolyte imbalances, hypermetabolic states
- Medications: digoxin, quinidine, central nervous system stimulants, thyroid medications

Treatment:

- Treatment depends on severity and duration of dysrhythmia and patient's response to the rhythm (asymptomatic versus symptomatic)
- Sustained ventricular tachycardia is considered a medical emergency; immediate intervention is required
- Investigation and correction of underlying electrolyte imbalance (e.g., hypokalemia)
- Medications: lidocaine, bretylium, procainamide
- Electrical cardioversion necessary for hemodynamically unstable ventricular tachycardia or when patient is not responsive to drug therapy
- See Appendix: ACLS: Tachycardia Algorithm, Ventricular Fibrillation/Pulseless Ventricular Tachycardia Algorithm, Pulseless Electrical Activity (PEA) Algorithm, Electrical Cardioversion Algorithm
- Torsades de pointes: removal of offending drug, magnesium sulfate, overdrive pacing
- Implantable cardiodefibrillator for long-term prophylaxis

dysrhythmia. In addition to MI, ventricular tachycardia is associated with various clinical entities including myocardial ischemia, cardiomyopathy, and electrolyte imbalances (e.g., hypokalemia, hypomagnesemia). Certain antidysrhythmic medications may produce a *prodysrhythmic effect*, which causes an adverse reaction to the drug (within 30 days of its initiation) in which hemodynamically threatening ventricular tachycardia occurs. Ventricular tachycardia is considered the most dangerous of all ventricular dysrhythmias. Prolonged or sustained ventricular tachycardia may lead to ventricular fibrillation and cardiopulmonary arrest. Prompt identification and urgent intervention is critical in patients with sustained ventricular tachycardia.[28]

VENTRICULAR FIBRILLATION. Ventricular fibrillation is a chaotic ventricular rhythm without identifiable QRS complexes on the surface ECG (Figure 8–39 and Chart 8–26). Ventricular fibrillation is actually the quivering motion of the ventricles resulting from a lack of organized electrical activity. There is no forward blood flow and thus no cardiac output. The most frequent cause of this dysrhythmia is coronary artery disease, and it is the most common terminal event in sudden cardiac death.[27] The terms *coarse* and *fine* are used to describe the amplitude of ventricular fibrillation.

CHART 8–26

Ventricular Fibrillation

ECG criteria:

- Rate: rapid, chaotic; too rapid to count
- Rhythm: irregular and chaotic; ventricular rhythm lacks pattern
- Conduction: no organized conduction
- P waves: none
- PR interval none
- QRS complex: none; undulating, fibrillating baseline

Cause:

- See Ventricular Tachycardia (Chart 8–25)

Treatment:

- Ventricular fibrillation a medical emergency; immediate intervention is required
- Immediate direct-current defibrillation
- Immediate cardiopulmonary resuscitation
- See Appendix: ACLS: Ventricular Fibrillation/Pulseless Ventricular Tachycardia Algorithm

Coarse ventricular fibrillation is associated with a higher likelihood of responding to defibrillation. Fine ventricular fibrillation is often difficult to distinguish from asystole and must be confirmed in two leads. Therapy for ventricular fibrillation is immediate defibrillation. Defibrillation should never be delayed while waiting for pharmacologic therapy to take effect.

Asystole. Asystole is the total absence of electrical activity. Neither atrial nor ventricular activity is present on the ECG (Figure 8–40 and Chart 8–27). This may occur as a primary event, or it may follow ventricular fibrillation or pulseless electrical activity (see Appendix: ACLS: Pulseless Electrical Activity Algorithm). Intermittent escape beats may be present and are termed *agonal* beats. Intervention must occur immediately with asystole. The health care team must actively search for reversible causes of asystole while initiating resuscitation efforts.

Bundle Branch Block Patterns. The bundle branches are part of the specialized electrical conduction system of the heart located in the intraventricular septum. If one of the branches of the bundle of His is blocked by disease, the impulse travels down the healthy branch to the other ventricle first. Depolarization of first one ventricle and then the other takes longer than depolarization of both ventricles simultaneously. The result of this prolonged conduction is a widened QRS complex, commonly referred to as a bundle branch block pattern.

Conduction delays can occur in the bundle branches for the same reasons that they do in the AV node or bundle of His. Bundle branch blocks can occur in the healthy individual; however, they do occur more commonly in patients with coronary artery disease or hypertension. Treatment is directed toward the underlying cause rather than the block itself.

ECG changes associated with bundle branch block are best visualized in the precordial leads V_1 and V_6. Lead V_1 is most commonly used to differentiate between right and left bundle branch block. It is helpful to remember the normal configuration of lead V_1: a deep S wave preceded by a small R wave (see Figure 8–16). In addition, it is useful to understand the normal sequence of ventricular activation to understand the abnormal morphology associated with bundle branch block.

The electrical impulse generated in the SA node travels to the AV node nearly perpendicular to V_1's positive electrode. The P wave in V_1 can be entirely positive, entirely negative, or, most commonly, biphasic. The P wave in V_6 is usually completely positive because the positive electrode (located at the fifth intercostal space, left midaxillary line) is near the left atrium, which is depolarized from right to left by the impulse spreading from the SA node. Depolarization of the intraventricular septum occurs from *left to right*, resulting in an initial positive deflection of the QRS complex in V_1 and an initial negative deflection in V_6. Simultaneous depolarization of the right and left ventricles from endocardium to epicardium results in a *net* leftward vector resulting from the greater muscle mass of the left ventricle. The resultant deflection is a large negative deflection (S wave) in V_1 and a large positive deflection (R wave) in V_6 (Figure 8–41).

CHART 8–27

Asystole

ECG criteria:

- Rate: no atrial or ventricular activity
- Rhythm: none; either a straight, flat line or fine, chaotic and incomprehensible tracing
- Conduction: no atrial or ventricular activity
- P wave: none
- PR interval: none
- QRS complex: none; either a straight, flat line or fine, chaotic and incomprehensible tracing

Treatment:

- Immediate cardiopulmonary resuscitation
- Distinction necessary from fine ventricular fibrillation; check two leads
- See Appendix: ACLS: Asystole Treatment Algorithm

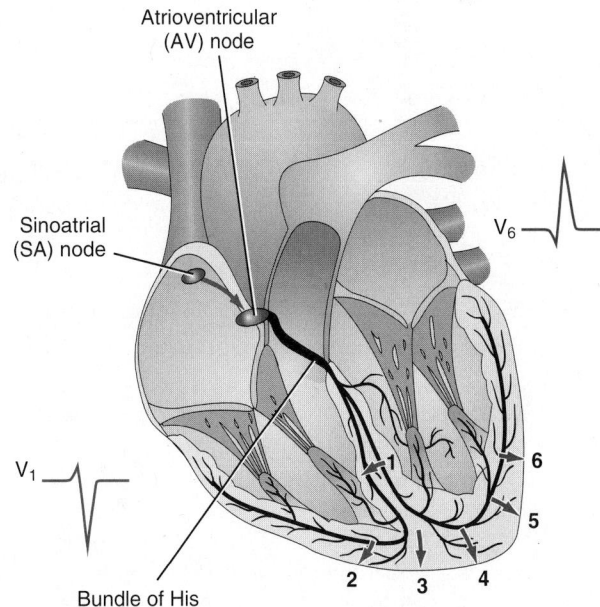

Figure 8–41

Normal sequence of the electrical activation of the ventricles (*arrows 1 to 6*). Electrical activation is depicted in leads V_1 and V_6.

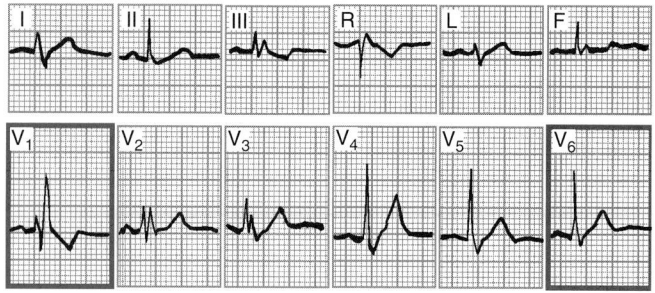

Figure 8–42

Morphology of right bundle branch block in precordial leads V_1 and V_6.

RIGHT BUNDLE BRANCH BLOCK. The characteristic triphasic QRS morphology of right bundle branch block is best observed from precordial lead V_1 because this electrode, located at the fourth intercostal space just right of the sternal border, "sees" the right ventricular free wall. Delayed right ventricular activation (conduction), which occurs in right bundle branch block, produces a primarily positive wide QRS complex with a large R wave in this lead. In right bundle branch block, the QRS complex broadens or slurs, and the QRS complex now looks like an "M" and is referred to as rSR[1]. In addition, the QRS complex is above the isoelectric line in right bundle branch block (Figure 8–42).

LEFT BUNDLE BRANCH BLOCK. The characteristic morphology of left bundle branch block can be observed in either precordial lead V_1 or V_6. Delayed left ventricular activation (conduction) in this condition produces a negative, wide QRS complex in precordial lead V_1. The S wave deepens, and most of the QRS complex in lead V_1 is below the isoelectric line. In lead V_6, a positive, wide R wave is visualized (Figure 8–43). ECG charac-

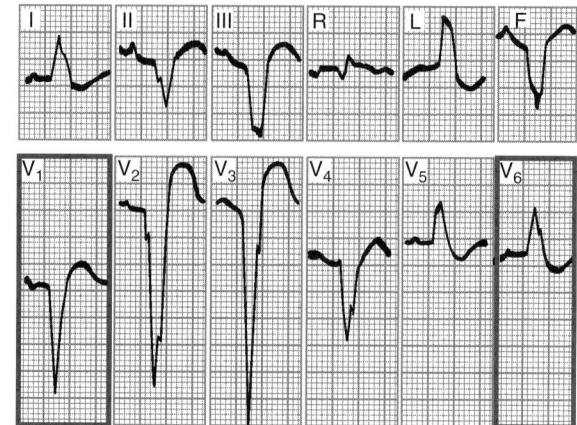

Figure 8–43

Morphology of left bundle branch block in precordial leads V_1 and V_6.

teristics of right and left bundle branch blocks are summarized in Chart 8–28.

ECG Changes Associated with Acute Myocardial Infarction

The ECG is the classic tool used in the rapid and accurate diagnosis of myocardial ischemia and AMI. The most common cause of AMI is occlusion of a coronary artery from a thrombus superimposed on atherosclerotic plaque. This thrombus obstructs coronary blood flow to the affected myocardium. Depending on the degree of oxygen deprivation caused by the obstruction to blood flow, various changes in myocardial tissue result. These changes are reflected on the surface

---

CHART 8–28

ECG Summary of Right Bundle Branch Block (RBBB) and Left Bundle Branch Block (LBBB) in Precordial Leads V_1 and V_6

RBBB

1. Wide QRS complex (>0.12 seconds)
2. Triphasic rsR[1] in MCL_1/V_1; triphasic qRs in MCL_6/V_6
3. ST segment and T wave slope away from the major deflection (i.e., negative in MCL_1/V_1 and positive in MCL_6/V_6)
4. If the QRS complex has the typical RBBB contour, but measures 0.09 to 0.11 seconds, the diagnosis of incomplete RBBB is made

LBBB

1. Wide QRS complex (>0.12 seconds)
2. Large Q in MCL_1/V_1 (about one-third of LBBBs have an initial little r wave in these leads that is not well understood, but it results in an rS complex with the S wave prolonged and large amplitude); a large R wave in MCL_6/V_6
3. ST segment and T wave slope away from the dominant wave of the QRS
4. Widened QRS complexes with LBBB contour measuring 0.10 to 0.12 seconds are all called incomplete LBBB or left intraventricular conduction delay

ECG. The location and type of AMI can be determined by examining the changes of the ST–T-wave segment as they occur in specific leads. ECG changes associated with AMI occur in the leads *facing* the damaged area of myocardium and reflect the stage of evolution of the infarct. The ECG must be interpreted in conjunction with the patient's history, physical examination, and laboratory data at the time of presentation. Rapid diagnosis of AMI is essential for early intervention and effective treatment aimed at limiting myocardial cell death (see Chapter 10).

Insufficient blood supply to the myocardium can result in *ischemia, injury, infarction,* or all three. This classic triad is the basis for recognizing and diagnosing AMI and is identified by careful monitoring of the ST–T-wave segment of the ECG. *Ischemia* is defined as a lack of sufficient blood supply from the coronary arteries to the surrounding myocardium. Ischemia is visualized on the ECG as inverted T waves or ST-segment depression. *Injury,* a more severe stage of ischemia, is brought about by continued lack of blood supply. Myocardial injury appears on the ECG as either ST-segment depression or ST-segment elevation, depending on the extent of tissue involvement. Both myocardial ischemia and myocardial injury are reversible conditions when blood flow is reestablished to the affected areas.

Actual necrosis of myocardial tissue is termed *infarction* and is caused by a prolonged lack of blood supply to myocardial tissue, most commonly resulting from an occlusive coronary thrombus. Myocardial necrosis is an irreversible state, which differentiates it from ischemia and injury. Myocardial necrosis is observed on the ECG as abnormal Q waves. ECG findings associated with myocardial ischemia, injury, and infarction are depicted in Figure 8–44.

The typical evolutionary ECG changes associated with an acute, Q-wave MI include tall T waves, ST-segment elevation, appearance of *abnormal* Q waves, decrease of ST-segment elevation with the beginning of T-wave inversion, and finally, an isoelectric ST segment with symmetric T-wave inversion.[34] Hyperacute or tall, peaked T waves are often seen in the first minutes and hours after the onset of chest pain in AMI. These changes are frequently *not* visualized by the health care team because patients often do not seek medical attention in this period, and the changes may be transient. Hyperacute T-wave changes are thought to be caused by subendocardial ischemia.[34]

The initial ECG change usually visualized in AMI is ST-segment elevation in the leads *facing* the area of infarction. ST-segment elevation indicates a zone of ischemic myocardial tissue. This is referred to as a "zone of injury" pattern. With myocardial injury, the area involved is depolarized incompletely. It remains electrically more positive than the uninjured area at the end of the depolarization, causing ST-segment ele-

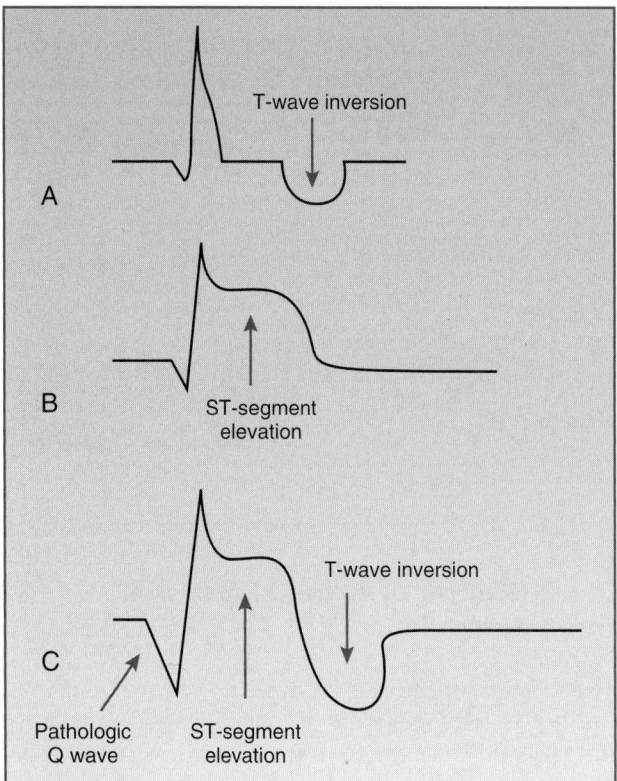

Figure 8–44

ST-segment and T-wave changes associated with myocardial ischemia (A), injury (B), and necrosis (C).

vation in the lead facing that region. ST-segment depression or T-wave inversion in the leads facing the opposite wall of the myocardium (180° from the area of infarction) are also commonly visualized. These ECG changes are referred to as *reciprocal changes.*

The next phase of evolution is the appearance of large Q waves in the leads facing the zone of infarction that indicate myocardial necrosis. The presence of Q waves is the most characteristic ECG finding of a transmural MI of the left ventricle. Pathologic or abnormal Q waves must be at least 0.04 seconds (1 mm or one small box) wide and at least one-fourth of the height of the QRS complex in the leads facing the infarction. Q waves may appear immediately or within the first few days after the onset of symptoms, and they may be present on the ECG indefinitely.

As the AMI continues to evolve, ST-segment elevation decreases, and the T waves begin to invert. The inverted T waves become progressively deeper as the ST-segment elevation subsides.[34] After several hours or days, the ST segment returns to baseline or becomes isoelectric. When the ST segment becomes isoelectric, the T waves are usually symmetrically inverted. The T-wave inversion may resolve within months or years, or it may persist indefinitely. Table 8–7 summarizes ECG changes that occur with AMI over time.

TABLE 8–7

Common Electrocardiographic Changes with Myocardial Infarction Over Time

Type of Infarction	ECG Changes
Acute infarction	ST-segment elevation hyperacute, coved, and often marked
	Q waves are small or absent
	Hyperacute or tall, peaked T waves
	Reciprocal ST-segment depression often present
Recent infarction	Pathologic Q waves
	ST-segment elevation minimal or absent
	T-wave inversion often present and possibly marked
	Reciprocal ST-segment depression minimal or absent
Old infarction	Q waves present
	ST-segment elevation absent
	T-wave inversion minimal or absent
	No reciprocal ST-segment changes

Identification of Acute Myocardial Infarction

The location of the site of MI or myocardial ischemia can be determined with considerable accuracy from the 12-lead ECG. Although many factors influence the diagnostic accuracy of the 12-lead ECG, the overall sensitivity of the ECG in determining AMI ranges from 48 to 82%.[34] When evaluating the 12-lead ECG for changes consistent with AMI, it is necessary to learn which leads reflect the various walls of the heart (see Table 10–1). Damaged myocardium is either transmural (Q wave), involving the full thickness of the ventricle, or nontransmural, involving only the partial thickness of the ventricle (subendocardial or non–Q wave). ST-segment elevation of at least 1 mm in two contiguous leads is considered significant evidence of AMI.

Once the ECG changes associated with myocardial ischemia, injury, or infarction have been identified, the next step is to localize the area of infarction. Limb leads II, III, and aVF view the inferior surface of the heart. Leads I, aVL, V_5, and V_6 reflect electrical activity of the lateral regions of the myocardium. Changes occurring at the anterior surface of the heart are observed by viewing leads V_1, V_2, V_3, and V_4. ECG changes associated with anterior and inferior AMI are depicted in Figures 8–45 and 8–46, respectively.

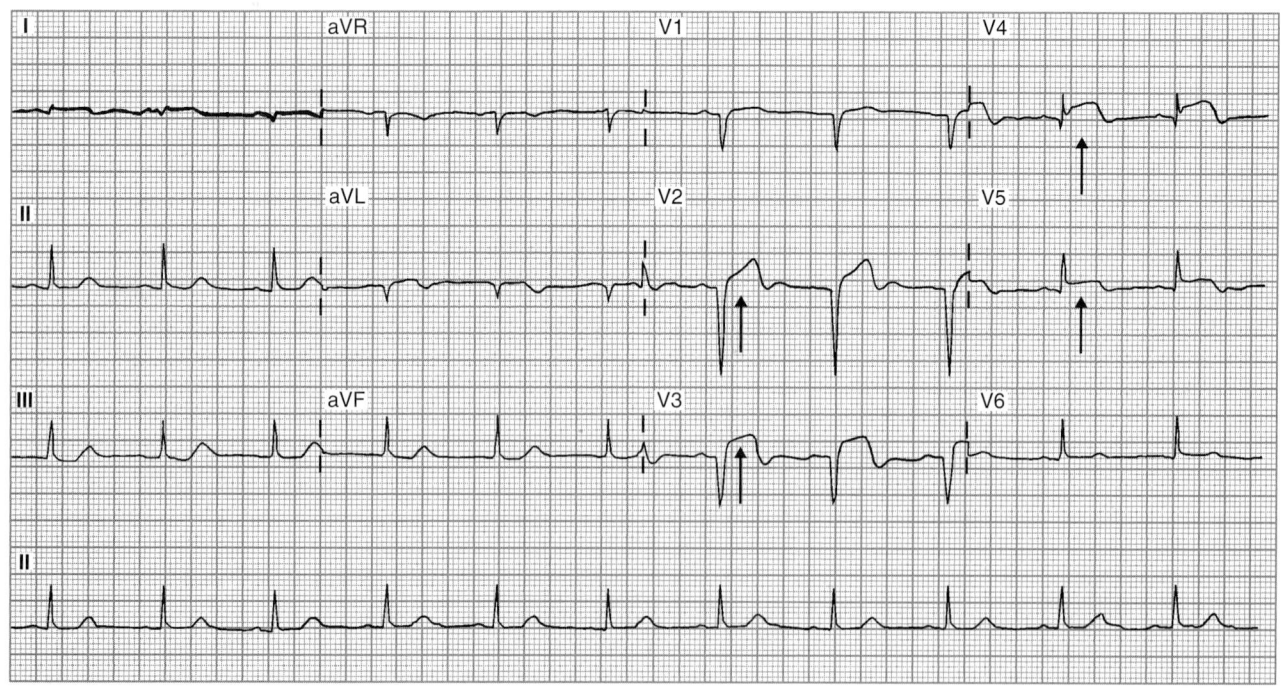

Figure 8–45

Electrocardiographic findings with anterior myocardial infarction. Note the ST-segment elevation in precordial leads V_2 to V_5 (*arrows*).

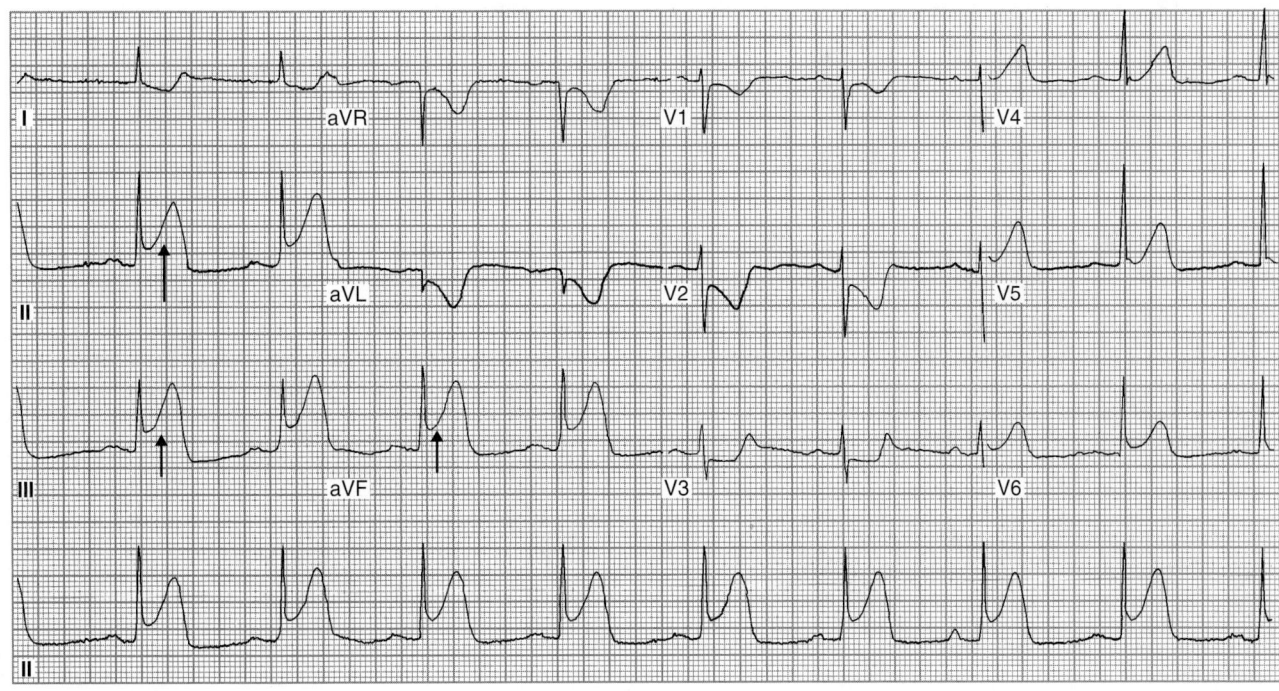

Figure 8–46

Electrocardiographic findings with inferior myocardial infarction. Note the ST-segment elevation in the inferior leads II, III, and aVF *(arrows)*.

The ECG changes seen with a posterior wall infarction are reciprocal changes reflected in leads V_1 and V_2, because the traditional 12-lead ECG does not have leads that view the posterior wall. Tall broad R waves (longer than 0.04 seconds), ST-segment depression, and upright T waves in leads V_1 and V_2 suggest a posterior infarct. These changes are often referred to as a *mirror image* of the posterior wall. When posterior infarction is suspected, additional leads may be placed at the fifth intercostal space, left posterior axillary line (V_7), left posterior scapular (midscapular) line (V_8), and to the left (V_9) and right (V_9R) of the spinal column. Expected changes that further point to posterior infarction in leads V_8 and V_9 are pathologic Q waves with ST-segment elevation.[35]

Up to 50% of all patients who present to a coronary care unit with an acute inferior MI have concurrent right ventricular infarction.[36] Nurses in these settings play an important role in the recognition of right ventricular infarction by performing the standard 12-lead ECG and incremental right ventricular leads when this disorder is suspected. With the standard 12-lead ECG, ST-segment elevation of 1 mm or more in leads II and III with a ratio of ST-segment elevation in leads III:II of more than 1 had an 88% specificity and 91% positive predictive value for right ventricular infarction.[34,35] In addition to the standard 12-lead ECG, six precordial chest leads can be placed on the right chest wall as a mirror image of the standard precordial leads to further confirm the diagnosis of right ventricular infarction (Figure 8–47). These incremental leads directly interrogate the right ventricular wall and may demonstrate ST-segment elevation associated with MI, if it is present. Lead V_4R is reported to be 70 to 100% sensitive for right ventricular infarction, with a predictive accuracy of 78 to 100%.

The prevalence of MI without Q waves is reported to range between 16 and 40%.[34] Non–Q-wave patterns are believed to involve only a partial thickness of the myocardium. The ECG changes associated with a non–Q-wave MI are usually ST-segment elevation, ST-segment depression, and deep T-wave inversion. A diagnosis of non–Q-wave MI can only be made if the ST-segment and T-wave changes are accompanied by other evidence of myocardial necrosis (e.g., elevation of cardiac enzymes).

ST Segment Monitoring

Various patients in the critical care unit are at risk of developing myocardial ischemia. With the use of continuous ST-segment monitoring, the nurse may more effectively evaluate patients with MI, those receiving thrombolytic therapy, those undergoing coronary angioplasty, and patients with a history of CAD who are at risk of developing myocardial ischemia. ST-segment monitoring detects ischemia more completely than the monitoring of cardiac symptoms, heart rate, and rhythm alone.[37] As previously discussed, elevation or depression of the ST segment is associated with myocardial injury and ischemia, respectively. ST-segment deviation is the number of millimeters the ST segment is displaced from the isoelectric line, measured at 60 or 80 msec after the J point (Figure 8–48). For the ST

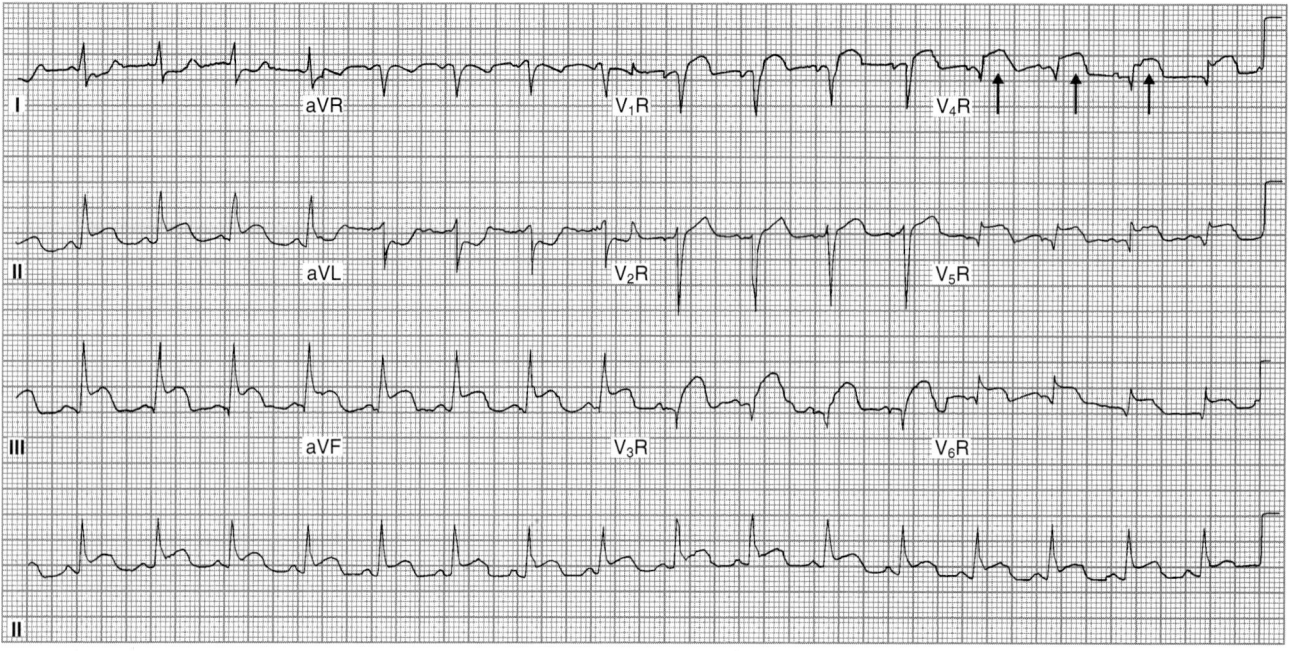

Figure 8–47

Electrocardiographic findings with right ventricular myocardial infarction. Note the ST-segment elevation in the right precordial lead (V₄R) *(arrows)*. The ratio of ST-segment elevation in lead III/lead II is greater than 1.

segment to be indicative of ischemia, it must be displaced a minimum of 1 mm from the patient's baseline or isoelectric line for at least 1 minute.

Many bedside monitors now have the capability to provide continuous ST-segment monitoring in one or more leads. The ST-segment software in the bedside monitor determines the patient's isoelectric line, the ST-segment measurement point, and default alarm parameters. Adjustments of these parameters can be made by the nurse. Alarms should be set 1 mm above and 1 mm below the defined ST-segment measurement point. The nurse is faced with the challenge of ac-

curately interpreting ST-segment variations because some conditions may alter the ST segment (e.g., bundle branch block, ventricular paced rhythms, electrolyte imbalances). It is also important for the nurse to evaluate changing trends of the ST-segment measurement rather than treating individual values.

According to Tisdale and Drew,[37] the most important challenge for the nurse when using continuous ST-segment monitoring is appropriate lead selection. Lead V₁ is recommended for monitoring whenever the capability exists. The patient's *ischemic fingerprint* should be obtained by documenting the patient's ST-segment patterns of ischemia with a 12-lead ECG. The nurse will then be able to select a multi-lead combination from the 12-lead ECG that best represents the patient's ischemic pattern (or "fingerprint"). Lead selection for patients for whom the ischemic fingerprint has not been identified or CAD has not been defined should include an anterior lead and an inferior lead.[37] For example, V₁ and lead II, III, or aVF are appropriate choices for both dysrhythmia detection and ischemia monitoring. Additional research is necessary to validate optimal bedside monitoring lead selection for use with continuous ST-segment monitoring.

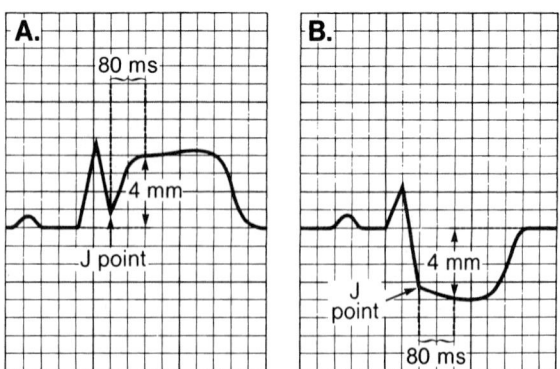

Figure 8–48

Measurement points used in ST-segment analysis. Typically, a point either 60 or 80 msec after the J point is used. A, ST-segment elevation of more than 4 mm above the J point. B, ST-segment depression of less than 4 mm below the J point. (Adapted from Tisdale LA, Drew BJ: ST segment monitoring for myocardial ischemia. AACN Clin Issues Crit Care Nurs 4:36, 1993.)

Holter Monitoring

Long-term ECG recording or Holter monitoring is widely used for the detection of cardiac dysrhythmias and myocardial ischemia.[34] The ECG is recorded over a given period while the patient assumes normal daily activities. The patient records these activities and any symptoms in a diary for correlation with the ECG. The correlation of symptoms and activities with the ECG is the most useful noninvasive method to document and quantitate the frequency and complexity of dysrhythmias, to correlate dysrhythmias with symptoms, and to evaluate the effect of antidysrhythmic therapy on spontaneous dysrhythmias.[38]

The Holter monitor records the ECG tracing continuously in two or three leads for reading and extraction of pertinent data at a later time by an experienced health care provider. The usual leads for ambulatory Holter monitoring are the bipolar leads (modified) V_1 and V_5, and if three channels are used, lead aVF is included.[34] Several modes of recording are available. When a tape recorder is used, the leads are connected to a portable ECG monitor, and the ECG is recorded on a magnetic tape for 10, 12, or 24 hours. The recorder may be patient activated and initiated only when the patient experiences symptoms. Finally, the recording may be dysrhythmia or "event" activated. Holter monitoring is a relatively inexpensive diagnostic tool and can be used on an outpatient basis and an inpatient basis.

Identification of cardiac dysrhythmias, both bradydysrhythmias and tachydysrhythmias, is the most common indication for Holter monitoring. Holter monitoring is indicated in patients with symptoms of suspected cardiac origin, that is, palpitations, dizziness, syncope, or angina. The Holter monitor is also a useful diagnostic tool for patients with known cardiac disease. For example, the identification of patients at high risk for ventricular dysrhythmias (e.g., after MI, in patients with cardiomyopathy) can be accomplished with Holter monitoring. Evaluation of the efficacy of antidysrhythmic drug therapy is another important indication for this type of monitoring. The Holter monitor may be used to evaluate pacemaker function, especially in patients who exhibit symptoms suggestive of pacemaker malfunction, such as dizziness and syncope. Finally, Holter monitoring is used to document conduction disturbances during sleep in patients with sleep apnea syndrome.

Patient Considerations

As with all diagnostic tests, the patient should be informed about the rationale for the test. The nurse should instruct the patient in the use of the Holter monitor by reviewing all components of the system. If a patient-activated monitor is used, the patient should be instructed in how and when to initiate a recording.

An essential component of Holter monitoring is the patient's diary. The nurse should instruct the patient to record the type and time of each daily activity and any symptoms that may be associated with the given activity. The nurse should explain to the patient that the information recorded in the diary allows for activities and associated symptoms to be correlated with findings on the ECG.

Instructions should be clear and specific regarding care of the monitor during the monitoring period. To facilitate reliable recordings, the nurse should instruct the patient not to remove the electrodes, to keep the electrodes dry, and to avoid damaging the monitor. Activities such as bathing and swimming are to be avoided. Finally, the nurse should instruct the patient when to return the Holter monitor for interpretation. Transtelephonic monitoring is often used with Holter monitoring and should be explained to the patient, if appropriate.

CARDIAC PACEMAKERS

The cardiac pacemaker is designed to treat patients with cardiac dysrhythmias, specifically bradydysrhythmias and tachydysrhythmias. Approximately 500,000 persons in the United States have had permanent pacemakers implanted.[39] As the demand for pacemakers continues to increase, the technology of these devices also continues to grow in complexity and diversity. The purpose of this section is to provide the nurse with a basic overview of pacemakers. Temporary pacemaker systems, specifically pacemakers used in the critical care unit, are emphasized.

Pacemaker Codes

Because of the increasing complexity and diversity of pacemaker technology, coding systems have been developed to identify the type of cardiac pacemaker implanted. The first pacemaker coding system was developed in 1974 by the pacemaker committee of the Inter-Society of Heart Disease and Resource Development. A three-position pacemaker code was developed indicating: the chamber or chambers in which pacing occurs (position I); the chamber or chambers in which intrinsic cardiac activity is sensed (position II); and the mode in which the pacemaker is operating (position III). For positions I and II, capital letters are used to denote the cardiac chamber involved: A, atrium; V, ventricle; and D, double (both atrium and ventricle). The pacing response to sensed intrinsic cardiac activity, referred to as the pacing *mode*, is depicted in position III. The pacing modes are: I, inhibited; T, triggered; and O, not applicable. When the pacemaker is programmed in the inhibited mode, it is inhibited from firing in response to a sensed intrinsic beat. In the triggered mode, the pacemaker fires in response to a sensed intrinsic beat or interval. The letter O in the third position indicates that the pacemaker does not fire in response to sensed intrinsic cardiac activity resulting in asynchronous cardiac pacing. For example, a pacemaker programmed to the *VVI* mode lets the nurse know that the device paces in the ventricle, senses intrinsic cardiac rhythm in the ventricle, and is inhibited by sensed intrinsic ventricular beats.

Over the past two decades, the three-position pacemaker code has been revised to keep up with the advances in pacemaker technology. In 1981, the three-position code was expanded to a five-position code. Two additional positions were added to the original code to denote programmability (position IV) and antitachycardia pacing (position V). In 1987, the North American Society of Pacing and Electrophysiology (NAPSE) and the British Pacing and Electrophysiology Group (BPEG) introduced the NAPSE/BPEG Generic Pacemaker Code, which is the most frequently used code today (referred to as the NBG code). The first three positions of the NBG code have retained all features of the original three-position pacemaker code and are intended for describing antibradycardia pacing functions. The letter D has been modified to signify dual (rather than double) and continues to denote activity of both the atrium and ventricles when used in the first two positions and to also indicate the use of both inhibited and triggered modes when used in the third position. The fourth position describes the presence or absence of programmable features of the pacemaker and the presence or absence of rate modulation. Finally, the fifth position of the code indicates the presence of one or more antitachycardia functions that can be initiated manually or automatically. Chart 8–29 depicts the NBG pacemaker code. In clinical prac-

tice, it is common to use the first three positions of the pacemaker code to identify the patient's pacemaker. The first three positions of the code are also applied to temporary cardiac pacing.

Indications for Cardiac Pacing

With the many different pacemaker programming options available, the type of pacemaker selected reflects the patient's clinical condition and underlying cardiac rhythm. Because of the increasing complexity of modern pacemakers and the need to evaluate patients in a more uniform manner, the Joint American College of Cardiology/American Heart Association Task Force established a classification system for pacemaker implantation.[40] Class I indicates all conditions for which it is generally agreed that a pacemaker should be implanted. Class II identifies conditions for which pacemakers are frequently used but for which there is disagreement about the need for their use. Conditions for which it is determined that permanent pacing is not required are identified as class III. Table 8–8 outlines the indications for permanent pacemakers according to the Joint American College of Cardiology/American Heart Association Task Force recommendations.[40,41]

Temporary pacing as the treatment of choice occurs whenever bradycardia or heart block contributes significantly to hypotension or a low cardiac output state that is refractory to pharmacologic therapy. In the critical care setting, various situations may warrant the need for temporary pacing to manage the hemody-

---

CHART 8–29

NAPSE/BPEG (NBG) Generic Pacemaker Code

Position*	I	II	III	IV	V
Letter Codes	0 = none	0 = none	0 = none	0 = none	0 = none
	A = atrium	A = atrium	T = triggered	P = simple programmable	P = pacing (antitachydysrhythmia)
	V = ventricle	V = ventricle	I = inhibited	M = multiprogrammable	S = shock
	D = dual (A + V)	D = dual (A + V)	D = dual (T + I)	C = communicating	D = dual (P + S)
				R = rate modulation	
Manufacturer's designation	S = single (A or V)	S = single (A or V)			

*Positions I through III are used exclusively for antibradydysrhythmia function.
From Bernstein AD, et al: The NAPSE/BPEG generic pacemaker code for antibradyarrhythmia and adaptive rate pacing and antitachyarrhythmia devices. PACE Pacing Clin Electrophysiol 10:794–799, 1987.

TABLE 8–8
Indications for the Implantation of a Permanent Cardiac Pacemaker

Disorder	Class of Indication
Sinus node dysfunction	I. Sinus node dysfunction with documented symptomatic bradycardia
	II. Sinus node dysfunction with heart rates <40 beats per minute; no clear association between symptoms and bradycardia
	III. No symptoms
Atrioventricular (AV) block	I. Symptomatic complete or second-degree AV block with heart rates 40 beats per minute or consequence of His bundle ablation
	II. Asymptomatic second-degree type II or complete heart block with heart rates >40 beats per minute
	III. First-degree AV block or asymptomatic type I AV block
Bifascicular or trifascicular block	I. Fascicular block with intermittent complete heart block associated with symptoms or second-degree type II AV block with or without symptoms
	II. HV intervals >100 msec or fascicular block associated with syncope that cannot be ascribed to other causes
	III. Asymptomatic fascicular block or fascicular block with associated first-degree AV block
Neurogenic syncope	I. Recurrent syncope provoked by carotid sinus stimulation; pauses of >3 seconds induced by minimal carotid sinus pressure
	II. Syncope associated with bradycardia reproduced by head-up tilting
	III. Recurrent syncope in the absence of a cardioinhibitory response
Cardiomyopathy	I. None
	II. Severely symptomatic patients with hypertrophic cardiomyopathy refractory to drug therapy (may become class I in the future)
	III. Severely symptomatic patients with dilated cardiomyopathy (may become class II in the future)

HV interval, conduction interval between the His bundle and the ventricular myocardium. (From Kusumoto FM, Goldschlager N: Cardiac pacing. N Engl J Med 334:90, 1996. Reprinted, by permission, from the New England Journal of Medicine.)

namic sequelae associated with rhythm disturbances, such as profound bradycardia, heart block, and dysrhythmias associated with MI. Temporary pacing may also be used as a prophylactic measure in those patients who are at high risk of conduction disturbances. Patients at high risk of developing lethal bradycardias, such as bundle branch block in the setting of AMI that may progress to asystole or complete heart block, may benefit from the prophylactic use of a temporary transvenous pacemaker. Prophylactic temporary pacing may be indicated in patients with left bundle branch block who will undergo catheterization of the right side of the heart, to provide a backup measure in the event of right bundle branch block. Temporary pacing is also used to prevent tachydysrhythmias, such as ventricular tachycardia, associated with a prolonged QT interval or sinus bradycardia. *Overdrive pacing* refers to the termination of tachycardia in an attempt to restore sinus rhythm. Termination of hemodynamically compromising tachycardias may be accomplished by pacing the atria or ventricle at a rate *higher* than that of the tachycardia. Finally, temporary pacing wires may be attached to the ECG and used as a diagnostic tool to determine the origin of a cardiac rhythm that is difficult to diagnose when characteristic ECG findings cannot be distinguished on the 12-lead ECG, for example, atrial flutter with 2:1 conduction.

Pacemaker System

Cardiac pacing may be accomplished with the use of permanent or wholly implantable systems or with the use of temporary systems that can be easily removed from the patient when the need for pacing no longer exists. The nurse must become familiar with the various types of devices that may be in use. A pacing system, whether permanent or temporary, is composed of a pulse generator, electrodes, and leads.

The pulse generator contains the electronic circuitry and the power source (battery) that initiate electrical impulses. The pulse generator may be located either inside (permanent) or outside (temporary) the patient's body. The lithium iodide battery is the power source of choice for most permanent pacemakers. Life expectancy of the lithium iodide battery is anywhere from 4 to 15 years, depending on how the pacemaker is programmed and the degree to which the pacemaker is used.[26]

Pacing electrodes deliver electrical energy to the heart that results in myocardial contraction. A lead or leads connect the electrodes, located at the tip of the lead, to the pulse generator. In general, pacing leads contain one (unipolar) or two (bipolar) electrodes at their distal tip that are in contact with the surface of the heart. Electrical current flows from the negative electrode (cathode) to the positive electrode (anode). In a unipolar system, the impulse is sent to the negative electrode, which is in contact with the heart. After stimulating the myocardium, the impulse travels to the positive electrode, which, in the unipolar system, is the metal casing of the pulse generator. In a bipolar system, both the negative and positive electrodes are located at the distal tip of the lead; thus, the "pathway" in which the electrical current travels is much smaller than that of the unipolar system. Today, bipolar leads are used more frequently than unipolar systems.

Temporary Pacemakers

Various types of pacing systems may be used in the critical care unit to optimize hemodynamic status resulting from either temporary or permanent alterations of heart rate and rhythm. Temporary pacing provides patients with a consistent cardiac rhythm as their own conduction system recovers or serves as a bridge to permanent pacing.[26] The temporary pacing systems most commonly used in the critically ill include transvenous pacing, epicardial pacing, and transcutaneous pacing systems. Although considerable differences are apparent among these systems, each system is composed of a pulse generator that is external to the patient, pacing leads, and electrodes.

TRANSVENOUS PACING SYSTEM. Transvenous pacing uses a pacing catheter or lead placed, through a percutaneous route, in the right ventricle or right atrium for pacing the endocardial surface of the heart. The most common access sites for transvenous pacing include the internal or external jugular vein, the antecubital vein, the subclavian vein, and the femoral vein. The transvenous pacing lead is usually guided into position with the aid of fluoroscopy. The proximal end of the pacing lead is attached to the pulse generator. Once proper position of the lead is established, all noninsulated components of the pacing system, that is, the lead connections to the pulse generator, should be secured and insulated to protect the patient from environmental electricity, which can be directed to the patient's heart through these components.

Complications associated with the temporary transvenous pacing system are rare, but they do occur. Complications associated with insertion of the lead include infection, pneumothorax, air embolism, myocardial perforation, hematoma, dysrhythmias, and accidental electrocution.

TRANSTHORACIC EPICARDIAL PACING SYSTEM. Transthoracic epicardial pacing is accomplished through electrodes that are loosely attached to the epicardial surface of the heart during cardiac surgery. Electrodes are placed on both the atrium and the ventricle while the proximal ends of the leads are brought through the chest wall. The leads are then attached to an external pulse generator. Complications with the epicardial system are few. Infection and perforation of vascular structures are rare; however, the epicardial system is limited by the feature that the electrodes must be placed during cardiac surgery and may become dislodged from the epicardial surface, thus rendering them ineffective.

TRANSCUTANEOUS PACING SYSTEM. The transcutaneous temporary pacing system is composed of two adhesive conducting pads that are placed externally on the chest wall. One pad is placed anteriorly to the left of the sternum as close to the point of maximal impulse as possible. The posterior pad is placed directly behind the anterior pad, to the left of the thoracic spine. The electrodes are incorporated into the pad and cover a large surface area over the skin. The pads are connected to an external pulse generator and function primarily in the VVI or VVO mode. Transcutaneous pacing or external pacing is commonly used in emergency situations (e.g., cardiac arrest, complete heart block with low cardiac output) until a transvenous pacing system can be placed. The use of the transcutaneous pacemaker has expanded and may also be used for standby or prophylactic use in cardioversion, for electrophysiologic studies, and during induction of anesthesia. Use of the transcutaneous pacemaker system causes stimulation of skeletal muscle and the diaphragm because more energy is required to pace the heart externally. Thus, the transcutaneous pacemaker may be painful and uncomfortable for some patients and may require the administration of analgesics and sedatives.

Monitoring the Function of a Pacemaker

The nurse is responsible for monitoring the patient's physiologic response to treatment with a pacemaker. Monitoring the ECG is an important component of the nurse's assessment to ensure appropriate functioning of the pacemaker. The nurse should be able to recognize normal paced beats and common ECG criteria indicative of pacemaker malfunction. ECG evaluation of multiprogrammable permanent pacemaker systems is beyond the scope of this chapter, and the student is referred to the references for additional reading.[26]

The pacemaker impulse is recognized on the ECG by a pacemaker *artifact* or *spike*. The pacemaker spike is a sharp, narrow vertical line with a duration normally less than 2 msec.[34] The morphology of the waveform of the chamber paced is distorted after the pacemaker impulse because of alteration of the normal conduction pathway (e.g., the QRS complex of a paced ventricular beat is >0.12 msec).

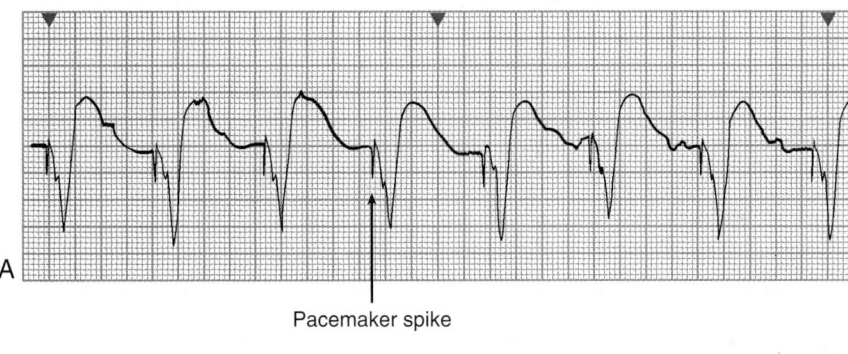

A

Pacemaker spike

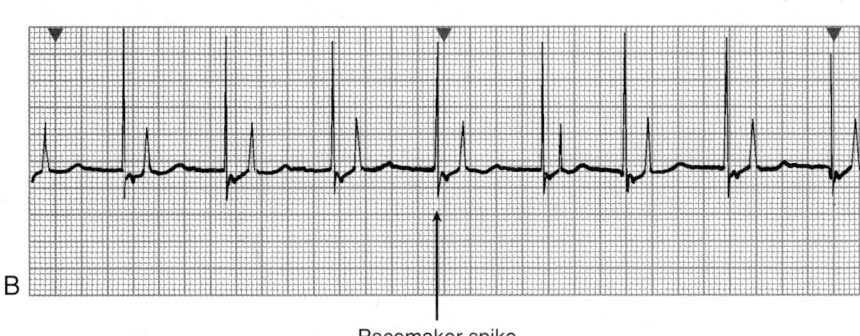

B

Pacemaker spike

Figure 8–49

A, Ventricular (depolarization) capture secondary to a pacemaker lead in the right ventricle. Note the left bundle branch block pattern after the pacemaker spike that demonstrates delayed conduction through the ventricle. *B,* Atrial (depolarization) capture secondary to a pacemaker lead in the right atrium. Note the inverted P wave and the normal conduction of the impulse through the ventricles.

Pacemaker Capture

The first step in the assessment of the paced rhythm is to evaluate the pacemaker's ability to *capture.* Capture refers to the depolarization of the atria or ventricle in response to a pacing stimulus.[39] With appropriate capture, the depolarization (contraction) of the chamber being paced follows the pacemaker spike on the ECG. Thus, capture of the atria is indicated by a P wave after the pacemaker spike, and capture of the ventricle is indicated by a wide QRS complex after the pacemaker spike (Figure 8–49).

Failure to capture is evident on the ECG when a pacemaker spike is visible on the ECG, but the appropriate complex does not follow (Figure 8–50). The pacing output from the pulse generator has not resulted in depolarization of the heart. Failure to capture may be related to dislodgment or improper placement of the pacing lead, excess fibrosis at the catheter tip, fracture of the lead, MI at the site of the electrode, severe electrolyte imbalances, inappropriate programming of the pulse generator, and battery failure.

Pacemaker Sensing

Once appropriate capture has been determined, the nurse must establish that the pacemaker is sensing the patient's intrinsic rhythm appropriately. To evaluate pacemaker sensing, the nurse must know in which mode the pacemaker is programmed (position III in the pacemaker code). If the pacemaker does not sense intrinsic cardiac activity and does not inhibit pacemaker output, inappropriate pacemaker stimuli may appear during intrinsic complexes. This problem is called *undersensing* (Figure 8–51). Undersensing may result from an inadequate cardiac signal (e.g., low voltage secondary to AMI), ectopic beats, inappropriate programming of the pacemaker's sensitivity, electromagnetic interference, loss of lead integrity, and poor lead connections.

Oversensing occurs when the pacemaker senses activity other than cardiac activity and inhibits pacing output. This situation results in pauses in the ECG and a rate that is lower than the set rate of the pacemaker. Sources that may inhibit the pacemaker's ability to

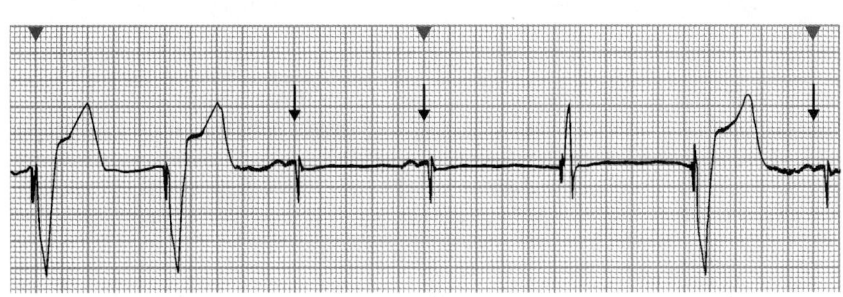

Figure 8–50

Pacemaker malfunction with failure to capture. Pacemaker spikes are present on the electrocardiogram, but they are not followed by a QRS complex *(arrows).*

Figure 8–51

Pacemaker malfunction with failure to sense. The pacemaker does not sense the intrinsic (sinus) beats leading to the inappropriate firing of the pacemaker (arrows). These pacemaker spikes do not capture the ventricles because they occur during the refractory period of the cardiac cycle.

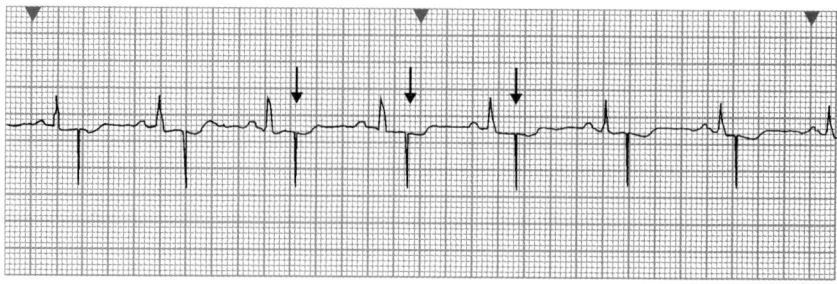

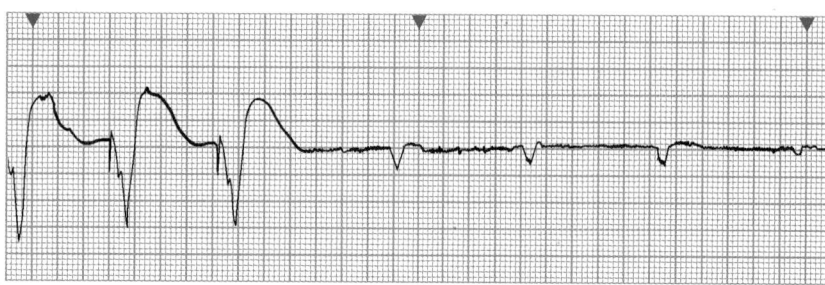

Figure 8–52

Pacemaker malfunction with failure to pace. Note the sudden cessation of pacemaker spikes, leaving only the underlying (intrinsic) bradycardic rhythm.

sense appropriately include electrical signals or myopotentials generated by skeletal muscle, electromagnetic interference (e.g., microcircuitry blood warmers, electrocautery, or radar), T-wave sensing, improper position of the catheter tip, lead dislodgment or fracture, and inappropriate programming of the pulse generator.

Pacemaker Failure

Pacemaker failure is easily recognized because no pacemaker activity (spike or capture) is evident on the ECG when pacing should be occurring (Figure 8–52). Pacemaker failure should addressed immediately, and, if hemodynamic deterioration is evident, transcutaneous pacing should be initiated. Pacemaker failure is commonly due to fracture of a lead wire, lead dislodgment, disconnections between the lead and the pulse generator, battery failure, and possible perforation of the ventricular wall.

Patient Considerations for Pacemaker Implantation

The nurse plays a vital role in educating the patient and family when pacemaker therapy, temporary or permanent, is indicated. Preprocedure instruction for the patient and family should include the purpose and indications for pacemaker implantation, as well as the associated benefits and risks of the procedure. Informed consent should be obtained by the appropriate personnel. During the preprocedure discussion, the nurse should describe the type and mode of pacemaker to be used, the method of insertion, and the use of local anesthesia with IV sedation during the procedure. Many

different written and audiovisual patient education materials are available to supplement information provided by the nurse when educating the patient. Written guidelines for preprocedure and postprocedure care are a valuable component to patient education and should be provided for the patient and family before discharge if a permanent pacemaker is implanted.

Key Concepts

- Diagnosing cardiovascular disorders presents a challenge to the nurse and the multidisciplinary team. Understanding various diagnostic and laboratory tests allows the nurse to deliver safe and comprehensive care to the critically ill cardiac patient.

- Electrolytes assist in regulating body fluid water balance, help to regulate acid–base balance and enzyme reactions, and contribute to cardiac and neuromuscular activity. Sodium, potassium, calcium, and magnesium are the key ions involved in cardiac electrophysiology.

- Serum parameters of renal function include the BUN and creatinine. These tests also provide an indication of the patient's hydration status. BUN and creatinine should be evaluated together, and a normal BUN-to-creatinine ratio is 10:1.

- Important values included in the complete blood count that affect the cardiovascular system are red blood cells, white blood cells, hemoglobin, hematocrit, and platelet count. Anemia, an abnormally low number of red blood cells or an abnormally low hemoglobin count, or both, may lead to worsening of some cardiovascular conditions (e.g., CAD, CHF) by increasing myocardial demand for oxygen.

➡ The lipid profile is a crucial serum test in the treatment of cardiovascular disease. Prevention and treatment of cardiovascular disease is aimed at achieving specific target levels of total cholesterol, LDL, HDL, and triglycerides through diet, exercise, and in some cases, medication.

➡ Cardiac enzymes are necessary to diagnose AMI in conjunction with other laboratory tests and the patient's history. CPK, or CK, is the most widely used serum marker of AMI. CK elevations begin to appear in the blood stream within 4 to 6 hours of AMI and usually peak at 12 to 24 hours. CK is not specific for cardiac damage because it is found in other body tissues; therefore, the use of CK-MB is required. CK-MB is released from the myocardium during AMI and provides a definitive diagnosis. Troponin I has been added to the diagnostic arsenal of AMI. Troponin I appears earlier than CK-MB in patients with AMI. It is considered to have greater specificity and sensitivity for AMI and thus facilitates early identification and treatment.

➡ Monitoring coagulation status is of vital importance with cardiac conditions such as unstable angina, AMI, atrial fibrillation, and prosthetic heart valves. The PTT is a measure of the intrinsic coagulation system and is used to assess the coagulation status of patients receiving heparin therapy. The PT is monitored for patients who require oral anticoagulation with warfarin. The INR mathematically corrects the PT to standardize interpretation of the PT.

➡ Radiographic studies are often used in the diagnosis of cardiovascular disease. The chest radiograph is used to determine heart size and configuration, changes in individual chambers, and various cardiac abnormalities and conditions (e.g., CHF, pulmonary edema).

➡ CT scans produce a planar image of the heart. Advances in imaging technology allow for acquisition of clear images of the heart and lungs by improving the ability of the CT scan to detect and quantify coronary artery calcification. In addition, ultrafast CT can be used to delineate cardiac structures and wall thickness and to derive chamber volumes and stroke volume.

➡ MRI uses a powerful magnetic field and pulses of radiofrequency to obtain images of the heart and related structures. MRI provides detailed images used to evaluate cardiac structural abnormalities (congenital defects or valve disease), regions of myocardial infarction, cardiac masses, and abnormal or unusual blood flow. MRI is an expensive noninvasive test.

➡ Echocardiography is an imaging test that records the structures of the heart using the transmission of ultrasonic high-frequency sound waves. A transducer, placed externally on the chest, sends out sound waves to the heart and receives "echoes" that are reflected back from the structures of the heart and recorded. Doppler color flow imaging can be added to the echocardiogram for visualization of blood flowing through the heart. TEE uses a miniature transducer placed in the patient's esophagus to derive images of nearby cardiac structures. TEE is commonly used to evaluate valvular heart disease, congenital heart disease, and cardiac masses.

➡ The exercise treadmill test, the most commonly used test to detect CAD, attempts to induce myocardial ischemia and to document electrocardiographic changes that may correlate with the patient's symptoms. Echocardiography may be added to the stress test to provide more information such as ejection fraction and wall motion response to exercise. For patients unable to exercise, pharmacologic agents such as dobutamine may be used to simulate the cardiovascular response to exercise.

➡ Nuclear imaging studies use radioactive imaging agents in conjunction with exercise treadmill testing to evaluate ischemic heart disease and myocardial perfusion. Tl-201 and Tc 99m sestamibi (Cardiolite) are radioactive imaging agents commonly used. For patients unable to exercise, pharmacologic simulation of exercise is achieved with dipyridamole or adenosine.

➡ Cardiopulmonary exercise testing provides information about exercise capacity and maximal oxygen consumption that is valuable for the diagnosis and management of patients with heart failure, dyspnea, and previous myocardial infarction, and for patients who are undergoing or have undergone heart transplantation.

➡ Cardiac catheterization is a widely used invasive diagnostic test. Cardiac catheterization involves a variety of invasive procedures using intravascular catheters that evaluate the coronary circulation and structures of the heart, determine intracardiac pressures, and sample cardiac tissue for biopsy.

➡ An electrophysiology study (EPS) is an invasive test performed to evaluate the electrical conduction system of the heart, identify the origin of dysrhythmias, and evaluate the effect of antidysrhythmic therapies. EPS involves intravascular catheters that attempt to stimulate a tachydysrhythmia to locate its origin.

➡ The ECG is a simple, inexpensive and commonly used diagnostic tool in the evaluation of cardiovascular disease. The ECG, both bedside and 12 lead, provides a recording of the electrical activity of the heart. The ECG is used to diagnose various cardiac conditions (e.g., AMI, cardiac rhythm abnormalities). Nursing research demonstrates that appropriate lead placement is crucial in promptly detecting and documenting cardiac rhythm abnormalities in the critical care unit.

➡ The nurse caring for monitored patients must be competent in the identification and interpretation of basic rhythms and life-threatening dysrhythmias.

References

1. Porth C: Pathophysiology, 4th ed. Philadelphia, J.B. Lippincott, 1994.
2. Fischback F: A Manual of Laboratory and Diagnostic Tests, 5th ed. Philadelphia, J.B. Lippincott, 1996.
3. Felver L: Fluid and electrolyte balance and imbalances. In: Underwood SL, Froelicher ES, Halpenny CJ, et al (eds): Cardiac Nursing. Philadelphia, J.B. Lippincott, 1995, pp 121–138.
4. Ricciuti CG, Radke L: Laboratory tests. In: VanRiper S, VanRiper J (eds): Cardiac Diagnostic Tests: A Guide for Nurses. Philadelphia, W.B. Saunders, 1997, pp 105–134.
5. Grundy SM, Bilheimer D, Chait A, et al: Summary of the second report of the national cholesterol education program (NCEP) expert panel on detection, evaluation, and treatment of high blood cholesterol in adults, panel II. JAMA 269:3015–3023, 1993.
6. Marcus AO: Rationale for effective treatment of hypercholesterolemia. Am J Cardiol 78 (Suppl 6A):4–12, 1996.
7. Goe M: Laboratory tests using blood. In: Woods SL, Froelicher ES, Halpenny CJ, et al (eds): Cardiac Nursing. Philadelphia, J.B. Lippincott, 1995, pp 259–277.
8. Roberts R, Kleiman NS: Earlier diagnosis and treatment of acute myocardial infarction necessitates the need for a "new diagnostic mind set." Circulation 89:872–881, 1994.
9. Adams JE III, Budor GS, Davila-Roman VG, et al: Cardiac troponin I: a marker with high specificity for cardiac injury. Circulation 88:101–106, 1993.
10. Mair J, Dienstl F, Puschendorf B: Cardiac troponin T in the diagnosis of myocardial injury. Crit Rev Clin Lab Sci 29:31–57, 1993.
11. Hamm CW, Ravkilde J, Gerhardt W, et al: The prognostic value of serum troponin T unstable angina. N Engl J Med 327:146–150, 1992.
12. Hirsh J, Dalen J, Deykin D, et al: Oral anticoagulants: mechanism of action, clinical effectiveness and optimal therapeutic range. Chest 108 (Suppl 4):231S–246S, 1995.
13. Felner JM, Martin RP: The echocardiogram. In: Schlant RC, Alexander RW (eds): Hurst's The Heart, 8th ed. New York, McGraw-Hill Information Services, Health Professions Division, 1994, pp 375–422.
14. Feigenbaum H: Echocardiography. In: Braunwald E (ed): Heart Disease: A Textbook of Cardiovascular Medicine, 5th ed. Philadelphia, W.B. Saunders, 1997, pp 53–107.
15. Nanda NC: Doppler Echocardiography, 2nd ed. Philadelphia, Lea & Febiger, 1993.
16. Roelandt J: Multiplane Transesophageal Echocardiography. New York: Churchill Livingstone, 1996.
17. Labovitz A: Transesophageal Echocardiography: Basic Principles and Clinical Applications. Philadelphia, Lea & Febiger, 1993.
18. Oka Y, Goldiner P: Transesophageal Echocardiography. Philadelphia, J.B. Lippincott, 1992.
19. Wackers FJ, Soufer R, Zaret BL: Nuclear cardiology. In: Braunwald E (ed): Heart Disease: A Textbook of Cardiovascular Medicine, 5th ed. Philadelphia, W.B. Saunders, 1997, pp 273–316.
20. Pellikka PA, Roger VL, Oh JK, et al: Stress echocardiography. Part II. Dobutamine stress echo: techniques, implementation, clinical applications and correlations. Mayo Clin Proc 70:16–27, 1995.
21. Ricciuti CG: Cardiac catheterization. In: Van Riper S, Van Riper J (eds): Cardiac Diagnostic Tests: A Guide for Nurses. Philadelphia, W.B. Saunders, 1997, pp 265–296.
22. Baim DS, Grossman WS: Cardiac Catheterization, Angiography, and Intervention, 5th ed. Baltimore, Williams & Wilkins, 1996.
23. Peppine CJ, Hill JA, Lambert CR (eds): Diagnostic and Therapeutic Cardiac Catheterization, 2nd ed. Baltimore, Williams & Wilkins, 1994.
24. Kern MJ (ed): The Cardiac Catheterization Handbook, 2nd ed. St. Louis, Mosby–Year Book, 1994.
25. Wagner GS: Mariott's Practical Electrocardiography, 9th ed. Baltimore, Williams & Wilkins, 1994.
26. Jones MC: Pacemakers. In: Clochesy JM, Breu C, Cardin S, et al (eds): Critical Care Nursing. Philadelphia, W.B. Saunders, 1996, pp 167–202.
27. Conover MB: Understanding Electrocardiography, 7th ed. St. Louis, Mosby–Year Book, 1996.
28. Cummins RO (ed): Advanced Cardiac Life Support. Dallas, TX: American Heart Association, 1994.
29. Drew BJ, Ide B, Sparacino PSA: Accuracy of bedside electrocardiographic monitoring: a report on current practices of critical care nurses. Heart Lung 20:597–609, 1991.
30. Drew BJ, Scheinman MM: Value of electrocardiographic leads MCL_1, MCL_6 and other selected leads in the diagnosis of wide complex tachycardia. J Am Coll Cardiol 18:1025–1033, 1991.
31. Drew BJ: Bedside electrocardiogram monitoring. AACN Clin Issues Crit Care Nurs 4:25–33, 1993.
32. Drew BJ: Bedside electrocardiographic monitoring: state of the art for the 1990's. Heart Lung 20:610–623, 1991.
33. Boyer MJ: Lippincott's Need-To-Know ECG Facts. Philadelphia, Lippincott-Raven, 1997.
34. Chou T, Knilans TK: Electrocardiography in Clinical Practice: Adult and Pediatric, 4th ed. Philadelphia, W.B. Saunders, 1996.
35. Hearns P: Differentiating ischemia, injury, infarction: expanding the 12-lead electrocardiogram. Dimensions Crit Care Nurs 13:172–183, 1994.
36. Stewart S, Kucia A, Poropat S: Early detection and management of right ventricular infarction: the role of the critical care nurse. Dimensions Crit Care Nurs 14:282–291, 1995.
37. Tisdale LA, Drew BJ: ST segment monitoring for myocardial ischemia. AACN Clin Issues Crit Care Nurs 4:34–43, 1993.
38. Zipes D: Genesis of cardiac arrhythmias: electrophysiological considerations. In: Braunwald E (ed): Heart Disease: A Textbook of Cardiovascular Medicine, 5th ed. Philadelphia, W.B. Saunders, 1997, pp 588–627.
39. Morton PG: The pacemaker and defibrillator codes: implications for critical care nursing. Crit Care Nurse 17:50–59, 1997.
40. Dreifus LS, Fisch C, Griffin JC, et al: Guidelines for implantation of cardiac pacemakers and antiarrhythmia devices: a report of the American College of Cardiology/American Heart Association Task Force on Assessment of Diagnostic and Therapeutic Cardiovascular Procedures (Committee on Pacemaker Implantation). J Am Coll Cardiol 18:1–13, 1991.
41. Kusumoto FM, Goldschlager N: Cardiac pacing. N Engl J Med 334:89–98, 1996.

9

Coronary Artery Disease

Deborah Becker

Objectives

After completing this chapter, the student will be able to:

1. Relate the pathogenesis of coronary artery disease (CAD) to assessment findings.
2. Differentiate among the various types of angina.
3. List the risk factors associated with the development of CAD.
4. Plan collaborative care extending across the health care continuum for patients with CAD.
5. Evaluate the outcomes of the collaborative management of patients with CAD, comparing what is expected with what actually occurs.

CAD is a leading cause of death in the United States. Researchers have been addressing the risk factors, causes, symptoms, and treatments of CAD since the early 1940s. Despite this research, little has changed in its prevalence.[1] CAD is a progressive disease. As nurses, it is our responsibility to educate, treat, and manage not only the people who develop CAD, but also those who are at risk. The following chapter provides the information and tools necessary to set forth on this quest.

ETIOLOGY AND PATHOPHYSIOLOGY

Cardiovascular disease accounts for more than 930,000 deaths in the United States annually. This number includes approximately 500,000 deaths due to CAD, most of which are sudden deaths. More than 156,000 cardiovascular deaths occur annually before the age of 65 years, and more than half of these deaths occur in women.[2]

In the late 1960s, the United States government started a nationwide initiative to increase the public's awareness of the causes of heart disease. As a result of this initiative, the death rates due to cardiovascular disease have declined. In the decade between 1980 and 1990, the death rate from CAD disease alone decreased 32.6%.[2]

Despite the increase in public awareness about the risk factors and suggested modifying activities, the prevalence of CAD in the United States has remained steady.[1] This statement seems alarming in light of how health conscious Americans like to believe they are. This relative stability in the rate of patients diagnosed with CAD has provided nurses with the opportunity to play an integral role in the identification, assessment, and evaluation of current educational programs. It also affords nurses with the opportunity to develop new programs that teach risk factor identification as well as the management of modifiable factors. Opportunities to be instrumental in the treatment of CAD in both the short term and the long term, and in more community-based settings, have increased over the past decade. Nurses can provide care in various settings across the health care continuum because of the pervasiveness of this disease.

Definition of Atherosclerosis

CAD is defined as the narrowing of the lumen of the coronary artery caused by the accumulation of cholesterol, calcium, and other minerals. The proliferation of cells within the artery lumen also decreases the diameter of the lumen.

Pathogenesis of Coronary Artery Disease

The cause of CAD is still not definitely known. However, two widely accepted theories attempt to explain what happens within the coronary artery that results in plaque formation and the functional narrowing of the artery.

The first theory is described as the response-to-injury theory. This theory suggests that an endothelial injury within the intimal layer of the artery occurs from factors such as hypertension, vasoconstriction, hyperlipidemia, and the accumulation of fats (Figure 9–1). This injury from the force of blood flow against the irregularly shaped interlumen of the artery results in a tear in the intimal wall of the artery. This tear, in turn, causes platelet formation and aggregation at the site of the injury and smooth muscle proliferation and lipid deposition, all in an effort to repair the site.[3]

The second theory is the thrombogenic theory. This theory describes the atherosclerotic process in which three levels of plaque lesions form. The first lesion formed is known as the fatty streak. The second lesion is known as the fibrous plaque. The fibrous plaque is a yellowish, gray lump that protrudes into the intima from the medial layer and sometimes obstructs blood flow. It is the result of the accumulation of lipids and collagen and the proliferation of smooth muscle. This lesion is thought to be the culprit in CAD. The third lesion that can be formed is the complicated lesion. This lesion is caused by hemorrhage into a fibrous plaque, and the clot becomes calcified. This plaque is commonly associated with myocardial infarction (MI).[3]

A third theory combines the first two. This theory suggests rupture of the plaque from the intimal wall of the artery. This rupture, caused by the stress on the plaque from hypertension, stress hormones, and cell proliferation, activates the clotting cascade in an effort to repair the site. Platelet formation and aggregation are also activated. The resultant clot causes significant narrowing, if not complete occlusion of the interlumen of the artery, that, in turn, results in the signs and symptoms of ischemia.

A study conducted in Boston reports findings that atherosclerosis may be precipitated by inflammation within the arteries of patients who go on to develop CAD.[4] This inflammation is thought to occur much like the inflammation that develops at the site of a cut that becomes red and infected. The study also claims that the presence of this inflammation may be detected through a blood test that measures C-reactive protein concentrations.[4] C-reactive protein is present in a person's serum when an inflammatory process is present. This study, however preliminary in its findings, may give great promise to the quick identification of those at risk of atherosclerosis as well as a clue to the prevention of this disease.

Etiology

The Framingham Heart Study, which began in 1948 and continues today, found the correlation between certain risk factors and the development of CAD. Several studies performed since the initiation of the Framingham Heart Study have found similar results. Hypertension, hyperlipidemia, smoking history, activity levels, stress levels, obesity, hyperinsulinemia, age, gender, race, and family history have all been identified as risk factors in CAD. These risk factors are further categorized into modifiable and nonmodifiable. Investigators have also found that the more risk factors one person possesses, the greater is the probability for the development of CAD.

Nonmodifiable Risk Factors

The risk factors identified as nonmodifiable are age, gender, heredity, and race. CAD develops over time. Fatty streak lesions have been noted in infants. Plaque formation is believed to develop gradually and to become significant typically after the age of 40 years.

Gender is a risk factor receiving much attention by the medical community at present. Men are six to eight times more likely to have CAD than women who are premenopausal. However, once women are postmenopausal, the incidence of CAD in women is almost equal to that in men.[2] As stated earlier, more than half the deaths that occur due to cardiovascular disease annually are in women. Most of the research performed in the area of CAD has been done with primarily male subjects. The causes, manifestations, and treatment for

Figure 9–1

Lesions of the atherosclerotic process: damage to the intimal layer (A) and to the fibrous plaque (B); a complicated lesion (C).

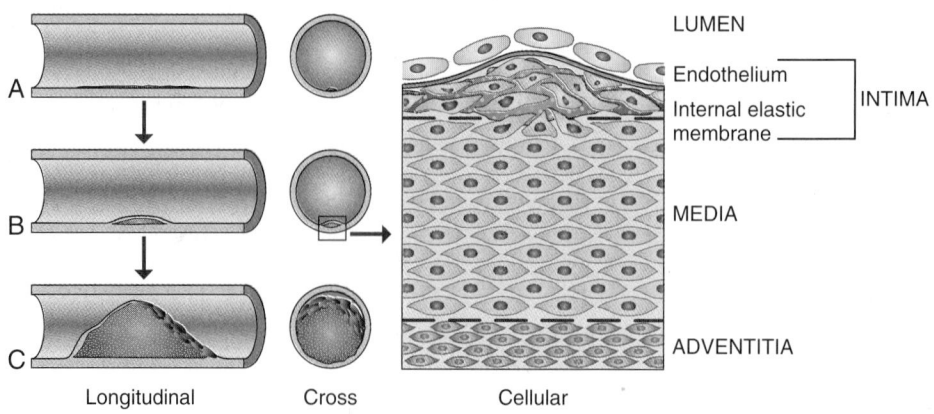

LUMEN
Endothelium
Internal elastic membrane — INTIMA
MEDIA
ADVENTITIA

Longitudinal   Cross   Cellular

CAD in women have been extrapolated from this research. Only in the past few years has research been done that concentrated on the way women are affected by CAD. Some of the preliminary results of this female-based research have shown that women do not manifest CAD in the same ways as do men. Moreover, women do not respond in the same way to some of the treatments.

Heredity is also a factor that cannot be changed. A positive family history for CAD appears to increase the risk of CAD development. This increase may be related to the familial link found in hypertension, hyperlipidemia, and diabetes.

White men die more frequently from CAD than nonwhite men, and white women die slightly less frequently from CAD than do nonwhite women. Although nothing can be done about these risk factors, some risk factors can and should be modified, particularly by persons who have one or more of the unmodifiable risk factors.

Modifiable Risk Factors

Hyperlipidemia is the leading risk factor responsible for atherosclerosis. Cholesterol, triglycerides, and free fatty acids are all plasma lipids carried in the blood. High levels of these plasma lipids greatly increase the chances of CAD. Investigators have suggested that close attention be paid to these levels, over a person's lifetime, and modifications be made to reduce and control them.

Cholesterol is a steroid that is synthesized endogenously by the liver and obtained exogenously from the diet. Triglycerides consist of three fatty acids connected to a glycerol molecule. Fatty acids are classified into two categories based on their level of saturation with hydrogen. Saturated fatty acids, such as lard, are unable to absorb more hydrogen and tend to be solid at room temperature. Unsaturated fats can absorb additional hydrogen and are usually in liquid form at room temperature.

Serum cholesterol levels under 200 mg/dL are associated with minimal risk of CAD. Studies such as the Cholesterol Lowering Atherosclerosis Study (CLAS), the Lifestyle Heart Study, and the Stanford Coronary Risk Intervention Project (SCRIP) have shown that a dietary reduction of fat and cholesterol can retard the progression of coronary artery narrowing and may have a favorable effect on regression of CAD.[5] Cholesterol and triglycerides are carried in the blood by lipoprotein complexes. These lipoprotein complexes are categorized into four major classes based on the percentage of protein they carry. High density implies a high protein content, and low density implies a low protein content. Low-density lipoproteins (LDLs) carry 60 to 70% of the total serum cholesterol. High-density lipoproteins (HDLs) are composed of 25% phospholipid, 20% cholesterol, 50% protein, and 5% triglycerides. HDLs are believed to take cholesterol to the liver for clearance. HDLs are associated with a decrease risk of heart disease. Both children and premenopausal women have high levels of HDLs. HDLs also rise in response to stress reduction, exercise, weight loss, and cessation of smoking.

Cigarette smoking is a major risk factor for CAD. Smoking increases the levels of LDLs and decreases the levels of HDLs. Smoking increases heart rate and causes vasoconstriction, thereby impairing oxygen transport by the blood and increasing myocardial oxygen demand. Smoking also facilitates atherosclerosis by making the endothelium more porous, a condition that leads to the activation of the clotting cascade and increases thrombosis. One positive aspect is that with the cessation of smoking, the ill effects of cigarette smoking can be reversed, with an almost 50% reduction in ill effects within the first year.[2]

Hypertension is considered a risk factor because of the probability of blood vessel damage and the increased likelihood of atheroma formation. Systolic hypertension higher than 160 mm Hg and diastolic hypertension higher than 95 mm Hg increase the risk of CAD two to three times. Hypertension is affected by sodium intake, obesity, sedentary lifestyle, and oral contraceptive use. These factors, along with other medical conditions, may affect the renin-angiotensin-aldosterone system and may decrease the effectiveness of intrinsic mediators, thereby affecting the development of CAD.

Diabetes and obesity are also considered modifiable risk factors. Diabetes is a stronger risk factor in women than in men. If diabetes is kept under control, CAD risk is abated, although not completely eliminated. Obesity is a long-range risk factor for CAD, related to diet, sedentary lifestyle, and hormonal imbalances, all risk factors themselves. Obesity may also be associated with the development of diabetes, hypertension, and increased cholesterol, triglyceride, and fatty acid levels.

All the risk factors listed previously should be considered when evaluating the patient who presents for health care. This may be the person who comes for blood pressure screening in the community or the patient who is having a cardiovascular assessment before surgery. No matter what the setting is, we must assess for the presence of risk factors, their effects on the patient's present health status, and their long-term potential effects.

Hemodynamic Effect of Coronary Artery Disease

The decrease in lumen size secondary to atherosclerosis causes a reduction in the amount of blood that can pass through the narrowed area during a given period.

If oxygen demand exceeds oxygen supply, then the narrowing is considered hemodynamically significant. The supply of blood and oxygen to the heart muscle is vital to maintain its function and viability. If blood and oxygen are significantly reduced, the heart tissue has the potential to become ischemic or even necrotic. The potential exists for a decrease in the function of the heart muscle resulting in a reduction in the amount of blood ejected from the left ventricle (ejection fraction), the development of irregularities in both heart rate and rhythm, and the potential for a secondary reduction in blood pressure.

The presence of atherosclerosis in a coronary artery alters the artery's ability to respond to increased oxygen demand by decreasing compliance of the arterial wall. The stiffening of the wall does not allow for an increase in blood flow to the distal region of heart muscle, beyond the plaque region. This diminished blood flow to heart muscle can force the myocardium to shift from aerobic to anaerobic metabolism. The consequences of anaerobic metabolism occurring in the myocardium are less efficient energy production, lactic acid buildup, intracellular hypokalemia, intracellular acidosis, intracellular hypernatremia, and interference with the release of calcium from the sarcoplasmic reticulum.[6] Again, the end result becomes a decrease in left ventricular function. This impaired function leads to an increase in left ventricular end-diastolic volume (LVEDV) and in left ventricular end-diastolic pressure (LVEDP). The patient experiencing these hemodynamic changes should be monitored closely for signs and symptoms of hypotension, diminished peripheral pulses, and changes in level of consciousness.

Angina

Angina pectoris (chest pain) is the classic symptom of CAD and is not a disease itself. Angina is a perceived sensation caused by a decrease in oxygen supply to the myocardium. Angina is usually manifested when the coronary artery occlusion is equal to or greater than 75% of the lumen. Several classifications of angina are recognized, depending on the frequency of symptoms and causes.[6]

Classic effort or exertional angina, also known as chronic stable angina, is an effort-induced discomfort that has not changed in duration, intensity, or frequency for at least 2 months. It may be mild or debilitating. The angina occurs as a result of exercise or exertion. The exertion causes an increase in demand beyond the arteries' ability to supply the heart muscle with adequate oxygen.

Unstable or acute angina is described as angina that is changing from the previous stable type of angina or a new onset of severe pain. It is usually more intense than stable angina and often is described as pain, rather than discomfort. Unstable angina is also referred to as preinfarction angina, acute coronary insufficiency, or crescendo angina. Unstable angina is often referred to as a clinical syndrome because of its ill-defined borders with chronic stable angina and the presentation of acute MI.[7] Preinfarction angina or angina associated with acute coronary insufficiency is associated with or can lead to MI. The blood supply to the myocardium is so greatly diminished that the myocardium is at risk of necrosis. The pain is usually described as severe. The use of beta blockers appears to reduce the risk of MI, but not of overall mortality.[8] Nitrate therapy decreases the frequency and duration of myocardial ischemia and the development of angina, but it is usually prescribed in combination with other medications.

Crescendo angina is an effort-induced pain that occurs with increasing frequency and with decreasing provocation. This angina requires aggressive management, or it may lead to preinfarction angina.

The third major type of angina is known as Prinzmetal's or variant angina. In this case, the angina occurs without an increase in exercise or exertion and without any warning. This type of angina is believed to be caused by vasospasm of the coronary artery. This type of angina seems to occur in a cyclic fashion, occurring at similar times each day. Studies have shown an increased number of cardiac events, including anginal attacks, within the first 3 hours of awakening from sleep.[9] This type of angina can occur in patients with atherosclerosis or in patients with normal or near-normal coronary arteries. The hallmark sign of variant angina is ST-segment elevation with chest pain that resolves when the pain subsides. Table 9–1 summarizes the types of angina.

Assessment

The nurse's role in the physical assessment of a patient with angina is vital. Obtaining an accurate account of the patient's symptoms along with a health history facilitates the diagnosis and treatment of the patient with CAD. The nurse must know what questions to ask as well as what the answers indicate. A systematic approach to chest pain assessment can assist the nurse in data gathering and interpretation.

A common method for chest pain assessment to describe the attributes of symptoms is the use of the P-Q-R-S-T acronym. This acronym helps the clinician to obtain both subjective and objective data from the patient.[10]

P—Precipitating factors: What was the patient doing when the pain occurred? Was the chest pain provoked by exercise or stress? Do temperature ex-

TABLE 9–1
Types of Angina

Type	Description
Acute coronary insufficiency	Angina that is changing or unstable, often increasing in intensity and duration; this angina can lead to a myocardial infarction, if left untreated
Angina decubitus	Angina associated with lying in the recumbent position
Crescendo angina	Angina that is increasing with frequency with less intense precipitating factors
Nocturnal angina	Angina that has its onset associated with the REM (rapid eye movement) phase of sleep
Preinfarction angina	Unstable angina that progresses to myocardial infarction
Prinzmetal's, or variant, angina	Angina associated with the vasospasm of one or more of the coronary arteries; it is often severe and not induced by effort; it may occur at or around the same time of day; it may or may not occur in the presence of atherosclerosis
Progressive angina	Angina that is newly diagnosed and increasing in severity
Stable (chronic) angina	Angina that has not changed in intensity, duration, or frequency for at least 2 months; often it is exercise or exertion induced; it can be mild or severe
Unstable (acute) angina	Angina that is changing or unstable, often increasing in intensity and duration; this angina can lead to a myocardial infarction if left untreated

tremes, deep sleep, straining to have a bowel movement, deep breathing, or positional changes precipitate chest pain? What are the vital signs at rest? And after activity?

Q—Quality: What does the chest pain feel like? Is it a throbbing, stabbing, crushing, burning, pressure, heaviness, aching, or "strange feeling"?

R—Region: Is the chest pain isolated or does it radiate? Ask the patient to locate the origin of the pain. Does the patient use his or her finger to show an isolated region or the hand to show a more broad area of involvement? What areas are involved? The pain may radiate to the jaw, teeth, or neck, to one or both shoulders, arms, or elbows, or to the back. If the pain radiates down the arm, it may cause a sensation of numbness or tingling. Sometimes, no pain is associated with the attack, but the patient may have a feeling of fatigue or weakness.

S—Severity: Ask the patient to rate the severity of the pain. Use a self-reporting pain scale of 0 to 10 where 0 is no pain at all and 10 is the worst pain the patient has ever experienced. Remember the rating is subjective. The rating can be used to compare subsequent episodes of chest pain and can also help to determine whether the treatment being administered is helping to alleviate or worsen the pain.

T—Time: What is the frequency and duration of attacks? What did the person do to alleviate the pain? The patient may have taken sublingual nitroglycerin or over-the-counter medications (e.g., Mylanta) before seeking help. Did rest help alleviate the discomfort? What was the response to the action(s) taken?

The use of this acronym can assist the nurse in obtaining much needed information (Table 9–2). Much more information, however, is needed to determine the full extent of the patient's symptoms.

TABLE 9–2
Using the P-Q-R-S-T Acronym to Assess Angina

P: precipitating factors	Emotional upset
	Exercise or exertion
	Eating a large meal
	Temperature extremes
	Sexual intercourse
Q: quality of discomfort	Substernal or left-sided pain or pressure
	Burning, throbbing, or stabbing pain
	Heaviness like an elephant sitting on chest
	Tightness like a vise around chest
	Shortness of breath
	Worse pain ever experienced
R: region of discomfort	Substernal or left-sided chest pain
	Pain radiating down left arm
	Intrascapular discomfort
	Pain radiating into jaw and neck
	Epigastric discomfort
	Numbness or tingling in left arm
	Left shoulder or left axillary region discomfort
	Any combination of the above
S: severity	Use a scale from 0 to 10, with 10 representing the worse pain ever experienced by the patient; a subjective scale helps clinicians to determine the patient's perception of pain as well as the effects of interventions
T: time	Investigate the frequency and duration of attacks: When did the chest pain start? Stop? What did the patient do before seeking help and did it work?

Signs and Symptoms Associated with Coronary Artery Disease

The nurse should inquire about the presence of other symptoms that accompanied the angina. Did the patient experience shortness of breath, palpitations, diaphoresis, nausea or vomiting, or anxiety? Did the patient experience any lightheadedness or dizziness or a momentary loss of consciousness? The presence of these symptoms may indicate the degree of atherosclerosis and the extent to which the myocardium was threatened.[7]

Shortness of breath or dyspnea is frequently associated with angina. The increase in oxygen demand and the decrease in supply activate the body's response to increase respirations in an effort to meet the demand. The shortness of breath can also indicate an increase in LVEDV, secondary to left ventricular dysfunction, that can result in the development of congestive heart failure. Therefore, one must obtain a full description of when the shortness of breath started, how long it lasted, and whether it occurred on exertion (dyspnea on exertion) or at rest. Does the patient sleep in an upright or semivertical (orthopnea) position because he or she cannot tolerate lying flat? All these points can help the clinician to determine the patients' clinical syndrome.

Syncope or fainting is a momentary loss of consciousness resulting from a reduction in cerebral blood flow. A patient who reports a loss of consciousness or a near loss of consciousness must be evaluated for dysrhythmias or a change in circulatory hemodynamics. The patient who complains of syncope requires close monitoring to determine the cause.[7]

Finally, a discussion of the patient's past medical history and lifestyle should occur. This discussion can identify risk factors, explore the health history of the patient and family members, and provide clues to the cause and extent of cardiovascular disease the patient may be experiencing. A review of the medications the patient is taking should also be included in this discussion. It may be necessary for the family to bring the patient's medication for review.

After obtaining all the information described previously, a physical examination should be performed. The patient's physical appearance should be noted, comparing symptomatic times with nonsymptomatic times. The presence of associated symptoms and their effect on the patient's examination should be considered. Heart rate, blood pressure, pulse strength and quality, location of point of maximal impulse, and level of distress should all be evaluated. Cardiovascular problems also affect the pulmonary, neurologic, and renal systems, so an examination should include these systems as well. Inspection, auscultation, and palpation of the patient with regard to these systems is essential.[7]

A few special considerations should be mentioned before continuing. Patients with diabetes, elderly persons, females, and patients who abuse cocaine manifest symptoms of angina differently.

Patients who are elderly, with or without diabetes, may have a decreased perception, or no perception at all, that they are experiencing myocardial ischemia because of the neuropathies that often coexist. It takes a more probing and focused examination of the patient to discover the presence and extent of angina, as well as determining the effect of treatment. It also requires the clinician to realize that the elderly patient who is restless or agitated may be experiencing angina, but may be unable to communicate that information because of the neurologic changes that often occur with advanced age.[6]

More than 80% of those who have diabetes die from some form of heart disease.[2] The American Heart Association recommends that people with diabetes who want to delay or avoid heart disease should control other risk factors. The particular factors suggested are weight, cholesterol levels, blood pressure, and smoking. The risk of heart attack in diabetic women is more than double that in nondiabetic women of the same age. The precise reasons for this prevalence are unknown.[2]

Women manifest CAD differently from men, primarily because of the physiologic differences between men and women. Women have higher percentage of body fat. Cholesterol levels are higher in women than in men beginning at age 55 years.[2] Women also have smaller hearts with smaller coronary arteries. Because of this, the coronary arteries of women can become occluded more easily.

Estrogen in women is thought to increase the concentration of HDLs and to reduce LDLs. Once menopause occurs, however, this protective mechanism is lost, and the incidence of CAD greatly increases. This fact helps to explain the notion that when women present to the health care system with angina, they tend to be sicker because of their advanced age.

Women with CAD typically present with angina. However, other reasons for chest pain in women are more common. These are mitral valve prolapse, rheumatic heart disease, and variant angina.[11]

The use of oral contraceptives is a major risk factor for CAD in women. The effects of smoking while taking oral contraceptives are even more dangerous. The American Heart Association recommends that all women who smoke avoid oral contraceptives. Studies have shown that the newer, low-dose oral contraceptives may be less harmful and can actually be used to protect against heart disease.[2]

The patient who abuses cocaine may experience Prinzmetal's angina. Cocaine can induce coronary artery spasm. This spasm decreases the coronary artery oxygen supply and causes angina. Many times, because of a misunderstanding of the patient's presenting symptoms, the patient may not receive the care that the situation demands. Clinicians should put aside any prejudices they may have regarding drug abuse and should treat the patient and his or her symptoms. The coronary artery spasm is real, and so is the threat to myocardial tissue. This patient's pain must be managed as an emergency. Patients who experience coronary artery spasm may also have atherosclerosis. These patients should be treated in the same manner, with investigative measures performed to determine the extent of CAD. Chart 9–1 explores a hypothetic situation in which the level and extent of care provided were questioned.

Differential Diagnosis

Once the nurse has examined the patient and has obtained all the information possible regarding the patient's health status as it relates to CAD, it is important to determine whether these problems are truly cardiac. Therefore, the nurse must understand other disorders that can manifest themselves as angina-like pain and the symptoms associated with them. Such disorders as costochondriasis (muscle and chest wall pain), dissecting aortic aneurysm, pericarditis, pulmonary embolism, and anxiety states can exhibit similar symptoms. Table 9–3 lists some of the other

conditions that can resemble angina and the way in which one can make a differential diagnosis.

Laboratory and Diagnostic Tests

A diagnostic workup includes tests that help to differentiate angina from other types of chest pain and tests to determine the severity of CAD. Descriptions of several commonly prescribed diagnostic tests follow.

Electrocardiogram

An electrocardiogram (ECG) may document persistent or transient ischemic changes during an angina attack. Ischemia is evidenced by ST-segment depression or T-wave inversion. Prinzmetal's angina appears as marked ST-segment elevation during pain. Transient Q waves may also be seen. Depending on the setting, the nurse may be responsible for obtaining the ECG tracing as well as interpreting the results. If responsible for interpreting the ECG tracing, the nurse will determine the extent of ischemia present and will collaborate with a physician regarding the treatment required. Typically, serial ECGs are obtained, at least daily, as well as with each episode of angina (see Chapter 8).

Laboratory Studies

Serum levels of cardiac enzymes are assessed to determine whether the angina has resulted in actual

---

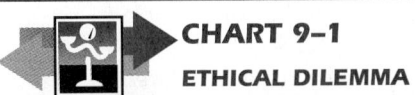 **CHART 9–1**

ETHICAL DILEMMA

A 43-year-old obese man presents to the emergency department complaining of severe substernal and left-sided chest pain. The patient reports that this pain is 10 on a scale of 0 to 10. He has shortness of breath and diaphoresis with this chest pain. On further questioning, he admits to having recently used cocaine. He is unable to convey any past medical history at this time. The patient's vital signs are as follows: blood pressure, 180/92; heart rate, 136 beats per minute and regular; respiratory rate, 28.

The physician examines the patient and, after an assessment of the 12-lead ECG, orders sublingual nitroglycerin and oxygen to be administered. After three sublingual nitroglycerin tablets, the patient reports full relief of his symptoms. His vital signs are stable, and a serial 12-lead ECG without chest pain is found to be normal. The physician now orders the patient to be discharged. You are surprised by this decision. You confront the physician, stating that this patient just had an acute episode of angina and that he should be monitored for any further

episodes of angina, as well as have blood work drawn to determine whether he had a myocardial infarction with this episode.

The physician states that the episode was drug induced, and if this patient stopped using drugs, he would stop having chest pain.

1. What do you perceive as being the major areas of conflict between the nurse and the physician?
2. What additional information, beyond that provided, would assist in defining the conflict?
3. What ethical principles do you believe are guiding the nurse's requests?
4. What ethical principles do you believe are guiding the physician's decisions?
5. What is the role of the nurse in this dilemma at this point?
6. What role should the patient have in this conflict?
7. Should other care issues be addressed in this situation?

TABLE 9–3
Differential Diagnosis of Angina-like Discomfort

Condition	Related Symptoms
Angina	Increasing episodes, ECG changes, presence of atherosclerosis
Costochondriasis	Chest wall pain due to inflammation that increases in quality on palpation of area
Myocardial infarction	Acute ECG changes, chest pain lasting longer than 15 minutes
Pericarditis	Sharp, stabbing pain aggravated by deep breathing, rotating chest, or supine position and relieved by sitting up and leaning forward; presence of pericardial friction rub.
Dissecting aortic aneurysm	Anterior chest pain, radiating to thoracic area of back or abdominal pain; described as tearing pain; lower blood pressure in one arm, absent pulses, murmur in aortic region
Mitral valve prolapse syndrome	Substernal stabbing pain that may radiate to left arm, back, or jaw; variable palpitations, dizziness, or dyspnea
Pulmonary hypertension	Substernal pain, aggravated by effort; pain usually associated with dyspnea, right ventricular lift
Spontaneous pneumothorax	Unilateral pain that is sharp and well localized; painful breathing; dyspnea, cough, fever, dull to flat percussion; occasional pleural rub
Gastrointestinal disorders	Lower substernal area, epigastric, right or left quadrant burning, colic-like, aching pain; precipitated by meals or lying down; nausea, regurgitation, food intolerance

damage to myocardial cells. Creatinine kinase (CK) is a nonstructural muscle enzyme that is secreted by cardiac muscle cells on cell damage. CK occurs in three isoenzyme forms: skeletal muscle (MM), brain (BB), and MB (predominantly cardiac). CK-MB, the most sensitive and specific diagnostic test for acute MI, begins to rise within 6 hours of myocardial injury and peaks at 10 to 18 hours. Total CK begins to rise at about 12 hours after the onset of symptoms and peaks at 12 to 24 hours. Because of the rapid rise and clearance of CK-MB and total CK, timing of blood sampling is crucial in achieving maximal detection of acute MI. CK and isoenzymes are commonly obtained every 6 hours until they begin to decline, and then they are obtained every day.

Lactate dehydrogenase (LDH) is a widely distributed cellular enzyme that is also secreted by the cardiac cells on injury. It has five isoenzymes. LDH_1 is most common in myocardium, red blood cells, and the kidney. Elevation of LDH_1 is usually seen within 12 to 24 hours of myocardial necrosis and may fall to nondiagnostic levels by 72 hours.[7]

More sensitive cardiac markers have been identified. Myoglobin, troponin I, and C-reactive protein are markers that can be detected in the blood of patients who have experienced myocardial cell injury. Myoglobin is released more rapidly than CK-MB, rising in the blood within 2 to 4 hours in most patients with acute MI. This timing helps in the diagnosing of patients with anginal symptoms without ECG changes and in direct care for those who are actively having an MI.[12]

Cardiac troponin I is a serum protein that is highly specific for myocardial tissue, is not detectable in the blood of healthy persons, and may remain elevated for 7 to 10 days after an episode of myocardial necrosis.[13] Studies are currently being conducted to determine the exact sensitivity of the laboratory studies examining serum levels of cardiac troponin I and its clinical applications.

C-reactive protein is an acute-phase reactant that is a marker for underlying systemic inflammation. Elevated plasma concentrations of C-reactive protein have been reported in patients with acute ischemia or MI. C-reactive protein levels are also associated with a risk of MI among those with unstable angina. Based on the results of studies, investigators have found that C-reactive protein is not only a short-term marker of risk, but is also a long-term marker of risk, up to 6 years before the first ischemic attack.[4]

Serum lipid levels should be measured within 24 hours of admission unless patients have had a recent lipid determination or are receiving long-term therapy for hyperlipidemia.[7] These measurements can help to direct the care of the patient in the discharge phase of management more than the acute phase.

Additional laboratory tests can be obtained, such as complete cell count, electrolyte levels, and coagulation profiles. These values can help determine whether the angina experienced can be easily corrected by replacing electrolytes, by administering blood products, or by decreasing the viscosity of the blood.

The nurse's role in the diagnostic workup thus far is to be involved in educating the patient about the studies being done, including what each test measures, the normal values, and what those values mean to the patient's care. It may also be the nurse's role to draw the blood for the actual test.

Noninvasive Studies

An echocardiogram may be performed. Echocardiograms use ultrasound waves to obtain and display images of cardiac structures. This test is performed to rule out aortic valvular disease, idiopathic hypertrophic subaortic stenosis, or other structural malformations. It can also help to determine the extent to which left ventricular wall motion has been affected and to estimate ejection fraction.

Two-dimensional echocardiograms provide a cross-sectional view of the area imaged. The two-dimensional echocardiogram provides better quantification of valvular stenosis and a greater ability to detect ventricular aneurysms. The two-dimensional echocardiogram is better able to provide pictures of the location of cardiac structures as well as the size of dyskinetic wall segments. The results of a two-dimensional echocardiogram may be useful in determining whether the patient presenting with anginal symptoms has had any myocardial damage and may help to identify patients at risk of having complications.

Doppler echocardiography uses pulsed or continuous sound waves, showing velocity and direction of blood flow relative to the transducer. Doppler echocardiography is extremely useful in determining the function of valves as well as in estimating cardiac output.

Transesophageal echocardiography (TEE) uses a transducer mounted on a flexible shaft similar to an endoscope. This transducer is advanced down the patient's throat, into the esophagus. TEE provides high-quality pictures of intracardiac structures and the thoracic aorta. TEE can be used for the same reasons as transthoracic echocardiograms. The nurse is often responsible for positioning the patient in the left lateral decubitus position and for administering the conscious sedation in preparation for a TEE. The back of the patient's throat is anesthetized before advancing the TEE probe. The patient is typically placed on a cardiac monitor with pulse oximetry capability. The patient's oxygenation status, vital signs, and overall ability to tolerate the procedure are monitored throughout the study as well as during the recovery phase. The recovery phase is complete when the effects of the sedation have worn off, the patient's gag reflex has returned, and oxygenation status and vital signs have returned to baseline values.

Stress testing can also be performed. A stress test is used to reproduce anginal episodes by increasing the patient's exertion while monitoring the patient for symptoms and for ECG changes. Several types of stress tests are performed. The traditional exercise stress test requires the patient to walk on a treadmill. The speed and incline of the treadmill increase with time. As the patient exercises, heart rate and rhythm are monitored by ECG, and blood pressure is monitored. ECG and blood pressure are recorded every minute and whenever any symptoms occur. The test is stopped when a certain predetermined heart rate is achieved or when symptoms such as angina or dysrhythmias occur. The results are determined by examining the ECG tracings and any symptoms that occurred during the study. If ST-segment depression or elevation occurs or if the patient has frequent premature ventricular contractions, the test is considered positive. These results may indicate the need for further noninvasive studies or angiographic evaluation. The decision is based on the patient's clinical presentation and the results of all studies performed.

In pharmacologic stress testing, medications such as disopyramide or dobutamine are administered to produce the same effect as exercise stress testing. An echocardiogram is used to determine the effects on wall motion, the ejection fraction, and the presence of atherosclerosis. ECG and blood pressure monitoring are the same. Pharmacologic stress testing is done in patients who are unable to perform exercise. If the patient experiences anginal symptoms during a stress test, then the clinician can determine the extent and location of the ischemia.[7]

Thallium scans are used to determine the presence of perfusion defects in cardiac muscle. A thallium scan is indicated for patients who have known or suspected CAD in whom exercise stress testing may be difficult to interpret. The thallium is injected into the patient, and subsequent radiographic films are taken. The films show how the coronary arteries perfuse the myocardium. If an area of myocardium is infarcted, the thallium will not be taken up or absorbed, and the areas on the film will appear as "hot" spots.

Nuclear imaging can also be performed to determine the extent of wall motion abnormalities and coronary artery perfusion both at rest and during exercise. A radiopaque dye is injected into the patient, and several films are taken. The films obtained from these scans show "hot" spots or white spots that indicate areas of ischemia.

The nurse's role in caring for the patient who is undergoing a noninvasive cardiology study focuses on educating the patient about the procedure. The nurse caring for the patient in the preprocedure phase ensures that the patient has been properly prepared for the procedure. This may be as simple as notifying the patient that a study is to be done, or it may include completing a preprocedure checklist. In many cases, the patient is to take nothing by mouth (NPO) after midnight the night before the procedure, and a patent intravenous access line is in place.

Invasive Studies
Cardiac catheterization or coronary angiography is a procedure used to document the actual extent of CAD through direct visualization of the arteries by use of radiopaque dye and radiographic equipment. The patient is brought into a special laboratory, referred to as a catheterization laboratory or cath lab, designed for the performance of this procedure. The patient is placed on an x-ray table and is connected to the heart monitor and blood pressure machine. The patient is then draped with sterile drapes, and the selected area

to be used for the placement of the introducer sheaths is washed with an antimicrobial agent. When this preparation is finished, the physician begins the procedure. The physician locally anesthetizes the entry site, typically either the right or left femoral vein and artery areas or the antecubital region. The physician then places a large-bore (7- or 8-French) catheter or sheath into the femoral artery. This sheath is used as the introducer site for the catheterization wire. The wire is threaded through the introducer sheath, up the femoral artery, the descending aorta, up to the aortic arch, at the level of the coronary sinuses. The radiopaque dye is then injected into both the right coronary artery and the left coronary artery. The flow of dye through these arteries and their branches is recorded on film. The extent of coronary artery perfusion can be accurately determined by analyzing these films. Blockages appear as narrowing or total occlusion to the flow of dye (see Figure 8–7). This procedure assists the clinician in determining the best treatment for the extent of disease present.

When preparing the patient for cardiac catheterization, the nurse has several responsibilities. The time line for these responsibilities is dictated by whether the patient is an inpatient or an outpatient. The patient is maintained NPO from midnight the night before the procedure. The site chosen for the placement of introducer sheaths must be prepared. This preparation typically consists of shaving the sites and washing the area with an antimicrobial agent. A peripheral intravenous access line is inserted. A consent form must be signed by the patient. Obtaining this consent is the responsibility of the physician. The responsibility of the nurse is to ensure that consent is obtained and the signature is witnessed before sending the patient to the laboratory. An ECG, chest radiograph, electrolyte panel, coagulation profile, and a complete blood count are also usually required. Any allergies the patient may have must be ascertained. If the patient is allergic to intravenous pyelography dye, shellfish, or iodine, it will be necessary to premedicate the patient to prevent or to limit an allergic reaction during the procedure. The physician will order specific medications (e.g., antihistamine) to be given.

The patient will be awake for the procedure. A sedative is administered to help to alleviate some of the anxiety the patient may have. Ensuring that the patient understands how the procedure is done, the possible complications, why it is being done, and what occurs during the postprocedure recovery phase is an important part of the nurse's role. The physician provides this information when obtaining consent; however, the patient often requires reinforcement and clarification of the material. The nurse's role is to provide emotional support to the patient and family. The possible risks of the procedure and the possible need for open heart surgery based on the findings may upset the patient. It

is important that, in the rush to prepare the patient for the procedure, the need for emotional support is not overlooked.

The nurse's role during the postprocedure recovery phase is to monitor the patient's vital signs, to assess the sheath's entry site for bleeding, and to check the circulation quality distal to the entry site to ensure that having the large-bore catheter in place has not compromised circulation to the limb. The patient is required to maintain bed rest for at least 4 hours after the procedure. This period varies, depending on whether the arterial sheaths have been removed and on the extent of anticoagulation present. Unless contraindicated, it is necessary to hydrate the patient after the procedure because of the high-ionic content of the dye. If the dye is not completely excreted from the body, renal dysfunction may ensue. Specific orders written by the physician are to be followed after the procedure. These orders may be written on an individual basis, or there may be unit-specific standing orders for the management of the patient after cardiac catheterization. Addressing psychosocial needs is crucial. The patient may be surprised by the results received and by the recommended course of treatment and may need emotional support in coping with them. The results of any or all of these diagnostic procedures assist the clinician in determining the most appropriate method of treatment or management for that particular patient's CAD.

Nursing Diagnoses

Nursing care of the patient admitted with CAD or angina focuses on continuous assessment of the patient's symptoms, administration of antianginal medications, monitoring the effects of all interventions, and documentation of all episodes of chest pain. Providing the patient with a calm and restful environment and providing the patient and family with reassurance are major responsibilities of the nurse. The patient with angina is admitted to a monitored setting, most likely an intermediate care or telemetry unit. The nurse who admits this patient is responsible for obtaining a baseline ECG and for the continuous monitoring of the patient's heart rate and rhythm. Any angina that the patient may be experiencing on admission should be addressed immediately, with the goal of total pain relief. Once pain is relieved, an ECG should be obtained to determine whether the changes noted on the ECG during the angina episode have returned to baseline. The assessment for the return of angina and its associated symptoms is continual.

Nursing diagnoses need to be identified and individualized (Table 9–4). Care that is solely within the realm of nursing is provided, as well as care that includes other members of the health care team. This

TABLE 9–4
Nursing Diagnoses

Problem Statement	Etiologic Factors
Pain	Inadequate flow of oxygen to the myocardium
Knowledge deficit, learning need	Disease process; diagnostic workup; treatment strategies; risk factor reduction; discharge information
Anxiety (mild, moderate, severe)	Unknown diagnosis and/or prognosis; sudden hospitalization; pain; fear of dying
Altered tissue perfusion (myocardial)	Atherosclerotic changes in coronary artery vascular system
Activity intolerance	Imbalance between myocardial oxygen supply and demand

effort is collaborative and is not the sole domain of any one discipline. A discussion of the care associated with the priority nursing diagnoses for a patient with angina follows.

Pain and Chronic Pain

The patient with angina has pain, whether it is new in onset or chronic. The pain is a manifestation of the somatic, muscular, and visceral perception of impulses secondary to myocardial ischemia. The nurse should recognize that the pain exhibited by the patient with CAD may be life-threatening. It is essential to recognize that if prompt and efficient treatment is not instituted immediately, the patient could have an MI. Many institutions have adopted clinical pathways. These pathways are designed to provide the nurse and other health care team members with a definitive plan of care for the patient with angina. The pathway is instituted on the patient's admission to the nursing unit. When the patient exhibits angina, a sequence of actions is performed to document and manage the pain, with the ultimate goal of pain relief and the abatement of an MI. Figure 9–2, a chest pain clinical pathway and outcome record, and the ACLS: Ischemic Chest Pain algorithm (see Appendix) are used for the management of the patient with angina presenting to the emergency department. Both examples involve members from several disciplines, all in an effort to provide the best care to the patient. Nurses must work collaboratively in the effort to provide quality care, given the short time the patient is in the health care system.

Knowledge Deficit

It has always been the goal of nursing to include the patient and family in the plan of care. The patient's participation is essential to a successful outcome.

Therefore, knowledge deficit is a nursing diagnosis that should be addressed. The patient needs accurate information about the disease process, its progression, ways to reduce risk factors, diagnostic workup, and the management to expect.

Several health care team members provide information to the patient and family. The physician provides an analysis of diagnostic studies and management options. The cardiac rehabilitation nurses provide information on strategies to perform activities of daily living (ADLs), progression of activity level, and risk factor management. Dietary concerns are discussed by a nutritional support nurse or dietitian.

The nurse provides information regarding treatment, diagnostic tests to be performed, management of symptoms, and medications administered. The nurse assists the patient with understanding the information provided from all sources and provides clarification and further explanations as needed. If this information is provided in a positive manner, the patient and family will be more likely to accept the information and to decide to incorporate the changes suggested into their lifestyle.

Anxiety

The patient with CAD may be anxious about having pain, about being hospitalized, about the diagnosis, about the possibility of having an MI, and especially about dying. Recognizing the causes of anxiety and allowing the patient to verbalize concerns are critical to alleviating the anxiety and opening up an avenue for communication. Developing a rapport with the patient allows for the opportunity to obtain accurate information about the disease process. Involving other team members such as a psychiatric liaison nurse or psychiatrist may help the patient more fully to understand his or her feelings and ways of coping with the disease process. Spiritual support can be provided by a chaplain or priest, if available and desired by the patient. Encouraging the patient to discuss his or her concerns creates a dialog with the health care team, which in many cases seems to be the entity with all the power. The nurse should stress that the patient is an integral piece of the puzzle, and participation and cooperation are required.

Altered Myocardial Tissue Perfusion

The patient who exhibits angina is suffering from an alteration in myocardial tissue perfusion. The plan of care for this patient should include the management of the symptoms of angina, as discussed before, as well as the potential and actual alterations that occur as a result of the decrease in myocardial tissue perfusion.

An atherosclerotic plaque interrupts normal blood flow through the artery. The decrease in blood flow to a particular area of the myocardium is recognized by

EMERGENCY DEPARTMENT PROTOCOL
AND CLINICAL PATHWAY

Case type:
    Chest Pain, Possibly
    Cardiac Origin

Exception:
    IV NTG
    IV Heparin

INSTRUCTIONS:
- Review pathway each shift.
✓ - Mark in appropriate box when outcomes are met.
* - Asterisk outcomes not met and document on patient record.
- Review physicians' orders daily. Activities without a physician's order, cross out with a straight line.
- Transcribe additional physician orders onto pathway.
- If activity discontinued, draw a straight line through and write d/c.

20521 S (15525)(0497)

ADDRESSOGRAPH

DATE					
INTER-VENTION	**0 - 1 Hour**	MN/DY/EV	**1 - 6 Hours**	MN/DY/EV	**6 - 8 Hours**	MN/DY/EV

Assessments/Consults

0 - 5 min assess:
    Chest pain, using pain scale 0-10
    Diaphoresis, nausea, vomiting, anxiety, bilateral blood pressures

Medical
Assess for presence of symptoms presumptive of MI
Call cardiology if PMH - MI, Angioplasty, by-pass surgery, or presenting under care of cardiologist

Reassess q 2 hr
Consult Cardiology for recurrent chest pain

Reassess q 2 hr

No recurrent CP

No recurrent CP

Specimens/Tests

EKG
CXR
Urinanalysis
CPK on arrival and 06, 12, 18, and 2400 hrs
CK-MB Profile as needed
PT
PTT
CBC
SMA6
Glucose

EKG

STAT EKG with chest pain
CPK (06, 12, 18, and 2400 hrs)

Treatments

Cardiac monitoring
NPG: Cardiac dysrhythmia
ST segment monitoring if indicated
Oxygen therapy if indicated
Pulse Oximetry

Cardiac monitoring
NPG: Cardiac dysrhythmia
ST segment monitoring if indicated
Oxygen therapy if indicated

Cardiac monitoring
NPG: Cardiac dysrhythmia
ST segment monitoring if indicated
Oxygen therapy, if indicated
Vital signs q 2 hr while awake, as indicated

No life threatening dysrhythmias

No life threatening dysrhythmias
Vital signs within specified limits

Medications/IV

Medicate for chest discomfort
IV access
ASA, unless allergic

Relief of cardiac ischemic signs and symptoms without narcotics or IV NTG

No signs of phlebitis or infiltration of IV

Medicate for chest discomfort, headache, sleep, indigestion
IV access

Relief of cardiac ischemic signs and symptoms without narcotics or IV NTG

No signs of phlebitis or infiltration of IV

Medicate for chest discomfort, headache, sleep, indigestion
IV access

Relief of cardiac ischemic signs/ symptoms without narcotics or IV NTG

No signs of phlebitis or infiltration of IV

Nutrition

NPO

4 GM Na, low cholesterol, low saturated fat diet

4 GM Na, low cholesterol, low saturated fat diet

Tolerating prescribed diet

Tolerating prescribed diet

Safety/Activity

Bedrest
NPG: Fall Precautions, if appropriate

No injuries

Dangle
NPG: Fall Precautions, if appropriate

Tolerates activity without chest pain
No injuries

OOB to bathroom with assistance if no recurrent chest pains
NPG: Fall Precautions, if appropriate

Tolerates activity without chest pain
No injuries

Teaching

Instruct patient/family of signs/ symptoms of cardiac ischemia and need to notify nurse
Explain procedures

Patient/family verbalizes understanding of signs/symptoms of cardiac ischemia and when to notify nurse

Instruct patient/family of signs/ symptoms of cardiac ischemia and need to notify nurse
Explain procedures
Diagnostic/Tests
    •Explain diagnostic testing
    •Give test information if applicable
    •Give Change of Heart Booklet

Patient/family verbalizes understanding of signs/symptoms of cardiac ischemia and when to notify nurse
Patient family/verbalizes use of Change of Heart Booklet as a resource

Instruct patient/family of signs/ symptoms of cardiac ischemia and need to notify nurse

Patient/family verbalizes understanding of signs/symptoms of cardiac ischemia and when to notify nurse

Figure 9–2

An example of a clinical pathway and outcome record for chest pain. (Courtesy of Christiana Care Health Services, Newark, DE.)

DATE								
INTER-VENTION	**8 - 12 hours**		MN/DY/EV	**12 - 16 hours**		MN/DY/EV	**16 - 24 hours**	MN/DY/EV
Assessments/ Consults	Reassess q 2 hr			Reassess q 2 hr			Reassess q 2 hr	
	No recurrent chest pain		☐☐☐	No recurrent chest pain		☐☐☐	No recurrent chest pain	☐☐☐
Specimens/ Tests	EKG CPK Schedule stress test for 13-24 hours post ED admission, if indicated						Stress test To consider stress test post discharge Prescription for post discharge stress test received by patient	☐☐☐
	Lab results within acceptable limits		☐☐☐				Stress test within acceptable limits	
Treatments	Cardiac monitoring NPG: Cardiac dysrhythmia ST segment monitoring if indicated Pulse Oximetry Discontinue O$_2$			Cardiac monitoring NPG: Cardiac dysrhythmia ST segment monitoring if indicated			Cardiac monitoring NPG: Cardiac dysrhythmia ST segment monitoring if indicated	
	Vital signs within specified limits No life threatening dysrhythmias		☐☐☐	Vital signs within specified limits No life threatening dysrhythmias		☐☐☐	Vital signs within specified limits No life threatening dysrhythmias	☐☐☐
Medications/ IV	Medicate for chest discomfort, headache, sleep, indigestion IV access			Medicate for chest discomfort, headache, sleep, indigestion IV access			Discontinue IV	
	Relief of cardiac ischemic signs/ symptoms without narcotics or IV NTG		☐☐☐	Relief of cardiac ischemic signs/ symptoms without narcotics or IV NTG		☐☐☐	Relief of cardiac ischemic signs/ symptoms without narcotics or IV NTG	☐☐☐
	No signs of phlebitis or infiltration of IV		☐☐☐	No signs of phlebitis or infiltration of IV		☐☐☐	No signs of phlebitis or infiltration of IV	
Nutri-tion	4 GM Na, low cholesterol, low saturated fat diet			4 GM Na, low cholesterol, low saturated fat diet			4 GM Na, low cholesterol, low saturated fat diet	
	Tolerating prescribed diet		☐☐☐	Tolerating prescribed diet		☐☐☐	Tolerating prescribed diet	☐☐☐
Safety/ Activity	OOB to bathroom NPG: Fall precautions, if appropriate			OOB ad lib NPG: Fall precautions, if appropriate			OOB ad lib NPG: Fall precautions, if appropriate	
	Tolerates activity without chest pain No injuries		☐☐☐	Tolerates activity without chest pain No injuries		☐☐☐	Tolerates activity without chest pain No injuries	☐☐☐
Teaching	Information on smoking cessation (PMRI brochure)			Instruct patient/family of signs/ symptoms of cardiac ischemia and need to notify nurse Review MCD and Community Resources in Change of Heart Booklet Review activity guidelines			Instruct patient/family of signs/ symptoms of cardiac ischemia and need to notify nurse Review emergency planning: •Use of sublingual NTG •911 system	
	Patient/family verbalizes understanding of signs/ symptoms of cardiac ischemia and when to notify nurse		☐☐☐	Patient/family verbalizes understanding of signs/symptoms of cardiac ischemia and when to notify nurse		☐☐☐	Patient/family verbalizes understanding of signs/symptoms of cardiac inschemia	☐☐☐
	Patient/family verbalizes: Risks of smoking and heart disease and need for smoking cessation		☐☐☐	Patient/family verbalizes understanding of: •MCD and community resources •Activity guidelines		☐☐☐☐	Patient/family verbalizes understanding of: •signs and symptoms of cardiac ischemia •use of sublingual NTG •911 system •Discharge instructions •Follow-up visits	☐☐☐☐☐☐
Discharge Coordination							Consult physician for decision to admit or discharge	
							Patient / family have understanding of disposition plans	☐☐☐

S I G N A T U R E S	**Health Care Team Signatures** Signature/Initial/Print Name/Shift		**Health Care Team Signatures** Signature/Initial/Print Name/Shift		**Health Care Team Signatures** Signature/Initial/Print Name/Shift	
	Signature	Initial	Signature	Initial	Signature	Initial
	Print Name	Shift	Print Name	Shift	Print Name	Shift
	Signature	Initial	Signature	Initial	Signature	Initial
	Print Name	Shift	Print Name	Shift	Print Name	Shift
	Signature	Initial	Signature	Initial	Signature	Initial
	Print Name	Shift	Print Name	Shift	Print Name	Shift

Figure 9–2 *Continued*

Illustration continued on following page

CLINICAL PATHWAY

OUTCOME RECORD

Addressograph

Chest Pain Observation

Clinical Pathway

Patient off pathway because: ❏ Ruled In
❏ Other Diagnosis of _____

If patient falls off pathway, do not complete questions 1 through 3

Start Date: _____

1. Did patient receive narcotics for pain?
   ❏ Yes   ❏ No   ❏ IM   ❏ IV
2. Was Stress Test ordered?

Stop Date: _____

   ❏ Yes   ❏ No
3. If Stress Test was ordered, was it completed

Discharge Date: _____

   ❏ during 23-hour stay   ❏ scheduled after discharge
   ❏ not ordered   (outpatient basis)

MI Clinical Pathway

DRG 121 Uncomplicated
DRG 122 Complicated

Start Date: _____

Stop Date: _____

Discharge Date: _____

Patient not placed on pathway because:
❏ Complex co-morbidity   ❏ Transfer from another facility 5 days post MI
❏ Physician Order   ❏ Other: _____

Patient off pathway due to:
❏ MI Ruled Out   ❏ CABG   ❏ CVA
❏ CHF   ❏ Other: _____

If patient not placed on pathway or falls off pathway
DO NOT complete questions 1 through 12

		Yes	No
1.	Was patient transferred from another hospital?	❏ Yes	❏ No
2.	Was pre-printed Adult Critical Care Orders Set used?	❏ Yes	❏ No
3.	Was patient able to verbalize signs and symptoms of cardiac ischemia?	❏ Yes	❏ No
4.	Was patient able to verbalize use of 911 system?	❏ Yes	❏ No
5.	Was patient able to verbalize use of SL NTG?	❏ Yes	❏ No
6.	Patient referred to Inpatient Cardiac Rehab?	❏ Yes	❏ No
7.	Patient referred to Outpatient Cardiac Rehab?	❏ Yes	❏ No
8.	Did patient exceed LOS?	❏ Yes	❏ No
	If yes, why? _____		

"PHARMACY WILL COMPLETE CONTRAINDICATION BOX FOR QUESTIONS 9-12 IF APPROPRIATE"

			Yes	No	N/A	Contra
9.	Received aspirin during hospitalization?		❏ Yes	❏ No		❏ Contra
10.	Discharged on Beta-blocker?		❏ Yes	❏ No		❏ Contra
11.	Discharged on ACE Inhibitor if EF < 40%?	❏ Yes		❏ No	❏ N/A	❏ Contra
12.	Discharged on Aspirin?		❏ Yes	❏ No		❏ Contra

Cardiac Cath/PTCA/Stent/
PCA/Rotoblator

Procedure Date: _____

Stop Date: _____

Patient:
❏ from ED   ❏ Referral from another hospital

❏ Inpatient at MCD   ❏ From physician's office

Figure 9–2 *Continued*

the muscle in that area. The muscle becomes ischemic, and the nerves pick up the signals of decreased perfusion and manifest them as angina. The extent of occlusion necessary for symptoms to occur is thought to be at least 75%. With the decrease in blood flow to the myocardium comes a decrease in left ventricular function. Depending on the area involved, several hemodynamic changes can occur. Cardiac output is the amount of blood ejected from the left ventricle per minute. Cardiac output is a function of heart rate and stroke volume. If the volume ejected decreases, the heart rate will increase as a compensatory mechanism to maintain the same cardiac output. If the heart rate is unable to maintain the same level of cardiac output, blood pressure will drop. The body has mechanisms to compensate for this drop in blood pressure, but if blood flow to the heart is altering perfusion, then these compensatory mechanisms may also be affected.

If blood does not leave the left ventricle, then the fluid will back up into the lungs and cause congestive heart failure. This can be exhibited by shortness of breath, dyspnea, or crackles on auscultation of the lung fields. If this condition is allowed to persist, then the patient may develop a productive cough of frothy, pink sputum resulting from pulmonary edema.

A decrease in myocardial tissue perfusion can also result in dysrhythmias. If the myocardial tissue is not receiving adequate blood and oxygen supply, the tissue becomes irritable. This may be demonstrated by changes in heart rate or rhythm. If the heart muscle becomes extremely ischemic, the cells can become damaged, and electrolyte imbalances can occur, which can also lead to cardiac dysrhythmias. The development of dysrhythmias also decreases the patient's cardiac output. This decrease in cardiac output can be life-threatening, depending on the type of dysrhythmia.

Careful monitoring and treatment of the patient with an alteration in myocardial tissue perfusion are essential. The development of cardiogenic shock or cardiopulmonary arrest could be the end point if the disorder is not managed correctly.[7] Monitoring the patient's response to treatment does not rely solely on the nurse. Cardiologists, respiratory therapists, pharmacists, and other health care team members are involved in managing the clinical situation. It is the nurse's responsibility to coordinate team activities and to convey information that directly affects the course of treatment to appropriate team members.

Activity Intolerance

The patient with angina may exhibit pain at rest or on exertion. The patient who develops pain at rest is directed to stay on strict bed rest until management of the symptoms has been adequate to prevent recurrence of pain at rest. Then, a gradual increase in the patient's activity is ordered. The acute care nurses, cardiac rehabilitation nurses, and physical therapists are responsible for monitoring the patient's activity level and tolerance. The collaborative efforts of all team members provide the patient with the program that best allows for the gradual and safe return to independence. The patient must be involved in the plan of care, to allow an understanding of the need for a gradual return to independence. Evaluation of the patient's ability to perform ADLs and the need for periods of rest should be included in the nurse's documentation.

Collaborative Management

The patient with angina and its associated symptoms should be monitored closely during the evaluation and treatment phase. The Agency for Health Care Policy and Research (AHCPR) and the National Heart, Lung and Blood Institute (NHLBI) convened a panel to develop clinical practice guidelines for the diagnosis and treatment of unstable angina. These guidelines are recommendations and cover all aspects of care, in both inpatient and outpatient settings.[7]

Initial management of unstable angina is to place the patient on bed rest. Patients with obvious cyanosis, respiratory distress, or high-risk symptoms should receive supplemental oxygen. A finger pulse oximetry or arterial blood gas determination should be used to confirm adequate arterial oxygen saturation and continued need for supplemental oxygen. The nurse and respiratory therapist are involved in this phase of management.

The patient should also be placed on continuous cardiac monitoring for ischemia and dysrhythmia detection (see Chapter 8). These actions are recommended in the patient who is at risk of developing symptoms of unstable angina as well as the person who is actively having pain.

Pharmacotherapeutics

Once these initial actions are taken, the next part of management includes pharmacologic treatment. Drugs to be considered for use at the time of *initial* treatment include aspirin, heparin, nitrates, analgesics, and beta-blockers. The certainty of diagnosis, the severity of symptoms, the hemodynamic state, and the patient's medication history determine the choice and timing of drugs. The dosage of medications depends on the severity of symptoms and on the patient's response to the medications. The use of intravenous thrombolytic therapy, such as tissue plasminogen activator (tPA) or streptokinase, is *not* indicated in patients who do not have evidence of acute MI.

Aspirin
Regular aspirin, in either 160- or 324-mg strength, is recommended to be administered as soon as possible after the presentation of symptoms, unless a definite contraindication is present. It is suggested that the patient chew the aspirin to enhance the onset of action of the drug. Aspirin directly inhibits the formation of thromboxane A_2, thereby inhibiting platelet aggregation. Because platelets are one of the main participants in the thrombotic consequences of disruption of a coronary plaque, platelet inhibition is a plausible mechanism for clinical benefit.[7]

Newer research claims that aspirin's usefulness is more pronounced in the reduction of inflammation in the blood vessels involved in the progression of atherosclerosis than in the inhibition of platelet aggregation.[4] Whichever theory is correct, aspirin should be given for angina.

Other antiplatelet medications, such as ticlopidine (Ticlid) and dipyridamole (Persantine), are used in the treatment of CAD, but aspirin remains the most frequently recommended agent.

Heparin

Heparin exerts its anticoagulant effect by accelerating the action of circulating antithrombin III. Antithrombin III inhibits thrombin and several other activated factors in the clotting cascade. Heparin therefore acts to prevent thrombus propagation. Intravenous heparin should be initiated as soon as possible. The suggested initial dose is 80 U/kg by intravenous bolus, followed by a constant infusion of 18 units/kg hourly, maintaining the activated partial thromboplastin time (aPTT) at 1.5 to 2.5 times control values.[7]

Several studies have documented the benefits of starting both heparin and antiplatelet medications in combination. The results of these studies show a decrease in death rate and MI incidence. Early initiation of both heparin and aspirin has also been shown to decrease the incidence of recurrent angina.

Nitrates

The patient who complains of angina is typically treated with sublingual nitroglycerin. Each sublingual tablet provides a bolus of up to 400 µg nitroglycerin. The patient's response to the nitroglycerin should be documented, along with the patient's vital signs. Nitroglycerin has both peripheral and coronary artery vascular effects. It increases venodilation, thereby decreasing the amount of blood returning to the heart and hence decreasing LVEDV (preload). Nitroglycerin vasodilates both normal and atherosclerotic vessels. Nitrates also promote coronary collateral flow. Therefore, a decrease in preload, along with promotion of collateral flow, should decrease the myocardial oxygen demand and hence decrease angina. A drop in blood pressure is probable and should be monitored for closely. If the patient's systolic blood pressure is already low, it may be inappropriate to administer nitrates. The nurse must collaborate with the physician to determine whether other measures should be used to relieve the angina.

If a patient has not obtained relief from three sublingual nitroglycerin tablets, administered 5 minutes apart, an intravenous infusion of nitroglycerin should be initiated. Again, the nurse should monitor the patient for any contraindications, including hypotension, before beginning an infusion. If there appears to be a reason not to begin therapy, the nurse should notify the physician as soon as possible, so alternate therapies can be prescribed.

Once the patient's acute episode has passed, the nitrates should be switched to oral or topical agents for their long-term use. It is important to teach the patient how to take sublingual nitroglycerin pills when at home, if needed. When to call the emergency medical system should also be reviewed with the patient who is being treated for CAD.

Analgesics

The use of intravenous morphine sulfate is recommended for patients who are having angina that is unrelieved by nitrates. Morphine sulfate has potent analgesic and anxiolytic effects, as well as hemodynamic effects (reduction in preload), that are potentially beneficial in unstable angina. Meperidine hydrochloride (Demerol) can be substituted for morphine in patients who are allergic to morphine sulfate. Morphine causes significant venodilation. It may also produce modest reductions in heart rate and systolic blood pressure. One of the significant side effects that should be monitored for is hypotension. Naloxone can be used to reverse the effects of morphine if necessary. Respiratory depression is the most serious complication of morphine use and should be monitored for closely when administering morphine sulfate for any reason.

Beta Blockers

Beta blockers such as propranolol (Inderal) and metoprolol (Lopressor) are competitive antagonists to catecholamines that exert their effects on the beta receptors of cell membranes. Beta$_1$ receptors are located primarily in the myocardium. Inhibition of catecholamines (e.g., epinephrine) at these sites reduces cardiac contractility, sinus node rates, and atrioventricular node conduction velocity. In unstable angina, the primary benefits of beta blockers on the beta$_1$ receptors are to decrease oxygen consumption of the myocardium by decreasing heart rate, blood pressure, and myocardial contractility. The actions of nitrates and beta blockers appear to complement each other.

Some concerns with the use of beta blockers should be considered. The patient with known chronic obstructive pulmonary disease or asthma may have exacerbations of the disorder with the use of beta blockers. If other medications are as effective with these patients, then beta blockers should be avoided.

The patient with diabetes may have variations in the effectiveness of his or her antihyperglycemic medications or insulins. Adjustments may need to be made to regain control of blood sugar levels.

Some beta blockers are more cardioselective, with primarily beta$_1$ effects. However, these medications have a more profound negative inotropic effect, meaning that they reduce the contractility of the heart muscle. This characteristic is significant in patients who have a reduction in their ejection fraction from myocardial damage. An ejection fraction of greater than 45% should be present before these medications are prescribed.[7]

Calcium Channel Blockers

Calcium channel blockers are effective against angina because they produce coronary and systemic arterial vasodilation. Calcium channel blockers reduce the myocardial cell transmembrane influx of calcium, which, in turn, affects myocardial and vascular smooth muscle contraction, as well as atrioventricular conduction. The agents, such as diltiazem (Cardizem), reduce afterload, heart rate, and contractility. The calcium channel blockers have been shown to be more effective in the treatment of variant or Prinzmetal's angina than the beta blockers.

Angiotensin-Converting Enzyme

Angiotensin-converting enzyme inhibitors (ACE inhibitors) are agents that block the conversion of angiotensin I to angiotensin II. Angiotensin II is a potent vasoconstrictor. By using ACE inhibitors, successful reduction in the patient's blood pressure and hence in afterload occurs without causing a reflex increase in heart rate or a change in cardiac output. The use of these agents is becoming more popular in patients with unstable angina. The agents in this category are captopril (Capoten), enalapril (Vasotec), lisinopril (Zestril), and quinapril (Accupril). Studies have shown that patients who exhibit left ventricular dysfunction have improved mortality and morbidity rates from major cardiovascular events when these drugs are used. These drugs have also been found to relieve symptoms and to slow the progression to overt left ventricular dysfunction symptoms. With their administration, hypotension is a common side effect, particularly at the beginning of therapy. Close monitoring of blood pressure and heart rate should be done to ensure that the patient is not having any adverse effects from the medication.

Cardiac Glycosides

Digoxin is a cardiac glycoside agent that is used to increase the force of myocardial contraction, to prolong the refractory period of the atrioventricular node, and to decrease conduction through the sinoatrial and atrioventricular nodes. The therapeutic effects of this agent are increased cardiac output and slowing of the heart rate. These effects can be beneficial to the patient experiencing unstable angina. The goal of treatment is to reduce the myocardial oxygen demand and to relieve pain. If the patient receives digoxin, the patient's heart rate is reduced, thereby decreasing workload and, hence, oxygen demand. It also increases the force of contraction (positive inotropic effect), emptying the left ventricle more effectively with each contraction. This effect should reduce the possibility of congestive heart failure in patients with left ventricular dysfunction. It is important to monitor serum levels of digoxin and potassium. Normal potassium levels are essential to achieve the positive effects of digoxin. Toxicity can occur, with many detrimental side effects, including dysrhythmia formation and worsening left ventricular dysfunction.

Antidysrhythmic Agents

As stated earlier, one of the adverse effects of a decrease in myocardial blood flow is the occurrence of dysrhythmias. Dysrhythmias can be life-threatening at worst and bothersome at best (see Chapter 8). The development of tachycardias can increase the oxygen demand in patients who are already having trouble meeting the demands. Bradycardias can result in the development of congestive heart failure. Irregular beats can disrupt proper contraction and may enhance left ventricular dysfunction effects. If left untreated, dysrhythmias can cause hypotension, congestive heart failure, or even death. A patient who is experiencing dysrhythmias with hemodynamic compromise should be treated with an antidysrhythmic agent as quickly as possible, particularly during the acute phase. These antidysrhythmic agents may include the beta blockers, calcium channel blockers, and digoxin already mentioned, or they could include other agents such as procainamide, lidocaine, and adenosine, which inhibit the ectopic focus and restore the normal heart rhythm.

Table 9–5 summarizes the medications frequently used in the treatment of angina. The nurse, physician, and pharmacist collaborate on the best medication regimen for the patient.

Cardiac Monitoring

During the course of treatment, the patient requires close cardiac monitoring (see Chart 8–7). The patient most likely requires only a short visit to the intensive care unit, if at all. Therefore, the nurse in the intermediate care and telemetry units must be familiar with the manifestations and treatments for unstable angina. Continuous cardiac monitoring is prescribed until an effective therapeutic regimen has been found. Until that time, the nurse assesses the patient's condition, evaluates the medical regimen prescribed, and documents any further episodes of angina. Complaints of chest pain must be evaluated quickly. Chest pain represents myocardial ischemia. Assessment criteria should include documentation of the characteristics of the chest pain (see Table 9–2), the patient's heart rate and rhythm, and the presence of any dysrhythmias. Blood pressure readings, overall perfusion status (skin temperature and color and presence of pulses), mentation, and urine output should also be noted. Obtaining a 12-lead ECG and quickly notifying the physician are paramount to the treatment of anginal episodes. The ability to determine the patient's response to new or additional medications and to recognize adverse effects is necessary to provide the patient with safe and effective management. Once the goal of effective management of anginal episodes has been obtained, the patient is discharged from the hospital. It then becomes the responsibility of the patient to manage his or her own signs and symptoms. Before this can happen, the nurse, along with other members of the health care team, must prepare the patient for this

TABLE 9–5
Medications Used in the Treatment of Coronary Artery Disease

Medication	Mechanism of Action
Aspirin	Inhibition of platelet aggregation; anti-inflammatory agent
Heparin	Prevention of thrombus propagation
Nitrates	
Nitroglycerin (sublingual)	Peripheral and coronary vasodilation
Nitroglycerin (IV)	Peripheral and coronary vasodilation
Analgesics (IV)	
Morphine sulfate	Analgesia, anxiolysis, vasodilation
Meperidine	Analgesia, anxiolysis, vasodilation
Beta Blockers	
Propranolol	Reduction of oxygen consumption by reducing cardiac contractility, decreases in sinoatrial and atrioventricular node velocity, and reduction in blood pressure
Metoprolol	Same as above
Calcium Channel Blockers	
Diltiazem	Coronary and peripheral vasodilation; reduction in afterload, heart rate, and contractility
ACE Inhibitors	
Captopril, enalapril, lisinopril, quinapril	Vasodilation, reduction in afterload
Cardiac Glycosides	
Digoxin	Increase in cardiac output, decreases in sinoatrial and atrioventricular conduction, and reduction in oxygen consumption
Antidysrhythmia Agents	
Lidocaine, Pronestyl, adenosine, beta blockers, calcium channel blockers, digoxin	Restoration of normal heart rhythm

eventuality. However, this preparation is often difficult because of shorter lengths of stays in hospitals.

Coronary Angioplasty and Related Procedures

If the patient continues to have episodes of angina, it may be necessary to consider more aggressive means to achieve relief. The means most commonly employed are the catheter-based interventions such as the percutaneous coronary transluminal angioplasty (PTCA), directional coronary atherectomy, rotoblader, or placement of a coronary stent. These interventions require the patient to undergo radiographic studies similar to cardiac catheterization discussed earlier. Typically, the patient has had cardiac catheterization previously, and the results are such that an interventional procedure would be beneficial. In some situations, the patient may have diagnostic cardiac catheterization immediately before the interventional procedure. In either situation, the interventional cardiologist has a clear idea of the location, extent, and qualities of the occlusion. The cardiologist considers these issues and decides which intervention best suits the situation. The patient is prepared for the procedure in much the same way as when a cardiac catheterization is to be performed. The differences are that the patient undergoing an interventional procedure has a cardiothoracic surgery consultation. This is in the event of an untoward complication, such as complete dissection of the coronary artery, that would require emergent coronary artery bypass grafting. The patient's blood is typed and crossmatched in case a transfusion would be necessary secondary to a bleeding incident. Otherwise, the preparation for the procedures is the same as for cardiac catheterization (Chart 9–2).

Percutaneous Transluminal Coronary Angioplasty

The PTCA is a catheter-based procedure that uses a guidewire with an inflatable balloon on its tip. The patient is prepared for the procedure much the same way as for cardiac catheterization. Instead of using a catheter that only allows dye to be injected through it, this catheter has the capability of having the balloon

CHART 9–2

RESEARCH UTILIZATION: NURSING CONSIDERATIONS FOR CARE OF THE PATIENT UNDERGOING AN ANGIOPLASTY

Abstract: The number of patients undergoing an angioplasty annually is approximately 300,000. Much of the research has focused on perfecting the procedure, improving outcomes, and promoting comfort in the recovery period. There is little research available investigating patients' responses to the entire experience. Nursing care for these patients has been driven by physician protocols and responses to the potential and actual complications associated with this procedure. This study was designed to elicit patients' descriptions of the angioplasty experience. The questions were designed to investigate patient's angioplasty experience in a variety of settings such as the intensive care unit, telemetry unit, outpatient admitting area, holding area, cardiac catheterization laboratory, and community rehabilitation settings.

Critique: The study identified several areas of nursing care that can be improved throughout many critical care settings. Considering the large number of patients who undergo angioplasty annually, the sample size is small (N = 45). A focus group of patients recounting their experiences and emotions regarding such a potentially dangerous procedure may not have been the most appropriate format. The information received from the study indicates the general concerns of patients who undergo angioplasties. Further studies investigating nursing interventions to promote positive experiences are suggested.

Nursing Considerations: Patients who undergo an angioplasty are cared for in various settings: the preprocedure area, intensive care units, telemetry units, holding areas, and cardiac catheterization laboratories. Critical care nurses are the most likely providers of care to these patients. The patient who is waiting for an angioplasty, who is having one performed, or who is recovering from one has many concerns. Some of the concerns identified by this study are unexplained and long periods of waiting before a procedure is performed, the situation regarding whether family members are informed of delays and are given updates on the patient's condition, lack of attention to the patient, dehumanization, lack of control over the decision to have an angioplasty or other interventional procedure, discomfort in the back and leg, and feeling cold. Positive issues identified from the focus groups included attentive nurses, warm blankets, background music, compassion, respect, attention to needs, and a

patient-focused environment. Several of the negative issues can be addressed easily by the nurses caring for the patient at the different phases of the procedure. Following are general guidelines that are recommended for nurses who care for patients who are undergoing an angioplasty.

1. Evaluate the patient's understanding of the procedure and his or her feelings regarding the need for the angioplasty.
2. Recognize that the patient is looking for a positive and supportive approach to care. Provide compassionate and respectful care to the patient at all times.
3. When delays occur, convey the reasons for the delay to the patient as soon as possible.
4. Reassure the patient that the family members waiting are being updated on the progress of the study.
5. Remember that care should be patient focused.
6. Patients generally have discomfort in their back and affected leg during and after the procedure. Comfort measures, other than medication, should be considered (e.g., music therapy) to help to alleviate the discomfort and to reduce the anxiety associated with it.

In addition, the specific desire of the patient to remain an active participant throughout the procedure must also be addressed. Considering the nature of the procedure, nurses should promote the patient's participation whenever possible. If the patient can feel valued, remain educated regarding the expectations and possible outcomes, and not be overlooked or disregarded, positive outcomes can be achieved, and a win–win situation results. The way to achieve this is to

1. Treat each patient with the respect every person deserves. Remember that even patients who have had a previous angioplasty require emotional support and education regarding the procedure.
2. Provide the patient with options to promote a feeling of power and control.
3. Assess the patient, throughout all stages of the process, for discomfort. The possibility of discomfort is the greatest fear of patients who are undergoing angioplasty.

More research is needed regarding the specific interventions that can be performed to help reduce patients' discomfort associated with angioplasty.

(From Gulanick M, Bliley A, Perino B, et al: Patients' responses to the angioplasty experience: a qualitative study. Am J Crit Care 6:25–32, 1997.)

inflated. The physician performing the procedure passes the guidewire through the aorta, through the coronary sinus, and down the occluded coronary artery. When the wire reaches the occlusion, if possible, the wire is passed through the center of the blockage. The balloon catheter is then advanced over the guidewire. Once in place, the balloon is inflated, and the plaque causing the blockage is compressed against the wall of the vessel.[14] While the balloon is inflated, blood flow distal to the blockage is reduced. The patient may experience angina, usually similar to the angina that required this intervention. Because the patient's ECG tracing is being recorded during the procedure, if angina occurs, the extent of ischemia is documented. One can determine whether the vessel that is being occluded is the same one that has caused the angina attacks. The patient may receive sublingual nitroglycerin, intracoronary nitroglycerin, or other medications to alleviate the discomfort. If necessary, the balloon may be deflated. The balloon is usually left inflated for a short period to promote stabilization of the plaque now compressed against the wall.

Once the physician has determined that the dilatation is complete, the balloon is deflated, and blood flow is restored to the distal portion of the artery. Dye is again injected into the artery to determine the amount of reduction in the stenosis achieved. The patient is monitored for approximately 10 minutes to determine whether the compressed plaque appears to be stable or whether additional inflations are required. Again, dye is injected to determine the amount of

stenosis reduction achieved. If it is decided to be adequate, the guidewire and catheters are removed from the patient, and the patient is transferred to the intensive or intermediate care unit. Preprocedure and postprocedure patient care guidelines are described in the sample pathway for PTCA (Figure 9–3).

Directional Coronary Atherectomy

Directional coronary atherectomy involves a specialized catheter that has a cylindrical steel cutting blade housed at the distal tip of a rigid cylinder.[14] The premise for the atherectomy is that removal of the obstructing atheroma in a coronary artery should provide a better relief of the stenosis, resulting in improved flow, greater predictability of the result, fewer complications such as dissection, and a lower rate of restenosis than is achieved by the conventional balloon angioplasty (Figure 9–4).

During the atherectomy, the device is advanced over the guidewire and positioned so its cutting window is within the coronary stenosis. Once in place, the motor is started, and the spinning cutter is slowly advanced to shave off the atheroma and to push it into the nosecone for storage. Angiographic pictures are taken to determine the extent of the stenosis reduction. The limitations to the use of this device are related to the rigidity of the catheter. This property limits the ability to maneuver the device around curves. This device must also pass through the lumen of the atheroma to be placed into position to cut it away. A

PTCA/INTERVENTION ALGORITHM		
	PRE INTERVENTION **DATE:** ___	**POST INTERVENTION** **DATE:** ___
ASSESSMENTS & CONSULTS	CT SURGEON STANDBY	
LABS, DIAGNOSTICS & INTERVENTIONS	CBC, CHEM 7, TYPE & HOLD, PTT, ACT SHAVE & PREP BILATERAL GROINS INTERVENTION CARE PER STANDARD*	PTT & WITH HEPARIN CHANGES, ACT 4H POST AND TILL BASELINE WITH SHEATH PULL NEXT DAY: CK, H&H IF STENT: ACT'S PER STANDARD INTERVENTION CARE PER STANDARD* D/C SHEATH BEDREST X 48 HOURS IF STENT GROIN CARE*
MEDICATIONS & IV'S	HOLD MEDS FOR INTERVENTION AS ORDERED PRE INTERVENTION MEDS* IV ACCESS*	RESUME MEDS POST SHEATH REMOVAL D/C HEPARIN PRE SHEATH PULL
DIET & ACTIVITY	NPO POST MIDNIGHT	RESUME DIET OOB TO CHAIR AND AMBULATE PER INTERVENTION & SHEATH PULL STANDARDS*
TEACHING & FOLLOW-UP	INSTRUCTIONS & CONSENT	GROIN CARE* POST INTERVENTION INSTRUCTIONS*

NURSING CARE PERFORMED
 	
KEY: *NSG
Activities
V = Variance
N = No Var.
	△ 1. V
	   N _____
	△ 2. V
	   N _____
	△ 3. V
	   N _____
		△ 1. V
		   N _____
		△ 2. V
		   N _____
		△ 3. V
		   N _____

NSG;AMI:01C Rev. 4/95
This pathway was developed as a guideline only. It is not intended to be used as a substitute for clinical judgment. Acceptable medical practice generally does include a variety of responses to a particular problem.

Figure 9–3

Critical path algorithm for PTCA. (Courtesy of Graduate Hospital, Philadelphia, PA.)

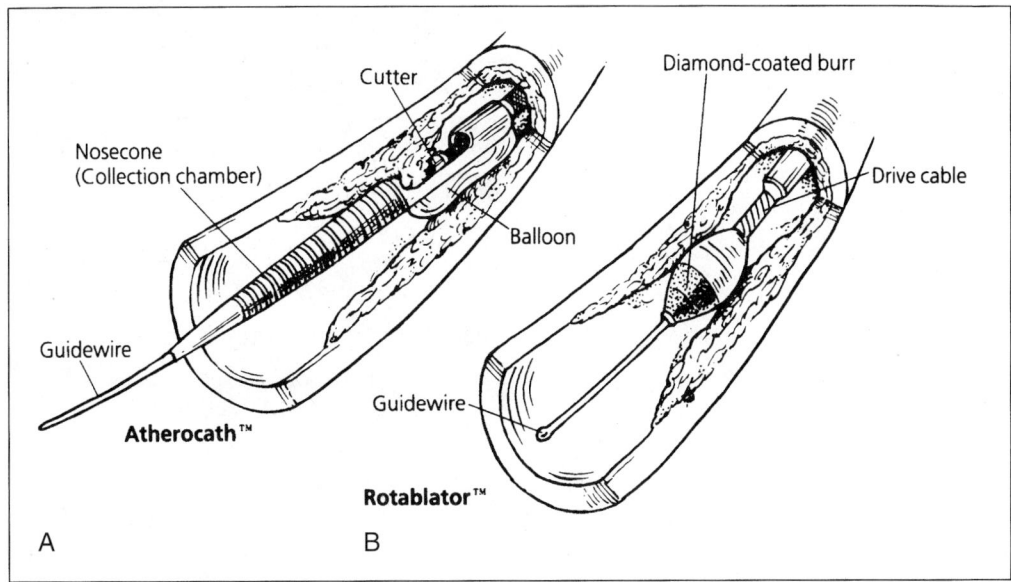

Figure 9–4

Atherectomy devices. A, Simpson AtheroCath. B, Rotablator. (From Herrmann HC, Hirshfeld JW Jr: Coronary angioplasty and related techniques. In: Baum S, Pentecost MJ (eds): Abrams' Angiography, vol. 3. Boston: Little, Brown, 1997, p 378.)

balloon angioplasty may have to be performed first, with the atherectomy catheter used next.[14] This can be risky depending on the condition of the patient's coronary architecture. The results of this procedure have been shown to be comparable to the results of traditional balloon angioplasty.

Rotational Atherectomy

The rotational atherectomy or Rotablator is a device that has a diamond burr on the distal tip of the catheter. The catheter is advanced in the same way as with the directional coronary atherectomy, but it does not have to pass through the lumen of the atheroma.[15] When the Rotablator catheter is proximal to the lesion, the Rotablator motor is started. The Rotablator performs differential cutting. Differential cutting allows the elastic materials, such as the vessel wall, to deflect away from the blade, whereas inelastic materials are ablated by the cutting edge.[15] The cardiologist can also direct the placement of the burr to ablate areas of the atheroma (see Figure 9–4).

Angiographic pictures are taken during the cutting process to determine the extent of the cutting, to direct the burr, and to determine when the procedure should be completed.[15] Results are generally favorable. However, the complication and restenosis rates are comparable to those with balloon angioplasty.

Laser Ablation

The use of laser ablation to improve coronary lumen size has been limited. The current systems use pulsed high-energy waves to ablate plaque with minimal thermal damage to surrounding tissue. The tip of the catheter is encapsulated within a metal cap to prevent perforation of the coronary artery. However, the success of laser angioplasty is still limited by the small channel size created. The high cost of laser systems and catheters is a further obstacle to the widespread adoption of lasers.[14]

Coronary Stenting

Coronary stenting consists of deploying an expandable prosthesis, called a stent, at an atheroma site. The use of stents over a balloon angioplasty attempts to solve two principal dilemmas of coronary angioplasty: inadequate lumen enlargement of the target site and acute occlusion resulting from dissection flaps. The stent acts as a scaffold to hold the stenotic area open.[14] Several stents are in use. The Palmaz-Schatz stent and the Gianturco-Roubin Stent are two of the stents that are approved by the United States Food and Drug Administration (FDA) for use (Figure 9–5). Others are currently being evaluated to determine their efficacy and safety in research studies.

The procedure for the placement of a coronary artery stent is similar to the balloon angioplasty procedure. The catheter used for the placement of stents has a balloon on the distal end with a stent placed over it. The catheter is advanced through the coronary artery and into the center of the atheroma. When the catheter is properly positioned, the balloon is inflated. The stent has small "feet" or hooks that latch on to the intimal wall of the vessel. The balloon is then deflated, and the stent remains in place. Angiographic pictures are taken to determine the position of the stent as well

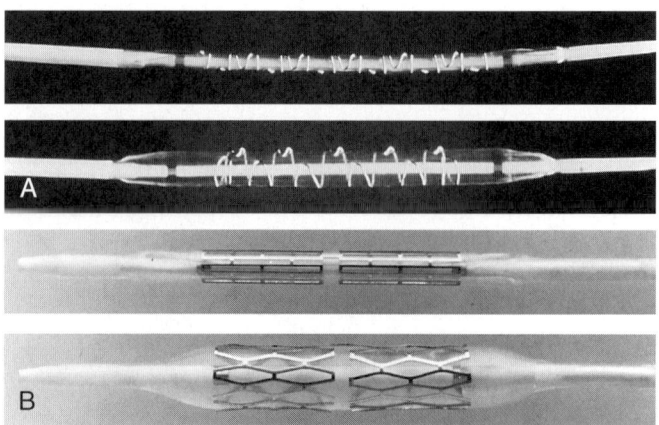

Figure 9–5

A, Gianturco-Roubin balloon-expandable coil stent. *Top,* Undeployed, wrapped around delivery balloon. *Bottom,* Deployed by expansion of delivery balloon. (Courtesy of Cook, Inc., Bloomington IN.) *B,* Palmaz-Schatz balloon-expandable slotted tube stent. *Top,* Undeployed, wrapped around delivery balloon. *Bottom,* Deployed by expansion of delivery balloon. (Courtesy of Cordis, a Johnson and Johnson Company, Warren, NJ.)

as the amount of reduction in the stenosis. On arrival to the patient's room, an ECG is obtained to assess whether any periprocedural changes have occurred and to serve as a baseline.[14] In the patient with a clean, successful result, free of thrombus or dissection, no further anticoagulation is required. In these patients, activated clotting times (ACT) are taken serially until it is determined that the sheaths can be removed. Once the ACT is within an acceptable range, the sheaths are removed, at the bedside. Manually or with the help of a mechanical device, pressure is applied to the sheath removal site until hemostasis is obtained. Typically, the patient resumes intravenous heparin after the sheaths are removed, in an attempt to prevent abrupt closure of the site.

Patients who have a difficult procedure, dissection flaps, or angiographically visible thrombus are treated with intravenous heparin for 12 to 18 hours, after which the sheaths are removed.[14] The nurse's role during the recovery phase is to monitor the patient's vital signs, sheath insertion site for any bleeding or hematoma formation, distal limb circulation, and recurrence of anginal symptoms. The patient is maintained on bed rest for at least 6 hours after the sheaths are removed. Anticoagulation may be reinstituted after hemostasis is achieved. The nurse must administer the intravenous heparin and monitor its effects. Typically, the patient has some level of discomfort both in the back and legs during this time. It is important to assess for this discomfort and to treat it. Back rubs, repositioning, relaxation techniques, and analgesics and sedatives may be helpful in this endeavor.[16] The patient has been NPO for a long time. Food and fluids should be given to the patient as soon as possible. Attention to basic needs such as eating, elimination, and comfort will promote a sense of well-being in the patient.

The patient who has a stent placed requires antiplatelet agents or anticoagulation for a time after the procedure. Because of the anticoagulation required, bleeding complications can occur after stenting. Before the procedure, a careful history should identify those patients at high risk of bleeding.[16] For patients with stents, antiplatelet medications may be given the day before the procedure. Patients are typically given aspirin and ticlopidine hydrochloride in varying dosages. These medications are given to reduce the amount of platelet aggregation that will occur at the site of the new stent in response to the perceived injury. Heparin is given as a bolus to the patient at the beginning of the procedure. During the procedure, the level of anticoagulation is closely monitored by means of ACT. Patients may receive intravenous heparin for 1 to 5 days after stent placement.[16] Heparin therapy is briefly interrupted for sheath removal and is restarted after hemostasis is achieved. Warfarin (coumadin) therapy is started on the day of the procedure. When an international normalized ratio (INR) between 2 and 4 is achieved, the heparin is discontinued, and the warfarin therapy is continued. The aspirin and ticlopidine hydrochloride are continued for a period determined by the physician.

The patient who requires warfarin therapy must be carefully instructed about the potential dangers inherent in anticoagulation. The need for routine blood work (coagulation studies), careful adherence to the medication schedule, and instructions to call the physician with any questions must be emphasized. Signs of bleeding such as blood in the urine, black stools, frequent nosebleeds, unusual weakness or pain, skin discoloration and bruising, and persistent headaches should be conveyed. Factors that affect the action of warfarin should be discussed. These factors include the use of alcoholic beverages, multivitamins, vitamin K, antibiotics, diuretics, antacids, and nonsteroidal anti-inflammatory drugs. Certain physical conditions such as cancer, congestive heart failure, diarrhea, hepatic disorders, and poor nutritional status may also affect the therapeutic effects of warfarin. If the patient has any of these conditions or develops any while receiving warfarin, the physician should be notified. Patients should notify other physicians and dentists that they are taking warfarin. Written information outlining all these items should be given to the patient for reference after discharge.

Cardiac Rehabilitation

Preparation for the patient's eventual discharge from the inpatient setting should start as early in the patient's hospital stay as feasible. The patient may have little knowledge of what has just happened and may require extensive education and support. It is the responsibility of the health care team—nurses, doctors, therapists, and counselors—to assist the patient and family in understanding the disease process. Such topics as what angina is, how it occurs, and how episodes can be prevented need to be addressed. Identification of the patient's risk factors and a discussion of what the patient can do to either reduce or eliminate those factors must ensue. The patient needs to know what the prescribed medication regimen includes. A review of the type of medication, dose, route, frequency, expected effects, and adverse side effects should be included in the discharge process. Diet and exercise program as well as a weight control program should be discussed to assist the patient in selecting one that meets the individual needs.[17] Education regarding the patient's ability to resume sexual activity should also be given because this issue is of concern to many patients and their partners.

Patient and family education may not be completed within the short inpatient stay. Therefore, these topics can be addressed in several additional settings. Several health maintenance organizations (HMOs) have programs that send home health care nurses into patients' homes to address patients' individual needs and concerns. These programs are designed to promote a sense of continuity between the inpatient setting and the home. They are also designed to address issues that may not have been addressed earlier and to reinforce those that have been discussed. The goal is to prevent the patient from reentering the acute care setting for a recurrence of angina.

Outpatient cardiac rehabilitation programs, either directly associated with hospitals or free standing, have seen a resurgence. The goals of these programs are to educate the patient on risk factor modification and to provide the patient with a place to go to receive the much needed positive reinforcement to continue the changes. Several of these programs include classes on risk factor modification, nutritional counseling, and medication teaching. Exercise programs and other activities are also provided to those interested in improving their exercise tolerance and managing their weight. Only approximately one-third of eligible patients continue risk factor interventions over the long term. In addition, a significant increase in that number can be achieved if a multidisciplinary team approach that includes doctors, nurses, and dietitians manages risk reduction therapy by using follow-up techniques that include office or clinic visits and telephone contacts.[18] In many cases, a multidisciplinary team is available at these cardiac rehabilitation facilities (see Chart 9–3).

Risk Factor Modification

It is essential to instruct patients who smoke to quit. Smoking reduces the supply of oxygen to the myocardium and can precipitate an anginal episode. Providing the patient with information on different programs as well as providing emotional support will assist the patient in the quest to become smoke free.

Management of the patient's hypertension by both medication and diet is equally important. Educate the patient that hypertension may have no outward manifestations, but it is essential to continue therapy to maintain that sense of well-being.

Encourage the patient to participate in a regular exercise program. This effort will assist the patient in improving coronary circulation, managing weight, and indirectly controlling hypertension.

Instruct the patient on dietary modifications. Educate the patient regarding the foods that are high in cholesterol, triglycerides, and LDLs. Encourage the patient to lose weight if needed. Inform the patient that foods high in fiber decrease the appetite, prevent constipation, help to reduce weight, and decrease anginal attacks by lowering cholesterol and triglyceride levels. CAD is less common among patients with high intake of dietary fiber than in those with lower fiber intake. High-fiber diets also reduce hypertension.

Encourage the patient to decrease stress. Recommend that the patient take brief rest periods throughout the work day, have a good night's rest, and take vacations to help reduce the amount of catecholamines and stress hormones circulating in the blood, thereby reducing anginal attacks.

Advise patients who appear anxious and nervous to seek counseling. Instruct the patient in the use of relaxation techniques such as guided imagery or music therapy. Suggest to the physician that antianxiety medications be prescribed to those patients who could benefit from a reduction in anxiety levels.

Instruct the patient to avoid factors known to precipitate anginal attacks. Factors such as eating large meals, smoking cigarettes, going out in the cold, having an argument, or doing strenuous exercise should be avoided if at all possible. If an attack occurs, instruct the patient to stop the activity and rest.

Educate the patient about the prescribed medications. Ensure that the patient understands how to use the sublingual nitroglycerin that has been prescribed. Instruct the patient that if the pain does not subside or worsens after using three sublingual pills, the emergency medical system should be activated. Emphasize that the patient should not drive himself or herself to the hospital.

Additional information about medications should include course of action if a dose is skipped, monitoring for adverse side effects, and the need to store medications in a cool, dry place.

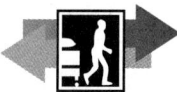

CHART 9–3

BEYOND THE ICU: CRITICAL CARE NURSING ACROSS SETTINGS

Patients with coronary artery disease (CAD) are treated in a variety of health care arenas. The nurse has the opportunity to provide care in many of these settings. Several nursing opportunities can be identified by following the "typical" patient with CAD through a health care experience.

The patient is at home in a usual state of health when an angina attack occurs. Emergency medical services are called, and emergency medical technicians and, at times, a nurse respond. The patient's condition is stabilized in the home, but the technicians believe that a visit to the emergency department of the local hospital is warranted. The patient is then taken to the hospital.

When the patient arrives in the emergency department, the angina returns. The emergency department nurses begin to care for the patient. A health history and physical assessment are taken by one nurse while another connects the patient to the cardiac monitor, obtains a set of vital signs, inserts an intravenous line, and draws blood for laboratory studies. The physician is present, and the ECG technician is obtaining a 12-lead ECG. The patient is treated appropriately, and pain relief is achieved. It is decided to admit the patient to the hospital for observation because the ECG showed ischemic changes during the angina episode. A nursing report is given to the nurse in the intermediate care unit where the patient is to be admitted.

The nurse admits the patient to the room, takes a set of vital signs, connects the cardiac monitor, and does a thorough physical assessment. The patient is oriented to the hospital room environment, the usual routine of the unit, and what to expect during this hospitalization. The patient is encouraged to report all episodes of angina as soon as they occur so that swift management can be initiated.

The patient has several episodes of angina over the next couple of days. Several diagnostic studies are conducted including cardiac catheterization. The patient has a blockage in the right coronary artery and coronary angioplasty is recommended. The patient consents to the procedure, which is scheduled for the next day.

The patient is prepared for the angioplasty. When it is time for the procedure, the patient is transported to the cardiac catheterization laboratory's holding area. The nurses in this area ensure that all the paperwork is completed, the patient has received premedications as ordered, and the consent form has been signed and witnessed. A general assessment is performed by the nurses, and the patient is told that there will be a short delay because of complications that occurred with an earlier procedure.

About 15 minutes later, the patient is taken into the laboratory, placed on the table, and draped and prepared. The nurses who work in the cardiac catheterization laboratory physically prepare the patient, and educate the patient on what to expect during the procedure. Appropriate emotional support is also provided by the nurses. The nurses assist the physician during the study, and when the procedure is over, the patient is transported to the intensive care unit (ICU), where the recovery phase of the process is monitored.

The ICU nurse admits the patient to the room, assesses the patient's condition, administers the appropriate treatment, and provides the patient with comfort measures, education, and information as necessary. The patient's family is included in the process. When it is apparent that the patient's condition is stable, the cardiac rehabilitation nurse is consulted so that issues regarding reentry into the community are addressed. It is determined that the patient would benefit from support from home health nurses to ensure proper adherence to medication schedules and to promote risk factor modification on discharge.

The patient is discharged, and the home health nurse schedules a visit for the next day. On arrival, the home health nurse assesses the patient and evaluates the home situation. In collaboration with the patient and the family, the home health nurse determines that the patient needs information on medications, diet modification, and exercise. At the nurse's suggestion, the patient agrees to enroll in a cardiac rehabilitation program. An appointment is made with the cardiac rehabilitation nurse specialist at a nearby facility.

Evaluate the patient's situation individually and provide information and support in whatever manner that will best benefit the patient. Remember that the goal of cardiac rehabilitation is to prevent recurrence of anginal symptoms and to increase myocardial oxygen supply.

Multidisciplinary Outcomes

Multidisciplinary outcomes for patients experiencing angina can be differentiated based on the area of the health care continuum considered. Throughout the health care continuum, the objective is to balance myocardial oxygen supply and demand and to reduce angina attacks. Table 9–6 summarizes outcomes starting with the emergency department, continuing through the intensive care unit and the intermediate care unit, through to discharge, and follow-up in the community.

Critical Thinking Exercise

A 72-year-old obese woman is one of the patients in the telemetry unit today when her call bell rings. When asked what she needs, the patient complains of left-sided chest pain, over the breast area and into the left axilla. Associated symptoms include shortness of breath, diaphoresis, and generalized weakness. The patient states that the pain radiates into her neck and jaw. The patient's past medical history is positive for a cerebrovascular accident 4 years ago, with no residual deficits now, although she reportedly had dysphagia and left-sided weakness at first. Her past medical history also includes diet-controlled diabetes mellitus and increased cholesterol. She was recently placed on metoprolol, 50 mg twice daily 3 weeks before this hospitalization. The patient cannot tell you why she is taking this medication. The patient reports that the pain has been intermittent for the past 2 days, and that's the reason she was admitted to the hospital. This morning, the pain woke her up from her sleep, and it is the worst she has ever experienced. The patient's vital signs are as follows: blood pressure, 164/88 mm Hg; heart rate, 102 beats per minute and regular; and respiratory rate, 28 to 30.

1. From the information provided here, what would the patient's diagnoses be at this time?
2. Discuss the interventions that should be performed at this time. Provide rationales for each.
3. List the risk factors that can be identified from the information provided that would place this patient at risk for CAD.
4. Discuss the classes of medications this patient should be receiving and the rationale for each.
5. The pain is relieved after efforts made by the health care team. List the knowledge deficit issues that can be identified at this time.

TABLE 9–6
Multidisciplinary Outcomes

Phase of Recovery	Outcome
Emergency department	Relief of angina by conventional treatment (e.g., oxygen, sublingual nitroglycerin)
	Normalization or stabilization of the ECG
	Stabilization of the patient for transfer to the ICU or intermediate care unit
Intensive care unit	Relief of angina by use of advanced methods (e.g., IV nitroglycerin or IV morphine)
	Abation of the myocardial infarction process
	Restoration of myocardial blood flow
	Normalization or stabilization of the ECG
	Preservation of myocardial contractility
	Preparation of the patient for transfer to the intermediate care unit
Intermediate care unit	Maintenance of myocardial perfusion
	Maintenance of adequate cardiac output
	Maintenance of adequate oxygenation
	Reduction in the frequency of angina episodes
	Management of angina with oral or topical medications
	Education of the patient and family regarding the disease process, risk factors, and treatment modalities
	Restoration of the patient's psychological well-being
	Preparation of the patient for discharge and cardiac rehabilitation
Community	Initiation of a cardiac rehabilitation program
	Control of angina episodes
	Maintenance of adequate cardiac output
	Management or reduction of identified modifiable risk factors
	Restoration of previous role functions
	Maintenance of psychological well-being

Key Concepts

➡ CAD is a progressive disease that is defined as the narrowing of the lumen of the coronary artery.

➡ CAD is caused by the accumulation of cholesterol, minerals, and cells that causes the decrease in the diameter of the lumen of the artery.

➡ Modifiable and nonmodifiable risk factors contribute to the development of CAD.

➡ Gender, age, race, and heredity are the nonmodifiable risk factors.

➡ Smoking, hypertension, diabetes, activity level, cholesterol level, and obesity are modifiable risk factors.

➡ CAD causes a reduction in the supply of oxygen to the myocardium inadequate to meet demand.

➡ Angina (chest pain) is the manifestation of the imbalance between myocardial oxygen supply and demand.

➡ Unstable angina has the potential to lead to an MI if left untreated.

➡ Angina has many manifestations and associated symptoms.

➡ A differential diagnosis is essential to treat the disorder correctly.

➡ Nursing responsibility focuses on the continual assessment and quick intervention of the symptoms of angina.

➡ Collaborative management focuses on providing relief of the symptoms as well as management of the causes of CAD.

➡ Pharmacotherapeutics are a major part of the management of CAD.

➡ Invasive treatment strategies for CAD include PTCA, coronary atherectomy, and coronary stenting.

➡ The focus of cardiac rehabilitation is providing additional education and support to the patient's lifestyle changes.

➡ The objective of the collaborative management of CAD is the reduction in myocardial oxygen demand and the subsequent reduction in angina episodes.

References

1. US Department of Health and Human Services: Cardiac Rehabilitation. AHCPR Publication No. 96–0672. Rockville, MD, US Department of Health and Human Services, 1995.

2. American Heart Association Heart and Stroke Facts: 1996 Statistical Supplement. Granville, TX, American Heart Association, 1996.

3. Huether SE, McCance KL: Understanding Pathophysiology. St. Louis, Mosby–Year Book, 1996, pp 627–648.

4. Ridker PM, Cushman M, Stampfer MJ, et al: Inflammation, aspirin and the risk of cardiovascular disease in apparently healthy men. N Engl J Med 336:973–979, 1997.

5. Fair JM, Berra K: Lifestyle changes and coronary heart disease: the influence of nonpharmacologic interventions. J Cardiovasc Nurs 9:12–24, 1995.

6. Braunwald E (ed): Heart Disease: A Textbook of Cardiovascular Medicine, 5th ed. vols. 1 and 2. Philadelphia, W.B. Saunders, 1997, pp 1150–1151, 1202–1204, 1289–1349.

7. US Department of Health and Human Services: Unstable Angina: Diagnosis and Management. AHCPR Publication No. 94–0602. Rockville, MD, US Department of Health and Human Services, 1994.

8. McClellan JR: Unstable angina: prognosis, noninvasive risk assessment and strategies for management. Clin Cardiol 17:229–238, 1994.

9. Willich SN, Lewis M, Lowell H, Arntz HR, Schubert, F, Schroder R. (1993) Physical exertion as a trigger of acute myocardial infarction. N Engl J Med 329(23):1684–1690.

10. Reynolds A: The Skidmore-Roth Outline Series: Critical and High Acuity Nursing Care, El Paso, TX, Skidmore-Roth, 1995, pp 73–74.

11. Jensen L, King K: Women and heart disease: the issues. Crit Care Nurs 17:45–53, 1997.

12. Montague C, Kircher T: Myoglobin in the early evaluation of acute chest pain. Am J Clin Pathol 104:472–476, 1995.

13. Antman EM, Tanasijewic MJ, Thompson B, et al: Cardiac-specific troponin I levels to predict the risk of mortality in patients with acute coronary syndromes. N Engl J Med 335:1342–1349, 1996.

14. Herrmann HC, Hirshfield JW Jr: Coronary angioplasty and related techniques. In: Baum S, Pentecost, MJ (eds): Abrams' Angioplasty, vol. 3. Boston: Little, Brown, 1997, pp 366–385.

15. Reisman M: Technique and strategy of rotational atherectomy. Cathet Cardiovas Diagn 3(Suppl):2–14, 1996.

16. Gardner E, Joyce S, Iyer M, et al: Intracoronary stent update: focus on patient education. Crit Care Nurs 16:65–75, 1996.

17. US Department of Health and Human Services: Cardiac Rehabilitation as a Secondary Prevention. AHCPR Publication No. 96–0673. Rockville, MD, US Department of Health and Human Services, 1995.

18. Pearson TD, Rapaport E, Criqui M, et al: Special report: American Heart Association medical/scientific statement. Circulation 90:3125–3133, 1994.

10

Acute Myocardial Infarction

Linda Bucher

Objectives

By completion of this chapter, the student will be able to:

1. Relate the pathophysiology of an acute myocardial infarction (AMI) to the anticipated plan of care for a patient experiencing an AMI.
2. Identify assessment strategies for patients presenting with signs and symptoms of an AMI.
3. Describe the elements of the diagnostic workup specific to patients presenting with signs and symptoms of an AMI.
4. Plan collaborative care that extends across the health care continuum for patients experiencing an uncomplicated AMI.
5. Select appropriate interventions for patients experiencing an uncomplicated or complicated AMI.
6. Evaluate effects of collaborative care on anticipated outcomes for a patient experiencing an AMI.

The number of deaths from an AMI has declined in the United States over the past three decades, yet the rate of cardiovascular disease among Americans has remained relatively constant. Each year, over 1.5 million persons experience an AMI, and of these almost 500,000 die.[1] The role of the nurse in the care of patients experiencing AMIs has dramatically evolved over this period. Some of the diverse needs of the population at risk of an AMI include community education regarding early symptom recognition and hospital access, prompt initiation of treatment in the emergency department, close observation and rapid intervention during the initial hours after the event, continued monitoring and early discharge planning on step-down units, and cardiac rehabilitation with community follow-up. Nurses have an important part in providing care to these patients that stretches across the health care continuum.

ETIOLOGY AND PATHOPHYSIOLOGY

AMI refers to necrosis of some segment of myocardial tissue. Atherosclerosis remains the primary condition responsible for the development of an AMI because it produces a narrowing of the lumen of a coronary artery and a subsequent decrease in blood flow through the artery. This decrease in coronary blood flow can be the result of thrombosis at the site of the atherosclerotic plaque or of sustained, local vasospasm.[2] Regardless of the mechanism, the primary consequence is a decrease in the oxygen delivered to some portion of the myocardium. Cellular death occurs when the amount of oxygen delivered to the myocardium is unable to meet the cellular demand (Figure 10–1).

The ultimate damage to the heart is influenced to a great extent by the degree of collateral circulation embedded within the heart. Normally, almost no communication exists among the major coronary arteries, but many anastomoses do exist among the smaller arteries (Figure 10–2). During times of acute coronary occlusion, these anastomoses dilate within seconds. Although the amount of blood initially delivered through these collateral vessels is approximately half that required to keep the myocardium viable, the diameters of these vessels enlarge further for 8 to 24 hours after the occlusive event. The development of these collateral vessels continues over the next 2 to 3 days and can ultimately provide normal blood flow to previously ischemic myocardium within 1 month. The amount of collateral circulation varies among individuals and plays an important role in determining the size of the infarction. In some instances, patients may recover with little or no residual damage to the myocardium.[2]

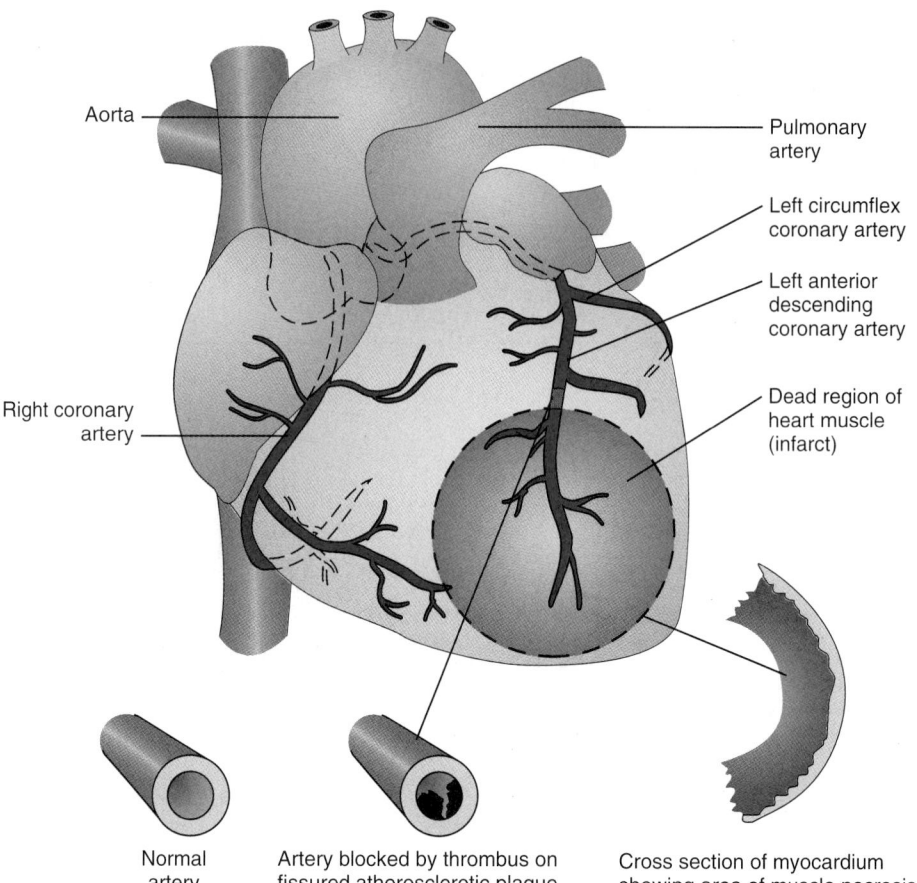

Figure 10–1

Interrelationship of chronic athero- sclerotic obstruction, acute plaque change, superimposed thrombus, and myocardial injury resulting from acute myocardial infarction. (From Shoen FJ: The heart. In: Cotran RS, Kumar V, Robbins SL [eds]: Pathologic Basis of Disease, 5th ed. Philadelphia, W. B. Saunders, 1994.)

Aorta

Pulmonary artery

Left circumflex coronary artery

Left anterior descending coronary artery

Dead region of heart muscle (infarct)

Right coronary artery

Normal artery

Artery blocked by thrombus on fissured atherosclerotic plaque

Cross section of myocardium showing area of muscle necrosis (infarct)

Zones of Infarction, Injury, and Ischemia

When myocardial tissue death does occur, the area involved is referred to as the zone of infarction. This zone is most frequently identified by the development of a pathologic Q wave on the electrocardiogram (ECG), as discussed in Chapter 8. This development reflects the electrical changes in the surface of the myocardium that is involved in the infarction process. Necrotic cells are unable to depolarize, and, as healing takes place (usually within 6 weeks), scar tissue replaces the damaged area. The Q wave, when seen on the ECG, usually persists as lifelong evidence of an AMI.

The zone of infarction is surrounded by potentially viable myocardial tissue that comprises the zone of injury. Cells in this zone are not fully capable of con- tracting because of the reduced blood supply to this area. ECG evidence of this property is reflected by ST- segment elevation.

The outermost area, referred to as the zone of is- chemia, represents the most viable cells. Repolariza- tion in this area is impaired and is evidenced by T-wave inversion on the ECG.

During the period of reduced blood flow, the cells in the zones of injury and ischemia revert to anaerobic

metabolism. The subsequently increased lactic acid is released into the extracellular fluid. In addition, as the cells in the zone of infarction begin to die, their cell membranes are disrupted, and their intracellular con- tents, particularly potassium, are released into the sur- rounding extracellular fluid. This combination of local changes in the pH and in potassium predispose the cells in the zones of injury and ischemia to conduction defects and dysrhythmias.

Classification of Infarctions

Myocardial infarctions (MIs) can be classified into two subgroups based on ECG changes. Traditionally, the development of a pathologic Q wave was thought to indicate involvement of all three layers of the heart muscle, and, consequently, these infarctions were labeled transmural (or full-thickness) MIs. Conversely, when no abnormal Q waves were present, it was thought that the area of necrosis was limited to the subendocardium, and these infarctions were termed nontransmural (or partial-thickness) MIs.

Infarctions that do not involve the full thickness of the heart muscle are usually restricted to the subendo-

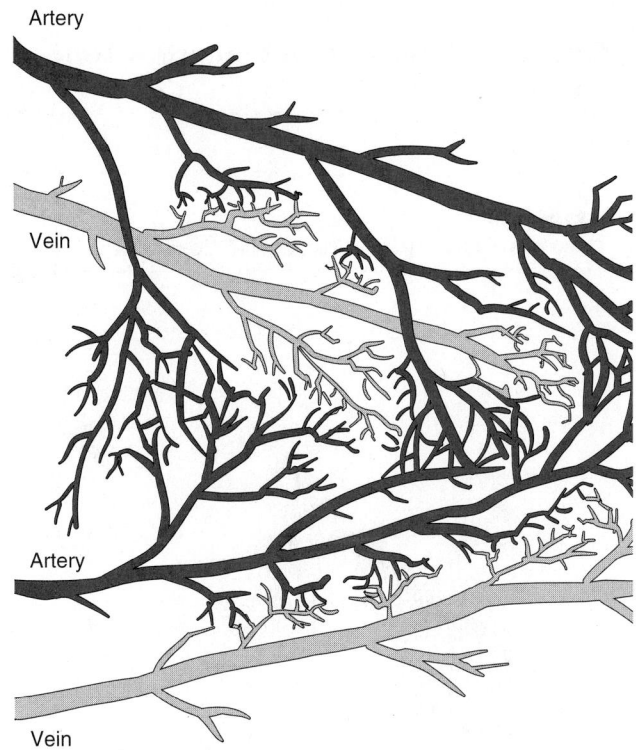

Figure 10-2

Anastomoses of the coronary arterial system. (From Guyton AC, Hall JE: Textbook of Medical Physiology, 9th ed. Philadelphia, W. B. Saunders, 1996, p 260.)

necrotic myocardium can impede the heart's ability to contract during systole and can result in dyskinetic or akinetic areas of the myocardium. The ejection fraction, which evaluates the amount of blood pumped with each contraction, is often used as a prognostic measure after an AMI. Ejection fractions less than 40% are more often related to poorer outcomes.[4]

AMIs can be classified further according to the location of the infarction, as determined by the changes in the 12-lead ECG (see Chapter 8). Specifically, Q waves and ST-segment–T-wave abnormalities are correlated with groups of ECG leads. By examining the ECG in this way, not only can the location of the infarction be identified, but also the potential electrical and mechanical complications can be determined (Table 10–1). For example, knowing that the right coronary artery supplies blood to the sinoatrial (SA) node, the atrioventricular (AV) node, and the posterior papillary muscle of the mitral valve can alert the nurse to monitor the patient experiencing an inferior MI for conduction disturbances or new heart murmurs. An occlusion in the left anterior descending coronary artery precipitates changes in the leads overlooking the anteroseptal portion of the left ventricle (LV). These changes should direct the nurse to observe the patient for signs of mechanical problems such as pump failure as well as for signs of electrical problems such as complete heart block.

Hemodynamic Consequences of an Acute Myocardial Infarction

The hemodynamic consequences of an AMI are directly related to the size and location of the infarction. Most infarctions involve some portion of the LV, the main pumping chamber of the heart. As recovery takes place, fibrous scar tissue replaces the necrotic tissue. This scar tissue lacks the contractile, elastic, and conductive properties of healthy myocardial tissue.

If the infarcted area is large enough, it can interfere with the functioning of the LV. Consequently, stroke volume and ultimately cardiac output may be reduced. In approximately 40% of patients who experience a transmural MI, especially in the anterior LV region, an event known as ventricular remodeling occurs during the weeks and months that follow the acute incident. During remodeling, the now hypercontractile healthy myocardium stretches and thins the infarct area, further limiting the efficiency of ventricular contraction. This regional expansion and dilation is thought to precede aneurysm formation.[5]

If LV function is significantly compromised, aortic pressure and coronary perfusion pressure may decrease and may contribute to additional ischemia. Pa-

cardial muscle. Normally, the subendocardial muscle has difficulty in obtaining an adequate blood supply because of the intense compression of the blood vessels in this area during systole. Therefore, any situation that reduces the blood supply to the myocardium damages the subendocardial area first. Continued ischemia causes the damage to extend outward toward the epicardium.[2]

However, research has shown that classifying MIs as transmural or nontransmural is imprecise and is often incorrect. Patients with pathologic Q waves can have nontransmural infarctions, whereas patients with normal Q waves can have transmural infarctions.[3] Consequently, the terms Q-wave and non–Q-wave MI represent the most appropriate terminology and imply clinical and prognostic significance.

Patients experiencing non–Q-wave infarctions generally sustain smaller areas of necrosis, demonstrate lower levels of cardiac enzymes, and suffer fewer incidences of congestive heart failure (CHF). However, these patients have higher rates of postinfarction angina and reinfarction compared with patients with Q-wave MIs.[3]

Patients with Q-wave infarctions usually experience a greater loss of heart tissue, and, consequently, they are at greater risk of ventricular dysfunction. In addition, approximately 70% of patients with Q-wave MIs demonstrate a pericardial friction rub. Areas of

TABLE 10–1

Acute Myocardial Infarction: Infarct Area, ECG Evidence, Associated Coronary Arteries, and Potential Complications

Area of Infarct	ECG Evidence		Associated Coronary Artery	Potential Complications
	Leads Reflecting Infarct Area Directly	Leads Reflecting Reciprocal Changes		
Left Ventricle				
Lateral wall, high	I, aVL	II, III, aVF	Left circumflex	Pump failure, conduction disturbances
Inferior wall	II, III, AVF	I, aVL, V_5, V_6	Right coronary, possibly left circumflex	Sinoatrial and atrioventricular nodal conduction disturbances; valve dysfunction
Septal wall	V_1–V_2	II, III, aVF	Left anterior descending	Pump failure, conduction disturbance
Anterior wall	V_2–V_4	II, III, aVF	Left anterior descending	Pump failure, conduction disturbance
Lateral wall, low (apical area)	V_5–V_6	II, III, aVF	Left anterior descending	Pump failure, conduction disturbance
Posterior	V_7–V_9*	V_1–V_3	Posterior descending, right coronary, or left circumflex	Atrioventricular nodal conduction disturbance
Right Ventricle†	V_4R	—	Right coronary	Atrioventricular nodal disturbance, valve dysfunction, hypotension

*Leads are placed on the left posterior chest wall at the fifth intercostal space, beginning at the left posterior axillary line.

†Right ventricular infarction is present in approximately one-third of patients with inferior myocardial infarctions and assessment of this lead should be routinely performed in all patients diagnosed with an acute inferior myocardial infarction.

tients experiencing a loss of 40% or more of functional LV almost always develop cardiogenic shock, and death occurs in approximately 85% of these patients.[5]

Similarly, hemodynamic alterations can result if the infarcted portions of the myocardium involve significant amounts of conductive tissue. If the conduction defects are serious enough, such as complete heart block, cardiac output may be compromised. Because hemodynamic consequences of an AMI depend on the size and location of the infarction, initial treatment strategies are aimed at halting or limiting the infarction process.

Assessment

The diagnosis of an AMI is determined by the clinical history of the chest pain, the physical examination findings, changes on the ECG, and the presence of serum cardiac enzymes. "Time is muscle" when treating patients who are experiencing AMIs. Initiation of treatment strategies within 6 hours of the onset of symptoms has shown to reduce mortality significantly in these patients. Ideally, treatment should be initiated within 60 to 90 minutes of the onset of symptoms, to produce optimal benefit.[6] Approximately 60% of persons who die of an AMI do so before ever reaching a hospital. These deaths usually occur within 1 hour of the onset of symptoms and result from lethal dysrhythmias.[7]

The three major components of delay in treatment of an AMI are 1) patient decision making once symptoms develop, 2) responding to and transporting the patient to the emergency department, and 3) initiation of treatment once the patient reaches the hospital. Prehospital delay times range from 2 to 6.5 hours, with many people delaying beyond 6 hours and even days.[8] This component of delays in treatment represents the largest source of delay time. To develop strategies to reduce prehospital delay time, it is important to explore the nature of people who experience symptoms of an AMI and postpone obtaining care.

The literature revealed that delay times were increased in persons experiencing symptoms of an AMI who were female, older, African-American, Hispanic, or extremely economically disadvantaged.[8,9] Persons with known risk factors for an AMI, such as hypertension, diabetes, or angina, also demonstrated longer delay times. In addition, persons who consulted with a spouse or a physician regarding their cardiac symptoms experienced increased prehospital delay times. However, if the person consulted an unrelated individual, delay times were significantly shorter. The effects of time of day, day of week, and place where symptoms occur appear to be interrelated with other factors, particularly with the person whom the patient was with when symptoms first occurred. Finally, Dracup and colleagues found that persons who initiated self-treatment measures, such as over-the-counter medications, experienced significantly longer prehospital delays. Unfortunately, a previous history of heart disease or even an MI was not related to a decrease in prehospital delay.[8]

In general, prehospital delay times were shorter in persons who were hemodynamically unstable, who had large infarctions, and who identified their symptoms as being cardiac in origin.[8] In addition, persons who called 911 had shorter time to hospital arrival than persons who selected other means of transport.[10]

The National Heart Attack Alert Program (NHAAP) was established to reduce both patient-related and treatment-related delays associated with AMIs.[11] A major goal of this program is to increase public awareness of the signs and symptoms of an AMI, especially for persons at risk and for those close to these people. Nurses can play a major role in educating patients, families, and communities about the importance of early recognition and treatment of cardiac symptoms. Table 10–2 suggests a collaborative approach aimed at reducing prehospital delay time.

Signs and Symptoms of Acute Myocardial Infarction

In spite of the numerous advances in the laboratory detection of an AMI, the patient's history continues to contribute substantial information toward establishing a definitive diagnosis. A prodromal history can be obtained in as many as 60% of patients with an AMI.[12]

Persistent chest pain is the most frequently reported prodromal symptom associated with an AMI. This pain generally lasts more than 30 minutes and is unrelieved by rest or nitrates. Typical chest pain associated with an AMI is described as a burning, crushing, tightness, or squeezing sensation in the chest. Many patients describe the sensation as a feeling that an "elephant" is standing on their chest. Often patients attribute the pain to indigestion and attempt to treat themselves with antacids. The pain is usually located in the substernal or left precordial region of the chest. The pain may radiate to the shoulders, neck, back, jaws, ears, or arms. Atypical signs of an AMI include

TABLE 10–2
Collaborative Approach to Reducing Prehospital Delay Time

Goals	Strategies	Implementation
Increase community awareness of signs and symptoms of AMI and benefit of prompt action	Educational campaigns using mail, radio, television, and public service announcements	Professional nursing organizations (e.g., emergency nurses, critical care nurses), physicians, community leaders, emergency medical technicians/paramedics
Target high-risk individuals (e.g., older individuals, females, African-Americans, and persons with hypertension, diabetes, or heart disease)	Education in primary care providers' offices and at senior citizen health fairs, church-sponsored screenings, and clinics	Primary care providers (physicians, nurse practitioners), professional nursing organizations
Target bystanders (families and friends) of high-risk individuals to recognize and respond promptly to cardiac symptoms	Group meetings in community centers, churches, and nursing centers	Professional nursing organizations, nurse practitioners, emergency medical technicians/paramedics
Increase use of emergency medical system (911) for transporting individuals with cardiac symptoms	Media campaign to inform community of benefits of using emergency medical system	Community leaders, professional nursing organizations, physicians, emergency medical technicians/paramedics
Modify CPR curriculum to emphasize early symptom recognition and rapid access to emergency medical system	CPR instructor programs to stress process of identifying a potential AMI and actions to be taken as well as CPR technique; CPR community programs to focus on behavior of witnesses to reduce delays in accessing care	American Heart Association/American Red Cross CPR instructor-trainers and instructors
Identify community educational programs that bridge knowledge–behavior gap	Development of research studies to determine the most effective educational strategies	Nurse/physician researchers

AMI, acute myocardial infarction; CPR, cardiopulmonary resuscitation.

nausea, vomiting, and diaphoresis, and these frequently accompany the pain of an AMI. It is recommended that a 10-point rating scale, with 0 equal to "no pain" and 10 equal to "the worst pain imaginable" be used to assess changes in the patient's pain.

Patients over the age of 65 years who are experiencing an AMI may not report the classic descriptions of chest pain or the associated nausea, vomiting, and diaphoresis. Rather than a crushing or squeezing pain, elderly patients may describe their pain as a vague ache or discomfort that is often poorly localized. The incidence of atypical chest pain and even the absence of chest pain in the presence of an AMI increases with age, especially in patients 85 years old and older. One explanation for this phenomenon may be that the coexistence of diabetes or other diseases causing neuropathies may conceal the sensations and perceptions of cardiac pain. In this population, shortness of breath, syncope, or acute confusion may be the primary presenting symptom of an AMI.[13]

Several gender-related differences exist in the development and presentation of an AMI. Women have a delayed onset of coronary heart disease by 10 years, making them older than their male counterparts at time of diagnosis. More often, women present with angina than an AMI as the first manifestation of coronary heart disease. However, when women do present with an AMI (usually 20 years later than men), mortality rates are higher than for men.[14]

Women experiencing an AMI may present with typical chest pain symptoms, although, compared with men, women experience more "silent" MIs. The most likely reason for this presentation is that women are generally older when they experience their first MI. In addition, women report more atypical signs of an AMI, such as nausea, vomiting, and shortness of breath.[15]

Although studies examining differences in ethnic pain styles in AMI are limited, some evidence indicates that African-American men have atypical presentations of an AMI. African-American men are more likely to report shortness of breath as a symptom of AMI than their white counterparts.[16] This difference may be explained in part by the higher incidence of hypertension among African-Americans, and this disorder may predispose them to CHF and ultimately an AMI. Information regarding age, gender, and ethnic differences in onset of AMI symptoms needs to be included in educational programs aimed at reducing prehospital and treatment delays.

In about one-half of patients experiencing an AMI, precipitating factors can be identified. Most often, patients relate some degree of physical exertion to the onset of chest pain. Emotional stress, such as that associated with major life events, has also been noted as an important trigger of an AMI. Figure 10–3 depicts the hypothetic chain of events that may precipitate an AMI in the presence of exertion or mental stress.

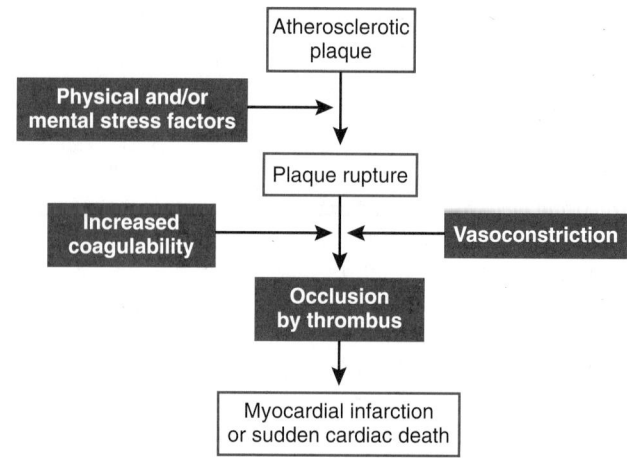

Figure 10–3

Hypothetic blueprint for understanding the manner in which daily activities may trigger coronary thrombosis. Three mechanisms may be involved in triggering the process, including stress (physical or mental) leading to hemodynamic changes that cause plaque rupture, activities that lead to coagulability increase, and stimuli that lead to vasoconstriction.

Finally, evidence indicates that the onset of an AMI is related to circadian rhythm. The peak incidence of onset of AMI symptoms occurs between the hours of 6:00 AM and noon. The early morning increases in circulating catecholamines and cortisol, as well as increases in platelet aggregability, are believed to contribute to plaque rupture and subsequent thrombosis.[12] Patients who are taking beta blockers or aspirin before the onset of AMI do not demonstrate this characteristic circadian peak.

Rapid assessment of the patient experiencing an AMI is integral to the correct diagnosis and selection of treatment strategies for these patients. The nurse should use a focused approach when obtaining the history of chest pain. The "P, Q, R, S, T" method of collecting data regarding the history of the chest pain is one such approach (see Chapter 9).

Clinical Presentation

Patients experiencing an AMI demonstrate various physical findings that are mostly influenced by the severity and location of the infarct. Patients with uncomplicated MIs involving small areas of infarction often have a normal physical examination. Abnormal physical findings are frequently associated with large infarcts complicated by heart failure or dysrhythmias. A rapid head-to-toe assessment is recommended and provides the nurse with important baseline information. Table 10–3 provides a summary of clinical findings often associated with an AMI.

Laboratory and Diagnostic Tests

The initial and serial ECGs are the most useful tools for the diagnosis of an AMI. Ideally, a baseline 12-lead

TABLE 10–3
Clinical Presentation of Acute Myocardial Infarction

System	Possible Findings
Neurologic Patients >85 yr	Restlessness Acute confusion* Syncope* Stroke*

Cardiovascular	Chest pain
	ECG findings:
	  Bradycardia
	  Tachycardia
	  Ventricular ectopy
	  Atrioventricular blocks
	Normotension or hypotension
	S_3 or S_4
	Systolic murmur
	Decreased cardiac output:
	  Diminished capillary refill
	  Diminished peripheral pulses
	Jugular venous distention
	Peripheral edema

Respiratory
  African-American Males,
  patients >85 yr, female
  patients
	Shortness of breath*
	Orthopnea
	Tachypnea
	Crackles
	Frothy sputum

Integumentary	Diaphoresis Pallor
Gastrointestinal Female patients	Nausea* Vomiting*
Genitourinary	Diminished urine output
Psychosocial	Anxiety Agitation Anger Denial

*Indicates physical findings that are often the primary presenting symptoms for *certain* populations, but may also be associated symptoms for anyone experiencing acute myocardial infarction.

ECG should be obtained as soon as possible after chest pain develops, either in the field by emergency medical personnel or immediately on arrival to the emergency department. Continuous ECG monitoring should be initiated and maintained to document changes in the evolution of the AMI. As discussed earlier, initial 12-lead ECG changes associated with AMIs include unique patterns of ST-segment–T-wave abnormalities. The development of a pathologic Q

wave varies and, when present, is often associated with an increase in post-MI complications.[5]

Although the ECG is readily available, easy to use, and noninvasive, it has limitations. Many patients report to the emergency department with a history of chest pain but no diagnostic changes in the ECG. Elderly patients presenting with signs and symptoms of an AMI often have preexisting cardiac abnormalities that may complicate ECG interpretation and may delay treatment.[13] Finally, interobserver variability can contribute to delays in treatment as well as the number of undiagnosed AMIs.

As many as 50% of patients presenting to the emergency department with chest pain and who are in fact having an AMI initially have normal or nondiagnostic ECGs. Consequently, serologic markers for detecting or ruling out an AMI are useful. When myocardial necrosis occurs, large proteins (enzymes) escape from the cells and enter the circulation. Serial measurements of these cardiac enzymes, total creatine kinase (CK) and lactate dehydrogenase (LDH) and their respective cardiac-specific isoenzymes ($CK-MB$, LDH_1, and LDH_2), are obtained every 8 hours for 1 to 2 days (see Chapter 8 for review).

Cardiac enzyme profiles may be atypical in the elderly population. Baseline CK levels may be significantly lower than normal in this group because of the overall decrease in total body muscle mass. In the presence of an AMI, CK-MB levels may be increased in spite of normal CK levels. Consequently, one should always evaluate CK-MB levels in the elderly who are at risk of an AMI; otherwise, important diagnostic information may be overlooked.[13]

Elevations in cardiac enzymes only provide adjunctive data to the diagnosis of an AMI because several other clinical conditions, such as pericarditis and recent cardioversion, can precipitate similar increases in serum CK and LDH levels. In addition, the earliest rise in CK-MB isoenzymes is often not seen until 4 hours after the onset of infarction.

Several new immunoassay techniques are currently in use and may provide important diagnostic information as early as 1.5 to 3 hours after the onset of symptoms. Two isoforms or subforms of CK-MB isoenzymes ($CK-MB_1$ and $CK-MB_2$) have been isolated, and abnormal elevations of $CK-MB_2$ have been demonstrated as early as 2 hours after the onset of AMI symptoms. Investigators have reported that CK-MB isoforms have greater prognostic value than CK isoenzymes within the first 2 to 4 hours and after 8 hours of the onset of symptoms.[17]

Other studies have examined the role of myoglobin (Mgb), carbonic anhydrase, and cardiac troponin in the early diagnosis of AMI. During an AMI, Mgb is released from the necrotic cells more rapidly than CK-MB because of its lower molecular weight. Serum Mgb levels can increase to twice their normal values within 2 hours and can peak within 4 hours after an AMI. Serial evaluations of Mgb have shown high sensitivity for AMI, particularly during the early hours after the onset of symptoms.[18]

Carbonic anhydrase III (CA-III) is a protein found in skeletal muscle, but not in cardiac muscle. During cellular injury, CA-III is released from skeletal muscle in a fixed ratio to Mgb. In an attempt to increase the specificity of Mgb in the diagnosis of an AMI, serum Mgb and the ratio of Mgb to CA-III (Mgb/CA-III) were measured. Early work demonstrated that twice as many patients with an AMI can be accurately diagnosed within 3 hours of symptoms by this method compared with measurement of CK-MB.[19]

Cardiac troponin T (cTnT) and cardiac troponin I (cTnI) are additional proteins unique to the myocardium. Comparisons of the sensitivity and specificity for an AMI between cTnT or cTnI values and CK-MB isoforms have been found to be similar.[20] cTnT appears in the circulation 2 to 6 hours after the onset of AMI symptoms and remains elevated for 6 to 20 days, making it potentially useful in the confirmation of an AMI when the patient's arrival at the hospital is significantly delayed.[21]

Nurses need to be aware of the evolving changes in assessment strategies for patients presenting with symptoms of an AMI. Rapid and accurate diagnosis and treatment of these patients result in improved physiologic outcomes and more efficient use of health care services.

Nursing Diagnoses

The care of patients presenting with an AMI is challenging, and nurses are required to execute superior observational and assessment skills to intervene appropriately and to detect complications quickly. Patients diagnosed with uncomplicated AMIs are usually treated in the emergency department for the first 1 to 3 hours, quickly transferred to an intensive or coronary care unit for 1 to 2 days, then moved to and discharged from an intermediate care or step-down unit on day 4 or 5. As members of a multidisciplinary health care team, nurses are guided by both nursing and medical diagnoses when planning care for these patients and their families. A priority list of actual or potential diagnoses for the various phases of hospitalization is presented in Table 10–4.

Collaborative Management

The management of patients experiencing an AMI involves a multidisciplinary team approach and usually

TABLE 10–4
Nursing Diagnoses According to Phase of Hospitalization

Phase of Hospitalization	Actual or Potential Diagnoses
Emergency department	Pain related to myocardial ischemia
	Decreased cardiac output related to impaired left ventricular function; dysrhythmias
	Anxiety related to sudden change in health status, threat to life, or unknown prognosis
	Ineffective denial related to acceptance of diagnosis
	Activity intolerance related to changes in cardiac status
	Powerlessness related to change in environment and health status
	Sensory/perceptual alterations related to visual and auditory overload in emergency department
	Knowledge deficit, learning need, related to emergency treatment activities or role in plan of care
Intensive care unit	In addition to the above:
	High risk of fluid volume deficit (bleeding) related to thrombolytic or anticoagulation therapy
	Sleep pattern disturbance related to frequent interruptions or change in environment
	Ineffective individual coping related to change in health status or unknown future
	Impaired adjustment: depression related to sudden change in health status
	Ineffective family coping related to sudden change in family roles or unknown future
	Sensory/perceptual alterations related to sensory overload/deprivation in the intensive care unit
	Knowledge deficit, learning need, related to ongoing treatment activities or role in plan of care
Intermediate care unit	In addition to the above:
	Altered role performance related to change in physical capacity
	Self-esteem disturbance related to change in physical capacity or role
	Altered sexuality patterns related to change in physical capacity or fear of death
	Knowledge deficit, learning need, related to modifying risk factors and discharge information, including cardiac rehabilitation

CLINICAL PATHWAY

Case type:
Acute MI

Exception:
None

ADDRESSOGRAPH

DATE		0 - 1 hr If direct admission (not through ED) initiate this column MN/DY/EV	1 - 24 hr MN/DY/EV	INFARCT SIZING/STABILIZATION PHASE 1 MN/DY/EV
		ISCHEMIA CONTROL / INFARCT SIZING PHASE		
ASSESSMENTS	**CONSULTS**	**0-5 Minutes** Assess for presence of symptoms presumptive of CAD Identify cardiologist of record Assess pain by using pain scale 0-10 Assess bilateral blood pressures **5-15 Minutes** Medical Patient assessment completed by physician Determine eligibility for thrombolytics/emergent PTCA Consult cardiologist	Cardiac Rehabilitation Consult Cardiac Rehabilitation Consult for Smoking Cessation Program Clinical Dietitian Consult for diet education Home Health Care/Social Work referral	
SPECIMENS	**TESTS**	EKG Draw red top tube and hold for SMA-12 or Cholesterol, HDL, Triglycerides CBC SMA-6, Mg, Glucose Baseline CPK, then CPK q 6h [06-12-18-24] until CPK peak defined CK-MB profile as needed PT, PTT, Heparin protocol PCXR	Urinalysis Heparin protocol Continue CPK until peak defined	EKG Heparin protocol
TREATMENTS		**0-5 Minutes** Cardiac monitoring ST segment monitoring if indicated Oxygen therapy	Cardiac monitoring ST-segment monitoring if indicated NPG: Cardiac dysrhythmia Oxygen therapy Admission height and weight I&O	Cardiac monitoring NPG: Cardiac dysrhythmia Discontinue oxygen therapy Consider daily weight/I&O for patients on diuretics and/or positive inotropes
MEDS	**IV**	IV access Aspirin Nitroglycerin Heparin Beta Blockers unless contraindicated Consider Morphine for pain control	IV access Aspirin Nitroglycerin Continue Heparin Continue Beta Blocker Continue Morphine Consider ACE Inhibitor Consider anti-anxiety medication Acetaminophen PRN headache Stool softener	IV access Aspirin Nitroglycerin Continue Heparin Continue Beta Blocker Continue ACE Inhibitor Continue anti-anxiety medication Acetaminophen PRN headache Stool softener
		Relief of cardiac ischemic signs/symptoms No signs of phlebitis or infiltration of IV	Relief of cardiac ischemic signs/symptoms No signs of phlebitis or infiltration of IV	Relief of cardiac ischemic signs/symptoms No signs of phlebitis or infiltration of IV
INITIALS	**TIME**			

Figure 10–4

An example of an acute myocardial infarction pathway. (Courtesy of Christiana Care Health Services, Newark, DE.)

Illustration continued on following page

includes physicians, nurses, cardiac rehabilitation specialists, dietitians, clergy, social workers, and community nurses. Clinical nurse specialists and case managers may also be included in this team. Elements of the care required by these patients extend from the community, to various units within the acute care setting, to rehabilitation facilities, and finally back to the community. Nurses can select from various essential roles that intersect all these settings. The acute MI pathway (Figure 10–4) is an example of one pathway that is used to direct collaborative care for patients hospitalized with an AMI. See Chapter 9 for the outcome record for this pathway.

CLINICAL PATHWAY

The Clinical Pathway represents best clinical practice as defined by a multidisciplinary team. It is not intended to replace good medical judgement, clinical decision making, or critical thinking. The Pathways are intended for use as a guide and tool for collaborative practice.

ADDRESSOGRAPH

DATE	0 - 1 hr If direct admission (not through ED) initiate this column MN/DY/EV	1 - 24 hr MN/DY/EV	INFARCT SIZING/STABILIZATION PHASE 1 MN/DY/EV
	ISCHEMIA CONTROL / INFARCT SIZING PHASE		
NUTRITION	NPO	Cardiac diet (300 mg Cholesterol,3-4GM Na, caffeine restricted) Cardiac, no concentrated sweets (300mg Cholesterol, 3-4GM, Na,diabetic) Low Cholesterol, Low saturated fat (300 mg Cholesterol, No Na+restriction) Cardiac Reversal (10-15% saturated fat, < 200 mg Cholesterol) Cardiac Clear Liquids	Continue prescribed diet
		Tolerating prescribed diet	Tolerating prescribed diet
SAFETY / ACTIVITY	NPG: Fall prevention / fall precautions NPG: Bleeding precautions Bedrest	NPG: Fall prevention / fall precautions NPG: Bleeding precautions Bedrest Dangle Bedside commode	NPG: Fall prevention / fall precautions NPG: Bleeding precautions OOB to chair for meals Active ROM in chair as tolerated
	No injuries No uncontrolled bleeding	No injuries No uncontrolled bleeding	No injuries No uncontrolled bleeding Tolerating prescribed activity level without signs/symptoms of cardiac ischemia
TEACHING	<u>Nursing</u> Instruct patient/family of signs & symptoms of cardiac ischemia and need to notify nurse Explain immediate procedures	<u>Nursing</u> Instruct patient/family of signs & symptoms of cardiac ischemia and need to notify nurse Diagnosis/Tests: ♥ Explain diagnosis ♥ Give Change of Heart Booklet ♥ Give test info re: PTCA, cardiac Cath, etc if applicable	<u>Nursing</u> Instruct patient/family of signs & symptoms of cardiac ischemia and need to notify nurse Medications/MI vs Angina: ♥ Review Micromedex drug information ♥ Review angina vs MI and SL nitroglycerin <u>Cardiac Rehabilitation</u> Review of Day 1 cardiac Rehab risk factor assessment Initiate Smoking Cessation Protocol <u>Registered Dietitian</u> Cardiac diet teaching on appropriate diet
			pt/family verbalizes understanding of signs and symptoms of cardiac ischemia and when to notify nurse pt/family verbalizes use of Change of Heart Booklet as a resource pt/family verbalizes Signs and symptoms of overexertion Inpatient activity guidelines Rationale of diet principles
		pt/family verbalizes understanding of signs and symptoms of cardiac ischemia and when to notify nurse	
DISCHARGE COORDINATION		<u>Nursing</u> Assess initial discharge needs Identify initial discharge plan	Continuing care needs assessment
		pt/family participates in discharge plan Needs for discharge resources identified	pt/family verbalizes understanding of updated discharge plan
SIGNATURES	**Health Care Team Signatures** Signature/Initial/Print Name/Shift Signature ___ Initial Print Name ___ Shift Signature ___ Initial Print Name ___ Shift Signature ___ Initial Print Name ___ Shift	**Health Care Team Signatures** Signature/Initial/Print Name/Shift Signature ___ Initial Print Name ___ Shift Signature ___ Initial Print Name ___ Shift Signature ___ Initial Print Name ___ Shift	**Health Care Team Signatures** Signature/Initial/Print Name/Shift Signature ___ Initial Print Name ___ Shift Signature ___ Initial Print Name ___ Shift Signature ___ Initial Print Name ___ Shift

Figure 10–4 *Continued*

Emergency Department

As discussed earlier, prehospital delays represent the largest component of delay time in treating patients with an AMI. Consequently, time to treatment once a patient arrives at the emergency department is critical because patient outcomes after an AMI are significantly improved the closer treatment is to the onset of symptoms. The NHAAP recommends a 30-minute "door-to-drug" time frame.[11] Many emergency departments have developed specific strategies to decrease time to treatment for these patients. Critical pathways, chest pain emergency departments, and code "H" (for heart attack) are some examples.

Management of these patients on arrival to the emergency department begins with a rapid assess-

DATE		INFARCT SIZING/STABILIZATION PHASE 2	MN/DY/EV	RISK ASSESSMENT / DISCHARGE PHASE	MN/DY/EV	RISK ASSESSMENT / DISCHARGE PHASE	MN/DY/EV
A S S E S S M E N T S	C O N S U L T S	Medical To consider discharge to home for uncomplicated MI's with follow-up by homecare					
S P E C I M E N S	T E S T S	Heparin protocol		Heparin protocol		Heparin protocol	

	T R E A T M E N T S	Cardiac monitoring
		NPG: Cardiac dysrhythmia
		Weight and I&O for patients on
		   diuretics / positive inotropic agents
				Cardiac monitoring
				NPG: Cardiac dysrhythmia
				Weight and I&O for patients on
				   diuretics / positive inotropic agents
						Cardiac monitoring
						NPG: Cardiac dysrhythmia
						Weight and I&O for patients on
						   diuretics / positive inotropic agents	

M E D I C A T I O N S	I V	IV Access Aspirin Nitroglycerin Continue Heparin Continue Beta Blocker Continue ACE Inhibitor Continue anti-anxiety medication Acetaminophen PRN headache Stool softener		IV Access Aspirin Nitroglycerin Continue Heparin Continue Beta Blocker Continue ACE Inhibitor Continue anti-anxiety medication Acetaminophen PRN headache Stool softener		IV Access Aspirin Nitroglycerin Continue Heparin as indicated Continue Beta Blocker Continue ACE Inhibitor Continue anti-anxiety medication Acetaminophen PRN headache Stool softener	

		Relief of cardiac ischemic signs/
		   symptoms
		No signs of phlebitis or
		   infiltration of IV
			☐☐☐
			☐☐☐
				Relief of cardiac ischemic signs/
				   symptoms
				No signs of phlebitis or
				   infiltration of IV
					☐☐☐
					☐☐☐
						Relief of cardiac ischemic signs/
						   symptoms
						No signs of phlebitis or
						   infiltration of IV
							☐☐☐
							☐☐☐

N U T R I T I O N		Continue prescribed diet		Continue prescribed diet		Continue prescribed diet	
		Tolerating prescribed diet	☐☐☐	Tolerating prescribed diet	☐☐☐	Tolerating prescribed diet	☐☐☐
I N I T I A L S	T I M E						

Figure 10–4 *Continued*   *Illustration continued on following page*

ment of the chest pain history and the 12-lead ECG. Continuous ECG monitoring is established, and baseline serum cardiac enzymes are drawn, although the availability of the results varies and often exceeds 30 minutes. Overall, treatment strategies are aimed at preserving the myocardium and reducing mortality and morbidity. (See Appendix, ACLS: Acute MI algorithm.)

Reperfusion Strategies

Various reperfusion strategies are available to treat patients experiencing an AMI. Selection depends, in part, on the physician's preference and on the technology available within the treating facility.

Thrombolytic Therapy

Dissolution of clots with thrombolytic agents has shown to reperfuse the affected coronary artery and continues to be a standard practice for treating patients with an AMI, especially in facilities without invasive cardiology laboratories and open heart surgical suites. Three agents are currently in use: 1) streptokinase (SK); 2) recombinant tissue plasminogen activator (rt-PA); and 3) anisoylated plasminogen streptokinase activator (APSAC). Basically, these agents convert plasminogen to plasmin (an enzyme), which catalyzes the fibrin clot and produces fibrin degradation products. Although the exact mechanism of each agent varies, the end result is clot lysis. Table 10–5 has further comparisons among these agents.

DATE							
	INFARCT SIZING/STABILIZATION PHASE 2 MN/DY/EV		**RISK ASSESSMENT / DISCHARGE PHASE** MN/DY/EV		**RISK ASSESSMENT / DISCHARGE PHASE** MN/DY/EV		

SAFETY / ACTIVITY

NPG: Fall prevention / fall precautions NPG: Bleeding precautions Ambulate 110 ft with assistance Assess hemodynamic stability	NPG: Fall prevention / fall precautions NPG: Bleeding precautions Ambulate independently TID if asymptomatic	NPG: Fall prevention / fall precautions NPG: Bleeding precautions Ambulate ad lib if asymptomatic

No injury
No uncontrolled bleeding
Tolerating prescribed activity
   without signs/symptoms of cardiac ischemia
	No injury
	No uncontrolled bleeding
	Tolerating prescribed activity
	   without signs/symptoms of cardiac ischemia
		No injury
		No uncontrolled bleeding
		Tolerating prescribed activity
		   without signs/symptoms of cardiac ischemia

TEACHING

Nursing
Instruct patient/family of signs
  and symptoms of cardiac
  ischemia and need to notify nurse
Review Micromedex drug information
Review angina vs MI
Review SL nitroglycerin
 	
Cardiac Rehabilitation
Activity guidelines
Signs and symptoms of overexertion
Reinforce smoking cessation
Registered Dietitian
Cardiac diet teaching on
  appropriate diet and printed diet information
	Nursing
	Instruct patient/family of signs
	  and symptoms of cardiac ischemia
	  and need to notify nurse
	Emergency planning:
	♥ Use of sublingual NTG
	♥ 911 System
	
	Cardiac Rehabilitation
	Home walking program
	Discuss phase II
	Reinforce smoking cessation
		Nursing
		Instruct patient/family of signs
		  and symptoms of cardiac
		  ischemia and need to notify nurse
		Review community resources
		Review final medication schedule
		Discharge instructions
		Emergency planning:
		♥ Use of sublingual NTG
		♥ 911 System
		
		Cardiac Rehabilitation
		Reinforce previous cardiac rehabilitation teaching
		Reinforce smoking cessation

pt/family verbalizes:
• Understanding of signs and
  symptoms of cardiac
  ischemia and when to notify nurse
• Rationale of diet principles
• Medication rationale and side effects
• Risks of smoking and heart
  disease and need for smoking cessation
• Use of sublingual NTG
	pt/family verbalizes:
	• Understanding of signs and
	  symptoms of cardiac ischemia
	  and when to notify nurse
	pt/family able to verbalize rationale
	for:
	• Home walking program
	• Signs and symptoms of
	  overexertion at home
	• Activity guidelines at home
	• 911 System
	• Use of sublingual NTG
		pt/family able to verbalize
		  rationale for:
		• Signs and symptoms of cardiac ischemia
		• Use of sublingual NTG
		• 911 System
		pt/family able to explain home medication schedule
		pt/family able to verbalize
		  community resources and understanding of discharge
		  instructions

DISCHARGE COORDINATION

Order home equipment if indicated
Notify homecare of early
  discharge if ordered
	Referral to phase II Cardiac Rehabilitation
	Notify homecare of discharge, if indicated
		Schedule entry into phase II
		  Cardiac Rehabilitation
		Notify homecare of discharge, if indicated

pt/family demonstrates
  equipment competencies
pt/family verbalizes rationale for
  homecare, if applicable
	pt/family verbalizes rationale for
	  Cardiac Rehabilitation
		pt/family verbalizes rationale for
		  Cardiac Rehabilitation

SIGNATURES

Health Care Team Signatures Signature/Initial/Print Name/Shift		**Health Care Team Signatures** Signature/Initial/Print Name/Shift		**Health Care Team Signatures** Signature/Initial/Print Name/Shift	
Signature	Initial	Signature	Initial	Signature	Initial
Print Name	Shift	Print Name	Shift	Print Name	Shift
Signature	Initial	Signature	Initial	Signature	Initial
Print Name	Shift	Print Name	Shift	Print Name	Shift
Signature	Initial	Signature	Initial	Signature	Initial
Print Name	Shift	Print Name	Shift	Print Name	Shift

Figure 10–4 *Continued*

Several large, multisite, international, randomized clinical trials have been conducted and support the efficacy of early use of thrombolytic agents in the treatment of AMI. Findings have consistently demonstrated the beneficial effects of thrombolytic therapy on patient outcomes and survival, particularly for patients treated within 1 hour of the onset of symptoms.[22] These effects include limiting the size of the infarct and often yielding a non–Q-wave MI with a borderline rise in CK enzymes. It has been predicted that 25 to 33% of patients presenting with an AMI would benefit from thrombolysis, yet as few as 18% actually receive a thrombolytic agent.[23] Some evidence indicates that older patients, African-American pa-

tients, and female patients are treated less aggressively with thrombolysis than other patients.[10,23] Chart 10–1 depicts a hypothetic situation that evolves around some of these factors.

Selection criteria for thrombolytic therapy include persistent chest pain that is typical of an AMI and is less than 6 hours in duration. In addition, ECG evidence is required and includes ST-segment elevation of 1 mm or more in two contiguous leads.[6] Several exclusion criteria exist and are based on the propensity of thrombolytic agents to precipitate severe bleeding, notably intracerebral hemorrhage. Although this complication occurs in only 0.3 to 0.7% of patients, the results are often catastrophic.[22] Chart 10–2 describes

TABLE 10–5
Comparisons of Major Thrombolytic Agents

Feature	Drug		
	Streptokinase	Recombinant Tissue Plasminogen Activator*	Anisoylated Plasminogen Streptokinase Activator
Dose	1.5 million IU in 60 min (750,000 IU over first 10 min)	100 mg in 90 min (15 mg over 1–2 min, then 50 mg over next 30 min, then 35 mg over next 60 min)	30 U in 2–5 min
Route	IV†	IV†	IV‡
Peak effect	1–2 hr	20–120 min	45 min
Duration of effect	Up to 12 hr	Up to 3 hr	4–6 hr
Elimination (half-life)	Biphasic: initially, 18 min; subsequent, 83 min	Rapid, >80% cleared within 10 min	90–120 min

*Accelerated dosage schedule for patients >67 kg.
†Should be administered through a dedicated intravenous (IV) line, using a volumetric infusion pump. After infusion, the line should be flushed with 25–30 mL normal saline solution.
‡Directly into a vein or by a free-flowing IV infusion of normal saline solution.

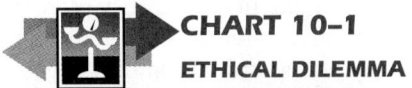

CHART 10–1
ETHICAL DILEMMA

A 76-year-old woman was admitted to the emergency room by ambulance from an assisted-living, retirement community. It was reported that the patient had complained of vague aches and pains for several hours. In the past hour, the patient became increasingly confused, and the ambulance was called. On admission, the patient was assessed and found to be a well-nourished, hydrated woman who was not oriented to time or place and was not in any apparent distress. Vital signs included the following: blood pressure, 156/90 mm Hg; heart rate, 62 beats per minute; and respiratory rate, 20. An initial ECG demonstrated a 1- 2-mm ST-segment elevation in leads II, III, and aVF. Baseline laboratory studies, including creatine kinase (CK) enzymes, are drawn, oxygen is started, and continuous ECG monitoring is maintained.

The patient's past medical history is positive for hypertension (for 23 years), mastectomy (8 years earlier), and recent onset of Alzheimer's disease (requiring assistance with activities of daily living and supervision). The patient does have an advance directive, although a copy did not accompany her to the hospital. A brother is listed as next of kin, and it is uncertain whether he has been notified.

The first CK result has returned and is normal. The physician elects not to evaluate the CK-MB. She states that, given the patient's age, past medical history of Alzheimer's disease, and the existence of an advance directive, she intends to treat the patient conservatively (with nitroglycerin and heparin). You are the nurse caring for this patient and believe that she would benefit from more aggressive therapy such as thrombolysis. You present your thoughts to the physician, and she emphasizes that the patient has an advance directive, indicating that she does not want any heroic measures. She also reminds you of the patient's history of Alzheimer's disease.

1. What do you believe is the basis of the conflict between the nurse and the physician?
2. What additional information would be helpful in defining this conflict?
3. Could any additional care decisions be considered for this patient?
4. Is the patient capable of making her own health care decisions? If not, what other options for decision makers are available?
5. What ethical principles do you believe are guiding the nurse's and physician's decisions?
6. What is the role of the nurse in this dilemma at this point?

CHART 10–2

Absolute Contraindications to Thrombolysis

Active or recent (4 weeks) internal bleeding

Intracranial neoplasm or recent head trauma

Prolonged, traumatic cardiopulmonary resuscitation

Suspected aortic dissection

History of hemorrhagic cerebrovascular accident

Sustained systemic blood pressure over 200/120 mm Hg in spite of medication

Trauma or surgery that is a potential bleeding source in the past 4 weeks

From Morris DC: Treatment of acute myocardial infarction by invasive cardiology techniques. Semin Thorac Cardiovasc Surg 7:185, 1995.

the absolute contraindications to the use of thrombolytics.

Thrombolysis for patients who are candidates is usually initiated in the emergency department, although this approach may change in the future. In one study, time from symptom onset to treatment was reduced from 110 to 77 minutes when prehospital-initiated thrombolytic therapy was compared with hospital-initiated therapy.[10] In preparation for administration of the thrombolytic agent, three large-bore (18-gauge) peripheral intravenous lines are started, and additional baseline laboratory studies (coagulation studies, complete blood count, blood chemistry) are obtained. Blood for future studies is obtained through one of the intravenous sites because venipunctures and intramuscular injections are contraindicated in patients receiving thrombolytics.

Bleeding precautions are initiated for all patients receiving thrombolytics because bleeding may be a major or minor complication of this therapy. Results of the Global Utilization of Streptokinase and Tissue Plasminogen Activator for Occluded Coronary Arteries (GUSTO-1) trial indicated that women experience serious bleeding as a complication of thrombolytic therapy significantly more often than men.[24] Table 10–6 provides nursing guidelines for monitoring patients on bleeding precautions.

Patients are generally transferred to a coronary or intensive care unit once thrombolytic therapy has been initiated. Patency of the infarct-related artery should be achieved in 60 to 85% of patients.[22] A major role of the nurse during this time is to observe the patient for signs of reperfusion. Monitoring includes resolution of chest pain, early peaking of CK-MB enzymes because of recanalization of the infarcted area and early removal of enzymes, reperfusion dysrhythmias such as accelerated idioventricular rhythm, ventricular tachycardia (VT), and AV blocks, and normalization of ST segments (see Chapter 8). Changes in the ST segment have been shown to be highly predictive of successful thrombolysis and preservation of the LV.[25] These changes should be noted within 2 to 3 hours after initiating the thrombolytic therapy.[26] Complete resolution of the ST segment is associated with smaller infarct areas and lower mortality rates, whereas no ST-segment resolution, indicating failed reperfusion, is predictive of high early mortality rates.[25] Unfortunately, presentation of these clinical findings after thrombolysis varies, and approximately 50% of patients with a patent infarct-related artery demonstrate none of the clinical signs of reperfusion.[27]

TABLE 10–6

Monitoring a Patient on Bleeding Precautions for Complications: Laboratory, Physical Assessment, and Subjective Data

Laboratory Data	Physical Assessment Data	Subjective Data
Reduction in hemoglobin, hematocrit	Ecchymosis, petechiae	Anxiety
	Bleeding gums	Palpitations
Coagulation studies exceeding therapeutic goals (aPTT, ACT)	Gross blood in stool, urine, emesis, nasogastric drainage, sputum	
Reduced platelets	Bleeding from IV sites, previous venipuncture or IM injection sites	
Occult blood in stool, urine, emesis, nasogastric drainage, sputum	Changes in mentation, level of consciousness	
	Changes in vital signs:	
	Decrease blood pressure	
	Increase heart rate	
	Cool, clammy skin	

aPTT, activated partial thromboplastin time; ACT, activated clotting time.

Invasive Techniques

Despite the widespread use of thrombolytics, problems do exist with the currently available agents. Resistance to reperfusion within 2 hours occurs in 15 to 40% of patients, and acute reocclusion of the involved artery occurs in 5 to 25% of patients.[22] Advances in angiography have led physicians to consider "rescue" angioplasty after failed thrombolysis.[27,28] Widespread use of this procedure has been limited because of the difficulty in determining failed thrombolysis, as discussed earlier. Current recommendations for rescue angioplasty include the situations in which clinical signs, ECG, and cardiac enzymes indicate continued occlusion of the left anterior descending coronary artery.[27]

The role of direct or primary angioplasty in patients who are eligible for thrombolytic therapy remains controversial. A review of the literature suggests that angioplasty should be considered as a primary treatment approach for the following patients: 1) those who are older or who are ineligible for thrombolytic therapy; 2) those presenting within 12 hours of an acute anterior infarction to a facility with an experienced team to perform angioplasty; and 3) those experiencing signs of cardiogenic shock (CHF, severe hypotension, and tachycardia).[6,27] See Chapter 9 for the preprocedure and postprocedure care of a patient undergoing angioplasty.

Surgical Techniques

Before the advent of thrombolytics and angioplasty, patients undergoing emergency surgical revascularization within 6 hours of an AMI demonstrated improved survival rates compared with those treated medically.[29] Currently, coronary artery bypass graft (CABG) surgery is recommended for patients who remain symptomatic after thrombolytic therapy or angioplasty or who have evidence of major multivessel disease.[27,30] Optimal outcomes are achieved when surgery is scheduled at least 48 hours after a Q-wave MI and at any time in symptomatic patients with non–Q-wave MIs.[30] See Chapter 13 for care of a patient undergoing CABG surgery.

Treatment Adjuncts

Certain treatment adjuncts are established concurrently with reperfusion strategies, whereas others are initiated in the hours, days, and weeks that follow successful reperfusion. These adjuncts include pharmacologic support, including oxygen therapy, continuous ECG monitoring, monitoring for complications, psychosocial support, risk factor modification, cardiac rehabilitation considerations, and preparation for discharge. The nurse works collaboratively with other members of the health care team to provide these elements of care to patients with an AMI and to their families.

Pharmacotherapy

Many of the harmful structural changes that occur in the myocardium after an AMI can be diminished by the administration of various pharmacologic agents. Most of these agents work to either increase myocardial oxygen supply or reduce myocardial oxygen demand. Table 10–7 provides a summary of the pharmacologic agents commonly used as adjuncts for patients with an AMI.

Nitrates. Nitroglycerin (NTG) has been in use for more than 100 years, and it remains the drug of choice for both angina and AMI. With both venodilation and arterial vasodilation effects, NTG effectively dilates the epicardial arteries, increases collateral blood flow, and decreases preload and afterload. Evidence suggests that NTG may also trigger an antiplatelet effect, a reduction in infarct size, and an improvement in ventricular remodeling.[6]

Sublingual (Nitrostat) or translingual (Nitrolingual) NTG is usually administered every 5 minutes for a total of three doses in the field or in the emergency department to patients with chest pain. The chest pain associated with an AMI is usually persistent and is not relieved with these forms of NTG. Intravenous NTG (Tridil) is initiated at a starting dose of 5 to 10 μg per minute and is titrated in 5- to 10-μg increments every 5 to 10 minutes until the patient is pain free or becomes hypotensive (systolic blood pressure <90 mm Hg). Special care should be taken with elderly patients who are receiving nitrates. This population is particularly sensitive to the hypotensive effects of nitrates because of age-related impairments of the baroreceptor reflex.[13] In addition, nitrates are used cautiously in patients with a right ventricular (RV) infarction because the resultant decrease in preload can exacerbate the hypotension that accompanies this type of infarct.

Intravenous NTG is usually tapered off in the intensive care unit when the patient is stable and is no longer experiencing chest pain. During this time, oral (e.g., Nitro-Bid), topical (e.g., Nitrol), or transdermal (e.g., Nitro-Dur) forms of NTG are initiated. Because of the propensity for nitrate tolerance to develop with the longer-acting forms of NTG, intermittent dosing is recommended and is usually accomplished by providing a 10- to 12-hour nitrate-free period. Antianginal protection is usually achieved during this time by the concurrent administration of other agents, such as beta blockers.

Assessment of the patient for persistent or recurrent chest pain is important throughout the period of hospitalization. Some evidence exists that patients may underreport or may fail to report chest pain to nurses. Explanations for this phenomenon include decisions by patients to see whether the pain would resolve spontaneously, a lack of patient awareness that all episodes of chest pain should be reported, and decisions by the patient that the pain is not serious enough

TABLE 10-7

Pharmacotherapeutic Adjuncts and Nursing Considerations for Patients Experiencing an Acute Myocardial Infarction

Drug	Recommended Dose	General Nursing Considerations
Nitrates		
Nitroglycerin (NTG):		Monitor effectiveness of drug by assessing patient for chest pain using standardized pain scale
		For IV, SL, and TL routes, monitor BP every 5 min until stable; for other routes, monitor BP per orders and assess for orthostatic hypotension
Sublingual (SL)	0.4 mg every 5 min × 3	Consider interactive effects on BP if administered with other hypotensive agents
Translingual (TL)	1 spray (0.4 mg) every 5 min × 3	Administer acetaminophen if headache develops
Intravenous (IV)	Begin at 5–10 µg/min and titrate (5–10 µg/min every 5–10 min) until pain is relieved or patient becomes hypotensive (systolic pressure <90 mm Hg); maximum dose not established	Monitor for s/s of methemoglobinemia* (pallor, dyspnea, cyanosis, coma) with prolonged use of high doses of IV NTG
When tapering IV NTG, consider conversion to:		Use infusion pump to deliver IV NTG
Oral	2.5 mg TID–QID to maximum of 26 mg/day	Dilute drug in compatible solution and use glass or nonabsorbable container; use non-PVC administration sets (to limit absorption of drug by tubing)
Topical	1–2 inches every 8 hr to maximum of 5 inches every 3–6 hr	When tapering IV NTG, reduce dose gradually to limit rebound chest pain or hypertension
Transdermal	0.2–0.4 mg/hr for 10–12 hr/day to maximum of 0.8 mg/hr for 10–12 hr/day	
Antiplatelet Agents		
Aspirin (ASA)	80–160 mg/day	Administer with meals to limit gastrointestinal distress
If unable to tolerate ASA: Ticlopidine hydrochloride	250 mg BID	Consider interactive effects on risk for bleeding if administered with other anticoagulants
		Therapeutic response for ticlopidine hydrochloride may take 2–3 mo to achieve
Anticoagulants		
Heparin	80 U/kg IV bolus, then 18 U/kg/hr infusion to keep aPTT 1.5–2 × patient control	Initiate bleeding precautions per policy
		In case of severe bleeding, administer protamine sulfate to neutralize heparin
		Monitor for interactive effects: NTG decreases anticoagulant effect; ASA increases anticoagulant effect
		Monitor for s/s of heparin-induced thrombocytopenia (HIT or white clot syndrome)†: impaired peripheral perfusion, pulmonary embolism, AMI, stroke)
		Use infusion pump to deliver dose
Analgesics		
Morphine	2–5 mg IV every 5–15 min	Administer dose slowly and observe for drop in BP, respiratory rate, central nervous system effects (sedation, confusion)
If RVMI, consider meperidine	10–50 mg IV every 2–4 hr	Consider interactive effects on BP when administered with other hypotensive drugs
		Assess the effectiveness of drug in relieving chest pain by using standardized pain scale
		Severe hypotensive effects most likely when dose is administered rapidly
		Administer naloxone for s/s of severe hypotension or respiratory depression
		Consider reduced dose in elderly patients and in those with hepatic or renal impairment

TABLE 10–7

Pharmacotherapeutic Adjuncts and Nursing Considerations for Patients Experiencing an Acute Myocardial Infarction (Continued)

Drug	Recommended Dose	General Nursing Considerations
Beta Blockers		
Metoprolol	5 mg IV every 5 min × 3, then 50 mg PO 15 min after completion of IV dosing, repeat PO dose every 6 hr for 48 hr	Administer IV dose slowly and monitor patient for symptomatic bradycardia, hypotension, and s/s of CHF and heart block
Atenolol	5 mg IV every 10 min × 2, then 50 mg PO 10 min after completion of IV dosing, repeat PO dose every 12 hr for 7 days	Monitor for interactive effects: increase in lidocaine levels may mask hypoglycemic symptoms in patients taking antidiabetic agents, additive effect on BP in patients receiving other hypotensive medications
		Consider reduced dose in elderly patients and in those with hepatic (metoprolol) and renal (atenolol) impairment
		Abrupt cessation of drug may precipitate chest pain, ventricular dysrhythmias, or AMI
ACE Inhibitors		
Captopril	6.25 mg PO as a test dose, then titrate to 50 mg TID	Assess BP and heart rate 1 to 2 hours (peak effect) after administering test dose
		Severe allergic reactions include angioedema and stridor
		Monitor patient for symptomatic hypotension, orthostatic hypotension
		Monitor for interactive effects: increase in serum digoxin levels, additive effects on BP in patients receiving other hypotensive medications
		Consider reduced dose in elderly patients and in those with renal impairment; may see hyperkalemia in patients with renal insufficiency and hypoglycemia in those with diabetes
		Administer 1 hr before or 2 hr after meals
		Abrupt cessation of drug can precipitate hypertension
Antidysrhythmics		
Lidocaine	Bolus dose of 1–1.5 mg/kg; may repeat dose (0.5 mg/kg) every 5–10 min, not to exceed a total dose of 3 mg/kg	Monitor ECG for effectiveness in controlling ventricular ectopy; may worsen dysrhythmias
	Initiate maintenance infusion of 2–4 mg/min	Assess BP every 5 min during loading dose and every 15–60 min once stable
		Use lower bolus doses in the elderly and in patients with liver disease and CHF
		Assess for adverse central nervous system effects (tremors, confusion, and agitation) and s/s of toxicity (somnolence, seizures, respiratory depression, hypotension, cardiac arrest); rapid injection often associated with seizures
		Monitor for interactive effects: increase risk of hypotension, bradycardia, and toxicity when administered with beta blockers
		Monitor serum lidocaine levels
		Use infusion pump to deliver continuous dose

Table continued on following page

TABLE 10–7

Pharmacotherapeutic Adjuncts and Nursing Considerations for Patients Experiencing an Acute Myocardial Infarction (Continued)

Drug	Recommended Dose	General Nursing Considerations
Others		
Magnesium	1–4 g IV bolus over 5–20 min, then 0.5–1 g/hr × 24 hr	Rapid injection may cause hypotension, heart block, or cardiac arrest Monitor vital signs every 15 min after bolus dose Assess respiratory status: rate, rhythm, quality Monitor for s/s of hypermagnesemia (loss of deep tendon reflexes, heart block, respiratory paralysis) Treat toxicity with calcium gluconate to reverse respiratory depression and heart block
Oxygen	2–4 L/min by nasal cannula	Titrate as needed and based on appropriate laboratory or assessment data Discontinue once patient's condition stabilizes

AMI, acute myocardial infarction; BP, blood pressure; CHF, congestive heart failure; RVMI, right ventricular myocardial infarction; s/s, signs and symptoms.

*Methemoglobinemia is a rare side effect that results from the oxidation of the heme iron by nitrates to the ferric state (methemoglobin), making it incapable of transporting oxygen.

†HIT is found in approximately 10% of patients receiving heparin therapy and is thought to be a result of the production of antiplatelet antibodies that induce clotting.

to report or to bother staff.[31] The nurse's ongoing evaluation of patients for chest pain should include an explanation of the importance of reporting all episodes of chest pain and the use of patients' own descriptors for chest pain when performing assessments.

Aspirin. The role of aspirin in the treatment of patients with AMIs has been clearly demonstrated.[4,6] Aspirin inhibits platelet aggregation and provides a rapid antithrombic effect in the presence of an AMI. Doses as low as 80 to 160 mg per day are recommended for patients diagnosed with an AMI and as a preventive measure for patients at risk of an AMI. Aspirin is usually administered to all patients with symptoms of an AMI either in the field or immediately on arrival to the emergency department.

For patients who cannot tolerate aspirin, other antiplatelet agents are available, such as ticlopidine hydrochloride (Ticlid) and dipyridamole (Persantine), although their immediate and maximal effects require a significantly longer time compared with the rapid onset (within 15 minutes) of aspirin's effects.

Anticoagulants. The administration of anticoagulants, specifically heparin sodium (Liquaemin), is recommended for all patients experiencing an AMI who do not receive thrombolytic therapy. The use of heparin in these patients has shown to reduce the complications of an AMI and to decrease reinfarction and mortality rates.[4,6]

Reocclusions, usually occurring within the first 12 to 24 hours after thrombolytic therapy, are problematic and represent a limitation of thrombolytic agents.[22] The administration of heparin during and after thrombolytic therapy is thought to reduce early reocclusion of the infarct-related artery and other complications such as deep vein thrombosis, pulmonary embolism, early reinfarction, and death.[32] Heparin works by inhibiting free thrombin, but it does not inactivate thrombin that is bound to fibrin.[22] Results of various trials exploring the efficacy of adding heparin to the treatment regimen after the use of thrombolytic agents have been ambiguous.[22,32] In addition, further controversy exists regarding heparin dosing and route of administration.

Current recommendations for the initiation of heparin vary according to the thrombolytic agent used. For patients receiving rt-PA, intravenous heparin should be initiated concurrently, using a weight-based dosing schedule (Table 10–8) and maintained for 24 to 72 hours. Studies have shown that non–weight-based heparin dosing is generally ineffective in achieving therapeutic levels of anticoagulation, especially in the first 24 hours of therapy.[6,32] Lower-dose or subcutaneous heparin therapy is probably adequate for patients receiving SK, and no added benefit has been noted with the administration of heparin in patients receiving APSAC.[32]

Several newer anticoagulants have been developed and may help to resolve some of the controversies surrounding heparin. Unlike heparin, hirudin and bivalirudin (Hirulog) are angiotensin III–independent thrombin inhibitors that work by accessing and inactivating thrombin that is bound to fibrin.[22] Early studies have shown promising results.

TABLE 10–8
Heparin Dosing Nomograms

Weight-based Doses		Non–Weight-based Doses	
Initial dose: 80 U/kg bolus, then 18 U/kg/hr		Initial dose: 5000 U bolus, then 1000 U/hr	
aPTT* (sec)	Dosage Adjustment	aPTT* (sec)	Dosage Adjustment
<35 (<1.2 × control)	80 U/kg bolus, increase maintenance dose by 4 U/kg/hr	<35 (<1.2 × control)	5000 U bolus, increase maintenance dose by 200 U/hr
35–45 (1.2–1.5 × control)	40 U/kg bolus, increase maintenance dose by 2 U/kg/hr	35–45 (1.2–1.5 × control)	2500 U bolus, increase maintenance dose by 100 U/hr
46–70 (1.5–2.3 × control)	No change	46–70 (1.5–2.3 × control)	No change
71–90 (2.3–3 × control)	Decrease maintenance dose by 2 U/kg/hr	71–90 (2.3–3 × control)	Decrease maintenance dose by 100 U/hr
>90 (>3 × control)	Hold infusion for 1 hr, then decrease maintenance dose by 3 U/kg/hr	>90 (>3 × control)	Hold infusion for 1 hr, then decrease maintenance dose by 200 U/hr

*Activated partial thromboplastin time, assessed from blood drawn 6 hours after the initial dose and every 6 hours after dosage adjustment. From Bowlby H, Hisle K, Clifton GD: Heparin as adjunctive therapy to coronary thrombolysis in acute myocardial infarction. Heart Lung 24:299, 1995.

Certain low-molecular-weight heparins (LMWHs) have been developed, and one, enoxaparin sodium (Lovenox), has been approved for use in the United States by the Food and Drug Administration. Although these agents are currently used to prevent venous thrombosis in high-risk patients, studies of the use of LMWHs in the treatment of an AMI should be anticipated. These newer forms of heparin have the potential to achieve antithrombotic activity while reducing bleeding complications.[32]

Patients receiving heparin therapy in conjunction with thrombolytics are at greater risk of bleeding complications and require close observation (see Table 10–6). Therapeutic levels of anticoagulation with heparin are achieved when the activated partial thromboplastin time (aPTT) is 1.5 to 2 times the patient control. Evidence indicates that subtherapeutic levels of heparin have a minor effect on reducing reinfarction and mortality rates after thrombolysis.[22,32] Consequently, the nurse must carefully evaluate the patient's aPTT and must initiate adjustments in collaboration with the physician. Table 10–8 presents two possible nomograms for heparin dosing.

The use of activated clotting time (ACT) to assess the therapeutic levels of heparin has been advocated. The automated ACT on whole blood is easy to perform, can be done at the bedside, and may provide a more accurate picture of the anticoagulant effect of heparin.[32]

Patients experiencing an AMI are frequently receiving intravenous NTG and heparin. Concurrent administration of these drugs produces an antagonistic effect on the function of heparin, resulting in difficulty in achieving therapeutic levels of anticoagulation. These patients may require larger doses of heparin to achieve therapeutic goals. Conversely, nurses must monitor aPTTs closely when discontinuing NTG.

Analgesics. In the early hours of an AMI, chest pain is usually severe and may not be relieved by intravenous NTG. The drug of choice to treat the pain of an MI is morphine sulfate (Duramorph). In addition to pain relief, morphine reduces both preload and afterload and decreases myocardial oxygen demand. A reduction in anxiety and in the sensation of dyspnea may be additional benefits of morphine and may lead to a decrease in circulating catecholamines and, possibly, ventricular irritability.[6] Morphine is administered in 2- to 5-mg intravenous bolus doses and may be repeated every 5 to 15 minutes. Patients receiving morphine must be monitored frequently for signs of hypotension and respiratory depression. Like nitrates, morphine is generally contraindicated in patients with a RV infarction because the resultant decrease in preload can also exacerbate the hypotension that accompanies this type of infarct. Meperidine hydrochloride (Demerol) should be considered for pain control in these patients.

Beta Blockers. As many as 32 randomized clinical trials have studied the efficacy of beta blockers in the treatment of patients with AMIs. Analyses of data have confirmed that the use of these agents results in decreases in infarct size and reductions in reinfarction and mortality rates.[6,33] These effects appear to be more pronounced in older patients (≥65 years) and in patients with larger infarcts.[33] Beta blockers work by selectively blocking beta$_1$-adrenergic receptors located primarily in cardiac muscle, thus rendering the receptors inaccessible to circulating catecholamines. The net result is a decrease in heart rate and contractility, which ultimately increases coronary blood flow, decreases myocardial oxygen demand, and decreases the incidence of cardiac rupture and ventricular fibrillation (VF). When beta blockers are combined with thrombolytics, reinfarction rates and recurrent ischemia are reduced.

Beta blockers should be administered to patients experiencing an AMI within 2 hours of presentation. Intravenous metoprolol (Lopressor) or atenolol (Tenormin) should be initiated in the emergency department or the intensive care unit and followed with an oral dosing schedule (see Table 10–7). Contraindications include bradycardia, hypotension, moderate to severe CHF, advanced AV blocks, and certain pulmonary disorders (e.g., severe chronic obstructive pulmonary disease and asthma).[6] Although beneficial to elderly patients, beta blockers are also used cautiously in this population because many present with preexisting low resting heart rates resulting from a decrease in the cardiac response to beta-adrenergic stimulation. In addition, the elderly demonstrate a diminished baroreceptor sensitivity.[13] These age-related changes may intensify the likelihood of side effects related to beta blockers such as postural hypotension, bradycardia, and syncope.

Angiotensin Converting Enzyme (ACE) Inhibitors. Soon after an AMI, changes in the size and shape of the myocardium begin to occur through a process described as ventricular remodeling. This slow, progressive process extends over the first year and results in a ventricular dilatation that predisposes patients to CHF and premature death.[33] Data from the Survival and Ventricular Enlargement (SAVE) trial demonstrated that captopril (Capoten), and angiotensin-converting enzyme (ACE) inhibitor, reduced ventricular dilatation, prevented CHF, and reduced mortality related to an AMI.[33]

The renin–angiotensin system is activated shortly after an AMI. The resultant production of angiotensin II, a potent vasoconstrictor, increases both preload and afterload, which then enhances ventricular remodeling. By blocking the conversion of angiotensin I to angiotensin II with ACE inhibitors, LV dilatation is reduced, as are the subsequent complications associated with ventricular remodeling.[34]

Recommendations for the initiation of ACE inhibitor therapy varies depending on the particular agent selected. For example, oral captopril therapy should begin with an initial test dose of 6.25 mg 3 to 16 days after an AMI is confirmed. Therapy should be titrated over the next several weeks until the target dose of 50 mg three times daily is achieved.[33] Patients are usually in a step-down or intermediate care unit when this therapy is initiated. Nurses must monitor patients carefully for changes in blood pressure or ischemia when administering the test dose and subsequent doses. Maximal effects on blood pressure occur 60 to 90 minutes after administration, and concomitant therapies that also reduce blood pressure (e.g., ni-

trates) can precipitate symptomatic hypotension.[33] Therapy with ACE inhibitors is usually well tolerated by the elderly, is used cautiously in patients with renal impairment, and is contraindicated in patients with symptomatic LV dysfunction.

Magnesium. The role of magnesium in the treatment of AMI has received renewed interest. The second Leicester Intravenous Magnesium Intervention Trial (LIMIT-2) examined the effect of an intravenous regimen of magnesium in patients with an AMI. Early results of this therapy included reduced mortality and reduced incidence of LV failure.[35] The first minutes of reperfusion of an infarcted coronary artery have been associated with increases in intracellular calcium, depletion of high-energy phosphates, and contractile dysfunction. Magnesium is thought to moderate these negative effects by preserving contractile function, but the window of opportunity is limited to the minutes surrounding reperfusion.[35] For patients experiencing an AMI and who are not candidates for thrombolysis, magnesium should be considered. Recommendations include initiating a loading dose of intravenous magnesium in the emergency department and maintaining a continuous infusion for 24 hours (see Table 10–7). For patients receiving thrombolytic therapy, the use of magnesium remains questionable. If considered, magnesium therapy should be initiated before thrombolytics.[6, 35]

Oxygen. The routine use of oxygen therapy in patients with uncomplicated MIs has been challenged. Currently, supplemental oxygen by nasal cannula at 2 to 4 L per minute is ordered for most patients and is initiated in the emergency department. The rationale for this therapy is based on the premise that these patients demonstrate some degree of hypoxemia, probably because of a ventilation–perfusion mismatch.[6] Other sources suggest that the primary use of oxygen is to prevent or to maximize myocardial oxygenation to prevent or to minimize the development of dysrhythmias. Oxygen therapy can usually be discontinued once the patient is clinically stable and is transferred to the step-down or intermediate care unit.

ECG Monitoring

For patients with an AMI, continuous ECG monitoring is established in the field and is maintained throughout the period of hospitalization. Nurses in the emergency department, intensive care unit, and intermediate care unit need well-developed ECG interpretation skills. Early recognition of ECG evidence of infarction, dysrhythmias, reperfusion, and reocclusion is necessary to plan treatment strategies, to prevent or detect complications, to evaluate interventions, and to achieve optimal patient outcomes. Refer to Chapter 8 for information on ECG interpretation.

As mentioned earlier, patterns of 12-lead ECG changes, particularly ST-segment–T-wave changes, provide important data regarding the presence and location of an AMI. Patients with an AMI have an "ischemic fingerprint," that is, a 12-lead ECG pattern unique to the patient and related to the anatomic location of the infarcted artery.[36] This fingerprint is readily apparent in the ECGs recorded early in the MI process and before reperfusion therapy is initiated. Investigators have suggested that resolution of ST-segment elevation is an excellent prognostic indicator of reperfusion.[25, 26] Similarly, evidence of acute reocclusion after successful reperfusion therapy can be documented by a return of the "ischemic fingerprint" with or without additional clinical manifestations.[36] Newer bedside ECG monitors and telemetry monitors are equipped with ST-segment monitoring capability as well as multichannel capability. It has been recommended that nurses monitor one of the six limb leads in addition to one of the recommended dysrhythmia leads (V_1 or V_6) in patients with an AMI.[36] Selection of the limb lead should be guided by the patient's ischemic fingerprint. When this information is unknown, nurses should select leads V_1 and III or V_1 and aVF to obtain the best dual-lead combination for detection of dysrhythmias or ischemia (see Chart 8–7).[36]

Monitoring for Complications

Complications of an AMI can be categorized as electrical, structural, hemodynamic, or inflammatory. Complications are related to the size and location of the infarction and occur most often within 2 to 3 days of the event, although some complications may evolve over weeks. The role of the nurse in the prompt detection of post-MI complications requires superior observational and assessment skills as well as technologic competence.

Electrical: Dysrhythmias

Successful thrombolysis has been associated with the development of transient "reperfusion rhythms," specifically, accelerated idioventricular rhythm (AIVR), VT, and AV blocks, within the first 2 hours of initiation of thrombolytic agents. The nurse should recognize these rhythms because AIVR is usually tolerated well and is not treated. Treatment for sustained VT and symptomatic AV blocks is usually according to Advanced Cardiac Life Support (ACLS) guidelines (see Appendix). Careful and frequent evaluation of the patient's vital signs during these episodes is critical.

Most patients develop some dysrhythmias after an AMI. The most common cause of these dysrhythmias is ischemic injury, resulting in changes in membrane excitability and in the conduction and refractory periods of myocardial cells. Prompt attention to dysrhythmias is paramount because the ischemic myocardium has a lower fibrillatory threshold, and, consequently, few dysrhythmias are considered benign after an infarct.

The risk of sudden cardiac death from VT or VF after an AMI and unrelated to reperfusion usually occurs during the first few hours after the onset of symptoms. Unfortunately, this period is often when patients are deciding on a course of action relative to their symptoms. The risk of VT or VF after an AMI decreases over the first 24 hours. Treatment involves the prompt initiation of ACLS guidelines (see Appendix). Nursing considerations for the care of patients after successful resuscitation that are often underemphasized are described in Chart 10–3.

Implantable Cardioverter Defibrillator. Survivors of sudden cardiac arrest may be assessed further with electrophysiologic studies and treated prophylactically with antidysrhythmic agents, and, in some cases, they may be candidates for an implantable cardioverter defibrillator (ICD). Care of patients requiring an ICD involves a team approach. Physicians, nurses, advanced nurse practitioners, and pacemaker representatives are needed to met the diverse needs of these patients and their families.

INDICATIONS. Patients who have survived an episode of sudden cardiac arrest or who have documented life-threatening, medication-refractory ventricular dysrhythmias are candidates for an ICD. Research supports the efficacy of this therapy because mortality rates are decreased in patients who receive ICDs when compared with patients treated with conventional therapy.[37] Currently, more than 15,000 patients in the United States have an ICD.

DEVICE. Like a pacemaker, the ICD is composed of a pulse generator and a lead system. The pulse generator, powered by a lithium battery with a life expectancy of more than 5 years and about the size of a deck of cards, is usually placed in a subcutaneous pocket in the patient's abdomen. The endocardial lead system is possible for most patients and involves the insertion of the lead into the right ventricle through the left subclavian vein. The lead end is then tunneled to the pulse generator, where it is connected. The Endotak lead system (CPI) consists of a tripolar lead tip. Two of the electrodes are dedicated to dysrhythmia detecting and delivering a shock; the remaining electrode is dedicated to sensing the heart rate.[38]

FUNCTIONS. The functions of the newer, third-generation ICDs include antitachycardia pacing (ATP), cardioversion, defibrillation, and antibradycardia pacing (ABP). These ICDs can be programmed to provide "tiered therapy." On sensing dysrhythmias, a tailored treatment program can be initiated and can include different combinations of the unit's functions.

CHART 10–3

RESEARCH UTILIZATION: NURSING CONSIDERATIONS FOR CARE OF PATIENTS AFTER A NEAR-DEATH EXPERIENCE

Abstract: Many people who survive a near-fatal crisis report some variant of a phenomenon known as the near-death experience (NDE). These numbers are expected to increase because of advances in technology. This study examined critical care nurses' knowledge about and attitudes toward the NDE. A self-administered questionnaire was distributed to 1000 participants at a national critical care nursing conference. Six research questions exploring nurses' interest, knowledge, attitudes, and interventions related to patients reporting an NDE were posed in this descriptive, comparative study. Findings (N = 448) indicated high levels of interest in the NDE but minimal knowledge about the phenomenon itself. Most respondents reported believing in the phenomenon and desired educational programs about the NDE. Finally, critical care nurses identified interventions for patients "surviving" an NDE.

Critique: Because of the nature of nonprobability and convenience sampling, the results of this survey are limited and are best used cautiously beyond the sample. The sample demographics are suggestive, however, of the larger critical care nursing community. Further work on the development of research-based therapeutic nursing interventions for this patient population is recommended.

Nursing Considerations: Patients survive near death and experience NDEs in various settings: community, emergency department, intensive care unit, and intermediate care unit. Nurses are the most likely providers of care to survivors of NDEs. First, the nurse must properly identify patients to extend physical and psychological support. The nurse must also be able to facilitate communication about the NDE among patients, their families, and other health care providers. The following general **guidelines** are recommended for nurses who care for patients who report an NDE:

1. Evaluate one's own knowledge and attitudes about NDEs. An open and inquiring mind is essential to recognize the possibility of an NDE.
2. Include NDE in patient assessments. The nurse must be alert to the subtle signs of an NDE by being an active listener and careful observer. Patients may seem distracted or may mention an unusual dream. Use open-ended statements such as "Tell me what you remember about the event" when assessing patients.
3. After collecting data regarding the NDE, several nursing diagnoses may be appropriate. These could include alterations in sensory perception, knowledge deficit, and ineffective family coping.

Specific guidelines for nursing interventions can be discussed from two perspectives: care **during** the near-death event and care **after** the event. Appropriate interventions to use while a patient is experiencing a near-death event follow:

1. Place a care giver near the patient's head.
2. Avoid threatening or suggestive language, and, if possible, have someone hold the patient's hand during the resuscitation.
3. Allow a family member, if possible, in the resuscitation room.

When the patient has regained consciousness, different nursing interventions are necessary. After resuscitation, the nurse should focus equally on the patient's psychological and critical physiologic needs for at least 4 hours. Some postevent interventions follow:

1. Begin a systematic orientation to reality.
2. Develop a trusting relationship with the patient and the family.
3. Encourage the patient to discuss any recollections about the event. Discussions should also involve the family at some point.
4. Offer verbal and nonverbal reassurance.
5. Document the patient's report of the NDE.

Limited information about the NDE is available in the current professional literature. This gap in information presents a dilemma for the nurse who practices in an area where death is frequently imminent and where holistic care is crucial. The increasing number of persons reporting NDEs, coupled with the similarities of these reports, should encourage nurses to be more receptive, inquisitive, and supportive of this group of patients. Nurses must learn from these patients in order to identify the specific, therapeutic nursing interventions that best meet these patients' needs.

Source: Bucher L, Wimbush F, Hardie T, et al: Near death experiences: critical care nurses' attitudes and interventions. Dimensions Crit Care Nurs 16:194–201, 1997.

Lower-rate tachycardias may be treated first with ATP, pacing at a rate that exceeds the native rate, in an effort to abolish the tachydysrhythmia. One advantage of this treatment is that it is not generally perceived by the patient. If the tachycardia persists or accelerates, the ICD may attempt a low-energy, synchronized cardioversion; if the rhythm disintegrates into VF, the ICD could deliver a series of increasingly powerful shocks to defibrillate the patient. Patients' reports of these shocks vary from mildly uncomfortable to severely painful. Bradycardiac rhythms often result from this sequence, and, consequently, the patient may require a short period of ventricular pacing after conversion.[37]

Like pacemakers, ICDs can sense, pace, capture, or shock inappropriately or ineffectively. To facilitate troubleshooting these problems, ICDs have advanced memory capabilities for sensed events and subsequent therapies and telemetry capabilities for programming adjustments.

PERIOPERATIVE MANAGEMENT. Patients and families should be provided with appropriate education and emotional support before the implantation of the ICD. These patients have often experienced sudden cardiac arrest, and denial, anxiety, disbelief, confusion, and distress have been noted in these patients after the event.[39]

The ICD is implanted while the patient is under general anesthesia. During the procedure, the physician, in consultation with the pacemaker representative, determines stimulation and sensing thresholds. Malignant dysrhythmias are induced, and the defibrillation threshold is established. The device is usually left inactive for 2 to 3 days after the procedure because the transient dysrhythmias that often develop postoperatively may falsely trigger a shock.[38]

Patients are usually ambulatory on postoperative day 1 and are discharged by postoperative day 3. ECG monitoring is necessary while the ICD is inactive. Should the patient require external defibrillation, an anteroposterior paddle placement should be used.

DISCHARGE CONSIDERATIONS. Patients and their families need information on the care of the implant site, including signs and symptoms of complications, anticipated sensations should the device fire, documentation of device-related events, actions to take should the device deliver a shock, and importance of carrying device identification as well as MedicAlert identification.[38] Cardiopulmonary resuscitation (CPR) training for family members may be recommended, although some research has indicated that it could contribute to higher levels of anxiety and depression.[39]

Patients also need information on the effects of external magnets on the device. External magnets are used by health care providers to activate and deactivate ICDs. However, inadvertent exposure to environmental magnets or magnetic fields may deactivate the device and may leave the patient unprotected. In most cases, the device emits tones signaling activation or deactivation.

Finally, activity guidelines should be defined for these patients. Because patients with ICDs could experience syncope or even loss of consciousness with a device-related event, it is often recommended that they do *not* drive. Adjustment to life after receiving an ICD can be challenging for these patients and their families. Nurses should inform patients and families of support groups that may be available and can provide a means for improving quality of life after ICD implantation.[37]

Ventricular ectopy is also common and transient in the early hours of an AMI. Intravenous lidocaine hydrochloride (Xylocaine) continues to be the drug of choice for rapidly treating patients with persistent or complex ventricular ectopy, such as more than six premature ventricular contractions (PVCs) per minute, R on T phenomenon, and multifocal PVCs. The prophylactic use of lidocaine is not recommended for patients experiencing an AMI.

Various etiologic factors may precipitate ventricular ectopy later in the course of recovery and include hypoxia, ischemia, acid–base imbalances, electrolyte imbalances (e.g., hypokalemia and hypomagnesemia), and drugs (e.g., digoxin [Lanoxin]). Treatment modalities (e.g., oxygen therapy and electrolyte replacement) are usually dictated by the cause. If these factors are ruled out or are treated and ventricular ectopy persists, then treatment with oral antidysrhythmic agents, such as procainamide hydrochloride (Pronestyl), quinidine sulfate (Quinidex), and amiodarone hydrochloride (Cordarone) is often indicated.[4] The development of postinfarction dysrhythmias over the days after the event can be categorized as either bradydysrhythmias or tachydysrhythmias (see Chapter 8). Bradycardiac rhythms can result from both inferior and anterior MIs. Occlusions in the right coronary artery, which supplies the SA and AV node, result in inferior wall infarctions that often precipitate sinus node dysfunction. This condition can be manifested by sinus bradycardia, sinus arrhythmia, sinus pauses, or atrial fibrillation. In most patients, sinus node dysfunction is benign and transient, resolving within 4 hours of onset.

Inferior MIs also result in major AV blocks in 15 to 33% of patients. These blocks are usually second-degree AV blocks, Mobitz type I (Wenckebach), and usually resolve within 2 weeks. For patients who develop complete heart block, the onset is usually within 72 hours of an AMI, with an earlier onset (within 6 hours) causing severe bradycardia. When the onset occurs after 6 hours of an AMI, the block generally progresses slowly through first-degree block, second-degree block, and so forth, before ending in complete heart block. The role of the nurse in the surveillance of patients and their rhythms cannot be overemphasized.

The pharmacologic management of patients with inferior MIs who experience symptomatic sinus bradycardia or high-grade AV blocks with bradycardia should include the careful administration or delay of medications that could further depress the sinus or AV node (beta blockers). Treatment of symptomatic bradycardia should be according to ACLS guidelines and may include atropine or temporary pacing (see Chapter 8).

Occlusions in the left anterior descending coronary artery, which supplies the myocardial tissue that contains the bundle of His, bundle branches, and Purkinje system, result in anterior wall infarctions that can also precipitate heart block. These heart blocks are a result of intraventricular conduction defects, and when they occur, mortality rates are increased. Some investigators believe that prophylactic temporary pacing (either transcutaneous or transvenous) may be appropriate in these patients, although most deaths in this population are attributed to ventricular failure rather than to conduction defects.[40] However, for patients who do survive, permanent pacing is reserved for those in whom heart block does not resolve.

Tachydysrhythmias occur most frequently in the presence of anterior MIs and include sinus tachycardia, atrial fibrillation, atrial flutter, and paroxysmal supraventricular tachycardia. The deleterious effect of these rapid rhythms on myocardial oxygen consumption cannot be overstated. Various causes precipitate these rhythms and include pain, anxiety, hypovolemia, atrial distention from fluid overload, and CHF. Rapid and accurate assessment of these patients by the nurse is integral to the proper selection of treatment modalities. For example, if patients are experiencing sinus tachycardia because of anxiety or pain, then they should receive appropriate anxiolytics or analgesics. If tachydysrhythmias develop in response to the injured myocardium and no signs of CHF are present, beta blocker therapy is effective in reducing heart rates and in preserving myocardial tissue.

Premature atrial contractions in the presence of an AMI are often an early warning sign of CHF. The further development of supraventricular tachydysrhythmias often reflects LV dysfunction and impending CHF.[40] Initiation of diuretic and digoxin therapy is usually effective in treating overt CHF (see Chapter 11).

Structural Defects After Acute Myocardial Infarction

Structural defects after an AMI are often devastating and include papillary muscle rupture, ventricular septal rupture, and ventricular aneurysm. The risk of these complications is generally greatest within the first week of an AMI.

Papillary muscle rupture may be either partial or complete and results from prolonged ischemia to the area surrounding the mitral valve. Complete rupture usually presents with severe sudden mitral regurgitation, shock, and death in 95% of patients experiencing this defect. Patients with a partial rupture also present with mitral regurgitation, but they may be stabilized with the intra-aortic balloon pump and inotropic agents (e.g., dobutamine hydrochloride [Dobutrex]) in preparation for emergent mitral valve replacement surgery. Nurses need to assess patients carefully for evidence of pulmonary edema or a sudden holosystolic heart murmur because these clinical manifestations represent the onset of physiologic decline associated with this defect.

Like papillary muscle rupture, ventricular septal rupture results from prolonged ischemia to the intraventricular septum. The end result of ventricular rupture is biventricular failure due to the shunting of blood from the LV to the RV through the septal defect. This shunting increases RV pressure, pulmonary blood flow, and left preload and decreases cardiac output. These hemodynamic consequences present in patients as sudden hypotension, chest pain, loud S_2, and a new holosystolic murmur. Diagnosis is easily confirmed with bedside echocardiography or when blood samples from a pulmonary artery catheter demonstrate elevated levels of partial pressure of oxygen. The patient's condition is stabilized first with afterload reducers (e.g., nitroprusside sodium [Nipride]) and the intra-aortic balloon pump, although emergency correction of the defect is required and is foremost to the patient's survival.

Ventricular aneurysms are thin-walled, noncontractile outpouchings of the ventricle (usually the left) and are commonly located in the apex region of the heart (Figure 10–5). Ventricular aneurysms are suspected in patients with persistent ST segment elevation, distortion of the cardiac image on the chest radiograph, and the presence of a holosystolic, apical thrust. Diagnosis is easily confirmed with bedside echocardiography. Pathophysiologic consequences of ventricular aneurysms depend on the amount of myocardium involved and, in general, include CHF, LV thromboembolism, VT, and chest pain.[41] Management involves prevention (e.g., early reperfusion to limit infarct size) and treatment according to the clinical manifestations. Patients with mild CHF are treated with usual pharmacologic agents, such as digoxin and diuretics; patients with thromboembolism are treated with anticoagulation therapy, specifically heparin followed by warfarin sodium (Coumadin) for 3 months after the infarct. Patients with ventricular tachydysrhythmias are treated with antidysrhythmics as determined by electrophysiologic studies and, if necessary, implantable cardiodefibrillator or ablative therapy. Chest pain in these patients is treated primarily with nitrates, with beta blockers used cautiously in patients with LV dysfunction in the nonaneurysmal segments. Surgical inter-

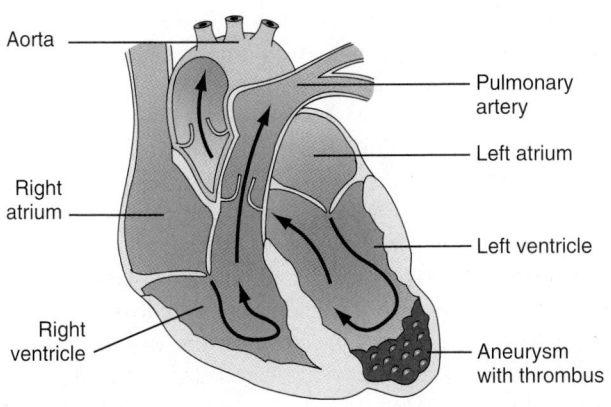

Figure 10–5

Structural complication of an acute myocardial infarction: left ventricular aneurysm.

ventions are considered for patients with refractory angina and high-risk coronary anatomy, with aneurysmectomy performed secondary to the revascularization procedure.[41]

Hemodynamic Alterations After Acute Myocardial Infarction

The development of CHF or cardiogenic shock after an acute AMI is intimately related to the size of the infarction. As previously described, CHF is a common sequela of an AMI that involves the LV, and hemodynamic alterations can range from mild (e.g., bibasilar rales responsive to diuretics) to severe (e.g., severe hypotension, hypoperfusion, and tissue hypoxia leading to cardiogenic shock). See Chapters 11 and 47 for complete descriptions of the pathophysiology and management of CHF and cardiogenic shock.

RV infarctions are present in approximately one-third of patients with inferior wall MIs because the right coronary artery supplies the inferior wall of the LV and the RV. These patients should be monitored for RV failure. Clinical manifestations include increases in RV end-diastolic, right atrial, and central venous pressures and a decrease in RV output. Reduced pulmonary blood flow precipitates a decrease in left end-diastolic pressure and, consequently, a drop in cardiac output. Patients demonstrate hypotension, distended jugular veins, clear chest radiographs, and a murmur related to tricuspid regurgitation. In this situation, the patient is experiencing relative hypovolemia, and fluids are administered to increase preload. Nitrates should be used cautiously in these patients, and morphine should be replaced with meperidine for pain control. If fluids do not correct the failure, dobutamine should be considered.

The role of the nurse in monitoring patients for hemodynamic changes after an AMI is paramount and can influence the patient's prognosis. Accurate and frequent patient assessments (e.g., vital signs, heart and breath sounds, peripheral pulses, capillary refill, and chest pain) often provide timely clues to the onset of CHF or impending shock.

Inflammatory Responses After Acute Myocardial Infarction

Pericarditis, an inflammation of the pericardial membrane lining the area of infarction, can occur 2 to 4 days after an AMI. Clinical manifestations include precordial pain different from the presenting chest pain that increases during deep inspiration, a pericardial friction rub that can be auscultated in some, but not all, cases, and persistent ST-segment elevation. Treatment with nonsteroidal, anti-inflammatory agents (e.g., indomethacin [Indocin]) for 3 to 5 days is highly effective and usually brings rapid relief of symptoms. Late pericarditis, called Dressler's syndrome, occurs anywhere from 1 week to several months after an AMI and is almost always accompanied by a pericardial friction rub. Chest pain similar to the pain of early pericarditis, diffuse ST-segment changes, fever, arthralgias, and pericardial effusion may also be present in these patients. Treatment is similar to that of early pericarditis, although oral corticosteroids (e.g., prednisone) may be considered.

In summary, the nurse needs to be aware of the various complications that can develop after an AMI, as well as the time frames in which they are likely to occur. Diligent and ongoing assessment of the patient's heart, lungs, periphery, and ECG throughout all phases of the hospitalization alerts the nurse to the onset of these complications and assists the physician in determining appropriate interventions. Evaluating the effects of subsequent interventions becomes equally important. Continued assessment for complications or evaluation of interventions by nurses can extend beyond hospitalization to the outpatient clinic and the home care setting.

Psychosocial Support

The onset of an AMI is usually sudden and often occurs in persons who previously believed they were healthy. Further, many persons believe that an AMI places them close to death, and, in spite of advances in treatment and improvement of outcomes, these persons view damage to the heart as ominous to their future health.[4] Throughout the care of a patient experiencing an AMI, the nurse should offer verbal and nonverbal reassurance and should provide direct and simple explanations of all procedures, including the patient's role in these procedures.

Anxiety, Denial, and Depression

The admission to an emergency department of a person with a presumptive diagnosis of an AMI is a psychophysiologically stressful event that affects the patient and the family. Acute, situational anxiety is the most frequent psychological response to an AMI and typically occurs at several points throughout hospitalization (i.e., admission, transfer from the intensive care unit to the intermediate care unit, and discharge).[4,42] Denial may also be manifested by the patient, and later in the hospitalization and in the weeks that follow, depression may develop. The nurse is the one member of the health care team in constant contact with the patient and family and thus is positioned best to facilitate psychosocial adjustment by recognizing the need for and initiating appropriate and timely interventions.

Frequent causes of anxiety in patients experiencing or recovering from an AMI include the threat or fear of death, pain, loss of control, and the unknown (e.g., related to the environment, treatment plan, their role in treatment plan, or prognosis). The consequences of anxiety can have deleterious effects on the cardiovascular system. Anxiety, fear, and pain trigger the stress response, and the subsequent release of catecholamines can place further demands on the injured myocardium. Because of this connection, physicians frequently order anxiolytics (e.g., alprazolam [Xanax]) for these patients. Nurses need to assess the appropriateness of these pharmacologic agents carefully for patients and to document the response to the medications. For some patients, the sedative effect of many anxiolytics contributes to a increased sense of loss of control and greater anxiety.

Patients and their families should be encouraged to express their feelings and emotions as one way of identifying and reducing anxiety. In addition, nonpharmacologic interventions, such as music therapy, aromatherapy, prayer, and relaxation have shown promise as nontraditional, alternative approaches to managing stress and anxiety and should also be considered[43] (see Chapter 4).

Denial, as a response to an AMI, can certainly be demonstrated as early as the onset of the initial symptoms of an infarction and can contribute to a delay in treatment as well as physiologic outcomes. In certain patients, denial can persist throughout the patient's hospitalization. This can be manifested as denial of the diagnosis, denial that the diagnosis will change their lives, denial of feelings surrounding the event (anxiety, fear, and depression), and denial of chest pain.[42] Explanations for the use of denial by these patients include adaptation when self-esteem or life is threatened, a defense mechanism useful in controlling the overwhelming anxiety that accompanies an MI, and a means of controlling events by minimizing the seriousness of the MI.[42] Research on the harmful or helpful benefits of denial is inconclusive and conflicting. Rather than support or confront the patient expressing denial, the nurse should establish effective interpersonal relationships with the patient and the family and use open-ended communication techniques. Evidence indicates that when patients are encouraged to express their thoughts and feelings about their illness, anxiety is the underlying issue, not denial.[42]

Depression in the post-MI patient can evolve from various psychosocial issues such as feelings of hopelessness or powerlessness, changes in self-esteem and role, and insecurity regarding future financial and physical health. The most frequent cause of depression in these patients emerges from a sense of loss of control regarding the events surrounding the disease. When depression is present, nurses should design interventions that focus on assisting the patient to regain control. The use of antianxiety agents (e.g., imipramine hydrochloride [Tofranil]) is usually considered only if depression was present before the infarction.[6]

Patterns of emotional reactions to an AMI vary among patients and are likely to continue well into the weeks and months that follow discharge. Nurses need astute skills for assessing patients for signs of psychosocial distress. When necessary, collaboration with clinical nurse specialists, social workers, clergy, or psychiatrists may be helpful in facilitating psychosocial adjustment.

Needs of Families

Nurses must remember that the families of patients experience emotional crises concurrently with the patient. These crises usually evolve from the perceived threat to family roles and functioning related to the sudden illness. Family members may experience feelings of anxiety, denial, anger, frustration, and hopelessness when a loved one is hospitalized with a critical illness.[44]

Families should be assessed by nurses to uncover their needs from the health care team. Research has revealed that information represents the foremost need of families. To enhance family coping, nurses should intervene proactively by communicating information frequently with the family, integrating the family into the health care team, facilitating hope, and encouraging families to retain their life-role positions (see Chapter 4).[44]

Controlling the Hospital Environment

The nurse plays an important role in manipulating the patient's environment so that it is conducive to healing after an MI. Monitoring for and reducing high levels of noise, limiting interruptions in sleep and rest, balancing sensory overload with sensory deprivation, and providing appropriate access to the patient by the family represent major nursing goals relative to this issue. The importance of family access to patients in the intensive care unit has been well documented and cannot be overestimated. At all times, visiting policies should be designed to provide the most humane critical care possible.

The words and actions of nurses throughout all phases of the patient's hospitalization are important. According to the American Association of Critical-Care Nurses (AACN), the health care system should be driven by the needs of patients and their families. Nurses can make their optimal contribution to patients and families by providing caring and competent nursing practice.

Risk Factor Modification and Cardiac Rehabilitation

Risk factor modification after an AMI has been linked to a regression or halting of the underlying disease process, atherosclerosis (see Chapter 9). The initiation of patient and family teaching during the acute phase of an MI may not always be appropriate or effective because of the presence of various psychophysiologic stressors. In addition, patients are usually discharged within 5 days of an uncomplicated MI, leaving little time for intensive education on modifying cardiac risks.

Education concerning risk factor modification during this time is most effective if the topics are selected by the patient and family. Most often, discussions develop around diet and activity. Arranging a consultation with the dietitian for the patient and the care giver who normally purchases and prepares the food is highly recommended. In addition, patients may be ordered lipid-lowering medications such as lovastatin (Mevacor) as an adjunct to the diet regimen.

The initiation of phase I of the cardiac rehabilitation process usually begins with range-of-motion exercises and activities of daily living (bathing and toileting) in the intensive care unit and progresses throughout the period of hospitalization. Early and progressive activity has been shown to provide both physiologic and psychological benefits to patients recovering from an AMI. Recommendations for exercise during the period of hospitalization are usually established by the cardiac rehabilitation specialist. The patient's response to the exercise regimen is monitored (pulse, blood pressure, ECG, and chest pain), and adjustments in the regimen are made accordingly.

Phase II of cardiac rehabilitation occurs outside the hospital, usually within 4 to 6 weeks of an uncomplicated MI. The components of rehabilitation during this phase include exercise training, risk factor modification, counseling, and behavioral interventions.[1] The cardiac rehabilitation team is multidisciplinary and usually consists of physicians, nurses, dietitians, and exercise physiologists, with pharmacists, social workers, and psychologists consulted as needed. The overall benefits of cardiac rehabilitation consist of an improvement in exercise tolerance, reduction in symptoms, improvement in blood lipid studies, and a reduction in cigarette smoking.[1] In spite of this benefit,

cardiac rehabilitation services are grossly underused. Results from the GUSTO trial revealed that only 38% of the study participants enrolled in a cardiac rehabilitation program after discharge. Additionally, elderly patients and, in particular, elderly female patients are referred to and participate in cardiac rehabilitation programs less frequently than their younger, male counterparts.[1] Benefits of exercise training for elderly patients have been shown to be comparable to those for younger patients. Financial support for costs related to cardiac rehabilitation programs has increased with Medicare, and most insurance companies provide some degree of reimbursement. Nurses should strongly encourage all patients with AMIs to consider participation in a cardiac rehabilitation program. A unique, home-based approach to cardiac rehabilitation that uses the nurse as a case manager is described in Chart 10–4.[45]

Patient Education and Discharge Planning

Patient education and discharge planning start on hospital admission and continue to discharge. As mentioned earlier, patients should be provided with simple explanations of all procedures throughout the hospitalization. Specific educational topics for discussion (e.g., disease process, risk factors, and medications) should be selected based on the patient's expressed "desire to know." In addition, information that patients "need to know" to be discharged "safely" should be identified and provided. These generally include actions to take if chest pain should reoccur, activity limitations, information on the prescribed medication regimen, and instructions for follow-up. Whenever possible, the family should be included in the education process.

One area of education frequently overlooked relates to sexual counseling, and this may be related to a degree of discomfort among nurses regarding this topic.[46] The resumption of a preinfarct level of sexual activity has been identified as a measure of a patient's psychosocial adjustment.[42, 46] Patients are not always ready to discuss sexual concerns when approached in the acute care setting. In addition, shorter hospital stays may impede patients from reaching a level of comfort regarding this topic. Minimally, nurses should assess patients regarding their interest in this topic before hospital discharge. Ongoing assessment in the recovery phase is recommended. If necessary, nurses should make appropriate referrals to health care professionals, especially if sexual concerns persist.[46]

Overall discharge goals for patients with an AMI can be described as follows: 1) improve prognosis by assessing residual ischemia, selecting medications aimed at improving LV function, and treating risk factors; and 2) maximize functional level by prescribing appropriate rehabilitation and addressing psy-

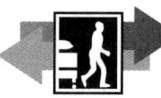

CHART 10–4

BEYOND THE ICU: HOME-BASED CASE MANAGEMENT APPROACH TO CARDIAC REHABILITATION

Nurses have opportunities to provide care to patients recovering from an acute myocardial infarction (AMI) in various acute care settings and, most recently, in community settings. Systematic modification of coronary risk factors for patients discharged after an AMI remains a challenge, and nurses, with their specialized knowledge base, can make a difference. In 1994, DeBusk and colleagues reported on a physician-directed, nurse-managed, home-based, case-management system in which a nurse case manager, working with a variety of health care professionals (psychiatrist, cardiologist, lipid specialist, and nutritionist) managed coronary risk factors for a group of patients who had experienced an AMI.[45]

Nurse case managers enrolled patients in this program while these patients were still hospitalized, usually on day 3 unless the patients were in a medically unstable condition. At this time, patients completed self-reports on smoking, diet, and exercise. Scheduled interactions with case managers consisted of nurse-initiated telephone contacts, mailed progress reports based on questionnaires completed by the patients, and patients' visits to the nurse case manager.

Depending on the individual patient's risk factor profile, specific interventions were prescribed to assist with behavioral changes. A smoking intervention program was available and included emphasis on smoking cessation and relapse prevention. Nurse case managers provided individual counseling and telephone follow-up.

Nutritional counseling was provided to all patients and was based on their responses to a food frequency questionnaire that was completed in the hospital and at 6, 11, and 26 weeks after discharge. Detailed strategies for achieving a diet low in cholesterol and saturated fat were individualized and were mailed to patients within 48 to 72 hours of receiving the patients' self-reports. Nurse case managers provided additional reinforcement of the information and the patient's progress during scheduled visits.

For patients with plasma low-density lipoprotein (LDL) cholesterol values of more than 95 mg/dL, drug therapy was initiated. During visits with the nurse case manager, education and counseling regarding the rationale for lipid-lowering medications and ways to maximize drug efficacy and to minimize side effects were provided. In addition, after consultation with a physician lipid specialist, changes in therapy were coordinated by nurse-initiated telephone contacts.

Exercise training programs were based on patients' heart rate responses during treadmill testing. Patients were initially instructed to exercise (e.g., walking, jogging, biking, or swimming) at the prescribed heart rate for 30 minutes per day for 5 days per week. Nurse case managers instructed patients on warm-up exercises, regulation of exercise intensity with heart rate monitoring, and recognition of and response to cardiac symptoms during scheduled visits. The patients' home-based exercise training prescriptions were increased after 4 weeks, and instructions for exercise maintenance were provided between 6 and 12 months after infarction. Up to this time, nurse case managers telephoned patients at regular intervals to detect or correct any problems with the training prescription.

Results of this program demonstrated reductions in plasma LDL cholesterol levels, enhanced functional capacity, and reductions in cigarette smoking among the patients who participated. It was further determined that a single care giver, the nurse case manager, aided by telephone consultations with experts, as needed, could provide cost-effective, individualized home-based, rehabilitative services. Nurse case managers were selected to coordinate patient activities because their experience in cardiac care provided them with the requisite knowledge to guide patients through their medication, exercise, nutritional, and smoking cessation regimens.

chosocial concerns.[4] Patients with uncomplicated MIs are scheduled for a low-level, thallium exercise stress test before discharge. Echocardiography or multiple gated acquisition scanning may also be ordered as a means of evaluating LV function and ejection fraction. These strategies aid in evaluating the effectiveness of ordered medications and provide guidance to the

physician and rehabilitation team in determining patient goals (see Chapter 8).

Patients who experience complicated recoveries from an AMI may need to consider a short-term stay in a skilled nursing facility as a bridge to home. Minimally, a referral for follow-up with community nursing should be considered. These patients are generally discharged with greater physical limitations, more complex medication regimens, and more serious psychosocial concerns.

Multidisciplinary Outcomes

Multidisciplinary outcomes for patients experiencing an AMI can be differentiated according to the phase of hospitalization and recovery. Table 10–9 summarizes these outcomes, starting in the emergency department and moving through the intensive and intermediate care units, to discharge and follow-up in the community.

TABLE 10–9
Multidisciplinary Outcomes

Phase of Recovery	Outcome
Emergency department	Preservation of myocardium by rapid diagnosis and initiation of appropriate reperfusion strategies and treatment adjuncts
	Stabilization of the patient for transfer to the intensive care unit
Intensive care unit	Restoration of perfusion to the infarct-related vessel
	Stabilization of cardiac rhythm
	Stabilization of cardiac functioning
	Restoration and maintenance of adequate oxygenation
	Prevention and detection of complications
	Stabilization of psychosocial health
	Preparation of the patient for transfer to the intermediate care unit
Intermediate care unit	Maintenance of perfusion to the infarct-related vessel
	Maintenance of cardiac rhythm
	Improvement of cardiac functioning
	Maintenance of adequate oxygenation
	Prevention and detection of complications
	Improvement of psychosocial health
	Preparation for discharge and cardiac rehabilitation
Community	Prevention and detection of complications
	Initiation of a cardiac rehabilitation program
	Return to previous or improved level of health
	Restoration and maintenance of psychosocial health

Critical Thinking Exercise

A 56-year-old, overweight man with no significant medical history arrives at the emergency department by car with his wife. The patient complains of excruciating chest pain that radiates to his jaw and left arm. The pain began approximately 3 hours ago while he was mowing the lawn. Attempts to treat the pain with antacids and rest were unsuccessful. The patient is short of breath and diaphoretic. Vital signs are as follows: blood pressure, 146/92 mm Hg; heart rate, 110 beats per minute and regular; respiratory rate, 28. Sublingual NTG is administered; oxygen is started by nasal cannula at 4 L per minute; a 12-lead ECG is ordered; and blood for baseline laboratory studies, including CK-MB isoenzymes, is drawn. A tentative diagnosis of an AMI is made.

1. Discuss the clinical signs and symptoms that contribute to the tentative diagnosis of an AMI for this patient.
2. Provide rationales for the interventions ordered at this point.

The 12-lead ECG reveals 2- to 3-mm ST-segment elevation in leads V2 to V4; the patient reports no relief from sublingual nitroglycerin after 5 minutes. Because the onset of pain is less than 6 hours, a decision to start thrombolysis is made.

3. How does this new information support the decision to initiate thrombolysis?
4. Identify the concurrent therapies that you would expect for this patient at this time and defend your decisions.

The patient is transferred to the coronary care unit with rt-PA infusing. Vital signs are as follows: blood pressure, 146/92 mm Hg; heart rate 121 beats per minute, with rare isolated PVCs; respiratory rate, 26. The patient continues to complain of severe chest pain (8 on a scale of 0 to 10). Intravenous NTG is titrated to relieve pain and to maintain systolic blood pressure above 95 mm Hg. rt-PA has been infusing for approximately 1 hour. The first CK-MB isoenzymes have returned and are positive for an AMI. The patient is apprehensive, concerned about his condition, and asking to see his wife.

5. Nursing diagnoses of pain, potential alteration in cardiac output, decreased, and anxiety have been made. What nursing interventions would you anticipate relative to these diagnoses?

The patient shows definitive evidence of reperfusion within 90 minutes of the thrombolytic therapy (ST-segment resolution, brief episode of nonsustained VT). He reports that his chest pain has resolved. His aPTT has returned and is 95 seconds.

6. What would be your response to this laboratory information and why?

The patient remains hemodynamically stable over the next 24 hours, and transfer to an intermediate care unit is planned for the morning of day 2. Nitroglycerin is titrated, and the patient remains pain free. An ACE inhibitor will be added to the medication regimen on day 3.

7. What is the rationale for the addition of ACE inhibitors to the postinfarction drug regimen?
8. What are the major nursing considerations for patients at this phase of recovery?

Key Concepts

➡ An MI is the result of an acute occlusion of a coronary artery, usually resulting from a thrombosis at the site of an atherosclerotic plaque.

➡ The primary consequence of an AMI is cellular death of some portion of the myocardium leading to some degree of ventricular dysfunction.

➡ The zone of infarction is frequently associated with the development of a Q wave on the ECG, the zone of injury by ST-segment elevation, and the zone of ischemia by T-wave inversion.

➡ The location of the infarction and the artery involved can be determined by patterns of changes on the 12-lead ECG.

➡ The diagnosis of an AMI consists of a clinical history of persistent chest pain, serial changes in the ECG, and the presence of serum cardiac enzymes.

➡ Delays in the treatment of an AMI can contribute to physiologic outcomes. In general, the greatest delays to treatment are those caused by patients.

➡ Typical chest pain associated with an AMI is prolonged (>30 minutes in duration) and described as a burning, crushing, tightness, or squeezing sensation in the substernal region of the chest. This pain may radiate to the shoulders, neck, jaw, or arms and may be associated with nausea, vomiting, shortness of breath, and diaphoresis.

➡ Age, gender, and ethnicity may contribute to differences in chest pain associated with an AMI.

➡ Treatment of a patient with an AMI should be instituted within 30 minutes of arrival in the emergency department and is directed at reperfusion of the infarcted artery.

➡ Reperfusion can be accomplished by thrombolytic agents, invasive techniques, or surgical revascularization.

➡ In addition to reperfusion strategies, treatment adjuncts for a patient with an AMI include various pharmacotherapeutic agents (nitrates, aspirin, anticoagulants, analgesics, beta blockers, antidysrhythmics, ACE inhibitors, magnesium, and oxygen).

➡ Pharmacologic agents (e.g., beta blockers and ACE inhibitors) administered after infarction have been shown to decrease mortality.

➡ Patients receiving thrombolytics and anticoagulants are at increased risk of minor and major bleeding.

➡ Continuous ECG monitoring is maintained throughout the period of hospitalization and provides important information on reperfusion, the detection of complications, and the effectiveness of pharmacologic agents.

➡ ST-segment monitoring in specific groupings of ECG leads can contribute significantly to the early detection of reocclusion.

➡ Complications after an AMI depend on the size and location of the infarct and can be classified as electrical (dysrhythmias), structural (papillary muscle rupture, ventricular septal rupture, and ventricular aneurysm), hemodynamic (right ventricular failure, CHF, cardiogenic shock), and inflammatory (pericarditis).

➡ Common dysrhythmias after an AMI are either bradydysrhythmias (e.g., sinus bradycardia, atrial fibrillation, AV blocks) or tachydysrhythmias (e.g., sinus tachycardia, PVCs, VT, VF, premature supraventricular tachycardia, rapid atrial fibrillation).

➡ Most dysrhythmias after an AMI are self-limiting; persistent dysrhythmias are treated with pacing, antidysrhythmic agents, or implantable cardioverter defibrillators.

➡ Structural defects are usually catastrophic, manifested by sudden physiologic decline, require rapid intervention, and associated with high rates of mortality.

➡ Hemodynamic defects after an AMI range from mild degrees of CHF to cardiogenic shock.

➡ Pericarditis, an inflammatory condition, can occur early or late in the aftermath of an AMI and is usually treated with nonsteroidal anti-inflammatory agents.

➡ Psychosocial support for patients after an AMI is aimed at identifying and treating anxiety, denial, and depression.

➡ Needs of families of patients with AMIs include information needs, psychosocial support, and access to family members.

➡ Cardiac rehabilitation programs have been shown to reduce cardiac risk factors and to improve exercise tolerance and symptoms. Phase I of cardiac rehabilitation occurs during hospitalization, and phase II occurs after discharge.

➡ Patient and family education in the acute care setting should be a balance of what the family "wants to know" with what the nurse believes they "need to know" to return home safely.

➡ Outcomes after an AMI revolve around preserving myocardium and cardiac function, preventing and detecting complications, and restoring patients to their previous level of functioning.

References

1. US Department of Health and Human Services: Cardiac Rehabilitation as Secondary Prevention (AHCPR Publication No. 96–0673). Rockville, MD, US Department of Health and Human Services, 1995.

2. Guyton AC, Hall JE: Textbook of Medical Physiology, 9th ed. Philadelphia, W. B. Saunders, 1996.

3. Keller KB, Lemberg L: Q and non-Q wave myocardial infarctions. Am J Crit Care 3:158–161, 1994.

4. Havranek EP: Managing patients with myocardial infarction after hospital discharge. Am Fam Physician 49:1109–1119, 1994.

5. Riegel B: Myocardial infarction. In: Clochesy JM, Breu C, Cardin S, et al (eds): Critical Care Nursing, 2nd ed. Philadelphia, W. B. Saunders, 1996, pp 354–373.

6. Sirois JG: Acute myocardial infarction. Emerg Med Clin North Am 13:759–767, 1995.

7. US Department of Health and Human Services: Morbidity and Mortality: Chartbook on Cardiovascular, Lung, and Blood Diseases. Bethesda, MD, National Heart, Lung, and Blood Institute, 1992.

8. Dracup K, Moser DK, Eisenberg M, et al: Causes of delay in seeking treatment for heart attack symptoms. Soc Sci Med 40:379–392, 1995.

9. Dempsey GA, Seidman RN: Women's decision to seek care for symptoms of acute myocardial infarction. Heart Lung 24:444–456, 1995.

10. Maynard C, Weaver WD: Streamlining the triage system for acute myocardial infarction. Cardiol Clin 13:311–320, 1995.

11. National Heart Attack Alert Program Coordinating Committee, 60 Minutes to Treatment Working Group: Emergency department: rapid identification and treatment of patients with an acute myocardial infarction. Ann Emerg Med 23:311–329, 1994.

12. Pasternak RC, Braunwald E, Sobel BE: Acute myocardial infarction. In: Braunwald E (ed): Heart Disease, 4th ed. Philadelphia, W. B. Saunders, 1992.

13. Thompson L, Wood C, Wallhagen M: Geriatric acute myocardial infarction: a challenge to recognition, prompt diagnosis, and appropriate care. Crit Care Nurs Clin North Am 4:291–299, 1992.

14. Romeo KC: The female heart: Physiological aspects of cardiovascular disease in women. Dimensions Crit Care Nurs, 14(4): 170–177, 1995.

15. Jensen L, King KM: Women and heart disease: the issues. Crit Care Nurs 17:45–53, 1997.

16. Lee H-O: Typical and atypical clinical signs and symptoms of myocardial infarction and delayed seeking of professional care among blacks. Am J Crit Care 6:7–13, 1997.

17. Puleo FR, Meyer D, Wathen C, et al: Use of a rapid assay of subforms of creatine kinase MB to diagnose or rule out acute myocardial infarction. N Engl J Med 331:561–566, 1994.

18. Brogan GX, Vuori J, Friedman S, et al: Improved specificity of myoglobin plus carbonic anhydrase assay versus that of creatine kinase-MB for early diagnosis of acute myocardial infarction. Ann Emerg Med 27:22–28, 1996.

19. deWinter RJ, Koster RW, Sturk A, et al: Value of myoglobin, troponin T, and CK-MB$_{mass}$ in ruling out an acute myocardial infarction in the emergency room. Circulation 92:3401–3407, 1995.

20. Williams K, Morton PG: Diagnosis and treatment of acute myocardial infarction. AACN Clin Issues 6:375–386, 1995.

21. Tietz NW (ed): Clinical Guide to Laboratory Tests. Philadelphia, W. B. Saunders, 1995.

22. Agnelli G: Thrombolytic and antithrombotic treatment in myocardial infarction: main achievements and future perspectives. Int J Cardiol 49(Suppl):S77–S87, 1995.

23. Pashos CL, Normand S-L, Garfinkle JB, et al: Trends in the use of drug therapies in patients with acute myocardial infarction. J Am Coll Cardiol 23:1023–1030, 1994.

24. Weaver WD, White HD, Wilcox RG, et al: Comparisons of characteristics and outcomes among women and men with acute myocardial infarction treated with thrombolytic therapy. JAMA 275:777–782, 1996.

25. Schroder R, Wegscheider K, Schroder K, et al: Extent of early ST segment elevation resolution: a strong predictor of outcome in patients with acute myocardial infarction and a sensitive measure to compare thrombolytic regimens. J Am Coll Cardiol 26:1657–1664, 1995.

26. Buszman P, Szafranek A, Kalarus Z, et al: Use of changes in ST segment elevation for prediction of infarct artery recanalization in acute myocardial infarction. Eur Heart J 16:1207–1214, 1995.

27. Morris DC: Treatment of acute myocardial infarction by invasive cardiology techniques. Semin Thorac Cardiovasc Surg 7:184–190, 1995.

28. McKendall GR, Forman S, Sopko G, et al: Value of rescue percutaneous transluminal coronary angioplasty following unsuccessful thrombolytic therapy in patients with acute myocardial infarction. Am J Cardiol 76:1108–1111, 1995.

29. Coleman WS, DeWood MA, Berg R, et al: Surgical intervention in acute myocardial infarction: an historical perspective. Semin Thorac Cardiovasc Surg 7:176–183, 1995.

30. Braxton JH, Hammond GL, Letsou GV, et al: Optimal timing of coronary artery bypass graft surgery after acute myocardial infarction. Circulation 92(Supply II):II-66–II-68, 1995.

31. Mackintosh C: Non-reporting of cardiac pain. Nurs Times 90:36–40, 1994.

32. Bowlby H, Hisle K, Clifton GD: Heparin as adjunctive therapy to coronary thrombolysis in acute myocardial infarction. Heart Lung 24:292–302, 1995.

33. Connors KF, Lamas GA: Postmyocardial infarction patients: experience from the SAVE trial. Am J Crit Care 4:23–28, 1995.

34. Fara AM: The role of angiotensin-converting enzyme inhibitors in reducing ventricular remodeling after myocardial infarction. J Cardiovasc Nurs 8:32–48, 1993.

35. Woods KL, Fletcher S: Long-term outcome after intravenous magnesium sulphate in suspected acute myocardial infarction: the second Leicester intravenous magnesium intervention trial (LIMIT-2). Lancet 343:816–818, 1994.

36. Drew BJ, Tisdale LA: ST segment monitoring for coronary reocclusion following thrombolytic therapy and coronary angioplasty: identification of optimal bedside monitoring leads. Am J Crit Care 2:280–292, 1993.

37. Witherell CL: Cardiac rhythm control devices. Crit Care Nurs Clin North Am 6:85–101, 1994.

38. Jones MC: Pacemakers. In: Clochesy JM, Breu C, Cardin S, et al (eds): Critical Care Nursing, 2nd ed. Philadelphia, W. B. Saunders, 1996, pp 167–202.

39. Dougherty CM: Longitudinal recovery following sudden cardiac arrest and internal cardioverter defibrillator implantation: survivors and their families. Am J Crit Care 3:145–154, 1994.

40. Granrud GA, Vatterott PJ: Arrhythmias and acute myocardial infarction. Postgrad Med 90:85–96, 1991.

41. Friedman BM, Dunn MI: Postinfarction ventricular aneurysms. Clin Cardiol 18:505–511, 1995.

42. Malan SS: Psychosocial adjustment following MI: current views and nursing implications. J Cardiovasc Nurs 6:57–70, 1992.

43. Guzzetta CE: Effects of relaxation and music therapy on patients in a coronary care unit with presumptive acute myocardial infarction. Heart Lung 18:609–616, 1989.

44. Byrd JA: Critical waiting: families in crisis. UltraSTAT Essential Issues Adv Crit Care Nurs 1:1, 3–6, 1994.

45. DeBusk RF, Miller NH, Superko RS, et al: A case-management system for coronary risk factor modification after acute myocardial infarction. Ann Intern Med 120:721–729, 1994.

46. Steinke EE, Patterson P: Sexual counseling of MI patients by cardiac nurses. J Cardiovasc Nurs 10:81–87, 1995.

11

Heart Failure

Catherine Nuss Kotecki

Objectives

After completing this chapter, the student will be able to:

1. Correlate hemodynamic changes in heart failure to patients' signs and symptoms.
2. Categorize pharmacotherapeutic interventions according to a target physiologic compensatory mechanism.
3. Select nursing interventions for patients with heart failure across a continuum of critical care.
4. Identify compensatory physiologic mechanisms characteristic of acute and chronic heart failure.
5. Discuss nursing interventions that ameliorate fatigue and dyspnea in patients in heart failure.
6. Differentiate between assessment findings for a diagnosis of right-sided or left-sided heart failure.
7. Describe outcomes expected across care settings to meet the physical, social, and psychological needs of patients with heart failure.

Heart failure manifests itself in acute and chronic forms, across the life span, and as a sequela of different disease entities. Heart failure presents a nursing care challenge across various critical care settings and into the home. The nurse may care for patients with a single episode of heart failure or for those whose heart failure is the final stage of disease. Heart failure is a syndrome that occurs as an individual experiences increased limitation in activities, dyspnea, and fatigue as a result of increased diastolic volumes, decreased ventricular ejection, and decreased tissue and organ oxygenation. During an event of heart failure, multiple physiologic compensatory events occur, many of which exacerbate the problem. Treatment is directed at manipulating the compensatory mechanisms of the body, so that they contribute to physiologic balance, rather than harm the patient. Nursing interventions focus on assisting the patient to overcome fatigue and dyspnea, managing multiple symptoms, and educating the patient and care givers about drug and treatment regimens. Simply, heart failure can be defined as the inability of the myocardium to meet the oxygen demands of the body.

ETIOLOGY AND PATHOPHYSIOLOGY

Heart failure has become a major health problem in the United States. Overall, deaths from coronary artery disease, myocardial infarction (MI), and stroke are decreasing.[1] However, as individuals survive initial cardiac insults and depend on medication and technology to support their ailing hearts, chronic complications, such as heart failure, have become more prevalent. Thirty to 50 years ago, hypertension and valvular disease were the most frequent causes of heart failure. Now, left ventricular dysfunction from coronary heart disease is the most common cause. Currently, it is estimated that more than 4.7 million Americans have a medical diagnosis of heart failure.[2] Further, the American Heart Association estimated in 1996 that 400,000 new cases are diagnosed each year. After adjusting for age, the survival rate for women with heart failure is better than that for men. Estimates of death from heart failure are 50% higher in African-American populations than in white populations, with the greatest differences in mortality found in younger age groups and the smallest differences found in the age group over 75 years.[3,4] Hypertension increases the risk of heart failure threefold. Other subtle predictors include diabetes, elevated ratio of total cholesterol to high-density lipoprotein, abnormally high or low hematocrit levels, and proteinuria.[5] Whatever the related risk and precipitating factors, primary symptoms of heart failure are fatigue and dyspnea causing an alteration in activities of daily living.[3,6] Predictors of mortality include decreased functional capacity, poor cardiac output, spontaneous dysrhythmias, and laboratory evidence of neurohormonal activation.[7] In summary, a brief review of etiologic factors associated with heart failure has been presented. A more comprehensive review of pathophysiology related to conditions associated with heart failure, hemodynamic and compensatory mechanisms of heart failure, classification of heart failure, and review of acute and chronic heart failure is considered.

Conditions Precipitating Heart Failure

Heart failure occurs as the "final common pathway in a variety of cardiovascular disorders such as coronary heart disease, long standing hypertension, valve deformities and cardiomyopathy."[3] It can occur as a result of infection, immune and connective tissue disorders, and endocrine imbalance. Heart failure can strike a woman who is pregnant or young children with congenital cardiac disorders, but it is most common during advanced age. Table 11–1 lists conditions known to precipitate heart failure.

Heart failure occurs as a result of disorders that may be classified as occurring from decreased myocardial contractility or increased myocardial workload. The primary disease states contributing to decreased myocardial contractility are MI and coronary artery disease (see Chapter 10 for a discussion of MI). Cardiomyopathy, characterized by changes in the cellular structure of the myocardium, also leads to symptoms of heart failure. Infiltrative diseases and collagen vascular disease that invade the cardiovascular system can cause symptoms of heart failure. The problem in cardiomyopathy is the inability of the myocardium to contract in a manner sufficient to meet a person's oxygen demands. Increased myocardial workload is characterized by increased need for oxygen by the myocardium. Disease states causing heart failure that occur as a result of increased myocardial workload include high-output states, valvular heart disease, and hypertensive states. High-output states include diseases such as thyrotoxicosis or states in which increased blood volume causes increased cardiac output. In high-output states, increased myocardial workload occurs as a result of increased pressures within the heart and of decreased myocardial contractility.

Cardiomyopathy is a contributing factor to heart failure. Cardiomyopathy consists of three different classifications of a disease state of the myocardium: dilated, restrictive, and hypertrophic. Despite differing

TABLE 11–1

Precipitating Factors and Disease States Leading to Heart Failure

Precipitating Factor	Disease State
Infections	Systemic viral or bacterial infection
	Pericarditis
Endocrine imbalances	Hyperthyroidism
	Thyroid toxicosis
	Pheochromocytoma
Nutritional disorders	Beriberi (thiamine disorder)
	Kwashiorkor (protein deficiency)
Pregnancy	Preeclampsia
Alcoholism	Alcoholic cardiomyopathy
Musculoskeletal disorders	Myasthenia gravis
	Muscular dystrophy
	Myotonic dystrophy
Autoimmune disorders	Amyloidosis
	Sarcoidosis
	Lupus
Heredity (non–sex-linked autosomal dominant trait)	Hypertrophic cardiomyopathy
Myocardial muscle damage	Coronary artery disease
	Myocardial infarction
Hemodynamic pressure changes	Hypertension
	Valve disease (regurgitation or stenosis)
	Dysrhythmias

pathologic features and treatment regimens, all the cardiomyopathies lead to symptoms of heart failure. Dilated cardiomyopathy, the most common type, results from destruction by toxic, infectious, or metabolic agents. It also occurs as a result of endocrine, electrolyte, and nutritional disorders. In dilated cardiomyopathy, the ventricles dilate without proportional compensatory hypertrophy, causing the heart to take on a globular shape and subsequently to contract poorly during systole, thus affecting cardiac output.[8]

Restrictive cardiomyopathy is characterized by restricted ventricular filling as a result of left ventricular hypertrophy, endocardial fibrosis, and muscle thickening. Amyloidosis is a rare disease that causes endomyocardial fibrosis. As in constrictive pericarditis, diastolic filling is decreased as a result of a stiff ventricle.[8]

Hypertrophic cardiomyopathy (HCM), formerly known as idiopathic hypertrophic subaortic stenosis or asymmetric septal hypertrophy, is characterized by left ventricular hypertrophy and thickening of the ventricular septum without dilatation. HCM is thought to be genetically linked, but it may also have other causes. Patients with HCM may experience sudden death related to exercising. The thickened myocardium may present signs and symptoms that initially mimic coronary artery disease such as angina, syncope, or ventricular dysrhythmias. If sudden death does not result, a patient may progress to symptoms of heart failure.[9]

Hemodynamic Changes in Heart Failure

Hemodynamic events in heart failure focus on meeting myocardial and peripheral oxygen demands by maintaining adequate cardiac output. Essentially, the heart can be viewed as two pumps separated by the low pressure system of the lungs. A brief discussion of factors affecting cardiac output in heart failure assists the reader in understanding classifications of heart failure and compensatory mechanisms. Normal adult cardiac output is between 4 and 6 L per minute and is represented by the following equation

$$\text{Cardiac output} = \text{heart rate} \times \text{stroke volume.}$$

The stroke volume is the amount of blood ejected from the heart with each beat. Stroke volume is influenced by three factors: preload, afterload, and contractility of the heart muscle. Not all the blood is ejected with each heart beat. The percentage of blood normally ejected with each heart beat is approximately 60 to 75%. This is known as ejection fraction. Some blood always remains in the left ventricle, to influence the next systolic event. The total volume of blood in the left ventricle at the end of diastole is approximately 75 mL.

Thus, left ventricular end-diastolic pressure (LVEDP), represented by the concept of preload, influences the stroke volume. Preload is a term used to describe the stretch of myocardial muscle fiber by the volume of blood at the end of diastole. The principle of the Frank–Starling law states that subsequent systolic contraction is influenced by the end of diastolic stretch caused by ventricular volume. Afterload is described as the force against which the ventricle must pump. Afterload is measured by the derived value of systemic vascular resistance and is regulated in part by adrenergic receptors of the sympathetic nervous system. The final factor affecting stroke volume is contractility. Contractility refers to the contraction of the myocardial muscle fibers, the slipping of sarcomere over the myofibril. For an adequate stroke volume to be maintained, myocardial muscle fibers must be intact and able to contract.[10]

In the usual situation, heart failure results in a decreased cardiac output as a result of myocardial injury or MI. A damaged ventricle makes effortless contractility impossible and unleashes a series of hemodynamic consequences that offset a drop in cardiac output.

Preload increases as the damaged ventricle is unable to contract in a forceful manner. Concomitantly, stroke volume and ejection fraction are decreased, negatively affecting the cardiac output. The ejection fraction may be decreased to 40% before a diagnosis of heart failure is made.[6] Compensatory mechanisms to stabilize cardiac output result in increased heart rate and increased afterload, mechanisms under control of the sympathetic nervous system. The benefit of sympathetic stimulation comes with a price: increased demand for oxygen by the myocardium.

Right-Sided and Left-Sided Heart Failure

Hemodynamic changes throughout the body can be characterized by determining whether the heart failure is right sided or left sided. This is only one way to classify heart failure; other ways include forward or backward and high output or low output.[11] Table 11–2 describes the signs and symptoms of left-sided and right-sided heart failure. Left-sided failure occurs when a person has sustained myocardial damage to the left ventricle. This may occur after an anterior or lateral wall MI. Increase in preload in the left side of the heart results in an increase in intraventricular pressure. A numeric value representative of the preload may be obtained by the measuring the LVEDP or "wedge pressure" by the pulmonary artery catheter. The wedge pressure is expected to increase in left-sided heart failure.

TABLE 11–2

Signs and Symptoms of Right-Sided and Left-Sided Heart Failure

Right-Sided Failure	Left-Sided Failure
Elevated central venous pressure and right atrial pressure	Elevated pulmonary artery wedge (wedge) pressure and left atrial pressure
Jugular venous distention	Dyspnea, paroxysmal nocturnal dyspnea, dyspnea on exertion
Hepatojugular reflex	
Splenomegaly	
Ascites	
Nausea and vomiting	Orthopnea
Abdominal distention and anorexia	Adventitious lung sounds: crackles, wheezes, rhonchi
Peripheral edema	
Weight gain	Cough, hemoptysis
Nocturia	Cyanosis
	Cheyne–Stokes breathing
	Palpitations, cardiac dysrhythmias, tachycardia
	Pulsus alternans
	Extra heart sounds: S_3, S_4
	Diaphoresis, nocturia

On the left side of the heart, increased pressure is ultimately transferred to the normally low-pressure system of the lungs. As volume of blood increases, pulmonary artery capillary pressure increases. If the pressure in the pulmonary capillary bed rises above a value equal to the colloid osmotic pressure of the plasma, fluid begins to filter out of the capillaries into the interstitial spaces in the lungs. Therefore, a consequence of left-sided heart failure is manifested as symptoms involving the patient's lungs. Signs may range from adventitious lung sounds to pulmonary edema. Interstitial edema causes impaired gas exchange, which is associated with symptoms of dyspnea, orthopnea, and anxiety.[12]

When the right ventricle has sustained injury or infarction, such as in inferior wall MI, signs and symptoms of right-sided heart failure are manifested. Signs and symptoms of right-sided heart failure involve the systemic circulation and an increase in peripheral edema. Because the right side of the heart is a low-pressure system, increased right ventricular pressure is referred back to the right atrium and subsequently to the inferior and superior vena cava. The low-pressure venous system is able to accommodate the higher cardiac pressures. In right-sided heart failure, central venous pressure measurements are expected to be higher than normal as the blood volumes and pressure within the right side of the heart increase. In extreme cases, right-sided heart failure may occur as a result of left-sided failure. Cor pulmonale is a type of right-sided heart failure that results because of pulmonary hypertension or recurrent pulmonary emboli.[13]

Hemodynamic changes in dilated cardiomyopathy are similar to the changes in left-sided heart failure. In HCM, cardiac out put is low, normal, or high, depending on whether stenosis is obstructive or nonobstructive.[8] Cardiac output may be high as a result of the hyperdynamic systolic contraction of the hypertrophied myocardium. Obstructive stenosis of the mitral valve increases intraventricular pressures, increases myocardial workload, and decreases cardiac output. As a result of the high systolic output state in HCM, treatment differs from traditional treatment of heart failure.[9]

Further, hemodynamic changes in heart failure affect every system of the body. As cardiac output falls, poor perfusion to the brain results in anxiety, confusion, and altered cognitive processes. When the body senses that vascular blood volume is decreased through poor perfusion to the kidneys, compensatory physiologic mechanisms are instituted to counteract the low blood volume. The primary result of this process is sodium and water retention, which serves to increase preload. Unfortunately for the failing heart, the increased blood volume contributes to a scenario of decompensation.

In summary, hemodynamic changes in heart failure can be generally described in terms of an increased preload of the right or left ventricle, increased afterload in the peripheral vascular system, and decreased myocardial contractility resulting in decreased cardiac output. Next, compensatory mechanisms that affect the hemodynamics of heart failure are described.

Compensatory Mechanisms in Heart Failure

In response to changes in cardiac output resulting from the onset of heart failure, two compensatory mechanisms are initiated: cardiovascular and neurohormonal. The compensatory mechanisms are interrelated and initiated immediately; they can have a long-term effect and are not always beneficial to patients. If the nurse understands compensatory mechanisms of heart failure, then the treatment of heart failure is easily understood.

Neurohormonal Mechanisms

Neurohormonal compensatory mechanisms include the influence of the sympathetic nervous system on adrenergic receptors in the cardiovascular system, the activation of the renin–angiotensin–aldosterone system, and the influence of atrial natriuretic hormone on volume control. Activation of a sympathetic response occurs when baroreceptors in the carotid arteries respond to a decrease in arterial pressure and circulating volume as cardiac output falls. The sympathetic nervous system is alerted to changes in pressure and releases epinephrine and norepinephrine. Sympathetic stimulation of beta$_1$-adrenergic receptors in the myocardium by the neurohormone results in increased heart rate and contractility. This increase in heart rate contributes a stabilizing effect to cardiac output. It takes 30 seconds to 1 minute for sympathetic activation and stabilization of cardiac output. This situation is temporary because, in heart failure, myocardial contractility is impaired. Thus, the nervous system stimulates a damaged heart. With sympathetic stimulation, the myocardial oxygen demand increases, at times extending the area of infarction.[11]

Further increasing the myocardial workload is the effect of the sympathetic nervous system on the peripheral vascular nervous system. Sympathetic stimulation of alpha$_1$-adrenergic receptors in the peripheral vasculature promotes vasoconstriction, thereby increasing afterload. The overall effect of sympathetic nervous system compensation in heart failure is to improve cardiac output while increasing myocardial oxygen demand and myocardial workload.

A second neurohormonal compensatory mechanism initiated during falling cardiac output is the renin–

angiotensin–aldosterone system, which has several effects on fluid volume and blood pressure. The kidneys respond to a decreased blood flow and increased vasoconstriction (caused by sympathetic stimulation) and respond to these events by the initiation of the renin–angiotensin–aldosterone compensatory mechanism. Initially, renin is secreted by the juxtaglomerular cells of the kidney. Renin is transported through the plasma, where it acts on the liver substrate angiotensinogen, producing angiotensin I. As angiotensin I passes through the lungs, it is converted by an enzyme to angiotensin II. Angiotensin II acts as a vasopressor, contributing to vasoconstriction. It also initiates water retention through the secretion of aldosterone. Increased levels of aldosterone increase sodium retention. The overall effect of this compensatory mechanism in heart failure is to increase blood pressure by fluid volume retention and vasoconstriction.[11]

An inhibitory hormonal mechanism that counteracts the fluid conservation effects of the renal system is found in the natriuretic systems, particularly atrial natriuretic factor (ANF). ANF is stimulated by an increase in atrial pressure, as commonly occurs in heart failure. After being released by the atria, ANF enters the systemic circulation and acts on the kidneys to promote increased filtration and decreased reabsorption of sodium. The result is increased excretion of salt and water that compensates for the overall fluid retention occurring in heart failure. In heart failure, circulating blood volumes of ANF increase 5 to 10 times higher than normal in an effort to manage fluid volume excess. However, in acute heart failure, this increase is not enough to reverse the trend of water conservation.

Cardiovascular Mechanisms

Cardiac compensatory mechanisms focus on cellular changes in the myocardium that affect contractility and initiate other compensatory mechanisms. Hypertrophy of individual myocytes occurs in response to myocardial injury and leads to cardiac dilatation. The death of individual myocytes as a result of MI contributes to the activation of the sympathetic nervous system and to increased levels of circulating norepinephrine, ANF, and arginine vasopressin. These same substances contribute to myocyte growth, promoting hypertrophy. Ventricular remodeling occurs as myocardial cell hypertrophy and chamber dilatation adapt to the reduction in contractile strength in an attempt to maintain stroke volume.[12] Hypertrophy is not only an acute response, but also one that happens over a period of months.

Acute Versus Chronic Heart Failure

Physiologic compensatory mechanisms initiate an acute compensation and chronic compensation. The primary mechanism in an acute response to MI is activation of the sympathetic nervous system. Over time, chronic compensation is managed by the renal system. Retention of fluid in chronic heart failure is a significant clinical problem. Decompensation of the heart occurs when the heart is severely damaged and when compensation by neurohormonal and cardiac effects can no longer sustain cardiac output. In decompensation, continued fluid retention taxes the cardiovascular system, the patient develops increasing edema, and death results. Clinicians generally agree that patients with cardiac decompensation incompatible with life have a cardiac output that is less than 2.5 L per minute and a right atrial pressure greater than 16 mm Hg.[11]

Classification of Heart Failure

Physiologic changes in cardiovascular status in heart failure result in myriad symptoms that inhibit the ability to perform activities of daily living. The New York Heart Association (NYHA) functional classification of heart failure has been used consistently to measure functional level for the last 20 years. The classification describes the activity of individuals in relation to cardiac disease and places a number on activity related to symptoms (Table 11–3). Researchers and clinicians have used this tool to describe outcomes and quality of life of persons with heart failure. Persons with an NYHA classification of IV have an annual mortality rate of 50%.[14]

Assessment

Assessment of the patient with heart failure includes a comprehensive health history and physical examination. Clinical presentation of acute heart failure may be dramatic, with the patient exhibiting signs of pulmonary edema and impending shock. In the case of worsening chronic heart failure, symptoms may be more subtle, occurring over time. Patients in heart failure need to be evaluated by physical examination both for acute symptoms and for those that represent changes in physical trends, such as increased weight gain. Finally, functional assessment provides valuable information about the patient's activities of daily living and provides the nurse with a baseline for future teaching.

Health History

In taking as comprehensive a health history as the patient's condition will allow, the nurse gathers information that illuminates the patient's current state of health and past level of health, reviews systems for clinical signs and symptoms, and performs a func-

TABLE 11–3
New York Heart Association Functional Classification of Heart Failure

Functional Class	Definition	Manifestation
I	Persons with cardiac disease, but without resulting limitations of physical activity	Ordinary physical activity causing no undue fatigue, palpitations, dyspnea, or angina
II	Persons with cardiac disease resulting in slight limitation of physical activity, but comfortable at rest	Ordinary physical activity resulting in fatigue, palpitations, dyspnea, or angina
III	Persons with cardiac disease resulting in marked limitation of physical activity, but comfortable at rest	Less than ordinary physical activity causing fatigue, palpitations, dyspnea, or angina
IV	Persons with cardiac disease resulting in an inability to carry out any physical activity without discomfort	Symptoms of cardiac insufficiency or of angina often present even at rest

Data from The Criteria Committee of the New York Heart Association. Nomenclature and Criteria for Diagnosis of Diseases of the Heart and Great Vessels. Boston, Little, Brown, 1979.

tional assessment, as delineated in any health assessment and physical examination text.[15] Specific risk factors associated with the onset of acute or chronic heart failure include coronary artery disease, MI, hypertension, and valvular disorders. Onset of disease process and symptoms should be noted. Events that precipitated the current state of heart failure should be investigated for intervention and future teaching.

Clinical Presentation

Surprisingly, many persons with limited left ventricular function have no symptoms of heart failure. It has been reported that individuals with ejection fractions of 30 to 40% have had no reported clinical symptoms. Generally, the first clinical symptom of heart failure is dyspnea on exertion. Other symptoms such as orthopnea and paroxysmal nocturnal dyspnea are highly suggestive of heart failure, and evaluation should proceed along these diagnostic lines. These symptoms are related to vascular volume overload. Additionally, these symptoms in conjunction with known MI, poorly controlled hypertension, and other heart disease are strongly indicative of heart failure.[4] Similarly, heart failure secondary to cardiomyopathy includes presentation of symptoms such as fatigue, dyspnea on exertion, angina, mental status changes, and dysrhythmias. Low cardiac output states can precipitate changes in mental status such as confusion, lethargy, forgetfulness, and disorientation.[9,16]

Physical Examination

Assessment of heart failure should proceed through all systems, because clinical signs and symptoms can be both pervasive and elusive. Signs and symptoms can be characterized according to left-sided and right-sided occurrences (see Table 11–2). Palpation of the point of maximal impulse (PMI) may yield information about cardiomegaly or cardiomyopathy. In left-sided heart failure, the PMI may shift left from the fifth left intercostal space on the midclavicular line to a position closer to the axilla. It may also be palpated as larger than the normal nickel-size area. In right-sided heart failure, the enlarged right ventricle and atrium may rotate to the rear, resulting in a shift of the location of the PMI to a more medial position.

Auscultation of cardiac sounds may be made difficult by loud lung sounds. The characteristic sign of heart failure is the S_3 gallop. This additional heart sound is heard early in diastole, after S_2. It is frequently characterized as Ken-tuck-y, with the first two syllables representing S_1 and S_2. In the person with heart failure, the sound is produced as blood rushes into a stiff, noncompliant ventricle. It is heard best at the apex, with the bell of the stethoscope, with the patient in the left lateral position.[15]

An additional heart sound, S_4, may also be heard in heart failure, although S_4 is not as characteristic of heart failure as S_3. S_4 occurs late in diastole and represents reverberation of blood as a result of a stiff and noncompliant atrium. This sound is characterized as Ten-nes-see, with the second and third syllables representing S_1 and S_2. S_4 may also be heard in coronary artery disease, cardiomyopathy, hypertension, and aortic stenosis. Heard together, S_3 and S_4 are often called the summation gallop and may be heard in either right-sided or left-sided heart failure, at the apex of the heart.[15]

Dysrhythmias frequently occur with heart failure and may be evidenced as an irregular pulse and a mismatched apical and radial rate. The apical rate should be counted for a full minute in the presence of dysrhythmias. In heart failure, the most common dysrhythmias are atrial, such as atrial fibrillation and premature atrial contractions. Atrial fibrillation is present in 10 to 15% of patients in heart failure, with an estimate as high as 50% of patients in the heart failure population. Premature ventricular contractions, ventricular tachycardia, and sudden death from dysrhythmias are also common (see Chapter 8). The nurse should ask the patient whether he or she experiences palpitations, lightheadedness, or fainting spells, to determine whether the patient is experiencing dysrhythmias.

Signs of systemic vascular involvement are associated with both right-sided and left-sided heart failure. Left-sided failure with associated low cardiac output may be characterized by a weak, thready pulse. The nurse may also palpate a peripheral pulse that is strong and bounding, but alternates with a weak, thready pulse. This pattern is called pulsus alternans and may be palpated in association with an S_3 heart sound.

Signs and symptoms of left-sided heart failure are usually in evidence in the respiratory system. Adventitious lung sounds, such as crackles, that do not clear with cough are nonspecific signs. Taken into account with other, stronger signs, such as an S_3, they contribute to the overall picture of heart failure. Crackles may vary in intensity and location of the lung and should be evaluated in conjunction with medication and oxygen therapy. Variations in symptoms of dyspnea often provide an indication of a patient's condition. Orthopnea that changes from using two pillows to sleeping in a recliner is an example of change in a patient's condition. Additionally, paroxysmal nocturnal dyspnea may occur. At night, as the patient lies down, fluid that has been sequestered in the third space or in the peripheral vasculature returns to the circulating volume. When a critical point has been reached, volume overload occurs and fluid is shifted from the circulating blood volume to the lungs. The person wakes from sleep, unable to breathe.

In right-sided heart failure, jugular venous distention may be apparent. As a result of increased pressure within the right side of the heart, the low-pressure jugular vein accommodates the backflow of pressure. As the patient reclines in a sitting position at no less than 45°, the normally flat jugular veins can be seen to fill and pulsate. Finally, jugular venous distention may be present in right-sided heart failure, evidenced as the hepatojugular reflex, which can be demonstrated when the nurse palpates the patient's liver. Assessment findings in the gastrointestinal system are usually associated with right-sided heart failure. Symptoms of nausea, bloating, anorexia, and feelings of fullness are common. In extreme instances of right-sided heart failure, ascites may be evident. As pressure increases in the gastric system, fluid leaks into the peritoneum. Ascites may be assessed through evaluation of a fluid wave. The patient places his or her hand in the midline of the abdomen. The nurse taps one side

of the abdomen near the flank area. The patient's hand in the middle of the abdomen stops the transmission across the skin. If the nurse feels the tap on the other flank area, fluid is in the abdomen.

Cardiac output can be evaluated by assessing urinary output. Urinary output that is between 30 and 50 mL/hour is indicative of adequate cardiac output and circulating extracellular volume. Urinary color and volume are evaluated with the patient's medication regimen in mind. After a dose of a loop diuretic, such as furesomide (Lasix), the nurse expects to see an increase in volume of urine. The urine should change to light yellow or almost clear after taking a diuretic. Changes in weight are the most accurate indicator of changes in fluid status. The patient should be weighed at the same time each day, wearing the same amount of clothing. A weight gain of 1 lb is equal to 1 L of water gain.

The final system to assess is the skin. Patients in heart failure may have various findings, from skin that is cool, pale, sweaty, to normal in appearance. In dark-skinned patients, decreased oxygen is indicated by an ashen quality to the skin.[15] Peripheral edema may be severe, in excess of 3 to 4+ in right-sided and chronic heart failure. Edema may be prevalent in the upper arms, as well as the legs. In advanced heart failure, as decompensation occurs, skin at the periphery becomes cold, purplish, and mottled.

Functional Assessment

When assessing persons with a potential or actual diagnosis of heart failure, evaluation of daily activities, medication regimen, fluid and salt intake, and sleep patterns provides the nurse with important information. Evidence indicates that persons in heart failure are frequently uninformed about or noncompliant with their regimen; therefore, questioning patients about the prescribed regimen and their actual practices is also essential. Psychosocial issues, body image, and care giving issues need to be explored with the patient and significant others, to provide holistic care. Couples can expect a change in the sexual libido of the partner with heart failure, with a decrease in sexual interest and frequency of sexual relations.[17] Patients are assigned to an NYHA class to evaluate their functional status over time. Although assessment findings can be suggestive and helpful, definitive diagnosis is based on diagnostic testing and assessment of left ventricular function.[4]

Diagnostic Workup

Diagnostic workup should be performed to evaluate the patient's ejection fraction and to differentiate between cardiac and pulmonary dysfunction. One of the earliest diagnostic tests that should be performed is a chest radiograph, because a normal chest radiograph is not usually found in heart failure. The chest radiograph demonstrates left ventricular enlargement, cardiomegaly, or pulmonary congestion. Cardiomegaly is a sign of heart failure, especially when it occurs in the presence of pulmonary congestion. An electrocardiogram (ECG) is performed to assess whether the patient has had ischemia, dysrhythmias, prior MI, left ventricular hypertrophy, and pulmonary disorders. The ECG may be nonspecific in heart failure. Two common occurrences in the patient with left ventricular enlargement in heart failure are an increased amplitude of R waves in the precordial leads over the left ventricle and a reflective increase in the S wave of precordial leads closest to the right ventricle. The most accurate criterion for a diagnosis of left ventricular enlargement is an increased R-wave amplitude in lead V_5 or V_6 in association with an increased S-wave amplitude in lead V_1 or V_2 that exceeds 35 mm.[18]

Blood work must be evaluated on several fronts: complete blood count, serum electrolytes, serum creatinine, serum albumin, liver function tests, and urinalysis. Abnormalities such as decreased hemoglobin, hematocrit, and red blood cell count; alterations in electrolytes and creatinine; and decreased albumin levels contribute to the picture of heart failure. Decreased hemoglobin, hematocrit, and red blood cell count may occur as a result of hemodilution because of fluid volume overload. These changes may also result from anemia of chronic illness. Decreased albumin levels are common in elderly and chronically ill patients. Once

again, electrolytes, especially sodium, chloride, and potassium levels, change depending on fluid status and on diuretic and other medication administration. Additionally, all persons over the age of 65 years should have their thyroid function evaluated.[4] Hyperthyroidism can influence metabolism, increasing heart rate and dysrhythmias, which further increase myocardial workload. Hypothyroidism can decrease heart rate and metabolic rate, resulting in a decrease in preload, which increases myocardial workload. Table 11–4 summarizes the recommended tests for persons with suspected heart failure.

After the diagnosis of heart failure is confirmed, additional information regarding the quality of left ventricular function must be obtained. Echocardiography or radionuclide ventriculography is needed to distinguish among left ventricular systolic and diastolic dysfunction, valvular heart disease, and disease of noncardiac origin. Distinguishing among different causes of heart failure allows the physician to prescribe the correct medication regimen. It is especially important for elderly patients to have echocardiograms or ventriculography because medications may have untoward side effects if prescribed incorrectly. The decision regarding which test to order is made by the cardiologist and depends on availability of equipment and the reliability of interpretation of test findings. A comparison between the two tests is presented in Table 11–5. The diagnostic workup in heart failure assists the physician in uncovering treatable causes of heart failure, obtaining a measure of ejection fraction for future comparison, and

TABLE 11–4
Recommended Tests for Patients With Signs or Symptoms of Heart Failure

Test Recommendation	Finding	Suspected Diagnosis
Electrocardiogram	Acute ST–T-wave changes	Myocardial ischemia, infarction
	Atrial fibrillation, other tachydysrhythmias	Thyroid disease or heart failure due to rapid ventricular rate
	Bradydysrhythmias	Heart failure due to low heart rate
	Previous MI (e.g., Q waves)	Heart failure due to reduced left ventricular performance
	Low voltage	Pericardial effusion
	Left ventricular hypertrophy	Diastolic dysfunction
Complete blood count	Anemia	Heart failure due to or aggravated by decreased oxygen-carrying capacity
Urinalysis	Proteinuria	Nephrotic syndrome
	Red blood cells or cellular casts	Glomerulonephritis
Serum creatinine	Elevated	Volume overload due to renal failure
Serum albumin	Decreased	Increased extravascular volume due to hypoalbuminemia
T_4 and TSH (obtain only if atrial fibrillation, evidence of thyroid disease, or patient age >65)	Abnormal T_4 or TSH	Heart failure due to or aggravated by hypothyroidism or hyperthyroidism

T_4, thyroxine; TSH, thyroid-stimulating hormone; MI, myocardial infarction.
From Konstam M, Dracup K, Baker D, et al: Heart Failure: Evaluation and Care of Patients With Left-Ventricular Systolic Dysfunction. Clinical practice guideline no 11. AHCPR publication no. 94-0612. Rockville, MD, Agency for Health Care Policy and Research, Public Health Service, US Department of Health and Human Services, 1994.

TABLE 11–5
Echocardiography and Radionuclide Ventriculography Compared in Evaluation of Left Ventricular Performance

Test	Advantages	Disadvantages
Echocardiogram	Permits concomitant assessment of valvular disease, left ventricular hypertrophy, and left atrial size Less expensive than radionuclide ventriculography in in most areas Able to detect pericardial effusion and ventricular thrombus More generally available	Difficult to perform in patients with lung disease Usually only semiquantitative estimate of ejection fraction provided Technically inadequate in up to 18% of patients under optimal circumstances
Radionuclide ventriculogram	More precise and reliable measurement of ejection fraction Better assessment of right ventricular function	Requires venipuncture and radiation exposure Limited assessment of valvular heart disease and left ventricular hypertrophy

From Konstam M, Dracup K, Baker D, et al: Heart Failure: Evaluation and Care of Patients With Left-Ventricular Systolic Dysfunction. Clinical practice guideline no 11. AHCPR publication no. 94-0612. Rockville, MD, Agency for Health Care Policy and Research, Public Health Service, US Department of Health and Human Services, 1994.

prescribing a medication regimen matched to the underlying cause of the heart failure.

Nursing Diagnoses

The potential and actual problems of patients may be presented in an acute or chronic manner or over time (Table 11–6). Patients may present to the emergency department with worsening symptoms of fatigue and dyspnea, they may be admitted to the hospital from a physician's office, or they may develop heart failure as a complication of acute MI while in a critical care unit. The actual severity of a patient's problem may occur over a continuum and can be related to the severity of the physiologic event. Patients with both acute and

TABLE 11–6
Nursing Diagnoses Grouped by Acute or Chronic Classification

Classification	Nursing Diagnosis
Acute	Activity intolerance related to insufficient oxygen levels in vital organ systems to meet activities of daily living Anxiety related to uncertain outcomes Ineffective breathing pattern related to imbalance between oxygen supply and demand Decreased cardiac output related to ventricular damage, ischemia, or restriction Fatigue related to imbalance between oxygen supply and demand Fear related to current hospitalization Fluid volume excess related to decreased urinary output secondary to decreased cardiac output Impaired gas exchange related to decreased pulmonary blood supply secondary to decreased cardiac output Knowledge deficit, learning need, related to new medical regimen, new diagnosis Self-care deficit related to endurance, environment, or imposed restrictions Sleep pattern disturbance related to environmental noise Risk for impaired skin integrity related to immobility Altered tissue perfusion, myocardial, related to imbalance between oxygen supply and demand
Chronic	Body image disturbance related to perceived change in cardiac status Ineffective individual coping related to health care demands in chronic illness Diversional activity deficit related to change in activity pattern, burdens of medical regimen Altered health maintenance related to complicated medical regimen, decrease in energy level Hopelessness related to deteriorating cardiac and physical condition Altered nutrition: less than body requirements related to increased nutritional demands, decreased ability to provide for nutrition Personal identity disturbance related to changes in perception of self precipitated by chronic illness Powerlessness related to lifestyle changes, multiple care givers, and health care providers Altered sexuality patterns related to change in physical capacity, medication side effects Social isolation related to chronic illness, changes in lifestyle

chronic heart failure have similar symptoms that vary in intensity; those with chronic heart failure also experience functional deficits. Fatigue and dyspnea are the primary symptoms that must be addressed.[13]

In a national study on the use of nursing diagnosis in specific populations of patients, Carpenito[19] identified diagnoses used frequently (75–100% of the time) to often (50–74%) in the care of patients with heart failure. Carpenito[19] reported that activity intolerance, anxiety, and high risk of fluid volume excess are the nursing diagnoses most frequently identified by nurses in the care of patients in heart failure. Further, the diagnoses of altered nutrition, altered peripheral tissue perfusion, sleep pattern disturbance, powerlessness, and high risk of ineffective management of the therapeutic regimen are used by nurses often. Dahlen and Roberts[13] suggest the use of the following diagnoses: decreased tissue perfusion, impaired gas exchange, fluid volume excess, ineffective breathing pattern, and activity intolerance.

Decreased cardiac output is a nursing diagnosis that has been used by nurses to manage and evaluate the care of patients in heart failure. This diagnosis is useful to the nurse in providing collaborative care with the physician. Major subjective defining characteristics of the nursing diagnosis include fatigue and dyspnea. Objective defining characteristics include dysrhythmias, changes in skin color and temperature, decreased peripheral pulses, jugular venous distention, oliguria, orthopnea, rales, restlessness, and fluctuating blood pressure.[20] Other collaborative problems managed by nurses and physicians include hypoxemia, deep vein thrombosis, dysrhythmias, and cardiogenic shock.[19]

Collaborative Management

The importance of collaborative management across the continuum of critical care settings into the home has been emphasized by authors discussing the Agency for Health Care Policy and Research (AHCPR) guidelines for heart failure.[21] These guidelines serve as a standard for treatment of heart failure and incorporate care provided by physicians, nurses, pharmacists, dietitians, social workers, and cardiac rehabilitation specialists. Goals of treatment are focused on preventing the progression of existing disease, preventing exacerbations of episodes of heart failure, relieving symptoms, and preventing mortality.[22] The focus of collaborative management includes maintaining fluid and electrolyte balance, balancing oxygen availability and activity demands on the myocardium, selecting and optimizing pharmacologic treatments, and selecting appropriate surgical interventions when fluid, oxygen, and pharmacologic treatments fail.

Maintaining Fluid and Electrolyte Balance

Reduction of dietary sodium is an initial step in the therapy of patients in heart failure. Reduction in dietary sodium to 2 g per day or less promotes diuresis and enables diuretics and angiotensin-converting enzyme (ACE) inhibitors to function more effectively. With a 2-g sodium limitation, the patient is instructed to avoid high-sodium foods such as processed meats, pickles, and foods with salt on them, such as snack foods and chips. Patients must also be made aware that the packaging of food may result in a higher sodium content. For example, canned and frozen prepared vegetables have a higher sodium content than fresh vegetables. If the patient's condition is severe enough, the allowance of sodium may be as low as 200 mg per day.

Free water restriction may not be advisable, especially when the patient is taking diuretics and ACE inhibitors. However, in severe heart failure, increased circulating levels of antidiuretic hormone may impair the excretion of free water and may thus contribute to hyponatremia. In this situation, a water restriction of 1.5 to 2 L per day is recommended. The patient is weighed at the same time each day while wearing the same amount of clothes. In general, a 1-lb weight gain equals a 1-L gain in water. The exception is in the elderly, in whom significant body mass may be lost as water weight is gained. Therapeutic interventions are reevaluated when the patient experiences a 2- to 3-lb weight gain in a week. During the hospital stay, as patients are weighed daily, they should be taught the significance of weight gain and what to do about it. Fluid overload in heart failure can be managed through pharmacologic means as well as by fluid and dietary sodium restriction.

Balancing Oxygen Availability and Activity Demands

Patients with acute heart failure are kept on bed rest to minimize their oxygen demands and to maximize availability of oxygen to the failing myocardium. Fatigue and dyspnea are two common symptoms that result from decreased oxygen. Nursing management includes promotion of rest, spacing activities, and not allowing the patient to become overtired as a result of care activities. Chart 11–1 describes a nursing research study that evaluated patients' fatigue in heart failure.

As the cardiac output declines, supplemental oxygen at 2 to 4 L per minute may be needed to support the patient. In acute heart failure, the patient may require mechanical ventilation (see Chapter 17). Mechanical ventilation is instituted to increase the arterial partial pressure of oxygen (PaO_2), to decrease or manage the carbon dioxide (CO_2), and to maintain the acid–base balance. Various modes of ventilation can be

CHART 11-1

RESEARCH UTILIZATION: APPLYING LEVINE'S CONSERVATION MODEL TO PERSONS WITH FATIGUE ASSOCIATED WITH HEART FAILURE

Abstract: Fatigue is a prevalent symptom reported by patients with heart failure. The study's aim was to refine and extend findings of a previous study that described fatigue associated with heart failure. A descriptive methodology was used based on Levine's Conservation Model. The model explains how individuals respond to internal and external environments through the principles of conservation: energy conservation, structural integrity, personal integrity, and social integrity. The purposes of the study were to describe the fatigue experience in patients who had heart failure as a result of myocardial injury or valvular disorder and to determine the relationship between selected objective parameters and the severity of fatigue in the same population of patients. Thirty-eight patients were interviewed using a Fatigue Interview Schedule (FIS) developed by the researchers. Data describing vital sign measurements were obtained from the nursing assessment form. The findings of the study indicate that 71% of the subjects were fatigued on admission to the hospital, and 55% of the subjects said that their fatigue was intermittent. A positive correlation was demonstrated between age and severity of fatigue ($R = 0.39$, $p<.01$). No relationship was found between the severity of fatigue and the physiologic measures recorded. The researchers concluded that subjects experienced more subjective fatigue than suggested by their physiologic data.

Critique: The researchers did not include information on the original development of the FIS or on its reliability and validity. Therefore, it is difficult to ascertain the relationship between the FIS used in this study and that of the previous study. Minimal description of the subscales of the FIS are included in the description of the instruments, making it difficult to ascertain their appropriateness. By name alone, the areas of the subscale seemed to correlate with the key conservation areas of Levine's Conservation Model.

Nursing Considerations: Clearly pinpointing the correlates of fatigue remains difficult, although fatigue is a pervasive phenomenon in the heart failure population. Reasons for fatigue as identified by the patients fell into four categories: stress, physical activity, disease, and cigarettes.

The researchers identified nursing interventions correlated to the conservation principles identified by Levine. Energy conservation is described as the balance of energy supply and demand to avoid excessive fatigue. The principle of energy, which was expressed as feelings of tiredness in individuals, can be ameliorated through the nursing interventions of promoting rest, activity, and distraction therapy. The conservation of structural integrity is aimed at maintaining or restoring the structure of the body. In conserving structural integrity in the patient in heart failure, the nurse monitors responses to drugs and provides a balance of rest and activity. Careful evaluation of oxygen levels also promotes structural integrity. Evaluating the skin for breakdown as a result of edema and inactivity is a part of maintaining structural integrity. Conservation of personal integrity involves overcoming feelings of frustration and depression in the patient in heart failure. Nursing interventions that can assist the patient include teaching, acknowledging problems, and affirming and supporting the patient through lifestyle changes. Conservation of social integrity acknowledges that the patient is a social being. Social interaction must be balanced through the preplanning of activities and interventions. Adequate rest must also be provided to the patient. The authors of this study concluded that fatigue "remains a clue to other possible difficulties and requires nursing interventions."

Source: Schaefer KM, Potylycki MJ: Fatigue associated with congestive heart failure: use of Levine's Conservation Model. J Adv Nurs 18:260–268, 1993.

employed: continuous positive airway pressure (CPAP), positive end-expiratory pressure (PEEP), intermittent mandatory ventilation (IMV), and pressure support ventilation (PSV). The goal of ventilation in acute heart failure is to support spontaneous inspiration with positive airway pressure.[23] Patients with left ventricular dysfunction take a longer time to wean from mechanical ventilation than those who do not have left ventricular dysfunction. This finding may be related to poor inspiratory muscle strength and decreased ventilatory capacity. Other contributory factors are increased venous return to the heart and increased afterload, which occur with positive-pressure mechanical ventilatory support. These factors are postulated to work against the incapacitated left ventricle, thus setting the stage for pulmonary edema and making weaning even more difficult.[24]

Further support to the oxygen-deprived myocardium can be supplied through the intra-aortic balloon pump (IABP) and by left ventricular assist devices (LVAD). These mechanical interventions are short term, serving as a bridge to surgical interventions and heart transplantation. The IABP is most commonly used in cardiogenic shock to support the failing myocardium. It consists of a sausage-shaped balloon mounted on a catheter inserted through the femoral artery and placed in the descending thoracic aorta. As the balloon inflates in systole, blood is pushed into the aortic root, thus supplying the coronary arteries with oxygen-rich blood. Deflation of the balloon immediately before systolic ejection creates a negative intra-aortic pressure, which serves to decrease afterload. The role of the IABP in heart failure is to increase myocardial oxygen availability while decreasing myocardial workload through the reduction of afterload. The LVAD is an external mechanical assist device that serves as a left ventricle. The left atrium of the patient is cannulated, and blood is removed and reinfused into the aortic root, allowing perfusion of the myocardium and systemic circulation of blood. The LVAD is a temporary measure used in patients who are awaiting heart transplantation (see Chapter 13).

Selecting and Optimizing Pharmacologic Treatments

Treatment of heart failure involves various different classifications of drugs that work in tandem to optimize cardiac output. Agents may be administered through multiple routes, depending on the severity of heart failure. Classifications of drugs used in heart failure include diuretics, ACE inhibitors, vasodilating agents, inotropic agents, and beta-adrenergic agonists.

Diuretics

Diuretic agents are a first-line treatment in acute and chronic heart failure for fluid volume overload. In the emergency department, coronary care unit, and intermediate care unit, intravenous infusion or bolus of diuretics can reverse the symptoms of acute heart failure in a short period. When the patient exhibits the signs of adventitious lung sounds, S_3 gallop, or peripheral edema, intravenous diuretics are likely to be prescribed. Classification of diuretics primarily used in heart failure include loop diuretics, proximal tubule diuretics, and thiazide diuretics. A fourth type, potassium-sparing diuretics, is used with caution in patients who receive ACE inhibitors. The action of diuretics is to increase elimination of sodium and water by the kidney, thus reducing vascular volume and pulmonary artery pressures. Loop diuretics such as furosemide (Lasix) can be used in patients with impaired renal function. Doses may be doubled and administered once a day, an approach that may be more effective than doubling the dose and administering it twice a day. Initial dosing may begin at 20 to 40 mg/day, orally or intravenously, depending on the severity of the patient's symptoms and whether or not he or she was taking a diuretic previously.[25] Efforts at diuresis with furosemide need to be evaluated at doses greater than 160 mg/day. When loop diuretics do not have the desired effect, or when they have lost their effectiveness through repeated use, drugs that act on the distal tubule, such as thiazide diuretics, may be used.[26]

The problems associated with diuretic administration occur as a result of fluid and electrolyte imbalance. Hypokalemia results from increased potassium excretion secondary to increased sodium and water delivery to the distal tubule. Symptoms of hypokalemia include lethargy, weakness, somnolence, muscle cramps, and dysrhythmias. Potassium is inevitably lost with the administration of loop diuretics and must be replaced, either orally or intravenously. In acute heart failure, when a large fluid volume is undergoing diuresis, potassium levels are checked daily. Administration of potassium supplements occurs when the potassium level falls below 4.0 mEq/L. Hyponatremia may also occur as a result of overdiuresis. Symptoms of hyponatremia include lethargy, weakness, and mental status changes.[25]

With shifts in fluid volume status and electrolytes comes the possibility of acid–base imbalance. Metabolic alkalosis occurs when hypokalemia is accompanied by depletion in the extracellular fluid volume and the subsequent absorption of bicarbonate. Alkalotic states can be reversed by decreasing diuresis or by changing the diuretic to a carbonic anhydrase inhibitor such as acetazolamide (Diamox). Acetazolamide prevents the reabsorption of bicarbonate ions from the proximal tubules and thus reverses the alkalotic state. Metabolic acidosis may occur if acetazolamide is used continuously or if potassium-sparing diuretics induce a hyperkalemic state.[27]

Angiotensin-Converting Enzyme Inhibitors

ACE inhibitors are used as first-line treatment in patients with fatigue and dyspnea who do not have signs of fluid volume overload. ACE inhibitors are available in oral form. Two commonly used agents are captopril (Capoten) and enalapril (Vasotec). Diuretics may be used in conjunction with ACE inhibitors, if symptoms persist, or in acute heart failure. The mechanism of action of ACE inhibitors is to block the conversion of angiotensin I to angiotensin II, thereby inhibiting the renin–angiotensin–aldosterone system. ACE inhibitors are the treatment of choice in heart failure and have been reported to be underused.[28] ACE inhibitors are contraindicated in patients who have a history of

TABLE 11–7

Nursing Interventions for Adverse Reactions to Angiotensin-Converting Enzyme (ACE) Inhibitors

Adverse Reactions to ACE Inhibitors	Nursing Interventions
Hypotension	Monitor the patient's blood pressure on a regular basis. Blood pressure monitoring is required with the addition of an ACE inhibitor to a regimen that includes diuretics. Instruct the patient that taking the drug at night may reduce the effect of hypotension. Dizziness, fatigue, or light headedness should be reported to the patient's practitioner.
Hyperkalemia	Potassium levels should be monitored during the initiation of therapy and continued on a regular basis after discharge. Evaluate the relationship between drug therapy and fluid and electrolyte balance. Desired potassium level is 4.0 to 5.5 mg/mL. Potassium levels greater than 5.5 mg/L need to be reported the practitioner.
Persistent cough	Evaluate the patient's airway for signs of angioedema and obstruction in which the practitioner needs to be notified. Some coughing is to be expected. Anticipate a dose adjustment when coughing is present.
Skin Rash	Report skin rash to practitioner. Anticipate a dose adjustment.
Renal insufficiency	Monitor creatinine levels in light of electrolyte balance. Creatinine levels greater than 1.5 mg/dL need to be reported.

adverse reaction, potassium levels greater than 5.5 mEq/L that cannot be reduced, and symptomatic hypotension. Because of the possibility of renal failure in persons who take ACE inhibitors, patients with a creatinine clearance of less than 30 mL/minute should be closely monitored or given a reduced dose. A major concern in patients who take ACE inhibitors is the potassium-sparing nature of the drug. ACE inhibitors may appropriately be given with loop diuretics, which are potassium wasting, but not with aldosterone-blocking agents, which are potassium sparing, such as spironolactone (Aldactone).

Results of several drug trials over the last 10 years have demonstrated that patients with heart failure who take ACE inhibitors have a reduction in mortality and an improvement in functional classification.[28, 29] These studies suggest that the side effects of low blood pressure without orthostatic hypotension, moderate renal insufficiency, and mild hyperkalemia are not contraindications to ACE inhibitors. Nursing interventions for patients taking ACE inhibitors are given in Table 11–7.

Vasodilating Agents

Vasodilating agents are a classification of drugs that reduce preload and afterload, thereby improving cardiac output. Vasodilating agents do not directly affect the myocardium, but have their effect in the systemic vasculature. Vasodilating agents commonly used in heart failure include the combination of hydralazine (Apresoline) and isosorbide dinitrate (Isordil) and nitrates. Nitrates are discussed in Chapter 10.

When ACE inhibitors are not tolerated by patients, the oral drug regimen of hydralazine and isosorbide dinitrate is recommended. The combination of hy-

dralazine and isosorbide dinitrate has been demonstrated to reduce mortality.[4] Hydralazine is a vasodilating agent that has its primary effect on arteriole smooth muscle, causing relaxation, and a subsequent reduction in preload and afterload. Side effects associated with the administration of this combination include headaches, palpitations, and nasal congestion. If the side effects are severe enough, patient noncompliance may result. See Table 11–8 for a summary of these medications.

Inotropic Agents

Inotropic agents play an important role in heart failure because they work directly on cardiac tissue to improve contraction. Inotropic agents are available in oral and parenteral forms and have different sites of action, thereby allowing their concomitant use. Three classifications of inotropic agents used in heart failure are discussed in this section: cardiac glycosides, catecholamines, and bipyrimidine derivatives.[26, 30]

Cardiac Glycosides. Digitalis glycosides have been used for more than 200 years in the treatment of cardiac problems. Digoxin (Lanoxin) is the most commonly used digitalis glycoside, and as such it is considered the prototype. Also available is the preparation digitoxin (Crystodigin), which has a longer half-life, thereby predisposing patients to toxicity.[31] As a result of potential toxicity and because it is biotransformed in the liver, this product is prescribed less frequently. Digoxin is useful in heart failure because it is available in oral or parenteral form and has positive inotropic, negative chronotropic, and negative dromotropic effects.[27] As a result of the positive inotropic effect on the myocardium, myocardial contractility is

TABLE 11–8

Summary of Medications Commonly Used in Heart Failure

Drug Classification	Generic (Trade) Name	Initial Dose (mg)	Target Dose (mg)*	Recommended Maximum Dose
Diuretics				
Loop	Furosemide (Lasix)	20–40 QD	*	240 BID
Thiazide	Hydrochlorothiazide (Esidrix)	25 QD	*	50 QD
Potassium sparing	Spironolactone (Aldactone)	25 QD	*	100 BID
Carbonic anhydrase inhibitors	Acetazolamide (Diamox)	250–375 QD	*	*
Angiotensin-Converting Enzyme (ACE) Inhibitors				
	Captopril (Capoten)	6.25–12.5 TID	50 TID	100 TID
	Enalapril (Vasotec)	2.5 BID	10 BID	20 BID
Vasodilators				
Nitrates	Intravenous nitroglycerin (Nitro-Bid)	5 μg/min	titrated as needed	200–400 μg/min
	Isosorbide dinitrate (Isordil)	10 TID	40 TID	80 TID
Other	Hydralazine (Apresoline)	10–25 TID	75 TID	100 TID

*As needed; QD, once a day; BID, twice a day; TID, three times a day.

improved. The effects of digoxin are to improve the strength of contraction, to improve stroke volume, and subsequently to improve cardiac output. As a negative chronotropic agent, digoxin works on the sinoatrial node to decrease the rate of impulse formation. The result is to improve stroke volume further because ventricular filling time is improved with a slower heart rate. The negative dromotropic effect decreases the conduction time of the electrical impulse through the atrioventricular node. Automaticity is decreased, thereby decreasing atrial dysrhythmias, which can be problematic in heart failure. In patients who have heart failure and atrial fibrillation, digoxin is usually the drug of choice.[4,31]

The pharmacodynamic action of digoxin is to alter the balance of intracellular sodium and extracellular potassium. By inhibiting the sodium–potassium pump, it allows for increased intracellular sodium, which stimulates a release of calcium from the sarcoplasmic reticulum. An increase in availability of calcium promotes stronger myocardial contraction.

Although the effect on mortality is not clear, digoxin is estimated to improve physical function and to decrease symptoms in at least some patients with heart failure. Digoxin should be initiated in patients with severe heart failure and used in conjunction with diuretics and ACE inhibitors in patients with persistent heart failure. Table 11–9 displays the dosing schedule of digoxin.

"Digitalization is the saturation of body tissues with enough digitalis glycoside to cause the signs and symptoms of heart failure to disappear."[27] Therapeutic serum digoxin concentration is 0.5 to 2.0 ng/mL. To reach therapeutic ranges, patients may be digitalized rapidly or slowly. Rapid digitalization involves the intravenous administration of the drug and may occur in any critical care setting in which the patient is monitored for toxicity. The goal of treatment in rapid digitalization is to obtain the maximum therapeutic effect as rapidly as possible. Factors that must be considered in rapid digitalization include renal and liver function, electrolyte balance, particularly potassium and magnesium, and the age of the patient. The slow method of digitalization may occur on an outpatient basis, with the use of oral preparations, and is appropriate for patients in chronic heart failure.

As a result of this drug's multiple actions and long half-life (36 hours), patients who take digoxin must be closely monitored for adverse reactions and toxicity. Specifically, the elderly, patients in renal failure, and those with electrolyte imbalances must be closely monitored. Cardiac adverse reactions include dysrhythmias. Monitoring for toxicity may be accomplished as the nurse evaluates the patient's telemetry monitor or 12-lead ECG for dysrhythmias such as first-degree atrioventricular block, depressed ST segments, short QT intervals, flat T waves, increase or decrease in rate, and premature ventricular contractions (see

TABLE 11–9
Digoxin Dosing in Heart Failure

	Oral	Intravenous
Onset of action	½–2 hr	5–30 min
Peak effect	2–6 hr	1–4 hr
Plasma half-life	32–48 hr	32–48 hr
24-hour loading dose	Slow: 0.5–1 mg once a day for 7 days	
	Rapid: 0.75–1.25 mg divided into 2 or more doses administered at 6–8 hr intervals	Rapid: 0.4–0.6 mg initially, then 0.1–0.3 mg every 6–8 hr as needed
Daily maintenance dose	0.125–0.5 mg single or divided doses	0.125–0.5 mg single or divided doses
Therapeutic plasma levels	0.5–2 ng/mL	0.5–2 ng/mL

From McKenry L, Salerno E: Mosby's Pharmacology in Nursing. St Louis, C.V. Mosby, 1995.

Chapter 8). In the absence of ongoing ECG evaluation, careful monitoring of the apical and radial pulse for at least 1 minute is recommended, particularly in relation to the patient's symptoms. Gastrointestinal adverse reactions are common and include upset stomach, stomach pain, and anorexia. Visual disturbances such as blurred vision, green or yellow halos around objects, or other visual disturbances should prompt the nurse to evaluate the patient for toxic drug levels. Weakness, confusion, headaches, and skin rashes are also symptoms associated with toxicity.[27] A major cause of digitalis toxicity is hypokalemia because patients in heart failure are inevitably taking potassium-wasting diuretics. When hypokalemia is present, hypomagnesemia may also be present.

Catecholamines. Two catecholamine medications are useful in acute and chronic heart failure: dobutamine hydrochloride (Dobutrex) and dopamine hydrochloride (Intropin). Once found only in coronary care units, dobutamine is now part of the long-term home care of the chronically ill patient in heart failure. Although these two drugs are of the same classification, their actions and indications are sufficiently different that they must be considered separately.

The action of dobutamine is directly on the beta$_1$-adrenergic receptors of the myocardium to increase the force of contraction. This occurs with minimal action on alpha or beta$_2$ receptors. Cardiac output is improved, with limited elevation in heart rate and increased peripheral vascular resistance. Dobutamine is used in acute and chronic heart failure across critical care settings. In the acute phase of heart failure, the patient may have hemodynamic monitoring of arterial and pulmonary pressures for titration of dobutamine to a desired cardiac output. Dobutamine is now administered in the home to chronically ill patients who are not responding to digoxin, diuretics, or ACE inhibitors. In long-term situations, dobutamine may be administered for a set time and then withdrawn. Patients who are dependent on dobutamine are at the

end of their treatment options. Urinary output is monitored as a determinant of cardiac output. Dobutamine is contraindicated in patients with HCM. Before initiating the drug, the patient's fluid volume status must be assessed and hypovolemia must be corrected. Table 11–10 describes the dosing administration and adverse effects of dobutamine.[32]

Dopamine hydrochloride (Intropin) is an adrenergic nervous system stimulant with multiple effects on the heart and general circulation. In low doses, dopamine is useful in promoting renal vasodilatation, thereby increasing urine production. As the dose of dopamine increases, it has more of a beta$_1$ and alpha$_1$ effect, resulting in increased cardiac contractility and systemic vasoconstriction. For these reasons, dopamine is used in low doses in heart failure and is a second choice to dobutamine.[30] Table 11–10 provides information on the dose, effect, and adverse effects of dopamine.

Bipyrimidine Derivatives. The bipyrimidine derivatives amrinone (Inocor) and milrinone (Primacor) are positive inotropic vasodilating agents. They are administered intravenously and have a quick effect that makes them useful in acute heart failure that is unresponsive to diuretics, digoxin, or ACE inhibitors. Amrinone and milrinone are inhibitors of cyclic adenosine monophosphate phosphodiesterase (cAMP) activity, which increases cellular concentrations of cAMP. The exact role of amrinone and milrinone in producing an inotropic effect is not fully known. These drugs appear to have a dilating effect on vascular smooth muscle.[33]

Nursing assessment of patients receiving bipyrimidine derivatives for sensitivity to sulfites is crucial, because amrinone lactate injection contains sodium metabisulfite, which may cause an allergic reaction. Additionally, amrinone should not be used in patients who have severe aortic or pulmonary valve disease. Additionally, amrinone may exacerbate HCM and should be used with caution in patients who have heart failure secondary to this disease. Milrinone has

TABLE 11–10
Dose, Effect, and Adverse Reactions of Catecholamines Used in Heart Failure

Drug	Administration Guidelines	Dose	Effect	Adverse Reaction
Dopamine hydrochloride (Intropin)	Acute failure: 1–5 μg/kg/min Chronic refractory failure 0.5–2 μg/kg/min	Low: 0.5–2 μg/kg/min	Low doses result in primary simulation of dopaminergic receptors in the renal and mesenteric arteries. Vasodilatation results, promoting increased urinary output	Angina, chest pain, respiratory distress, tachycardia, palpitations, increased heart rate and blood pressure, premature ventricular contractions As dose increases, so does likelihood of peripheral vasoconstriction, resulting in pain, mottling, coldness of extremities
		Moderate: 2–10 μg/kg/min	Moderate doses result in primary stimulation of beta$_1$-adrenergic receptors in the heart, resulting in a positive inotropic effect leading to improved cardiac output	Extravasation of peripheral IV requiring administration of phentolamine mesylate (Regitine) to prevent tissue necrosis
		High: >10 μg/kg/min	High doses result in primary stimulation of alpha$_1$-adrenergic receptors, promoting increased peripheral resistance and improved blood pressure	
Dobutamine hydrochloride (Dobutrex)	2.5–10 μg/kg/min	2.5–10 μg/kg/min	Primary effect is on beta$_1$-adrenergic fibers promoting a positive inotropic effect, improving cardiac output	Angina or chest pain, respiratory difficulties, increased heart rate and blood pressure

been reported to cause precipitate in the line when it is infused with furosemide.[33]

Amrinone and milrinone are indicated for short-term treatment of heart failure and should be administered when the patient is in the coronary care or intermediate care unit. The patient receiving these medications is in a critical situation that warrants close monitoring of blood pressure and heart rate and rhythm, hemodynamic parameters, and laboratory values. Hypotension, thrombocytopenia, hepatotoxicity, and nausea and vomiting are adverse reactions that must be reported to the physician.[27]

Beta-Adrenergic Agonists
Beta-adrenergic receptor agents may be used cautiously in patients in heart failure. Beta$_1$ agonists with intrinsic sympathetic activity (ISA), such as pindolol (Visken), are the drug classification of choice. Agents with ISA do not totally block the sympathetic activity of the beta$_1$ receptors. As a result, the heart rate is not slowed as much as when agents without ISA are used. Patients with heart failure may benefit from improved ventricular function and exercise tolerance as a result of beta-agonist therapy. Therapy with beta-adrenergic agonists is initiated after standard therapy is maximized. Submaximal doses are initiated and titrated up to patient tolerance. Beta-adrenergic agonists are not recommended in patients with bradycardia, heart block, chronic obstructive pulmonary disease, asthma, or diabetes. Agents such as pindolol are prescribed in heart failure.[22]

Surgical Interventions for the Failing Myocardium

Cardiac failure may progress to such a point that, without mechanical intervention, the patient will die. The IABP may be used in acute heart failure when the patient has sustained an MI. The purpose of the IABP is to reverse ischemia and to preserve the myocardium. If the patient's condition further deteriorates, an LVAD may be used. The patient may be placed on an LVAD to maintain cardiac output while the patient is waiting for a heart transplant. This situation is discussed more fully in Chapter 13. Mechanical interventions are not intended to be an end point of treatment, but they are usually initiated as a bridge to a surgical treatment. Surgical options for the patient in heart failure have become more prevalent in the last decade. Initially, revascularization of the myocardium by coronary artery bypass grafting (CABG) is considered. Other surgical options include heart transplantation, cardiomyoplasty, and left ventricular myotomy and myectomy.

Revascularization

The decision to undertake a revascularization procedure in the patient in heart failure rests on several issues. First, the primary cause of heart failure is myocardial ischemia. The goal of revascularization is to prevent further ischemic injury to remaining functional myocardium or to restore function to the hibernating myocardium. The hibernating myocardium is a term used to describe cardiac muscle that is underperfused, but still viable. Three subgroups of patients in heart failure have been identified by the AHCPR panel on heart failure as likely to have ischemia: those with angina, those without angina but a past history of MI, those with neither MI nor angina. Patients with nonischemic causes of heart failure do not benefit from revascularization.[4]

The benefits of undergoing revascularization are not clearly delineated by random control trials. It has been the practice to exclude patients in heart failure, or those with poor left ventricular function, from studies comparing medical treatment with surgical treatment; therefore, benefits are extrapolated on what is known from the general population of patients who have undergone CABG. There is increased risk of mortality in patients with ejection fractions less than 20% and NYHA class IV. Further, risk determinants can be correlated to age, sex, concomitant disease before cardiothoracic surgery, emergency surgery, and concomitant valve surgery.[4] However, innovations in cardiac surgery have improved the outlook for patients in heart failure who have cardiac surgery. One development that benefits patients with a poorly perfused myocardium is warm retrograde cardioplegia. Warm retrograde cardioplegia has been demonstrated to protect the myocardium in a more consistent manner than cold cardioplegia, by delivering continuous fluid to the heart through the coronary sinus. This and other techniques have improved the survival rate for persons with heart failure who undergo high-risk CABG.[34] See Chapter 13 for additional information on CABG.

Heart Transplantation

Heart transplantation is now within the realm of conventional treatment for heart failure. Currently, patient selection encompasses a broad scope with respect to age, concomitant illness, and the use of mechanical assist devices. About half of the adult patients who need heart transplants have heart failure as a result of coronary artery ischemia. Other causes of heart failure in this population include idiopathic, inflammatory, toxic, and familial cardiomyopathy.[35] The overriding impairment in nonischemic cardiomyopathy is systolic dysfunction. The decision to undergo heart transplantation is based on multiple criteria, including the patient's severity of disease, adequacy of current therapy, coexisting conditions, and other conditions that may preclude heart transplantation. The greatest difficulty lies in ascertaining the severity of disease. Measures of hemodynamics, including cardiac output, cardiac index, ejection fraction, pulmonary artery pressure, and systemic vascular resistance, are gathered as indices of the severity of disease. Ejection fractions below 20 to 25% are common in patients being evaluated for a heart transplant.[36] Patients who have an NYHA functional classification of less than III are not generally candidates.[37] Diagnostic testing is aimed at projecting prognosis. Patients with a prognosis of survival of less than 1 year are preferred candidates. Patients admitted into heart transplant programs may require intermittent or continuous infusions of dobutamine or amiodarone, and they may be maintained on mechanical assist devices. Chapter 13 further explains cardiac transplantation.

Cardiomyoplasty

Cardiomyoplasty is a surgical procedure that has emerged as an alternative to cardiac transplantation. In cardiomyoplasty, the patient's own latissimus dorsi flap is freed surgically and is wrapped around the heart. A cardiomyostimulator is implanted in the anterior chest wall and provides low-frequency electrical stimulation to the latissimus dorsi muscle. Over time, the muscle responds to the electrical stimulation by beating with increased force. Thus, the failing cardiac muscle has been augmented by a skeletal muscle in training. Cardiomyoplasty is indicated in patients with cardiomyopathy due to both ischemic and nonischemic causes. Patients who undergo cardiomyoplasty may do so when a donor heart is not available, because of patient preference, or because of concomitant illness. The results of cardiomyoplasty are not seen until muscle training has occurred, and this process often takes several months. Therefore, patients must have an adequate ventricular ejection fraction to see them through the training period. Patients with poor ejection fractions who are hemodynamically unstable are not candidates for cardiomyoplasty. Patients in the age range of 18 to 80 years have been accepted as cardiomyoplasty candidates.[38,39]

Before the surgical procedure, extensive testing is done to validate the patient's condition and to uncover problems that would preclude the patient from undergoing the operation. Cardiac testing includes evaluation of left ventricular performance through M-mode and two-dimensional echocardiography, multigated acquisition studies, and Doppler flow studies. Stress testing and left and right heart catheterization are also performed. The patient's NYHA classification is reviewed.[40]

The role of the nurse during the testing and evaluation phase is one of support and education. The nurse provides the patient and family with information about the procedure, answers questions, and directs the patient to the appropriate person to answer questions. Further, because of the limited activity tolerance of patients who are considered for this procedure, the nurse coordinates the testing in a way that enhances the patient's energy conservation.[38] Depending on the severity of the patient's illness, he or she may be in the intensive care or intermediate care unit.

The surgical procedure has two components. First, the latissimus dorsi muscle is isolated, and second, the muscle is wrapped around the myocardium and is set up for cardiac stimulation (Figure 11–1). Initially, the patient is positioned in the right lateral decubitus position with the left arm extended and elevated. An incision is made from the axilla to the posterior iliac crest. The muscle is released from the left vertebrae, ribs,

and iliac crest, but the thoracodorsal neurovascular supply is maintained. Next, pacing leads are inserted into the muscle flap, and the flap is threaded through the thorax at the second rib. The next phase of the operation begins as the patient is placed into the dorsal recumbent position, and the cardiothoracic surgeon performs a median sternotomy. Although cardiopulmonary bypass is available, it is not usually required. After the sternum is opened, the posterior ventricle is sutured to the latissimus dorsi muscle. The latissimus dorsi muscle is wrapped around the heart, and the walls of the left and right ventricle are sutured to the borders of the muscle. Next, a sensing electrode is positioned inside the heart to synchronize the heart with the latissimus dorsi muscle. The muscle is connected to leads of the cardiomyostimulator, which is placed in a pocket in the anterior abdomen. When the chest is closed, the patient has pleural chest tubes in place.[39,41]

Nursing care is geared to three phases: the intensive phase, the prestimulation phase, and the stimulation phase. The intensive phase of nursing care begins when the patient is admitted to the intensive care unit from the operating suite. An initial goal is to stabilize the patient's cardiac rhythm and hemodynamic parameters. This goal is accomplished through inotropic agents such as dobutamine. Nitrates and epinephrine may also be infused, particularly if the cardiac index is less than 2.0 L/m^2. Ventricular dysrhythmias may be present and treated with lidocaine. The patient's pulmonary artery pressure is monitored, and diuretics are ordered based on the wedge pressure.[38] By way of

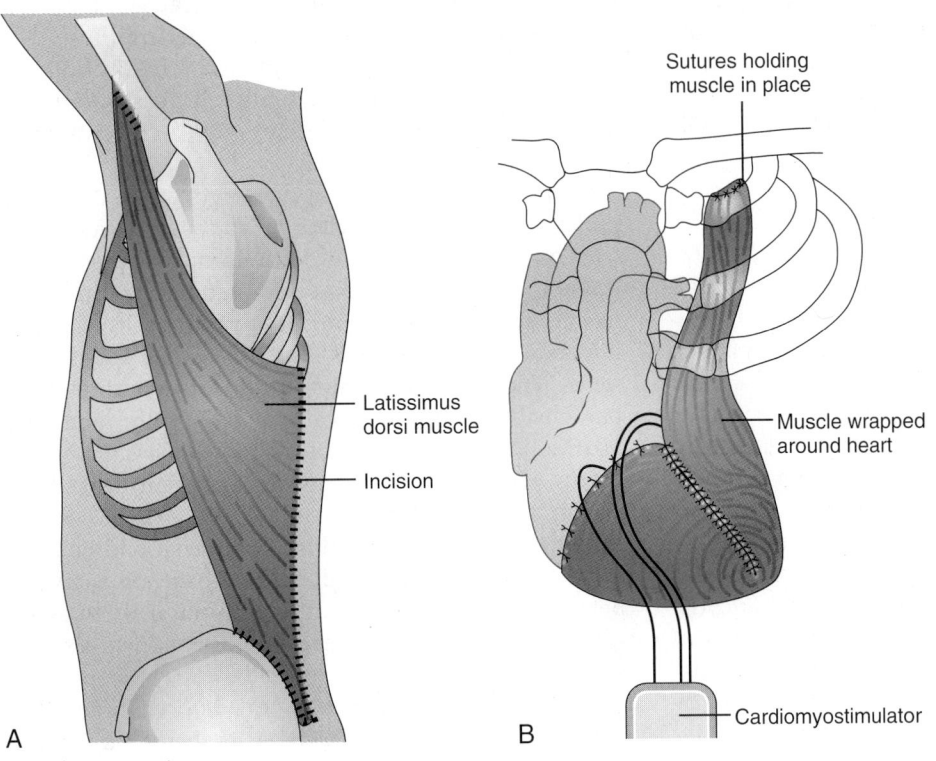

A   B

Latissimus dorsi muscle

Incision

Sutures holding muscle in place

Muscle wrapped around heart

Cardiomyostimulator

Figure 11–1

Two-part procedure for cardiomyoplasty includes (A) isolating the latissimus dorsi muscle and (B) wrapping the muscle around the myocardium.

contrast to the patient who has CABG, the patient undergoing cardiomyoplasty may be more prone to decreased cardiac output and does not experience the massive fluid shifts seen after CABG.[41] Pain is a collaborative management problem that is initially managed through morphine administration. After the initial 12 hours, and when the patient is hemodynamically stable, ventilator weaning is considered.

In the initial 2 weeks after surgery, the latissimus dorsi muscle is not stimulated, to allow healing to occur. The patient remains in the intensive care unit until extubated and hemodynamically stable, and until all inotropic and vasodilator intravenous medications have been discontinued. The patient is restarted on the appropriate preoperative medication regimen including ACE inhibitors, diuretics, and oral inotropic agents. Cardiac monitoring continues until the patient has been stable in the intermediate care unit for 5 to 6 days.[38] During this postoperative period, respiratory and wound infections and ventricular dysrhythmias are of concern. During the initial 2-week prestimulation phase, the patient increases his or her activities of daily living with the assistance of physical therapy. The patient limits strenuous exercise to the left arm.

Stimulation of the latissimus dorsi muscle begins 2 weeks after the patient's operation. During the stimulation phase, the impulse timing and amplitude are increased gradually. Over time, the muscle's strength of contraction increases as it is trained. During the stimulation phase, the patient's ECG resembles the ECG rhythm of someone with a pacemaker. In approximately 6 to 8 weeks after the surgery, the patient begins to experience an improvement in condition. The patient continues to be closely monitored and evaluated. Optimistically, the patient can expect a one-step improvement in NYHA functional class.[41]

Left Ventricular Myotomy and Myectomy

Left ventricular myotomy and myectomy (LVMM) may be performed on patients with HCM. This surgical procedure is appropriate for patients not responding to medical treatment. Improvement has been demonstrated in functional class and symptoms for patients enrolled in a retrospective 20-year study of the procedure.[42] In the procedure, the chest is opened, and the patient is placed on cardiopulmonary bypass. An aortotomy is made and the intraventricular septum is exposed. Incisions are made into the septum, below the aortic annulus and directed to the left ventricular apex. The incisions are parallel to each other, and the intervening muscle is excised in order to relieve outflow obstruction. During the procedure, patients may have CABG performed and a mitral valve replacement. The care following the procedure is similar to that given a patient undergoing CABG.

Adjunctive Therapy

Nonpharmacologic, adjunctive therapies such as exercise, behavior modification, and the promotion of self-care activities have been demonstrated to improve quality of life and to reduce symptoms in patients with heart failure. In a reversal of an earlier trend to keep these patients on bed rest, exercise is now an option for these persons. Even patients with left ventricular ejection fractions as low as 13 to 25% can increase their exercise performance after an exercise program, without untoward effects.[43]

One goal of exercise therapy is to improve the quality of life of patients in heart failure. Rehabilitation programs for these patients may occur in association with an established cardiac rehabilitation program or in specialized heart failure clinics. Duke University in North Carolina has been a pioneer in studying the effect of exercise on patients with heart failure over time. After patients participated in a bicycle exercise program of 4 hours per week for up to 6 months, several improvements in functioning were noted. First, patients improved their functional class by one grade. They also had an improvement in peak oxygen consumption.[44] No change was noted in cardiac function or size after the period of exercise training. Sullivan and Hawthorne[44] concluded that "exercise training may improve both submaximal and maximal exercise capacity in patients with mild to moderate heart failure and systolic left ventricular dysfunction." Other studies suggest that neuroendocrine effects of sympathetic stimulation are decreased after exercise training. This finding is important because it has been demonstrated that beneficial therapies are those that decrease sympathetic stimulation.[22] Additionally, long-term exercise may actually decrease afterload and may thereby delay progressive left ventricular dysfunction in heart failure.

Before undergoing a supervised exercise program, patients with active ischemia and severe left ventricular dysfunction should undergo angioplasty and possibly myocardial revascularization. At the minimum, a stress test should be performed to obtain a maximal heart rate with attending signs and symptoms. The best candidates for exercise training are patients who are medically stable with moderate heart failure, as indicated by an NYHA classification of I to III, with systolic left ventricular impairment. Exercise training is stepped and occurs over weeks to months (Chart 11–2). Further, exercise should be used as part of a total program including psychological and behavioral interventions and promotion of self-care activities to effect the greatest changes in functional status.

Psychological and behavioral interventions that may be beneficial to patients with heart failure are diverse, and selection depends on patient activity

CHART 11–2

General Guidelines for Exercise Training of Patients With Heart Failure

Step I: Screen patient for relative contraindications:

- Symptomatic ventricular tachycardia (VT)
- Active myocarditis
- Pseudoaneurysm

Step II: Exercise testing to set training range and evaluate safety of exercise. Training may be contraindicated in patients with the following:

- Exertional hypotension
- Severe ischemia at low levels of exercise (if possible should have revascularization before exercise)
- Sustained exercise-induced VT

Step III: Begin patient's choice of low-level exercise as tolerated 3 to 4 times a week:

- Walking
- Exercise bicycle
- Low-level weightlifting with 15 repetitions

Step IV: Accelerate program as tolerated with goal set at 45 min at 75% Vo_2; more strenuous forms of exercise such as jogging and water aerobics can be added as tolerance improves.

Note: It is not uncommon for patients who have been exercising for approximately 6 weeks to need an increase in diuretic dosage. Care should be taken that this does not discourage the patient from continuing exercise training.
Adapted from Sullivan M, Hawthorne M: Nonpharmacologic interventions in the treatment of heart failure. J Cardiovasc Nurs 10:47–57, 1996.

---

level, cost, accessibility, and individual preference. These interventions are aimed at reducing the stress of chronic illness through the promotion of relaxation, reduction of anxiety and depression, and promotion of feelings of support and belonging. Specific strategies to promote relaxation may include progressive relaxation, biofeedback, hypnosis, imagery techniques, music therapy, and meditation. Depression is a known predictor of mortality in cardiac patients. Therefore, recognizing the symptoms and initiating treatment are crucial elements of adjunctive therapy. Support groups for individuals and their families can aid in reducing feelings of isolation and in providing useful information and assistance.[44] Additionally, complementary therapies such as nutritional medicine, acupuncture, and homeopathy have been suggested as appropriate for the chronically ill person with heart disease.[45]

Self-care activities promote the patient's well-being through an understanding of the disease process and a willingness to follow the treatment regimen. Early recognition of a change in physiologic status by the patient can lead to early intervention if the patient has been properly educated.[16] Elements of self-care include the ability to recognize and to interpret symptoms, a caregiver to provide support, close professional follow-up, and treatment plans that address comorbidities.[44] Self-care strategies encompass activity, diet, and treatment plans, and they depend on the knowledge and support of caregivers.[46] Charts 11–3 and 11–4 present information related to self-care strategies for patients with heart failure. Additionally, end-of-life decisions

related to advanced directives should be made evident to all parties involved (Chart 11–5).

Clinical pathways are often used to direct the multidisciplinary contributions to the process of care of a patient with heart failure (Figure 11–2). Pathways are often used in conjunction with case management and have been instituted in hospital settings to decrease cost, to improve the coordination and quality of care, and to decrease length of stay.[47] In a coordinated manner, a clinical path serves as a guide for the care of the patient through the course of illness. A practical example of how clinical pathways can serve to improve care relates to the timely administration of diuretics in patients in heart failure. A hospital quality improvement team evaluated treatment and outcomes for patients in heart failure. The hospital team concluded that patients exhibited a higher mortality when intravenous diuretics were delayed and when daily weights and other indicators of fluid status, such as electrolytes, were not monitored appropriately.[48] Clinical pathways that prompt the health care team to attend to a patient's fluid balance can remedy this situation.

Adjunctive therapies may be continued in the community, through the support and guidance of heart failure clinics, home health services, and case managers.[4] Recently, clinical pathways have been used in home care agencies and heart failure clinics in an effort to improve patient outcomes. When the clinical pathway follows the patient after discharge into the home care setting, communication regarding the patient's treatment plan is enhanced. The focus of

0 – 48 Hours	/ /	/ /
LOS = 5 days **Emergency OR** **Direct Admit**	**Physicians Office**	**Emergency Department** **OR ICU / CCU / tele / floor** **(if direct admit)**	**Telemetry / Floor**
Key Pt. Outcomes	*Notify ED or Central Scheduling (CS) or JFMA resident of pts. arrival.* **[YES] [NO]** If direct admit, call CS x6464; if pt to go to ED, call x 6840.	• Responds to diuretics with adequate diuresis. • Improved hemodynamic monitoring parameters. • Pt. reports less dyspnea. • Pt. initiated on critical pathway.	• Lung sounds improved from admission. • Breathing pattern at baseline or improved. • Adequate urine output. • Adequate oxygenation. • Pt. requires lower intensity monitoring with clinical improvement. • Verbalize signs and symptoms to report.

Laboratory/ Diagnostic Tests	ECG (send copy with pt. to ED/unit).	SMA- 7 **Consider:**
		SMA 12 CK with MB
		CBC LDH with iso
		CXR ABG
		Access old record ECG (if not done in MD office.)
			Access old records
			Consider: SMA7 ECG
			      CBC CXR
			      ABG Echo
			      CK-MB

Assessment	Social History: compliance-med and diet (send copy with pt. to ED or pt care unit). VS H & P **Cause of CHF.** ADL history. NYHA Classification _____	VS **Cause of CHF** Tx. PTA to ED H & P PMH Is the patient chronic or acute? I & O Cardiac monitor Pulse ox. NYHA Classification _____	VS, pulse ox., Weight (on admission & each day before breakfast), I & O, Physical exam, Delirium assessment for those over age 75.(done by Case Manager), **D/C cardiac monitor.** **[YES] [NO]** NYHA Classification _____

Treatment(s)	O2	O2
		Consider: ETT and mechanical ventilation
		      C-PAP or Bi-PAP.
			Titrate O2 to maintain pulse ox ≥ 90%,
			Consider: C-PAP
			      Bi-PAP.

Medications / IV's	IV/hep lock	IV/hep lock
		Consider: • diuretics (IV)
		      • nitrates
		      • ACE Inhibitors
		      • K replacement
		      • Morphine sulfate
		      • Calcium or beta blocker (if diastolic dysfunction is known to be the cause).
			IV/hep lock
			Consider: • diuretics
			      • nitrates
			      • digoxin
			      • ACE Inhibitors (If ACE inhib. contra-indicated, hydralazine + nitrates)
			      • K replacement
			      • sq heparin
			      • Calcium or beta blockers (if diastolic dysfunction known to be cause)
			      • IV free water restriction.

Consultations/ Other Department Interventions		*Call Case Managers if pt. to be admitted:* **[YES] [NO]** M - F: 8:00 am - 4:30 pm (beeper 4551 or 4552) M - F: after 4:30 pm & weekends and holidays (x8946 or x8408). Call PCP.	Home Health Referral [ ] Yes [ ] No Cardiology Consult [ ] Yes [ ] No Nutrition Referral [ ] Yes [ ] No Pastoral Care [ ] Yes [ ] No Social Work Referral [ ] Yes [ ] No
Activity		Bedrest, commode	OOB to chair / commode as tolerated. Advance as tolerated.
Nutrition		NPO until evaluated then 2 GM sodium. **Consider** other diet modifications based on medical condition (i.e., diabetic or low cholesterol).	2 GM. sodium with appropriate other restrictions as needed (i.e. diabetic or low cholesterol), Nutrition/Education screen, **Consider:** dietary fluid restriction.
Pt. Teaching/ Discharge Planning		Orient to unit and call bell use. Explain meds/tests. Explain monitor. Teach pt. to report worsening or new signs and symptoms immediately.	Orient to unit/call bell Identify learning needs Give pt. path Explain meds/tests equipment if applicable & initial plan of care. Teach to report worsening/new S/S immediately Provide emotional support Begin D/C plan assmt Give CHF education booklet.
Select variance Facts/analysis ** Please document variance interventions in daily progress note or patient teaching record	A. MAR and/or ED unaware of patient's transfer from office B. Other (specify)	C. MAR unaware of contact D. CM not available E. Pt discharged from ED B. Other (specify)	F. New dysrhythmia G. Uncontrolled dysrhythmia B. Other (specify) If No, Why?_____

Figure 11–2

An example of a clinical pathway for congestive heart failure (CHF). (Courtesy of the Thomas Jefferson University Hospital, Jefferson Health System, Philadelphia, PA.)

48 – 72 Hours	**Day 4 / /**	**Day 5 / /**	**Home / /**
Telemetry / Floor	**Telemetry/Floor**	**Telemetry/Floor**	**Post Discharge Care / Home Health**
• Lung sounds improved from admission. • Breathing pattern at baseline or improved. • Decreased peripheral/sacral edema. • Adequate urine output. • Adequate oxygenation. • Pt. requires lower intensity monitoring with clinical improvement. • Verbalize importance of taking medicine as prescribed.	• Decreased wt. from admission. • Decreased edema from admission. • Drugs stabilized. • Self or baseline ADL performance. • Verbalize foods to avoid.	• Sustantial improvement in signs (rales/edema/body weight) and symptoms (dyspnea/orthopnea) of CHF. • Drugs stabilized. Baseline ADL performance. • Verbalize when to call the health care provider. • Verbalize some foods to avoid.	• Maintain appropriate weight. • Contact health care professional as appropriate. • Keep appointments with physician. • Return to baseline activity level. • Maintain compliance with meds and diet.
Consider: SMA7(if actively diuresing &/or change in ACE inhibitor), ECG (if changed from ED or event related), CXR.	**Consider:** SMA7(if actively diuresing &/or change in ACE inhibitor), ECG (if changed from ED or event related), CXR.		Labs per MD order
VS, pulse ox, weight (before breakfast), I & O, Physical exam, D/C cardiac monitor. Referral to sub acute care. NYHA Classification _____	VS, weight (before breakfast), I & O, Physical exam. Assess effectiveness and side effects of medication. **Consider:** referral to subacute care **Weight obtained.** \[YES \] \[NO \] NYHA Classification _____	VS, weight (before breakfast), I & O, Physical exam. Assess effectiveness and side effects of medication. NYHA Classification _____	Home Health/Case Management • weight (before breakfast) • edema • shortness of breath • chest pain • other signs and symptoms of heart failure • VS/ physical exam • Assess effectiveness and side effects of meds NYHA Classification _____
Consider: D/C O2 if pulse ox ≥ 90%.	Titrate medications with aim to arrive at out-pt. regimen.	Titrate medications with aim to arrive at out-pt. regimen.	

IV/hep lock
Consider: • diuretics
 • nitrates
 • digoxin
 • ACE Inhibitors
  (If ACE inhib. contra-indicated, hydralazine + nitrates)
 • K replacement
 • sq heparin
 • Calcium or beta blockers (if diastolic dysfunction known to be cause)
 • IV free water restriction.
	IV/hep lock
	Consider: • diuretics
	 • nitrates
	 • digoxin
	 • ACE Inhibitors
	  (If ACE inhib. contra-indicated, hydralazine + nitrates)
	 • K replacement
	 • sq heparin
	 • Calcium or beta blockers (if diastolic dysfunction known to be cause)
	 • IV free water restriction.
		D/C IV/hep lock
		Consider: • diuretics
		 • nitrates
		 • digoxin
		 • ACE Inhibitors
		  (If ACE inhib. contra-indicated, hydralazine + nitrates)
		 • K replacement
		 • sq heparin
		 • Calcium or beta blockers (if diastolic dysfunction known to be cause)
		 • IV free water restriction.
			• Review medications.
			• Set up med schedule via mediplan or calendar.
			• Communicate medication changes after first physicians office visit

If subacute care indicated, page admissions coordinator at **401-1017**.	If subacute care indicated, page admissions coordinator at **401-1017**.		Home Care visits. Case Management follow up phone calls.
Advance activity as tolerated.	Advance activity as tolerated.	Advance activity as tolerated.	• As tolerated. • Exercise protocols. • Reinforce limitations. • Consider cardiac rehab
2 GM. sodium with appropriate other restrictions as needed (i.e. diabetic or low cholesterol), **Consider:** dietary fluid restriction. Follow / implement dietary care plan.	2 GM. sodium with appropriate other restrictions as needed (i.e. diabetic or low cholesterol), **Consider:** dietary fluid restriction. Follow/implement dietary care plan. Refer to out-pt. nutrition **x5077**.	2 GM. sodium with appropriate other restrictions as needed (i.e. diabetic or low cholesterol), **Consider:** dietary fluid restriction. Follow/implement dietary care plan. Refer to out-pt. nutrition **x5077**.	Reinforce prescribed diet. Start a diet diary. Refer as necessary to out-patient dietitian **x5077**.

Review/reinforce pt. pathway
Weight diary,
Explain meds/tests, monitor, plan of care.
Encourage watching CHF video on pt. education channel.
Orient to unit as needed, Nutrition education as appropriate.
Consolidate D/C plan.
 	
Able to verbalize importance of taking meds.
\[YES \] \[NO \]
	Same as previous day plus:
	Teach foods to avoid,
	  S/S of CHF,
	  when to contact health care professional
	  when to call for follow up appt.(s),
	  how to activate Emergency Medical System(EMS).
	  Home Health protocol.
	Teach D/C meds.
	Nutrition education as appropriate.
		Same as previous day plus:
		Review pt. educational materials.
		Reinforce D/C instructions and previous teaching.
		Clarify exercise limitations.
		
		State some foods to avoid.
		\[YES \] \[NO \]
			Reinforce diet and med teaching via home health care pathway.
			Weight diary.

J. Pt./Family unavailable for teaching K. Pt./Family not instructed L. Pt./Family instucted, but unable to verbalize M.Refused instruction B. Other (specify)	N. Information not charted O. No measuring tool available P. Pt refused B. Other (please specify)	J. Pt./Family unavailable for teaching K. Pt./Family not instructed L. Pt./Family instucted, but unable to verbalize M.Refused instruction B. Other (specify)	

Figure 11–2 *Continued*

CHART 11–3

Self-Care Lesson Plan

Gerontologic nurses teach patients with congestive heart failure (CHF) self-care in hospitals, long-term care facilities, clinics, or private homes. After nursing instruction, patients can do the following:

CHF: Identify CHF and problems related to cardiac reserve to decrease the heart workload.

Weight: Weigh-in every morning before eating, wearing the same clothes and using the same scale.
  Report a weight gain of more than 3 lb to the primary care provider (physician or nurse practitioner) if diet has not changed.

Nutrition: Identify high- and low-salt foods. Keep a daily journal of foods for the gerontologic nurse to reinforce a low-salt diet.

Symptoms: Identify CHF symptoms (e.g., weight gain, shortness of breath, exercise intolerance,

edema, sensation of heart pounding, increased fatigue, confusion, polyuria, and stomachache).
  Report any of these symptoms to the primary care provider.

Medication Regimen: Identify all prescribed medications, discuss the reason why they were prescribed and their side effects, and identify the correct dosage. Take medications as prescribed and document information on a self-care medication sheet (drug name, dosage, and time and date taken). Report drug side effects to the primary care provider (physician or nurse practitioner).

Activity Tolerance: Identify activity level (e.g., number of stairs or blocks walked without experiencing CHF symptoms). Identify ways to conserve energy (e.g., dress in the bathroom after a shower rather than in the bedroom). Set limits to decrease cardiac workload.

From Bushnell F: Self care teaching for heart failure patients. J Gerontol Nurs 18:27–32, 1992.

CHART 11–4

Self-Care Activities for Patients With Congestive Heart Failure

Weigh myself daily on waking, before breakfast, in the same clothes, and using the same scale
If I have gained more than 3 lb in a week and have not changed my diet, I will call my health care provider and report the weight gain.
I will maintain a low-salt diet. I will know the foods low in salt and will include them in my diet. I will avoid foods high in salt.
I will take all medications as prescribed and know the names, dosages, side effects, and action of each medication.
I will call and report any side effects or problems with my medication.

I will know the symptoms of congestive heart failure, and if I have shortness of breath, increased fatigue, swelling, the need to go to the bathroom frequently, or frequent colds, I will not wait but will call the health care provider as soon as possible.
I will conserve energy and think about what I will be doing and plan ways to save my heart from having to work hard. I will ask others to help me if needed.

From Bushnell F: Self care teaching for heart failure patients. J Gerontol Nurs, 18:27–32, 1992.

CHART 11–5

ETHICAL DILEMMA

Frank B. is a 73-year-old widower who lives alone in a small house with two dogs. He has a history of hypertension, myocardial infarction (MI), and left ventricular heart failure. Frank manages his day-to-day activities with the support of visiting nurses, his neighbors, a local church, and periodic visits from a daughter who lives in a different state. Frank has been hospitalized twice in the last 6 months with episodes of failure that responded to medication treatment. Again, Frank is admitted to the hospital, this time with an anterior wall MI and recurrent left ventricular failure. Efforts to stabilize Frank hemodynamically are more difficult because of the MI. His medication regimen includes angiotensin-converting enzyme inhibitors, diuretics, digoxin, and nitroglycerin. During his stay in the cardiac step-down unit, Frank continues to exhibit signs of failure: tachycardia with S_3, adventitious lung sounds, dyspnea, fatigue, and peripheral edema. He is dependent on 2 L of oxygen continuously. Frank is begun on a dobutamine infusion, to which he responds. Over the course of several days, his vital signs improve, edema is reduced, and some energy returns. When the dobutamine is tapered down, symptoms return. Based on Frank's medical history,

the doctor believes the dobutamine may be needed at intervals, but not continuously. Discharge plans are begun for intermittent home dobutamine infusion. Unfortunately, no one is available to be a care giver at home to monitor the dobutamine infusion, as is the protocol of the visiting nurse agency. Thus, the visiting nurse agency is inclined to refuse Frank as a patient and suggests he be referred to hospice. Frank refuses to move to his daughter's home to receive treatment. He states that he would rather "Go home to die" than leave his beloved dogs. Overall, the physician and nurses on the step-down unit are inclined to believe that Frank would be able to lead a satisfactory life at home with intermittent dobutamine support, that death is not the only option.

1. What personal and organizational conflicts can be identified in this situation?
2. What ethical principles are evident in this situation?
3. What other options may be available to Frank?
4. What can nursing do to facilitate communication between organizations and individuals in this situation?

the home health clinical path is education and monitoring of patient's status and laboratory values. Key elements of home care for the patient in heart failure include education regarding the disease process and treatment protocols, assessment and evaluation of cardiovascular status, and administration of intravenous furosemide to thwart episodes of heart failure. Home care can include the continuous or intermittent monitoring of infusions of inotropic agents such as dobutamine.[32,49]

Further, home care can extend to hospice care as the end of life draws near. Hospice care is indicated for patients in NYHA class IV who have an ejection fraction of 20% or less with optimal treatment. Additionally, mortality is further increased with a history of dysrhythmias, cardiac arrest, unexplained syncope, cerebrovascular accident, and human immunodeficiency virus. These concomitant disease processes suggest the need for hospice care for the patient in heart failure.[50]

Heart failure clinics may also be used as a way to extend the monitoring and education patients receive in the hospital and to promote adaptive behavior (see Chart 11–6). Patients who are candidates for the clinic are visited by a nurse while they are in the hospital. Patients are made aware of the services of the clinic,

which include assessment, medication instruction, dietary planning, exercise, and counseling.

Case management identifies an accountable person to ensure that the patient receives the care outlined in the clinical pathway. Case managers for patients in heart failure are found across the continuum of care from critical care to home care. In a critical care setting, the case manager assumes authority for the implementation of the critical pathway, or other standard of care, ensuring that the patient meets benchmarks of care through the critical care experience. Case management is especially crucial for those patients who are chronically critically ill, such as ventilator-dependent patients with heart failure. These patients are most likely to suffer from a loss of continuity of care. The case manager ensures that the care they receive is appropriate and timely, according to the standard of care of the institution.[51]

Multidisciplinary Outcomes

At the current writing, heart failure represents the number 1 admitting diagnosis of Medicare patients. Hospital readmission rates for patients with heart

CHART 11-6

BEYOND THE ICU: HEART FAILURE CLINICS

Clinical pathways, case management, and the desire to improve patient outcomes have contributed to a need to develop an organized approach to the management of persons with heart failure. Essentially, the question has become, How can the continuum of care for the person in heart failure be expanded from the ICU experience through discharge to home, to prevent readmission to the hospital? A growing solution is found in the heart failure clinic. Heart failure clinics are potentially one way patients can find day-to-day assistance with complicated regimens at minimal cost.

The purpose of such clinics is to assist patients in adapting to the demands of their chronic illness and to stabilize or improve functional capacity. This goal is achieved through a multidisciplinary approach in which advanced practice nurses and registered nurses play a key role. Patients may enter a heart failure clinic as part of the clinical pathway initiated during their hospital stay. In one setting, patients were identified by clinical nurse specialists acting as case managers and were invited to participate in an introductory session prior to discharge.[53] In another report, the heart failure clinic was a nurse-managed clinic operating under a managed care contract in conjunction with a physician practice.[5] The heart failure clinic may serve as a bridge between home health care and complete independence, and may be associated with a hospital, a home health care agency, a nurse-run clinic, or a cardiac rehabilitation center. Patients must be ambulatory, have transportation to the clinic, and be motivated to participate in the program.

The time the patient spends in the program varies. The patient may visit the clinic 1 hour biweekly for 1 month. Other programs last for a minimum of 6 weeks up to 4 to 6 months, depending on progress in the program. When electronic databases are shared between hospital and clinic, the patient may be followed by acute care and clinic providers as he or she progresses through the health care system.

A major strength of the heart failure clinic is that the patient has someone to assess and evaluate his or her condition on a frequent basis before symptoms become acute. Thus, small gains in weight, attributed to water retention, can be managed before the situation becomes a crisis. Additionally, education can be provided and evaluated in a timely manner, offering the patient and family the opportunity to change behavior in response to what they have learned. Assessment of vital signs and of general status occurs with each visit. Signs and symptoms of heart failure are reviewed with the patient and are correlated to patient status. Additionally, medication side effects are evaluated and are correlated to symptoms.

Teaching areas include diet, medication, and lifestyle changes. Additionally, counseling and social support are established to assist the patient and family through the chronic illness. Diet counseling may be provided by nutritionists and covers sodium and fluid restriction. Additionally, cholesterol education is addressed. Medication teaching allows the patient the time to understand the complex medication regimen fully. If side effects of medication cannot be controlled, the physician is notified. Exercise is usually a part of each session. This may occur in conjunction with an existing cardiac rehabilitation program. Exercise increases stamina and contributes to the well-being of the patient. Finally, the heart failure clinic affords the patient an opportunity to discuss end-of-life issues and to face death with support. This occurs through interaction with staff. Grief work, counseling, and a caring attitude are provided by social workers and nurses alike.

Outcomes from one heart failure clinic demonstrated that out of 2 years of operation, and a total of 84 patients, no one was readmitted to the hospital. Costs of the program may be offset by the associated hospital or through managed care contracts. Third-party payers do not reimburse participation in heart failure clinics. This may change in the future, as the need for such clinics grows.

failure are estimated at 17% within 30 days of discharge. Nursing home admissions after discharge are estimated at 8 to 12%, and the death rate is 13%.[52] As a result of the financial drain on acute care settings, strategies have been suggested to decrease the incidence of readmission. Suggestions by health care providers across the United States include the imple-

mentation of clinical pathways, heart failure clinics, home health care, community-based case management programs, telemanagement of patients, cardiac rehabilitation programs, emergency department observation units, and subacute care units for patients with heart failure.[53] The most promising of these strategies, clinical pathways, heart failure clinics, and home man-

CHART 11–7

Multidisciplinary Outcomes Grouped by Acute or Chronic Classification

Acute:

Restoration of adequate cardiac output
Achievement of optimal level of functioning
Restoration of fluid balance
Restoration and maintenance of adequate oxygenation
Stabilization of psychosocial health
Self-Management of therapeutic regimen:
    knowledge of
    Medications
    Nutritional needs and restrictions
    Early signs of congestive heart failure

Chronic:

Achievement and maintenance of adequate nutrition
Restoration and maintenance of psychosocial health, including
    Role function
    Sexuality patterns
    Social interactions
    Diversional activities
Maintenance of optimal level of functioning
Prevention of complications related to chronic illness
Continuation of therapeutic regimen
Delineation of end-of-life decisions

agement of patients with heart failure, recognize that the patient is on a continuum, fluctuating between acute and chronic episodes. These strategies track patients through many different areas of care while incorporating a multidisciplinary approach. Outcomes along the continuum are measured in terms of quality of life, functional status, and costs. The multidisciplinary outcomes that can be anticipated for patients with acute and chronic heart failure can be found in Chart 11–7.

Critical Thinking Exercise

Ann is a 67-year-old white woman who had an anterior wall MI 3 days ago. She is currently in the step-down unit. Her vital signs are: blood pressure, 110/60 mm Hg; heart rate, 65 beats per minute; monitor showing sinus rhythm; respira-

tory rate, 18. A brief assessment of systems follows: neurologic: pupils equal, reactive to light and accommodation, conversant, alert, awake, oriented to person, place, and time; cardiovascular: pulses are equal bilaterally, no chest pain since admission, normal S_1, S_2 heart sounds; respiratory: lungs have fine crackles in bilateral bases, with no cough or dyspnea. Current medications include the following: isosorbide mononitrate (Imdur), 60 mg, once daily; aspirin, 1 tablet daily; metoprolol (Lopressor), 50 mg once daily.

In the afternoon of the third day, Ann calls the nurse because she notes "my pulse is racing, and I can't catch my breath." Assessment findings reveal a blood pressure of 90/60 mm Hg, coarse crackles in bilateral bases, and a rhythm of atrial fibrillation, rate of 110 beats per minute. Oxygen, 2 L/min, is begun.

1. What nursing diagnosis and related interventions are appropriate for Ann at this time?
2. What assessment finding suggest a diagnosis of left-sided heart failure?
3. What other assessments must the nurse make?
4. What hemodynamic changes occurred as a result of the dysrhythmia?
5. What additional medications could be indicated for Ann related to this episode of heart failure?
6. List the diagnostic tests that are indicated to determine the extent and cause of Ann's heart failure.

Key Concepts

⟹ Heart failure manifests in acute or chronic forms, occurs as a result of different etiologic factors, and presents a care challenge to a multidisciplinary team.

⟹ As deaths decrease from coronary artery disease, MI, and stroke, the incidence of heart failure is increasing.

⟹ Heart failure can occur as a result of infection, immune and connective tissue disorders, endocrine imbalance, and pregnancy.

⟹ Hemodynamic events in heart failure focus on meeting myocardial and peripheral oxygen demands by maintaining an adequate cardiac output.

⟹ Left-sided heart failure occurs when a person has sustained myocardial damage to the left ventricle. Signs include adventitious lung sounds and an S_3 gallop. Symptoms include dyspnea, orthopnea, and fatigue.

⟹ Right-sided heart failure occurs as a result of insult to the right ventricle, lungs, or left ventricle. Signs are jugular venous distention, hepatomegaly, and gastric distention. Symptoms are abdominal discomfort and fatigue.

⟹ Hemodynamic changes in heart failure have the potential to affect every organ in the body.

⟹ In response to changes in the cardiac output, two compensatory mechanisms are initiated: neurohormonal and cardiac compensatory mechanisms.

➡ Neurohormonal compensatory mechanisms include the influences of the sympathetic nervous system on adrenergic receptors in the cardiovascular system, the activation of the renin–angiotensin–aldosterone system, and the influence of atrial natriuretic hormone on volume control.

➡ Cardiovascular compensatory mechanisms focus on cellular changes in the myocardium that affect contractility and initiate hypertrophy.

➡ Frequently used nursing diagnoses include activity intolerance, anxiety, fluid volume excess, and alteration in cardiac output.

➡ Diuretics used in heart failure include loop, proximal tubule, thiazide, and potassium sparing. Loop diuretics have the best action against high-volume heart failure.

➡ Classification of vasodilating agents used in heart failure include nitrates and the combination of hydralazine and isosorbide dinitrate. Hydralazine and isosorbide dinitrate are used when a patient does not tolerate ACE inhibitors.

➡ ACE inhibitors are preferred over digoxin as the drug of choice in heart failure, especially when the person is not in high-volume heart failure.

➡ Dobutamine is a catecholamine that may be used to improve quality of life when other medication options have been maximized.

➡ Surgical treatment for heart failure includes revascularization, heart transplantation, myoplasty, and myectomy and myotomy.

➡ Adjunctive therapies such as exercise, behavior modification, and self-care can improve the quality of life and can decrease symptoms in patients with heart failure.

References

1. American Heart Association: Heart Facts. Dallas, American Heart Association, 1996.
2. Williams JF, Bristow M: Guidelines for the evaluation and management of heart failure. J Am Coll Cardiol 26:1376, 1995.
3. Funk M, Krumholz H: Epidemiologic and economic impact of advanced heart failure. J Cardiovasc Nurs 10:1–10, 1996.
4. Konstam M, Dracup K, Baker D, et al: Heart Failure: Evaluation and Care of Patients with Left-Ventricular Systolic Dysfunction. Clinical practice guideline no 11. AHCPR publication no. 94-0612. Rockville, MD, Agency for Health Care Policy and Research, Public Health Service, US Department of Health and Human Services, 1994.
5. Brass-Mynderse N: Disease management for chronic congestive heart failure. J Cardiovasc Nurs 11:54–62, 1996.
6. Dracup K: Heart failure secondary to left ventricular dysfunction: therapeutic advances and treatment recommendations. Nurse Pract 21:56–68, 1996.
7. Gradman A, Deedwnia P: Predictors of mortality in patients with heart failure. Cardiol Clin 12:25–35, 1994.
8. Vitello-Cicciu J, Johantgen M: Cardiomyopathy. In: Kinney MR, Packa DL, Dunbar SB, (eds): AACN'S Clinical Reference for Critical Care Nursing. St. Louis, Mosby, 1993, pp 571–582.
9. Uszenski H, Booker S, Goliash I, et al: Hypertrophic cardiomyopathy: medical, surgical, and nursing management. J Cardiovasc Nurs 7:13–22, 1993.
10. Meyer M: Congestive heart failure: meet the challenge. Medsurg Nurs 4:341–351, 1995.
11. Guyton AC, Hall JE: Textbook of Medical Physiology, 9th ed. Philadelphia, W. B. Saunders, 1996.
12. Oka R: Physiologic changes in heart failure: "what's new." J Cardiovasc Nurs 10:11–28, 1996.
13. Dahlen R, Roberts S: Acute congestive heart failure: pathophysiological alterations. Intensive Crit Care Nurs 11:210–216, 1995.
14. Shocken D, Arieta M, Leaverton P: Prevalence and mortality of congestive heart failure in the United States. J Am Coll Cardiol 20:301–306, 1992.
15. Jarvis C: Physical Examination and Health Assessment, 2nd ed. Philadelphia, W. B. Saunders, 1996.
16. Janowski M: Managing heart failure. RN 59:34–38, 1996.
17. Jaarsma T, Dracup K, Walden J, et al: Sexual function in patients with advanced heart failure. Heart Lung, 25:262–269, 1996.
18. Magdic K, Saul L: ECG interpretation of chamber enlargement. Crit Care Nurse 17:13–25, 1997.
19. Carpenito LJ: Nursing Care Plans and Documentation: Nursing Diagnosis and Collaborative Problems, 2nd ed. Philadelphia, J. B. Lippincott, 1995.
20. Wilkinson J: Nursing Diagnosis and Intervention Pocket Guide, 6th ed. Redwood City, CA, Addison-Wesley, 1995.
21. Dunbar S, Dracup K: Agency for health care policy and research: clinical practice guidelines for heart failure. J Cardiovasc Nurs 10:85–88, 1996.
22. Moser D: Maximizing therapy in the advanced heart failure patient. J Cardiovasc Nursing 10:29–46, 1996.
23. Dahlen R, Roberts S: Nursing management of congestive heart failure. Part 2. Intensive Crit Care Nurs 11:322–328, 1995.
24. Sereika S, Clochesy J: Left ventricular dysfunction and duration of mechanical ventilatory support in the chronically critically ill: a survival analysis. Heart Lung 25:45–51, 1996.
25. Byers J, Goshorn J: How to manage diuretic therapy. Am J Nurs 95:38–44, 1995.
26. Yacone-Morton L: First-line therapy for CHF. RN 58:38–44, 1995.
27. McKenry L, Salerno E: Mosby's Pharmacology in Nursing. St. Louis, C. V. Mosby, 1995.
28. SOLVD Investigators: Effect of enalapril on survival in patients with reduced left-ventricular ejection fractions and congestive heart failure. N Engl J Med 325:293–302, 1991.
29. SOLVD Investigators: Effect of enalapril on mortality and the development of heart failure in asymptomatic patients with reduced left-ventricular ejection fractions. N Engl J Med 327:685–691, 1992.
30. Brown K: Boosting the failing heart with inotropic drugs. Nursing 23:34–44, 1993.
31. Meissner J, Gever L: Reducing the risks of digitalis toxicity. Nursing 23:47–51, 1993.
32. Berkland D: Creative solutions: home dobutamine infusions. AACN Clin Issues 6:443–451, 1995.
33. Yacone-Morton L: Inotropic agents and nitrates. RN 58:22–29, 1995.
34. Brown K: Surgical therapy of chronic heart failure and severe ventricular dysfunction. Crit Care Nurs Q 18:45–55, 1995.
35. Hosenpud JD, Novick R, Breen J, et al: The registry of the International Society for Heart and Lung Transplantation: eleventh official report—1994. J Heart Lung Transplant 13:561–570, 1994.
36. Ventura HO, Stapleton DD, Van Meter CH, et al: Cardiac transplantation: clinical aspects of recipient selection. Med Clin North Am 76:1196–1206, 1992.
37. Grady K: When to transplant: recipient selection for heart transplantation. J Cardiovasc Nurs 10:58–70, 1996.
38. Bove L: Now! Surgery for heart failure. RN 58:26–30, 1995.

39. Bove L, Mancini M, Duris L, et al: Nursing care of patients undergoing dynamic cardiomyoplasty. Crit Care Nurse 15:96–104, 1995.

40. Futterman L, Lemberg L: Cardiomyoplasty: a potential alternative to cardiac transplantation. Am J Crit Care 5:80–86, 1996.

41. Stewart J, Hicks S, Leflar K, et al: Cardiomyoplasty: treatment of the failing heart using the skeletal muscle wrap. J Cardiovasc Nurs 7:23–31, 1993.

42. Robbins R, Stinson E: Long term results of left ventricular myotomy and myectomy for obstructive hypertrophic cardiomyopathy. J Thorac Cardiovasc Surg 111:586–594, 1996.

43. Sullivan M, Hawthorne M: Exercise intolerance in patients with chronic heart failure. Prog Cardiovasc Dis 38:1–22, 1995.

44. Sullivan M, Hawthorne M. Nonpharmacologic interventions in the treatment of heart failure. J Cardiovasc Nurs 10:47–57, 1996.

45. Ivker R: Holistic medicine in action: the treatment of chronic disease. Beginnings: Official Newslett Am Holistic Nurses Assoc 15:1, 3, 1995.

46. Bushnell F: Self care teaching for CHF patients. J Gerontol Nurs 18:27–32, 1992.

47. Jungkind K, Shaffer R: CHF path cuts length of stay, saves $2,300 per case. Hosp Case Manage 4:119–122, 1996.

48. Lauver L: Bench marking: improving outcomes for the congestive heart failure population. J Nurs Care Qual 10:7–11, 1996.

49. Hall H: Dobutamine therapy in the home. J Home Health Care Pract 7:6–15, 1994.

50. Stuart B, Alexander C, Arnella C, et al: Medical Guidelines for Determining Prognosis in Selected Non-cancer Diseases. Arlington, VA, National Hospice Organization, 1996.

51. Briones J, Thompson K, Daly B: Case management of patients with chronic critical illnesses. Crit Care Nurse 15:59–66, 1996.

52. Reiley P, Howard E: Predicting hospital length of stay in elderly patients with congestive heart failure. Nurs Econ 13:210–216, 1995.

53. Venner G, Seelbinder J: Team management of congestive heart failure across the continuum. J Cardiovasc Nurs 10:71–84, 1996.

12

Infectious Cardiac Disorders

Catherine Nuss Kotecki

Objectives

After completing this chapter, the student will be able to:

1. Identify common pathologic organisms and the treatment of these organisms in infectious cardiac diseases.
2. Relate the effects of structural damage of the myocardium, pericardium, and endocardium to cardiovascular functioning.
3. Identify common risk factors associated with three types of infectious cardiac disease.
4. Differentiate among assessment findings in selected infectious cardiac disease states.
5. Formulate nursing diagnoses for patients experiencing the sequelae of infectious cardiac diseases.
6. Compare and contrast selected nursing and medical interventions in the collaborative management of infectious cardiac disease.

This chapter presents the etiology, pathophysiology, assessment, and collaborative care of patients with diseases of the myocardial muscle and structures that occur as a result of infections. Pericarditis, myocarditis, and endocarditis are differentiated from the perspectives of infectious agents causing the disease, assessment data, and outcome of the disease process on cardiovascular functioning. Infection is a primary cause of damage to the endocardial structures and myocardium of the heart. Multiple organisms proliferate, making detection difficult and treatment even more so. Further, because of the use of invasive techniques in intensive care, critically ill patients are at risk of acquiring infectious cardiac disease from sources such as pulmonary artery catheters, invasive procedures, and implanted vascular devices. Surgical procedures to alleviate structural damage, as in heart valve replacement, have resulted in new causes of infection. Finally, because of intravenous drug use and the rise in the acquired immunodeficiency syndrome (AIDS), the introduction of infectious organisms in groups of people not at risk by age has increased.

Data obtained through assessment vary by type of infectious disease of the heart, and distinctive characteristics can be found in each of the three types. Cardiac assessment of heart sounds provides valuable information for the clinician. Pain is part of cardiac in-fectious disease and should be differentiated from the pain of angina or of myocardial infarction (MI). A final consideration in infectious cardiac disease is the effect of the disease on cardiovascular functioning. Myocarditis is a contributing factor to dilated cardiomyopathy, with resultant signs and symptoms of left heart failure. Pericarditis can lead to constriction and cardiac tamponade. Endocarditis may be far advanced before regurgitation of the aortic or mitral valve leads to signs of heart failure.

VIRAL MYOCARDITIS

ETIOLOGY AND PATHOPHYSIOLOGY

A categorization schema of myocarditis suggested by Mason[1] lists the following causes of the disorder: acute viral myocarditis, lymphocytic postviral myocarditis, giant cell myocarditis, other infectious causes, hypersensitivity to drugs, and autoimmune disease reactions. The primary cause of acute viral myocarditis is Coxsackievirus B1 to B5, which can be diagnosed through myocardial biopsy. Other enteroviruses that cause myocarditis are Coxsackievirus A, echoviruses, and hepatitis. Table 12–1 contains the Mason cate-

TABLE 12–1

Mason's Categories of Myocarditis and Related Organisms

Category	Representative Example
Acute Viral Infection	
Common	Coxsackievirus A, B1 to B5
	Echovirus
	Human immunodeficiency virus
	Influenza virus
Less Common	Adenovirus
	Epstein–Barr virus
	Rubeola virus
	Respiratory syncytial virus
	Rubella virus
	Varicella-zoster virus
Other Infectious Causes	
Bacterial	*Corynebacterium diphtheriae*
	Beta hemolytic streptococci
	Neisseria meningitidis
	Mycoplasma pneumoniae
	Mycobacterium tuberculosis
Protozoal	*Trypanosoma cruzi*
	Toxoplasma gondii
Metazoal	*Trichinella*
	Echinococcus
Fungal	*Aspergillus*
	Candida
	Histoplasma
Hypersensitivity to Drugs	
Anti-infective agents	Amphotericin B
	Isoniazid
	Streptomycin
	Sulfonamides
	Tetracycline
Antihypertensive agents	Methyldopa
Autoimmune Disease	
	Systemic lupus erythematosus
	Kawasaki's syndrome
Lymphocytic Myocarditis (Postviral)	
Giant Cell Myocarditis	

gories of myocarditis-related organisms: this table further presents viruses that cause viral myocarditis. Acute viral myocarditis can occur at any age, but it is most prevalent in young to middle-aged populations ranging from infants to school-age children, young adults, and the middle aged. Slightly more males than females contract the disease.[2] Clinical signs and symptoms of acute viral myocarditis can range from flulike symptoms, including fever, to more dramatic signs of cardiac involvement including chest pain, dysrhythmias, MI, and left and right ventricular failure. Symptoms of Coxsackievirus B infection include respiratory and gastrointestinal symptoms, headache, myalgia,

rash, muscle tenderness, lymphadenopathy, and splenomegaly.[3]

The course of illness in myocarditis varies, including chronic and acute components. The condition may be chronic and self-limiting, and the patient's symptoms may subsequently resolve. Individuals with chronic viral myocarditis suffer from flulike symptoms, including fatigue and fever. In the fulminant form, acute viral myocarditis may initially be identified as heart failure and can subsequently lead to death. Unlike idiopathic dilated cardiomyopathy, spontaneous improvement of left ventricular ejection fraction is not uncommon in persons with viral myocarditis. Investigators have suggested that viral myocarditis is a predisposing illness to idiopathic dilated cardiomyopathy, although epidemiologic data do not fully bear out this suggestion.[3,4] Acute viral myocarditis must be differentiated by myocardial biopsy from other types of myocarditis, particularly lymphocytic myocarditis, because the treatment is different.

Viral myocarditis occurs as viral organisms infiltrate the myocardium and cause necrosis or degeneration of adjacent myocytes. After myocardial injury, cellular and humoral responses can result in further myocardial cell destruction.[3] The primary cause of myocarditis is Coxsackievirus B, although a myriad of viruses have been associated with viral myocarditis. The estimated rate of disease is 1 in 10,000 annually. Myocarditis emerges in cycles, making tracking of data difficult. An increased incidence of the disease was observed in 1993 and 1994. During the Myocarditis Treatment Trial of the late 1980s to early 1990s, it has retrospectively been postulated that the incidence was low.[3,4] Epidemiologic tracking of the disease is difficult because of the waxing and waning of the disease.

In addition to the Coxsackievirus B group, other infectious causes of myocarditis include bacterial, protozoal, and fungal agents. Group A hemolytic streptococcus has been found to cause myocarditis in much younger populations of patients in association with pharyngitis.[5] Protozoal infection with *Trypanosoma cruzi* is the primary cause of Chagas' disease, a prevalent cause of heart failure in Central and South America. Chagas' disease involves the gastrointestinal system and causes toxic megacolon. Fungal organisms implicated in myocarditis include *Aspergillus* and *Candida*.

In viral myocarditis, a sequence of physiologic events is initiated that contributes to the complexity of the disease and confounds diagnosis and treatment. In the acute phase of myocarditis, a virus invades myocardial cells and produces myocardial necrosis over 4 to 7 days. The virus may also invade surrounding cells such as cardiac interstitial cells, vascular endothelium, and myocardial fibroblasts. One sees many diffuse areas of myocyte loss, as well as calcification of the cardiac muscle. This feature makes diagnosis by myocardial biopsy limited, because the biopsy must be taken from an affected area. Subsequent to localized cell damage, an immune response is mounted by macrophages, leukocytes, and B lymphocytes in an effort to eliminate the virus. Eventually, the virus replicates inside the myocardial cell to become part of the cell's DNA/RNA. The humoral T-cell response to the virus serves to inflame the myocardium further through the initiation of autoantibodies that attack the foreign antigens incorporated in the cell's DNA/RNA. "Autoantibodies to cardiac myosin have been found in post viral myocarditis, supporting the hypothesis of a viral trigger of an autoimmune response that extends the initial damage produced by the viral attack."[4] Further, viral RNA is postulated to continue in the myocardial cell. Patients with chronic dilated cardiomyopathy have been found to have viral DNA/RNA in the cardiac myocyte. Spontaneous remission of the disease may occur if the body's defense system is successful.

Lymphocytic myocarditis is the type most commonly indicated by the unmodified term "myocarditis." It occurs most frequently in Europe and North America and is caused by an immune-mediated response after a viral illness. It may acutely represent a continuation of illness from acute viral myocarditis. Giant cell myocarditis is postulated to be a more virulent form of lymphocytic myocarditis, associated with dramatic left ventricular decline and high mortality.[6]

Noninfectious causes of myocarditis arise when the patient is given specific drugs that cause an inflammatory response in the myocardium. Drugs such as sulfonamide, streptomycin, isoniazid, and methyldopa have been known to cause myocarditis in rare instances. Autoimmune diseases that have been associated with myocarditis include systemic lupus erythematosus and Kawasaki's syndrome.[7]

Assessment

Assessment includes health history, physical examination, and diagnostic workup. "Acute viral myocarditis should be suspected in any patient with a recent or recurrent flulike illness or respiratory infection who has persistent signs of left ventricular dysfunction."[3] Thus, the history of viral illness is a crucial element to be determined from the health history. Because viral myocarditis needs to be distinguished from myocardial infarction, idiopathic dilated cardiomyopathy, and other cardiac illnesses, a complete cardiac history should be obtained from the patient.

Physical Examination

The presentation of the patient may vary from vague symptoms of flu to an acute state of heart failure.

When the patient presents in heart failure, all the usual manifestations of heart failure are in evidence, including dyspnea, fatigue, tachycardia, palpitations, and fluid retention.[3] Children typically present with signs of a viral illness, such as malaise, runny nose, fever, vomiting, and diarrhea that starts to improve as symptoms of heart failure appear. Signs of heart failure in children include the foregoing in addition to tachypnea, respiratory distress, pulmonary edema, anorexia, tiredness, and changes in activity level. Children may also present with signs of cardiogenic shock and sudden death.[4]

Assessment findings depend on the degree of cardiac involvement resulting in heart failure. See Chapter 11 for a full discussion of assessment findings in heart failure. Case reviews of patients with viral and bacterial myocarditis have shown that findings associated with left-sided and right-sided heart failure may be anticipated.[4–8] Heart sounds that may be encountered include the characteristic S_3 gallop of heart failure, as well as the S_4 heart sound. Depending on the extent of the myocardial damage, murmurs as a result of mitral or tricuspid regurgitation may also be present.[7] Atypical chest pain, which requires differential diagnosis with chest pain of myocardial infarction, may also be encountered. Pericarditis may also occur as a result of inflammation, and auscultation for a pericardial friction rub may or may not be positive. A final finding associated with viral myocarditis is systemic or pulmonary thromboembolic disease, found in both adults and children.[4]

Diagnostic Workup

The diagnosis of viral myocarditis is made based on clinical presentation, confirmation of myocardial necrosis by endomyocardial biopsy, and laboratory data and by ruling out other appropriate diagnoses, such as myocardial infarction.[6] A myocardial biopsy can confirm the disease by demonstrating myocardial necrosis and inflammation without myocardial ischemia or suspected drug reaction. The presence of viral genome in biopsy samples of myocardial tissue after a viral illness provides a positive diagnosis. Negative aspects of obtaining a biopsy include the instability of the patient and difficulty in obtaining a specimen reflecting cellular changes. Because the cellular changes that occur in myocarditis are focal, a false-negative biopsy result may be obtained. Contraindications to the procedure include bleeding, the use of anticoagulant therapy, and intramural thrombosis.

There are many different approaches to myocardial biopsy; the one most commonly used in the United States is the Stanford method of percutaneous myocardial biopsy. In this approach, a no. 9 French 50-cm Stanford bioptome is inserted through a sheath in the right internal jugular vein. The bioptome has a jaw at the end and a handle controlling the jaw in the surgeon's hand. The procedure is done in the cardiac catheterization laboratory or in another room where fluoroscopy is available. The patient's electrocardiogram (ECG) is monitored and the cardiac structures are visualized by fluoroscopy or two-dimensional echocardiography as the bioptome is advanced to the ventricle. The physician takes three to five biopsy samples from the septum, which is thicker than the free wall of the ventricle. Complications of the procedure include palpitations, dysrhythmias, discomfort at insertion site, pneumothorax, and air embolism.

Nursing care after a biopsy procedure is similar to care rendered after cardiac catheterization. The patient is monitored for cardiac dysrhythmias, hematoma formation at the bioptome insertion site, and changes in fluid status. A rare complication is ventricular rupture and subsequent tamponade. The nurse is observant for signs of tamponade such as narrowing pulse pressure, low blood pressure, muffled heart sounds, and tachycardia. The patient may appear anxious and apprehensive.

Laboratory data obtained in viral myocarditis indicate the presence of a viral infection. Table 12–2 offers a summary of the laboratory tests and results expected in infectious cardiac disease. Frequently, the sedimentation rate is elevated. Less frequently, cardiac enzymes are elevated. The ECG may demonstrate normal rhythm, sinus tachycardia, or nonspecific ST-segment and T-wave changes as a result of infection. A pseudoinfarct pattern may mimic a pattern of myocardial injury; this pattern coupled with an increase in cardiac enzymes may confound the diagnosis. Case studies have also cited dysrhythmias such as wide complex tachycardia, atrioventricular block, third-degree heart block, and bundle branch block as occurring in viral myocarditis.[4,9] Echocardiograms demonstrate structural heart disease, increased heart size, and diminished cardiac function. Diffusely hypokinetic chambers and segmental wall motion abnormalities provide a visual image of a boggy, failing heart.

Nursing Diagnoses

A list of commonly encountered nursing diagnoses found in persons with infectious cardiac diseases is provided in Table 12–3. Because disease can occur across the life span, developmental considerations are essential in planning care. In considering aspects of health perception, it is recognized that persons who have acute myocarditis may progress from a high state of wellness to illness rapidly. Changes in functional ability and the need for diagnostic testing, medications, and treatments influence the individual's perception of health. The nurse can be instrumental in assisting the patient to incorporate the medical regimen into a plan for health for the future. Recognizing that the outcome of the disease is variable, the nurse also teaches the patient about healthy living patterns, such

TABLE 12–2
Laboratory Findings in Infectious Cardiac Disease

Laboratory Findings	Pericarditis	Endocarditis	Myocarditis
White blood count	Normal or elevated	Normal or elevated	Elevated
Erythrocyte sedimentation rate	Elevated	Elevated	Elevated
Antibody titers	Antistreptolysin O titers indicated to detect rheumatic fever	+ Antistreptolysin O titer in evidence 6 wk after onset of disease; hypergammaglobulinemia, circulating immune complexes, low level of serum complement	Antistreptolysin O titers indicated to detect rheumatic fever
Cardiac enzymes CK/MB fraction	Slightly elevated, especially if in association with myocarditis	Normal	Elevated
Blood urea nitrogen	May be elevated in uremic pericarditis	Normal	Normal
Tuberculin test	May be positive if tuberculous pericarditis	Normal	Normal
Cultures	Indicated for pericardial fluid, chest tube drainage	3 or more blood cultures in 24–48 hr identify causative organisms in 90% of patients; negative cultures suggest fungal infection	Stool, throat, pharyngeal washes, and blood to identify bacterial or viral causative organism

TABLE 12–3
Nursing Diagnoses

Problem Statement and Etiologic Factors	Type of Infectious Cardiac Disease		
	Myocarditis	Pericarditis	Endocarditis
Decreased cardiac output related to inflammation or infection of the lining of the heart and surrounding structures including pericardium and valves	X	X	X
Anxiety related to sudden hospitalization, changes in health status, uncertain diagnosis, treatment plan	X	X	X
Pain related to inflammatory process	X	X	
Altered tissue perfusion (cardiopulmonary) related to embolic interruption of arterial flow			X
Activity intolerance related to imbalance between O₂ supply and demand	X	X	X
Knowledge deficit, learning need related to condition, medical regimen, recommended changes in lifestyle, discharge needs	X	X	X

as smoking cessation, exercise, weight management, stress reduction, and decreasing sodium in the diet, which will benefit the patient no matter what the outcome.

In responding to altered nutritional metabolic patterns, the nurse evaluates the nutritional status and implements a plan to assist the patient to meet individual nutritional requirements. Consultation with a registered dietitian to determine an adequate nutritional plan for the patient is vital in critical illness. This is especially crucial for the child experiencing myocarditis, because ensuring adequate nutritional intake can be a challenge. In children, an early sign of myocarditis may be decreased appetite and nausea. Further, the child may be nutritionally depleted from the viral episode predating the myocarditis.[4] The management of fluid volume is an important nursing function in the patient who has myocarditis. As with the patient in heart failure, weights and careful monitoring of intake and output are recommended. Fluid restrictions may be ordered by the physician, depending on the severity of heart failure.

Fatigue and dyspnea are symptoms of cardiac disease that contribute to a patient's inability to maintain usual activity levels. An increase in activity in the person with myocarditis can be fatal. A concern exists about adults who exercise after viral illness regarding the risk of sudden death.[3] Multiple nursing diagnoses under this pattern of health can be used, depending on the patient's unique situation. Nursing interventions aimed at promoting rest and sleep are needed for the patient in the intensive care unit.

Interventions for the cognitive and perceptual areas of pain and knowledge deficit are important in the patient with myocarditis. Pain needs to be alleviated, and patients must be educated regarding their illness and expected outcomes. The nurse can support criti-

cally ill patients and their families by assisting patients in maintaining their self-concept and role relationships. Through the use of appropriate communication techniques, time spent with the patient and family, and the use of a caring approach, the nurse can do much to support the patient through a life-threatening illness.

Collaborative Management

Collaborative problems in myocarditis include infection, pain, and decreased cardiac output; interventions are aimed at alleviating these problems. Standard therapy for myocarditis includes the provision of oxygen, ECG monitoring, activity restrictions, and pharmacotherapeutics. In the event of shock, the patient should be afforded mechanical assist devices such as the intra-aortic balloon pump and left ventricular assist devices. Despite a gloomy hemodynamic picture, myocarditis can resolve, with a resulting improvement in the patient's condition. In the young patient without systemic involvement, a heart transplant may be considered (see Chapter 13). Heart transplantation is a last resort, because the myocarditis may spontaneously resolve, despite a poor hemodynamic picture. Another consideration in heart transplantation is the high rate of organ rejection in patients after myocarditis. This complication is postulated to occur as a result of an already activated autoimmune response.[4]

As with the patient in heart failure, the person with myocarditis experiences a compromise in cardiac output and is able to meet the oxygen demands of the body with varying ability. Case reports of myocarditis indicate that the patient may initially present with normal oxygen saturations.[5,6,8] Depending on the course of the illness, the patient may require supplemental oxygen or even mechanical ventilation. Promoting rest and restriction of activity supports cardiac output through conservation of energy and decreased myocardial oxygen consumption and should continue until signs of inflammation have subsided.

ECG monitoring occurs from the time of admission until the physician is satisfied that life-threatening dysrhythmias such as third-degree heart block will not occur. It is estimated that 25% of patients with viral myocarditis have runs of nonsustained ventricular tachycardia. Treatment of this dysrhythmia should be approached cautiously with agents that do not suppress ventricular function. As myocarditis improves, dysrhythmias may resolve, although residual occurrences are possible. Temporary pacing should be considered for atrioventricular block. Implantable cardioverter defibrillators (ICDs) and permanent pacemakers are used for residual dysrhythmias.[9]

The goal of initiating pharmacotherapeutics is to maximize myocardial oxygen availability and contractility, to control infection, to manage pain, and to minimize the inflammatory response. This goal is initially realized through prescription of a regimen similar to or the same as for heart failure. Agents used in heart failure such as angiotensin-converting enzyme inhibitors, vasodilating agents, and inotropic agents may also be used in myocarditis, depending on the severity of the illness (see Chapter 11). Additional therapy in myocarditis includes anti-infective agents for specific causative organisms. Cephalosporins are commonly used for beta-hemolytic streptococci. The efficacy of antiviral agents has not been demonstrated in humans. Data from animal trials suggest that a decrease in viral titers occurs when these agents are administered at the onset of the disease process.[10] Usually, by the time antibody titers rise to a detectable level, the subclinical phase of the illness is over, and the chronic or acute phase has begun, making the administration of antiviral agents less effective. Finally, some controversy exists over the use of nonsteroidal anti-inflammatory drugs (NSAIDs) for management of pain and inflammation and the use of immunosuppressive agents such as corticosteroids.

NSAIDs may be useful for pain relief in various situations, especially if the patient experiences concomitant pericarditis. The primary action of NSAIDs occurs through the inhibition of the biosynthesis and the release of prostaglandins. The result is a decrease in the inflammatory response and the inhibition of substances that sensitize pain receptors to stimuli. Locally, NSAIDs inhibit leukocyte migration and lysosomal enzyme release and activation. NSAIDs also exhibit an antipyretic effect. Caution is advised in administering NSAIDs early in the infectious process of myocarditis, because animal studies have demonstrated a worsening of pathophysiologic changes. When NSAIDs are administered later in the illness, these changes have

not been observed. The conclusion drawn from this information is that NSAIDs should be administered later in the course of illness, in conjunction with signs and symptoms of pericarditis.[10]

The continuing process of inflammation and the formation of antiheart antibodies has led researchers to study whether immunosuppressant agents such as corticosteroids and cyclosporine could be useful in preventing the progression of ventricular damage. Animal models demonstrate that treatment with prednisone early in the course of the illness contributes to overall myocardial necrosis and inflammation. Therefore, the use of prednisone or other immunosuppressive agents should be reserved for extreme cases. The guiding principle in administration of immunosuppressant agents is to administer them later in the course of illness, after 2 weeks to 18 days, rather than at the beginning of the illness.[3,4] The rationale behind this approach is that immunosuppression at an early stage allows for more rapid viral replication.

Controversy exists over the efficacy of the administration of corticosteroids in viral myocarditis because of the difficulty in obtaining randomized clinical trials in humans. In addition to the uncertainty of the timing of administration of prednisone, patients who receive corticosteroids experience complications that are dose related. These complications include the worsening of cardiac symptoms (e.g., decreased blood pressure, increased heart rate, and dysrhythmias) and side effects (e.g., hyperglycemia, gastrointestinal hemorrhage, and mental status changes).[4] The use of cyclosporine in the Myocarditis Control Trial[1] produced problematic side effects such as hypertension and renal failure. Other drugs with less severe side effects, such as methotrexate (amethopterin) and azathioprine (Imuran), were not available at the start of the trial, and thus they have not been adequately studied.[10] See the section on multidisciplinary outcomes for outcomes anticipated for a patient with myocarditis.

PERICARDITIS

Pericarditis is the second infectious cardiac disease considered in this chapter. Like viral myocarditis, it has an inflammatory component, causing pain and alteration in cardiac output. Moreover, like myocarditis, pericarditis has multiple causative factors, resulting in acute and chronic conditions. Pericarditis has a different pathophysiologic course than myocarditis; it occurs as a result of complications of acute or chronic inflammation that restrict the pericardium. Pericarditis, an infectious process, can occur alone or concomitantly with pericardial effusion. Pericardial effusion, a buildup of fluid in the pericardium, can be hemorrhagic or exudative. Cardiac tamponade can occur insidiously or acutely, resulting in death. Cardiac tamponade occurs when blood or exudate builds up in the pericardial space and restricts movement of the atria and ventricles, resulting in low cardiac output. Assessment is centered on determining causative factors of pericarditis and identifying the cardiac and pulmonary signs and symptoms of pericarditis. Treatment goals are aimed at the reduction of pain, the maintenance of cardiac output, and the resolution of infection.

ETIOLOGY AND PATHOPHYSIOLOGY

Diseases of the pericardium encompass various disorders arising from different causative factors, including infection, cardiac injury such as MI and cardiac surgery, renal disease, neoplasms, and collagen vascular diseases. Pericarditis involves inflammation and infection of the visceral, parietal, and fibrous pericardium (see Chapter 6). The visceral pericardium encases the heart and extends several centimeters onto the great vessels. The parietal pericardium is fused to the fibrous pericardium to form a fibrous layer. The parietal pericardium is attached by ligaments to the manubrium, xiphoid process, vertebral column, and diaphragm. The two pericardial surfaces are lined by smooth serous tissue, separated by 15 to 50 mL of fluid. When the fluid exceeds the expected amount or when it becomes purulent or hemorrhagic, a pericardial effusion exists.

Changes in the pericardium occur related to inflammation and the buildup of excess fluid. In pericarditis without effusion, sometimes called "dry" pericarditis, the visceral and parietal structures surrounding the heart have an intense inflammatory response characterized by adhesions, increased vascularity, and fibrin deposits.[11] In pericardial effusion, the constrictive outcome is related to the quantity and rapidity with which the effusion develops. If the effusion develops slowly, the pericardial space may accommodate up to 2 L of fluid, accompanied by a little increase in intrapericardial pressure. When fluid develops rapidly, such as in trauma, as little as 100 to 200 mL of fluid may cause cardiac tamponade. Large effusions lead to findings such as muffled heart sounds, elevated jugular venous pressure, fatigue, adventitious lung sounds, and decreased blood pressure.[12]

Pericarditis is usually self-limiting, but it can manifest as the first symptom of a systemic illness, such as cancer. Pericarditis is classified as acute or constrictive. Acute pericarditis is associated with infection and cardiac trauma or injury. Constrictive pericarditis usually results from chronically occurring episodes of pericarditis in patients with cancer and those who are receiving renal dialysis. The slow onset of fluid buildup allows for accommodation by the pericardial

walls; as a result, symptoms may not be apparent until a volume of fluid greater than 250 mL has accumulated.

Acute Pericarditis

The diagnosis of acute pericarditis is estimated to occur in less than 0.1% of hospitalizations. It has been found in 2 to 6% of postmortem cases in persons without signs of the disease.[11] Of cases of acute pericarditis, 86% are estimated to have an idiopathic cause. Idiopathic pericarditis is usually associated with a viral cause, although other organisms, such as bacteria or fungi, have been suggested.[11] Viral causes occur most frequently in North Americans and Europeans. Viral organisms that cause acute pericarditis include Coxsackievirus group B and echovirus, common causative organisms in viral myocarditis. Similar to the infectious process in myocarditis, these viruses are cyclic and experience a resurgence in the fall and spring.[12] The course of acute viral pericarditis is generally self-limiting, lasting from 1 to 3 weeks. Treatment is directed at alleviating symptoms. Two complications that must be monitored include acute myocarditis and cardiac tamponade.

Pericarditis is increasingly becoming a cardiovascular complication of AIDS. Pericarditis may be the first cardiac sign in a patient with AIDS, and it may occur with or without pericardial effusion.[13] In a study conducted in the San Francisco area, 30% of human immunodeficiency virus (HIV)-infected patients had pericardial effusion as documented by echocardiography, with tamponade developing in approximately 8% of those patients.[14]

Bacterial causes of acute pericarditis include organisms such as *Mycobacterium tuberculosis* and *Mycoplasma pneumoniae*. *Mycobacterium tuberculosis* is the most common cause of acute pericarditis in developing areas such as India and Africa.[12] A second cause of acute pericarditis is related to cardiac injury or trauma, such as occurs in myocardial infarction or cardiac surgery. Acute pericarditis in this situation is mediated by an autoimmune response and is known collectively as postcardiac injury syndrome and, respectively, as Dressler's syndrome and postpericardiotomy syndrome. The exact mechanism by which the patient develops pericarditis is unclear, but it is postulated that after cardiac injury, a release of cardiac antigens leads to the formation of antiheart antibodies. Subsequent to their development, an inflammatory response is mounted, causing inflammation in the pericardium, lungs, and pleura.

Pericarditis after MI, or Dressler's syndrome, can occur 2 to 11 weeks after MI and has been reported as occurring as early as 1 week and as late as several months after MI. The incidence has been reported to be between less than 5% and up to 25% of patients with MI.[11, 15] This syndrome is associated with transmural infarction, anterior and right ventricular infarctions, and left pleural effusion. Pericarditis associated with MI is reduced when thrombolytic agents are used. Dressler's syndrome is usually self-limiting, but it rarely becomes chronic, occurring up to 1 year after MI.

Postpericardiotomy syndrome includes a clinical picture of fever, eosinophilia pericarditis, and pleuritis. Pleural effusions are present, as demonstrated on a chest radiograph. This syndrome is estimated to occur in 10 to 40% of cardiac surgical cases.[15] Syndromes occurring as a result of autoimmune activity after cardiac injury or surgery must be differentiated from postperfusion cardiac syndrome, which occurs as a result of cytomegalovirus infection during the surgical procedure. Other factors associated with acute pericarditis are presented in Table 12–4.

Constrictive Pericarditis

Constrictive pericarditis frequently arises from chronic inflammation of the pericardium occurring over a period of months or years. Initially, pericardial fluid produced during an acute infection is reabsorbed. Subsequently, the visceral and parietal pericardium thicken and fuse. Finally, calcification of the pericardium inhibits cardiac movement altogether. This process may occur symmetrically around the heart or locally. Constriction of the heart occurs with subclinical symptoms and is associated with previous cardiac surgery or radiation therapy for cancer including Hodgkin's disease. Treatment is surgical removal of all or part of the pericardium.[12]

Assessment

Assessment of the patient with pericarditis focuses on differentiating this illness from other cardiac illnesses, especially angina or MI, and determining the type of pericarditis present. The PQRST method of assessment is again helpful in evaluating the patient (see Chapter 9). In focusing on the questions of the history, the nurse takes into consideration whether the patient has had a viral syndrome or bacterial infection, previous cardiac surgery, cancer or other immunosuppressive diseases, or renal failure. New immigrants to the United States must be suspected of having tuberculosis pericarditis. The possibility of gastrointestinal disease must be evaluated as well.

Clinical Presentation

The assessment of signs and symptoms of pericarditis is aimed at differentiating between acute or constrictive with or without a pericardial effusion. The classic presentation of acute pericarditis is of a patient with severe chest pain. The medical history is initially focused on evaluating the patient's pain and differentiating it from other causes, especially angina or MI. Table 12–5 compares the pain of pericarditis to pain in angina or MI. Pain is the most common acute symptom and is frequently manifested as retrosternal or left substernal, radiating to shoulder, neck, or arm. The characteristic of the pain is more sharp or burning, and it is exacerbated by deep breathing, coughing, or lying down. The patient presents in a characteristic upright, bent-forward position.[16]

Physical Examination

Assessment should proceed in a systematic manner, starting with general appearance and evaluation of the patient for signs of infection and cardiac status. Signs of infection that may be evident include fever, chills, and weakness. Patients may exhibit signs of dyspnea, which must be investigated to determine whether they are related to pain or lack of oxygen due to tamponade. The nurse evaluates the patient for the classic sign of pericardial friction rub. This cardiac sound is heard as a high-pitched, scratching sound and can be described as two pieces of sandpaper being rubbed together.[17] It is heard best at the lower left sternal border, where the pericardium lies close to the chest wall, or at the location of inflammation, as inflamed pericardial and epicardial surfaces come together. A pericardial friction rub is differentiated from a pleural friction rub by having a person initially hold his or her breath and listening and then releasing the breath and listening. A rub of cardiac origin continues, whereas a pleural friction rub ceases during respiration. A pericardial friction rub is heard best during forced expiration and may be heard intermittently.[18]

Because the patient with acute pericarditis may experience a sudden increase in the amount of fluid surrounding the heart, the nurse is alert for signs of tamponade. Cardiac tamponade occurs in response to constriction around the heart that prevents contraction of the myocardium. Characteristic signs include low blood pressure with a narrowing pulse pressure, elevated jugular venous distention, and pulsus paradoxus (see Chapter 7). Pulsus paradoxus is a characteristic increasing and decreasing of the pulse pressure that may be viewed on the arterial waveform. This pattern of higher pulse pressure with lower pulse pressures can be seen in concert with the patient's respiratory pattern.

By way of contrast, signs of chronic pericarditis closely resemble those of right-sided heart failure. This similarity relates to an increase in intracardiac pressure that forces increased system pressure. Thus, jugular venous distention is a characteristic sign of

TABLE 12–4
Summary of Causes of Acute Pericarditis

Classification	Etiology	Organism	Disease Course	Population
Infectious				
Idiopathic or viral	Peak in fall and spring; viral symptoms, fever, chills, fatigue	Coxsackievirus group B, echovirus type B, in AIDS patients, cyto-megalovirus, herpes	Self-limiting 1–3 wk course, associated with pain; serious complications inclu-ding acute myocar-ditis and cardiac tamponade	Opportunistic infection in immunosup-pressed patients, e.g., cancer or AIDS
Bacterial	Associated with medi-astinitis after cardiac surgery	*Staphylococcus epi-dermidis, Staphy-lococcus* sep-ticemia	Occurring within a week of surgery, chest tubes for drainage of puru-lent material possi-bly required	Patients experiencing chest trauma or cardiac surgical procedures involving the mediastinum
Postcardiac Injury Syndrome				
Pericarditis after MI (Dressler's syndrome)	Mediated by an immune response after MI; less than 5% of MI up to 25% of MI; common findings fever, fatigue, pericarditis, leukocytosis		2 to 11 weeks after MI, as early as 1 week, late occurrences up to 1 year, possibly becoming chronic	After MI
Postericardiotomy syndrome	Mediated by immune re-sponse; 10 to 40% of post cardiac surgery		Occurring within a week of surgery or trauma	Cardiac surgical pa-tients and patients who experience trauma of pericardium
Neoplastic	Most common cause of hemorrhagic pericardi-al effusion; occurs as a result of direct exten-sion of mediastinal tu-mor, e.g., breast, or through seeding as in leukemia, lymphoma, or melanoma		Varying depending on the length of time the tumor has been growing	Tumor of mediastinum, breast cancer, leukemia, lymphoma, melanoma
Uremic	Seen in renal dialysis pa-tients related to azote-mia, develops when blood urea nitrogen > 100 mg/dL, small effusions may be a re-sult of volume over-load		Occurs between dial-ysis; can last 1 to 2 weeks with large pleural effusions	Patients on renal dialysis

MI, myocardial infarction.

constrictive pericarditis. Also evident are clinical signs of edema, anasarca, gastric fullness, and anorexia. As the disease progresses, left heart involvement becomes apparent, and the patient demonstrates symptoms such as dyspnea, cough, and orthopnea. Auscultation may or may not reveal the sound of "cardiac knock." This early diastolic sound corresponds to the sudden cessation of rapid filling that occurs as a result of con-striction. It is similar to S_3, but with a higher pitch.

Diagnostic Workup

Diagnostic workup includes evaluation of laboratory values (see Table 12–2), ECG, chest radiograph,

TABLE 12–5

Comparison of Pain in Pericarditis, Angina, and Myocardial Infarction

Causes	Location	Characteristic Symptoms	Duration
Pericarditis	Retrosternal, radiating to arms, neck, back	Stabbing or burning, increasing with inspiration, aggravated by coughing, deep breathing, or lying down; auscultation of a pericardial friction rub	Intermittent
Angina	Substernal, radiating to arms, shoulders, neck, back, or jaw	Burning, squeezing, or pressure that is mild to severe; onset related to activity, emotional upset, eating a large meal	Short duration, < 30 minutes, relieved by nitroglycerin
Myocardial infarction	Substernal pain radiating to arms, shoulder, neck, back, or jaw, particularly on the left side	Heavy pressure, burning, associated with dyspnea, sweating; onset can be related to above, also can be sudden	Prolonged pain > 30 min unrelieved by nitroglycerin

echocardiogram, and cardiac catheterization. In acute pericarditis, the rhythm is usually sinus rhythm or sinus tachycardia. During the acute phase, the ECG goes through characteristic changes that distinguish the condition from myocardial infarction. Initially, the ECG demonstrates increased ST-segment elevation in a concave pattern in the leads with prominent R waves. This pattern occurs in the presence of chest pain. The ST-segment elevation is diffuse across leads, without the specificity of patterns that emerge in myocardial infarction. Concomitant with ST-segment elevation is PR depression (Figure 12–1). After a few days, the ST segment returns to the isoelectric line, with T-wave flattening and then inversion. Finally, T waves revert to normal weeks or months after the illness. The ECG with signs of pericardial effusion often demonstrates a reduction of QRS voltage or T-wave flattening.

Diagnostic imaging of the heart provides the most useful information in pericardial effusion. Pericardial effusion can be visualized on chest radiograph, magnetic resonance imaging (MRI), and echocardiogram. The chest radiograph of pericarditis presents with a characteristic bottleneck appearance of the heart, indicating a widened mediastinum. MRI is useful in distinguishing between hemorrhagic and serous exudate and pericardial thickening. The most definitive tool for diagnosis of pericardial effusion is the echocardiogram, which demonstrates an echo-free space between the ventricular wall and the pericardium (Chart 12–1). Constrictive pericarditis demonstrates calcified thinning of the pericardium with normal left ventricular function. Cardiac catheterization may complete the cardiac workup. Catheterization documents right-sided and left-sided heart pressures, and it can aid in diagnosing constrictive pericarditis.[11]

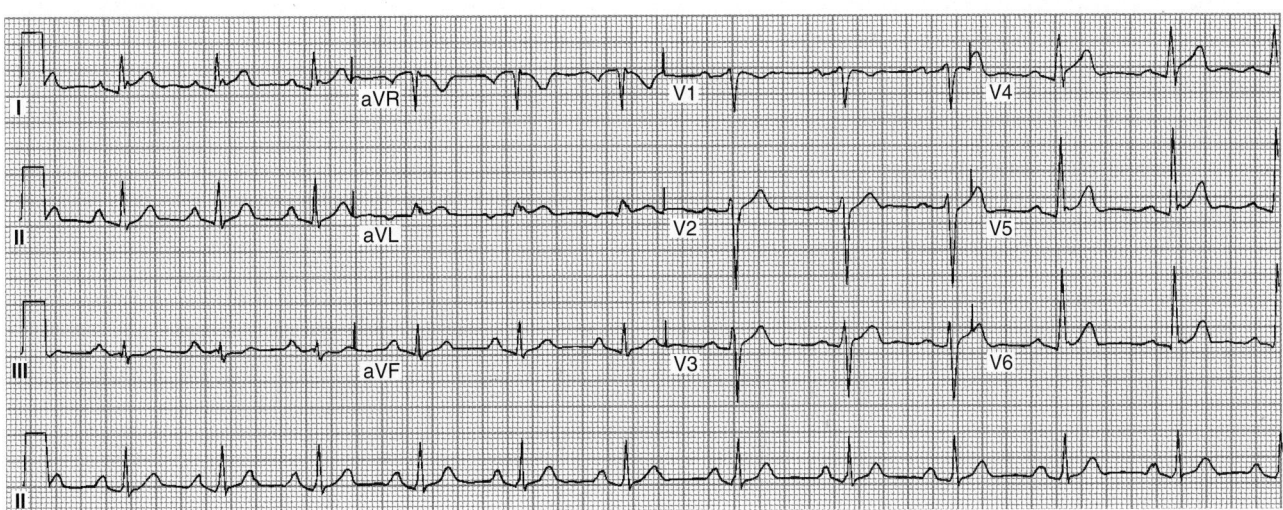

Figure 12–1

ECG evidence of pericarditis. Note the depression of the PR segment in leads I, II, aVF, V$_4$, V$_5$, V$_6$ and the 0.5-mm ST elevation in leads V$_2$, V$_3$, and V$_4$.

CHART 12-1

RESEARCH UTILIZATION: PERICARDIAL INVOLVEMENT DURING MYOCARDIAL INFARCTION

Abstract: The purpose of this study was to investigate the long-term course of infarct-related pericarditis and pericardial effusion. The objectives of the study were as follows: 1) to describe the incidence of pericarditis and pericardial effusion during the initial 3 weeks and following 3 years after acute myocardial infarction (AMI), 2) to describe the timing, size, and hemodynamic consequences of pericardial effusion, 3) to determine the extent of the relationship between clinical signs of pericarditis and echocardiographic findings, and 4) to evaluate the effect of thrombolytic or anticoagulant therapy on the consequences of pericardial effusion. The study was a prospective study of 192 patients, 158 male, 34 female, experiencing AMI for the first time. Patients were followed from 1 day to 3 years after AMI; follow-up was 100%. The clinical diagnosis of pericarditis was made when 2 cardiologists confirmed the presence of a friction rub or when inspiratory pericardial pain appeared. Patients were evaluated twice a day for the first 5 days and then daily for 3 weeks. Echocardiography using two-dimensional, M-mode, and Doppler techniques was performed at day 1, 5, 10, and 21, and at year 1, 2, and 3. Coronary arteriography was performed at 3 weeks. Nonparametric statistical analysis was used.

Critique: The study clearly stated the criteria for enrollment, using accepted clinical parameters of pericarditis. No attempt was made to quantify subjective measures of a patient's pain or to evaluate for gender-based differences in the population. Further, the hemodynamic parameters evaluated were limited to the extremes of cardiac tamponade and heart failure. By leaving a 3-day gap between the first echocardiogram and the second, the study could not determine when the onset of pericarditis began. The study was undertaken in the Czech Republic and reflects the practice of retaining patients for 3 weeks after MI. Overall, the study was well reported and internally consistent.

Nursing Implications: Pericardial effusion was detected at least once in 43% of the study population. This percentage is higher than that in other reports and may reflect international practice differences. The higher incidence may also be related to the fact the patients remained in the hospital and thus could undergo frequent evaluations. The finding points to the need for all nurses, including those in critical care, home care, and cardiac rehabilitation coming in contact with AMI patients during the initial 3 weeks of recovery to be alert for signs and symptoms of pericarditis and effusion. This is further supported by the finding that pericardial effusion was diagnosed initially in 25% of the population on day 5, 30% of the population on day 10, and 28% of the population on day 21. In 3 patients, the effusion persisted for up to 3 years.

The size of the pericardial effusion was described as small. Evaluation of hemodynamic consequences focused on cardiac tamponade, which did not occur in the study. This gives an indication for nurses about the likelihood of this unwanted sequela. It does not suggest, however, that nurses should decrease their vigilance in evaluating the patient for the signs and symptoms. A finding that could not be confirmed for prognostic value was the relationship among heart failure, mortality, and pericardial effusion. The authors postulated that the mortality associated with pericardial effusion was more a function of the heart failure than of the pericardial effusion.

Of interest to nurses in various settings is the relatively low incidence (8%) of pericarditis diagnosed through clinical signs and symptoms compared with echocardiographic findings of pericardial effusion (43%). The results were not statistically significant. This finding suggests that nurses must compare echocardiographic results with clinical findings because pericardial effusions may be subclinical.

Finally, thrombolytic and anticoagulant therapy was not associated with increased frequency or size of pericardial effusion. Nurses can be assured that the common use of these agents after AMI will not place patients at increased risk. In conclusion, pericarditis and pericardial effusion may be more widespread than previously thought after AMI. The incidence of this disease is greatest in the first 3 weeks after MI and subsequently resolves over time. A few cases are not resolved by 3 years. Regular assessment and correlation to echocardiograms will assist the nurse in evaluating for this complication after AMI.

Source: Widimsky P, Gregor P: Pericardial involvement during the course of myocardial infarction: a long term clinical and echocardiographic study. Chest 108:89–93, 1995.

Nursing Diagnoses

Diagnosis of pericarditis is aided by a complete history, evaluating for related factors, and differentiating signs and symptoms of pericarditis from other cardiac diseases. Diagnosis can be confounded by inconclusive ECGs and laboratory studies, as well as symptoms that elude the diagnostician. The role of the nurse in diagnosis is to gather data, continually assessing and evaluating the patient's status in light of a potential diagnosis. The nurse meets the patient's needs through identification of nursing diagnoses, such as those listed in Table 12–3.

Collaborative Management

Collaborative management for the patient with pericarditis is focused on maintaining cardiac output, eradicating infection, and ameliorating pain. Cardiac output is maintained through providing oxygen, maintaining rest and limited activity, and implementing pharmacologic and surgical interventions. Oxygen therapy is required to overcome the high demands for oxygen resulting from infection and constriction of cardiac muscle. Pharmacologic therapy depends on the cause of the pericarditis. Viral pericarditis and pericarditis of an immune origin may be treated with NSAIDs and corticosteroids. Generally, NSAIDs are initiated as first-line therapy. Indomethacin (Indocin) is the drug of choice. Corticosteroids are used if NSAIDs have failed and infection is not present. Bacterial infections are treated with the appropriate antibiotics.

To maintain cardiac output, it may be necessary to relieve pleural effusion and pressure through surgical interventions. The surgical interventions include pericardiocentesis, pericardiectomy, and thoracoscopic pericardial resection. Pericardiocentesis is a diagnostic procedure that is also used to remove accumulating fluid in the pericardial sac. Ideally, the patient is prepared for the procedure, which can occur in the cardiac catheterization laboratory or the radiography department. The procedure can also be done on an emergency basis at the patient's bedside. During pericardiocentesis, the physician accesses the pericardial space with a large-bore needle and withdraws blood or fluid. Visualization of the effusion, through echocardiogram or fluoroscopy, enables the cardiologist to access the fluid while avoiding the myocardial surface. Two-dimensional echocardiography is used most frequently for visualization of the pleural effusion. When the effusion is visualized, an 18- to 21-gauge spinal needle, 6 inches long, filled with anesthetic solution, is advanced to the fluid. The ideal puncture site is selected, based on ease of access and avoiding cardiac

and pulmonic structures. A V lead is connected to the aspiration needle. Several areas of entry are possible. The most popular approach is the xiphocostal approach, in which the needle is inserted in the angle between the left costal margin and the xiphoid process. Alternative approaches include the parasternal (insertion of the needle between the fifth and sixth intercostal space to the left of the sternum) and the apical areas. These approaches are used less frequently without visualization because the risk of puncturing a vital organ is greater. If the heart is entered, ST-segment elevation is seen on the ECG. Resistance may be encountered as the needle passes through the pericardium. If the fluid aspirated is grossly bloody, in likelihood a heart chamber has been entered. Clots in the aspirate further confirm this finding. Fluid aspirated is sent to the laboratory for evaluation. After fluid is removed, air may be injected to visualize the pericardial space in relation to cardiac structures. In the case of malignancy or recurrent effusion, a plastic intrapericardial catheter may be left in place to facilitate drainage.

Pericardiotomy may be performed when pericardiocentesis is not feasible or for biopsy and drainage. Pericardiotomy is the opening of the pericardium through a surgical incision for the purpose of biopsy or resection. A subxiphoid approach may be used for biopsy when viral pericarditis is suspected. Under surgical asepsis, with the patient under local anesthesia with appropriate sedation, a small 6- to 8-cm incision is made at the tip of the xiphoid process. The incision extends down 3 cm below the tip of the xiphoid process. Using this procedure, 3 to 4 cm of the pericardium can be resected. Through this incision, video endoscopic thoracic resection of the pericardium may also be performed. When constrictive pericarditis is suspected, an approach through the left fourth or fifth intercostal space is preferred.

Nursing interventions for the patient undergoing pericardiocentesis and pericardiotomy can be addressed before, during, and after the procedure. Before the procedure, the patient should be informed and educated about what the procedure entails and his or her role in it. Patients may have to assume a specific position for the physician to able to access the fluid. Patients should be informed of this ahead of time, and the patient and the nurse should work out an arrangement of supports so the patient is comfortable. Before the procedure, the patient's chest is prepared. During the procedure, the nurse evaluates the patient's oxygen status and monitors the ECG. The ECG is observed for increase in ectopy, especially premature ventricular contractions and elevation of the ST segment, PR interval, or QRS complex. Elevations indicate that the needle is touching the myocardium. The nurse further assesses for signs of cardiac tamponade. After the procedure, the patient's vital signs are evaluated frequently. A rise in blood pressure can be anticipated if a large amount of fluid has been aspirated. The patient's ECG is evaluated for changes in the ST segment and further ectopy. The patient is also evaluated for returning tamponade.[19]

Pericardiectomy is the surgical removal of the parietal or visceral pericardium. In general, the parietal pericardium is removed when effusion is a recurrent problem and no constriction is present. The visceral pericardium is removed when inflammation and infection have caused constriction. If the visceral pericardium is removed sooner rather than later, fewer complications will arise after surgery. The most common complications of pericardiectomy are heart failure, dysrhythmias, infection, bleeding, and post-pericardiotomy syndrome. Nursing interventions are aimed at maintaining cardiac output, assessing for complications, maintaining the patency of chest tubes, and preventing infection.[19] Sudden cessation of chest tube drainage may indicate tamponade. See the multidisciplinary outcomes section for outcomes for patients with pericarditis.

INFECTIOUS ENDOCARDITIS

The causes of infectious endocarditis have changed since the widespread use of antibiotics for group A beta-hemolytic streptococcal infections has dramatically decreased the incidence of rheumatic heart disease in the industrialized world. Infectious endocarditis has been characterized as a disease in transition, as a result of widespread availability of antibiotics, increases in intravenous drug use, and previous cardiac disease. The etiology and pathophysiology of infectious endocarditis and rheumatic heart disease are considered. Then, assessment, diagnosis, and collaborative management of both diseases are presented.

ETIOLOGY AND PATHOPHYSIOLOGY

Infectious endocarditis is defined as a microbial infection of the lining of the heart, primarily the heart valves. Before the use of antibiotics, endocarditis primarily affected adults under the age of 40 years. Currently, it is seen most frequently in adults over the age of 60 years, with men afflicted five times more frequently than women. The disease rarely occurs in children.[20] Risk factors associated with the incidence of infectious endocarditis include a preexisting cardiac illness, bacteremia induced by surgical, dental, or invasive procedures, and intravenous drug use. Since the advent of prosthetic valve cardiac surgery, the relationship between valve replacement and infectious endocarditis has been established. Prosthetic valve endo-

carditis is associated with *Staphylococcus epidermidis* and *Staphylococcus aureus* in early onset (within 60 days of valve replacement) and with alpha-hemolytic streptococci in late-onset disease.[20] Additionally, degenerative heart diseases such as aortic valve calcification, mitral valve prolapse, asymmetric septal hypertrophy, and hypertrophic cardiomyopathy have been increasingly recognized as predisposing conditions to infectious endocarditis. In the hospital setting, nosocomial infections of the endocardium occur in patients with systemic bacteremia and invasive lines, such as pulmonary artery catheters and arterial lines. It is estimated that 10 to 20% of cases of infectious endocarditis are of nosocomial origin. Elderly patients, immunocompromised patients, and patients with burns may develop infectious endocarditis. Finally, a growing number of patients with endocarditis have no definable underlying cardiac lesion. This group includes the population of intravenous drug users, who may introduce foreign material into the vascular system.[21]

Infectious endocarditis is fatal if untreated. The interval between the onset of symptoms and death varies, with a median time of 6 months. Infectious endocarditis and heart failure are indicative of a poor prognosis. Other negative indicators of prognosis include renal failure, culture-negative disease, Gram-negative or fungal infection, and the development of valve abscesses. Positive indicators of prognosis include young age, early diagnosis and treatment, and penicillin-sensitive streptococcal infection.[22]

Previously, endocarditis was classified as acute, subacute, or chronic. Currently, classifications are based on etiologic agents. This is because causative organisms are more easily tied to outcomes, and confusing overlap of symptoms is avoided. Organisms associated with infectious endocarditis include Gram-positive organisms of the streptococcal, enterococcal, and staphylococcal groups. Gram-negative organisms include *Pseudomonas aeruginosa*, *Serratia marcescens*, and the HACEK group (*Haemophilus sp.*, *Actinobacillus actinomycetemcomitans*, *Cardiobacterium hominis*, *Eikenella corrodens*, and *Kingella kingae*). Fungal organisms that have been known to cause infectious endocarditis include *Candida albicans* and *Candida parapsilosis*. Additionally, spirochetes, rickettsiae, chlamydia, viruses, and parasites have been noted clinically to cause infectious endocarditis.[20] Table 12–6 presents common organisms in infectious endocarditis.

Early in the antibiotic era, group A beta-hemolytic streptococcal organisms caused rheumatic fever, a predisposing factor to rheumatic heart disease. Rheumatic fever is a systemic disorder in which streptococcal organisms damage collagen fibrils in connective tissue. The disorder is characterized by inflammatory lesions that invade connective and endothelial tissue and is associated with untreated streptococcal infections. Rheumatic heart disease occurs as a sequela to

TABLE 12–6
Common Organisms in Infectious Endocarditis

Organism	Associated Risk
Gram-Positive Bacteria	
Streptococci	
Alpha-hemolytic streptococci	Native valve endocarditis, prosthetic valve endocarditis
Streptococcus bovis	Gastrointestinal malignancies
Enterococci	
Streptococcus faecalis	
Streptococcus durans	
Staphylococci	
Staphylococcus aureus	Intravenous drug abuse
Staphylococcus epidermidis	Intravenous drug abuse
Gram-Negative Bacteria	
Pseudomonas aeruginosa, Serratia marcescens	Intravenous drug abuse, immunocompromised patients, nosocomial infection
HACEK (*Haemophilus sp., Actinobacillus actino-mycetemcomitans, Cardiobacterium hominis, Eikenella corrodens, Kingella kingae*)	Usually culture negative
Fungal	
Candida albicans, Candida parapsilosis	Intravenous drug abuse, prosthetic valve endocarditis, cardiac surgery, intravenous catheters, immunosuppression

rheumatic fever and can involve the pericardium, myocardium, and endocardium. Laboratory findings associated with rheumatic fever include an elevated antistreptolysin O titer, increased erythrocyte sedimentation rate, and C-reactive protein. Clinical signs of acute rheumatic fever include fatigue and malaise, polyarthritis, erythema marginatum, abdominal pain, and subcutaneous nodules over bony prominences.

Various factors contribute to the development of the vegetative lesions on heart valves that are characteristic of infectious endocarditis. First, turbulent blood flow at valve leaflets encourages damage of endothelial surfaces, resulting in a murmur. Second, endothelial trauma can result because of immune complex deposition, such as occurs in autoimmune disease. Once endothelial trauma occurs, epithelial damage sets up an environment conducive to platelet aggregation. Platelet aggregation encourages fibrin deposits, which form a sterile vegetation. Finally, the valves become colonized with pathogens that have an affinity for the endothelial surface of the heart.

Infection progresses through a state of bacteremia, local infiltration of tissue, embolization, and the formation of immune complexes. When organisms are introduced into the blood on a continual basis, the infection is perpetuated in the valve tissue. Intravenous drug users, critically ill patients with invasive lines, or patients undergoing dental procedures are all at risk for continuous bacteremia. Organisms can also infiltrate the valve tissue, thus precipitating rupture of the chordae tendineae or aneurysm. As a result of organ-ism infiltration, heart failure, pericarditis, and conduction disturbances may occur. Signs of infection peripheral to the cardiac system are evident when embolization occurs. Emboli may cause problems with peripheral blood flow to the extremities and vital organs, or they may precipitate stroke. Emboli are associated with organisms that produce large, mobile vegetations, such as Gram-negative bacilli, fungi, and variant forms of alpha-hemolytic streptococci.[21] Further, embolization is associated with vegetations on the mitral valve, particularly when these vegetations are large and mobile.[23] Vasculitis may also occur, as a result of peripheral emboli of infectious organisms. Immune complexes activated in response to invading organisms contribute to systemic signs of infection.[24]

Assessment

Assessment of the patient with infectious endocarditis includes a careful health history to uncover causative factors, a review of systems for signs and symptoms, and the use of diagnostic tests, particularly blood cultures, and echocardiography to confirm bacteremia and to visualize vegetation on valves. Items for review in the health history include uncovering a possible source of infection. In the critical care setting, the nurse must consider invasive lines and procedures as a source of bacteremia. The nurse investigates whether the patient has had invasive lines and procedures: Was sterile and aseptic technique maintained during dressing changes, and during the procedure itself? Have intravenous lines been dressed properly, with sites rotated according to agency policy? Nosocomial infectious endocarditis can arise in elderly patients in critical care settings. Because patients present from the community through the emergency room with signs and symptoms that appear to be those of infectious endocarditis, the carefully obtained history can assist in making the diagnosis. The patient in the emergency department needs to be asked about intravenous drug use, recent or past dental procedures or infections, urinary tract infections, invasive procedures involving the skin or mucous membranes such as body piercing or tattooing, and lesions or infections of the bowel or respiratory system (Chart 12–2). Additionally, patients should be questioned about recent hospitalizations and the events of the hospitalization. Patients should be questioned if they have implantable venous access devices or dialysis shunts in place.

Clinical Presentation

Signs and symptoms of infectious endocarditis are changing. The characteristic lesions of skin, nails, and eyes, petechiae, and subungual hemorrhages, termed respectively Osler's nodes, Janeway lesions, and Roth's spots, are rarely seen. Current clinical presentation of signs and symptoms depend on systemic and local effects, systemic emboli, and abnormal immunoglobulin levels. The systemic signs are manifested in fever, sweats, chills, anorexia, fatigue, weight loss, arthralgia, and arthritis. Local symptoms include back pain, dyspnea, pleuritic chest pain, and cough. Diagnostic clues to infectious endocarditis include a prior cardiac lesion and vague constitutional symptoms. Signs include heart murmurs, mucosal, cutaneous, and retinal changes, and metastatic infections such as septic arthritis, osteomyelitis, and purulent pericarditis. One-third of the patients have neurologic symptoms such as stroke and transient ischemic attacks. Signs and symptoms are frequently elusive, making the endocarditis

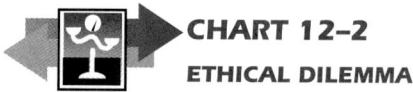 **CHART 12–2**
ETHICAL DILEMMA

S.B. is a 38-year-old woman who has used intravenous heroin for 18 years. S. was admitted through the emergency department with acute sepsis secondary to bacterial endocarditis. She had a stay in the intensive care unit, where she was managed with multiple antibiotics for her acute infection and inotropic agents for cardiac failure. Currently, she is in your intermediate care unit. S. is managed on methadone in lieu of heroin. She has been through detoxification programs and rehabilitation in the past, but has always returned to her drug use. Physically, S. exhibits signs of cardiac failure, she has an S_3 and grade V murmur of mitral regurgitation, adventitious lung sounds are present, and she exhibits grade IV pitting edema in her legs. Her vital signs have been stable, with a sinus tachycardia of 125 beats per minute with ventricular ectopy. Her blood pressure is 100/60 mm Hg, and her respiratory rate is 18. She is maintained on oxygen at 3 L, with orders to titrate to an oxygen saturation of 92%. S. has been verbalizing her desire to leave the hospital. Recently, she has been found in the stairwell, short of breath, and has had to be escorted back to her room. S. has been referred to the cardiac surgical group for mitral valve replacement and to the hospital social worker for placement in drug rehabilitation.

1. How can the nurse act as an advocate for this patient in light of her substance abuse, desire to leave the hospital, and need for cardiac surgery?
2. The ethical principle of beneficence is the obligation to do good and to avoid doing harm. In this situation, what is identified as "good" and "harm" from the perspectives of the health care team and the patient?
3. If S. refuses cardiac surgery, can this decision be accepted by health care providers in light of her drug abuse?
4. What legal responsibility does the health care team have to ensure that S. does not leave the hospital in her current condition?
5. What nursing diagnosis is operative in this situation, and what nursing interventions should be provided to S. at this time?

Two articles which would provide a helpful adjunct to the discussion of this case are as follows:

Maupin CR: The potential for noncaring when dealing with difficult patients: strategies for moral decision making. J Cardiovasc Nurs 9:11–22, 1995.
Omery A: Care: the basis for a nursing ethic? J Cardiovasc Nurs 9:1–10, 1995.

difficult to diagnose. Subclinical signs associated with alpha-hemolytic streptococcal infections include vague symptoms such as low-grade fevers, night sweats, weight loss, and other flulike symptoms. A more acute picture includes high fever, bacteremia, sepsis leukocytosis, and heart failure.[20,25]

Physical Examination

Murmurs are encountered up to 90% of the time in patients with infectious endocarditis, but they may be initially absent. Murmurs that are present in the early stages of the disease may be present because of preexisting cardiac disease. Endocarditis results in structural damage to the valve. As a result, damage such as tears, deformities, and rupture of chordae tendineae often leads to murmurs of regurgitation of the mitral, aortic, or tricuspid valve. The most common murmurs are aortic and mitral, which may be associated with signs of heart failure. Murmurs arising from the tricuspid valve are common to intravenous drug users.[22] Murmurs that change in character, intensity, or timing are diagnostic and may signal impending valve rupture.[24] Symptoms associated with murmurs of regurgitation depend on the ability of the chamber in the retrograde position to handle an increased volume of blood. In aortic regurgitation, the left ventricle responds to an increased volume of blood by becoming hypertrophied. Patients can have minimal symptoms as long as the left ventricle is able to accommodate increased blood volume. When systolic pressures increase, causing pulmonary signs and symptoms, surgical intervention is warranted. Table 12–7 categorizes heart murmurs of infectious endocarditis.

Diagnostic Workup

Diagnosis of infectious endocarditis hinges on the triad of fever, cardiac murmur, and positive blood cultures. Diagnostic workup includes laboratory tests such as blood cultures, echocardiography, and cardiac catheterization. Infectious endocarditis may be associated with leukocytosis, thrombocytopenia, or leukopenia associated with splenomegaly. Hyperglobulinemia is common, and rheumatoid factor is present in 50% of patients with infection of at least 6 weeks' duration. Laboratory findings reverse after appropriate treatment. Two or three blood cultures are collected over a 24-hour period. The collection of three venous blood cultures over a 24-hour period is usually sufficient to isolate the offending organism in persons who have not had antimicrobial therapy 2 weeks before culture collection. When venous blood cultures have not yielded results in 3 days, and the diagnosis seems likely, then an additional two venous cultures and an arterial culture should be obtained.[22] Blood cultures can be falsely negative when a patient has a fastidious organism such as alpha-hemolytic streptococci or a slow-growing organism from the HACEK group. Blood cultures can also be falsely negative when the patient has received a previous course of antibiotic therapy. However, cultures are positive within a few days after stopping antibiotics. Patients who have a diagnosis of endocarditis with persistently negative cultures have culture-negative endocarditis, the incidence of which is reported to be between 5 and 20%.

Echocardiograms are a major diagnostic tool in individuals with infectious endocarditis. Because the hallmark of infectious endocarditis is vegetation adhering to the endocardium, echocardiography offers the clinician the opportunity to visualize the vegetation and to determine its size and relation to cardiac structures. Different types of echocardiograms are used in the diagnostic workup, including M mode, two-dimensional, Doppler, and transesophageal. Sensitivity of echocardiography for diagnostic value varies. The echocardiogram can detect vegetations larger than 2 to 3 cm on valves. Sensitivity is between 40 and 70% with the two-dimensional transthoracic mode and increases to with 95% with transesophageal studies. Transesophageal studies are particularly helpful in diagnosing small lesions less than 10 cm, vegetations on prosthetic valves, and abscesses. Initially, the patient has a transthoracic two-dimensional echocardiogram, with a transesophageal echocardiogram if needed.[25]

Chest radiographs and cardiac catheterization lend additional information to the diagnosis of infectious endocarditis. A chest radiograph documents the extent to which heart failure is present. In intravenous drug users, patchy infiltrates revealed on a chest radiograph suggest a process of embolism. Cardiac catheterization is indicated as a prelude to cardiac surgery or in those with heart failure. Cardiac catheterization demonstrates valvular lesions, congenital defects, coronary artery disease, and other structural abnormalities not evident on the echocardiogram.

Clinicians agree that making the diagnosis of infectious endocarditis can be difficult and elusive.[22,26] Different diagnostic criteria have been proposed to facilitate making a firm diagnosis. The von Reyn criteria were utilized in the 1970s, before the widespread use of echocardiograms. Therefore, these criteria are of limited usefulness at present. However, the von Reyn criteria established a systematic way to evaluate the patient in terms of pathologic and clinical criteria in light of the probability that the patient had the disease. Current criteria proposed by physicians at Duke University Medical Center in North Carolina incorporate the following concepts: echocardiographic data, distinctive criteria of major and minor elements, pathogens, the use of intravenous drugs, and the definition of a "rejected category."[26]

TABLE 12-7
Common Heart Murmurs Found in Infectious Endocarditis

Type	Timing	Location	Configuration	Intensity	Pitch	Quality	Radiation
Aortic stenosis	Systole; sound begins shortly after S_1, ends before S_2	Second right intercostal space (loudest). Erb's point (third left intercostal space along the sternal border). Apex	Crescendo/decrescendo	Sometimes soft, often loud, with a thrill, heard best with patient sitting and leaning forward	Medium at apex	Harsh, may be more musical at apex	Carotid arteries, usually the right; down left sternal border, even to apex
Aortic regurgitation	Early diastole, immediately after S_1	Second to fourth left intercostal space	Decrescendo	Grades I–III, best heard with patient sitting, leaning forward with breath held in exhalation	High	Blowing	Lower left sternal border
Mitral regurgitation	Systole, begins with S_1 and continues to S_2	Apex	Holosystolic	Soft to loud; does not become louder on inspiration	Medium to high	Blowing	Left axilla, less often to left sternal border
Mitral valve prolapse	Mid to late systole, clicks are heard in midsystole (position changes will affect timing)	Apex, often lateralized	Crescendo	Varies with position changes; squatting may intensify	High	Whooping, honking	Varies
Mitral stenosis	Diastole, between S_1 and S_2	Apex	Decrescendo/crescendo	Grade I–IV: louder in left lateral supine position or after exercise; heard better in exhalation	Low	Rumbling	Little or none

From Matthews D: The prevention and diagnosis of infective endocarditis. Nurse Pract 19:55, 1994. © Springhouse Corporation, Springhouse, PA.

Nursing Diagnoses

Nursing diagnoses for the patient with infectious endocarditis are included in Table 12–3. Nursing diagnoses appropriate for the patient with a medical diagnosis of infectious endocarditis may be found in all functional health pattern categories. Initial presentation of symptoms may include signs of infection that warrant a diagnosis of hyperthermia. As with the patient in heart failure, the patient with infectious endocarditis is likely to manifest symptoms of breathlessness, dyspnea, and fatigue. Therefore, nursing diagnoses of activity intolerance, fatigue, decreased cardiac output, and ineffective breathing pattern are likely to be appropriate.

Collaborative Management

Goals of collaborative management of infectious endocarditis are to eradicate the infecting organism as soon as possible, to prevent complications, and to initiate surgical intervention as appropriate. Treatment with antibiotics is the primary therapy. Oxygen therapy is initiated by nasal cannula to maintain adequate oxygen levels. The ECG is monitored for tachydysrhythmias and for conduction disturbances that may manifest as first-, second-, or third-degree heat block. See the multidisciplinary outcomes section for outcomes for patients diagnosed with endocarditis.

Pharmacotherapeutics

Antibiotics are selected on the basis of identification of the infecting organism. The time of eradication of the organism may be as short as 2 weeks or as long as 6 weeks. Several principles of drug therapy are considered when the clinician selects antimicrobial therapy. First, parenteral antibiotics are used for their bactericidal effect. The bactericidal effect of antibiotics is to cause bacterial cell death and lysis, acting in place of the host's immune mechanism. Bacteriostatic antibiotics inhibit bacterial growth and allow host defense mechanisms time to remove the invading organism. In infectious endocarditis, bactericidal antibiotics are chosen over bacteriostatic antibiotics. Occasionally, these types of antibiotics are used in combination for their synergistic effect. If the patient's symptoms are not severe, and if initiation of antibiotic therapy can wait, it is best to delay until positive blood cultures identify the offending organism. When the patient cannot wait, the physician will most likely order antibiotics effective against *Staphylococcus aureus* and enterococci.

Antimicrobial agents may exert their bacteriostatic or bacteriocidal effects in one of four ways. First, they may inhibit cell wall synthesis, causing the cell to lyse and causing cell death. Second, they may disrupt or alter cell membrane permeability, resulting in the leakage of the cell interior. Third, they may inhibit protein synthesis, causing the formation of defective cells. Finally, antimicrobial agents may inhibit the synthesis of essential metabolites.[27]

In general, Gram-positive organisms causing infectious endocarditis of the native valve are treated with penicillin derivatives such as penicillin G, ampicillin, and nafcillin. An aminoglycoside, such as gentamicin, is added to the early part of the treatment regimen in relatively resistant strains of streptococci. Vancomycin is the drug of choice in methicillin-resistant *Staphylococcus aureas* and native valve infection with *Staphylococcus epidermidis*. Prosthetic valves infected with this organism usually require a 2-week course of vancomycin and gentamicin. The HACEK group of organisms responds well to penicillin and aminoglycosides or a first-line cephalosporin. Gram-negative organisms require a broad-spectrum penicillin or third-generation cephalosporin with an aminoglycoside.

Patients undergoing intravenous therapy with antibiotics for a protracted period may develop side effects with these drugs. Allergic reactions of skin rashes, diarrhea, and gastrointestinal upset may occur. More severe side effects such as hearing loss and kidney failure may also occur. The patient is educated about side effects of the drug, because he or she is likely to be discharged with intravenous therapy at home (Chart 12–3). Patients also need to be aware of situations that require prophylactic treatment for infectious endocarditis. Patient conditions that necessitate treatment when certain high-risk procedures are undertaken include prosthetic cardiac valves, previous history of endocarditis, congenital heart disease, rheumatic or acquired valvular heart disease, and mitral valve prolapse with valvular regurgitation. High-risk dental procedures include dental cleaning or other procedures likely to induce gingival bleeding. Procedures of the respiratory system that require prophylaxis include surgery of the upper respiratory tract and bronchoscopy. Gastrointestinal and genitourinary surgery or instrumentation such as gallbladder surgery, urethral dilatation, and urethral catheterization require prophylactic antibiotics. Patients must be instructed to inform physicians of their history of infectious endocarditis and related cardiac history before undergoing any of these procedures, so an appropriate course of antibiotics may be ordered.[24,25]

Anticoagulant therapy during the acute phase of infectious endocarditis in persons with prosthetic valves should be accomplished through the use of warfarin. Patients with native valve endocarditis are not routinely anticoagulated. The use of heparin and antibiotics has been demonstrated to carry a higher risk of fatal intracerebral hemorrhage. In patients

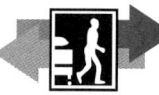

CHART 12–3

BEYOND THE ICU: MANAGING HOME INTRAVENOUS ANTIBIOTIC THERAPY

To provide long-term intravenous antibiotic therapy in the patient with endocarditis, a peripherally inserted central catheter (PICC) is likely to be used. PICC is a generic term for one of many catheters that may be inserted centrally for the delivery of fluids and medications. The catheter is inserted in either the basilar or the cephalic vein, with the tip resting in the superior vena cava. The median cubital vein may also be considered. PICCs are made of silicone or polyurethane and are available in single-lumen or double-lumen configurations. Their size ranges from 16 to 28 gauge. The PICC comes with a radiopaque stripe recognizable on a chest radiograph.

PICCs possess low thrombogenicity and phlebitis rates and are less costly than other central venous access devices They are not surgically placed, but are usually placed by specially trained nurses. A variation of the PICC is the midline catheter (MLC), which is placed between the antecubital fossa and the head of the clavicle. Antibiotics may be easily infused through the MLC. Further, the MLC may be a choice for antibiotic therapy that lasts longer than 6 weeks.

Patients are selected for insertion of a PICC to be used during home therapy based on several criteria: vein availability, patient compliance, hygiene, and home resources. The home care nurse caring for the patient with a PICC needs to involve the patient and the family in the care of the catheter. After placement, the catheter is secured, and the insertion site is cleansed with iodine, covered with sterile 2-inch by 2-inch dressings, and then covered with a transparent dressing. The dressing is changed initially every 24 hours and then weekly as needed. If appropriate, the family may be taught to redress the catheter. In addition, the patient and family are taught to identify the signs and symptoms of catheter-related complications and to notify the nurse should any of these occur.

The PICC may remain in place for several months. Complications of PICCs include phlebitis, occlusion, fever, thrombosis, and accidental removal. Occlusion of the catheter can be avoided by flushing the catheter with a heparin solution after each use or daily. Further, occlusion can be avoided by maintaining positive pressure on the flush syringe as it is withdrawn form the injection port.

The use of these catheters for home administration of antibiotic therapy for patients with infectious cardiac disease has reduced the patient's length of stay in the acute care setting as well as the overall costs related to the treatment of the disease. By incorporating the advanced skills of nurses who manage patients with these devices, holistic care can be provided in the comfort of the patient's home.

Additional readings are as follows:

Macklin D: How to manage PICCs. Am J Nurs 97:26–33, 1997.
Steinhuser M: Vascular access device: choices for home care patients. Caring 14:14–16, 1995.

with intracranial complications, anticoagulant therapy should not be used.[22]

Surgical intervention may be required in certain patients in whom a course of antibiotics fails, or in those whose symptoms indicate a need. Surgical intervention may be the replacement of a valve, either native or prosthetic, débridement of vegetation, valvuloplasty, or valve repair. Valve replacement may be the only way to correct bacteremia in a patient who remains infected despite antibiotic treatment, especially in endocarditis affecting a prosthetic valve. Surgical intervention is considered when the patient exhibits complications such as embolization, heart failure, or renal failure.

The timing of surgery is critical in the treatment of endocarditis. The patient should be allowed sufficient time for the antibiotics to reduce the number of circulating and vegetative organisms. Consideration to the type of organism and outcome of treatment must be given before surgical intervention. For example, intravenous drug users respond well to courses of penicillin, and surgery is not indicated unless signs of heart failure are present. If time allows, symptoms of heart failure and renal failure should be corrected to improve the operative risk.[28]

Multidisciplinary Outcomes

Infectious cardiac diseases, specifically myocarditis, pericarditis, and endocarditis, have been discussed from a broad perspective of etiology and pathophysiology, assessment, diagnosis, and collaborative management. The care of patients with infectious cardiac

TABLE 12–8
Multidisciplinary Outcomes

Phase of Recovery	Outcome
Emergency department	Assessment of patient's history, physical status, and functional status leading to diagnosis of illness
	Initiation of appropriate laboratory tests to assist in diagnosis of infection
	Initiation of course of antibiotics, as appropriate
	Initiation of measures to decrease or alleviate patient pain
	Stabilization of cardiac output through oxygen therapy, pharmacologic means, and restriction of physical activity
Intensive care unit	Maintenance of cardiac output through oxygen support, pharmacologic means, and restriction of physical activity
	Reduction in temperature
	Completion of appropriate diagnostic modalities including ECG, echocardiogram, cardiac catheterization, myocardial biopsy, pericardial tap
	Management of pain through pharmacologic and nonpharmacologic means
	Implementation of appropriate treatment regimen to eradicate infectious process and minimize cardiac damage
Intermediate care unit	Stabilization or improvement in cardiac output through continued oxygen support, pharmacologic means, and restriction of physical activity
	Prevention of complications
	Preparation for surgical interventions of treatment
	Continued management of pain and infection
	Preparation for discharge and cardiac rehabilitation
	Education on disease process, pharmacotherapeutics, and course of home therapy
	Consultation with appropriate home agency for follow-up care
	Acknowledgment of psychosocial issues related to new disease or onset of chronic illness
Community	Initiation of cardiac rehabilitation.
	Prevention of relapse or recurrent infection through education
	Return to previous level of perceived health and functional ability
	Acceptance in changes in body image secondary to altered level of health

disease involves a concerted, multidisciplinary approach that usually crosses various health care settings (Table 12–8). Achievement of these outcomes can best be accomplished using a holistic approach to identifying and meeting the needs of the patient and family.

Critical Thinking Exercise

A 32-year-old woman is admitted to the emergency department with a chief complaint of chest pain lasting several hours. The pain is centered under the "breast bone" and does not radiate. She has been unable to rest in bed. The patient's past medical history includes a fractured femur 5 years ago and systemic lupus erythematosus, which is in remission. Recently, she has complained of having a "cold" a "couple of weeks ago" for which she was treated with a course of a cephalosporin. Vital signs are as follows: temperature, 99.0°F; monitor showing sinus tachycardia at a rate of 115 beats per minute with no ectopy; blood pressure 100/70 mm Hg; O_2 saturation, 92%. Physical examination yields a well-nourished woman, in moderate distress, alert, awake,

and oriented to person, place, and time. Her cardiovascular assessment reveals normal S_1 and S_2, with no murmurs. No adventitious lung sounds are heard.

1. What additional data related to history and physical assessment need to be obtained before a diagnosis can be made?
2. What are possible causes of the chest pain?
3. What diagnostic tests are anticipated for this patient? Given the accompanying 12-lead ECG (Figure 12–2), what conclusions can be drawn?
4. What is the priority nursing diagnosis for this patient?
5. The patient's chest pain intensifies without change in vital signs or heart rhythm. What assessment signs should the nurse evaluate?
6. What medications may the nurse anticipate will be prescribed for the patient?

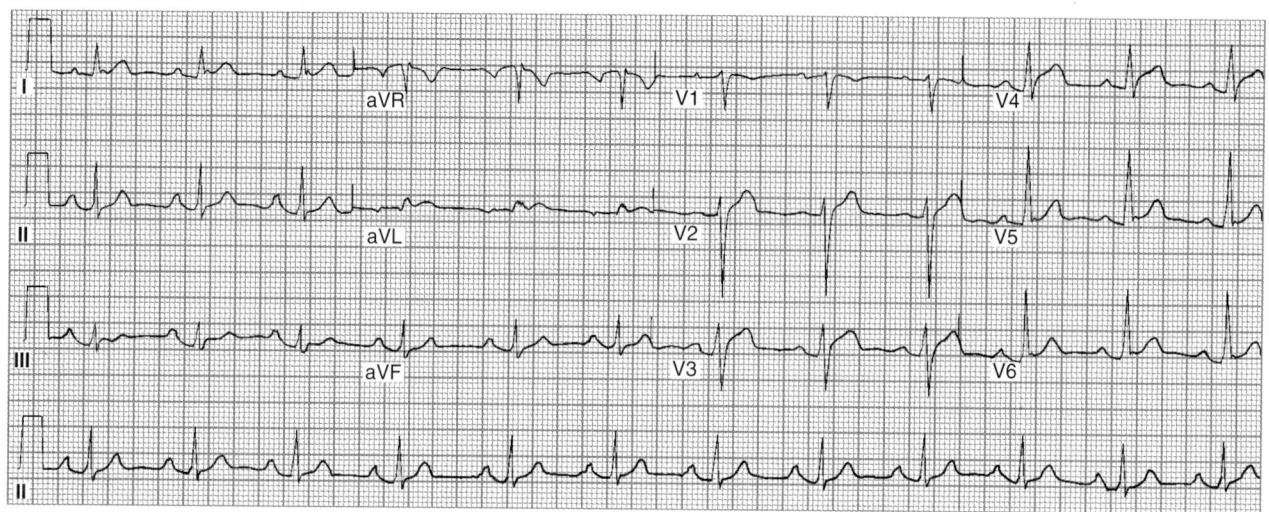

Figure 12–2

A 12-lead ECG of a 32-year-old woman admitted to the emergency department with chest pain.

Key Concepts

➠ The primary cause of viral myocarditis is the B group of Coxsackieviruses; as a result of the waxing and waning of the disease, epidemiologic tracking of the disease is difficult.

➠ Symptoms of low cardiac output and heart failure in viral myocarditis may resolve spontaneously or may lead to a permanent state of heart failure with a low ejection fraction.

➠ Diagnosis of viral myocarditis is made based on clinical presentation, confirmation of myocardial necrosis by endomyocardial biopsy, laboratory data, and ruling out of other appropriate diagnosis.

➠ Collaborative problems in myocarditis include the management of infection, pain, and decreased cardiac output.

➠ Agents used in the treatment of heart failure, such as angiotensin-converting enzyme inhibitors, vasodilating agents, and inotropic agents may also be used in myocarditis, depending on the severity of the illness. NSAIDs may be used for pain management late in the illness.

➠ Disease of the pericardium encompasses various disorders arising from different causative factors including infection, cardiac injury such as myocardial infarction and cardiac surgery, renal disease, neoplasms, and collagen vascular diseases.

➠ Pericarditis involves inflammation and infection of the visceral, parietal, and fibrous pericardium.

➠ Idiopathic pericarditis occurs in 86% of cases of the disease, usually arising from a viral cause.

➠ Pericarditis is increasingly becoming a cardiovascular complication of AIDS.

➠ Pericarditis after MI, or Dresslers' syndrome, can occur 2 to 11 weeks after MI and has an autoimmune component.

➠ Syndromes occurring as a result of autoimmune activity after cardiac injury or surgery are to be differentiated from postperfusion cardiac syndrome, which occurs as a result of cytomegalovirus infection during the surgical procedure.

➠ Pain is the most common acute symptom associated with pericarditis and manifests itself as retrosternal or left substernal, radiating to shoulder, neck, or arm.

➠ The classic sign of pericarditis is the pericardial friction rub, heard as a high-pitched scratching sound, that can be described as sandpaper rubbed together. It is heard best at the lower left sternal border, where the pericardium is close to the chest wall.

➠ Cardiac tamponade occurs in response to constriction around the heart and prevents the contraction of the myocardium. Characteristic signs include low blood pressure with a narrowing pulse pressure, elevated jugular venous distention, and pulsus paradoxus.

➠ ECG signs of pericarditis are evident in the depressed PR interval and increased ST segment occurring diffusely across multiple leads.

➠ Collaborative management for the patient with pericarditis is focused on maintaining cardiac output, eradicating infection, and ameliorating pain.

➠ Cardiac output may be restored through pericardiocentesis, the removal of fluid from the pericardial space.

➠ Infectious endocarditis has been characterized as a disease in transition, as a result of widespread availability of antibiotics, increases in intravenous drug use, and persons with a previous cardiac history.

➠ Before the use of antibiotics, endocarditis primarily affected adults under the age of 40 years. Currently, it is seen most frequently in adults over the age of 60 years, with men afflicted five times more frequently than women.

➡ Diagnostic clues to infectious endocarditis include a prior cardiac lesion and vague constitutional symptoms.

➡ Murmurs are encountered up to 90% of the time in infectious endocarditis. The most common are regurgitation murmurs of the aortic and mitral valves. Tricuspid murmurs are evident in intravenous drug users.

➡ Echocardiograms are the major diagnostic tool in patients with infectious endocarditis, and transesophageal studies provide the greatest sensitivity.

➡ Treatment of infectious endocarditis is centered on the selection of appropriate antibiotics administered intravenously for 2 to 6 weeks.

References

1. Mason J, Billingham ME, Ricci D: Treatment of acute inflammatory myocarditis assisted by endomyocardial biopsy. Am J Cardiol 45:1037–1044, 1980.

2. Myocarditis Treatment Trial (MTT) Investigation: incidence and clinical characteristics of myocarditis. Circulation 84 (Suppl II):11–12, 1991.

3. Francis G: Viral myocarditis: detection and management. Physician Sportsmed 23:63–68, 1995.

4. Suddaby E: Viral myocarditis in children. Crit Care Nurse 15:73–82, 1996.

5. Gill M, Klein N, Cunha B: Nonrheumatic poststreptococcal myocarditis. Heart Lung 24:425–426, 1995.

6. Friend L, Hancock W: Myocarditis or acute myocardial infarction? Hosp Pract 28:109–110, 1993.

7. Kantrowitz N, Smith R: Myocarditis update. Emerg Med Clin North Am 25:69–70, 1993.

8. Barron G, Senechal P: Case and comment. Primary care: the heart of the problem—acute myocarditis. Patient Care 29:61–63, 1995.

9. Butt A, Solsi A, Khan M, et al: Complete heart block and cardiogenic shock with Coxsackevirus B4 myocarditis requiring permanent pacing and intra-aortic balloon pump counterpulsation. Am J Crit Care 4:319–321, 1995.

10. Kontos C, Hess M: Today's approach to managing severe myocarditis. J Crit Illness 9:152–158, 1994.

11. Dehmer G, O'Meara J: Update on acute pericarditis. Hosp Med 31:39–44, 52–54, 1995.

12. Porterfield J: Pericardial disease. In: Stobo J, Hellmann D, Ladenson P, et al (eds): The Principles and Practice of Medicine, 23rd ed. Stamford, CT, Appleton & Lange, 1996, pp 83–91.

13. Bondmass M: The cardiac manifestations of acquired immune deficiency syndrome and nursing implications. Medsurg Nurs 3:42–48, 1994.

14. Kaul S, Fishbein MC, Siegal RJ: Cardiac manifestations of acquired immune deficiency syndrome: a 1991 update. Am Heart J 8:535–543, 1991.

15. Prince S, Cunha B: Case studies in infectious disease: postpericardiotomy syndrome. Heart Lung 26:165–168, 1997.

16. Maish B: Pericardial diseases, with a focus on etiology, pathogenesis, pathophysiology, new diagnostic imaging methods and treatment. Curr Opin Cardiol 9:379–388, 1994.

17. Fabius D: Solving the mystery of heart murmurs. Nursing 24:39–44, 1994.

18. Fabius D, Stunkard J: Uncovering the secrets of snaps, rubs, and clicks. Nursing 24:45–50, 1994.

19. Miller J: Surgical management of pericardial disease. In: Schlant RC, Alexander RW, O'Rourke RA, et al (eds): The Heart, Arteries and Veins, 8th ed. New York, McGraw-Hill, 1994, pp 1675–1679.

20. Amin NM: Infective endocarditis: the picture is changing. Will you recognize the face? Consultant 34:319–324, 1994.

21. Nunley DL, Perlman P: Endocarditis: changing trends in epidemiology, clinical and microbiologic spectrum. Postgrad Med 93:235–238, 241–247, 1993.

22. Durack D: Infective and noninfective endocarditis. In: Schlant RC, Alexander RW, O'Rourke RA, et al (eds): The Heart, Arteries and Veins, 8th ed. New York, McGraw-Hill, 1994, pp 1681–1705.

23. Shanewise J, Martin R: Assessment of endocarditis and associated complications with transesophageal echocardiography. Crit Care Clin 12:411–427, 1996.

24. Matthews D: The prevention and diagnosis of infective endocarditis: the primary care provider's role. Nurse Pract 19:53–60, 1994.

25. Amin NM: Infective endocarditis: timely diagnosis and treatment of a great mimic. Consultant 34:331–333, 337–338, 341–343, 1994.

26. Lukes A, Bright D, Durack D: Diagnosis of infective endocarditis. Infect Dis Clin North Am 7:1–8, 1993.

27. McKenry L, Salerno E: Mosby's Pharmacology in Nursing. St Louis, C.V. Mosby, 1995.

28. Fortuin N: Valvular heart disease. In: Stobo J, Hellmann D, Ladenson P, et al (eds): The Principles and Practice of Medicine, 23rd ed. Stamford, CT, Appleton & Lange, 1996, pp 59–70.

13

Cardiac Surgery and Heart Transplantation

Debra Lynn-McHale and Catharine Dorozinsky

Objectives

After completing this chapter, the student will be able to

1. Identify the most common vessels used for coronary artery bypass graft surgery.
2. Differentiate the indications and patient implications for using mechanical and biologic heart valves.
3. Relate the physiologic effects of cardiopulmonary bypass to the patient's postoperative recovery.
4. Select appropriate nursing interventions for managing the care of patients undergoing cardiac surgery.
5. Plan appropriate interventions for patients experiencing a complicated postoperative course after cardiac surgery.
6. Evaluate the criteria for listing heart transplant patients.
7. Compare the relative versus absolute contraindications in the heart transplant process.
8. Analyze the impact of health care reform and the donor shortage on the current and future care of heart transplant patients.
9. Select appropriate interventions to address the psychosocial needs of the heart transplant patient during the pretransplant and posttransplant phases.
10. Evaluate the effects of the postoperative immunosuppressive medications on the recovery of the heart transplant patient.

CARDIAC SURGERY

CORONARY ARTERY REVASCULARIZATION

Significant strides have been made in attempts to revascularize the ischemic myocardium. Thrombolytic therapy and interventional procedures, such as percutaneous transluminal angioplasty, stents, atherectomy devices, intravascular laser therapy, and angiojet therapy have all played an important role in reperfusing jeopardized areas of the myocardium. These advances have offered new hope for many patients with coronary artery disease. These therapies have often been effective in relieving angina and, for other patients, have delayed the timing for surgical revascularization.

Coronary Artery Bypass Graft Surgery

Coronary artery bypass surgery was first performed in 1967. Today, only 32 years later, it is one of the most frequently performed operations. Almost half a million coronary artery bypass graft surgeries are performed annually in the United States.[1] Initially, the saphenous vein was used most frequently to bypass diseased coronary arteries. However, the use of arteries has become more popular for bypassing blocked coronary arteries. Arteries currently used include the internal thoracic artery (also referred to as the internal mammary artery), the gastroepiploic artery, the inferior epigastric artery, and the radial artery. The most common artery used for bypassing blocked coronary arteries is the internal thoracic coronary artery. Arteries have patency rates superior to those of vein grafts.

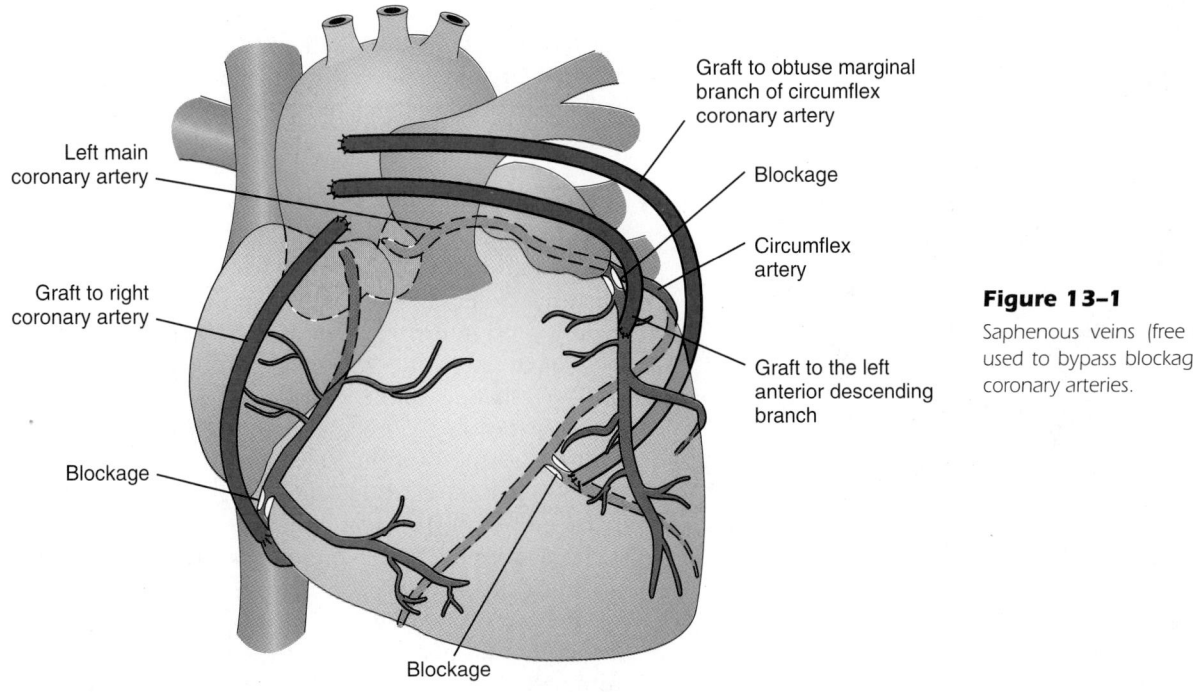

Left main
coronary artery

Graft to right
coronary artery

Blockage

Blockage

Graft to obtuse marginal
branch of circumflex
coronary artery

Blockage

Circumflex
artery

Graft to the left
anterior descending
branch

Figure 13–1

Saphenous veins (free grafts) are
used to bypass blockages in three
coronary arteries.

The most common vein used for bypassing blocked coronary arteries is the saphenous vein. If a vein or a detached artery (free graft) is used to bypass a diseased coronary artery, the vessel simply goes around or bypasses the blockage. The surgeon places a small incision in the diseased coronary artery above the blockage and another small incision below the blockage. Thus, blood flows around the blockage, thereby taking blood and oxygen to the heart. Figure 13–1 demonstrates saphenous veins used to bypass blockages in three coronary arteries.

The Cleveland Clinic Foundation has reported 5-year patency data of 82% for saphenous vein grafts. If an artery is used, the artery's site of origin usually remains intact (an in situ graft), and the distal end of the artery is dissected. The distal end of the artery is then used to bypass the diseased coronary artery. Figure 13–2 demonstrates use of the internal thoracic artery to bypass a blockage of the left anterior descending coronary artery. The Cleveland Clinic Foundation has reported that 97% of internal thoracic artery grafts are patent at 5 years, and 90% are patent at 15 years. From 85 to 95% of internal thoracic artery grafts are patent 10 years after cardiac surgery. Arteries that remain attached to their original site of origin continue to maintain properties that are unique to arteries, the most important being the ability to respond to cellular needs. Thus, arteries can dilate in response to ischemic myocardium.[2]

The right gastroepiploic artery lies along the greater curvature of the stomach. The artery is dissected and is brought through the diaphragm, in front of the stomach and the liver. This artery is commonly used as an in situ (origin still attached) graft to bypass block-ages in the right coronary artery or the posterior descending coronary artery. Figure 13–3 demonstrates use of the gastroepiploic artery to bypass a blockage of the right coronary artery. It can also be used as a free graft, in which the artery is completely dissected from

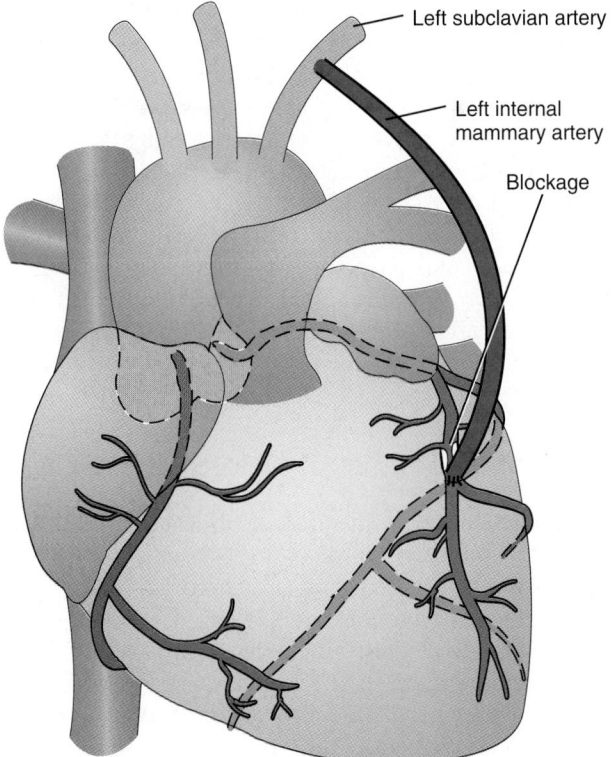

Left subclavian artery

Left internal
mammary artery

Blockage

Figure 13–2

Anastomosis of the distal end of the left internal mammary artery to the
left anterior descending artery, below the area of blockage.

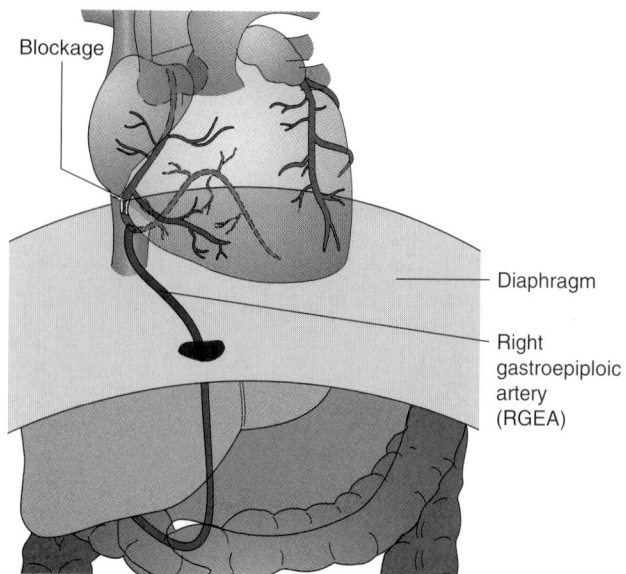

Figure 13–3

The use of the gastroepiploic artery to bypass a blockage of the right coronary artery.

its previous source. When used as a free graft (depending on its length), the gastroepiploic artery can be used to bypass any blocked coronary artery.

Another artery used for bypass surgery is the inferior epigastric artery, which is the continuation of the internal thoracic artery. When this artery is selected, it is used only as a free graft because it is not long enough to use as an in situ graft.

The radial artery was used early in the history of cardiac surgery. Over time, cardiothoracic surgeons stopped using the radial artery because of its poor patency rates. However, interest in using the radial artery has been renewed. The surgical technique has changed slightly. Instead of dissecting only the radial artery to use for the bypass, the surgeon dissects the radial artery and its pedicle as a unit. The pedicle is thought to provide additional structural support to the radial artery. Favorable early patency data using this new technique have been reported.

Minimally Invasive Cardiac Surgery

A more recent trend in cardiac surgical procedures is minimally invasive cardiac surgery, which involves using small incisions and microscopic technology. Minimally invasive cardiac surgery is usually performed in patients with single-vessel disease of the left anterior descending (LAD) coronary artery (see Figure 13–2). Several small incisions are made between the ribs, instead of using the traditional median sternotomy approach. Some centers are performing minimally invasive cardiac surgery through small ports and with video-assisted technology. Candidates for

minimally invasive cardiac surgery include patients who have totally occluded or tightly stenotic LAD lesions not amenable to percutaneous coronary artery angioplasty or patients with lesions resulting from failed percutaneous coronary artery angioplasty or stents.[3]

During minimally invasive cardiac surgery, the heart is not stopped for suturing of the bypass graft. The heart rate can be slowed with a beta blocker or calcium channel blocker to minimize movement during graft suturing.[4] Stabilizing devices have been developed, negating the need for beta blocker and calcium channel blocker therapy. These stabilizing devices, such as the Access Platform and Stabilizer, in addition to the Octopus, provide stabilization of the heart, so that the cardiothoracic surgeon can suture the distal end of the bypass graft to the coronary artery without stopping or slowing the heart rate.

Minimally invasive cardiac surgery is often performed without the use of cardiopulmonary bypass. Currently, more and more surgeons are performing minimally invasive cardiac surgery; however, data are not yet available to demonstrate its benefits over standard cardiac surgery. It is anticipated, however, that the patient's need for blood transfusions will be reduced, incisional pain will be less, length of stay will be decreased, and recovery will be quicker than with standard coronary artery bypass surgery.[4]

Transmyocardial Laser Revascularization

Transmyocardial laser revascularization is an experimental procedure for patients with severe coronary artery disease. In the operating room, laser therapy is used to pierce small channels through ischemic areas of the heart. It is not uncommon for 30 to 40 channels to be created in an effort to improve blood flow to the myocardium. The channels provide a means for blood to flow from the ventricle through the endocardium, through the myocardium, and toward the epicardial surface of the heart. The exact mechanism for improving oxygenation to the heart is unknown. It may be due to the direct channels created or due to angiogenesis. Angiogenesis, the growth of new blood vessels, may occur in response to the myocardial tissue injury caused by the laser energy.[5] Although this procedure is experimental, it offers a surgical option for patients who are not candidates for coronary artery bypass surgery because of diffuse, extensive coronary artery disease.

Data demonstrate that angina is improved, as is the patient's functional status. It is anticipated that, in the future, coronary artery bypass surgery may be performed on repairable vessels, whereas transmyocardial laser revascularization may be done to ischemic yet viable areas of the myocardium that are not amenable to bypass grafts.

CARDIAC VALVE SURGERY

Ten percent of all cardiac operations are performed for valvular heart disease. Cardiac valve surgery extends life expectancy in patients with progressive valve dysfunction. Valve dysfunction is most commonly caused by rheumatic heart disease, degenerative disease, or endocarditis (see Chapter 12). Valves on the left side of the heart, the mitral and aortic valves, are diseased more frequently than valves on the right side of the heart. The reason is the significant amount of pressure against which the mitral and aortic valves open and close. The exact timing of surgery is often difficult to determine. Usually, patients are medically managed until symptoms develop or until patients begin to develop ventricular dysfunction.

Cardiac Valve Replacement

Approximately 2 million people have had an artificial cardiac valve inserted.[6] Table 13–1 lists prosthetic valves currently available for insertion in the United States.[7] Both mechanical and bioprosthetic valves are available for valve replacement. The two types of mechanical valves that are most widely used today are the caged ball design and the tilting disc design. The caged ball mechanical valve consists of a ring, a cage, and a ball (Figure 13–4). The ball moves back and forth within the cage as pressure changes within the heart. If the valve is placed in the aortic position, during systole the blood flows from the left ventricle and pushes the ball forward, and blood flows around the

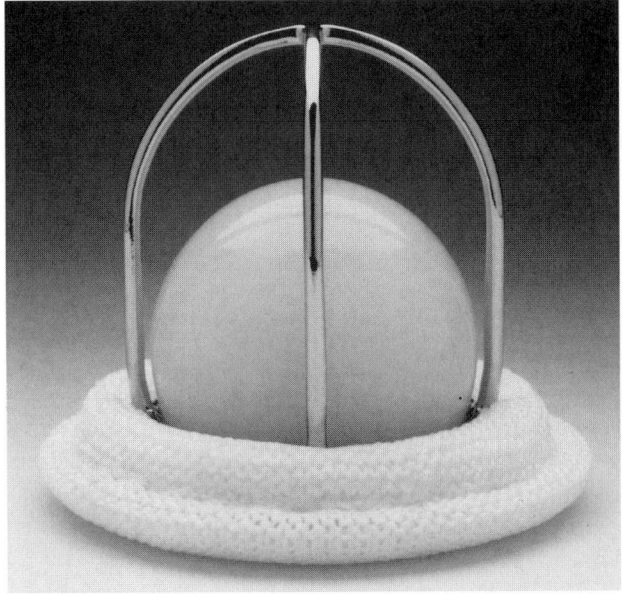

Figure 13–4

The Starr–Edwards ball and cage mechanical valve. (Courtesy of Baxter Healthcare Corp., Edwards CVS Division, Santa Ana, CA.)

ball into the aorta. As pressure in the aorta decreases, the ball falls back into the ring, and diastole occurs.

Another mechanical valve is the tilting disc valve. The tilting disc valve consists of a single disc or a bileaflet valve design. The single disc valve opens to a 60 or 80° angle as pressure pushes the valve open during systole (if placed in the aortic position) (Figure 13–5). The bileaflet valve opens both its leaflets as pressure pushes the valve open during systole (Figure 13–6). Both types of tilting disc valves close as pressure in the aorta decreases and the valve discs passively close.

Bioprosthetic valves are also called biologic valves. The three types of biologic valves are porcine, bovine,

TABLE 13–1
Prosthetic Valves Currently Available for Use in the United States

Category	Type of Valve	Manufacturer
Mechanical valves	Caged ball	Starr–Edwards
	Tilting disk	Medtronic Hall
		Omniscience
	Bileaflet	St. Jude
Biologic valves	Porcine	Hancock modified orifice
		Carpentier Edwards
	Bovine	Carpentier Edwards

Adapted from Whitman GR: Valve repair and replacement. In: Urban NA, Greenlee KK, Krumberger JM, et al (eds): Guidelines for Critical Care Nursing. St. Louis, C.V. Mosby, 1995, p 227.

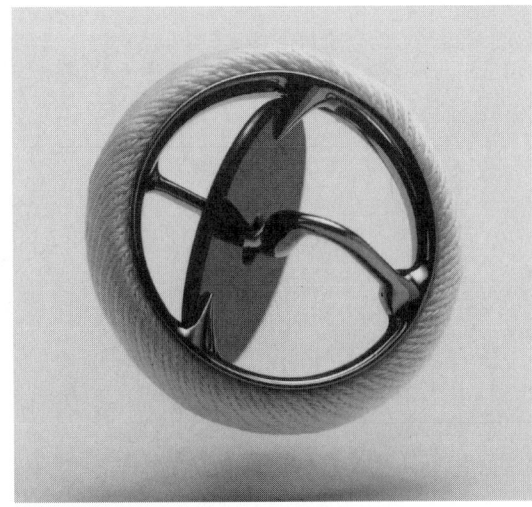

Figure 13–5

Medtronic-Hall single tilting disc valve. (Courtesy of Medtronic, Inc., Minneapolis, MN.)

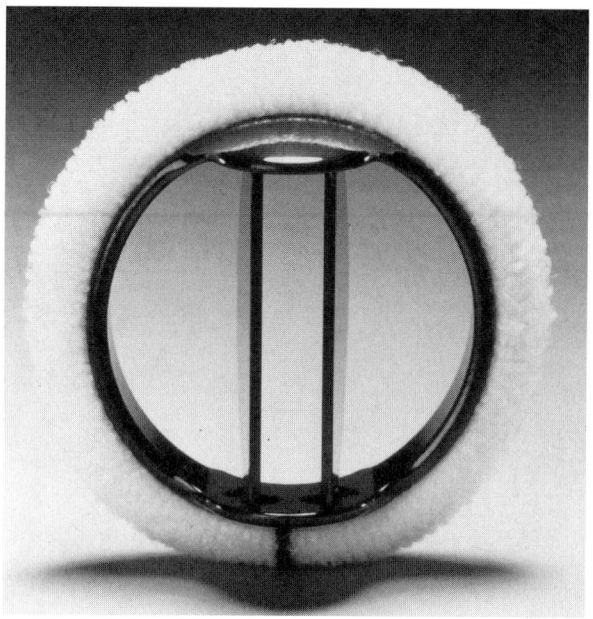

Figure 13–6

St. Jude Medical mechanical heart valve. (St. Jude Medical is a registered trademark of St. Jude Medical, Inc. Courtesy of St. Jude Medical, Inc., Saint Paul, MN. All rights reserved.)

and homografts. A porcine valve is a pig aortic valve that is mounted on a stent (Figure 13–7). A bovine valve is constructed from the pericardial tissue of calves. The pericardial tissue is used to form the valve leaflets, which are then mounted on a stent. Homografts are valves that are retrieved from human hearts within 24 hours of cardiac arrest. Homograft valves fit well in small aortic valve areas.

A new valve that has received approval by the United States Food and Drug Administration (FDA) is the Toronto stentless valve. This porcine valve is not mounted on a supporting structure or stent.

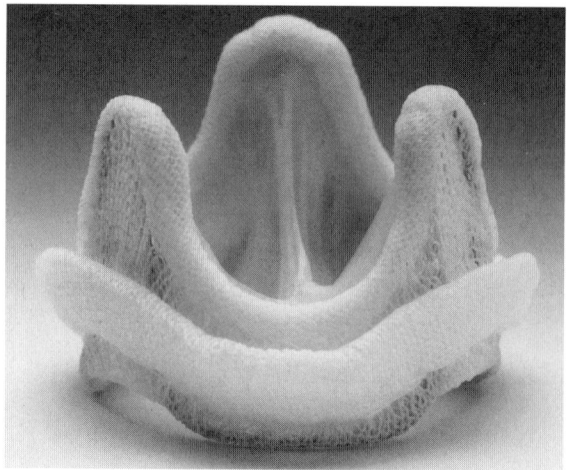

Figure 13–7

Carpentier–Edwards porcine valve. (Courtesy of Baxter Healthcare Corp., Edwards CVS Division, Santa Ana, CA.)

The patient, the cardiologist, and the cardiothoracic surgeon determine which prosthetic valve would be best suited, based on the location of the valve and the patient's age, lifestyle, and past medical history. Biologic valves are durable for 7 to 14 years and thus are more commonly placed in elderly patients. Although mechanical valves are durable, they necessitate lifelong anticoagulation therapy. If prospective patients have a history of coagulopathy, bleeding disorders, or hepatic disorders, or if they anticipate involvement in contact sports, a biologic valve would be preferred, because anticoagulation therapy would be contraindicated. Patients who have been noncompliant with past medications are not ideal candidates for a mechanical valve, because daily anticoagulation therapy is essential. A mechanical valve necessitates frequent testing of coagulation levels to guide anticoagulation doses. Mechanical valves are usually selected if a long life expectancy is likely (e.g., >15 years), if no contraindication to anticoagulation exists, or if the patient is already receiving anticoagulation therapy.

Cardiac Valve Repair

In the 1950s, valve reconstruction was the original technique used to repair damaged cardiac valves. After prosthetic valves were developed, the frequency of operations to repair valves decreased significantly. Because numerous complications can occur with valve replacement, valve repairs are once again gaining popularity.

Although valve reconstruction can be performed to improve the function of insufficient or stenotic valves, most surgical procedures are performed for valve insufficiency. Surgical repairs can be performed for damaged commissures, valve leaflets, chordae tendineae, and papillary muscles.

Open mitral commissurotomy is a procedure in which the cardiothoracic surgeon excises the patient's fused commissures in an effort to increase the valve orifice size and to improve leaflet mobility (Figure 13–8). This technique is performed if the valve leaflets are thin and pliable.

An insufficient cardiac valve may be repaired by the surgeon by inserting an annuloplasty ring (Figure 13–9). During valve annuloplasty, a flexible ring is sewn to the valve annulus in an attempt to reshape the valve orifice so that the mitral valve leaflets or the aortic valve cusps coapt.[7]

Tears in valve leaflets can be patched with pericardial tissue. The excessive or redundant portion of the valve leaflet can be resected in an effort to improve valve leaflet function. Ruptured papillary muscles can also be reattached to the endocardium.

Shortened chordae tendineae can be longitudinally excised in an effort to lengthen the chordae. Elongated chordae tendineae can be folded onto themselves, or the folded chordae tendineae can be tucked into the papillary muscle in an effort to shorten the chordae

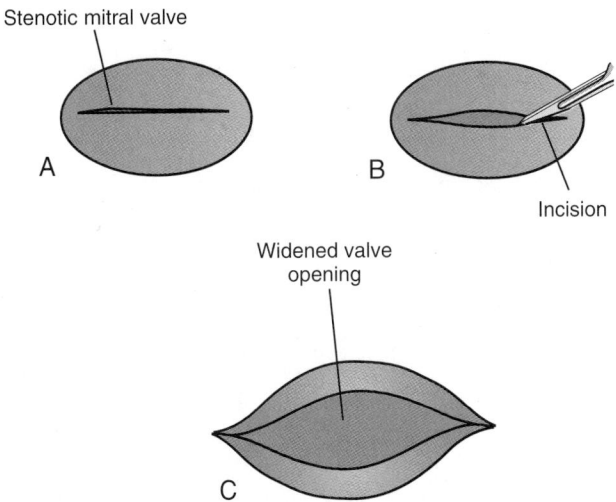

Figure 13–8

Open mitral commissurotomy. *A,* Severely narrowed valve opening. *B,* Surgical incision. *C,* Improved valve opening.

(Figure 13–10). Shortening or lengthening of the chordae tendineae may preserve valve leaflet function.

Investigators estimate that 80% of all dysfunctional mitral valves can be repaired. A much smaller percentage of aortic valves can be repaired. Aortic valve repair may include valve resuspension to decrease or eliminate the amount of valve regurgitation. Thickened leaflet edges can be shaved in an attempt to improve or eliminate aortic insufficiency.[8]

Assessment

Cardiac surgery may be scheduled as an elective procedure, yet commonly it is planned under urgent or emergency conditions. Cardiac catheterization pro-

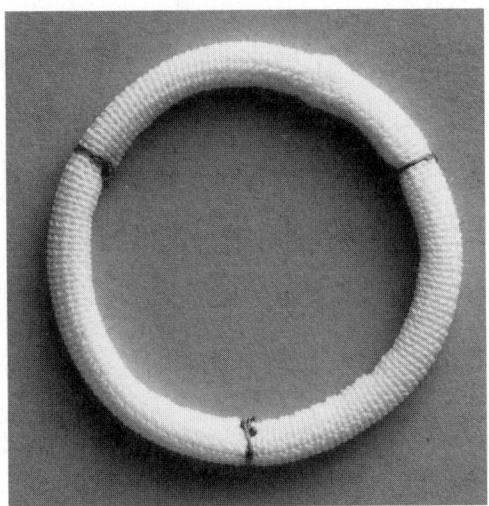

Figure 13–9

Annuloplasty ring. (Courtesy of Medtronic, Inc., Minneapolis, MN.)

vides definitive information regarding cardiac function. Information provided includes condition of the coronary arteries, degree of coronary artery stenosis, condition of the cardiac valves, degree of stenosis or insufficiency of the cardiac valves, cardiac pressures, and ejection fraction.

The decision to undergo cardiac surgery is usually made after treatment options are discussed among the patient, family members, the cardiologist, and the cardiac surgeon. Timing of surgery depends on the severity of the disease state.

Preoperative Phase

Preparation of the patient and family is an important phase of the cardiac surgical experience. Meeting educational needs is important, because preoperative preparation increases knowledge, decreases anxiety, and promotes patient and family involvement. Both patients and their family members must be as physically and emotionally prepared for cardiac surgery as possible.

Educational Preparation

Preoperative preparation is essential so that patients understand the entire surgical process. Although patients may be hospitalized preoperatively, most patients are admitted to the hospital the morning of the surgical procedure. This approach challenges health care professionals to have a coordinated system in place to meet the educational needs of patients and their family members in both inpatient and outpatient settings.

Patients and family members should be prepared for what to expect before, during, and after cardiac surgery. During the preoperative phase, most teaching focuses on what to expect during the hospitalization with just a preliminary discussion regarding home expectations. Postoperatively, emphasis is placed on discharge planning.

Preoperative anxiety levels are usually elevated for both patients and family members. Because anxiety decreases retention of information, attempts should be made to decrease the anxiety felt by patients and family members before teaching essential information. Research has demonstrated that family members' anxiety levels are higher than patients' levels before cardiac surgery.[9] Thus, family members must be included in the educational process. See Chart 13–1 for content to include in preoperative teaching.

Educational programs for patients may include individual teaching, group classes, videotape presentations, or computer-assisted programs. Educational booklets can also be helpful. Often, the booklets contain diagrams of the heart, valves, and coronary anatomy. The patient's own disease process can be drawn on the diagrams and thus can enhance under-

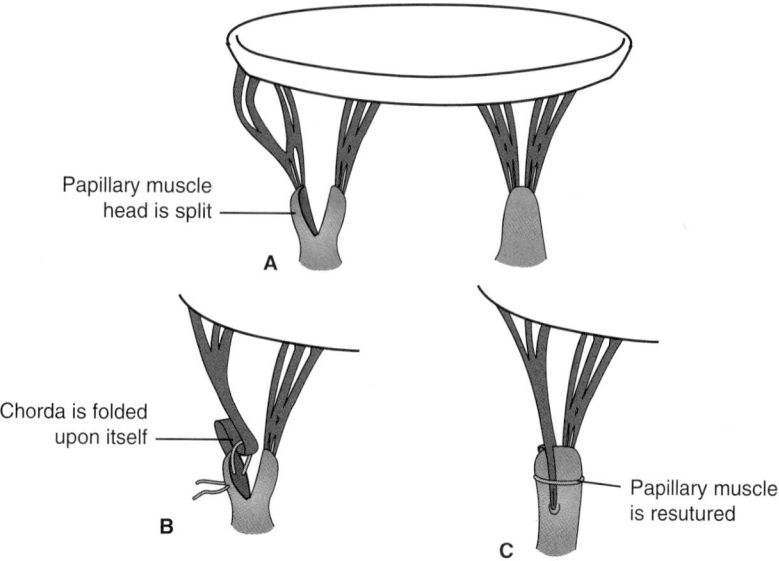

Figure 13–10

Chordae tendineae shortening. A, Note the elongated chorda and the surgically incised papillary muscle. B, The chorda is folded upon itself and is tucked into the papillary muscle. C, The papillary muscle is resutured and the repair is completed.

standing by the patient and family members of the cardiac dysfunction and the anticipated plan for surgical intervention.

In addition, as a part of the educational process, many hospitals offer patients and their family members a tour of the intensive care unit (ICU). ICU tours help patients know what to expect after surgery.[9] An ICU tour usually includes touring the patient and family members through the ICU, the intermediate cardiac care unit, and the family waiting room. The equipment and the sights and sounds of the ICU can be explained. Patients and their family members can be given the opportunity to see a patient recovering in the initial hours after cardiac surgery and to see patients in the ICU or intermediate cardiac care unit, who may be out of bed and walking or in a chair. Chart 13–2 describes a study that was conducted on the effectiveness of ICU tours.

CHART 13–1

Preoperative Educational Content

Expectations before cardiac surgery
  Diagnostic tests (chest radiograph, laboratory studies)
  Skin preparation
  Nothing by mouth at least 8 hours preoperatively
  Ability to demonstrate effective cough and deep breathing, using splint for sternal or chest support
  Ability to demonstrate use of incentive spirometry
  Ability to demonstrate leg exercises (foot flexion and extension)
  Time family members should be at the hospital to visit preoperatively
Expectations during cardiac surgery
  Type of procedure anticipated
  Anticipated time in the operating room
  Convenient location for family to wait during surgery
  How family will be contacted at intervals during surgery or after surgery is completed

Expectations after cardiac surgery
  Name and location of the ICU
  External devices to expect and their purpose
    Endotracheal tube and ventilator
    Nasogastric tube
    ECG electrodes and monitoring
    Hemodynamic monitoring (pulmonary artery and arterial lines)
    Epicardial pacing wires and external pulse generator
    Chest tubes and drainage system
    Foley catheter
  Procedures to expect
    Endotracheal suctioning, if intubated
    Pain management plan
    Blood administration
    Activity progression
  Additional expectations
    Sounds of ICU
    Family involvement

CHART 13–2

RESEARCH UTILIZATION: BENEFITS OF ICU TOURS BEFORE CARDIAC SURGERY

Abstract: This study investigated the benefit or potential benefit of offering a tour of the ICU to patients and family members of patients before cardiac surgery. The effect of an ICU tour on the anxiety levels of patients (N = 92) and family members (N = 91) before and after cardiac surgery was studied. Using a pretest–posttest quasiexperimental design, patients and family members were assigned to a control group, which received preoperative teaching, or to an experimental group, which received preoperative teaching with an ICU tour. Patients and family members completed two measures of anxiety, the State Trait Anxiety Inventory and a visual analog scale, before and after the intervention. Family members completed the anxiety tools again after their first postoperative visit. Patients also completed the Patient Perception of the ICU Tour Questionnaire after transfer from the ICU.

Both patients and family members had a decrease in anxiety after cardiac surgery teaching, yet this decrease was not due to the ICU tour. However, most patients who toured the ICU perceived the tour as beneficial and recommended a tour for future patients. Patients found the tour helped them to feel more prepared, to know what to expect, and be better able to cope with what was ahead.

Critique: This study was conducted in a university medical center. A convenience sample of participants was used. Generalization beyond the sample is limited. Subjects were placed into the control or experimental group based on predetermined criteria, a procedure that may have led to selection bias. Some of the patients and family members were taught individually, and others were taught in group settings. Anxiety levels may have been influenced by the different settings.

This is the first published study on the effectiveness of ICU tours. Thus, the effect of an ICU tour for patents about to have cardiac surgery remains unknown, and additional studies are needed.

Nursing Implications: Patients and family members are usually anxious as they await the surgical day. The importance of preoperative preparation of patients and family members was reinforced in this study. Adequate teaching and preparation can assist patients and their family members with this process. Although the preoperative ICU tour did not significantly decrease patient and family member anxiety levels, patients who received a tour of the ICU perceived a benefit from the tour. Thus, a tour of the ICU should be considered and offered to patients and family members as they are prepared for cardiac surgery. Individual patients and family members may not want to go on an ICU tour, and their preferences should be respected.

Preoperative teaching must be given a high priority. Adequate time needs to be given to prepare patients and family members for what they can expect before, during, and after cardiac surgery. Patients and family members should be encouraged to ask questions and to participate actively in the plan of care.

Source: Lynn-McHale DJ, Corsetti A, Brady-Avis E, et al: Preoperative ICU tours: are they helpful? Am J Crit Care 6:106–115, 1997.

Patients and their family members can also be offered the opportunity to talk with other patients whom have experienced cardiac surgery. Talking with someone who has already been through the experience can be extremely helpful. Members of the Zipper Club can be formally asked to see prospective patients. The Zipper Club is a national organization that assists patients and family members with the cardiac surgical process. If a formal Zipper Club consultation is not possible, patients currently hospitalized who have experienced a cardiac operation are often willing to speak with prospective patients and family members and to answer their questions.

Preoperative preparation should be initiated as early as possible. If patients are admitted on the day of surgery, cardiac surgical education can be included in the preadmission process. Educational videotapes that patients can take home with them to view again can help to reinforce information taught.

Additional Preparation for Cardiac Surgery

Results of preoperative laboratory studies should be within normal limits preoperatively. Common laboratory studies include a complete blood cell count, Sequential Multiple Analysis 12 (SMA 12), and coagulation studies. A preoperative arterial blood gas determination may be obtained if patients have a comorbid pulmonary condition. Blood is also sent for type and screen or type and cross to prepare standby blood replacement products. A chest radiograph is also obtained.

Patients are usually asked to bathe or shower with an antibacterial soap the evening before and also the morning of surgery. Patients are usually allowed nothing by mouth (NPO) for at least 8 hours before surgery. Essential oral medications may be prescribed the morning of the operation. If oral medications are prescribed, patients should be encouraged to take the minimal amount of water necessary to swallow the medications.

Nursing Diagnoses

Care of the patient having a cardiac operation is challenging and often complex. Nursing diagnoses can be identified for the preoperative phase, the intensive phase, and the intermediate care phase (Table 13–2). The plan of care must be individualized for each patient and specific for each procedure.

Priority nursing diagnoses during the preoperative phase relate to knowledge deficit and anxiety regarding the anticipated cardiac surgery. Provision of education may decrease the anxiety that patients and their family members may be experiencing. However, it is unrealistic to expect that no anxiety will be present. Patients and their family members need to be knowledgeable about what they can expect to occur before, during, and after a cardiac operation. The specific cardiac surgical procedure must be explained, and questions must be answered. In addition, patient recovery is often facilitated if patients are given opportunities to demonstrate the ability to splint an incision, to cough and breathe deeply, and to use incentive spirometry.

Several nursing diagnoses are present during the intensive care phase of cardiac surgery. Nursing diagnoses include, but are not limited to, acute pain, alteration in cardiac output, fluid volume deficit, sensory or perceptual alterations, and sleep pattern disturbances. Nursing is instrumental in assisting patient recovery through this phase. Patients may experience hemodynamic stability or instability during this phase. Nurses constantly are assessing patients' status and patients' responses to interventions.

During the intermediate care phase of cardiac surgery, nursing diagnoses include alteration in cardiac output, activity intolerance, potential ineffective coping, knowledge deficit, and altered sexuality patterns. Nurses assist patients as they begin to increase their activity and to resume activities of daily living. Patients' responses to activity need to be evaluated carefully. Coordination of discharge planning is important.

Collaborative Management

A collaborative effort among multidisciplinary health care professionals is essential in coordinating the care of patients undergoing cardiac surgery. This multidisciplinary team often includes nurses, advance practice nurses, physicians, physician assistants, and case managers. Corsetti and Perry[10] demonstrated that positive patient outcomes can be achieved when the multidisciplinary cardiac surgical team works together to develop protocols and to create system changes.

TABLE 13–2
Nursing Diagnoses

Problem Statement	Etiologic Factors
Preoperative Phase	
Knowledge deficit (learning need)	Expectations before, during, and after cardiac surgery
Anxiety	Anticipated cardiac surgery
Intensive Care Phase	
Pain	Trauma of cardiac surgery
Decreased cardiac output	Myocardial hypothermia, edema, stunning, left ventricular dysfunction, or dysrhythmias
Fluid volume deficit	Effects of cardiopulmonary bypass, postoperative fluid loss, bleeding, or temperature changes
Sensory/perceptual alterations	Sensory overload and sensory deprivation in the ICU setting
Sleep pattern disturbance	Frequency of nursing care activities after cardiac surgery
Ineffective family coping	Stressors of cardiac surgery and change in family dynamics
Intermediate Care Phase	
Decreased cardiac output	Dysrhythmias
Activity intolerance	Recovery from cardiac surgery
Ineffective individual coping	Stressors of recovery after cardiac surgery
Knowledge deficit (learning need)	Self-care, risk factor modification, and discharge planning
Altered sexuality patterns	Change in physical capacity and discomfort

Intraoperative Phase

Before the initiation of cardiac surgery, the patient is prepared for the procedure in the operating room holding area or in the operating room itself. While the patient is still awake, yet drowsy, several large-bore intravenous (IV) lines are placed. Electrocardiographic (ECG) electrodes are placed for ECG monitoring of heart rate and rhythm. A central line is inserted, and a pulmonary artery catheter is positioned through the central line. The pulmonary artery catheter provides essential data regarding the pressures within the heart. An arterial line is usually placed in the radial artery to monitor the patient's blood pressure. In addition, a Foley catheter is inserted. The anesthesiologist inserts the endotracheal tube and initiates anesthesia. A nasogastric tube may also be inserted.

The skin is cleansed with povidone–iodine (Betadine), and the patient's sternum is opened using a surgical saw. At the same time, the patient's leg is cleansed (if a saphenous vein will be used) with povidone–iodine, and surgical excision of the saphenous vein is initiated. Usually, two surgical teams are present, one working on the patient's chest and one working on the patient's leg (again, if a saphenous vein will be used).

During cardiac surgery, blood is diverted from the heart to provide a bloodless field. Cardiopulmonary bypass is achieved by placing a venous cannula in the right atrium and by placing an arterial cannula in the aorta. Thus, the blood is diverted from the venous system to the cardiopulmonary bypass machine and back to the arterial system (Figure 13–11). The cardiopulmonary bypass machine oxygenates the blood as it flows through the system. The patient is always anticoagulated to prevent thrombus development during cardiopulmonary bypass. Until recently, cardiopulmonary bypass was used routinely during all cardiac operations. However, because this technique has numerous untoward effects, attempts are being made to use alternative techniques.

The aorta is clamped, and the heart is arrested by instilling a cardioplegic solution into the aorta. The solution is usually cooled and consists of an electrolyte solution with a large amount of potassium. The cardioplegic solution infuses into the coronary arteries. The hypothermic, hyperkalemic solution produces a decrease in tissue temperature and cardiac arrest.[11] The cardioplegic solution can also be infused through the coronary sinus to infuse into the coronary venous system. In addition, the same solution is poured around the heart to cause cardiac standstill.

Once the heart is arrested and blood is diverted from the heart, the surgeon can begin the operation. If the patient is undergoing coronary artery bypass surgery, the vessels (arteries or veins) are dissected and are used to bypass the areas of blockage within the coronary artery. If the patient is undergoing valve surgery, the diseased valve is either repaired or replaced. If the patient is having both coronary artery bypass surgery and cardiac valve surgery, usually the bypass is completed, and then the valve is repaired or replaced. When surgery is complete, heparin is reversed with protamine sulfate, cardiopulmonary bypass is removed, and the heart is allowed to restart.

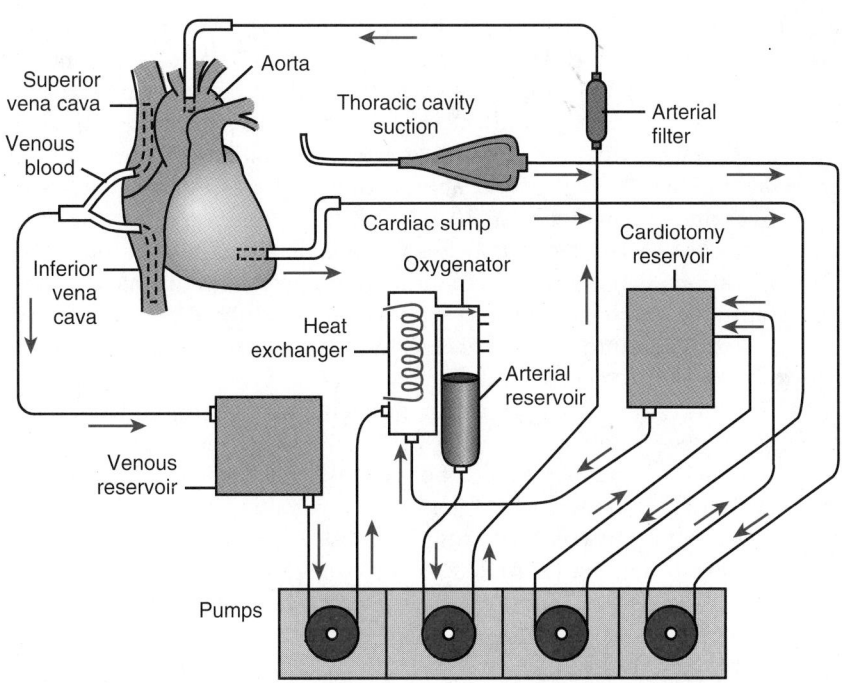

Figure 13–11

Cardiopulmonary bypass system.

Postoperative Phase

Collaborative management of patients after cardiac surgery is essential. Priority goals include early extubation, achievement of hemodynamic stability, and effective management of pain. Table 13–2 provides an overview of nursing diagnoses and collaborative problems that are common in patients who are undergoing cardiac surgery. A clinical pathway can also be used as a guideline for the necessary interventions and collaborative goals of care (Figure 13–12). Individualization of the clinical pathway is important.

Intensive Care Unit

Most patients are admitted directly to the ICU from the operating room. Because the patient has multiple needs simultaneously, most critical care units have an organized system developed to facilitate smooth patient admission and rapid assessment. This system may involve two nurses working together for the first 30 to 45 minutes. An anesthesiologist usually accompanies the monitored patient to the ICU. After initial vital signs, cardiac rhythm, hemodynamic parameters, and chest tube outputs are assessed, the anesthesiologist provides a thorough report of the patient's status during and immediately after the operation. This report builds on the report given by telephone by the operating room nurse before the patient leaves the operating room.

Neurologic Status. Patients may return to the ICU from the operating room while they are still under anesthesia. The patient's pupils should be midline and should react to light and accommodation. Limbs are flaccid, and motor and sensory checks are unnecessary during the immediate postoperative period. Neurologic assessments should be performed hourly until the patient is alert and then every 4 hours. If abnormalities are detected, neurologic assessments should be continued hourly.

Most patients regain consciousness within the first few postoperative hours. As consciousness is regained, patients should be told that the operation is over and that they are in the ICU. In addition, it may ease patient's anxiety to know exactly what the operation entailed (e.g., "The surgeon performed four bypasses") and whether family members are nearby. After patients awaken, it is important to determine movement and strength of upper and lower extremities. These features can be assessed by asking patients to squeeze the nurse's hands as firmly as possible and by asking patients to push against the nurse's hands with their feet. If any abnormalities are assessed, the surgeon should be notified, and frequent neurologic examinations should be continued.

While patients are intubated, the nurse should ask simple yes-or-no questions that patients can respond to by nodding their heads. After patients are extubated, the nurse should assess their orientation to person, place, and time. Many patients have little or no recall of the day of the operation and may need frequent reorientation to the day and time.

Ventilation and Oxygenation. Most patients return to the ICU anesthetized, intubated, and ventilated by a mechanical ventilator. The inspired flow of oxygen (FIO_2) is usually at 50%, the tidal volume is usually set at 10 to 15 mL/kg, and the rate may be 10 to 12. It is not uncommon for patients to receive 5 cm of positive end-expiratory pressure (PEEP). PEEP is pressure delivered by the ventilator to enhance oxygenation. PEEP expands alveoli that may have collapsed during surgery. As PEEP expands alveoli, surface area is increased, and the exposure time for the diffusion of oxygen is improved.[12] Changes in ventilator settings are made based on arterial blood gas values and patients' responses.

Pulse oximetry and mixed venous oxygen saturation are closely monitored to assess that each patient's oxygen needs are being met. Normal mixed venous oxygen saturation levels (60–80%) are desired, and usually a pulse oximetry level greater than 94% is expected. As soon as the patient is hemodynamically stable, the head of the bed can be elevated slightly to facilitate lung expansion.

The length of time during which patients receive mechanical ventilation is variable. Patients may return from the operating room extubated, or they may remain intubated for a time, even extending to the morning after the operation. Anesthesiologists are more commonly administering short-acting anesthetic agents in an effort to allow the patient to wake up quickly after surgery so that the weaning process can begin. A recent trend is early extubation, in which an effort is made to extubate patients within 2 to 4 hours after surgery. Before extubation, patients need to be awake and alert, assisting the ventilator, able to demonstrate a negative inspiratory pressure of −25 mm Hg, and able to demonstrate a vital capacity of greater than 10 mL/kg. In addition, early extubation protocols may necessitate that patients are hemodynamically stable and that chest tube drainage is less than 200 mL per hour before extubation.[10] Additional information on weaning from mechanical ventilation can be found in Chapter 17.

After extubation, patients may be placed for a short period on a 50% face mask, which is usually rapidly weaned to 6 L of oxygen by nasal cannula. Patients are assessed for tolerance of weaning by respiratory rate, auscultatory lung sounds, color, pulse oximetry (>94%), mixed venous oxygen saturation (60–80%), and their own sense of comfort with the weaning process (e.g., absence of distress and ease of breathing).

The critical pathway is meant to serve as a guideline for routine patient care. When the condition of the patient warrants, treatment decisions must be dictated by the skill and judgement of the health care professional.

MR#

ENC.#

NAME

Key: M = Met
      N = Not Met

COMPLETE OR IMPRINT WITH ADDRESS-O-PLATE

CABG PATHWAY	Day of Surgery Transfer to SCCU	Date M	N	Post Op Day 1 Transfer to ICCU	Date M	N
Consults/ Other Therapies	Cardiology					
Tests	Post-op: CBC, calcium, Mg, SMA-7			SMA-7		
	Chest x-ray			CBC		
	ECG, ABG			ECG		
Treatments	Extubate per standard of care			Daily weights		
				D/C Foley		
				D/C chest tube		
				D/C Swan Ganz		
				Incentive spirometer		
				Coughing/deep breathing		
				Cap pacer wires		
				Cap IV		
				O_2/pulse OX		
				Wound care		
Medication Reminders	Medications per order sheet					
	PCA morphine			Medications per order sheet		
	D/C vasopressors/vasodilators			D/C PCA morphine		
Nutrition	NPO			Liquids and advance to low fat, low cholesterol diet as tolerated		
Activity/ Safety	Bed rest			Partial care for bathing		
				Out of bed		
Teaching	Family orientation			Orient to telemetry		
				Incentive spirometer, coughing, deep breathing		
				Pain management		
				Wound care		
				Activity		
Desired Outcomes	Extubation			D/C Foley, chest tubes, Swan		
	D/C vasopressors/vasodilators			Pain relief		
	No bleeding			OOB, ambulation		
	Pain relief			Tolerating diet		
	No malignant dysrhythmia			No malignant dysrhythmia		
				Pacing not necessary		
				Transfer to ICCU		
Variance	Remains intubated			Requires Foley, chest tubes, Swan		
	Requires vasopressor/vasodilator			Inadequate pain relief		
	Chest tube bleeding >100 cc/hr			Not out of bed or ambulating		
	Inadequate pain relief			Malignant dysrhythmia		
	Malignant dysrhythmia			Requires epicardial pacing		
				Diet not tolerated		

Initials	Signature	Initials	Signature	Initials	Signature

Figure 13–12

Coronary artery bypass graft surgery clinical pathway. (Courtesy of Thomas Jefferson University Hospital, Philadelphia, PA.)

Figure 13-12 Continued

CABG PATHWAY	Post Op Day 2/3	Date M	Date N	Post Op Day 4/5	Date M	Date N
Consults/ Other Therapies	PT/Rehab consult day 3			D/C telemetry on day 4		
	Home health care consult day 2					
Tests				CXR PA & LAT;		
				CBC, ECG on day 4		
Treatments	Daily weights			Incentive spirometer		
	D/C pacing wires on day 3			Coughing/deep breathing		
	Incentive spirometer			D/C IV on day 4		
	Coughing/deep breathing					
	IV INT					
	O₂/pulse OX					
	Wound care					
	D/C O₂ on day 3					
Medication Reminders	Medications per order sheet			Medications per order sheet		
Nutrition	Low fat, low cholesterol diet as tolerated			Low fat, low cholesterol diet		
Activity/ Safety	OOB and ambulate as tolerated			Ambulate ad lib		
				Shower after monitor and pacing wires D/C		
				Discharge		
Teaching	Medication teaching (cards & calendar)			Medication teaching (cards & calendar)		
	Risk factor booklet			Reinforce teaching for discharge including medications, diet, activity, wound care		
	Reinforce teaching for discharge					
	Pain management					
	Diet			Discharge medications and prescriptions		
	Wound care					
	Activity			Discharge instructions		
Desired Outcomes	D/C pacer wires			No signs of infection		
	No signs of infection			No malignant dysrhythmias		
	No respiratory difficulty			Adequate nutrition		
	Pain relief			Independent in mobility and activities of daily living		
	Ambulation					
	Tolerating diet			Pain relief		
	No malignant dysrhythmia			Discharge needs met		
	No complication after pacer wires D/C					
Variance	Requires epicardial pacing			Evidence of infection present		
	Inadequate pain relief			Malignant dysrhythmia		
	No ambulation			Inadequate nutrition		
	Diet not tolerated			Inadequate ambulation		
	Malignant dysrhythmia			Dependent on assistance for activities of daily living and mobility		
				Inadequate pain relief		
				Discharge needs not met		

Initials	Signature	Initials	Signature	Initials	Signature

Figure 13–12 *Continued*

While patients are intubated, removal of secretions is essential to adequate oxygenation. Patients are suctioned through the endotracheal tube when lung sounds are abnormal, obvious secretions are noted in the endotracheal tube, patients are coughing, or oxygen saturation is not adequate. Hyperoxygenation and hyperventilation are always necessary before, during, and after suctioning. Incentive spirometry should be initiated soon after extubation. Patients should perform at least 10 incentive spirometry breaths every hour when they are awake. Nurses should instruct patients to inhale as deeply as possible and to hold each breath in as long as possible. Incentive spirometry should be performed at the patient's own rate of comfort. Patients commonly begin coughing while performing incentive spirometry. Nurses should ensure that patients are adequately medicated for pain and have a pillow to support their chests during coughing. Placing pressure on the pillow usually helps to decrease the amount of sternal discomfort experienced during coughing.

Hemodynamic Monitoring. Most patients who undergo cardiac surgery have a pulmonary artery catheter placed and an arterial line. On rare occasion, a low-risk, stable patient does not have a pulmonary artery catheter, but has a central line catheter placed instead.

Myocardial performance is enhanced if preload, afterload, and contractility are optimized. Myocardial hypoxemia and acidosis should be avoided and treated immediately in an effort to preserve myocardial functioning. Myocardial stunning is severely ischemic myocardium that produces ventricular dysfunction.[13] Myocardial stunning may occur during cardiac surgery and may lead to suboptimal myocardial functioning in the postoperative period.

The major tenets of patient management center on optimizing preload, enhancing contractility, and reducing afterload.[7] Fluid replacement may be necessary to optimize preload, inotropes may be necessary to improve contractility, and afterload reduction may be needed to decrease systemic vascular resistance.

The arterial catheter is usually placed in the radial artery. It is attached to a fluid-filled pressurized system and is connected to the bedside monitor. The pressure in the artery is measured by the transducer, and a waveform is displayed on the bedside monitor; a digital display of the patient's systolic, diastolic, and mean arterial pressures is also on the monitor. It is commonly desirable to maintain the patient's mean arterial blood pressure between 65 and 75 mm Hg for the first 12 postoperative hours. A stable mean arterial pressure provides a constant low pressure on the newly bypassed artery or vein grafts, as well as on any additional suture lines for patients undergoing valve surgery. By decreasing stress on the suture lines, postoperative bleeding may be minimized. After 12 hours, the mean arterial pressure is commonly maintained below 90 mm Hg. Variation in desired mean arterial pressures may be prescribed by the physician. Hypotension may be managed by administering intravenous fluids, inotropic agents, vasoconstricting agents, or a combination of these therapies. Hypertension may be treated with sedation, analgesics, and vasodilators. Common vasodilator therapy may include nitroglycerin (Tridil), sodium nitroprusside (Nipride), or nicardipine (Cardene) infusions.

The pulmonary artery catheter is usually placed through the right superior vena cava or the right internal or external jugular vein. The pulmonary artery catheter is attached to a fluid-filled pressurized system and is connected to the bedside monitor. The pressure at the distal tip of the pulmonary catheter is measured by the transducer, and a waveform is displayed on the bedside monitor. A digital display of the patient's systolic, diastolic, and mean pulmonary artery pressures is also visible on the monitor. In addition, the proximal tip of the pulmonary artery catheter is also connected to a fluid-filled transducer system and measures pressure in the right atrium (see Chapter 6). Hemodynamic

parameters are usually kept within normal range. Table 13–3 contains normal values for hemodynamic parameters. Although normal ranges exist for hemodynamic monitoring parameters, hemodynamic values may vary among patients.

Pulmonary artery systolic and diastolic pressures and right atrial pressures are observed continuously. More important than a single set of hemodynamic parameters is the trend in data. If a patient's pulmonary artery pressures (PAPs) and right atrial pressures gradually decrease (preload decreases), the patient will probably benefit from fluid replacement. If, on the other hand, a patient's PAPs and right atrial pressures gradually increase (preload is increased), the patient may benefit from a decrease in fluid replacement, an inotropic agent, or a vasodilating agent.

Cardiac output and cardiac index can readily be obtained by the thermodilution method through the pulmonary artery catheter or by a continuous cardiac output technology through the pulmonary artery catheter. Cardiac output, cardiac index, and systemic vascular resistance are obtained in the immediate postoperative period and as needed to guide initiation, titration, and discontinuation of vasoactive therapy. If a patient's cardiac index is below 2.4 L per minute, inotropic agents, such as epinephrine (Adrenalin), dopamine (Intropin), and dobutamine (Dobutrex) are initiated. If the cardiac index is low and systemic vascular resistance is high, a vasodilator may dilate the arterial system and may allow the heart to propel blood more easily, thus improving myocardial functioning. It is not uncommon for patients to receive both an inotropic agent and a vasodilating agent. The inotropic agent (e.g., dobutamine) increases cardiac contractility, and the vasodilating agent (e.g., sodium nitroprusside) decreases afterload. A new classification of medications includes the phosphodiesterase inhibitors. A phosphodiesterase inhibitor or inodilator, such as am-

TABLE 13–3
Hemodynamic Parameters

Parameter	Value
Pulmonary artery systolic pressure (PAS)	15–25 mm Hg
Pulmonary artery diastolic pressure (PAD)	8–15 mm Hg
Pulmonary artery mean pressure (PAM)	10–20 mm Hg
Pulmonary artery occlusive pressure (PAOP)	6–12 mm Hg
Right atrial pressure (RAP)	1–7 mm Hg
Cardiac index	>2.4 L/min
Systemic vascular resistance (SVR)	900–1500 dynes/sec
Pulmonary vascular resistance (PVR)	100–250 dynes/sec

Note: Pulmonary artery pressure (PAP) is frequently recorded as PAS/PAD.

rinone (Inocor) or milrinone (Primacor) increases contractility and at the same time causes vasodilation. Thus, two essential effects can be achieved by using one medication (a phosphodiesterase inhibitor), instead of by using two medications (e.g., an inotropic agent and a vasodilating agent).

Mechanical Support. Cardiac mechanical support may be needed after cardiac surgery. Often, chemical support (vasoactive medications) is used after surgery to augment cardiac output. When chemical support is unable to attain or to maintain an adequate cardiac index, mechanical support is then initiated. Mechanical support can be provided by an intra-aortic balloon pump, the hemopump, or by a ventricular assist device.

An intra-aortic balloon pump is usually inserted through the femoral artery, but it may be inserted in the operating room through the thoracic aorta. The intra-aortic balloon is positioned in the thoracic aorta and is timed to inflate and deflate with the cardiac cycle. It is usually timed by the ECG waveform or the arterial waveform. The intra-aortic balloon is timed to inflate during diastole and to deflate during systole. During diastole, the intra-aortic balloon inflates in the thoracic aorta. As the balloon inflates, it displaces blood anteriorly toward the coronary arteries and distally toward the aortic periphery. The blood displaced to the coronary arteries improves oxygenation to the heart. The blood displaced toward the periphery improves perfusion to the entire body. Just before systole, the intra-aortic balloon deflates, creating a "potential" space and allowing the heart to eject blood more easily and against less resistance. Because resistance is decreased, myocardial workload is also decreased. Thus, the intra-aortic balloon pump can help to increase cardiac output, to decrease afterload, and to decrease preload.[14]

The Hemopump is a more recent device that may also be inserted for patients who require mechanical assistance to improve cardiac output. The Hemopump is inserted through the femoral artery. The catheter is advanced under fluoroscopy into the aorta, through the aortic valve, and is placed in the left ventricle. The catheter is connected to an external pump. The Hemopump contains a motor that creates a spinning motion. This spinning motion pulls blood out of the left ventricle and into the aorta. The Hemopump does not require timing with the cardiac cycle. It can augment cardiac output by 0.5 to 3.5 L per minute.

Ventricular assist devices are placed in patients at the end of the cardiac operation when the patient's cardiac output is not adequate and one of the foregoing two devices is not effective in increasing cardiac output. Patients may receive a right ventricular assist device, a left ventricular assist device, or biventricular assist devices. A right ventricular assist device is

placed in patients with poor function of the right ventricle. The outflow port is placed in the right atrium. The inflow port is placed in the pulmonary artery. Thus, blood is diverted from the right ventricle as it flows from the right atrium to the pulmonary artery. The exact cardiac output can be set by the controls on the external console.

The left ventricular assist device is placed in patients with poor function of the left ventricle. The outflow port is placed in the left atrium. The inflow port is placed in the aorta. Thus, blood is diverted from the left ventricle as it flows from the left atrium to the aorta. As with the right ventricular assist device, the exact cardiac output can be set by the controls on the external console.

A biventricular assist device combines both the right and left ventricular assist devices. Thus, blood is diverted from the right ventricle as it passes from the right atrium to the pulmonary artery, and blood is diverted from the left ventricle as it passes from the left atrium to the aorta. Cardiac outputs for both the right and left side of the hearts can be set by the external device.

Despite the type of mechanical device, meticulous monitoring and care need to be provided. The mechanical device should be gradually weaned as contractility of the patient's heart improves. Close observation of hemodynamic monitoring parameters is essential to assess the patient's need for and response to weaning of the device.

Cardiac Rhythm. Cardiac rhythm disturbances are common in the postoperative period after a cardiac procedure. Potential causes of rhythm disturbances include electrolyte disturbances, hypothermia, and edema of the conduction pathways. Damage to the conduction pathways can occur during valve surgery because the mitral, tricuspid, and aortic valves lie in close proximity to the conduction pathways. In the initial hours after a cardiac operation, bradycardia or asystole may occur. Continuous ECG monitoring is essential for several days postoperatively.

Toward the end of the cardiac surgical procedure, epicardial pacing wires are placed on the heart and exit through the chest wall. Usually, two epicardial pacing wires are placed on the atria, and two epicardial pacing wires are placed on the ventricle. The atrial wires commonly exit the chest to the right of the sternum, and the ventricular wires commonly exit the chest to the left of the sternum. These pacing wires can be used to initiate temporary epicardial pacing if necessary.

Atrial pacing is commonly used for patients with asystole, bradycardia, or relative bradycardia. To initiate atrial pacing, the atrial epicardial pacing wires need to be connected to the temporary pacemaker. A rate is set, and the milliamps are set at a level that elicits a pacing impulse followed by capture of the atria. Atrioventricular pacing can be initiated if the atrial impulses are inhibited from conducting to the ventricles. Atrioventricular pacing sends an impulse to the atria and another impulse to the ventricles. The advantage of atrial pacing and of atrioventricular pacing is that the atria are stimulated to conduct an electrical impulse that elicits atrial contraction. Atrial contraction and synchrony between the atria and the ventricles are important, because atrial contraction contributes 20 to 30% to cardiac output.

After the patient's normal rate and rhythm returns, it is common to connect the temporary pacemaker to the patient's ventricular pacing wires. If the sensitivity of the pacemaker is good, the pacemaker can be set in the demand mode, and the rate is set at a rate lower than the patient's inherent rate. This system allows the pacemaker to elicit a pacing impulse only if the patient's inherent rate falls below the rate set on the temporary pacemaker.

Because the pacing wires are in direct contact with the epicardium, patients can receive microshocks. To avoid microshocks, certain safety precautions should be observed. Precautions include wearing gloves when handling the pacing wires, placing the pacing wires in an insulated nonconductive container (e.g., needle cover), ensuring that equipment is grounded, and avoiding the use of electric shavers.

Ventricular dysrhythmias may occur after cardiac surgery. Dysrhythmias may be due to electrolyte imbalances. If electrolyte levels are below normal, electrolyte replacements should be prescribed and administered. Life-threatening ventricular dysrhythmias, although rare, should be treated according to advance cardiac life-support protocols (see Appendix: ACLS Algorithms).

In the event of cardiac arrest, temporary epicardial pacing usually is effective in establishing a cardiac rhythm. In the event that it does not, cardiopulmonary resuscitation (CPR) is initiated. A priority in resuscitating a patient after mediastinal cardiac surgery is to open the chest. This procedure is important because the sternal edges are not healed, and external CPR causes displacement of the sternal edges; the sternal edges may lacerate the heart. Chest trays in the ICU are used during resuscitation efforts. The chest tray contains the instruments necessary for the cardiac surgeon, resident, or nurse practitioner to open the patient's chest quickly if necessary. Once the chest is opened, internal cardiac massage is initiated. A new sterile suction system should be set up for chest suction. In addition, a sterile environment should be encouraged (use of sterile gowns, masks, caps, boots) in an effort to minimize the risk of infection.

Internal defibrillator paddles are usually readily available in the ICU in the event that internal defibrillation is necessary. Internal defibrillator paddles connect easily to standard cardiac defibrillator machines. Decreased energy levels are needed to defibrillate internally, and the defibrillator machines have safety cutoff limits for the voltage that can be used safely for internal defibrillation.

Fluid Status (Fluid Shifts or Bleeding). Achieving fluid balance is a significant priority in the immediate postoperative period. Hemodynamic monitoring parameters are useful for assessing fluid status and for guiding fluid replacement. Patients are commonly fluid depleted in the initial hours after a cardiac operation. Several consequences of cardiopulmonary bypass affect fluid status. As the patient's blood passes through the cardiopulmonary bypass circuitry, cells are damaged. Damaged cells release vasoactive substances such as bradykinin and serotinin, which cause vasodilatation. When this change occurs, fluid leaks into the interstitial tissue. Although the patient may receive what would seem to be a sufficient amount of fluid replacement, much of this fluid leaks into the interstitial spaces, leaving an insufficient amount in the intravascular space.

Renin is also released because of the nonpulsatile flow created by the cardiopulmonary bypass machine during cardiac surgery. Renin stimulates angiotensin II, which causes vasoconstriction and further decreases the vascular space.

Patients also commonly experience diuresis in the immediate postoperative period. This change results from hemodilution and the osmotic effect of mild hyperglycemia. Urinary output should be measured hourly.

Fluid replacement should be administered to avoid hypovolemia. A combination of crystalloid and colloid replacement is common postoperatively. Crystalloids, such as normal saline or Ringer's lactate, may be infused. In addition, colloid replacement with albumin or hetastarch (Hespan) may also be periodically infused. The amount of fluid replacement is guided by hemodynamic parameters (see Table 13–3). If hemodynamic parameters (preload or filling pressures) are low (e.g., PAP 15/8, PAM 9, PAOP 4, RAP 2), fluids are needed.

Another factor that contributes to fluid volume deficit is postoperative bleeding. All dressings should be assessed frequently for signs of bleeding. Chest tube drainage needs to be monitored meticulously after cardiac surgery. Chest tube drainage of more than 200 mL per hour should be reported immediately to the cardiothoracic surgeon. In addition, hemoglobin and hematocrit counts and coagulation studies are obtained in the immediate postoperative period and frequently if chest tube bleeding continues. The international normalized ratio (INR) is frequently elevated because patients are anticoagulated during cardiopulmonary bypass. Platelet levels are also commonly decreased, because platelets are damaged as they pass through the cardiopulmonary bypass circuitry. Red blood cell replacement is usually prescribed if the hemoglobin falls below 8.0, yet this procedure may vary depending on the surgeon or the institution.

Postoperative blood loss may be due to inadequate hemostasis or disruption of the sutures, yet more commonly it is due to coagulopathy after cardiopulmonary bypass. Maintaining mean arterial pressure between 65 and 75 mm Hg minimizes the stress placed on the new cardiac suture lines and aids in efforts to decrease suture line bleeding. Often, PEEP is increased if patients are bleeding postoperatively. Additional PEEP (added at 2.5-cm increments) is gradually added in an effort to increase the intrathoracic pressure in an attempt to "tamponade" bleeding. High levels of PEEP (>10 cm PEEP) may not be tolerated by many patients. When PEEP is added, close observation of the patient's blood pressure and cardiac output is essential. As PEEP is increased, intrathoracic pressure is increased, and preload is decreased. A decrease in preload can have negative effects on blood pressure and cardiac output.

Postoperative bleeding may necessitate blood replacement therapy. Possible blood replacement products include autologous blood and donor blood (whole blood, packed red blood cells, platelets, and fresh frozen plasma). Autologous blood may include blood that was donated by the patient before the operation, blood that was collected during the operative procedure, and blood that drains postoperatively into the chest tube system. Mediastinal chest tubes are placed anterior and posterior to the heart. A tube connects the chest tubes to the autotransfusion system, which is attached to a chest drainage system. Figure 13–13 depicts an autotransfusion system. Blood collected in such a system should be infused within 6 hours of initiating the collection.[15] When infusing autotransfused blood, a 40- to 60-μm blood filter should be used to reduce the potential administration of debris or microaggregates.[16] Table 13–4 describes the pharmacologic agents that can be used with blood replacement products to correct abnormal coagulation studies.

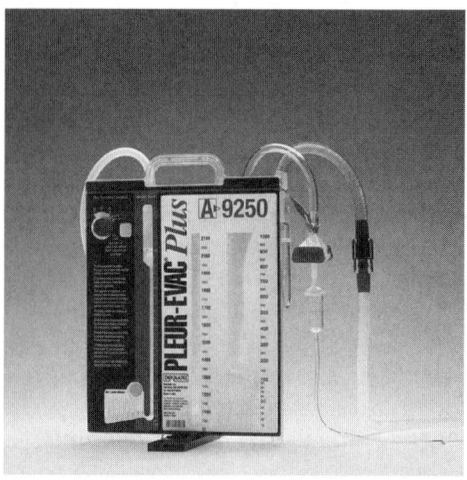

Figure 13–13

Autotransfusion system. (Courtesy of Deknatel Product Group, Genzyme, Inc., Fall River, MA.)

Restoration of Temperature. During cardiac surgery, patients are often cooled by the heat exchanger in the cardiopulmonary bypass pump oxygenator to 28 to 32°C. This procedure is done in an effort to decrease metabolism and to minimize cellular requirements during surgery. In addition, a cold cardioplegic solution is often used to arrest the heart. Hypothermia causes myocardial depression, ventricular dysrhythmias, increased blood viscosity, and increased systemic vascular resistance.[17] Because hypothermia has many undesirable consequences, some centers no longer use hypothermia. Instead, normothermia is maintained in an effort to minimize the effects of hypothermia.[18]

When hypothermia is used, rewarming is initiated toward the end of the operation through the heat exchanger in the cardiopulmonary bypass machine. Rewarming is continued in the postoperative period. Methods used to rewarm patients include the use of warm humidified oxygen, covering the patient's head, thermal blankets, warming infrared lamps, and convective air mattresses. Usually, patients are rewarmed to 36°C and then are allowed to stabilize their temperature passively to 37°C.

TABLE 13–4

Pharmacologic Agents Used to Control Postoperative Bleeding

Medication	Action	Dosage
Desmopressin (DDAVP)	Increases release of factor VIII and improves platelet function	0.3–0.4 μg/kg in 50 mL normal saline over 15–30 min
Aprotinin (Trasylol)	Antifibrinolytic; stabilizes fibrin clots, preserves platelet function	15,000–20,000 KIU/kg loading; 50,000 KIU/hour infusion
Aminocaproic acid	Antifibrinolytic; stabilizes fibrin clots	5 g loading over 1 hour; 1–1.25 g/hour infusion (maximum dose 30 g in 24 hours)
Tranexamic acid	Antifibrinolytic; stabilizes fibrin clots	10–15 mg/kg or 0.5–1 g IV every 4–6 hours

Adapted from Auer IK: The role of pharmacologic agents in blood conservation. AACN Clin Issues 7:262, 1996.

When patients return hypothermic to the ICU, they usually are vasoconstricted. This vasoconstriction often leads to elevated systemic vascular resistance, which may decrease cardiac output. Vasodilating agents (e.g., nitroprusside) may be necessary to decrease the systemic vascular resistance and to improve cardiac output.

As rewarming occurs, the patient begins to vasodilate. As vasodilatation continues, systemic vascular resistance decreases, preload decreases, and cardiac output decreases. As this occurs, the vasodilating agent usually needs to be titrated down until it is discontinued. Inotropic and vasoconstrictor agents may need to be added (e.g., epinephrine and dopamine) at the same time fluid replacement therapy is infused.

While patients are still hypothermic, they commonly shiver. Shivering is a compensatory response of the body to cold. Shivering attempts to rewarm the body. Unfortunately, shivering has several untoward consequences. Shivering increases the body's metabolic needs by 300 to 800%, increases carbon dioxide production, increases heart rate, depresses myocardial contractility, increases myocardial workload, and increases systemic vascular resistance. When shivering occurs, pharmacologic agents are usually administered to stop and to prevent additional shivering. These agents include meperidine (Demerol), 12.5 mg IV, repeated once. If shivering continues, morphine sulfate, 2 to 4 mg IV, may be used. Although paralyzing agents (e.g., pancuronium [Pavulon]) can be administered, they are usually administered only if shivering continues and patients are severely hemodynamically compromised.

Renal Status. Intake and output are monitored closely. Urine is usually collected by a Foley catheter for at least 24 hours. Urine output is measured hourly and should be at least 0.5 mL/kg per hour. As fluid is mobilized from the interstitial fluid, it is gradually reabsorbed into the intravascular space. The increased amount of fluid reabsorbed is filtered by the kidneys and is excreted. Patients commonly experience diuresis for at least 24 hours postoperatively. In addition to monitoring electrolytes, blood urea nitrogen and creatinine levels are usually followed for at least 2 postoperative days.

Potassium levels need to be closely observed during diuresis because potassium wasting occurs. Serum potassium levels are maintained at more than 4.0 mEq/L. IV potassium replacements are given to maintain normal potassium levels.

Pain. Postoperative pain should be assessed and managed effectively for patients after cardiac surgery. Depending on the type of operation, patients may experience discomfort of the sternal incision, anterior thoracotomy incision, or minimally invasive incisions or discomfort at the vein harvest sites. A short-acting anesthetic agent used frequently for sedation immediately after cardiac surgery is propofol (Diprivan). Propofol is initiated in the operating room and is administered intravenously at a rate of 10 to 50 µg/kg per minute. Propofol can be titrated down until discontinued in a relatively short time, so that patients can awaken rapidly when it is time for extubation.[19]

Some centers routinely prescribe patient-controlled anesthesia for pain management, whereas other centers prescribe analgesics as needed. Protocols for pain management after cardiac surgery include IV morphine sulfate for the first 24 to 48 hours postoperatively, followed by oral oxycodone with acetaminophen (Percocet).[20] It is recommended that a nonsteroidal anti-inflammatory agent, such as ketorolac tromethamine (Toradol), be given along with analgesics to manage postoperative pain effectively.[21]

Frequent turning and range of motion can also promote comfort. Patients should use a pillow to splint their chest incisions during coughing. This support often decreases discomfort during coughing.

Activity. Patients are turned within the first hour in the ICU to assess posterior lung sounds and to assess skin integrity. Patients should be turned every 2 hours if they are hemodynamically able to tolerate turning. Patients are encouraged to begin foot, ankle, and leg exercises soon after awakening from the cardiac procedure. Hemodynamically stable patients may dangle their feet at the side of the bed the evening of the operative day. Some may even be encouraged to sit up in a chair for a short while. Most patients are up in a chair the day after the operation. Ambulation begins as soon as patients are free from hemodynamic monitoring lines.

Intermediate Cardiac Care Unit

Patients' length of stay in the ICU continues to shorten. Most patients spend 1 day in the ICU and then transfer to an intermediate cardiac care unit. Often patients are discharged to home from this unit. Patient care in this phase requires the nurse to monitor the patient's progress diligently.

Neurologic Status. Neurologic assessments should be performed every 8 hours and as needed. Sudden neurologic changes in mental status could indicate a stroke or embolic phenomena and should be reported immediately to the physician.

After cardiac surgery, patients may find that they experience difficulty with fine motor dexterity. Memory losses may also occur. Some patients do not recall preoperative teaching,[9] and they need repeated education.

Cardiovascular (Cardiac Rhythm and Hemodynamic) Status. ECG monitoring is usually continued for 3 to 5 days postoperatively. Postoperative dysrhythmias, specifically atrial dysrhythmias, are common within the first 3 days after a cardiac procedure (see Chapter 8). Postoperative atrial fibrillation occurs in 20 to 40% of patients after cardiac operations and often delays discharge.[22] Studies are currently being conducted to determine which pharmacologic agents may be most effective in preventing and treating postoperative atrial dysrhythmias.

Vital signs are monitored at least every 4 hours. Heart sounds are auscultated, and peripheral circulation is assessed at the same frequency. Pericardial friction rubs are common because of pericardial inflammation in response to surgery. Usually, the pericardial friction rub is transient and requires no specific treatment. Patients' responses to activity are monitored as their activity levels gradually progress.

Pulmonary Status. Prevention of pneumonia is important during the entire postoperative period. Aggressive pulmonary care is continued. Because patient discomfort increases during coughing and deep breathing, patients may take shallow breaths and may avoid coughing. Patients should be encouraged to continue incentive spirometry and to perform coughing and deep breathing exercises. To limit discomfort with these activities, patients should be encouraged to use pain medications appropriately and to splint their incisions with a pillow. Incentive spirometry should be encouraged every hour that patients are awake. Expectorated secretions should be clear or white. If expectorated secretions are discolored, a sputum culture should be obtained.

Oxygen saturation can be assessed by pulse oximetry. Lung sounds should be auscultated at least every 4 hours. Oxygen therapy is gradually weaned.

Mediastinal or pleural chest tubes may be discontinued in the ICU, or they may remain in place connected to a closed drainage system and to wall suction. The chest tubes should be monitored for patency, drainage, and the presence of an air leak. Chest tubes are commonly removed when drainage is less than 100 mL in an 8-hour period, no air leak is noted, and the lung is fully expanded (pleural chest tube), as observed by chest radiograph. The patient should be assessed for ease of breathing and respiratory rate after chest tube removal. In addition, the nurse should assess the site for presence of crepitus, bleeding, or hematoma formation. A follow-up chest radiograph is not usually obtained.

Pain. Pain management is important, especially as patients increase their activity. Pain may be managed with epidural pharmacologic agents, patient-controlled analgesia, or intermittent pain-relieving analgesics. Nonsteroidal anti-inflammatory agents are usually continued.

Patients have reported that removal of the chest tubes is one of their worst memories after cardiac surgery.[23] Thus, patients must be premedicated before chest tube removal. In addition, patients often fear becoming addicted to pain medications and may avoid requesting them, especially before painful activities (e.g., ambulating, self-care activities, coughing, and deep breathing exercises). The nurse needs to educate patients on the proper use of medications (e.g., before pain becomes severe), so that cooperation with recovery-related activities is enhanced.

Gastrointestinal Status. A nasogastric tube may be placed in the operating room. It is connected to low, intermittent suction until bowel sounds return. The nasogastric tube is usually discontinued the day after the operation. If the gastroepiploic artery is used for bypass, the nasogastric tube may remain in place for an additional day. Until blood flow is redistributed to the stomach, patients may experience nausea, vomiting, and gastrointestinal symptoms.

A histamine blocker may be prescribed to decrease the risk of gastric irritation and bleeding until patients resume adequate dietary intake. Liquids are usually offered soon after extubation, and meals are advanced to a low-fat, cardiac diet as tolerated. Although patients often have no appetite after the operation, they are encouraged to eat in an effort to promote good nutrition and wound healing. A nutritionist may be consulted to evaluate the patient's diet at home and to assist with dietary teaching.

Renal Status. Intake and output are monitored until discharge. Daily diuretics may be necessary in an effort to mobilize interstitial fluids. Potassium levels should be assessed daily if diuretics are continued.

It is ideal if fluid status is balanced before discharge. When the postoperative length of stay was longer (10–14 days), the achievement of preoperative weight was optimal. Although with shorter length of stays this goal may not be possible, patients should be weighed every day, and progress toward this goal should be realized.

Integumentary System. Operative incisions should be assessed at least daily. Incisions should be clean and dry, with edges well approximated. Dressings on incisions are usually removed on the first postoperative day, and the incisions are left open to air. Chest tube sites are usually covered with a dry sterile dressing, which is removed after the chest tubes are removed. The site is then covered with a bio-occlusive dressing. Often serosanguineous drainage oozes for 1 to 3 days from the saphenous site incisions. Usually, a dry, sterile dressing is maintained on the leg incisions, until oozing ceases. It is not uncommon to cleanse incisions with normal saline. However, institutional standards for incision care should be followed. Any signs of infection should be reported to the surgeon. Usually, patients are receiving short-term antibiotic therapy postoperatively to prevent infection.

Infection. After cardiac surgery, the incidence of sternal wound and infection of the leg after saphenous vein removal is less than 3%. Temperature assessments are monitored, and white blood cell counts are followed. Antibiotics are administered as prescribed.

Musculoskeletal Status and Activity. Patients are assisted to the chair on the first postoperative day, and activity is gradually increased as tolerated. Patients are encouraged gradually to increase the distance they walk each day. Stair climbing is initiated before discharge.

Shoulder and arm exercises can be initiated in an attempt to minimize or relieve musculoskeletal discomfort of the arms, chest, and back. A cardiac rehabilitation specialist is often consulted to assist with exercises and walking and to initiate cardiac rehabilitation protocols.

Multidisciplinary Outcomes

If a clinical pathway is used to guide patient care after cardiac surgery (see Figure 13–12), it should be individualized as appropriate for each patient and their family. Unanticipated care needs and complications can arise at any point in the patient's recovery. Interventions to address these problems can be added as necessary.

It is essential that patient progress is closely monitored and that progress toward optimal outcomes is achieved. If patients are not meeting anticipated outcomes, the patient's plan of care must be revised, and interventions must be initiated in an attempt to meet positive outcomes. Goals include maintaining adequate oxygenation, hemodynamic stability, and achievement of optimal activity level. Prevention and early detection of complications are important (Table 13–5).

Maintaining Adequate Oxygenation

Patients must be well oxygenated after a cardiac operation. Adequate oxygenation is essential to meet the oxygen requirements of the healing heart and also to meet the body's oxygen needs. The patient's respiratory rate should be within normal limits, and the patient's breathing should be effortless. In addition, arterial blood gas results should be within normal limits. Ideally, they should be compared with preoperative blood gas results. However, preoperative blood gases are usually only obtained if the patient has a history of pulmonary disease or when pulmonary problems are anticipated.

Oxygenation can be assessed by monitoring the oxygen saturation by pulse oximetry. Oxygen saturation as measured by pulse oximetry should be at least 94%. Oxygen saturation levels may be difficult to assess in the immediate postoperative period. Hypothermic patients are usually vasoconstricted. This vasoconstriction can decrease blood flow to the periphery, often making it difficult for the pulse oximeter to detect adequate blood flow and to provide an accurate oxygenation level. This may also occur if patients are receiving vasoconstrictor agents (e.g., epinephrine). Placing the pulse oximeter probe on the patient's earlobe may improve accuracy instead of attempting to use a patient's finger or toe.

Oxygenation can also be assessed by mixed venous oxygenation. Mixed venous oxygen saturation levels can be obtained through the pulmonary artery catheter. Intermittent levels or continuous levels can be assessed depending on the type of pulmonary artery catheter placed. A normal mixed venous oxygenation level should be between 60 and 80%. Mixed venous oxygen saturation levels will decrease with activity (e.g., turning, suctioning), but they should rapidly return to baseline.

Maintenance of Hemodynamic Stability

Optimization of preload, contractility, and afterload is essential in the postoperative period. Postoperative preload is commonly maintained as close as possible to baseline values. Thus, attempts should be made to maintain postoperative right atrial pressures and pulmonary artery occlusive pressures (PAOPs) as close as possible to preoperative and intraoperative values.

Afterload should be frequently assessed during the initial postoperative period. Afterload can be determined by measuring the systemic vascular resistance. Systemic vascular resistance should be maintained between 900 and 1500. Because an increase in afterload inhibits myocardial unloading and increases myocardial oxygen consumption, aggressive treatment with vasodilator therapy is necessary.

Adequate cardiac contractility is essential. Enhancing preload and afterload often optimizes cardiac contractility. The patient's systolic blood pressure should be more than 95 mm Hg or comparable to trends in preoperative blood pressure. Another important sign of an adequate cardiac output is a cardiac index more than 2.4 L/min. In addition, strong peripheral pulses (2+ to 3+), brisk capillary refill (<2 seconds), and adequate urine output (>0.5 mL/kg/hour) are positive signs that the myocardium is working effectively.

Restoration of Fluid and Electrolyte Balance

Intake and output are measured throughout the patient's hospital stay. The patient is also weighed

TABLE 13–5
Multidisciplinary Outcomes of Cardiac Surgery Patients

Phase		Outcome
Preoperative	Preadmission testing or intermediate cardiac care unit	Assessment of patient's history, physical status, and functional status leading to diagnosis of illness
		Initiation of appropriate laboratory tests to prepare the patient for cardiac surgery
		Initiation of appropriate diagnostic tests to prepare the patient for cardiac surgery
		Patient and family education regarding what to expect before, during, and after cardiac surgery
		Initiation of measures to decrease or alleviate patient and family anxiety
		Initiation of appropriate consults (e.g., dental clearance before cardiac valve surgery)
Intraoperative	Operating room	Maintenance of cardiac output through cardiopulmonary bypass
		Initiation of vasoactive agents
		Maintenance of oxygenation by mechanical ventilation
		Maintenance of hypothermia
		Completion of transesophageal echocardiography for patients having valve surgery
Immediate postoperative	Surgical cardiac care unit	Maintenance or improvement of oxygen status
		Maintenance of cardiac output through oxygen support, vasoactive agents, or mechanical assistive devices
		Completion of appropriate diagnostic modalities including ECG, chest radiographs, and laboratory tests
		Management of pain through pharmacologic and nonpharmacologic means
		Achievement of optimal activity level
		Prevention or management of complications (dysrhythmias, pneumonia, emboli, myocardial infarction, cardiac tamponade, infection)
	Intermediate cardiac care unit	Stabilization or improvement in cardiac output through continued oxygen support, pharmacologic means, and progressive activity
		Continued management of pain
		Prevention of complications
		Preparation for discharge and cardiac rehabilitation
		Education regarding coronary artery disease, medications, risk factor reduction, dietary regimen, activity prescription, incision care, and follow-up
		Consultation as appropriate with home care agency for necessary follow-up care
		Acknowledgement of psychosocial issues related to recovery after cardiac surgery
Long-term postoperative	Community	Initiation of cardiac rehabilitation
		Return to work or to optimal level of functioning
		Acceptance in changes in body image related to surgical scars and altered level of health

daily. It is anticipated that the patient will be discharged as close as possible to his or her admission weight. As discussed, diuretics may or may not be necessary to meet this goal. Electrolytes are also maintained within normal values. Table 13–6 highlights essential electrolyte values for the patient after cardiac surgery.

Achievement of Optimal Activity Level

The patient's activity is slowly increased after cardiac surgery. Patients gradually increase the time and frequency of being out of bed and in the chair. Patients should also be able to increase their walking distance daily and also should begin stair climbing before

TABLE 13-6
Essential Electrolyte Values for Patients After Cardiac Surgery

Electrolyte	Desired Value
Potassium	>4.0 mEq/L
Ionized calcium	>4.5 mg/dL
Magnesium	>2.0 mEq/L

leaving the hospital. Patients should also be able to increase their ability to meet their activities of daily living before discharge. It is critical that patients are hemodynamically stable during activity. Heart rate and blood pressure are closely monitored, and activity can be increased if changes are not noted.

Maintenance of Nutritional Status

Patients often have a poor appetite after cardiac surgery. A temporary alteration in taste may be the reason for the appetite change. Although patients do not feel hungry, they should be encouraged to eat. Small, frequent meals or snacks may be more appetizing.

Prevention of Complications

Complications after cardiac procedures should be prevented to the greatest extent possible. Complications of cardiac surgery include pneumonia, emboli, myocardial infarction, tamponade, and infection. Although complications cannot always be prevented, early detection and management are essential.

Dysrhythmias occur frequently after cardiac surgery. The most common dysrhythmias are atrial dysrhythmias (tachycardia, atrial fibrillation, and atrial flutter). Atrial dysrhythmias occur in 11 to 40% of patients after coronary artery bypass graft surgery.[24-26] Dysrhythmias are more common after valve surgery than after cardiac bypass surgery and occur in more than 50% of patients having cardiac valve procedures.[24] Dysrhythmias may result from electrolyte imbalances, hypothermia, elevated catecholamine levels, inflammation, or myocardial stunning. Medications such as digoxin, beta blockers, and calcium channel blockers are commonly used to treat atrial dysrhythmias. Pharmacologic agents such as beta blockers and calcium channel blockers are also being administered perioperatively in an effort to prevent postoperative atrial dysrhythmias.[22,27] Research is being conducted to determine which pharmacologic agents have the greatest efficacy.

Stroke occurs in 1 to 6% of patients after coronary artery bypass graft surgery.[24,28] Patients after coronary artery bypass surgery are usually prescribed one aspirin per day.

Thrombus formation and emboli occur more commonly in patients after valve surgery than after cardiac bypass surgery. Anticoagulation is usually initiated within 48 hours of valve operations and after the epicardial pacing wires are removed. Patients with mechanical valves are at a much higher risk of developing thrombi than patients with biologic valves. In addition, valves placed in the mitral position are at a greater risk of developing thrombi because of the wider valve orifice and lower rate of blood flow as compared with valves placed in the aortic position.[7] Anticoagulation therapy is recommended for all patients after cardiac valve procedures, in an effort to decrease the incidence of thrombus and emboli formation. Usually, anticoagulation therapy is initiated with warfarin (Coumadin) within 48 hours of cardiac valve replacement. The 1992 Guidelines of the American College of Chest Physicians recommend that patients with biologic valves be anticoagulated for 3 months, followed by lifelong aspirin (325 mg/day) therapy.[29] These guidelines also recommend lifelong anticoagulation therapy for patients with mechanical valves in addition to patients with atrial fibrillation and left atrial thrombi, and those patients with a history of embolism.

From 5 to 15% of patients undergoing coronary artery bypass surgery may experience a perioperative myocardial infarction.[30,31] A 12-lead ECG is obtained immediately postoperatively and usually for 2 additional postoperative days, to assess for significant ECG changes. New and persistent Q waves accompanied by new, persistent, and evolutionary ST–T-wave abnormalities aid in diagnosing an acute myocardial infarction.[32] In addition, measurement of creatine phosphokinase and isoenzymes is obtained for at least 24 hours postoperatively. A long cardiopulmonary bypass time (>75 minutes) and a long aortic cross-clamp time (>50 minutes) correlate with an increased incidence of perioperative myocardial infarction.[32]

Cardiac tamponade occurs in 3 to 7% of patients after cardiac surgery.[33] It occurs most commonly in the immediate postoperative period, yet it also may occur after epicardial pacing wire removal. Signs and symptoms of cardiac tamponade include minimal or sudden cessation in chest tube drainage, tachycardia, hypotension, equalizing pulmonary artery pressures, narrowed pulse pressure, distended neck veins, muffled heart sounds, and pulsus paradoxus. Cardiac tamponade is a life-threatening emergency. Emergency sternotomy is necessary.

Strict aseptic technique should be used in an effort to prevent postoperative infection. Antibiotic therapy is initiated just before a cardiac operation and is continued for 24 hours postoperatively.[34] Intravenous catheters and additional tubes (e.g., central lines, epicardial pacing wires, Foley catheter) should be discontinued as soon as possible.

CHART 13–3

Educational Content for Patients Preparing for Home After Cardiac Surgery

Pain management

Incision care

Rest and activity program, including initiation of a cardiac rehabilitation program, if appropriate

Low-fat, low-cholesterol diet (sodium restrictions may or may not apply)

Medications

Signs and symptoms to report to physician (e.g., increase in weight, chest pain, dyspnea, nocturnal dyspnea, cough, edema)

Risk factor modification

Self-Management of Therapeutic Regimen (Home Issues)

Preparing the patient for discharge actually begins in the preoperative phase. Additional teaching is initiated early in the postoperative period. Chart 13–3 describes the essential educational content to prepare the patient and family for discharge.

Patients having cardiac valve replacement also need information regarding anticoagulation therapy. Patients need to know the medication, the dosage, and the importance of blood tests to assist in dosage adjustment. In addition, patients need to know signs and symptoms that may alert them to the presence of too much medication (e.g., bruising, bleeding).

Patients with replaced cardiac valves also need to be informed of the need for lifelong prophylactic antibiotic therapy before undergoing oral, urogenital, or invasive procedures. The American Heart Association has published specific recommendations regarding prevention of bacterial endocarditis (see Chapter 12).[34]

Patients must know whom they can call if they have questions after they are discharged. It is also important that they clearly understand their discharge care and necessary follow-up appointments (Chart 13–4).

HEART TRANSPLANTATION

Approximately 400,000 people are newly diagnosed with heart failure each year.[35] The longitudinal data from the Framingham study indicate that the 1-year survival rate for newly diagnosed heart failure is 57% for men and 64% for women. The mean 1-year survival is 1.7 years for men and 3.24 years for women.[36] Heart transplantation is a favorable option for treatment of congestive heart failure. According to the 1997 Registry of the International Society for Heart and Lung Transplantation (ISHLT), the survival rates for patients who undergo heart transplantation is 79% at 1 year, 63% at 5 years, and 43% at 10 years.[37] However, heart transplantation has several extraordinary hurdles for patients to overcome to benefit truly from this surgical procedure. First, the discrepancy between the number of organs for transplant and the cost-containment issues of health care reform are addressed. Second, factors that affect long-term survival are also discussed. Heart transplantation is still a relatively new field needing additional research to improve survival further.

The number of patients with end-stage heart disease continues to grow, and increasing numbers of patients are being placed on the transplant waiting list. With advances in medications, surgical technique, and mechanical assist devices, these patients are kept alive longer. According to the United Network for Organ Sharing (UNOS), approximately 4000 patients are waiting for a suitable donor.[38] The problem is no significant increases have occurred in the donor pool, despite the increased use of older donor hearts.[37] UNOS reported that 3048 heart transplants were performed in 1996, a number that demonstrates the discrepancy between supply and demand. Organ transplantation centers are continually reevaluating standards for recipients listed for a heart transplant to provide solutions for this crisis.[39]

The Uniform Anatomical Gift Act (UAGA) was a federal law passed in 1972 and allowed any person over 18 years of age to donate organs. Pennsylvania State Legislation Act 102 is an amendment to the UAGA and was signed December 1, 1994. It charges health care workers to contact the local organ procurement agency with the death or impending death of any patient. The amendment was added to increase the number of referrals in the hope of increasing the number of potential donations. Nurses have a key role in reporting a potential patient for donation to their local donor agency. The act also increases public education opportunities to learn about organ donation. A curriculum specifically designed to teach nurses about organ transplantation was formalized in 1995.[40] In addition, prime time television programs and radio broadcasts began national advertising for donor awareness. The issue of mandated choice as a means to increase the education and number of potential organ donors is another topic under discussion.[41] Individuals must make a decision, thereby removing the anxiety of a decision from family members. Public education and favorable legislation will need to continue if there is any hope of increasing the donor pool.

> ## CHART 13–4
>
> ### BEYOND THE ICU: MANAGEMENT OF PATIENTS DISCHARGED EARLY AFTER CARDIAC SURGERY
>
> Many patients after cardiac surgery are "fast tracked." Fast tracking refers to using guidelines or protocols that streamline the care of patients after cardiac surgery. The Division of Cardiac Surgery at Baystate Medical Center, Springfield, Massachusetts has been a leader in developing the fast-track concept. Since the fast-track concept has been developed, patient length of stay has been shortened after cardiac surgery. Before fast tracking, it was not uncommon for patients to be hospitalized 7 to 10 days after cardiac surgery. Many fast-track protocols now discharge patients 3 to 6 days after cardiac surgery.
>
> Patients are discharged from the hospital sooner and are completing their recuperation at home. Although some patients may feel prepared for this early discharge, others may still feel unprepared. Anxiety among patients and family members may be heightened. It is essential that patients and family members have adequate resources available to assist them during home recuperation from cardiac surgery.
>
> Discharge planning is essential to fast tracking, and anticipated patient and family needs are discussed before cardiac surgery. Corsetti and Perry at Baystate Medical Center stress that both the patient and family need to be emotionally prepared for the early discharge, should feel comfortable with the process, and should feel well prepared for the anticipated follow-up care. Before discharge, patients and family members view an educational videotape and are also asked to view the inpatient television channel for information regarding postcardiac surgery discharge and home care. Detailed written instructions given to each patient provide information on discharge medications, wound care, activity progression, dietary requirements, and emergency and follow-up care. Before discharge, the nurse evaluates the patient and family members for their understanding of the discharge teaching. If the patient and family members do not adequately understand the necessary information, a referral is made to a visiting nursing agency for home care and further teaching. At Baystate Medical Center, the home care nurses are experienced cardiac nurses.
>
> Patients discharged after cardiac surgery should be aware of available resources. Corsetti and Perry discuss resources they provide to patients and their family members. Patients and family members are given a 24-hour telephone number to call should they have any problems or questions after discharge. In addition, each patient receives a telephone call within the first 24 to 72 hours from the cardiothoracic nurse practitioner. During this telephone call, the nurse practitioner evaluates the patient's progress, reinforces discharge teaching, reviews medications, schedules follow-up appointments, and answers questions. At Baystate Medical Center, patient follow-up appointments are made with the cardiothoracic nurse practitioner 1 week and 3 weeks after hospital discharge. If problems occur, patients are seen as frequently as needed or until the problem resolves.
>
> According to Corsetti and Perry, outpatient cardiac rehabilitation is coordinated before hospital discharge and is usually initiated 1 month after surgery. Before the initiation of cardiac rehabilitation, patients are encouraged to increase their activity gradually.
>
> Early discharge after cardiac surgery can occur if protocols are in place to facilitate this process. The patient's recovery can be supported if an organized system is in place to help answer patient and family questions and to assist with problems should they arise.
>
> Data from Corsetti AL, Perry D: A comprehensive approach to facilitating the recovery of cardiac surgery patients. J Cardiovasc Nurs 12:82–90, 1998.

Another hurdle that affects the heart transplant population is managed care. Measures to achieve cost-effective health care continue to affect the management of heart transplant patients. Increasing costs to maintain patients in an ICU until they undergo heart transplantation may force changes to be made in legislation. UNOS is currently reevaluating current waiting criteria and reviewing proposals to allow these patients to accumulate time on the waiting list in less formal, but monitored, settings. Possible alternatives are to care for stable patients in less acute care settings or in the home.

Follow-up care typically occurs in the transplant center. However, health care reform is evaluating the cost-to-benefit ratio of the transplant center versus the local physician. Local primary care physicians may be asked to take a more active lead in follow-up care as dictated by insurance company policies. Debate exists on the appropriateness of the local physician as the primary caretaker in the *immediate* postoperative period. This population of patients needs experts in cardiology, immunology, infectious disease, renal disease, nutrition, physical therapy, and social work, who are all readily accessible in a heart transplant center. Favorable outcomes have been reported when patients are monitored by the heart transplant team, despite the distance to a transplant center.[42,43] There is also competition among transplant centers because of health care reform. Centers of excellence, based on numbers of transplants performed, may determine insurance contracts with a facility. Insurance contracts then dictate the transplant facility for which the patient is financially covered for treatment and care, thus removing the patient's choice from the process.

INDICATIONS

Heart transplantation is indicated for the treatment of end-stage heart disease when all other medical or surgical options have been exhausted. Treatment may have included maximal medical therapy, clinical drug trials, or surgical interventions, such as cardiomyoplasty or the Batista procedure.[44] Cardiomyoplasty is a surgical wrapping of the latissimus dorsi muscle around the cardiac muscle (see Figure 11–1). A retraining period of the muscle during which electrical impulses duplicate those of a normal functioning heart muscle.[45] One study suggests that cardiomyoplasty can passively reverse the remodeling of dilated hearts in addition to decreasing symptoms of heart failure.[46] The Batista procedure is the surgical removal of a wedge of heart muscle from the apex of the ventricle to the mitral annulus.[47] It literally reduces the size of the heart to decrease the workload of the heart. The Batista procedure shows some benefits to performing a mitral valve repair as part of the procedure. The advantage of both operations over heart transplantation is that immunosuppressant medications are not needed postoperatively. However, neither one of these operations is approved by the FDA, and outcomes will need to be evaluated through multicenter research trials. At present, most patients chosen for these studies are also transplant candidates. If the operation fails, then a heart transplant is still a backup option for the patient.

Cardiomyopathy is a disease state caused by the abnormal function of the heart muscle. It is characterized by severe dilatation of the heart, usually involving all four chambers. Myocardial contractility decreases, leading to low cardiac output, stroke volume, and ejection fraction. Congestive heart failure develops, leading to pulmonary edema, liver congestion, or peripheral edema.

The primary indication for heart transplantation is dilated cardiomyopathy. This type of myopathy has several causes: coronary artery disease, hypertension, toxins (alcohol and chemotherapy), infection, metabolic disorders (thiamin or protein deficiency), pregnancy, neuromuscular disorders (muscular dystrophy), connective tissue disorders (lupus erythematosus, rheumatoid disease, or scleroderma), and infiltrative disorders (sarcoid or amyloid) (see Chapter 11). Ischemic dilated cardiomyopathy is the primary diagnosis in 43.5% of the population awaiting heart transplantation.[48] This trend will continue as procedures to treat coronary artery disease continue to improve survival. Idiopathic dilated cardiomyopathy is the primary diagnosis in another 41.8% of patients awaiting heart transplants, congenital disease about 7%, and valvular disease 4%.

Some of these disease states are reversible if diagnosed and treated promptly.[49] Reversible causes of myocardial dysfunction include the following: atrial fibrillation, thyroid disease, postpartum cardiomyopathy, hibernating myocardium, stunned myocardium, myocardial dysfunction after bypass surgery, myocarditis, and sepsis. In addition, the use of positron emission tomography (PET) scanning has assisted in the diagnosis of viable tissue that can be surgically bypassed, thus postponing the need for a heart transplant.

Assessment

Selection Process

Selecting the appropriate patients for heart transplantation requires extensive evaluation. The two objectives are the determination that the end-stage heart disease is not reversible and the identification of any comorbidities that would preclude the patient from safely undergoing heart transplantation. The current standard for selecting the appropriate candidates for heart transplantation is the metabolic (V_{O_2}) stress test. This is the best predictor of survival because patients with a peak V_{O_2} less than 10 mL/kg per minute, equivalent to New York Heart Association (NYHA) class IV, have a 50% 1-year survival rate.[50] Patients with a peak $V_{O_2} < 10$ mL/kg per minute, in conjunction with a decreased cardiac output, have only a 38% 1-year survival.[51]

Hemodynamic pressures are measured by a right heart catheterization to assess for further failure or decompensation. Typically, an elevated pulmonary artery occlusive pressure (PAOP) and an elevated PAP indicate fluid overload. In addition, measurement of the cardiac output will determine whether the patient needs IV inotropic support. Pulmonary vascular resistance (PVR) is then calculated to determine the patient's risk for a heart transplant. PVR is a measure to determine the likelihood of immediate postoperative right heart failure. If the patient has a PVR of more than 250, agents such as nitroprusside (Nipride), prostaglandin E_1 (Prostin VR), or nitric oxide (NO) are used to reverse the elevated pulmonary pressures (see Table 13–3).[52] If the pressures remain elevated despite these agents, the chance of right heart failure after heart transplantation is high. The donor heart would have difficulty pumping blood against the fixed, high pulmonary pressures, and the new donor heart would also fail.[53]

Another prognostic factor to determine survival is the transpulmonary gradient (TPG):

$$TPG = mean\ PAP - PAOP$$

If the patient has a TPG of more than 12 mm Hg, then mortality is greater at 6 and 12 months after the transplant.[54] The standards vary from program to program, but a nonreversible PVR of more than 600 is an absolute contraindication to heart transplantation. One way transplant centers have been successful in operating on higher-risk patients (PVR >250) is to accept donor hearts that are larger than the recipient's. Larger hearts can pump against these high pulmonary pressures to lower the risk of right heart failure.

Ventricular size, function, and ejection fraction are assessed and can be obtained by several measures: echocardiogram, multigated acquisition study (MUGA), or radionuclide ventriculography. Left ventricular ejection fraction (LVEF) helps to determine the patients at highest risk of death who should be listed for a heart transplant. LVEF less than 30% is typically used as an indication to evaluate the patient for heart transplantation. However, it has less predictive value when the patient has symptoms of refractory heart failure.[55] Patients with no symptoms and with stable hemodynamic pressures may go on for years maintaining their present lifestyle, despite their low LVEF. However, an LVEF less than 10% is a marker of end-stage heart failure indicating a need for a heart transplant.[56]

The other part of the evaluation process is the identification of comorbidities that may prevent the patient from doing well after heart transplantation. Standard testing is done to diagnose end-organ damage and underlying comorbidities. Table 13–7 lists the evaluation testing the patient must undergo to allow the physicians to determine the patient's appropriateness for heart transplantation.

Contraindications

The size of the program (the number of transplants done each year) may determine the relative contraindications established for a program's protocol for patient acceptance. Small transplant centers are generally not aggressive in accepting high-risk patients with relative contraindications. The many contraindications to heart transplantation need to be distinguished as relative versus absolute contraindications (Chart 13–5). The extent and number of relative contraindications a patient has are factors in the decision to accept a patient for heart transplantation.[57]

Age is a controversial relative contraindication. People are living longer, and patients may medically fit the selection criteria. However, the donor shortage behooves centers to place restrictions on the acceptance of older patients, thus precipitating many difficult ethical dilemmas. At present, common practice is to choose patients selectively over the age of 60 years.[58] The percentage of heart transplant candidates registered nationally over the age of 65 years is only 3.4%, yet the percentage of patients between the ages of 50 and 64 years is 50.9%. Outcomes in older patients

---

CHART 13–5

Contraindications for Listing Heart Transplant Patients

Absolute Contraindications
  Malignancy
  Positive HIV test
  Sepsis
  End-organ disease due to uncontrolled diabetes
  Major chronic disabling illness (e.g., lupus or stroke with
    residual deficits)
  Active mental illness
  Fixed pulmonary vascular resistance >600
  Nonreversible vital organ impairment (e.g., primary pul-
    monary, liver, kidney disease not due to low-output state)

Relative Contraindications
  Age
  Pulmonary infarction in the past 8 weeks
  Diabetes
  Vascular disease
  Obesity
  Drug, tobacco, or alcohol use
  Peptic ulcer disease

TABLE 13–7
Standard Evaluation Testing for Determination of Heart Transplant Candidacy

Evaluation Tests	Indications
Metabolic Vo_2 stress test	Evaluate heart failure class to predict survival
Echocardiogram/multigated acquisition study	Evaluate heart function, degree of regurgitation, and left ventricular ejection fraction
Left heart catheterization	R/O reversible coronary artery disease
Right heart catheterization	R/O nonreversible elevated pulmonary vascular resistance
Pulmonary function test	R/O obstructive disease, primary lung disorder
Vascular studies (peripheral and carotid)	R/O arterial stenosis in lower extremities or carotid arteries
Ultrasound (abdomen and retroperitoneum)	R/O masses, abdominal aortic aneurysm, and gallstones, and evaluate kidney size
Posteroanterior lateral chest radiograph	R/O masses or effusions
Mammogram (females)	R/O masses
Dental medicine consultation	R/O infection
Psychosocial consultation	R/O unstable psychiatric history and evaluate compliance, transportation, and support systems
Finance consultation	R/O need for financial assistance, fund raising
Physical therapy consultation	R/O disabling factors and evaluate rehabilitation needs
Dietary consultation	R/O morbid obesity or cachexia
Purified protein derivative test	R/O tuberculosis exposure
Gynecologic examination	R/O cancer
Laboratory Testing	
HIV, hepatitis screen	R/O active or chronic infection
Type and screen	R/O donor incompatibility
Cytomegalovirus, herpes simplex virus, varicella-zoster virus, Epstein–Barr virus, *Toxoplasma* titers	R/O active infections, susceptibility to infection after transplantation
Prostate surface antigen (males)	R/O prostate cancer (screening)
Tissue typing	R/O need for prospective crossmatch
Urinalysis/urine culture	R/O infection
24-hour urine collection	R/O renal insufficiency

R/O, rule out.

do not show an increase in death or rejection, but they do show that these patients may be more subject to infections, renal side effects, or gastrointestinal complications.[48]

A patient's pulmonary function can be difficult to assess because of coexisting congestive heart failure and related symptoms. Most program directors agree that chronic obstructive pulmonary disease diagnosed with an FEV_1 less than 50% may be a contraindication for heart transplantation because these patients may be difficult to wean from mechanical ventilation postoperatively.[57]

Listing

The evaluation results are compiled and are reviewed by the transplant team, consisting of cardiologists, surgeons, transplant coordinators, staff nurses, social workers, nutritionists, physical therapists, financial counselors, psychiatrists, and infectious disease physicians. Based on the patient's clinical history, test results, consultation recommendations, and relative versus absolute contraindications, the transplant team recommends whether or not the patient should be placed on the transplant waiting list. Based on the recommendation, the patient is then informed by the cardiologist or transplant coordinator, and the patient gives permission to be placed on the regional waiting list. The regional waiting list is run by personnel unrelated to the local hospitals and is monitored by the national organization, UNOS. This organization ensures the fair and appropriate allocation of organs. Patients currently await transplants under two criteria. The higher priority is status 1, and the lower priority is status 2 (Table 13–8). There is also a status 7 for those on hold for a heart transplant. Status 7 patients would not lose the time accrued on the waiting list but have contraindications to transplant at the time (medically doing too well or need resolution of a recent event such as infection or smoking).

Patients need to be evaluated continually to determine those at higher risk of death shown by worsening heart failure symptoms, a decrease in Vo_2, a decrease in cardiac output, or elevation in PAPs.[59] In addition nonsustained ventricular tachycardia in patients in heart failure is a marker for increased mortality from sudden death.[60] These patients also qualify as status 1 if these dysrhythmias are not amenable to medication, ablation, or internal defibrillation despite their lack of need for inotropic support. The donor organs are offered to the patient with the most status 1 time and with a compatible blood type. UNOS is working to address the problems with the current policies that were implemented back in 1989.[61] Because of longer waiting times for donor organs, the main efforts are focused on improving the categories of medical urgency of patients awaiting heart transplantation (see Table 13–8).

Nursing Diagnoses

Preoperative Issues Related to the Recipient

By the time a patient is ill enough to be listed for a heart transplant, he or she is typically receiving standard triple-drug therapy: digoxin (Lanoxin), diuretics (furosemide), and angiotensin-converting enzyme (ACE) inhibitors (captopril). These medications are titrated by the cardiologist in accordance with the patient's symptoms and hemodynamics. It is often difficult for the nurse to diagnose an increase in fluid overload or a decrease in cardiac output in this group of patients because they are chronically decompensated. Therefore, with the physician's collaboration, right heart catheterizations are periodically performed to assist in the diagnosis. In addition, Vo_2 stress tests are carried out to determine the patient's NYHA classification.

When maximal triple-drug therapy is no longer adequate, patients may present to the emergency room with acute signs of heart failure. Applicable nursing diagnoses are the same as for any patient with heart failure and can be found in Chapter 11. Table 13–9 lists nursing diagnoses specific to the heart transplant patient. The physician typically orders IV diuretics for immediate relief of symptoms. IV inotropes may be appropriate if the patient is demonstrating signs of decreased cardiac output. Dobutamine (Dobutrex) and milrinone (Primacor) are two IV medications frequently used to facilitate cardiac output and to decrease vascular resistance. Nurses need to be cautious when initiating inotropes because of the potential for tachycardia and dysrhythmias. Either of these side effects can be life-threatening in this patient population. Patients listed for a heart transplant have little reserve, and they can acutely deteriorate. Milrinone has the added benefit of lowering PVR. This drug can facilitate the failing right heart by making it much easier to pump against higher pulmonary artery pressures. Whichever inotrope is chosen, it must be assessed for adequate dosing. Patients can become tolerant to the inotrope dose, and the medication may need titration. It is vital that nurses obtain daily weights and accurate intake and output records to determine whether fluid overload exists despite the inotropes.

In addition, results of blood tests need to be followed to assess for signs of heart failure (Table 13–10).

TABLE 13–8
United Network for Organ Sharing (UNOS) Current and Proposed Criteria for Listing Patients for Heart Transplant

	Status	Criteria
Current	1	Intravenous inotropes and in an intensive care unit
	Must meet one criterion	Mechanical support (IABP, ventricular assist device, or ventilator) and in the intensive care unit
		Thermo Cardiosystems Internal left ventricular assist device in the hospital or at home
	2	Intravenous inotropes but not in the intensive care unit (including home-bound patients)
	Must meet one criterion	Intensive care bound but not on intravenous inotropes or mechanical support
		Maintained on oral medications at home or in the hospital
Proposed	1a	Admitted in the listing transplant center or hospital
	Must meet all three criterion	Hemodynamic monitoring
		Cardiac support (intravenous inotropes, IABP, ventricular assist device)
	1b	Circulatory assist device (these patients can be at home)
	Must meet one criterion	Intensive care unit with intravenous inotropes
	2a	Intravenous inotropes not in an intensive care unit (can be at home)
	Must meet one criterion	Intensive care, no support
	2b	All other patients listed, typically patients at home on oral medications

IABP, intra-aortic balloon pump.
From the United Network for Organ Sharing (UNOS). Policy and by-law proposals. Richmond, VA, UNOS, 1997.

TABLE 13–9
Nursing Diagnoses for the Heart Transplant Recipient and Family Throughout the Transplant Process

Phase	Patient	Family
Preoperative		
Diagnosis	Fear related to diagnosis of end-stage heart disease	Anxiety related to potential death of partner
Evaluation	Anxiety related to uncertain outcomes Knowledge deficit related to evaluation and listing process for transplantation	Ineffective family coping related to emotional and financial needs of the family
Listing	Fear related to acceptance versus denial for transplantation Hopelessness related to lack of treatment options	Social isolation related to lifestyle changes
Waiting	Decreased cardiac output related to dysrhythmias or tachycardias secondary to chronic low output state or IV inotropes Fatigue related to anemia secondary to heart failure and frequent blood draws Anxiety related to waiting away from home as status 1 Self-care deficit related to structure of nursing unit and environmental restrictions in the hospital Powerlessness related to waiting for someone to die for one's own survival	Anxiety related to performing new tasks or maintaining home or family independently
Intraoperative		
Surgery	Fear related to own mortality	Fear related to donor compatibility and success of surgery
Intensive and Intermediate care	Fluid volume excess related to sodium retention secondary to steroids	Anxiety related to participating in care of patient
Recovery	Decreased cardiac output related to denervation of the heart Self-care deficit related to dependence on health care staff and impending discharge from hospital Knowledge deficit related to new diagnosis of immunocompromised state and related medical regimen	
Community	Sleep pattern disturbance related to use of steroids to prevent rejection	Altered sexuality patterns related to fear of harming partner
Long-term	Altered nutrition related to anorexia or overeating secondary to side effects of immunosuppressant medications Risk of impaired skin integrity related to side effects of immunosuppressant medications Personal identity disturbance related to characteristics of the donor and donor's cause of death Fear related to lifelong threat of rejection and infection	

Once the patient has been stabilized, it is generally sufficient to obtain blood values only one to three times a week. These patients have a tendency to have lower hemoglobin levels; therefore, frequent blood collection needs to be avoided. In addition, blood collection is kept to a minimum for the patient's comfort. These patients can potentially be waiting in the hospital for months before they receive a compatible donor. It is

TABLE 13–10
Nursing Guidelines for Status 1 Heart Transplant Patients

Assessments	Interventions
Weight	Monitor ideal body weight
	Reassess need for diuresis if weight gain > 2 lb/day
Blood pressure	Monitor for symptomatic drop in blood pressure
	Adjust inotropes, angiotensin-converting enzyme inhibitors, diuretics
Heart rate	Monitor for tachycardia or dysrhythmias
Sodium intake	Maintain maximum of 2 g/day; individualize per patient; most require 1–1.5 g/day
Fluid intake	1500 mL/day, adjusted to individual patient
Blood work	Note blood work for trends and subtle changes:
	Sodium <130; K >5 or <3.5; creatinine >2.0; total bilirubin >1.5

beneficial that the nurse becomes the patient's advocate in coordinating anticipated blood collections and discussing the possibility for long-term intravenous access (i.e., peripherally inserted central catheter [PICC]).

Occasionally, these patients may require blood transfusions because of anemia secondary to frequent blood collection or heart failure. It is critical that heart transplant patients receive filtered blood transfusions to decrease the foreign lymphocytes that may stimulate an antibody reaction. Circulating antibodies may also occur as a result of previous transfusions, previous pregnancies, or a ventricular assist device. Patients should not develop increased antibodies or they will require a prospective blood match with the donor (it requires a longer waiting time to obtain an exact blood match with the donor). Patients with a panel-reactive antibody (PRA) reaction of more than 11%, despite a prospective crossmatch, may have earlier and more severe rejection.[62] In addition, patients with a PRA of more than 25% at the time of the transplant procedure may be at risk of decreased long-term survival.[63] Chart 13–6 gives an example of an ethical dilemma faced by a heart transplant patient and caregivers.

Psychosocial Issues Related to the Recipient

The recipient has a multitude of psychosocial factors to address throughout the entire transplantation process. At each phase, the patient may have feelings of fear, grief, and anxiety. Nurses need to be sensitive to these stages to care for the patient best and to meet his or her needs at each phase of transplantation. Heart transplantation is unique in that the operation does not bring closure to many of the physical or psychological factors associated with the transplant. See Table 13–9 for the complex psychosocial issues that these patients and their families experience throughout assessment, diagnosis, and treatment.

The initial diagnosis of severe cardiomyopathy may be new, or the patient may have a chronic disease that is not amenable to medical treatment options. This period may be met with anger or "why me," especially if the disease is newly diagnosed (e.g., idiopathic, postpartum, or recent acute myocardial infarction). This patient population and their families need emotional support. In addition, the patient may be acutely ill and may have difficulty in processing the information.

During the evaluation, patients sometimes ask whether they are going to pass or fail. There is also the burden of waiting for test results and the final approval by the heart transplant committee. Patients may have feelings of hopelessness if they are turned down for a heart transplant. There may be relief if they are determined to be too healthy for a transplant. Some patients, especially those with a new diagnosis of cardiomyopathy, may need time to accept the recommendation that heart transplantation is their best option. Once the patient accepts the deteriorating health condition, there is relief that an option other than death exists.

The waiting period is an anxious time period for both the recipient and the family. A unique factor for recipients awaiting heart transplant surgery is another human will die in order for the recipient to live. The role of the nurse is to allow these feelings to be verbalized and to assure the patient that these emotions are normal and appropriate. The patient needs to be reassured that he or she does not have control over the tragic events related to the donor and that the donor or his or her family has turned the tragedy into a positive event.

When the recipient and family are told that an appropriate donor has been found and the patient is going to the operating room for the transplant, there is a flurry of emotions and excitement that the waiting is finally over. The patient and family may also have feelings of uncertainty, because they know that the recipient may be brought back from the operating room without a new heart if the donor's heart becomes unstable or unsuitable for transplantation. The recipient will need support and time to accept the loss if this situation does occur.

A common request of the recipient or family is for information about the donor. Philosophies and clinical practice vary on the time, appropriateness, and

CHART 13–6

ETHICAL DILEMMA

A 47-year-old woman is on the heart transplant waiting list in the coronary intermediate care unit and is dependent on intravenous milrinone for treatment of heart failure symptoms. Her blood type is O+, and she has waited in the hospital as a status 1 patient for more than 5 months. She was previously on the waiting list as a status 2 patient for about a year. She has reached the top of the transplant list for her blood type and has the potential for receiving the next suitable donor in the region. However, she has developed a positive panel-reactive antibody of 60% secondary to blood transfusions for treatment of anemia from her worsening heart failure. She is requiring prospective crossmatching with all potential donor offers, a process that will make her wait longer because she needs an exact blood match with the donor. She is deteriorating further and requires transfer to the coronary care unit for a pulmonary artery catheter for hemodynamic monitoring. After 2 months and 16 unsuccessful donor prospective blood matches, she has had a successful crossmatch. The donor had good cardiac function; however, the donor had a questionable social history and was positive for hepatitis C. The cardiologist and surgeon have decided to use the donor heart after discussion with the patient and her significant other about the potential risk factors. The nurse caring for the patient is unaware of the donor's history and is preparing the patient for the operating room.

1. Should this recipient have been taken off the list because she developed a contraindication to transplantation? Defend your answer.
2. What are the psychosocial factors involved with someone who has waited this long and then has developed a contraindication?
3. How does this affect the other patients waiting and the staff caring for these patients?
4. Should the patient have been involved in the decision process and told the donor information? Defend your answer.
5. Should the donor organ have been accepted in light of the clinical history of both the donor and the recipient? Defend your answer.
6. Should the nurse have been informed of the donor situation, and would it have affected her preoperative care?

amount of information given to the recipient about the donor. Most programs adopt the philosophy that only anonymous factors are relayed to the recipient, such as sex, age, and or race. Interaction between organ donor families and recipients is controversial. Direct contact between the two parties has historically not been supported by transplant professionals. Yet, one survey of donor families and recipients revealed that 70% of the donors and 75% of the recipients favored direct contact; 93% of the recipients reported that their reason for wanting direct contact was to express their gratitude toward the donation.[64] Nurses can facilitate the needs of both donors and recipients by encouraging the recipient or significant other to write an anonymous thank you note when emotionally ready.

Collaborative Management

Preoperative Management of the Donor

When a potential donor for transplantation is found, the regional procurement agency is typically contacted by the nurse caring for the patient. Nurses can be strong advocates of this process. They see first hand when a patient they are caring for is being assessed by the medical team for brain death. Contact is made to the procurement agency, and nurses begin the donor evaluation. The donor patient goes through a battery of tests similar to those performed on the recipient. Once brain death has been declared, the procurement nurse can approach the potential donor's family. Consent is still obtained from the next of kin, despite a donor card or written intentions, and the process begins. The procurement nurse gathers information about the patient from the family, the chart, and the nurse and physician caring for the patient. The donor must have the same blood type and be within the specified size restrictions of the recipient. The procurement coordinator calls the recipient's center to relay the information. If the donor information is acceptable to the recipient team physician, the transplant coordinator or transplant surgeon on call coordinates the preparation of the recipient for the surgical procedure. If the first donor is not acceptable, then the procurement coordinator calls the next center on the list, and so on. Chart 13–7 gives pertinent information needed for the recipient physician to determine an acceptable donor.

CHART 13-7

Donor Information Used to Determine Acceptable Candidates

- Brain death criteria met with corresponding consent for donation
- Cause of death
- Past medical history: no evidence of cancer
- Social history: no heavy alcohol, smoking, or drug use
- Recent hospital course events: no septicemia
- Hemodynamics: no circulatory arrest or minimal interruption of cardiac output
- Laboratory data: negative for HIV and hepatitis B; recipient patients who are hepatitis C positive can receive hepatitis C–positive donor hearts
- Blood type
- Donor size (height and weight)
- Electrocardiogram
- Echocardiogram
- Cardiac catheterization (requested if the donor is older than 50 years or has a history of smoking, diabetes, or hypertension)

If other organs are being donated, specific tests for that organ are requested by the procurement coordinator in conjunction with the recipient team physicians. The nurse needs to assist the procurement coordinator to ensure that all these interventions are carried out in a timely manner. Nurses need to be aware that some of the interventions may be conflicting. The abdominal transplantation teams (liver, kidney, and pancreas) request the donor to be well hydrated. However, the lung transplantation team prefers the donor patient to be as dry as possible. Cardiac team members want the patient on minimal inotropic support to evaluate heart function fully. The procurement coordinator assists the nurse in keeping the donor stable and in maintaining a fluid balance acceptable by all teams. In addition, the nurse caring for a donor patient is also managing the physiologic consequences of brain death such as diabetes insipidus, neurogenic pulmonary edema, and vasomotor and temperature instability. The collaborative work with the physicians, staff nurses, and coordinators contributes to the successful retrieval of donor organs.

Psychosocial Issues Related to the Donor

Organ transplantation is intertwined with psychosocial issues at all phases of the transplantation process.

Donor issues and recipient issues are unique and are addressed individually. The role of the nurse during the donor process includes the care of the patient and the family. The nurse assists with tests to determine brain death and appropriateness for donation, manages a potentially unstable patient, and provides education and support to the grieving family. Nurses need to assess the family for their level of understanding of all phases of the procurement process. Interventions and support of the family need to define two separate issues clearly. First, the family must be educated about brain death. Interventions to determine brain death can vary but ultimately need to demonstrate no upper central nervous system activity. Until this step is acknowledged, it may be difficult for the family to discuss organ donation. Second, family members need to be educated about organ donation to assist them in making a decision with which they will be comfortable. This step is especially important when the deceased has not passed on his or her intents about donation. Finally, the donor family needs to be supported while they grieve. Organ donation frequently revolves around a tragedy. Donor families may find comfort in the fact that something positive has resulted from such a tragedy. The procurement coordinator is responsible for these discussions, but nurses initiate the donation process and need to provide the necessary emotional support.

Intraoperative Management

The recipient is prepared as for other cardiac surgical cases. One difference is the recipient may receive preoperative, immunosuppressive medications. Programs vary as to the agents used, if any, before the operation. The second difference is the timing of the operation. Unlike other cardiothoracic operations, transplant surgery depends on the arrival of the donor heart. Coordination of the two procedures by the recipient and procurement heart surgeons is critical for heart transplant patients. Donor operating room times often change for a multitude of reasons: waiting for another organ team to arrive, being bumped by another surgical case or trauma, or the donor's becoming unstable. The nurse must keep the recipient's family updated along the way with any time changes.

The goal is for close communication between the receiving facility's two teams to shorten the ischemic time of the heart. Ischemic time is the time from the cross-clamp of the donor heart to the removal of the recipient's new heart from bypass. Ischemic time should be less than 4 hours for better outcomes. In the recipient operating room, the patient is prepared by the anesthesiologist with the appropriate IV lines and catheters, but the patient is not placed under anesthesia until the donor team calls to say that they are accepting the heart. In the donor operating room, the heart is visually and manually inspected by the recipient's procurement surgeon for any signs of disease. If the donor heart has disease or damage and is unacceptable, then the recipient team will be called and the surgery will be canceled. If the donor heart is accepted, anesthesia is induced and the recipient's mediastinum is opened in preparation for the heart transplant. This procedure typically takes 1 to 1½ hours. If the recipient is a reoperative patient who had a previous mediasternotomy secondary to bypass, valve, or ventricular assist surgery, then more time is needed because of adhesions or removal of the ventricular assist device.

The surgeon inspects the donor heart when it arrives and trims the great vessels and atria. Cardiopulmonary bypass is then initiated, and the aorta is cross-clamped. The recipient's native heart is resected, leaving plenty of area on the atrial cuffs and great vessels to attach the donor heart. The donor heart is placed in the same position and space as the native heart and is referred to as an orthotopic heart transplant. The donor organ is sutured in the following sequence: left atrium, right atrium, pulmonary artery, aorta (Figure 13–14). On removal of bypass, isoproterenol hydrochloride (Isuprel) is initiated to maintain an adequate heart rate.

Postoperative Management

The immediate postoperative management of the heart transplant patient is similar to the care of other cardiac surgical patients. Management of oxygenation and mechanical ventilation, pacer wires, chest tubes, wound care, and urinary catheter care are all part of nursing interventions for the cardiac surgical patient. Factors unique to transplantation, such as denervation and rejection, and complications that may be accentuated after transplantation, such as right heart failure, hemostasis, and renal dysfunction, are discussed. Lifelong complications, such as infection and chronic rejection, are also addressed. Strict hand washing is the primary precaution against infections, and nurses need to educate both hospital staff and visitors to the importance of this practice. Positive-pressure flow rooms are recommended to limit the transfer of airborne pathogens, and sick visitors are asked to stay at home or to wear masks.

Denervation

Denervation results from the loss of the sympathetic and parasympathetic nervous system at the time of the surgical removal of the recipient's heart. The intrinsic heart rate is commonly increased because of the loss of the parasympathetic nervous system or vagal tone. However, it may take some time for the new heart to achieve a stable intrinsic rhythm. Isoproterenol hydrochloride is the agent of choice because of the beta$_1$ (inotropic) and beta$_2$ (chronotropic) effects. The inotropic effects decrease PVR and systemic vascular resistance, thus making it easier for the donor heart to recover. The chronotropic effect increases heart rate and is typically needed for the first 3 postoperative days to increase preload and cardiac output. In addition, the atrial pacing wires can be used to augment the heart rate to increase cardiac output. Atropine

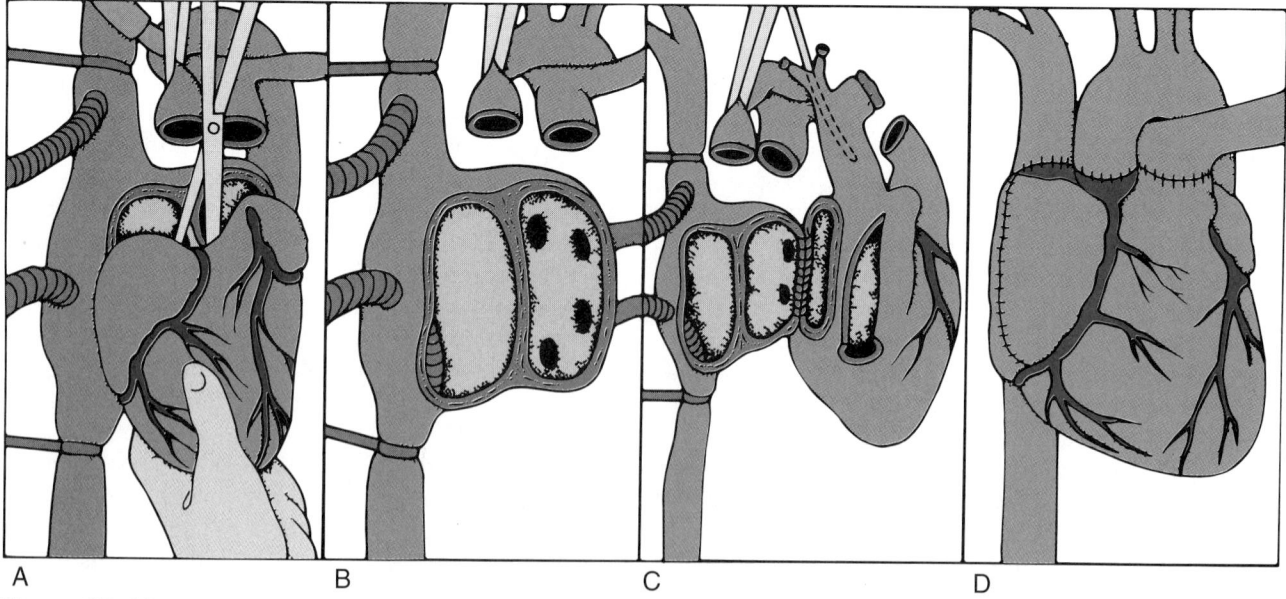

Figure 13–14

Illustration of the surgical procedure of heart transplantation. *A,* After the recipient is placed on cardiopulmonary bypass, the heart is removed. *B,* The posterior walls of the recipient's left and right atria are left intact. *C,* The left atrium of donor heart is anastomosed to the recipient's residual heart tissue. *D,* Postoperative result. (From Ignatavicius DD, Workman ML, Mishler MA: *Medical-Surgical Nursing Across the Healthcare Continuum,* 3rd ed. Philadelphia, W.B. Saunders, 1999.)

sulfate (Atropine) and other vagal agonists or lytics are not effective in heart transplant recipients because of the loss of vagal tone. Digoxin is partially effective: the inotropic effect remains intact, but the vagotonic effect is absent. Carotid massage and the Valsalva maneuver for treating dysrhythmias are also ineffective.

Rehabilitation starts postoperative day 1. The Frank–Starling mechanism remains intact, but reflex tachycardia is absent in response to orthostatic changes. Therefore, the nurse should assist the patient in the immediate postoperative period to sit, stand, and then walk or pivot to the chair the first few times out of bed. The nurse needs to educate the patient to perform this deliberate three-step procedure to allow catecholamines time to circulate and to increase the heart rate, to keep the patient from losing consciousness. Exercise and stress also require increased cardiac output, and cardiac output is preload dependent. Venous pooling may affect preload, so warm-up and cool-down periods should be initiated with any form of exercise. The response to circulating catecholamines is intact but slower. Therefore, in response to stress or exercise, the increase in heart rate takes longer because the patient does not have an intact sympathetic nervous system.

Heart transplant patients can have interesting ECG strips to analyze that can easily be misread. The ECG or rhythm strip needs to be evaluated by the cardiologist and nurse to determine the donor versus recipient P waves. The P waves may be the atrial electrical activity from the recipient's old sinoatrial (SA) node. This electrical activity cannot cross over the surgical suture line. These remnant P waves are visible, but they do not correlate with the ventricular electrical activity. If the patient is in sinus rhythm, two P waves may be seen. One P wave belongs to the recipient, and one P wave belongs to the donor. This rhythm may be mistaken for atrial fibrillation. Only the donor P wave can conduct an electrical response, leading to a contraction of the heart. Because of the surgical incision across the atria, it is possible that the donor SA node can be cut. In this situation, no donor P waves will be present, and the patient will be in a junctional rhythm. This pattern can be misdiagnosed as heart block if there are visible remnant P waves from the native heart (Figure 13–15).

Right Heart Failure

Right heart failure is the most common cause of cardiac dysfunction postoperatively. Four common causes of immediate right heart failure are a history of elevated PVR preoperatively, donor size mismatch in which the donor heart is too small for the recipient, long ischemic time of more than 4 hours, and acute rejection.[64] The nurse needs to monitor cardiac output, PVR, and SVO_2 for trends and to note any abrupt changes. Specifically, the nurse needs to assess for early signs of right heart failure. Early signs may be seen as an increase in right atrial pressure and PAP or a narrowing of the gradient (mean PAP − right atrial pressure).

Surgeons treat the recipient with right heart failure by providing longer time on mechanical ventilation. The goal is a $PaCO_2$ of 25 to 30 mm Hg because hyperventilation decreases the PVR. Pharmacologic support is typically required for a longer period. Agents used include isoproterenol hydrochloride, milrinone, and prostaglandin E_1 to reduce pulmonary pressures, thus making it easier for the right heart to pump. These medical interventions typically are successful in reducing the PVR. From 4 to 25% of cases of acute heart failure could be due to early cardiac allograft failure or biventricular failure of the donor heart. Mechanical and pharmacologic assistance is highly recommended in these patients to salvage the new heart.[65]

Hemostasis

Besides the typical postbypass anticoagulation problems, additional circumstances in the heart transplant patient may cause postoperative bleeding. Transplant recipients generally have passive liver congestion due to chronic congestive heart failure. Liver congestion can increase the risk of bleeding. Second, many patients are receiving anticoagulation preoperatively to prevent the risk of thrombus or emboli in a stagnate "pump." Inadequate heparin reversal (heparin rebound) can occur. Nurses need to monitor chest tube drainage and laboratory results closely. Treatment varies, depending on the severity, but it can include fresh frozen plasma, platelets, protamine, cryoprecipitate (Cryo), aminocaproic acid (Amicar), or desmopressin acetate (DDAVP).

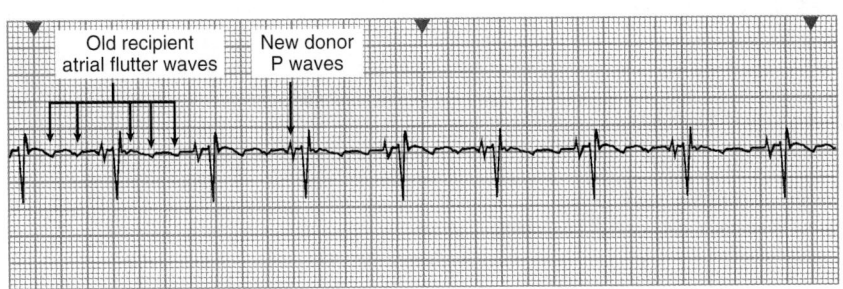

Figure 13–15

Postoperative ECG tracing of a heart transplant recipient. The recipient demonstrates normal sinus rhythm at a rate of 80 beats per minute with old recipient atrial flutter waves at a rate of 300 per minute (lead V_1). The new donor P waves are distorted by the old recipient flutter waves.

Renal Dysfunction

In addition to the effects of bypass and circulatory arrest, patients have additional reasons for renal dysfunction. Because of their low cardiac output state preoperatively, they commonly have preexisting renal insufficiency. The long-term use of diuretics may also play a part in the pretransplant borderline renal insufficiency in these patients. After the operation, the use of cyclosporine (Neoral) can then put these borderline patients into renal failure secondary to drug toxicity. Physicians withhold cyclosporine preoperatively when patients have a creatinine level higher than 2.5 and reduce the dose when creatinine is between 2.0 and 2.5. In addition, surgeons may withhold IV cyclosporine postoperatively until the patient is taking oral medications. Another option is to give IV cytolytics, which are typically used only for acute rejection, just until the creatinine concentration is stable. Muromonab-CD3 (OKT-3) or lymphocyte immune globulin (Atgam) are two different cytolytics that may be administered.

Long-Term Management

Immunosuppressant Medications

Immunosuppressant medications are required in the postoperative patient. The normal functioning immune system recognizes the newly transplanted heart as foreign and mounts a cellular or humoral response. This attack on the heart ultimately damages the heart and needs to be prevented or treated with immunosuppressants. Oral agents are maintained for the patient's lifetime to prevent rejection from occurring. IV methylprednisolone (Solu-Medryl) and cytolytics are typically prescribed to treat rejection.

Patients in the immediate postoperative period are commonly placed on three agents: cyclosporine IV,

methylprednisolone IV, and azathioprine (Imuran) IV. If the patient has known renal insufficiency, intravenous cytolytics may be used, as discussed earlier. Cyclosporine IV is more nephrotoxic than oral medication. Therefore, as soon as the patient is extubated and has bowel sounds, medications are switched over from the IV to the oral route. Cyclosporine IV is approximately three times as potent as oral medication. Azathioprine is close to a 1:1 conversion from IV to oral form. Methylprednisolone IV after the first 24 hours changes to prednisone (Deltasone) once the patient is taking oral medications. If not, the patient will need to receive the IV equivalent, which is a 5:4 conversion ratio. For every 5 mg of prednisone the patient is ordered, 4 mg of methylprednisolone IV would be administered.

Patients are typically maintained on triple immunosuppression for the first year (cyclosporine, azathioprine, and prednisone). Some programs are using newer alternatives such as tacrolimus (Prograf) instead of cyclosporine and mycophenylate mofetil (CellCept) in place of azathioprine. Clinical trials of heart transplant patients are needed to compare the effectiveness and side effects of these drugs with traditional therapy. Programs vary on the amount of steroids given and the rate they are tapered. Table 13–11 lists the goals of long-term immunosuppressive management.

Medication Side Effects

Immunosuppressants are required for life to prevent rejection of the transplant. Patients must be taught, from the onset of their evaluation, that their compliance is an absolute necessity. If patients stop their immunosuppressant medications, they will have rejection. If the rejection is undetected and they continue not taking their medications, death will result.

TABLE 13–11
Long-Term Immunosuppression

Medication	Pill Strength	Laboratory Levels
Cyclosporine (Sandimmune or Neoral)	100-mg and 25-mg gel capsules (cannot be broken)	Maintain cyclosporine trough level at: 250–300 µg/L, the first year 200–250 µg/L, the second year 150–200 µg/L, thereafter Monitor for increase in creatinine, liver function tests
Tacrolimus (Prograf)	4-mg, 2-mg, and 1-mg capsules (cannot be broken)	Tacrolimus trough level, 15–20 µg/L
Azathioprine (Imuran)	50-mg tablets (can be broken in half)	WBC, 4,000–8,000 Monitor for drop in WBC, hemoglobin, or platelets
Mycophenylate mofetil (CellCept)	500-mg and 250-mg capsules (cannot be broken)	WBC, 4,000–8,000 Monitor for drop in WBC, hemoglobin, or platelets
Prednisone (Deltasone)	10-mg, 5-mg, 2-mg, and 1-mg pills (can be broken in half)	Per program taper protocol Monitor fasting glucose for signs of steroid-induced diabetes

However, the medications used to treat and prevent rejection have multiple side effects and can make compliance a challenge.[66] Patients should be taught the various side effects, to minimize fear of these symptoms (Table 13–12). Immunosuppressant medications can also cause many chronic side effects or complications, specifically, hypertension, hyperlipidemia, diabetes, and renal dysfunction. The 1997 report from the Registry of the ISHLT reported that hypertension occurs in 64.8% of heart recipients 1 year postoperatively. In addition, hyperlipidemia occurs in 29.8% of recipients, renal dysfunction in 10%, and diabetes in 18.5% at the 1-year follow-up.[37]

Biopsies. The current standard for detecting rejection of the donor heart is endomyocardial biopsy. It is an invasive procedure by entry through the right subclavian vein with an IV catheter that has a bioptome on the end of the sheath to enable tiny pieces of the right ventricle to be taken. The procedure generally takes about 15 to 30 minutes and is performed under fluoroscopy. These tissue samples are sent to a pathologist to diagnose rejection (see Figure 8–9). The first biopsy is done 1 week after transplantation, while the patient is still hospitalized. Subsequent biopsies occur weekly for approximately 4 weeks and are typically done as outpatient procedures. The frequency of biop-

TABLE 13–12
Side Effects From Immunosuppressive Therapy for Heart Transplant Patients

Medication	Side Effects	
Cyclosporine (Sandimmune, Neoral)	Hypertension Nephrotoxicity Hypercholesterolemia Hepatotoxicity Hyperkalemia Hyperglycemia	Tremors Seizures Headache Gingival hyperplasia Hirsutism Nausea Vomiting
FK506 Tacrolimus (Prograf)	Hypertension Nephrotoxicity Hyperkalemia Hyperglycemia Headache	Tremors Seizures Nausea Diarrhea
Prednisone (Deltasone)	Joint pain Muscle weakness Increased appetite Salt and water retention Increased weight Hypertension Hyperglycemia/diabetes Cushingoid appearance (moon face)	Mood swings Insomnia Night sweats Gastrointestinal ulceration Cataracts Hirsutism Acne Ultraviolet rays sensitivity (need > SPF 15 sunscreen)
Azathioprine (Imuran)	Bone marrow suppression (particularly WBC and occasionally RBC)	Bruising Alopecia Hepatotoxicity
Mycophenylate (CellCept)	Abdominal pain Nausea Vomiting Diarrhea	Leukopenia Neutropenia Sepsis (typically cytomegalovirus)
OKT3	Rigors Malaise Pyrexia Diarrhea	Hypertension Hypotension Pulmonary edema Meningitis
Antilymphocyte preparation (Atgam)	Fever Chills Serum sickness Inflammatory reactions	Bone marrow suppression Thrombocytopenia Anaphylaxis

TABLE 13–13
Heart Transplant Rejection and Treatment

ISHLT Grade	Rejection	Treatment
0	None	None
1-A	Focal, mild acute	None
1-B	Diffuse, mild acute	None
2	Focal, moderate acute	Maximize oral medications Biopsy in 2–4 weeks
3-A	Multifocal, moderate acute	Maximize oral medications, if asymptomatic and more than 3 months after transplant Steroids or IV cytolytics, if symptomatic, decreased heart function, or less than 3 months after transplant Biopsy 7–10 days after treatment
3-B	Diffuse, borderline severe acute	Steroids or IV cytolytics Biopsy 7–10 days
4	Severe acute	IV cytolytics Biopsy 1 week

ISHLT, International Society for Heart and Lung Transplantation.
Adapted from Billingham ME, Cary NRB, Hammond ME, et al: A working formulation for the standardization of nomenclature in the diagnosis of heart and lung rejection: Heart rejection study group. The International Society for Heart Transplantation. J Heart Transplant 9:587–593, 1990.

sies depends on the patient's symptoms, the pathology report of any rejection, previous rejection, and the program's steroid-tapering protocol. The minimum number of biopsies in stable patients 1 year after heart transplantation, is one or two per year.

Rejection

At the time of the endomyocardial biopsies, the tissue samples are examined for any signs of rejection. Rejection commonly occurs in small areas throughout the heart. Therefore, the physician should obtain four to six samples to decrease the chance of sampling error. The number of samples and the frequency of biopsies are particularly important in the immediate postoperative period because acute rejection is most common in the first 3 months.[67] To standardize the diagnosis of rejection, the ISHLT grading system was formulated as a means to categorize the severity of rejection objectively (Table 13–13). Signs and symptoms of rejection are vague and need to be correlated with biopsy results before treatment decisions are made. The most common symptom reported by the patient is fatigue or malaise that may or may not correlate with clinical assessment. Dysrhythmias, ventricular gallop (S_3), or an elevated central venous pressure can be associated with rejection. An increased central venous pressure can be noted by an elevated jugular venous pressure on physical assessment or an elevated right atrial pressure seen when a biopsy is obtained. Typically, if rejection is suspected based on clinical examination or the patient's symptoms, a right heart catheterization is done at the time of the biopsy to determine fluid overload and decompensation. Treatment of rejection varies depending on clinical symptoms, prior rejection episodes, any active infection, prednisone lev-

els, compliance, and cyclosporine levels. Physicians and coordinators work collaboratively to maximize the immunosuppressant drugs as much as the patient's renal function and white blood cell count will allow.

Infection

Patients who have had a heart transplant are at higher risk for infections throughout their lives because of their immunocompromised state. Chart 13–8 lists the

CHART 13–8

Common Infections After Heart Transplantation

Viral
    Cytomegalovirus
    Epstein–Barr virus
    Herpes simplex virus
    Varicella-zoster virus
Bacterial
    Nosocomial
    Pneumococcal pneumonia
    Nocardia
Protozoal and Fungal
    Candida
    Pneumocystis
    Aspergillus
    Toxoplasma
    Cryptococcus

more common infections seen in heart transplant patients. Prophylaxis is given for up to 1 year to prevent common infections. Trimethoprim–sulfamethoxazole (Bactrim) is given for the first year to prevent *Pneumocystis* pneumonia. Acyclovir (Zovirax) is used for 3 months to 1 year for recipients who had a positive herpes simplex virus titer done on the original screening test for the transplant evaluation. Clotrimazole troche (Mycelex troche) tablets or nystatin (Mycostatin) mouthwash is recommended to prevent thrush, a common fungal infection in the mouth. Patients are at highest risk for infection during the first 3 months after the heart transplant, but they remain at high risk for a full year for less common infections, such as aspergillosis or candidiasis. Cytomegalovirus (CMV) is potentially the most important and devastating viral pathogen seen. About 60 to 90% of patients show laboratory evidence of CMV infection 1 to 6 months after heart transplantation. Of special concern is the recipient who tests negative for CMV before the heart transplant and receives a CMV-positive donor heart. Seroconversion generally occurs about 3 months after heart transplantation and may mimic viral symptoms. Research is being conducted to determine the most appropriate prophylaxis to prevent an active infection from occurring in this patient population. At present, ganciclovir (Cytovene) IV is started immediately postoperatively and then is switched to high-dose acyclovir for the first year. In addition, patients receiving cytolytic therapy are at higher risk for CMV and will be treated with ganciclovir.

Any time patients are fighting a virus or are being treated for an infection, an endomyocardial biopsy should be obtained, especially if the patient presents with symptoms of fatigue, malaise, vomiting, or diarrhea. The immune system responds, and excess white blood cells circulate to fight off the invading organism. If a patient is vomiting or has diarrhea, he or she may not have therapeutic immunosuppressive drug levels. Both these factors can place the patient at higher risk of transplant rejection.

Posttransplant Lymphoproliferative Disease

All immunosuppressants place the patient at risk of infection and malignancy.[68] This disease is uncommon, but it is more prevalent with patients several years after the heart transplant. Again, because of the immunocompromised state of the patient, lymphoproliferative disorders can occur. Immediate diagnosis is needed so the immunosuppressants can be decreased rapidly. Depending on the location of the disease and the expedience of diagnosis, this process can be resolved with substantial reduction in immunosuppressants alone. More progressive, nodal involvement may need surgical node removal, chemotherapy, and or radiation therapy.

Accelerated Graft Vessel Disease

Accelerated graft vessel disease is the most critical risk factor associated with late death in the heart transplant population.[69] One of the drawbacks to transplantation is that *all* patients develop this type of atherosclerosis or vasculopathy. Scientifically, it is not well known how it occurs, but it is assumed to be due to the long-term use of immunosuppressant agents that damage the endothelium. Cyclosporine may specifically play a role in the development of endothelial cell dysfunction leading to the vasculopathy.[70] This type of atherosclerosis affects all the coronary vessels, including the minute coronary vessels. It is referred to as chronic rejection of the endothelium, although acute rejection may also contribute to the development of vasculopathy.[71] In addition, these patients are more likely to suffer dysrhythmias and sudden death. Aggressive antidysrhythmic therapy may be warranted in this subgroup of patients.[72] In addition, dobutamine echocardiography should be considered part of the annual evaluation to determine those patients at higher risk of ischemic events.[73,74]

The main coronary arteries also develop a long narrowing of the arteries, all the way down the vessel, as opposed to a single area of blockage. Because the nerves were cut during the operation, symptoms of chest pain do not typically occur. Patients undergo cardiac catheterization yearly after the heart transplant to diagnose the onset and progression of the disease in the main coronary arteries. This type of atherosclerosis is not amenable to standard treatment (thrombolytics, angioplasty, or coronary artery bypass). Rather, conservative treatment, with medications, or, on rare occasions, retransplantation is recommended. Postoperative hyperlipidemia is common as a result of immunosuppressant use, specifically cyclosporine. Research has suggested that aggressive treatment of hyperlipidemia may lead to lower cholesterol levels, a decrease in graft vessel disease, and a higher long-term survival rate.[75] Research to stall or prevent the onset of this type of vessel disease is the key to longer survival after a heart transplant.

Multidisciplinary Outcomes

Heart transplant patients generate various needs for nursing care throughout all phases of transplantation. Table 13–14 lists the multidisciplinary outcomes in the care of the transplant patient throughout the process. As is typical for nursing, many roles overlap, and some roles are unique. The goal of the nurse is to guide the patient competently through the various transplant phases. The ultimate goal for the patient with advanced heart failure is successful treatment with heart transplantation. It is not a simple process. There are physical,

TABLE 13–14
Multidisciplinary Outcomes of Heart Transplant Patients

Phase		Outcome
Preoperative	Emergency room	Assessment of patient for timely and accurate diagnosis of heart failure
		Initiation of intravenous diuretics to alleviate acute symptoms of heart failure
	Intensive care unit	Stabilization of patient with intravenous inotropes or mechanical support
		Initiation of transplant evaluation tests, blood work, and consultations
		Education of the patient and family about the evaluation and listing process
	Intermediate care unit	Management of heart failure symptoms, diet, fluid intake, and medication
		Completion of transplant evaluation
		Maintenance of measures to decrease anxiety
		Implementation of discharge teaching about new medications and follow-up care
Intraoperative	Intensive care unit	Stabilization of donor patient
	Operating rooms	Coordination of procurement and recipient teams to decrease ischemic time
		Initiation of immunosuppressants
Immediate postoperative	Surgical intensive care unit	Management of immediate postoperative complications
		Initiation of immunosuppressant medications
		Prevention of infection
		Implementation of rehabilitation of the patient with a denervated heart
	Intermediate care unit	Maintenance of immunosuppressant medications
		Education of patient and family about medications, infection, rejection, activity, and follow-up
		Preparation for discharge and follow-up requirements related to rejection and infection
		Acknowledgment of psychosocial issues related to transplanted heart and life-long need for medication and follow-up
Long-term postoperative	Community	Initiation of cardiac rehabilitation
		Acknowledgment of long-term complications and potential need for readmission

psychosocial, and financial considerations for the patient, the family members, and the health care team. Because of the shortage of donors in comparison with the number of patients that could benefit from heart transplantation, optimal selection of this patient population is necessary. Evaluation of outcomes after a heart transplant is useful to determine the benefit-to-risk ratio. The Registry of the ISHLT reports that the highest percentage of deaths in the first month is due to nonspecific graft failure. In the first year, infection and rejection are the two most common causes of death. In the late phases of heart transplantation, the most common reasons for mortality are accelerated graft atherosclerosis, malignancy, and acute rejection.[37]

Rehabilitation is the patient's primary goal after heart transplantation. Despite the side effects and the complications, 79.8% of patients report no activity limitations the first year after heart transplantation.[3] Whether or not these patients return to the work force depends on their insurance benefits and prescription coverage. Many of these patients lose their disability benefits by returning to work. Their new insurance may not cover their follow-up care or their prescriptions, and the patient may be financially at risk for noncompliance with medications. When patients say they are having trouble paying for their medications, nurses must initiate consultations with social services and financial counseling services. Care of the transplant patient is both complex and rewarding. For the patient to achieve optimal outcomes after heart transplantation, responsibilities must be shared by the patient and the health care team.

Critical Thinking Exercise

Mrs. S., a 48-year-old woman, was admitted to the hospital with mitral valve insufficiency. She had bacterial endocarditis 5 years ago and has had increasing difficulty with shortness of breath and fatigue. She went to the operating room the next day for a mitral valve replacement.

Mrs. S. is admitted to the ICU after surgery. She had a size 23 St. Jude valve inserted. She is not receiving any vasoactive medications.

Mrs. S.'s vital signs are: blood pressure, 122/74 (mean arterial pressure, 90); heart rate, 82; R = 12; T = 36.5. She is in normal sinus rhythm according to the monitor. Her hemodynamic parameters are: right atrium, 12; pulmonary artery, 35/25; PAOP 24; cardiac output, 4.8; cardiac index, 1.9; systemic vascular resistance, 2100. Her pulse oximeter is 98% saturated, and her SvO_2 is 52% saturated. Her hemoglobin is 10. Her lungs are clear, and you are easily able to hear the clicking of her mechanical valve.

Mrs. S. is started on amrinone (Inocor) at 5 μg/kg per minute. You repeat parameters in 1 hour and find: right atrium, 10; pulmonary artery, 35/24; cardiac output, 5.5; cardiac index, 2.2; systemic vascular resistance 1400. Her SvO_2 is 60% saturated.

1. What considerations would be given in determining which type of valve to insert in Mrs. S.?
2. What information will you include in your assessment of Mrs. S.?
3. What immediate interventions do you believe Mrs. S. needs? Provide rationales.
4. What additional interventions do you think Mrs. S. may need?
5. Before Mrs. S.'s discharge, what discharge teaching would she need specific to her valve replacement?

Key Concepts

⇒ Coronary artery bypass graft surgery improves blood flow to areas of ischemic myocardium.

⇒ If a vein or a detached artery is used for coronary artery bypass surgery, the section of vein or artery is used to bypass or go around the diseased area of the coronary artery.

⇒ If an in situ artery is used for coronary artery bypass surgery, the distal end of the artery is dissected and is used to bypass the diseased area of the coronary artery.

⇒ Minimally invasive cardiac surgery minimizes the size of the incisions and may or may not involve the use of cardiopulmonary bypass. This procedure is performed in selected patients.

⇒ Transmyocardial laser revascularization is an experimental procedure for patients with ischemic, yet viable areas of the myocardium that are not amenable to bypass grafts. It involves the use of laser energy to pierce small channels through the myocardium in an effort to improve myocardial blood flow.

⇒ Mechanical and biologic valves are available for implantation in patients with cardiac valve disease.

⇒ Valve repair can be performed in an effort to improve the hemodynamic function of the patient's native valve.

⇒ Patients receiving mechanical heart valves need lifelong anticoagulation therapy.

⇒ A primary goal after cardiac surgery is early extubation.

⇒ Myocardial function is enhanced if preload, afterload, and contractility are optimized.

⇒ Cardiac output, cardiac index, and systemic vascular resistance are frequently determined after cardiac surgery to guide the initiation, titration, and discontinuation of vasoactive drug therapy.

⇒ Cardiac mechanical support for the failing heart can be provided by an intra-aortic balloon pump, a hemopump, or ventricular assist devices.

⇒ Temporary pacing may be necessary using the epicardial pacing wires after cardiac procedures to initiate a cardiac rhythm or to increase heart rate.

⇒ Patients commonly experience diuresis after cardiac surgery in response to the physiologic effects of cardiopulmonary bypass.

⇒ Postoperative bleeding through chest tubes can be treated by applying PEEP, by reducing mean arterial pressure, by administering blood products, or by correcting abnormal coagulation values.

⇒ Restoration and maintenance of normothermia is essential to reduce myocardial workload after cardiac surgery.

⇒ Postoperative pain should be managed with analgesics, nonsteroidal anti-inflammatory agents, and nonpharmacologic pain-reduction interventions.

⇒ Atrial dysrhythmias are the most common dysrhythmias after cardiac surgery.

⇒ Cardiac tamponade after cardiac procedures is a medical emergency and needs to be treated immediately by opening the patient's sternum.

⇒ Heart transplantation is a treatment option for end-stage, nonreversible heart disease when all other medical and surgical options have been exhausted.

⇒ The primary indication for heart transplantation is ischemic dilated cardiomyopathy and idiopathic dilated cardiomyopathy.

⇒ The evaluation of a patient for a heart transplant has two objectives: determination of nonreversible end-stage heart disease and identification of any comorbidities that would preclude the patient from safely undergoing the procedure.

➡ The primary diagnostic factors for listing a patient on the heart transplant list include a metabolic stress test with Vo_2 less than 10 mL/kg per minute, ejection fraction less than 10%, and elevated PAPs.

➡ The absolute contraindications to listing patients for transplant include elevated, fixed pulmonary vascular resistance, positive HIV status, malignancy, and nonreversible vital organ disease.

➡ Patients with the highest priority status waiting the longest are considered first for a donor organ. The donor heart is accepted if the blood type matches, the size is acceptable, and heart function is adequate.

➡ Denervation of the newly transplanted heart results from the loss of the innervation of the sympathetic and parasympathetic nervous system during the operation.

➡ ECG tracings may demonstrate extraneous atrial activity from the patient's old SA node. These P waves do not cross over the suture line and do not correlate with ventricular activity.

➡ Endomyocardial biopsies are performed to rule out organ rejection. Symptoms do not always accompany rejection because of the masking effects of the immunosuppressant medications.

➡ Patients are maintained on immunosuppressant therapy for life and are always at risk of organ rejection and infection. In essence, heart trans-plant recipients are trading one disease (end-stage heart disease) for another (immunocompromised state).

➡ Many complex psychosocial issues relate to heart donors and their families as well as heart recipients and their families. The transplant team and the nurse must work together to address these needs and to facilitate adjustment throughout the heart transplantation process.

References

1. American Heart Association: Heart and Stroke Facts: 1998 Statistical Supplement. Dallas, TX, American Heart Association, 1997.
2. Singh RN, Beg RA, Kay EB: Physiological adaptability: the secret of success of the internal mammary artery grafts. Ann Thorac Surg 41:247–250, 1986.
3. Vitello-Cicciu J, Fitzgerald C, Whalen D: On the horizon: minimally invasive surgery. J Cardiovasc Nurs 12:1–16, 1998.
4. Vaca KJ, Drake CJ, Lambrecht DS: Nursing care of patients undergoing thoracoscopic minimally invasive bypass grafting. Am J Crit Care 6:281–286, 1997.
5. Lynn-McHale DJ, Hambach C, Carter T, et al: Transmyocardial laser revascularization. J Cardiovasc Nurs 12:17–28, 1998.
6. Grunkemeier GL, Starr A, Rahimtoola SH: Prosthetic heart valve performance: long-term follow-up. Curr Probl Cardiol 17:329–406, 1992.
7. Whitman GR: Valve repair and replacement. In: Urban NA, Greenlee KK, Krumberger JM, et al (eds): Guidelines for Critical Care Nursing. St. Louis, C.V. Mosby, 1995.
8. Lytle BW: Impact of coronary artery disease on valvular heart surgery. Cardiol Clin 9:301–314, 1991.
9. Lynn-McHale DJ, Corsetti A, Brady-Avis E, et al: Preoperative ICU tours: are they helpful? Am J Crit Care 6:106–115, 1997.
10. Corsetti AL, Perry D: A comprehensive approach to facilitating the recovery of cardiac surgery patients. J Cardiovasc Nurs 12:82–90, 1998.
11. Seifert PC: Advances in myocardial protection. J Cardiovasc Nurs 12:29–38, 1998.
12. Greenlee KK: Mechanical ventilation. In: Urban NA, Greenlee KK, Krumberger JM, et al (eds): Guidelines for Critical Care Nursing. St. Louis, C.V. Mosby, 1995.
13. Braunwald E (ed): Heart Disease: A Textbook of Cardiovascular Medicine, 4th ed. Philadelphia, W.B. Saunders, 1997.
14. Lynn-McHale DJ, McGrory: Intraaortic balloon pump management. In: Boggs RL, Wooldridge-King M (eds): AACN Procedure Manual for Critical Care. Philadelphia, W.B. Saunders, 1993.
15. Gross SB: Current challenges, concepts, and controversies in chest tube management. AACN Clin Issues 4:260–275, 1993.
16. Ley SJ: Intraoperative and postoperative blood salvage. AACN Clin Issues 7:238–248, 1996.
17. Barden C, Hansen M: Cold versus warm cardioplegia: recognizing hemodynamic variations. Dimensions Crit Care Nurs 14:114–126, 1995.
18. Earp JK, Mallia G: Myocardial protection for cardiac surgery: the nursing perspective. AACN Clin Issues 8:20S–32S, 1997.
19. Staples JR, Ramsay JG: Advances in anesthesia for cardiac surgery: an overview for the 1990s. AACN Clin Issues 8:41–49, 1997.
20. Gylys KH: Pharmacology. J Cardiovasc Nurs 12:39–43, 1998.
21. Watt-Watson J, Stevens B. Managing pain after coronary artery bypass surgery. J Cardiovasc Nurs 12:44–56, 1998.
22. Kern LS: Management of postoperative atrial fibrillation. J Cardiovasc Nurs 12:57–77, 1998.
23. Puntillo K: Dimensions of procedural pain: analgesic management in critically ill surgical patients. Am J Crit Care 3:116–122, 1994.
24. Creswell LL, Schuessler RB, Rosenbloom M, et al: Hazards of postoperative atrial arrhythmias. Ann Thorac Surg 56:539–549, 1993.
25. Hashimoto K, Ilstrup DM, Schaff HV: Influence of clinical and hemodynamic variables on risk of supraventricular tachycardia after coronary artery bypass. J Thorac Cardiovasc Surg 101:56–65, 1991.
26. Leitch JW, Thomson D, Baird DK, et al: The importance of age as a predictor of atrial fibrillation and flutter after coronary artery bypass grafting. J Thorac Cardiovasc Surg 100:338–342, 1990.
27. Ommen SR, Odell JA, Stanton MS: Atrial arrhythmias after cardiothoracic surgery. N Engl J Med 336:1429–1433, 1997.
28. Reed GL III, Singer DE, Picard EH, et al: Stroke following coronary artery bypass surgery: a case-control estimate of the risk from carotid bruits. N Engl J Med 319:1246–1250, 1988.
29. Stein PD, Alpert JA, Copeland J, et al: Antithrombotic therapy in patients with mechanical and biological prosthetic heart valves. Chest 102:445S–455S, 1992.
30. London MJ, Hollenberg M, Wong MG, et al: Intraoperative myocardial ischemia: localization by continuous 12-lead electrocardiography. Anesthesiology 69:232–241, 1988.
31. Slogoff S, Keats AS: Does perioperative myocardial ischemia lead to postoperative myocardial infarction? Anesthesiology 62:107–114, 1985.
32. Antman EM: Medical management of the patient undergoing cardiac surgery. In: Braunwald E (ed): Heart Disease: A Textbook of Cardiovascular Medicine, 4th ed. Philadelphia, W.B. Saunders, 1997, pp 1715–1740.
33. Kern LS: Emergency exploratory sternotomy: the nurse's role. AACN Clin Issues Crit Care Nurs 1:148–157, 1990.
34. Dajani AS, Taubert KA, Wilson W: Prevention of bacterial endocarditis: recommendations by the American Heart Association. JAMA 277:1794–1801, 1997.
35. Smith WM: Epidemiology of congestive heart failure. Am J Cardiol 55:3A–8A, 1985.

36. Ho KL, Anderson KM, Kannel WB, et al: Survival after the onset of congestive heart failure in Framingham Heart Study Subjects. Circulation 88:107–115, 1993.

37. Hosenpud JD, Bennett LE, Keck BM, et al: The registry of the International Society for Heart and Lung Transplantation: fourteenth official report—1997. J Heart Lung Transplant 16:691–712, 1997.

38. United Network for Organ Sharing (UNOS): The UNOS Bulletin. Richmond, VA, UNOS, 1997. (Available from UNOS, 1100 Boulders Parkway, Suite 500, PO Box 13770, Richmond, VA 23225–8770.)

39. Stevenson LW, Warner SL, Steimle AE, et al: The impending crisis awaiting cardiac transplantation: modeling a solution based on selection. Circulation 89:450–457, 1994.

40. Helderman JH, Goral S: Update in transplant 1995. In: Cecka JM, Terasaki PI (eds): Clinical Transplants 1995 Los Angeles, UCLA Tissue Typing Laboratory, 1995, pp 323–350.

41. Spital A: Mandated choice for organ donation: time to give it a try. Ann Intern Med 125:66–69, 1996.

42. Hosenpud JD, Breen TJ, Edwards EB, et al: The effect of transplant center volume on cardiac transplant outcome: a report of the United Network for Organ Sharing Scientific Registry. JAMA 271:1844–1849, 1994.

43. Rodkey SM, Hobbs RE, Goormastic M, et al: Does distance between home and transplantation center adversely affect patient outcomes after heart transplantation? J Heart Lung Transplant 16:496–503, 1997.

44. Kao W, Costanzo MR: Prognosis determination in patients with advanced heart failure. J Heart Lung Transplant 16:S2–S6, 1997.

45. Furnary AP, Jessup M, Moreira L: Multi-center trial of dynamic cardiomyoplasty for chronic heart failure. J Am Coll Cardiol 28:1175–1180, 1996.

46. Kass DA, Baughman KL, Pak PH, et al: Reverse remodeling from cardiomyoplasty in human heart failure: external constraint versus active assist. Circulation 91:2314–2318, 1995.

47. Batista RJ, Santos JL, Takeshita N, et al: Partial left ventriculectomy to improve left ventricular function in end-stage heart disease. J Card Surg 11:96–97, 1996.

48. Keck BM, Bennett LE, Fiol BS, et al: Worldwide thoracic organ transplantation: a report from the UNOS/ISHLT international registry for thoracic organ transplantation. In: Cecka JM, Teraski PI (eds): Clinical Transplants 1995. Los Angeles, UCLA Tissue Typing Laboratory, 1995, pp 35–39.

49. Hollenberg SM, Parrillo JE: Reversible causes of severe myocardial dysfunction. J Heart Lung Transplant 16:S7–S12, 1997.

50. Mancini DM, Eisen H, Kussmaul W, Mull, et al: Value of peak exercise oxygen consumption for optimal timing of cardiac transplantation in ambulatory patients with heart failure. Circulation 83:778–786, 1991.

51. Chomsky DB, Lang CC, Rayos GH, et al: Hemodynamic exercise testing: a valuable tool in the selection of cardiac transplantation candidates. Circulation 94:3176–3183, 1996.

52. Loh E, Stamler JS, Hare JM, et al: Cardiovascular effects of inhaled nitric oxide in patients with left ventricular dysfunction. Circulation 90:2780–2784, 1994.

53. Costard-Jäckle A, Fowler MB: Influence of preoperative pulmonary artery pressure on mortality after heart transplantation: testing of potential reversibility of pulmonary hypertension with nitroprusside is useful in defining a high risk group. J Am Coll Cardiol 19:48–54, 1992.

54. Erickson KW, Costanzo-Nordin MR, O'Sullivan J, et al: Influence of preoperative transpulmonary gradient on late mortality after orthotopic heart transplantation. J Heart Transplant 9:526–537, 1990.

55. Costanzo MR, Augustine S, Bourge R, et al: Selection and treatment of candidates for heart transplantation: a statement for health professionals from the committee on heart failure and cardiac transplantation of the Council on Clinical Cardiology, American Heart Association. Circulation 92:3593–3612, 1995.

56. Cintron G, Johnson G, Francis G, et al: Prognostic significance of serial changes in left ventricular ejection fraction in patients with congestive heart failure: the V-HeFT VA Cooperative Studies Group. Circulation 87(Suppl VI):VI-17–VI-23, 1993.

57. Miller LW, Kubo SH, Young JB, et al: Medical management of heart and lung failure and candidate selection: report of the consensus conference on candidate selection for heart transplantation—1993. J Heart Lung Transplant 14:562–570, 1995.

58. Bull DA, Karwande SV, Hawkins JA, et al: Long-term results of cardiac transplantation in patients older than sixty years. J Thorac Cardiovasc Surg 111:423–428, 1996.

59. Frigerio M, Gronda EG, Mangiavacchi M, et al: Restrictive criteria for heart transplantation candidacy maximize survival of patients with advanced heart failure. J Heart Transplant 16:160–168, 1997.

60. Doval HC, Nul DR, Grancelli HO, et al: Nonsustained ventricular tachycardia in severe heart failure: independent marker of increased mortality due to sudden death. Circulation 94:3198–3203, 1996.

61. United Network for Organ Sharing (UNOS): Policy and by-law proposals. Richmond, VA, UNOS, 1997. (Available from UNOS, 1100 Boulders Parkway, Suite 500, P.O. Box 13770, Richmond, VA 23225–8770.)

62. Kobashigawa JA, Sabad A, Drinkwater D, et al: Pretransplant panel reactive-antibody screens: are they truly a marker for poor outcome after cardiac transplant? Circulation 94(Suppl II):II-294–II-297, 1996.

63. Loh E, Bergin JD, Couper GS, et al: Role of panel-reactive antibody cross-reactivity in predicting survival after orthotopic heart transplantation. J Heart Lung Transplant 13:194–200, 1994.

64. Lewino D, Stocks L, Cole G: Interaction of donor families and recipients. J Transplant Coordination 6:191–195, 1996.

65. Hauptman PJ, Aranki S, Mudge GH, et al: Early cardiac allograft failure after orthotopic heart transplantation. Am Heart J 127:179–186, 1994.

66. Jalowiec A, Grady KL, White-Williams C, et al: Symptom distress three months after heart transplantation. J Heart Lung Transplant 16:604–614, 1997.

67. Billingham ME, Cary NRB, Hammond ME, et al: A working formulation for the standardization of nomenclature in the diagnosis of heart and lung rejection: heart rejection study group. The International Society for Heart Transplantation. J Heart Transplant 9:587–593, 1990.

68. McGiffin DC, Kirklin JK, Naftel DC, et al: Competing outcomes after heart transplantation: a comparison of eras and outcomes. J Heart Lung Transplant 16:190–198, 1997.

69. Akosah KO, Olsovsky M, Kirchberg D, et al: Dobutamine stress echocardiography predicts cardiac events in heart transplant patients. Circulation 94(Suppl II):II-283–II-288, 1996.

70. Khalil A, Carrier M, Latour J, et al: Cyclosporine-A induced coronary artery vasoconstriction through myogenic and endothelium-dependent mechanisms. Circulation 94(Suppl II):II-308–II-311, 1996.

71. Perrault LP, Bidouard J, Janiak P, et al: Time course of coronary endothelial dysfunction in acute untreated rejection after heterotopic heart transplant. J Heart Lung Transplant 16:643–657, 1997.

72. Patel VS, Lim M, Massin EK, et al: Sudden cardiac death in cardiac transplant recipients. Circulation 94(Suppl II):II-273–II-282, 1996.

73. Kwame OA, Olsovsky M, Kirchberg D, et al: Dobutamine stress echocardiography predicts cardiac events in heart transplant patients. Circulation 94(9)(Suppl II):II-283–II-288, 1996.

74. Lewis JF, Selman SB, Murphy JD, et al: Dobutamine echocardiography for prediction of ischemic events in heart transplant recipients. J Heart Lung Transplant 16:390–393, 1997.

75. Wenke K, Meiser B, Thiery J, et al: Simvastatin reduces graft vessel disease and mortality after heart transplantation. Circulation 96:1398–1402, 1997.

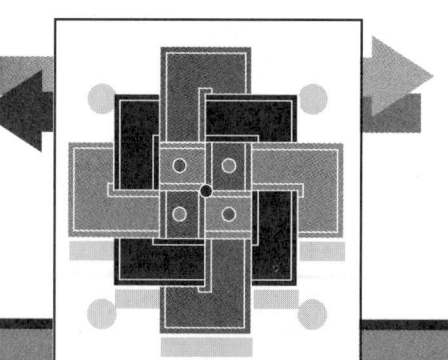

Respiratory Disorders

Nurturing the Will to Live Taught Important Lessons

M. had been in the surgical intensive care unit (ICU) for 2 months after a mitral valve replacement. Postoperatively, she developed sepsis, acute respiratory distress syndrome, and pneumonia. Dependent on the ventilator the entire time, she was unable to talk, eat, drink, or move independently. She also was being restrained intermittently to prevent self-extubation. After many unsuccessful attempts to wean her from the ventilator, M. was transferred to my medical ICU for pulmonary management. It was our job to wean her from the ventilator. I assumed the role of her care manager.

M. was awake when she was transferred to the unit, but she had a look of terror in her eyes and a deep red color to her face. Her hands were shaking as she gripped the bed rails. Her heart rate, blood pressure, and respiratory rate were elevated. She was trying to communicate her needs and feelings, but she could not speak.

Many departments and staff members outside of nursing were involved in M.'s care, including respiratory therapy, pharmacology, medicine, and physical therapy. The medical ICU clinical nurse specialist was also involved. The team evaluated both her physical and her psychosocial readiness to be weaned from the ventilator before developing an effective plan of care. The nursing staff focused on her psychosocial readiness by addressing sleep and rest patterns, tolerance to activity, coping strategies, and mindset. M. had a history of zealousness and had been a dynamic, independent, and active person before her surgery. Her family described her as "always joking and laughing, but very sensitive." She preferred to be in control of her surroundings.

However, in her present situation, M. was demonstrating extreme mood shifts. One minute, she was anxious and experiencing panic attacks; the next minute, she was withdrawn and depressed. During these episodes, M. was neither communicating with us nor cooperating with the plan of care. The only intervention that calmed her was to have someone sit at her bedside and reassure her while stroking her forehead and holding her hand. Her family members expressed concerns that she was "shutting them out and didn't care anymore," which was so unlike the cheerful, easygoing, head of the household they knew. Working with M. day after day was frustrating.

After 5 days as her primary care giver, I saw no improvement in her emotional outlook or progress toward her weaning. As M.'s care manager, I felt defeated and ineffective. M. had obviously lost the ability to control her environment. Her dependence on the ventilator was the factor contributing most to this loss. After reassessing the situation, I began to understand that the most pressing problems interfering with M.'s emotional recovery were her loss of control and feelings of powerlessness. By addressing and resolving these problems, she would have a better chance being weaned from the ventilator.

I explained to M. that if she got involved in her care, we could work together to wean her from the ventilator. We developed an activity schedule that included daily goals. By allowing her to identify activity choices on an hourly basis, she got back a measure of control. We decided on the times she would rest and the times she would be active. M. understood that sufficient rest and a positive frame of mind would improve her chance of weaning when her underlying disease improved. It was wonderful when M. started to interact with me and to become involved. However, she still displayed a degree of doubt in her ability to succeed. To keep M. devoted to the plan, I needed to prove to her that she could be successful.

We needed more structure and a tangible way for M. to identify her daily progress, so we developed a list of goals for 5 consecutive days. Each day, M. was expected to do a little more than the previous day. If she could not meet a particular day's goals, they would be repeated the following day. There was no pressure or negative feedback if the goals were not achieved.

Notes on M.'s progress, daily goals, and activity schedule were hung at the foot of the bed, where they could be visualized at all times. This constantly reminded M. of her accomplishments as well as of the anticipated activities and goals for the next day. Our plan also fostered consistent care among health care personnel. Although this method of scheduling activities and setting daily goals had not been tried in our unit, M. and I found it effective.

After following the plan for 4 days, M. showed significant progress. She had progressed from sleeping most of the day to taking steps with a walker and sleeping only during scheduled nap times. Most important, she was once again smiling, laughing, and looking forward to her family's visits. At the same time, M. broke through her communication barrier by writing notes, nodding yes and no, and interacting as she actively participated in the plan of care. To further her sense of independence, her tube feedings were discontinued once her tracheotomy had healed sufficiently, and she began a regular diet. Giving M. back the ability to eat had a tremendous effect on her already positive mood. The basic things we took for granted meant a lot to M.

Everything seemed promising at this point. I felt good about how our patient–nurse team had shed new light on the situation. Working as a team to help this patient provided the continuity needed to achieve the desired outcomes. Everybody provided encouragement and positive reinforcement to her. The key in this process was involving the patient in planning her own care, instead of dictating her daily activities. Once M. realized that she had a say in what happened, her emotional state improved dramatically.

Unfortunately, just as we were looking forward to recovery and potential weaning from the ventilator, M. suffered respiratory distress and, subsequently, cardiac arrest. Although she was revived, the cardiac arrest was prolonged and the duration of anoxia rendered her neurologically unresponsive.

It is difficult to express what I felt when I came to work the next morning. As I walked past M.'s bed to the conference room, I knew something had happened. I could not believe it, until I heard the report at the bedside myself. Why M.? Why now? I was crushed, disappointed, shocked, and, most of all, angry. I felt as if I had deserted M. I felt I should have been able to somehow prevent this from happening. How could this have happened to a woman who was walking, smiling, laughing, and beginning to realize her potential for recovery? We had made so much progress.

A nurse is supposed to anticipate the unexpected and to be emotionally prepared for this type of outcome, but somewhere along the way, I and many others who were influenced by M.'s situation lost sight of how ill she actually was, because on the surface she had come so far. She radiated hope and success. At the beginning of our nurse–patient relationship, M. wanted to give up on life. Just when she started fighting back toward recovery, she was stripped of her rewards.

M.'s wishes had been made clear in previous patient–family discussions. She did not want to remain on life-support machines and be dependent on the people around her without hope of recovery. Because she had openly discussed life support with her loved ones, their decision was reluctant and painful, but selfless. After several days of watching and waiting, M. showed no signs of neurologic recovery. The family, wishing to abide by M.'s wishes, requested the withdrawal of life support.

It was difficult to work with M. and her family through these last days. To see her lack of neurologic response and her struggle to breathe was especially difficult after the triumphs she and I had experienced. The realization that everyone involved did their professional and personal best to help M. during her cardiac arrest eased the feeling of injustice that I was experiencing. The support of my coworkers helped me to cope and to adjust to her eventual death.

Even though this was a trying case, I am grateful to have had this opportunity. Too often, nurses take themselves for granted. We are true professionals, do an outstanding job, and make a difference in patients' lives. I was touched deeply by M. and her family. Some could say that I became too involved. However, if I had to do it over, I would not change a thing. I have learned a great deal about myself as a person and as a professional. My role as a care manager provided me the opportunity to be intimate with a patient's and family's personal space and to make a difference, even if for a brief time. It was a reminder of the care and compassion that the professional nurse possesses. I will remember this patient for the rest of my nursing career and hope to share the knowledge I gained from the experience with other professionals.

Tracy A. Creechan, RN, BSN, CCRN
Medical ICU
Henry Ford Hospital
Detroit, Michigan

1997 AACN/3M Health Care Excellence in Clinical Practice Award Recipient.

14

Respiratory Anatomy and Physiology

Jo Ann Brooks-Brunn

Objectives

After completing this chapter, the student will be able to

1. Identify the basic structures of the thoracic cage.
2. Describe the muscles of respiration.
3. Discuss the mechanisms for oxygen and carbon dioxide transport.
4. Explain the relationship of ventilation and perfusion in gas exchange.
5. Describe the influence of aging on the respiratory system.

Besides the skin, the respiratory system is the only organ system that is directly exposed to the outside environment. The major function of the respiratory system is gas exchange, to provide oxygen (O_2) to nourish the cells and to remove carbon dioxide (CO_2), the byproduct of aerobic metabolism. Other functions of the respiratory system include acid–base balance, production of enzymes, phonation, water balance, and protective functions.

This chapter first describes the anatomy of the respiratory system, beginning with the most external structures (bony thorax) and then moving inward through the differing structures to the airways and lung tissue. The discussion of the physiology of the respiratory system focuses on the concepts of ventilation, diffusion, and perfusion and the relationships among these concepts as they relate to critical care.

ANATOMY

Bony Thorax

The lungs and mediastinum are located within the chest cage or bony thorax. The bony thorax provides protection to structures of the thoracic cage and is the functional structure necessary for the process of breathing. The chest cage is composed of the sternum, 12 pairs of ribs, and the thoracic vertebrae (Figure 14–1). The sternum is divided into three parts: manubrium, body, and xiphoid process. The top of the manubrium is concave and forms the suprasternal notch that serves as a landmark for the origin of the clavicles laterally. The junction between the manubrium and the body of the sternum is a slightly raised area called the sternal angle or angle of Louis. This anatomic landmark is the approximate location of the carina (bifurcation of the trachea). The carina is discussed in more detail in the section of this chapter on the lower airways. Lateral to the sternal angle is the origin of the second rib. This landmark is important when the critical care nurse needs to count ribs or to locate a certain area of the chest wall.

Ribs 1 to 7 are called the true ribs because they articulate directly with the sternum by the costal cartilages. Ribs 8 through 10 are called the false ribs and articulate with the rib above and not directly with the sternum. Finally, ribs 11 and 12 are called false or floating ribs. These ribs have no skeletal attachment with the sternum, only with the vertebrae. The space between each rib is called the intercostal space and is named by the rib that is superior to or above the space (e.g., second rib, second intercostal space and third rib, third intercostal space).

The 12 thoracic vertebrae form the posterior bony thorax. The posterior basilar aspect of each lung lies at the level of thoracic vertebrae 9 and 10 (T9-T10). Other bony structures, the scapulae, cover a large portion of

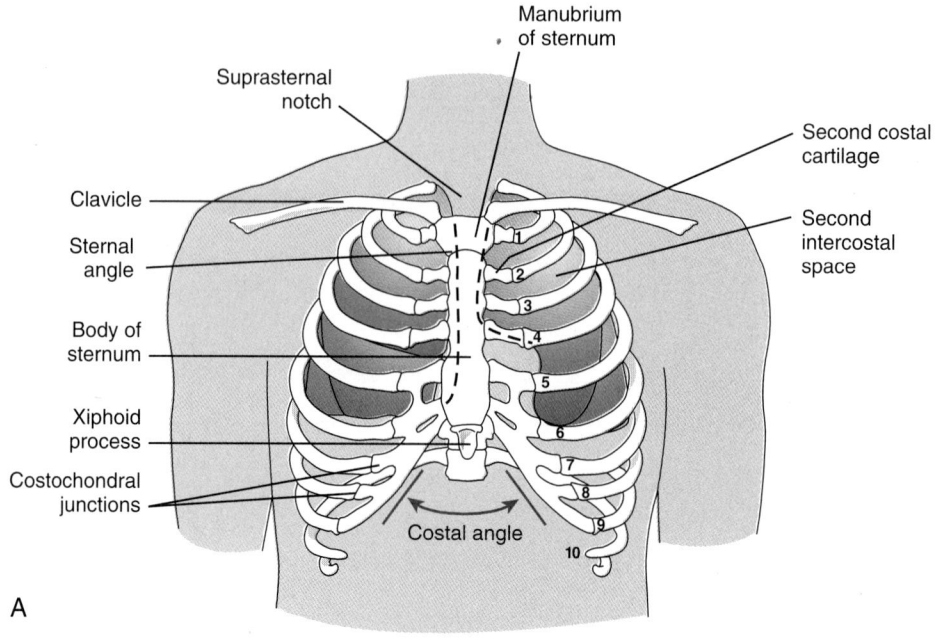

A

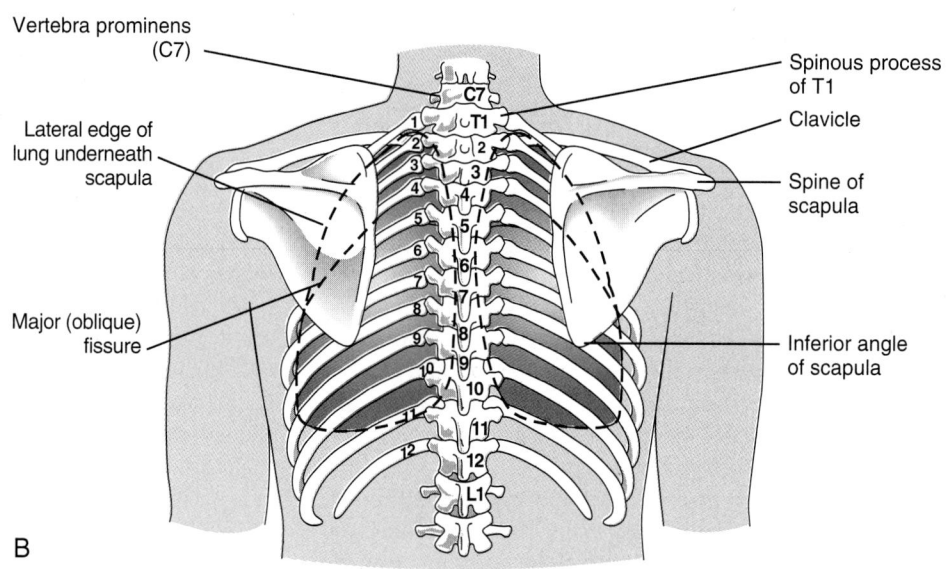

B

Figure 14–1

Structures of the bony thorax. A, Anterior view. B, Posterior view. (Redrawn from Kersten LD: Comprehensive Respiratory Nursing. Philadelphia, W.B. Saunders, 1989, p 12.)

the posterior thorax on each side at the level of ribs 2 through 7.

Clinical applications involving problems or changes in the bony thorax include broken ribs or flail chest from blunt trauma (e.g., steering wheel injury causing a traumatic breakage of two or more ribs in a vertical fashion). With blunt chest trauma, the patient is at risk of injury to lung tissue (pulmonary contusion) and also to the heart, including cardiac contusion and pericardial tamponade. Another clinical example involving the bony thorax is the median sternotomy surgical approach (sternum cut lengthwise with a vertical incision). The median sternotomy is the most widely used thoracic incision. After the procedure, sternal closure is accomplished by wiring the two pieces of the sternum

together. Postoperatively, these wires are visible on chest radiographs.

Respiratory Muscles

Inspiration

Normally, inspiration is an active process (requiring muscular contraction), whereas expiration is a passive process (Table 14–1). The diaphragm and the external intercostal muscles accomplish the major muscular work of ventilation. The diaphragm is a dome-shaped muscle that lies between the thorax and the abdomen and is composed of striated muscle fibers. The right

TABLE 14–1
Muscles of Inspiration and Expiration

Action	Process	Muscles Used
Inspiration	Active, requiring muscular contraction	Diaphragm External intercostals Scalene Sternocleidomastoid Pectoralis major Trapezius
Expiration	Passive, accomplished by relaxation of inspiratory muscles	
	Forced (e.g., cough)	Internal intercostals Abdominal wall muscles

hemidiaphragm is more cephalad or higher in location than the left, because of the position of the liver on the right side.

Anatomically, the diaphragm is considered one muscle; however, it is divided into two hemidiaphragms by a central tendon. Each hemidiaphragm has separate innervation by the phrenic nerves that arise from the third to fourth cervical segments (C3-4). With normal diaphragmatic function, both hemidiaphragms contract synchronously to initiate inspiration. During normal, quiet breathing, the diaphragm descends 1 to 1.5 cm, and with a maximal effort, it descends up to 10 cm.

The diaphragm descends with contraction, resulting in an increased volume of the thoracic cavity. The external intercostal muscles assist in the outward movement of the rib cage during inspiration, as do the scalene, sternocleidomastoid, pectoralis major, and trapezius muscles (muscles known as the accessory muscles of inspiration). These muscles help to elevate the first and second ribs and the sternum, increase the anteroposterior diameter, and elevate the thoracic cage. Accessory muscles are used to assist the diaphragm in the inspiratory process and are frequently used by patients with severe obstructive lung disease or those in acute respiratory distress.

Expiration

In contrast to the active process of inspiration, expiration is normally a passive process accomplished by relaxation of the inspiratory muscles. The normal elastic properties of the lungs and chest wall bring the thorax to its normal resting position at end-expiratory volume when all forces are equal and in opposition. When expiration is forced or labored, the internal intercostal muscles contract and have a net effect of lowering the ribs, thereby assisting with the expiration of

air. The muscles of the abdominal wall are also powerful expiratory muscles. The muscles of expiration are used to generate the expulsive pressure needed to produce a cough or a maximal expiratory effort (e.g., in pulmonary function testing).

Problems or abnormalities of the respiratory muscles that may be seen include phrenic nerve and diaphragmatic dysfunction. After cardiac surgery involving a median sternotomy, the left hemidiaphragm is frequently elevated. Postulated reasons for this elevation are exposure of the phrenic nerve to the hypothermic environment caused by the iced solution sometimes used for myocardial preservation, nerve damage during mobilization of the internal mammary artery, and compression of the phrenic nerve during the operation. Other causes of phrenic nerve dysfunction include crushing traumatic or surgical damage to the nerve. Diaphragmatic paralysis occurs after a high spinal cord injury at C3-4 (loss of phrenic nerve innervation). Finally, diaphragmatic weakness may occur result from nutritional depletion, muscle wasting, or muscular diseases (e.g., amyotrophic lateral sclerosis, muscular dystrophy, Guillain–Barré syndrome).

The mechanical properties of the lung and chest wall are important in a discussion of ventilation. Respiratory muscles generate forces or pressures that produce mechanical alterations in the dimensions of the thoracic cage. To produce these alterations, opposing forces or the resistance of the lung must be overcome (Figure 14–2). During inspiration, air moves by bulk flow from the external environment into the lungs because of pressure differences or gradients within the system (gas moves from an area of higher pressure to one of lower pressure). For air to move from the environment into the lungs, the pressure within the lungs and airways (intrapulmonary pressure) must be lower than the atmospheric pressure.

Compared with spontaneous ventilation, air movement into and out of the lungs occurs differently with positive-pressure mechanical ventilation (the most common type of mechanical ventilation in the critical care unit). With spontaneous breathing, air moves into the lung because of a negative pressure gradient generated by the contraction of the diaphragm. Conversely, with positive-pressure mechanical ventilation (or differing variants of positive-pressure ventilation), air is forced into the lungs by positive pressure. With positive-pressure ventilation, expiration normally occurs as a passive process and is the same as in spontaneous ventilation. Additional information on mechanical ventilation is located in Chapter 17.

Pleural Space

Each lung is covered with two membranes—the parietal pleura, which is the outer membrane, and the vis-

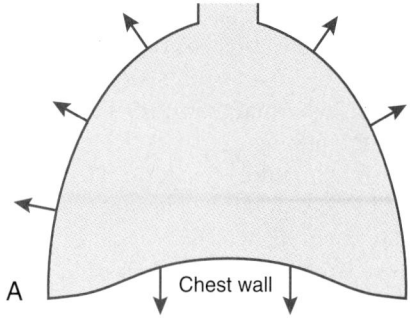

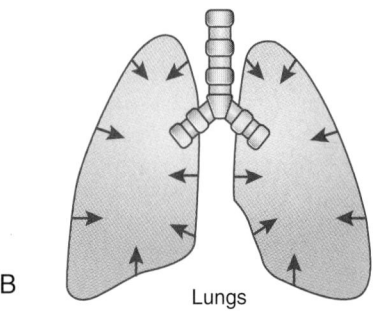

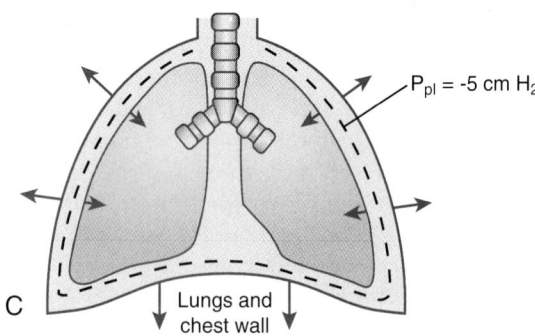

$P_{pl} = -5$ cm H_2O

Figure 14–2

Opposing forces of the chest wall and lungs. These opposing forces are responsible for the negative (subatmospheric) pressure in the pleural space. A, Chest wall. B, Lungs. C, Lungs and chest wall. P_{pl}, pleural pressure. (Redrawn from Kersten LD: Comprehensive Respiratory Nursing. Philadelphia, W.B. Saunders, 1989, p 7.)

ceral pleura, which covers each lung like a sac (Figure 14–3). Both layers join at the root of the lung (hilum) near the center of the mediastinum. The space between the two pleurae is called the pleural space or pleural cavity and is only a potential space. The two pleural surfaces are held together by a thin film of serous fluid that is secreted by the parietal pleura and is absorbed by the visceral pleura in a dynamic fashion. This small amount of fluid allows the two pleurae to slide across each other during the process of breathing.

The natural tendency of the rib cage is to spring outward and that of the lungs is to collapse. To overcome this, the parietal pleura is attached to the rib cage and the visceral pleura is attached to the lung. Thus, a negative or subatmospheric pressure (negative intrapleural pressure, also called pleural pressure or intrathoracic pressure) is created between the two pleurae. This negative intrapleural pressure keeps the lung inflated and against the chest wall during the process of inspiration and expiration (see Figure 14–2).

Pathophysiologic changes in the pleural space are commonly observed in the critical care setting. If air, blood, or other fluid enters the pleural space, the two pleurae will separate. The pleural space is exposed to atmospheric pressure during thoracic surgery or in the presence of a bronchopleural fistula, which is an opening between the bronchus or airways and the pleural space. Disorders or interventions related to the pleural space include pneumothorax, pleural effusion, and chest tube placement. With a pneumothorax, the pleural space is violated or opened to atmospheric pressure, and the subatmospheric intrapleural pressure is lost. The lung collapses either partially or totally. A tension pneumothorax occurs when atmospheric air continues to enter the pleural space. This increasing positive pressure pushes or shifts the trachea and other mediastinal structures away from the affected side. Anatomically, the pleural space for each lung is separate, so both lungs do not collapse if atmospheric pressure enters one of the pleural spaces. Another example

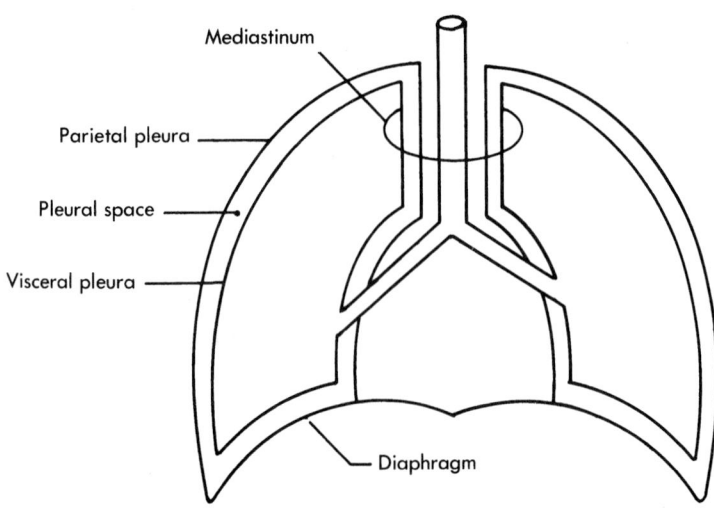

Figure 14–3

The parietal pleura covers the internal portion of the chest cage, diaphragm, and lateral mediastinum. The visceral pleura covers each lung. (From Scanlan CL, Spearman CB, Sheldon RL (eds): Egan's Fundamentals of Respiratory Care, 6th ed. St. Louis, Mosby–Year Book, 1995, p 181.)

is a pleural effusion in which fluid accumulates in the pleural space. Pleural effusion may be due to a disease process, and it is sometimes observed in patients after cardiac or thoracic surgery. Finally, chest tubes are placed in the pleural space to drain fluid or air and to reestablish the negative intrapleural pressure. This procedure allows the lung to reexpand.

Mediastinum

Although not part of the respiratory system, the mediastinum contains organs and tissues in the center of the thoracic cage. These structures include the trachea, the heart, the major or great blood vessels to and from the heart, various nerves, portions of the esophagus, the thymus gland, and lymph nodes. The mediastinum is bordered anteriorly by the sternum, posteriorly by the thoracic vertebrae, and laterally by the right and left lungs.

Clinical situations involving the mediastinal space include surgery for resection of a mediastinal mass or tumor, open heart surgery, and placement of a mediastinal chest tube for postsurgical drainage. A shift of the mediastinal structures may occur with a tension pneumothorax or a large hemothorax. With a tension pneumothorax, positive pressure in the pleural space increases with each breath. The trachea and mediastinal structures are pushed or shifted away from the affected side. Tracheal deviation away from the affected side is a hallmark sign of tension pneumothorax. The increased intrapleural pressure and mediastinal shift may severely compromise cardiac output by compressing both the heart and the great vessels. This condition has the potential to cause cardiac arrest if left untreated.

Lungs

The top portion of each lung is termed the apex and is located approximately 2.5 cm above the clavicles. The base or bottom portion of the lung is located at about the level of the sixth rib. The left lung is divided into 2 lobes (upper and lower), whereas the right lung has three lobes (upper, middle, and lower) (Figure 14–4). The left lung is slightly smaller than the right because of the area of the mediastinum occupied by the heart. Lobes of the lung are further subdivided into a total of 18 segments (8 segments on the left and 10 on the right). One respiratory intervention used in critical care is chest physical therapy or segmental drainage of the lung. Patients are positioned and are treated to optimize drainage of differing segments of the lung.

Thoracic surgical patients are frequently cared for in the critical care setting. Clinical examples of surgical procedures in which differing amounts of lung tissue are removed include wedge resection (removal of a small portion of a segment), segmentectomy (removal of a segment), lobectomy (removal of a lobe), bilobectomy (removal of two lobes on the right side), and pneumonectomy (removal of the entire lung).

Airways

Upper Airway

The upper airway starts at the nose and mouth and ends at the larynx or voice box. The functions of the nose are to warm, to filter, and to humidify inhaled air. The mouth also serves as an entry into the upper respiratory system and offers half the airway resistance of the nose. Thus, breathing through the mouth increases the speed or velocity of air as it moves through the upper airway. The next portion of the upper respiratory system is the pharynx. The pharynx is about 12.5 cm in length and extends from the nose to the esophagus. Artificial airways such as an endotracheal tube or tracheostomy tube bypass the normal humidification mechanism of the upper airway. Thus, additional humidification (cascade humidifier, artificial nose, tracheostomy mask) must be provided when the patient has an artificial airway.

The larynx (voice box) is the transitional area to the lower airway and functions as a conducting channel between the upper and lower airway. It is composed of the glottis (the opening into the larynx), the thyroid cartilage, the cricoid cartilage, the arytenoid cartilage, and the true and false vocal cords. The cricoid cartilage, the only laryngeal cartilage to form a complete ring, is the narrowest portion of the upper airway in infants and small children, whereas the narrowest area in adults is the vocal cords.

Dead space is defined as a portion of the inspired breath that does not participate in gas exchange. The types of dead space are shown in Figure 14–5. The upper airway is considered part of the anatomic dead space ventilation ($V_{D_{an}}$). Anatomic dead space ventilation is that amount of the tidal volume (V_T) that remains in the conducting airways and does not participate in gas exchange. A normal $V_{D_{an}}/V_T$ is less than 0.3, or less than 30% of the tidal volume is dead space ventilation. The conducting airways include the upper airway, trachea, and bronchi to the level of the respiratory bronchioles. Alveolar dead space is described in the section on ventilation and perfusion. A normal $V_{D_{an}}$ is approximately 1 mL/lb (2.0 mL/kg) of ideal body weight. Often, a value of 150 mL is used as an estimate in the adult.

Lower Airway

Trachea. The trachea is the beginning of the lower airway. In the adult, the trachea is 10 to 12 cm in length and 1.5 to 2.5 cm in diameter. It is composed of approximately 20 C-shaped cartilaginous rings with cartilage on the anterior and lateral surface and a thin fibroelastic membrane forming the posterior wall. The

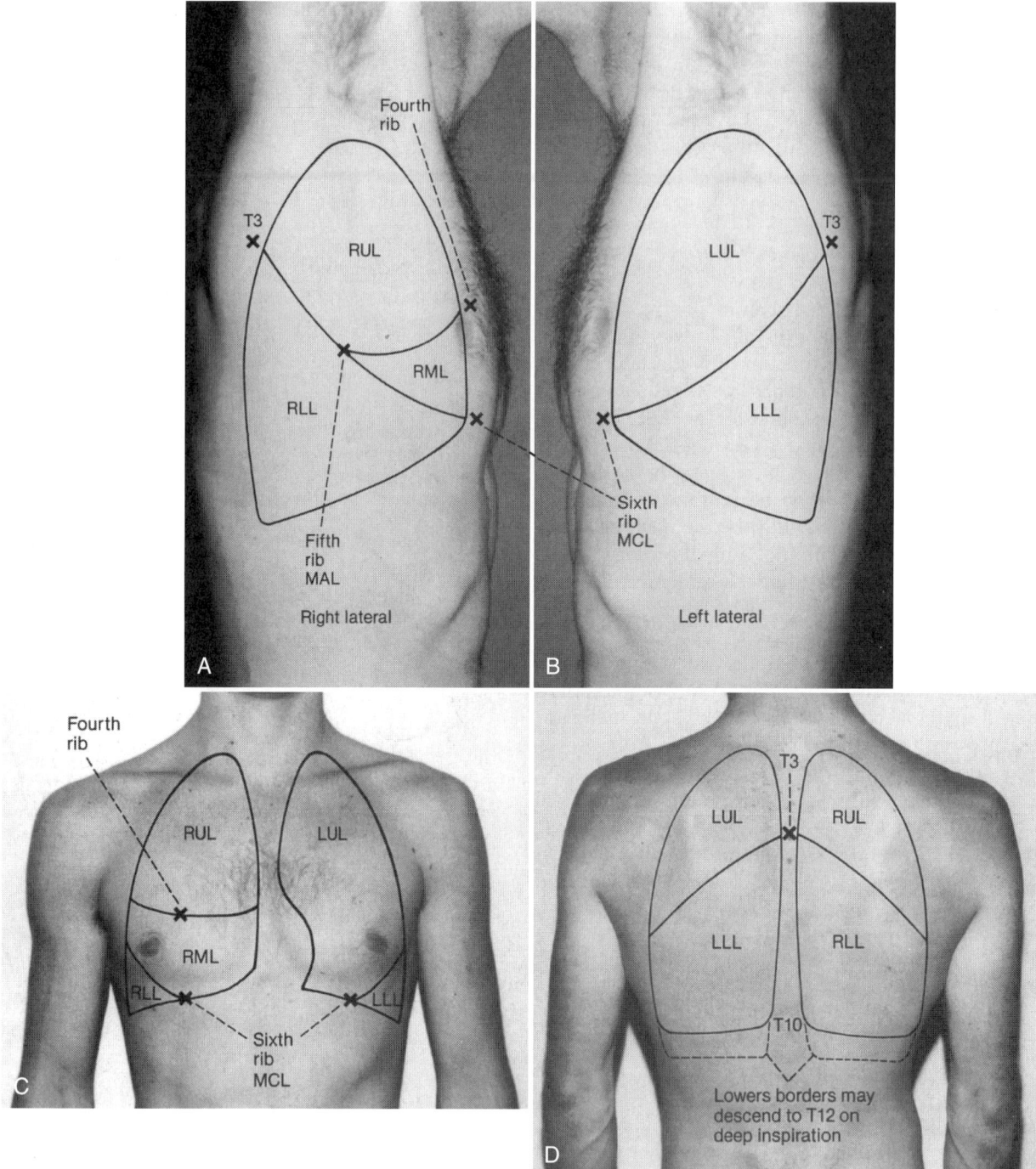

Figure 14–4

Lobes of the lung. A, Right lateral view. B, Left lateral view. C, Anterior view. D, Posterior view. LLL, left lower lobe; LUL, left upper lobe; MAL, midaxillary line; MCL, midclavicular line; RLL, right lower lobe; RML, right middle lobe; RUL, right upper lobe. (From Kersten LD: Comprehensive Respiratory Nursing. Philadelphia, W.B. Saunders, 1989, pp 258–259.)

trachea bifurcates into the left and right main stem bronchus. The point of bifurcation is termed the carina. The left main stem bronchus is angled more sharply (40 to 60°) than the right (25°), is slightly narrower, and is longer by approximately 5 cm (Figure 14–6). This difference in the angle and anatomic structure of the left main stem bronchus is important. Aspiration and accidental intubation of the right main stem

bronchus occurs more frequently because of the lesser anatomic angle on the right side.

Airway Branching. The function of the tracheobronchial tree is to conduct gas down to the alveoli. This structure is formed by 23 to 24 generations of dichotomously branching airways that become sequentially smaller in diameter.[1,2] Generations 0 (the trachea) through 16 are termed the conducting zone because they do not par-

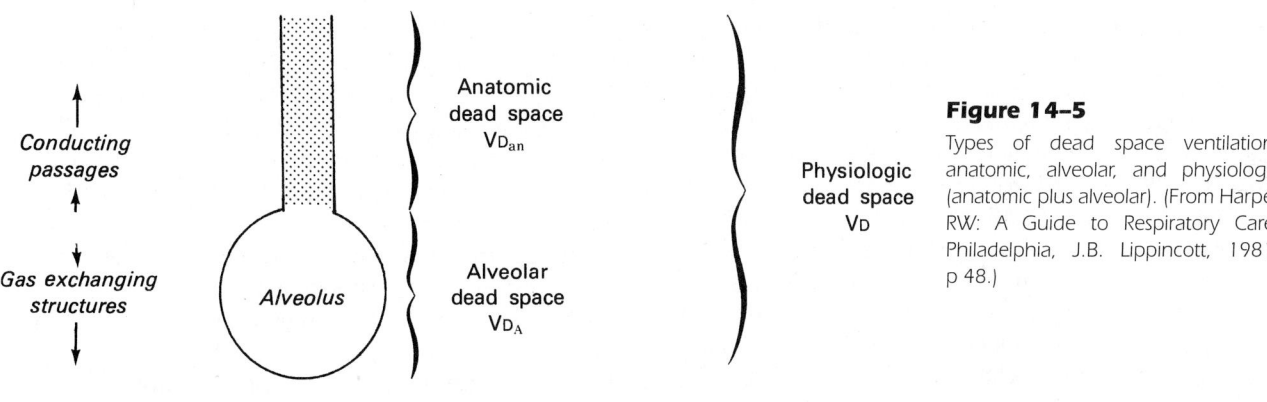

Conducting passages

Gas exchanging structures

Alveolus

Anatomic dead space $V_{D_{an}}$

Alveolar dead space V_{D_A}

Physiologic dead space V_D

Figure 14–5

Types of dead space ventilation: anatomic, alveolar, and physiologic (anatomic plus alveolar). (From Harper RW: A Guide to Respiratory Care. Philadelphia, J.B. Lippincott, 1981, p 48.)

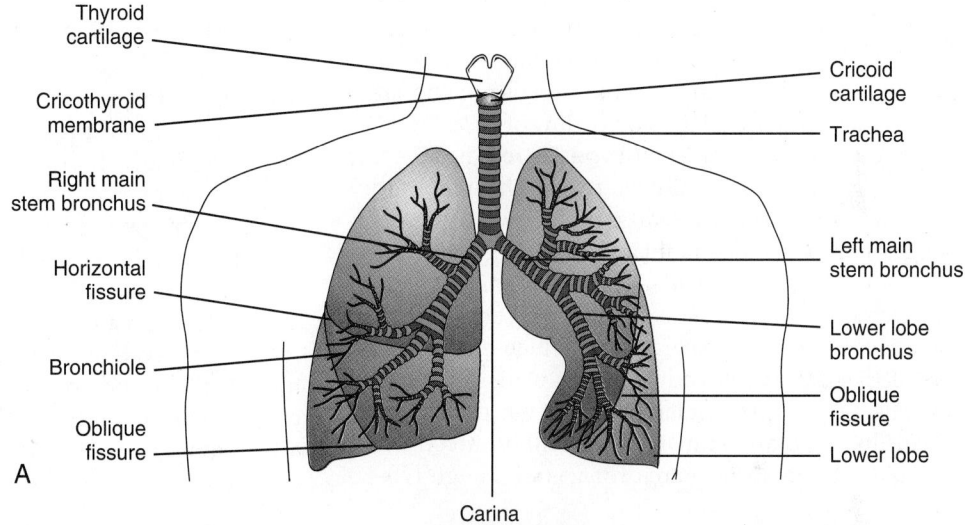

Thyroid cartilage

Cricothyroid membrane

Right main stem bronchus

Horizontal fissure

Bronchiole

Oblique fissure

Cricoid cartilage

Trachea

Left main stem bronchus

Lower lobe bronchus

Oblique fissure

Lower lobe

A

Carina

Figure 14–6

The carina or bifurcation of the trachea. *A,* The trachea is shown in relation to other structures. The left main stem is angled more sharply and is slightly longer than the right main stem. *B,* The trachea is shown in relation to the anterior chest wall. (A. From Jacob SW, Francone CA: Elements of Anatomy and Physiology, 2nd ed. Philadelphia, W.B. Saunders, 1989, p 230; B, From Bates BA: Guide to Physical Examination and History Taking, 6th ed. Philadelphia, Lippincott-Raven, 1995, p 235.)

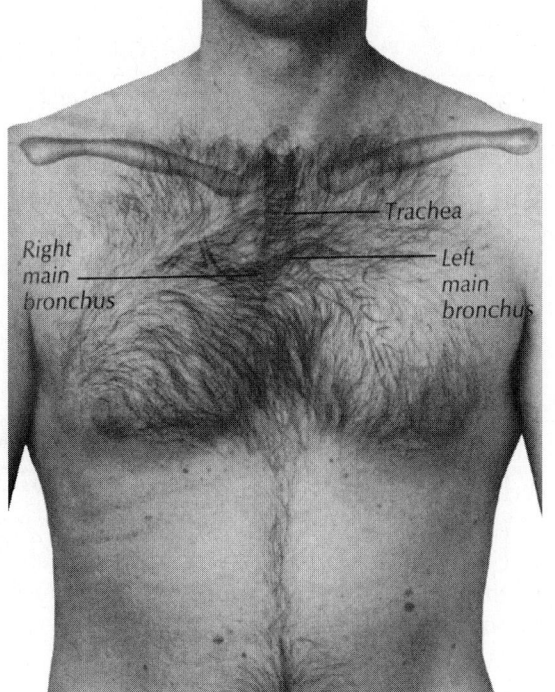

Right main bronchus

Trachea

Left main bronchus

B   ANTERIOR VIEW

ticipate in gas exchange. The conducting zone is composed of the trachea, bronchi, bronchioles, and terminal bronchioles. Generations 17 to 19 are termed the transitional zone and are composed of the respiratory bronchioles that have scattered alveoli throughout their walls. Finally, generations 20 to 28 are considered the respiratory zone where gas exchange takes place and include the alveolar ducts and alveolar sacs (generations 24–28) (Figure 14–7).

It is important to understand the anatomic significance of the numerous generations of branching airways. Airway diameter becomes increasingly smaller with each generation, whereas the total cross-sectional area of airway lumen increases. This configuration provides a rationale for the differing breath sounds heard over the lung. In the larger airways, air flow is more turbulent because of the smaller cross-sectional area and the high air flow (e.g., bronchial breath sounds are loud and coarse). In the numerous smaller airways in the periphery of the lung, sounds heard are laminar (e.g., the soft, rustling vesicular breath sounds) because of the large cross-sectional area and the slower flow of gases.

Respiratory or Gas Exchange Zone. The alveolar ducts serve as a transition between the respiratory bronchioles and the alveolar sacs. The walls are composed of alveoli and contain approximately 50% of the lung alveoli. The alveolar sacs are responsible for approximately 35% of gas exchange. The end points of the airways are the alveolar sacs, which exist in clusters of 15 to 20 alveoli with common walls. This area is responsible for approximately 65% of gas exchange.[3]

Adults have an estimated 300 million alveoli that provide a huge surface area for gas exchange (70–80 m²).[4] The alveoli are composed of type I, type II, and type III (macrophage) cells. Type I cells provide the structure for the alveoli and are composed of a single layer of squamous epithelial cells. Type II cells are cuboidal and produce the fluid lining the alveoli, surfactant. Type III cells are called macrophages and serve a protective function.

For optimal gas exchange to occur, alveoli that are ventilated must be perfused by the pulmonary capillaries. If alveoli are ventilated but not perfused with blood, this is termed alveolar dead space (V_{D_A}) (see Figure 14–5). An example of a disease process causing alveolar dead space is pulmonary embolism. Ventilation to the lung continues, but a blood clot or some other type of obstruction impairs perfusion to an area of the lung.

Defense Mechanisms

The respiratory system has several defense mechanisms to filter and remove particles inhaled with the 10,000 to 30,000 L of air inspired each day.[1] Particles that are more than 5 μm in diameter are usually filtered out in the nasopharynx or oropharynx, whereas particles less than 1 μm in diameter are trapped in the tracheobronchial tree or distal airways.

Cough is an important defense mechanism of the respiratory system. Irritation or stimulation of receptors in the upper or lower respiratory system may cause a sneeze or cough. The explosive expiration of air with a sneeze or cough helps to move the irritant and mucus out of the respiratory system. Cough may

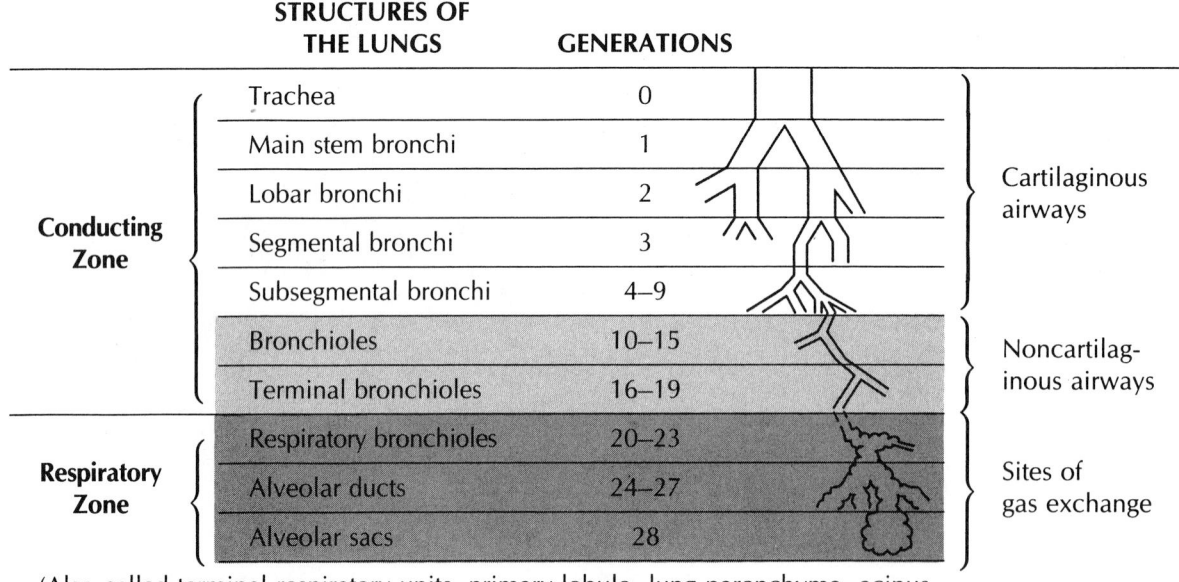

STRUCTURES OF
THE LUNGS   GENERATIONS

		GENERATIONS	
Conducting Zone	Trachea	0	Cartilaginous airways
	Main stem bronchi	1	
	Lobar bronchi	2	
	Segmental bronchi	3	
	Subsegmental bronchi	4–9	
	Bronchioles	10–15	Noncartilaginous airways
	Terminal bronchioles	16–19	
Respiratory Zone	Respiratory bronchioles	20–23	Sites of gas exchange
	Alveolar ducts	24–27	
	Alveolar sacs	28	

(Also called terminal respiratory units, primary lobule, lung parenchyma, acinus, and functional units)

Figure 14–7

Major structures and generations of the airways from the trachea to the alveolar sacs. (From Des Jardins T: Cardiopulmonary Anatomy and Physiology, 2nd ed. Albany, NY, Delmar Publishers, 1993, p 21.)

be impaired in the critically ill patient because of an artificial airway, excessive sedation, or pain.

The mechanism to remove the filtered particles in the lower airway is called the mucociliary transport system (also known as the mucociliary escalator). The area from the upper airway to the level of the terminal bronchioles is lined with mucus-covered epithelium. Normally, 100 mL of mucus is produced per day by the goblet cells and mucus-secreting glands in the lower airway. This mucus serves a protective mechanism because inhaled particles are trapped in the mucus lining the airways. The mucous blanket is moved continuously toward the upper airway by the cilia lining the airways. There are approximately 200 cilia per cell. These tiny, hairlike projections beat or move at frequencies between 1000 and 1500 beats per minute to move the mucus toward the upper airway, where it is swallowed, expectorated, or removed by blowing the nose.[4] The mucous blanket moves rapidly (1–2 cm/min) and allows clearing of normal, healthy adult lungs in less than 20 minutes.[3] In the critically ill patient, mechanisms that may impair normal mucociliary clearance include artificial airways, impaired cough, decreased level of consciousness, general anesthesia, excessive amounts of secretions, and supine positioning. Finally, particles that reach the terminal respiratory units may be removed through engulfment or ingestion by alveolar macrophages, through enzymatic breakdown by lysozymes, through removal by the lymphatic system, or through immunologic reactions (antibody-mediated or cell-mediated responses).[1]

Blood Supply

Pulmonary Circulation

The pulmonary circulation is defined as the vascular system that conducts blood flow from the right side of the heart through the lungs (Figure 14–8). Although the primary function of the pulmonary circulation is gas exchange, other functions include a reservoir for the left side of the heart, protection (to filter emboli before they reach the systemic circulation), and nourishment to the alveolar tissue. The pulmonary circulation is composed of the following: outflow of the right ventricle, two pulmonary arteries (one to each lung), a pulmonary capillary bed, and two pulmonary veins from each lung into the left atrium. The pulmonary arteries carry deoxygenated (poorly oxygenated) blood to the lungs, and the pulmonary veins deliver oxygenated blood to the left side of the heart. The total amount of blood in the pulmonary circulation is 250 to 300 mL/m^2 of body surface area, with 60% located in the pulmonary veins, 30% in the pulmonary arteries, and 10% in the pulmonary capillary bed at any point in time. More than 280 billion pulmonary capillaries are available for gas exchange.[4]

Two examples of abnormalities or problems related to the pulmonary circulation are pulmonary edema and pulmonary embolism. Pulmonary edema occurs when the pulmonary capillary bed becomes engorged because of excessive fluid overload or left ventricular dysfunction that causes a backup of blood in the pulmonary circulation. Pulmonary embolism is discussed in detail in Chapter 19.

Bronchial Artery Circulation

The bronchial artery circulation is the second circulatory system of the respiratory system, but it is not involved in gas exchange. The blood flow of the bronchial artery circulation involves about 1 to 2% of the output of the left ventricle and arises from the aorta or intercostal arteries.[5] The bronchial artery circulation provides arterial blood to nourish the tracheobronchial tree down to the level of the terminal bronchioles and also provides partial blood flow to the hilar lymph nodes, visceral pleura, and esophagus.

Figure 14–8
The relationship between the pulmonary and systemic circulation. (From Leff AR, Schumacker PT: Respiratory Physiology: Basics and Applications. Philadelphia, W.B. Saunders, 1993, p 57.)

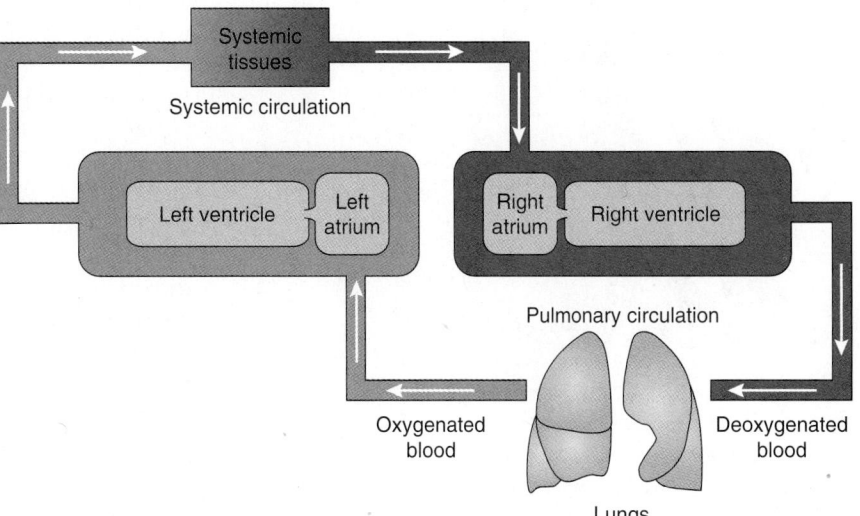

The bronchial circulation is one source of extrapulmonary shunt. A shunt is blood that bypasses the normal gas exchange process. Bronchial venous blood (deoxygenated) drains into the pulmonary circulation downstream (or after it has left the gas exchange–alveolar area). Thus, the deoxygenated bronchial venous blood mixes with the well-oxygenated blood in the pulmonary veins. This process is called venous admixture or anatomic shunt and involves 3 to 5% of the cardiac output. Thus, 3 to 5% of the cardiac output does not participate in gas exchange in the normal lung.

Alveolar–Capillary Unit

Given the 300 million alveoli and 280 billion capillaries in the normal adult, there are approximately 1000 capillaries per alveolus. Diffusion of gases is optimized by the huge surface area for gas exchange along with the relatively thin barrier (0.04 μm) between the alveolar wall and the capillary. Oxygen must transverse the following barriers to reach the pulmonary capillary: surfactant, alveolar epithelium, basement membrane, and capillary endothelium (Figure 14–9). Carbon dioxide moves through these barriers in the opposite direction.

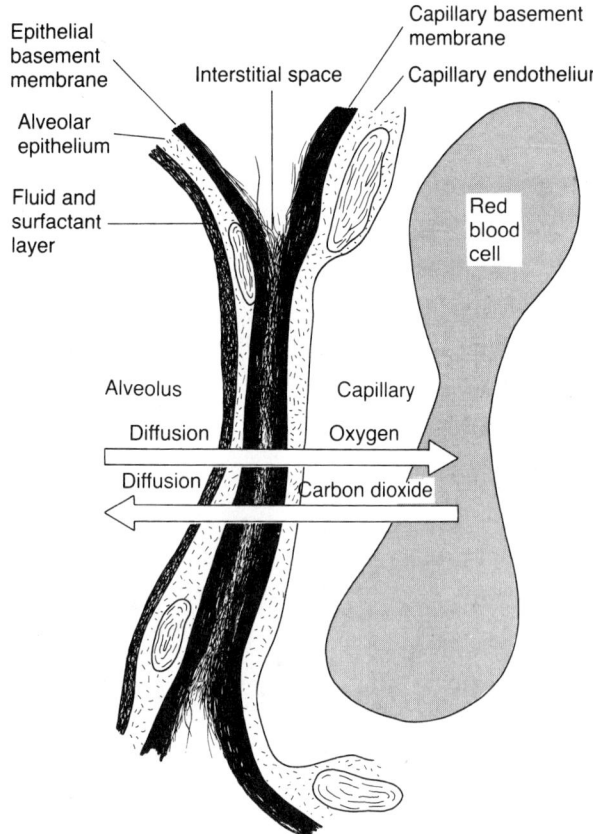

Figure 14–9

Alveolar–capillary unit and the movement of oxygen and carbon dioxide. (From Guyton AC: Textbook of Medical Physiology, 8th ed. Philadelphia, W.B. Saunders, 1991, p 429.)

PHYSIOLOGY

Ventilation

Ventilation is the process by which air moves into and out of the lungs. Alterations in ventilatory control or lung mechanics may cause problems in the normal process of ventilation. The act of breathing is spontaneous and is normally accomplished without effort or voluntary awareness. The process of diaphragmatic movement to accomplish the movement of air into and out of the lung is described earlier in the section on respiratory muscles.

Control of Breathing

Central Control

Control of breathing refers to the generation and regulation of breathing by the respiratory center in the brain stem, with modification by the input from higher brain centers and systemic receptors.[1] The control of breathing (rate and pattern) is composed of numerous complex interactions and the integration of neural impulses and chemical responses.

Unlike the spontaneous contraction of the muscles of the heart, the muscles of respiration require a neural innervation for each breath. Groups of neurons located in the medulla and pons generate spontaneous breathing. In the medulla oblongata is the respiratory control center, with several groups of nerve cells that act to generate or modify the basic rhythmic ventilatory pattern. The dorsal group of neurons provides rhythmic drive to the contralateral phrenic motor neurons. The ventral group provides input into the accessory muscles and intercostal muscles.

Chemoreceptors

The two types of chemoreceptors involved in the control of breathing are central and peripheral. The central chemoreceptors account for 70 to 80% and are hypothesized to be located below the ventrolateral surface of the medulla. They detect changes in hydrogen ion (H^+ ion) concentration and pH of the brain stem interstitial fluid. Neither H^+ ion nor bicarbonate (HCO_3^-) can cross the blood–brain barrier or the blood–cerebrospinal fluid barrier. However, carbon dioxide easily crosses these barriers and goes through an interaction with final dissociation into H^+ and HCO_3^-. The H^+ ion concentration in the brain interstitial fluid parallels carbon dioxide levels.[1] Increased levels of carbon dioxide (>45 mm Hg) and thus increased H^+ ion levels stimulate respiratory drive, whereas lower than normal levels (<35 mm Hg) decrease the drive to breathe.

Peripheral chemoreceptors are located in the aortic arch (aortic bodies) and at the bifurcation of the carotid arteries in the neck (carotid bodies). These peripheral chemoreceptors sense partial pressure of arterial oxygen (PaO_2), partial pressure of arterial carbon dioxide ($PaCO_2$), and pH of arterial blood. Information regarding high or low amounts of PaO_2, $PaCO_2$, and pH are transmitted back to the medulla by the cranial and vagus nerves, to modulate breathing pattern and depth further.

Lung Volumes and Capacities

The amount of air that the lungs can accommodate is divided into four volumes: tidal volume, inspiratory reserve volume, expiratory reserve volume, and residual volume. Combinations of differing lung volumes are termed capacities. Definitions of these volumes and capacities are described in Figure 14–10.

Distribution of Ventilation

The distribution of the gases with each breath has regional differences. When a patient is in the standing, upright position, alveoli in the upper portions (apices) of each lung are partially distended because of gravitational pull. In contrast, the alveoli at the base of each lung are less distended. Thus, the uppermost alveoli can expand less with inspiration during a normal breathing cycle than can the alveoli in the lower portions of each lung (Figure 14–11). In the supine posi-

tion, the distribution of ventilation is equal in the apical and basilar areas.

Lung Mechanics

Airway Resistance. Airway resistance is defined as the resistance produced in the airways by the movement of air from the environment through the upper and lower respiratory system to the alveolar level. Approximately 25 to 40% of resistance to air flow is located in the upper airway. The small airways have a large cross-sectional area for flow, and at this level, airway resistance is extremely low during normal breathing. The airways that provide the greatest resistance during normal breathing are the medium-sized bronchi.

Physical factors for airway resistance include changes during inspiration and expiration and lung volume. During inspiration, airway resistance is lower because the airways widen or dilate as a result of the lung expansion. During expiration, airway resistance is increased as the airways narrow. Resistance is also related to lung volume. As lung volume increases, airway resistance decreases. Other factors that may increase airway resistance include inflammation of the mucosa, accumulation of secretions, bronchospasm, and the presence of a foreign body or an artificial airway.

Elastic Recoil. Elastic recoil is the property of the lung that allows it to return to its resting volume. During inspiration, the muscular forces of the chest

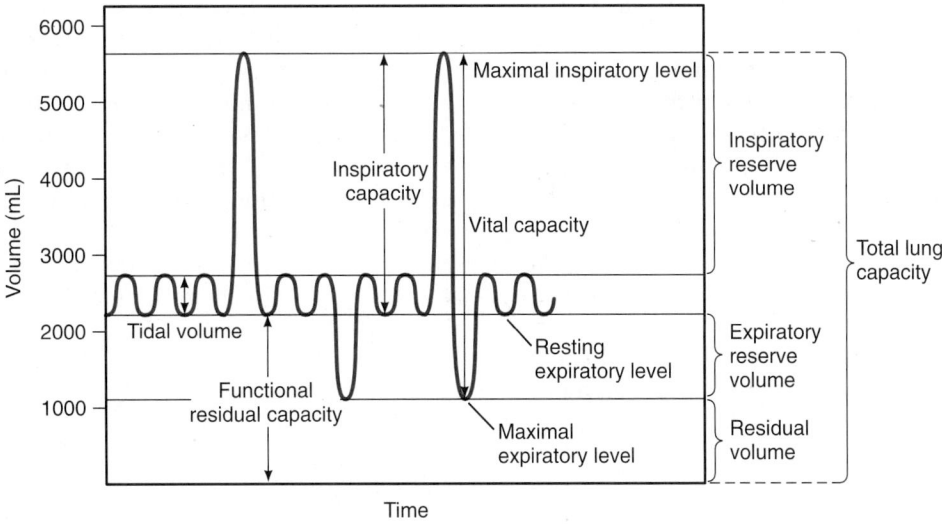

Figure 14–10

Spirometric graph demonstrating lung volumes and capacities. The pulmonary capacities are calculated as follows: inspiratory capacity = tidal volume (TV) + inspiratory reserve volume (IRV); functional residual capacity = expiratory reserve volume (ERV) + residual volume (RV); vital capacity (VC) = IRV + TV + ERV; and total lung capacity = IRV + TV + ERV + RV. TLC (total lung capacity): total amount of air in the lungs after a maximal inspiration; TV (tidal volume): volume of air inhaled or exhaled with each breath during normal breathing; VC (vital capacity): total amount of air exhaled after a maximal inspiration; IC (inspiratory capacity): maximal amount of air that can be inspired after a normal exhalation; IRV (inspiratory reserve volume): maximal volume of air inspired after a normal inspiration; FRC (functional residual capacity): volume of air left in the lungs at the end of a normal expiration; ERV (expiratory reserve volume): maximal volume of air expired after a normal expiration; RV (residual volume): volume of air left in the lungs after a maximal expiration. (From Hansen M: Pathophysiology. Philadelphia, W.B. Saunders, 1998, p 450.)

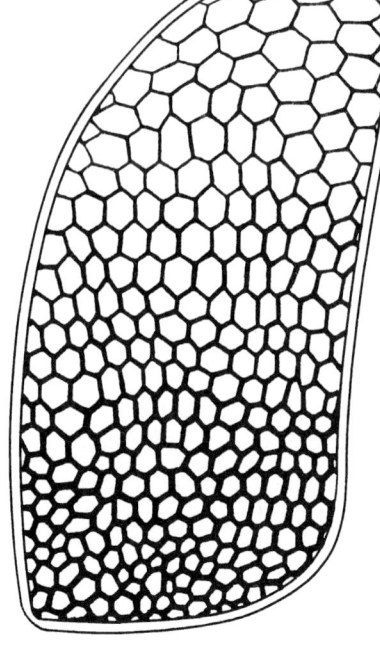

Ventilation

Intrapleural pressure more negative

Greater transmural pressure gradient

Alveoli larger, less compliant

Less ventilation

Perfusion

Lower intravascular pressures

Less recruitment, distention

Higher resistance

Less blood flow

Figure 14–11

Regional differences in ventilation and perfusion in the normal upright lung. (From Levitszky MG: Pulmonary Physiology, 3rd ed. New York, McGraw-Hill, 1991, p 116. Copyright © by McGraw-Hill, Inc. Used by permission of McGraw-Hill Book Company.)

Intrapleural pressure less negative

Smaller transmural pressure gradient

Alveoli smaller, more compliant

More ventilation

Greater intravascular pressures

More recruitment, distention

Lower resistance

Greater blood flow

wall must overcome the elastic recoil for lung expansion to occur (see Figure 14–2). The elastic recoil properties of the lung are referred to in terms of lung compliance. Elastic recoil properties of the lung and lung compliance have an inverse relationship. Lung compliance can be defined as the distensibility of the lung and is measured as the amount of volume change per unit of pressure change across the lung. As the elastic recoil of the lung is decreased, lung compliance is increased (less pressure is needed to generate a specific volume).

The total compliance of the respiratory system has two components: the chest wall and the lungs. Chest wall compliance is influenced by the characteristics of the thoracic cage and respiratory muscles, and lung compliance is characterized by the elastic properties of the lung as well as the airflow resistance. An example of a disease that increases total compliance (less pressure needed to generate a specific volume) is chronic obstructive lung disease. Examples of diseases or problems that decrease total compliance (increased pressure needed to generate a specific volume) are acute respiratory distress syndrome, pulmonary edema, restrictive lung diseases, and morbid obesity.

Perfusion

Control

The dense networks of pulmonary capillaries around the alveolus provide an efficient arrangement for gas exchange. The capillaries have thin walls and only a small amount of smooth muscle, features that make

them subject to collapse or distention, depending on the pressures within or around them. During exercise or in diseases causing increased cardiac output, the pulmonary capillary bed is able to accommodate these increases in blood flow because of distensibility and recruitment. As perfusion pressure increases, the capillary walls distend to accommodate blood flow. Recruitment refers to the opening of capillaries that are collapsed or closed under normal conditions. Recruitment is thought to occur with small increases in pulmonary vascular pressure and distention at higher pressures.[4] The pulmonary vasculature is responsive to neural and humoral stimuli. Both the sympathetic and parasympathetic arms of the autonomic nervous system influence the pulmonary vasculature, with greater innervation of the larger vessels as compared with the smaller vessels. Substances such as epinephrine, norepinephrine, serotonin, histamine, and prostaglandins all influence pulmonary vascular resistance. In addition, low oxygen levels (hypoxemia) and increased carbon dioxide levels (hypercapnia) increase pulmonary vasculature resistance.

Distribution

Perfusion of the lung depends on gravity, cardiac output, and pulmonary vascular resistance. As in ventilation, the distribution of perfusion in the lungs is not equal at the apex and the base. In the upright position, most blood flow goes to the lung base rather than the apex (see Figure 14–11). When a patient is in the supine position, blood flow is preferential to the dependent or posterior segments of the lung. When a patient is in the side-lying or lateral position, perfusion is increased to the dependent (down) lung.

In addition, perfusion may be changed by either an increase or a decrease in pulmonary artery pressure or alveolar pressure. Other factors that may alter the distribution of perfusion are intermittent positive-pressure breathing, positive end-expiratory pressure, continuous positive-pressure breathing, removal of lung tissue, or a change in cardiac output.

Ventilation–Perfusion Matching

Perfect matching of ventilation and perfusion (V/Q) would mean that each alveolus would receive an equal amount of ventilation and perfusion (V/Q = 1.0). In reality, total alveolar ventilation is approximately 4 L per minute, whereas capillary blood flow is approximately 5 L per minute, thus producing an overall ratio of ventilation to perfusion of 0.8 (greater perfusion than ventilation). However, differences in V/Q ratios occur throughout the lung. Factors that influence the matching of V/Q include gravity, positioning of the patient, the amount and distribution of ventilation to the alveoli (alveolar ventilation), and the amount and distribution of perfusion to the pulmonary capillary bed (cardiac output).

Optimal matching of V/Q enhances gas exchange. If either perfusion or ventilation is altered, interference with normal gas exchange results. This condition is referred to as a V/Q imbalance or mismatch. The spectrum of V/Q matching is shown in Figure 17–1. Intrapulmonary shunting is one extreme of this spectrum and results when blood perfuses unventilated (collapsed) alveoli; thus, perfusion is wasted, and no gas exchange occurs. A V/Q imbalance can occur when blood perfuses poorly ventilated alveoli. Clinical examples of this include increased airway secretions or bronchospasm.

On the other end of the spectrum is wasted ventilation, also known as alveolar dead space (V_{D_A}). This situation occurs when alveoli are ventilated but not perfused. Thus, ventilation to the area is wasted (dead space ventilation), and no gas exchange takes place. A clinical example of this condition is pulmonary embolism. A V/Q imbalance can also occur when alveoli are ventilated but perfusion to the area is decreased.

The respiratory system attempts to compensate for areas of V/Q imbalance in the lung to improve the overall exchange of oxygen and carbon dioxide between the alveoli and capillaries. A formal method used to assess V/Q matching in the lung is V/Q radioisotope scanning. Methods used at the bedside include calculation of the A–a oxygen gradient (alveolar–arterial oxygen difference), shunt studies to quantify the amount of blood bypassing the normal gas exchange units, and measures of dead space ventilation (the proportion of each breath not participating in gas exchange).

Diffusion

Diffusion refers to the passive transfer of gases to and across the alveolar capillary membrane. It is a passive process because no extra energy is required for the transfer of gas to occur from an area of higher partial pressure to an area of lower partial pressure. The major determinant of the rate of diffusion is the partial pressure gradient (the larger the gradient or difference, the faster the diffusion). Another factor that influences diffusion is the diffusing properties of the gas. Carbon dioxide diffuses approximately 20 to 24 times more rapidly than does oxygen because of the solubility of carbon dioxide.[4–6] Therefore, clinical problems with carbon dioxide diffusion at the alveolar capillary level are seen less frequently than are problems with oxygen (see Figure 14–9).

The surface area of the membrane is also important in diffusion. Factors affecting the surface area for diffusion include changes in lung volume, changes in pulmonary capillary perfusion, and loss of lung tissue. The thickness of the membrane must also be considered, because increasing the thickness of the membrane impairs the diffusion of gases. Two clinical examples that impair diffusion of gases are interstitial edema and fibrotic thickening of the alveolar–capillary membrane.

Gas Transport

Oxygen Transport Mechanisms. Oxygen moves through the alveolar–capillary membrane, where it combines with hemoglobin or remains dissolved in the plasma. Transport of oxygen by either method depends on the Pa_{O_2}. Hemoglobin combined with oxygen is called oxyhemoglobin, and unoxygenated hemoglobin is referred to as deoxyhemoglobin or reduced hemoglobin. Hemoglobin accounts for approximately 97% of the total amount of oxygen carried in the blood. Each gram of hemoglobin can combine with 1.34 mL of oxygen at 37°C. The amount of oxygen carried in combination with hemoglobin is described by the saturation of hemoglobin with oxygen (Sa_{O_2}). Factors that can influence oxygen transport by hemoglobin include decreased hemoglobin level (anemia), carbon monoxide (binds more quickly with hemoglobin than does oxygen), methemoglobin (does not combine with oxygen), and variant hemoglobins (those other than hemoglobin A or adult hemoglobin).

The amount of oxygen dissolved in the plasma is small (3%) compared with the amount carried by the hemoglobin and is described by the Pa_{O_2}. At a temperature of 37°C, normal arterial blood with a Pa_{O_2} of 100 mm Hg contains only about 0.003 mL of oxygen per milliliter of blood (0.3 mL of oxygen per 100 mL of blood). The blood oxygen content is expressed in milliliters of oxygen per 100 mL of blood (referred to as volumes percent). Terms used to describe aspects of oxygen content are similar, but they have unique differences. Additional information on assessment of oxygen is located in Chapter 16.

Oxyhemoglobin Dissociation Curve. The amount of oxygen carried in physical solution is a linear relationship, whereas the amount of oxygen carried with hemoglobin (oxyhemoglobin) is nonlinear. The relationship between the PaO_2 and the SaO_2 is described as the oxyhemoglobin dissociation curve (Figure 14–12). This curve is derived by plotting incremental PaO_2 values versus the amount of oxygen in combination with hemoglobin (percentage of saturation). The **S** or sigmoidal shape of this curve is important to understand. The flat upper portion demonstrates that, for small decreases in the PaO_2, the SaO_2 remains relatively constant. However, as shown on the steep midportion of the curve, for a PaO_2 that is less than 60 mm Hg, a significant drop in SaO_2 will occur.

The position of the oxyhemoglobin dissociation curve is not fixed and may be affected by many factors, as shown in Figure 14–12. A shift to the right (decreased affinity of hemoglobin and oxygen) reflects that oxygen is unloaded rapidly by hemoglobin at the tissue level, and the hemoglobin at the lung level picks up less oxygen. A shift to the left (increased affinity of hemoglobin and oxygen) means that less oxygen is released at the tissue level, but increased oxygen is loaded on the hemoglobin at the lung level. Either of these conditions affects oxygen transport and delivery.[7]

Diffusion of Oxygen. At sea level and room temperature, the partial pressure of alveolar oxygen (PAO_2) is about 100 mm Hg, whereas the partial pressures of mixed venous blood oxygen (PvO_2) is 40 mm Hg. Thus, a large diffusion gradient of 60 mm Hg

between the alveolar gas and returning venous blood facilitates the movement of oxygen from the alveolus into the pulmonary capillary (Figure 14–13).

As blood leaves the lung and enters the systemic capillaries, it is exposed to lower PO_2 levels of the tissues, and the oxygen is released. Tissues have varying oxygenation needs. Unloading at the tissue level is also facilitated or impaired by the position of the oxyhemoglobin dissociation curve.

Carbon Dioxide. Carbon dioxide and water are the major end products of cellular metabolism and are continuously produced by all cells in tissues. The average person produces carbon dioxide at a rate of approximately 200 to 250 mL per minute.[4] In the critically ill patient, carbon dioxide production may be greatly increased.

Carbon dioxide is transported by three methods: 1) being dissolved in the plasma (5–10%); 2) being chemically combined to amino acids in blood proteins (5–10%); and 3) as HCO_3^- (70–90%) (Figure 14–14). Carbon dioxide is 20 to 24 times more soluble in plasma than is oxygen. Thus, dissolved carbon dioxide plays a significant role in transport, as compared with the role of dissolved oxygen in oxygen transport. Each 100 mL of blood contains about 2.4 mL of carbon dioxide in physical solution.[4]

Carbon dioxide transported as HCO_3^- is formed through a chemical reaction. While in the plasma, the

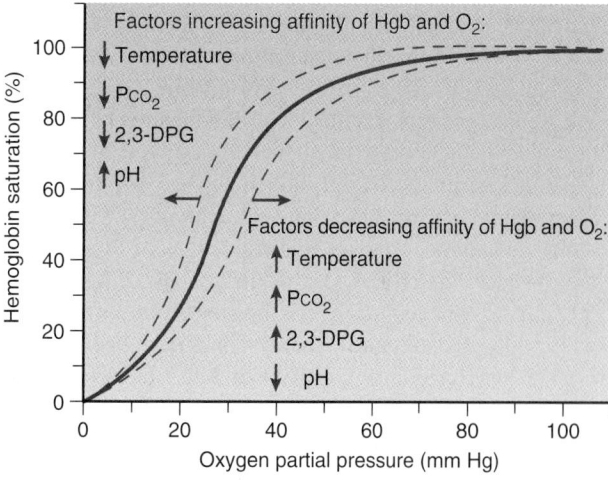

Figure 14–12

Oxyhemoglobin dissociation curve and situations that cause a left shift (increased affinity of oxygen and hemoglobin) and right shift (decreased affinity of hemoglobin and oxygen). 2,3-DPG, 2,3-diphosphoglycerate; Hgb, hemoglobin; O_2, oxygen; PCO_2, partial pressure of carbon dioxide. (From Leff AR, Schumacker PT: Respiratory Physiology: Basics and Applications. Philadelphia, W.B. Saunders, 1993, p 78.)

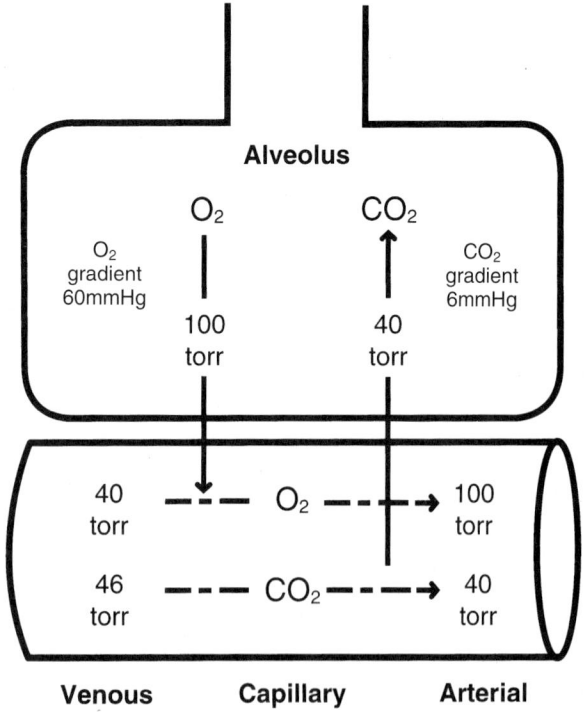

Figure 14–13

Diffusion gradients for oxygen (O_2) and carbon dioxide (CO_2) from the venous to arterial side of the capillary. (From Scanlon CL, Spearman CB, Sheldon RL (eds): Egan's Fundamentals of Respiratory Care, 6th ed. St. Louis, Mosby–Year Book, 1995, p 268.)

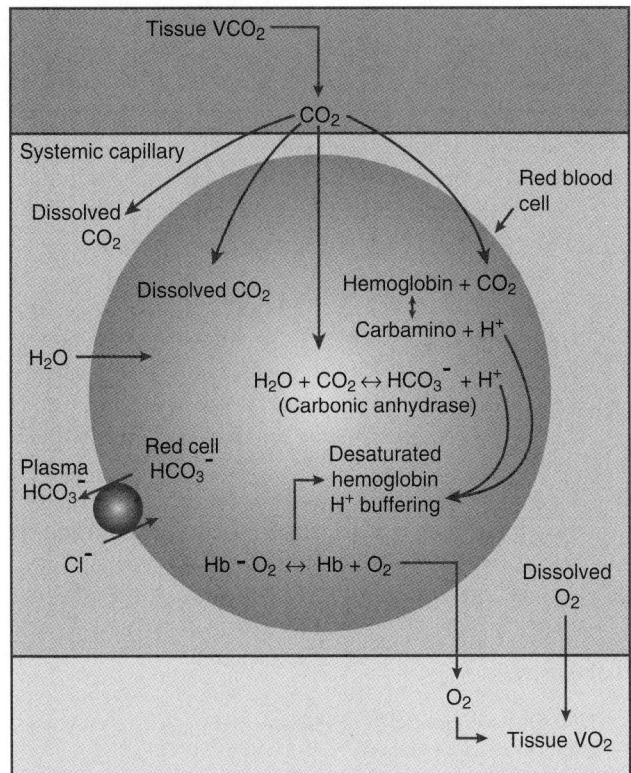

Figure 14-14

Mechanisms of oxygen (O_2) and carbon dioxide (CO_2) transport in the blood. Hb, hemoglobin; V_{CO_2}, carbon dioxide output. (From Leff AR, Schumacker PT: Respiratory Physiology: Basics and Applications. Philadelphia, W.B. Saunders, 1993, p 81.)

carbon dioxide enters the red blood cell, and under the influence of carbonic anhydrase (CA), it forms carbonic acid (H_2CO_3), which then dissociates to form H^+ and HCO_3^-. Carbonic anhydrase is an enzyme present in high concentrations in the red blood cell that serves as a catalyst to make this reaction occur quickly.

The formation for transport of CO_2 to the lung for removal is as follows:

$$CO_2 + H_2O \xrightarrow{\hspace{1.5cm}} H_2CO_3 \leftrightarrow HCO_3^- + H^+$$

As H^+ and HCO_3^- are formed, an accumulation of HCO_3^- occurs within the red blood cell. Some HCO_3^- diffuses into the plasma, where it is carried in this form. To maintain electron neutrality, as HCO_3^- diffuses into the plasma, chloride anions move into the red blood cell (the chloride shift). At the lungs, the equation moves in the opposite direction, and carbon dioxide is released.

The reverse of the equation, for release of carbon dioxide at lung level, is as follows:

$$CO_2 + H_2O \xleftarrow{\hspace{1.5cm}} H_2CO_3 \leftrightarrow HCO_3^- + H^+$$

The chloride shift once again occurs, this time into the plasma, to maintain electron neutrality (see Figure 14-14).

The carbamino compounds are formed when carbon dioxide combines with the terminal amine groups in blood proteins. Most of the carbon dioxide is bound to the amino acids of hemoglobin. As the venous blood returns to the lung, the hemoglobin picks up oxygen and releases carbon dioxide from the terminal amine groups.

The diffusion time course for carbon dioxide movement from the capillary to the alveolus is similar to that of oxygen; equilibrium is achieved in about 0.25 seconds. Although the diffusion gradient for carbon dioxide is only about 6 mm Hg (capillary P_{VCO_2} 46 mm Hg → alveolar P_{ACO_2} 40 mm Hg), as previously stated, the solubility coefficient of carbon dioxide is 20 to 24 times that of oxygen. Perfusion, rather than problems with diffusion, usually limits carbon dioxide transport. However, in some circumstances with abnormal alveolar–capillary membranes, carbon dioxide transport may be limited by diffusion.

AGING AND THE LUNG

With the aging process, the lung undergoes identifiable and predictable changes. The shape of the chest wall changes, with an increase in the anteroposterior diameter. This configuration is similar to the "barrel chest" observed in the patient with chronic obstructive lung disease.

Physiologically, pulmonary function decreases with advancing age. Both static and dynamic properties of the lung undergo changes. The elasticity of the lung tissue decreases, and compliance increases. Because of these changes, lung volumes also change. The vital capacity decreases to approximately 70% of the baseline (age 17) value by the time a person reaches age 80 years. The residual volume increases nearly 50% during the same time span. Overall, the total lung capacity may remain constant or may decrease slightly because of the usual decrease in body height resulting from flattening of the vertebral discs. The dynamic properties of the lung also change with aging. Because of the decrease in elasticity, maximal air flow rates decrease with advancing age, especially at low lung volumes.[8]

The distribution of ventilation is also altered with advancing age. This change is primarily due to the earlier airway closure or elevated closing volume. In the elderly, the closing volume may be larger than the functional residual capacity. Therefore, some dependent airways may be closed, and the respiratory units supplied will not be continuously ventilated during normal tidal breathing. In the critical care setting, this phenomenon may be exaggerated by supine positioning, decreased tidal volume due to muscular weakness, analgesics, or sedatives. Elderly persons may be prone to altered drug metabolism and analgesic effects that may exacerbate respiratory depression.

The efficiency of gas exchange decreases progressively with age. These changes are due to a small increase in anatomic dead space, but, more important, they result from V/Q mismatching and the decrease in diffusing capacity across the alveolar–capillary membrane. Alveolar dead space increases with advancing age, probably because of the decreased cardiac index associated with aging and structural changes in the pulmonary capillaries.

Changes in the mechanisms of gas exchange lead to a reduction of the normal arterial oxygen tension with aging. At sea level, an acceptable range for persons between 60 and 90 years of age can be calculated by subtracting 1 mm Hg from the minimal P_{O_2} level of 80 mm Hg for every year over age 60. This new "normal" Pa_{O_2} level must be interpreted along with the person's clinical status for acceptable oxygenation. A decreased hemoglobin level may impair oxygenation. Anemia is a common finding in the elderly. Factors that may contribute to anemia include slowed absorption of iron, poor nutrition, and changes in the red bone marrow. In comparison, the Pa_{CO_2} remains constant throughout the life span. This phenomenon can be explained by the increased ability of carbon dioxide to diffuse across the alveolar–capillary membrane.

Key Concepts

➥ The primary function of the respiratory system is gas exchange of oxygen and carbon dioxide.

➥ The main function of gas exchange occurs at the alveolar–capillary level by the process of diffusion. With diffusion, gases move from an area of higher pressure to one of lower pressure.

➥ Oxygen is transported primarily in combination with hemoglobin. The saturation of hemoglobin and oxygen is influenced by the partial pressure of oxygen in the arterial blood (dissolved form of oxygen). This relationship is called the oxyhemoglobin dissociation curve and is influenced by numerous factors such as temperature, pH, and acid–base balance.

➥ The three processes that are vital to gas exchange are ventilation, diffusion, and perfusion. The interrelationship of these three processes influences gas exchange.

➥ Problems with V/Q matching in the lung are common in critical care. V/Q ratios differ, depending on the area of the lung and factors such as positioning, pathophysiologic processes that influence ventilation or perfusion, and mechanical ventilation.

➥ Intrapulmonary shunting occurs when perfusion is present in an area of the lung, but ventilation is absent. Dead space ventilation occurs when ventilation is present in an area, but perfusion is absent.

References

1. Leff AR, Schumacker PT: Respiratory Physiology: Basics and Applications. Philadelphia, W.B. Saunders, 1993.
2. Dantzer DR, MacIntyre NR, Bakow ED: Comprehensive Respiratory Care. Philadelphia, W.B. Saunders, 1995.
3. Shapiro BA, Kacmarek RM, Cane RD, et al: Clinical Application of Respiratory Care, 4th ed. St. Louis, Mosby–Year Book, 1991.
4. Levitzky MG: Pulmonary Physiology, 3rd ed. New York, McGraw-Hill, 1991.
5. Malik AB, Feustel PJ: Pulmonary circulation and lung fluid and solute exchange. In: Murray JF, Nadel JA (eds): Textbook of Respiratory Medicine, vol 1. Philadelphia, W.B. Saunders, 1994, pp 139–174.
6. West JB: Ventilation, blood flow, and gas exchange. In: Murray JF, Nadel JA (eds): Textbook of Respiratory Medicine, vol 1. Philadelphia, W.B. Saunders, 1994, pp 51–89.
7. Dantzker DR, Scharf SM: Cardiopulmonary Critical Care, 3rd ed. Philadelphia, W.B. Saunders, 1998.
8. Plopper CG, Thurlbeck WM: Growth, aging, and adaptation. In: Murray JF, Nadel JA (eds): Textbook of Respiratory Medicine, vol 1. Philadelphia, W.B. Saunders, 1994, pp 36–49.

15

Respiratory Assessment

Jo Ann Brooks-Brunn

Objectives

After completing this chapter, the student will be able to

1. Obtain a thorough health history and symptom assessment from a patient with a respiratory problem.
2. Apply the four components of the physical assessment process to the respiratory system.
3. Identify areas to assess in the inspection of the chest.
4. Differentiate normal from abnormal (adventitious) breath sounds.
5. Correlate assessment findings in the physical examination of the respiratory system with related dysfunctions.

The total assessment of the respiratory patient includes an integration of historical, laboratory, and physical assessments. This chapter discusses the historical and physical assessment of the respiratory system. The laboratory assessment is discussed separately in Chapter 16. As an introduction, several terms are used in the assessment process and in the description of syndromes and diseases. A symptom is a subjective abnormality perceived by the patient and is a departure from the normal or usual function, sensation, or appearance (e.g., chest pain, dyspnea). A sign is an observable or measurable manifestation that indicates an abnormality or disease. It may be a subjective or objective abnormality perceived by the examiner (e.g., tachypnea, cyanosis, crackles). Finally, a finding is the objective or subjective result of a laboratory or radiology test (e.g., leukocytosis, decreased forced expiratory volume in 1 second, decreased arterial partial pressure of oxygen).

The competent nurse brings knowledge, skills, and experience to the bedside of the critically ill patient. The nurse is able to 1) quickly identify acute respiratory clinical symptoms and signs, 2) anticipate changes and findings related to acute and chronic disease processes, 3) understand the pathophysiologic basis for these signs, symptoms, and findings, and 4) develop an individualized plan of care for the patient. Given the fast pace of the critical care unit, it is not feasible to conduct a total respiratory assessment of every patient. The experienced nurse identifies and monitors key components specific to a patient's individual disease process and presentation.

HEALTH HISTORY

Although it may be difficult to obtain a patient's complete respiratory history on admission to the unit, this history remains an important part of the assessment process. The person providing the medical history may not be the patient, but a family member or friend. The patient's previous medical record may also be helpful in completing the historical assessment. An overview of information to obtain in the historical assessment is shown in Chart 15–1.

Review of Symptoms

The complete respiratory history includes a discussion of the patient's past respiratory problems and hospitalizations. First, the nurse should assess whether the patient has a history of an acute or chronic respiratory problem (Chart 15–2). Is respiratory disease the primary reason for the critical care admission, or is it a complication or a consequence of another condition or a comorbid condition? These answers will help to identify key components of the remaining assessment process and to tailor the assessment to guide the planning and evaluation of care.

CHART 15–1

Respiratory Historical Assessment

Chief complaint
Medication allergies
History of present illness: critical care admission related to
    Acute versus chronic respiratory problem
        Duration of problem or disease process
        Previous hospitalization for a similar problem
    Respiratory complication of surgery or another disease process
    Respiratory comorbidity
Past respiratory history
    Chronic obstructive pulmonary disease (emphysema, chronic bronchitis, bronchiectasis, cystic fibrosis)
    Asthma
    Frequent infections (sinusitis, upper respiratory or lower respiratory infections)
    Pneumonia
    Tuberculosis: date of the patient's most recent TB test
Past surgical history
    Any previous surgeries related to the lung or thorax
    Problems with general anesthesia, lung problems after surgery, or the need for mechanical ventilation
Medications
    Present medications (prescription, nonprescription or over the counter, inhalers, cutaneous patches, oxygen, nebulizer treatments, home remedies)
        Indication, dosage, schedule, time since last dose
    Recently discontinued medications
    Recent vaccines (flu, pneumococcal pneumonia, others)
Allergies
Social history
    Smoking history
        Nonsmoker, active smoker, or exsmoker
        Type of smoking history (cigarettes, cigars, pipe)
        Duration of smoking history (years) and packs per day
        Pack-year history (duration in years times average number of packs per day)
        Smoking cessation history
    Ethyl alcohol (ETOH) intake
Family history of respiratory problems
Symptom assessment
    Breathlessness, shortness of breath
    Cough
    Sputum production
    Hemoptysis
    Chest pain

CHART 15–2

Assessment of History of Acute or Chronic Respiratory Problems

1. Have you ever been treated by a doctor or health care provider for a lung problem (outpatient, emergency room, inpatient)?
2. Have you ever been attached to a breathing machine (ventilator) or had a tube placed into your mouth or nose to help you breathe?
3. Have you ever had any breathing tests in which the amount of air in your lungs is measured or a blood test to look at the amount of oxygen in your blood?
4. Do you take any medications to help your breathing?

Medication History

Establishment of the patient's past and present medication history is important, as well as a history of any medication allergies. It is important to assess the present medications and the time since the last dose. This evaluation includes prescription and nonprescription medications, oxygen, and inhalers. The nurse should ask specific questions regarding nonprescription, over-the-counter medications and home remedies. The nurse should ask whether the patient has recently stopped taking any medications (e.g., completed a course of antibiotics, stopped a medication because of side effects, or stopped because a prescription was not refilled). In addition, the nurse should ask whether the patient has received any vaccines recently (flu, pneumococcal pneumonia) and whether the patient has ever had a tuberculin skin test? Last, the nurse should inquire regarding any medication allergies or other types of allergies (e.g., tape, latex).

History of Respiratory Diseases

It is important to assess the patient's history of respiratory disease, both acute and chronic. A common respiratory disease is chronic obstructive pulmonary disease (COPD), also known as chronic obstructive lung disease or chronic airway obstruction. This disease is strongly related to acute cardiopulmonary failure in the critical care setting and may account for up to 15% of all cases of respiratory failure.[1] COPD encompasses various respiratory problems: emphysema, chronic bronchitis, bronchiectasis, and cystic fibrosis.

The nurse must also assess the patient for a history of asthma, which may affect up to 6% of the population.[2] It is important to elicit information on the history of asthma episodes: how often these occur, possible seasonal patterns, detailed information on the most recent episode, use of medications (over the counter and prescribed), emergency room visits, hospitalizations, critical care admissions requiring intubation, and potential "triggers" of asthma attacks. In addition, a pulmonary infection history must be assessed. This includes information on upper airway infections including sinusitis and lower airway infections (bronchitis). Specifically, a question should be asked about a history of pneumonia. Last, the nurse must assess the patient for a history of tuberculosis, a positive skin test, or exposure to a person with diagnosed tuberculosis.

Surgical History

It is important to question the patient regarding any type of surgical procedures performed on the lung, thoracic cage, or upper airway. In addition to information on thoracic operations or procedures, the patient should be asked about other previous surgical procedures and any history of lung complications related to general anesthesia, surgery, or the postoperative period (e.g., aspiration, pneumonia, pulmonary embolism).

Social History

Smoking

Smoking history is an important part of the respiratory assessment. Smoking is strongly associated with numerous pulmonary diseases (e.g., lung cancer, COPD) and is a risk factor for complications.[3–5] The following questions should be asked: 1) Does the patient have a history of smoking (often defined as >100 cigarettes in a lifetime)? 2) Is the patient currently a smoker, and what is the patient's pack-year history (PYH)? The PYH is calculated by multiplying the number of years of smoking by the average number of packs of cigarettes per day (20 cigarettes per pack). For example, if a patient has smoked for 20 years and has averaged 1.5 packs of cigarettes per day, the PYH is 30 pack years. In addition, for an exsmoker, it is important to also assess the PYH and time since smoking cessation.

If the patient has an active history of smoking, the nurse should obtain information regarding the patient's interest and past history in attempting smoking cessation. Although the critical care unit is not the optimal setting for implementing a formal smoking cessation program, it may be important to begin educating and encouraging the patient regarding smoking cessation. This information can then be reinforced throughout the hospitalization and in the outpatient setting.[6,7]

Ethyl Alcohol

It is important to assess the patient's ethyl alcohol (ETOH) intake history. This includes average number of drinks per day or per week, the type of ETOH consumed, and any history of ETOH abuse. If the patient has a strong ETOH intake history, this is important to know because it may affect laboratory values and the medical or surgical treatment of the patient. The nurse must assess the patient for potential withdrawal symptoms and must be prepared to intervene.

Family History

The nurse must assess the patient for any family history of respiratory problems. This may include asthma, COPD, tuberculosis, lung cancer, or recurrent pulmonary infections. Although family respiratory problems are not frequently related to the critical care admission, this information is important.

Symptom Assessment

Each of the key respiratory symptoms should be assessed in a systematic way with specific questions relating to the characteristics, as shown in Chart 15–3. The patient's pulmonary history should focus on primary pulmonary symptoms including breathlessness, cough, sputum production, hemoptysis, and chest pain. In addition, the presence of fever, chills or night sweats, and weight loss must also be assessed.

Breathlessness (Shortness of Breath)

Breathlessness or shortness of breath is a common pulmonary symptom. Dyspnea is a medical term for the *subjective* report of breathlessness or shortness of breath experienced by a patient.[8] Often, the terms of

CHART 15–3

Respiratory Symptoms: Specific Characteristics to Assess

Key Pulmonary Symptoms	Characteristics to Assess for Each Symptom
Breathlessness (dyspnea, shortness of breath)	Location
	Quality
	Related symptoms
Cough	Severity
Sputum production	Timing
Hemoptysis	
Chest pain	

CHART 15–4

Specific Questions to Ask Regarding Breathlessness (Dyspnea, Shortness of Breath)

Location	Where is it located?
Quality	How does the breathlessness feel?
	Is it an acute or a chronic symptom?
	Is it increasing, decreasing, or staying the same?
Related symptoms	Are other signs of respiratory distress or problems present (e.g., pursed-lip breathing, use of accessory muscles, central cyanosis, increased respiratory rate, change in inspiratory/expiratory ratio, chest pain)?
Severity	Is the patient able to complete a sentence or to speak only in short phrases?
	Is the patient reluctant to speak, and is it due to the breathlessness?
	What position is the patient assuming?
	Is the patient able to lie flat in bed?
	How many pillows does the patient use at night?
	Has the patient ever used supplemental oxygen?
Timing	How long has the patient experienced shortness of breath?
	Is it intermittent or continuous?
	Is the patient short of breath at rest or with exercise (quantify the amount: e.g., number of feet walked, number of stairs)? Attempt to differentiate between shortness of breath and fatigue as a limiting factor.

dyspnea, breathlessness, and shortness of breath are used interchangeably. The nurse should not assume that a patient is experiencing breathlessness just because he or she is tachypneic (breathing faster than normal) or appears to have labored breathing.

Dyspnea may be described in numerous ways by the patient (e.g., breathless, short of breath, winded, unable to get air in). It is important to communicate with the patient using simple terms. Key questions to be asked in assessing breathlessness are shown in Chart 15–4. The patient may describe specific types of dyspnea. *Paroxysmal nocturnal dyspnea* (sudden awakening with shortness of breath) may be brought on by asthma, chronic left ventricular failure, airway obstruction due to secretion retention, or sleep apnea. Some patients may describe shortness of breath while lying flat and may find relief in a sitting position (*orthopnea*). A key question refers to the number of pillows used at night (sometimes referred to as pillow orthopnea). The need for multiple pillows (to raise the head and thorax) may be due to congestive heart failure, mitral valve disease, asthma, COPD, ascites, or pregnancy. *Trepopnea* is a condition in which a patient is more comfortable breathing in a lateral position. Examples of diseases causing trepopnea are congestive heart failure and unilateral lung disease.

Dyspnea is common in the mechanically ventilated patient; however, it is not routinely assessed.[9] The nurse should assess the mechanically ventilated patient for the symptom of shortness of breath. This evaluation may be accomplished by asking the patient, by using a scale of some type, and also by integrating other findings that may be associated with shortness of breath (e.g., increased heart rate, "fighting" the ventilator, anxiety, agitation). As yet, reliable and valid measures to assess dyspnea during mechanical ventilation and weaning from mechanical ventilation have not been established.[10, 11] Continued research in this area is important to enhance patient care.

Cough

Cough is a common symptom of acute and chronic respiratory disease. However, cough may also be associated with aspiration, gastroesophageal reflux, or the use of certain medications (e.g., angiotensin-converting enzyme inhibitors). As with breathlessness, the nurse should establish certain characteristics about the cough (Chart 15–5). For some patients, the chronicity of a cough becomes integrated into the daily routine, and they may not be aware of the frequency of this symptom. Family members may be able to provide additional information about the symptom of cough because of heightened awareness that the cough sometimes interrupts sleep or is apparent or distracting to others.

If the patient reports a productive cough, it is important to distinguish specific characteristics of the sputum: amount (best described by the patient in simple terms, e.g., teaspoon, tablespoon, number of tissues used per day), color, consistency, and smell. The nurse should also ask whether there has been a recent change in the characteristics of the sputum and whether the patient has recently taken antibiotics for respiratory symptoms. This factor may be key in the early identification of an infection or an exacerbation of an ongoing infection. Acute onset of cough along with other constitutional symptoms may represent a serious or potentially life-threatening condition such as pneumonia, pulmonary embolism, congestive heart failure, tuberculosis, or aspiration. The concurrent constitutional respiratory symptoms include those in Chart 15–3, and the nurse should also assess the patient for fever, chills, night sweats, and weight loss.

Hemoptysis (Coughing Up of Blood)

Hemoptysis is the coughing of blood from the airways. The nurse must establish whether the patient is expectorating blood from the lung, vomiting blood from the gastrointestinal system (hematemesis), or experiencing a posterior nosebleed (epistaxis). In the critical care setting, traumatic intubation or frequent suctioning may cause blood-tinged sputum; however, this condition is usually not described as hemoptysis.

As with sputum production, the patient should be asked to describe the properties of the expectorated blood. This includes the amount of blood described in simple terms that are easily understood. The color and characteristics of the expectorated blood should be described—blood-tinged sputum, fresh blood (bright red), or old blood (dark red, brownish). The description of color can help to distinguish whether the blood is old and has finally been expectorated or whether it is new, an ominous sign.

The patient may describe sensations relating to the episode of hemoptysis. These descriptions include a warm feeling, gurgling in the airway, vague discomfort, and chest pain in an area. Often, these sensations allow the patient to describe the approximate origin of bleeding from the airways. Examples of diseases or situations that predispose a patient to hemoptysis include chronic pulmonary diseases (bronchitis, bronchiectasis, cystic fibrosis), lung cancer, necrotizing pneumonia, recent surgery, administration of blood thinners (warfarin, thrombolytic agents), tuberculosis,

---

CHART 15–5

Characteristics to Assess Regarding the Symptom of Cough

Location	Location more upper airway (throat clearing) or deeper, lower airway
Quality	Type: Dry or "hacky" versus productive
	Productivity: amount, color, characteristics of sputum; recent changes in characteristics of the sputum
Related symptoms	Accompanying signs or symptoms (breathlessness, fever, night sweats, weight loss, nausea, vomiting, chest pain, dizziness, wheezing)
Severity	Presence of paroxysms of cough (uncontrollable spasms of cough)
	Impairment of activities of daily living, quality of life
	Medications associated with cough or taken to relieve the cough (over the counter versus prescribed)
Timing	Duration of the cough; acute onset or a chronic problem
	Frequency, occurrence during the day versus at night
	Association with an activity or event (eating, drinking fluids, lying flat)
	Relationship with any environmental factors
	Recent instrumentation of the airway (intubation, bronchoscopy, surgical procedure involving airways)

and an increased bleeding tendency or coagulation disorder.[12]

As with other pulmonary symptoms, symptoms related to hemoptysis must also be assessed. These include breathlessness, cough, chest pain, and fever. Assessment of the severity of the hemoptysis includes frequency of occurrence, amount of blood, and type of secretions expectorated. The spectrum of hemoptysis ranges from minor, blood-tinged sputum to massive hemoptysis (>200 mL/24-hour period).

Last, the timing of the symptom of hemoptysis should be evaluated by establishing the onset, frequency, and duration of the blood expectoration. It is important to establish when the last episode of hemoptysis occurred.

Chest Pain

Chest pain is a nonspecific symptom that must be reviewed in detail. Diseases of the lungs may produce chest pain or discomfort, but it is often difficult to distinguish the origin of the chest pain. Chest pain related to the respiratory system may be superficial (related to the bony thorax, muscular structures) or related to the pleurae, airways, or lung parenchyma. Table 15–1 describes different types of chest pain related to the respiratory system. For assessment of other types of chest pain, see Chapter 9.

The chest pain may be musculoskeletal in origin and may develop as a result of thoracic incisions or muscle–ligament strains brought on by severe coughing spasms or trauma. Pain may also be felt in the costochondral or chondrosternal junctions (where the ribs attach to the sternum) or in the anterior chest wall muscles. Usually, chest pain resulting from a chest wall problem is sharply localized and exhibits point tenderness. It may be made worse by tensing the muscles, coughing, or sneezing.

Rib fractures also cause chest pain. This type of chest pain exhibits point tenderness, and may be caused by trauma to the ribs or by severe paroxysms of coughing. Other causes of chest pain related to the bony thorax and muscular structures are lesions and tumors of the chest wall, including primary lesions on the ribs or tumors of the pleurae or lung that have spread to the chest wall.

Chest pain may also be pleuropulmonary in origin. Chest pain can be caused by inflammation or stretching of the parietal pleura (called pleurisy). The visceral pleura is not sensitive to pain. Pleuritic pain is usually described in the lateral aspects of the chest wall and is sharply localized. Pleuritic pain is described as sharp and is exacerbated with deep breathing and movements of the trunk region (e.g., bending over, turning). Diaphragmatic pleural pain is often referred to the shoulder or is described as shoulder pain. This chest pain is of sudden onset and may be aggravated by deep breathing, coughing, and positioning.

Chest pain may also be related to the airways and lung parenchyma. Some disease processes, such as acute tracheobronchitis, may also cause chest pain perceived as soreness or burning high in the retrosternal area. Last, pulmonary chest pain that mimics cardiovascular pain and is described as crushing or constricting may be due to acute pulmonary embolism. This pain is caused by acute pulmonary artery hypertension (high arterial pressure in the pulmonary artery).

PHYSICAL EXAMINATION

The four methods used to examine the respiratory system are inspection, palpation, percussion, and auscultation. A systematic approach in assessing the patient helps to prevent oversight of any aspect of the examination. Although the nurse does not perform a

TABLE 15–1

Description of Types of Chest Pain Related to the Respiratory System

Location	Characteristics	Possible Causes
Musculoskeletal	Sharply localized point tenderness worsened by deep breathing, cough, movement, or sneezing	Thoracic incision; muscle, ligament strains; rib fracture; lesions on the ribs; tumors
Pleuropulmonary	Sharply localized "stabbing" in lateral aspect of chest; may be sudden in onset aggravated by movement, cough, deep breathing; may radiate to the shoulder or abdomen	Pleurisy; pneumothorax
Airways	Sudden-onset, crushing midsternal pain may be pleuritic as well; mimics myocardial pain	Acute pulmonary embolism; depending on the severity of the embolism, chest pain possibly located over the affected side or area of the lung
	Burning, soreness in the midsternal area	Acute tracheobronchitis

complete physical assessment each time the patient is examined, it is important to remember the essential aspects of each step of the examination. In addition to physical examination data, one must also incorporate laboratory data in the assessment. Laboratory evaluations pertinent to the respiratory patient are discussed in Chapter 16.

Proper body positioning of the patient is crucial in the physical assessment process. The upright, sitting position is preferred for the respiratory assessment process. However, in the critical care setting, adjustments must be made to position the patient for the assessment without compromising respiratory function. The nurse should assess the anterior, posterior, and lateral aspects of the patient's chest.

Anatomic Landmarks

Before beginning the respiratory physical assessment, the nurse must be familiar with the anatomic landmarks of the thorax that help to describe the position of the underlying structures and the location of abnormalities in relation to the anterior, lateral, and posterior surfaces. See Figure 14–1 for anatomic landmarks. Figure 14–4 demonstrates the underlying location of the lungs in the anterior, posterior, and lateral positions.

Inspection

The inspection process of the examination can be divided into specific anatomic locations. Each nurse develops a personal preference and a process for conducting this aspect of the examination. This discussion describes the inspection process in the following order: general appearance of the patient, extremities, head and neck region, and thorax. Chart 15–6 summarizes areas to assess during the inspection process.

General Appearance

Inspection or observation of the patient is perhaps the most underrated aspect of respiratory assessment. The nurse should make an overall assessment of the level of consciousness, general nutritional status, musculoskeletal development, and skin turgor of the patient. The patient's position should be assessed, and the nurse should determine whether turning the patient impairs or enhances the respiratory effort. In addition, the nurse should evaluate whether the patient is able to speak in sentences or whether shortness of breath impairs the patient's speech pattern.

The patient's extremities should be examined for signs of peripheral cyanosis, edema, and clubbing. Peripheral cyanosis is seen in the extremities as a result

---

CHART 15–6

Specific Areas to Assess During the Inspection Process

General	Level of consciousness
	General nutritional status (cachexia, obesity)
	Skin turgor
	Musculoskeletal development
	Positioning of patient
	Speech pattern, ability to speak in sentences
	Hoarseness
	Scars
Extremities	Edema
	Peripheral cyanosis
	Clubbing
Head and Neck	Type of breathing (mouth versus nose)
	Rate, pattern of breathing; inspiratory to expiratory ratio
	Nasal flaring
	Pursed-lip breathing
	Central cyanosis
	Tracheal positioning
	Use of accessory muscles of shoulders and neck
Thorax	Rate and pattern of breathing
	Symmetry of chest wall movement
	Synchrony of chest, abdominal movement
	Chest wall deformities
	Bulging, retraction of interspaces

---

of cooling of the area, lack of circulation, or hypoxia of the tissues. Edema is an excessive accumulation of interstitial fluid that is commonly associated with congestive heart failure. However, it may also be secondary to chronic hypoxemia and pulmonary hypertension leading to cor pulmonale. For the bedfast critical care patient, edema should be assessed in the presacral area and more dependent areas of the body.

Clubbing is described as the bulbous enlargement of the fingernails or toenails. It is often described as drumstick nails and is best appreciated by comparing normal nail beds with those of the patient. The earliest sign of clubbing is sponginess or mobility of the fixed end of the nail plate; as clubbing enters advanced stages, the nail becomes thickened, ridged, and curved. Clubbing can be seen in various respiratory diseases: pulmonary neoplasms, bronchiectasis, lung abscess, interstitial fibrosis, and cystic fibrosis. It is also observed with cardiovascular (cyanotic congenital heart disease, subacute bacterial endocarditis) and gastrointestinal diseases (liver disease, inflammatory bowel disease, infections). Several theories exist regarding the cause of clubbing; however, the exact cause is unknown.[12]

Head and Neck

After the general appearance of the patient, the next area for assessment is the head and neck region. The nurse should note whether the patient is breathing primarily through the nose or through the mouth. Adults are usually nose breathers at rest. In addition, one may observe the use of pursed-lip breathing in the patient with obstructive airway disease, especially if he or she is sitting in an upright position. This technique is thought to help prolong the expiratory phase of ventilation, which helps to decrease resistance to airflow and reduces the work of breathing. Therefore, the patient can increase the amount of air exhaled with each breath. This technique may help to decrease air trapping in the patient with COPD. Last, the patient's mouth and throat should be inspected for any signs of inflammation or problems with the tongue or teeth that could cause airway obstruction.

Evaluation of the patient for central cyanosis is important in the pulmonary examination and is best observed in the lips or buccal mucosa (circumoral cyanosis). The bluish discoloration of central cyanosis occurs secondary to unoxygenated hemoglobin (reduced hemoglobin) in the capillaries. Central cyanosis is not perceptible until the patient has at least 5 g of reduced hemoglobin per 100 mL of blood, and it signifies a late sign of hypoxemia. Factors that alter the observation of cyanosis may include the practitioner's color perception, lighting conditions, and patient's skin pigmentation. When assessing for central cyanosis, the patient's hemoglobin level is taken into consideration. Extremely high or low levels of hemoglobin in the body alter the patient's presentation of cyanosis. Peripheral cyanosis alone does not signify central cyanosis. The nurse must specifically assess the patient for central cyanosis.

The position of the trachea should be noted and evaluated for a shift or deviation from the normal midline position (Figure 15-1). Conditions causing tracheal deviation include a loss of lung volume or tissue that causes the trachea to shift toward the affected side (e.g., atelectasis, pneumonectomy). Conditions that push or shift the trachea away from the affected side include tension pneumothorax, mediastinal mass, lung tumor, and large pleural effusion.

Finally, the nurse should note whether the patient is using the accessory muscles of the neck and shoulders and whether there are retractions of the suprasternal notch and supraclavicular spaces. These are all signs of respiratory distress and increased work of breathing. These signs, in addition to skin color, facial expression, positioning of the patient, and impaired patterns of speech, may all signify respiratory distress.

Thorax

Respiratory Rate and Pattern. The first step in the inspection of the chest is to assess the respiratory rate. If the patient is on a ventilator and has sponta-

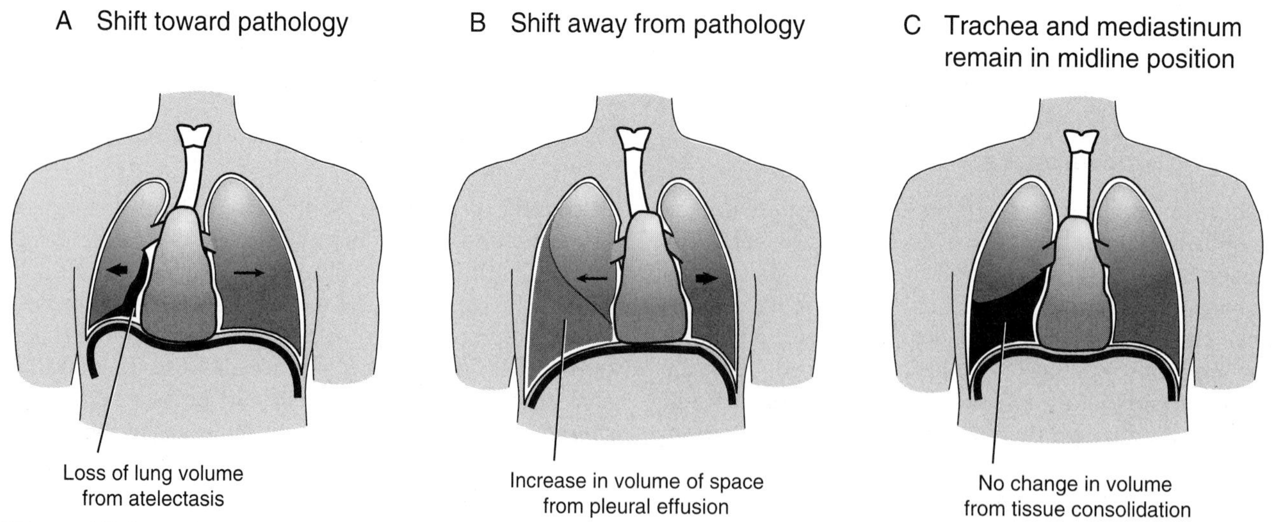

A   Shift toward pathology

B   Shift away from pathology

C   Trachea and mediastinum remain in midline position

Loss of lung volume from atelectasis

Increase in volume of space from pleural effusion

No change in volume from tissue consolidation

Figure 15-1

Examples of conditions causing tracheal and mediastinal shift. *A* and *B,* The large arrow indicates the direction of the shift. *C,* Pleural pressures remain about equal for the left and right lungs. (From Cherniack R, Cherniack L: Respiration in Health and Disease, 3rd ed. Philadelphia, W.B. Saunders, 1983.)

neous respirations, the patient's spontaneous rate along with the ventilator rate should be noted. Several terms are used to describe the rate, depth, and pattern of breathing and are described in Table 15–2.

In addition, other types of chest movement and breathing patterns are recognized. Paradoxic chest wall movement is seen with a flail chest. This condition occurs when two or more ribs are broken on one side of the chest wall, often in two or more places, with a resulting distortion of the structural aspect of the thoracic cage. The affected side of the chest wall moves asynchronously on inspiration and expiration. On inspiration, the affected area moves inward, and on expiration, it bulges outward. A flail chest may be accentuated and more easily visualized by 1) having the patient take a spontaneous deep breath (the patient will be reluctant to take a deep breath due to pain), 2) observing during the inspiratory cycle if the patient is receiving mechanical ventilation, or 3) observing the patient during inflation of the lungs with a manual resuscitator bag. Repositioning a patient may also accentuate a flail chest if the flail segment has been splinted or held in place by a specific position.

Asynchronous breathing is observed when the respiratory muscles become discoordinated because of fatigue. The rib cage and abdomen do not move outward at the same time. Asynchronous breathing may progress to a more disruptive pattern called paradoxic breathing. With this pattern, the abdomen moves outward while the lower rib cage moves inward during inspiration. This abdominal movement works in opposition to the contraction of the diaphragm. Finally, a breathing pattern called respiratory alternans occurs when the patient alternates between rib cage breathing and abdominal breathing.[12]

Symmetry of Chest Wall Movement. The symmetry of movement of the chest wall should be observed. The two sides of the chest should move in a synchronous and equal fashion. The chest wall configuration should be noted, and an assessment should be made of the anteroposterior diameter. The normal adult thorax is elliptic. Alterations in the shape of the thorax may include a barrel chest or an increase in the ratio of the anteroposterior to lateral diameter of the chest (>1:2). This change is frequently observed in the

TABLE 15–2
Abnormal Breathing Patterns

Type	Spirogram	Description
Tachypnea		Breathing rate faster than 20 breaths per minute; nonspecific finding that may be due to various causes including pain, anxiety, fever, hypercapnia, or hypoxemia
Bradypnea		Breathing pattern slower than 10 breaths per minute; nonspecific finding that may be due to various causes including excessive use of sedatives or narcotics, metabolic disorders, or brain disorders
Apnea	> 15 seconds	Disruption and cessation of air flow to the lungs; usually considered pathologic if longer than 15 seconds; prolonged apnea may result from respiratory arrest due to acute upper airway obstruction, stroke, or depression of the respiratory center
Cheyne–Stokes	Apnea	Crescendo–decrescendo cyclic pattern of breathing of progressively deeper respirations followed by progressively shallower respirations, followed by a period of apnea; then the cycle repeats itself: periods of apnea may last up to 15–20 seconds; caused by changes in blood flow to the respiratory center or impairment in the control of breathing
Kussmaul's		Deep, regular breaths at a rate greater than 20 breaths per minute; caused by the respiratory system's reacting to a severe metabolic acidotic state; respiratory system attempts to compensate by excreting carbon dioxide in response to the metabolic acidosis
Biot's	Apnea	Irregular breathing pattern with an unpredictable rate, pattern, and depth of breathing; may include periods of apnea; caused by CNS disorder affecting the central control of breathing (head trauma, stroke); this pattern is not compatible with life and requires intubation and mechanical ventilation

Modified from Kersten LD: Comprehensive Respiratory Nursing. Philadelphia, W.B. Saunders, 1989, p 279.

patient with severe COPD, but it also occurs as a normal aspect of aging. Kyphosis is a forward curvature of the spine, and scoliosis is a lateral curvature of the spine. Other potential chest wall deformities include pectus excavatum (sinking in of the sternum) and pectus carinatum (bulging out of the sternum). Usually, these chest wall deformities do not impair the patient's gas exchange, but they may alter chest wall excursion.

Assessment of the patient's work of breathing is accomplished by inspection. Bulging or retraction of the intercostal spaces should be noted. Intercostal retractions are inward movements of the tissues between the ribs of the chest wall noted on inspiration. This condition indicates an obstruction to inspiratory airflow. Bulging of the interspaces may occur with massive pleural effusion or tension pneumothorax and may be seen during expiration.

Palpation

Palpation is use of the fingertips to evaluate areas of tenderness and chest wall abnormalities, to assess the structural integrity and movement of the chest wall, to assess the position of the trachea, and to assess for tactile fremitus. Posteriorly, thoracic excursion or expansion can be better appreciated by palpation than by simple observation. However, it may prove difficult to assess with the critically ill patient in a supine position. The anterolateral and posterolateral aspects of the rib cage should be palpated during both quiet breathing and deep breathing. Disorders that interfere with lung expansion or that cause decreased lung volume or diaphragmatic dysfunction can produce asymmetric chest movement. Examples of these disorders include pneumothorax, atelectasis, pneumonia, resection of

lung tissue, and diaphragmatic disorders or phrenic nerve injuries.

Crepitation or subcutaneous emphysema may be palpated when air escapes into the planes of subcutaneous tissue. Crepitus or a popping sensation can be felt by compression of the affected tissues. This condition is harmless and resolves on its own; however, it may be bothersome or frightening to the patient. These crepitations may result from thoracic trauma or leaking of air around a chest tube or tracheostomy tube site.

The nurse may also assess the presence and quality of vocal or tactile fremitus. Fremitus can be assessed in the patient who is spontaneously breathing and is able to follow instructions and to communicate. Fremitus is the sensation of sound vibrations produced in the airways when the patient phonates. In a patient with patent airways, the vibrations are felt on the chest wall by the palm of the hand or the fingertips (Figure 15–2). To elicit vocal fremitus, the patient is instructed to say words or phrases that cause increased resonance or vibrations (e.g., "1, 2, 3," "99"). The patient should be instructed to speak in a normal voice so as not to increase or decrease the intensity of the fremitus. The nurse systematically compares the areas of each side of the chest for symmetry of fremitus by placing the palm of the hand or the fingertips on differing areas of the chest wall in a systematic fashion.

In general, tactile or vocal fremitus is more prominent in areas where the large airways are closest to the thoracic wall. Alterations of tactile fremitus include increased, decreased, or absent fremitus (Chart 15–7). Differences in fremitus felt in areas of the thoracic cage are due to differing media and their ability to conduct vibrations. Solid media or uniform structures conduct vibrations better than do porous structures composed of solids and air. Additional media such as air or fluids may distort the vibrations.

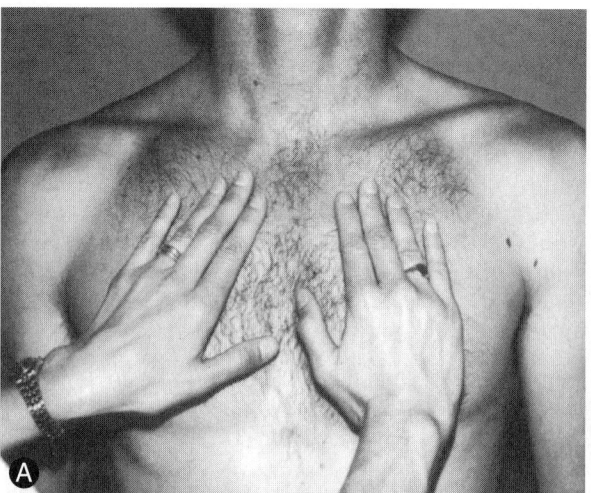 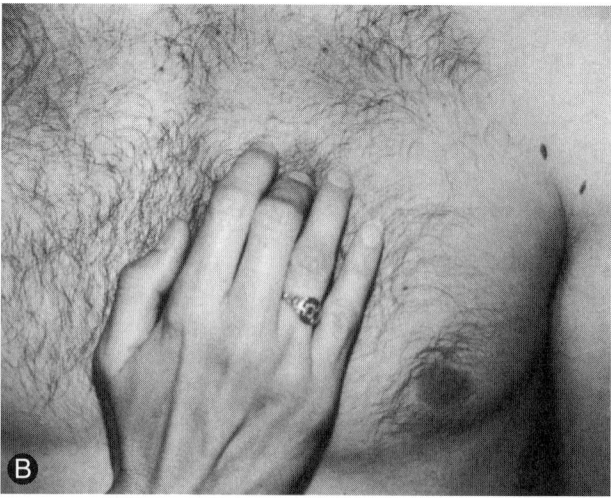

Figure 15–2
Fingertip techniques for general palpation and assessing fremitus through the chest wall. *A,* General assessment of an area. *B,* Focused assessment of an area of the chest wall. (From Kersten LD: Comprehensive Respiratory Nursing. Philadelphia, W.B. Saunders, 1989, p 286.)

CHART 15–7

Factors Influencing Tactile Fremitus

Normal intensity of fremitus	Location of bronchi to chest wall
	Thickness of chest wall
	Conditions that increase density of lung tissue
Increased fremitus	Thin chest wall
	Lung consolidation, pneumonia
	Severe atelectasis
	Lung mass
Decreased fremitus	Obesity
	Muscular chest wall
	Conditions with air trapping (chronic obstructive pulmonary disease, asthma)
	Pleural effusion
	Pneumothorax
	Pleural thickening

Percussion

The third step in the assessment process, percussion, is not frequently used by nurses in the critical care setting. Percussion is difficult to master and takes a great deal of practice. It is the art of tapping the chest wall in a systematic way to elicit a sound. Over the lungs, sonorous percussion is usually performed to evaluate the density of underlying tissues. The sounds produced by percussion probably do not penetrate more than about 4 to 5 cm below the chest wall surface.[12] Percussion helps to determine whether the underlying tissues are air filled, fluid filled, or solid.

The most common type of percussion used is mediate percussion. The middle pleximeter finger of the left or right hand is hyperextended and is placed firmly on the surface to be percussed. It is important to avoid contact by any other part of the hand on the chest wall because to do so will dampen the vibrations produced. Next, the opposite hand should be placed near the hand that is placed on the patient's chest wall. The middle finger of the "striking" hand should be poised partially flexed, but with a relaxed wrist above the hand on the chest wall. With a sharp but relaxed motion, the pleximeter finger is struck on the chest wall with the right middle finger of the opposite hand. Use of the fingertip and not the finger pad produces the most distinct percussion note. The motion should be done smoothly and quickly so as not to dampen the percussion note (Figure 15–3).

Percussion should be done on all aspects of the patient's chest wall in a systematic fashion. The sounds produced should be noted and compared with the sounds from the contralateral side. Percussion sounds are influenced by the character of the immediate underlying structures. Percussion over solid structures such as the heart, liver, or scapulae produces a dull sound, whereas percussion over normal, air-filled lungs (a porous structure) produces a vibration referred to as normal resonance. Figure 15–4 shows normal percussion notes over differing structures in the chest. Percussion over fluid (pleural effusion, hemothorax) or consolidated lung tissue (pneumonia, extensive atelectasis) produces a dull sound. Percussion over a large pneumothorax is hyperresonant or tympanic. Table 15–3 describes differing percussion sounds and their characteristics.

Positioning of the patient may affect the percussion note obtained. The anterior and anterolateral walls of the chest may be satisfactorily examined with the patient in the supine position. If the patient is in the lateral recumbent position, several factors may change the sound. The surface of the patient's bed may dampen the percussion sounds. The hemidiaphragm on the side next to the bed may be elevated because of pressure from the abdominal contents. Proper body alignment will help to minimize these changes.

Auscultation

Auscultation is the most widely used step in the respiratory physical assessment. It is the art of listening to the sounds produced within the airways, and the nurse listens for both normal breath sounds and adventitious (abnormal) breath sounds. Breath sounds result from air moving through the tracheobronchial tree and are produced by turbulence in the airways. Breath sounds are described relative to location, duration, pitch, and quality.

Procedure

The diaphragm or flat side of the stethoscope piece is used to listen to lung sounds. The diaphragm should be placed firmly on the patient's chest wall with equal contact of all parts of the diaphragm with the skin. The nurse should auscultate the patient's lungs in a systematic fashion starting in the apical areas and listening to both sides of the chest for comparison. The anterior, posterior, and lateral aspects of each lung should be examined (Figure 15–5). It is best to perform auscultation with the patient sitting erect. This position may

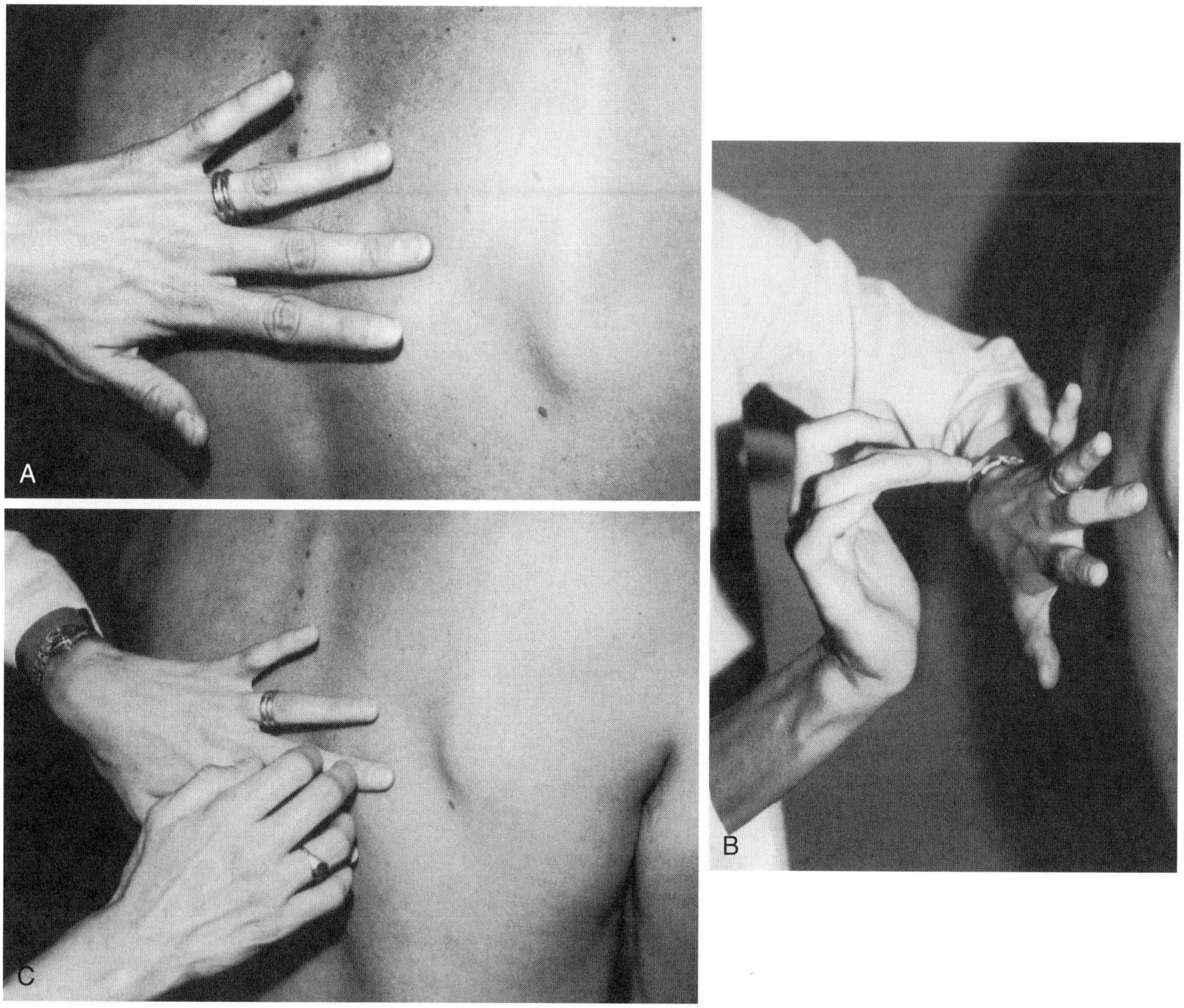

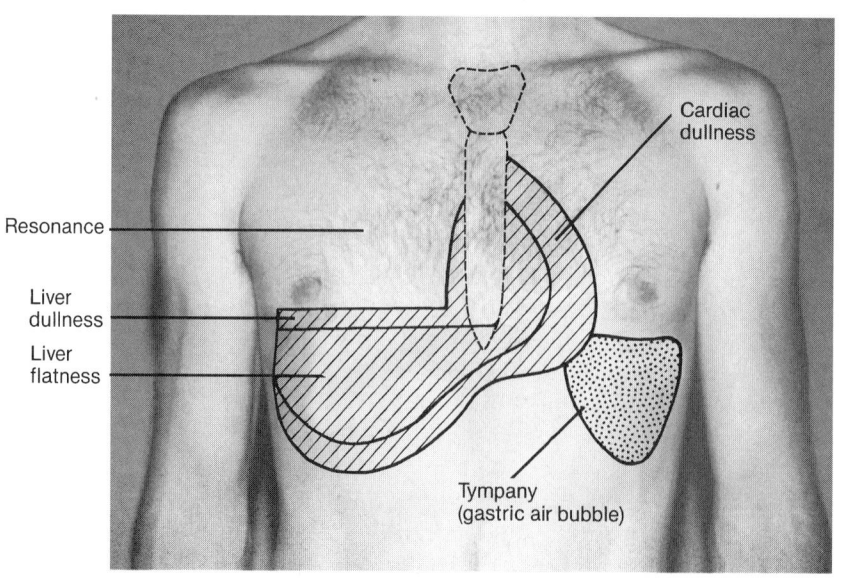

Figure 15–3

Technique for percussion of the chest wall. *A,* Place the middle pleximeter finger (distal joint) firmly on the patient's chest wall; elevate the hand. *B,* Cock the wrist and arch middle pleximeter finger of the opposite hand. *C,* Strike the pleximeter finger on the patient's chest wall. Let the plexor finger bounce off the distal joint. (From Kersten LD: Comprehensive Respiratory Nursing. Philadelphia, W.B. Saunders, 1989, p 292.)

Figure 15–4

Normal percussion notes over areas of the anterior chest. Most of the anterior chest is resonant to percussion, except the heart, liver, and stomach. The size of the gastric air bubble varies among individuals, in different positions, and at different times of the day. (From Kersten LD: Comprehensive Respiratory Nursing. Philadelphia, W.B. Saunders, 1989, p 295.)

TABLE 15–3
Percussion Notes and Their Characteristics

Type	Amplitude	Pitch	Quality	Duration	Sample Location
Resonant	Medium loud	Low	Clear, hollow	Moderate	Over normal lung tissue
Hyperresonant	Louder	Lower	Booming	Longer	Normal over child's lung; in the adult, over lungs with increased amount of air, as in emphysema
Tympanic	Loud	High	Musical and drumlike (like the kettle drum)	Sustained longest	Over air-filled viscus, e.g., stomach and intestine
Dull	Soft	High	Muffled thud	Short	Relatively dense organ, e.g., liver or spleen
Flat	Very soft	High	Dead stop of sound, absolute dullness	Very short	When no air is present, over thigh muscles, bone, or tumor

From Jarvis C: Physical Examination and Health Assessment, 2nd ed. Philadelphia, W.B. Saunders, 1996, p 164.

be difficult to achieve in the critical care setting. A supine patient should be rolled first on one side while the nurse listens to the anterior, posterior, and lateral sounds of the "up" side. Then the patient should be rolled to the opposite side-lying position. Placing the patient in the lateral position helps to minimize compression of the lung on the nondependent side. The patient should be instructed to breathe normally through the mouth. Mouth breathing provides less airway resistance of the upper airway than does breathing through the nose. If the examiner is having a difficult time hearing the breath sounds, the patient should be instructed to take deeper breaths. Breath sounds are the result of airflow through the airways, and increasing the flow augments the sounds.

Auscultation is an art of selective listening and must be practiced. Although it may be difficult to filter out some of the extraneous noises of an active critical care unit, the nurse should minimize these noises as much as possible while listening to the patient's chest. In addition, differing interventions and therapies may alter the auscultative findings in the critical care patient. If the patient has a nasogastric tube or a chest tube attached to suction, the sounds from the suction may interfere with listening. Mechanical ventilation changes the characteristics of breath sounds. Although mechanical ventilation of the lungs does not produce abnormal breath sounds, it amplifies or distorts breath sounds. In addition, high-flow oxygen devices may also interfere with listening to breath sounds.

On completing the auscultation assessment, the nurse should clean the diaphragm of the stethoscope with an alcohol swab. The stethoscope provides an excellent medium for transmission of nosocomial infections among patients and among health care staff members.

Auscultation of the chest is a systematic process. An understanding and an appreciation of distinguishing slight changes in chest sounds come with practice and experience. Although auscultation is widely used, this part of the examination is not always done correctly, with resulting incorrect information and interpretation or failure to obtain all available information about the breath sounds. The most common errors made during the auscultation process include listening to breath sounds through the patient's gown, allowing the stethoscope tubing to rub against the bed rails, interpreting chest hair sounds as "abnormal" crackles, quickly moving to different parts of the chest during a respiratory cycle, and listening only to one area of the chest or only to convenient areas of the chest wall.[13] Table 15–4 describes patient situations that may produce false-positive breath sounds.

Breath Sounds

Normal Sounds

Bronchial (tracheal) and vesicular breath sounds are considered normal breath sounds. Characteristics of these normal breath sounds are described in Table 15–5. A third sound, bronchovesicular, is referred to in some textbooks and indicates transitional areas between bronchial and vesicular breath sounds.

The nurse should note the location and intensity of the patient's normal breath sounds. If a normal sound

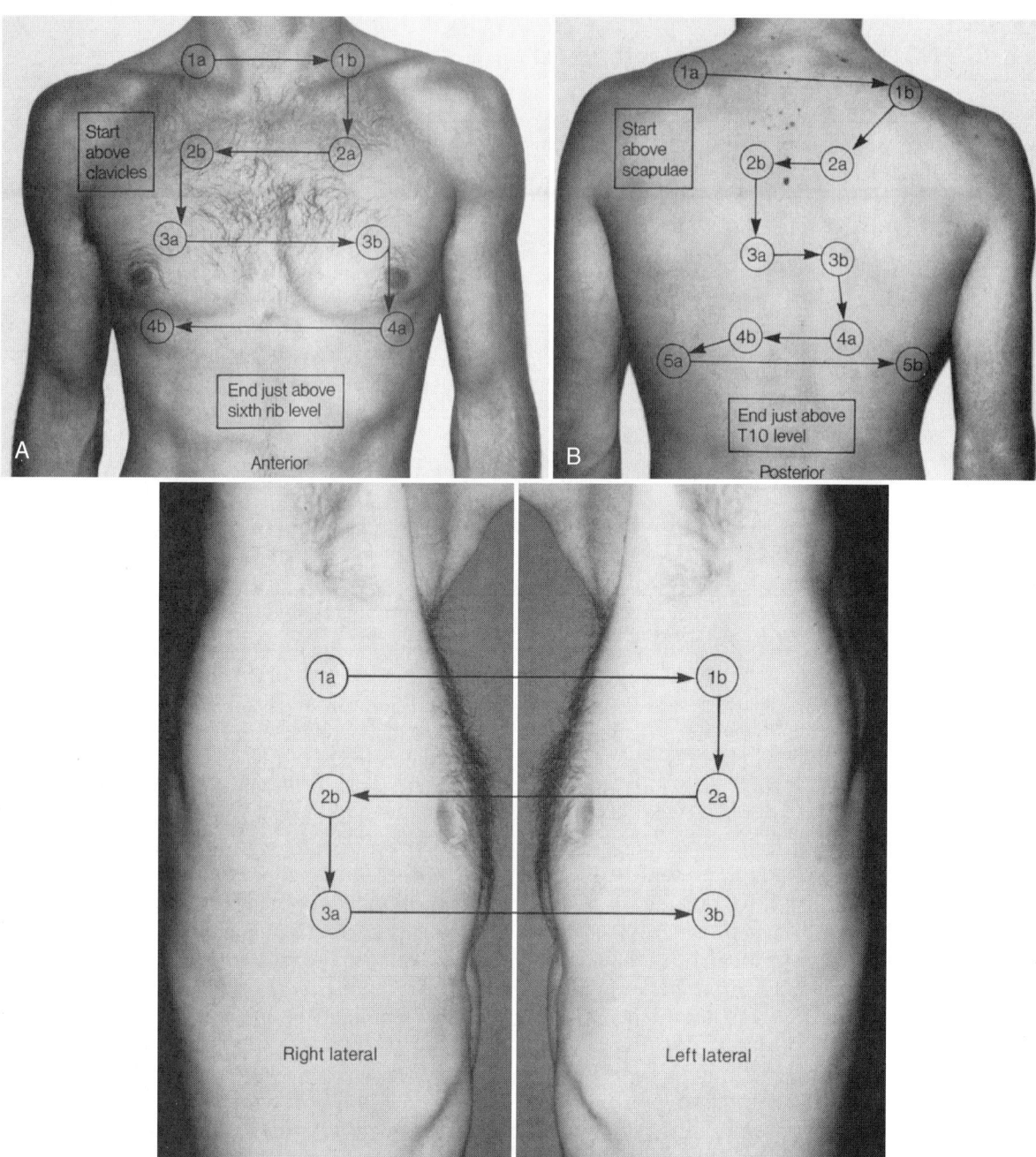

Figure 15–5

Systematic method of ausculating all aspects of the chest wall starting at the top and moving downward. This stepwise approach allows the examiner to assess for symmetry of breath sounds. A, Anterior chest wall. B, Posterior chest wall. C, Right lateral chest wall. D, Left lateral chest wall.

is heard somewhere other than in its usual location, this sound is considered abnormal. An example is a bronchial breath sound found in an area where vesicular breath sounds should be heard. This finding is typical over an area of consolidation or atelectasis.

Several factors and diseases may cause breath sounds to be decreased or absent. This feature is also important to note in the assessment of breath sounds. Table 15–6 describes disorders that may cause breath sounds to be decreased or absent.

Adventitious Sounds

Adventitious or abnormal breath sounds are those sounds other than the bronchial, tracheal, or vesicular sounds. It is easiest to identify the characteristics of abnormal sounds as being continuous or intermittent and inspiratory or expiratory. Although some attempt has been made to standardize the nomenclature of abnormal breath sounds, many different descriptions are used in the clinical setting.[14–16] Table 15–7 describes the characteristics of adventitious sounds.

TABLE 15–4
Examples of Patient Situations Leading to False-Positive Lung Sounds

Patient Situation	False-Positive Lung Sound	Explanation	To Eliminate Sound
Mechanical ventilation	Rhonchi, usually expiratory	Water bubbling in ventilator tubings	Empty ventilator tubing before auscultation
Pursed-lip breathing	Decreased breath sounds (expiration almost absent)	Mouth almost closed during expiration	Instruct patient to exhale with mouth wide open
Nasogastric tube	High- or low-pitched squeak audible on anterior chest	Varies with intermittent suction	Clamp nasogastric tube during auscultation
Chest hair	Crackles or other extraneous sounds	Hair moves against diaphragm during chest movement	Select areas free of hair or wet chest hair before auscultation
Stethoscope contact with patient's gown, bedsheets, etc.	Crackles or other extraneous sounds	Articles rub against stethoscope diaphragm or tubing	Do not listen over clothes or allow any part of stethoscope to touch articles of clothing
Muscle tension, as in Shivering	Crackles or other extraneous sounds	Increased surface tension	May be unavoidable
Muscle twitching Pain Use of accessory muscles of respiration	Decreased breath sounds	Breathing is not free and easy	Listen after sedation or pain medication Instruct tense patient to relax shoulders

Modified from Kersten LD: Comprehensive Respiratory Nursing. Philadelphia, W.B. Saunders, 1989, p 325.

Continuous Sounds. Before attempting to summarize auscultatory findings in specific pulmonary conditions, it is helpful to discuss the general relationships of the adventitious sounds mentioned previously. Continuous sounds usually reflect abnormalities of the airways, whereas discontinuous or intermittent sounds reflect abnormalities of the parenchyma or airways. High-pitched continuous, musical sounds (wheezes) are associated with narrowing of the airways.

Wheezes may be caused by bronchospasm, edema of the airway lining, mucous plugging and foreign bodies, or tumors. A high-pitched, crowing, continuous sound that is confined to inspiration or is accentuated during inspiration, is called stridor. Stridor is commonly associated with extrathoracic obstruction. Lower-pitched continuous sounds (rhonchi) are usually associated with secretions of the large, central airways. These rhonchi change significantly after cough and expectoration.

TABLE 15–5
Characteristics of Normal Breath Sounds

	Pitch	Amplitude	Duration	Quality	Normal Location
Bronchial (Tracheal)	High	Loud	Inspiration < expiration	Harsh, hollow, tubular	Trachea and larynx
Bronchovesicular	Moderate	Moderate	Inspiration = expiration	Mixed	Over major bronchi where fewer alveoli are located: posterior, between scapulae especially on right; anterior, around upper sternum in first and second intercostal spaces
Vesicular	Low	Soft	Inspiration > expiration	Rustling, like the sound of the wind in the trees	Over peripheral lung fields where air flows through smaller bronchioles and into alveoli

From Jarvis C: Physical Examination and Health Assessment, 2nd ed. Philadelphia, W.B. Saunders, 1996, p 479.

TABLE 15–6
Disorders Causing Decreased or Absent Breath Sounds

Decreased	Absent	Decreased or Absent
Hypoventilation	Respiratory arrest	Pleural effusion
Pleural thickening	Pneumonectomy	Hemothorax
Obesity	Elevated diaphragm	Pneumothorax
Chest cage deformity	Large abdomen	Empyema
Emphysema	Stomach distention	Malpositioned endotracheal tube
Pulmonary embolism	Paralyzed diaphragm	Partial to complete airway obstruction
Partial airway obstruction	Large lung resection	Tumor
Tumor	Atelectasis	Foreign object
Foreign object	Complete airway obstruction	Pneumonia
Left ventricular failure	Tumor	Upper airway obstruction
Pneumonia	Foreign object	Atelectasis
Atelectasis	Laryngeal spasm	Pulmonary cavitation
	Mucous plugs	
	Collapsed lung	

From Kersten LD: Comprehensive Respiratory Nursing. Philadelphia, W.B. Saunders, 1989, p 304.

TABLE 15–7
Characteristics of Abnormal or Adventitious Lung Sounds

Sound*	Description	Mechanism	Clinical Example
Discontinuous Sounds			
Crackles—Fine (Rales) Inspiration Expiration	Discontinuous, high-pitched, short crackling, popping sounds heard during inspiration that are not cleared by coughing; you can simulate this sound by rolling a strand of hair between your fingers near your ear, or by moistening your thumb and index finger and separating them near your ear	Inhaled air collides with previously deflated airways; airways suddenly pop open, creating crackling sound as gas pressures between the two compartments equalize	Late inspiratory crackles occur with restrictive disease: pneumonia, congestive heart failure, and interstitial fibrosis Early inspiratory crackles occur with obstructive disease: chronic bronchitis, asthma, and emphysema
Crackles—Coarse (Coarse Rales)	Loud, low-pitched, bubbling and gurgling sounds that start in early inspiration and may be present in expiration; may decrease by suctioning or coughing, but reappear shortly; sounds like opening a Velcro fastener	Inhaled air collides with secretions in the trachea and large bronchi	Pulmonary edema, pneumonia, pulmonary fibrosis, and the terminally ill, who have a depressed cough reflex
Atelectatic Crackles (Atelectatic Rales)	Sound like fine crackles, but do not last and are not pathologic; disappear after the first few breaths; heard in axillae and bases (usually dependent) of lungs	When sections of alveoli are not fully aerated, they deflate and accumulate secretions; crackles are heard when these sections reexpand with a few deep breaths	In aging adults, bed-ridden persons, or in persons just aroused from sleep

Table *Continued*

TABLE 15–7
Characteristics of Abnormal or Adventitious Lung Sounds—(Continued)

Sound*	Description	Mechanism	Clinical Example
Pleural Friction Rub	Superficial sound that is coarse and low-pitched; has a grating quality as if two pieces of leather are being rubbed together; sounds just like crackles, but close to the ear; sounds louder if you push the stethoscope harder onto the chest wall; sound is inspiratory and expiratory	Caused when pleurae become inflamed and lose their normal lubricating fluid; their opposing rough-ened pleural surfaces rub together during respiration; heard best in anterolateral wall, where greatest lung mobility exists	Pleuritis, accompanied by pain with breathing (rub disappears after a few days if pleural fluid accumulates and sep-arates pleurae)
Continuous Sounds			
Wheeze—High-Pitched (Sibilant)	High-pitched, musical squeaking sounds that sound polyphonic (multiple notes as in a musical chord); predominate in expiration but may occur in both expiration and inspiration	Air squeezed or compressed through passageways narrowed almost to closure by collapsing, swelling, se-cretions, or tumors; the pas-sageway walls oscillate in apposition between the closed and barely open po-sitions; the resulting sound is similar to a vibrating reed	Diffuse airway obstruc-tion from acute asthma or chronic emphysema
Wheeze—Low-Pitched (Sonorous Rhonchi)	Low-pitched; monophonic (single note), musical snoring, moaning sound heard throughout the cycle, although more prominent on expiration; may clear by coughing	Airflow obstruction as de-scribed by the vibrating reed mechanism above; the pitch of the wheeze can-not be correlated to the size of the passageway that generates it	Bronchitis, single bron-chus obstruction from airway tumor
Stridor	High-pitched, mono-phonic, inspiratory, crowing sound, louder in neck than over chest wall	Originating in larynx or trachea, upper airway ob-struction from swollen, in-flamed tissues or lodged foreign body	Croup and acute epiglot-titis in children, post-extubation edema, and obstructed airway may be life-threatening

*Although nothing in clinical practice seems to differ more than the nomenclature of adventitious sounds, most authorities concur on two cat-egories: discontinuous, discrete crackling sounds; and continuous, or musical sounds.
From Jarvis C: Physical Examination and Health Assessment, 2nd ed. Philadelphia, W.B. Saunders, 1996, pp 502–503.

Discontinuous Sounds. Intermittent sounds (crackles or rales) are usually heard on inspiration and reflect abnormalities in the peripheral airways and lung parenchyma. Crackles are explosive sounds caused by vibrations from the sudden release of energy stored in the elastic or surface forces in the lung. The coarse crackles of pulmonary edema or other conditions characterized by fluid accumulation in the airways are hypothesized to be caused by rupture of fluid films or bubbles. These crackles often occur during both inspiration and expiration and may change after a cough or a change in position. Com-pared with the coarse crackles of pulmonary edema, the fine crackles heard in pulmonary fibrosis or early congestive heart failure are not a result of fluid in the airways. These crackles are the result of the delayed opening of airways during inspiration that have closed at the end of the previous expiration. These sounds are heard primarily on inspiration.

Other Adventitious Sounds. Three other adventi-tious sounds are pleural friction rub, referred breath sounds, and mediastinal crunch. The pleural friction rub is a discontinuous, grating sound heard on both inspiration and expiration. It has frequently been de-scribed as a localized, low-pitched, creaking sound. It indicates distortion of the normal anatomy of the pleural surface, usually from inflammation. It may be heard around a chest tube insertion site. Deep breathing exacerbates this sound. A pleural friction rub can be distinguished from a pericardial friction rub in several ways. Both cause a scratchy, scraping sound; however, the pleural friction rub is heard on inspiration and expiration, and the pericardial rub is louder on expiration. In addition, each sound is extremely localized, the pleural friction rub to an area of the chest and the pericardial rub to a cardiac area. Another way to distinguish the two is to listen to the chest while the patient holds his or her breath.

Referred breath sounds are sounds heard over an area where no sounds are expected (e.g., complete pneumothorax, pneumonectomy). These sounds are referred or transmitted from other areas of the chest and are heard because sound travels through fluid and tissue. Last, although not a true "breath sound," a mediastinal crunch (Hamman's sign) is a precordial crackling or crunching sound heard over the mediastinal area. It is associated with each heartbeat, but not with respiration, and it is best heard in the left lateral

TABLE 15–8

Summary of Physical Assessment Findings in Common Respiratory Diseases

Problem	Inspection	Palpation	Percussion	Auscultation
COPD Exacerbation	Increased anteroposterior diameter of chest; if hypoxemic, central cyanosis; most comfortable in sitting position with stabilization of shoulder girdle (tripod position); use of accessory muscles; labored respiration; pursed-lip breathing; prolonged expiration	↓ Movement ↓ Fremitus with air trapping	Hyperresonant	Distant breath sounds if not moving air well; crackles, rhonchi, or wheezes
Asthma Exacerbation	If hypoxemic, most comfortable in sitting position with stabilization of shoulder girdle (tripod position); use of accessory muscles; labored respiration; pursed-lip breathing; central cyanosis	↓ Movement ↓ Fremitus with air trapping	Hyperresonant	Wheezes Distant breath sounds if not moving air well
Atelectasis	Symmetry of chest wall movement unless segment or lobe involved; depending on severity, respiratory rate may be increased	Minor, no change; major, asymmetry of chest wall movement	Dull over affected area	Crackles
Pneumonia	Tachypnea, labored breathing, use of accessory muscles; may have cough, sputum production, fever; depending on respiratory compromise, may have central cyanosis	Asymmetric chest wall movement; ↑ fremitus over affected area	Dullness	Bronchial breath sounds over area of consolidation; crackles, rhonchi
Pneumothorax	Tachypnea, labored breathing, possible central cyanosis, use of accessory muscles	↓ Movement affected side ↓ Fremitus	Hyperresonant	Diminished, absent over area of collapse
Tension Pneumothorax	Tachypnea, labored breathing, central cyanosis, use of accessory muscles; tracheal shift	↓ Movement affected side ↓ Fremitus	Tympany	Diminished, absent over affected area
Pulmonary Edema	Tachypnea, labored breathing, frothy sputum production	Normal or decreased chest wall movement	Normal or dull (depends on severity)	Fine, coarse crackles (initially in dependent areas of lung)
Pleural Effusion	Tachypnea, labored breathing	↓ Movement affected side ↓ Fremitus	Dull	Diminished, absent over area of effusion

COPD, chronic obstructive pulmonary disease.

position.[17] This sound is due to air in the mediastinum, also called pneumomediastinum.

NORMAL VARIATIONS ASSOCIATED WITH AGING

The elderly critically ill patient presents additional challenges when conducting the respiratory assessment. The assessment process may need to be modified or adapted to meet special needs of this population. Prior to beginning the process, the nurse must assess the patient for any sensory and functional impairments that may alter the process (e.g., hearing or vision loss, impaired movement). If the patient requires assistive devices such as eyeglasses or hearing aids, these should be made available in the critical care setting if at all possible.

The historical assessment of the elderly patient may require additional time due to length of the health history. During the assessment of respiratory symptoms, the interview process may require more in-depth questioning to detail symptoms and determine functional changes due to aging versus specific respiratory symptoms. For example, the elderly patient may report shortness of breath and fatigue with activity. The nurse must ask probing questions to determine whether these symptoms are due to lack of cardiopulmonary fitness and decreased functional ability or if they are due to a respiratory disease.

Age-related changes in respiratory structure and function must be considered during the inspection phase of the physical examination. Aging causes structural changes in the thoracic cage with an increase in the outward elastic recoil of the chest wall. This leads to an increase in the anterior-posterior diameter. Also, calcification of the costal cartilages, decreased spaces between the spinal vertebrae, and increasing spinal curvature will change the normal configuration of the thoracic cage.

Increased static lung compliance and decreased volumes and flow rates lead to changes that are assessed during the physical examination. On inspection, chest wall movement will be decreased as compared with that in a younger individual. Changes in lung volumes and flow rates may be noted during chest auscultation. Breath sounds may seem more distant and difficult to hear. These changes are exacerbated in the supine position. The patient must be instructed to breathe through the mouth and take deeper breaths to increase the flow rates and enhance the breath sounds. Last, small airway closure is increased in the aged patient, especially in the supine position. Fine crackles may be heard on end-inspiration when the patient is asked to take a deep breath. This is due to the popping open of small airways. These changes are more prominent in the dependent portions of the lung.

In summary, the respiratory physical assessment is a comprehensive process that involves inspection, palpation, percussion, and auscultation. By integrating all these data along with historical and laboratory data, the nurse is better able to provide comprehensive care to the critically ill patient. Table 15–8 provides a summary of diseases and typical findings during the assessment process. Although a complete respiratory assessment (historical, laboratory, physical assessment) may be time consuming and involved, the nurse should be skilled in all facets of this evaluation and must be able to apply these skills selectively in the clinical setting.

Key Concepts

➠ The examination of the respiratory system includes an integration of the history, laboratory, and physical assessment data for the patient.

➠ The two most frequent symptoms related to respiratory disease are dyspnea and cough.

➠ It is important to conduct the respiratory physical examination systematically (inspection, palpation, percussion, and auscultation) and to adapt the approach to the clinical situation.

➠ In the physical examination process, the inspection and auscultation steps provide most of the respiratory information on the critically ill patient. More advanced skills such as palpation and percussion are helpful, but they take time to learn.

➠ The presence of central cyanosis indicates at least 5 g of desaturated hemoglobin. It is a late sign of hypoxemia.

➠ Signs and symptoms of respiratory distress include tachypnea, breathlessness, difficulty with speech, leaning forward, use of accessory muscles, pursed-lip breathing, central cyanosis, diaphoresis, paradoxic breathing, and decreased air movement.

➠ Consolidation due to pneumonia may cause increased fremitus and bronchial breath sounds over the affected area. Fine or coarse crackles may also be heard.

➠ Pulmonary edema may cause tachypnea, breathlessness, use of accessory muscles, pursed-lip breathing, central cyanosis, diaphoresis, and decreased air movement. Crackles are initially heard in the dependent areas of the lung. In the supine position, these are the posterior bases.

References

1. Berger, KI, Rapoport DM: Chronic obstructive pulmonary disease. In: Dantzker DR, Scharf SM (eds): Cardiopulmonary Critical Care, 3rd ed. Philadelphia, W.B. Saunders, 1998, pp 593–609.

2. Ahmed T, Chediak AD: Status asthmaticus. In: Dantzker DR, Scharf SM (eds): Cardiopulmonary Critical Care, 3rd ed. Philadelphia, W.B. Saunders, 1998, pp 529–591.

3. Buist S, Vollmer WM: Smoking and other risk factors. In: Murray, Nadel (eds): Textbook of Respiratory Medicine 2nd ed. vol. 1. Philadelphia, W.B. Saunders, 1994, pp 1259–1287.

4. Greenblatt MS, Reddel RR, Harris CC: Carcinogenesis, and cellular and molecular biology of lung cancer. In: Roth JA, Ruckdeschel JC, Weisenburger TH (eds): Thoracic Oncology, 2nd ed. Philadelphia, W.B. Saunders, 1995, pp 5–25.

5. Brooks-Brunn JA: Postoperative atelectasis and pneumonia: risk factors. Am J Crit Care 4:340–349, 1995.

6. Wewers M, Bowen JM, Stanislaw AE, et al: A nurse-delivered smoking cessation intervention among hospitalized postoperative patients—influence of smoking-related diagnosis: a pilot study. Heart Lung 23:151–156, 1994.

7. Taylor CB, Miller NH, Herman S, et al: A nurse-managed smoking cessation program for hospitalized smokers. Am J Public Health 86:1557–1560, 1996.

8. Stulbarg MS, Adams L: Dyspnea. In: Murray JF, Nadel JA (eds): Textbook of Respiratory Medicine, 2nd ed. vol. 1. Philadelphia, W.B. Saunders, 1994, pp 511–528.

9. Lush MT, Janson-Bjerklie S, Carrieri VK, et al: Dyspnea in the ventilator-assisted patient. Heart Lung 17:528–535, 1988.

10. Clochesy JM, Daly BJ, Montenegro HD: Weaning chronically critically ill adults from mechanical ventilatory support: a descriptive study. Am J Crit Care 4:93–99, 1995.

11. Carrieri-Kohlman V: Dyspnea in the weaning patient: assessment and intervention. AACN Clin Issues 2:462–473, 1991.

12. Murray JF: History and physical examination. In: Murray JF, Nadel JA (eds): Textbook of Respiratory Medicine, 2nd ed. vol. 1. Philadelphia, W.B. Saunders, 1994, pp 563–584.

13. Wilkins, RL: Bedside assessment of the patient. In: Scanlon CL, Spearman CB, Sheldon RL (eds): Egan's Fundamentals of Respiratory Care, 6th ed. St. Louis: Mosby–Year Book, 1995, pp 361–390.

14. American Thoracic Society Ad Hoc Committee on Pulmonary Nomenclature: Updated nomenclature for membership reaction. ATS News 3:5–6, 1977.

15. Joint Committee of the American College of Chest Physicians and American Thoracic Society: Pulmonary terms and symbols. Chest 67:583–593, 1975.

16. Wilkins RL, Dexter JR, Murphy RLH, et al: Lung sound nomenclature survey. Chest 98:886–889, 1990.

17. Harold CE, Harvey J (eds): Expert 10-Minute Physical Examinations. St. Louis, Mosby–Year Book, 1997.

16

Respiratory Laboratory and Diagnostic Tests

Jo Ann Brooks-Brunn

Objectives

After completing this chapter, the student will be able to:

1. Compare the four primary states of acid–base imbalance according to the underlying causes and mechanisms of correction.
2. Identify the basic thoracic structures assessed in a portable chest radiograph.
3. Describe three diagnostic procedures used for pulmonary disorders.

Various laboratory and diagnostic tests are performed to assess the respiratory status of the critically ill patient. This chapter provides information on frequently ordered tests, bedside monitoring of respiratory status, and diagnostic procedures.

LABORATORY TESTING

Arterial Blood Gas

The arterial blood gas (ABG) is used to determine both the acid–base status and the arterial oxygenation status of the body. The ABG is a limited analysis in that 1) it provides a point estimate or snapshot analysis of the patient's acid–base and oxygenation status; 2) indications for drawing a sample are often vague; and 3) samples are frequently drawn after a deleterious event has occurred.[1] Results must be interpreted in conjunction with the patient's clinical presentation and are most helpful when previous ABG values are available. Trending analysis helps to assess the results of interventions and the progress of the patient.

The ABG sampling procedure is not without risk. Hazards of arterial puncture include arteriospasm, bleeding, hematoma formation, thrombosis, nerve damage, infection, pain, and anxiety. The nurse should assess a patient's clotting ability before drawing a percutaneous sample from either the radial or the femoral site. Blood coagulation disorders and medications that

may interfere with the clotting mechanism should be assessed before performing this procedure. A low platelet count or abnormal prothrombin time (PT), partial thromboblastin time (PTT), or activated clotting time (ACT) may result in significant bleeding after the procedure. Sampling of blood from a patient with a coagulation defect (e.g., hemophilia, thrombocytopenia, liver failure) leads to greater bleeding at the puncture site and the potential for large hematoma formation. The nurse must also assess the patient for any anticoagulant therapy (heparin, warfarin, aspirin) or thrombolytic medications (streptokinase, tissue plasminogen activator). These potent thrombolytic agents are used to lyse vascular occlusive clots (e.g., acute myocardial infarction, stroke), and they place the patient at a greatly increased risk of bleeding. The elapsed time since infusion of these drugs must be assessed before proceeding with an arterial puncture.

Additional patient parameters to be assessed before drawing an ABG include the patient's diagnosis, infectious disease status, vital signs and noninvasive monitoring values, current fraction of inspired oxygen (FIO_2) if on supplemental oxygen (O_2), current respiratory care modalities in use, and amount of time the patient has been in a steady state (e.g., in one position, time since last suctioning procedure or respiratory intervention). Besides the patient's ventilatory and acid–base status, other factors may influence the ABG results obtained. These include puncture technique or access from the indwelling catheter, handling or processing of the specimen, the patient's response to the procedure, and other parameters (e.g., temperature, spontaneous versus assisted ventilation, supplemental O_2).[2] Patients' responses are often overlooked when obtaining an ABG. Increased respiratory rate due to pain or anxiety and breath holding are two examples of factors that may influence the results.

Most commonly, an ABG sample is drawn from the radial artery, brachial artery, femoral artery, or arterial catheter (see Figure 6–9). A percutaneous arterial blood sample is obtained by inserting a 25-gauge needle into the artery (Figure 16–1). In addition to the normal, universal precautions when drawing blood, several key factors are important to remember when drawing and processing an ABG. For a percutaneous puncture, the nurse must apply pressure over the puncture site for 2 to 5 minutes. For patients receiving anticoagulants, pressure may be needed for up to 20 minutes. The sample must be carefully processed by expelling all air bubbles, gently rotating the tube to mix heparin with the blood to prevent clotting, appropriately labeling the specimen, and quickly placing the sample on ice to minimize metabolic changes. In addition, the nurse should check the percutaneous puncture site 2 minutes after relieving pressure for evidence of bleeding or hematoma formation.

An indwelling arterial catheter (an "A" line) provides direct access for ABG sampling. Often, the critically ill patient has an arterial catheter in place for continuous blood pressure monitoring and simplified access for blood sampling. Whether the ABG is being drawn by percutaneous puncture or through an arterial catheter, the nurse should consult the institutional manual for specific steps of each procedure.

Acid–Base Homeostasis

The acid–base interpretation of the ABG result requires not only knowledge of basic chemistry, but also a foundation in basic physiology. First, basic knowledge of the definitions of acid–base status is necessary (Chart 16–1). One of the most important factors in the cellular environment is hydrogen ion (H^+) activity. *Acids* are defined as substances that tend to donate H^+, whereas *bases* are substances that remove or accept H^+ from solution. By definition, pH stands for the negative logarithm of the H^+ concentration (pH = $-$log H^+). Therefore, the pH is inversely proportional to the H^+ concentration (as H^+ ion increases, pH decreases, and vice versa).

Acids can be divided into volatile and nonvolatile types. The lung can remove volatile acids, whereas nonvolatile acids are removed by the kidneys. The respiratory system is responsible for the clearance of the volatile acids or 98 to 99% of the total acid products generated by the body during a 24-hour period.[3] Carbonic acid ($H_2CO_3^-$) is a volatile acid that can be dehydrated into carbon dioxide (CO_2) and water (H_2O). These end products are the result of normal aerobic metabolism. The nonvolatile or fixed acids account for 1 to 2% and are composed of inorganic and organic anions.[3] The kidneys are responsible for elimination of nonvolatile acids.

The regulation of acid–base balance means the regulation of H^+ concentration of the body fluids. The overall goal of acid–base homeostasis is to maintain the arterial blood pH between 7.35 and 7.45. A slight change in H^+ concentration from the normal value can cause significant alterations in the rates of chemical reactions in the cells. Some reactions are depressed,

Figure 16–1

The radial artery puncture. The wrist is extended approximately 30° over a rolled towel, and the puncture is made at a 45° angle, with the bevel of the needle up and directed into the oncoming arterial flow. (From Malley WJ: Clinical Blood Gases: Application and Noninvasive Alternatives. Philadelphia, W.B. Saunders, 1990, p 16.)

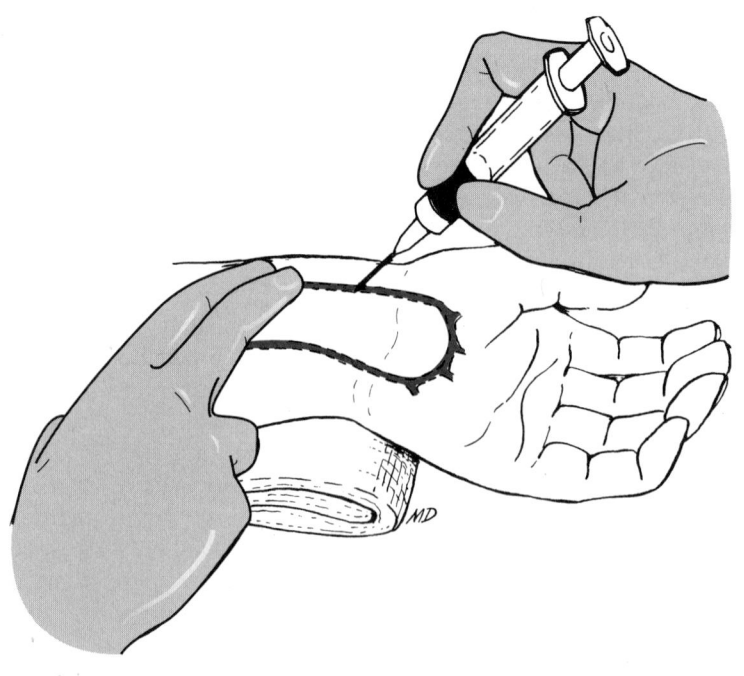

CHART 16-1

Acid–Base Definitions

Acid	Ion that releases H^+ in solution
Base	Ion that combines with H^+ and removes them from solution
pH	Symbol used to express the concentration of H^+; pH is the negative logarithm of H^+ ion concentration; an inverse relationship
Acidemia	pH < 7.35
Alkalemia	pH > 7.45
Acidosis	Process leading to state of excess addition of H^+ or a loss of basic ions from a solution: ↓ pH
Alkalosis	Process leading to state of excess removal of H^+ or the addition of basic ions to solution: ↑ pH
Compensatory mechanisms	Responses of chemical buffers, respiratory, or renal systems

whereas others are accelerated in the presence of acid–base disturbances.

The regulation of H^+ concentration is the most important aspect of homeostasis of the system. Three mechanisms are available to minimize pH change in response to an excessive acid or base load in the system: 1) chemical buffering mechanisms; 2) lung regulation; and 3) kidney regulation.

Chemical Buffers. Chemical buffers are substances that act to minimize changes in the pH of a solution when an acid or base is added. Buffers do not prevent changes in pH when strong acids or strong bases are added to solutions; they simply minimize these changes. The two primary types of chemical buffers can be divided into the total bicarbonate (HCO_3^-) buffers (53%) and the total non–HCO_3^- buffers (47%). The total HCO_3^- system is composed of plasma HCO_3^- and red blood cell HCO_3^-, whereas the total non–HCO_3^- system includes hemoglobin (Hgb), organic and inorganic phosphates, and the plasma proteins. Both the total HCO_3^- and the total non–HCO_3^- buffer systems respond immediately to any change in H^+ concentration. These buffer systems function in harmony to maintain acid–base homeostasis.

Respiratory Regulation. Respiratory regulation plays an important role in acid–base balance by controlling the arterial CO_2 tension of blood through changes in ventilation. Alveolar ventilation is normally controlled, so that blood pH changes are kept to a minimum. Small changes in the partial pressure of arterial CO_2 ($Paco_2$) are quickly sensed by the chemoreceptors in the medulla. These chemoreceptors respond by causing an increase or decrease in ventilation. CO_2 is a volatile acid (an acid that releases H^+ in solution). Increasing or decreasing alveolar ventilation indirectly affects the H^+ level through changes in CO_2. Specifics of CO_2 transport (dissolved in the plasma and in the red blood cells) are described in Chapter 14.

If alveolar ventilation is decreased, this allows CO_2 to accumulate in the blood at higher than normal levels. This process leads to an increase in H^+ ion level and a decrease in pH (pH = $-\log H^+$ concentration). If alveolar ventilation is increased, larger amounts of CO_2 are eliminated (loss of the volatile acid). This causes a decrease in H^+ concentration, and the pH rises. Any change in alveolar ventilation may profoundly influence pH.

Renal Regulation. The lungs cannot regulate nonvolatile or fixed acids. Concentrations of these acids are changed through the kidney. The renal system influences the blood H^+ ion concentration by excretion of either acidic or basic urine. This is accomplished by changing the concentrations of H^+ and HCO_3^- through urinary excretion or conservation. In an acidotic state (pH < 7.35), the kidneys may respond by increasing urinary excretion of H^+ and conservation of HCO_3^- (a base); in an alkalotic state (pH > 7.45), there is increased urinary excretion of HCO_3^- and conservation of H^+ (acid). For every H^+ ion excreted in the urine, an HCO_3^- ion is reabsorbed along with sodium. In addition, phosphate and ammonium ions play a role in the regulation of H^+ ion concentration by the kidney.

The renal control mechanism is the most powerful of the systems to regulate H^+ ion concentration and pH, but it has a slower response time than does the respiratory system. It may take 48 to 72 hours for the renal system to reach its maximum potential to return the pH to a near-normal range.

Acid–Base Parameters of Arterial Blood Gas

In this section, the parameters of acid–base are discussed. Assessment of the oxygenation parameters is described in a later section on oxygenation.

pH. The pH describes the patient's general acid–base status. The pH is proportionate to the ratio of HCO_3^- ion (controlled by the kidney) and CO_2 (controlled by the lung). The normal arterial pH (7.35–7.45) is described by a ratio of 20:1 base to acid in

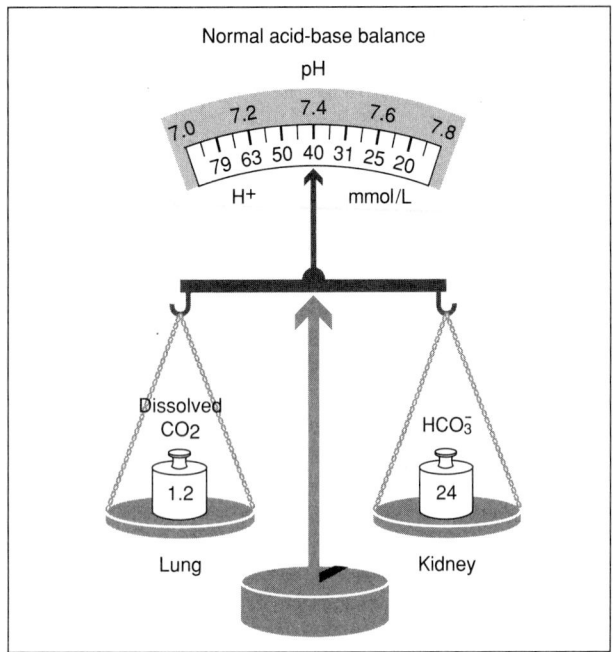

Figure 16–2

The balance between bicarbonate (HCO_3^-) (24 mEq/L) and dissolved carbon dioxide (CO_2) (1.2 or $Paco_2$, 40 mm Hg) is normally 20:1. This ratio is usually associated with a pH of approximately 7.40. (From Cherniack RM: Pulmonary Function Testing, 2nd ed. Philadelphia, W.B. Saunders, 1992, p 96.)

the arterial blood (Figure 16–2). Changes in this ratio change the pH of the arterial blood. An arterial pH of less than 7.35 indicates *acidemia* (high H^+ concentration), whereas a pH greater than 7.45 indicates *alkalemia* (low H^+ concentration) (Chart 16–2). The body responds to abnormal pH by buffering excess acid or base and attempts to compensate until the abnormality naturally resolves or is medically treated.

The nurse must be aware of the body's physiologic responses to the states of acidemia and alkalemia

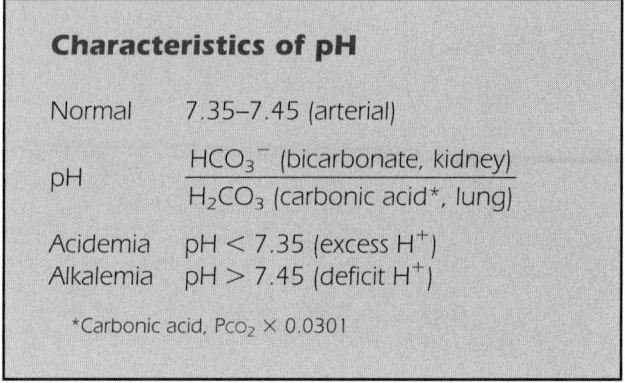

CHART 16-2

Characteristics of pH

Normal	7.35–7.45 (arterial)
pH	$\dfrac{HCO_3^- \text{ (bicarbonate, kidney)}}{H_2CO_3 \text{ (carbonic acid*, lung)}}$
Acidemia	pH < 7.35 (excess H^+)
Alkalemia	pH > 7.45 (deficit H^+)

*Carbonic acid, $Pco_2 \times 0.0301$

(Table 16–1). Critically ill patients are often physiologically unstable, and the body's responses to acid–base abnormalities may exacerbate or may cause additional medical problems.

Partial Pressure of Arterial Carbon Dioxide. The respiratory parameter of the ABG is $Paco_2$. A normal range for $Paco_2$ is 35 to 45 mm Hg (Chart 16–3). This parameter is controlled by the lungs and reflects the adequacy of alveolar ventilation. The $Paco_2$ value is inversely related to the alveolar ventilation. A respiratory acid–base disorder occurs when alveolar ventilation is inappropriate for the production of CO_2.

An increased $Paco_2$ indicates hypoventilation or inadequate ventilation at the alveolar level. When the $Paco_2$ is more than 45 mm Hg, this condition is called *hypercapnia* or *hypercarbia*. Likewise, a decreased $Paco_2$ (<35 mm Hg) indicates hyperventilation or excessive alveolar ventilation (alveolar ventilation is in excess of CO_2 production). A $Paco_2$ less than 35 mm Hg is termed *hypocapnia* or *hypocarbia*. Both alveolar hyperventilation and alveolar hypoventilation are not reflected directly by the respiratory rate and cannot be

TABLE 16–1
Physiologic Effects of Acidemia and Alkalemia

System	Effects of Acidemia (pH < 7.35)	Effects of Alkalemia (pH > 7.45)
Cardiopulmonary	Pulmonary vascular constriction Myocardial irritability, decreased contractility Systemic vasodilatation	Bronchoconstriction Pulmonary vascular dilatation Myocardial irritability Systemic vasoconstriction
CNS	Depressed cortical function Dilatation of cerebral vessels Changes in respiratory control center	Constriction of cerebral vessels Increased excitability of neuromuscular system
Associated symptoms	Headache Slow responses Asterixis (flapping tremor) Confusion Nausea, vomiting Kussmaul's respirations	Dizziness Tingling of fingers or toes Muscle weakness or spasm Sweating Dysrhythmias

CHART 16–3

> ## Characteristics of $Paco_2$
>
> Normal: 35–45 mm Hg
> Respiratory/ventilatory parameter
> Regulated by the lung
> Think of CO_2 as an acid
> Alveolar hypoventilation: ↑ CO_2 (hypercarbia, hypercapnia)
> Alveolar hyperventilation: ↓ CO_2 (hypocarbia, hypocapnia)

diagnosed by observation. These terms describe processes at the alveolar level and can only be directly assessed by the results of an ABG and the $Paco_2$ parameter.

Bicarbonate. HCO_3^- is primarily regulated by the kidneys and is the metabolic or nonrespiratory parameter (Chart 16–4). A normal range for arterial HCO_3^- is 22 to 26 mEq/L. Natural changes in this parameter are slow (kidney regulation) as compared with changes in the $Paco_2$ (respiratory regulation). However, HCO_3^- can be manipulated quickly by intravenous administration of sodium bicarbonate ($NaHCO_3$).

As a beginning foundation in the interpretation of the ABG, HCO_3^- can be considered a base. As a primary disorder, an increase in HCO_3^- (>26 mEq/L) causes alkalemia (pH > 7.45), and a HCO_3^- less than normal (<22 mEq/L) causes acidemia (pH < 7.35). However, as shown later in this section, the nurse must consider all the acid–base parameters (pH, $Paco_2$, and HCO_3^-) in the interpretation of the patient's acid–base balance status.

Base Excess. Base excess (BE) is another metabolic or nonrespiratory parameter. It describes the total amount of buffering or base in solution. It is expressed in milliequivalents per liter above or below the normal buffer base range (0 ± 2 mEq/L). A negative value describes a base deficit or excess of acid, whereas a posi-

tive value signifies an excess base or loss of acid. It is analyzed in relation to the pH as an index of total buffering. Therapeutically, the BE may be used to calculate the amount of exogenous HCO_3^- needed to compensate for a metabolic acidosis. However, use of exogenous HCO_3^- in correcting a metabolic acidosis remains controversial.[4]

Acid–Base Imbalances

In analyzing the acid–base status, the nurse must understand the meaning of each parameter and the way in which these parameters vary in relation to one another. Chart 16–5 describes the normal ranges for each blood gas parameter in the arterial and venous blood. Information regarding venous blood gas parameters and assessment of the parameters of oxygenation (Pao_2 and Sao_2) are discussed in later sections of this chapter.

To begin to analyze the acid–base status, the nurse should consider three parameters: pH, $Paco_2$, and HCO_3^-. First, one must interpret the pH. Even if the pH is within the normal range, this does not always indicate normal acid–base balance. The nurse must also assess the $Paco_2$ and HCO_3^-. The primary cause of an abnormal pH must be determined: a respiratory process ($Paco_2$), a metabolic process (HCO_3^-), or a combination of these two. Once the primary cause is determined, then the nurse must assess whether or not compensation has taken place or is in progress.

Compensation. Assessment of the compensatory response to an acid–base imbalance is an important part of the interpretation process. Each acid–base disorder is described as a primary disorder (e.g., respiratory or metabolic or nonrespiratory) and whether compensation has occurred. The compensatory parameter is the secondary parameter. For example, if a respiratory acid–base disorder (primary process, abnormal

CHART 16–4

> ## Characteristics of HCO_3^-
>
> Normal: 22–26 mEq/L
> Metabolic/nonrespiratory parameter
> Regulated by the kidneys
> Think of HCO_3^- as a base

CHART 16–5

> ## Normal Arterial and Venous Blood Gas Values*
>
> | Arterial | Venous |
> |---|---|
> | pH 7.35–7.45 | pH 7.30–7.40 |
> | $Paco_2$ 35–45 mm Hg | $P\bar{v}co_2$ 46 mm Hg |
> | HCO_3^- 22–26 mEq/L | HCO_3^- 22–26 mEq/L |
> | Pao_2 80–100 mm Hg | $P\bar{v}o_2$ 40 mm Hg |
> | Sao_2 >95% | $S\bar{v}o_2$ 70–76% |
> | BE −2 to +2 | |
>
> *Values based on sea level; $\bar{v}$, mixed venous

PaCO₂) is described, then the compensatory parameter is HCO_3^-. The condition may be described as acute or chronic with compensation in progress. Examination of serial ABG results assists in determining the acuity of the process and the amount of compensation that has taken place.

The compensatory parameter changes in the same direction as the primary cause of the acid–base imbalance. This is the body's attempt to maintain the pH at the 20:1 ratio between base (HCO_3^-) and acid ($PaCO_2$). As an example, in the face of increased $PaCO_2$ resulting from alveolar hypoventilation, the HCO_3^- begins to rise. The body does not overcompensate, so despite respiratory or renal compensation, the pH remains slightly abnormal in the direction of the primary disturbance. Table 16–2 describes each acid–base disorder, the compensatory response, and the expected compensation.

Unfortunately, iatrogenic overcompensation can occur in the critical care setting. Changes in the settings (rate or tidal volume) on the mechanical ventilator may cause abrupt changes in the $PaCO_2$, as will inadequate or excessive ventilation with a manual resuscitator bag. Administration of medications (e.g., $NaHCO_3$) may also cause abrupt changes in the acid–base status.

Respiratory Acidosis. Acute respiratory acidosis is caused by alveolar hypoventilation that results in an increase in $PaCO_2$ and a decrease in pH. In an acute state, the HCO_3^- is usually within normal limits because the kidneys have not had time to respond or to compensate. Potential causes of acute respiratory acidosis include acute respiratory failure, congestive heart failure, pulmonary edema, severe pulmonary infections, and CNS depression (drug overdose, head trauma, sedation, anesthesia). Signs and symptoms include palpitations, flushed skin, muscular twitching, and mental cloudiness. Causes of chronic respiratory acidosis include COPD, cystic fibrosis, obesity, and chronic neuromuscular diseases. Signs and symptoms include hyperpnea, weakness, headache, stupor, and irritability. Laboratory findings consistent with alveolar hypoventilation and respiratory acidosis include the following:

- **pH 7.4 to 7.0**
- **PCO₂ 45 to 120 mm Hg**
- CO_2 content upper normal or above
- HCO_3^- is normal or slightly elevated
- BE upper normal
- Elevated serum potassium (K+)

If the respiratory acidosis is chronic, compensation will be in process or maximized, depending on the time frame and severity of the abnormality. The description of compensated respiratory imbalance is termed chronic if the body has begun to respond or to compensate. In compensated respiratory acidosis, the pH is near normal or slightly acidotic, and the $PaCO_2$ remains elevated (Figure 16–3). Compensation for respiratory acidosis occurs by the kidney, which increases the excretion of H^+ and reabsorbs and releases HCO_3^- into the blood (HCO_3^- increases). Simultaneously, chloride (Cl^-) is eliminated by the kidney in the form of hydrochloric acid or ammonium chloride. The compensatory process begins immediately, but it does not reach its maximum response for 48 to 72 hours. Table 16–3 shows examples of acute and chronic or compensated respiratory acidosis.

Treatment of respiratory acidosis is focused on improving alveolar ventilation. For the spontaneously

TABLE 16–2

Compensatory Responses in Acid–Base Disorders

Primary Disorder	Primary Abnormality	Compensatory Response	Expected Compensation*
Metabolic acidosis	↓ HCO_3^- ↓ pH	↓ $PaCO_2$	$\Delta PaCO_2 = 1.2 \times \Delta HCO_3^-$
Metabolic alkalosis	↑ HCO_3^- ↑ pH	↑ $PaCO_2$	$\Delta PaCO_2 = 0.7 \times \Delta HCO_3^-$
Respiratory acidosis			
Acute	↑ $PaCO_2$ ↓ pH	↑ HCO_3^-	$\Delta HCO_3^- = 0.1 \times \Delta PaCO_2$
Chronic	↑ $PaCO_2$ ↓ pH	↑ ↑ HCO_3^-	$\Delta HCO_3^- = 0.35 \times \Delta PaCO_2$
Respiratory alkalosis			
Acute	↓ $PaCO_2$ ↑ pH	↓ HCO_3^-	$\Delta HCO_3^- = 0.2 \times \Delta PaCO_2$
Chronic	↓ $PaCO_2$ Normal to ↑ pH	↓ ↓ HCO_3^-	$\Delta HCO_3^- = 0.5 \times \Delta PaCO_2$

*$\Delta PaCO_2$ and ΔHCO_3^- are the changes in concentration from normal. $PaCO_2$ is 38–42 mm Hg. HCO_3^- is 24–28 mEq/L. Double arrows indicate a profound change.

From Dantzker DR, MacIntyre NR, Bakow ED: Comprehensive Respiratory Care. Philadelphia, W.B. Saunders, 1995, p 73.

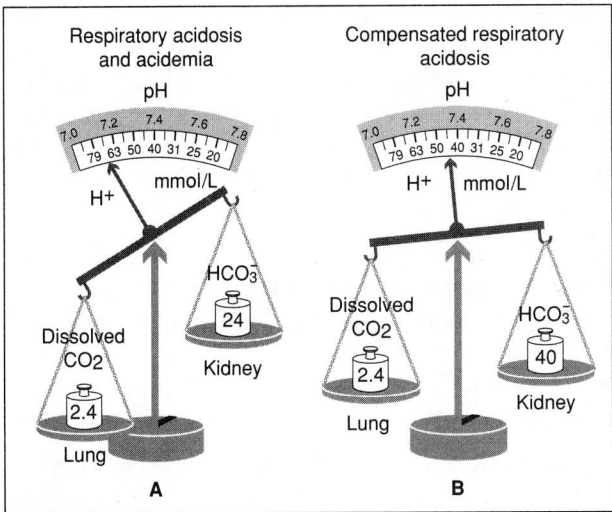

Figure 16-3

An elevated arterial carbon dioxide pressure (Pa_{CO_2}) constitutes respiratory acidosis. *A*, In the acute condition, the balance between bicarbonate and dissolved carbon dioxide is less than 20:1, so that the pH is low (acidemia) and the H^+ concentration is elevated. *B*, With compensation by the kidney, bicarbonate is retained, so that the ratio of bicarbonate to dissolved carbon dioxide is closer to 20:1, and the pH and H^+ concentration are almost normal (but on the acidemic side). (From Cherniack RM: Pulmonary Function Testing, 2nd ed. Philadelphia, W.B. Saunders, 1992, p 99.)

breathing patient, treatments may include repositioning of the patient, enhancing the respiratory drive, clearance of secretions, clearance of other airway obstruction, or alleviation of bronchoconstriction. In severe cases of alveolar hypoventilation (e.g., drug overdose or head injury with decreased respiratory drive), the patient may require intubation and mechanical ventilation. Acute respiratory failure is a broad clinical example of alveolar hypoventilation caused by a dysfunction in the respiratory system leading to an increase in CO_2 and inadequate O_2 delivery. Acute respiratory failure has multiple causes (see Chapter 17). Three of the criteria used to define acute respiratory failure are partial arterial pressure of oxygen (Pa_{O_2}) less than 50 mm Hg on room air, Pa_{CO_2} more than 50 mm Hg, and arterial blood pH compatible with significant respiratory acidosis.[5]

In the critical care setting, the nurse should assess the patient with chronic respiratory acidosis (increased CO_2, compensatory increase in HCO_3^-). If the patient is intubated and requiring mechanical ventilation, the ABG parameters should be monitored closely. Often, the Pa_{CO_2} is decreased by mechanical ventilation. The patient then develops rebound metabolic alkalosis because of the increased HCO_3^- from the compensation for the chronic respiratory acidosis. Remember that the kidneys respond slowly, so it will take hours for the kidneys to begin to excrete the excess HCO_3^-.

Respiratory Alkalosis. Acute respiratory alkalosis is caused by alveolar hyperventilation in excess of CO_2 production. This results in a decrease in Pa_{CO_2} and an increase in pH. In an acute state, the HCO_3^- is within normal limits because the kidney has not had time to respond or to compensate. Potential causes of alveolar hyperventilation and respiratory alkalosis include hyperventilation, hypoxemia, excessive mechanical ventilation, hypermetabolic states, toxic stimulation of the respiratory center, pregnancy, and Gram-negative septicemia. Signs and symptoms include dizziness, lightheadedness, numbness of fingers, tinnitus, palpitations, sweating, feeling of panic, muscle cramp, tetany, tightness of chest, dry mouth, and blurred vision. Laboratory findings consistent with alveolar hyperventilation and respiratory alkalosis include the following:

- **pH greater than 7.45**
- **P_{CO_2} less than 35 mm Hg**
- CO_2 content low
- HCO_3^- normal or low
- Base excess normal in acute, and low in chronic alkalosis
- Decreasing calcium (Ca^{++}) and K^+

The renal system compensates for respiratory alkalosis. If the respiratory alkalosis is chronic, compensation will be in process or completed. In compensated respiratory alkalosis, the pH is near normal or slightly alkalotic, the Pa_{CO_2} remains decreased, and the HCO_3^- is decreased. The kidney attempts to compensate for the respiratory alkalosis by excreting more HCO_3^- (base) to balance the decreased Pa_{CO_2} (acid) in the blood (Figure 16-4). At the same time, the kidney

TABLE 16-3
Respiratory Acidosis and Alkalosis

		Examples	
Disorder	**Compensatory Response**	**Acute**	**Chronic or Compensated**
Respiratory acidosis ↑ CO_2 (>45 mm Hg) ↓pH (<7.35)	Hypoventilation; decreased effective alveolar ventilation; reduced CO_2 elimination	pH 7.27 P_{CO_2} 56 HCO_3^- 24	pH 7.36 P_{CO_2} 55 HCO_3^- 39
Respiratory alkalosis ↓ CO_2 (<35 mm Hg) ↑pH (>7.45)	Hyperventilation; increased effective alveolar ventilation; excessive CO_2 elimination	pH 7.58 P_{CO_2} 18 HCO_3^- 24	pH 7.49 P_{CO_2} 30 HCO_3^- 21

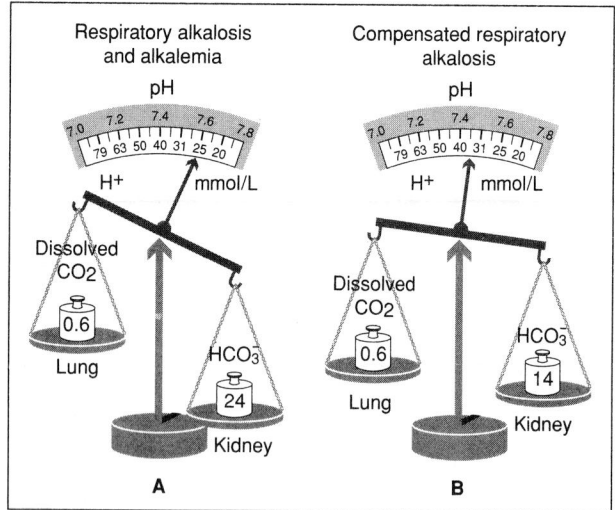

Figure 16–4

A reduced $Paco_2$ constitutes respiratory alkalosis. *A,* In the acute condition, the balance between bicarbonate and dissolved carbon dioxide is greater than 20:1, so that the pH is high (alkalemia) and the H^+ concentration is low. *B,* With compensation by the kidney, bicarbonate is excreted, so that the ratio of bicarbonate to dissolved carbon dioxide is closer to 20:1, and the pH and H^+ concentration are closer to normal (but on the alkalemic side). (From Cherniack RM: Pulmonary Function Testing, 2nd ed. Philadelphia, W.B. Saunders, 1992, p 100.)

conserves Cl^-. Table 16–3 shows examples of acute and chronic or compensated respiratory alkalosis. As shown, complete compensation by the renal system is not likely, and the pH usually remains above the normal range with slight alkalosis.

Treatment of respiratory alkalosis focuses on the underlying cause of the alveolar hyperventilation. In the patient with respiratory alkalosis, the nurse must closely assess the patient for the cause of the problem and must intervene. In the critical care setting, hypoxemia, anxiety, and pain are frequent causes of alveolar hyperventilation and the resulting respiratory alkalosis. If the patient is mechanically ventilated by a control mode, a decrease in the rate or tidal volume will help to correct the respiratory alkalosis. Usually, the rate is adjusted because the tidal volume is set according to body weight. If the patient is mechanically ventilated by a mode that allows spontaneous breaths as well as machine-generated breaths or assistance, the nurse should assess the patient's spontaneous rate and estimated depth of breathing. ABG determinations help to determine the alveolar ventilation ($Paco_2$ level). Nursing interventions focus on nonpharmacologic or pharmacologic methods to decrease the rate or depth of ventilation.

Metabolic Acidosis. Metabolic acidosis is defined as a gain of fixed or nonvolatile acids or excess loss of a base (HCO_3^-) by the kidney or intestinal tract. Various problems may cause metabolic acidosis. The most common causes include renal failure, ketoacidosis, acute myocardial infarction, starvation, salicylate

intoxication, anaerobic metabolism, prolonged diarrhea, intestinal fistulas, ureterosigmoidostomy, and renal tubular acidosis. Signs and symptoms include headache, confusion, Kussmaul's respirations, weakness, nausea, stupor, delirium, dysrhythmias, and warm, flushed skin. Laboratory findings include the following:

- **pH less than 7.35**
- **HCO_3^- less than 22 mEq/L**
- Pco_2 less than than 35 mm Hg (compensatory)
- BE negative
- Increased K^+
- Decreased Ca^{++} in some

Causes of metabolic acidosis are classified as either an increased anion gap or a normal anion gap. An increase or retention of an unmeasured anion (e.g., lactate or ketones) causes an increased anion gap. Metabolic acidosis related to normal anion gap is related to an excessive loss of HCO_3^-, an inability of the kidney to excrete H^+, or the addition of an exogenous acid.[4] In metabolic acidosis, the pH is decreased, and the primary abnormality is a decrease in HCO_3^-. Because the lungs respond rapidly to try to compensate, an increase in ventilation occurs almost immediately in response to the increased fixed body acids (H^+ ion concentration). However, the response of the respiratory system to compensate by decreasing CO_2 is limited (Figure 16–5). Table 16–4 provides examples of acute and compensated metabolic acidosis.

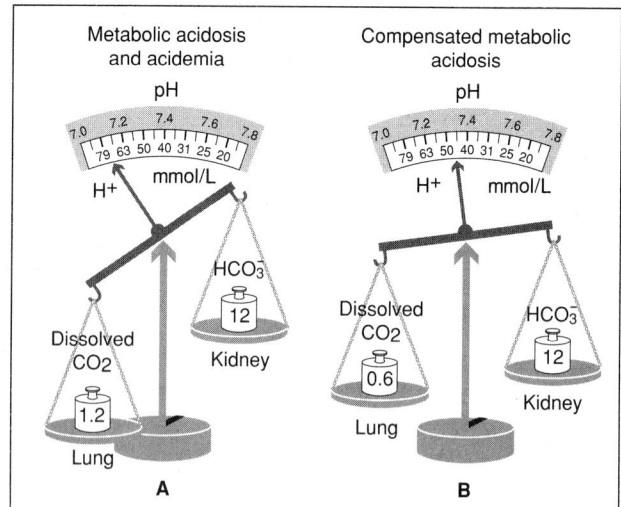

Figure 16–5

A reduced bicarbonate concentration constitutes metabolic acidosis. *A,* In the acute condition, the balance between bicarbonate and dissolved carbon dioxide is less than 20:1, so that the pH is low (acidemia) and the H^+ concentration is high. *B,* With compensation by the respiratory system, carbon dioxide is eliminated, so that the ratio of bicarbonate to dissolved carbon dioxide is closer to 20:1, and the pH and H^+ concentration are closer to normal (but on the acidemic side). (From Cherniack RM: Pulmonary Function Testing, 2nd ed. Philadelphia, W.B. Saunders, 1992, p 102.)

TABLE 16–4
Metabolic Acidosis and Alkalosis

Disorder	Cause	Examples Acute		Chronic or Compensated	
Metabolic acidosis $\downarrow HCO_3^-$ (<22 mEq/L) $\downarrow$ pH (<7.35)	Excessive loss of HCO_3^- or excessive load of an acid in the body	pH $Paco_2$ HCO_3^-	7.11 40 12	pH $Paco_2$ HCO_3^-	7.40* 20 12
Metabolic alkalosis $\uparrow HCO_3^-$ (>26 mEq/L) $\uparrow$ pH (>7.45)	Gain of HCO_3^- or excessive loss of an acid from the body	pH $Paco_2$ HCO_3^-	7.57 40 36	pH $Paco_2$ HCO_3^-	7.40 60 36

*If the metabolic acidosis is severe, the lungs may not be able to blow off enough CO_2 to compensate. In metabolic acidosis, the body does not fully compensate to return the pH back to 7.40.

Treatment of metabolic acidosis is targeted at the underlying cause. Serum K^+ is elevated with a metabolic acidosis because of the flux of K^+ into the extracellular fluid in response to H^+ and Cl^- moving into the intracellular space. Depending on the severity of the acidosis, it may be necessary to correct the acidosis partially with administration of $NaHCO_3$. $NaHCO_3$ administration may be indicated if the pH is less than 7.20.[6] However, correction of metabolic acidosis with an HCO_3^- infusion is controversial.[4] This correction should be done slowly to avoid rapid movement of K^+ back into the cells and resulting hypokalemia (low K^+). Determining the amount of HCO_3^- to administer is calculated by the following equation[4]:

$$HCO_3^- \text{ deficit} =$$
$$(\text{desired } HCO_3^- - \text{actual } HCO_3^-) \times HCO_3^- \text{ space}$$

$$HCO_3^- \text{ space} = 0.6 \times \text{body weight (kg)}$$

Thus, for a 70-kg person with an actual HCO_3^- of 10 mEq/L and a desired HCO_3^- of 25 mEq/L, the HCO_3^- deficit is: $(25 - 10) \times 0.6 (70 \text{ kg}) = 15 \times 42$ or 630 mEq of HCO_3^-.

Metabolic Alkalosis. A loss of a strong acid (e.g., hydrochloric acid from the stomach) or a gain of a strong base (HCO_3^-) in the extracellular fluid causes metabolic alkalosis. Increased pH and increased HCO_3^- characterize this imbalance. A common cause of metabolic alkalosis in the critical care setting is K^+ depletion. Other causes include the following: acute loss of hydrogen ions resulting from vomiting or nasogastric suction; K^+ or Cl^- loss, resulting from diuretics, corticosteroids, or liver disease; or the addition of base, caused by excess use of HCO_3^-, lactate, and administration in dialysis. Signs and symptoms include tingling of fingers and toes, dizziness, nausea, vomiting, lethargy, coma, paralytic ileus, disorientation, convulsions, weakness, muscle cramps, tetany, depressed respirations, and electrocardiographic changes. Laboratory findings include the following:

- **pH greater than 7.45**
- **HCO_3^- greater than 26 mEq/L**
- BE positive
- Pco_2 normal or high
- Normal or low K^+
- Low Ca^{++}
- Urinary Cl^- low with vomiting, higher with K^+ loss

The respiratory system is responsible for compensation in metabolic alkalosis. The decreased H^+ concentration in metabolic alkalosis causes a compensatory inhibition of ventilation, so that alveolar ventilation decreases and CO_2 increases (Figure 16–6). This compensatory response begins quickly. However, this

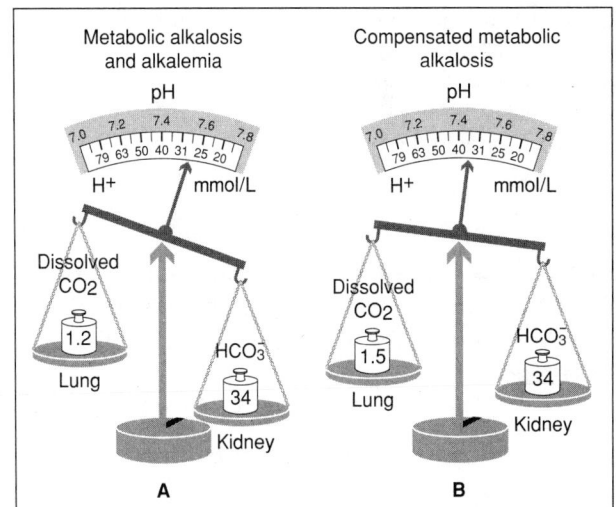

Figure 16–6

An elevated bicarbonate concentration constitutes metabolic alkalosis. *A,* In the acute condition, the balance between bicarbonate and dissolved carbon dioxide is greater than 20:1, so that the pH is high (alkalemia) and the H^+ concentration is low. *B,* With compensation by the respiratory system, carbon dioxide is retained, so that the ratio of bicarbonate to dissolved carbon dioxide is closer to 20:1, and the pH and H^+ concentrations are closer to normal (but on the alkalemic side). (From Cherniack RM: Pulmonary Function Testing, 2nd ed. Philadelphia, W.B. Saunders, 1992, p 102.)

compensatory response is limited, and the $Paco_2$ usually does not increase above 50 mm Hg regardless of the severity of the metabolic alkalosis.[7]

Treatment of metabolic alkalosis is focused on the underlying cause, and K^+ repletion is often necessary. In addition, the nurse must monitor the fluid volume of the patient. Inadequate fluid volume along with loss of H^+, Cl^-, and K^+ may lead to a severe metabolic alkalosis.

Mixed Acid–Base Disorders. More than one acid–base disorder may occur simultaneously, especially in the critically ill patient. In general, the direction of the pH usually indicates the dominant disorder. An example is the patient who is lethargic, has alveolar hypoventilation (respiratory acidosis), and has had severe episodes of vomiting (metabolic alkalosis, acute loss of H^+ ions). To determine the dominant disorder, the nurse should first examine the pH. In this case, if the pH is alkalotic (>7.45), the dominant disorder is the metabolic alkalosis. However, the pH is not excessively abnormal because of the concurrent respiratory acidosis. Another example of a mixed disorder may be in a patient with chronic obstructive lung disease (chronic respiratory acidosis) and acute ketoacidosis (metabolic acidosis). This situation would cause a severe drop in the pH because of both these processes. However, the metabolic acidosis would probably be the dominant disorder.

Interpretation of the Acid–Base Status. The nurse should first quickly scan the ABG results for values that are severely abnormal and may require immediate intervention. These values have been termed "panic values" by some investigators and are shown in Table 16–5.[7] Before reporting or acting on a "panic value," the nurse should always assess the patient to determine whether the clinical picture is congruent with the abnormal parameter.

TABLE 16–5

Suggested "Panic Values" Ranges (Values That May Require Immediate Therapeutic Intervention) for Arterial Blood Gas Results*

pH	<	7.20 pH
pH	>	7.60 pH
Pco_2	>	65 mm Hg†
Po_2	<	50 mm Hg

*Clinicians should remember to interpret all blood gas values collectively and with regard to the patient's underlying condition because an accurate diagnosis seldom depends on a single measured parameter.

†Only in cases with a marked decrease in pH; check HCO_3^- to see whether renal compensation has occurred.

Adapted from Burton GG, Hodgkin JE, Ward JJ: Respiratory Care: A Guide to Clinical Practice, 4th ed. Philadelphia, Lippincott–Raven, 1997, p 261.

After this quick screen, a systematic, stepwise approach should be used in assessing the patient's acid–base status. These steps are described in Chart 16–6, and an algorithm is shown in Figure 16–7. In addition, the patient's clinical status, physical assessment findings, and previous ABG results should be integrated into the overall interpretation of acid–base status. Table 16–6 provides examples of clinical situations and ABG results.

Oxygenation Parameters

To assess the basic oxygenation parameters in the critically ill patient, the nurse must assess the Pao_2, Sao_2 (percentage of saturation of hemoglobin with oxygen), Hgb level, and Fio_2. As described in Chapter 14, 97% of O_2 is transported in combination with Hgb, and the oxyhemoglobin dissociation curve describes the rela-

CHART 16–6

Steps in the Interpretation of an Acid–Base Disorder

Acid–Base Status

1. Evaluate the pH. Is it normal (7.35–7.45), low (<7.35 [acidemia]), or high (>7.45 [alkalemia])?
2. Evaluate the Pco_2. Is it normal (35–45 mm Hg), low (<35 mm Hg), or high (>45 mm Hg)?
3. Evaluate the HCO_3^-. Is it normal (22–26 mEq/L), low (<22 mEq/L), or high (>26 mEq/L)?
4. Determine the primary disorder. Is it respiratory or metabolic (nonrespiratory)?
5. Determine whether compensation is present. Is the secondary parameter trending in the same direction as the primary parameter?

Disorder	pH	Primary	Compensation
Respiratory acidosis	↓	↑ CO_2	↑ HCO_3^-
Respiratory alkalosis	↑	↓ CO_2	↓ HCO_3^-
Metabolic acidosis	↓	↓ HCO_3^-	↓ CO_2
Metabolic alkalosis	↑	↑ HCO_3^-	↑ CO_2

6. Compare with previous arterial blood gas measurements.

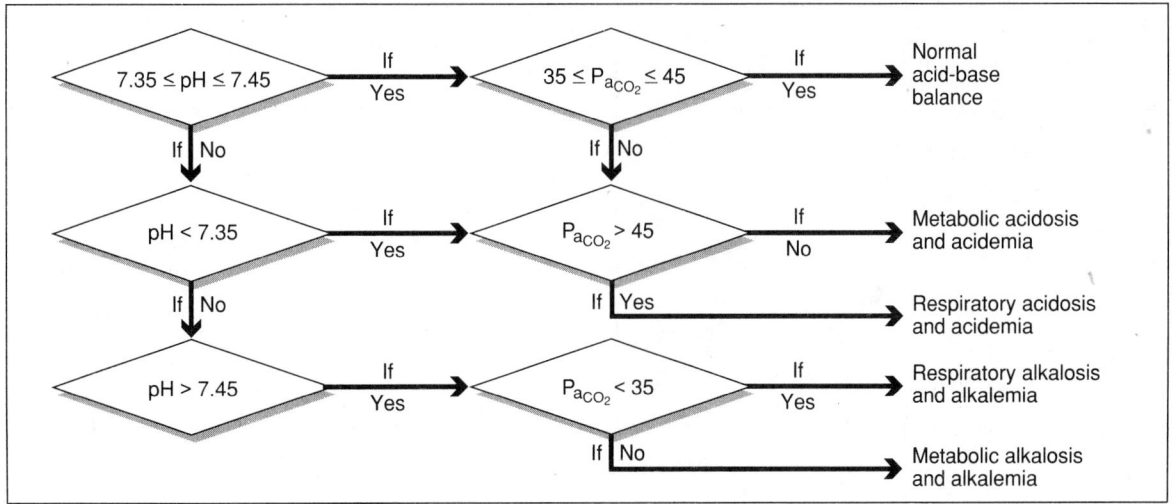

Figure 16–7

Algorithm for interpretation of acid–base balance. (From Cherniack RM: Pulmonary Function Testing, 2nd ed. Philadelphia, W.B. Saunders, 1992, p 244.)

tionship between oxyhemoglobin and O_2 carried in the dissolved state (Pa_{O_2}).

Two terms used when describing a patient's oxygenation status are hypoxia and hypoxemia. *Hypoxia* means that O_2 delivery to the *tissues* is inadequate to meet the tissues' metabolic needs. No laboratory test directly assesses tissue hypoxia. *Hypoxemia* exists when O_2 is inadequate in the *arterial* blood (<80 mm Hg for the adult at sea level) and can be assessed from the ABG. The five causes of hypoxemia are ventilation–perfusion mismatch, anatomic right-to-left shunt, ambient hypoxemia (altitude), alveolar hypoventilation, and diffusion abnormality. As shown in Chart 16–7, hypoxemia causes several physiologic effects and symptoms. The severity of these effects depends on the degree of hypoxemia and the patient's underlying condition and comorbid problems.

Figure 16–8 describes the various processes leading to tissue oxygenation and methods used to evaluate each process. Table 16–7 provides definitions of terms frequently used in describing the oxygenation status of the critically ill patient. Although Pa_{O_2} and Sa_{O_2} are the most commonly used, more in-depth evaluations

are also available to assess the adequacy and efficiency of oxygenation at the lung and tissue levels.

Partial Pressure of Arterial Oxygen. The two oxygenation values obtained with the ABG are Pa_{O_2} and Sa_{O_2}. The "normal" Pa_{O_2} depends on age and altitude and is affected by changes in ventilation and perfusion. The Pa_{O_2} represents the amount of oxygen carried in the dissolved state. To calculate the amount of O_2 carried in the dissolved state, the Pa_{O_2} is multiplied by 0.003. Only a small fraction of O_2 is carried by this method.

A "normal" Pa_{O_2} is 80 to 100 mm Hg on room air (Fi_{O_2} .21 or 21%). However, oxygenation is adequate if the Pa_{O_2} can be maintained between 60 and 100 mm Hg and adequate amounts of Hgb are available. When the Pa_{O_2} falls below 60 mm Hg, there is a sharp decrease in the Sa_{O_2} and impairment in gas transport, as seen in the oxyhemoglobin dissociation curve (see Chapter 14). A Pa_{O_2} less than 60 mm Hg is termed hypoxemia, and a value of 60 to 80 mm Hg is termed relative hypoxemia.

Both the Pa_{O_2} and Sa_{O_2} must be interpreted in relation to the amount of supplemental O_2 the patient is

TABLE 16–6

Examples of Arterial Blood Gas (ABG) Results and Clinical Situations

Clinical Situation	pH	Paco$_2$	HCO$_3^-$	Pao$_2$
Acute alveolar hyperventilation with hypoxemia	7.54	29	21	63
Acute ventilatory failure with hypoxemia	7.15	91	28	57
Chronic ventilatory failure with hypoxemia	7.38	88	33	62
Acute alveolar hyperventilation superimposed on chronic ventilatory failure	7.54	57	29	53
Acute ventilatory failure superimposed on chronic ventilatory failure	7.18	103	39	46

From Burton GG, Hodgkin JE, Ward JJ: Respiratory Care: A Guide to Clinical Practice, 4th ed. Philadelphia, Lippincott–Raven, 1997, p 175.

CHART 16–7

Physiologic Effects of Hypoxemia and Signs or Symptoms

Physiologic Effects

Pulmonary vasoconstriction
Altered CNS function
Anaerobic metabolism

Signs and Symptoms

Mild–Moderate Hypoxemia
  Tachypnea
  Hyperventilation
  Dyspnea
  Tachycardia
  Mild hypertension
  Peripheral vasoconstriction
  Mild changes in intellectual function
  Headache
  Restlessness
Severe Hypoxemia
  Tachypnea
  Hyperventilation
  Dyspnea
  Cyanosis
  Tachycardia early stage, leading to
    bradycardia and dysrhythmias
  Hypertension early stage, leading to
    hypotension
  Somnolence
  Confusion
  Loss of coordination

receiving. For each 20% rise in FIO_2, the acceptable PaO_2 level rises by approximately 100 mm Hg. Conversely, the acceptable PaO_2 for a given FIO_2 can be estimated by multiplying the $FIO_2 \times 5$. Thus, for a person with normal lungs, no gas exchange impairment, and who is receiving an FIO_2 of 0.40 (40% oxygen), the PaO_2 should be approximately 200 mm Hg.

A clinical example is a patient admitted to the critical care unit with vomiting, dehydration, and lower respiratory infection who has a PaO_2 of 50 mm Hg on 30% (FIO_2 0.30). This patient has unacceptable oxygenation, is hypoxemic, and needs increased supplemental O_2. The predicted PaO_2 for this patient on 30% supplemental O_2 would be 150 mm Hg (30% × 5).

Oxygen Saturation. SaO_2 describes the percent of Hgb bound or saturated with O_2 in the arterial blood. It may either be a calculated parameter of the ABG, directly measured from the blood by a method called co-oximetry, or noninvasively estimated by pulse oximetry (SpO_2). The details of SpO_2 are discussed later in this chapter.

A normal SaO_2 value is greater than or equal to 95%. In the critically ill patient, a value greater than or equal to 90% is usually acceptable. Given adequate Hgb, a SaO_2 of 90% represents a PaO_2 of 60 mm Hg (see Chapter 14). The SaO_2 value describes *the available* Hgb, the percentage of Hgb bound with O_2. To assess oxygenation, the SaO_2 *must always be interpreted in relation to the Hgb level* of the patient. For example, a patient may have an adequate saturation (>90%) in the presence of a low Hgb. If the Hgb is 8 g and the SaO_2 is 96%, this means that 96% of the 8 g Hgb (normal, 14–16 g/dL in males and 12–15 g/dL in females) is saturated with O_2. Even though the SaO_2 is adequate (>90%), oxygenation is inadequate because of the low Hgb.

Hemoglobin. An evaluation of Hgb goes hand in hand with evaluation of the SaO_2. Although not a parameter of the ABG, the patient's Hgb *must* be considered when evaluating the other oxygenation parameters. A normal Hgb value for men is 14 to 16 g/dL and for women it is 12 to 15 g/dL. Each gram of Hgb can maximally carry 1.34 mL of O_2 in the blood. If the body were devoid of Hgb, the cardiac output would have to be 83.3 L per minute at a PaO_2 of 100 mm Hg to meet the tissues' demand for O_2 *at rest*.[8] A normal cardiac output is approximately 5 L per minute. Because Hgb is critical in O_2 transport, it is important to monitor this parameter in the critically ill patient.

Total Oxygen Content of Arterial Blood. The total arterial oxygen content (CaO_2) describes the amount of O_2 carried in combination with Hgb and in the dissolved form in the arterial blood. It is described in milliliters per 100 mL blood or volumes percent. The CaO_2 is calculated as follows:

$$CaO_2 = (Hgb \times 1.34 \times SaO_2) + (.003 \times PaO_2)$$

    (carried in   (dissolved state)
    combination
    with Hgb)

Thus, it is easy to see that a decrease in any of the oxygenation variables may affect the CaO_2. Table 16–8 shows how a decrease in the Hgb level decreases the CaO_2. For the example in this table, the PaO_2 remains at 100 mm Hg, and only the Hgb is varied.

Mixed Venous Oxygen Monitoring. Although the primary type of blood gas analyzed is the ABG, the nurse should also understand the monitoring of parameters of the venous blood gas. Mixed venous O_2 monitoring is invasive. Intermittently, a mixed venous blood sample may be drawn from the distal port of a pulmonary artery catheter and analyzed. A mixed venous sample implies that the blood reflects a mixing of all the venous blood and is obtained from the pulmonary artery or the area just proximal to

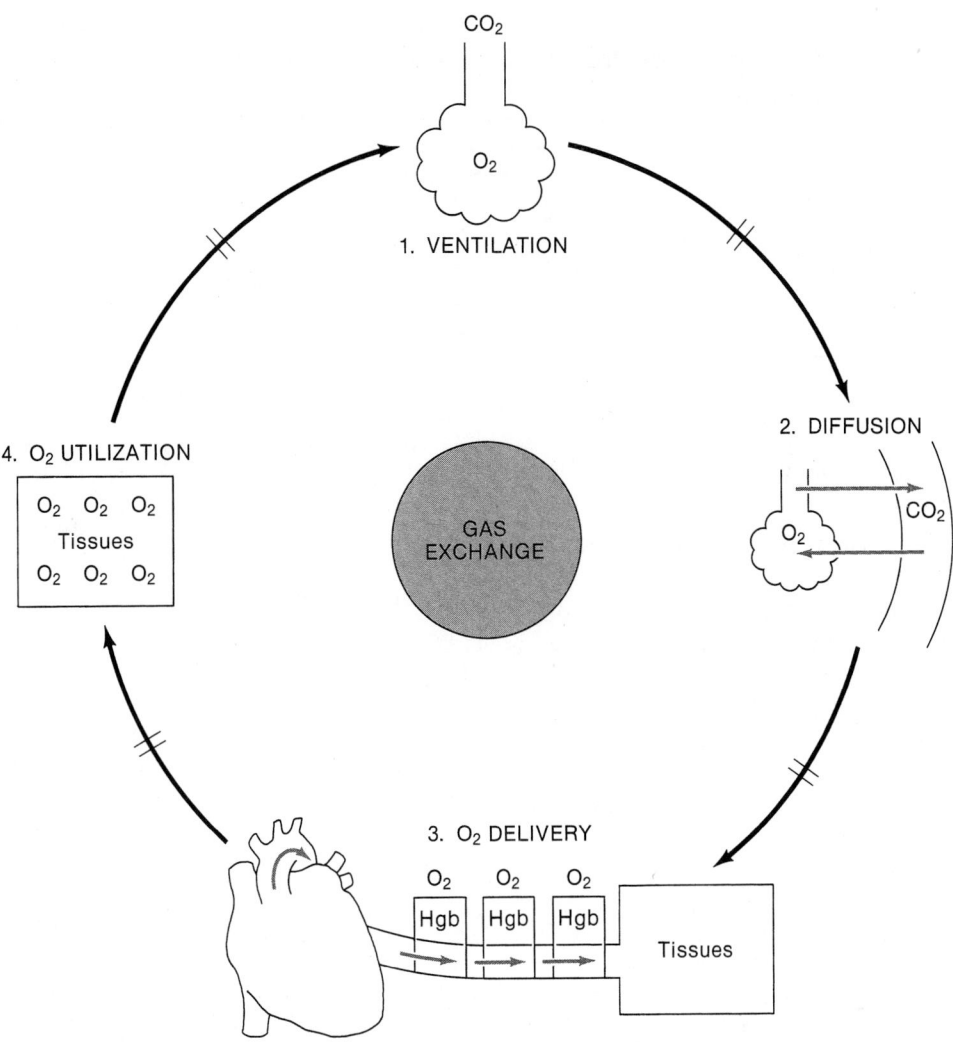

Figure 16–8

Process of gas exchange leading to tissue oxygenation and measurements used to assess each step. An interruption at any point in the cycle will lead to acute respiratory failure. (From Clochesy JM, Breu C, Cardin S, et al: Critical Care Nursing, Philadelphia, W.B. Saunders, 1993, p 529.)

TABLE 16–7
Measurements of Oxygenation

Oxygenation Measurement	Definition	Normal Range or Values
Pao_2	Partial pressure of oxygen in arterial blood	80–100 mm Hg
Sao_2	Percent saturation of hemoglobin with oxygen in arterial blood	>95%
A-ao_2 gradient	Oxygen pressure difference between alveoli and arterial blood; also written as $P(A-a)o_2$, and $A-aDo_2$	5–20 mm Hg
Cao_2	Content of oxygen in arterial blood expressed as milliliters per 100 mL blood or volume %	16–20 mL/100 mL blood
Q_S/Q_T	Shunted cardiac output (L/min) divided by total cardiac output (L/min), expressed as a percent	3–5%
$P\bar{v}o_2$	Partial pressure of oxygen in mixed venous blood drawn from a pulmonary artery catheter	35–40 mm Hg
$S\bar{v}o_2$	Percent saturation of hemoglobin with oxygen in mixed venous blood	70–76%
$C(a-\bar{v})o_2$	Difference in oxygen content between arterial blood and mixed venous blood, expressed in milliliters per 100 mL blood; also written as $Cao_2 - C\bar{v}o_2$ (volume %)	3.5–5 mL/100 mL blood

From Kersten LD: Comprehensive Respiratory Nursing. Philadelphia, W.B. Saunders, 1989, p 343.

TABLE 16–8

Comparing Effects of Normal and Reduced Hemoglobin (Hgb) Levels on Arterial Oxygen Content

	Normal Volume of Hemoglobin (15 g/dL)	Reduced Volume of Hemoglobin (10 g/dL)
O_2 Content: (Hgb × 1.34) × % saturation	19.5 vol % (15 × 1.34) × 97.5%	13 vol % (10 × 1.34) × 97.5%
Dissolved oxygen	0.3 vol % (100 mm Hg × 0.003)	0.3 vol % (100 mm Hg × 0.003)
Total oxygen content	19.8 vol %	13.3 vol %

Note: Volumes percent = mL oxygen/100 mL blood
Adapted from Harper RW: A Guide to Respiratory Care. Philadelphia, J.B. Lippincott, 1981, p 128.

alveolar–capillary gas exchange (Figure 16–9). Venous blood gas values are shown in Chart 16–5.

- $P\bar{v}O_2$. A normal $P\bar{v}O_2$ is 40 to 46 mm Hg. O_2 delivery at the tissue level is considered adequate if the $P\bar{v}O_2$ is between 38 and 42 mm Hg.[9] A value less than 35 mm Hg may indicate that O_2 extraction is increased or O_2 delivery is inadequate.
- $S\bar{v}O_2$. More commonly, a fiberoptic pulmonary artery catheter may be used to assess oxygenation by continuously monitoring the oxygen saturation of venous blood ($S\bar{v}O_2$). This parameter is the counterpart to the SaO_2. The SaO_2 describes the percent saturation of Hgb in the arterial blood, and the $S\bar{v}O_2$ is the percent saturation of Hgb in the venous blood. The difference between these two values ($SaO_2 - S\bar{v}O_2$) estimates the amount of O_2 delivered at the tissue level. A normal $S\bar{v}O_2$ value is 70 to 76%. Hgb returns to the lung 70 to 76% saturated with O_2. This means that, in the normal state, only a portion of the O_2 carried is released at the tissue level, and Hgb returns to the lung 70 to 76% saturated.

Mixed venous O_2 monitoring is used to assess O_2 delivery or uptake (extraction) at the tissue level. Delivery to the tissue level depends on CaO_2 (ability to transport O_2 in combination with Hgb plus the dissolved form) and cardiac output. The amount of O_2 remaining after tissue extraction is the mixed venous O_2 content ($C\bar{v}O_2$). The $C\bar{v}O_2$ can also be calculated much the same as CaO_2, only the venous $P\bar{v}O_2$ and $S\bar{v}O_2$ values are used. A normal $C\bar{v}O_2$ is approximately 14 volumes percent assuming an Hgb of 14 g/dL, $P\bar{v}O_2$ of 40 mm Hg, and $S\bar{v}O_2$ of 75%. It is calculated by the following formula:

$$(C\bar{v}O_2) = (Hgb \times 1.34 \times S\bar{v}O_2) + (P\bar{v}O_2 \times 0.003).$$

Oxygen Transport Measurements. Oxygen transport or delivery (DO_2) is calculated from the cardiac output (Q) and CaO_2:

$$DO_2 = Q \times CaO_2 \times 10.$$

The value of 10 is a conversion factor to change CaO_2 from deciliters to liters. Normal O_2 delivery is 600 to 1000 mL per minute or 500 to 600 mL per minute/m^2. In the critically ill patient, several factors may separately or in combination affect O_2 delivery, such as decrease in cardiac output or decrease in the parameters of CaO_2 (Hgb, SaO_2, PaO_2).

O_2 utilization (VO_2) is calculated by multiplying the cardiac output times the amount of O_2 extracted at the tissue level. The amount of O_2 extracted is the arterial–venous O_2 content difference ($Ca-\bar{v}O_2$). A normal $Ca-\bar{v}O_2$ is 3.5 to 5 mL/100 mL blood or 3.5 to 5 volumes percent.

A measure of the efficiency of oxygenation is the intrapulmonary shunt (Q_S/Q_T). A true or physiologic shunt is defined as that percentage of the cardiac

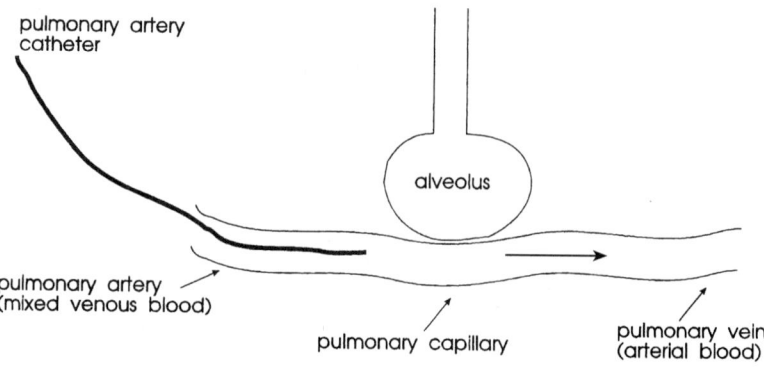

Figure 16–9

Tip of a pulmonary artery catheter in the pulmonary circulation. (From Burton GG, Hodgkin JE, Ward JJ: Respiratory Care: A Guide to Clinical Practice, 4th ed. Philadelphia, Lippincott-Raven, 1997, p 328.)

output that is returned to the left atrium without passing by functioning alveoli. Thus, this portion of the blood remains poorly oxygenated. A normal physiologic shunt is 3 to 5% of the cardiac output and is caused by blood from the bronchial circulation and thebesian veins draining into the left ventricle. This is considered a normal anatomic shunt.

A true shunt or capillary shunt results from pulmonary capillary blood being in contact with unventilated alveoli and may result from numerous conditions. A true shunt may become clinically significant at more than or equal to 15%. In the critical care unit, the most common causes are alveolar collapse, pulmonary consolidation associated with infection, and segmental or lobar collapse of the lung. This condition is called a true shunt because the hypoxemia caused by the shunt does not respond to increasing supplemental O_2 therapy.

Pulmonary Function Testing

Various tests may be done both in the pulmonary function laboratory and at the patient's bedside to assess lung volumes, flow rates, and pulmonary mechanics. Basic lung volumes and capacities are described in Chapter 14 (see Figure 14–10).

Spirometry. The most common pulmonary function test is called basic spirometry. This test measures lung volumes, lung capacities, and flow rates and may be performed at the patient's bedside or in the pulmonary function laboratory. Spirometry may be performed before and after bronchodilator medication to assess for airway bronchoconstriction. To perform spirometry, the patient is asked to inhale and exhale normally through a mouthpiece (with noseclips on). The tidal volume (TV) is recorded. Then the patient is asked to breathe in as deep a breath as possible. After this deep breath, the patient is instructed to quickly and forcefully blow as much air out of the lungs as possible. This is called a forced vital capacity maneuver (FVC). The FVC maneuver requires considerable cooperation from the patient. So, all results must be interpreted in relation to the estimated patient effort.

The amount of air that the patient can exhale in the first second is called the forced expiratory volume in 1 second (FEV_1). This value reflects airflow in the large airways, and a decreased value indicates the presence of airway obstruction. An FEV_1 value less than 1.0 L represents severe obstruction, 1.0 to 2.0 L represents moderate obstruction, and more than 2.0 L indicates low normal volumes. In addition, the ratio of FEV_1 to FVC is also recorded (FEV_1/FVC%), with a normal value being approximately 75% of the FVC. This means that the patient is able to exhale approximately 75% of the FVC during the first second of exhalation. A decreased FEV_1/FVC% indicates airway obstruction, and an increased FEV_1/FVC% may indicate restrictive disease. Figure 16–10 compares spirograms of the normal lung, the obstructive lung, and the restrictive lung. Given the results of the spirometry, more extensive pulmonary function tests may be ordered. Examples of additional tests include body plethysmography, flow volume loops, measurement of diffusing capacity, and exercise testing. A description of these tests is beyond the scope of this chapter, and the reader is referred to specific texts on pulmonary function testing.

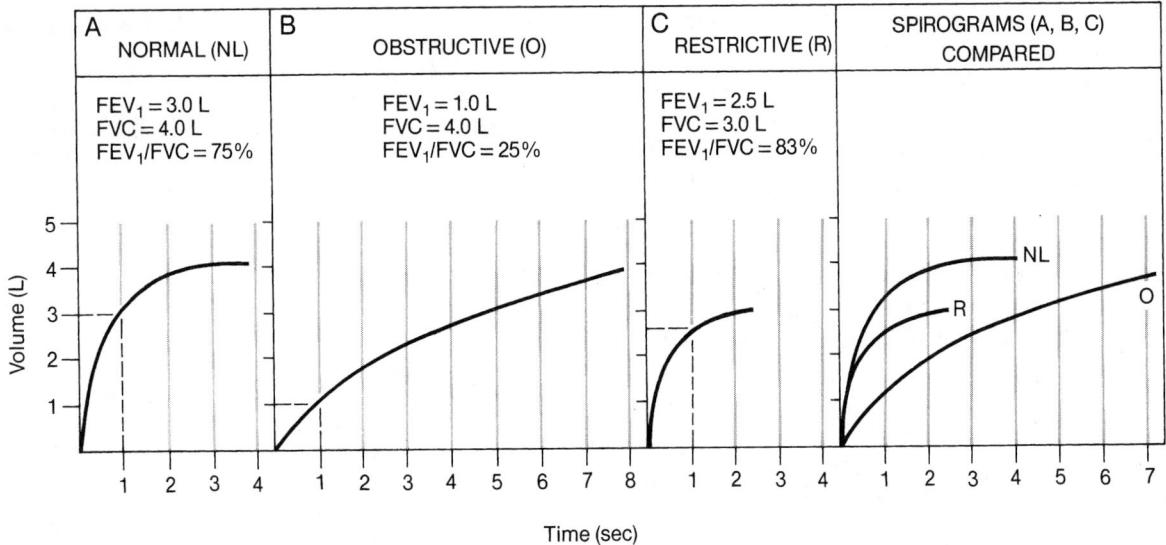

Figure 16–10

Examples of spirograms and flow rates for A, normal lungs (NL), B, obstructive disease (O), and C, restrictive disease (R). Spirograms represent one forced vital capacity breathing maneuver. FEV₁, forced expiratory volume in 1 second; FVC, forced vital capacity. (From Kersten, LD: Comprehensive Respiratory Nursing. Philadelphia, W.B. Saunders, 1989, p 376.)

Peak Expiratory Flow. Peak expiratory flow is the maximum flow that can be achieved during an FVC maneuver. It is measured with a peak expiratory flow meter. Measurement of peak expiratory flow is a quick evaluation of airway patency and is often used to assess and monitor the asthmatic patient or the patient with bronchospasm.

The patient is instructed to inhale to total lung capacity and then quickly and forcefully exhale into a mouthpiece attached to the expiratory flowmeter. Noseclips are usually applied just before the expiratory phase of the maneuver. The peak flow achieved during exhalation is measured. Usually, three maneuvers are done, and the highest value is recorded. If the patient is experiencing bronchospasm, the peak expiratory flow maneuver may cause coughing and may be difficult to perform. Normal peak expiratory flow is based on sex, age, and height. The normal range of values is available from a nomogram found in pulmonary function textbooks. Peak expiratory flow monitoring is done both in the hospital setting and the outpatient setting. It is an easy and inexpensive way for asthmatic patients to monitor signs and symptoms of the disease. Medications and treatment plans can be adjusted based on peak expiratory flow values and symptoms.

Bedside Pulmonary Function Tests. Pulmonary function tests are also done at the patient's bedside. In the critical care setting, these tests are frequently done to assess the patient's respiratory mechanics, ventilation, and readiness to be weaned from mechanical ventilation. Some of these parameters are discussed in Chapter 17 in the section on mechanical ventilation.

The measurements of TV, vital capacity (VC), and minute ventilation (V_E) are routinely monitored in the critically ill patient on mechanical ventilation. These parameters may be monitored as part of the mechanical ventilator-generated patient data, or they may be monitored manually using a hand-held respirometer. These include pulmonary function tests for VC, FEV_1, minute ventilation, maximum voluntary ventilation, maximal inspiratory force or inspiratory effort, dead space, effective dynamic compliance, effective static compliance, and shunting.

Dead space ventilation is the ratio of physiologic deadspace ventilation (V_D) to TV. This concept is discussed in Chapter 14. Physiologic dead space is composed of anatomic dead space (V_{an}, that portion of the TV in the conductive zone of the lung) and alveolar dead space (V_A, that portion of the TV at the alveolar level that does not participate in gas exchange). Normal V_{an} accounts for approximately one-third or 33% of the TV. It is calculated as 2 mL/kg body weight. V_A occurs when ventilation is wasted at the alveolar level because the inspired air does not interface with the pulmonary capillary blood. Any problem that decreases pulmonary capillary blood flow to any area of the lung potentially causes V_A. Acute pulmonary em-

bolism and low cardiac output are examples. In general, V_D must be less than 0.55 or 55% for effective alveolar ventilation and adequate oxygenation of venous blood.

Other Laboratory Tests

Complete Blood Count. A complete blood count (CBC) includes red blood cell (RBC) and white blood cell (WBC) counts as well as evaluation of various components and types of the RBC and CBC (Table 16–9). Only those tests specific to the pulmonary laboratory assessment are discussed here.

RED BLOOD CELL COUNT. A normal RBC count is 4.6 to 6.26 million/mm^3 in men and 4.2 to 5.4 million/mm^3 in women. Anemia is characterized by a low RBC count and a below normal Hgb and hematocrit; polycythemia is characterized by an increased concentration of RBC, usually more than 6 million/mm^3 or Hgb more than 18 g/dL. Polycythemia may be seen in patients with chronic hypoxemia. The body attempts to increase O_2 transport by increasing the production of Hgb. Unfortunately, higher than normal Hgb levels increase blood viscosity and strain the heart. Oxygenation is not improved dramatically because the cause of hypoxemia is at the lung level versus the ability to transport.

Hgb is the most important parameter of the RBC count in the pulmonary assessment. Several types of Hgb are recognized. The predominant Hgb in adults is

TABLE 16–9

Normal Adult Values for the Complete Blood Count

Test	Normal Values
Red blood cell count (RBC)	
Men	4.6–6.2 × 10^6/mm^3
Women	4.2–5.4 × 10^6/mm^3
Hemoglobin (Hgb)	
Men	13.5–16.5 g/dL
Women	12.0–15.0 g/dL
Hematocrit (Hct)	
Men	40–54%
Women	38–47%
White blood cell count (WBC)	4500–11,500 cells/mm^3
Differential of white blood cells	
Segmented neutrophils	40–75%
Bands	0–6%
Eosinophils	0–6%
Basophils	0–1%
Lymphocytes	20–45%
Monocytes	2–10%
Platelet count	150,000–400,000 platelets/mm^3

From Burton GG, Hodgkin JE, Ward JJ: Respiratory Care: A Guide to Clinical Practice, 4th ed. Philadelphia, Lippincott–Raven 1997, p 178.

HgbA, which carries O_2. Carboxyhemoglobin and methemoglobin are Hgb derivatives that are *unable* to bind O_2. Normal levels of both of these Hgb derivatives are usually less than 1.5% of the Hgb in the body. However, carboxyhemoglobin levels may be as high as 10% in the smoking adult. Thus, O_2 transport is impaired. Carbon monoxide has a high affinity for Hgb as compared with O_2 and binds quickly with Hgb. Thus, in carbon monoxide poisoning, one sees a decrease in the ability of O_2 to bind with Hgb that leads to severe hypoxemia. In addition, carbon monoxide changes the configuration of the Hgb molecule. This change further decreases the release of O_2 at the tissue level.

LEUKOCYTE COUNT (WHITE BLOOD CELL COUNT). The total WBC count and differential are important parameters in assessing patients for infection. A normal WBC value is 4500 to 10,000/mm^3. The total WBC count provides an estimate of the patient's ability to fight infection. Leukocytosis means an elevated WBC count, and leukopenia means a low WBC count. Agranulocytosis is characterized by an almost complete absence of granulocytes. The patient is at great risk of infection.

The differential WBC count provides specific percentages of each type of WBC that comprise the total WBC. Table 16–9 describes the normal values for a WBC differential count. The six types of WBCs found in the blood are divided into two distinct categories, the granulocytes and nongranulocytes. The granulocytes (also called polymorphonuclear leukocytes or PMNs) include the neutrophils, eosinophils, and basophils. The segmented neutrophils (called polys or segs) constitute 40 to 75% of the circulating WBCs. Their primary function is the destruction and elimination of microorganisms. An increased neutrophil count indicates a bacterial infection or inflammation. Bands are immature granulocytes and usually account for only a small percentage (<6%) of the WBC differential. An increase in bands is termed a "shift to the left" and is seen in response to a bacterial infection. Eosinophils increase in relation to an allergic reaction or parasitic infection. Last, an increase in the basophil count may indicate a myeloproliferative disorder.

The nongranulocytic WBCs are the monocytes and lymphocytes. Monocytes account for 2 to 10% of the WBC, and lymphocytes account for 20 to 45%. Lymphocytes are produced primarily in the lymph nodes and lymphoid tissues. An increase in lymphocytes may indicate a viral infection. Last, monocytes are produced by the bone marrow, and an increase may indicate a chronic infection or a malignant disease.

In summary, the differential WBC count may be used to determine whether an infection is an acute bacterial infection or a viral infection. A bacterial infection causes an increase in granulocytes with a release of immature cells (bands). Conversely, an elevation of lymphocytes or monocytes indicates a viral infection or allergy and is called a "shift to the right."

Sputum Studies. A sputum culture and sensitivity study is used to assess for pulmonary infection and is used in conjunction with other diagnostic data (e.g., chest radiograph), clinical signs, and symptoms. Various tests may be done on the specimen including Gram stain, culture and sensitivity, acid-fast smear or culture, and cytologic examination. A *Gram stain* allows a quick classification of bacteria into Gram-negative or Gram-positive types. This classification provides guidance for the initial antibiotic therapy. A *culture and sensitivity test* of a sputum specimen provides diagnostic information on the type of bacteria and its sensitivity to various antibiotics. A specimen for *acid-fast bacilli* (AFB culture) is used to diagnose tuberculosis and for the specific classification of the bacteria. Last, a *cytologic examination* may be done on the sputum specimen. This examination is used to assess for malignant cells. For this examination, a special fixative solution is used for the specimen.

A sputum culture may be obtained by various methods (voluntary cough, suction from the intubated patient, bronchoscopy). The quality of the specimen is critical. The collection of a high-quality specimen means the difference between clinically useful information to guide patient care and a waste of valuable time and resources in the diagnostic evaluation of the patient.[10] Poor specimens contain predominantly the oropharyngeal organisms and are not helpful in determining the cause of a lower respiratory infection.

In the critical care setting, a sputum specimen may be obtained by expectoration, by suctioning, or by bronchoscopy. Transtracheal aspiration was used in the past, but the widespread use of bronchoscopy has almost eliminated this method. The optimal specimen obtained by expectoration should be obtained in the early morning from a deep cough and should be free of saliva. It may be helpful to have the patient rinse his or her mouth before obtaining the specimen. If the patient is receiving some type of respiratory treatment (chest physical therapy, bronchodilator therapy), it may be helpful to obtain the specimen after these treatments, when the secretions are mobilized. Specimens obtained by suctioning or bronchoscopy (a flexible scope into the airway) should be collected in a sterile container and sent promptly to the laboratory for processing.

RADIOLOGIC DIAGNOSTIC PROCEDURES

Chest Radiograph

Chest radiographs (chest x-rays) are frequently ordered in the critically ill patient. Most frequently, a posteroanterior (PA) chest radiograph is taken. This means that the beam is shot from the back (posterior) to the front (anterior). Along with this view, a lateral view is taken. However, in the critical care setting, a bedside, portable anteroposterior (AP) radiograph is taken with the patient in a semisitting or supine position. Bedside chest radiographs are obtained to monitor changes in the lung's pathologic condition, to assess line or catheter placement, to identify or monitor abnormalities of the pleural space (pleural effusion, pneumothorax), to assess the chest after a procedure, or to check for artificial airway (endotracheal tube) placement. Limitations of the portable chest radiograph include poor visualization of mediastinal structures, magnification of the cardiac silhouette, and difficulty in visualizing lung bases, as well as impairment by supine positioning of assessment of vascula-

ture or effusions. Besides the AP radiograph, other types of radiographs may be ordered, such as a lateral decubitus study in which the patient lies on the right or left side to assess for free fluid (pleural effusion, blood).

Figure 16-11 shows the normal anatomic structures or "landmarks" observed on a PA chest radiograph. The nurse must be able to identify the normal structures of the chest radiograph. The four densities identified on the radiograph from most dense to least dense include bones or metal, fat, water, and air. Bones or metal are dense and appear white on the radiograph. These entities include ribs, clavicles, metal clips, and wires. Often the tip of a tube has a radiopaque marker so it can be identified on the radi-

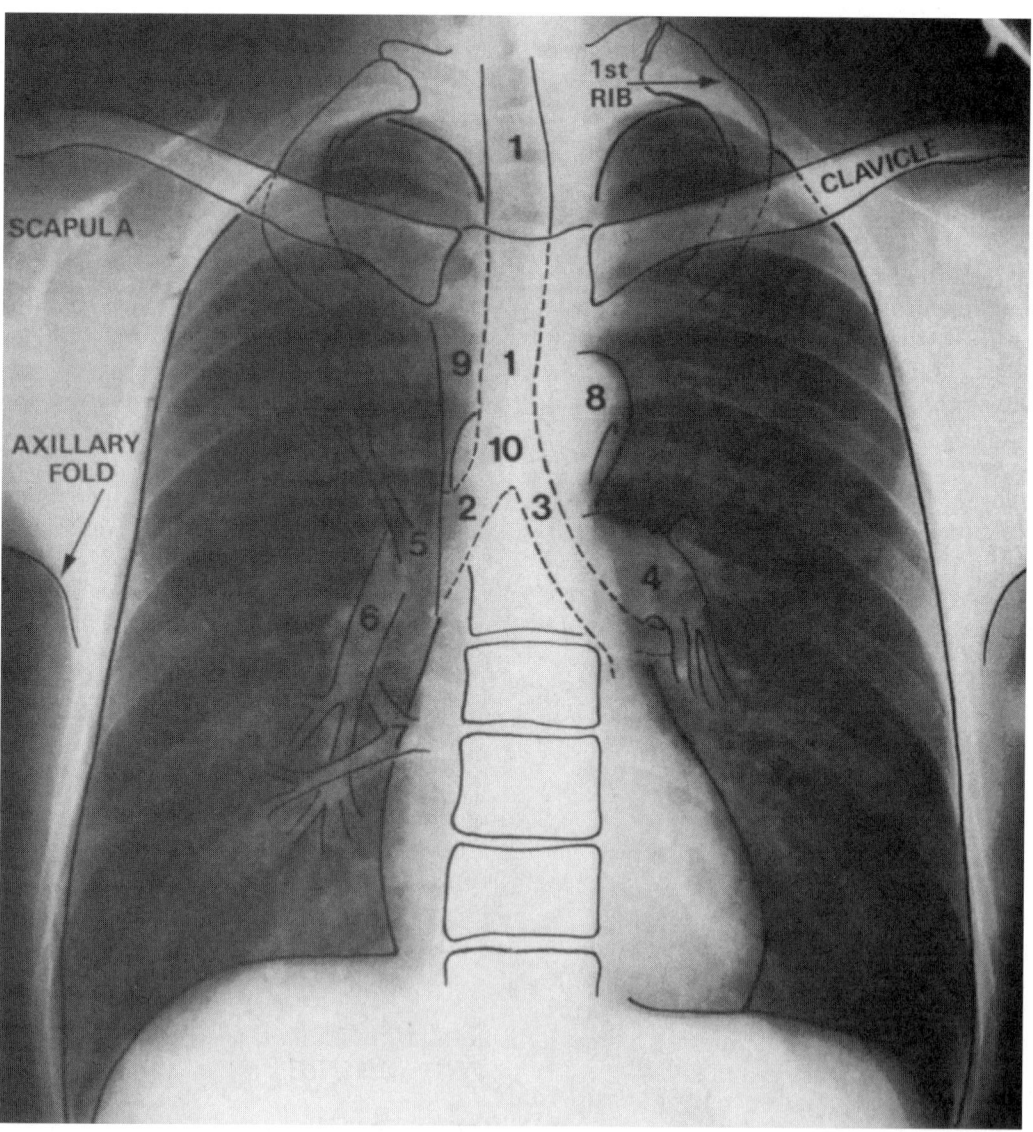

Figure 16–11

Normal posteroanterior chest radiograph with outlining and labels of basic anatomic structures. (1) trachea, (2) right main bronchus, (3) left main bronchus, (4) left pulmonary artery, (5) right upper lobe pulmonary vein, (6) right interlobar artery, (7) right lower and middle lobe vein, (8) aortic knob, and (9) superior vena cava, (10) carina. (From Fraser RG, Paré JA: Diagnosis of Diseases of the Chest, vol. I, 3rd ed. Philadelphia, W.B. Saunders, 1991, p 288.)

ograph. Fat is less dense and appears off white. Examples of fat are breast tissue or the tissue surrounding the rib cage. Water is also less dense than bone and is off white. Examples of water density are blood in the heart and blood in the vessels. Lung tissue is filled with air and is radiolucent. Therefore, it should appear dark or black on the chest radiograph.

A systematic approach should be used to examine the chest radiograph. Table 16–10 describes a process for examining the chest radiograph. Although it is not practical for the beginning nurse to have expertise in interpreting a chest film, the nurse should have the knowledge to identify normal patterns, gross abnormalities, and normal placement of artificial airways and catheters. Over time, the nurse becomes experienced in assessing the chest radiograph along with the clinical findings to determine changes in the patient's condition.

Two examples of abnormalities seen on chest radiographs are shown in Figures 16–12 and 16–13. Figure 16–12 shows a patient with congestive heart failure and a right pleural effusion. Note the increased vascular markings. Figure 16–13 shows a right main stem intubation of the endotracheal tube.

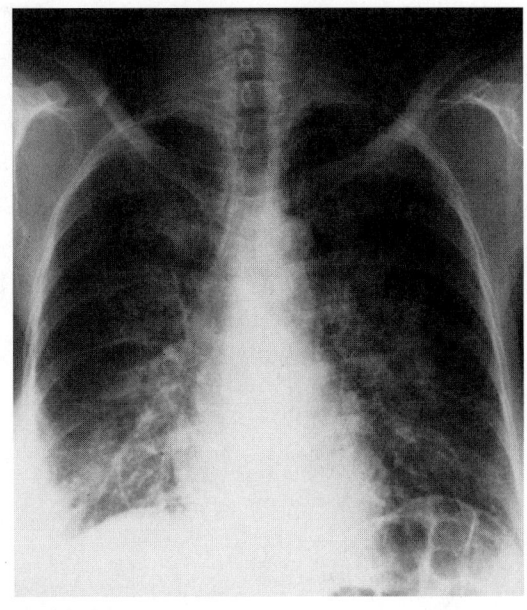

Figure 16–12

Posteroanterior chest radiograph of congestive heart failure with effusion. (From Meholic A, Ketai L, Lofgren R: Fundamentals of Chest Radiology. Philadelphia, W.B. Saunders, 1996, p 155.)

TABLE 16–10
Systematic Assessment of the Chest Radiograph

Area to Assess	Observations
General	Determine whether the film is adequate; all structures of the thoracic cage visible Assess for gross abnormality not present on previous film (if available) Compare with previous film if possible
Soft tissues (neck, shoulders, axillary area, breast tissue	Overall physique of patient (overweight, underweight) Nipple shadows
Trachea	Tracheal deviation Tracheal stenosis Position of endotracheal tube
Bony Thorax	Ribs, clavicles, scapulae, spine Symmetry of bony structures Absence of bony structures
Intercostal Spaces	Symmetry of intercostal spaces Width of spaces; wider space indicates increased lung volume
Diaphragm	Normal; right diaphragm slightly higher than left because of liver (in upright individual); may not be apparent with portable radiography Flattened diaphragms (lower than normal) seen in chronic obstructive pulmonary disease because of air trapping
Pleural spaces	Lung tissue should extend out laterally to rib margins
Mediastinum	Assess heart and great vessels
Lung fields	Compare sides for symmetry and equal density Vascular markings should be evident out to lateral rib margins Prominence of vascular markings associated with pulmonary edema Assess for haziness, distribution of different densities in lung parenchyma Assess for infiltrate or haziness especially in basilar areas

Assess for placement of lines, tubes

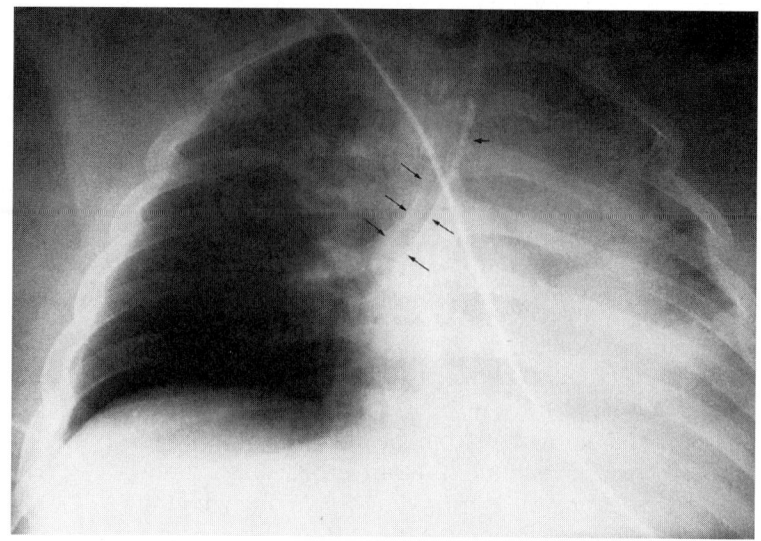

Figure 16–13

Anteroposterior chest view of right mainstem intubation of endotracheal tube. The endotracheal tube extends into the right mainstem bronchus (arrows). The right lung is hyperaerated and the left lung is almost fully collapsed. (From Meholic A, Ketai L, Lofgren R: Fundamentals of Chest Radiology. Philadelphia, W.B. Saunders, 1996, p 41.)

Chest Computed Tomographic Imaging

Chest computed tomographic imaging (CT scan) allows the visualization of cross sections of the chest. These multiple, cross-sectional anatomic pictures or "cuts" provide an excellent mechanism to assess areas that are difficult to visualize with a conventional chest radiograph (mediastinal structures, pleurae, small lesions in the lung parenchyma). The test may also be done with the infusion of contrast material that provides a higher resolution of specific structures in the thoracic cage. No special preparation of the patient is necessary for a chest CT scan; however, this scan must be done in the radiology department.

Ventilation–Perfusion Scan

A ventilation–perfusion scan or study is a scintigraphic study of the lung using radiolabeled gases for assessment of ventilation and radiolabeled particles in solution to assess perfusion of the lung. This test provides an assessment of the matching of ventilation and perfusion in different areas of the lung. A normal scan shows homogeneity of the radiolabeled gas and particles throughout the lung fields.

The scan may be used diagnostically for various purposes. Most commonly, it is used to assess for the presence of a pulmonary embolism. A ventilation–perfusion scan may also be used in the preoperative assessment of a patient before thoracic surgical resection, lung transplantation, or lung volume reduction surgery. When comparing the matching of ventilation to perfusion in the lung, there is decreased uptake or absence of the radiolabeled solution in the area of a pulmonary embolism (decreased perfusion), whereas the ventilation remains relatively normal or slightly decreased.

This examination is usually done in the radiology department, and no special preparation is necessary. For the ventilation scan, the patient inhales a radiolabeled gas and air mixture through a mask or endotracheal tube. The perfusion portion of the scan is performed by injecting a radioisotope. Scintillation cameras record the distribution of gamma radiation images during the ventilation and perfusion scanning.

Pulmonary Angiography

Pulmonary angiography is an invasive test done in the radiology department to assess the pulmonary vasculature. Pulmonary vasculature narrowing or obstruction is commonly due to a blood clot or emboli, but it may also be anatomic. Pulmonary angiography is most frequently used diagnostically to confirm the presence of a pulmonary embolism. However, it may be used therapeutically to remove a blood clot from the pulmonary artery or to instill medications directly.

A radiopaque dye is injected through a catheter into the right side of the heart or into the pulmonary arteries. Serial radiographs or films are taken to assess the vasculature for obstruction. No special preparation of the patient is needed for this test; however, the contrast dye may cause flushing, coughing, a warm sensation, nausea, or vomiting. During angiography, the patient is closely monitored for possible complications relating to the pulmonary embolism or to the instrumentation and procedure itself. If possible, a patient should have nothing by mouth for 2 to 3 hours before the procedure. However, this test is frequently done as an emergency, to diagnose and treat a pulmonary embolism. After the procedure, the nurse should monitor the patient's bedside pulmonary parameters, vital signs, catheter insertion site, and peripheral pulses.

BEDSIDE DIAGNOSTIC AND MONITORING PROCEDURES

Pulse Oximetry

Pulse oximetry (SpO_2) is a noninvasive method of estimating arterial O_2 saturation and is frequently used as a method to monitor patients continuously. This technology uses two wavelengths of light shown through a capillary bed to detect the amount of unsaturated Hgb; however, results are described as saturation values. It is an estimate of SaO_2 because not only is oxyhemoglobin assessed, but other types of saturated Hgb are assessed as well (e.g., carboxyhemoglobin). A transcutaneous sensor is usually placed on the fingertip in the adult, but it can be placed on the earlobe or toe.[11] An acceptable SpO_2 value is greater than or equal to 90%. The SpO_2 has been shown to have an excellent correlation with SaO_2 measured by co-oximetry (directly from a sample of blood) over the range of 70 to 100% with an accuracy of $\pm2\%$ (±1 standard deviation).[11, 12]

The SpO_2 has added a new dimension to monitoring the critically ill patient continuously and is also used in numerous other settings. As with the SaO_2, the nurse should assess the SpO_2 in relation to the patient's available Hgb. A patient can have a low Hgb level and impaired O_2 transport and still have a "normal" SpO_2.

End-Tidal Carbon Dioxide Monitoring

Capnometry is the measurement of CO_2 at the patient's airway during the ventilatory cycle. A capnometer is a noninvasive instrument used to assess the partial pressure of CO_2 in the end-tidal gas ($PetCO_2$), and the waveform produced during inspiration and expiration is called the capnogram.

$PetCO_2$ monitoring may be assessed in the intubated or nonintubated patient. The $PetCO_2$ is not equal to the $PaCO_2$, but it is useful in monitoring trends in patients who have a stable hemodynamic status. End-tidal gas is defined as the last portion of the exhaled breath and is assumed to contain primarily alveolar (A) gas. It approximates the $PaCO_2$ and, thus, the $PaCO_2$ under conditions of normal ventilation and perfusion matching. The normal $PetCO_2$ gradient ($PaCO_2 - PetCO_2$) is approximately 1 to 5 mm Hg.[13]

Various factors may cause an increase or decrease in the $PetCO_2$. To use this tool effectively and safely in patient care, these factors along with the patient's clinical status must be taken into account when interpreting the $PetCO_2$. Examples of conditions causing an increase in the $PetCO_2$ include fever, sepsis, increased metabolic rate, respiratory center depression, alveolar hypoventilation, and rebreathing of gases. A decreased $PetCO_2$ may be caused by hypothermia, pulmonary hypoperfusion, cardiac arrest, hypotension, alveolar hyperventilation, ventilator disconnection, esophageal intubation, or complete airway obstruction.

Bronchoscopy

Bronchoscopy is an endoscopic procedure used to visualize the trachea and the large bronchi. In the critical care setting, flexible fiberoptic bronchoscopy may be used diagnostically to assess the airways and as a therapeutic tool for patients on mechanical ventilation.[14] Bronchoalveolar lavage may be done by instilling small aliquots of sterile saline (30 mL) through the scope and into the airways. The solution is then withdrawn or is suctioned. The lavage fluid is sent for cellular examination in the laboratory. Bronchoscopy may also be used in secretion management. If the airways cannot be cleared by routine measures (positioning, coughing, deep breathing, suctioning), then bronchoscopy may be performed to remove excessive mucus or mucous plugs.

Bronchoscopy may be done by inserting the scope through the nose or, if the patient is intubated, through the artificial airway with a bronchoscope adapter. The patient should have nothing by mouth for a minimum of 6 hours before the procedure. Sedation is used before the procedure for patient comfort and to reduce the cough reflex. During the procedure, vital signs, heart rhythm, and pulse oximetry are monitored. In most institutions, both the respiratory care practitioner and the nurse assist with the procedure. The most common effects of bronchoscopy on gas exchange and pulmonary mechanics are hypoxemia, hypercarbia, decreased TV, decreased flow rates, increased positive end-expiratory pressure, increased peak inspiratory pressure, and increased intratracheal pressure.[14] The nurse should monitor the patient after the procedure for any signs of bleeding, respiratory distress, hypoxemia, or increases in airway pressures if the patient is receiving mechanical ventilation. Airway management is important because the gag and cough reflexes may be suppressed. This suppression puts the patient at risk of aspiration.

Thoracentesis

A thoracentesis is done as either a diagnostic or a therapeutic procedure. A pleural effusion is an abnormal collection of fluid in the pleural space. A needle is inserted through the chest wall and into the pleural space. Diagnostically, fluid may be aspirated or removed for laboratory analysis. Therapeutically, if excessive fluid in the pleural space is causing respiratory distress, then the fluid may be removed by this procedure. Depending on the amount of fluid, a chest tube may be inserted for drainage.

Before a thoracentesis, the patient should be assessed for any bleeding disorders or coagulopathies. These conditions would place the patient at increased risk of bleeding after the procedure. The nurse is responsible for preparing the patient for the procedure and for obtaining the correct procedural tray and equipment. The patient is positioned in a sitting position over the side of the bed with arms supported by a bedside table. If the patient is unable to sit up, the patient is assisted into a side-lying position with the affected side down. A local anesthetic is used to numb the area for insertion of the thoracentesis needle. Preemptive pain medication may be used, depending on the assessment of the nurse and the preference of the physician. The patient is instructed not to move or cough during the procedure. Specimens are sent to the laboratory for analysis.

During and after the procedure, respiratory assessment parameters are monitored including SpO_2, respiratory rate, and signs and symptoms of respiratory distress. After a thoracentesis, a chest radiograph may be ordered. Possible complications of a thoracentesis include pain, pneumothorax, infection, bleeding, and reexpansion pulmonary edema (if a large pleural effusion is removed).

Key Concepts

➡ CO_2 is a volatile acid and is excreted by the lung by ventilation; nonvolatile acids are regulated by the kidney.

➡ A normal arterial pH is 7.35 to 7.45 and represents a balance between acid and base in the blood. A pH of less than 7.35 indicates acidemia (excess of acid or deficit of base); a pH of more than 7.45 represents alkalemia (deficit of acid or an excess of base).

➡ Respiratory acidosis is caused by alveolar hypoventilation (increased $PaCO_2$, decreased pH). Respiratory alkalosis is caused by alveolar hyperventilation (decreased $PaCO_2$, increased pH). The adequacy of alveolar ventilation can only be assessed directly by the $PaCO_2$. $PETCO_2$ is an indirect method of assessing the adequacy of alveolar ventilation.

➡ Metabolic or nonrespiratory imbalances include metabolic acidosis (decreased HCO_3^-, decreased pH) and metabolic alkalosis (increased HCO_3^-, increased pH).

➡ The body does not overcompensate for an acid–base disorder.

➡ The hemoglobin must always be considered when assessing oxygenation.

➡ The SaO_2 or SpO_2 evaluate the saturation of the available Hgb with O_2. A value greater than or equal to 90% is acceptable.

➡ Dead space ventilation is wasted ventilation that does not participate in gas exchange. Shunt is wasted perfusion or the percentage of cardiac output that does not interface with functioning alveoli.

➡ Hypoxemia is defined as insufficient O_2 in the arterial blood, whereas hypoxia means insufficient O_2 at the tissue level.

References

1. Tobin MJ (ed): Principles and Practice of Intensive Care Monitoring. New York, McGraw–Hill, 1998.
2. Van Hooser T: Analysis of gas exchange. In: Scanlon CL, Spearman CB, Sheldon RL (eds): Egan's Fundamentals of Respiratory Care, 6th ed. St. Louis, Mosby–Year Book, 1995, pp 391–405.
3. Harrison RA: Acid–base balance. Respir Care Clin North Am 1:7–21, 1995.
4. Thompson CS: Acid–base disorders and electrolyte imbalance. In: Dantzker DR, MacIntyre NR, Bakow ED (eds): Comprehensive Respiratory Care. Philadelphia, W.B. Saunders, 1995.
5. Bone RC: Acute respiratory failure. In: Burton G, Hodgkin JE, Ward JJ (eds): Respiratory Care: A Guide to Clinical Practice, 3rd ed. Philadelphia, J.B. Lippincott, 1991.
6. Beachey W, Scanlan C: Acid–base balance and the regulation of respiration. In: Scanlan CL, Spearman CB, Sheldon RL (eds): Egan's Fundamentals of Respiratory Care, 6th ed. St. Louis, Mosby–Year Book, 1995, pp 303–340.
7. Mahoney JJ, Hodgkin JE, Van Kessel AL: Arterial blood gas analysis. In: Burton GG, Hodgkin JE, Ward JJ (eds): Respiratory Care: A Guide to Clinical Practice, 4th ed. Philadelphia, J.B. Lippincott, 1997, pp 249–280.
8. Levitzky MG: Pulmonary Physiology, 3rd ed. New York, McGraw–Hill, 1991, p 135.
9. Scanlan CL: Patient monitoring and management. In: Scanlon CL, Spearman CB, Sheldon RL (eds): Egan's Fundamentals of Respiratory Care, 6th ed. St. Louis, Mosby–Year Book, 1995, pp 920–967.
10. Papasian CJ, Kragel PJ: The microbiology laboratory's role in life-threatening infections. Crit Care Nurs Q 20:44–59, 1997.
11. Grap MJ: Pulse Oximetry. Technology series. Aliso Viejo, CA, American Association of Critical-Care Nurses, 1996.
12. Yelderman M, New W Jr: Evaluation of pulse oximetry. Anesthesiology 59:349–352, 1983.
13. St. John RE: End-Tidal CO_2 Monitoring. Technology series. Aliso Viejo, CA, American Association of Critical-Care Nurses, 1996.
14. Jones WS, Byrd RP, Lukeman RW: Flexible fiberoptic bronchoscopy in mechanically ventilated patients. J Respir Care Pract 10:95–98, 1997.

17

Acute Respiratory Failure

Bonnie R. Sakallaris

Objectives

After completing this chapter, the student will be able to:

1. Relate the specific pathophysiologic derangement to the plan of care for a patient with acute respiratory failure.
2. Identify assessment findings consistent with acute respiratory failure.
3. Describe common diagnostic tests useful in the diagnosis of acute respiratory failure.
4. Identify assessment findings consistent with resolution of acute respiratory failure.
5. Identify appropriate nursing diagnoses for the patient experiencing acute respiratory failure.
6. Develop a plan of care for the patient requiring mechanical ventilatory support.
7. Relate nursing interventions to specific desired patient outcomes.
8. Discuss current pharmacology used in the treatment of acute respiratory failure.
9. Identify the care of patients experiencing respiratory failure in a nontraditional setting.
10. Relate research findings to current nursing interventions in the care of the patient experiencing acute respiratory failure.

ETIOLOGY AND PATHOPHYSIOLOGY

The primary function of the respiratory system is to supply the body tissues with oxygen, to support aerobic metabolism, and to remove the by-product of metabolism, carbon dioxide (CO_2). To accomplish these goals, air must move between the external environment and the alveoli (*ventilation*), and gas exchange then occurs between the alveoli and the mixed venous blood entering the lungs (*oxygenation*). Oxygenated blood is delivered to the body tissues through the arterial circulation (*oxygen delivery*), and gas exchange takes place across the capillary membranes and diffuses to the body tissues. Finally, the tissues utilize the oxygen delivered (*oxygen utilization*), and by-products of metabolism, such as CO_2, are transported in the blood by the venous system to the lungs for disposal through the movement of air between the alveoli and the external environment (see Figure 14–8). Effective respiration hinges on optimal functioning of the central nervous system, airways, lungs, heart, arterial and venous circulation, and viable tissues. Failure in any of the components described—ventilation, oxygenation, delivery, or utilization—may lead to acute

respiratory failure. Table 17–1 lists disease processes that contribute to respiratory failure.

Acute respiratory failure is the sudden and severe impairment in the lung's ability to maintain adequate oxygenation and ventilation. In 1965, Campbell defined respiratory failure as a condition in which the patient's arterial partial pressure of oxygen (PaO_2) is below 60 mm Hg or the arterial partial pressure of CO_2 ($PaCO_2$) is above 50 mm Hg while breathing air at sea level.[1] This definition continues to be used with modification based on the patient's age and chronic conditions (Table 17–2). Respiratory failure is classified as *acute* if the abnormalities develop too rapidly for compensation to occur, or if the abnormality has overwhelmed compensatory mechanisms. The diagnosis of acute respiratory failure requires a change from the patient's baseline to a degree that causes significant potential for mortality or morbidity.[2] Acute respiratory failure due to ventilatory failure is termed *hypercapnic respiratory failure* (e.g., >normal $PaCO_2$), and respiratory failure due to abnormalities of oxygenation is called *hypoxemic respiratory failure* (e.g., <normal PaO_2). Respiratory failure involves the whole body and the psyche. Throughout this chapter, the connections

TABLE 17-1

Disease Processes that Cause Failure of Ventilation, Oxygenation, Perfusion, or Oxygen Utilization

Systems, Structures, and Conditions	Causes of Respiratory Failure
Central nervous system	Drug overdose
	Pickwickian syndrome
	Cerebrovascular accident
	Ondine's curse
	Cerebral trauma ($\uparrow$ intracranial pressure)
	Central sleep apnea
	Tumors
	Myxedema
Peripheral nervous system	Multiple sclerosis
	Poliomyelitis
	Amyotrophic lateral sclerosis
	Guillain–Barré syndrome
	Botulism
	Tetanus
	Drugs
	Spinal cord injury
	Myasthenia gravis
	Electrolyte imbalance
Musculoskeletal and pleural functions	Muscular dystrophy
	Kyphoscoliosis
	Flail chest
	Ankylosing spondylitis
	Morbid obesity
	Restrictive pleural diseases
	Pleural effusion
	Pneumothorax
	Hemothorax
Conducting airways	Epiglottitis
	Laryngotracheitis
	Trauma
	Tracheal stenosis
	Foreign body aspiration
	Tumors
	Asthma
	Bronchospasm
Lungs	Chronic obstructive pulmonary disease
	Cystic fibrosis
	Pneumonia
	Pulmonary emboli
	Aspiration
	Inhaled toxins
	Pulmonary edema
	Adult respiratory distress syndrome
	Interstitial lung disease
	Near drowning
	Inhaled toxins
	Trauma
	Radiation pneumonitis
	Oxygen toxicity
Nonpulmonary conditions	Sepsis
	Myocardial infarction
	Eclampsia
	Anaphylaxis
	Shock
	Disseminated intravascular coagulation
	Fat embolism
	Systemic inflammatory response syndrome

TABLE 17–2
Patient Factors Influencing Expected Arterial Blood Gas Values

Patient Factors	Pao$_2$ Norms on Room Air	Paco$_2$ Norms
Newborn infants	40–70 mm Hg	32–41 mm Hg
Children and adults	80–100 mm Hg	35–45 mm Hg
Elderly adults (>60 yrs)	60–80 mm Hg	35–45 mm Hg
	[103.5 − (0.42 × age) ± 4]*	
High altitudes	↓	Normal
Chronic obstructive pulmonary disease	Low normal	↓

*Formula for calculating Pao$_2$ norms for adults >60 yrs.

among mind, nonpulmonary function, and pulmonary function are explored.

Acute Ventilatory Failure

The hallmark of acute ventilatory failure is an elevated Paco$_2$; the exchange of air between the alveoli and the atmosphere is inadequate to clear the CO$_2$ delivered to the lungs from the tissues. Acute ventilatory failure may result from trauma, neurologic depression, musculoskeletal abnormalities, or airway obstruction. In these examples, the patient's minute ventilation (VE), the amount of air in liters exchanged each minute, is abnormally low. This condition may be caused by a decreased respiratory rate, as in neurologic depression, or by decreased tidal volume, as in severe pneumothorax or airway obstruction. The common pathophysiologic feature is the inability to inflate and deflate perfused alveoli so that adequate gas exchange can take place.

A mismatch between ventilation (V) and perfusion (Q) may cause ventilatory failure, as in pulmonary emboli. The normal V/Q ratio equals 1. When the amount of air volume flowing through the lungs (VE) is equal to the amount of blood flow through the lungs

(Q), the ratio is 1:1. V/Q ratios are not equal everywhere in the lung fields. Areas in which air exchange is present but blood flow with gas exchange is absent are called dead space or wasted ventilation. Examples of normal, physiologic dead space are the right and left main stem bronchus and bronchioles, in which airflow occurs but gas exchange does not. Increased dead space, as in pulmonary emboli, can cause ventilatory failure with resultant hypercapnia as diffusion of CO$_2$ from the pulmonary capillaries into the alveoli is impaired. Initial Paco$_2$ may be normal as the body compensates with an elevated respiratory rate, termed tachypnea. Figure 17–1 illustrates normal and abnormal V/Q relationships. Often, ventilatory failure leads to failure to oxygenate the blood adequately. Hypoxemia does not occur immediately if normal gas exchange occurs in the ventilated areas and if the volume of ventilated areas is great enough.

Failure of Arterial Oxygenation

Oxygenation occurs when oxygen diffuses from the alveoli, across the capillary membrane into the blood. The oxygen is carried by the blood in dissolved form measured by the Pao$_2$ and bound to hemoglobin, mea-

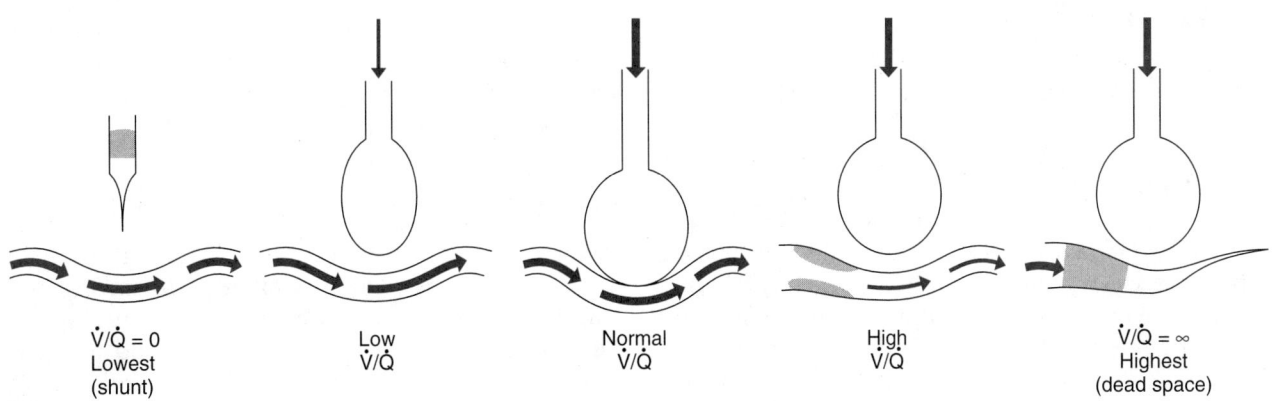

$\dot{V}/\dot{Q} = 0$
Lowest
(shunt)

Low
$\dot{V}/\dot{Q}$

Normal
$\dot{V}/\dot{Q}$

High
$\dot{V}/\dot{Q}$

$\dot{V}/\dot{Q} = \infty$
Highest
(dead space)

Figure 17–1

Ventilation–perfusion ($\dot{V}/\dot{Q}$) ratios in the lung. (From Hanson M: Pathophysiology: Foundations of Disease and Clinical Intervention. Philadelphia, W.B. Saunders, 1998, p 458.)

sured by arterial oxygen saturation (SaO_2) or with pulse oximetry (SpO_2). Failure of arterial oxygenation results from conditions that impair the ability of oxygen to diffuse across the alveolar–capillary membranes such as pulmonary edema or adult respiratory distress syndrome (ARDS). A V/Q mismatch is the most common cause of hypoxemic respiratory failure in the critically ill patient (see Figure 17–1). When underventilated alveoli are well perfused, severe hypoxemia results, for example, in patients experiencing mucus plugging, atelectasis, bronchospasm, chronic obstructive pulmonary disease (COPD), or severe asthma. The most severe form of V/Q mismatch is shunting. Shunting occurs when nonventilated alveoli are perfused, no gas exchange takes place, and unoxygenated blood returns to the arterial circulation, thus significantly lowering the arterial oxygen content. An example of pathologic shunting occurs in ARDS, in which alveolar collapse occurs, causing massive atelectasis. Normal anatomic shunting occurs when bronchial and thebesian veins empty into the left side of the heart, and it accounts for 3 to 5% of normal cardiac output.

Failure of Oxygen Delivery

The delivery of oxygen to the tissues depends on oxygen content, cardiac output, and effective circulation (see Chapter 14). Any condition that affects the ability of hemoglobin to carry oxygen to the tissues may result in acute respiratory failure; examples include severe anemia and carbon monoxide poisoning. Conditions that impair cardiac output such as myocardial infarction, dysrhythmias, severe hypertension, or hypovolemia may profoundly affect oxygen delivery and may precipitate acute respiratory failure. Finally, circulatory deficits such as profound hypotension, severe peripheral vasoconstriction, or local emboli disrupt oxygen delivery to the tissues.

Failure of Oxygen Utilization

Utilization of oxygen at the tissue level (oxygen consumption) depends on intact cellular membranes and on pressure gradients among the capillary system, interstitial fluids, and intracellular fluids. Conditions such as sepsis or systemic inflammatory response syndrome cause capillary and cellular membrane damage, impair the cells' ability to utilize oxygen, and ultimately result in acute respiratory failure. Normally, oxygen delivery is driven by oxygen consumption at the cellular level; for example, with exercise, oxygen consumption increases dramatically. The body responds by increasing delivery through an increased respiratory rate and increased cardiac output. When

oxygen delivery drops to dangerously low levels, usually because of low oxygen content, consumption of oxygen by the cells becomes dependent on delivery, and oxygen utilization by the tissues is less than actual need. Decreased oxygen consumption by the cells is associated with a poor prognosis.

Assessment

Critically ill patients typically experience multisystem problems leading to acute respiratory failure. Holistic assessment is vital because dysfunction in one system usually affects the function of others; for example, inadequate ventilation with hypercapnia may cause local vasoconstriction and a resultant V/Q mismatch with hypoxemia. Decreased oxygen content resulting from an arterial oxygenation deficit may lead to decreased tissue consumption, anaerobic metabolism, and severe metabolic acidosis. These situations are common in the critically ill and require astute assessment to determine the primary cause and appropriate treatment.

History

A complete medical and social history obtained from the patient or family member is helpful in determining baseline respiratory functioning as well as in discriminating among conflicting physical findings. Important social facts include history of smoking, occupational and recreational exposure to known respiratory irritants such as asbestos or pesticides, travel history, alcohol and drug consumption, and lifelong exercise patterns. Sleep history is important to determine position-related respiratory issues as well as any history of sleep apnea.

A complete medical history should include the family history of respiratory diseases or allergies, childhood diseases and immunizations, personal allergies, asthma, past surgical procedures, and traumatic injuries. The chief complaint, such as cough, sputum production, or shortness of breath, and details about the precipitating events such as trauma, infections, flu, colds, or allergin exposure are helpful in determining the cause and in planning treatment.

Physical Examination

Acute respiratory failure is life-threatening; therefore, the physical examination is often performed in conjunction with lifesaving treatment measures, specifically, maintenance of a patent airway and adequate ventilation. The examination must be organized to conserve the patient's energy, and information should be obtained through the medical record, the family interview, and the physical examination.

Neurologic System

The brain has a high requirement for oxygen and is therefore sensitive to changes in arterial oxygen content. The neurologic abnormalities demonstrated by patients with acute respiratory failure may be manifestations of hypoxia, or they may be the root cause of the acute respiratory failure. Early signs of hypoxia include subtle personality changes, restlessness, headache, anxiety, and may progress to confusion and loss of consciousness. An arterial blood gas (ABG) determination may be warranted at this point in the assessment to detect hypoxemia.

Patients with a decreased level of consciousness may be unable to protect their airway, or they may experience a profoundly decreased respiratory rate with decreased VE or apnea. Increased intracranial pressure may precipitate various ventilation abnormalities causing hypercapnia and hypoxia, which, in turn further increase intracranial pressure. Medications that cause neurologic depression are associated with respiratory depression (Table 17–3). It is important to monitor respiratory function closely when using anesthetic agents, sedatives, paralytics, and analgesics, even if these agents are short acting.

Cardiovascular System

The cardiovascular system is responsible for oxygen delivery. Cardiovascular abnormalities seen in patients with acute respiratory failure are often the body's attempt to compensate for low oxygen content, or hypercapnia ($\uparrow Pa_{CO_2}$). Early compensation includes tachycardia and vasoconstriction as the body attempts to increase cardiac output. If oxygen content remains low, the patient's blood pressure eventually falls, and the patient becomes profoundly hypotensive. As the body extracts more and more of the available oxygen from hemoglobin, cyanosis becomes apparent. The nurse should check the patient's nail beds and mucous membranes for color and should measure capillary refill on the patient's fingers and toes. The heart has a high requirement for oxygen for normal functioning. Hypoxemia may lead to decreased cardiac output, dysrhythmias, ischemia, and, potentially, death. Hypoxia is a leading cause of frequent premature ventricular contractions, and hypercapnia exacerbates vasoconstriction and is a myocardial irritant, causing multiple dysrhythmias.

Cardiovascular pathophysiologic features that contribute to acute respiratory failure include congestive heart failure, myocardial infarction, lethal dysrhythmias, and embolic processes. Careful assessment of the cardiac system is vital to determine the effectiveness of oxygen delivery to all tissues as well as to diagnose any cardiovascular causes of the acute respiratory failure.

Pulmonary System

A systematic and thorough assessment of the pulmonary system is vital to the diagnosis and treatment of acute respiratory failure. Table 17–4 describes the physical assessment findings in common pulmonary problems. Determination of a patent airway is the first step in assessing the patient. Airflow in and out of the nose, mouth, and throat should be silent and natural. Evidence of stridor, barking, nasal flaring, or unusual head positions indicates potential obstruction of the airway. Lack of air movement or respiratory rate requires immediate initiation of emergency procedures to relieve airway obstruction and to provide ventilation.

Observation of the patient's breathing pattern should include respiratory rate, pattern, and depth. Tachypnea, use of accessory muscles, nasal flaring, and diaphoresis all indicate that the patient is experiencing excessive work of breathing and may need supplemental oxygen or airway or ventilatory assistance. A depressed respiratory rate may indicate hypocapnia, neurologic depression, or pharmacologic depression. If drug overdose is suspected, intravenous naloxone hydrochloride (Narcan) will reverse the effects of opiate overdose. The patient must be closely monitored because the half-life of naloxone hydrochloride is less than that of many opiates, so respiratory-depressant effects of the opiates may reappear.

Chest wall abnormalities may be obvious because of trauma or chronic respiratory disease. The nurse should observe the patient's chest for the barrel shape typical of patients with COPD, asymmetric chest movements, flail chest associated with rib fractures, chest wounds, or tracheal deviation. Sucking chest

TABLE 17–3
Common Drugs that May Cause Respiratory Depression

Drug Class	Drugs*
Anesthetic agents	Sufentanil citrate (Sufenta)
	Remifentanil hydrochloride (Ultiva)
	Propofol (Diprivan)
Sedatives	Pentobarbital
	Pentobarbital sodium (Nembutal)
	Secobarbital (Seconal)
	Midazolam hydrochloride (Versed)
	Diazepam (Valium)
Paralytics	Pancuronium bromide (Pavulon)
	Succinylcholine chloride
	Tubocurarine chloride (Tubarine)
Analgesics	Codeine
	Fentanyl (Sublimaze)
	Hydromorphone hydrochloride (Dilaudid)
	Meperidine hydrochloride (Demerol)
	Morphine sulfate
	Oxycodone hydrochloride (Percocet)

*Commonly used drugs only, not an exhaustive listing.

TABLE 17–4

Physical Presentation of Common Pulmonary Problems Leading to Acute Respiratory Failure

Disease	Inspection	Palpation	Percussion	Auscultation	Definitive Diagnosis
Pneumonia	Coughing Tachypnea Nasal flaring Use of accessory muscles Purulent sputum	↑ Tactile fremitus	Dullness	Bronchial breath sounds Crackles	CXR Sputum cultures Fever
Emphysema	Pursed-lip breathing Barrel chest	↓ Chest excursion	Hyper-resonance	Crackles Prolonged expiration	CXR Pulmonary function tests
Atelectasis	Tachypnea Anxiety Diaphoresis	↓ Tactile fremitus	Dull	Crackles Diminished breath sounds at bases	CXR Fever
Pulmonary edema	Tachypnea Anxiety Orthopnea Diaphoresis Copious frothy sputum Distended neck veins	↓ Chest excursion	Normal to dull	Dependent Crackles Wheezing S_3, S_4 gallop	CXR Fever

CXR, chest radiograph

wounds and tracheal deviation require immediate treatment, usually decompression with a chest tube.

Auscultation is performed to determine the presence of breath sounds throughout the lung fields and to identify adventitious sounds. Diminished or absent breath sounds usually indicate collapsed alveoli, as in atelectasis, pleural effusions, pneumothorax, or hemothorax. The presence of fine crackles may indicate pulmonary edema, and coarse crackles usually indicate the buildup of secretions. Bronchospasm or severe pulmonary edema may cause wheezing. The presence of bronchial breath sounds over peripheral lung fields usually indicates an area of consolidation, as in pneumonia. A harsh, grating sound associated with respiration is called a pleural friction rub and is usually associated with pleural inflammation or loss of pleural fluid.

Percussion may be used to identify areas of hyperresonance, as in pneumothorax versus dullness over consolidated areas in patients with pneumonia. Palpation can help to identify tactile fremitus, abnormal chest excursion, or tracheal deviation.

Other Body Systems

Total physical assessment is necessary to detect problems with other body systems that result from poor tissue oxygenation. This assessment may be deferred until the patient's cardiopulmonary status has been stabilized, but it should be performed as soon as possible and then routinely. Patients in acute respiratory failure are at high risk of developing an ileus, stress ulcers, and nutritional deficits. Daily assessment of bowel sounds, gastric drainage, and bowel movements is important to detect these problems. Fluid and electrolyte balance, as well as urine output, should be assessed initially and frequently, to detect abnormalities and to guide treatment. The prevention of acute renal failure is vital to the survival of the patient with acute respiratory failure. Maintenance of adequate oxygen supply to the kidneys should be a key priority. An initial assessment of skin integrity and then subsequent inspections assist in the prevention and early treatment of skin breakdown.

Psychosocial Assessment

Critical illness and particularly acute respiratory failure are associated with panic, anxiety, loss of control, and crisis functioning. The patient and family are in crisis, and a complete psychosocial assessment is necessary to plan support measures and to reinforce positive coping.

Patients' manifestations of anxiety or panic may be physical, such as hypertension, tachypnea, tachycardia, and manic behavior. Each of these signs also signals hypoxia, and a differential diagnosis is crucial. Once adequate oxygenation is established, assessment of previous coping mechanisms is helpful in planning care to alleviate anxiety and panic. Patients with a history of claustrophobia, panic disorder, bipolar disease, and depression have greater difficulty in tolerating the interventions commonly used in the treatment of acute respiratory failure, for example, mechanical ventilation, suctioning, or oxygen masks. Patients receiving neuromuscular blocking agents are particularly vulnerable in the intensive care unit (ICU) because they are unable to express the anxiety or panic they are experiencing. Astute physical assessment and routine reversal of the agents are essential to determine the patient's psychological state.

Assessment of the patient's family and friends is crucial to providing appropriate support. Positive coping mechanisms include seeking clinical information from appropriate health care professionals, gathering support from significant others, communicating with the patient verbally and through touch, accepting the need to rest, and planning for the future care of the patient. Families often need assistance to gather support and to identify resources, and they need permission to rest. Assisted visiting hours are often beneficial in facilitating communication between the patient and family members (Table 17–5).

Diagnostic Testing

The physical examination often yields nonspecific signs and symptoms related to hypercapnia, hypoxia, increased work of breathing, and anxiety. Diagnosis and treatment of acute respiratory failure are usually based on laboratory findings and diagnostic testing in conjunction with physical assessment findings.

Blood Gas Measurements

ABGs may be monitored intermittently by drawing arterial blood from an arterial monitoring line or peripheral arterial puncture and sending the blood to the laboratory for analysis. Point-of-care testing systems have been developed to decrease the delay between blood sampling and test results, and continuous monitoring systems are available using optical sensors that allow the nurse to monitor PaO_2, $PaCO_2$, pH, and bicarbonate (HCO_3^-) at the bedside. Oximetric pulmonary artery catheters are available to monitor venous oxygen saturation, and noninvasive monitors include SpO_2 and end-tidal capnography. Frequent monitoring of ABG parameters is essential to determine adequacy of ventilation ($PaCO_2$, end-tidal CO_2 tension [$PETCO_2$]), oxy-

TABLE 17–5
Assisted Visiting

Suggestion*	Desired Outcomes	
Negotiate visiting time and number of people	Family:	Increased control and planning
	Patient:	Planned rest periods
	Nurse:	Assistance in planning of care
Develop communication plan and tools	Family:	Improved communication
Pictures		Involvement with care
Flash cards		Increased trust
Alphabet board	Patient:	Improved communication
Symbol board	Nurse:	Individualized communication tools
Read to patient	Family:	Feeling of accomplishment and purpose
Newspaper	Patient:	Entertainment, distraction
Short articles		Kept in touch with the world
Stories		Familiar voices
		Stress reduction
	Nurse:	Assistance in orienting patient
Provide care (if comfortable)	Family:	Involvement with care
Bath	Patient:	Care from loved ones
Feed	Nurse:	Assistance with care
Give permission to touch	Family:	Involvement with care
Hand holding		Improved communication
Gentle massage face, feet, and shoulders	Patient:	Relaxation
		Stress reduction
	Nurse:	Assistance with care
Bring in comfort items	Family:	Involvement with care
Pictures	Patient:	Comfort
Music		Personalized environment
Blanket		Stress reduction
Stuffed animal	Nurse:	Personalized care

*These suggested interventions have not been researched. This is an area of research opportunity.

TABLE 17–6
Arterial Blood Gas Assessment of Simple Acid–Base Disorders

	pH 7.35–7.45	$Paco_2$ 35–45 mm Hg	HCO_3^- 22–25 mm Hg	Compensation Respiratory $Paco_2$	Metabolic HCO_3^-
Respiratory					
Acidosis	↓	↑			↑
Alkalosis	↑	↓			↓
Metabolic					
Acidosis	↓		↓	↓	
Alkalosis	↑		↑	↑	

↑, above normal range; ↓, below normal range.

genation (Pao_2, Sao_2, Spo_2), and the degree of compensation (pH, $Phco_3^-$) present (Table 17–6; see also Table 17–2).

Ventilation. Adequacy of ventilation is determined by the $Paco_2$ level from the ABG sample. Capnography can be used to measure CO_2 in intubated patients' expired air. The measurement is $Petco_2$ and rarely correlates exactly with the patient's $Paco_2$. In healthy volunteers, $Petco_2$ is usually 1 to 5 mm Hg less than the $Paco_2$. A widened gap between $Paco_2$ and $Petco_2$ may be due to increased dead space, positive end-expiratory pressure (PEEP), tachypnea with a low tidal volume (Vt), pulmonary embolus, right-to-left shunting (ventricular septal defect, atrial septal defect), decreased blood volume, or cardiac arrest. In the critically ill, $Petco_2$ is used to monitor the patient's CO_2 level continuously. Capnography is the monitoring of the waveform produced by $ETCO_2$ monitoring and is used to demonstrate endotracheal tube placement, to identify obstruction, and to monitor the effectiveness of ventilation (Figure 17–2).

Hypercapnia (high $Paco_2$) indicates hypoventilation, a Ve inadequate to clear the CO_2 returning to the lungs from the tissues, and it indicates respiratory acidosis if the blood pH is less than 7.40. Hypercapnia may be caused by a depressed respiratory drive, as in anesthesia, drug overdose, loss of consciousness, or low Vt generated if the lung fields are collapsed, such as in pneumothorax, hemothorax, atelectasis, or pneumonia. Iatrogenic hypercapnia occurs if the Vt or respiratory rate set on the ventilator is too low to clear CO_2 produced.

Hypocapnia (low $Paco_2$) indicates hyperventilation, a high Ve, and it may be due to anxiety, hypoxia, or too high a Vt or rate set on the ventilator. Respiratory alkalosis is delineated by $Paco_2$ of less than 35 mm Hg with a blood pH of more than 7.40. Compensation for ventilatory abnormalities is demonstrated if the patient's pH is close to normal despite an abnormal $Paco_2$ (see Table 17–6). This compensation is accomplished by raising or lowering the HCO_3^- in response to the blood pH. Hypocapnia may result as the patient's respiratory system compensates for meta-

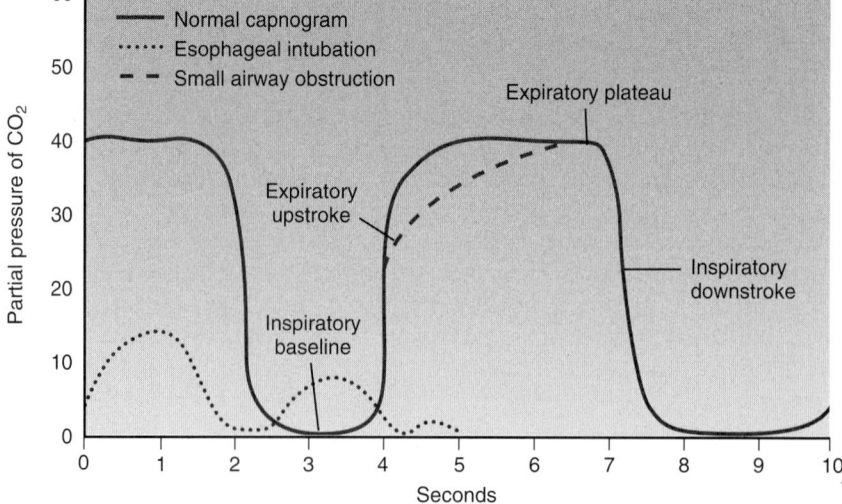

Figure 17–2

Normal and abnormal capnograms.

CHART 17–1

Mixed Acid–Base Disorders

The following are rules to follow in patients with mixed acid–base disorders:

- A mixed acid–base disorder is present if either the $Paco_2$ or the HCO_3^- does not follow its predicted value ($\uparrow$ or $\downarrow$) or is not close to its predicted compensatory activity.
- Metabolic changes are predictable: for every 10-mEq/L change in HCO_3^-, there should be a 0.15 change in pH.
- Respiratory changes are predictable: for every 20-mm Hg increase in $Paco_2$ above 40 mm Hg, the pH will decrease by 0.10 unit, and for every 10-mm Hg decrease in $Paco_2$ under 40 mm Hg, the pH will increase by 0.10 unit.
- The $Paco_2$–HCO_3^- relationship is predictable: for every 10-mm Hg increase in $Paco_2$ there is a corresponding increase of 1 mEq/L of HCO_3^-.

bolic acidosis, as in septic shock. Critically ill patients often manifest mixed respiratory and metabolic problems. These conditions are difficult to analyze and require practice (Chart 17–1).

Oxygenation. Oxygenation is assessed by the Pao_2, Sao_2, and Spo_2. Normal Pao_2 values depend on the patient's age, the disease process, and the fraction of inspired oxygen (Fio_2) administered (see Table 17–2). Hypoxemia may be due to hypoventilation, diffusion deficits as in pulmonary edema or ARDS, or V/Q mismatches and shunting. Pao_2 measures the amount of dissolved oxygen in the plasma, which accounts for approximately 3% of the patient's total oxygen content. The remaining 97% of oxygen is bound to hemoglobin and is measured by the Sao_2. Sao_2 is measured directly with ABGs or can be measured peripherally (Spo_2) with a pulse oximeter (Figure 17–3). The oxygen–hemoglobin dissociation curve represents the relationship be-

tween Pao_2 and Sao_2 and is used to predict Pao_2 from the Sao_2 (see Figure 14–12). The patient's temperature or CO_2 level affects the ease of oxygen dissociation from the hemoglobin; for example, patients who are hyperthermic give up oxygen more readily, shifting the dissociation curve to the right, whereas patients who are hypothermic have tighter bonds between the oxygen and hemoglobin, shifting the curve to the left. Arterial oxygen content (Cao_2) can be calculated as follows:

$$Cao_2 = (Pao_2 \times 0.003) + (1.34 \times \text{hemoglobin} \times Sao_2)$$

$$\text{Normal } Cao_2 = 20 \text{ vol\%}$$

Continuous venous measurements of oxygen saturation (Svo_2) provide the percentage of oxygen returned to the lungs after tissue utilization (normal = 60–80%). A low Svo_2 may indicate inadequate oxygen content to meet the patient's metabolic needs. Venous oxygen content (Cvo_2) can be calculated using the same formula as arterial content, substituting venous gases:

$$Cvo_2 = (Pvo_2 \times 0.003) + (1.34 \times \text{hemoglobin} \times Svo_2)$$

$$\text{Normal } Cvo_2 = 15 \text{ vol\%}$$

Oxygen Utilization. Oxygen consumption (Vo_2) can be calculated by subtracting Cvo_2 from Cao_2; under normal conditions, it equals 5 vol%. The oxygen extraction ratio is the relationship between oxygen content and oxygen utilization. It is calculated by dividing Vo_2 by Cao_2; normal is 1/4. Problems with oxygen utilization are not demonstrated directly with ABGs; however, low HCO_3^- levels indicating metabolic acidosis are often associated with inadequate oxygen utilization. When the cells convert to anaerobic metabolism, the acids produced require increased utilization of the buffering system, lowering the HCO_3^-. The patient may experience tachypnea with hypocarbia as the body tries to compensate for the metabolic acidosis. Other measures include a high serum lactate level and a high Svo_2 (>80%).

Chest Radiograph

Chest radiographs are used frequently to confirm physical examination findings or to differentiate among conflicting findings. Chest radiographs are also used to confirm invasive line placement such as central lines, to confirm appropriate placement of endotracheal, gastric, and chest tubes, and to rule out adverse effects of line placement, placement of chest tubes, and intubation. Typically, the patient in the ICU receives an anteroposterior portable chest radiograph, which is done while the patient sits as upright as clini-

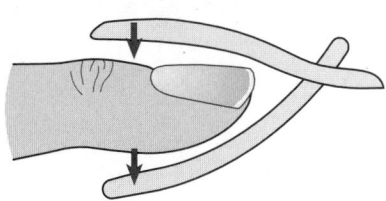

Figure 17–3

Pulse oximetry.

cally possible with the x-ray plate behind his or her back. The ideal anteroposterior chest radiograph requires the patient to stand, a position usually impossible in a critical care unit.

On the anteroposterior view of the chest, radiopaque lines, tubes, and intravenous lines are visible and are marked against anatomic landmarks to determine placement. Anatomic landmarks include the heart borders, vascular markings, rib cage, clavicles, sternal notch, and diaphragm. Air-filled lungs are dark, and the lung borders can be determined against the rib cage and diaphragm (Figure 17–4). Air, blood, or fluid in the pleural space impinges on the lung borders and is noted on the chest radiograph. Areas of consolidation such as atelectasis or pneumonia are white and often follow a lobar pattern. Patchy, lacy patterns usually indicate fluid or vascular areas and indicate pulmonary edema. Effusions cause blunting of the costophrenic angle on the anteroposterior chest radiograph, but they are often difficult to diagnose.

To determine the presence and size of effusions, right or left lateral decubitus films are needed. The patient is placed on the left or right side and is propped with pillows, with the x-ray plate behind the patient. The patient is usually left in this position for at least 30 minutes before the radiograph is obtained. If free fluid is present, it will layer horizontally on the dependent side.

Pulmonary Function Tests

Pulmonary function tests measure lung volumes, lung capacities, flow of gases through the airways, and the ability of the lungs to diffuse gases. Pulmonary function tests are useful to determine the degree of pulmonary disease or disease reversibility, to assess postoperative risk of severe pulmonary compromise before surgery, to determine the degree of disability due to pulmonary disease, and to evaluate the effectiveness of treatments, particularly bronchodilators. Pulmonary function studies are rarely performed in critically ill patients in acute respiratory failure because these tests require an alert, cooperative patient, and can be physically stressful. Modified pulmonary measurements can be performed at the bedside or calculated from measurements obtained on the ventilator. Table 17–7 lists the common measurements obtained at the bedside. Weaning parameters are pulmonary function measurements performed at the bedside used to predict readiness to wean the patient from ventilator support.

Bronchoscopy

Bronchoscopy is performed by inserting an endoscope into the bronchi for visualization or removal of secretions or foreign objects. The main objectives of a bronchoscopy are diagnosis through direct visualization and provision of therapy. Bronchoscopy may be used to facilitate endotracheal intubation, to remove airway secretions, aspirated foreign bodies, or malignant tumors causing tracheal or bronchial obstruction, and to provide local radiation therapy or laser phototherapy.

Bronchoscopy causes significant patient discomfort, so sedation is recommended, with close monitoring. Patient preparation usually includes numbing of nasal passages and airways with lidocaine (Xylocaine) gel and misted lidocaine. Sedation combinations include midazolam hydrochloride (Versed) with an analgesic such as meperidine hydrochloride (Demerol). Hypoxemia may occur during bronchoscopy and is treated with oxygen therapy. Bronchospasm may be problematic, particularly in asthmatic patients, and it is prevented or blunted with premedication with bronchodilators. It is important to monitor the patient's recovery from the sedation used during the procedure and particularly to verify the return of the patient's

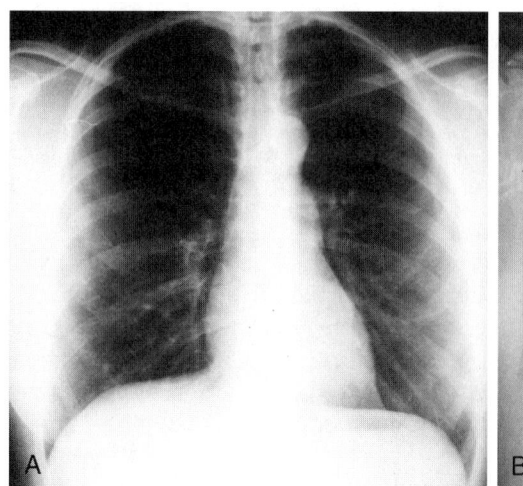 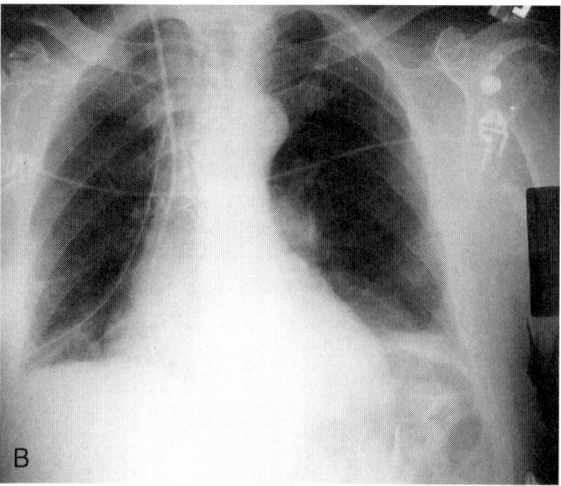

Figure 17–4

Normal (A) and abnormal (B) chest radiographs. (Courtesy of Cheryl Hyde Davia, RN.)

TABLE 17-7
Bedside Pulmonary Measurements

Respiratory Parameter	Normal Value	Weaning Predictor
Volumes		
Tidal volume (VT): volume inhaled or exhaled per breath	350–600 mL	>5 mL/kg
Minute ventilation (VE): volume exhaled per minute	4–8 L/min	5–10 L/min
Vital capacity (VC): maximal exhaled volume after a maximal inspiration	60–80 mL/kg*	>15 mL/kg
Forced vital capacity (FVC): maximal forceful exhaled volume after a maximal inspiration	<20 mL/kg may indicate need for support	(>1000 mL)
Dead space to tidal volume ratio (VD/VT): the portion of VT that does not participate in gas exchange: $VD/VT = PaCO_2 - (PETCO_2 \div PaCO_2)$ (must be corrected if ventilated)	25–35% but position dependent	<60%
Airway Pressures		
Peak inspiratory pressure (PIP): maximal pressure during inspiration	Individually trended	
Static pressure: pressure required to maintain delivered VT during a period of no gas flow	Individually trended	>30–33 mL/cm H_2O
Compliance (C_{dyn}): calculated value indicating volume change per unit of pressure change; measures lung distensibility: $C_{dyn} = VT \div$ (plateau pressure − PEEP)	60–100 mL/cm H_2O (60–80 mL/cm H_2O if ventilated)	
Mean airway pressure: average pressure recorded during positive pressure and spontaneous phases of a respiratory cycle	Individually trended	
Fractional Gas Concentrations		
Exhaled carbon dioxide (PETCO$_2$): measures carbon dioxide elimination	Usually 0–5 mm Hg lower than PaCO$_2$	
Alveolar to arterial oxygen gradient {P(A − a)O$_2$}: indicates gas exchange efficiency: $PAO_2 = FIO_2(Pb - PH_2O)^\dagger - (PaCO_2 \div 0.8)$ $P(A - a)O_2 = PAO_2 - PaO_2$	5–10 mm Hg on room air or 0.4 × patient's age, <65 mm Hg on 100% O$_2$	
Ratio of arterial to alveolar PO$_2$ (a/A ratio): proportion of oxygen going from alveoli to blood; indicates gas exchange efficiency: $a/A = PaO_2 \div PAO_2$	0.74 in elderly, 0.9 in young adults (90%)	
Ratio of arterial partial pressure of oxygen to inspired fractional concentration of oxygen (P/F ratio): assesses efficiency of oxygenation; yields a constant value for a given degree of shunting regardless of FIO$_2$: $P/F = PaO_2 \div FIO_2$	>200	
Respiratory index (RI): ratio of alveolar arterial oxygen tension gradient to the arterial partial pressure of oxygen; measure of efficiency of gas exchange: $RI = P(A - a)O_2 \div PaO_2$	<1.0 (1–5 suggests V/Q imbalance treatable with O$_2$)	
Respiratory Mechanics		
Negative inspiratory force or pressure (NIF, NIP): maximum inspiratory pressure the patient is capable of generating against a closed airway	−80 to −100 cm H_2O (60–80 if ventilated)	−30 cm H_2O
Maximum voluntary ventilation (MVV): averaged minute ventilation when breathing as deeply and rapidly as possible in 12 to 15 seconds (measures ventilatory reserve)	120–180 L/min	>twice VE
Rapid-shallow breathing index (f/VT ratio): weaning index: $f/VT =$ spontaneous resp. rate (f) $\div$ average VT in liters	Threshold is 100 breaths/min/L	100 breaths/min/L
Work of breathing index (WOB): measures actual work of breathing	>1.8 kg·m/min	1.6 kg·m/min
Oxygen cost of breathing (OCB): difference between whole-body oxygen consumption (VO) during spontaneous breathing versus that obtained during controlled ventilation: OCB = VO (spontaneous) − VO (controlled)	Threshold is 15%	15%
CROP score: combines measures of compliance, rate, oxygenation, and maximum inspiration pressure (MIP): $CROP = (C_{dyn} \times MIP \times a/A) \div f$	≥18	≥18

*10–15 mL/kg necessary for effective deep breathing and cough.
†Pb Barometric pressure; PH$_2$O water vapor pressure; Pb − PH$_2$O = 713

gag reflex after the procedure. Patient monitoring guidelines should be delineated in the hospital's conscious sedation standard of care.

Angiography

Angiography is the procedure of cannulating an artery or vein and injecting contrast medium to diagnosis a vascular abnormality. In the patient with acute respiratory failure, angiography may be used to diagnosis a pulmonary embolism (PE). Although angiography is the most accurate diagnostic test for PE, these patients are often too unstable to tolerate the procedure. A V/Q scan performed in the nuclear medicine department can provide information on the probability of a PE. Results are graded as low, intermediate, or high probability of PE.

Drug Screen

Patients who present in acute respiratory failure with a decreased level of consciousness require a drug screen to detect the presence of respiratory-depressant drugs. Drug screening is further indicated if the patient presents with dilated or pinpoint pupils, confusion, or a history of drug use or suicide attempts. A toxicology screen can determine the type of drug as well as the level, so that appropriate treatment can begin.

Nursing Diagnoses

The diagnosis of acute respiratory failure is made based on evidence of the patient's inability to maintain adequate oxygenation, ventilation, oxygen delivery, or the inability to utilize oxygen delivered to the tissues. A complete diagnosis list must be made to identify the cause and to guide treatment. The diagnostic process, pathophysiology, and treatment generate several nursing and collaborative diagnoses, which are listed in Table 17–8.

Collaborative Management

Identification and treatment of the precipitating condition are primary goals of collaborative management of patients in acute respiratory failure. Physical examination, history, and diagnostic testing guide the identification of the precipitating condition. Effective management of acute respiratory failure depends on a multidisciplinary approach to diagnosis and treatment as well as coordination across the continuum of care from home through emergency systems, the hospital, and the community.

Treatment priorities are guided by the acute nature of the patient's distress; therefore, initiation of therapy to treat the primary condition may be delayed to ensure adequate airway, breathing, and circulation. The treatment of ARDS, PE, pneumothorax, and hemothorax are discussed at length in Chapters 18 and 19. Treatment of common disorders leading to acute respiratory failure includes antibiotic or antiviral medication for pneumonia, initiation of bronchodilators, and mucolytics, inotropic support, diuretics, and other vasoactive medications. Table 17–9 delineates common pharmacologic agents used in the treatment of acute respiratory failure. Patients with neurologic depression, traumatic

TABLE 17–8
Nursing Diagnoses

Problem Statement	Etiologic Factors
Activity intolerance	Inadequate oxygenation to the tissues
Ineffective airway clearance	Depressed neurologic status, presence of an artificial airway, muscle weakness or atrophy, copious secretions or thick, tenacious secretions
Anxiety	Disease process, unknown diagnosis, hypoxia, pain, fear of dying
Ineffective breathing pattern	Disease process, depressed neurologic status, administration of analgesics or sedatives
Acute confusion	Hypoxemia, sensory overload, sleep deprivation
Dysfunctional ventilatory weaning response	Depressed neurologic status, muscle weakness or atrophy, anxiety, or mismatch of ventilatory weaning plan to patient's physiology
Ineffective family coping	Grief response, anxiety, lack of knowledge regarding prognosis and treatment plan, loss of control, separation from loved one, dysfunctional family patterns
Impaired gas exchange	Disease process, respiratory-depressant medications, neurologic depression, inappropriate ventilatory settings, airway clearance problems, inadequate cardiac output
Altered nutrition, less than body requirements	Presence of artificial airway, neurologic depression, risk of aspiration
Risk for infection	Presence of artificial airway, ineffective airway clearance, presence of invasive lines
Knowledge deficit, learning need	Disease process, diagnostic workup, treatment strategies, discharge plan

TABLE 17–9

Respiratory Pharmacology: Action and Side Effects of Drugs Commonly Used in Acute Respiratory Failure

Drug	Action	Side Effects
Bronchodilators*		
Epinephrine (Bronkaid, AsthmaHaler)	Adrenergic stimulation; alpha, beta$_1$, beta$_2$ stimulation	Anxiety
Ephedrine sulfate		Tremors
Isoproterenol (Isuprel)		Hypertension
Metaproterenol (Alupent)		Tachycardia
Albuterol (Proventil)		Nausea and vomiting
Terbutaline sulfate (Brethine, Bricanyl)		Dizziness
Atropine sulfate	Parasympathetic antagonism	Tachycardia
		Urinary retention
		Pupil dilation
		Dry mouth
Ipratropium bromide (Atrovent)	Parasympathetic antagonism	Slight decrease in mucous clearing
Theophylline, aminophylline (Primatene, Theo-Dur, Slo-Bid)	Inhibition of phosphodiesterase, adenosine antagonism	Central nervous system stimulation
		Diuresis
		Cardiac stimulation
		Pulmonary vasodilation
Prostaglandins, (PGE$_1$, PGE$_2$)	Increase in cellular cAMP	Vasodilation
Mucolytics		
N-acetylcysteine (Mucomyst)	Disruption of molecular structure of mucus and lowering of viscosity	Nausea
		Bronchospasm
		Rhinorrhea
		Hemoptysis
Steroids		
Dexamethasone sodium phosphate (Decadron)	Anti-inflammatory action inhibiting production and release of histamine and decreasing bronchospasm	Hyperglycemia
		Osteoporosis
		Increased fat production
Prednisone, prednisolone (Orasone, Deltasone, Meticorten)		Decreased resistance to infection
Methylprednisone (Medrol, Solu-medrol)		Hypertension
Beclomethasone dipropionate (Vanceril)		Minimal systemic effects
		Fungal infection in oropharynx or larynx
Flunisolide (AeroBid)		
Triamcinolone acetonide (Aristocort)		
Diuretics		
Furosemide (Lasix)	Loop diuretic	Hypovolemia
		Hypokalemia
		Ototoxicity
Antibiotics/Antivirals	Treatment of bacterial or viral infections	Ototoxicity
		Nausea and vomiting
		Varies
Vasoactive Drugs	Various actions: inotropic support, vasodilation, vasoconstriction	See Chapter 11

*Not all bronchodilators represented.

Data from Peters J, Peters B: In: Scanlan CL, Spearman C, Sheldon RL (eds): Fundamentals of Respiratory Care. St. Louis, Mosby–Year Book, 1995.

injuries, or space-occupying lesions may require surgical intervention as well as medical management of their precipitating condition.

Airway Management

The first priority in the management of the patient experiencing respiratory problems is the *establishment and maintenance of a patent airway.* The need for airway support and monitoring is particularly important for patients with a decreased level of consciousness, patients experiencing partial or complete airway obstruction, patients in need of assistance with secretion management, and patients who require mechanical ventilation.

The head tilt with chin lift or jaw thrust is the first step in establishing a patent airway (Figure 17–5). This maneuver relieves airway obstruction by the tongue, which occurs with the loss of muscle tone. This position should be maintained until any foreign body obstructions are removed, spontaneous ventilation is restored, or an artificial airway is in place and assisted ventilation is established.

Many types of artificial airways are used in critical care and emergency situations (Table 17–10). The most commonly used in critical care are oropharyngeal and nasopharyngeal airways, endotracheal tubes (ETTs), and tracheostomy tubes (Figure 17–6). The most invasive forms of airway support are endotracheal intuba-

tion and tracheal intubation. Intubation is indicated for 1) persistent airway obstruction despite intervention, as in airway edema, 2) the need for frequent suctioning to clear secretions, 3) protection from aspiration in the neurologically depressed, and 4) the need for mechanical ventilation support.

Endotracheal intubation is accomplished by the nasal or oral route. The nurse assists a qualified anesthesiologist, nurse anesthetist, or certified respiratory therapist during intubation. Critical care units and emergency rooms usually have an intubation box containing all the equipment necessary for emergency intubation (Chart 17–2).

When assisting with intubation, the nurse should first prepare the patient and family by explaining what will happen and the steps necessary to ensure safety (restraints, sedation) and then provide reassurance. Before and during intubation, it is vital to provide adequate oxygenation. This can be accomplished utilizing the manual resuscitation bag and mask. As the patient responds to sedation and paralytics, manual resuscitation is vital. During the procedure, the nurse monitors the SpO_2 continuously to ensure adequate oxygenation. The nurse should inform the intubating professional if the SpO_2 is falling or if the time without respiration is lengthy. Holding your breath while the patient is not ventilated is a way of tracking time without respiration. If you are uncomfortable, your patient needs a manual breath. Once intubation is ac-

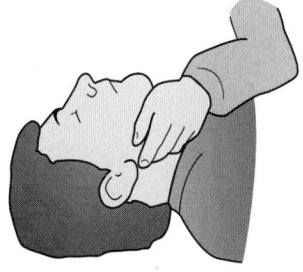

A Jaw thrust

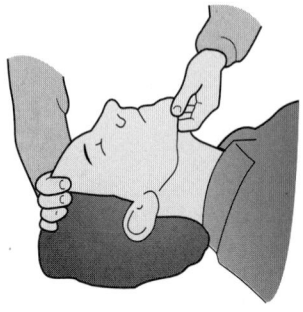

B Chin lift

Figure 17–5

A, Head tilt with jaw thrust. *B,* Head tilt with chin lift.

CHART 17–2

Equipment Necessary for Emergency Intubation

- Endotracheal tubes
- Oropharyngeal airway
- Tongue depressor
- 10-mL syringe for cuff inflation
- Plastic-coated malleable stylet
- Magill forceps
- Laryngoscope with curved and straight blades with functioning light
- Water-soluble lubricant
- Spray topical anesthetic
- Manual resuscitation bag and mask
- Oxygen source, flowmeter, and tubing
- Suction equipment and flexible and rigid (Yankauer) suction catheters
- Tape
- Stethoscope
- Gloves, masks, and goggles
- Anesthesia induction medications

TABLE 17–10

Airways Most Commonly Used in Acute Respiratory Failure: Indications, Contraindications, and Complications

Airway	Indications	Contraindications	Complications
Oropharyngeal airway	Unconscious patient Prevention of biting during seizures or biting on endotracheal tube	Conscious patient	Gagging Vomiting Discomfort Trauma to palate and oral soft tissues
Nasopharyngeal airway	Unconscious patient Facial injuries Need for frequent naso-tracheal suctioning	Sinusitis Closed head injury Basilar skull fracture Coagulopathy	Discomfort Skin breakdown at nares
Oral endotracheal tube	Inability to maintain patent airway Emergency intubation Mechanical ventilation	Caution with spinal cord injury Caution with facial injuries	Greatest risk of self-extubation or inadvertent extubation Tube occlusion by biting or trismus Injury to lips, teeth, tongue, palate, and oral soft tissues Retching, gagging, and aspiration Inability to swallow oral secretions Greatest risk of main stem bronchus intubation Laryngeal or tracheal erosion or necrosis
Nasal endotracheal tube	Inability to maintain patent airway Nonemergency intubation Mechanical ventilation Preferred with cervical spinal cord injury	Caution with facial injuries Basilar skull fracture Sinusitis	Greater discomfort during intubation Sinusitis Epistaxis Otitis Laryngeal or tracheal erosion or necrosis Injury to nares Smaller tube required, so greater suctioning difficulty and increased work of breathing
Tracheostomy tube	Inability to maintain patent airway Facial trauma Airway obstruction Cervical spinal cord injury Long-term mechanical ventilation to facilitate weaning, oral feedings, and communication	Patients requiring high ventilatory pressures	Hemorrhage Infection Aspiration Voice change Mediastinal emphysema Tracheoinnominate artery fistula Tracheoesophageal fistula Tracheal stenosis Persistent stoma

complished, the ETT cuff is inflated, and tube placement is evaluated by

- Assessing bilateral breath sounds (diminished or absent breath sounds on the left indicates right main stem intubation)
- Checking for the presence of exhaled CO_2 with a hand-held meter or capnogram
- Confirming symmetric chest movement
- Chest radiography

The importance of chest radiographic confirmation of ETT placement can not be overstated. It is extremely easy to intubate the right main stem bronchus. Signs of right main stem intubation are diminished or absent breath sounds on the left, asymmetric chest movements, and hypoinflation of the left lung on the chest radiograph. After confirmation of placement, the ETT is secured to the patient's face with tape or commercially available ETT security devices. Steps taken to ensure that the patient does not pull out the ETT (self-extubation) include sedation, paralytics, and wrist restraints. The ETT is connected to the oxygen source or mechanical ventilation circuit.

Endotracheal intubation is not without risk of complications. The tube can inadvertently move up or down, so frequent assessment of breath sounds is important along with daily chest radiographs. Patients are at risk of aspiration if vomiting should occur, and often a gastric tube (nasal or oral) is indicated for gastric decompression. A properly inflated cuff maintains appropriate ETT placement and helps to prevent aspiration of oral secretions. Cuff inflation is assessed by auscultating the patient's neck; a minimal leak of air should be heard on inspiration. If the patient can

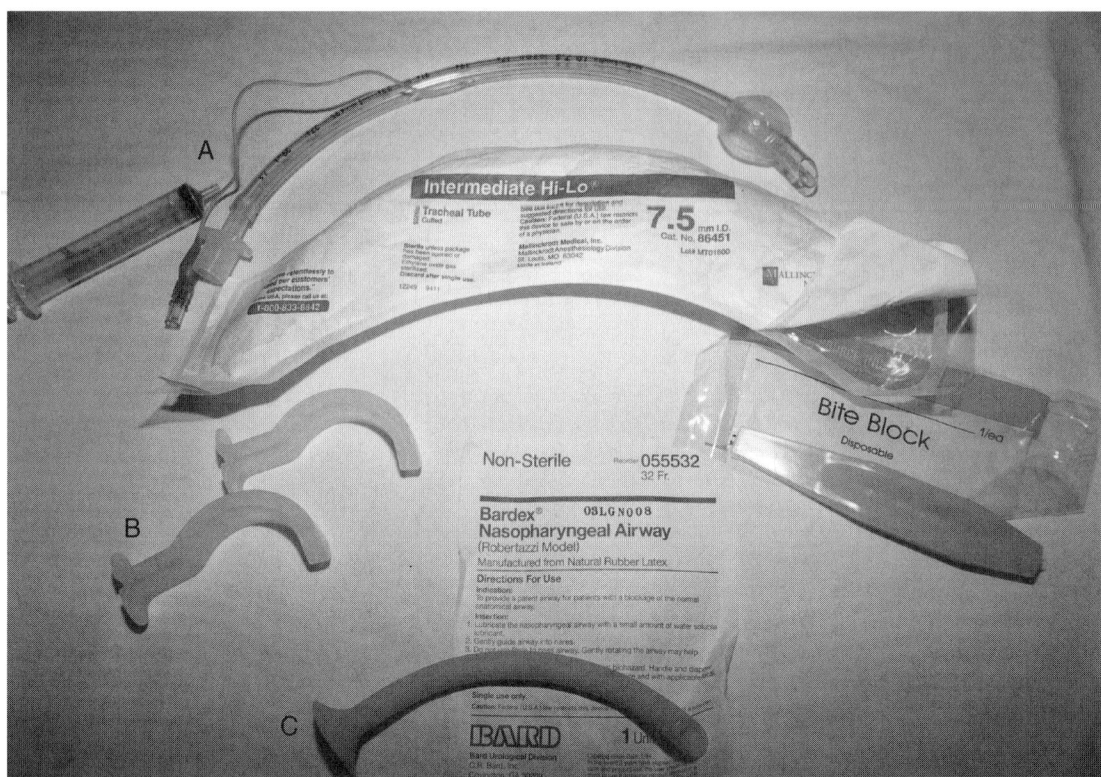

Figure 17–6

Common artificial airways used in critical care. A, Endotracheal tube; B, oropharyngeal airway; C, nasopharyngeal airway. (Courtesy of Cheryl Hyde Davia, RN.)

speak, or if a loud leak is heard, then the cuff is not inflated or more air is needed. An overinflated cuff causes laryngeal or tracheal erosion and necrosis. Measurements of cuff pressures and appropriate inflation help to prevent this problem. Maximum cuff pressure recommendations range from 20 to 25 mm Hg.[1] The pressure of the tube on the nares or lip can cause ulceration. This complication is prevented by frequent repositioning and retaping to relieve pressure and meticulous skin care at the site.

The longer the patient experiences endotracheal intubation, the higher is the risk of serious complications such as sinusitis, otitis media, pneumonia, laryngeal stenosis, laryngeal spasm or edema on extubation, and vocal cord paresis or paralysis. In patients requiring long-term mechanical ventilation or secretion management, placement of a tracheostomy tube should be considered. Other indications for tracheostomy tube placement include obstruction preventing endotracheal intubation and airway protection from aspiration. Tracheostomy tubes are placed surgically, preferably in an operating room, or with a percutaneous puncture and dilators. Patients report that tracheostomy tubes are more comfortable than ETTs because they are away from the face and allow for better oral hygiene, oral intake, and, with some tube designs, talking. They are more securely fixed, prevent further laryngeal injury, and facilitate ventilator weaning by decreasing dead space and airway resistance. Placement of a tracheostomy tube often facilitates transfer of the patient from the ICU to an intermediate care unit.

Ensuring Adequate Arterial Oxygenation

Most patients experiencing acute respiratory failure require supplemental oxygen to maintain appropriate oxygenation of body tissues. Arterial oxygenation can be monitored both continuously or intermittently as mentioned earlier in the discussion of ABGs. The use of supplemental oxygen should be guided by careful monitoring of oxygenation parameters and by consideration of the patient's underlying pathophysiologic features and psychologic state. Table 17–11 delineates the various oxygen delivery systems and clinical applications. Supplemental oxygen should always be provided at the lowest concentration appropriate, to decrease the risk of oxygen toxicity. Patients who retain CO_2 are at risk of respiratory depression when they are given high concentrations of supplemental oxygen. These patients depend on hypoxic stimulation to breathe. This trigger may be lost if these patients are placed on supplemental oxygen.

TABLE 17–11
Supplemental Oxygen Delivery Systems

Oxygen Delivery System	Description	Theoretic F_{IO_2}	Comments
Variable Performance, Low-Flow Systems	Provides a portion of inspired gas needs	Varies with patient's minute ventilation	Limited to stable patients Limited O_2 delivery for mouth breathers if nasal delivery used
Nasal cannula		0.24–0.44	Flows >6–8 L/min by nasal cannula
Nasal catheter		0.24–0.60	uncomfortable for patients
Simple face mask		0.40–0.60	Face masks require flows >
Partial rebreathing mask		0.65–0.80	5 L/min to avoid CO_2 rebreathing
Nonrebreathing mask		0.85–1.0	
Fixed Performance, High-Flow Systems	Meets patient's inspired flow needs	Constant	Best for short-term therapy because of patient discomfort (mask)
Venti-mask		0.24–0.40	May cause mucal drying unless humidity is added
Fixed-Performance, Reservoir Systems	Meets patient's volume needs	Constant	Must be tightly sealed around patient's face
Leak-free nonrebreathing mask		0.57–0.70	Risk of vomiting and aspiration with tight masks
Air entrapment nebulizers or oxygen blending systems used with T-piece systems, tracheostomy collar, aerosol masks, and face tents		0.50–0.86	Reservoir length on T piece must be adjusted to prevent rebreathing Output flows must meet or exceed inspiratory demands to ensure constant F_{IO_2}

F_{IO_2}, fraction of inspired oxygen.

Mechanical Ventilation

Mechanical ventilation is considered if the patient's respiratory failure worsens despite measures to treat the underlying cause and despite the provision of supplemental oxygen. If the patient is experiencing life-threatening hypoxia and respiratory acidosis, the decision will be made to intubate the patient and to place the patient on mechanical ventilatory support (Figure 17–7). Exact PaO_2 and $PaCO_2$ thresholds are difficult to determine and should be based on the patient's respiratory history, as well as on the ABG trends and physical signs and symptoms. Mechanical ventilation does not treat the primary problem causing the respiratory failure, but it supports the patient with adequate oxygenation and ventilation until appropriate treatment can be applied and healing can occur.

Positive-pressure ventilators are used in the acute setting and can provide two types of breaths: spontaneous breaths and mandatory breaths. A spontaneous breath is initiated and ended by the patient. Mandatory breaths are initiated and terminated by the ventilator. Ventilators can provide full support, for example, in continuous mandatory ventilation (CMV), in which all breaths are mandatory, or partial support, as in intermittent mandatory ventilation (IMV), in which some breaths are spontaneous and some are mandatory. In addition, ventilator settings can be manipulated to control pressure, volume of gases, flow of gases, and timing of inspiration and expiration. To understand the impact of mechanical ventilation, it is helpful to examine each phase of the patient's breath.[3]

On most ventilators, a breath may be triggered either by the machine or by the patient. If the machine triggers the breath, the initiating event is usually time. A preset rate is programmed; at the set time intervals, a breath is triggered regardless of the patient's efforts. This method is called controlled ventilation. When the patient initiates the ventilator breath, the ventilator must sense the effort, usually through negative pressure, but flow and volume may also be used. Patient-induced triggering is often called assisted ventilation. A combination of time and patient triggering is called assist/control (A/C) ventilation. In this mode, a preset rate is determined, but the patient may trigger over that rate.

With the trigger event, the breath may be delivered by a set pressure with flow fluctuations from the ventilator or by constant airflow from the ventilator with pressure fluctuations. Flow and pressure during inspiration are limited by set parameters that, when reached, are maintained throughout inspiration. Limits that may be set include pressure, flow, and volume.

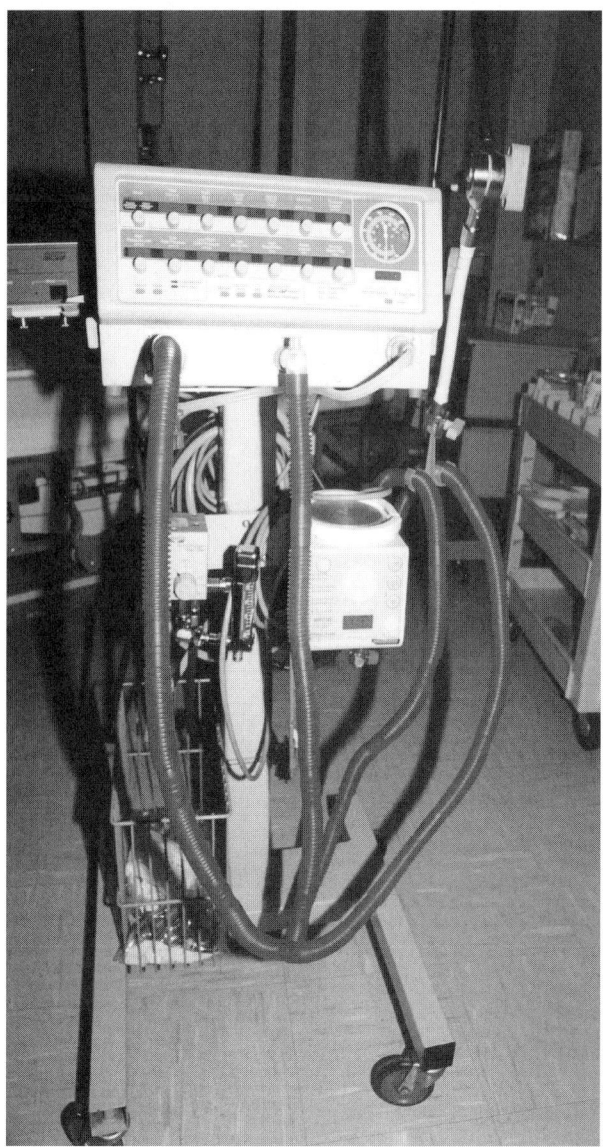

Figure 17–7

Mechanical ventilator. (Courtesy of Cheryl Hyde Davia, RN).

A cycle variable is the parameter that, when reached, ends inspiration by cycling off the ventilator. Inspiration ends when the ventilator senses preset pressure, volume, time, or flow parameters. Most ventilators have a manual cycle button, allowing the operator to end inspiration when necessary.

Expiration is a passive event as air is expelled through the pressure gradient created during inspiration in combination with the elastic recoil of the lungs. Expiratory pressure is set relative to atmospheric pressure, so if expiration pressure is to be equal to atmospheric pressure, it is set at zero, or zero end-expiratory pressure (ZEEP). PEEP is the application and maintenance of pressure above atmospheric pressure throughout expiration. Many experts theorize that physiologic PEEP is present during expiration because of airway structures, such as the glottis, that close, thus maintaining pressure slightly above atmospheric pressure.

Artificial airways bypass these physiologic structures, making ZEEP possible. PEEP is frequently set at 5 cm H_2O (physiologic), but it may be increased to 20 cm H_2O in some clinical situations. When PEEP is maintained during totally spontaneous breaths, for example, in the treatment of sleep apnea, it is termed continuous positive end-expiratory pressure (CPAP). Finally, expiratory time may be manipulated to change the normal inspiratory to expiratory relationship (I:E ratio). In spontaneous breathing, expiration is usually longer than inspiration. If the I:E ratio is reversed, inspiratory time is longer than expiration, and oxygenation is improved in some clinical situations such as ARDS.

Each of the ventilation variables—pressure, flow, time, and volume—can be manipulated to improve ventilation and oxygenation. In addition, FIO_2 and rate can be changed in response to variations in the patient's respiratory parameters. It is important to differentiate between primary oxygenation problems and ventilation problems, to determine the appropriate ventilator manipulations.

Basic Ventilator Adjustments

Primary *oxygenation problems* are evidenced by decreasing PaO_2, SaO_2, and SpO_2. Adjusting the FIO_2 or the PEEP should improve oxygenation. Conversely, when the patient begins to improve, weaning of the FIO_2 and the PEEP is possible. In most settings, the patient is placed on a high FIO_2 initially (0.7–1.0) and then is weaned utilizing ABGs or SpO_2. If simple FIO_2 adjustments do not improve oxygenation, PEEP is increased. It is thought that 5 cm of PEEP mimics normal end-expiratory pressure caused by airway structures. These structures are bypassed by the ETT causing a ZEEP situation. At PEEP levels greater than 5 cm H_2O, the patient is at risk of barotrauma.

Barotrauma is alveolar injury or rupture, in this case caused by pressure. The air escapes by the route of least resistance and moves to the mediastinal space (pneumomediastinum), the pleural space (pneumothorax), or the subcutaneous spaces in dependent areas, with subcutaneous emphysema resulting in crepitus. Of the consequences mentioned, pneumothorax is the most serious because it compresses lung tissue and compromises ventilation. If the air has no escape route, tension pneumothorax develops, compressing the heart, great vessels, and major airways and causing tracheal deviation, rapid cardiovascular decompensation, and death. Patients requiring 10 cm H_2O of PEEP or greater should be monitored by a pulmonary artery catheter to determine cardiovascular stability. Pneumothorax should be suspected if breath sounds disappear over a specific lung field, ABGs deteriorate, and the patient exhibits increasing signs of respiratory distress. The diagnosis is made by chest radiograph. Tension pneumothorax causes rapid deterioration of respiratory status and cardiovascular collapse because of displacement of the heart and great vessels. No breath sounds are heard over the affected lung, and, if the disorder is severe, tracheal deviation may be noted. Tension pneumothorax requires immediate and emergency decompression by chest tube.

Problems with ventilation are demonstrated by abnormal $PaCO_2$, $PETCO_2$, and pH values. VE is the amount of air expired each minute and is calculated by multiplying the VT times the respiratory rate. Therefore, if the patient is experiencing respiratory acidosis, increasing the respiratory rate or the VT on the ventilator will increase the VE and decrease the patient's $PaCO_2$. Conversely, if the VT or respiratory rate is set too high, the patient will experience respiratory alkalosis and should have the respiratory rate or VT turned down. When initiating mechanical ventilation, the VT is usually set at 10 to 15 mL/kg and then is adjusted using the patient's ABG values. Initial VT should be significantly lower for patients with obstructive or restrictive lung disease.[4] The respiratory rate is set depending on the ventilator mode and the patient's condition. Excessive peak inflation volume can also cause alveolar injury and is termed volutrauma. To prevent or treat volutrauma, one should decrease set volumes or change the ventilator mode.

When manipulating ventilator settings, clinicians should adjust one parameter at a time, allow at least 20 minutes for physiologic effect, and then look for improvement. Clinicians frequently err by performing multiple adjustments without allowing time for improvement.

Modes of Mechanical Ventilation

The mode of mechanical ventilation determines the way in which the patient and ventilator interact throughout the respiratory cycle. Modes are classified by the inspiratory trigger: ventilator initiated and controlled or patient initiated and assisted. The amount of control over the respiratory cycle exerted by the ventilator determines the degree of work of breathing experienced by the patient. The choice of a ventilator mode is determined by the pathophysiologic process causing the acute respiratory failure as well as the ability of the patient to assume the work of breathing and to tolerate the ventilatory pattern (Table 17–12).

Controlled Mandatory Ventilation
During CMV, the patient receives a set respiratory rate at specific time intervals and a consistent VT. The inspiratory trigger is time, the cycle variable is usually volume, and inspiration limits include pressure and flow. PEEP is often added as an expiratory variable. This mode is usually poorly tolerated by patients because patient efforts do not trigger a breath, and breath delivery is not coordinated with these efforts. This mode is rarely used, and only in conjunction with sedation and often paralytics. This mode is used when the patient must experience no work of breathing.

Assist/Control Mode
A more common highly supportive mode of ventilation is the A/C mode. In this mode, the trigger is time, but the ventilator sensitivity is set to allow patient-assisted breaths. The ventilator delivers preset VT at specific time intervals, but when a patient effort is sensed between breaths, the preset VT is also delivered to the patient. This mode guarantees a specific minimum VE and therefore decreases the patient's work of breathing. The cycle variable is usually volume, with inspiratory pressure and flow limits set, and PEEP is added as an expiratory variable. This mode is useful when patients are recovering from anesthesia because it allows some respiratory effort, but it guarantees a minimum minute ventilation. As the patient recovers, hyperventilation may occur, requiring a change in ventilator mode.

Synchronized Intermittent Mandatory Ventilation
Synchronized intermittent mandatory ventilation (SIMV) provides a preset respiratory rate at a set VT, but it allows spontaneous breathing between breaths. If the machine senses a spontaneous breath close to the time trigger for a mandatory breath, the spontaneous breath is augmented to the preset VT. Spontaneous breaths occurring between the time window for mandatory breaths are not augmented. This mode increases the patient's work of breathing because the VT of the spontaneous breaths depends solely on the patient's respiratory effort. The inspiratory cycle variable is volume; inspiratory limits include pressure and flow, with the usual addition of PEEP to the expiratory phase. This mode is well tolerated because of the synchronized effort of the machine and the patient, and it facilitates the accessory muscle conditioning in patients with chronic debilitating pulmonary disease. This mode differs from A/C in that the preset number of breaths is at the mandatory VT, but VT of the additional breaths is generated by the patient's respiratory efforts (Figure 17–8). This is the most frequently utilized ventilation mode during the supportive phase, and the preferred mode for short-term weaning.

Continuous Positive Airway Pressure
CPAP is a spontaneous breath mode with the baseline pressure elevated above zero. CPAP may be used to improve oxygenation when the patient has adequate respiratory drive and muscle strength. CPAP is used intermittently during long-term weaning to increase respiratory muscle strength or as the final step before extubation to determine readiness to extubate. All breaths are generated by the patient, and VT is com-

TABLE 17–12

Comparison of Ventilator Modes

Ventilator Mode	Indication	Specific Patient Monitoring*	Comments
CMV	Precise control of V_E or Pa_{CO_2} (closed head injuries) Perioperative period Patients with minimal or no respiratory effort	Level of sedation Asynchronous breathing Acid–base balance PIP Hemodynamic stability	Use with caution in patients with obstructive disorders Sedation needed to tolerate this mode May worsen hemodynamic status because of positive pressure with each breath Respiratory muscle atrophy
A/C	Perioperative period Complete ventilatory support	Patient comfort PIP Acid–base balance V_E	May worsen air trapping in patients with COPD Hyperventilation problematic if patient is anxious Respiratory muscle atrophy
SIMV	Synchronous partial ventilatory support Smooth transitions for weaning	RR PIP Exhaled V_T spontaneous and ventilator breaths Patient comfort	Improves patient comfort Less respiratory muscle atrophy Increased work of breathing with initiation of spontaneous breaths from demand flow system
PS	Spontaneous breathing mode May be combined with SIMV Unloading of respiratory muscles (COPD, long-term ventilator-dependent patients) Weaning	Exhaled V_T RR Airway cuff leaks (patient does not achieve full V_T) Hemodynamic parameters	Most comfortable mode for patients Effect on hemodynamic status from positive pressure Patient control over V_T and respiratory pattern V_T increased by increasing PS Combine with SIMV if patient has periods of apnea
PC	Full ventilatory support Patients with noncompliant lungs, ARDS Poor oxygenation on volume-cycled ventilators Often used in conjunction with inverse I:E ratio	Inspiratory pressure level RR Acid–base balance Auto-PEEP PIP should = PC plus set PEEP Cuff pressures Hemodynamics I:E ratio Patient sedation	Not tolerated without sedation and paralytics Hemodynamic stability often affected Reduced probability of barotrauma Frequent adjustment of pressures required
MMV	Weaning Often used with PS	RR Acid–base balance	Preset V_E does not ensure efficient respiratory pattern Patients usually comfortable Early computerized process
CPAP	Patients with adequate respiratory drive with oxygenation defect Weaning	RR V_T Patient comfort Oxygenation and ventilation Assessment of readiness to extubate	Patient assumes all work of breathing Usually last step before extubation May be used without intubation to improve oxygenation

*Patient monitoring and documentation should always include all ventilator settings, pressures, flows, and volumes per unit standards.

A/C, assist/control; ARDS, adult respiratory distress syndrome; CMV, controlled mandatory ventilation; COPD, chronic obstructive pulmonary disease; CPAP, continuous positive airway pressure; MMV, mandatory minute ventilation; PEEP, positive end-expiratory pressure; PIP, peak inspiratory pressure; PC, pressure control; PS, pressure support; RR, respiratory rate; SIMV, synchronized intermittent mandatory ventilation; V_E, minute ventilation; V_T, tidal volume.

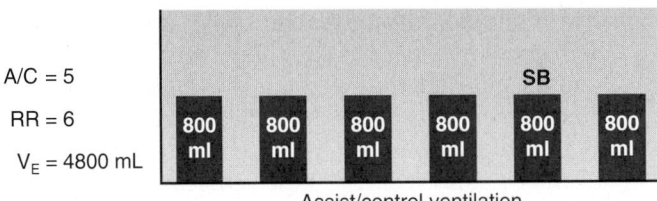

A/C = 5

RR = 6

V_E = 4800 mL

Assist/control ventilation

Figure 17-8

Assist/control (A/C) versus synchronized intermittent mandatory ventilation (SIMV) tidal volumes. RR, respiratory rate; SB, spontaneous breath; V_E, minute ventilation.

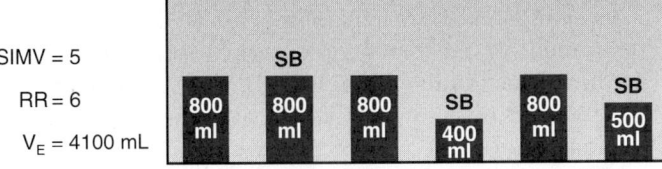

SIMV = 5

RR = 6

V_E = 4100 mL

Synchronized intermittent mandatory ventilation

pletely patient determined. The ventilator supplies continuous baseline pressure, FIO_2, and apnea alarms. The patient must have an adequate respiratory drive and the ability to generate adequate V_T. The baseline pressure enhances oxygenation and maintains open alveoli. CPAP can be delivered through a specially designed mask and therefore can be used to prevent intubation in some patients.

Pressure Support

Pressure support (PS) ventilation augments the patient's spontaneous respiratory effort with preset inspiratory positive pressure. The patient triggers the inspiratory cycle, and the inspiratory cycle ends when a preset flow criterion is reached. The patient's V_T varies, depending on patient effort and lung compliance. Positive pressure throughout inspiration augments airflow into the lungs, decreasing the work of breathing. The higher the inspiratory pressure provided, the more respiratory support the patient is receiving. PS ventilation may be used alone if the patient's respiratory drive is adequate or in conjunction with SIMV. Weaning occurs by decreasing the SIMV rate, then decreasing the amount of PS applied. Because the patient has control over respiration, this mode is usually well tolerated. For patients receiving long-term ventilation, PS prevents severe respiratory muscle wasting because the patient must expend some respiratory effort. PS is often the weaning mode of choice for long-term gentle weaning when respiratory muscle compromise is evident (e.g., COPD) or cardiac reserve is limited.

Pressure Control or Pressure Assist/Control

Pressure control (PC) or pressure A/C (PA/C) ventilation is time triggered with a preset inspiratory pressure. V_T varies, depending on lung compliance and set pressure. The patient's spontaneous respiratory rate may be assisted if the ventilator sensitivity is set to recognize patient effort. Gas flow is delivered in a decelerating pattern as the lungs fill, but the cycle variable

is time. The patient has no control over the ventilatory pattern. This mode is useful in situations such as ARDS in which complete control is vital and lung compliance is problematic because adequate V_T is usually achieved at lower peak inspiratory pressures. PEEP may be added to the expiratory phase, and because timing of inspiration is controlled, the I:E ratio may be reversed. If the I:E ratio is reversed, air trapping occurs as a result of the shortened expiratory times, thus preventing alveolar collapse and enhancing oxygenation. This air trapping is often called auto-PEEP and must be monitored closely. PC ventilation and manipulation of the I:E ratio are uncomfortable for patients. Most patients require sedation and paralytics to tolerate this form of ventilatory support.

Several other modes of ventilation are used to provide support in unusual circumstances. These modes are beyond the scope of this chapter and include high-frequency jet ventilation and simultaneous independent lung ventilation.

The patient in acute respiratory failure requires varying degrees of support as the differential diagnosis is made, treatment is begun, and healing occurs. During the treatment phase of acute respiratory failure, the goals of ventilator manipulation are to optimize ventilation, to optimize tissue oxygenation, and to rest respiratory muscles to allow healing while minimizing complications associated with mechanical ventilation. Using ventilator modes and settings appropriately is vital to this process. As healing occurs and the patient is able to increase the work of breathing, the ventilator mode should be changed to allow the patient to assume more ventilatory responsibility.

Complications

Complications associated with mechanical ventilation are related to 1) the artificial airway, 2) ventilator management, 3) interventions for secretion management, 4) infection, and 5) physiologic changes associated with assisted ventilation.

Airway

Airway problems mentioned earlier include, sinusitis, otitis media, laryngeal stenosis, laryngeal spasm or edema on extubation, and vocal cord paresis or paralysis. Self-extubation is a problem for most patients receiving long-term ventilation. The ETT is uncomfortable, and even oriented patients reflexively reach to pull the tube in their airway. Patients often need wrist restraints for a time to prevent self-extubation. Research is needed to develop alternative strategies to prevent self-extubation. Patients are unable to eat while an ETT is in place and are at high risk of aspiration of gastric contents as well as the development of stress ulcers. Most require placement of a gastric tube, either by the oral or nasal route. During the acute phase, the gastric tube is used for removal of gastric contents to prevent aspiration. Enteral feedings should be started within 48 hours of intubation, and tolerance should be monitored. Placement of a tracheostomy tube should be considered for patients requiring long-term mechanical ventilation or secretion management.

Ventilator

Incorrect pressure and volume settings on the ventilator can cause barotrauma or volutrauma and can be prevented by careful calculation of pressure and volume settings and alarms. Patients with COPD and other chronic lung problems are more vulnerable to lung trauma resulting from mechanical ventilation. Consideration of the patient's history and pathologic process when choosing an appropriate ventilation mode can prevent traumatic injury. Iatrogenic respiratory acidosis or alkalosis results when the V_T or respiratory rate parameters are not set appropriately. These abnormalities are usually easily corrected with setting changes. Loss of ventilator support can be devastating to some patients. Power outlets in critical care units are normally connected to an emergency generator system in the event of power failure. Portable oxygen sources and a bag–valve ventilation system should be available for manual ventilation in emergency situations. Patients become disconnected from the ventilator when they move or are moved in the bed or the chair. Ventilators have alarms to alert care providers of a disconnection. The low-pressure alarm usually signals a disconnection somewhere in the system (Table 17–13). Ventilator modes vary in their synchrony with the patient's efforts to breathe. Attention to the patient's comfort and anxiety level in choosing appropriate ventilatory modes will assist in minimizing the physical and psychological discomfort and the panic associated with mechanical ventilation.

Secretion Management

Artificial airways and mechanical ventilation inhibit the patient's ability to clear secretions. Patients need endotracheal suctioning to remove secretions. An increase in peak inspiratory pressures, sounding of the high-pressure alarm, coughing, or coarse breath sounds indicate the need for suctioning. Complications associated with endotracheal suctioning include hypoxemia, airway trauma, infection, and incomplete clearance of secretions. These problems are avoidable with meticulous suctioning techniques (Chart 17–3). Abundant research evidence supports preoxygenation of patients before suctioning as well as the abolishment of the practice of normal saline instillation during suctioning (Table 17–14). Normal saline instillation has not shown to be effective in increasing secretion removal and has a negative effect on oxygenation. The procedure of instilling normal saline through the ETT was shown to dislodge a significantly larger number of colonized bacteria when compared with use of a suction catheter.[5] The detrimental effects of normal saline instillation far outweigh any perceived benefit.

Infection

Patients receiving mechanical ventilation face an increased risk of respiratory infection. Sources of infection include colonized ETT, sinusitis, and contaminated suction catheters. Natural barriers to lung infections are bypassed by the ETT, as well as by changes in humidification of air by the natural airways. Patients experiencing mechanical ventilation are more vulnerable to infection resulting from impaired host resistance, nutritional deficits, inadequate hydration, oxygen toxicity, and potential for aspiration. Meticulous attention to sterile procedure, hand washing, and equipment maintenance are vital in the prevention of infection. Sputum cultures should be monitored if changes in sputum amount, color, or consistency are noted, and antibiotics should be administered as necessary.

Physiologic Changes

Several physiologic changes are associated with mechanical ventilation. Positive-pressure ventilation increases intrathoracic pressure, decreasing preload. Patients with cardiac compromise often experience decreased cardiac output while receiving positive-pressure ventilation. These effects are more pronounced in patients experiencing hypovolemia or patients with poor cardiac reserve. Some patients experience decreased cardiac output when they are disconnected from positive-pressure ventilation, as in a weaning trial. This effect is thought to be due to a sudden increase in venous return that overwhelms the cardiac capacity. The patient's normal respiratory physiology is changed by both the precipitating condition causing acute respiratory failure and mechanical ventilation. Work with animals and healthy subjects suggests that adverse changes in respiratory muscle

TABLE 17-13
Ventilator Alarms

Ventilator Alarm	Usual Cause	Treatment
Oxygen	FiO_2 changed,	Reset FiO_2
	Oxygen analyzer error	Recalibrate
	Oxygen source failure	Reconnect
High pressure (usually set at 10 cm H_2O above average peak inspiratory pressure)	Airflow obstruction: mucus, biting, fighting ventilator, water or kinks in tubing	Suction patient
		Fix kinks in tubing
		Empty water in tubing
		Evaluate airway
		Prevent biting
		Sedate patient
	Decreased pulmonary compliance: adult respiratory distress syndrome, pneumothorax, hemothorax, pulmonary edema, atelectasis, pneumonia, splinting	Insert chest tube
		Suction patient
		Assess chest radiograph
		Consider diuresis
		Increase positive end-expiratory pressure
		Control pain
Low inspiratory pressure (usually set 5–10 cm H_2O below average peak inspiratory pressure)	Ventilator disconnection	Reconnect ventilator to patient
	Air leak	Check cuff pressure and replace air in endotracheal or tracheostomy cuff if necessary
High exhaled tidal volume or minute ventilation	Increased respiratory rate or tidal volume	Determine and treat cause (anxiety, pain, hypoxemia)
	Inappropriate setting	Reset alarm, tidal volume, or respiratory rate
	Ventilator self-cycling	Decrease sensitivity setting
Apnea (no ventilation for a set time period, 20 sec)	Apnea or respiratory arrest	Provide manual ventilation with bag valve mask
		Determine and treat cause
	Loose connection to exhalation flow sensor	Reconnect
Ventilator inoperative	Loss of electrical power	Manually ventilate, reconnect to power source
	Loss of air or oxygen pressure	Check hoses and reconnect, provide manual ventilation until problem corrected
	Internal hardware malfunction	Manually ventilate and replace ventilator; send defective ventilator for servicing

FiO_2, fraction of inspired oxygen.

function occur within 72 hours of mechanical ventilation.[6]

Noninvasive Positive-Pressure Ventilation

To overcome some of the inherent problems associated with endotracheal intubation and the complications of mechanical ventilation, noninvasive methods of positive-pressure ventilation (NIPPV) have been developed and are gaining popularity. Studies comparing NIPPV with traditional mechanical ventilation requiring endotracheal intubation have suggested similar or decreased mortality rates, shortened length of stay, and avoidance of intubation.[7] Candidates for NIPPV are listed in Table 17–15. Contraindications include hemodynamic instability, inability to clear secretions, uncooperative behavior, risk of aspiration, or inability to remove the mask in the event of vomiting. NIPPV is the application of positive-pressure ventilation through a form-fitting oronasal or nasal mask. NIPPV can be used with any positive-pressure ventilator, but the trend is to use time- or patient-triggered, pressure-limited, flow-cycled devices. Some units available on the market are made specifically for NIPPV. Other forms of noninvasive ventilatory support include nasal CPAP and bi-level positive airway pressure (BiPAP). Both methods are utilized to treat sleep apnea and to prevent complications associated with sleep apnea. CPAP provides a continuous baseline pressure, whereas BiPAP allows for different pressures set for the inspiratory and expiratory phases of respiration. Nursing care of patients with the noninvasive forms of ventilatory support includes the same monitoring as in patients with invasive respiratory

CHART 17–3

Endotracheal Suctioning Technique

Endotracheal suctioning is necessary to remove secretions when a patient is intubated. Nosocomial injury, infection, hypoxia, and airway trauma can be prevented with excellent technique. The following steps must be taken each time suctioning is performed:

- Determine the need for endotracheal suctioning (breath sounds, coughing, high-pressure alarm on ventilator).
- Wash your hands.
- Explain the procedure to your patient and the family (if present).
- Gather equipment (suction kit, suction tubing to collection canister and gauge, manual resuscitation bag to 100% oxygen, or set ventilator to 100% oxygen).
- Using aseptic technique, open the sterile suctioning kit.
- Don sterile gloves.
- Determine your nonsterile hand.
- Connect the suction catheter to the suction tubing with your nonsterile hand.
- Preoxygenate the patient with 100% oxygen. You may use manual breaths with the ventilator or the manual resuscitation bag. Maintain the sterility of one hand. It is usually best to have another health care provider oxygenate the patient.

- Gently insert the suction catheter into the endotracheal tube or tracheostomy tube. Insert until the patient coughs. Stop immediately if you feel resistance.
- Apply suction only during withdrawal of the catheter.
- Hyperoxygenate the patient. Monitor the pulse oximetry (SpO_2) to avoid hypoxia.
- Repeat the suctioning. Note the color, consistency, and amount of sputum.
- Oxygenate until the patient's oxygenation status returns to baseline.
- Reassess the patient.
- Determine the need to send a sputum culture if sputum assessment findings have changed.
- Wash your hands.
- Document your intervention and assessment findings.

The American Association of Respiratory Care has delineated the following criteria for a successful suctioning outcome:

1. Improvement in breath sounds
2. Decreased peak inspiratory pressure
3. Decreased airway resistance
4. Increased tidal volume
5. Improvement in arterial blood gases or SpO_2

Outcome data from Ackerman MH, Ecklund MM, Abu-Jumah M: A review of normal saline instillation: implications for practice. Dimensions Crit Care Nurs 15:31–38, 1996.

support, as well as the prevention of complications resulting from the tight-fitting masks required. Frequent assessment of tolerance of the treatment, examination of skin condition, and prevention of aspiration are priorities of nursing care.

Ventilatory Weaning

Removal from mechanical ventilation support is complex and requires multidisciplinary planning (Figure 17–9). Ventilator weaning takes place in multiple stages including preweaning, weaning process, and weaning outcome.[8]

Preweaning

The first step in weaning a patient from the ventilator is the ongoing assessment of readiness to wean. The primary cause of the acute respiratory failure must

have been effectively treated. For example, if the patient has pneumonia, appropriate antibiotic therapy should have begun, therapy should have been given to enhance mobilization of secretions, and the patient should demonstrate improvement on chest radiograph. Assessment then focuses on the patient's ability to support ventilation and oxygenation. Neurologically, the patient must have a sufficient level of consciousness to maintain a patent airway, to produce adequate V_E, and to cough up secretions. The patient must have adequate cardiac output, heart rate, blood pressure, and hemoglobin to ensure oxygen delivery, and finally, the patient must be able to utilize oxygen at the tissue level. Other important areas to consider before and during weaning include the patient's nutritional status, body temperature, and psychological readiness. If all body systems have achieved the stability to support respiration, weaning may begin. Condi-

TABLE 17–14

Clinical Research: Normal Saline Instillation Versus No Instillation During Endotracheal Suctioning

Dependent Variable	Authors	Measurement	Result Summary
Oxygenation	Bostick, Wendelgass	Arterial blood gas	NSD
	Ackerman, Gugerty	SpO_2	Decreased SpO_2 after saline instillation
	Gray, Macintyre, Kronenberger	Arterial blood gas and SpO_2	NSD
	Reynolds, Hoffman, Schlichtig, Davies, Zullo	SpO_2	NSD
	Ackerman	SpO_2	Decreased SpO_2 after saline instillation
Sputum recovered	Bostick, Wendelgass	Sputum weights	Increase with saline instillation NSS
	Ackerman, Gugerty	Sputum weights	SS increase with saline instillation
	Gray, Macintyre, Kronenberger	Sputum weights	SS increase with saline instillation
	Reynolds, Hoffman, Schlichtig, Davies, Zullo	Sputum volume	No increase in sputum volume with saline instillation
Other respiratory parameters	Reynolds, Hoffman, Schlichtig, Davies, Zullo	Peak inspiratory pressure, tidal volume, compliance	No difference in any of the parameters with saline instillation
	Gray, Macintyre, Kronenberger	Minute ventilation, peak inspiratory pressure, forced vital capacity	NSD in any of the parameters with saline instillation
Contamination	Rutala, Stiegel, Sarubbi	Cultured saline vials after opening and nurses' hands	25% of vials were contaminated; 6 organisms were in common with nurses' hand cultures
	Hagler, Traver	Number of bacteria dislodged when saline and suction catheter passed through an endotracheal tube	SS larger number of bacteria dislodged by saline instillation

SpO_2, pulse oximetry; NSD, no significant difference; NSS, not statistically significant; SS, statistically significant.

Data from Raymond SJ: Normal saline instillation before suctioning: helpful or harmful? A review of the literature. Am J Crit Care Nurs 4:267–271, 1995; and Copnell B, Ferguson D: Endotracheal suctioning: time-worn ritual or timely intervention? Am J Crit Care Nurs 4:100–105, 1995.

tions that interfere with the patient's ability to wean from the ventilator are listed in Table 17–16.

Weaning parameters are physiologic measurements that may predict weaning success. Traditional weaning parameters include measurement of vital capacity, maximum inspiratory pressure, which is also known as negative inspiratory force, VE, and maximum voluntary ventilation (MVV) (see Table 17–7). In addition, the amount of support required to maintain acceptable oxygenation and ventilation is considered. The correlation of these traditional measurements with successful weaning has not been well documented in the research

TABLE 17–15

Clinical Conditions that Benefit Most from Noninvasive Positive-Pressure Ventilation

Hypercapnic Respiratory Failure	Hypoxemic Respiratory Failure
Exacerbation of COPD	Postoperative respiratory failure
Chronic respiratory failure with COPD	Hemodynamically stable cardiogenic pulmonary edema
Cystic fibrosis with decompensation	Opportunistic pneumonia in AIDS patients
End-stage lung disease awaiting lung transplantation	Patients inappropriate for intubation (DNR order, terminally ill with reversible acute respiratory failure)
Patients inappropriate for intubation (DNR order, terminally ill with reversible acute respiratory failure)	

AIDS, acquired immunodeficiency syndrome, COPD, chronic obstructive pulmonary disease; DNR, do not resuscitate.

VENTILATOR DEPENDENT: TRACHEOSTOMY OR ENDOTRACHEAL TUBE

DRG 483/475

Addressograph

Completed by Pulmonary Outcomes Manager after
Discharge:
Total Ventilation Days _____
Trach days post Ventilation _____
Total LOS _____
Discharge / on Ventilation? _____ (Y/N)
Initial Intubation Date _____

DRG 483 Health Care Financing Administration (HCFA)
Length of Stay (LOS) = 41.9
Pulmonologist and Date of Consult: _____
Discharge Date: _____
Discharge Where? _____
Re-intubation _____ # of times

	Phase I: Acute Ventilatory Support	Phase II: Ventilatory Support	Phase III: Weaning	Phase IV: Resolution
Consultations	Pulmonologist consultation if patient still intubated after 72 hours or if reintubation required Swallow or speech consultation considered Nutritional support dietitian Pulmonary outcomes manager Respiratory care clinician	Physical medicine and rehabilitation consultation considered Physical therapy Occupational therapy Swallow or speech consultation	Physical medicine and rehabilitation consultation considered	
Diagnostic Tests	ABG CXR SMA-7 Sputum culture and sensitivity after 72 hr of ETT Blood culture as needed (PRN) Phosphorus 4 times daily if patient on TF or TPN for first week Prealbumin PRN Pulse oximetry Complete blood count (CBC) SMA-12 ECG	Pulmonary mechanics ECG PRN SMA-7 ABG PRN 24-hr urinary urea nitrogen (if no renal failure) PRN Prealbumin PRN CBC SMA-12 weekly Pulse oximetry CXR	Pulmonary mechanics ECG PRN CXR SMA-12 weekly 24-hr urinary urea nitrogen (if no renal failure) PRN Prealbumin PRN CBC PRN SMA-7 Pulse oximetry ABG PRN	Pulmonary mechanics Pulse oximetry PRN
Treatments	SvO_2 PRN Mechanical ventilation Tracheostomy after ETT in place × 7 days Gastrointestinal protection with histamine blockers/carafate Sedation PRN Diuretics PRN Vasopressors Vasoactive infusions Respiratory treatments	Respiratory treatments Packed cells PRN Secretion management Antibiotics PRN Sedation PRN Diuretics PRN Tracheostomy care	Respiratory treatments PRN Packed cells PRN Secretion management Antibiotics PRN Diuretics PRN Tracheostomy care	Tracheostomy collar or decannulation or extubation or continued ventilatory management and slow weaning

Interventions	Secretion management IV medications Packed cells PRN Antibiotics PRN Paralytics PRN Daily weight Special bed PRN Foley catheter Swallow or dysphagia screening Social services: supportive counseling and crisis intervention I&O hourly Suction PRN	Daily weight Suction PRN Evaluate need for permanent IV access Social services: supportive counseling and crisis intervention. I&O Foley catheter	Daily weight Suction PRN If prolonged TFs, evaluate need for percutaneous endoscopic gastrostomy Evaluate continued need for IV access Social services supportive counseling	Daily weight I&O every 8 hr Suction PRN
Activity	Bed rest Passive range of motion every 4 hr Increased activity as tolerated	Up on side of bed with assistance Foot support Up in chair if tolerated Active range of motion	Up in chair 3 × daily Increased ambulation	Up in chair 3 times daily for increased time Increased ambulation Decreased involvement in self-care activities
Nutrition	Nutritional assessment TPN/TF; attempt TF to preserve gut integrity	If patient on TPN, transition to tube feedings Nutritional reassessment every 10 days	Transition to oral diet if no dysphagia Nutritional reassessment every 10 days	Continued oral diet or TF
Teaching	Orientation of patient/family to intensive care unit (ICU): visiting policy, tests, procedures, disease process, changes in care Establishment of a communication mode with patient	Education of patient and family regarding changes in care, procedures, and improvements/changes in patient's condition	Education of patient and family regarding weaning process	Education of patient and family regarding discharge plan, any new equipment or procedures
Discharge Planning	Social services: high-risk screening and initiate assessment of resources	Social services: continued assessment of resource needs	Social services: evaluation of patient for placement options; initial discharge referrals	Social services: finalized arrangements for transportation to discharge destination, home, equipment, home health
Outcomes	Patient or family verbalizes knowledge of surroundings, tests, visitation policy, and disease process. Patient demonstrates understanding of need for ETT, suctioning, and alarms	Patient demonstrates improved/stable ventilatory status as evidenced by improved CXR, ABGs	Patient demonstrates improved ventilatory status as evidenced by decreased ventilatory support and increased activity without respiratory signs and symptoms of distress	Patient or family verbalizes knowledge of discharge plans, follow-up care, and all new equipment, procedures, and medications

Figure 17–9

Clinical pathway for patients requiring long-term ventilation. (© St. Luke's Episcopal Hospital, Houston, TX, 1996: used with permission; From Kite-Powell DM, Sabau D, Ideno KT, et al: Optimizing outcomes in ventilator-dependent patients: challenging critical care practice. Crit Care Nurs Q 19:77–90, 1996.)

TABLE 17–16

Conditions that Hinder Weaning from Ventilators

Condition	Problem
Neuromuscular disorders	Decreased vital capacity
Age	
Malnutrition	
Electrolyte imbalance	
Muscle atrophy	
Drug therapy:	Decreased inspiratory force
Paralytics	
Sedation	
Hypothyroidism	
Sepsis	Abnormally elevated tidal volume
Fever	
Overfeeding	
Abdominal distention	Inadequate tidal volume
Pain	
Anxiety	
Malpositioning	
Pneumothorax	
Hemothorax	
Pulmonary embolism	Increased dead space
Emphysema	
Adult respiratory distress syndrome	
Small endotracheal tube	Increased work of breathing
Auto-positive end-expiratory pressure	
Ventilator circuitry	
Atelectasis	Ventilation–perfusion mismatch
Pulmonary embolism	
Pneumonia	
Pulmonary edema	
Bronchospasm	

literature.[6,9,10] More advanced parameters include combinations of respiratory mechanics and oxygenation measures such as the CROP index (compliance, rate, oxygenation, and pressure) and the rapid shallow breathing index (f/V_T ratio). Because research demonstrates the complex nature of ventilatory support weaning, more tools are needed to assist bedside clinicians in the assessment of readiness to wean as well as the patient's progress in the weaning process. An example of a multiparameter assessment tool is the Burns' Weaning Assessment Program (BWAP) designed to integrate the impact of general, pulmonary, and mechanical factors on weaning.[11] The BWAP bedside assessment checklist includes 26 physiologic parameters identified from the literature as important to weaning (Figure 17–10).

Before the weaning process may begin, measures should be taken to correct issues identified in the preweaning assessment. For example, nutritional support should be adequate for the energy needs of healing, increased respiratory muscle demands, and increased mobility. Consultation with a dietitian assists the team in providing a balanced mixture of carbohydrates and fats at a rate slightly higher than baseline requirements. Overfeeding increases CO_2 production and ventilatory workload. The optimal method of feeding is the oral route, which occasionally is possible if the patient has a tracheostomy tube. More commonly, the patient requires enteral tube feedings with commercial preparations that are readily available. Monitoring the patient's serum albumin level weekly is important to ensure nutritional balance.

Fluid and electrolyte imbalance often results from the precipitating clinical event or treatment. This im-

TABLE 17–17

Laboratory Values

Laboratory Test	Normal Value	Comment
Serum Electrolytes		
Blood urea nitrogen	5–20 mg/L	Renal failure delays recovery
Creatinine	0.5–2.0 mg/L	
Magnesium	1.5–2.5 mEq/L	Electrolytes involved in muscle contraction and relaxation as well as
Potassium	3.5–5.0 mEq/L	acid–base balance
Sodium	135–145 mEq/L	
Calcium	9–11 mg/dL	
Carbon dioxide	23–30 mEq/L	Acid–base balance
Glucose	70–105 mg/dL	Hyperglycemia delays recovery
Lactate	0.5–2.0 mEq/L	Elevated serum lactate levels may indicate inadequate tissue perfusion
Hematology		
Hematocrit	38–49%	Oxygen is transported by red blood cells bound to hemoglobin
Hemoglobin	13–17 g/dL	
White blood count	4500–11,000 cells/mm^3	Elevation may indicate infection
Carboxyhemoglobin	<25%	Indicative of carbon monoxide poisoning
Toxicology Screening	Varies	Toxins, narcotics, sedatives, or paralytics may cause respiratory depression

Burns' Weaning Assessment Program (BWAP)

Patient name _____   Patient history number _____

Yes	No	Not assessed	

General assessment

1. Hemodynamically stable (pulse rate, cardiac output)?
2. Free from factors that increase or decrease metabolic rate (seizures, temperature, sepsis, bacteremia, hypo/hyperthyroid)?
3. Hematocrit >25% (or baseline)?
4. Systemically hydrated (weight at or near baseline, balanced intake and output)?
5. Nourished (albumin >2.5, parenteral/enteral feedings maximized)? (If albumin is low and anasarca or third spacing is present, score for hydration should be "no").
6. Electrolytes within normal limits? (including Ca^{++}, Mg^+, PO_4).
   * Correct Ca^{++} for albumin level.
7. Pain controlled? (subjective determination)
8. Adequate sleep/rest? (subjective determination)
9. Appropriate level of anxiety and nervousness? (subjective determination)
10. Absence of bowel problems (diarrhea, constipation, ileus)?
11. Improved general body strength/endurance (i.e., out of bed in chair, progressive activity program)?
12. Chest roentgenogram improving?

Respiratory assessment

Gas flow and work of breathing

13. Eupnic respiratory rate and pattern (spontaneous respiratory rate <25, without dyspnea, absence of accessory muscle use).
    * This is assessed off the ventilator while measuring #20-23.
14. Absence of adventitious breath sounds (rhonchi, rales, wheezing)?
15. Secretions thin and minimal?
16. Absence of neuromuscular disease/deformity?
17. Absence of abdominal distention/obesity/ascites?
18. Oral endotracheal tube >#7.5 or trach >#7.5

Airway clearance

19. Cough and swallow reflexes adequate?

Strength

20. Negative inspiratory pressure <-20
21. Positive expiratory pressure >+30

Endurance

22. Spontaneous tidal volume >5 mL/kg?
23. Vital capacity >10-15 mL/kg?

Arterial blood gases

24. pH 7.30-7.45
25. $Paco_2$ approximately 40 mm Hg (or baseline) with minute ventilation <10 L/min (evaluated while on ventilator).
26. Pao_2 >60 on Fio_2 <40%

Figure 17–10

Burns' Weaning Assessment Program bedside assessment checklist. (Courtesy of Suzanne M. Burns, MSN, RN, RRT, CCRN. Copyright by the University of Virginia Patent Foundation, Charlottesville, VA.)

balance must be corrected if the patient is to be weaned from the ventilator. Treatment may include fluid resuscitation, blood transfusion, electrolyte replacement, or diuretic therapy, depending on the disorder. Patients receiving long-term ventilation should be weighed frequently to determine fluid balance trends. Intake and output measurements are important monitoring tools, as are laboratory values (Table 17–17). Adequate hematocrit and hemoglobin are vital for oxygen delivery and must be corrected if deficient. Electrolytes important to muscle contraction include potassium, magnesium, and calcium.

Other abnormalities that contribute to difficulty in weaning from the ventilator include impaired thyroid functioning, metabolic acidosis, renal failure, and hyperglycemia. Measures should be taken to correct or improve these abnormalities before and during weaning.

Weaning Process

Weaning the FIO_2 required by the patient to maintain adequate oxygenation is usually the first step in the weaning process, and it is a good indicator of successful treatment of oxygenation deficits contributing to the patient's acute respiratory failure. Although ABG values may be used to wean the patient's FIO_2, the real-time oxygenation parameter, SpO_2 has been found to be as valuable and has cost and comfort advantages.[9] When the FIO_2 has been successfully weaned to less than or equal to 0.4, and PEEP levels have been decreased to less than or equal to 5 cm, weaning of ventilatory support may begin.

Multiple methods are used to wean patients from ventilator support; none has clear advantages supported by research. Methods used to wean include abrupt trials of spontaneous breathing utilizing a T-tube delivery of oxygen, or CPAP mode, gradual decreasing support as in SIMV and PS weaning, and computerized controlled weaning as in MMV weaning. The choice of weaning method depends on the patient's underlying respiratory disorder, as well as on the patient's physical and psychological response to the weaning process. Consistency in weaning method is important for the patient to achieve complete independence from the ventilator (Chart 17–4).

Spontaneous breathing trials are effective for the patient experiencing short-term ventilation, such as the patient under anesthesia. As the anesthesia is reversed and neuromuscular control returns, evidence of spontaneous breathing is documented, and a spontaneous breathing trial is begun. If the patient demonstrates adequate VT, positive gag and cough reflexes, appropriate respiratory rate, oxygenation, and $ETCO_2$, ventilation is discontinued, and the patient is extubated. Spontaneous breathing trials are utilized in the patient receiving long-term ventilation to build respiratory muscle strength and to assess readiness for discontinuance of ventilatory support. Typically, ventilatory support is alternated with spontaneous breathing trials of increasing length until the patient tolerates spontaneous breathing for 24 hours at a time with no periods of ventilatory support. The spontaneous breathing trials may be as short as 15 minutes four times per day, increasing to all day with rest at night and then to 24 hours.

To decrease ventilator support gradually, the patient is placed on SIMV mode. The ventilator respiratory rate is gradually decreased, and patient's tolerance is assessed. Usually, when the ventilator rate is weaned to 4 to 6 breaths per minute, the patient is placed on CPAP and is reassessed for an ability to discontinue the ventilator and potentially to be extubated. This method is commonly successful in patients experiencing short-term ventilation such as cardiac surgical patients. Patients who are anesthetized or sedated after surgery and are extubated within 4 to 10 hours usually are successfully weaned with this method. SIMV weaning is associated with an increased work of breathing at lower respiratory rates imposed by the ETT and ventilator circuitry.

Patients with neuromuscular dysfunction, COPD, and limited cardiac reserve lack the respiratory muscle strength to wean successfully on SIMV and may need the addition of pressure support to help unload respiratory muscles. Every spontaneous breath is assisted with pressure, thus overcoming airway impedance and augmenting VT. The respiratory muscles experience high-volume, low-pressure work that promotes endurance conditioning. PS may be used to supplement SIMV, or it may be the sole weaning mode. When used as the sole weaning mode, PS is set to ensure VT of 10 to 12 mL/kg and then is decreased as the patient is able to generate adequate spontaneous VT. At PS of 5 cm H_2O, the patient can usually be extubated. Studies suggest and patients report greater comfort and ventilatory synchrony on PS ventilation than with other modes.[10]

Computer-assisted weaning modes are in the developmental phase. MMV weaning is a crude example. In the MMV mode, VE is preset, and the patient is allowed to breath spontaneously. If the spontaneous VE drops below the preset VE, the machine will automatically provide the support needed to achieve the VE goal. More sophisticated computer-assisted modes enter more than one preset parameter into an algorithm that allows breath-by-breath monitoring and assistance as needed. These systems have not been widely tested to date.

Patients experiencing difficulty in weaning from the ventilator may benefit from facilitative therapies and techniques such as inspiratory resistance training, physical therapy, hypnosis, biofeedback, and pharmacologic support. Inspiratory resistance training involves the use of a device that requires the patient to breathe through an increasingly narrowed orifice.[12] The theory behind the exercise is that the increase in airway resistance causes inspiratory muscle training that increases muscle bulk and endurance. Research support for facilitative therapies is inconclusive because of the lack of control group methods and the small numbers of subjects.[10] Case reports suggest that hypnosis and biofeedback are helpful to control anxiety and dyspnea after physiologic causes have been eliminated. Physical therapy to improve overall muscle tone, to mobilize secretions, and to improve mobility is important for the patient experiencing long-term mechanical ventilation.

Weaning Outcome

The desired outcome of ventilatory weaning is complete independence from ventilatory support, with extubation or decannulation if the patient has a tra-

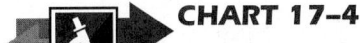

CHART 17–4

RESEARCH UTILIZATION: A RANDOMIZED, CONTROLLED TRIAL OF PROTOCOL-DIRECTED VERSUS PHYSICIAN-DIRECTED WEANING FROM MECHANICAL VENTILATION

Abstract: A significant portion of nurses', respiratory therapists', and physicians' time and energy is devoted to ventilator weaning in the ICU. In addition, time spent on mechanical ventilation is uncomfortable for patients and distressing for families. No conclusive studies have delineated the optimal weaning method, despite the focus of many studies on identifying the best technique for weaning patients from mechanical ventilation. This study compared protocol-directed weaning from mechanical ventilation implemented by nurses and respiratory therapists with traditional physician-directed weaning. The study design utilized a randomized, controlled trial in four intensive care units located in two university-affiliated teaching hospitals. Patients requiring mechanical ventilation were randomly assigned to receive either protocol-driven (N = 179) or physician-driven (N = 178) weaning from mechanical ventilation. Within the protocol-driven group, four specific protocols were utilized and compared. The primary outcome measured was length of time on mechanical ventilation from tracheal intubation until discontinuation of mechanical ventilation. Other outcomes measured included the need for reintubation, length of stay in the hospital, mortality rate, and hospital costs. Findings: ". . . nurses and respiratory therapists, using protocol guidance, weaned patients from mechanical ventilation safely and more quickly than the team following the traditional practice of physician-directed weaning." Patients who had protocol-directed weaning had statistically significant shorter durations of mechanical ventilation as compared with patients randomized to physician-directed weaning. Cox proportional-hazards regression analysis showed that the rate of successful weaning was significantly greater for patients receiving protocol-directed weaning compared with patients receiving physician-directed weaning. No statistically or clinically significant difference was noted among the four protocols utilized, and the secondary outcomes—reintubation, mortality, hospital length of stay, and costs—did not show a statistically significant difference. Patient demographics were similar for both the protocol-directed group and the physician-directed group. Total hospital costs for the protocol-directed weaning group were $42,960 less than costs for the physician-driven weaning group.

Critique: This study is timely and important to the nursing profession as well as to critically ill patients. The study design was scientific and was adapted appropriately to the clinical arena. The study is limited by its inclusion of only university-affiliated hospitals with physicians in training. Some variability occurred among the four units used in the study, a finding suggesting that differences in structure and processes of medical care as well as protocol implementation may account for some of the variability. This study's findings of no difference among protocols is supported by previous research, as well as the findings of decreased mechanical ventilation duration. This study contributed to the evidence that timing and consistency of weaning decisions are more important than a specific weaning protocol. Unique to this study is its use of a control group as well as the large sample size.

Nursing Considerations: The efficacy and superiority of teamwork among bedside professionals, nurses, and respiratory therapists were demonstrated by this study. The ability of these highly trained professionals to use appropriate judgment and skill in the timely weaning of patients was demonstrated clearly and reinforced the findings of other studies in a more scientific manner. Advantages to protocol-driven weaning include

- Patient-driven, real-time weaning decisions
- Facilitation of teamwork between respiratory therapy and nursing staff
- Physicians' freedom to perform duties that cannot be delegated to nonphysicians
- Positive weaning outcomes

Protocol-directed weaning demands more complex thinking and skill from the nurse. Critical care nurses must be prepared to demonstrate expertise in

- Respiratory assessment
- Respiratory mechanics
- Development of trusting, professional relationships with other disciplines
- Communication with patients, families, and other professionals
- Confident problem solving

More studies are needed to determine the effectiveness of weaning teams, the importance of consistent weaning protocols, and nursing's unique contribution to positive weaning outcomes.

Source: Kollef MH, Shapiro SD, Silver P, et al: A randomized, controlled trial of protocol-directed versus physician-directed weaning from mechanical ventilation. Crit Care Med 25:567–574, 1997.

cheostomy. The definition of successful weaning varies in the literature, with the most commonly accepted definition being 24 hours without distress after extubation.[8] Utilization of a clinical pathway is thought to improve outcomes. Figure 17–9 is an example of a clinical pathway used in patients requiring long-term ventilation.[13] After successful weaning from mechanical ventilation, the patient requires close monitoring for airway patency, oxygenation issues, adequate ventilation, and oxygen delivery. The patient is particularly vulnerable in the first 48 hours after long-term ventilation weaning to problems with respiratory muscle fatigue, laryngedema, aspiration, and anxiety or panic. The critical care nurse must be particularly vigilant for exacerbation of the precipitating problem and for airway issues. If the patient has a tracheostomy, airway management will gradually progress with downsizing and eventual decannulation.

Some patients experience incomplete weaning and require partial intermittent ventilatory support, commonly as nocturnal periods of rest on the ventilator. The focus for these patients shifts from critical care to intermediate care or long-term care placement. Patients who require nocturnal ventilatory rest periods may benefit from the NIPPV techniques mentioned earlier. More study is needed in this area to guide planning of care.

Another outcome of the weaning process may be the determination that the patient requires long-term full ventilatory support. At this point, the patient and family need to plan for long-term care placement with the aid of social services (Chart 17–5).

The fourth outcome possibility is the decision to wean the patient terminally. Terminal weaning is the withdrawal of mechanical ventilatory support when the patient is not expected to survive.[12] Terminal weaning is considered when death is anticipated because of the nature of the illness, or when permanent dependence on ventilator support is anticipated and is against the patient's expressed wishes through an advanced directive or discussions with the family. The decision to wean a patient terminally is difficult for the health care team and the family. Many institutions have a biomedical ethics committee offering assistance in decision making for both the family and the health care team.[14]

Care priorities shift to the alleviation of pain and suffering when the decision is made to wean the patient terminally from the ventilator. The nurse uses narcotics to relieve the patient's dyspnea and pain, and anxiolytics such as lorazepam (Alzapam) or midazolam (Versed) are given to relieve the patient's anxiety. Bronchodilators and diuretics may be utilized to relieve dyspnea. The shift from using pharmacologic agents to

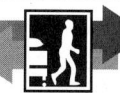

CHART 17–5

BEYOND THE ICU: VENTILATED PATIENTS IN LONG-TERM CARE FACILITIES OR AT HOME

For years, a criterion for continuing ICU services was mechanical ventilation. With advances in simple ventilators, remote alarm systems, and airway management, patients requiring long-term ventilator support are no longer confined to ICUs. Patients are now managed in intermediate care units, long-term care facilities, and at home. Most long-term ventilator-dependent patients can be cared for out of the ICU if the following conditions are met:

- The patient's condition has stabilized; all system problems are adequately treated.
- The patient has a stable airway, usually a tracheostomy tube.
- The patient is receiving optimal nutritional support by enteral feedings through a secure gastric tube, or oral intake is not aspirated.
- The patient has stabilized on the ventilator model and settings used in the alternate care facility.
- The patient and family are emotionally prepared for the transfer.

- The care providers have been educated in the care of a long-term ventilator-dependent patient and have established contact with the patient and family.

Long-term care facilities across the United States are upgrading their institutions and are educating their staff to care for ventilator-dependent patients. Families who wish to care for the patient at home require tremendous amounts of support emotionally. In addition, these families need extensive education on ventilator technology and management as well as information on supportive services such as respite.

The critical care nurse can play a key role in the preparation of the patient and family for transfer and with outreach education for the long-term care facilities. Career opportunities abound in long-term care and home care with this expanding patient population.

> ## CHART 17–6
> ### ETHICAL DILEMMA
>
> The determination that a patient will never support independent ventilation or will not survive the present illness is difficult for professionals and almost impossible for families to accept.
>
> Mrs. S. was a 50-year-old wife and mother of two teenage children. She had been diagnosed with lung cancer a year earlier and had spent the year in and out of the hospital for surgery, chemotherapy, and radiation treatments.
>
> During her last admission, she had two separate surgical repairs of a broncopulmonary fistula. After the second repair, she deteriorated into acute respiratory failure. Despite chest tube drainage, continuous BiPAP, and massive medical support, Mrs. S. had to be intubated and placed on mechanical ventilation. Mrs. S.'s condition deteriorated over many weeks in the ICU. Her family and friends visited daily, always speaking with her, praying for her, and often singing and playing music. The nurses, doctors, social worker, and family met frequently to discuss her condition, and each time the prognosis grew worse.
>
> Despite advanced ventilatory support (simultaneous independent lung ventilation), Mrs. S.'s respiratory status worsened. Her family made funeral arrangements and tried to say good-bye, but they were not ready to let go. Mrs. S. was continuously sedated and unresponsive to her surroundings.
>
> When the family was ready, they gathered with special friends in her room. Mrs. S. was weaned from her sedation and was medicated for pain. Mrs. S. was dressed in a special nightgown, her hair combed, and lipstick applied. Her primary nurses stayed over from their shifts to be with her and her family. She seemed to recognize each person but was unable to communicate. The F_{IO_2} was weaned from 1.0 to .21, and the pressure support to 0. With her friends, family, and nurses with her, she died peacefully and comfortably.
>
> 1. How do you determine that a family is ready to accept the death of a loved one who is maintained on life support?
> 2. What role should teenage children play in life-and-death decisions?
> 3. There are often marked differences in philosophies regarding withdrawal of ventilator support among physicians, nurses, and family members. What resources are available to resolve these differences and to provide compassionate care to the dying?
> 4. What are your feelings toward participation in terminal weaning?
> 5. Are there legal ramifications to terminal weaning of patients?

treat disease to using drugs for the relief of symptoms is difficult for critical care nurses as the priority of monitoring for improvement shifts to monitoring for comfort. The family should be permitted to comfort the patient, to complete leave taking, and to begin grieving. A chaplain, social worker, or family member is often the lead team member at this time. In this situation, the desired outcome is a peaceful death under circumstances chosen by the patient (Chart 17–6).

Multidisciplinary Outcomes

Successful management of the patient in acute respiratory failure is a multidisciplinary process involving physicians, nurses, respiratory therapists, social workers, family members, physical therapists, and pastoral care. Multidisciplinary management is focused on identification and treatment of the precipitating clinical event, maintenance of a patent airway, optimization of oxygenation and ventilation, and provision of adequate oxygen delivery for tissue utilization. The psychosocial needs of the patient and family in crisis must be considered, to ensure optimal outcomes. The use of highly invasive treatments such as mechanical ventilation demands increased attention to relief of anxiety and facilitation of communication. Skilled clinicians make a tremendous difference in the lives of these patients and their families. Table 17–18 lists the phase of multidisciplinary management and expected outcomes for patients experiencing acute respiratory failure.

Critical Thinking Exercise

Mr. S. is a 78-year-old man with a history of emphysema, coronary artery disease, and arthritis. At home, Mr. S. usually spends his day in a recliner chair watching television and smokes approximately 2 packs of cigarettes per day. Mr. S. was admitted to the ICU after coronary artery bypass grafting on 4 vessels. He was unstable postoperatively and

TABLE 17–18

Multidisciplinary Outcomes

Phase of Recovery	Outcome
Emergency room	Establishment of patent airway
	Establishment of adequate breathing pattern
	Establishment of adequate circulation
	Stabilization of patient for transport to appropriate unit
Intensive care unit	Appropriate respiratory support to maintain adequate tissue oxygenation and waste removal
	Definititive diagnosis
	Appropriate treatment of underlying cause of respiratory failure
	Prevention of complications of treatment
	Weaning from supportive therapy
	Initiation of disease teaching
Intermediate care unit	Maintenance of adequate respiratory functioning
	Increase in activity tolerance
	Return to premorbid level of self-care
	Understanding of self-care and treatment
Community/Home management	Maintenance of optimal respiratory function
	Establishment of a risk-reduced lifestyle
	Restoration of previous role functions

required dobutamine for low cardiac output (inotropic support), low-dose dopamine to improve renal perfusion, and norepinephrine (Levophed) to maintain adequate blood pressure. Mr. S. bled significantly from his chest tubes in the first 6 hours after surgery and is receiving his second unit of packed red blood cells. Mr. S.'s ventilator settings are as follows: FIO_2, 0.7, SIMV, 10, V_T, 1000 mL, and +5 of PEEP. The ICU standard of care allows the nurse to wean and extubate the patient utilizing a decreasing SIMV rate protocol. The usual time frame for weaning and extubation is 4 to 6 hours after surgery. As a novice critical care nurse, you consult with a more experienced peer and are advised not to wean Mr. S. within the usual time frame.

1. Why is this advice appropriate?
2. Identify the potential abnormalities in
   Ventilation
   Oxygen content
   Oxygen delivery
   Oxygen utilization
3. What treatment measures are currently used to treat the problems identified in number 2?

Mr. S. had ABGs drawn on the foregoing ventilator settings mentioned above: PaO_2, 106; $PaCO_2$, 25; HCO_3^-, 22; pH, 7.56; and SaO_2, 97%.

4. Discuss the foregoing ABGs in regard to oxygenation, acid–base balance, and compensation.
5. Recognizing that you would only make one ventilator change at a time, what are the two options available to correct the abnormality identified in number 3?
6. Which is the best option for Mr. S.?
7. It takes 48 hours for Mr. S. to achieve hemodynamic stability and to be weaned from vasoactive drugs. On morning rounds, you and the physician decide that a slow PS weaning would be most appropriate for Mr. S. Provide a rationale for this decision.

Key Concepts

➡ Acute respiratory failure is the sudden and severe impairment in the lung's ability to maintain adequate oxygenation and ventilation.

➡ Respiratory failure may be due to ventilatory failure, abnormalities of oxygenation, or both.

➡ Many disease processes contribute to acute respiratory failure, so it is important to assess all body systems and to correct the underlying causes while providing respiratory support.

➡ Adequate ventilation requires central nervous system stimulation, an intact pulmonary system, adequate perfusion to the lungs, musculoskeletal strength, and appropriate fluid and electrolyte balance.

➡ Adequate tissue oxygenation depends on oxygen diffusion in the lungs, adequate cardiac output, hemoglobin, and normal circulation.

➡ Acute respiratory failure is a crisis for both the patient and the family.

➡ Diagnostic testing assists in the differential diagnosis of acute respiratory failure and may identify the root cause. Common diagnostic tests include ABGs, chest radiographs, pulmonary function tests, bronchoscopy, angiography, and drug screening.

➡ Oxygenation may be assessed utilizing ABGs (PaO_2, SaO_2) or SpO_2.

➟ Ventilation may be assessed by ABGs (Pa_{CO_2}) and ETCO$_2$.

➟ Metabolic disturbances influencing respiratory status are determined through ABG analysis ($HCO_3{}^-$) and blood chemistry studies.

➟ The body compensates for acid–base imbalance through the respiratory system and the metabolic (buffer) system. The degree of compensation can be determined through ABG analysis.

➟ Priorities of care for the patient with acute respiratory failure are, first, to ensure a patent airway and, second, to provide adequate ventilation and oxygenation.

➟ Treatment modalities range from noninvasive supportive care such as supplemental oxygenation, medical management of underlying causes such as infection, congestive heart failure, or asthma, to full support on mechanical ventilation.

➟ Many modes of mechanical ventilation are available. The mode of ventilation must be matched to the patient's pathophysiologic process for optimal outcomes.

➟ Ventilator adjustments are made to ensure optimal oxygenation and ventilation. Adjustments should be made one at a time, with assessment and evaluation guiding each change.

➟ Many appropriate ways to wean patients from the ventilator are recognized. The method chosen should be appropriate to the patient's pathophysiologic features and should be consistent despite changes in bedside nurse and physician.

➟ Successful weaning of patients receiving long-term ventilation requires a multidisciplinary team to ensure adequate nutrition, muscle conditioning, medical management of infections, fluid and electrolyte shifts and imbalance, anxiety management, and constant encouragement.

➟ Possible weaning outcomes include 1) complete independence from ventilatory support with extu-bation, 2) incomplete weaning with intermittent support, 3) long-term ventilator care, or 4) terminal weaning and death.

➟ Patients requiring long-term ventilator support are cared for in various settings, such as ICUs, intermediate care units, long-term care facilities, and at home.

References

1. Scanlan CL, Spearman C, Sheldon RL (eds): Fundamentals of Respiratory Care. St. Louis, Mosby–Year Book, 1995.
2. Weiss SM, Hudson LD: Outcome from respiratory failure. Crit Care Clin 10:197–215, 1994.
3. Chatburn RL: Classification of mechanical ventilators. Respir Care 97:1009–1025, 1992.
4. Hess DR, Kacmarek RM: Essentials of Mechanical Ventilation. New York, McGraw-Hill, 1996.
5. Hagler DA, Traver GA: Endotracheal saline and suction catheters: sources of lower airway contamination. Am J Crit Care 3:444–447, 1994.
6. Hanneman SKG: Multidimensional predictors of success or failure with early weaning from mechanical ventilation after cardiac surgery. Nurs Res 43:4–10, 1994.
7. Abou-Shala N, Meduri UG: Noninvasive mechanical ventilation in patients with acute respiratory failure. Crit Care Med 24:705–715, 1996.
8. Knebel AR: Ventilator weaning protocols and techniques: getting the job done. AACN Clin Issues 7:550–559, 1996.
9. Clement JM, Buck E: 1996. Weaning from mechanical ventilatory support. Dimensions Crit Care Nurs 15 (3), p. 114–132.
10. Burns S, Clochesy JM, Hanneman SKG, et al: Weaning from long-term mechanical ventilation. Am J Crit Care 4:4–22, 1995.
11. Burns S, Burns JE, Truwit JD: Comparison of five clinical weaning indices. Am J Crit Care 3:342–352, 1994.
12. Pierce LNB: Mechanical Ventilation and Intensive Respiratory Care. Philadelphia, W.B. Saunders, 1995.
13. Kite-Powell DM, Sabau D, Ideno KT, et al: Optimizing outcomes in ventilator-dependent patients: challenging critical care practice. Crit Care Nurs Q 19:77–90, 1996.
14. Campbell ML: Managing terminal dyspnea: caring for the patient who refuses intubation or ventilation. Dimensions Crit Care Nurs 15:4–12, 1996.

18

Acute Respiratory Distress Syndrome

Janet Mulroy

Objectives

After completing this chapter, the student will be able to:

1. Define acute lung injury as a continuum of acute respiratory failure with emphasis on acute respiratory distress syndrome (ARDS).
2. Plan strategies that limit the iatrogenic effects of mechanical ventilation on the lung.
3. Compare and contrast the current supportive techniques in mechanical ventilation available for acute lung injury and ARDS.
4. Differentiate the current pharmacologic therapies available for acute lung injury and ARDS.
5. Evaluate future technologic and pharmacologic developments for supporting the patient experiencing acute lung injury and ARDS.
6. Select appropriate nursing interventions that support oxygenation and ventilation in the patient with acute lung injury.

Acute respiratory distress syndrome (ARDS) is not a disease but a syndrome or group of clinical manifestations associated with a serious insult to the body. This insult sets into motion a series of events that affect the lung. It is a particularly life-threatening form of acute respiratory failure. It was identified nearly 30 years ago during the Vietnam War because of the implementation of mobile army surgical hospital (MASH) units. Many injured soldiers survived the first several days after trauma only to develop acute respiratory failure and die. In those days, 1 in 10 survived. More recent medical advances have made it possible for people to survive an acute traumatic event and to undergo intensive care in a hospital setting. ARDS has many other names such as white lung, DeNang lung, shock lung, wet lung, high-permeability pulmonary edema, and noncardiogenic pulmonary edema. Despite the resources available to us in today's intensive care units (ICUs), the mortality rate for ARDS remains high.

INCIDENCE

Nearly 30 years have passed since the first reports of the strange phenomenon known as ARDS. The mortality rate is estimated to be 40 to 60% despite the advances made in recognition of triggering factors and management techniques. There have been many controversies in the management of the ARDS patient, and not until recently have we begun to see a decline in the mortality rate of ARDS.[1] The reason for the optimism in management of ARDS represents a return to basic hemodynamic and ventilatory support of the patient with ARDS. It also represents a recognition that many techniques of mechanical ventilation may actually be detrimental to the patient rather than helpful.

The incidence of ARDS reported in the literature varies from 150,000 cases[2] to 250,000 cases[3] per year. The disparity in the reported incidence may be due to the controversy surrounding the definitions of ARDS. For many years, ARDS was known as "adult respiratory distress syndrome." In 1927, Weed and McAffee[4] reported a syndrome of respiratory failure associated with wound shock after the First World War. It was described by Ashbaugh, Bigelow, and Petty[5] in 1967 as diffuse pulmonary infiltration on chest radiograph, impairment of oxygenation, and pulmonary congestion. In May and October of 1992, experts in pulmonary medicine met for the American–European Consensus Conference on ARDS to coordinate definitions, mechanisms, relevant outcomes, and clinical trials.[6] The consensus conference overcame much difficulty to create these recommendations:

1. ARDS is defined as "acute" rather than "adult" respiratory distress syndrome because it is widely recognized that ARDS is not limited to adults.
2. The clinical spectrum of respiratory failure should be represented on a continuum of acute lung injury (ALI). ALI describes the syndrome of inflammation and increased permeability that is associated with a constellation of clinical, radiographic, and physiologic abnormalities that cannot be explained by, but may coexist with, left atrial hypertension or pulmonary capillary hypertension. The term ARDS should be reserved for the most severe form of ALI or the most severe end of the continuum of respiratory failure.[6]

Jones and colleagues[7] added clarification to the concept of a continuum by stating: "All patients who develop ARDS initially have acute lung injury, but not all patients with acute lung injury develop ARDS." Moreover, as pointed out by Schuster[8] in 1995: "Not all patients with acute lung injury are equally ill." Clinicians accept that ALI can manifest as "mild ARDS," and the term ARDS needs to be reserved for those patients who progress beyond the mild stages despite appropriate treatment.

ETIOLOGY AND PATHOPHYSIOLOGY

Definitions of ARDS

The recommended definitions of ALI and ARDS by the 1992 American–European Consensus Conference on ARDS are represented in Table 18–1. Both conditions have an acute onset. The differentiation between ALI and ARDS is made using the measurements of the ratio of the arterial partial pressure of oxygen to fraction of inspired oxygen (PaO_2/FIO_2 ratio), pulmonary artery occlusive pressure (PAOP), and examination of chest radiographic findings. The PaO_2/FIO_2 ratio is calculated using the arterial oxygen reading from arterial blood gases (ABGs) and dividing it by the FIO_2 setting for the patient. The normal PaO_2/FIO_2 ratio is usually greater than 300. PAOP readings are performed with a pulmonary artery catheter. PAOP is considered normal between 5 and 15 mm Hg, with variations possible depending on the patient's diagnosis. Patients with worsening oxygenation despite appropriate therapy most likely progress to the ARDS end of the spectrum.[6]

Schuster[8] advocates that diffuse alveolar damage be included in the defining criteria for ARDS. He defines ARDS in both structural and functional aspects. The structural abnormalities are manifested in diffuse alveolar damage, and the functional abnormalities are manifested in the disturbance in gas exchange by the proteinaceous alveolar edema (Chart 18–1).

Systemic Inflammatory Response Syndrome

Systemic inflammatory response syndrome (SIRS) is an overly aggressive host defense response to insult or tissue damage in the body. The normally local response to injury becomes exaggerated and creates a "systemwide" or total-body response. It is proposed that the exaggerated inflammatory response is caused by macrophages, with granulocytes as the targeted tissues (see Chapter 47).

SIRS can be triggered by many insults to the body. The most common trigger is infection. Most patients with SIRS have a bacterial infection. Gram-negative infections have been found more frequently in hospital-acquired infections, and Gram-positive infections have

TABLE 18–1

Recommended Criteria for Acute Lung Injury (ALI) and Acute Respiratory Distress Syndrome (ARDS)

	Timing	Oxygenation (PaO_2/FIO_2)	Chest Radiograph	Pulmonary Artery Occlusive Pressure
ALI Criteria	Acute onset	$PaO_2/FIO_2 < 300$ mm Hg regardless of PEEP	Bilateral infiltrates	<18 mm Hg when measured or no clinical evidence of left atrial hypertension
ARDS Criteria	Acute onset	$PaO_2/FIO_2 < 200$ mm Hg regardless of PEEP	Bilateral infiltrates	<18 mm Hg when measured or no clinical evidence of left atrial hypertension

PEEP, positive end-expiratory pressure.
Adapted from Bernard G, Artigas A, Brigham K, et al: The American–European Consensus Conference on ARDS. Am Rev Respir Dis 149:818–824, 1994.

CHART 18-1

Diffuse Alveolar Damage

Alveolar epithelial cell necrosis
Inflammatory cell infiltration
Proteinaceous alveolar and interstitial edema
Alveolar hyaline membranes
Type II pneumocyte proliferation (later)
Intra-alveolar and interstitial fibrosis in varying
  degrees (later)

From Schuster D: What is acute lung injury? What is ARDS? Chest 107:1721–1726, 1995.

same triggering events do not develop SIRS and others do. Meduri[9] found a persistent and marked elevation of plasma and broncheoalveolar lavage fluid levels of inflammatory cytokines. In this study, the survivors of ARDS had a rapid reduction in inflammatory cytokines. Meduri[9] found that an overaggressive and protracted host defense response is the major factor influencing the outcome in ARDS. The continued production of inflammatory mediators prevents normal healing of the lung. There is also new injury to previously spared lung tissue. This finding helps to explain why patients with ARDS may not improve despite aggressive treatment of the precipitating disease. Many questions exist about measures to prevent or to treat patients prophylactically for the fulminant response.

been found to be more common in community-acquired infections. Infection is not the only cause of SIRS. The systemic responses to tissue injury have been reported in trauma, hypoxic states, pneumonitis, pancreatitis, hematomas, hemolysis, major surgical procedures, burns, and conditions of tissue necrosis such as retained fetus, infarcted bowel, or severe peripheral vascular disease.

Many patients experience repeated triggering events and repeated bouts of SIRS during their ICU stay. Using a burn patient as an example, each dressing change or each débridement procedure has the potential for triggering another SIRS response because of the release of chemotactic substances into the blood by tissue injury. Each episode of infection from the lungs, the bladder, the invasive lines, or other wounds has the potential for stimulating an exaggerated inflammatory response.

Critical care professionals are faced with the ongoing question of why some patients exposed to the

Precipitating Causes of ARDS

The hallmark of ARDS is accumulation of protein-rich fluid in the alveoli and interstitial spaces as a result of increased permeability of the alveolar–capillary membranes. The types of insults that can precipitate this syndrome are many and may be divided into direct and indirect pulmonary insults. A direct pulmonary insult may be the triggering event for ALI, ARDS, and a SIRS response that induces multiorgan failure. An indirect pulmonary insult may result from tissue damage or an insult to another part of the body that triggers a SIRS response. The ALI and ARDS develop as a secondary organ failure (Table 18–2).

The damage to the endothelial lining of the alveolar–capillary membrane increases its permeability. Fluid and large molecules such as proteins that are normally inside the capillaries leak into the alveoli and surrounding interstitial tissues and cause edema. This fluid inactivates surfactant, thus causing a decrease in

TABLE 18-2

Triggering Events for Acute Lung Injury, Acute Respiratory Distress Syndrome, or Systemic Inflammatory Response Syndrome

Direct Pulmonary Insults	Indirect Pulmonary Insults
Aspiration of gastrointestinal contents	Sepsis
Near drowning	Severe pancreatitis
Inhalation of toxic substances (pesticides, smoke)	Multiple trauma
Inhalation of drugs (cocaine)	Burns
Diffuse pneumonia (bacterial or viral)	Shock
Pulmonary contusion	Cardiopulmonary bypass
Pulmonary embolism	Multiple blood transfusions
End-stage chronic respiratory disease	Neurogenic states
Chronic obstructive pulmonary disease	Nonpulmonary systemic disease
Cystic fibrosis	Anaphylaxis
Oxygen toxicity	Eclampsia
	Tissue necrosis
	Disseminated intravascular coagulation

the surface tension of the alveoli, and they collapse. The normal balance between blood flow and ventilation of the alveoli is disrupted. The gas that normally remains in the alveoli and airways on exhalation is called the functional residual capacity (FRC). When alveoli collapse, fewer alveoli remain open and filled with gases to participate in gas exchange. This is called the ventilation–perfusion ratio or V/Q ratio. As the alveoli collapse, more blood passes through the lungs without exchanging carbon dioxide for oxygen. Unoxygenated blood reenters the circulation, and the tissues begin to suffer, a condition known as hypoxemia. The phenomenon of circulation of unoxygenated blood is a V/Q mismatch or shunt. The nurse may observe a V/Q mismatch when the patient's condition keeps worsening in spite of increases in oxygen. The alveoli are so full of debris that no gas exchange can take place. Failure to respond to oxygen therapy is the classic sign of ARDS. This condition is known as refractory hypoxemia. These changes in the lung activate the inflammatory process. As the lung tries to heal itself, hyaline membranes and fibrosis (scarring) further disrupt gas exchange on a long-term basis. This change also causes a decreased compliance or lung elasticity (Figure 18–1).

Mediators of Sepsis, SIRS, ALI, and ARDS

Much research continues to be done to identify the mediators responsible for the cascade of organ damage created by tissue injury. Meduri[9] described the components of the host defense response as inflammation, coagulation, modulation of the immune response, tissue repair, and activation of the hypothalamic–pituitary–adrenal axis.

Inflammation is characterized by local vasodilation, increased capillary permeability, clotting within the interstitial spaces related to fibrinogen and other plasma–protein leakage, migration of granulocytes and monocytes to the tissue, and edema of tissue cells. Some of the substances that mediate this phase of the response have been identified as bradykinin, histamine, prostaglandins, and products of the complement system.[10]

Tumor necrosis factor and interleukin-1 are stimulated by endotoxin release from the walls of the Gram-negative bacteria. These cytokines play a direct role in producing fever through stimulation of the hypothalmus and endothelial damage by activation of the neutrophils.

The complement system also attracts neutrophils to the pulmonary capillaries that damage the pulmonary capillary endothelial lining. This damage allows increased capillary permeability and perpetuates pulmonary edema in ALI. The endothelial damage caused

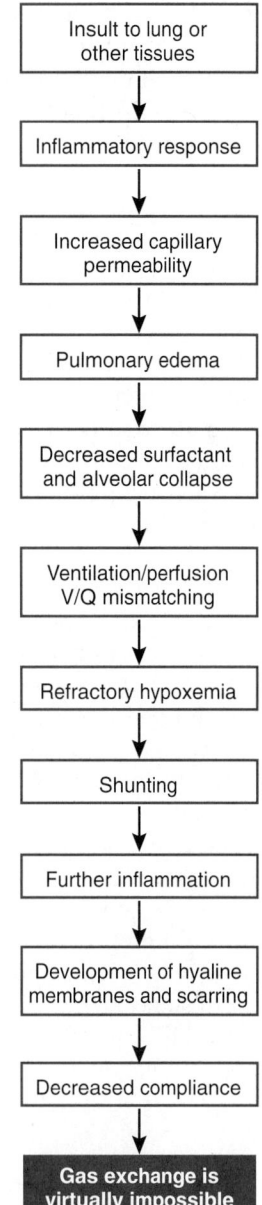

Figure 18–1

Pathophysiologic progression of ARDS.

by activated neutrophils is believed to create organ damage in other organ systems.[11]

Other mediators under study are arachidonic acid, prostacyclin, and thromboxane. Arachidonic acid is released from the cell membrane during injury. Arachidonic acid release leads to prostacyclin and thromboxane synthesis. Thromboxane, prostaglandins, leukotrienes, and platelet-activating factor are believed to be involved in smooth muscle constriction, pulmonary hypertension, increased airway resistance, and increased membrane permeability.[11, 12]

The coagulation system is believed to be involved in this process through the discovery of microthrombi and fibrin deposition in tissue samples of patients with ARDS. Petty[12] believed that although the coagulation system may be activated and involved, it is probably not a central pathogenetic mechanism responsible for ALI. Meduri[9] found that intravascular coagulation decreases the size of available pulmonary vascular beds, and intra-alveolar fibrin deposition leads to fibrosis and scarring.

The process of tissue repair involving regeneration of native parenchymal cells and filling in of the gaps with fibroblastic tissue creates persistent problems with gas exchange, decreased compliance, and reduced recruitment of alveoli by mechanical ventilation techniques. This condition necessitates prolonged mechanical ventilation, which causes the patient to be at risk of pneumonia, extrapulmonary infections, and sepsis. Meduri[9] suggested that the progression of fibroproliferation to extensive pulmonary fibrosis is directly responsible for death in 15 to 40% of patients with ARDS.

Activation of the hypothalamic–pituitary–adrenal axis during times of stress is important in the host defense response. The release of catecholamines such as epinephrine and the production of acute-phase reactants are under the influence of glucocorticoids. Catecholamine and glucocorticoid interactions play an important role in the maintenance of vascular tone. The hypothalamic–pituitary–adrenal axis is also important in regulating the termination of the host defense response. If the inhibitory signals are not present, the patient will have sustained inflammation, tissue injury, coagulation, and fibroproliferation.[9] The hypothalamic–pituitary–adrenal axis, combined with other anti-inflammatory substances, is therefore essential in preventing persistent SIRS, which can lead to ARDS and multiple organ dysfunction.

Stages

ARDS is often divided into three stages for ease of discussion. The first phase of ARDS is the early exudative phase. This stage is manifested by alveolar edema with fibrin and leukocyte debris and damage to type I pneumocytes and endothelial cells. The second phase is the proliferative phase or subacute ARDS. This stage is manifested by persistent capillary endothelial damage, type II cell proliferation, and the beginning of squamous cell transformation. The third phase is the fibroproliferative phase or chronic ARDS. This stage is manifested by thickening of the interstitium by an increased number of type II cells and fibrosis.[13]

Murray and colleagues[14] in 1988 published the now famous lung injury scoring system. It was developed to classify the extent of pulmonary damage in studies of patients with sepsis. It has been used to gauge improvement or worsening of the severity of pulmonary

disease. The lung injury score can be used for assessment of acute and chronic lung damage (Table 18–3). It can be calculated quickly and is recognized by many practitioners. Murray[13] recommended using the term ARDS for severe abnormalities, such as those with scores greater than 2.5. A lower score, such as 0.1 to 2.5, is designated as mild to moderate lung injury.

Another point made by Murray and colleagues[14] is that their tool does not require invasive hemodynamic monitoring or mechanical ventilation to determine the diagnosis. The practitioner must simply divide the score by the components available in the calculation of the score. Interest in noninvasive methods of assessment and support of the critically ill patient has increased.

Assessment

ARDS occurs between 24 and 72 hours after an insult to the body. The best assessment includes knowing the types of patients who are at risk for ARDS. The most common risk factors are sepsis, shock, pneumonia, and trauma. The early indications of the changes taking place in the alveolar–capillary membranes are not as easy to detect without comprehensive and frequent respiratory assessments. The patient at risk of ALI and ARDS tries to compensate for decreasing oxygenation levels. Most of the signs and symptoms of ALI and ARDS are created by activation of the normal compensatory mechanisms of the body. Thorough assessment of the patient with ALI may require cardiac monitoring, pulse oximetry, strict intake and output measurements, frequent ABG measurements, frequent blood pressure measurements using a noninvasive blood pressure device or an intraarterial catheter, and hemodynamic monitoring with or without fiberoptics for evaluation of oxygenation status. Laboratory and diagnostic assessment of the patient with ALI and ARDS may include ABGs, serum electrolytes, complete blood count with differential, blood cultures, serum lactate levels, cultures of other body fluids, chest radiographs, gallium scans, and ventilation–perfusion scans.

Neurologic System

Patients may exhibit a change in level of consciousness because of hypoxemia and changes in the acid–base balance. These patients may be restless, anxious, confused, disoriented, and frightened, and they may vocalize a sense of impending doom. As the hypoxemia progresses, these patients may become more lethargic and sluggish in their responses. The change from being restless and frightened to being lethargic and docile should be a sign to the nurse that the patient is decompensating quickly.

TABLE 18–3
Lung Injury Score*

Component	Ranges	Value
Chest radiograph score	No alveolar consolidation	0
	Alveolar consolidation confined to 1 quadrant	1
	Alveolar consolidation confined to 2 quadrants	2
	Alveolar consolidation confined to 3 quadrants	3
	Alveolar consolidation in all 4 quadrants	4
Hypoxemia score	Pao_2/Fio_2 >300	0
	Pao_2/Fio_2 225–299	1
	Pao_2/Fio_2 175–224	2
	Pao_2/Fio_2 100–174	3
	Pao_2/Fio_2 <100	4
Positive end-expiratory pressure (PEEP) score (when available)	PEEP >5 cm H_2O	0
	PEEP 6–8 cm H_2O	1
	PEEP 9–11 cm H_2O	2
	PEEP 12–14 cm H_2O	3
	PEEP >15 cm H_2O	4
Compliance score (when available)	Compliance >80 mL/cm H_2O	0
	Compliance 60–79 mL/cm H_2O	1
	Compliance 40–59 mL/cm H_2O	2
	Compliance 20–39 mL/cm H_2O	3
	Compliance <19 mL/cm H_2O	4
Total score	No lung injury	0
	Mild to moderate lung injury	0.1–2.5
	Severe lung injury (ARDS)	>2.5

*The final value is obtained by dividing the aggregate sum by the number of components that were used.
From Murray J, Matthay M, Luce J, et al: An expanded definition of the adult respiratory distress syndrome. Am Rev Respir Dis 138:720–723, 1988.

Respiratory System

One of the first signs in ARDS is an increase in respiratory rate. Dyspnea occurs along with the tachypnea to compensate for the loss of oxygen supply. Crackles occur as fluid shifts across the damaged alveolar–capillary membrane into the alveoli and interstitial spaces. The patient may begin to cough, and the sputum may become thick and foamy because of the large amounts of protein in the mucus. Hemoptysis may also develop as a result of inflammation of the microvasculature of the alveolar–capillary membrane.

The patient may become alkalotic from breathing so quickly. A patient may also exhibit nasal flaring, use of accessory muscles, orthopnea, and some hypoxemia. Safe pulse oximetry readings are considered to be greater than 90%. The nurse must keep in mind that accurate pulse oximetry is affected by temperature, pH, partial arterial pressure of carbon dioxide ($Paco_2$), tissue perfusion to the finger (or location of the sensor), anemia, the type of hemoglobin, and the use of vasopressors that create vasoconstriction. It can also be affected by incorrect application of the sensor, nail polish,

serum bilirubin level, skin color, and the amount of room light.[15] Considering these factors, the nurse needs to report declining oxygen saturation (Sao_2) quickly to the physician. As the syndrome progresses, the nurse and the respiratory therapist may see an increase in minute ventilation and a decreased FRC.

The chest radiograph may be normal during the first 24 hours. The chest radiograph then changes to a "white out" or "ground glass" picture that is diffuse. ARDS is not selective for one lobe or the other, a feature that differentiates ARDS from pneumonia. Pneumonia is frequently located in more dependent regions of the lungs and may be isolated to a particular lobe. As the hypoxemia worsens, the patient becomes less responsive and may even completely lose consciousness. Cyanosis, pallor, and diaphoresis may occur as hypoxemia continues. The nurse may hear more widespread crackles and wheezes. The breath sounds may become difficult to hear as alveoli collapse and as the patient fatigues into more shallow breathing. The nurse needs to be aware that hearing crackles is better than not hearing breath sounds at all. The collapse of alveoli is manifested in absent breath sounds.

This finding should be reported immediately to the physician.

At this time in the sequencing of this syndrome, the ABGs may be more acidotic, showing the creation of lactic acid as a by-product of anaerobic metabolism. Anaerobic metabolism occurs because of the lack of oxygen to the tissues. These patients may have combined metabolic and respiratory acidosis because of the production of lactic acid and the inability to excrete carbon dioxide at the alveolar level.

Cardiovascular System

The nurse may note tachycardia and other dysrhythmias. The tachycardia is a compensatory mechanism of the sympathetic nervous system to increase the heart rate and to increase the cardiac output to compensate for the drop in oxygen saturation.

Depending on the age and previous medical history of the patient, he or she may be able to keep up the rapid pace of compensatory mechanisms in the form of tachycardia and tachypnea. Many patients eventually fail at compensation and may begin to experience a decrease in cardiac output and dysrhythmias. Cardiac arrest is a possibility. Hemodynamic readings from a pulmonary artery catheter usually show an elevated pulmonary artery pressure with a normal PAOP. This finding indicates to the nurse that the patient is experiencing high pulmonary vascular pressures without an increase in vascular volume or total volume. This is one method of differentiating ARDS from congestive heart failure. Cardiac output is usually low in the later stages because the compensatory mechanisms of the sympathetic nervous system can no longer keep up with the demands.

Nursing Diagnoses

The nursing diagnoses in the patient with ALI and ARDS are focused on the oxygenation and comfort of the patient. The nurse must combine the available technology with astute assessment and monitoring, to reach successful outcomes for the patient with ALI and ARDS (Table 18–4).

Collaborative Management

Interventions for the patient with ALI and ARDS are primarily supportive because the damage to the alveolar–capillary membrane cannot be treated directly. The goals of therapy are to optimize oxygen delivery to the tissues, to facilitate restoration of alveolar–capillary membrane integrity, and to identify and treat the primary condition promptly (Figure 18–2).

Airway Management

Positive-pressure ventilation is the major supportive therapy for the patient with ALI (see Chart 18–2). To deliver positive-pressure ventilation consistently and safely, an endotracheal tube is required. In patients who require prolonged mechanical ventilatory support, a tracheostomy should be considered. Mechanical ventilation is considered prolonged if it lasts more than 7 days. A tracheostomy provides the advantages of improved comfort, better mouth care, more efficient suctioning of the tracheobronchial secretions, and the opportunity for the patient to communicate and eat normally.[12]

TABLE 18-4
Nursing Diagnoses

Problem Statement	Etiologic Factors
Altered respiratory function	
Impaired gas exchange	Atelectasis and pulmonary interstitial edema
Ineffective airway clearance	Thick secretions, endotracheal intubation, and parenchymal destruction
Ineffective breathing patterns	Pulmonary injury, mechanical ventilation settings, anxiety, or pain
Risk for Infection	Mechanical ventilation, retained secretions, and multiple invasive procedures
Anxiety	Dyspnea, air hunger, fear of dying, knowledge deficits regarding the disease process, multiple invasive procedures or sensory overload from the ICU environment
Decreased cardiac output	Altered fluid volume, decreased left ventricular function, effects of positive-pressure ventilation, hypoxemia-induced dysrhythmias, or myocardial ischemia
Altered tissue perfusion: peripheral	Increased capillary permeability, decrease in cardiac output, impaired gas exchange, and increased metabolic demands
Altered nutrition: less than body requirements	Debilitating lung disease, mechanical ventilation, nutritional deficits from enteral or parenteral sources, and increased metabolic demands
Activity intolerance	Labile oxygenation and hemodynamics, decreased cardiac output, and impaired gas exchange

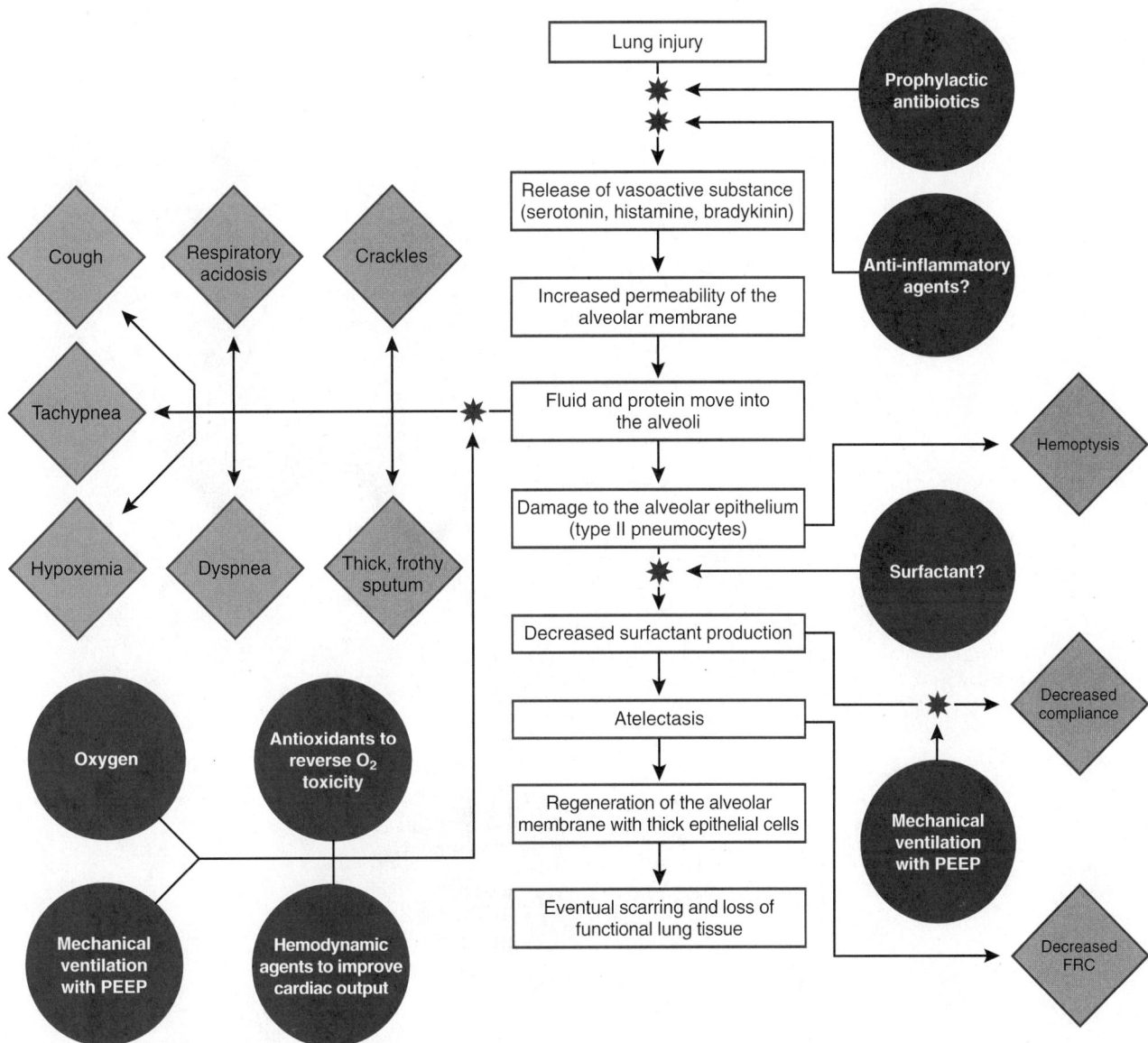

Items noted with a question mark are being researched. Their outcome looks promising.

Figure 18–2

Pathophysiology of ARDS and related treatments. Terms noted with a question mark are under study, and their outlook is promising. FRC, functional residual capacity; PEEP, positive end-expiratory pressure. (From Black JM, Matassarin-Jacobs E (eds): Medical-Surgical Nursing, 5th ed. Philadelphia, W.B. Saunders, 1997, p 1171.)

Mechanical Ventilation

Positive-pressure ventilation can be lifesaving for patients with acute severe hypoxemia or worsening respiratory acidosis. Positive-pressure ventilation can reverse and prevent atelectasis, reduce the work of breathing, and reverse respiratory muscle fatigue. The goals of mechanical ventilation are as follows:

- Improving pulmonary gas exchange by reversing hypoxemia and relieving acute respiratory acidosis
- Relieving respiratory distress by decreasing the oxygen cost of breathing and reversing respiratory-muscle fatigue

- Altering pressure–volume relationships by preventing and reversing atelectasis, improving compliance, and preventing further injury
- Permitting lung and airway healing
- Avoiding complications[16]

The major challenges in management of patients with ALI occur in the disorders that require high distending pressures to improve gas exchange. One of the major classifications of disorders that require high distending pressures is ARDS. ARDS is characterized by collapsed alveoli and increased endothelial permeability that floods the alveoli and surrounding interstitial

CHART 18–2

RESEARCH UTILIZATION: EXPLORING COMMUNICATION PATTERNS BETWEEN
NURSES AND PATIENTS ON VENTILATORS

Abstract: The American Association of Critical-Care Nurses has identified communication between nurses and patients on ventilators as an important area for research. Effective nurse–patient communication is essential to provide reassurance, comfort, and support to patients unable to speak due to intubation. The purpose of this study was to examine nurse actions and reactions with ventilated patients and the relationship between specific nurse characteristics and communication patterns. An analytical, cross-sectional design was used to study 30 RNs, each for a 30-minute interval while caring for a ventilated patient. The Categories of Nurse–Patient Interaction Content (CN-PIC) tool and the Glasgow Coma Scale (GCS) were used for data collection. Significant correlations were found between the nurse's perception of the patient's responsiveness and the number of interactions with the patient and between the length of time the nurse cared for the patient and the number of positive *reactions* from nurse to patient (p <.05). More positive reactions and fewer negative reactions from the nurse to the patient were observed with patients with higher GCS scores. Most of the interactions that were observed were *actions* (89%) and were positive (74%). No significant correlations were found among length of time the nurse cared for the patient, amount of ICU experience or educational level, and the number of positive or negative *actions* with the patient.

Critique: Research in patterns of nurse communication with ventilated patients is sparse, and information from this study contributes to the body of knowledge in this area. Specific information regarding the reliability and validity of the data-collection tools was not provided. Observational data were collected by one observer in order to limit variability among observations, but the reliability of the observer was not reported. Finally, the number of observations (one per RN) may have been insufficient to reveal a true picture of the nurse-patient interactions.

Nursing Considerations: Nurses must find effective means of communicating with patients who are ventilated. Patterns of communication identified in this study revealed that nurses most often explain procedures to patients (31% of observed positive *actions*) and less often (5% of observed positive *actions*) attempt to clarify a nonverbal patient message (the type most frequently transmitted by these patients). Nurses also spent less time reacting to their patients and made few attempts to communicate with patients who demonstrated limited responsiveness. Nurses need to reevaluate the type of interaction they have with this patient population. More emphasis should be placed on discovering what the patient needs versus simply supplying information to the patient. Similarly, nurses must remember to continue to communicate with patients regardless of their level of consciousness. Patient-centered care requires a focused effort on the part of the nurse to respond to the patient's needs. Patients with impaired communication due to intubation present a unique challenge to nurses. Efforts to become familiar with the patient's method of communication and sharing this information with all members of the health care team will result in greater patient satisfaction.

Source: Hall, D: Interactions between nurses and patients on ventilators. Am J Crit Care 5:293–297, 1996.

tissues with protein-rich fluid, which impairs gas exchange. This creates a situation in which unoxygenated blood is returned to the heart for circulation to the tissues, a condition known as shunting. It also creates poor elasticity or compliance of the lung tissues. This change is evident at the bedside by failure to respond or lack of improvement in the patient when the oxygen is increased again and again until the patient finally is intubated and is placed on mechanical ventilation.

Also inherent in ARDS is that many areas of the lung are spared the inflammatory responses and can function "normally." These areas receive most of the mechanical ventilation because the gas follows the "path of least resistance." The "normal or near-normal" areas of the lung are therefore overloaded and hyperinflated because the tidal volumes and pressures are too great for the small area that remains functional. This situation also results in high minute ventilation requirements.

Ventilator-Induced Lung Injury
Ventilator-induced lung injury occurs most often in situations of high pressures and large tidal volumes,

such as ARDS. Examinations of tissue have revealed an increase in microvascular pressure and an increase in microvascular permeability that cause fluid and protein leaks, leading to a decrease in compliance.[17] These changes are reminiscent of ARDS. These findings have occurred more often in dependent lung areas, and mechanical ventilation shifts more to the smaller, nondependent lung areas that are relatively normal or near-normal in function. Investigators have estimated that as little as one-third of the lung actually participates in gas exchange (the "small lung theory" or "baby lung theory").[18] The small area of the lung that is receiving the entire tidal volume and pressure is susceptible to hyperventilation and overdistention. In ARDS, the lungs may not be so "stiff," but may actually be just "small."

The lungs of the patient with ARDS have been described in three distinct lung zones by Marik and Krikorian[19]: 1) that portion of the lung that is diseased and not recruitable, 2) that portion of the lung that is diseased but recruitable, and 3) that portion of the lung that is normal. Marik and Krikorian[19] pointed out that a significant portion of the lung is consolidated and not recruitable, so only a small amount of the lung receives the full tidal volume.

Newer techniques in mechanical ventilation of the patient with ALI and ARDS are aimed at recruiting alveoli with positive pressure such as PEEP and minimizing the ventilator-induced lung injury to that portion of the lung that remains "near normal or normal." Problems associated with conventional mechanical ventilation include oxygen toxicity, hypotension and hemodynamic compromise, barotrauma, and volutrauma.

Oxygen Toxicity. Oxygen toxicity becomes a concern when oxygen percentages are set above 50% for longer than 12 to 24 hours. The known effects are increased pulmonary microvascular permeability, absorption atelectasis, impedance of tracheal cilia, decrease in surfactant formation, and surfactant inactivation.[20]

Hypotension. Hemodynamic compromise with hypotension and decreased cardiac output occurs most often in compliant lungs (young, fairly healthy lungs). Positive-pressure ventilation, in all forms, increases intrapulmonary pressures and intrathoracic pressures. This pressure compresses the great vessels and leads to a decreased venous return to the heart, or preload. Decreased stroke volume, decreased cardiac output, and hypotension result. For this reason, hypotension occurs most frequently with PEEP, alveolar distention, and auto-PEEP.

Barotrauma. Barotrauma is reported to occur in 5 to 15% of all mechanically ventilated patients. Death

from barotrauma is a real threat, with the reported incidence ranging from 13 to 77%.[18] Barotrauma is a general term that includes many situations such as pneumothorax, pneumomediastinum, pneumopericardium, pneumoperitoneum, and subcutaneous emphysema. These conditions are proposed to occur more often in patients with high ventilation pressures and alveolar overdistention.[18]

Volutrauma. Also implicated in ventilator-induced lung injury is the concept of "large shearing forces" that are created from repeated opening and closing of alveoli with each respiratory cycle,[20] or "volutrauma." Volutrauma is used to summarize all the elements of ventilator-induced lung injury (Chart 18–3).

The techniques of mechanical ventilation that are most famous for causing volutrauma are described by Wilmoth and Carpenter as high peak inspiratory pressures, high mean airway pressures, high PEEP, large tidal volumes, and rapid ventilator rates.[18]

Volutrauma is not easily corrected. Many of its causes are "necessary evils" and are required to manage the patient with ALI and ARDS. For example, high PEEP is implicated in creating volutrauma, but it has also been found to be a necessary technique for preventing the shearing forces by keeping alveoli open to prevent the repeated opening and closing of alveoli with each breath.[20]

The future of management of the patient with ALI and ARDS focuses on limiting or minimizing the damage caused by mechanical ventilation.

Future Management of ALI and ARDS

High-Frequency Jet Ventilation. High-frequency jet ventilation, pressure-controlled inverse-ratio ventilation (PCIRV), high PEEP, and pressure-controlled ventilation without inversing the ratio are all designed to recruit alveoli and to keep them open throughout the respiratory cycle.

CHART 18–3

Causes of Volutrauma

High peak inspiratory pressures
High mean airway pressures
High positive end-expiratory pressures
Large tidal volumes
Rapid ventilator rates

From Wilmoth D, Carpenter R: Preventing complications of mechanical ventilation: permissive hypercapnia. AACN Clin Issues 7:473–481, 1996.

High-frequency jet ventilation creates a constant airway pressure throughout the respiratory cycle that should lower peak airway pressures and allow for the use of smaller tidal volumes. High-frequency jet ventilation has been used with mixed reviews. It requires significant sedation and even paralysis for patient comfort, and it induces a continuous situation of auto-PEEP, which can be good for oxygenation but bad for barotrauma. It requires the purchase of a jet ventilator, and it also requires that the bedside staff be familiar with the concepts and monitoring of these patients.[7,21]

Pressure-Controlled Inverse-Ratio Ventilation. PCIRV is not a new mode of mechanical ventilation. It has been used with success in infants with respiratory distress syndrome for many years. It is designed to reverse the normal inspiratory time and expiratory time ratios (I:E ratios) to prolong inspiratory time and to deliver the gas at a preset inspiratory pressure. The normal I:E ratio is 1:2 or 1:3, with inspiration being shorter than expiration. PCIRV stretches out the inspiratory time to 2:1, 3:1, and even 4:1, which prolongs inspiratory time and allows initiation of the next breath before expiration is completed. The positive aspects of PCIRV are that it opens recruitable alveoli, allows for more consistent gas delivery, and can allow for reductions in FIO_2 and PEEP. It also is reported to reduce peak inspiratory pressures, to increase compliance, and to reduce minute ventilation in patients.[22] The negative aspects of PCIRV are just like those for high-frequency jet ventilation. It is not similar to normal breathing patterns and creates significant auto-PEEP or intrinsic PEEP. Although comfort has not been studied directly, many authors report the need for sedation and paralysis to ensure patient comfort. This technique also requires the purchase of a special ventilator and significant education of the bedside staff. A major drawback of PCIRV is its complexity.[23] Close monitoring and frequent adjustment of ventilator settings are required.

Super PEEP. Levels of PEEP greater than 15 cm H_2O have been dubbed "super PEEP." Conventional PEEP is described as PEEP between 5 and 15 cm H_2O designed to maintain a PaO_2 greater than 60 on an FIO_2 of less than 60. The use of high PEEP (PEEPs of 20–25 cm H_2O) with similar goals of a PaO_2 of 60 and a pulse oximetry reading of greater than 90% is described in Chart 18–4. These techniques enabled the researchers to achieve survival rates of 60 to 80% in patients with severe ARDS.[24] Titration of PEEP until $PEEP_{max}$ is reached is a labor-intensive and expensive protocol that requires intense monitoring.

Pressure-Controlled Ventilation Without Inverse Ratio. The method of using pressure-controlled ventilation without inversing the I:E ratio is called pressure-

---

CHART 18–4

Recommendations for Using High Levels of Positive End-Expiratory Pressure (PEEP)

1. Titrate the PEEP in increments of 2 to 3 cm H_2O until you achieve a level of reduced shunting of approximately 20% or less.
2. Maintain an FIO_2 of 40% or less.
3. Use tidal volumes of 10 to 15 mL/kg.
4. Use pressure support ventilation to enhance spontaneous breathing.
5. Use continuous hemodynamic monitoring (PA line) to monitor for side effects of PEEP and to calculate oxygen transport.
6. Treat the hemodynamic compromise of PEEP with blood, fluids, and inotropic infusions as needed.

From Safcasak K, Nelson L: High-level positive end expiratory pressure management in the surgical patient with acute respiratory distress syndrome. *AACN Clin Issues* 7:482–494, 1996.

---

controlled ventilation. In pressure-controlled ventilation, each breath is delivered to reach a preset pressure level. In volume-controlled ventilation, breaths are delivered to reach a prescribed tidal volume. With volume-controlled ventilation, achieving a certain volume is the priority. In pressure-controlled ventilation, keeping the peak inspiratory pressure below a prescribed level is the priority. Recall from the information on iatrogenic lung injury that preventing high peak pressures would, one hopes, minimize ventilator-induced lung injury. Most physicians agree that keeping the pressure level below 35 to 50 cm H_2O should be low enough so as not to damage lung tissue.[18]

Commonly used pressure-cycled ventilators are intermittent positive pressure breathing (IPPB) machines. Other forms of pressure ventilation are biphasic positive airway pressure (BiPAP) machines, continuous PAP (CPAP) machines, face mask ventilation, and pressure support ventilation. In pressure support ventilation, the level of pressure reached during a breath is lowered and is triggered only on spontaneous breaths.

The positive side of pressure-controlled ventilation is that it is well tolerated by patients and it is easy to monitor. The nurse and respiratory therapist need to be aware of the patient's tidal volume and minute ventilation. Normal tidal volumes in pressure-controlled ventilation range between 5 and 10 mL/kg, so they would be smaller than one would expect in volume-controlled ventilation. Normal minute ventilation ranges from 5 to 8 L per minute.

The negative side of pressure-controlled ventilation is that the tidal volume varies. When the ventilator reaches the preset pressure level, it ends inspiration and vents the remaining volume of gas. If the patient is agitated, or if secretions or bronchospasm create increased resistance in the airways, the patient's preset pressure level will be reached more quickly, and the patient could possibly be underventilated. The tidal volume will be inconsistent, but the lungs will be protected from increased pressure.[25] The other important parameter to monitor is the respiratory rate. In pressure-controlled ventilation, the patient is allowed to trigger the ventilator with every inspiratory effort. The patient can initiate a breath by generating a small level of negative pressure ranging from -1 to -2 cm H_2O. Most ventilators allow the therapist to set a high respiratory rate alarm as an indicator of respiratory distress. The nurse needs to be aware that increased respiratory rate and increased minute ventilation are signs of respiratory distress. The patient may need to be suctioned or medicated for pain, or he or she may not be tolerating the current settings.

Two other techniques that are combined with modes of ventilation are low tidal volume ventilation and permissive hypercapnia. These two techniques, combined with PCIRV or pressure-controlled ventilation, should also minimize injury to the lung tissues.

Additional Lung Protective Techniques

Low Tidal Volume Ventilation. Low tidal volume ventilation is defined as tidal volumes as low as 4 mL/kg up to about 10 mL/kg.[26,27] The tolerance of lower tidal volumes is based on the concept of "baby lungs" associated with ARDS and is advocated to minimize ventilator-induced lung injury. Lower tidal volumes may help to avoid overdistention of well-ventilated lung areas and high peak airway pressures and still support oxygen delivery.[28]

Permissive Hypercapnia. The goal of permissive hypercapnia is not to create hypercapnia with respiratory acidosis, but to limit the amount of stretch on the lungs by limiting the tidal volumes and pressures exerted on the lungs. Permissive hypercapnia is basically a change in philosophy that recognizes that most adults tolerate higher levels of carbon dioxide with few side effects. Using all the techniques described to minimize lung injury may ultimately cause the patient to retain carbon dioxide. Higher levels of carbon dioxide and a drop in pH are relatively well tolerated. The concept is to use the techniques to minimize lung injury and not to become overly concerned about rising carbon dioxide levels.[26,27,29]

Acute intracellular acidosis does have side effects. Most adults can compensate for the drop in pH within 3 hours using the buffering systems of the body. Acidosis is often associated with myocardial depression. In acidosis, a catecholamine surge also offsets the myocardial depression with increased cardiac output and increased oxygen delivery. Moderate hypercapnia actually increases the responsiveness to catecholamines. Hypercapnia may also cause an increase in peripheral vascular resistance that reduces shunt fractions and improves oxygenation.[18] Hypercapnia also causes vasodilation of cerebral vessels and can raise intracranial pressures. Metabolic compensation is possible within hours to days, depending on the integrity of renal function. If needed, sodium bicarbonate infusions may be used to prevent profound metabolic acidosis.

The nurse needs to be aware of the contraindications and side effects of permissive hypercapnia. The contraindications for permissive hypercapnia are listed in Chart 18–5. The side effects of hypercapnia are generally rare and are listed in Table 18–5.

Extracorporeal Membrane Oxygenation, Intravascular Oxygenation, and Extracorporeal Carbon Dioxide Removal. Extracorporeal membrane oxygenation (ECMO), intravascular oxygenation (IVOX), and extracorporeal carbon dioxide removal (ECO$_2$R) are invasive techniques used to supplement mechanical ventilation with direct oxygenation of the blood or to assist in removal of carbon dioxide wastes from the blood. These techniques can be used to rest the injured lung and to remove part of the lung's burden.[26] ECMO and IVOX have been used for years with varying degrees of success in infants and children. The basic difference between ECMO and IVOX is that ECMO

CHART 18-5

Contraindications for Permissive Hypercapnia

1. Anyone in whom a catecholamine surge would be potentially harmful, such as someone with impaired ventricular function, ischemic heart disease, or hypertension
2. Anyone with increased intracranial pressure or cerebral edema, such as head trauma or neurologic disease

Adapted from Simon R, Ivatury R: The expanding role of permissive hypercapnia in patients with ARDS. Trauma Q 12:257–271, 1996; and Wilmoth D, Carpenter R: Preventing complications of mechanical ventilation: permissive hypercapnia. AACN Clin Issues 7:473–481, 1996.

TABLE 18–5

Side Effects of Hypercapnia

System	Side Effects
Central nervous	Headache, drowsiness, coma, marked increase in cerebral blood flow that causes increased intracranial pressure, tremor, muscle twitching, a lowered seizure threshold, and weakness
Cardiovascular	Myocardial depression, vasodilation, elevated peripheral vascular resistance resulting in pulmonary hypertension, and surge of endogenous catecholamines with the potential for dysrhythmias
Metabolic	Hyperkalemia and impaired actions of some drugs
Respiratory	Hypoxemia caused by a decrease in oxygen-carrying capacity of the blood, possibly causing an increase in respiratory effort and distress

Adapted from Simon R, Ivatury R: The expanding role of permissive hypercapnia in patients with ARDS. Trauma Q 12:257–271, 1996; and Wilmoth D, Carpenter R: Preventing complications of mechanical ventilation: permissive hypercapnia. AACN Clin Issues 7:473–481, 1996.

uses arterial cannulation and IVOX uses venous cannulation. Their use in adults is still considered controversial and experimental. $ECO_2 R$ is used in conjunction with IVOX. $ECO_2 R$ assists in reduction of the workload of the lungs by removing carbon dioxide. Although there have been reports of success with these techniques in some centers, the consensus is that these techniques are invasive, expensive, and labor intensive for the small improvement in results (Chart 18–6).[30–32]

Advances in Pressure-Controlled Ventilation

Although the characteristics of pressure-controlled ventilation are favorable, many clinicians are concerned about the variability of the tidal volume. Several ventilator manufacturers have responded by designing mode options that guarantee the prescribed tidal volume while delivering the volume as a pressure breath. Volume-guaranteed pressure options (VGPOS) and volume-assured pressure support (VAPS) ventilation deliver a prescribed tidal volume while using a decelerating flow pattern. The modes include spontaneous and control options. In VGPOS, the pressure is adjusted automatically by the ventilator to attain the predetermined volume. In VAPS, the breath begins as a pressure breath and is completed, if necessary, as a volume breath to achieve the prescribed volume. When compared with conventional ventilation, VAPS ventilation was reported to decrease the patient's work of breathing by optimizing the inspiratory flow rate. VAPS ventilation was also reported to decrease auto-PEEP.[33,34] These technologies will allow for improved gas distribution while minimizing volume- and pressure-induced lung injuries.[25]

Pharmacologic Support

Several pharmacologic approaches to ALI and ARDS have been studied. Some of the preparations are receiving positive remarks in the literature and some are not. For example, use of liquid ventilation, surfactant infusions, and prostaglandin infusions are techniques studied in the early 1990s with little proven benefit.

These preparations are used in neonatal ICUs with some reported success.[35–39]

Nitric Oxide

Nitric oxide is a gas that is manufactured normally in the body and is released by endothelial cells. It diffuses easily across cell membranes into the cells of smooth

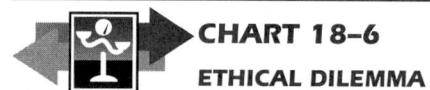

CHART 18–6

ETHICAL DILEMMA

Mrs. K. is a 45-year-old woman who suffered a gunshot wound to the abdomen as a result of a random shooting. She developed ARDS as a complication of her trauma and has been in the ICU for 19 days. Mrs. K. had been healthy prior to this illness. She has a history of hypertension that has been well controlled. Currently, conservative treatment strategies have not worked and Mrs. K. has been steadily deteriorating. Her family wants everything done that can be done. Mrs. K.'s physicians are considering extracorporeal membrane oxygenation (ECMO) to improve her oxygenation status. This procedure is highly controversial and extremely expensive.

1. Define the ethical issues in this scenario.
2. Mrs. K. has no health insurance. Should this information influence decisions regarding the selection of treatment strategies? Defend your response.
3. Should the circumstances leading to Mrs. K.'s injuries influence decisions regarding the selection of treatment strategies? Defend your response.
4. Discuss the nurse's role as an advocate for this patient. How might this role conflict with the family's desires?

muscle and causes relaxation. It has a short half-life that is approximated at less than 1 second up to 6 to 10 seconds. Therefore, any vasodilation effect is short-lived and selective to the pulmonary vasculature when inhaled. Results are encouraging for treatment of pulmonary hypertension and intrapulmonary shunting, especially in septic patients and those with high degrees of pulmonary hypertension.[30,40–43]

Use of nitric oxide is limited at this time because of problematic side effects and difficulties in controlling the administration of the gas. The side effects are methemoglobinemia, possible atherosclerosis, prolonged clotting times by inhibition of platelet aggregation, free radical formation, possible mutagenicity, and diversion of blood away from unventilated areas, which may delay lung healing and recovery.[43] These side effects can be minimized with administration of small concentrations of the gas. It has also been reported that nitric oxide converts to nitrogen dioxide even in small doses. Nitrogen dioxide causes pneumonitis and fulminant pulmonary edema. Controlling the concentration of the gas has also been problematic. The gas must be administered in the inspiratory circuit in a continuous flow. Controlling the exposure of the hospital staff during disconnections of the ventilator circuits has also been a concern. Woodrow's recommendations for the administration of nitric oxide are listed in Chart 18–7.

Antioxidants

Ketoconazole. Ketoconazole is a thromboxane A_2 synthetase inhibitor, and investigators have proposed that if the agent is given within the first 24 hours after diagnosis, it can actually prevent the progression of ALI to ARDS. Yu and Tomasa[44] showed that administration of 400 mg of ketoconazole early in the septic course decreased the mortality rate in septic patients at high risk of ARDS.

The side effects of ketoconazole are elevated liver function tests, fulminant hepatitis, worsening platelet aggregation, reduced fungal colonization, renal failure, and suppression of cortisol and androgen levels. Yu and Tomasa[44] reported no morbidity in terms of hepatic toxicity or decreased platelet aggregation related to ketoconazole therapy. Ketoconazole may be an approach for controlling the biochemical processes in multiple organ system dysfunction in the future.

Procysteine and N-*Acetylcysteine.* Lung injury is caused by a cascade of chemical mediators, a few of which have been identified as toxic oxygen radicals. Three major antioxidants—superoxide dismutase, catalase, and glutathione—help to neutralize free radicals and to prevent their damaging effects. Procysteine and *N*-acetylcysteine have been found by Bernard and colleagues[45] to be effective in repletion of glutathione

CHART 18–7

Recommendations for the Administration of Nitric Oxide

1. Atmospheric levels should be controlled by measuring exhaled nitric oxide and nitrogen dioxide levels.
2. Methemoglobin levels should be measured routinely.
3. Pulse oximetry readings must be watched more closely.
4. Delivery must be continuous, and disconnections should be avoided. Closed-circuit suction systems should be utilized.
5. Nitric oxide needs to be weaned slowly, or rebound pulmonary hypertension may occur.
6. Staff, patients, and significant others should be informed of the risk of exposure to nitric oxide.
7. Administration of nitric oxide must comply with local environmental pollutant levels, and air quality surveys may be required.

From Woodrow P: Nitric oxide: some nursing implications. Intensive Crit Care Nurs 13:87–92, 1997.

levels to potentially combat oxidant-induced damage. These medications may be another beneficial treatment for the patient of the future who has ARDS.

Steroids. The use of corticosteroids in late stages of ARDS may decrease mortality rates by reducing fever, neutrophilia, gallium uptake in the lungs, and lung injury scores.[46] Because reports of steroid use have yielded mixed results, however, further studies must be done.[47–52]

Fluid Therapy

The most important goal of fluid management in the patient with ALI and ARDS is to maintain adequate circulating blood volume with a sufficient red blood cell mass to help maximize oxygen-carrying capacity and tissue oxygen delivery.[12] This requires careful monitoring of the hemodynamic parameters. A negative fluid balance has been beneficial in reducing hydrostatic forces in the lungs to reduce pulmonary edema and to improve gas exchange. Using diuretics to induce a negative fluid balance must be done with caution. Hypovolemia can lead to a decrease in cardiac output and impaired tissue perfusion. Fluid replacement is guided by measurements of PAOP and cardiac

TABLE 18–6
Decision Making Regarding Prone Positioning

Assessment Step	Purpose
1. Identify time interval from injury to position change	The nurse is actively involved in determining when the patient is most likely to benefit from prone positioning. Once resuscitation and stabilization of the patient are satisfactorily accomplished, the nurse may initiate the discussion regarding prone positioning with the physician.
2. Assess hemodynamic stability	The nurse assesses the patient to determine whether the patient will be able to tolerate the position change. To assess potential problems, the nurse should perform a trial of a 45° angle turn on the right side. If the parameters return to baseline in 5 minutes, the patient will most likely tolerate prone positioning.
3. Assess mentation	Agitation can have a negative effect on the prone position. Patient injury, employee injury, and loss of tubes and lines can occur if agitation and anxiety are not managed effectively before the turn. Careful explanations and sedation may be used.
4. Size up the patient	Lifting and turning the patient requires at least five people. The technique is awkward, and the potential for losing lines and tubes is high. Vollman has created a support frame to make the process easier for prone positioning. She also recommends that a large patient be moved to a stretcher while supine and then positioned prone as he or she is moved back onto the bed.

Adapted from Vollman K: Prone positioning for the ARDS patient. Dimensions Crit Care Nurs 16:184–193, 1997.

output. PAOP usually ranges between 5 and 15 mm Hg. Patients with ARDS are frequently kept on the low side of normal ranges. Kollef and Schuster[30] recommend restricting fluid intake and adding diuretics as necessary to achieve the lowest PAOP consistent with an adequate cardiac output. With the recent emphasis on less invasive monitoring of patients, central venous pressure monitoring may be used as well. Central venous pressure readings usually range from 1 to 6 mm Hg or 3 to 12 cm H_2O. Again, the patient with ARDS is maintained on the low end of normal ranges.

In addition to fluid, the patient with ALI and ARDS may require inotropic support for cardiac output and tissue perfusion. The use of dopamine may be beneficial in offsetting the side effects of positive-pressure ventilation causing a decreased cardiac output. The patient must be adequately monitored for adequate volume before vasoconstricting agents are added, to ensure appropriate tissue perfusion.

Sedation and Pain Management

From 53 to 70% of all ICU patients receive some type of sedation. Medication choices include sedatives, anxiolytics, analgesics, or a combination of these. Morphine is the most commonly used narcotic in ICUs. It is indicated for moderate to severe pain with or without anxiety. It also reduces preload and promotes vasodilation. The patient receiving morphine should be monitored for respiratory depression and decreased gastrointestinal motility.

Neuromuscular blockade medications may also be used to promote ventilator synchrony in patients with high minute ventilation requirements, such as in ARDS. Administration of neuromuscular blockade requires mechanical ventilation because all muscles are paralyzed. Patients receiving neuromuscular blockade must also receive concurrent analgesia and sedation because all their sensory function remains intact; only the motor responses are impaired with blockade. Patients may experience a frightening "locked in" sensation from inadequate sedation. Sources recommend that periodically, such as once every 24 hours, the paralytics be allowed to wear off, to perform extensive neurologic assessment of the patient and to assess for the need to continue paralytic medications.[54]

Nutrition

The normal defense mechanisms of the body are necessary to survival of patients with ALI. ALI and ARDS are often associated with sepsis and trauma. The infection must be eradicated, and the reparative processes must be encouraged with adequate nutrition. Preventing catabolism can also be challenging for the acutely ill patient. In addition to providing nutrition for immune function, something must be left of the patient to work with once the ALI is resolved. Weaning will be successful if the muscles of the diaphragm have maintained some degree of integrity during the catastrophic stage of the illness.

Body Positioning

In patients with pulmonary disease, differences in body positioning can produce clinically significant changes in ventilation and perfusion. In the dependent areas of the lung, perfusion is greater than ventilation because of gravity. In nondependent areas of the lung, ventilation is greater than perfusion, also because of gravitational forces. Numerous studies using prone positioning have reported positive results in oxygenation. The improvement in oxygenation is believed to be the result of greater perfusion to the healthier, better-ventilated lung segments of the anterior chest.[55–58]

Contraindications to prone positioning include an inability to tolerate a head-down position, hemodynamic instability, weight over 90 kg, and an abdominal girth greater than 50 inches. The nurse is actively involved in monitoring the physical cues of tolerance of the procedure such as respiratory rate and effort, heart rate, blood pressure, and SaO_2. The patient with ARDS may benefit from a simple, inexpensive practice for improving gas exchange (Table 18–6).

Preventing Infection

It is important to the care of the acutely ill patient to prevent infection, central line sepsis, and nosocomial pulmonary infection. Strict aseptic technique should be used with all access devices. ALI and ARDS often require many invasive procedures with the potential of inducing sepsis. Strict surveillance for infection is advocated for all ICU patients. As pointed out by Meduri and colleagues[53] in their work with ARDS and sepsis, many infections are not detected except with bronchoscopy, especially if patients are receiving steroids. Preventing sinusitis by using oral gastric tubes for feedings is a relatively new practice in some

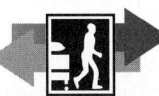

CHART 18–8
BEYOND THE ICU: ICU SURVIVORS OF ACUTE RESPIRATORY DISTRESS SYNDROME (ARDS)

Acute lung injury and ARDS are always secondary to some catastrophic event. At present, no method of truly preventing acute lung injury or ARDS exists. The patient may spend many days to weeks recovering in the ICU before transfer to the next level of care. Management of acute lung injury and ARDS in the recovery phases often takes place outside the ICU environment. "As few as 5 to 10% of ICU patients require prolonged mechanical ventilation, and this patient group consumes an estimated 35 to 50% of ICU patient days and ICU resources."[59] The patient who has survived the first few weeks of ARDS may be transferred to a subacute or transitional unit for continuation of therapy. Nurses who care for "ICU survivors" of ARDS need to be alert for complications during the reparative and remodeling processes of recovery. Fibroproliferation and fibrosis are common in "chronic ARDS" and can lead to irreversible lung failure. Nutritional support is essential for weaning and restoration of immune function. Long-term mechanical ventilatory support often requires efforts to restore the patient's interest in life and recovery. Efforts should be made to provide visitation, activities of daily living, and appropriate mental stimulation. Activity should be encouraged with chair sitting and progression to walking if possible.

Many ideas about the best method of weaning from mechanical ventilation have been offered. Petty[12] has advocated simple tube breathing without mechanical ventilation for supervised periods such as a T-tube or T-piece. Each exercise period is followed by a period of rest.[12] Other options are synchronized intermittent mandatory ventilation, pressure support ventilation, and combi-

nations of all three. Pressure support ventilation alone or in combination with synchronized intermittent mandatory ventilation or T-piece trials reduces the work of breathing, promotes respiratory muscle training, and improves patient–ventilator interactions.[59] Regardless of the technique, the patient must be monitored closely during the weaning process for changes in heart rate, respiratory rate, blood pressure, and arterial oxygen saturation by pulse oximetry. The periods of exercise or removal from the ventilator are gradually increased each day until the ultimate goal of independent ventilation is achieved. As pointed out by Schuster[60] in 1990, "The specific weaning technique employed is often less important than the care with which it is applied."

Survivors of ARDS may have long-term mechanical abnormalities of the lung as a result of fibrosis. Most patients who recover from ARDS lead normal lives without significant symptoms from their mild to moderate residual effects.

Despite all the controversy on managing the patient with acute lung injury and ARDS, there is improvement in the mortality rate. The reason for the improvement in management of ARDS represents a return to basic hemodynamic and ventilatory support of the patient with ARDS. It also represents the awareness that mechanical ventilation can be harmful and should be titrated carefully to achieve maximum benefit and to minimize harm. In addition, none of the conventional or unconventional therapies can improve the outcomes of acute lung injury alone. The combination of appropriate therapies with excellence in nursing care improves the survival rate of acute lung injury and ARDS.

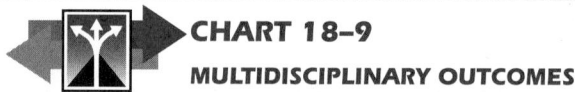

CHART 18–9

MULTIDISCIPLINARY OUTCOMES

Improvement of arterial oxygen saturation

Improvement of oxygen delivery and consumption

Return of fluid and electrolyte balance

Maintenance of adequate nutritional balance

Maintenance of adequate respiratory rate, rhythm, and tidal volume

Achievement of successful weaning from mechanical ventilation

Follow-up treatment plan with the patient and support systems

ICUs. If the patient is to be supported using enteral feedings, the nurse should monitor gastric residuals closely because aspiration pneumonia is a leading cause of ALI, ARDS, and SIRS.

Multidisciplinary Outcomes

The mortality rate for patients with ALI and ARDS remains high. Despite the many advances that have been made in the last 30 years, the outcomes of these phenomena are not always positive. The nurse needs to be aware that small improvements in the oxygenation of the patient are steps that need to be celebrated, and every effort needs to be made to maintain a positive outlook and a sense of hope for recovery for the patient, the significant others, and the nursing staff (Chart 18–8). The desired outcomes for the patient with ALI and ARDS are listed in Chart 18–9.

Critical Thinking Exercise

A 34-year-old white woman is admitted to the critical care unit with a history of flulike symptoms, including nausea, vomiting, diarrhea, and high fever for several days. She is admitted in moderate respiratory distress and is placed on an aerosol face mask at 60%. She is placed on ECG monitoring, pulse oximetry is performed, and a peripheral intravenous line is started of dextrose in half normal saline (D-5½ NS) at 50 mL per hour. Her arterial blood gases reveal the following: pH, 7.35; Po_2, 73; Pco_2, 35; and Fio_2, 60%.

Her oxygen is increased to 100% by face mask, and a pulmonary artery catheter is inserted, with the following readings: blood pressure, 98/60; pulse, 118; pulmonary artery, 44/25; PAOP, 12; central venous pressure, 4; cardiac output, 5.6; and cardiac index, 3.1. A chest radiograph is

completed after insertion of the pulmonary artery catheter. The chest radiograph showed diffuse infiltrates bilaterally, but no pneumothorax.

Three hours later, she is intubated and placed on mechanical ventilation. The settings are as follows: assist/control rate, 16; Fio_2, 1.0; PEEP, 10; pressure support, 20; and tidal volume, 800.

After mechanical ventilation, her blood gases are as follows: pH, 7.33; Po_2, 66; Pco_2, 50; and Fio_2, 1.0. Vital signs and pulmonary artery catheter values are as follows: blood pressure, 90/50; pulse, 124; pulmonary artery, 46/27; PAOP, 10; central venous pressure, 3; cardiac output, 4.6; and cardiac index, 2.4. Her PEEP is increased to 15 cm H_2O. An infusion of dopamine is begun at 5 μg/kg per minute.

1. Based on the preceding data, is this patient a candidate for developing ARDS? If so, what are the indications?

2. What treatment is mostly likely to support the pathophysiologic process indicated after mechanical ventilation?

3. What complication of mechanical ventilation is evident in the set of vital signs after mechanical ventilation?

4. What measurements help practitioners to differentiate between ARDS and cardiac failure–induced pulmonary edema?

Key Concepts

➡ ARDS is not a disease, but a syndrome or group of clinical manifestations that are always secondary to a serious insult to the body. This insult sets into motion a particularly life-threatening form of acute respiratory failure.

➡ Despite the advances made in recognition of the triggering factors and the management techniques, the mortality rate of ARDS remains between 40 and 60%.

➡ ALI is used to describe the syndrome of inflammation and increased permeability that cannot be easily explained by the underlying disease process. ARDS is used to describe the most severe forms of acute lung injury that do not respond well to treatment.

➡ Research has discovered that an overaggressive and protracted host defense response is the major factor in the progression and the outcomes in ALI and ARDS.

➡ The hallmark signs of ARDS are accumulation of protein-rich fluid in the alveoli and interstitial spaces as a result of increased permeability of the alveolar–capillary membrane and refractory hypoxemia, which is hypoxemia that does not respond to appropriate treatment.

➡ The best assessment includes knowing the patient's risk factors for the development of ALI and ARDS, which are sepsis, shock, pneumonia, and trauma.

➡ The goals of therapy for the patient with ARDS are to optimize oxygen delivery to the tissues, to facilitate restoration of the alveolar–capillary membrane integrity, and to identify the primary condition promptly.

➡ Information has revealed that mechanical ventilation with positive pressure can induce ventilator-related lung injury similar to ARDS. It creates increased microvascular pressure and increased microvascular permeability that causes fluid and protein leakage at the alveolar–capillary membrane level.

➡ The newest techniques of mechanical ventilation are aimed at recruiting alveoli with positive pressure such as PEEP and minimizing ventilator-induced lung injury.

➡ Many aspects of astute collaborative management of the critically ill patient can minimize ALI and may actually prevent ARDS.

References

1. Lemaire F: The prognosis of ARDS: appropriate optimism? Intensive Care Med 22:371–373, 1996.
2. Brandstetter R, Kailash S, DellaBadia M, et al: Adult respiratory distress syndrome: a disorder in need of improved outcome. Heart Lung 26:3–14, 1997.
3. Cutler L: Acute respiratory distress syndrome: an overview. Intensive Crit Care Nurs 12:316–326, 1996.
4. Weed F, McAffee L: Wound shock. The Medical Department of the United States Army in World War II, 1927, pp 185–213.
5. Ashbaugh D, Bigelow D, Petty T: Acute respiratory distress in adults. Lancet 2:319–323, 1967.
6. Bernard G, Artigas A, Brigham K, et al: The American–European consensus conference on ARDS. Am Rev Respir Dis 149:818–824, 1994.
7. Jones M, Hoffman L, Delgado E: ARDS revisited: new ways to fight an old enemy. Nursing 94. 24 (12):34–45, 1994.
8. Schuster D: What is acute lung injury? What is ARDS? Chest 107:1721–1726, 1995.
9. Meduri U: The role of the host defense response in the progression and outcome of ARDS: pathophysiological correlations and response to glucocorticoid treatment. Eur Respir J 9:2650–2670, 1996.
10. Guyton A: Basic Human Physiology. Philadelphia, W.B. Saunders, 1991.
11. Surratt N, Troiano N: Adult respiratory distress in pregnancy: critical care issues. J Obstet Gynecol Neonatal Nurs 23:773–780, 1994.
12. Petty T: Acute respiratory distress syndrome (ARDS). Dis Mon 36(1):7–58, 1990.
13. Murray J: Conference report: mechanisms of acute respiratory failure. Am Rev Respir Dis 115:1071–1078, 1977.
14. Murray J, Matthay M, Luce J, et al: An expanded definition of adult respiratory distress syndrome. Am Rev Respir Dis 138:720–723, 1988.
15. Dettenmeirer P, Johnson T: The art and science of mechanical ventilator adjustments. Crit Care Nurs Clin 3:575–583, 1991.
16. Tobin M: Mechanical ventilation. N Engl J Med 330:1056–1061, 1994.
17. Parker J, Hernandez L, Peevy K: Mechanisms of ventilator-induced lung injury. Crit Care Med 21:131–143, 1993.
18. Wilmoth D, Carpenter R: Preventing complications of mechanical ventilation: permissive hypercapnia. AACN Clin Issues 7:473–481, 1996.
19. Marik P, Krikorian J: Pressure-controlled ventilation in ARDS: a practical approach. Chest 112:1102–1106, 1997.
20. Tuxen D: Permissive hypercapnia. In: Tobin, M (ed): Principles and Practice of Mechanical Ventilation. New York, McGraw-Hill, 1994, pp 391–392.
21. Gluck E, Heard S, Patel C, et al: Use of ultrahigh frequency ventilation in patients with ARDS: a preliminary report. Chest 103:1413–1420, 1993.
22. Juarez P: Mechanical ventilation for the patient with severe ARDS: PC-IRV. Crit Care Nurse 12:34–39, 1992.
23. Lessard M, Guerot E, Lorino H, et al: Effects of pressure controlled with different I:E ratios versus volume controlled ventilation on respiratory mechanics, gas exchange, and hemodynamics in patients with adult respiratory distress syndrome. Anesthesiology 80:983–991, 1994.
24. Safcsak K, Nelson L: High-level positive end expiratory pressure management in the surgical patient with acute respiratory distress syndrome. AACN Clin Issues 7:482–494, 1996.
25. Burns S: Understanding, applying, and evaluating pressure modes of ventilation. AACN Clin Issues 7:495–506, 1996.
26. East T: The magic bullets in the war on ARDS: aggressive therapy for oxygenation failure. Respir Care 38:690–704, 1993.
27. Simon R, Ivatury R: The expanding role of permissive hypercapnia in patients with ARDS. Trauma Q 12:257–271, 1996.
28. Kiiski R, Takala J, Kari A, Milic-Emili J: Effect of tidal volume on gas exchange and oxygen transport in the adult respiratory distress syndrome. Am Rev Respir Dis 146:1131–1135, 1992.
29. Hickling K, Henderson S, Jackson R: Low mortality associated with low volume pressure limited ventilation with permissive hypercapnia in severe adult respiratory distress syndrome. Intensive Care Med 16:372–377, 1990.
30. Kollef M, Schuster D: The acute respiratory distress syndrome. N Engl J Med 332:27–37, 1995.
31. Mira J, Brunet F, Belghith M, et al: Reduction of ventilator settings allowed by intravenous oxygenator (IVOX) in ARDS patients. Intensive Care Med 21:11–17, 1995.
32. Hudson L: New therapies for ARDS. Chest, 106:79S–91S, 1995.
33. Amato M, Barbas C, Bonassa J, et al: Volume assured pressure support ventilation: a new approach for reducing respiratory muscle fatigue and workload during acute respiratory failure. Chest 102:1225–1234, 1995.
34. Amato M, Barbas C, Medeiros D, et al: Effect of a protective-ventilation strategy on mortality in the acute respiratory distress syndrome. N Engl J Med 338:347–354, 1998.
35. Dirkes S: Liquid ventilation: new frontiers in the treatment of ARDS. Crit Care Nurse 16:52–58, 1996.
36. Anzueto A, Baughman R, Guntupalli K, et al: Aerosolized surfactant in adults with sepsis induced acute respiratory distress syndrome. N Engl J Med 334:1417–1421, 1996.
37. Slotman G, Kerstein M, Bone RC, et al: The effects of prostaglandin E_1 on non-pulmonary organ function during clinical acute respiratory failure. J Trauma 32:480–489, 1992.
38. Abraham E, Park Y, Covington P, et al: Liposomal prostaglandin E_1 in acute respiratory distress syndrome: a placebo controlled, randomized, double-blind, multicenter clinical trial. Crit Care Med 24:10–15, 1996.
39. Walmrath D, Schneider T, Schermuly R, et al: Direct comparison of inhaled nitric oxide and aerosolized prostacyclin in acute respiratory distress syndrome. Am J Respir Crit Care Med 152:991–996, 1996.
40. Woodrow P: Nitric oxide: some nursing implications. Intensive Crit Care Nurs 13:87–92, 1997.

41. Rossetti M, Guenard H, Gabinski C: Effects of nitric oxide inhalation on pulmonary serial vascular resistances in ARDS. Am J Respir Crit Care Med 154:1375–1381, 1996.
42. Krafft P, Fridrich P, Fitzgerald R, et al: Effectiveness of nitric oxide inhalation in septic ARDS. Chest 109:486–493, 1996.
43. Morris G, Rich G: Inhaled nitric oxide as a selective pulmonary vasodilator in clinical anesthesia. J Am Assoc Nurse Anesth 65:59–67, 1997.
44. Yu M, Tomasa G: A double-blind, prospective, randomized trial of ketoconazole, a thromboxane synthetase inhibitor, in prophylaxis of the adult respiratory distress syndrome. Crit Care Med 21:1635–1642, 1993.
45. Bernard G, Wheeler A, Arons M, et al: A trial of antioxidants N-acetylcysteine and procysteine in ARDS. Chest, 112:164–172, 1997.
46. Meduri U, Belenchia J, Estes D, et al: Fibroproliferative phase of ARDS: clinical findings and effects of corticosteroids. Chest 100:943–952, 1991.
47. Luce J, Montgomery A, Marks J, et al: Ineffectiveness of high-dose methylprednisolone in preventing parenchymal lung injury and improving mortality in patients with septic shock. Am Rev Respir Dis 138:62–68, 1988.
48. Lefering R, Neugebauer E: Steroid controversy in sepsis and septic shock: a meta-analysis. Crit Care Med 23:1294–1303, 1995.
49. Cronin L, Cook D, Carlet J, et al: Corticosteroid treatment for sepsis: a critical appraisal and meta-analysis of the literature. Crit Care Med 23:1430–1439, 1995.
50. Ashbaugh D, Maier R: Idiopathic pulmonary fibrosis in adult respiratory distress syndrome: diagnosis and treatment. Arch Surg 120:520–525, 1985.
51. Hooper R, Kearl R: Established ARDS treated with a sustained course of adrenocortical steroids. Chest 97:138–143, 1990.
52. Martinot A, Fourier C, Cremer R, et al: Short-course, high-dose corticosteroid treatment in six children with late ARDS. Pediatr Pulmonol 23:314–318, 1997.
53. Meduri U, Headley A, Golden E, et al: Prolonged methylprednisolone treatment improves lung function and outcome in patients with unresolving acute respiratory distress syndrome: results of a randomized, double-blind, placebo-controlled trial. Memphis, TN, University of Tennessee Clinical Research Center and Baptist Memorial Health Care Foundation, unpublished manuscript, 1997.
54. Bizek K: Optimizing sedation in critically ill, mechanically ventilated patients. Crit Care Nurs Clin 7:315–325, 1995.
55. Swanland S: Body positioning and the elderly with adult respiratory distress syndrome: implications for nursing care. J Gerontol Nurs 22(2):46–50, 1996.
56. Gattinoni L, Presenti A: The nonhomogeneous lung: facts and hypothesis. Intensive Crit Care Diagn 6:1–4, 1987.
57. Vollman K: Prone positioning for the ARDS patient. Dimensions Crit Care Nurs 16:184–193, 1997.
58. Cohen I, Booth F: Cost containment and mechanical ventilation in the United States. New Horizons 2:283–290, 1994.
59. Weilitz P: Weaning from mechanical ventilation: old and new strategies. Crit Care Nurs Clin 3:585–590, 1991.
60. Schuster D: A physiologic approach to initiating, maintaining, and withdrawing mechanical ventilatory support during acute respiratory failure. Am J Med 88:268–278, 1990.

19

Common Respiratory Problems: Pulmonary Embolism, Pneumothorax, and Thoracic Pulmonary Surgery

M. Lynne Rodgers

Objectives

After completing this chapter, the student will be able to:

1. Describe the etiology of pulmonary embolism (PE), pneumothorax, and thoracic pulmonary surgery.
2. Discuss the pathophysiology of PE, pneumothorax, and thoracic surgery.
3. Differentiate assessment findings for the patient experiencing PE, pneumothorax, and thoracic pulmonary surgery.
4. Outline diagnostic approaches to confirm the presence of PE and pneumothorax.
5. Plan the collaborative management and interventions for the patient experiencing PE, pneumothorax, and thoracic pulmonary surgery.
6. Relate the impact of collaborative care on expected clinical outcomes for the patient experiencing PE, pneumothorax, and thoracic pulmonary surgery.

PULMONARY EMBOLISM

PE is a potentially fatal disorder that, as often as 30% of the time, is only identified on postmortem examination. More than 630,000 patients in the United States each year develop pulmonary embolism, resulting in approximately 200,000 deaths per year.[1] Approximately 2 million Americans experience deep vein thrombosis (DVT) each year, all of which are at risk for PE. In fact, PE is present in 50% of those with diagnosed DVT as demonstrated by perfusion lung scan. Conversely, 70% of those with symptomatic PE confirmed by lung scan have asymptomatic DVT. Without treatment, 20 to 30% of symptomatic distal leg thrombi will extend into more proximal leg veins. Such extensions are associated with the development of clinically significant PE 40 to 50% of the time.[2] Clearly, the association of DVT and PE is close and has strong implications for health care in the prevention, recognition, and treatment of PE.

The mortality from PE has changed little since the 1960s. To be certain, health care has changed. Diagnostic abilities, advanced treatments, and pharmacologic interventions have developed at a phenomenal rate over the past 30 years. However, diagnosis of PE can be complicated. No one basic assessment is definitively sensitive for PE; signs and symptoms often are not specific for PE. Key predisposing factors are prevalent in many patient populations. The patient may present through the emergency department, in the postpartum unit, in the intensive care unit (ICU), in a postsurgical unit, or at an extended care facility.

The problem in identifying patients with PE first starts with the initial failure to suspect the diagnosis clinically. Identifying those at risk for PE and recognizing the vague signs and symptoms are the key considerations for diagnosing and treating the patient with PE.[3] Once the *possibility* of PE is considered, today's advanced technology can be implemented. The nurse must be astute in all areas of the health care continuum when confronted with the possibility of this often illusive disorder.

ETIOLOGY AND PATHOPHYSIOLOGY

PE occurs when the pulmonary vasculature is completely or partially occluded by nonsoluble material. Although this material may be amniotic fluid, fat, a foreign object, air, migrated tumor cells, calcium, or septic emboli, most cases of PE are caused by a dislodged venous thrombus. Sixty-five percent of PE occur in both lungs, 25% in the right lung only, and 10% in the left lung only. Lower lung lobes are affected four times as often as upper lung lobes because of sluggish blood flow.[4] Results of PE depend on the vessels occluded and the patient's overall cardiovascular function. From 60 to 80% of PE are small and are clinically silent.[5] Even these cases of PE should be considered clinically significant. PE should alert the health care professional that a thrombus exists somewhere in the venous system of the patient. Predisposing risk factors rarely disappear, and patients with PE have a 30% chance of developing an additional PE.

The origins of PE are varied (Table 19–1). Patients who are elderly, traumatized, immobilized, or seriously ill have the highest occurrence. This occurrence proportionally increases with age and duration of illness. Women are affected more often than men in most instances, and in fact PE is the most frequent cause of death associated with pregnancy and childbirth. The presence of factor V:Q506, a gene mutation responsible for resistance to activated protein C, is high in patients with DVT resulting in PE.[6] Thrombi in the popliteal, femoral, iliac, and deep lower leg veins account for 95% of PE. Axillary, subclavian, calf muscle, pelvic, and superficial leg veins are less common sources.[7] Although PE can be caused by substances other than blood clots, the overwhelming risk factor that should alert the nurse to the presence or development of PE is DVT or the potential to develop DVT.

Deep Vein Thrombosis

In 1856, Virchow theorized that venous thrombosis was a result of three variances, since known as Virchow's triad. These factors are alterations in: vein

TABLE 19–1
Origins of Pulmonary Emboli

Embolism	Origin
Deep vein thrombosis	Venous stasis
	Hypercoagulability
	Vein wall damage
Fat embolism	Fracture of long bones
	Orthopedic surgery
	Sternal splitting
Air embolism	IV catheters
	Trauma: open chest wounds
	Diagnostic procedures
	Surgery: cardiovascular, abdominal, neurologic
	Decompression
Amniotic embolism	Amniotic fluid or sac
	Fluid clots
	Placental or embryonic tissue
Septic embolism	Massive infection
	Endocarditis
	Implanted devices
Tumor embolism	Malignant cells
Right heart embolism	Atrial clots or atrial fibrillation
	Ventricular clots
	Prosthetic valve debris
	Central line or port clots
	Dialysis
	Extracorporeal perfusion
	Valvular calcium
Foreign materials	IV catheters or pulmonary artery/ intra-aortic balloon pump
	Deliberate injection
	IV drug abuse
	Non-IV drugs given IV
	Missiles or bullets
	Parasitic infestation

wall, blood flow, and blood.[8] Approximately 2 million Americans experience DVT each year. The illness is often missed or misdiagnosed. Table 19–2 lists specific causes related to each of the three variances that act in the development of DVT and consequently PE.

Abnormal vein walls can be due to direct injury to the vein or surrounding tissues. Vein wall disruption can initiate an inflammatory response to injury to the intima of the vein wall, with associated clot development. However, *most* occurrences of DVT *are not* in response to inflammation. Instead, most instances of phlebitis occur in response to the presence of a thrombus. In other words, a clot initiates the inflammation, rather than inflammation initiating the clot. Thrombi in the veins are composed predominately of red blood cells that are trapped in a fine fibrin web with few platelets present and therefore are considered "red thrombi." In contrast, arterial thrombi are considered "white thrombi" and are composed predominately of platelets trapped in a fibrin mesh with few red cells.

TABLE 19–2
Etiology of Deep Vein Thrombosis

Location of Disorder	Causes	Location of Disorder	Causes
Vein Wall	IV catheters, sheaths, ports, or shunts	**Blood (cont'd)**	Excessive coagulation factors: fibrinogen, prothrombin, disorder of plasminogen activators
	Inflammation around vein		Irrigation of clotted IVs
	Infection around vein		Warfarin-induced hypercoagulability in first few days of therapy
	Varicose veins		Heparin-induced thrombocytopenia
	Long-term IV drug abuse		Hemolytic anemia
	Direct vessel trauma	**Blood Flow**	Prolonged bed rest
	Prior thrombophlebitis		Restricted leg activity
	Postthrombotic syndrome		Dependent leg position
	Mechanical manipulation		Venous compression
	Autoimmune disorders		Diabetes
	Major body burns		Obesity
	Prolonged standing or sitting		Sickle cell anemia
	Atherosclerosis		Prolonged surgery
	Familial hyperlipidemias		Peripheral vascular disease
	Blood type A		Low-flow states
	Sports or occupational stress thrombosis		Congestive heart failure
Blood	Hyperviscosity		Myocardial infarction
	Dehydration		Dysrhythmias
	Polycythemia		Shock
	Surgery		Impaired right atrial emptying with atrial fibrillation
	Trauma or fractures		Invasive devices: ports, intra-aortic balloon pumps, IV catheters, pacemakers
	Pregnancy and childbirth		Thoracic outlet syndrome
	Oral contraceptive use		
	Estrogen therapy		
	Autoimmune disorders: lupus erythematosus, ulcerative colitis, AIDS, Behçet's syndrome		
	Cancer		
	Deficient anticoagulation factors: protein C and S, heparin cofactor II, antithrombin III		

Thrombi may also be formed as a result of sluggish blood flow. Stasis of blood most often occurs in the valve cusps of the veins and in the venous sinuses of the leg muscles, but it can also occur around indwelling catheters or ports. When blood pools in the deep veins, clearance and dilution of activated coagulation factors are impaired, activity of coagulation factor inhibitors is decreased, and access to endothelial protective substances is limited. Hypercoagulability ensues.

Hypercoagulability of the blood can lead to clot formation. In some situations, this condition occurs as a protective or reparative mechanism for some other disorder, only to contribute to the development of DVT. Activation of blood coagulation can also occur in response to chemical mediators released at other distant sites of tissue damage. Cytokines such as interleukin-1 and tumor necrosis factor are released and stimulate the vessel endothelial cells to produce plasminogen activator inhibitor-1 and tissue factor. These actions reduce amounts of thrombomodulin, thereby enhancing the clotting activity of thrombin. The damaged vein endothelium is unable to exert its normal protective properties, and further thrombosis occurs.[8]

Once a patient has been diagnosed with DVT, recurrence depends on many factors. If causative risk factors are decreased or reversed, recurrence is generally less likely, reported in some studies to be less than 4% in the first year. However, patients who continue to have the same risk factors are more likely to have a recurrence, the rate of which is estimated to be 10% in the first year. Development of postthrombotic syndrome places the patient at an even higher risk of recurrence. Postthrombotic syndrome is a chronic condition that occurs after DVT and is characterized by recanalization of the thrombus, hypertension in the deep veins of the involved leg, venous valvular incompetence, and outflow obstruction. All these events result in the shunting of blood flow into superficial leg veins during muscular contraction. This condition leads to swelling, calf pain with activity, pigmentation and induration around the lower leg and ankle, impaired viability of superficial tissues, and, in severe cases, ulceration. The size and location of the original DVT have no significant relation to the development of postthrombotic syndrome. The rate of recurrence of DVT in postthrombotic syndrome increases each year and has been reported to be as high as 33% after 8 years.[2]

Relationship of Deep Vein Thrombosis and Pulmonary Embolus

Once a DVT develops, it can become dislodged and may travel as an embolism to the pulmonary vasculature. Dislodging of the thrombus can occur in various ways. Sudden jarring or movement, especially with first ambulations after several days of inactivity, can literally loosen the thrombus from its venous bed. Extremes in vascular pressure changes such as occur during activity, Valsalva maneuvers, coughing, sneezing, unstable hemodynamic blood pressure swings, or fluid challenges can dislodge the thrombus.[9] Vigorous deep leg muscle massage can mobilize the thrombus, as well the normal mechanism of clot dissolution that occurs in 7 to 10 days. The embolus travels through the venous system into the inferior vena cava, enters the right atrium of the heart, continues to the right ventricle, and finally enters the pulmonary artery. The embolus continues to travel as far into the pulmonary vasculature as its diameter allows.

Bronchial and Alveolar Changes

On occlusion of a pulmonary vessel, blood flow to distal lung tissues is impaired. Because no alveolar–capillary gas exchange can occur, carbon dioxide from the systemic circulation cannot enter the alveoli. This alveolar hypocarbia causes the smooth muscle of the bronchi to contract. The alveoli shrink, bronchoconstriction occurs, and atelectasis of alveolar air sacs results. Unfortunately, these actions are not limited to nonperfused alveoli, but they also involve perfused functional alveoli in the surrounding areas. Consequently, the extent of damage is greater than the original process. Some alveolar units are perfused but not ventilated, some are ventilated but not perfused, and some have no perfusion or ventilation and are considered silent units. When perfusion of alveoli decreases, ventilatory dead space or "wasted ventilation" occurs. Ventilating nonperfused alveoli results in a ventilation–perfusion (V/Q) mismatch, local tissue hypoxia, systemic hypoxemia, and eventually hypercapnea. Within 2 to 3 hours of decreased alveolar blood flow, production of surfactant by type II alveolar cells begins to decrease, and within 12 to 15 hours, levels are severely curtailed.[7] Surfactant allows alveolar sacs to remain open under low pressures. Inadequate amounts of surfactant result in decreased alveolar surface tension, causing alveolar units to collapse. Further pulmonary atelectasis develops, and interstitial fluid then enters the alveoli. The lungs' response to these nonfunctional alveoli is to shunt the blood to functional alveoli and to increase respiratory effects. Although these are protective compensatory measures, they usually are not sufficient to correct the V/Q mismatch, and in fact they can contribute to increased pulmonary vascular resistance. In addition, vasoactive substances such as thromboxanes, histamine, prostaglandin, and serotonin are released. If the PE is caused by air emboli, activation of the clotting cascade occurs in the small pulmonary vessels.

If fat emboli are the cause of the PE, interactions with free fatty acids and platelets cause further release of vasoactive substances. All these chemical mediators contribute even more to the constrictive response of the bronchioles and terminal alveolar units producing bronchospasm and asthma-type symptoms, often making diagnosis on initial presentation difficult. Finally, these chemical mediators exacerbate pulmonary vasoconstriction and have further undesirable hemodynamic effects.[2]

Hemodynamic Effects

The overall hemodynamic effects of PE depend on the patient's prior cardiopulmonary status and the impedance to blood flow caused by the PE. Impedance to blood flow is determined by the size and location of the PE and by the amount of pulmonary vasoconstriction caused by response to local controls and chemical mediators. As pulmonary vascular resistance increases and pulmonary hypertension develops, workload of the right ventricle increases. Pulmonary artery pressures increase and necessitate the right ventricle to contract harder to overcome the elevated pressures. If the patient's heart and lungs were previously healthy and the impedance to blood flow is not severe, this compensation may be adequate to prevent critical consequences. In patients with major vessel obstruction and no preexisting heart disease, pulmonary artery diastolic and systolic pressures are increased, whereas pulmonary artery occlusive pressure, which indicates left heart pressure, is normal. Massive PE is associated with widening of the pulmonary artery diastolic–occlusive pressure gradient, reflecting the precapillary pulmonary hypertension created by the obstruction.[9] Table 19–3 lists the typical hemodynamic profile of severe PE. If coexisting cardiopulmonary disease is present or if the extent of the PE is great, eventually the

TABLE 19–3
Hemodynamic Profile of Severe Pulmonary Embolism

Hemodynamic Value	Finding
Arterial pressure	Normal
	Decreased (with cor pulmonale)
Systemic vascular resistance	Increased
Peripheral vascular resistance	Increased
Central venous pressure/right atrial pressure	Increased
Pulmonary artery diastolic/ pulmonary artery systolic pressure	Increased
Pulmonary artery occlusive pressure	Normal
	Decreased
	Increased (with coexisting left ventricular dysfunction)
Pulmonary artery diastolic/ pulmonary artery occlusive pressure gradient	Widened
Cardiac output/cardiac index	Decreased
Mixed venous oxygen saturation	Decreased

right ventricle cannot compensate, and right ventricular failure occurs.

Right ventricular failure has both backward and forward effects. The backward effects occur simply by causing a backup of pressures and volumes in the areas before the right ventricle. Excessive pressure in the right ventricle can lead to right ventricular hypertrophy or strain. The enlarged right ventricle works harder and uses more oxygen. The right atrium must also work harder to send blood into the higher pressure of the right ventricle. As right atrial pressure increases, systemic signs of right-sided heart failure become apparent. Neck vein distention, hepatomegaly, hepatojugular reflex, peripheral edema, and ascites may occur.

The forward effects of right ventricular failure are caused by a decrease in right ventricular cardiac output. The left ventricle does not receive as much blood from the right ventricle, and a decrease in left ventricular filling and cardiac output occurs. In addition, right ventricular overload can cause a bulging of the interventricular septum into the left ventricle, thus affecting left ventricular chamber size and cardiac output. As a direct result of decreased left ventricular cardiac output, a decrease in perfusion of the coronary arteries, brain, and kidneys develops. Baroreceptors, sympathetic nervous system, chemoreceptors, and other compensatory mechanisms are stimulated, and this process leads to the development of other assessment findings, as discussed later.

Pulmonary Infarction

Pulmonary infarction is rare because of the great network of pulmonary collateral circulation. However, 10 to 15% of cases of PE do occur in terminal small pulmonary vessels and result in pulmonary infarction. These usually occur in patients whose circulation is already compromised by cardiopulmonary disease. Pulmonary infarction usually affects the lower lobes and involves the outer periphery of the lung, with well over half involving multiple areas within the lung. Sometimes, pulmonary infarction results when variances in blood flow and pressures cause larger, more proximal PE to break off small emboli and to occlude the distal end branches. Pronounced pulmonary consolidation resulting from hemorrhage or effusion develops. These areas can develop necrosis and abscess, and they usually result in pulmonary scarring and fibrosis. Large cavitary lesions after pulmonary infarction may require pulmonary resection, because mortality rates can be high if these lesions are left unresected.[10] From 10 to 15% of PEs involve midsize nonterminal pulmonary arteries and usually do not result in pulmonary infarction unless prior cardiopulmonary disease coexists. Nevertheless, these cases of PE can still result in severe symptoms and poor clinical outcomes.

Sudden Death

When 50 to 60% of the pulmonary vasculature is occluded by a large embolus or by many small emboli, acute right heart failure, cardiovascular collapse, or sudden death can occur. A saddle embolus occurring at the main pulmonary artery bifurcation is an example of such a PE that can result in instantaneous death with no warning symptoms.[7] Massive occlusion of the pulmonary vasculature prevents any blood flow to the left side of the heart. During resuscitative efforts, these patients frequently demonstrate electrical activity with no electrical response, commonly known as "pulseless electrical activity" or "electromechanical dissociation." Two-thirds of patients with fatal PE die within 1 hour of the onset of symptoms.[11] It is rare for a PE to pass into the systemic circulation. This phenomenon, known as paradoxic embolism, can only occur if a clot passes through an atrial or septal wall defect when right heart pressures exceed left heart pressures. These paradoxic emboli can result in massive stroke and sudden death as well.

Assessment

Signs and symptoms of acute-onset chest pain, dyspnea, fever, tachycardia, tachypnea, cough, and altered breath sounds can indicate numerous cardiopulmonary problems, especially in a population of patients with underlying cardiopulmonary disease. Myocardial infarction, pneumonia, dissecting aortic aneurysm, acute bronchitis, pneumothorax, and even severe anxiety can all initially present with some of the same symptoms as PE. It is especially important to make an accurate and quick diagnosis, because implementing the correct therapies is crucial to survival for those with substantial PE. Several assessment findings in conjunction, rather than just one or two, help to indicate the presence of PE. By adding a thorough investigation for positive risk factors, the identification of pulmonary embolism becomes easier.

History

Suspicion plays a key role in diagnosing PE. Identifying positive risk factors for the development of PE is the first step. During assessment of the patient's history, the nurse should obtain information concerning coagulopathies, recent or current pregnancy, use of birth control pills or high-dose estrogen therapy, recent illicit or prescribed intravenous drug use, coexisting major illnesses, age, recent immobility or trauma, exercise level, occupational activities, type A blood group, personal and familial history of DVT and PE, and recent surgery, especially prolonged surgery. The type of surgery affects the frequency of PE with the following percentages: thorax, 9.4%; abdomen, 15.8%; head and neck, 20%; and back and extremities, 40%.[12] Heart disease and venous thrombosis are by far the major risk factors for PE. Immobilized, very ill, elderly, traumatized patients have the highest incidence of PE. In fact, the older the patient and the longer the illness, the greater the incidence of PE. In hospitalized patients, the four main risk factors that contribute to the development of PE are DVT, prolonged immobilization of more than 7 days, postoperative state, and obesity.[13]

Physical Presentation

Signs and symptoms of DVT are often vague, minimal, or absent, but they may include swelling, warmth, redness, tenderness, and a palpable venous cord. A positive Homans' sign elicited when dorsiflexion of the foot causes calf pain is neither a specific nor a sensitive indication of DVT. Only 25% of DVTs are diagnosed by the physician based on clinical findings. If the DVT obstructs the vessels, swelling and differences in limb circumference may occur. Even with a strong clinical presentation, diagnosis of DVT is correct only 50% of the time.[8]

The most frequent clinical symptoms experienced with PE are sudden dyspnea, chest pain, cough, apprehension, and sweating (Table 19–4). Dyspnea may be the only symptom and can vary from mild to severe or intermittent to progressive. The pathophysiologic bronchoconstriction discussed earlier can cause increased work of breathing, increased airway resistance, bronchospasm, and wheezing. Pulmonary hypertension can disrupt capillary beds, and hemoptysis may accompany the cough. Pain can occur suddenly and may or may not be localized to the area of the PE. Pain may be pleuritic, may increase during inspiration, and may contribute to splinting or guarding of the area overlying the PE. Chest pain may be confused with that of a myocardial infarction because it can be described as substernal and crushing. Because of hypoxemia and decreased cardiac output, the sympathetic nervous system releases catecholamines, with resulting apprehension and sweating. Nausea, vomit-

TABLE 19–4
Signs and Symptoms in Confirmed Pulmonary Embolus

Symptoms	Percentage (%)	Physical Signs	Percentage (%)
Dyspnea	79.4	General signs	
Chest pain	64.9	Fever	53.6
Apprehension	63.0	Pallor	27.8
Sudden dyspnea	58.8	Cyanosis	17.5
Sweating	41.2	Cardiovascular signs	
Dyspnea and chest pain	40.0	Tachycardia > 100/min	41.2
Cough	39.2	Increased S_2	40.2
Palpitations	30.9	Hypotension	23.7
Pleuritic chest pain	27.8	Pulmonary artery systolic murmur	22.7
Altered mental status	25.0	Respiratory signs	
Progressive dyspnea	20.6	Breathing rate ≥ 25/min	58.8
Hemoptysis	13.4	Reduced diaphragm motion	41.2
Syncope	11.3	Decreased breath sounds	38.1
Crushing substernal pain	4.1	Crackles	23.7
		Pleural friction rub	22.7

ing, weakness, pallor, and palpitations may also occur. If the PE is large enough, severe hypoxemia, hypercapnea, cyanosis, syncope, or sudden death may occur.

Physical signs most prominent with PE are fever, tachycardia, increased second heart sound, neck vein distention, tachypnea, decreased breath sounds, and decreased diaphragm motion (see Table 19–4). Fever is attributed to the accompanying inflammatory response or is the result of a preexisting risk factor. A temperature of less than 101°F is most common. Pulmonary hypertension and vascular resistance result in a decrease in right ventricular output. Catecholamine release in response to this decrease in right ventricular output results in tachycardia, with heart rates most often over 100 per minute. Continued right ventricular heart failure causes right atrial strain, and atrial dysrhythmias such as atrial fibrillation develop. As pressures continue to increase in the right atrium and superior vena cava, neck vein distention becomes apparent. Because pressure in the pulmonary artery is high, pulmonic valve closure at the end of ventricular systole is accentuated. High pulmonary artery pressures also cause the pulmonic valve to close later than the aortic valve, resulting in a consistently widely split second heart sound. This situation is usually ominous because it indicates severe right ventricular failure. A systolic murmur of the pulmonary artery may be auscultated as a result of turbulence in the high-pressure pulmonary system during systole; a systolic regurgitation murmur of the tricuspid valve may occur if the right ventricle dilates to the point that the tricuspid valve is unable to close tightly. An S_3 or S_4 gallop indicates ventricular failure. If the PE is extensive or if the patient has severe preexisting cardiopulmonary disease, hypotension can develop and may lead to shock, cardiovascular collapse, and death. In a compensatory response to hypoxemia, use of respiratory accessory muscles and hyperventilation with respiratory rates higher than 25 breaths per minute develop. Decreased breath sounds over the affected area are a result of ventilation defects and splinting due to pain on breathing. Other findings may be crackles, wheezing, or a pleural friction rub heard most often in the lung bases, where most PEs occur. If the PE is caused by a fat embolus, petechiae are often seen on the anterior chest, the axilla, the neck, and the conjunctivae. Air embolus may produce a mill wheel murmur that sounds like a churning noise and may be audible without the use of a stethoscope.

Diagnostic Findings for Deep Vein Thrombosis

Because a direct relationship exists between DVT and PE, the presence of DVT is used as a clinical marker or indicator for thromboembolitic disorders. The annual incidence in the United States of DVT is estimated to be from 5 to 20 million,[14] with 25 to 50% of those

demonstrating PE on a V/Q scan.[8] From autopsy reports, 75% of those with DVT show pathologic signs of PE.[15] Other studies showed that 30 to 61% of patients with PE had no evidence of DVT on bilateral venograms; however, the researchers inferred that this finding could indicate total embolization of the DVT.[14] Because of this relationship, diagnostic tests for DVT are often used in high-risk patients to initiate anticoagulation therapy and to avert the possibility of PE.

Impedance Plethysmography

Plesthymography is a noninvasive method of measuring changes in volume in an extremity. Normally, pressure and volume in the leg veins increase during inspiration and decrease during expiration. Venous obstruction resulting from thrombi can impair venous outflow, resulting in changes in electrical resistance and impedance, detected by electrical impedance plethysmography. Limitations with this examination are that distal calf veins cannot be accurately evaluated, partial occlusions by thrombi are not detected, negative results can occur when collateral circulation is well established, and patient cooperation with respiratory maneuvers is required. Nevertheless, a positive finding is accurate 90% of the time, especially if serial studies are performed.[16]

Venous Duplex Doppler Studies

These noninvasive studies use the principle of sending and receiving sound waves to evaluate the patency of the deep veins from the inguinal ligament to the popliteal area. Characteristics of blood flow can indicate thrombosis, narrowing, compression, or occlusion of these venous vessels. The speed and direction of blood flow can also be determined. These studies have a 90 to 100% success rate in detecting above-the-knee DVT.[16] The success rate drops to 75% when identifying below-the-knee DVT, and this is troublesome because the venous sinuses of the calf muscle and the peroneal and posterior tibial veins are the most common sites of thrombus formation.

Venography

By injecting radiopaque dye into the dorsum of the foot, filling defects and diversion of flow in the leg veins can be demonstrated, as seen in Figure 19–1. Veins in the lower extremity and in the deep femoral area are often not visualized well, but still more than 90% of thrombi can be detected with this examination. Using radioisotopes instead of a radiopaque dye during venography has been shown to increase reliability and accuracy in detecting venous thrombi. Venography contrast dye can cause tissue sloughing if extravasation occurs. In 4% of patients, iatrogenic venous thrombosis can occur, and in 3% of patients, allergic dye reactions can develop.[8]

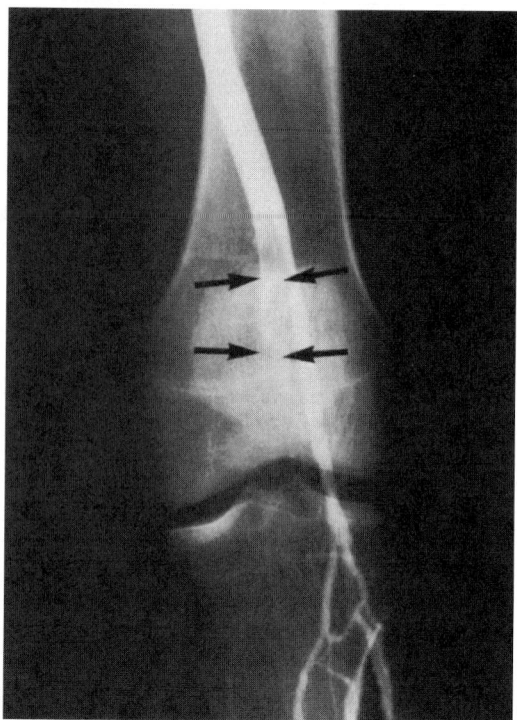

Figure 19-1

Contrast venogram. By injecting radiopaque dye into the dorsum of the foot, filling defects and diversion of flow in the leg veins can be seen. This contrast venogram shows a large filling defect (arrows) resulting from a thrombus in the politeal–femoral vein area, posing substantial embolic risk. (From Murray JF, Nadel JA: Textbook of Respiratory Medicine, 2nd ed. vol. 2. Philadelphia, W.B. Saunders, 1994, p 1654.)

Magnetic Resonance Imaging and Computed Tomography

Magnetic resonance imaging (MRI) of leg veins has been found to be an excellent diagnostic tool in visualizing DVT. MRI is not invasive and has a low incidence of complications. Accuracy has been shown to be comparable to that of contrast venography and venous duplex Doppler studies.[17] The use of MRI is limited in claustrophobic patients, those who have implanted metal devices, and the extremely obese. Spiral computed tomography (CT) scanning technology is used in some facilities with accuracy approaching that of pulmonary angiography. Spiral CT scanners are so rapid that a complete chest scan can be done while the patient holds his or her breath. This technique has some limitations, but results have been promising.[13]

Diagnostic Findings for Pulmonary Embolus

Routine diagnostic examinations such as blood tests, chest radiography, and electrocardiography (ECG) often are not specific enough to diagnosis PE. The most diagnostic examinations of lung scan and pulmonary angiography often require a high degree of suspicion for the disorder because of their specificity to PE (Figure 19–2). Again, we see that suspicion and identification of high-risk patients for PE are required to diagnosis this elusive disorder accurately.

Ventilation–Perfusion Lung Scan

The perfusion lung scan has long been used as the initial specific diagnostic examination for PE. Human albumin tagged with radioisotopes of technetium-99m or iodine-131 is injected intravenously, to allow the visualization of pulmonary arterial blood flow distribution from at least six different views. Ventilation scanning can be performed by inhalation of radioactive aerosol such as xenon to delineate ventilated and nonventilated areas. Typically, the areas involving the PE initially continue to be normally ventilated while demonstrating no or little perfusion on the perfusion lung scan. This V/Q mismatch, along with a high-probability perfusion scan, is 95% diagnostic for PE. Depending on the amount and distribution of segmental or lobar perfusion defects, the scan is reported as being of high (80–90% chance), intermediate (30–50% chance), or low (10–20% chance) probability for PE. In high-risk orthopedic surgical patients, some institutions perform baseline scans to use as a postoperative comparison.[18] This examination, along with clinical presentation, arterial blood gas analysis, chest radiograph, presence of risk factors, and absence of other possible diagnoses can be most helpful *if* the scan is abnormal. High-probability scans with high clinical suspicion are 96% diagnostic for PE; the rate drops to 80 to 88% if clinical suspicion is considered intermediate and to 50% if clinical suspicion is low.[2] However, false-positive results can occur in patients with atelectasis, neoplasm, pneumonitis, and emphysematous bullae, and a negative scan does not clearly rule out the diagnosis of PE. This situation validates the necessity of using the chest radiograph, past history, and physical examination in association with the scan results. The PIOPED (Prospective Investigation of Pulmonary Embolism Diagnosis) study indicated that 12% of patients with low-probability scans were shown to have PE as demonstrated by pulmonary angiography, and 12% of those with high-probability scans did not have PE as proven by angiography.[19] The diagnostic value of the lung scan is greatest when serial scans are performed, especially in patients with postoperative moderate-probability scan results, or when lung scans are used in conjunction with a ventilation scan. See Figure 19–2B for an example of a V/Q lung scan.

Pulmonary Angiography

The most specific test for PE is pulmonary angiography. During right heart catherization, a radiopaque dye is injected into the pulmonary vasculature to visualize filling defects in the lumen of the vessels or sudden cessation or "cutoff" of blood flow. Several different lung zones are injected, to identify any ab-

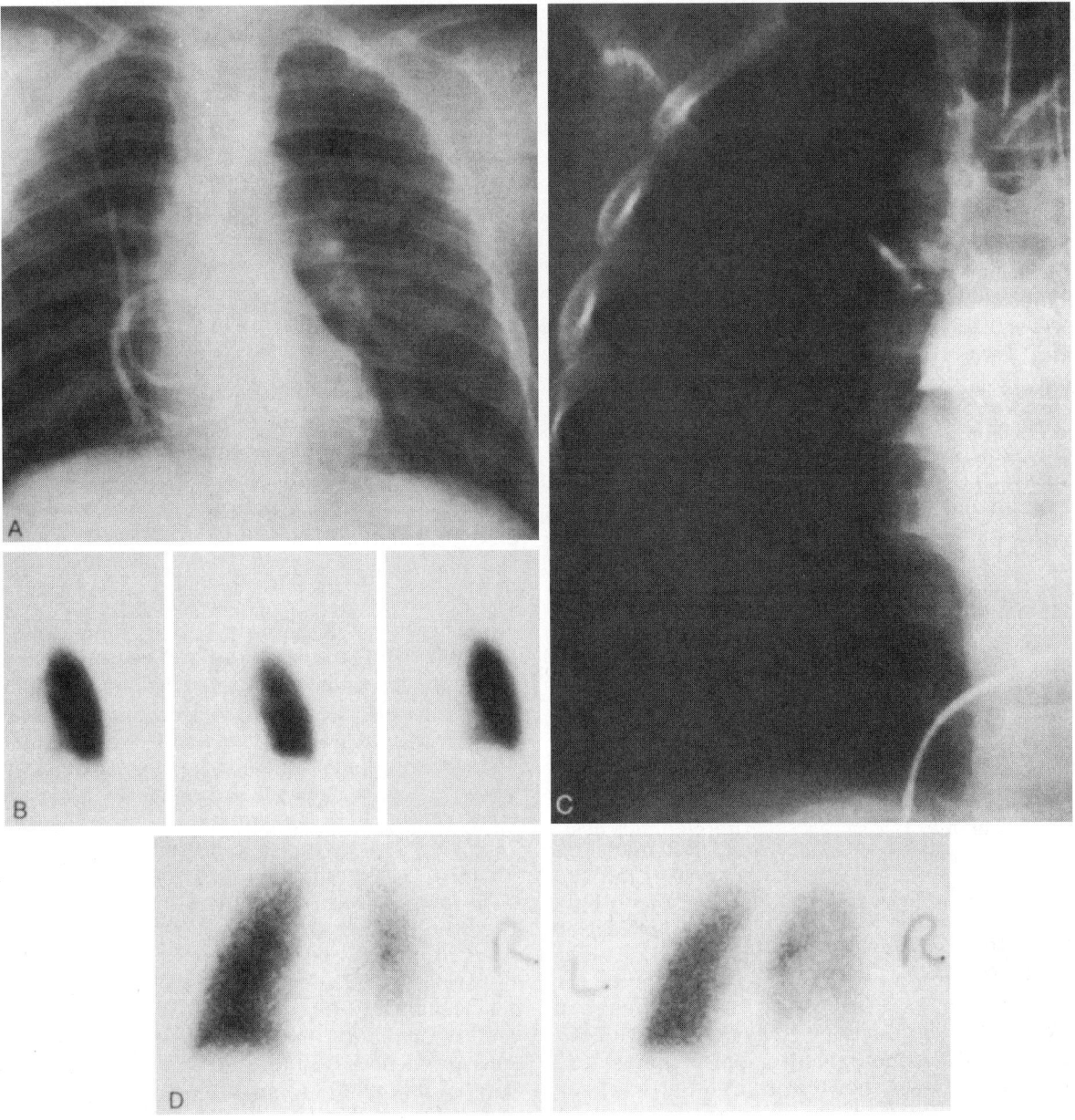

Figure 19–2

A, Plain chest film (child with long-term implantation of a hyperalimentation catheter in right atrium). Note the hypovascularity of the right lung compared with the left lung (Westermark's sign). *B,* Pulmonary radioactive scan showing no perfusion of the right lung. *C,* Pulmonary arteriogram confirming occlusion of the right main pulmonary artery. *D,* Pulmonary scan after intravenous streptokinase therapy showing great improvement in pulmonary arterial blood flow to the right lung. *(From Sabiston DC, Spencer FC: Surgery of the Chest, 6th ed. vol. 1. Philadelphia, W.B. Saunders, 1996, p 777.)*

normalities thoroughly. Because of its invasive nature, allergic possibilities, expense, and complications, angiography not used as a routine screening test. By selecting patients carefully, however, the complication rate for this test can be kept at less than 2%.[18] It is especially of value in those patients with high clinical suspicion but an intermediate or indeterminate scan or in those in whom anticoagulation is contraindicated. Figure 19–2C demonstrates typical findings of pulmonary angiography in a patient with PE. Patients who will require surgical intervention or placement

of an inferior vena caval filter or whose unstable conditions require immediate diagnosis also require pulmonary angiography. However, pulmonary angiography is considered unnecessary in patients with high-probability lung scans and high clinical suspicion. This approach has been confirmed by the findings of the Prospective Investigative Study of Acute Pulmonary Embolism Diagnosis (PISA-PED), which recommends angiography only in patients whose clinical assessments and perfusion scans are discordant.[20]

Chest Radiograph

The chest radiograph in the patient with PE may be normal, especially in the first 24 hours.[21] Eventually, abnormalities are demonstrated 80% of the time; however, the difficulty is that many of the abnormal findings are not clearly diagnostic for PE.[12] Nonspecific signs include increases in lung densities, effusions, and atelectasis, all of which can occur with many other cardiopulmonary diagnoses. Some characteristic changes in anatomic structures do indicate PE. In more than two-thirds of patients with PE, an enlarged descending pulmonary artery is apparent. Because of pulmonary hypertension, pressure in the pulmonary artery increases and dilatation of this artery occurs, so much so that "sausagelike" has been used to describe this enlargement. Elevation of the diaphragm, enlargement of the right heart shadow, and pleural effusion are the other most common radiographic findings, seen more than 50% of the time in confirmed PE. A wedge-shaped consolidation or a semicircular opacity at the peripheral pleural space known as "Hampton's hump" may also appear.[2] This is considered a late sign and may indicate pulmonary infarction.[13] Westermark's sign is a radiographic sign characterized by dilatation of pulmonary vessels proximal to the thrombus and drastic reduction of blood content and vascular markings in the pulmonary vessels distal to the thrombus. This sign almost always indicates PE, but it occurs in only 15% of cases.[12] Although the chest radiograph can be of value, further, more sensitive diagnostic tools are required to diagnose PE definitively. See Figure 19–2A for a demonstration of chest radiographic changes associated with PE.

Blood Tests

Routine blood tests do not have any definite value in assisting with the diagnosis of PE. Elevated bilirubin and lactate dehydrogenase with a normal AST is present in less than 15% of patients, but these findings clearly do not specify PE. An elevated white blood cell count may be present with pulmonary infarction or an associated infection. Dehydration may be a contributing factor in PE and can be indicated by an elevated hematocrit level, but this finding is certainly not specific to PE.

In symptomatic PE, however, arterial blood gas analysis often indicates the patient's efforts at compensating for the altered pulmonary ventilation and perfusion. Respiratory alkalosis and decreased partial arterial carbon dioxide pressure ($PaCO_2$) due to hyperventilation are often present. Even with compensatory hyperventilation and oxygen therapy, partial arterial oxygen pressure (PaO_2) is usually decreased. In fact, the triad of elevated pH, decreased PaO_2, and decreased $PaCO_2$ is classic for the suspicion of PE in patients without chronic respiratory disease. An additional indication of impaired gas exchange in PE is an assessment of the difference in alveolar oxygen pressure (PAO_2) and PaO_2 (A-a oxygen gradient). At sea level and on room air, the following formula can be used to calculate this gradient:

$$\text{A-a oxygen gradient} = 147 - [(1.2 \times PCO_2) + PaO_2]$$

A normal gradient should not be higher than 1/10 the patient's age in years plus 10. From 5 to 15% of patients with PE have a normal gradient, but not if hypotension or massive PE is present. An elevated gradient is not specific for PE because impaired gas exchange and elevated A-a oxygen gradient can be present in many pulmonary diseases. However, a suddenly elevated A-a oxygen gradient in a patient who has a clear chest radiograph and no wheezing is highly indicative of PE.[13]

Electrocardiography

One may see many changes in the ECG, or there may be none. Only 15% of patients with PE have ECG changes, but often these are nonspecific. The most common changes seen, in order of occurrence, are ST-segment depression, tachycardia, S slurred in V_1 or V_2, late R in aVR, PR-segment elevation or depression, and T-wave inversion in V_1 to V_4. The severity of PE is associated with the presence and extent of ST-segment depression and T-wave inversion. ECG changes indicating right ventricular hypertrophy are infrequent, although new development of right bundle branch block, P-pulmonale (peaked P waves in lead II), right axis deviation, and large R waves in V_1 and V_2 should give rise to the suspicion of this condition.[22] Atrial and ventricular ectopy are the most commonly observed dysrhythmias, with atrial fibrillation the most frequently sustained dysrhythmia. The pattern of $S_1Q_3T_3$ (deep S in lead I, Q in lead III, and inverted T wave in lead III) present in pulmonary infarction is seen in PE only about 15% of the time,[12] a percentage consistent with the occurrence of pulmonary infarct in patients with PE. Several of the changes discussed here can also be consistent with other cardiopulmonary disorders, so again, this diagnostic tool is not specific for PE.

Nursing Diagnoses

The key to managing the care of the patient presenting with symptoms of PE is first to suspect the possible diagnosis. As described previously, astute observations, assessments, and history taking are imperative. The initial diagnosis may occur in various settings. Depending on the patient's overall condition and the therapeutic interventions selected, initial definitive therapy may be started in the emergency department, in the critical care unit, or in the general nursing unit. Overall average length of stay of the patient with an

TABLE 19–5
Nursing Diagnoses: Pulmonary Embolism

Problem Statement	Etiologic Factors
Anxiety	Hypoxia, fear of unknown, pain
Altered tissue perfusion	PE: interruption of pulmonary blood flow
	DVT: hypercoagulability, stasis, inflammation
Decreased cardiac output	Right ventricular failure
	Stasis
	Dehydration
Ineffective breathing pattern	Pain
	Hypoxemia
	Anxiety and fear
Impaired gas exchange	Ventilation–perfusion mismatch
	Atelectasis
	Reembolization
Knowledge deficit	Lack of understanding of DVT and PE disease process, medications, and recovery or preventive care
Pain	Chest pain, inspiration, inflammation of the pleura, hypoxemia
Risk for injury	Anticoagulation therapy

DVT, deep vein thrombosis; PE, pulmonary embolism.

uncomplicated episode of PE is 7 days.[23] The nurse assists in the development of an overall plan of care utilizing a coordinated interdisciplinary team approach. Table 19–5 is a priority list of nursing diagnoses resulting from such team consultation.

Collaborative Management

Collaborative management of the patient with PE is imperative and often involves an interdisciplinary approach with physicians, nurses, paramedics, respiratory therapists, pharmacists, physical or occupational therapists, case managers, dietitians, clergy, and social workers. PE can develop almost immediately in high-risk patients, but it can occur as late as 3 to 4 months after the initial predisposing insult.[18] Because of such variances in the timing of the clinical presentation of PE, many different health care personnel in many different settings must be cognizant of this potential. From the prehospital setting to the emergency department, home health care agency, outpatient clinic, physician's office, extended care or rehabilitation facilities, any hospital unit, and even parish nursing, PE must be considered a viable possibility in high-risk patients when clinical evidence is highly suggestive of this disorder.

Nurses play a key role in all these settings to coordinate the care of these patients. The clinical pathway for PE in Figure 19–3 demonstrates the truly collaborative efforts required in the care of these patients.[23]

Maintaining Optimal Oxygenation

Stabilizing the respiratory system is of highest priority in the management of PE regardless of care setting. Adequate airway, ventilation, and oxygenation must be attained, and oxygen therapy must be started in an attempt to correct hypoxia and hypoxemia. The patient may require a 100% nonrebreathing mask to maintain oxygen saturation at 90% or greater as measured by pulse oximetry. Precaution must be taken to avoid depression of hypoxic drive in patients with chronic lung disease who are carbon dioxide retainers. However, oxygen is not withheld when airway support is available and the patient requires maximal oxygen levels. Because pulse oximetry only indicates the percentage of hemoglobin saturated, hemoglobin and hematocrit should be monitored, and blood and fluids should be given as needed. Pulse oximetry monitoring is especially valuable in trending oxygenation in a noninvasive manner. Inhaled or intravenous bronchodilators are used to decrease bronchoconstriction and wheezing. Chest physical therapy is avoided, to prevent further embolization of thrombi. Encouraging deep breathing, coughing, and use of incentive spirometry increases diaphragmatic excursion. Placing the patient in a high or semi-Fowler position optimizes lung expansion as well. Analgesics are given to reduce splinting, to allow deep breathing, and to decrease oxygen consumption. Morphine sulfate as the analgesic of choice has an additional therapeutic action of decreasing preload and afterload, thus decreasing pulmonary hypertension and right ventricular strain. The nurse must provide a restful, nonstressful environment to avoid anxiety, which can contribute to further respiratory difficulties. If air embolism occurs, the nurse should immediately turn the patient to a left-lying position with the head lower than the body, to prevent further migration of air into the lungs and left side of the heart. In instances of decompression air embolus, recompression protocols using hyperbaric oxygen therapy save hundreds of lives each year.[24]

If hemodynamic instability develops or if the patient's condition becomes critical, transfer to the ICU may be required. As respiratory efforts become more difficult, fatigue occurs, or clinical condition deteriorates, endotracheal intubation, mechanical ventilation, and positive end-expiratory pressure (PEEP) may be required. Short-term sedation and amnesia with continuous infusion low-dose midazolam (Versed) may be required or desirable during this difficult period to prevent ventilatory dysynchrony. These actions are assessed by frequent evaluation of

CLINICAL PATHWAY FOR PULMONARY EMBOLISM (WITHOUT MECHANICAL VENTILATION)

ICD-9 Code 415.1   ELOS 7 days

Nursing Diagnosis/ Collaborative Problem	Expected Outcome (The Patient Is Expected to . . .)	Met/ Not Met	Reason	Date/ Initials
Pain (chest)	State that pain is minimized following appropriate interventions			
Dyspnea, possible crackles	Have respiratory rate return to baseline; have no adventitious sounds; O_2 saturation >90%			
Potential for cardiac complications, such as dysrhythmias, abnormal ECG	Have normal sinus rhythm, pulse rate and quality return to baseline, and no S_3 or S_4 heart sounds present			
Anxiety and fear	Verbalize feelings regarding condition, especially dyspnea and chest pain			

Aspect of Care	Date ___ Day 1	Date ___ Day 2	Date ___ Day 3	Date ___ Day 4	Date ___ Day 5	Date ___ Day 6–7
Assessment	Systems assessment Chest pain assessment and respiratory assessment q1–2h Pulse oximetry VS q1–2h, depending on severity of condition Assess for cardiac complications Assess for bleeding tendencies	Same as Day 1	VS q4h with respiratory assessment Pulse oximetry Systems assessment Assess for bleeding tendencies	Same as Day 3	Same as Day 4	Same as Day 5

Aspect of Care	Date ___ Day 1	Date ___ Day 2	Date ___ Day 3	Date ___ Day 4	Date ___ Day 5	Date ___ Day 6–7
Teaching	Orient to hospital and unit routines Review clinical pathway/plan of care with patient and family Review diagnosis and answer questions	Same as Day 1	Teach measures to help prevent further thromboembolitic complications, such as increased mobility, weight loss, no oral contraceptives Teach early S/S of DVT	Review teaching from Day 3	Begin discharge teaching regarding • Anticoagulation therapy • Bleeding precautions • Need for follow-up laboratory work/diagnostic tests • Activity restrictions • Reduction of risk factors • S/S to report to MD	Reinforce discharge instructions (verbal and written)
Consults	Surgery (if indicated) Respiratory therapy	Dietitian, if indicated for weight reduction	N/A	N/A	N/A	N/A
Laboratory Tests	CBC with differential SMA-6, INR(PT)/APTT, ABGs	INR(PT)/APTT	INR(PT)/APTT ABGs	INR(PT)/APTT	Same as Day 4	Same as Day 5
Other Tests	ECG Chest x-ray Ventilation/perfusion scan Vascular studies (if DVT suspected) Pulmonary angiography (for nonconclusive ventilation/perfusion scan)	ECG	Same as Day 2	N/A	N/A	N/A

Figure 19–3

Sample clinical pathway for a patient experiencing pulmonary embolism without mechanical ventilation. (From Ignatavicius DD, Hausman KA: Clinical Pathways for Collaborative Practice. Philadelphia. W.B. Saunders, 1995, pp 270–273.)

Continued

CLINICAL PATHWAY FOR PULMONARY EMBOLISM (WITHOUT MECHANICAL VENTILATION) Continued

Aspect of Care	Date Day 1	Date Day 2	Date Day 3	Date Day 4	Date Day 5	Date Day 6–7
Medications	Continuous IV heparin via electronic device Stool softener QD PO analgesic PRN	Same as Day 1	Continuous IV heparin Start on oral anticoagulant (Coumadin) Stool softener QD PO analgesic PRN	Continuous IV heparin at decreased rate Coumadin dose based on laboratory values Stool softener PO analgesic PRN	Same as Day 4 (continue decreasing heparin rate per MD)	Same as Day 5
Treatments/ Interventions	I & O q8h Oxygen via N/C or mask Antiembolism stockings SCDs or Venodynes Emotional support Incentive spirometer q2h W/A	Same as Day 1	Same as Day 2	D/C I & O O₂ PRN Antiembolism stockings SCDs or Venodynes Incentive spirometer q2h W/A	Same as Day 4	Same as Day 5
Nutrition	DAT (unless need for calorie/fat restriction)	Same as Day 1	Same as Day 2	Same as Day 3	Same as Day 4	Same as Day 5
Lines/Tubes/ Monitors	Cardiac monitoring Continuous IV fluids at low rate	Same as Day 1 Convert IV to saline lock if adequate PO fluids	D/C cardiac monitor Saline lock	Saline lock	Same as Day 4	D/C saline lock

Aspect of Care	Date ___ Day 1	Date ___ Day 2	Date ___ Day 3	Date ___ Day 4	Date ___ Day 5	Date ___ Day 6–7
Mobility/Self Care	Bed rest HOB up at least 30° Leg exercises, such as ROM, quad sets, ankle pumps, q2h, *unless* DVT in LE If DVT suspected, elevated affected LE Assist with ADLs as needed	Same as Day 1	Same as Day 2	Up in chair BID with assistance as needed While in bed, keep HOB elevated 30° or higher Leg exercises q2h W/A If DVT, remain on bed rest with affected leg elevated Assist with ADLs as needed	Up in room ad lib unless DVT present Leg exercises while in bed	Up in hall ad lib unless DVT present Leg exercises while in bed
Discharge Planning	Assess home environment and personal support systems	Same as Day 1	Same as Day 2	Assess need for placement if patient unable to go home	Arrange for follow-up home health services if needed Arrange for transfer to LTC or other facility if needed	Arrange for follow-up appointment as MD specified Provide information for patient about lab services and availability

Figure 19–3 Continued

vital signs, pulse oximetry, cardiac rhythm, hemodynamic parameters, breath sounds, neurologic status, and tissue perfusion every 15 minutes to every 1 hour as indicated by the patient's condition.

Managing Thrombosis and Restoring Perfusion

Prevention

Prevention is the most important concept in the care of patients with PE, especially in those at high risk. Surprisingly, preventive measures are reported to be used in only one-third of patients with moderate or high thromboembolic risk.[25] Studies report that PE can occur anywhere from within the first week to as late as 3 to 4 weeks postoperatively.[18] Many approaches aimed at altering Virschow's triad of vein injury, blood stasis, and blood coagulability have been reported and are used in the prevention of DVT and PE. Simply keeping the patient properly hydrated and using diuretics judiciously can decrease blood stasis and coagulability. Anticoagulation therapy with heparin or warfarin is used to inhibit coagulation. Warfarin is given to some high-risk orthopedic patients the night before surgery and is continued daily on the first postoperative day to keep daily prothrombin time (PT) at 14 to 16 seconds.[18] Low-molecular-weight heparin preparations such as dalteparin (Fragmin), danaparoid (Orgaran), and enoxaparin (Lovenox) are being given subcutaneously to moderate- and high-risk postoperative patients before and after surgery, and these agents are often continued at home. Platelet function is altered by use of dextran and aspirin. Dextran interferes with platelet and coagulation protein functions, and when given to high-risk patients, it has some value in preventing PE. Aspirin has not been shown to be of significant value in preventing PE,[18, 26] although it is still used. Methods to counteract venous stasis and to promote venous return include thromboembolic compression stockings, pneumatic compression pumps, leg elevation, continuous passive leg movement, and early ambulation.

Anticoagulation Therapy

Anticoagulation therapy is used in DVT and PE to prevent further thrombi formation and to support the body's own natural ability to dissolve existing thrombi. Significant thrombus propagation can occur in seconds or minutes. Heparin is the drug of choice because it accelerates the action of antithrombin II and factor Xa, prevents further fibrin deposits, and inhibits the normal hemostatic mechanisms that support the clot by interfering with thrombin or platelet interactions on the clot itself. Platelets are prevented from releasing serotonin, thereby preventing hypotension and bronchoconstriction. Initiation of heparin therapy should begin as soon as possible even if thrombolytic therapy is eventually started. In the patient with inter-

mediate or high clinical suspicion of PE, it is advisable to start heparin therapy before the diagnosis is confirmed with more diagnostic definitive tests. In patients with high clinical suspicion and severe hemodynamic instability, heparin should be started immediately without delay, before any further diagnostic tests are performed.[25] If no contraindications exist for anticoagulation, the risk of a few hours of heparin therapy is low when compared with the risk of PE.[27] Many heparin dosing guidelines are used and have been published. Standard reported heparin therapy for DVT and PE is to administer an initial loading dose of 5000 to 10,000 U intravenously, followed by a continuous infusion of 1000 U per hour. This dosing standard may be subtherapeutic in many patients because effectiveness of heparin therapy is dose dependent, requiring adjustments based on patient weight and activated partial thromboplastin time.[28] Eighty percent of patients with PE receive no or inappropriate heparin therapy. Although heparin can be given by intravenous intermittent dosing and by subcutaneous administration, continuous infusion initially is desired to prevent complications of bleeding and to maintain consistent levels of anticoagulation. Weight-based dosing by continuous infusion is considered the most therapeutic method of administering heparin and should be used in all patients. Chart 19–1 gives an example of heparin orders that reflects such a weight-based heparin dosing regimen.

Warfarin therapy should be started within 24 hours of diagnosis of DVT or PE. It is unacceptable to start warfarin therapy in patients with thromboembolic disease without prior heparinization because of the clinical hypercoagulability and thrombogenetic state that can occur during early stages of warfarin use.[27] These effects occur because warfarin suppresses production of vitamin K–dependent *anticoagulation* factors before it depletes the desired *procoagulation* factors II, VII, IX, and X.[8, 29] Because it takes 3 to 5 days for the full therapeutic effect of warfarin to occur, warfarin administration is started before heparin therapy is stopped. An initial loading dose of warfarin 10 to 20 mg for the first 2 days, followed by 5 to 10 mg per day,[16] is usually adequate to bring the PT within a therapeutic range of 1.5 to 2.5 times control or the international normalized ratio (INR) within a therapeutic range of 2.0 to 3.0. In patients with documented DVT or PE or in those at high risk for developing these thromboembolic conditions, warfarin therapy is continued for 6 weeks to 3 months. In patients with reoccurring thromboemboli, warfarin therapy may be continued as long as a year. With two or more recurrences[8] or in patients with deficiencies of protein S or C or antithrombin III, anticoagulation therapy should be continued indefinitely.[16]

Complications or side effects of anticoagulation therapy mostly involve those of bleeding. Additionally,

CHART 19-1

Heparin Administration by Weight-Dosing Heparin Orders*

1. Record the patient's weight and height: wt _____ kg, ht _____ in
2. Weight-based heparin (verify bolus and infusion rate with pharmacy):
   Heparin bolus IV now: <u>80 U/kg</u>
   Heparin 25,000 U/250 mL D_5W at 18 U/kg/hr (if rate >1500 U/hr, pharmacist or physician may calculate rate using "dosing weight")
3. Laboratory studies
   a. Activated partial thromboplastin time (aPTT) 6 hours after heparin started
   b. aPTT 6 hours after each dosage adjustment until therapeutic
   c. If aPTT therapeutic, do daily morning aPTT
   d. If any aPTT is not therapeutic, follow dosage chart below (item no. 4 below) until aPTT is therapeutic, and then begin to do daily aPTT
   e. Complete blood count (CBC) every day; call physician if hemoglobin < 10 or platelets < 100,000

   f. Discontinue aPTT and CBC monitoring when heparin discontinued
4. With each aPTT result, adjust heparin infusion as follows:

aPTT result	Heparin dose adjustment
<25 sec	Call physician
25–34 sec	Bolus 3000 U; increase rate 200 U/hr (2 mL/hr)
35–49 sec	Bolus 2000 U; increase rate 100 U/hr (1 mL/hr)
50–70 sec	No change: therapeutic range
71–90 sec	Reduce rate 100 U/hr (1 mL/hr)
91–120 sec	Hold heparin for 1 hr; reduce rate 200 U/hr (2 mL/hr)
>120 sec	Stop infusion; call physician.

*The Pharmacy and Therapeutics Committee recommends use of weight-based dosing except with thrombolytic therapy.
Adapted with permission from standardized heparin orders at Deaconess Hospital, Evansville, IN.

heparin may cause thrombocytopenia within 1 to 20 days after initiation of therapy. Heparin does not cross the placental barrier, whereas warfarin does, and it can damage a developing fetus. Warfarin has the additional potential to interact with several different medications and to cause diarrhea. Nursing standards for the patient receiving anticoagulation therapy revolve around observation for and prevention of bleeding. Stool, urine, emesis, gastric drainage, skin, gums, intravenous sites, and incisions must all be monitored carefully. Antacids and histamine (H_2) blocking agents are given to decrease potential for gastric bleeding. Stool softeners are given to lessen chances of straining, vessel injury, and bleeding. Keeping systemic hypertension under control is essential. Initially keeping the patient on bed rest without excess movement decreases the possibility of embolizing further thrombi.[30] Care must be taken during this period of decreased activity and movement to prevent the hazards of immobility.

Thrombolytic Therapy

Thrombolytic therapy is used to dissolve the current emboli, to prevent formation of further thrombi, and to decrease long-term morbidity. Systemic or catheter-directed regional thrombolytic administration is indi-cated for those with severe DVT or extensive obstruction of venous outflow or in those patients for whom it is important to preserve venous circulation.[8] Currently, in the United States, no more than 10% of patients with PE are treated with thrombolytic therapy, even though a 2-week window of opportunity exists.[28] It has been a long-held position that thrombolytic therapy should be reserved for patients with massive PE with severely compromised hemodynamics or for nonsurgical candidates. This concept should be challenged because thrombolysis in acute PE not only affects immediate outcome, but can also affect long-term quality of life. According to the PIOPED study, the mortality rate for PE treated with anticoagulation alone was 19%; with thrombolytic therapy and anticoagulation, the mortality rate dropped to 9%.[19] Even small asymptomatic PEs can result in development of chronic pulmonary hypertension[27] with a decrease in functional ability. Patients who are hemodynamically stable but who have right ventricular hypokinesis can avoid right ventricular congestive heart failure by implementing thrombolytic therapy. See Figure 19–2D for radiologic results after thrombolytic therapy.

The decision of who *should not* receive thrombolytic therapy is easier than the decision of who *should* receive thrombolytic therapy. Relative contraindications for thrombolytic therapy include external bleeding, internal bleeding, major trauma or surgery, prolonged cardiac arrest resuscitation efforts, large arterial puncture, or pregnancy in the past 2 weeks or uncontrollable long-term hypertension of more than 180/110 mm Hg. Absolute contraindications include brain surgery, ocular surgery, solid organ biopsy, diabetic hemorrhagic retinopathy, or significant hemoptysis in the past 2 weeks or current uncontrolled active internal or external bleeding.[27] Thrombolytic therapy has been given within 24 hours of surgery for postoperative PE that was accompanied by a severe clinical presentation, poor systemic perfusion, profound hypoxemia, unstable hemodynamic status with pulmonary hypertension, and decreasing cardiac output despite vigorous vasoactive support. Although the incidence of postoperative bleeding was increased, certain death was avoided.[31]

Currently, three types of thrombolytic agents are used in PE. All three act by assisting plasminogen to become plasmin, which initiates fibrinolysis. Streptokinase and urokinase do this by systemically cleaving peptide bonds in plasminogen, thus converting it to plasmin. Recombinant tissue plasminogen activator (rtPA) binds to fibrin in a thrombus before converting plasminogen to plasmin, thus acting more locally. Chart 19–2 has Food and Drug Administration (FDA)–approved thrombolytic regimens for PE. In spite of the FDA and manufacturer's recommendations for rtPA, the current literature recommends a "front-loading" method of administration by giving 15 mg as an initial rapid intravenous bolus, followed by 50 mg over the next 30 minutes, with the remaining 35 mg given over the next hour. Dosage is adjusted for those patients less than 70 kg. Even though rtPA is expensive, many physicians believe that the cost is justified because rtPA is much faster acting than streptokinase and is safer than urokinase.[27] Chart 19–3 describes the administration of anticoagulants beyond the ICU.

Pharmacologic characteristics are similar for all three thrombolytic agents. Adverse reactions include severe spontaneous hemorrhage, hypotension, dysrhythmias, edema, nausea or vomiting, and hypersensitivity reactions. Hypersensitivity reactions are treated with epinephrine, antihistamines, and corticosteroids. Streptokinase and urokinase have added adverse reactions of bronchospasm and minor breathing difficulty. Patients who have ever received streptokinase or who have had a recent streptococcal infection will have developed resistance to the drug and antibodies that can result in a major allergic response. Hypersensitivity to streptokinase can be determined by giving 100 IU intradermally and observing for a wheal-and-flare response within 20 minutes. If a sensitivity reaction is not apparent, a higher loading dose may be required to adjust for resistance to the streptokinase. Increased risk of bleeding can occur if the patient receiving thrombolytic agents is taking anticoagulants, aspirin, dipyridamole, indomethacin, phenylbutazone, or other drugs affecting platelet activity. Bleeding during streptokinase and urokinase treatment can be reversed and treated with administration of aminocaproic acid, fresh frozen plasma, and cryoprecipitate. There is no direct reversal agent for rtPA. The incidence of intracranial bleeding resulting from PE treated with thrombolytic drugs is 1%.[28] Should severe bleeding or anaphylactic reactions occur, thrombolytic agents should be stopped, and the physician should be notified.

The standards of nursing care for the patient receiving thrombolytic therapy are similar to those for the patient receiving anticoagulation therapy. The nurse must monitor the patient for bleeding and must prevent tissue damage leading to bleeding. The patient should have at least one other intravenous access for administering other medications and drawing blood for laboratory tests. All venipuncture sites, incisions, and drains should be monitored for bleeding every 15 to 60 minutes. Pressure on venipuncture sites should be held for at least 10 minutes. Keeping the patient in bed with siderails up is preferred until thrombolytic therapy is over, to avoid injury. Blood pressure measurements should be taken as infrequently as possible while still maintaining adequate assessments. Automatic (noninvasive) blood pressure machines can be safely used during thrombolytic therapy with periodic inspection of the skin under the blood pressure cuff. Unnecessary handling of the patient should be avoided because it can

CHART 19–2

Food and Drug Administration–Approved Thrombolytic Regimens for Pulmonary Embolism*

Streptokinase: 250,000 IU as loading dose over 30 min followed by 100,000 IU/hr for 24–72 hr (approved in 1977)
Urokinase: 4400 IU/kg as loading dose over 10 min followed by 4400 IU/kg/hr for 12–24 hr (approved in 1978)
Recombinant tissue plasminogen activator (rtPA): 100 mg in continuous infusion over 2 hours (approved in 1990)

*Does not reflect current "front-loading" administration practices

CHART 19–3

BEYOND THE ICU: ANTICOAGULATION CLINICS

Warfarin sodium is the thirteenth most prescribed drug in the United States and is the fifth most prescribed cardiovascular drug. Patients with venous thromboemboli, pulmonary emboli, heart valve implants, atrial fibrillation, or dilated cardiomyopathy require anticoagulation therapy, sometimes for the rest of their lives. These patients are no longer kept or admitted in the hospital for many days to regulate doses to the appropriate levels. Outpatient management of this potentially dangerous drug has become the standard; however, careful monitoring of these outpatients is essential. Too much or too little medication can lead to serious and sometimes fatal hemorrhagic or thrombotic episodes. Frequent prothrombin time (PT) and international normalized ratio monitoring, extensive education, multiple dose adjustments, and intense follow-up are required. It is a time-consuming and costly effort. In fact, narrow therapeutic anticoagulation ranges and fear of complications have led to physicians' reluctance to prescribe anticoagulation therapy.

Anticoagulation Clinic Routine

A multidisciplinary anticoagulation clinic answers many concerns with anticoagulation therapy. Most programs are physician directed, but they are coordinated by an advance practice or registered nurse, a physician assistant, or a pharmacist. Usually, a patient is referred to an anticoagulation clinic by the primary care provider. The diagnosis and the reason for anticoagulation along with the therapeutic range and the expected duration of anticoagulation are communicated to the clinic. Patients are usually on a stable dose of anticoagulation, but many clinics do accept patients initially, to regulate their anticoagulation regimen. Patients continue to see their primary physicians for routine care and periodic evaluations. The anticoagulation clinic keeps in close contact with the primary physician by sending feedback reports on the patient's progress. The clinic makes appropriate referrals back to the primary physician if the patient's condition warrants.

Anticoagulation clinics not only adjust medication doses, but they also stress patient education and responsibilities. Anticoagulation classes taught by a nurse, dietitian, or pharmacist are required. Content in these classes includes reasons for anticoagulation therapy, anticoagulation effects, drug administration, drug–diet interactions, drug–drug interactions, lifestyle modifications, recognition of unusual signs and symptoms, and instructions on when to call the clinic. Patients' responsibilities are emphasized initially and during all clinic visits. Written contractual agreements are often used. Patients acknowledge their understanding of the teaching they receive, agree to take their medication as prescribed, come to the clinic as required, have their blood drawn as ordered, abide by recommended dietary restrictions, carry identification of anticoagulation therapy, and agree to notify all physicians, including their dentist, that they are taking anticoagulation therapy. Because patient responsibility is so important to compliance with treatment, many clinics include criteria for withdrawal of clinic services, including failure to attend scheduled clinic visits.

Anticoagulation Clinic Outcomes

Results of anticoagulation clinics are significant. Clinical outcomes are improved because therapeutic anticoagulation levels are achieved more easily and better with less hemorrhage and thromboembolism. A 21% reduction in major bleeding risk and a 30% reduction in thromboembolism risk have been reported when comparing anticoagulation clinic care with routine medical care. The literature reports that one-third or more of bleeding episodes occur within the first 90 days of anticoagulation therapy. Often, anticoagulation therapy unmasks a previously undetected and nonproblematic local bleeding source. In addition, dose adjustments are less tightly controlled and more frequent at the beginning of anticoagulation therapy, resulting in more episodes of bleeding. These early problems during anticoagulation therapy further validate the necessity of patient follow-up at an outpatient anticoagulation clinic.

Future of Anticoagulation Management

Future trends indicate that home patient-managed anticoagulation therapy is on the horizon. Although, at this time, instruments for home self-testing of PT levels are not approved or available in the United States, such self-management practices have become widespread in some parts of Europe. Ansell and colleagues reported a 7-year study of 20 patients who managed their anticoagulation therapy by fingerstick measurements of PT. Results indicate that this type of home management was as effective and safe as that of management of a control group of patients by an anticoagulation clinic, and

Continued

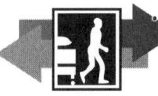

CHART 19–3

BEYOND THE ICU: ANTICOAGULATION CLINICS *(Continued)*

in some instances it was better. Complication rates between the two groups were no different. These home self-managed patients were within their target therapeutic PT range 88.6% of the time, as compared with 68% of the time in clinic-managed

patients. The rationale for these results includes fewer dosage changes and extremely high patient satisfaction and empowerment. Patients felt more in control of their illness, and compliance was improved.

Ansell JE, Hughes R: Evolving models of warfarin management: anticoagulation clinics, patient self-monitoring, and patient self-management [editorial]. Am Heart J 135:1095–1100, 1996.

Ansell J, Patel N, Ostrovsky D, et al: Long-term patient self-management of oral anticoagulation. Arch Intern Med 155:2185–2189, 1995.

Brosnan J: A patient-focused pathway for ambulatory anticoagulation care. J Nurs Care Qual 11:41–53, 1996.

Bussey HL, Chiquette E, Amato M: Anticoagulation clinic care versus routine medical care: a review and interim report. J Thromb Thrombolysis 2:315–319, 1996.

La Piana Simonsen L: Top 200 drugs. Pharm Times 61:17–23, 1995.

Palareti G, Leali N, Coccheri S, et al: Bleeding complications of oral anticoagulant treatment: an inception-cohort, prospective collaborative study (ISCOAT). Lancet 348:423–428, 1996.

result in minor tissue damage that causes large hematomas. Neurologic status should be assessed at least once a shift and more often should one suspect intracranial bleeding.[30]

Vena Caval Interruption

Interruption of the inferior vena cava is used in certain instances in an attempt to prevent lower extremity and pelvic vein thrombi from reaching the pulmonary vasculature. Surgical ligation can be done of the inferior vena cava just below the renal veins and of the ovarian and spermatic veins, although the formation of large retroperitoneal collateral vessels can make this a tempo-

rary solution. Patients with preexisting venous disease may develop venous insufficiency after vena caval ligation. Because of these sequelae, the preferred method of vena caval interruption is with an umbrellalike filter placed into the inferior vena cava. The most common stainless steel device used is the Greenfield filter (Figure 19–4), which is inserted through the internal jugular vein. This filter is used in high-risk patients in whom anticoagulation therapy is contraindicated, complications of anticoagulation prevent continued administration, or preoperative PE already exists.[18] It is also of value in the presence of paradoxic emboli, cor pulmonale with no tolerance for additional clots, a large floating thrombus

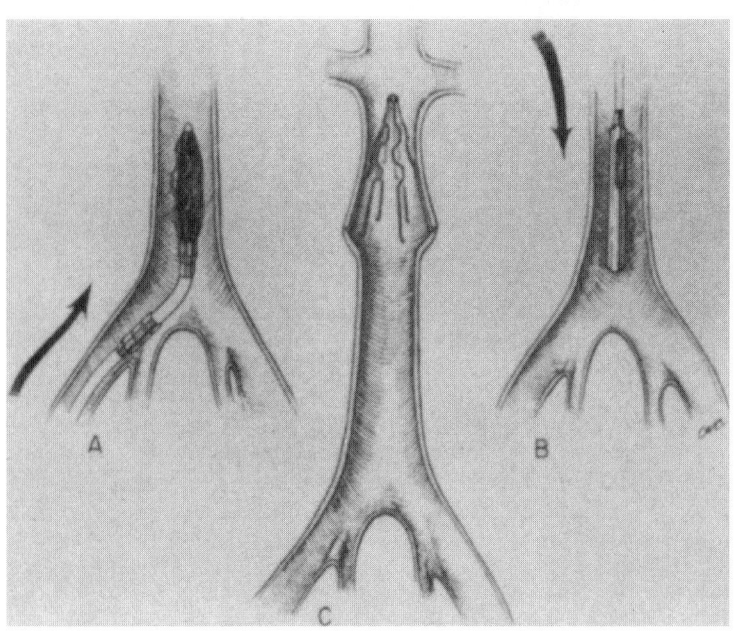

Figure 19–4

Greenfield filter. *A,* Insertion of the filter by means of a carrier catheter inserted from the femoral vein. *B,* Insertion of the filter in retrograde fashion from the jugular vein. *C,* Fixation is achieved as limbs spring open and the recurved hooks engage the wall of the inferior vena cava. (From Greenfield, LJ: Pulmonary embolism: diagnosis and management. Curr Probl Surg 13:1, 1976. Copyright © 1976 by Year Book Medical Publishers, Inc., Chicago.)

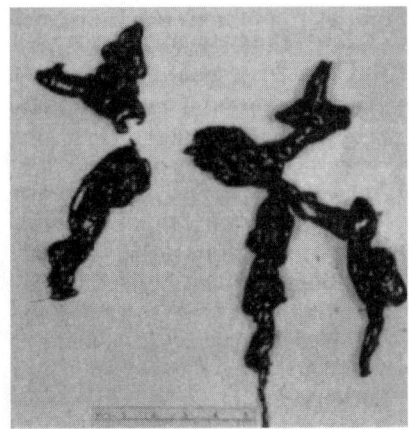

Figure 19–5

Emboli removed from pulmonary arteries. (From Sabiston, DC Jr: Pathophysiology, diagnosis, and management of pulmonary embolism. Adv Surg 3:351, 1968.)

in the deep proximal veins, or in chronic pulmonary hypertension resulting from chronic PE.[27] This filter can trap emboli larger than 3 mm and is most effective if used within the first week of diagnosis of PE. Long-term patency rate is 97%, with only a 4 to 5% PE recurrence rate. Efficacy of the filter continues until 80% of the filter is filled with thrombus. However, the body's normal thrombolytic mechanisms usually dissolve the clots collected in the filter, thereby making removal unnecessary and uncommon. The most common complication, migration of the filter, occurs in only 7% of patients.[18]

Embolectomy

In some situations, it may be necessary to perform a thoracotomy to remove PE surgically using low-flow hypothermic cardiopulmonary bypass. Embolectomy may be indicated in those patients for whom anticoagulation and thrombolytic therapies are contraindicated or have been ineffective, pulmonary vasculature is 50% occluded with thrombi, or sudden death is imminent. This acute surgical procedure carries an 11 to 36.5% mortality rate[32,33] and is most successful if it is performed within 24 hours of diagnosis of the PE.

Thromboendarterectomy in those patients with chronic pulmonary hypertension and cor pulmonale resulting from chronic PE can result in vastly improved pulmonary artery pressures, cardiac index, and functional class as measured by the New York Heart Association criteria.[34] Removal of the chronic clot only does not restore the pulmonary vessels' expandability. Instead, the pulmonary artery is peeled off the intact thrombi until the small branching ends pop out of the small subsegmental branches (Figure 19–5). Although it is technically more difficult to remove these chronic clots as compared with fresh clots,[35] because of a more stable preoperative clinical condition, operative mortality is 5 to 12.6%.[36] This operation should not be done until significant lifestyle impairment has occurred, and then only at centers that specialize in this difficult procedure.

Maintaining Hemodynamic Stability

Fluid Management

Volume expansion with normal saline or dextran is indicated to ensure adequate left ventricular filling pressures and thus to maintain left ventricular output and

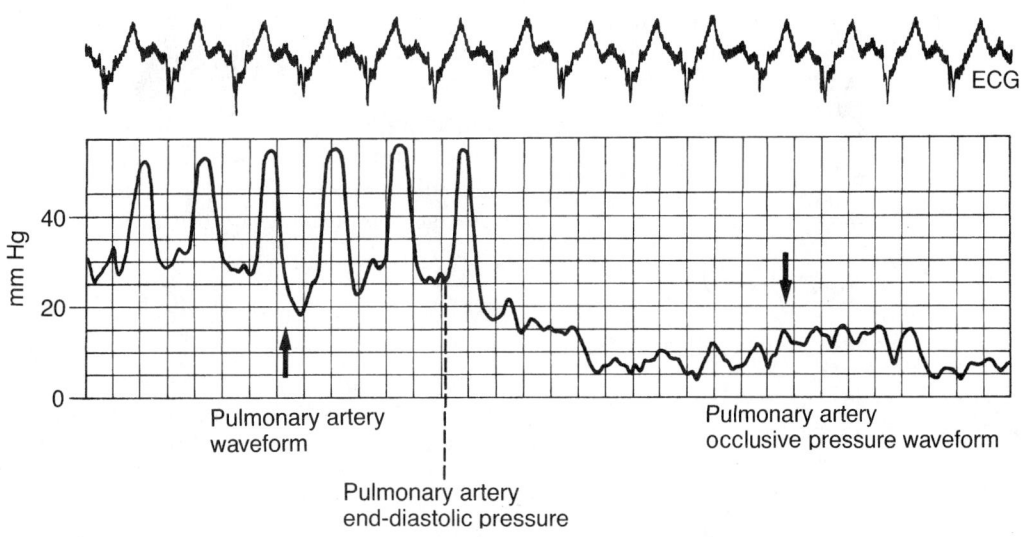

Figure 19–6

Pulmonary hypertension secondary to massive pulmonary embolism. Note the increased pulmonary artery diastolic to occlusive pressure (PAD-PAOP) gradient. Note also the respiratory-induced variation in the waveform baseline resulting from the patient's dyspnea. (From Darovic GO: Hemodynamic Monitoring, 2nd ed. Philadelphia, W.B. Saunders, 1995.)

systemic circulation. Dextran 40 or 70 decreases platelet aggregation and adhesion and results in copolymerization with fibrin, thus making it more susceptible to fibrinolysis. Fluid administration must be monitored carefully because aggressive therapy can result in pushing the already dilated right ventricle into complete collapse. When the right ventricle is in danger of serious failure, transfer to the ICU and placement of a pulmonary artery Swan–Ganz catheter are essential to monitor and treat this precarious hemodynamic profile (Figure 19–6). If the right ventricular end-diastolic pressures are high, diuresis may be required to decrease right ventricular preload, to increase pulmonary vessel compliance, and to remove interstitial fluid from the lungs.[1] Phlebotomy to keep the hematocrit below 50% may be used. Corticosteroid therapy may be instituted, especially if fat emboli are present.

Vasoactive Support

Vasoactive support is of particular importance when the patient develops pulmonary hypertension and acute cor pulmonale. Preload reduction decreases right ventricular pressures and unloads pulmonary vascular congestion. Because the systemic circulation is more sensitive to vasodilators than is the pulmonary circulation, it is difficult to decrease pulmonary vascular resistance without associated systemic hypotension. Hydralazine, nifedipine, captopril, prostaglan-

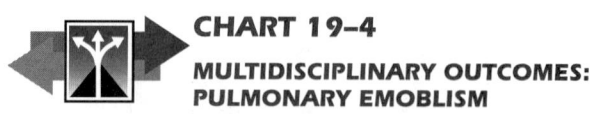

CHART 19–4

MULTIDISCIPLINARY OUTCOMES: PULMONARY EMOBLISM

Restoration of optimal and adequate oxygenation
Maintenance of hemodynamic stability
Achievement of a maximal comfort level
Prevention of recurrent pulmonary embolism and maintenance of health management
Reduction of the patient's anxiety and fear
Demonstration by the patient of an understanding of home care and follow-up instructions

dins, and aminophylline are helpful in achieving this goal, especially if dobutamine infusion is used to increase contractility. Trials with inhaled vasodilators of nitric oxide and prostacylin have been effective in further reducing pulmonary hypertension.[37] Suppression of microvascular inflammatory mediators by corticosteroids is useful in PE due to fat embolism or to prevent decompensation of chronic thromboembolic cor pulmonale.[38] Beta-adrenergic drugs are especially helpful because beta$_1$ stimulation results in positive inotropic support of the ventricles, whereas beta$_2$ stimulation results in decreases in pulmonary vascular resistance and pulmonary artery pressures. Epinephrine at low beta-agonist infusion rates can achieve these effects. Norepinephrine may be used in patients with profound decreases in systemic blood pressure and cardiac output.[27]

Observing for Complications

Complications can be extensive and require astute assessment skills. Primary complications occur in the cardiopulmonary system, but they can involve multiple organ systems as well. Table 19–6 has for a complete list of possible complications.

TABLE 19–6
Complications of Pulmonary Embolism

System	Complication
Cardiovascular	Recurrent thromboembolism
	Myocardial infarction
	Cardiogenic shock
	Dysrhythmias
	Sudden death
Pulmonary	Acute respiratory distress syndrome
	Pneumonia
	Atelectasis
	Pleural effusion
	Pulmonary hypertension
	Pulmonary infarction
Neurologic	Thromboembolic cerebrovascular accident
	Hemorrhagic cerebrovascular accident
Gastrointestinal	Bowel infarction
	Splenic infarction
	Liver failure
	Gastrointestinal bleeding
Metabolic or renal	Disseminated intravascular coagulopathy
	Thrombocytopenia
	Acute renal failure
	Renal infarction

Multidisciplinary Outcomes

Multidisciplinary outcomes are determined by the phase of the patient's care. Priorities are different, depending on the severity of the PE and the acuteness of the episode (Chart 19–4).

PNEUMOTHORAX

Pneumothorax is a disorder that most often initially occurs outside the clinical setting because of intentional or accidental trauma as a result of motor vehicle accidents, falls, or gunshots and stabbings. In the hospital, pneumothorax is seen as a complication arising from such therapeutic treatments as thoracentesis, central line placement, and mechanical ventilation. It can, however, accompany several different pulmonary and systemic diseases. Symptoms are similar to those of PE—chest pain and dyspnea. Often, time is of the essence in correctly identifying this situation. The nurse must be aware of which patients are more likely to experience this acute life-threatening condition, what are the accompanying symptoms, and what actions are essential when this problem arises.

ETIOLOGY AND PATHOPHYSIOLOGY

Pneumothorax is a condition in which air leaks into the pleural space and the lung collapses (Figure 19–7). The visceral pleura closest to the lungs and the parietal pleura closest to the chest wall are usually separated by a potential space containing a small amount of pleural fluid. The two pleurae are maintained in close proximity by the usual negative subatmospheric pressure in the pleural space. When the continuity of these pleurae is broken, atmospheric air rushes into the pleural space, with a resulting loss of the negative pressure. The visceral pleura is no longer held in place next to the parietal pleura by the suction of the nega-

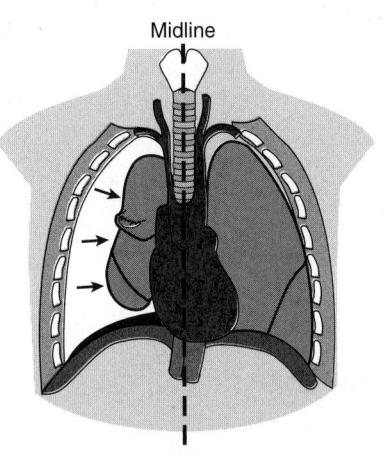

Midline

A CLOSED PNEUMOTHORAX

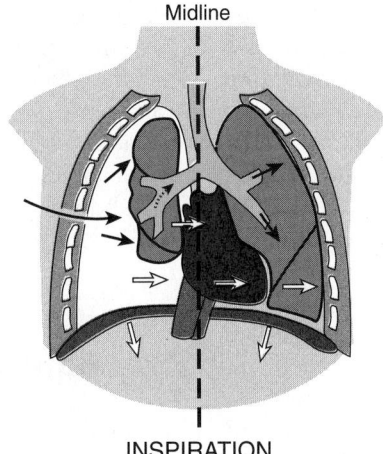

Midline

INSPIRATION

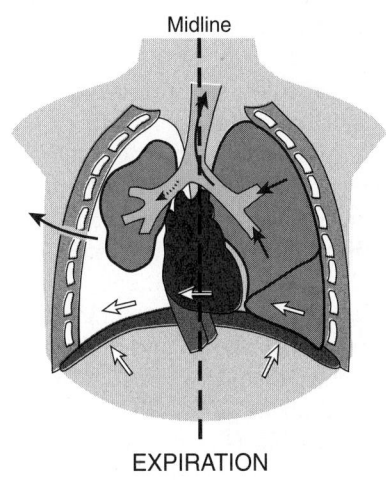

Midline

EXPIRATION

B OPEN PNEUMOTHORAX

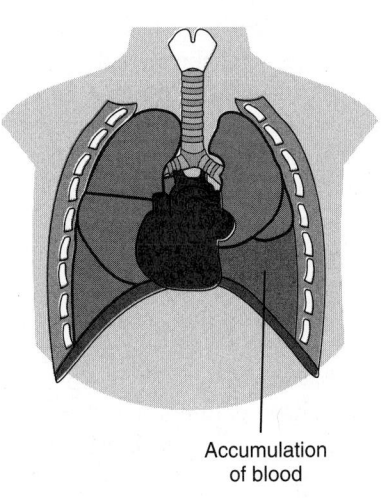

Accumulation of blood

C HEMOTHORAX

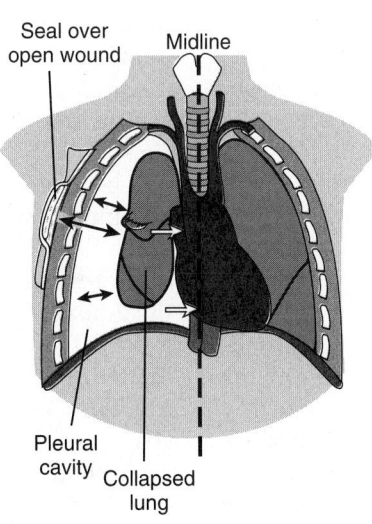

Seal over open wound Midline

Pleural cavity Collapsed lung

WITH SEALED WOUND

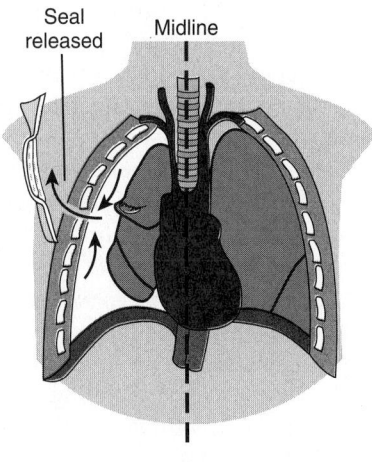

Seal released Midline

WITH SEAL RELEASED

D TENSION PNEUMOTHORAX

Figure 19–7

A, Closed pneumothorax. *B,* Open pneumothorax (sucking chest wound). *C,* Hemothorax. *D,* Tension pneumothorax. (Redrawn from Black JM, Matassarin-Jacobs E (eds): *Medical-Surgical Nursing,* 5th ed. Philadelphia, W.B. Saunders, 1997.)

tive pressure, and the lung collapses. Lung compliance, vital capacity, and total lung capacity are decreased. Hypoxia can result from V/Q mismatch.[39] Pneumo-thorax is more common on the right side, and in 10% of patients it occurs bilaterally.[39, 40] Pneumothorax can be classified as either spontaneous or traumatic, depending on its origin.

Spontaneous Pneumothorax

A spontaneous pneumothorax is either due to a primary idiopathic condition or a secondary disease process. The incidence of primary pneumothorax is 8.6 in 100,000 per year and is more common in males than females by a ratio of 6:1, with a peak age occurrence between 20 and 40 years. Spontaneous pneumothorax may have no underlying cause, or it may be caused by rupture of a previously undetected bulla, a small air- or fluid-filled sac in the lung, or of a bleb, a pleural blisterlike formation. There is a 20 to 50% recurrence rate of spontaneous pneumothorax, and 90% of these occur on the same side. After a second episode, the recurrence rate increases to 60 to 80%.[39]

Secondary pneumothorax is also more common in males and has an incidence of 6.3 in 100,000 per year. It is usually due to underlying pulmonary disease, which accounts for the second highest age group incidence of between 45 and 65 years.[39] Causes of secondary pneumothorax are varied. In chronic obstructive pulmonary disease (COPD), slow destruction of alveolar walls and poor pulmonary recoil result in slowly developing pneumothoraces. Signs and symptoms are frequently overlooked because the pain and dyspnea accompanying the pneumothorax appear to be an exacerbation of the primary COPD process. The mortality rate in these patients from pneumothorax is 16%.[39]

In malignant pulmonary disease, rapid neoplastic growth can cause pleural perforation from necrosis, or it can cause bronchial obstruction, alveolar distention, and bleb formation, again resulting in pleural destruction. Both mechanisms can result in pneumothorax. Patients with acquired immunodeficiency syndrome (AIDS) and *Pneumocystis carinii* pneumonia (PCP) have similar pathophysiologic features. Adhesions, nodules, blebs, and bullae occur more frequently in the lungs of AIDS patients with PCP. Diffuse necrotizing destruction of peripheral lung tissue occurs regardless of vigorous treatment with aerosol pentamidine. Active PCP infection is poorly penetrated in the lung periphery by the aerosol treatments, and the infection continues to proliferate, resulting in tissue destruction and pneumothorax. In these patients, the incidence of pneumothorax has been reported to be 4000 in 100,000,[41] a rate much higher than in the rest of the population. Hospitalized AIDS patients with PCP and

pneumothorax have a mortality rate of 50%. If these same patients require mechanical ventilation, mortality reaches 90%.[42]

Other pulmonary diseases resulting in secondary pneumothorax include cystic fibrosis, hyaline membrane disease and meconium aspiration in neonates, and cavitary tubercular disease. Patients with pulmonary tuberculosis can also develop pneumothorax and, eventually, tuberculous empyema. When a spontaneous pneumothorax is associated with weight loss, fever, and productive cough, tuberculosis should be suspected. Of those with spontaneous pneumothorax, 2 to 3% are found later to have tuberculosis and probably had it at the time of their pneumothorax.[39] Episodes of spontaneous pneumothorax also occur during menstruation, called catamenial spontaneous pneumothorax. This condition occurs most often within 2 to 3 days after menses begins. It is most prevalent in women in their thirties and forties and occurs 90% of the time on the right side. Theories for this unusual occurrence include pulmonary endometriosis, rupture of pulmonary bleb or alveoli due to elevated prostaglandin F_2 levels, and air entering the abdominal cavity through the fallopian tubes and finding its way to the pulmonary cavity by a diaphragmatic defect.[43]

Traumatic Pneumothorax

Traumatic pneumothorax occurs when a lung collapses as a result of physical injury and is either classified as an open sucking chest wound (see Figure 19–7B) or a closed blunt injury. The incidence is 300 in 100,000 people per year. Gunshot or knife wounds, motor vehicle accidents, and diving accidents are accidental causes of traumatic pneumothorax. High-risk medical procedures such as transbronchial biopsy, central line placement, thoracentesis, pleural biopsy, chest tube placement, intercostal needle anesthesia, and esphagoscopy are also associated with traumatic pneumothorax. Pneumothorax after thoracentesis in patients with COPD is so prevalent that some research indicates that such procedures should be done under the guidance of sonography[44] (Chart 19–5).

With traumatic pneumothorax, blood vessels can be injured, resulting in hemothorax or chylothorax. Hemothorax occurs when blood collects in the pleural space (see Figure 19–7C). These patients may lose significant amounts of blood and fluid, and hypotension and death can occur. If complete blood drainage from the chest cavity is not accomplished, fibrin will eventually deposit over the pleural surfaces, with resulting fibrothorax. The fixed trapped lung cannot reexpand well, and surgical intervention with decortication or removal of the peel that has developed must be done.

CHART 19-5

RESEARCH UTILIZATION: MONITORING FOR COMPLICATION AFTER THORACENTESIS

Abstract: Thoracentesis is a common procedure used for diagnostic and therapeutic measures. The pneumothorax complication rate has been reported to be 3 to 20%. This prospective study evaluated whether patients with chronic obstructive pulmonary disease (COPD) had a higher frequency of pneumothorax after thoracentesis compared with patients without COPD. Included in this study were 106 patients with radiologically documented pleural effusions, 70 patients without COPD, and 36 patients with COPD. Prior chest radiographs or pulmonary function tests determined the presence of obstructive airway disease. Utilizing a precise, fixed protocol, thoracentesis was performed by various physicians including third-year medical residents and pulmonologists. Within 2 hours, chest radiographs were taken to determine the therapeutic value of the thoracentesis and to assess for the presence of pneumothorax. Results showed that 28 of 106 patients or 26.4% developed a pneumothorax after thoracentesis; 13 of the 70 patients without COPD (18.5%) and 15 of the 36 patients with COPD (41.7%) developed a pneumothorax. Seven of the 9 patients who required chest tubes for this problem had COPD. There was no difference in the occurrence of pneumothorax when the thoracentesis was done for diagnostic or therapeutic purposes. No physician was responsible for more than one pneumothorax, and there was no difference in occurrence among the type of physicians. The overall conclusion was that a statistically significant difference $(P = .005)$ was noted in the occurrence of pneumothorax with thoracentesis in patients with COPD versus patients without COPD.

Critique: Although this study was well done with strict protocols, it was composed of a small population of convenience. The results are limited, but they do suggest a pattern with obvious implications. A larger study utilizing the same research design would be desirable.

Nursing Considerations: This study has implications for the nurse assisting with a thoracentesis or the acute care nurse practitioner performing a thoracentesis. Realizing that a patient with COPD is more at risk of pneumothorax during a thoracentesis alerts the nurse to observe the patient more closely during and after the procedure. Forewarned is forearmed by ensuring that a postthoracentesis chest radiograph is performed and by having oxygen and chest tube insertion equipment readily available. Patients with COPD have changes in lung parenchyma and in mechanical forces of the chest. Alveolar pressures are altered and may prevent the visceral pleura that is accidentally punctured from sealing over properly. In addition, peripheral blebs are common in the lungs of patients with COPD, as are recurrent inflammatory processes resulting in parenchymal fibrosis and air trapping. This study suggests that all these alterations increase the risk of pneumothorax during thoracentesis. Recommendations of the study suggest that a needle smaller than the 18 gauge used in this study be used for thoracentesis in these high-risk patients if at all possible. In addition, sonography-guided thoracentesis was suggested in patients with COPD, and this procedure has been shown to be safer than needle-catheter or needle-only methods.

Source: Brandstetter RD, Karetzky M, Rastogi R, et al: Pneumothorax after thoracentesis in chronic obstructive pulmonary disease. Heart Lung 23:67–70, 1994.

Chylothorax occurs when lymph fluid collects in the pleural space. Traumatic tearing of the thoracic duct or rupture of the thoracic duct by expanding tumors can cause the appearance of a white, creamy liquid in the chest tube.[39]

Tension Pneumothorax

Any pneumothorax can develop into a tension pneumothorax, in which air is trapped in the intrapleural space and causes pressures to be higher than those of the lung tissue. This situation occurs only in 2 to 3% of patients. Because of a "one-way" valve effect, air enters the pleural space during inspiration, but it cannot escape during expiration. The pleural space in effect is "blown up" like a balloon during inspiration, causing excessive pressure on surrounding areas. The remaining lung tissue and vascular structures including the heart are compressed, and the trachea is pushed toward the opposite side, resulting in tracheal deviation (see Figure 19–7D). Blood flow to and from the heart is decreased to the point of a critical emergency situation. This pressure must be released quickly, or death follows.

Assessment

Presentation of pneumothorax varies depending on its cause, the amount of lung collapsed, and the presence of prior lung disease. The nurse must make a careful assessment of the patient's history and clinical findings. Other diseases or disorders that may mimic pneumothorax include PE, myocardial infarction, acute aortic dissection, pericarditis, perforated gastric ulcer, pneumonia, and esophageal rupture. Because of the critical nature of acute pneumothorax, an accurate assessment of the situation with implementation of the correct therapeutic modalities must be done without delay.

History

The nurse should assess the patient for a history of asthma, COPD, cigarette smoking, chest trauma, pre-

TABLE 19–7
Risk Factors for Developing Pneumothorax

Type of Pneumothorax	Risk Factors
Spontaneous Pneumothorax	Bleb or bulla
	Emphysema
	AIDS
	Cystic fibrosis
	Tuberculosis
	Necrotizing pneumonia
	Malignancy
	Barotrauma or positive end-expiratory pressure
	Chest tube malfunction
	High altitudes
	Decompression diving injuries
	Ankylosing spondylitis
	Lymphangial myxomatosis
	Cocaine use
	Menstruation
Traumatic Pneumothorax	Chest surgery
	Insertion of central line
	Thoracentesis
	Gunshot wound
	Knife wound
	Penetrating foreign object
	Falls
	Motor vehicle accidents
	Blunt chest trauma
	Fractured rib

vious pneumothorax, rapid ascent to high altitudes, or histiocytosis, a condition caused by an overgrowth of histiocytes in the lungs. A familial history of pneumothorax is also a contributing factor because bleb or bulla formation may be genetic. Of patients with spontaneous pneumothorax, 11.5% have such a positive family history.[45] The nurse should also determine whether high-risk medical procedures or treatments associated with pneumothorax have been performed recently. It is common practice to obtain a chest radiograph after central line insertion and thoracentesis and during mechanical ventilation. The reported incidence of pneumothorax is 1 to 12% after central line insertion, 3 to 20% after thoracentesis,[46] and 3 to 4% in patients with mechanical ventilation. Risk factors for pneumothorax during mechanical ventilation include PEEP greater than 15 cm H_2O, tidal volume greater than 12 mL/kg, peak airway pressure higher than 60 cm H_2O, COPD, acute respiratory distress syndrome, (ARDS), subcutaneous emphysema, or pneumomediastinum.[47] Other risk factors for pneumothorax are listed in Table 19–7.

Physical Presentation

The primary presenting symptom in pneumothorax is the onset of sudden pain. This pain may be sharp and pleuritic, but later it may become dull and persistent. It often is worsened by deep breathing, coughing, or moving. The second most common symptom is shortness of breath. Rapid respiratory rate and easy fatigue may also be present. As expected, acute anxiety due to the pain, dyspnea, and hypoxia may develop. Asymmetric chest movement may occur, including splinting of ribs with breathing, little or no chest wall movement during breathing, or paradoxic chest movement, as demonstrated with a flail chest. Tympany and hyperresonance with percussion may be heard on the affected side. Breath sounds may be absent or decreased on the affected side. In chest trauma, when auscultation indicates abnormal or absent breath sounds, pneumothorax or hemothorax is almost certain. However, negative findings do not rule out the presence of these disorders. In one study on chest trauma, pneumothorax of up to 28% and hemothorax of 600 to 800 mL of blood were reported as missed by auscultation performed by experienced practitioners.[48]

If the pneumothorax is large, symptoms become more pronounced. Decreased tactile and vocal fremitus develops. The heart may shift in the chest, thus causing a shift in the point of maximal impulse (PMI) of the heartbeat. Air escapes into the surrounding soft tissues, with subcutaneous emphysema or crepitus developing to the point at which the patient's airway may be compromised. As torsion on the great vessels and bronchi increases, the neck veins become distended, tachycardia develops, cyanosis progresses, hypotension worsens, and cardiovascular collapse occurs. Sudden death with pulseless electrical activity from a nonpumping cardiac rhythm results.[49]

Diagnostic Findings

The most common immediate diagnostic tests performed for pneumothorax are chest radiography and arterial blood gas analysis. In clear-cut cases of pneumothorax with substantial clinical presentation, delaying treatment before these tests are done can be detrimental. Treatment must not be delayed for chest radiographic confirmation. When the diagnosis is in doubt or the patient's condition is not acute, chest radiography produces definitive findings. Pneumothorax is usually best visualized at the lung apex on an upright chest film, but it is clearest in the base or lateral lung area in a supine film.[50] Air in the pleural space appears black, whereas the compressed visceral pleura is identified by a thin line with areas of hyperlucency. If a hemothorax of greater than 250 mL is present, the costophrenic angle may be blunted. Widening of the mediastinum and the intercostal spaces and a depressed diaphragm may also be apparent.[51] Performing a chest radiograph at the end of expiration versus inspiration makes these changes even more pronounced.

Because the chest radiograph is a two-dimensional picture of the lung, which is a three-dimensional sphere within a sphere, a pneumothorax may be larger than radiographically evident. A small pneumothorax occurs when less than 15% of the pleural space is filled with air; 15 to 60% is considered medium, and more than 60% is considered large. Measuring the greatest distance from the pleural line to the chest wall is also a method by which to gauge the size of a pneumothorax. Less than 1 cm is small, 1 to 2 cm is medium, and wider than the deflated lung is considered large.[52] Chest radiography may not clearly indicate the extent of resolution of a hemothorax after several days. To better evaluate this situation, CT scanning of the chest is especially effective.[53]

Arterial blood gas analysis results depend on the extent of the pneumothorax and the degree of respiratory compensation. With a small pneumothorax, results may be normal or may even reveal a slight respiratory alkalosis due to hyperventilation. However, with a substantial pneumothorax, respiratory acidosis with a decrease in PaO_2 and an increase in $PaCO_2$ is expected. Although arterial blood gas analysis may be helpful to distinguish pneumothorax from PE, clinical presentation and physical assessment are of more value. Again, in cases of severe decompensation, waiting for time-consuming diagnostic tests before definitive treatment is implemented can have fatal results.

Nursing Diagnoses

Pneumothorax is truly a diagnosis requiring rapid, efficient collaborative efforts by all members of the health care team. Quick assessment of the situation with immediate decompression of the chest may be necessary, and advanced anticipatory planning is required. In prehospital or emergency department settings, this emergency is usually handled effectively without delay once the diagnosis has been made. Such may not be the case in other clinical settings, yet most care areas that have access to intravenous angiocatheterization equipment and oxygen therapy have all they need to handle this emergency quickly until more definitive therapy is implemented. Recognition of this potentially life-threatening disorder is imperative. Table 19–8 gives the nursing diagnoses indicated in the care of the patient with pneumothorax.

Collaborative Management

If initial emergency treatment is required, the paramedic, physician, nurse, and respiratory therapist are the key collaborative personnel needed to start oxygen therapy and to decompress the pneumothorax. Other team members such as the pharmacist, physical or occupational therapist, case manager, clergy, social worker, and dietitian are used as needs arise, especially if the initial pneumothorax is due to serious disease processes or environmental factors. The main focus must be to move the patient out of immediate

TABLE 19–8
Nursing Diagnoses: Pneumothorax

Problem Statement	Etiologic Factors
Anxiety	Pain
	Hypoxia
	Fear of unknown
Decreased cardiac output	Decreased circulating volume
	Compression of great vessels
Ineffective breathing pattern	Inadequate chest expansion
	Pain
	Hypoxemia
	Anxiety and fear
	Mechanical ventilation
Impaired gas exchange	Decreased lung capacity
Knowledge deficit	Lack of understanding of disease process, medications, and recovery or preventive care
Pain	Tissue trauma
	Chest tube insertion
Risk for infection	Trauma
	Pulmonary fluid collection

danger so that other assessments and interventions can be explored.

Oxygenation

Regardless of the cause of the pneumothorax, the nurse should start oxygen by nasal cannula at 5 L per minute unless this is contraindicated. For patients with COPD, oxygen should be given to maintain an oxygen saturation at 90% as measured by pulse oximetry. Unless hindered by other injuries, the patient assumes a position of comfort and optimal ventilation, which usually is a semi-Fowler or Fowler's position. While assessing the patient's initial vital signs and preparing for further interventions, the nurse is continually observing for clinical deterioration. In situations involving trauma, cervical spine stabilization, rapid intravenous access, and fluid resuscitation must all be considered.

Pulmonary Reexpansion

Treatment depends on the extent and cause of the pneumothorax and the severity of the patient's signs and symptoms. Spontaneous pneumothorax of 15 to 25% with no or few symptoms may be left untreated and resolves slowly on its own. Up to 1.25% of the pneumothorax absorbs daily. Administration of supplemental oxygen facilitates this resorption as the nitrogen gradient is increased from the lung to the pleura.[50] Simple aspiration of air with a Teflon catheter such as use of a 14- to 18-gauge angiocatheter occasionally is enough to reexpand the lung in 30 to 70% of the cases. This technique is also used in emergency situations until chest tube insertion can be accomplished. It is not always possible to evacuate the pneumothorax or hemothorax completely, but one can offer palliative treatment until chest tube insertion can be accomplished. Usually, needle aspiration is done on the affected side, either at the fourth or fifth intercostal space at the midaxillary line or at the second intercostal space at the midclavicular line.[54]

Chest tube placement in the pleura is done when the pneumothorax is large, when simple needle aspiration is not successful, or when pleural fluid or blood is to be evacuated. Insertion sites are the same as with needle aspiration. Reexpansion of the lung may take several days with the chest tube left in place. When complete lung expansion has occurred, the visceral and parietal pleurae come into close contact with each other, and ideally adhesion occurs, sealing any air leaks that are present. Chest tube drainage systems vary, but all operate with some type of one-way flow system. This drainage can be accomplished by underwater seal drainage or by a one-way valve device (Figure 19–8). Regardless of the system, the nursing responsibilities are the same, with modifications based on the type of system. Chart 19–6 describes nursing assessment and care of the patient with chest tubes in place.

Pleurodesis

Occasionally, the lung does not stay reexpanded with chest tube therapy alone. Adequate adhesion of the visceral and parietal pleurae does not occur, and surgical or chemical methods to create adhesion are used. Pleurectomy or pleural abrasion requires general anesthesia, thoracotomy, or thoracoscopy. A less traumatic method of creating adhesions is by pleurodesis. Pleurodesis is a bedside procedure that creates pleural adhesions by the introduction of irritating or sclerosing agents into the pleural space. Once such an agent is instilled through a chest tube, inflammatory reactions result in fibrous adhesions that obliterate the pleural space. Foreign body response with proliferation of fibroblasts and infiltration of macrophages resulting in visceral pleural thickening has been reported.[55] This method allows adhesions to seal off the pleura and is used when recurrent spontaneous pneumothoraces or pleural effusions develop.

Agents used for pleurodesis include talc, bleomycin, doxycycline, fibrin glue, and autologous blood. (Intravenous tetracycline had been used for 20 years as a pleurodesis agent, but this formulation is no longer manufactured, and tetracycline for intramuscular use is not a suitable substitute.) Instillation of these agents is done through a chest tube inserted into the affected side. If a chest tube is already in place for fluid drainage or lung expansion, the drainage must be no more than 100 mL per 24 hours, and the lung must be fully expanded before the pleurodesis agent can be instilled.[55]

Nursing implications of pleurodesis are great. The nurse either assists the physician with the procedure or may actual instill the pleurodesis agents through an existing chest tube as ordered by the physician. Almost all sclerosing pleurodesis agents cause pleuretic pain when instilled, and administration of narcotics and a benzodiazepine such as midazolam (Versed) to control the pain and to induce amnesia is indicated. The sclerosing agent is usually prepared in 25 to 50 mL of normal saline and is injected into the pleural space through the chest tube.[56] Instilling 1% lidocaine through the chest tube before the procedure or actually adding it to a compatible sclerosing agent is also reported to promote comfort. After flushing the chest tube with 30 to 50 mL of normal saline, the agent must not drain from the pleural space. Several methods to accomplish this goal have been used. Clamping the chest tube for 1 to 3 hours or looping the chest tube 40 to 60 cm above the chest for 1 to 3 hours ensures that the pleurae are in contact with the sclerosing agent. By changing the patient's position to that of sitting, lying,

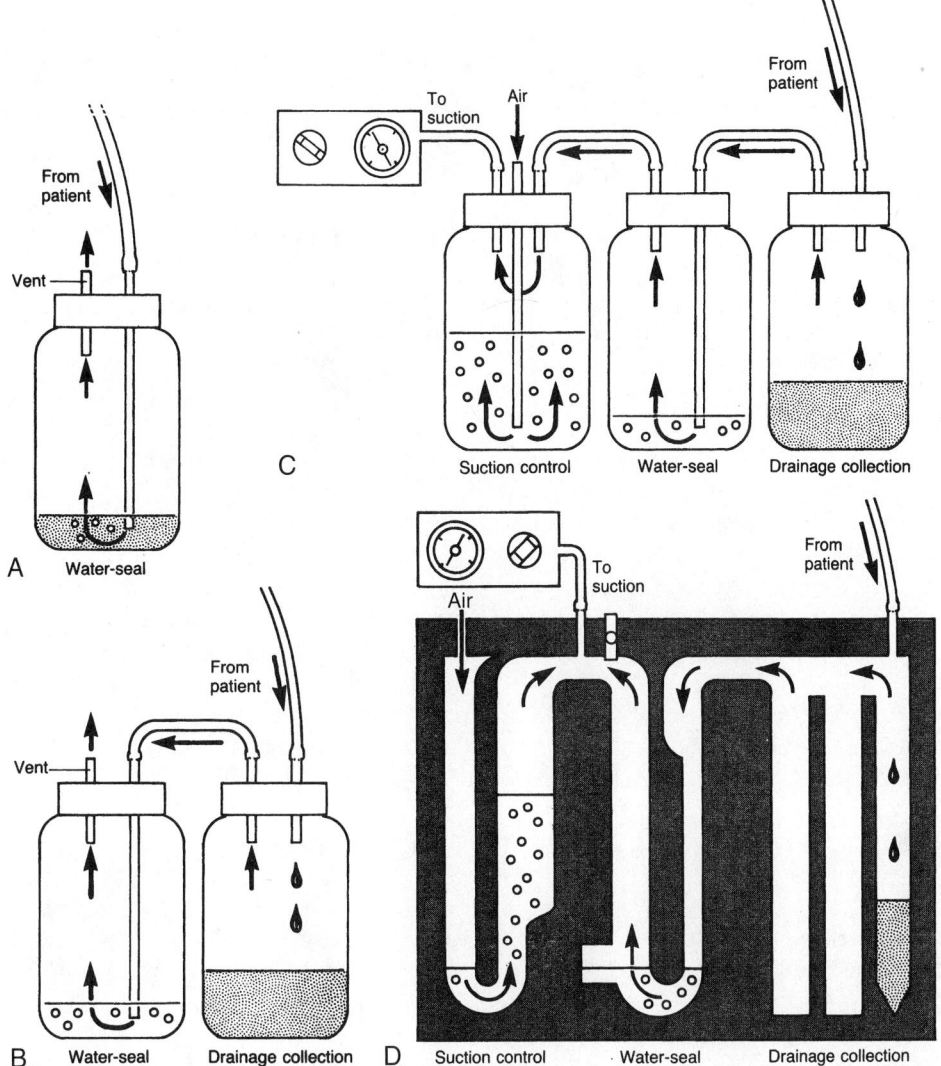

Figure 19–8

Several pleural drainage systems. A, One-bottle pleural drainage system. B, Two-bottle pleural drainage system. C, Three-bottle pleural drainage system. D, Pleur-evac pleural drainage system with air vent shown. (From Luce JM, et al: Intensive Respiratory Care, 2nd ed. Philadelphia, W.B. Saunders, 1993.)

both sides, prone, and Trendelenburg, even distribution of the sclerosing agent can be accomplished. Such position changes may be uncomfortable for the patient, and analgesia and amnestic agents should be continued as needed. The nurse should monitor respirations and pulse oximetry as well as breath sounds during this period. After 1 to 3 hours, the chest tube is allowed to resume underwater seal drainage for 2 to 4 days, after which time the chest tube is removed if the procedure was successful. Occasionally, periodic instillation at specified intervals may be required. During this time, careful observations should be made to assess whether the air leak or fluid accumulation has stopped, which would indicate that adequate pleurodesis had occurred. Observations for fever, pain, infection, embolization, and cardiopulmonary compromise should also be made because these condi-

tions indicate possible complications of the pleurodesis procedure.[55]

Intrapleural Fibrinolysis

Loculated hemothorax and empyema are often poorly evacuated by standard chest tube drainage. Fibrinolysis for these disorders has been used successfully for more than 40 years as an alternative to more invasive surgical therapy,[57] especially in patients with preexisting pulmonary disease who may poorly tolerate general anesthesia and surgery. Instilling urokinase or streptokinase into the chest tube, clamping the tube for 4 hours, and rotating the patient to various positions allow degradation of loculated fluids.[58] This treatment may be done by the nurse and may be repeated for several days until chest radiographic improvement is

CHART 19–6

Assessment of the Patient With Chest Tubes

Patient Assessment and Care

1. Assess the patient at least every 4 hours.
2. Auscultate breath sounds.
3. Note respiratory rate, quality, and depth.
4. Monitor pulse oximetry.
5. Assess for asymmetric chest excursion, hyperresonance, cyanosis, dyspnea, and decreased or absent breath sounds, which may indicate pneumothorax.
6. Assess for sudden sharp chest pain, anxiety, severe dyspnea, tachycardia, hypotension, dysrhythmias, tracheal deviation to the unaffected side, or neck vein distention, which may indicate tension pneumothorax.
7. Percuss the chest for dullness or flatness, which may indicate hemothorax or pleural effusion.
8. Palpate around the chest, neck, axilla, and back for subcutaneous emphysema.
9. Instruct the patient to cough, breathe deeply, and use incentive spirometry every 2 hours.
10. Ensure that the dressing is airtight, clean, dry, and covered with tape.

Tubing Assessment and Care

1. Check the chest tube to make sure it is secured to the chest.
2. Tighten and secure all chest drainage system connections.
3. Tighten caps on bottle setups.
4. Keep tubing free of kinks, looping, and obstructions to allow free flow of drainage.
5. Always keep two clamps with the chest tube drainage system.
6. Chest tubes should only be clamped under the following circumstances: when the physician orders it, to change a bottle, if the bottle breaks, or if tubing becomes disconnected from the system for any reason.

Drainage System Assessment and Care

1. Keep the drainage system below the level of the patient's chest.
2. Stabilize the system to prevent tipping or breakage.
3. Assess for fluctuation of drainage in the glass straw of a bottle setup or in the underwater-seal chamber of a disposable system.

4. Document the amount, color, and consistency of chest drainage.
5. Mark the level of drainage on the tape secured to the bottle or disposable system with the date and time every shift.
6. Ensure that the water seal is intact on a bottle setup by checking that the glass straw extends into the water half an inch and on a disposable system by assessing that the fluid level in the water-seal chamber is at the proper fluid line level.
7. Assess for air leaks in the patient and the drainage system.

Suction Assessment and Care

1. If the chest tube is to be drained by gravity with no suction, do not clamp the air vent. Remember: "no suction, no clamp."
2. If bottle setup is to use suction, connect it to a suction machine with an adjustable-centimeter and a suction dial that comes with one or two additional bottles. Clamp off the extra air vent tubing, turn the machine on, and adjust the dial until the ordered amount of suction is indicated.
3. If disposable system is to use suction, connect it to low continuous wall suction machine. The centimeters of suction ordered are adjusted by adding sterile water to the appropriate level in the suction-control chamber. Turn the control stopcock to allow gentle bubbling in the suction-control chamber and gentle rolling of the small ball in the water-seal chamber.
4. If a bottle system is to be converted from suction to gravity drainage, turn off the suction machine, disconnect the tube from the collection bottle from the bottles of the suction machine, and leave the air vent unclamped. If it is a disposable system, turn off the wall suction, disconnect the tube at the level of the stopcock, and keep the stopcock in the open position.

Assessing for Air Leaks

1. If there is continuous bubbling in the bottle setup glass straw or in the disposable water-seal chamber, you have a leak in the system and must clamp and unclamp the tubing in a systematic fashion to determine the source of the leak.

CHART 19–6

Assessment of the Patient With Chest Tubes *(Continued)*

2. Never clamp a chest tube for more than 1 to 2 minutes because this places the patient at risk of tension pneumothorax. Clamping to determine air leaks should not take more than 5 to 10 seconds.

3. Clamp tubing near the insertion site, and have the patient take several deep breaths while observing the glass straw of a bottle setup or the water-seal chamber of a disposable system for cessation of continuous bubbling. If bubbling stops, the air leak is at the chest tube insertion site or inside the patient. Unclamp the chest tube and redress and seal the insertion site with occlusive vaseline gauze, a large dressing, and tape. If continuous bubbling continues, the leak may be inside the patient. If patient is symptomatic, contact the physician immediately.

4. If the bubbling continues, clamp the tubing at 4- to 6-inch increments and check the water seal for continuous bubbling. When the bubbling stops, the leak is between your present position and the previous position. Tighten all connections in this area and try to seal a leak in the tube with tape.

5. If bubbling continues after checking the entire length of the tubing, the leak is in the drainage collection system itself. Prepare an additional drainage collection system according to the manufacturer's instructions. Clamp the chest tube, disconnect from the old system, reconnect to the new system, and unclamp the chest tube. Reassess again for air leaks.

---

demonstrated. A 92% success rate has been reported using this method of intracavitary fibrinolysis.[59] Complications of intrapleural thrombolytic agents are rare. Systemic absorption of fibrin degradation products during fibrinolysis has been associated with an increase in pulmonary capillary permeability and acute hypoxemic respiratory failure,[60] but this problem is not reported as a common event.

Video-Assisted Thoracic Surgery

When the methods discussed earlier do not result in adequate reexpansion of the lung or when chest and lung damage must be repaired, surgical treatment may need to take place. Video-assisted thoracic surgery (VATS) is a method of visualizing and repairing defects within the chest (Figure 19–9). Thoracoscopy is performed on the affected side with either neuroleptanalgesia allowing spontaneous ventilation[41] or with general anesthesia using double-lumen endotracheal intubation.[61] During this procedure, the lung surfaces and pleural cavity can be visualized and inspected for structural defects. Defects most often encountered are blebs, bullae, adhesions, cysts, and nodules. These lesions can be resected or sampled for biopsy through this videothorascopic procedure using wedge resection, stapler resection, endoloop ligation, electrocoagulation, neodymium–yttrium-aluminum-garnet (Nd–YAG) laser, or argon beam coagulation. Hemothorax evacuation of retained clots or fluid and coagulation of bleeding vessels can also be accomplished

with VATS.[62] This approach has also been used successfully in acute chest trauma. Hemostasis, removal of blood clots, and thoracic duct ligation have been performed that otherwise would require traditional thoracotomy. Even repair of lung and diaphragm lacerations and decortication can be accomplished.[63] Finally, pleurodesis using mechanical pleural brushing, chemical instillation, or pleurectomy has also been done with VATS.[61] The advantages of this endoscopic approach are obvious. The patient experiences less postoperative pain, a more rapid recovery, a shorter hospitalization, and a smaller chest wound.[64]

Surgical exploration of the chest by thoracotomy may be indicated in patients with multiple defects, extensive disease, severe bleeding, or trauma requiring extensive exploration and repair. See the later section on chest surgery for further description and care of these patients.

Observing for Complications

Complications of pneumothorax are related to incomplete chest decompression of air and fluid or sequelae from the treatment itself. Twenty percent of patients with spontaneous pneumothorax accumulate pleural fluid in the pleural space. A torn adhesion of the visceral pleura or subclavian vein accounts for hemothorax in 3% of these patients. Respiratory failure, pneumonia, lung abscess, atelectasis, ARDS, pulmonary edema, and recurrent pneumothorax may occur, depending on the initial injury or cause of the pneumo-

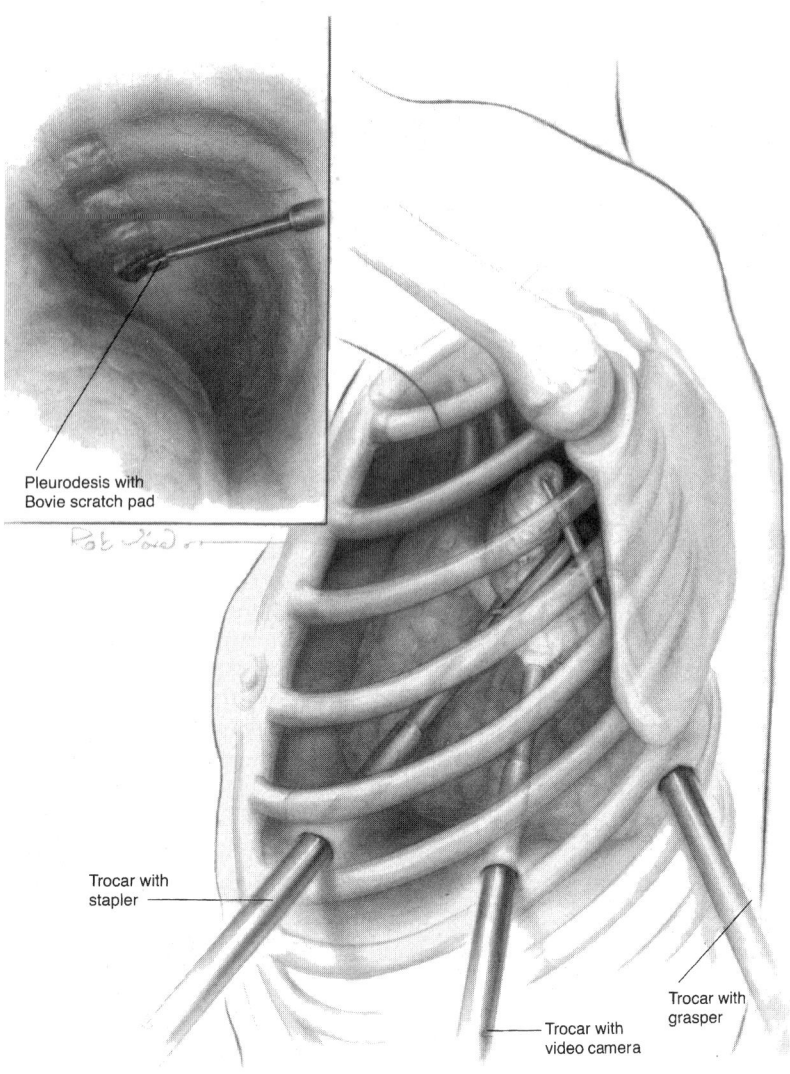

Pleurodesis with
Bovie scratch pad

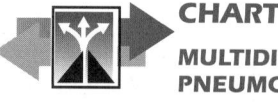

Trocar with
stapler

Trocar with
video camera

Trocar with
grasper

Figure 19–9

Pleurodesis is performed using video-assisted thoracic surgery to visualize and repair defects within the chest. (From Sabiston DC, Spencer FC: Surgery of the Chest, 6th ed. vol. 2. Philadelphia, W.B. Saunders, 1996, p 2156.)

thorax. In patients with preexisting chronic lung disease, respiratory reserves and compensation are poor, and pneumothorax can lead to severe respiratory failure and death if it is not quickly resolved. Empyema is a collection of purulent exudate in the pleural space. Although this condition is not common in patients with spontaneous pneumothorax, it has been associated with pneumothorax caused by tuberculosis, esophageal rupture, lung abscess, bronchopleural fistula, and congenital cyst rupture. Hemodynamic instability and death resulting from hemorrhage, shock, sepsis, and cardiovascular collapse are additional potential complications, again depending on the cause of the pneumothorax initially.[65]

Multidisciplinary Outcomes

Multidisciplinary outcomes are priority driven in the patient with pneumothorax. Obviously, emergency airway and oxygenation needs are of urgent concern.

Once the patient is out of immediate danger, additional outcomes are explored, depending on the cause of the pneumothorax. Outcomes are listed in Chart 19–7.

CHART 19–7

MULTIDISCIPLINARY OUTCOMES: PNEUMOTHORAX

Establishment and maintenance of an adequate airway, ventilation, and oxygenation
Maintenance of adequate perfusion and circulating volume
Achievement of an optimal comfort level
Control of the patient's anxiety and fear
Demonstration by the patient of an understanding of home care and follow-up instructions

THORACIC PULMONARY SURGERY

Thoracic pulmonary surgery is performed for various abnormalities, diseases, and injuries to the chest wall, pleurae, lungs, or trachea. Regardless of the initial cause, certain patient problems and care principles are common, and the nurse cares for these patients in various settings. Many thoracic surgical patients do not go to the ICU but still require "critical care." These patients often have many complex needs. The cooperation of the entire health care team makes meeting these needs easier and more complete.

Lung Surgery

Small peripheral disease processes may be removed by a wedge resection in which only a small peripheral part of a lung lobe is removed.[66] Segmental resection of the lung is required to remove an isolated disease process. Benign tumors, blebs, abscesses, bronchiectasis, or tuberculosis may involve only a segment and patients can benefit from such a resection. A lobectomy or removal of an entire lung lobe may be performed to resect even more lung tissue. Finally, when an abscess, tumor, or infection is extensive, removal of the entire lung or a pneumonectomy is performed. Depending on the extent of the operation, a thoracotomy may be performed, or a VATS approach may be taken. As many as three to four ports are placed in the chest to allow introduction of a thoracoscope, surgical stapler, plication device, or other surgical instruments as needed.[67]

Lung Volume Reduction Surgery

Lung volume reduction surgery is a palliative technique for severely symptomatic emphysematous patients. Chart 19–8 lists criteria for lung reduction in patients. In this procedure, sections of the diseased lungs are removed. The resected lung edges are resealed with a surgical stapling device and are reinforced with bovine pericardial buttressing. Lung volume is reduced by 20 to 30%, but lung function is improved. Increased efficiency in exchanging carbon dioxide and oxygen, greater exhaled air volumes, and improved breathing dynamics are achieved. Patients report less dyspnea, improved activity tolerance, and a reduced need for supplemental oxygen. Some patients who were ventilator dependent were able to achieve weaning from the ventilator after lung reduction surgery.[68] Although these clinical benefits are favorable, significant morbidity and mortality do occur

CHART 19–8

Criteria for Lung Reduction Surgery Candidates

Advanced emphysema
Unhappiness with emphysema limitations
Small amount of airway inflammation
Controlled or no active medical problems
No or low-dose systemic steroid use
Active participation in pulmonary rehabilitation program
No smoking in past year
Residual volume >150% predicted
Systolic pulmonary artery pressures <50 mm Hg

because of the median sternotomy approach used for this procedure. Minimally invasive no-cut thorascopic lung plication using VATS technology has virtually eliminated the problems associated with operative trauma of the surgical incision and air leaks arising from resecting emphysematous lung tissue. In most of these patients, an area of the upper lobe or the superior segment of the lower lobe is folded over itself and is stapled in place by a knifeless endoscopic stapler. Several folds can be made to effect concentric lung reduction. This method allows a double layer of lung tissue and four layers of visceral pleura to buttress the staple line, thus reducing possibility of air leaks greatly.[69] The need for prolonged postoperative mechanical ventilation and the ICU is decreased, if not eliminated, as compared with the traditional thoracotomy approach for lung reduction surgery.

Lung Transplantation

Lung transplantation has been a therapeutic option for end-stage lung disease since the advent of cyclosporine in 1981. Single-lung transplant (SLT) is indicated in patients with pulmonary fibrosis, pulmonary hypertension, and emphysema. Double-lung transplant (DLT) is indicated in patients with cystic fibrosis and end-stage lung disease complicated by bacterial colonization. SLT in these patients would result in overwhelming infection of the donor lung by the colonized remaining patient lung and is not recommended. Patients with a history of tuberculosis may warrant SLT or DLT.[70] Because healthy donor lungs are difficult to procure, many patients die while waiting for an appropriate lung donor. In young pa-

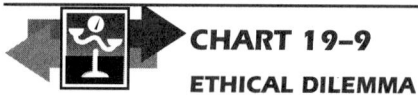

CHART 19-9

ETHICAL DILEMMA

G.R. is a 60-year old man with severe emphysema and pulmonary hypertension. He has an 80-pack-year history of smoking; he successfully quit smoking 3 years ago. In spite of strict compliance with current therapy, Mr. R. is in end-stage respiratory failure and has been told by his physician that lung transplantation is his only option. He requires aerosol breathing treatments every 4 hours and is on continuous oxygen therapy. He has right ventricular hypertrophy secondary to his pulmonary hypertension. He has been in the ICU three times over the past 6 months on a ventilator for acute exacerbation of his respiratory condition. He has become resistant to some antibiotics. Mr. R. has had excellent family support during his illness. Although he lives on a small, fixed income, his community and family have held several fund-raising activities to raise the money for his lung transplantation expenses. These efforts have earned more than half the expected costs.

E.W. is a 19-year-old college nursing student with cystic fibrosis. She is supposed to take pancreatic enzymes with every meal but occasionally "forgets." She now takes aerosol breathing treatments five times a day, but only recently has been compliant with this regimen. She has experienced pulmonary hemorrhage twice in the past few years that required bronchoscopy. Six months ago, she developed insulin-dependent diabetes as a complication of cystic fibrosis. She is in the hospital with pneumo-

nia every 3 months. During her last hospitalization, a venous access port was implanted for intravenous antibiotics. She, too, is on continuous oxygen therapy and requires lung transplantation. Ms. W. lives with her parents and is an only child. Her father farms several thousand acres, runs a successful grain processing company, and owns a farm equipment dealership.

1. What are each of these patients' advantages and disadvantages for surviving lung transplantation?
2. What role does compliance with therapy play in determining candidacy for lung transplantation?
3. Is ability to pay for transplant care a consideration in deciding who is appropriate for a lung transplant?
4. Should age be a factor in determining transplant candidacy?
5. If an appropriate donor becomes available that is suitable for both these patients, which of them should receive the lung transplant? Why?
6. Ms. W.'s parents are compatible lung donors for her, but her father is hesitant to become a living lung donor. He asks you whether he should do this. How do you respond?
7. Mr. R.'s wife has religious concerns regarding her husband's receiving a lung transplant. How do you address her concerns?

tients with cystic fibrosis, often a living lung donation of a lower lobe from each parent is performed (Chart 19–9).

Assessment

History

The nurse should assess the past medical history and the current health status of the thoracic surgical patient. Reviewing the origin and severity of the pulmonary problem, including prior pulmonary surgery and medical management of the pulmonary condition, allows the nurse to better determine possible postoperative care. Evaluating pulmonary secretions, chest discomfort, smoking history, and activity tolerance is necessary. An overall physical assessment with emphasis on pulmonary status is done. Rate and rhythm

of respirations, breathing patterns, and breath sounds give further evidence of the extent of the pulmonary disease.

Criteria for Surgery

The nurse must determine the patient's compliance with treatment and self-care with impending lung reduction or transplant surgery. In these patients, it is essential not only to evaluate their physical condition, but also to determine their psychological status, including motivation and emotional state. Specific criteria for both these surgical procedures are set, and an extensive multidisciplinary screening evaluation process is performed. See Chart 19–8 for selection criteria for lung reduction surgery. The inclusion and exclusion criteria for lung transplant candidates listed in Chart 19–10 are used to determine who *is* and who *is not* a candidate for lung transplantation.[71] Even so,

CHART 19-10

Criteria for Lung Transplant Candidates

Inclusion Criteria

Forced vital capacity <40% of predicted
FEV$_1$ (first second of expiration) <30% of predicted
Room air Pao$_2$ < 60 mm Hg at rest
Predicted survival <2 yr
Major pulmonary complications
Increased antibiotic resistance

Exclusion Criteria

Ongoing infection related to:
    AIDS
    Hepatitis B

Mycobacterium tuberculosis
Burkholderia cepacia
Methicillin-resistant Staphylococcus aureus
Aspergillus species
    Multiply resistant Pseudomonas aeruginosa
Hepatic, renal, or left ventricular failure
Diabetes with severe end-organ failure
Symptomatic osteoporosis
Inability to ambulate
Ventilator dependency
Significant psychiatric disorder

Adapted from Mallory GB, Yankaskas JR: Lung transplantation: concensus and controversies. In: Highlights: Selected Proceedings From the Tenth Annual North American Cystic Fibrosis Conference, October 24–27, 1996, p 20.

lung transplantation often involves resolution of various ethical and moral dilemmas (Chart 19–9). In addition, because many insurance companies consider lung transplantation experimental, adequate funding and finance must be secured for the transplant procedure, extensive postoperative care, and lifelong antirejection medications.[72]

Diagnostic Examinations

Various laboratory and diagnostic procedures are done preoperatively, depending on the thoracic surgical procedure. Arterial blood gas analysis, pulmonary function studies, bronchoscopy, chest radiograph, chest CT scan, and V/Q lung scan may be done. Cytologic examination of sputum, pleural fluid, lymph nodes, or lung tissue may be completed as well. The functional status of other body systems is evaluated as well.

Nursing Diagnoses

Management of the thoracic surgical patient is extensive. Many patient problems necessitate the collaborative efforts of the multidisciplinary health team. Table 19–9 contains a comprehensive list of possible patient problems and nursing interventions.

Collaborative Management

Care of the postthoracotomy patient requires interventions aimed at supporting adequate ventilation and

TABLE 19-9
Nursing Diagnoses: Thoracic Surgery

Problem Statement	Etiologic Factors
Anxiety	Hypoxia Fear of unknown Pain
Altered nutrition: less than body requirements	Poor preoperative nutritional status Chronic pulmonary disease Increased metabolic demand
Decreased cardiac output	Hemorrhage Circulatory overload Pulmonary hypertension Right ventricular failure Cardiac dysrhythmias
Ineffective breathing pattern	Pain Hypoxemia Anxiety and fear
Impaired gas exchange	Reperfusion injury Pulmonary edema
Ineffective airway clearance	Incisional pain Chest tubes Poor cough reflex
Impaired physical mobility	Surgical incision "Frozen shoulder"
Knowledge deficit	Lack of understanding of disease process, medications, and recovery or preventive care
Pain	Incisional pain Chest tubes

gas exchange, restoring hemodynamic stability, and preventing complications. Although specific surgical interventions have some specific postoperative management challenges, general overall management is similar.

Routine Care

Oxygenation

Oxygenation must be maintained during the postoperative period. Supplemental oxygen is required by most patients; however, many patients do not require mechanical ventilation after thoracic surgery unless complications occur. During the operation, patients undergoing SLT and other thoracic surgical patients may require a double-lumen endobronchial tube to allow different lung volumes and PEEP settings, which can continue into the early postoperative period. However, the patient who has undergone uncomplicated lung transplantation is often extubated within 24 hours.[70] Unless the patient has had a pneumonectomy, chest tubes are used to remove fluid and to reinflate the lungs. Air leaks may occur and may be expected in the early postoperative period until the pleura has had time to seal. Usually, the physician indicates whether such an air leak is to be expected or is serious. Chest

TABLE 19-10
Managing Problems of Chest Drainage

Problem	Nursing Intervention
Dislodged chest tube	Immediately place gloved hand over insertion site and call for assistance
	Secure occlusive vaseline dressing and dry gauze dressing over insertion site with tape
	Reassess patient and notify physician
Drainage system broken or tubing pulled apart and contaminated	Clamp chest tube
	Irrigate contaminated tubing with sterile water or saline and place end of tubing into sterile solution at least 2–4 cm below fluid surface; unclamp chest tube
	Stay with patient while another nurse obtains and sets up a new collection system
	Connect new system to chest tube
No fluctuation of fluid in glass straw of bottle setup or water-seal chamber of disposable system during respirations	Reposition patient and have him or her cough and deep breathe; assess for respiratory difficulty
	Gently milk or squeeze chest tubing
	Fluctuation will decrease as lung expands
	Fluctuation stops if lung is expanded and sealed
Dramatic increase in chest drainage of 200 mL in 1 hour 100 mL/hr × 3 hours 500 mL in 8 hours	Note activity before increase occurred; dumping of pockets of fluid can occur with position changes
	Note drainage color, amount, and consistency
	Assess vital signs for increased pulse rate, decreased blood pressure or orthostatic blood pressure changes that could indicate acute hemorrhage, and respiratory status
	Notify physician; recheck patient every 5–15 min
Continuous bubbling in glass straw of bottle setup or water-seal chamber of disposable system	Check for airleaks (see Chart 19–6)
Abnormal bubbling in suction-control chamber of disposable system	No bubbling: check for obstructions and that suction source is connected and turned on
	Vigorous bubbling: turn stopcock suction control until slow, gentle bubbling is visible
Too little or too much fluid in water-seal or suction-control chambers of disposable system	Pinch off to suction source to check for level of fluid in suction-control chamber
	If below required level, add more sterile water or saline to chamber though resealable diaphragm or with a syringe and needle or through the top filling port
	If above required level, remove excess fluid with a syringe and needle through resealable diaphragm; DO NOT tip over to remove fluid
Collection system turned over, placed higher than chest, or tubing obstructed	Place collection system in proper position
	Unkink tubing and gently milk if permitted
	Have patient take some deep breaths and cough

tubes should be carefully monitored for proper functioning because complications of pneumothorax or tension pneumothorax may occur. Chart 19–6 and Table 19–10 contain more information on the care of the patient with chest tubes.

Airway Clearance

Deep breathing and coughing every 1 to 2 hours for the first 2 days with the appropriate incisional splinting methods assist in preventing atelectasis and stasis of secretions. These measures are especially important in the patient undergoing lung transplantation because the allograft and airways do not have innervation below the anastomosis line, and cough reflexes and normal ciliary movements that assist in mobilizing secretions are absent or impaired. Gas exchange and compliance may be drastically hindered.[70] Adequate fluids and moisture can assist in keeping the secretions of the thoracic surgical patient thinner and easier to mobilize. Suctioning must be done carefully so that pulmonary suture lines are not disrupted. Aerosol treatments and chest physical therapy are ordered for some patients, especially after extubation. Incentive spirometry postoperatively also can assist in preventing atelectasis. Because many of these patients have preexisting underlying pulmonary disease or may be susceptible to infection, prophylactic antibiotics are begun preoperatively and are continued into the postoperative phase.

Pain Management

Careful attention must be given to avoid respiratory depression resulting from the use of pain medications. The use of intrapleural or epidural catheter administration of pain medication may cause less central respiratory depression than the intravenous route.[73] Patient-controlled analgesia is a favored method of pain medication administration. Planning activities to occur within 30 minutes of pain medication administration allows patients to participate in their care and to increase their activity postoperatively. Assessing the patient's pulse oximetry and respiratory effort, rate, and depth must be done before and after the administration of pain medications, as well as on a routine basis. Periodic evaluation of tidal volume is done in some institutions. Careful assessment of breath sounds, use of accessory muscles for breathing, and skin and mucous membrane color are also included in the routine postoperative assessment. Dyspnea can be associated with hypoxemia, secretions, pain, and hypoventilation.

Activity

Positioning of the patient can promote oxygenation and relieve pain. The nurse needs to know the extent of the surgical procedure to determine what patient positions are allowed. When in doubt, the nurse should consult with the physician. Generally, the patient who has undergone pneumonectomy should be turned with the unoperative side upward. This positioning prevents undesirable torsion and possible disruption of the bronchial stump suture line and offers splinting of the operative side.[73] For other patients, frequent turning and repositioning facilitate ventilation and perfusion in the lungs. Many patients show dramatic gas exchange improvement with repositioning of the operative side upward to decrease postoperative edema. Careful attention should be given to the patient's clinical condition, arterial and venous oxygen saturation, and hemodynamic parameters, to determine how well these position changes are tolerated. Mediastinal shift may occur, as evidenced by tracheal deviation, chest radiograph changes, and repositioning of the apex of the heart as determined by palpation or auscultation, and must be avoided. Usually, the day after the operation, the patient is able to dangle his or her legs at the bedside and progress to sitting in a chair. Early activity prevents further respiratory complications and thrombophlebitis. Planned range-of-motion exercises may be necessary to prevent surgical adhesions and stiffening of the shoulder on the operative side resulting in a "frozen shoulder." Usually, the physician orders a physical therapy consultation postoperatively to prevent this possibility, but the nurse can begin to encourage activity by keeping bedside items on the patient's operative side to encourage reaching.

Nutrition

The extent of the thoracic surgical procedure and the presence of mechanical ventilation determine when the patient will resume oral intake. Once bowel sounds have returned, oral fluids are started. Usually, this occurs by the first postoperative day if the patient has been extubated, followed by introduction of more solid foods by the second or third day postoperatively. For patients with chronic pulmonary diseases such as COPD, cystic fibrosis, and carcinoma, nutritional status may have been poor preoperatively, and this may affect postoperative progress. Postoperative activity, healing, and airway clearance are all delayed or hindered in patients with inadequate nutrition. Consultation with the dietitian and pharmacist should be made if total parenteral nutrition or tube feeding is to be instituted.

Postoperative Complications

Hemorrhage

Hemorrhage can occur as a postoperative complication of thoracotomy and depends on the extent of the surgical procedure. In patients who have undergone major thoracic surgery, blood loss may be substantial because blood vessels in the chest are large in diameter, and incisions frequently are large, to gain access to the surgical site. With lung transplantation, bleeding can occur from any of the vascular or airway anastomosis sites and from pleural adhesions severed when the native lung is removed. With some lung transplantations, the patient may need to be placed on cardiopulmonary bypass, and this procedure can increase the risk of bleeding even more. During the immediate postoperative period, chest tube drainage should be evaluated every 15 minutes for amount, color, and consistency. When chest tube drainage is more than 100 mL in 1 hour, when it changes to bright red, or when it suddenly increases in amount, hemorrhage should be suspected. However, many institutions do not tilt or turn their thoracotomy patients for the first 1 to 4 hours or until these patients are hemodynamically stable, and with this first turn, a "dumping" of pockets of chest drainage through the chest tubes may occur. Other signs of hypovolemic shock or hemothorax such as increased pulse, decreased blood pressure, increased respirations, cool, clammy, pale skin, decreased urinary output, and decreased level of consciousness or restlessness assist the nurse in determining whether this accumulation of fluid truly constitutes hemorrhage.[74] Because the patient who has undergone pneumonectomy does not have chest tubes, careful assessment for the development of tachycardia with a rate of 120 beats per minute or greater should alert the nurse to the possibility of early hemorrhage.[73]

Circulatory Overload

Circulatory overload with elevated central venous pressure can also occur after thoracic surgery. When part of the pulmonary tissue is removed or reexpansion of the remaining pulmonary tissue is delayed, the pulmonary vascular bed is reduced. This means that the right ventricle may be sending its blood to a much smaller pulmonary circulating area than before. Right ventricular failure may occur, as well as pulmonary hypertension and edema. With right pneumonectomy, this hemodynamic burden may be greater because the lung with the greater circulatory capacity has been removed. Other indications of circulatory overload and possible pulmonary edema are increased pulmonary artery occlusive pressure, pulmonary crackles, cyanosis, persistent cough, inadequate blood gas analysis, and increase in pulmonary secretions. The nurse should limit intravenous fluids to 125 mL per hour in most cases to prevent this circulatory overload. Urinary output of 20 to 30 mL per hour is acceptable when trying to limit postoperative fluids to prevent circulatory overload. Patients who have had SLT because of pulmonary hypertension or COPD have further alterations in pulmonary circulation. As much as 90% of the blood flow from the right ventricle may

go to the undiseased allograft,[70] which may or may not be able to accommodate the extra volume. In addition, when the thoracic lymphatic drainage system is disrupted by an extensive thoracic surgical procedure, the lung may be especially susceptible to pulmonary edema.

Cardiac Dysrhythmias

Cardiac dysrhythmias may occur in the postoperative period because of atrial enlargement or strain from previously described changes in pulmonary hemodynamics. The most common rhythm disturbances are atrial fibrillation, atrial flutter, and paroxysmal atrial tachycardia. Prophylactic digitalis is occasionally given to prevent such tachydysrhythmias.[70] Increased vagal tone, hypoxia, or acidosis may also account for other dysrhythmias such as sinus bradycardia, junctional rhythm, and premature ventricular contractions.

Pulmonary Complications

Respiratory failure, pulmonary edema, tension pneumothorax, and hemothorax are discussed previously as possible pulmonary postoperative complications in the thoracic surgical patient. Another complication is PE, which can be serious and is difficult to assess. The chest pain, dyspnea, hypoxia, tachypnea, hemoptysis, fever, tachycardia, and right-sided heart failure that indicate PE may be present for many other reasons already discussed. Subcutaneous emphysema can occur when a pleural leak causes air to enter the subcutaneous tissues around incisions and chest tubes. It produces a spongy or crackling sensation when pressed with the fingertips. This condition generally is not cause for alarm; however, the trachea can be compressed by severe subcutaneous emphysema around the neck, necessitating a tracheostomy. Progression of subcutaneous emphysema should be monitored by periodically marking its extent on the skin. If progression in 1 hour is more than one hand's width, a bronchial stump or large airway leak may have developed. The nurse should make the physician aware of the progress of this development.

Acute Graft Failure

Patients who have undergone lung transplantation can experience early dysfunction of the transplanted lung because of a "pulmonary reimplantation response." Even though the donor lung is ideally transplanted within 6 to 8 hours and is preserved with prostaglandin E_1 and cold glucose and electrolyte solution, it still remains ischemic during this time.[75] When the ischemic donor lung is exposed to molecular oxygen when reperfusion during transplantation occurs, a series of cytotoxic events develop, primarily as a result of the release of reactive oxygen metabolites. These oxidants interact with specific components

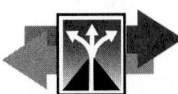

CHART 19–11

MULTIDISCIPLINARY OUTCOMES: THORACIC PULMONARY SURGERY

Establishment and maintenance of an adequate airway, ventilation, and oxygenation

Maintenance of adequate perfusion and circulating volume

Achievement of an optimal comfort level

Maintenance or improvement in nutritional status

Control of the patient's anxiety and fear

Demonstration by the patient of an understanding of home care and follow-up instructions

of extracellular fluid to generate substances that are chemotactic for leukocytes. These leukocytes adhere to the endothelium of the transplant lung and cause a severe, localized inflammatory-injury response.[76] This reperfusion pulmonary edema results in impaired oxygenation, reduced compliance, and pulmonary infiltration. Although this complication only occurs in about 20% of these patients, it is a major source of morbidity and mortality in the early postoperative period. Extended mechanical ventilation with high levels of PEEP may be required. In patients with severely deteriorating conditions, extracorporeal membrane oxygenation and inhaled nitric oxide have been used.[77]

Multidisciplinary Outcomes

The thoracic surgical patient requires a truly multidisciplinary team approach to ensure a positive outcome. The physician, respiratory therapist, dietitian, pharmacist, physical therapist, social worker, and nurse must all work together to care for this often long-term patient. Chart 19–11 lists expected outcomes.

Critical Thinking Exercise

S.D. was a 67-year-old woman admitted to the hospital for elective left total hip replacement. She had severe left hip pain and loss of range of motion because of progressive osteoarthritis. Mrs. D. was 5'10" tall and weighed 330 pounds. The debilitating condition of her left hip arthritic state required her to take numerous pain-relieving medications and inhibited her independence with activities of daily living. She had a sedate lifestyle and required a cane for ambulation. Mrs. D. had a history of heart disease and had a mild myocardial infarction 3 years earlier. In the past 2 years, she had experienced four episodes of congestive heart failure that had been controlled by digoxin and diuretics.

After her operation, Mrs. D. received prophylactic low-dose low-molecular-weight heparin. Antiembolism stockings and pneumatic compression devices were immediately applied to her lower extremities. Because of her weight and prior debilitated condition, postoperative activity and ambulation were slow. A large, firm hematoma developed around her left hip incision, and incisional dehiscence occurred. After evacuation of the hematoma, wound infection and delayed healing occurred. Aching and swelling of her lower extremities developed, and her diuretics were resumed. Postoperative activity and recovery were delayed. Intravenous antibiotics were given throughout her hospitalization, and she eventually was placed on warfarin. After 14 days of hospitalization, she had an episode of transient dyspnea and mild chest pain after ambulating in the hall. This problem subsided almost immediately with rest and was attributed to her heart disease. A chest radiograph and ECG were unchanged. The next day, Mrs. D. was transferred to an extended care facility, where her rehabilitation continued for another week before she was discharged to home.

Mrs. D. was able to ambulate with the assistance of a cane but with much difficulty. The first night she was home, her husband heard her call out and found her collapsed on the floor of the bathroom, where she had fallen off the toilet. He called 911 and began cardiopulmonary resuscitation. Paramedics started resuscitative efforts and transferred Mrs. D. to the local emergency department, where resuscitative efforts continued for 2 hours. Although a cardiac rhythm was restored, no pulse was ever felt. Resuscitative efforts were stopped, and Mrs. D. was pronounced dead. On autopsy, a large saddle embolus was found in her pulmonary artery.

1. What were Mrs. D.'s pre- and postoperative risk factors for developing PE?
2. Did Mrs. D. have a DVT? What therapeutic preventive measures were taken to prevent DVT and PE? Could further measures have been taken?
3. Should Mrs. D. not have had more signs and symptoms that would indicate a PE?
4. If a DVT had been discovered, what could have been done about it?
5. What happened to cause Mrs. D. to die suddenly? Could anything have saved Mrs. D.?
6. What can the nurse do to decrease the incidence of PE?

Key Concepts

→ PE occurs when a nonsoluble material in the venous system flows to the lungs and occludes one or several pulmonary vessels. Most PEs originate in the ileofemoral or popliteal deep veins, although nonthrombotic emboli of fat, air, calcium, foreign body, and amniotic fluid also occur.

→ Those patients at highest risk for development of DVT and PE are surgical patients and those with low cardiac output, coagulopathies, cancer, myocardial infarction, trauma, severe illness, chronic illness, varicose veins, and previous emboli, as well as persons who are elderly, pregnant, and receiving high-dose estrogen therapy and who are postoperative or immobile.

→ Untreated PE has a 50% recurrence rate, and half of these recurrences are fatal.

→ Virchow's triad of blood stasis, blood coagulation problems, and vein wall abnormalities favors development of DVT and PE.

→ Prophylaxis with antiembolism compression stockings, pneumatic compression pumps, early ambulation, elevation of lower extremities, and prophylactic anticoagulation therapy can reduce the incidence of PE.

→ The most common clinical presentation of PE includes sudden dyspnea, chest pain, and tachycardia. Other signs and symptoms that may occur are apprehension, sweating, cough, fever, increased S_2, rapid and shallow respirations, and decreased breath sounds.

→ Diagnosis of PE is usually made based on a high degree of clinical suspicion, arterial blood gas analysis with hypoxemia, hypocarbia, and increased A-a gradient, moderate-probability to high-probability lung scan, and diagnostic pulmonary angiography.

→ Pulmonary angiography is the most definitive test, but it is reserved for those patients whose clinical picture is highly suspicious but have an low or intermediate lung scan result.

→ Goals of treatment in the patient with PE are to maximize oxygenation and to restore tissue perfusion. Treatment with weight-based heparin therapy should not be delayed for further diagnostic evidence if no contraindications exist and clinical evidence indicates PE.

→ Thrombolytic therapy is grossly underused because even small, asymptomatic PEs can result in recurrence, decreased quality of life, increased incidence of chronic pulmonary hypertension and heart failure, and a rise in mortality rates. Reperfusion of pulmonary tissue can be accomplished with thrombolytic therapy and with surgical embolectomy in critical or certain-death situations.

→ Warfarin should be used only after heparin has been started.

→ The duration of anticoagulation therapy for treatment or prevention of DVT and PE may be up to 12 weeks. In patients with multiple continuing risk factors and two or more embolic episodes, the duration of therapy may be indefinite. Patients receiving anticoagulation or thrombolytic agents are at higher risk for minor and major bleeding complications. Anticoagulation therapy is most successfully managed in outpatient anticoagulation clinics.

→ Vena caval interruption with venous clips or intraluminary filters may be necessary in patients with past embolic events or a high number of risk factors.

→ Embolectomy or endarterectomy surgical procedures are limited to severely compromised patients with acute PE in whom thrombolytic therapy is contraindicated or not successful or with chronic PE, pulmonary hypertension, and heart failure.

→ Complications of PE include pneumonia, ARDS, pulmonary infarction, acute and chronic pulmonary hypertension, acute and chronic heart failure, severe hemodynamic compromise, multisystem organ failure, and sudden or prolonged death.

→ Pneumothorax results when the negativity of the pleural space is lost and the lung collapses. Spontaneous pneumothorax can occur for no known reason, or it may result from rupture of a weakened area in the lung from pulmonary disease. Traumatic pneumothorax is classified as an open sucking chest wound or a closed blunt trauma.

→ Hemothorax results when blood enters the pleural space, and it may or may not result in pneumothorax. Chylothorax results when lymph fluid enters the pleural space.

→ Tension pneumothorax occurs when air entering the pleural space during inspiration is trapped, resulting in excessive pressure on the surrounding tissues. It is considered a medical emergency in most situations.

→ Sudden dyspnea and inspiratory pain are the primary symptoms of pneumothorax. Chest radiographs can confirm the diagnosis of pneumothorax, but chest decompression should not be delayed when hemodynamic deterioration accompanies a strong clinical picture.

→ Pleurodesis is accomplished by chemical or physical adhesion of the visceral pleura to the chest wall and is used to prevent recurrent pneumothorax and pleural effusions.

→ Fibrinolysis of loculated hemothorax and empyema can be accomplished with instillation of thrombolytic agents through a chest tube.

⇒ VATS is a method of endoscopic thoracic surgery that allows visualization and correction of defects.

⇒ Thoracic surgery is done for various abnormalities, diseases, or injuries to the chest wall, pleura, lungs, or trachea. Types of resections commonly performed include wedge and segmental. A lobectomy is done to remove an entire lung lobe, and a pneumonectomy is removal of an entire lung.

⇒ Lung volume reduction surgery can be done with VATS or by thoracotomy to decrease the amount of tissue with resection or plication.

⇒ Lung volume reduction surgery improves pulmonary function and can result in decreased dyspnea, improved activity tolerance, and decreased need for supplemental oxygen.

⇒ Lung transplantation may be indicated in patients with pulmonary fibrosis, pulmonary hypertension, cystic fibrosis, and emphysema.

⇒ Supplemental oxygen is required by most thoracic surgical patients; however, many patients do not require mechanical ventilation unless complications occur or surgery is extensive.

⇒ Airway clearance of secretions by the thoracic surgical patient is done with frequent repositioning, coughing, use of incentive spirometry, and respiratory therapy treatments.

⇒ Pain management is essential in the postoperative thoracic surgical patient, to promote comfort, to allow increased activity, and to promote pulmonary toileting.

⇒ Encouraging activity in the postoperative thoracic surgical patient can prevent pulmonary complications and thromboembolic episodes.

⇒ Adequate nutrition is important for the thoracic surgical patient because preoperative nutritional status may have been poor.

⇒ Hemodynamic complications of thoracic surgery include hemorrhage, circulatory overload, and cardiac dysrhythmias.

⇒ Respiratory failure, pulmonary edema, tension pneumothorax, hemothorax, and subcutaneous emphysema are possible pulmonary postoperative complications of the patient with thoracic surgery.

⇒ Reperfusion injury resulting in pulmonary edema can cause acute graft failure in the immediate postoperative period after lung transplantation.

References

1. Layish DT, Tapson VF: Pharmacologic hemodynamic support in massive pulmonary embolism. Chest 111:218–224, 1997.

2. Hirsh J, Hoak J: Management of deep vein thrombosis and pulmonary embolism. Circulation 93:2212–2245, 1996.

3. Palla A, Petruzzelli S, Donnamaria V, et al: The role of suspicion in the diagnosis of pulmonary embolism. Chest 107(Suppl):21S–24S, 1995.

4. Alexander JK: Pulmonary embolism. In: Berkow R (ed): Merck Manual, 16th ed. Rayway, NJ, Merck Research Laboratories, 1992, pp 673–680.

5. Cotran RS, Rumar V, Robbins SL: Pathologic Basis of Disease, 5th ed. Philadelphia, W.B. Saunders, 1994, pp 111–116.

6. Martinelli I, Cataneo M, Panzeri D, et al: Low prevalence of factor V;Q506 in 41 patients with isolated pulmonary embolism. Thromb Haemost 77:440–443, 1997.

7. Kobzik L, Schoen FJ: The lung. In: Cotran RS, Rumar V, Robbins SL (eds): Pathologic Basis of Disease, 5th ed. Philadelphia, W.B. Saunders, 1994, pp 679–698.

8. Stephen JM, Feied CF: Venous thrombosis. Postgrad Med 97:36–47, 1995.

9. Darovic GO: Pulmonary disease (acute respiratory failure). In: Darovic GO (ed): Hemodynamic Monitoring: Invasive and Noninvasive Clinical Application, 2nd ed. Philadelphia, W.B. Saunders, 1995, pp 525–588.

10. Butler MD, Biscardi FH, Schain DC, et al: Pulmonary resection for treatment of cavitary pulmonary infarction. Ann Thorac Surg 63:849–850, 1997.

11. Layish DT, Tapson VF: Pharmacologic hemodynamic support in massive pulmonary embolism. Chest 111:218–224, 1997.

12. Manganelli D, Palla A, Donnamaria V, et al: Clinical features of pulmonary embolism. Chest 107(Suppl):25S–32S, 1995.

13. Miller GH, Feied CF: Suspected pulmonary embolism. Postgrad Med 97:51–58, 1995.

14. Evans AJ, Sostman HD, Knelson MH, et al: 1992 ARRS Executive Council Award. Detection of deep venous thrombosis: prospective comparison of MR imaging with contrast venography. J Roentgenol 161:131–139, 1993.

15. Havig O: Deep vein thrombosis and pulmonary embolism: an autopsy study with multiple regression analysis of possible risk factors. Acta Chir Scand Suppl 478:1–120, 1977.

16. Fontana GP, Sabiston DC: Pulmonary embolism I: acute pulmonary embolism. In: Sabiston DC, Spencer FC (eds): Surgery of the chest, 6th ed. Philadelphia, W.B. Saunders, 1995, pp 773–804.

17. Gefter WB, Hatabu H, Hollarn GA, et al: Pulmonary thromboembolism: recent developments in diagnosis with CT and MR imaging. Radiology 197:561–574, 1995.

18. Wolf LD, Hozack WJ, Rothman RH: Pulmonary embolism in total joint arthroplasty. Clin Orthop 288:219–233, 1995.

19. Miniati M, Pistolesi M, Marini C, et al: Value of perfusion lung scan in the diagnosis of pulmonary embolism: results of the prospective investigative study of acute pulmonary embolism diagnosis (PISA-PED). Am J Respir Crit Care Med 154:1387–1393, 1996.

20. Anonymous: Invasive and noninvasive diagnosis of pulmonary embolism. Preliminary results of the prospective investigative study of acute pulmonary embolism diagnosis (PISA-PED). Chest 107(Suppl):33S–38S, 1995.

21. Majoros KA, Moccia JM: Pulmonary embolism. Nursing 96 26:26–31, 1996.

22. Klein DG: Patients with trauma. In: Clochesy JM, Breu C, Cardin S, et al (eds): Critical Care Nursing, 2nd ed. Philadelphia, W.B. Saunders, 1996, pp 1352–1353.

23. Ignatavicius DD, Hausman KA: Clinical Pathways for Collaborative Practice. Philadelphia, W.B. Saunders, 1995, pp 270–273.

24. Lenart S: Decompression sickness and decompression air embolism: treatment with hyperbaric oxygen and nursing management. Crit Care Nurse 16:40–47, 1996.

25. Rosenow EC: Venous and pulmonary thromboembolism: an algorithmic approach to diagnosis and management. Mayo Clin Proc 70:45–49, 1995.

26. Sebastian MW, Sabiston DC: Pulmonary embolism. II. Chronic pulmonary embolism. In: Sabiston DC, Spencer FC (eds): Surgery of the Chest, 6th ed. Philadelphia, W.B. Saunders, 1995, pp 805–821.

27. Handler JA, Feied CF: Acute pulmonary embolism. Postgrad Med 97:61–72, 1995.

28. Goldhaber SZ: Contemporary pulmonary embolism thrombolysis. Chest 107(Suppl):45S–51S.

29. Evans DA, Wilmott RW: Pulmonary embolism in children. Respir Med 41:569–584, 1994.

30. Dressler DK: Patients with coagulopathies. In: Clochesy JM, Breu C, Cardin S, et al (eds): Critical Care Nursing, 2nd ed. Philadelphia, W.B. Saunders, 1996, pp 1147–1161.

31. Girard P, Baldeyrou P, Le Guillou J, et al: Thrombolysis for life-threatening pulmonary embolism 2 days after lung resection. Am Rev Respir Dis 147:1595–1597, 1993.

32. Meyer G, Tamisier D, Sors H, et al: Pulmonary embolectomy: a 20-year experience at one center. Ann Thorac Surg 51:232–236, 1991.

33. Schmid C, Zietlow S, Wagner TOF, et al: Fluminant pulmonary embolism: symptoms, diagnostics, operative technique, and results. Ann Thorac Surg 52:1102–1107, 1991.

34. Hartz RS, Byrne JG, Levitsky S, et al: Predictors of mortality in pulmonary thromboendartectomy. Ann Thorac Surg 62:1255–1260, 1996.

35. Shure D: Thromboendarterectomy: some unanswered questions. Ann Thorac Surg 62:1253–1254, 1996.

36. Jamieson SW, Auger WR, Fedullo PF: Experience results with 150 pulmonary thromboendartectomy operations over a 29-month period. J Thorac Cardiovasc Surg 106:116–127, 1993.

37. Bottinger BW, Motsch J, Dorsam J, et al: Inhaled nitric oxide selectively decreases pulmonary artery pressure and pulmonary vascular resistance following acute massive pulmonary microembolism in piglets. Chest 110:1041–1047, 1996.

38. Feied CF, Miller GH, Stephen JM, et al: Chronic pulmonary embolism. Postgrad Med 97:75–84, 1995.

39. Cohen RG, DeMeester TR, Lafontaine E: The pleura. In: Sabiston DE, Spencer FC (eds): Surgery of the Chest, 6th ed. Philadelphia, W.B. Saunders, 1995, pp 523–575.

40. Alfageme I, Moren L, Huertas C, et al: Spontaneous pneumothorax. Chest 106:347–350, 1994.

41. Slabbynck H, Kovitz KL, Vialette J, et al: Thoracoscopic findings in spontaneous pneumothorax in AIDS. Chest 106:1582–1586, 1994.

42. Walker WA, Pate JW, Amundsen D, et al: AIDS-related bronchopleural fistula. Ann Thorac Surg 55:1048, 1993.

43. Schoenfeld A, Ziu E, Zeelel Y, et al: Catamenial pneumonthorax: a literature review and report of an unusual case. Obstet Gynecol Surv 41:20–32, 1986.

44. Brandstetter RD, Karetzky M, Rastogi R, et al: Pneumothorax after thoracentesis in chronic obstructive pulmonary disease. Heart Lung 23:67–70, 1994.

45. Abolnik IZ, Lossos IS, Gillis D, et al: Primary spontaneous pneumothorax in men. Am J Med Sci 305:297–302, 1993.

46. Brandstetter RD, Karetzky M, Rastogi R, et al: Pneumothorax after thoracentesis in chronic obstructive pulmonary disease. Heart Lung 23:67–70, 1994.

47. Jantz MA, Pierson DJ: Pneumothorax and barotrauma. Clin Chest Med 15:75–91, 1994.

48. Chen S, Markmann JR, Kauder DR, et al: Hemopneumothorax missed by auscultation in penetrating chest injury. J Trauma 42:86–89, 1997.

49. Strohmyer LL: Nursing care of clients during medical-surgical emergencies. In: Black JM, Matassarin-Jacobs E (eds): Luckmann and Sorensen's Medical-Surgical Nursing, 4th ed. Philadelphia, W.B. Saunders, 1993, pp 2231–2237.

50. Wisner DH: Trauma to the chest. In: Sabiston DC, Spencer FC (eds): Surgery of the Chest, 6th ed. Philadelphia, W.B. Saunders, 1995, pp 456–493.

51. Spillane RM, Shepard JO, Deluca SA: Radiographic aspects of pneumothorax. Am Fam Physician 51:75–91, 1995.

52. Campolo S: Spontaneous pneumothorax. Am J Nurs 97:30, 1997.

53. Heniford BT, Carrillo EH, Spain DA, et al: The role of thoracoscopy in the management of retained thoracic collections after trauma. Ann Thorac Surg 63:940–943, 1997.

54. Davis JW, Mackersie RC, Hoyt DB, et al: Randomized study of algorithms for discontinuing tube thoracostomy drainage. J Am Coll Surg 179:553–557, 1994.

55. Kennedy L, Sahn SA: Talc pleurodesis for the treatment of pneumothorax and pleural effusion. Chest 106:1215–1222, 1994.

56. Samuel JR: Management of recurrent spontaneous pneumothorax and recurrent symptomatic pleural effusion with chest tube pleurodesis. Crit Care Nurse 17:28–32, 1997.

57. Tillett WS, Sherry S, Read CT: The use of streptokinase-streptodornase in the treatment of postpneumonic empyema. J Thorac Surg 21:275–297, 1951.

58. Moulton JS, Benkert RE, Weisiger KH: Treatment of complicated pleural fluid collections with image-guided drainage and intracavitary urokinase. Chest 108:1252–1259, 1995.

59. Jerjes-Sanchez C, Ramirez-Rivera A, Elizalde JJ, et al: Intrapleural fibrinolysis with streptokinase as an adjunctive treatment in hemothorax and empyema. Chest 109:1514–1519, 1996.

60. Frye MD, Jarratt M, Sahn SA: Acute hypoxemic respiratory failure following intrapleural thrombolytic therapy for hemothorax. Chest 105:1595–1596, 1994.

61. Janssen JP, Schramel FMNH, Sutedja TG, et al: Videothoracoscopic appearance of first and recurrent pneumothorax. Chest 108:330–334, 1995.

62. Landreneau RJ, Keenan RJ, Hazelrigg SR, et al: Thoracoscopy for empyema and hemothorax. Chest 109:18–24, 1996.

63. Liu D, Lui H, Lin PJ, et al: Video-assisted thoracic surgery in treatment of chest trauma. J Trauma 42:670–674, 1997.

64. Ryoo JY, Kim SW, Cho KH: Video assisted thoracic surgery of spontaneous pneumothorax. Korean J Thorac Cardiovasc Surg 30:512–516, 1997.

65. Andrivet P, Kjedaini K, Teboul J, et al: Spontaneous pneumothorax. Chest 108:335–339, 1995.

66. Douglas JM: Thoracoscopic surgery. In: Sabiston DE, Spencer FC (eds): Surgery of the Chest, 6th ed. Philadelphia, W.B. Saunders, 1995, pp 2149–2174.

67. Jacques LF: Videothoracoscopic operations for bullous lung disease. Chest Surg Clin North Am 5:751–763, 1995.

68. Bagley RH, Davis SM, O'Shea M, et al: Lung volume reduction surgery at a community hospital. Chest 111:1552–1559, 1997.

69. Swanson SJ, Mentzer SJ, DeCamp MM, et al: No-cut thoracoscopic lung plication: a new technique for lung volume reduction surgery. J Am Coll Surg 185:25–32, 1997.

70. George EL, Large AA, Boujoukos AJ, et al: Respiratory care of the postoperative lung transplantation patient. Crit Care Nurs Q 19:59–69, 1996.

71. Mallory GB, Yankaskas JR: Lung transplantation: concensus and controversies. In: Highlights: Selected Proceedings From the Tenth Annual North American Cystic Fibrosis Conference, October 24–27, 1996, p 20.

72. Stockwell N: The transplant world: getting listed. CF Life 1:1, 7, 1997.

73. Brenner ZR, Addona C: Caring for the pneumonectomy patient: challenges and changes. Crit Care Nurse 10:65–72, 1995.

74. Robinson CF: Thoracic cavity management. In: Boggs RL, Wooldridge-King M (eds): AACN Procedure Manual for Critical Care, 3rd ed. Philadelphia, W.B. Saunders, 1993, pp 165–198.

75. Cooper JD, Patterson GA: Transplantation. III. Lung transplantation. In: Sabiston DC, Spencer FC (eds): Surgery of the Chest, 6th ed. Philadelphia, W.B. Saunders, 1995, pp 2117–2134.

76. Granger N: Ischemic/reperfusion injury: role of leukocyte-endothelial adhesion. Sci Am 12:142–143, 1997.

77. MacDonald P, Mundy J, Rogers P: Successful treatment of life-threatening acute reperfusion injury after lung transplantation with inhaled nitric oxide. J Thorac Cardiovasc Surg 110:861–863, 1995.

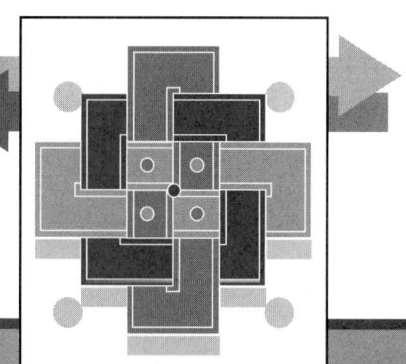

Renal Disorders

When Complications Divert the Patient and Challenge the Nurse

The medical intensive care unit (ICU) is a bustling place. The patients flow in and out, some for just an overnight stay. Others need our services for months at a time. I have worked in this unit for about 14 years, watching and assisting in its evolution to a high-quality unit.

The patient population is diverse, given the unique nature of the institution, which is a specialized, nonprofit, non–fee-charging hospital. This uniqueness presents many challenges on many levels. E. was a 63-year-old patient with unstable angina, who had had three invasive cardiac procedures before this admission at another institution. She was admitted to our unit with continuous chest pain unrelieved by nitroglycerin and morphine. She was immediately transferred to the cardiac catheterization laboratory. After undergoing heart catheterization, she was pain free, primarily because of the intra–aortic balloon pump (IABP) that was inserted during the procedure.

E. was nervous and anxious at our first meeting. I explained who I was and what she was to expect as I was settling her into the room. She stated that this was so different from the previous times she had the procedure done. On her assessment, I noted that her involved limb did not have pulses and then she stated that she had had problems with circulation. I notified the appropriate physicians about this development. In the meantime, the family came in and I explained the basics of the pump and the problems now being faced. The decision was made to remove the IABP. Again, more teaching with the patient and more reassurances about further pain were necessary. The IABP was removed without incident, and E.'s pulses returned. Later, the surgeons and the cardiologists saw E. and her family and explained the need for her to have open heart surgery.

The remainder of the day was spent explaining the operation and the patient and family's role in the recovery process. We also discussed living wills and health care representatives. E. had emphasized that her son was to make the decisions and not her husband: "He just can't handle this." In showing her the health care representative forms and in assisting her and her family in filling them out, E. was more able to focus on her upcoming surgery and not on her husband's anxieties. It also allowed her to feel more confident in that her family knew her wishes about prolonged health care.

I have been in ICU nursing for more than 16 years and have been a nurse for more than 17 years. I understood the options and the decisions that E. and her family were facing. These decisions are ones that I have assisted many other families to understand, so that they may comfortably choose the path that is right for them. Using a variety of educational materials, allowing and acknowledging patients' fears and concerns, and reminding patients that they have a choice in having the operation itself help patients and families to make a decision that is best for them. I have been on the "other side of the bed," having faced a similar experience with my own father, who required an interventional procedure and open heart surgery. This experience gave me a greater empathy and understanding about what the families are confronting. The decision to notify her son, who was from out of town, was a difficult one for E. Because I was once the child who was "out of town" and my family worried about notifying me, I was able to relate some of my feelings about being this child. It gave her and her family some insight on their decision without telling them what to do.

The next day, E.'s renal system started to show dysfunction and her surgical procedure was canceled. Later that night, her chest pain returned, and changes were noted on her electrocardiogram. After discussing the situation with the surgeons and the family, an emergency angioplasty was performed. This procedure was successful; however, the insult of the dye caused her renal system to shut down further. Over the next few days, as her urine output dropped and her blood urea nitrogen (BUN) and creatinine increased, she became increasingly confused and lethargic. Her oxygenation status became threatened because of congestive heart failure secondary to the renal failure and atelectasis resulting from prolonged bed rest. Many of her other systems were affected or were threatened (i.e., nutritional status, skin integrity, and neuromuscular status) by the renal dysfunction and the prolonged bed rest. My nursing colleagues and I worked with the physicians, specialists (in renal and infectious diseases), nutritionists, respiratory therapists, pharmacists, and physical therapists to promote and maintain as many body systems as possible. A thermal dilutional catheter was placed to monitor fluid status. E. was placed on renal dopamine, a furosemide drip, and afterload reducers. Total parenteral nutrition was started at a minimal rate. Chest physical therapy and incentive spriometry and eventually a nonrebreather mask were used to help with oxygenation. She was turned and positioned frequently.

E.'s family needed support during this time. Seeing E. so confused was frightening to them. We comforted them and kept them informed. Conferences were set up with the physicians, the specialists, and the nurses to allow the family members to hear and to attempt to understand the course of action and to allow them to voice their concerns. We invited them to assist with E.'s care and allowed them privacy whenever possible. We arranged for social services to speak with them and encouraged them to have their clergy visit.

The plan of action was to support E. while her kidneys recovered from the double insult of the catheterization dye. This usually takes approximately 5 days. If her renal status continued to worsen after that or if her other systems could not be maintained (e.g., if oxygenation was severely compromised), then dialysis would be started. The decision day arrived and dialysis was indicated. She would be unable to receive peritoneal dialysis because of previous abdominal operations, so continuous venous-to-venous hemofiltration

was to be started. This was a new form of dialysis for us, and it involved new equipment. We had done continuous arteriovenous hemofiltration (CAVH) in the past with a great deal of success. This new system promised to be more user and patient friendly and did not require arterial access. I was assigned to E. because I had written the policies and the procedure for CAVH and was the unit resource person for the procedure. I also have a strong understanding of the hemofiltration process and its effects on the patient.

E.'s renal status made a dramatic recovery at about the middle of the same day. The urine output increased to 200 mL per hour, and her BUN and creatinine started falling. Dialysis was not required. Over the next few days, she became less lethargic and her mentation improved. Her appetite returned, much to her husband's delight. For him, this was the best sign of improvement. As a team, physical therapy and nursing started working on her mobilization. Within a few days, her renal function returned to baseline, and we transferred her to a general cardiology unit, where she was discharged a few days later. This was such a great joy to all of us, especially me, because she had been so sick. To see her recover so completely was a testament to all the care we and her family had given her.

Our care and support of patients is ever changing and improving. As part of the health care team, I function as a resource person for others. I am a member of the policy and procedure committee that works to maintain a high level of care. I am also a preceptor for the new registered nurses who come to our unit. I feel that in these ways I am able to assist others in understanding and promoting our high standards of care for our patient population.

Katherine L. Klos, RN, BSN, CCRN
Deborah Heart and Lung Center
Browns Mills, New Jersey

1998 AACN-3M Health Care Excellence in Clinical Practice Nominee.

20

Renal Anatomy and Physiology

Susan A. Pfettscher

Objectives

After completing this chapter, the student will be able to:

1. Locate the kidneys in the body.
2. Identify the specific anatomic structures of the kidney.
3. Identify the three major types of function that the kidney performs.
4. Differentiate the functions of each portion of the nephron in the production of urine.
5. Differentiate the hormonal functions of the kidney.
6. Relate the normal variations associated with aging to the physiology of the kidneys.

The human kidneys are complex organs that perform multiple functions essential to the human body. Their overall activity is the maintenance of physiologic homeostasis for the entire body. The human kidney performs functions that are 1) excretory, 2) endocrine, and 3) regulatory; without any of these functions, a disease state develops. Specific functions of the kidney include the following:

- Excretion of end products of metabolism (uremic toxins)
- Excretion and reabsorption of electrolytes and water
- Acid–base balance
- Secretion of hormones
- Final metabolism of specific hormones
- Final metabolism and excretion of drugs

ANATOMY

Gross Structure of the Kidneys

The kidneys are paired, elongated, flattened organs that measure approximately 6 cm in width × 12 cm in length × 3 cm in thickness; they lie retroperitoneally on either side of the vertebral column. The left kidney is slightly higher in position than the right, with its upper border lying between the eleventh and twelfth ribs. The right kidney extends downward from the twelfth rib. Their lower borders are approximately at the level of the third lumbar vertebra (Figure 20–1A). The kidneys are embedded within a layer of perirenal fat that extends downward and surrounds the ureters. Both their physical location and the surrounding layer of fat protect these vital organs relatively well from direct injury or trauma (see Figure 20–1B). In addition, the surrounding fat anchors the kidneys in their retroperitoneal location.[1–3]

A pair of adult kidneys generally weighs 300 g.[1,2] Kidneys attain adult size and function (urine output) by adolescence. Kidney size is proportional to body size and may vary by gender, height, and bone structure.[2] In describing kidney size to a patient, it may be useful to equate it to the size of a person's fist.

The kidneys are covered by an indistensible collagenous layer of tissue called the *renal capsule.* The underlying tissues of the kidney adhere to this capsule covering. Two layers of renal tissue comprise the solid structure of the kidney (the renal parenchyma); these are the *cortex* and the *medulla.* Within these two layers reside the microscopic structures of the kidney. The cortex of the kidney is the outer, densest layer of tissues in which no functional structures can be grossly visualized. The medulla contains 10 to 15 wedge-shaped structures (pyramids), with the papil-

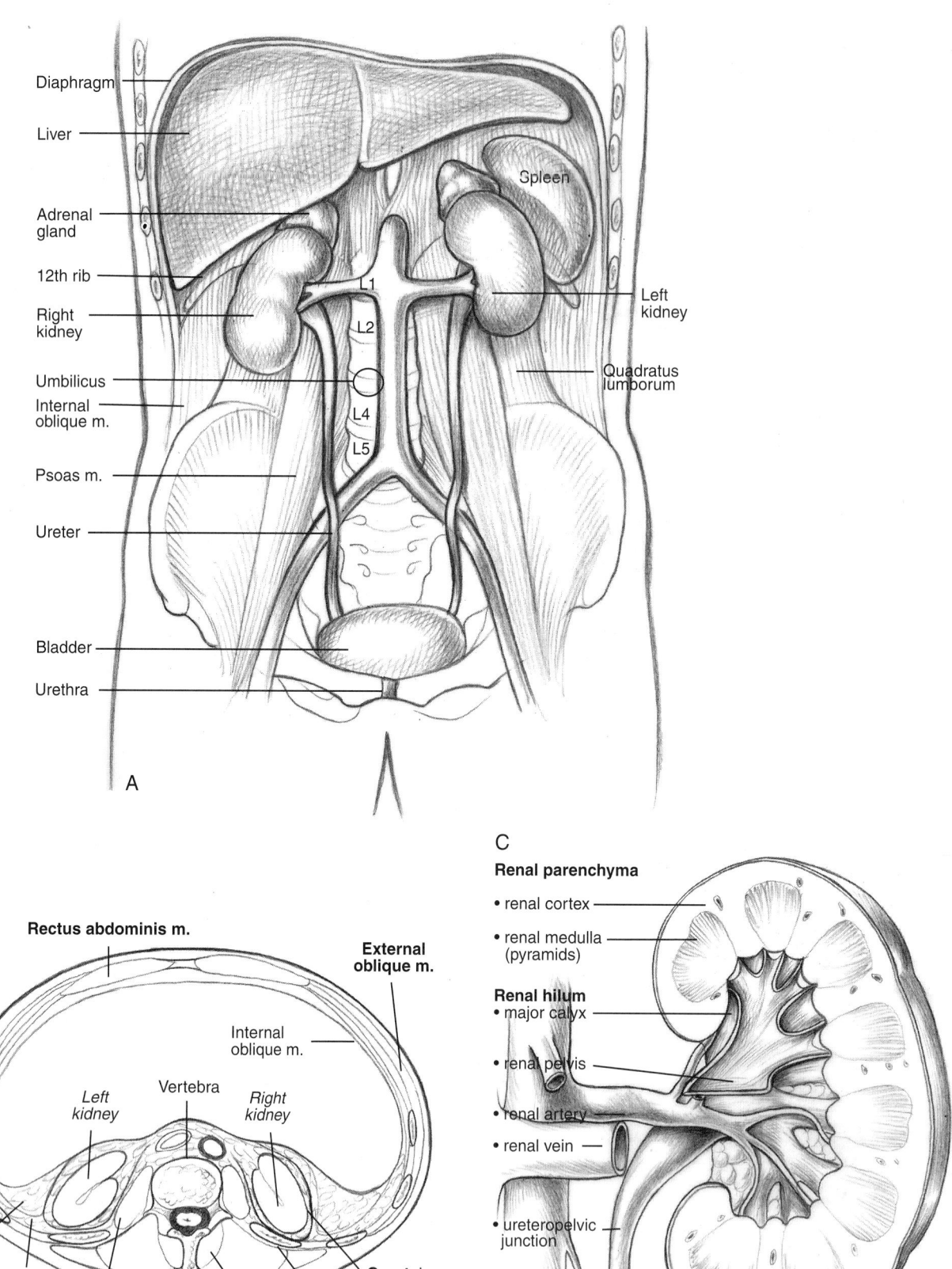

Figure 20–1

A, Location of the kidneys in the abdomen. *B*, Internal support and protection of the kidneys. *C*, Cross-sectional view of the kidney. (From *Saunders Manual of Nursing Care.* Philadelphia, W.B. Saunders, 1997, p 1174.)

lae (apices) of these structures facing inward (to the center of the kidney). The more central (innermost) area of the kidney (facing the vertebral column) is a slightly indented, hollow structure, the renal hilum, consisting of the *calyces* and the *renal pelvis* (see Figure 20–1C). These structures collect the urine formed in the structures of the outer two layers. From the renal pelvis, urine is transported in peristaltic waves down the ureter to the bladder. Urine is excreted from the bladder through the urethra.[1–4]

Vascular Structure of the Kidneys

Blood flow to the kidneys is supplied by a single renal artery that arises directly from the abdominal aorta, although duplicated renal arteries are present in approximately 20% of healthy individuals. Blood flows from the kidneys through a single renal vein that empties into the inferior vena cava; these veins may also be duplicated without adverse effect on renal function. (see Figure 20–1C). Blood flow to the kidneys is at high pressure and high flow to maintain its physiological functions. Approximately 1200 mL per minute (20% of cardiac output) is delivered to both kidneys. Compared with other vital organs such as the brain and heart, the tissue of the kidneys is relatively refractory to ischemia; the actual tissue does not suffer irreversible hypoxic damage easily.[1–4]

PHYSIOLOGY

Microscopic Structure and Function of the Kidney

The *nephron* is the microscopic structural and functional unit of the kidney (Figure 20–2); in describing the structure and function of one of these units, renal function is also essentially described. Within the nephron, the actions of filtration, reabsorption, and secretion take place to provide for the removal of end products of metabolism (toxic wastes), electrolyte and water balance, acid–base balance, hormonal secretion, and final metabolism and excretion of other substances such as hormones and drugs.

Approximately 1 million nephron structures are present in each kidney. Each nephron functions independently of the others. When individual nephrons are lost because of disease or surgical removal of a portion of or an entire kidney, the remaining nephrons undergo functional hypertrophy to maintain physiologic homeostasis of the body.

The structure of each nephron includes both vascular and tubular components. Each nephron is composed of the following segments:

- Glomerulus
- Proximal convoluted tubule
- Loop of Henle
- Distal convoluted tubule
- Collecting tubule

Most nephrons are located within the cortical layer of the kidney; a few nephrons begin deeper in the cortex and extend into the medulla of the kidney (juxtamedullary nephrons).[1–3]

Nephron Blood Flow

Blood flow to the nephron arises from the renal artery through branching into the interlobar, arcuate, and interlobular arteries. Blood enters the nephron through the *afferent arteriole*. This single vessel subdivides into a capillary tuft; the blood flows from this capillary structure through the *efferent arteriole*; one arteriole "goes to," and one "goes away from." This anomalous vascular structure (arterial–capillary–arterial) provides an important component of glomerular function in establishing pressure gradients or differences.

Renal blood flow and blood flow to the nephron through the afferent arteriole are controlled by various factors. In addition to cardiac output, systemic vascular volume, and systemic vascular resistance, renal blood vessels are affected by vasoactive substances. Norepinephrine specifically constricts both the interlobular and the afferent arterioles. Prostaglandins increase blood flow to the renal cortex, but they decrease flow to the medulla. Angiotensin II increases the glomerular filtration rate (GFR) by several actions, including efferent arteriolar vasoconstriction.[1,2,5]

Nervous system innervations also cause changes in renal and glomerular blood flow. When stimulated, the sympathetic noradrenergic nerves in the kidneys decrease renal blood flow. Stimulation of specific areas of the brain causes renal vasoconstriction, whereas stimulation of baroreceptors from decreased blood pressure also results in renal vasoconstriction. Direct stimulation of renal nerves may also stimulate renin secretion, resulting in vasoconstriction. However, these renal functions persist in a denervated kidney, so the nervous innervations of the kidney remain incompletely understood.[3,6,7]

Under normal conditions of blood flow and pressure to the kidneys, these vessels maintain a relatively constant blood flow and pressure through processes of autoregulation. The ability of the afferent and efferent arterioles of the glomerulus to dilate or constrict to maintain glomerular blood flow and pressure is one example of this autoregulation.[1–4]

The clinical significance of these mechanisms and their renal effects is particularly important to the ability to manipulate these mechanisms through the administration of drugs and other biologic agents in

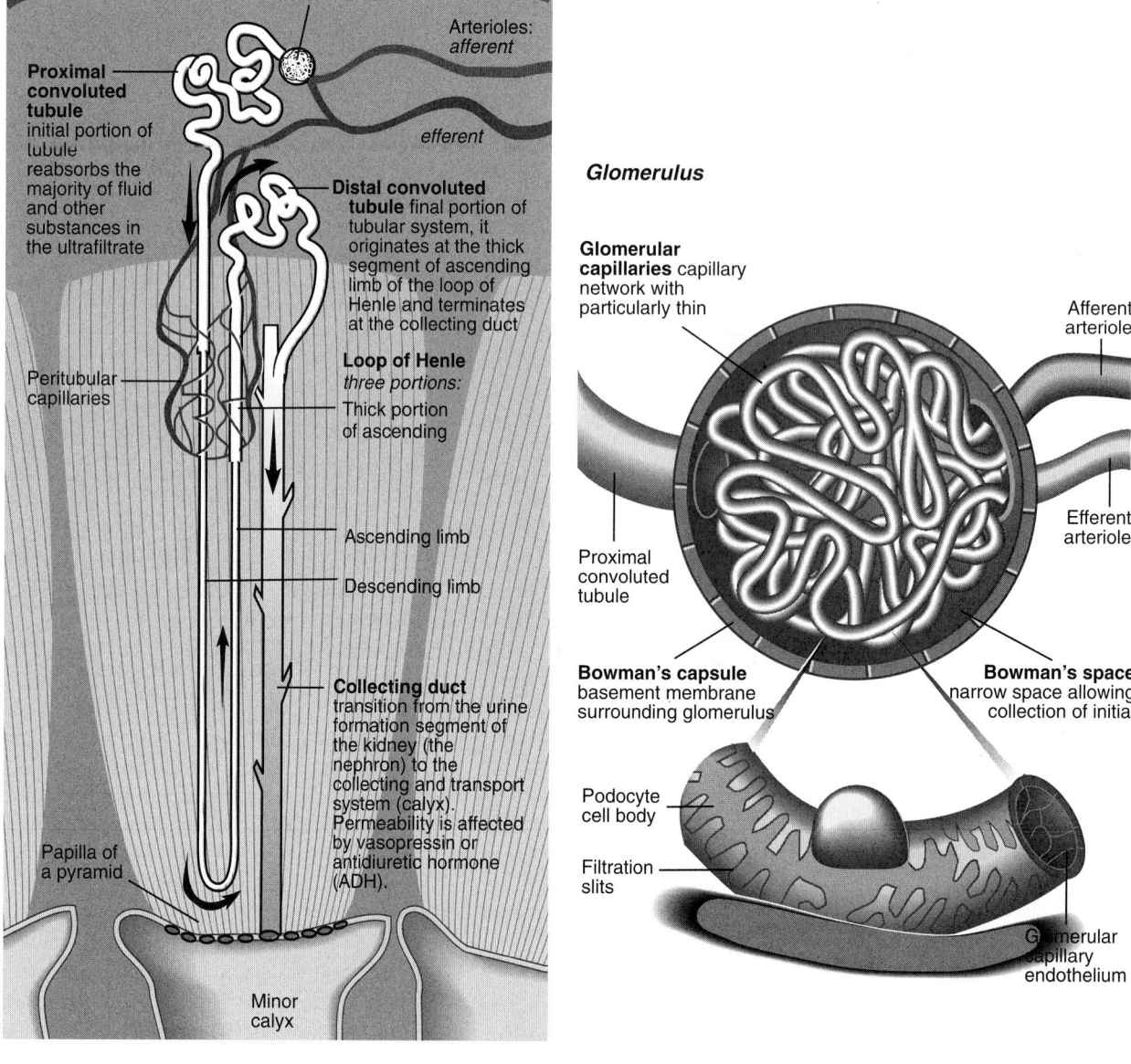

A

B

Figure 20–2

A, Microscopic apparatus of a nephron. B, Microscopic apparatus of a glomerulus. (From Saunders Manual of Nursing Care. Philadelphia, W.B. Saunders, 1997, p 1175.)

both the short-term and long-term management of patients.[1,5,7]

Glomerulus

Filtration of blood entering the glomerulus through the afferent arteriole is the primary function of this segment of the nephron (see Figure 20–2 A). The capillary bed of the glomerulus is a complex structure that creates an ultrafiltrate of plasma by functioning as a semipermeable membrane. Because of its semipermeability, this capillary structure allows for the filtration of particles of small molecular size (up to 8 nm), but it

retains larger molecules in the vascular compartment. Specifically, the small molecules that are filtered include water, end products of metabolism such as urea, nitrogen, and creatinine, electrolytes such as sodium (Na^+), potassium (K^+), and chloride (Cl^-), and glucose. The large molecules that are retained are exemplified by red and white blood cells and plasma proteins. Although size is a major determinant in this filtration, the electrical charge of an ion or molecule also determines whether it will be filtered across the capillary bed.[1,5,7]

The structure of the glomerulus includes two cellular layers that separate the capillary lumen from the final filtrate, which is collected in Bowman's capsule, the saucerlike structure surrounding the glomerular capillary tuft. These two layers, the capillary endothelium and the glomerular endothelium, are separated by a basal lamina. Mesangial cells reside between the basal lamina and the endothelium layers of the glomerular capillary; these cells are important to the function of the glomerulus because they are contractile and thus play a role in the regulation of glomerular filtration. These cells also take up immune complexes and thus are involved in the development of glomerular diseases[5,7] (see Figure 20–2B).

The amount and content of the ultrafiltrate produced in the glomerulus primarily determine the amount of final urine production. Although water is a small molecule that can pass freely across the glomerular capillary membrane, its passage is also controlled by pressure gradients. Because the blood flow entering the renal artery is at a high rate and pressure, the pressure and flow into the afferent arterioles and thus the glomerular capillary bed similarly remain higher than in other systemic capillaries. The difference between the intracapillary hydrostatic pressure and the pressure in Bowman's capsule also creates a gradient adequate to move large volumes of water from the glomerulus.

Two forces oppose the movement of water from the capillary bed; one is exerted by the oncotic pressure in the glomerular vascular compartment (opposing the movement of fluid from the blood), and the other is the hydrostatic pressure present in Bowman's capsule (Figure 20–3).

The net filtration pressure across the glomerular capillary bed is adequate to filter approximately 125 mL per minute of fluid into Bowman's capsule in all 2 million nephrons. In the fluid that crosses this membrane are the solutes that also have been filtered. This rate of filtrate flow is known as the *GFR*; it can be calculated by measuring the quantity of a substance that is filtered by the glomerulus and is excreted in the urine but is not reabsorbed or secreted in the rest of the nephron structure. The amount of this substance that remains in the vascular compartment (plasma) must also be measured to determine the amount that was not filtered. Finally, the total volume of fluid (urine) in which this amount of substance is excreted must be measured.

Calculation of the GFR is expressed as an equation:

$$\text{Clearance} = (U \times V)/P$$

with U = concentration of a substance in the urine

V = volume of urine collected over a certain time period (usually reported as volume/minute)

P = concentration of a substance in the plasma

Based on this equation, the GFR in healthy kidneys (all nephrons functioning) in a normal metabolic state is 125 mL per minute. Thus, 180 L of fluid are filtered through a healthy individual's nephrons in a 24-hour period.[1–4,6]

Clinical measurement of the GFR is performed as a creatinine clearance test. Although creatinine is an imperfect substance because minute amounts may be secreted or reabsorbed in the tubules, its almost complete filtration and excretion still exceed those of other substances. Other substances (e.g., inulin) may be injected venously and measured in the same manner as creatinine clearance to assess GFR more accurately.[1,2,5,6]

The glomerulus is an efficient structure and mechanism for initiating the process of urine formation through the creation of an ultrafiltrate of blood. If this ultrafiltrate were sampled, its solute concentrations would be similar to those of serum. The structure of the nephron is remarkable in its ability to maintain a steady state of function even when changes in hemodynamics occur; thus, the nephron plays a vital role in maintaining physiologic homeostasis.

Tubular Function

The tubular system of the nephron begins with Bowman's capsule, the saucerlike structure that collects the ultrafiltrate created in the glomerulus. It then extends into tubular structures known as the *proximal convoluted tubule*, the *loop of Henle*, the *distal convoluted*

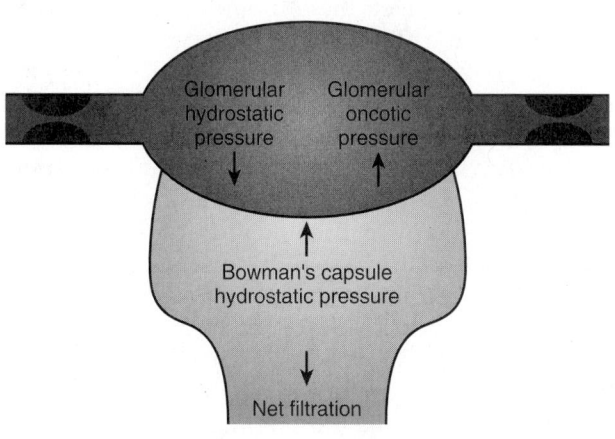

| Net filtration pressure (10 mm Hg) | = | Glomerular hydrostatic pressure (60 mm Hg) | − | Bowman's capsule hydrostatic pressure (18 mm Hg) | − | Glomerular oncotic pressure (32 mm Hg) |

Figure 20–3

Glomerular pressures and filtration. Net filtration pressure is the difference between the forces promoting and the forces opposing filtration. (Redrawn from Guyton A, Hall J: Textbook of Medical Physiology, 9th ed. Philadelphia, W.B. Saunders, 1996, p 322.)

tubule, and the *collecting tubule*. Although each of these structures has different functions, their overall function is dynamic balance of fluid and electrolytes through mechanisms that return these substances to the systemic vascular compartment or secrete additional substances into the tubules to be excreted (see Figure 20–2 A).

The tubular system is an active structure using the principles of active and passive diffusion, filtration, passive reabsorption, and active transport. In addition, the movement of substances through ion channels, pumps, exchangers, and cotransporters at the cellular level both explains and makes more complex the function of this system.

The vascular component of the tubular structure is known as the peritubular capillary network. This accompanying vascular system is responsible for the final absorption of the solutes and water that move or are transported out of the tubule for return to the systemic circulation. This movement is controlled by Starling's forces (osmotic and hydrostatic pressures) in the interstitium of the kidney and the capillary network. Thus, final reabsorption is a dynamic activity that responds to capillary hydrostatic and oncotic pressure.[1,5,7]

The *proximal convoluted tubule* receives the ultrafiltrate of plasma from the glomerulus through Bowman's capsule. The primary function of this structure is beginning reabsorption of solutes and water, primarily through physiologically active cellular functions. Approximately 65% of the solutes filtered by the glomerulus and 70% of the filtered water are reabsorbed in this tubular structure.[2,5,6]

Na^+ and Cl^- are ions of vital importance to maintenance of water and electrolyte balance in the human body. Reabsorption of these ions in the proximal convoluted tubule contributes to this homeostasis. Na^+ is actively transported out of the tubule by a Na^+/K^+ adenosine triphosphatase (ATPase) pump that also results in the transport of two K^+ ions into the tubular lumen for every three Na^+ ions actively reabsorbed; through this mechanism, excess K^+ ions are excreted, whereas Na^+ is retained.[6]

Glucose and amino acids are almost completely reabsorbed in the proximal convoluted tubule. These substances are reabsorbed by secondary active transport using the energy provided by the active transport of Na^+ out of the tubule.[6] Thus, amino acids are essentially completely transported by facilitated and passive diffusion into the interstitial fluid to be reabsorbed into the peritubular capillary system.

Glucose reabsorption is also an example of secondary active transport in which the amount reabsorbed depends on the amount filtered, the plasma level, and the GFR. In a euglycemic state, almost all the glucose filtered at the glomerulus is reabsorbed; only a few milligrams (not enough to be easily measured) are excreted in the urine. If larger amounts of glucose are excreted in the final urine, its *renal threshold* (the plasma concentration at which maximum reabsorption is exceeded and excretion begins) is reached or exceeded; this is also known as the transport maximum. Mathematically, the renal threshold of glucose is approximately 300 mg/dL; actually, it is approximately 200 mg/dL in arterial blood and 180 mg/dL in venous blood. Clinically, the result of this mechanism is known as "spilling sugar" or glycosuria.[1,2,5,6]

Other substances such as lactate, citrate, phosphate, hydrogen (H^+), and chloride (Cl^-) are also reabsorbed by secondary active transport. Finally, substances can be secreted from the surrounding interstitium into the proximal convoluted tubule; the best known of these clinically is penicillin.[6]

At the end of the proximal convoluted tubule, the solution contained within its lumen is still an isotonic, iso-osmotic fluid from which massive amounts of solutes and water have been removed. In its transit, however, no reabsorption of end products of metabolism (urea and creatinine) has occurred. Thus, this fluid has been manipulated to maintain physiologic homeostasis.

Loop of Henle. The loop of Henle is the continuing structure of the tubular system and extends from the proximal convoluted tubule, which resides in the cortical (outer) layer of the kidney. From there, the loop extends into the medullary layer of the kidney and is shaped in a long, narrow loop (often referred to as hairpin-shaped). The functions of each side of the loop of Henle are distinct and vital to the continued processing of the fluid that is becoming urine. In addition to the structure and function of the loop of Henle, the interstitium in which these tubules reside is also actively functioning tissue.

The *descending limb* of the loop of Henle consists of a cell wall that is permeable to water and relatively impermeable to the movement of other solutes; the *ascending limb* is impermeable to water but does transport solutes out of the tubule. The result of these functions is that the fluid in the descending limb becomes more concentrated (hypertonic) as it reaches the lowest point in the medulla; the fluid in the ascending limb actually becomes hypotonic as large amounts of Na^+ and Cl^- are transported out of the tubule into the surrounding interstitium. The transport of fluid out of the descending limb results in an osmolality of approximately 1200 mOsm/L at its lowest tip; in the ascending limb, the active transport of Na^+ and Cl^- is so efficient that the fluid at the upper end is hypo-osmolar (approximately 100 mOsm/L).[1,3,5,6]

Countercurrent Mechanism. The vascular structure and interstitial tissue of the cortex and medulla play an active role in achieving the dilute or hypo-osmolar state of the tubular filtrate. The vascular structure consists of a corresponding hairpin-shaped structure lying on either side of the loop of Henle; these vessels are known as the vasa recta (straight vessels). Along with the functions of the loop of Henle, the functions of these vasa recta comprise the countercurrent mechanism. The loops of Henle are known as the countercurrent multiplier, and the vessels are the countercurrent exchangers. The pumping of Na^+ and Cl^- from the ascending limb creates a hyperosmolar concentration in the surrounding interstitium. These solutes tend to recirculate in the medulla of the kidney, rather than immediately moving into the vasa recta. The vasa recta efficiently absorb the water that has been transported out of the loop of Henle into the interstitium and thus add it to the systemic vascular volume.

Urea has also been deposited in the medullary interstitium (early in renal development and beginning function); it remains in the interstitium unless alterations in renal blood flow or tubular function occur. This urea deposition in the medulla is facilitated by secretion of antidiuretic hormone (ADH, also known as vasopressin) and by its effect on the transport of urea out of the collecting tubule. Because the urea is not reabsorbed into the peritubular capillaries, it remains in the medullary interstitium to contribute to its hyperosmolar state, thus maintaining the countercurrent mechanism of osmolar gradients.

Although this countercurrent mechanism is a complex system in the kidney, it is easy to understand by describing its final effects. This mechanism is responsible for reabsorption of significant amounts of Na^+ and Cl^- (exceeding the amount that could be reabsorbed by other mechanisms). In addition, it allows for reabsorption of an additional 15% of the water that is in the filtrate presented to the loop of Henle. This system of Na^+ and water conservation is an important component of maintaining physiologic homeostasis in the sodium-rich human body.[1,3,5,6]

Distal Convoluted Tubule. The distal convoluted tubule receives a hypotonic, hypo-osmolar filtrate from the ascending limb of the loop of Henle. From the ascending limb which enters the cortex (outer layer) of the kidney, the distal convoluted tubule is positioned entirely in this outer layer. Much like the ascending limb of the loop of Henle, it is relatively impermeable to the reabsorption of water from its lumen. Solute reabsorption does continue in this structure. Active transport of Na^+ occurs along with secretion of K^+ although the opposite may occur based on the concentration of K^+ in the plasma. This active transport mechanism is the same as described for the proximal convoluted tubule.

A specific activity that occurs in the distal convoluted tubule is additional correction of K^+ balance. When the K^+ serum level rises, K^+ diffuses from the interstitium into the cell wall of the distal convoluted tubule; from there, the concentration gradient allows for diffusion of K^+ into the tubule lumen, with resulting excretion in the urine.

The increased excretion of K^+ is mediated by hormonal influences. In particular, aldosterone is secreted from the adrenal cortex when the serum and interstitial levels of K^+ are increased and stimulates this movement. In addition, the secretion of renin and its conversion to angiotensin II stimulate K^+ excretion, and decreased levels of Na^+ in the plasma and interstitial fluids also increase K^+ excretion. All these actions occur in states of physiologic stress.[1,3,5,6]

Calcium (Ca^{++}) may also be reabsorbed in the distal convoluted tubule in the presence of the active form of vitamin D (1,25-dihydroxycholecalciferol) or parathormone (parathyroid hormone or PTH).[1,5,6] Additional water reabsorption may occur in the distal convoluted tubule in the presence of ADH; this response further dynamically contributes to the correction or maintenance of systemic water balance. Final correction of acid–base balance occurs in the distal convoluted tubule through reabsorption of bicarbonate (HCO_3^-) out of the lumen and secretion of H^+ into the tubular lumen for subsequent excretion along with the excretion of other organic acids (e.g., phosphate and sulfate).[1,3,6]

Collecting Duct. The collecting duct or tubule is positioned in both the cortical and medullary layers of the kidney as it courses down to the innermost tip of the renal pyramid. The primary function of this portion of the nephron is the final correction of fluid–water balance. This dynamic process is controlled by the action of ADH on the cell wall of the collecting tubule. In the presence of ADH, water is reabsorbed from the lumen, enters the interstitium, and moves into the peritubular capillaries; the result is increased systemic vascular volume. The fluid in the collecting tubule is normally hypotonic; however, it can become isotonic or even hypertonic in the most severe conditions of excessive ADH secretion. Absence of ADH secretion results in such excessive urine excretion (massive losses of body water) that hypovolemic shock and death may quickly develop.[1,3,4,6]

The blood delivered to each nephron of the two kidneys undergoes the actions described earlier on a continual basis in the healthy individual. The urine produced contains end products of metabolism relative to diet and metabolic function, excess electrolytes, and water in amounts specific to maintain physiologic homeostasis for that individual.

Approximately 1.5 L of urine is produced in a 24-hour period by the healthy adult. This volume of urine contains almost all the urea, creatinine, and other end products of metabolic function that were formed; excess Na^+, K^+, Cl^-, and other ions are also excreted and can be measured in both aliquots and 24-hour collections of urine to measure kidney function.[1,3,5,6]

Metabolic and Endocrine Functions of the Kidney

The kidneys are metabolically active organs with functions that exceed the excretory function described earlier. Simultaneous to their excretory functions, the kidneys perform various metabolic and endocrine functions that contribute to the normal physiology of multiple organ systems and structures.

Acid–Base Balance

The kidneys play a vital role in the maintenance of acid–base balance in the human body. The kidneys' ability to serve as a buffering system in the presence of systemic acid–base imbalance is a powerful metabolic activity.

Although the body has other buffering systems, normal renal function *must* be present to maintain normal acid–base balance; without renal function, a state of metabolic acidosis occurs that cannot be corrected by other organ systems. Although the lungs function quickly to correct acid–base imbalance through respiratory changes, their function is generally insufficient and usually cannot be sustained. Renal function to reestablish normal acid–base balance is a slower process than the pulmonary system can achieve; it may take several hours before the response begins and several days to correct imbalances.

The kidneys regulate acid–base balance in two ways. Excess H^+ ions (acids) are secreted into the tubules and are then excreted in the final urine; HCO_3^- ions are reabsorbed from the filtrate in the tubules and are also regenerated by cells in the tubule wall. The kidneys also excrete fixed (nonvolatile) acids that cannot be removed through the lungs; fixed acids include sulfuric, phosphoric, and lactic acids, which are formed from general metabolic activities.

Because acids and bases are present in the body as products of nutritional or digestive and cellular metabolic activity, their production is constant and individual. Dietary intake, medication administration, and physical activity may alter acid–base formation.

The tubular structures (proximal convoluted, distal convoluted, and collecting tubules) of the nephron are the primary sites of acid–base regulation in the kidney. The chemical reactions that maintain acid–base balance occur in the cell walls of the these structures using molecules in the fluid in the tubule and the surrounding vasculature. Blood and urine pH and other measures of acid–base balance in the blood (arterial blood gases) reflect the work of the chemical buffers in body fluids, the pulmonary system, and the kidneys. If alterations in metabolic acid–base balance persist, one can assume that the kidneys are not functioning appropriately to correct this imbalance within the appropriate period (usually 48 hours).

H^+ ions are excreted after their secretion into the proximal tubule, the thick ascending limb of the loop of Henle, the distal tubule, and the collecting tubule. Regeneration of HCO_3^- in the tubular system also occurs; these ions combine with Na^+ and diffuse out of the renal tubule into the interstitial fluid and enter the vascular compartment through the peritubular capillaries.

Through several chemical reactions, represented by the following equation, reabsorption of filtered HCO_3^- is achieved across the tubular membrane:

$$HCO_3^- + H^+ \xleftrightarrow{CA} H_2CO_3 \xleftrightarrow{CA} CO_2 + H_2O$$

in which H_2CO_3 is carbonic acid and CA is carbonic anhydrase. Approximately 80% of filtered HCO_3^- is reabsorbed from the proximal convoluted tubule through these chemical reactions. Carbonic anhydrase is an enzyme required within the tubular epithelial cells to drive these chemical reactions.

Tubular buffers are also used to excrete excess H^+ ions. The combination with the weak acids (buffers) of phosphate and ammonia allow for excretion of large amounts of H^+ ions as well as these weak acids, thus contributing to acid–base balance. Acid phosphates are by-products of metabolism that are buffered by HCO_3^- in the extracellular fluid (vascular compartment); this reaction creates Na_2HPO_4, which then combines with H^+ and reacts in the tubule to form sodium biphosphate (NaH_2PO_4) + Na^+. The NaH_2PO_4 can then be excreted.

Ammonia (NH_3) is produced in tubular cells primarily from the amino acid glutamine. Ammonia diffuses into the tubule and combines with an H^+ ion to become NH_4, which then chemically combines with a negatively charged ion (usually Cl^-) to form ammonium chloride and is then excreted.

Renal correction of acidosis occurs by increasing the secretion of H^+ ions and thereby also increasing their excretion and simultaneously increasing the regeneration and reabsorption of more HCO_3^- in the tubules. In alkalosis, H^+ secretion is diminished; HCO_3^- is not regenerated or reabsorbed, thus reestablishing the ratios of H^+ to HCO_3^-.[1-6]

Regulation of Blood Pressure

The renin–angiotensin system, which originates in the juxtaglomerular apparatus of the kidney, is responsible for maintaining systemic blood pressures and extracellular fluid volume. This apparatus consists of specialized cells in the walls of the afferent and efferent arterioles and the distal convoluted tubule; as the name suggests, these two structures lie next to each other in the cortical layer of the kidney (Figure 20–4). Specialized cells in this apparatus are known as the macula densa; from the cells, the substance *renin* is secreted. This substance has been described as a

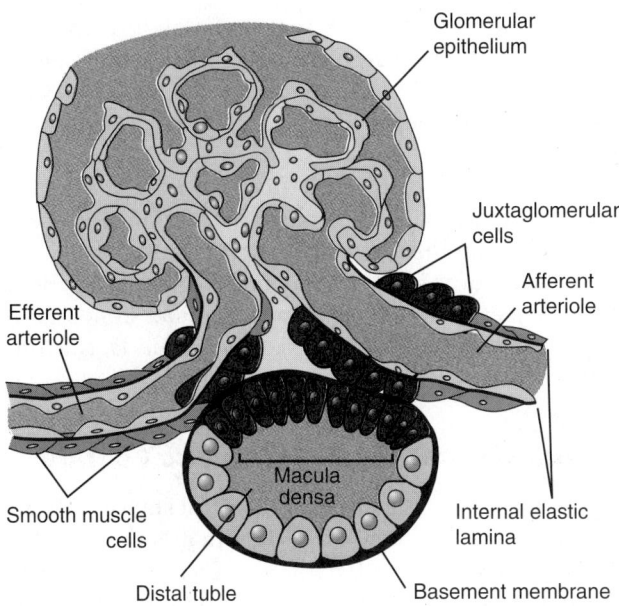

Glomerular epithelium

Juxtaglomerular cells

Afferent arteriole

Efferent arteriole

Internal elastic lamina

Smooth muscle cells

Macula densa

Distal tuble

Basement membrane

Figure 20–4

Juxtaglomerulus apparatus. (From Guyton A, Hall J: Textbook of Medical Physiology, 9th ed. Philadelphia, W.B. Saunders, 1996, p 328.)

hormone, but it is probably more accurately described as an enzyme or a prohormone because it exerts no direct actions in this form.

The anatomic location of this apparatus allows a baroreceptor mechanism to monitor the vascular pressure or volume in the afferent arteriole as blood flows into the glomerulus. Thus, these baroreceptors are able to respond to changes in the pressure and volume of blood entering the glomerulus. When pressure and volume remain at normal levels, little renin is secreted; when pressure or volume (blood flow) decreases in the afferent arteriole, renin secretion increases. Renin secretion is also stimulated by the transport of Na^+ and Cl^-; the macula densa responds to the amount of these ions in the filtrate as it reaches the distal convoluted tubule. When Na^+ and Cl^- concentrations are in-

creased in this fluid, the filtrate is perceived by the macula densa as being in a concentrated state reflecting systemic volume depletion; thus, renin is secreted to increase blood flow to the kidneys.[1,5,6]

After its secretion, renin acts on angiotensinogen, which is synthesized in the liver and is present in the general circulation. This reaction creates the substance angiotensin I. The next reaction on this inert substance occurs when angiotensin I is exposed to the angiotensin-converting enzyme (ACE), which is present in endothelial cells. The primary site for this conversion reaction is during blood flow through the pulmonary bed, although the reaction can occur in other parts of the body; when angiotensin I is exposed to ACE, it is converted to angiotensin II, its metabolically active form. Although angiotensin II has a short half-life (1–2 minutes), it is a potent vasoconstrictor.[5,6] Angiotensin II has several systemic reactions, which are all directed to protecting renal blood flow and its nephron function (Table 20–1).

Angiotensin III, a substance thought to be a biologically active metabolite of angiotensin II, appears to be primarily responsible for aldosterone secretion. These mechanisms are powerful and are often effective in their ability to protect kidney function in events of decreased perfusion. However, these mechanisms can be exhausted or may become ineffective over an extended period of renal hypoperfusion.[1,4–6]

Regulation of Red Blood Cell Production

Erythropoietin is a glycoprotein produced by the endothelial cells of the peritubular capillaries in the renal cortex of the kidney. It is often referred to as a hormone, with its receptor site being the bone marrow. Secretion of erythropoietin is primarily stimulated by conditions resulting in hypoxia, although secretion may be stimulated by cobalt salts, androgens, adenosine, and catecholamines. At the bone marrow site,

TABLE 20–1
Systemic Reactions of Angiotensin II

Action	Consequence
Produces peripheral vasoconstriction	Causes a rise in systolic and diastolic blood pressure; increases renal blood flow; increases afferent arteriolar blood flow and pressure; increases glomerular pressure; increases or maintains GFR; corrects or maintains renal function
Stimulates secretion of aldosterone	Causes reabsorption of water, Na^+, Cl^- in distal convoluted tubule, which increases systemic blood pressure; increases renal blood flow; increases or maintains GFR; corrects or maintains renal function.
Stimulates ADH (vasopressin)	Causes an increase in reabsorption of water in collecting tubule, which increases systemic blood volume and pressures; increases renal blood flow; increases or maintains GFR; corrects or maintains renal function
Stimulates postsympathetic neurons to release norepinephrine	Causes an increase in vasoconstriction, which increases systemic blood pressure; increases renal blood flow; increases or maintains GFR; corrects or maintains renal function

GFR, glomerular filtration rate.

erythropoietin stimulates the conversion of stem cells to red blood cells (erythrocytes). Although 15% of erythropoietin is produced in the liver, this source does not appear to be a biologically active site in stimulating red blood cell production when renal secretion of erythropoietin is lost.[1,5,6]

Regulation of Vitamin D, Calcium, and Phosphorus Metabolism

Along with other endocrine organs and body systems, the kidney plays a vital role in the maintenance of serum levels of calcium and phosphorus. This activity involves vitamins, minerals, hormones, digestion, and renal function. A description of all these mechanisms and components follows.

Vitamin D normally enters the body in the form of skin absorption from sunlight or dietary ingestion. It is converted to cholecalciferol, a metabolically inactive form, in the liver; the kidney is the organ that converts vitamin D to the metabolically active form of 1,25-dihydroxycholecalciferol. PTH stimulates this final conversion by the kidney. In the presence of the active form of vitamin D, Ca^{++} is absorbed from the gastrointestinal tract after its ingestion through foods or supplements.

Ca^{++} is a vitally important mineral or ion for physiologic homeostasis. Most (99%) of the body's Ca^{++} is deposited in the bones to provide rigidity to the skeleton. In this form, Ca^{++} is combined with phosphorus to form a salt. In addition, Ca^{++} is present in the extracellular fluid (the blood) and controls various cellular activities including blood clotting, neuromuscular excitability, cell membrane permeability, and secretory activities.

Although Ca^{++} is freely filtered at the glomerulus, approximately 98% of it is reabsorbed in the tubular structure of the nephron. PTH directly affects the reabsorption or excretion of Ca^{++} by the kidney; a decrease in serum Ca^{++} stimulates PTH release and calcium reabsorption, whereas an increase similarly suppresses PTH release and increases Ca^{++} excretion. Because Ca^{++} is stored in bone, it is an available source of Ca^{++} (in the presence of PTH) to the circulation when intake or absorption is diminished.

Phosphorus is a metabolic end product of dietary intake and is found in the forms of $H_2PO_4^-$ (biphosphate), $HPO_4^=$ (diphosphate), and PO_4^{+++} (phosphate). Approximately 75% of these phosphates are reabsorbed by active transport after their filtration at the glomerulus. When PTH is not present in the kidneys, phosphate reabsorption is controlled by a transport maximum (refer to the discussion of glucose reabsorption); excess amounts are excreted.

In the presence of PTH, phosphate transport is inhibited, thus maintaining appropriate ratios of calcium and phosphorus in the vascular compartment. This balance both controls the integrity of formed bone (none is resorbed) and prevents the deposition of calcium phosphate salts in the soft tissues, as occurs when excess amounts of both are in the vascular compartment.

These complicated mechanisms, achieved by interrelated organ systems and metabolic activities, successfully maintain the physiologic homeostasis of calcium and phosphorus in the human body. Alteration in renal function, even in the presence of other functioning systems (PTH secretion, intake of vitamin D, calcium, phosphorus), changes this homeostasis.[1,5,6]

Regulation of Atrial Natriuretic Peptide

Atrial natriuretic peptide (ANP) is a substance (also referred to as a hormone or factor) that is described in texts in the context of renal, cardiac, and endocrine systems. The kidney is the target organ of this substance after its secretion from the heart. It is secreted from secretory granules in the muscle cells of the atria; these granules apparently increase in number when extracellular fluid volume expands and NaCl content in the extracellular fluid increases. Investigators hypothesize that the rate of ANP secretion is proportional to the degree of stretch generated by the volume of blood in the atria and thus is responsive to increases in central venous pressure.[5,6]

Several mechanisms of action of ANP have been studied, although findings are still tentative. The actions described include the following:

1. Direct increase in GFR
2. Direct action on the tubules to promote Na^+ excretion
3. Lowering of blood pressure by inhibition of the renin–angiotensin system
4. Inhibition of aldosterone secretion
5. Neural regulation of the cardiovascular system in the brain resulting in the lowering of blood pressure and increased excretion of Na^+

From a clinical perspective, this substance may play a vital role in the treatment of patients with volume alterations, cardiac disease, and renal diseases.[4-6]

Other Metabolic Functions

The previous discussion is limited to the major substances handled by the kidney. Some other end products of metabolism can be identified and are clinically measured, although their values may be altered by dietary intake or metabolic activity. One must consider alterations in these substances within the context of a patient's medical condition.

An increasingly important aspect of metabolism and excretion by the human kidney is this organ's ability to handle modern pharmacologic agents. The kidney may serve as an organ of drug metabolism; it is the *major route* for drug excretion. In addition to the processes of renal function previously described, drugs presented to the kidney may be bound to proteins, thus preventing their excretion (these complexes are too large to be filtered at the glomerulus). In addition, drugs may be reabsorbed by passive diffusion of water or by active transport; they may also be secreted into the tubular lumen from the surrounding interstitium. Drugs that are weak acids or bases are also reabsorbed or excreted, depending on the pH of the formed urine in the nephron. Because drug action may depend on pH, manipulation of urine pH may be required to enhance drug excretion or to ensure pharmacologic activity.[1,6]

Finally, drugs may be toxins to the kidney structures (nephrotoxicity). These chemical agents may damage peritubular cells or their microscopic structures. Drugs may increase in their amounts when urine is concentrated within the tubular structure of the kidney or when renal blood flow is decreased; these drugs may become nephrotoxic because of their increased concentrations. Thus, the use of drugs may depend on renal function, and renal function should be assessed during the administration of many drugs.[6,7]

Other ions and trace metals are also presented to the kidney for filtration, reabsorption, and excretion. These substances may also be altered by dietary intake, metabolic activity, or specific disease states and should be interpreted relative to the patient's health status or treatment.[1,6]

NORMAL VARIATIONS ASSOCIATED WITH AGING

Like other vital organs, the kidneys are subject to the vascular and tissue changes attributed to the aging process. Currently, about one-third of the healthy elderly have essentially normal renal function, as studied over a 15- to 22-year follow-up. Improvements in the general health status of the elderly should increase this percentage.

Most elderly persons undergo a 30% deterioration in renal function (GFR) by their eightieth year. In persons with cardiovascular diseases or primary renal diseases, this deterioration may be even more extensive. Although the duplicated system of kidneys (most people have two separate kidneys) provides a large amount of reserve, in that 75% of renal function can be lost before a person shows signs of renal dysfunction, measurement of creatinine clearance identifies this functional loss earlier. The bedside mathematic calculation of GFR provides an estimate of renal function, but it should be interpreted cautiously and confirmed with creatinine clearance measurements.[6,7]

Chart 20–1 describes changes in renal function related to the aging process. Because of these renal changes and the systemic alterations of body water and fat or muscle mass ratio, the elderly person is especially sensitive to drug disposition. Because healthy kidneys efficiently metabolize and excrete drugs, loss of these functions places the elderly person at risk of drug overdose, nephrotoxicity, or increased drug accumulation, resulting in systemic adverse effects.[1,6,7]

CHART 20–1

Alterations in Renal Function Resulting From Aging

1. A decreased perception of thirst results in changes in blood volume. In situations of actual shifts in hydration resulting from heat, diarrhea, or decreased food and fluid intake, this alteration may become clinically significant.

2. Renal blood flow is decreased, resulting in a decreased glomerular filtration rate. In persons with systemic vascular disease, which may also contribute to decreased renal blood flow (e.g., atherosclerosis, congestive heart failure), this combination may be clinically significant.

3. Decreased renin response to volume loss prevents the aged kidney from increasing renal blood flow and systemic blood pressures through stimulation of the renin–angiotensin system.

4. Both maximum concentration and dilution of urine decrease by the seventh decade of life. These changes add to the aged person's risks of hypovolemia and hypervolemia in the face of changes in vascular volume. In combination with the altered renin response, these changes make the elderly especially vulnerable to hypotension when fluid losses occur or to overhydration and hyponatremia when vigorous hydration is required.

5. Decreased ammonia secretion also decreases the aged person's ability to maintain or correct a state of metabolic acidosis. This decrease in function may contribute to and may exacerbate other acid–base abnormalities.

In summary, the human kidneys are complex organs performing various functions that are directed at maintaining the normal physiologic features of the body. The kidneys govern water, electrolyte, and acid–base balance and the removal of metabolic wastes through actions of excretion and reabsorption that occur in the nephron. In addition, the kidneys regulate red blood cell formation through the secretion of erythropoietin, they maintain calcium and phosphorus balance, and they regulate vascular tone and volume balance through the renin–angiotensin system.

The kidneys' constant and dynamic functions allow an individual to lead a healthy life with safely enjoyed physical activities and a diverse intake of foods and fluids. Through their elaborate feedback systems, the kidneys protect other vital organ systems including the heart, lungs, and brain from the effects of decreased vascular volume or the accumulation of metabolic wastes and excessive concentrations of electrolytes. The complexity of the kidneys' structure and function continues to defy technologic (artificial) replication or replacement.

Key Concepts

➡ The kidneys perform the following functions to maintain or restore physiologic homeostasis: 1) excretion of end products of metabolism, including those generated by nutritional intake, cellular function, and drug administration; 2) excretion and reabsorption of water to maintain fluid balance; 3) excretion and reabsorption of electrolytes to maintain homeostasis; 4) maintenance of metabolic acid–base balance through excretion and regeneration or reabsorption of metabolic products; 5) secretion of erythropoietin to stimulate red blood cell production; 6) maintenance of calcium–phosphorus balance through excretion and reabsorption of metabolic products and the conversion of vitamin D to its active metabolite; and 7) control of systemic blood pressure and blood volume by the secretion of renin.

➡ Compared with other vital organs such as the brain or the heart, the tissues of the kidneys do not suffer irreversible hypoxic damage easily. If the cause of the decreased blood flow is diagnosed early, loss of function can be prevented.

➡ The nephron is the functioning unit of the kidney. Within the nephron, filtration, reabsorption, and secretion take place to provide for the removal of end products of metabolism, electrolyte and water balance, acid–base balance, hormonal secretion, and metabolism and excretion of other substances such as hormones and drugs.

➡ Each nephron is composed of a glomerulus, proximal convoluted tubule, loop of Henle, distal convoluted tubule, and collecting tubule.

➡ The primary function of the glomerulus is to allow for the filtration of small molecules. The amount and content of the ultrafiltrate produced in the glomerulus primarily determine the amount of final urine output.

➡ The tubular system of the nephron begins with Bowman's capsule and extends into the structures of the proximal convoluted tubule, the loop of Henle, the distal convoluted tubule, and the collecting tubule. Although each structure has different functions, the overall purpose is to establish a balance of fluid and electrolytes and to return these substances to the systemic vascular compartment.

➡ The renin–angiotensin–aldosterone system, which originates from the juxtaglomerular apparatus of the kidney, is responsible for maintaining systemic blood pressures and extracellular fluid volume.

➡ Along with other endocrine organ and body systems, the kidneys play a vital role in the maintenance of serum levels of calcium and phosphorus. This activity involves vitamins, minerals, hormones, digestion, and renal function.

References

1. Brenner B: Brenner and Rector's The Kidney, 5th ed. Philadelphia, W.B. Saunders, 1995.
2. Pfettscher S: Renal disorders. In: Holloway NM (ed): Nursing the Critically Ill Adult, 4th ed. Menlo Park, NJ, Addison-Wesley, 1993.
3. Marieb EN: Human Anatomy and Physiology. Redwood City, CA, Benjamin Cummings, 1995.
4. Hudak CM, Gallo BM (eds): Critical Care Nursing: A Holistic Approach, 6th ed. Philadelphia, J.B. Lippincott, 1994.
5. Lancaster LE (ed): ANNA Core Curriculum for Nephrology Nursing. Pitman, NJ, American Nephrology Nurses Association, A.J. Janetti, 1995.
6. Ganong WF: Review of Medical Physiology, 17th ed. Norwalk, CT, Appleton & Lange, 1995.
7. Lonergan ET: Handbook of Geriatrics. Stamford, CT, Appleton & Lange, 1996.

21

Renal Assessment

Rebecca S. Sloan

Objectives

After completing this chapter, the student will be able to:

1. Identify three clinical presentations of renal failure (acute, chronic, acute superimposed on chronic renal failure).
2. Identify the body systems involved in acute or chronic renal failure.
3. Describe the elements of the patient's health history that are important to the renal assessment.
4. Describe the elements of the physical assessment of patients with or at risk of renal compromise.
5. Identify important health history and physical assessment findings across the life span.

The kidneys perform various complex functions for the body including the elimination of waste products, electrolyte and water homeostasis, acid–base balance, and hormone regulation. When the kidneys do not function adequately, patients experience renal insufficiency resulting in various conditions such as hypertension, edema, anemia, and uremia. When kidney function is reduced to low levels (approximately 10% of full function), renal failure occurs. Patients then require dialysis treatment with an artificial kidney machine if they are to survive. For some patients, dialysis therapy provides short-term support while the body heals and renal function returns to normal or, at least, adequate levels. For others, the kidneys do not recover, and patients are diagnosed with end-stage renal disease for which lifelong dialysis therapy or renal transplantation offers the only means of survival.

Based on the American Nurses Association's description of the scope of nursing practice, nurses are charged with attending to the "real or potential health care problems" of patients.[1] The nurse's ability to anticipate a patient's risks for development of renal problems and diagnosis of actual renal compromise can be extremely important for the patient's short- or long-term outcome. Physical assessment of patients experiencing or at risk for renal compromise includes a comprehensive health history and physical examination, supported by findings from laboratory tests and radiographic studies.

HEALTH HISTORY

The nurse is likely to encounter patients at risk of renal compromise in three distinct groups: 1) patients who have no known history of renal failure, but who experience a sudden and devastating injury or toxic exposure resulting in the development of *acute renal failure;* 2) patients who have known *chronic renal insufficiency,* such as persons who have a history of hypertension or diabetes; and 3) patients who have *acute renal failure superimposed on chronic renal insufficiency,* as can occur when patients with chronic renal failure experience a sudden trauma or toxin exposure. The health history is vital in anticipating renal failure in patients in critical care settings, in outpatient clinic facilities, and in home care. The health history includes questions that the nurse explores with the patient or the patient's family when the patient is unable to provide information because of his or her condition. Although a general health history provides useful information regardless of the patient's presenting illness, historical data specific to the development of renal compromise are delineated in the following sections.

Risk Factors Associated With Renal Disorders

Family History of Renal Problems

The family health history explores a minimum of three generations surrounding the patient, including the patient and his or her siblings, parents, and grandparents. When the patient has children, it is important to assess their health histories as well. Of particular interest are questions about a family history of known renal disease.[2] Often, patients describe family members who have had renal transplants, are receiving dialysis, or have renal problems. The nurse should explore the family history for cardiovascular problems, such as hypertension, myocardial infarction, and heart failure. Errors of metabolism such as diabetes mellitus or gout are often seen in families of patients who have renal insufficiency, as are problems with kidney stones, urinary strictures, or congenital absence of one kidney. Polycystic kidney disease is a genetically inherited renal disease that can be identified from the family history.

Patient Health History

The personal health history of the patient includes the history of the present illness that resulted in the patient's seeking care. If the patient was admitted to the intensive care unit (ICU) as a result of an automobile accident, gunshot wound, or serious burn, or if the patient had a recent surgical procedure such as open heart surgery or a bone marrow transplant, development of renal failure is a significant concern. If the patient is currently diagnosed with chronic renal insufficiency or acute renal failure, septicemia, excessive doses of antibiotics, radiopaque dyes, and hypotensive events can compromise renal function even more, resulting in acute renal failure superimposed on chronic renal failure.[3]

The personal history also includes the patient's health before this time. Especially noteworthy is a history of hypertension, diabetes mellitus, arthritis, gout, or toxemia of pregnancy. Patients are frequently admitted to critical care settings with previously known problems with the kidneys, such as Goodpasture's syndrome, polycystic kidney disease, or glomerulonephritis. Other times, the patient is vulnerable for development of renal failure some time after the diagnosis of infectious diseases such as streptococcal infection or infection with human immunodeficiency virus (HIV). For elderly patients, a history of dehydration or fluid overload, mental confusion, and change in medications are important components of the health history for assessing renal function.

Medications. As part of the patient's history, the nurse should obtain information about actual or potential renal compromise by reviewing the patient's current and past medication history. The nurse should assess the patient's current medications that are indicative of primary renal insufficiency (from the kidneys directly) or secondary renal insufficiency (a result of coexisting medical conditions). Diuretic medications (e.g., furosemide, bumetadine) provide information about previously diagnosed renal insufficiency resulting from primary renal disease or secondary to cardiac pump failure. The nurse should assess for medications (e.g., digoxin) that are used for cardiovascular conditions, such as reduced cardiac output (a prerenal condition), that affect kidney function. Antihypertensive medications indicate the need for cardiovascular regulation, which may be cardiovascular or renal in origin. The use of insulin or oral hyperglycemic control agents indicates the presence of diabetes mellitus, which is a considerable risk factor for development of renal compromise. When the patient has needed a recent change in the amount of insulin, particularly a decrease in insulin required to attain glucose control, a significant reduction in renal function needs to be considered.

In addition to consideration of the pharmacologic agents that the patient currently takes for various health conditions, the nurse should assess the patient's recent exposure to medications that are known to be nephrotoxic. Although antibiotics have saved countless lives, they have also caused some patients to develop renal compromise or even acute renal failure. In particular, the aminoglycoside antibiotics (i.e., gentamicin, tobramycin), rifampin, and amphotericin B cause acute renal insufficiency, especially in patients who had known chronic renal failure before the use of these powerful agents.

Some cancer chemotherapy agents (e.g., cisplatin) are highly nephrotoxic. Patients who have been or are currently receiving chemotherapy for solid organ or blood-related cancers are at serious risk of developing renal failure.

Arthritis medications also contribute to the development of renal failure, even when used for only short periods in vulnerable patients. Patients with rheumatoid arthritis frequently are prescribed heavy metal medications, such as oral gold therapy (auranofin), which can be directly harmful to the kidneys.[4] Common nonsteroidal anti-inflammatory agents (NSAIDs; e.g., aspirin, ibuprofen, naproxen, oxaprozin, nabumetone) are recognized as having serious side effects due to nephrotoxity even in patients who display no previous renal compromise. According to Hellmann,[5] "All of the NSAIDs, including aspirin, can produce renal toxicity, resulting in interstitial nephritis, nephrotic syndrome, reversible renal failure, and aggravation of baseline hypertension." Patients who are also diabetic are at even higher risk for development of NSAID-induced renal failure. Diabetic patients commonly receive prescribed or over-the-counter NSAID therapy for arthritis relief. The combination of renal insufficiency from diabetes and nephrotoxicity from NSAID use often pushes patients into complete renal failure, frequently requiring lifelong dialysis therapy.

Accidental or intentional medication overdose is a frequent cause of renal failure. Incomplete suicide attempts often include use of medications that can result in acute renal failure or end-stage renal disease. Any patient with a recent history of attempted suicide from medication overdose requires surveillance for renal compromise. Of particular importance are overdoses of aspirin and heroin. The elderly are particularly at risk of medication overdosage from additive pharmacologic effects from multiple medications. Poor vision and difficulty in remembering complex dosage schedules can further lead to overdose in the elderly. Further, unrecognized renal or liver compromise alters how the elderly person metabolizes medications, frequently resulting in toxic drug levels at "normal" medication dosages.

In addition to the nephrotoxic aspects of certain medications, the nurse should assess for side effects caused by the kidneys' inability to excrete medications appropriately, resulting in toxic levels of medications.[6] Figure 21–1 illustrates the pharmacokinetics of drug elimination in patients with renal disease. In particular, the nurse should assess medication levels of digoxin, phenytoin, antibiotics, and other medications that are primarily excreted by the kidneys. Elevated medication levels or physical manifestations of

medication overdose may be one of the first indicators of change in the patient's renal function. The opposite is also true; when kidney function begins to return, the patient may suddenly need more medication than before to replace medication excreted through improving renal function.

Exposure to Toxins and Traumas. In addition to the medication history, the health history also includes the patient's exposure to nonpharmacologic nephrotoxic agents and traumas. Potential toxins are found in the patient's natural environment and include exposure to farm and industrial chemicals, cleaning solvents, lead, or other heavy metals.

Various nonnatural environmental situations place persons at risk of developing renal problems. Soldiers and civilians are at risk of renal disease from various war-related, toxin-producing devices. Civilians and rescue workers are at risk of exposure to toxins from natural or man-made disasters. Again, persons who attempt suicide place themselves in "unnatural" environments. Those who survive frequently develop acute renal failure. Particular attention needs to be paid to carbon monoxide overdose or gunshot wounds or other actions that cause massive hemorrhage. Persons who attempt suicide involving purposeful ingestion of medications or home cleaning fluids in toxic doses may survive, but they can go on to develop acute renal failure. Street people are known to ingest various toxic products, such as antifreeze, window washer, and other solvents. Loss of renal function can be life-threatening in these situations.

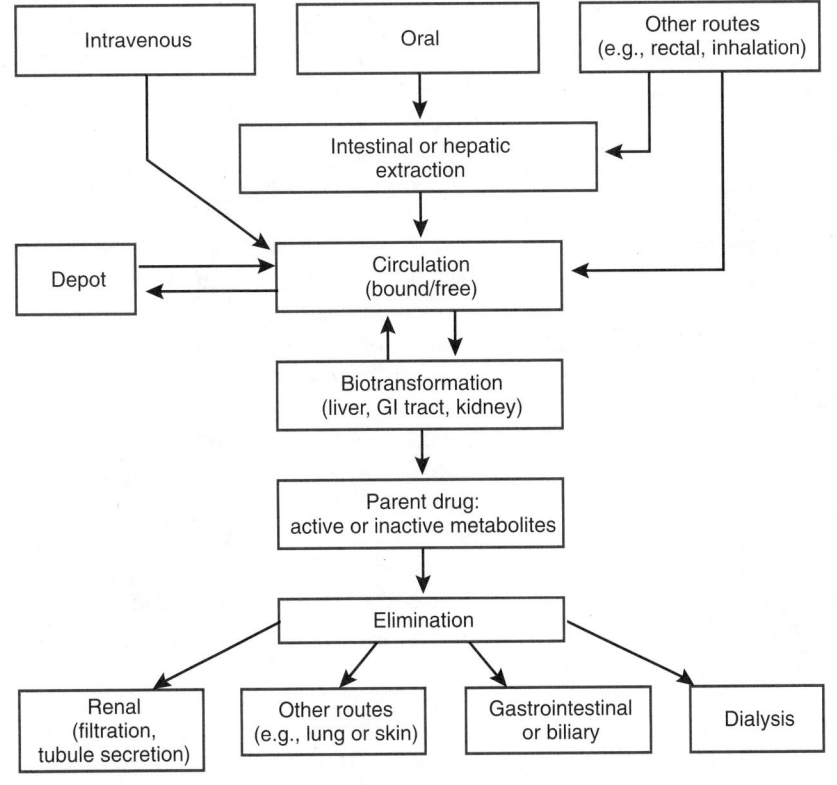

Figure 21–1

Schema of drug elimination in patients with renal disease. (From Shuler C, Golper TA, Bennett WM: Prescribing drugs in renal disease. In: Brenner BM (ed): Brenner and Rector's The Kidney, vol. 2. Philadelphia, W.B. Saunders, 1996, p 2654.)

A less dramatic, but still unnatural, environment is the hospital or health care setting. Patients are routinely exposed to nephrotoxic agents as they undergo diagnostic procedures such as intravenous pyelograms and cardiac catheterization procedures. Sometimes, nephrotoxicity can be avoided through careful maintenance of patient hydration; at other times, the toxic effects of radiopaque dyes and other agents cannot be ameliorated. Diabetic patients, again, are at increased risk of subsequent renal compromise resulting from exposure to iatrogenic nephrotoxic agents (such as radiopaque intravenous pyelography or cardiac catheterization dye).

Trauma plays an important role in the development of renal insufficiency. Historically, the need to help the many soldiers and civilians who suffered renal failure from massive crush injuries sustained during the bombings of London in World War II led to the development of today's hemodialysis therapies.[7] Although ICU patients who have sustained automobile accident injuries, gunshot wounds, or serious burns are highly likely to develop acute renal failure, patients in other health care settings must also be queried about trauma. Abused women and athletes need to be assessed for blunt trauma to the kidneys directly.

Trauma can also occur to the kidney as a result of obstruction.[8] Patients who have a history of urethral stricture, kidney stones, or spinal cord injury are often unable to empty their bladders in a natural fashion. The urine collects in the kidneys; the result is overfilling of the ureters (hydronephrosis) and possible damage to the nephrons themselves.

Renal ischemia, reduced blood flow to the kidney, can occur to a single kidney or to both kidneys as a consequence of systemic ischemia resulting from hypotension from cardiovascular failure, anaphylaxis, sepsis, or hemorrhage. The patient's need for intervention with medical devices can also contribute to the development of ischemia, such as use of the heart–lung machine during open heart surgery. Aortic aneurysm rupture or repair can also result in renal compromise from ischemia.

Signs and Symptoms Associated With Renal Disorders

Patients with renal problems present with signs and symptoms that vary across a continuum of severity based on the acute or chronic nature of the renal problem, as well as the degree of renal compromise. Patients with chronic renal failure may exhibit only mild physical symptoms such as trace to 2+ edema and hypertension, often controlled with medication. Some patients present with only laboratory findings of slowly increasing serum creatinine and blood urea ni-

trogen values to indicate that their kidney function is in jeopardy. Persons experiencing acute renal failure exhibit sudden loss of urine volume, significant weight gain and edema, rapidly increasing laboratory values for serum creatinine and blood urea nitrogen, and serious electrolyte imbalances. Some patients in acute renal failure present with congestive heart failure, shortness of breath, significant fatigue, abnormal cardiac rhythms, altered neurosensory status, or oliguria (scant or absent urine output). These findings occur in addition to symptoms directly related to the initiating cause of the acute or chronic renal failure, such as septicemia, diabetes, or trauma.

In addition to the physical signs and symptoms related to renal compromise, chronic and acute renal failure can also result in numerous psychosocial problems for patients. These include alterations in growth and development across the life span for persons who developed renal failure as children, as well as alterations in comfort, sleep, and nutrition for all patients who experience renal compromise.

As described earlier, renal compromise affects or is affected by multiple body systems: the skin, neurologic status, pulmonary function, cardiovascular status, musculoskeletal system, and endocrine function can all be involved. The nurse should query the patient about changes or problems with each of these systems.

Patients in acute or chronic renal failure frequently present with similar signs, but they differ in how rapidly the symptoms evolve and how serious the symptoms become. Early in the course of renal failure, patients exhibit symptoms related to elevated blood pressure and edema of the lower extremities. Periorbital edema and edema of the sacral area are common findings in patients confined to bed. Cardiopulmonary signs and symptoms include shortness of breath, the need for more than one pillow at night to facilitate breathing, cough, or easy fatigability. Patients describe decreased muscle strength and increased tiredness when doing normal activities such as climbing stairs, doing housework, and taking care of their children. When renal compromise becomes advanced, patients frequently describe memory loss, inability to concentrate, somnolence, and sometimes loss of consciousness.

Skin problems frequently occur in chronic or end-stage renal failure and include itching and a yellow–gray skin color indicating the presence of uremia.[2] Rarely seen outside the ICU, a classic skin manifestation is that of "uremic frost," in which levels of uremic toxins are so high that the body attempts to excrete them through the skin, resulting in a frostlike coating on the skin.

Signs and symptoms of renal problems can also be found in the endocrine system. Growth hormone production is affected in children who develop significant renal failure, resulting in short stature or delayed pubescence. Signs and symptoms related to anemia can be due to reduced erythropoietin activity that accompanies significant renal function loss.

Perhaps the clearest indicators of renal problems are found by thorough assessment of laboratory findings related to electrolyte balance, hydration, acid–base balance, and serum creatinine and blood urea nitrogen. These tests are described more fully in Chapter 22.

PHYSICAL EXAMINATION

Physical assessment of the patient at risk of renal problems, or with diagnosed renal insufficiency, requires expert physical examination techniques using all the nurse's senses, including what she or he sees, hears, smells, and feels during the examination.

Inspection

Inspection begins on the patient's entry to the ICU, hospital unit, or outpatient facility or on the nurse's entry to the home care patient's environment. The nurse observes for obvious physical signs of illness, difficulty with mentation or ambulation, and the patient's general ability to complete activities of daily living. The correlation between the patient's growth and development with the patient's stated age, such as short stature, is evaluated. In particular, children who experience chronic renal insufficiency frequently appear much younger than their stated ages because of alterations in growth hormone mediated by reduced renal function. Older patients may appear more aged or infirm than their stated age because of the ravages of acute or chronic renal insufficiency.

Specific physical assessment parameters for each body system are noted in the following sections and are pertinent to evaluation of both acute and chronic renal failure.

Skin

The patient's skin provides an excellent place to start the physical examination. The skin should be warm and intact. Normal variations based on racial or ethnic origins are considered when assessing skin color. Patients with renal disease frequently have a yellow–gray cast to their skin indicating uremia. Pallor is seen when patients experience anemia resulting from reduced erythropoietin production from long-standing renal insufficiency or renal failure. Erythema is seen in patients with infectious diseases that can cause acute renal failure. Hot, dry skin and fever can indicate the presence of infectious processes or dehydration.

The nurse assesses hydration status by pinching the skin of the patient's forearm between the nurse's thumb and index finger to test for skin turgor. If the skin turgor is brisk (returns to normal quickly), the patient is not dehydrated; if the skin remains in a "pinched" position for several seconds, the skin turgor is reduced, indicating dehydration. In babies, the nurse assesses the fontanelle for retraction or bulging as an early indicator of hydration status. Patients of all ages should be assessed for the presence of periorbital edema.

The skin is also assessed for bruises or injuries that could directly result in renal impairment from trauma. New surgical scars could indicate that the patient is at risk of postoperative complications of renal failure. Of particular interest are cardiovascular operations because of the potential renal damage from hemorrhage during surgery and the intraoperative use of the heart–lung bypass machine. The nurse also considers whether the patient was exposed to radiopaque dyes during the preoperative diagnostic period.

The presence of any skin rashes is also important. Systemic lupus erythematosus, an autoimmune disease with renal complications, frequently presents with a classic red "butterfly rash" over the cheeks. Kaposi's sarcoma is a frequent finding in patients with HIV infection, which can progress to include development of renal failure. Anaphylactic reaction to medications or other agents frequently presents with hives and perioral or generalized edema before the development of renal complications. Patients exposed to carbon monoxide frequently are unconscious and have a distinctive cherry red skin color; frequently, these patients develop acute renal complications.

As part of the skin assessment, the fingernails are also observed (Figure 21–2 and Table 21–1).

In addition to what the nurse sees and feels, she or he also attends to how the skin smells. Sometimes, a distinct urine smell can be noted as the body attempts to excrete urea through the skin when the kidneys can no longer perform this function. Patients with diabetic ketoacidosis have a distinct fruity smell on their breath (see Chapter 28).

Head, Ears, Eyes, Nose, and Throat

Headaches, blurry vision, and periorbital edema are frequent findings in patients with renal problems. Patients at risk of renal failure frequently have other problems evident in the physical examination of the mouth and eyes. Pallor of the mucous membranes and conjunctiva can indicate anemia due to renal problems or a recent hemorrhage. A funduscopic examination not only provides important knowledge about the vessels in the eyes, but also indicates how similar vascular beds (such as those in the kidney) have been affected by the presence of hypertension or diabetes.

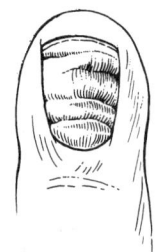 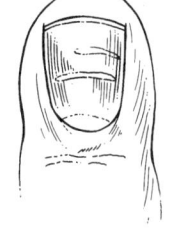 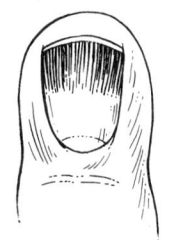 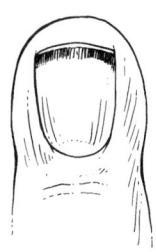

BEAU'S LINES MEES' BANDS LINDSAY'S NAILS TERRY'S NAILS

Figure 21–2

Common nail findings associated with renal disease. (From Swartz MH: Textbook of Physical Diagnosis: History and Examination, 2nd ed. Philadelphia, W.B. Saunders, 1998, p 99.)

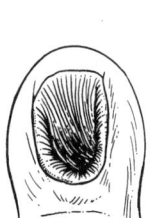 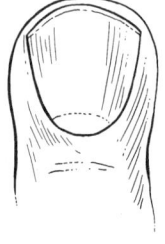 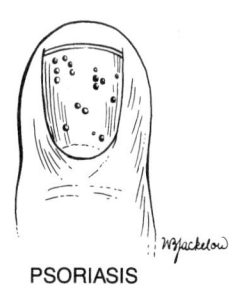

KOILONYCHIA CLUBBING PSORIASIS

For instance, eye grounds that indicate hypertensive changes of retinal hemorrhage, arteriovascular "nicking," or arterial spasm usually indicate that the same process is occurring in the vasculature of the kidney as well. Diabetic eye changes associated with hemorrhages, exudates, or "cotton-wool" patches indicate a similar process in the renal microvasculature.

Cardiac Status

Because of the direct connection between cardiac problems and renal disease, a thorough cardiac examination is necessary. The nurse observes for cyanosis of the lips, skin, or nail beds. Capillary refill is assessed by pressing lightly on the fingernails and toenails and observing for quick return of color (normal return is <3 seconds). The nurse monitors the patient's vital

signs for elevations in blood pressure, rapid or slow pulse rate, and fever. Patients with renal compromise frequently have observable jugular vein distention (see Chapter 7) resulting from fluid overload.

Pulmonary Status

The nurse observes the patient for shortness of breath (dyspnea) with normal activity, rapid breathing (tachypnea), or a feeling of "air hunger." Also assessed is whether the patient's breathing is even and rhythmic or ragged and labored. The presence of Kussmaul's breathing, or extremely deep breathing, can indicate the presence of metabolic acidosis often associated with renal compromise. Rapid or slow breathing and shallow or extra deep breathing are warning signs that the patient may be experiencing

TABLE 21–1
Fingernail Assessment

Finding	Characteristics	Cause
Beau's lines	Transverse grooves due to sporadic decrease in nail growth	Chronic renal or liver disease
Mees' bands	White transverse marks	Acute renal toxicities from poisonings or acute systemic disease
Lindsay's nails (or "half-and-half")	Proximal half of the nail whitish; distal portion reddish or pink	Renal disease
Terry's nails	White nail beds with small area of normal color in distal 1–2 mm border	Low albumin due to cirrhosis or renal disease
Koilonychia (spoon nails)	Nail indentation	Iron deficiency anemia, a common finding in patients with renal abnormalities
Clubbing	Broadened upper portion of finger and nail bed	Cardiovascular compromise
Pitted nails	Small pits in surface of nail	Psoriasis

pulmonary problems related to overhydration. The nurse observes the number of pillows the patient uses (orthopnea) or whether the patient breathes more easily when lying on one side (trepopnea), as commonly seen in patients experiencing congestive heart failure,[9] often of renal origin. The nurse observes for use of accessory muscles to assist the patient's breathing (see Chapter 15).

Muscloskeletal Status

The nurse observes the patient's stature and compares it with the normal range for the person's age and developmental status. Short stature frequently indicates a history of renal problems as a child. Electrolyte imbalance, particularly hyponatremia, hypercalcemia, and potassium imbalance, can result in neuromuscular weakness or involuntary "twitching" of the extremities.[10]

Neurologic Status

The critical care nurse who is caring for the conscious or unconscious patient in the ICU or hospice unit is well aware of the importance of the neurologic examination in assessing the patient's condition. Outpatient and home care patients also require neurologic assessment; alterations in neurologic examination findings can be early indicators of renal problems. These changes an be abrupt or may occur over a long period, and they can be immediately apparent or difficult to identify. Although loss of consciousness is easy to determine, it is more difficult to assess increased somnolence, difficulty in arousal after sleeping, and memory loss. Orientation to person, place, and time is a routine part of this examination. Short-term memory can be assessed by asking the patient to repeat a series of five to seven numbers. Patients who are experiencing neurologic problems associated with uremia have a difficult time doing this task.

The nurse observes the patient's gait and station to identify gross neurologic changes that could be the result of uremia, such as inability to perform tandem walking, inability to walk on the heels or toes, and increasing swaying with the Romberg test (see Chapter 39).

Renal Evaluation

Although laboratory evaluation provides specific and direct evaluation of renal function, nurses are able to evaluate some aspects of the patient's renal function at the bedside, home setting, or outpatient facility. Alterations in daily weight are important findings in the assessment of renal function. Patients need to be weighed at the same time of day and wearing the same amount of clothing each time for weight changes to be meaningful. Documentation of fluid intake and urine output is useful in the assessment of renal function. Intake includes all fluids administered by mouth or intravenously. Output includes all fluids excreted from the kidneys or bowels or through other losses, such as hemorrhage. Extreme care in measuring fluid intake and output is necessary to give an accurate picture of the patient's renal function. Urine color ranges from nearly colorless to extremely dark. More information on interpretation of the urine color can be found in Chapter 22. The nurse notes any changes in the color of the urine. Drugs can alter the color of the urine; for instance, phenazopyridine can cause the urine to be red-orange. The urine is also examined for clarity; the presence of blood, white blood cells, or bacteria results in cloudy urine.

Auscultation

The nurse uses his or her own auditory senses to assess the character of the patient's breathing. Frequently, the patient with renal problems presents with shortness of breath, rapid or irregular breathing patterns, or obvious oxygen deficit. The stethoscope is used to determine whether the patient has rales (crackles) or rhonchi (wheezes), which indicate a fluid imbalance (see Chapter 15). The stethoscope is used to assess for bruits over the major vessels including the carotid arteries, the abdominal aorta, the renal arteries, and the femoral arteries.[9]

The nurse assesses for the presence of extra heart sounds, which are indicative of cardiac overload. Extra heart sounds (S_3 or S_4) or murmurs are identified by listening at the aortic, pulmonic, Erb's point, mitral, and tricuspid areas (see Chapter 7). The presence of extra heart sounds when there previously were none is of particular importance.

Palpation

Skin

Regardless of the patient care setting, palpation of the skin provides the nurse with valuable information for assessing the patient's renal status. To begin, the nurse assesses whether the skin is feverish or feels clammy. The nurse assesses for edema of the lower extremities and sacral area by pressing the fingers into the patient's skin for 2 to 3 seconds.[9] Edema is recorded as 0 when no edema exists or from +1 to +4. "Pitting edema" is found when the fingers leave a deep depression in the skin after 30 seconds.[11] Figure 21-3 illustrates the technique of assessing the lower extremity (see Figure 7-5 for assessment of sacral edema).

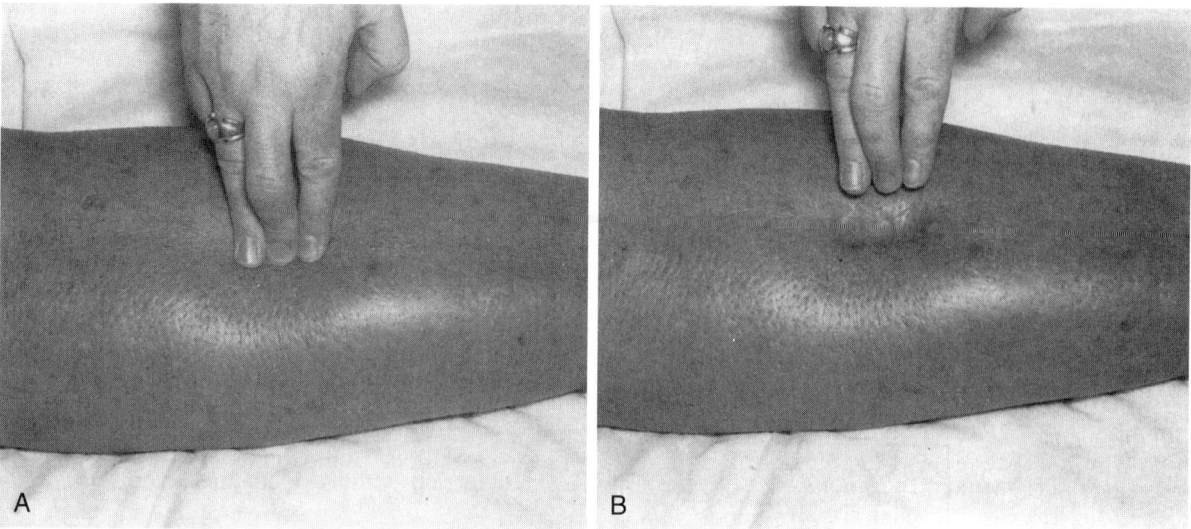

Figure 21–3

Technique for testing for pitting edema in the lower extremities. A, shows the examiner pressing into the shin area. B, shows the indentation that occurs after the fingers are lifted when pitting edema is present. (From Swartz MH: Textbook of Physical Diagnosis: History and Examination, 3rd ed. Philadelphia, W.B. Saunders, 1998, p 311.)

Cardiac Status

The nurse assesses the patient's cardiac status in various ways. Of significance to the patient with actual or potential renal problems is identification of cardiac size. In patients with renal insufficiency, it is not uncommon for the heart to be enlarged. The nurse assesses the size of the heart on a chest radiograph. When a chest radiograph is not available, such as in the home care environment, the nurse can assess cardiac size by palpating for the point of maximal impulse (the PMI). The nurse places a hand over the cardiac silhouette and feels for the PMI (Figure 21–4). It can be identified as approximately a 2 × 2 cm spot where the heartbeat is felt most strongly. Normally, the PMI is found in the left midclavicular line in the fifth intercostal space. In patients with congestive heart failure or cardiac insufficiency, a frequent finding in renal impairment, the heart is enlarged, and the PMI is found to the left of the midclavicular line or in the sixth or greater intercostal space. The nurse also observes the patient for neck vein distention from hypertension associated with fluid overload (see Chapter 7).

Abdomen

The abdomen is palpated to assess the kidneys. The kidneys are usually smooth and firm. Enlarged kidneys are associated with hydronephrosis or polycystic kidney disease, or they are a result of the kidneys' attempts to maintain renal function despite failing kidney function. Hard or lobular kidneys indicate a pathologic condition, such as polycystic kidney disease or a renal tumor. Frequently, the kidneys cannot be palpated,[9] although tenderness in the area where the kidneys are located can be assessed by palpation (Figure 21–5).

The bladder is also palpated for fullness, tenderness, or guarding. Occasionally, a patient displays "timid" bladder because of psychosocial reluctance to

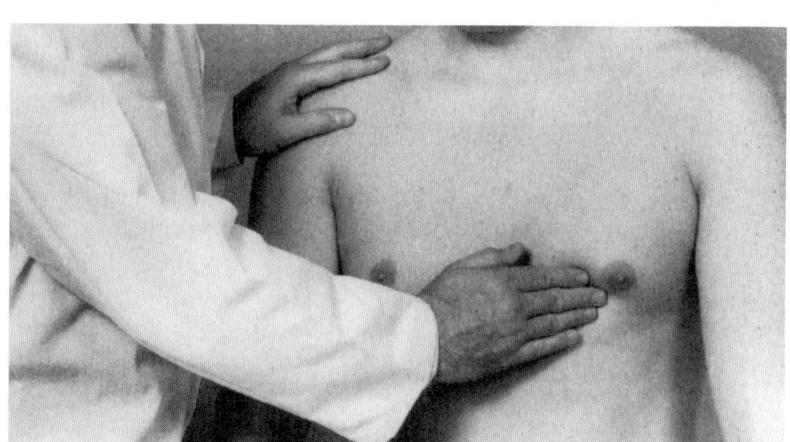

Figure 21–4

Technique for assessing the point of maximum impulse of the heart. (From Swartz MH: Textbook of Physical Diagnosis: History and Examination, 3rd ed. Philadelphia, W.B. Saunders, 1998, p 304.)

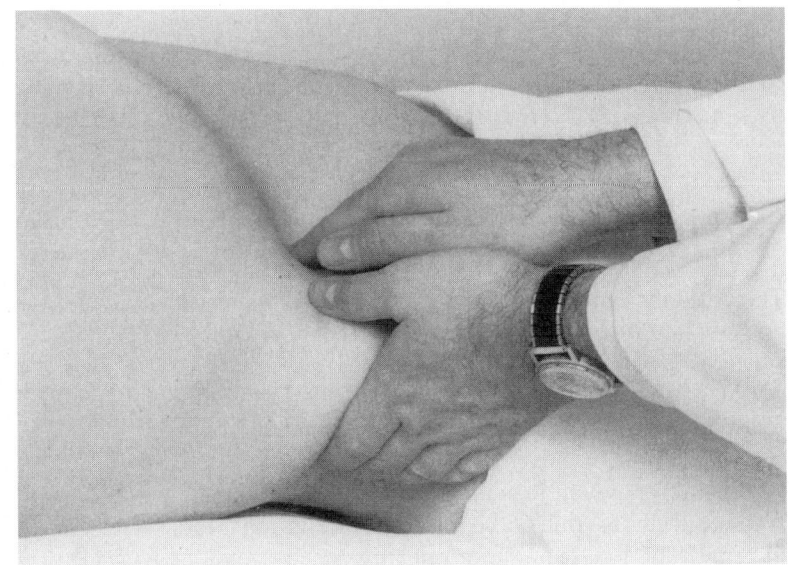

Figure 21–5

Technique for kidney palpation. (From Swartz MH: Textbook of Physical Diagnosis: History and Examination, 3rd ed. Philadelphia, W.B. Saunders, 1998, p 380.)

void in an unfamiliar or less than private setting. The nurse provides every opportunity for the patient to be comfortable in this situation. In other situations when the bladder is full and the patient is unable to void, neurogenic bladder or bladder–ureteral obstruction must be considered.

Percussion

The nurse uses percussion to identify whether the patient has cardiopulmonary signs of fluid in the lungs from congestive heart failure or pulmonary edema. If decreased breath sounds or the presence of rales or rhonchi are found on auscultatory examination, the nurse further assesses the patient's pulmonary status by percussing for dullness over all the lobes (see Chapter 15). A finding of dullness indicates a consolidation or fluid buildup in the lower respiratory tract.

Tenderness in the area where the kidneys are located is assessed by percussion. The same technique is useful in determining the presence of inflammation in the kidneys from infection or trauma. To perform this examination, percussion is done along the costal vertebral angle on both the right and left sides (Figure 21–6). The nurse increases the comfort of this maneuver by placing one palm against the patient's back just below the lowest rib (over the normal anatomic location of the kidney) and tapping with the fist of the other hand. This maneuver is repeated on the opposite side.

The reflex hammer is used to elicit neurologic function status through percussion (see Chapter 39). Because renal failure can result in imbalances of the body's sodium, potassium, and calcium concentrations, neuromuscular responses can be altered. Hyperreflexia is noted in patients who have hypernatremia as a result of small hemorrhages in the brain.[10] This condition is indicated by change in neurologic reflex responses over time. The Babinski test is performed by

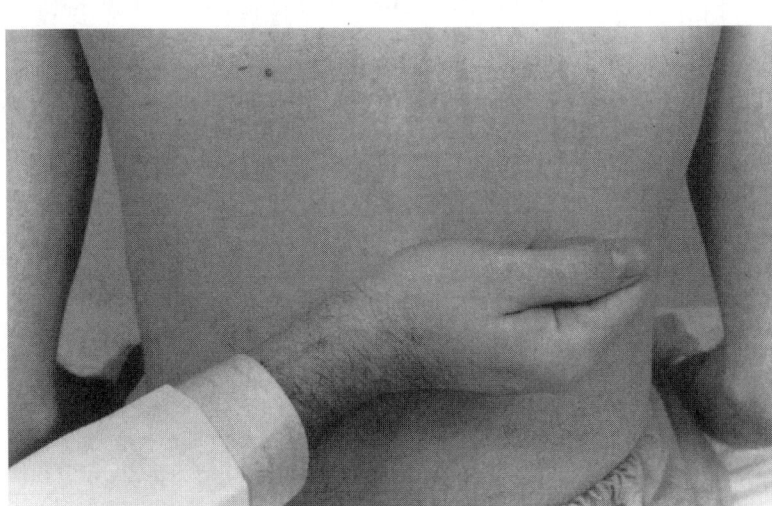

Figure 21–6

Technique for assessing costovertebral angle tenderness. (From Swartz MH: Textbook of Physical Diagnosis: History and Examination, 3rd ed. Philadelphia, W.B. Saunders, 1998, p 380.)

drawing the handle of the reflex hammer across the sole of the foot from the heel to the toes; curling of the toes inward is a normal finding, whereas flaring of the toes outward indicates a neurologic deficit.

Weight and Vital Signs

The patient's temperature, pulse rate, blood pressure, and weight provide important information during physical assessment of the patient diagnosed with or at risk of acute or chronic renal failure. Not only does fever indicate the presence of infection or dehydration, but also fever itself further dehydrates the body and results in hypovolemic renal ischemia.

Body weight is one of the most important indicators of renal function. It is important to weigh patients at the same time every day, on the same scale, and wearing the same amount of clothing to determine fluctuations in weight associated with fluid balance disturbances. Weight loss is a common finding in chronic illness, such as chronic renal failure. More commonly, however, patients with renal insufficiency experience weight gain because they are unable to excrete urine, and it is third spaced throughout the body as edema.[12] A change of more than 2 lb in 24 hours is a significant weight gain. Unfortunately, weight gain alone does not provide a broad picture of what is occurring. Patients at risk of dehydration or fluid overload require ongoing observation of their body weight.

Hypotension can indicate the presence of sepsis, hemorrhage, or other conditions that can cause renal ischemia. Hypertension can be the result of fluid buildup from poorly functioning kidneys. The pulse rate is frequently elevated in patients who are in fluid overload from acute or chronic renal failure because the heart must work extra hard to pump the blood or in patients who are entering a state of shock from sepsis or hemorrhage. When the heart begins to lose strength, the pulse rate may drop to low levels, indicating that all the organs including the kidneys may not be perfusing well enough to sustain the patient.

Intake and Output

In normal physiology, the amount of urine output is directly related to the amount of fluid intake. Normal urine output may vary from 750 to 1800 mL per day, depending on intake.[2] Urine output can also be reduced when patients are hyperventilating, running a fever, or losing fluid through emesis or the nasogastric tube and through seepage from massive burns or wounds (see Chapters 47 and 50). Seriously ill patients in various settings require daily evaluation of fluid

TABLE 21–2
Electrolyte Disturbances Associated with Acute or Chronic Renal Failure

Hypokalemia or hyperkalemia
Hyponatremia or hypernatremia
Hypocalcemia or hypercalcemia
Hypomagnesemia or hypermagnesemia
Hypochloremia or hyperchloremia
Hypophosphatemia or hyperphosphatemia

intake and urine output. When renal disease is present, however, urine output can fall drastically behind and contributes to the changes noted in vital signs, cardiopulmonary status, and body weight. A gain or loss of 500 mL of fluid is equal to 1 lb of body weight. In the ICU, the patient's condition may even warrant hourly calculation of intake and output. When fluid intake and urinary output are out of balance, electrolyte disturbances are seen (Table 21–2). These findings are discussed in Chapter 22.

NORMAL VARIATIONS ACROSS THE LIFE SPAN

Renal function undergoes distinct and normal changes as individuals move from one physical development stage to another. Under normal conditions, the kidney maintains a remarkable ability to support the body's functions. However, under the stress of disease, the kidneys of infants and the elderly[13] are at greatest risk of life-threatening complications. In newborn infants, losses of fluid due to fever or diarrhea frequently result in significant dehydration. The elderly also experience more problems with dehydration, electrolyte imbalance, and cardiovascular compromise that predispose these patients to renal compromise. Serum creatinine alone is not a good indicator of renal function in the elderly. With aging, muscle mass is lost, and this loss reduces the serum creatinine level.[13] This natural reduction in serum creatinine level may mask declining renal function. In these patients, measurement of the creatinine clearance is a more appropriate laboratory assessment of renal function. See Chapter 22 for more details on calculating creatinine clearance.

Key Concepts

- ⇒ A detailed health history including family history of cardiovascular problems, hypertension, kidney stones, urinary strictures, diabetes, arthritis, gout, or toxemia of pregnancy can assist in identification of patients at risk of acute renal failure.
- ⇒ A detailed medication history including antibiotic therapies used previously and any diagnostic tests

that could have included contrast media also assists in identifying patients at risk of acute renal failure.

➠ For the elderly, a history of dehydration, fluid overload, mental confusion, or change in medication is important information in the assessment of renal function.

➠ Renal failure exists in three different presentations: acute, chronic, and acute superimposed on chronic renal failure.

➠ Many antibiotics, particularly aminoglycosides, are nephrotoxic. Some chemotherapy agents and some arthritis medications can also contribute to the development of acute renal failure.

➠ Renal compromise affects the functioning of multiple body systems: the skin, neurologic status, pulmonary function, cardiovascular status, musculoskeletal system, and endocrine functions.

➠ Renal assessment includes auscultation of lungs and heart for signs of fluid accumulation, palpation of the bladder and kidneys, percussion of the chest walls and costal vertebral angle, weight and vital sign assessments, and intake and output evaluation.

➠ Prompt recognition and diagnosis prevent or limit irreversible damage and decrease the chance of advancement to renal failure.

References

1. American Nurses Association: Nursing: A Social Policy Statement. No. 27. Kansas City, MO, American Nurses Association, 1980.
2. Kernicki JG: Renal/urinary assessment. In: Ruppert SD, Kernicki JG, Dolan JT (eds): Critical Care Nursing: Clinical Management Through the Nursing Process. Philadelphia, F.A. Davis, 1996, pp 656–661.
3. American Society of Nephrology, National Kidney Foundation, and American College of Physicians: Acute renal failure and nephrotoxicity. In: Knochel JP (ed): Medical Knowledge Self-Assessment Program in the Subspecialty of Nephrology and Hypertension. Philadelphia, American College of Physicians, 1994.
4. Payan DG, Katzung BG: Nonsteroidal anti-inflammatory drugs; nonopioid analgesics; drugs used in gout. In: Kantzung BG (ed): Basic & Clinical Pharmacology, 6th ed. Norwalk, CT, Appleton & Lange, 1995, pp 536–559.
5. Hellman DB: Arthritis and musculoskeletal disorders. In: Tierney LM Jr, McPhee SJ, Papadakis MA (eds): Current: Medical Diagnosis and Treatment, 1997. Stamford, CT, Appleton & Lange, 1997, pp 750–799.
6. Shuler C, Golper TA, Bennett WM: Prescribing drugs in renal disease. In: Brenner BM (ed): Brenner & Rector's The Kidney, vol. 2. Philadelphia, W.B. Saunders, 1996, pp 2653–2702.
7. Peitzman SJ: Nephrology in the United States: from Osler to the artificial kidney. Ann Intern Med 105:937–946, 1986.
8. Curhan GC, Zeidel ML: Urinary tract obstruction. In: Brenner BM (ed): Brenner & Rector's The Kidney, vol. 2. Philadelphia, W.B. Saunders, 1996, pp 1936–1958.
9. Swartz MH: Textbook of Physical Diagnosis: History and Examination, 2nd ed. Philadelphia, W.B. Saunders, 1994.
10. Driver DS: Renal assessment: back to basics. Am Nephrol Nurses Assoc J 23:361–367, 1996.
11. Brasfield LK: Renal clinical assessment. In: Thelan LA, Davis JK, Urden LD, et al (eds): Critical Care Nursing, 2nd ed. St. Louis, C.V. Mosby, 1994, pp 593–598.
12. Kernicki JG: Fluid and electrolyte physiology and pathophysiology. In: Ruppert SD, Kernicki JG, Dolan JT (eds): Critical Care Nursing: Clinical Management Through the Nursing Process. Philadelphia, F.A. Davis, 1996, pp 662–707.
13. Palmer BF, Levi M: Effect of aging on renal function and disease. In: Brenner BM (ed): Brenner & Rector's The Kidney, vol. 2. Philadelphia, W.B. Saunders, 1996, pp 2274–2296.
14. North American Nursing Diagnosis Association (NANDA): Nursing Diagnoses: Definitions and Classification, 1997–1998. Philadelphia, NANDA, 1996.

22

Renal Laboratory and Diagnostic Tests

Rebecca S. Sloan

Objectives

After completing this chapter, the student will be able to:

1. *Discuss the importance of early identification of trends in laboratory and diagnostic data that suggest renal compromise.*
2. *Describe the concept of serum osmolality and its relevance to renal functioning.*
3. *Differentiate the systemic effects of common electrolyte disturbances.*
4. *Relate the impact of the normal variations in the aging process to the diagnostic assessment of the renal system.*
5. *Compare and contrast the diagnostic procedures of kidneys, ureters and bladder (KGB), renal arteriogram, intravenous pyelography (IVP), retrograde testing, renal computed tomography (CT), renal ultrasound, and renal biopsy, including indications, contraindications, and nursing considerations.*

Persons with acute or chronic renal failure experience biochemical alterations as a result of the kidney's inability to filter waste products and to regulate homeostasis. The causes of chronic and acute renal failure are varied and are the result of reduced blood flow to the kidney (prerenal failure), structural or functional changes within the kidneys themselves (intrarenal failure), or problems within the lower urinary tract (postrenal failure). In addition to findings directly related to urine production, the kidneys play important roles in multiple body systems. Therefore, laboratory and diagnostic tests related to hormone regulation, coagulation, erythropoiesis, respiratory function, and cardiac function frequently indicate abnormalities associated with reduced renal function. This chapter focuses on those laboratory and diagnostic tests that reflect renal function abnormalities.

Care providers have not always had the luxury of specific information provided through today's laboratory and diagnostic capabilities. Early in the history of medicine, physicians and nurses could only rely on the patient's symptoms to identify problems. By the 1820s, however, physicians were beginning to understand ways to categorize diseases based on anatomic and pathologic findings. During this period, Dr. Richard Bright of Guy's Hospital in London was following a group of patients who had been diagnosed with "dropsy," or congestive heart failure often associated with renal insufficiency.[1] He found that some of these patients had albumin in their urine. He discovered this by boiling a teaspoon of urine over a candle. Dr. Bright's discovery led to the renaming of "dropsy" to Bright's disease. This example highlights how, from simple beginnings, sophisticated laboratory and diagnostic tests continue to develop and to provide ever more specific understanding of acute and chronic renal insufficiency.

We now understand that substances enter the body by means of the foods and fluids we ingest (intake). Under normal conditions, the kidneys and gastrointestinal tract regulate which of those nutrients are used by the body and which are eliminated (output). When renal function is reduced, the delicate balance between intake and output is drastically altered. Laboratory tests are meaningful when one understands how the kidneys regulate blood levels of various substances through elimination of those substances in the urine (see Chapter 20). The following are some of the more common laboratory and diagnostic tests in use today for diagnosing renal disease and for monitoring renal function.

LABORATORY TESTS

Tremendous information is available to us from simple blood and urine tests performed at the bedside, in hospital or clinic laboratories, and sometimes even in the home setting. Although some patients require more specialized assessment, standard blood and urine testing remains relatively inexpensive and noninvasive, and results are available quickly. The student is reminded that each facility uses its own unique laboratory equipment, chemical reagents, collection methods, and laboratory procedures that result in variations in "normal" values from one institution to another.

Blood Assessment

Some tests, such as serum glucose concentration, require only a fingerstick drop of blood. Most blood tests require one or more test tubes of blood drawn from the antecubital or another suitable vein. The type of blood testing needed determines the type of test tube (e.g., heparinized, prepared with ethylene diaminetetra-acetic acid) used for sample collection. Although some tests require ice or immediate processing, most standard blood tests for renal function do not require special handling. Blood tests can be ordered to diagnose a condition or to determine the status of a known condition. Diagnostic tests include the complete blood count (CBC), which is further divided into the red blood cell count, white blood cell count, and differential, as well as hemoglobin and hematocrit. An elevated white blood cell count indicates the presence of inflammation or infection, which could affect the patient's renal function. A decreased hemoglobin or hematocrit is useful in identifying anemia, which often accompanies renal failure and is also frequently seen in acute care settings in which multiple blood samples are drawn to monitor a patient's condition. Blood samples that measure renal function directly include those obtained from serum chemistry panels: electrolytes (sodium, potassium, bicarbonate, and chloride), blood urea nitrogen (BUN), and serum creatinine (S_{Cr}). Additional information on some frequently performed serum laboratory tests in patients with or at risk of renal insufficiency is given in the following sections.

Serum Albumin

About 50% of the total plasma protein is albumin, which is manufactured in the liver.[2] Under normal conditions, the blood vessels do not permit proteins to escape, thus providing a means of colloid osmotic pressure that keeps fluid in the vascular space as well (see Chapter 20). However, when the vessel walls become permeable to proteins, such as occurs in diabetes mellitus, nephrotic syndrome, or serious burns, albumin can escape and can enter the interstitial space. A fluid shift results, causing peripheral edema. When this occurs, the patient's normal serum albumin level of 3.4 to 4.7 g/dL is reduced (hypoalbuminemia), a finding indicating that albumin is being lost from the blood.[3] Hypoalbuminemia is a common finding in patients with renal insufficiency, especially in nephrotic syndrome and glomerulonephritis, in which protein is lost through the urine.[4]

Blood Urea Nitrogen and Creatinine

BUN and S_{Cr} levels are standard markers of renal function. Each is a by-product of normal protein metabolism. BUN values are significantly influenced by protein intake and therefore are less reliable markers of renal function than S_{Cr} values.[4] Normal values for BUN are 8 to 20 mg/dL.[3] According to Brasfield[2] extrarenal causes of elevated BUN include infection, medication side effects, excessive protein intake, and dehydration. On the other hand, patients who are overhydrated or malnourished or who have liver failure and cannot make albumin sufficiently may present with BUN values lower than normal.[4]

Creatinine is found in the blood in amounts that are proportional to the patient's muscle mass. Because it is not influenced by protein intake, the S_{Cr} value provides a more sensitive indicator of renal function than BUN. S_{Cr} values are most useful when combined with a 24-hour urine creatinine measurement to determine the body's clearance of creatinine (C_{Cr}; see later). Normal S_{Cr} values are 0.6 to 1.2 mg/dL.[3] Elevated S_{Cr} values indicate decreased renal function.

Measurement of the BUN/Cr ratio is a useful tool in patients with renal failure. Normally 12:1 (BUN/S_{Cr}) to 20:1 (BUN/S_{Cr}), the BUN/Cr ratio is decreased in protein-losing conditions, such as nephrotic syndrome, liver disease, and malnutrition. The BUN/Cr ratio is elevated in fluid-losing conditions such as dehydration.[4]

Serum Osmolality

The serum osmolality is a measure of the concentration or dilution of the blood. Normal values are 285 to 293 mOsm/kg H_2O.[3] Antidiuretic hormone (ADH) plays an important role in regulation of serum osmolality (see Chapter 20). ADH works to concentrate the urine when the body needs to retain fluid. These values are important when attempting to determine whether a rise or fall in BUN or S_{Cr} is due to hydration status or to actual changes in renal function.

Hemoglobin and Hematocrit

Hemoglobin and hematocrit are indicators of intravascular fluid volume. Elevations in these values indicate hemoconcentration, while decreased values indicate fluid overload. Normal hemoglobin values are 13.6 to 17.5 g/dL for males and 12.0 to 15.5 g/dL for females. Normal hematocrit values also vary by gender and are 39 to 49% for males and 35 to 45% for females.[3] Hemoglobin and hematocrit levels are frequently low in patients with overhydration from reduced renal function or increased fluid intake. Hemoglobin and hematocrit values also are often low in persons with chronic renal failure because reduced renal function interferes with the normal release of erythropoietin (see Chapter 20) to stimulate the bone marrow to produce blood cells.

Serum Electrolyte Disturbances

As the kidney loses its ability to filter, secrete, and excrete various chemicals from the blood, either elevated or reduced concentrations of these chemicals are found by laboratory tests (Chapter 20). Found in the intracellular and extracellular fluids, electrolytes play important roles in the body's ability to maintain acid–base balance, body water homeostasis, crucial enzyme reactions, and neuromuscular activities. Alterations in electrolyte balance can result in life-threatening conditions (Table 22–1).[5] The following sections describe selected serum electrolyte disturbances related to acute or chronic renal failure.

Serum Potassium. Potassium can be lost from the body through vomiting, gastric suction, or diarrhea and with use of various medications, especially the diuretics. Hypokalemia (serum values less than 3.5 mEq/L) can result in muscle weakness, decreased peristalsis, and confusion.[6] Particularly important are the cardiac irregularities that can occur when potassium is depleted; these can result quickly in cardiac arrest (see Chapter 8).

Hyperkalemia is also life-threatening. Frequently the result of a failure of the kidneys to excrete potassium efficiently, hyperkalemia (>5.0 mEq/L) is also seen in patients who take potassium supplements and those who have serious burns or crush injuries.[6] Patients with hyperkalemia can present with symptoms as mild as muscle weakness, numbness, or tingling in the fingers or around the mouth, or they may have symptoms of serious cardiac irregularities that can result in cardiac arrest. Both hyperkalemia and hypokalemia can be seen in various abnormalities in renal function (see Chapters 23 and 24).

Serum Sodium. The serum sodium concentration varies, depending on whether the patient is actively losing or retaining sodium or water, conditions that cause the serum sodium level to be low (hyponatremia), normal, or elevated (hypernatremia).[5] Normal ranges for serum sodium are 135 to 145 mEq/L.[4] Loss of sodium from the gastrointestinal tract through vomiting or diarrhea can result in hyponatremia.[6] At other times, persons can become hyponatremic from drainage from large wounds or burns. Excessive sweating as seen in heat exhaustion can also result in hyponatremia. Diuretics can result in loss of sodium and potassium. The elderly are particularly vulnerable to conditions that result in hyponatremia.[5] In other cases, sodium levels may appear low in the serum, but the real problem is one of having comparatively too much water in the circulating volume, thus diluting the serum sodium value. These conditions include congestive heart failure, cirrhosis, and nephrotic syndrome, as well as side effects of many medications commonly given to patients with renal insufficiency (diuretics) or hypertension (angiotensin-converting enzyme medications). In patients with water intoxication, the release of ADH is inappropriate and causes the body to retain water that should be excreted (see Chapter 27). Clinically, the nurse observes for alterations in level of consciousness, dizziness, hypotension, lethargy, or the presence of nausea and vomiting. Patients can progress to convulsions, oliguria, and

TABLE 22–1
Concentration of Electrolytes in Various Body Fluids (mEq/L)*

Fluid	Sodium	Potassium	Chloride	Bicarbonate	Hydrogen
Plasma	135–145	3.5–5.0	98–106	25–29	7.35–7.45
Gastric juices	55–100	10–15	120	5–10	90
Pancreatic juices	145–160	5	65–90	50–80	—
Bile	130–145	5–9	75–100	10–45	—
Ileum	125	10–80	55	60	—
Sweat					
Insensible	8	10	15	—	—
Sensible	10–80	6	5–85	—	—

*Levels may vary depending on the physiologic state of the body.
From White B: Maintaining fluid and electrolyte balance. In: Bolander VB: (ed): Sorenson and Luckmann's Basic Nursing: A Psychophysiologic Approach, 3rd ed. Philadelphia, W.B. Saunders, 1994.

other life-threatening symptoms of sodium imbalance.

Hypernatremia (serum sodium >145 mEq/L) occurs when sodium is not excreted by the kidneys in a normal manner or when sodium intake is excessive.[6] The most frequent cause of this disorder is dehydration. Vomiting and diarrhea can result in the loss of excessive fluid from the body, thereby causing a more concentrated serum sodium level. Uncontrolled diabetes mellitus can result in excessive urination, which causes the serum sodium to be elevated as well. Symptoms of hypernatremia include thirst and elevated body temperature and can progress to neurologic signs such as altered level of consciousness and seizures. Medications that commonly contribute to the development of excessive sodium levels include steroids and oral contraceptives.[4]

Serum Calcium. Calcium is regulated by parathyroid hormone (PTH). PTH can mobilize calcium stored in the bones when the body needs additional calcium in the blood (see Chapter 25). Normal serum calcium values are from 8.5 to 10.5 mg/dL.[3] In renal failure, vitamin D metabolism is compromised, and calcium is not absorbed from the gastrointestinal tract efficiently. Other conditions that can cause reduced serum calcium levels are malnutrition, diarrhea, overuse of antacids, and defects in pancreatic function. Muscle cramps, tetany, mental confusion, and seizures can result. Hypocalcemia is present when serum calcium values are less than 8.5 mg/dL.[6] This value should not be confused with the test for *ionized serum calcium,* which has a normal value of 4.4 to 5.4 mg/dL and measures the physiologically active form of the total calcium concentration. According to Nicoll and colleagues,[4] "ionized calcium measurements are not needed except in special circumstances, e.g., massive blood transfusion, liver transplantation, neonatal hypocalcemia, and cardiac surgery." Ionized serum calcium values, however, are more useful than total serum calcium in patients who have renal failure, nephrotic syndrome, or other conditions associated with abnormal serum proteins.[4]

Hypocalcemia is seen in patients with renal insufficiency who present with hypoalbuminuria or low serum magnesium. Some patients with parathyroid disorders present with hypocalcemia, and others present with hypercalcemia, depending on the pathophysiologic features of the hormonal imbalance.[4]

Hypercalcemia (serum calcium >10.5 mg/dL)[4] occurs when calcium is released excessively from the skeletal system, such as in patients with multiple bone fractures or tumors of the bones. Renal cell carcinoma, multiple myeloma, and Addison's disease are associated with elevated total serum calcium levels. Immobilization can also affect how calcium is absorbed into the bones. Medications that contribute to hypercalcemia include antacids, thiazide diuretics, and lithium.[4] Thirst, lethargy, cardiac irregularities, and confusion are symptoms of calcium overload.

Serum Magnesium. Magnesium is essential for maintaining cellular permeability, neuromuscular function, and is necessary for many enzymatic reactions within the body. Normally 1.8 to 3.0 mg/dL,[4] low serum magnesium values (hypomagnesemia) are frequently seen in alcoholic patients because of their malnourished state. It is also seen in patients with dehydration, overuse of diuretics, and protracted diarrhea.[6] In renal disease, hypomagnesemia is seen in patients with chronic glomerulonephritis or diabetic ketoacidosis. Medications given to patients in renal failure, including diuretics and cyclosporine (used in renal transplantation), can cause hypomagnesemia. Various neuromuscular signs can be noted in patients with hypomagnesemia, including facial tics, spasticity, cardiac rhythm abnormalities, and confusion.

Hypermagnesemia is seen in patients who ingest large amounts of magnesium through antacids or laxatives.[6] Renal failure, dehydration, and serious trauma have been associated with elevated serum magnesium levels.[4] Central nervous system depression and cardiac rhythm changes (bradycardia) are frequent findings in patients with hypermagnesemia.

Serum Chloride. Chloride balance fluctuates in the same direction as sodium balance.[5] It is an important anion for maintenance of acid–base balance (see Chapter 20). Normal serum chloride values range from 98 to 107 mEq/L.[4] Hypochloremia is indicated when serum chloride levels fall below 98 mEq/L.[6] Vomiting, loss of electrolytes through diuretic use, and excessive sweating are common causes of hypochloremia. Excessive bicarbonate use, corticosteroids and diuretics contribute to development of hypochloremia. Slowed respiratory rate and tetany are frequently found in these patients.

Hyperchloremia is found in patients with chronic renal failure, renal tubular acidosis or acid–base disturbances from respiratory alkalosis, or metabolic acidosis from diarrhea.[4] Brasfield[6] noted hyperchloremia in patients who are given an aggressive regimen of parenteral isotonic saline. Diuretics can cause an elevation in chloride concentration through water loss. Kussmaul's respirations, altered level of consciousness, and muscle weakness are frequent symptoms.

Serum Phosphorus. Normal serum phosphorus values are 2.5 to 4.5 mg/dL.[3] Phosphorus metabolism is complex and includes PTH production, gastrointestinal absorption, vitamin D activity, nutritional status, and renal function capability. Conditions of hypophosphatemia result from excessive loss or reduced intake of phosphorus. Bone disease (e.g., rickets), chronic alcoholism, the need for nasogastric suction, and many other conditions contribute to reduced serum phosphorus values. Patients with renal failure are frequently restricted in foods that contain phosphorus. Malnutrition from alcoholism can cause phosphorus stores to become depleted. Excessive use of antacids can result in removal of phosphate through the gastrointestinal tract. Blood dyscrasias (e.g., hemolytic anemias, inadequate white cell function, or decreased platelet aggregation) are the most common results of reduced serum phosphorus levels.[6] Renal patients suffer long-term effects of calcium or phosphorus problems such as demineralization of bones, leading to fractures and mobility problems.

Hyperphosphatemia is indicated by excessive serum phosphate levels. Various chemotherapeutic agents can cause elevated serum phosphorus levels. Renal failure can result in decreased excretion of phosphorus. Muscle tetany is a common finding in hyperphosphatemia. Calcium deposits can be found in the soft tissues as the body attempts to correct the biochemical imbalance. At its extreme, hyperphosphatemia can cause tachycardia, hyperresponsive reflexes, tetany, and even paralysis.

Urine Assessment

The urinalysis serves as an excellent clinical diagnostic or monitoring test for many disease conditions, including acute or chronic renal failure. However, the findings must be interpreted in light of normal and abnormal variations in diet, medications, collection techniques, and variations in "normal" values from one laboratory to another.[7]

Urinalysis

Assessment of the urine begins with a determination of the urine's clarity, color, and odor. Urine is normally clear. Cloudy urine indicates the presence of particulate matter often associated with infection. Urine color varies from yellow to straw colored. Urine that is nearly colorless is often present with large volumes of diluted urine; dark yellow urine is frequently seen in highly concentrated urine samples. Urine can also be colored by medications such as rifampin (brown to dark red) and phenazopyridine hydrochloride (orange to red). Blood can also be seen in the urine as either bright red or dark (cola colored). The presence of bilirubin in the blood can cause the urine to appear dark red to brown. Greenish urine may indicate the presence of *Pseudomonas* bacteria or bile pigments in the urine.

Urine testing provides direct knowledge of what actually is filtered, reabsorbed, and eliminated through the kidney. Urine volume is frequently used in the critical care setting (from hourly collections to collections that reflect urine output over 8 to 24 hours) to assist in determining renal function and hydration status by comparing fluid intake and urine output. Urine volume measurements are also used to calculate mathematic determinations of renal clearance of toxins, metabolic by-products, and medications. These mea-

surements are discussed later, in the section on renal clearance measurements.

Specific Gravity

The specific gravity of urine is used to determine the dilution or concentration of a specific sample of urine. Pure water has a specific gravity of 1.000. Because of the chemical elements that generally are contained in urine, the specific gravity normally ranges from 1.003 to 1.030.[8] Urine that is more concentrated or has more elements than normal (i.e., glycosuria or proteinuria) has a higher specific gravity than dilute urine.[2] In some renal diseases, the body's ability to dilute or to concentrate urine is compromised, and the body cannot regulate homeostasis. Patients with diabetes mellitus, pyelonephritis, or acute tubular necrosis frequently display low specific gravity (<1.005). In normal kidneys, the specific gravity changes with the patient's need to remove water (high fluid intake) or to retain water (low fluid intake). In some renal diseases, such as chronic glomerulonephritis, the specific gravity becomes "fixed," and the kidneys can no longer regulate the dilution of the urine, regardless of fluid intake. Nephrotic syndrome, acute glomerulonephritis, and dehydration states are often accompanied by high urine specific gravity results.[7]

Urine pH

Additional information obtained from the urinalysis includes testing the pH of the urine sample. Normal urine pH ranges from 5.0 to 9.0.[4] Because the excreted by-products of normal metabolism are slightly acidic, normal urine is slightly acidic as well.[8] In the ICU setting, urine pH is useful in determining whether patients are experiencing respiratory or metabolic acidosis or alkalosis. In outpatient settings, urine pH is useful in identifying certain conditions, including urinary tract infection.

Renal conditions such as Fanconi's syndrome and urinary tract infections can cause the urine to become alkaline (pH > 7.0). Those consuming a vegetarian diet frequently have alkaline urine. Metabolic or respiratory alkalosis is also associated with alkaline urine. When the urine pH is below 7.0, the urine is termed "acidic." Renal tuberculosis and acidosis conditions are associated with acidic urine.[7] Diets high in protein also contribute to an acidic urine value. In patients who are prone to renal stones, the pathogenesis of stone formation as either calcium based (alkaline urine) or urate based (acidic urine) can be assisted by determination of urine pH.[9]

Urine Osmolality

Urine osmolality reflects the concentration of all dissolved particles in a liter of solution and normally ranges from 100 to 900 mOsm/kg H_2O.[3] Urine osmolality depends on the osmolality of the blood, an indicator of the patient's hydration status. When the body's ability to conserve or to dilute the urine is compromised, as in acute and chronic renal failure, the urine osmolality can become fixed, causing the patient to retain fluid or to overexcrete fluid from the body, with resulting homeostatic abnormalities. This highly complex process involves the interaction of renal, hormonal, and neurologic responses (see Chapter 20). In this minute-to-minute process, the kidney's juxtaglomerular complex affects the urine's sodium concentration through the renin–angiotensin–aldosterone hormonal system,[5] hypothalamic osmoreceptors respond to extracellular fluid osmolality, which activates the pituitary gland's release of ADH, and many other factors contribute to the concentration of fluid in the intracellular and extracellular fluid compartments (see Chapter 20).

Urine Electrolyte Concentration

Blood filtered by the kidneys contains numerous chemical electrolytes that are selectively reabsorbed or secreted by the tubules of the kidneys (see Chapter 20). Those electrolytes that are secreted appear in the urine and are measurable by simple laboratory tests on 24-hour urine collections. Commonly measured urine electrolytes are sodium, potassium, chloride, calcium, phosphorus, and magnesium. Abnormal findings indicate either excessive intake, which is then eliminated through the kidneys, or abnormalities in tubular reabsorption and secretion, which cause the body to retain or to eliminate electrolytes excessively.

In the critical care setting, random urine samples are frequently tested for *fractional excretion of sodium* (FE_{Na}). In patients with renal impairment, conditions associated with prerenal disorders (reduced renal perfusion from dehydration, trauma, or third spacing of fluids or reduced cardiac function) frequently result in low FE_{Na} levels ($<1\%$). In patients with intrarenal disorders of the glomeruli (associated with diabetic nephropathy, glomerulonephritis, or acute tubular necrosis), the renal tubules are unable to reabsorb sodium efficiently, and sodium is lost into the urine, resulting in high values of FE_{Na} ($>1\%$).[10] Table 22–2 provides more information about clinical laboratory values that help to differentiate prerenal from intrarenal disorders.[11]

Urine Protein

Under normal conditions, the kidneys do not allow protein, a large molecule, to be eliminated from the body. Therefore, normal urine protein values would be zero to trace on dipstick or less than 10 mg/100 mL in a collected sample.[12] However, certain disease states, such as diabetes mellitus or glomerulonephritis, alter the selective permeability of the tubules so that protein does escape into the urine. Once the condition is identified by dipstick or single sample testing, a 24-hour sample is needed to assess the significance of urinary protein loss adequately.

Glucose Levels

The body's natural function is to utilize all the glucose it receives, either initially as energy or stored as fat for later use. On occasion, stress or the ingestion of a par-

TABLE 22–2
Urine Indices Used in the Differential Diagnosis of Prerenal and Intrinsic Renal Azotemia

Diagnostic Index	Prerenal Azotemia	Ischemic Intrinsic Azotemia
Fractional excretion of Na^+ (%),* $\dfrac{U_{Na} \times P_{cr}}{P_{Na} \times U_{cr}} \times 100$	<1	>1
Urinary Na^+ concentration (mEq/L)	<10	>20
Urinary creatinine/plasma creatinine ratio	>40	<20
Urinary urea nitrogen/plasma urea nitrogen ratio	>8	<3
Urine specific gravity	>1.018	<1.012
Urine osmolality (mOsm/kg H_2O)	>500	<250
Plasma BUN/creatinine ratio	>20	$<10–15$
Renal failure index,* $U_{Na}/U_{cr}/P_{cr}$	<1	>1
Urine sediment	Hyaline casts	Muddy brown granular casts

*Most sensitive indices.

BUN, blood urea nitrogen; Na^+, sodium; P_{cr}, plasma creatinine concentration; P_{Na}, plasma Na^+ concentration; U_{cr}, urine creatinine concentration; U_{Na}, urine Na^+ concentration.

From Brady H, Brenner BM, Lieberthal W: Acute renal failure. In: Brenner BM (ed): The Kidney, 5th ed. vol. 2. Philadelphia, W.B. Saunders, 1997, p 1227.

ticularly high carbohydrate load can result in isolated findings of glucose in the urine (glucosuria). Under pathologic conditions, such as diabetes mellitus, the renal threshold is exceeded, and glucose spills over into the urine on a protracted basis. In addition to urine glucose loss, urine tests in diabetics can indicate the presence of proteinuria, one of the first indicators of direct renal damage from diabetes.

Urine Sediment

When a sample of urine is spun in the centrifuge, particulate matter collects in the bottom of the test tube as the urine sediment. When examined under the microscope, the urine sediment reveals physical evidence of certain physiologic conditions in the renal system. The presence of a few *epithelial cells* can be a normal finding; however, large numbers of epithelial cells can indicate inflammation of the nephrons themselves (nephritis). Another microscopic finding is the presence of *casts*. Casts are clumps of proteinaceous material that can be solid or shell-like and may take on various shapes. Casts are formed in the renal tubules and are washed out by the urine as it flows through the renal system. White blood cell casts are often seen when infection is present, such as in pyelonephritis. Red blood cell casts are seen with inflammation in the glomeruli themselves (glomerulonephritis) (Figure 22–1). Inflammation of the renal parenchyma or capillary membranes of the glomeruli is often indicated by the presence of hyaline casts in the urine.[13] Epithelial casts indicate renal tubular damage, heavy metal poisoning, or eclampsia.

Urinalysis samples are frequently assessed under the microscope for the presence of certain formed elements.

The presence of red blood cells (hematuria) indicates bleeding in the urinary tract, often the result of infection, mechanical irritation (placement of urinary catheters), or trauma to the kidneys directly or to the urinary tract. Renal conditions such as glomerulonephritis, lupus nephritis, renal hypertension, and renal stones, as well as blunt injury to the kidneys, are frequently followed by hematuria. White blood cells are seen in pyelonephritis and infections of the urinary tract. Microscopic analysis of the urinary sediment also provides information on the presence of bacteria or yeast in the urine, findings indicating a urinary tract infection.

Renal Clearance Studies

Although blood tests and urine tests provide important information about the status of renal function, even more useful information can be obtained by collecting both blood and urine samples at the same time. Combined blood and urine values are then correlated mathematically to determine exactly how well the kidneys are removing various substances from the blood and either reabsorbing or excreting those substances into the urine (renal clearance). An extremely important laboratory test for renal function is C_{Cr}. This test is described in the next section as an example of how all renal clearance studies are done.

Creatine Clearance

C_{Cr} is used to assess how well the kidneys function. As described earlier, creatinine is a by-product of protein metabolism and is produced consistently over time and is cleared consistently over time, thus providing a

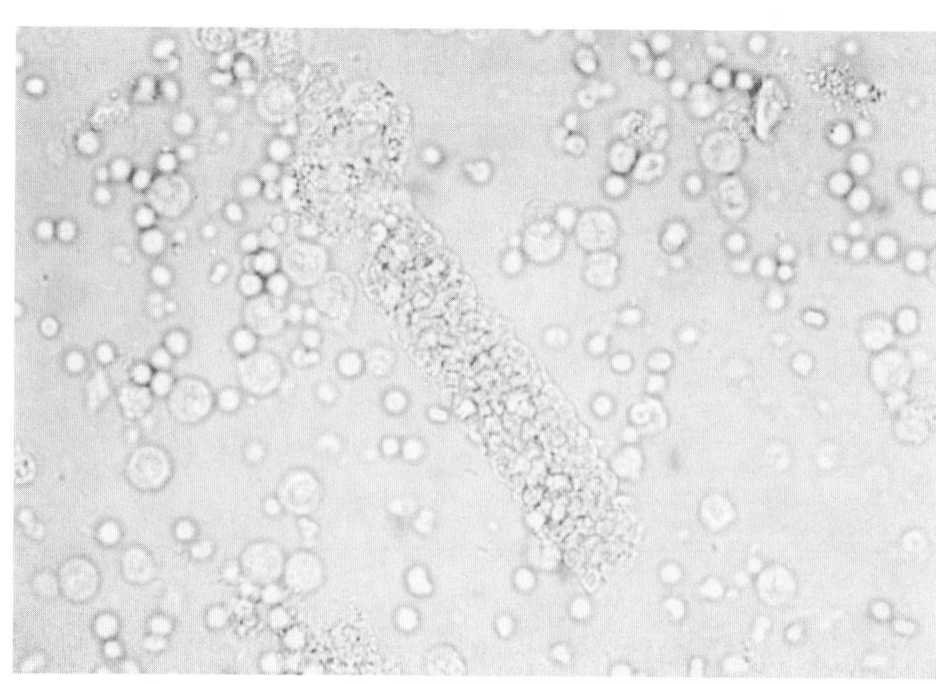

Figure 22–1

Red blood cell cast in a patient with acute nephritis (×430). (From Harrington JT: Assessment of the patient with renal disease. In: Levine DZ (ed): Caring for the Renal Patient, 3rd ed. Philadelphia, W.B. Saunders, 1997, pp 2–3.)

standard for measurement of renal function. A 24-hour urine specimen is usually collected for this test. In the urine collection, the first morning specimen of urine is discarded (although the time of collection begins with discarding this first sample), so that the patient begins the study with an empty bladder. All urine made during the next 24 hours is collected into one container for analysis. The sample is carefully measured for volume. The last sample is placed in the container exactly 24 hours later, thus providing a single sample containing all the urine produced by the kidneys in a 24-hour period. The exact time of collection (beginning and ending) must be noted on the specimen, because variations from the assumed 24-hour collection period can influence the accuracy of the C_{Cr} determination. Classically, a blood specimen is drawn at the midpoint of the urine collection (i.e., 12 hours after the initiation of a 24-hour urine collection). For practical reasons, however, the accompanying blood specimen is frequently drawn at the conclusion of the urine collection period.

The following equation is used to assess renal function based on C_{Cr} (mL/min): multiply the urine creatinine value (mg/dL) times the urine sample's volume (mL), divide that figure by the serum creatinine (mg/dL), and then divide that number by the total time (in minutes) for the urine sample collection period (Figure 22–2). Because variations in body size and muscle mass can affect the metabolism rate and production of end products of metabolism (such as creatinine), this calculation is often further refined by correcting for the patient's body surface area. Since 1916, the DuBois formula has been used to correct for differences in C_{Cr} by accounting for the patient's height and weight (reported in square meters). On laboratory reports, then, it is not uncommon for C_{Cr} to be reported as C_{Cr} (mL/min/1.73 m^2).[13]

When corrected for body surface area, normal C_{Cr} values are 90 to 130 mL/min/1.73 m^2 body surface area.[3] However, normal variations can occur based on age as well. The importance of accurate recording of time of collection and volume can be seen in the foregoing formula, in which slight variations in recording from what actually occurred are magnified by mathe-matic calculation of creatinine clearance. The result is either falsely elevated or falsely decreased values for renal function.

Glomerular Filtration Rate

Determination of the glomerular filtration rate (GFR) measures the amount of blood filtered through all the glomeruli in a given period and provides for a more specific clinical picture of what is actually occurring in the glomerular structures of the kidney.[9] A normal GFR is approximately the same as the C_{Cr}. The GFR depends on three factors: 1) the permeability of the glomerular capillary membrane, 2) the systemic blood pressure, and 3) the filtration pressure through the glomerulus itself. Alterations in any one of these process can affect the GFR.[14]

Clearance of Medications

Medications are cleared from the body by various routes of elimination, including the kidneys, liver, lungs, and other organs.[15] When renal function is compromised, the rate of elimination of medications can be dangerously prolonged, resulting in drug accumulation, prolonged exposure of drugs to sensitive organs, and toxicity.

Renal clearance studies are frequently done to determine appropriate dosage levels of medications in critically ill patients. Dosing is based on the difference between the delivered dose of medication (as determined by blood levels) and the clearance of the medication by the renal system. Pharmacy professionals are frequently involved in calculating the appropriate dosages of medications based on these combined blood and urine samples.

Clearance Studies Used in Research

Although serum, urine, and combined calculated measurements of renal clearance are frequently adequate for clinical determination of renal function in inpatient and outpatient settings, research studies often require more sophisticated and revealing studies of renal function. This is especially true in development of new medications when the effects on the kidneys are unknown or when researchers have reason to believe that similar medications have caused side effects involving renal function abnormalities. These tests are also useful in assessing whether preexisting renal function abnormalities play a role in the metabolism, toxicity, or effectiveness of new medications.

In these cases, expensive, time-consuming, and sometimes invasive tests of renal function may be warranted. A popular means of assessing renal function in the inpatient or outpatient research laboratory is to determine clearances of inulin and *para*-aminohippurate

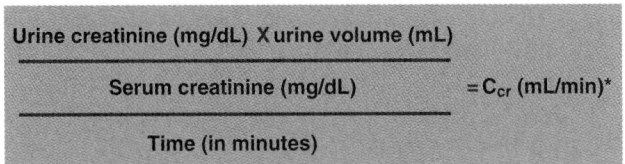

$$\frac{\dfrac{\text{Urine creatinine (mg/dL) X urine volume (mL)}}{\text{Serum creatinine (mg/dL)}}}{\text{Time (in minutes)}} = C_{cr}\ \text{(mL/min)*}$$

* A more accurate picture of renal function is obtained when the creatinine clearance is adjusted for the patient's body surface area (C_{Cr} = mL/min/1.73 m^2 BSA).

Figure 22–2

Formula for assessment of renal function based on creatinine clearance.

(In/PAH). In/PAH clearance studies are done in a fashion identical to that of C_{Cr} studies described earlier. In this test, however, after a loading dose, an infusion of combined In/PAH is administered by vein continuously throughout the renal function study period. Strict timing of blood and urine samples over 1- to 6-hour increments provides useful information for determining the effects of new or experimental medications on renal function. Of particular value is the ability of this test to elucidate the effects on GFR (as measured by inulin) separately from the effects on renal plasma flow (as measured by PAH). Researchers are then able to describe the effects of experimental medications and to make recommendations about side effects, dosing, interaction effects, and contraindications for use by particularly vulnerable groups of patients.

DIAGNOSTIC TESTS

Although blood and urine samples assessed in the inpatient and outpatient laboratory provide important information, additional diagnostic testing procedures are useful in assessing renal function. These tests can also be performed in inpatient or outpatient settings, but they require highly sophisticated technology. Selected tests are described in the following sections.

Kidneys, Ureters, and Bladder

The kidney, ureter, and bladder test (KUB) is a radiographic study in which a flat-plate radiograph is used to determine the size, location, structure, and position of the organs (kidneys) and the urinary tract (ureters and bladder). Abnormalities such as strictures or obstructions in the ureters, large cysts in the bladder or kidneys, and enlarged or misshapen organs can be elicited. This test is usually one of the earliest done in the diagnostic workup of the patient with renal problems.

Renal Arteriography

In this radiologic procedure, radiocontrast medium is used to visualize the renal arterial structure and is useful in identifying obstructions and masses within the kidneys. In some cases, the radiocontrast dye is injected systemically through intravascular administration; at other times, specific arteries can be targeted, and dye is selectively injected intra-arterially.

Intravenous Pyelography

The internal structures of the kidney including the parenchyma, renal pelvis, ureters, and bladder can be visualized by the intravenous pyelogram (IVP). In this diagnostic test, an intravenous injection of contrast dye is followed by radiologic study of the renal structures. Renal tumors or other obstructions are frequently visualized with this diagnostic examination.

Unfortunately, tests using radiocontrast dye are not without risks. Patients who are sensitive to iodine or other components of the contrast dye can experience a significant allergic reaction to the contrast dye. In addition, patients who are dehydrated or diabetic have an increased risk of toxic reaction within the kidneys themselves to the contrast dye. In these cases, significant acute renal failure can occur, which is sometimes nonreversible. These patients require specific intervention before testing, to ensure adequate hydration and protection of functioning nephrons before administration of contrast dye.

Retrograde Radiologic Testing

Like the IVP described earlier, the retrograde pyelogram uses contrast dye to visualize structures of the renal system for radiographic study. In this test, however, contrast dye is injected through the ureteral system and moves backward (retrograde) through the renal system. It is especially useful when the presence of stones, clots, or strictures of the urinary structures is suspected. An advantage is less exposure of the nephrons to the contrast dye, thus reducing exposure to toxic contrast medium. Brasfield[2] indicated advantages to using this diagnostic test over intravenous injection when patients are allergic to contrast dye.

Renal Computed Tomography

In some cases, a radiologic isotope is administered intravenously before the diagnostic procedure. After traveling by the circulation through the renal system, multiple radiologic films are taken that show a cross-sectional view of the kidneys. Through computer reconstruction, these images can indicate the presence of tumors, cysts, areas of necrosis, and other structural abnormalities in the renal system. Patients who are dehydrated or diabetic are at increased risk of radiocontrast-induced acute renal failure, which can limit the usefulness of this test in some settings.

Renal Ultrasound

The renal ultrasound scan is a noninvasive diagnostic test that is useful for determining the size and structure of the kidneys. In this test, high-frequency sound waves are transmitted through the abdomen, and echos are converted into electrical impulses that are visible on an oscilloscope screen. These images are then analyzed for abnormalities. Normal adult kidneys are approximately 12 cm long. The renal ultrasound scan is also useful in diagnosing the presence of cysts, obstructions, or fluid accumulation around the kidneys. Doppler studies, available with newer equipment, provide a mechanism for assessing arterial patency as well as more sophisticated studies of direction, volume, and speed of blood flow to the kidneys.[19] Because of its noninvasive nature and reduced cost, renal ultrasound has replaced more expensive and invasive tests such as the excretory renal urogram.

Renal Biopsy

When a definitive diagnosis of underlying pathologic lesions is needed, the renal biopsy provides the most complete and direct information. In this diagnostic test, a small piece of tissue is removed directly from the kidney for examination by a pathologist. The sample can be obtained either from an open surgical procedure or through a closed biopsy technique. In the open surgical procedure, an incision is made, and the kidney is exposed. A small specimen is removed for examination in the laboratory. In the closed procedure, a biopsy needle is inserted through the flank into the kidney, and a small sample of tissue is removed with the needle. These procedures are done while the patient is under general or local anesthesia.

Renal biopsies provide useful information for diagnosing the type of acute or chronic renal disease, for determining the course of treatment based on the type of lesions discovered, and for predicting long-term outcome for particular patients. Renal biopsies are also important diagnostic aids in determining acute and chronic rejection of transplanted kidneys. Transplanted kidneys are frequently positioned in the lower abdomen for several reasons, one of which is ease of access to the kidney for repetitive biopsy procedures.

Patients at risk of complications from renal biopsy are those with bleeding disorders, massive obesity, or only a single kidney. Therefore, renal biopsies are usually not the first diagnostic procedures undertaken.

NORMAL VARIATIONS ASSOCIATED WITH AGING AND GENDER

Creatinine production comes from metabolism of creatine and phosphocreatine, both of which are found nearly exclusively in muscle. In general, renal function undergoes distinct and normal changes over the life span. Interpretation of renal function using standard normal ranges can be misleading in determining renal function in the elderly. Kasiske and Keane[8] describe it in the following way:

For example, a serum creatinine level that falls in the normal range may indicate a normal glomerular filtration rate in a young, healthy individual. However, the same serum creatinine level in an elderly individual could indicate a twofold reduction in glomerular filtration rate as a result of a comparable reduction in muscle mass.

In addition, persons who are of extremely small stature normally have a lower S_{Cr} than large, muscular persons. Women tend to have lower S_{Cr} values than men, because women have smaller muscle mass than men who weigh the same amount. However, any person who experiences an increase in S_{Cr} of 0.5 mg/dL at one time or a series of increases of 0.2 mg/dL over time must be assessed for renal compromise.

Under normal conditions across the life span, the kidney maintains a remarkable ability to support the body's functions. However, under the stress of disease, the kidneys of infants and the elderly[16] are at greatest risk of life-threatening complications. In newborn infants, losses of fluid from fever or diarrhea frequently result in significant dehydration problems that are renally mediated. The elderly also experience more problems with dehydration, electrolyte imbalance, and cardiovascular insufficiency, all of which predispose the patient to renal compromise. The S_{Cr} level alone is not a good indicator of renal function in the elderly. With aging, muscle mass is lost and is reflected in a lower S_{Cr} level that may erroneously reflect normal values despite reductions in renal function.[16] It is possible that normal S_{Cr} values may be reported in elderly patients who experience up to a 60% reduction in GFR.[17] In these patients, measurement of the C_{Cr} provides a more appropriate laboratory assessment of renal function than S_{Cr} alone.

When C_{Cr} tests are not available, an estimate of age-related glomerular filtration can be done for male patients by using the Cockcroft–Gault formula, in which C_{Cr} (mL/min) is determined by subtracting the patient's age from 140 and multiplying that number by the patient's weight (kg), then dividing that number by 72 times the patient's S_{Cr} or plasma creatinine in milligrams per deciliter. For female patients, who have a lower muscle mass per body weight, C_{Cr} is estimated by using the same formula, but multiplying the result by 0.85[17] (Figure 22–3).

In addition to changes reflected in the C_{Cr}, age and race have also been shown to result in changes in how the kidney manages sodium balance. Luft, Weinberger, and Fineberg[18] conducted a study to determine the effects of age and race on the kidney's ability to provide salt and water balance by comparing young white men (<40 years of age) and older white men (>40 years of age) with young black men and older black men. In this study, these investigators found that

Figure 22-3

Cockcroft-Gault formula for estimating creatinine clearance for male and female patients when urine creatinine values are not available.

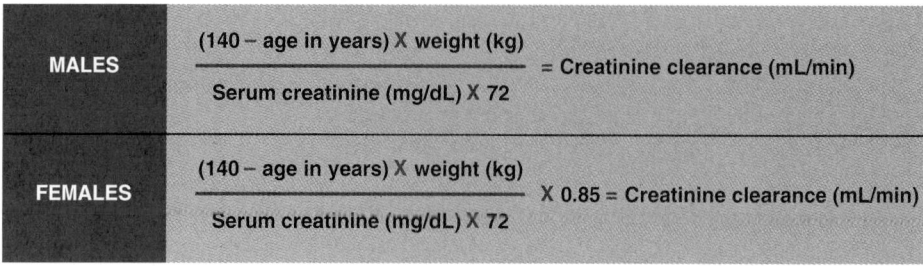

older white men excreted sodium less efficiently than young white men. Even more interesting were the findings that young black men cleared sodium in a fashion similar to that of older white men, and sodium homeostasis in older black men was the most compromised of all the groups tested. These findings have important implications in the development of hypertension in black men.

Key Concepts

➠ Laboratory assessment of blood and urine specimens provides specific information that is vital in the diagnosis and tracking of various renal impairments.

➠ BUN and creatinine are standard indicators of renal function. BUN levels are less reliable because they may be influenced by different factors.

➠ Abnormalities of electrolytes must be recognized quickly because alterations can have life-threatening consequences.

➠ Variations that occur normally in the aging process must be considered, to prevent misinterpretation of diagnostic information.

➠ Patients requiring diagnostic tests that use contrast media can experience allergic reactions to the contrast dye.

➠ Patients who are dehydrated or diabetic are at increased risk of radiocontrast-induced acute renal failure.

References

1. Pietzman SJ: From Bright's disease to end-stage renal disease. Hosp Pract 27:192–221, 1992.
2. Brasfield K: Renal diagnostic procedures. In: Thelan LA, Davie JK, Urden LD, et al (eds): Critical Care Nursing: Diagnosis and Management. St. Louis, C.V. Mosby, 1994, pp 599–602.
3. Tierney LM, Jr, McPhee SJ, Papadakis MA (eds): Current Medical Diagnosis and Treatment, 36th ed. Stamford, CT, Appleton & Lange, 1997.
4. Nicoll D, McPhee SJ, Chou TM, et al: Common laboratory tests: selection and interpretation. In: Nicoll D, McPhee SJ, Chou TM, et al (eds): Pocket Guide to Diagnostic Tests, 2nd ed. Stamford, CT, Appleton & Lange, 1997, pp 35–189.
5. White B: Fluid and electrolyte disorders. In: Black JM, Matassarin-Jacobs E (eds): Illustrated Guide to Diagnostic Tests, 2nd ed. Springhouse, PA, Springhouse Corporation, 1997, pp 273–324.
6. Brasfield K: Renal disorders. In: Thelan LA, Davie JK, Urden LD, et al (eds): Critical Care Nursing: Diagnosis and Management. St. Louis, C.V. Mosby, 1994, pp 603–620.
7. Illustrated Guide to Diagnostic Tests, 2nd ed. Springhouse, PA, Springhouse Corporation, 1998.
8. Kasiske BL, Keane WF: Laboratory assessment of renal disease: clearance, urinalysis, and renal biopsy. In: Brenner BM (ed): The Kidney, 5th ed. vol. 2. Philadelphia, W.B. Saunders, 1996, pp 1137–1174.
9. Berg D: Handbook of Primary Care Medicine. Philadelphia, J.B. Lippincott, 1993.
10. Clive DM: Azotemia. In: Green HL, Fincher R-ME, Johnson WP, et al (eds): Clinical Medicine, 2nd ed. St. Louis, C.V. Mosby, 1996, pp 587–591.
11. Brady HR, Brenner BM, Lieberthal W: Acute renal failure. In: Brenner BM (ed): The Kidney, 5th ed. vol. 2. Philadelphia, W.B. Saunders, 1996, pp 1200–1252.
12. Kernicki JG: Renal/urinary assessment. In: Ruppert SD, Kernicki JG, Dolan JT (eds): Critical Care Nursing: Clinical Management Through the Nursing Process, 2nd ed. Philadelphia, F.A. Davis, 1996, pp 656–661.
13. Harrington JT: Assessment of the patient with renal disease. In: Levine DZ (ed): Caring for the Renal Patient, 3rd ed. Philadelphia, W.B. Saunders, 1997, pp 1–9.
14. Holford NHG, Benet LZ: Pharmacokinetics and pharmacodynamics: rational dose selection and the time of course of drug action. In: Katzung BG (ed): Basic and Clinical Pharmacology, 6th ed. Norwalk, CT, Appleton & Lange, pp 33–47.
15. Brasfield K: Renal anatomy and physiology. In: Thelan LA, Davie JK, Urden LD, et al (eds): Critical Care Nursing: Diagnosis and Management. St. Louis, C.V. Mosby, 1994, pp 579–592.
16. Palmer BF, Levi M: Effect of aging on renal function and disease. In: Brenner BM (ed): The Kidney, 5th ed. vol. 2. Philadelphia, W.B. Saunders, 1996, pp 2274–2296.
17. American College of Physicians: Medical Knowledge Self-Assessment Program in the Subspecialty of Nephrology and Hypertension. Philadelphia, American College of Physicians, 1994.
18. Luft F, Weinberger M, Fineberg M, et al: Effects of age on renal sodium homeostasis and its relevance to sodium sensitivity. Am J Med 82(Suppl 1B):9–15, 1987.
19. Hricak H, White SS: Radiologic Assessment of the Kidney. In: Brenner BM (ed): The Kidney, 5th ed. vol. 2. Philadelphia, W.B. Saunders, 1996, pp 1175–1199.

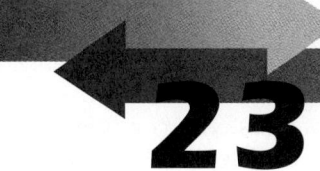

23

Acute Renal Failure

June Stark and Sheila Melander

Objectives

After completing this chapter, the student will be able to:

1. Correlate the high mortality rate seen in the critically ill patient with acute renal failure (ARF) to the nurse's role in prevention of ARF.
2. Compare and contrast the categories of ARF, including prerenal, intrarenal, and postrenal.
3. List the laboratory and diagnostic parameters used to differentiate the category of ARF present in a critically ill patient.
4. Differentiate between acute and chronic renal failure.
5. Describe the pathophysiologic and clinical characteristics of acute tubular necrosis (ATN), including the systemic manifestations.
6. Analyze the nurse's role in caring for the patient with ATN.
7. Formulate the appropriate nursing diagnoses for the patient diagnosed with ARF.
8. Compare and contrast the colloborative interventions implemented for the prerenal patient versus the patient who has developed ATN.
9. Evaluate the advantages and disadvantages of the three forms of dialysis available to the critically ill patient with ARF.
10. Describe other therapeutic modalities, besides dialysis, used to manage the critically ill patient with ATN.

ARF requiring dialysis is responsible for approximately 5 to 10% of patients in a critical care unit. Critically ill patients with ARF have a higher mortality rate than those patients with normal renal function. The mortality rate ranges from 50 to 80%; critically ill patients with the highest mortality rates are those with complex illnesses such as trauma, septic shock, or postpartum complications. Because of the high mortality rate, the prevention of ARF is the recommended intervention for the critically ill patient. When this is not possible and ARF is inevitable, then stabilization of the patient's condition as soon as possible, followed by the return and maintenance of the patient's homeostatic internal environment for the support and promotion of renal healing, is necessary.

ETIOLOGY AND PATHOPHYSIOLOGY

ARF is defined as the sudden deterioration in renal function usually associated with the loss of the kidney's ability to concentrate urine, as well as the retention and accumulation of nitrogen wastes. The presentation of this disorder can be associated with either an oliguric (<400 mL/day of urine output) or a non-oliguric (a normal or large volume of dilute urine output) pattern of urine output. As mentioned earlier, the mortality rate in critically ill patients who develop ARF is extremely high. This increase in mortality rate can be attributed to the finding that the loss of the body's biochemical regulator, the kidney, in the midst of a critical illness is a crucial factor associated with the patient's ability to survive. Because of the impact on the mortality rate of critically ill patients, the best intervention remains the prevention of ARF whenever possible.

ARF has many different causes (Table 23–1). For diagnostic purposes, the causes are organized into three categories: prerenal, renal, and postrenal.[1–5] Each category has unique characteristics that differentiate one group from another. These characteristics have clinical and therapeutic significance. The similarities among

TABLE 23–1
Common Causes of Acute Renal Failure

Category	Cause
Prerenal	Volume
	Dehydration
	Ischemia
	Hypotensive shock
	Cardiogenic shock
	Septic shock
	Hypoxemia
	Reduced cardiac output
Postrenal	Urethral
	Stricture
	Prostatic hypertrophy
	Ureteral
	Fibrosis
	Calculi
	Blood clots
	Bladder
	Neurogenic problems
	Neoplasms
	Obstruction
Renal	Glomerulus
	Acute glomerulonephritis
	Acute cortical necrosis
	Hepatorenal syndrome
	Tubule
	Acute tubular necrosis
	Acute pyelonephritis
	Nephrotoxins
	Heavy metals
	Antibiotics
	Radiographic contrast media
	Anesthetics
	Pigments
	Hemoglobin
	Myoglobin

causes of ARF in a single category often reveal common diagnostic indicators, symptoms, and medical or nursing interventions.

Postrenal Failure

Postrenal conditions are caused by an acute obstruction to urine flow from the kidney to the bladder. The usual sites of obstruction are the bladder neck, the urethra, or the prostate, whereas common causes include renal calculi, benign prostatic hypertrophy, urethral strictures, blood clots, sloughed necrotic tissue, and renal tumors. The presence of a postrenal condition should always be considered whenever an acute cessation of urine output presents in the critically ill, because this condition is easily reversible. The diagnosis can usually be determined by a flat plate radiograph of the abdomen. A flat plate of the abdomen on the initial examination reveals the size of the kidney and renal pelvis, as well as the patency of the urinary collecting system. The presence of a unilateral patent urinary tract rules out the presence of a postrenal condition, whereas a dilated renal pelvis is consistent with the diagnosis of obstruction; however, this finding can be absent in the presence of dehydration. If additional radiologic examination is necessary, one should consider ultrasonography followed by an intravenous pyelogram (IVP). The presence of a dilated renal pelvis on ultrasonography is diagnostic of obstruction. An IVP is an option if the patient does not have evidence of preexisting renal failure or a serum creatinine level higher than 3 mg/dL. The IVP dye needs to be administered in a hydrated patient, because administration of this agent has been associated with exacerbation of preexisting renal failure and nephrotoxicity, which can cause renal failure. A renal scan can also be considered, but it offers minimal additional information, except in the diagnosis of partial obstruction. Cystostomy performed by a urologist may reveal obstruction in the posterior urethra and bladder.

Children, women, and elderly men are the groups most vulnerable to a postrenal condition. Congenital abnormalities, such as anomalies in posterior or ureteropelvic function, are responsible for placing children at high risk. Cervical cancer in women can obstruct urinary flow, and elderly men often develop benign or malignant prostatic hypertrophy.

A postrenal condition results in the presence of an obstructed source in both kidneys or unilaterally in the patient with only one functioning kidney. A bilateral obstruction causes the cessation of urine flow and therefore the inability to excrete excess electrolytes and waste products. In this situation, the patient may present in a uremic state with blood urea nitrogen (BUN) and serum creatinine values in a 10:1 ratio. The patient usually complains of lower abdominal pain and a sudden decrease or absence of urine output. The patient's history, combined with a diagnostic examination, including physical, radiologic, and laboratory data, assists the health care team in determining whether the presenting renal failure is acute or chronic (Table 23–2). Early diagnosis and removal of the source of obstruction are important, because the risk of urinary tract infection or pyelonephritis increases in relation to the length of time the urinary flow is impaired.

Prerenal Failure

Prerenal conditions are the result of diminished renal perfusion without renal tubular damage. The intact nephron function is influenced by the decrease in renal blood flow; the glomerular filtration rate (GFR) decreases, resulting in an acute drop in urine output. Mul-

TABLE 23-2
Differences Between Acute and Chronic Renal Failure

Type of Renal Failure	Onset	Prognosis	Symptoms	Treatment
Acute	Sudden	Reversible	Dramatic	Treatment of imbalances, hemodialysis, peritoneal dialysis, and continuous renal replacement therapy
Chronic	Slow, progressive (3 or more years until end stage)	Irreversible	Gradual	Hemodialysis, peritoneal dialysis

tiple factors can be responsible for causing a prerenal condition, ranging from dehydration to altered cardiac output leading to an impairment in myocardial function to altered renal hemodynamics secondary to pharmacologic agents. The rapid reversal of these conditions usually results in the return of normal renal function. Correction is accomplished by volume replacement, improved cardiac function, and hemodynamic stability.

Dehydration is the most common cause of prerenal failure. The nurse initially observes a decrease in urine output, usually below 30 mL per hour (Table 23-3). A diagnosis of dehydration is confirmed by assessing for the presence of weight loss with a negative intake and output balance, hypotension, postural blood pressure changes, low central venous pressure, decreased pulmonary artery occlusive pressure, dry mucous membranes in the nose or mouth, poor skin turgor, absent neck veins, decreased or concentrated urine output, and possibly lethargy. Laboratory studies provide further diagnostic support, including an elevated BUN and a normal or slightly elevated creatinine in a ratio greater than 20:1 and a spot urine sodium of less 10 mEq/L. Once the presence of dehydration is established, a fluid challenge with a volume expander, such as the infusion of a crystalloid (i.e., normal saline) or a colloid (albumin), can result in the immediate reinstatement of urine output. When the urine output does not immediately return to normal, renal dopamine, at 2 to 5 $\mu g/kg$ per minute, as well as other types of vasopressors can be infused intravenously. When therapeutic intervention is not successful and the kidneys remain in a hypoperfused state for an extended period, the patient faces an increased risk of developing an intrarenal cause of ARF, ATN.

TABLE 23-3
Comparison of Laboratory Findings in Prerenal, Postrenal, and Intrinsic Renal Acute Oliguric States

Value	Prerenal	Postrenal	Intrinsic Renal (ATN)
Urine volume	Decreased	May alternate between anuria and polyuria	Anuria < 100 mL/24 hr Oliguria 100–400 mL/24 hr Nonoliguria > 400 mL/24 hr Isotonic (≤350 mOsm)
Urine osmolality	Increased (>500 mOsm)	Isotonic (≤350 mOsm)	Isotonic (≤350 mOsm)
Urine specific gravity	Increased (>1.020)	Fixed (1.008–1.012)	Fixed (1.008–1.012)
Urine sodium	<20 mEq/L	>40 mEq/L	>40 mEq/L
Fractional excretion of sodium (FE$_{Na}$)*	<1%	>1%	>1%
Urine failure index†	<1%	>1%	>1%
Urine pH	<6.0	>6.0	>6.0
Urine protein	Minimal	Minimal	Increased
Urine sediment	Normal, few casts	Normal, histiocytes and crystals	Granular casts, tubular epithelial cells
Urine/plasma creatinine ratio	>40	<20	<20
Blood urea nitrogen: serum creatinine	>20:1	10–15:1	10–15:1

*Fractional excretion of sodium = U/P sodium ÷ U/P creatinine × 100
†Renal failure index = U sodium ÷ U/P creatinine
Adapted from Brezis M, Rosen S, Epstein FH: Acute renal failure. In: Brenner BM, Rector FC (eds): The Kidney, 4th ed., Philadelphia, W.B. Saunders, 1991, pp 993–1061.

Hemodynamically unstable patients, such as those with hypotension or low cardiac output, who develop a prerenal condition are best treated with a combination of volume replacement, vasopressors, and diuretics. The most common diuretic used is furosemide (Lasix), administered either by intravenous push or at a constant infusion, which is preferred for its continual effect on kidney function.[6–10]

Intrarenal or Intrinsic Renal Failure

An intrarenal or intrinsic condition results in actual damage to the kidney tissue, including parenchymal and nephron damage. The multiple conditions responsible for this category of ARF may result in damage that targets either the glomerulus or the tubules. For example, glomerular damage can occur as a result of acute poststreptococcal glomerulonephritis or acute cortical necrosis. The damage to the tubules is frequently due to ATN, the most common cause of ARF. ATN is also the most common type of ARF seen in the intensive care unit (ICU). The cause of ATN is usually a prolonged or exacerbated prerenal condition, in which adequate perfusion to the kidney is not able to be reinstated in time; consequently, an ischemic or necrotic event occurs in the tubules. Other reasons for the onset of ATN include nephrotoxic injury to the tubules secondary to the administration of pharmacologic agents, such as the antibiotics gentamicin, amikacin, and carbenicillin. Exposure to heavy metals and endogenous toxins is another cause of tubular damage, by such agents as myoglobin secondary to rhabdomyolysis, septic endotoxins, and hemoglobin after a transfusion reaction. Contrast medium completes the list of sources contributing to the onset of ATN and actually ranks as the second most common cause. The injury to tubules presents in a "patchwork" pattern, with damage to the epithelial layer or basement membrane. The epithelial layer can regenerate, with scar tissue forming in the areas of the basement membrane as part of the healing process. The outcome is the resumption of renal tubular function leading in many cases to a normal to acceptable level of renal recovery free of medical intervention. The duration and extent of the acute tubular injury determine the likelihood of the kidney's ability to resume normal function.[6–11]

Systemic Manifestations

The systemic manifestations of uremia are most often associated with chronic renal failure rather than ARF. However, the patient with ARF who is experiencing uremia is also susceptible to uremic changes. The primary difference in the manifestations of the systemic effects of uremia in ARF versus chronic renal failure rests on the duration of time the patient is exposed to imbalances of uremia. Because ARF usually resolves quickly, the long-term problems associated with the chronicity of the renal failure do not occur. In addition, several problems are more commonly associated with ARF than with chronic renal failure.

Cardiovascular System

Renal failure has various effects on the cardiovascular system. The fluid volume excess associated with ARF creates an increase in preload, leading to an increase in cardiac output and, ultimately, elevated blood pressure even to the point of hypertension. If not treated, this overhydrated condition can contribute to the onset of congestive heart failure. Most electrolyte imbalances (hyperkalemia, hypokalemia, hypermagnesemia, hypocalcemia) can alter cardiac function, conduction, and contraction. In some instances, electrolyte imbalance can precipitate cardiac arrest. The patient with ARF is also susceptible to uremic pericarditis. Initially, the patient complains of precordial pain, usually in conjunction with a pericardial friction rub and an effusion visualized by radiologic examination. The pleural effusion may result from the buildup of the uremic toxins and often accompanies the pericarditis. The treatment for pericarditis is daily or continuous dialysis to remove the uremic toxins.

Respiratory System

The primary pulmonary complications of uremia include pleural effusion and pulmonary edema. Another complication is uremic lung or uremic pneumonitis, indicated on the chest radiograph by a "butterfly" pattern. The pulmonary system may try to compensate for the metabolic acidosis of renal failure by altering the respiratory pattern to Kussmaul's breathing pattern, which creates deep, slow respirations.

Gastrointestinal System

Changes in appetite secondary to anorexia, nausea, and vomiting are common manifestations of uremic syndrome. Malnutrition frequently follows, with significantly decreased serum protein and albumin levels that may contribute to the formation of edema. Uremic stomatitis may also further reduce the patient's ability to ingest adequate calories. A persistent uremic condition can cause the patient to be susceptible to stress or peptic ulcerations. The increased level of gastrin caused by the uremia is the explanation for the ulcer formation.

Neuromuscular System

The accumulation of uremic toxins may cause altered mental status, drowsiness, disorientation, delirium, coma, and psychosis. Other neurologic clinical manifestations include insomnia, apathy, lethargy, cognitive alterations (i.e., short-term memory loss, altered perceptions), and behavioral and even psychological changes. Peripheral neuropathy, often called restless leg syndrome, begins with footdrop and a burning sensation in the lower extremities. A more effective level of uremic toxin removal by dialysis is necessary to arrest or alleviate these symptoms. If this does not occur, then the peripheral neuropathy will advance to a progressive demyelination of the distal portion of the nerves from the lower to the upper extremities that may lead to paraplegia.

Endocrine or Metabolic System Changes

The metabolic abnormalities seen during uremia include carbohydrate intolerance, which presents as pseudodiabetes. This carbohydrate intolerance is caused by insensitivity to insulin. Hypocalcemia results from the lack of activated vitamin D and the binding of calcium with phosphate in the small intestine.

Hematologic System

The anemia of renal failure is caused by a lack of erythropoietin and is often accompanied by uremic bleeding abnormalities. The uremia causes a decrease in clotting factors, an alteration in platelet aggregation, and prothrombin consumption. These bleeding abnormalities cause an increase in bleeding time and a tendency to bleed. Thrombocytopenia is another uremic complication affecting anemia.

Integumentary System

Changes in skin integrity and texture and an increased susceptibility to bruising are common problems in the uremic patient. Pruritus contributes to the patient's discomfort, and frequently the multiple scratch marks further compound the skin problems by causing the patient to become more susceptible to localized infections. The buildup of uremic toxins on the skin is the cause of the pruritus. These toxins on the skin also lead to dryness and a thin, white film known as uremic frost. Skin pigments during uremia are varied and produce a yellow-orange hue that presents as a sallow appearance when combined with the pallor created by the anemic effect. In addition, the uremic bleeding abnormalities, compounded by the risk of falls caused by physical limitations, may lead to frequent episodes of bruising, ecchymosis, and petechiae.

Psychosocial Considerations

The acute onset of this form of renal failure usually leaves patients unprepared for the complexity of problems that face them, such as the increased mortality rate, the dialysis treatment, and the alterations in health caused by uremia. Because ARF can resolve, the patient and the family usually shift between hope and despair. In addition, a uremic condition can alter a patient's perceptions and interpretation of a situation.

Phases

Onset Phase

The onset phase of ARF can last from hours to days and should be thought of as the period in which the health care team attempts to prevent this disease process. Remember, because no known medical interventions can quickly reverse the tubular damage, prevention of ARF remains the best intervention at this time. During this phase, the renal oxygen consumption and the renal blood flow decrease to 25% of normal. The hemodynamic factors to watch during this stage are cardiac output, systemic blood pressure, and the renal response to these factors as expressed through urine output. Treatment is focused on determining the precipitating factors or events and correcting these conditions before any acute damage to the kidney develops. Once tubular damage is present, it cannot be reversed, and the healing process can range from a minimum of 8 to 14 days up to 3 months to 1 year.

Because renal function remains intact during the onset phase, the nephron responds to the alteration in hemodynamics by conserving fluid and sodium. The clinical presentation reveals a drop in urine output to 30 mL or less per hour and a urinary sodium of 10 mEq/L or less. The foregoing laboratory values provide the appropriate profile of a normal kidney attempting to conserve volume in a low-blood-flow state. The onset of the renal injury is characterized by the loss of tubule's ability to concentrate the urine. The loss of urinary concentrating ability is associated with the development of azotemia and an increase in the excretion of urinary sodium (>40 mEq/L). A comparison of urinary sodium levels that have not been influenced by the sodium-excreting properties of a diuretic can assist the critical care practitioner in determining the phase of ARF. The pattern of urine output, whether oliguria, nonoliguria, or, rarely, anuria, presenting at the beginning of ATN is helpful in providing prognostic and diagnostic predictors in each patient.

Oliguric/Anuric or Nonoliguric Phase

The pattern of urine output first seen during ATN determines the characteristics of the second phase, presenting as either oliguria or nonoliguria. Oliguria is the classic presentation form of ATN and is associated with a high mortality rate between 50 and 70% in critically ill patients. Nonoliguria generally reflects less severe nephron damage and is associated with a much lower mortality rate of 26%. The oliguric phase is discussed first.

Two pathophysiologic events are responsible for the oliguric phase: intratubular obstruction and backleak phenomenon. Intratubular obstruction results from both the sloughing off of ischemic tubular cells into the tubular space and the swelling of the remaining tubular cells. When present in a majority of the nephrons, this form of obstruction impedes the flow of urine and precipitates the oliguric phase. The backleak phenomenon also precipitates the onset of oliguria. Cracks or breaks form in the tubular wall secondary to the ischemic event and cause the glomerular filtrate actually to leak back into the renal tissue. The making of less filtrate contributes to the production of less urine output, hence the oliguria. The oliguric patient has a decreased urine output of less than 30 mL per hour and lacks the ability to concentrate the urine. As a result, the excreted urine is dilute, and has no excess fluid, electrolytes, or waste products. This patient, already facing a complex critical illness, is difficult to manage, and the situation becomes further compounded by the loss of the kidney's capacity to regulate the internal biochemical environment. The nurse should expect the following patient care issues: fluid overload, electrolyte and acid–base imbalances, azotemia, anemia, and increased risk of infection. Oliguric ATN has a recovery course usually ranging from a minimum of 12 to 16 days to a maximum of 3 to 12 months. Most patients do regain renal function, whereas a few do not.

Nonoliguria, in comparison with oliguria, is associated with a smaller amount and less severe form of tubular damage. The actual injury pattern is believed to be isolated to the epithelial layer, which has the ability to regenerate completely. Because of the confinement of the damage to one layer of the tubule, the primary defect observed is the loss of the nephron's capacity to concentrate the urine without the intratubular obstruction and the backleak phenomenon. The flow of a dilute filtrate moves freely along an intact, unobstructed tubule. The urinary output can vary form normovolemia to a diuretic response as large as 2L per hour. Because of the volume of urine output, fluid management problems are minimized or even absent during nonoliguria. The composition of the urine reflects the passive loss of electrolytes and waste products by virtue of the increase in flow of the glomerular filtrate, or the nonoliguric kidney retains the ability to concentrate the urine to some degree, and approximately 350 mOsm of solute is excreted daily. This contributes to a decreased need for dialysis.

The urinary creatinine clearance can be as high as 2 to 15 mL per minute; however, the potassium excretion is the same as in oliguria. Therefore, the critical care nurse must monitor the serum potassium level as needed and must be aware that the risk of symptomatic hyperkalemia still exists despite the presence of adequate urinary output. The recovery course of nonoliguria is short, varying from a minimum of 5 to 8 days.

Diuretic Phase

The diuretic phase follows oliguria and indicates that the patient is moving toward recovery. However, the nonoliguric phase is actually synonymous with the diuretic phase. This suggests that when a patient is starting the ARF process with nonoliguria, then that patient is only one step from recovery. The diuretic phase can last as long as 10 days and consists of a period of large urinary volumes, which is followed by a gradual decrease in urinary volumes approaching normal. The volumes can be high as 1 to 3 L per hour. Initially, the urine continues to be dilute, with the high glomerular flow rates contributing to the passive loss of electrolytes. Gradually, the urinary concentrating ability returns, but until then, occasional dialysis may be necessary to simply remove primarily solute. To maintain the hydration status of the patient during this phase of high volume loss, intravenous administration of crystalloids is necessary.

Recovery Phase

The final phase encompasses the time it takes for renal function to return to normal. This period may last as long as several months to 1 year. Serum and urinary studies, especially BUN and serum creatinine, are monitored on a periodic basis to determine the rate and degree of renal recovery. Patients must be informed that this phase may end with residual impairment of renal function, although renal function usually returns within normal limits. Patients who are likely to experience residual loss of renal function are those who with serious, prolonged, or repeated episodes of hemodynamic alterations during recovery from their critical illness or those whose course of recovery may have been further insulted by the use of a nephrotoxic agent. Other patients at risk of residual renal impairment are the elderly or those patients with preexisting renal disease at the onset of the ARF episode.

The recovery period is an extremely important phase for patient education. For example, compliance with the medical regimen is essential, to foster and maintain the returning renal function.[6–8,10] Frequent assessments of renal status are performed to determine the rate and extent of recovery. At the conclusion of the recovery phase, the health care team determines whether further medical or nursing intervention is required, based on the extent of the recovered kidney's ability to maintain homeostasis.

Assessment

The assessment of the renal system includes a patient and family history, physical examination, laboratory data analysis, and radiologic examination. The reason for the inclusion of these types of findings is to determine the presence of ARF versus chronic renal failure or a urinary tract disorder. On determining the presence of renal disease, the practitioner attempts to establish the duration, the severity, the cause, and possibly even the treatment of the disease.

Patient and Family History

The first step in the assessment process is to obtain data on the patient and family history. In approximately 30% of all azotemic patients, a relationship is found between the renal failure and a genetic predisposition. However, the type of renal problems that can be uncovered usually reflect chronic renal failure rather than ARF. Examples of some types of chronic renal failure that have a genetic component are polycystic kidneys, diabetes mellitus, hypertension, gout, malignant disease, hereditary nephritis, and cardiovascular disorders. A family history of renal calculi is significant in the search for a postrenal cause of ARF.

The patient's history reveals the presence and the predisposition to renal failure. The patient may reveal a previous episode of ARF or a diagnosis of chronic renal failure or urinary tract disease. A history of renal failure needs to be followed-up with the determination of the degree of residual renal function. An episode of renal calculi suggests a risk of recurrence. A second stone occurs in 40 to 50% of patients within a 5-year period and in 60 to 80% within 10 years.

A recent history of ingestion of antibiotics or exposure to environmental agents or toxins such a carbon tetrachloride causes the practitioner to look for a nephrotoxic renal insult. Tetracycline that is ingested past its expiration date is a common cause of nephrotoxic ATN. Other antibiotics associated with nephrotoxic ATN are gentamicin, amikacin, and carbenicillin.

A history of an upper respiratory infection in the past 1 to 2 weeks, especially a streptococcal infection, is compatible with the onset of acute glomerulonephritis. A recurrent history of urinary tract infection must be followed to determine whether the patient has a urinary tract abnormality. Repeated infections with the same organisms suggest kidney or prostate infection. Infections caused by different organisms indicate bladder infections. A history of cardiovascular disease

is significant, because a hemodynamic condition such as a drop in cardiac output or blood pressure is another cause of ischemic ARF. Diminished renal perfusion alone can cause the patient to present with oliguria. A recent allergic reaction has been known to cause acute interstitial nephritis. The patient with this disorder usually reports a history of recent drug ingestion followed by the occurrence of a fever and a skin rash. The medications most frequently associated with this problem are penicillin, diuretics, cephalothin, sulfa drugs, allopurinol, and phenindione.

Another cause of ARF is the onset of graft rejection in patients who have undergone renal transplantation. The patient reports signs and symptoms synonymous with the initiation of ARF or chronic renal failure, such as sudden onset of fatigue, decrease in the volume of urine, and change in the urine's color and concentration.

Physical Assessment

The purpose of the physical examination is to provide a review of all body systems, including general appearance, vital signs, edema if present, mucous membranes with eyes, ears, nose, and throat, muscle movement, activity level, and cognitive response to stimuli.[12] In this chapter, the overall focus is on obtaining a review of the renal and urinary tract. If renal or urinary problems are found to exist and have precipitated the onset of ARF, then the extent of the uremia and its systemic impact should be determined.

General Appearance

The patient with a renal or urinary tract disorder often presents with malaise, fatigue, and weight loss secondary to anorexia, nausea, and vomiting associated with a uremic state. A presentation of weight gain indicates overhydration and is supported by the presence of peripheral edema.

Vital Signs

Vital signs may be altered, especially blood pressure, by the systemic effects of renal or urologic disorders. The blood pressure may range from normal to hypotension or hypertension. Postural blood pressure measurement is essential to determine the impact of hydration status on hemodynamics. If the patient has a decrease in blood pressure during postural signs, one should consider hypovolemia secondary to vomiting without water replacement and excessive urinary losses in response to diuretic therapy or a renal disease, such as the diuretic phase of ARF. Hypertension indicates of overhydration or essential hypertension. The pulse rate may have a wide range of variations in response to hydration status, cardiovascular disease, or electrolyte imbalance. Overhydration is usually associated with a tachycardia, whereas the pulse rate during dehydration can vary from bradycardia to tachycardia, depending on the patient's compensatory mechanisms. The combination of cardiac failure and renal failure can produce a wide variation in pulse rate. The most common electrolyte imbalance during ARF is hyperkalemia, which contributes to the onset of bradycardia secondary to the myocardial depressant effects of increased extracellular potassium levels. Ultimately, if not treated, symptomatic hyperkalemia leads to asystolic cardiac arrest. All other electrolyte imbalances also have the potential to alter the regularity and the rate of the pulse (Table 23–4).

The patient's respiratory rate can present as normal or abnormal secondary to alterations resulting from acid–base imbalances or pulmonary compromise, such as uremic lung, or infection. Kussmaul's respirations, seen in severe metabolic acidosis, stimulate a slow, deep, and labored breathing pattern. Minimizing or correcting the metabolic acidosis eliminates the reason for this pattern of breathing. The practitioner who determines the presence of an abnormal respiratory rate or pattern needs to eliminate the possibility of a pulmonary infection because of the increased incidence of infection in the uremic patient.

TABLE 23–4
Electrolyte Imbalances: Impact on Cardiac Function

Electrolyte	Action on Myocardium
Hyperkalemia	↓ Contractility ↓ Conduction Asystole ECG changes: tall, peaked T wave, disappearance of P wave, widened QRS
Hypokalemia	Dysrhythmias Digoxin toxicity effect ECG changes: depressed ST segments, flat or inverted T wave, presence of U wave
Hypercalcemia	Enhanced digoxin effect ECG changes: shortened ST segment, increased incidence of heart block, cardiac arrest
Hypocalcemia	Dysrhythmias ECG changes: prolonged ST segment and QT interval
Hyperphosphatemia	ECG changes: prolongation of ST segment
Hypermagnesemia	Bradycardia ECG changes: peaked T waves similar to hyperkalemia Depressed contractility
Hypomagnesemia	Dysrhythmias ECG changes: flat or inverted T waves, possible ST-segment depression, prolonged QT interval

Integumentary: Skin

Renal failure, acute or chronic, leads to an alteration in skin color. A yellowish tone occurs secondary to the retention of carotenoids during uremic states. Pallor and a grayish tinge is often seen in anemia. Ecchymosis and bruises associated with complaints of easy bruising are common, as well as petechiae caused by increased capillary fragility. Scratch marks can alert the practitioner to assess for the presence of pruritus.

If the patient is undergoing dialysis, it is not unusual to observe a variation in the skin texture from scaly to rough changing from day to day. This variation can be associated with the changing degrees of uremia seen on days when the patient undergoes a dialysis procedure versus a nondialysis day. The uremia produces these alterations in skin texture by causing atrophy of the skin's oil and sweat glands. In severe uremic states, one may observe uremic frost, which is the passage of urate crystals through the skin's pore's. This condition is now rare because of the availability of effective and frequent forms of dialysis for critically ill patients. In the patient on bed rest, edema appears first in the sacral region, followed by edema in the extremities progressing from the lower to the upper limbs. Last, evidence of edema presents in the periorbital region. Edema in the extremities is evaluated from 1+ to 4+.

Ear, Nose, Mouth, and Throat

During renal failure, changes in the mucous membrane are usually seen in both the nose and the mouth. In the presence of uremia, the mucous membranes appear swollen, red, and often ulcerated. Changes in breath odor, called uremic fetor, may accompany these mucous membrane alterations. Pallor may be present, representative of anemia. Dehydration produces dry membranes.

Hearing loss during renal failure can be secondary to insult by a nephrotoxic antibiotic creating nerve deafness. The assessment of neck veins provides data on fluid status and its impact on cardiac status. Distended neck veins reflect overhydration and may indicate the onset of congestive heart failure.

Motor Movement and Activity Level

Mobility during renal failure is altered by the effects of progressive uremic symptoms. Both the neuromuscular system and the skeletal system can be affected by the uremia. Peripheral neuropathy is a segmental demyelination of the nerves progressing from the lower to the upper extremities. The physical findings may vary, depending on the stage in which the peripheral neuropathy is first detected. Early symptoms include complaints, as well as observations of the patient's periods of restlessness and discomfort, especially during bed rest. This phenomenon is called "restless leg syndrome." Next, the patient may complain of a "burning" pain of varying degrees of intensity, starting on the dorsal and ventral surfaces of the feet. Peripheral neuropathy can progress to footdrop and eventually paralysis.

Bone disease, such as osteomalacia and osteitis fibrosa, is more frequently associated with chronic renal failure than ARF. However, its onset is possible during cases of ARF when recovery occurs over a prolonged period. Bone disease results from the inability to maintain asymptomatic hypocalcemia, or it occurs when the patient is noncompliant about taking prescribed phosphate binders. The patient exhibits activity intolerance, problems with mobility, and bone pain with either of the foregoing problems. However, when faced with activity intolerance in the patient in renal failure, the practitioner must also assess the impact of anemia on the creation of this problem.

Cognition, Thought Processes, and Response to Stimuli

Uremia has various effects on an individual's cognition, thought processes, and responses. Assessment of the manifestations of these alterations in a patient is important, to be able accurately to assess a patient's level of understanding of explanations surrounding their present health status, their ability to retain teaching material, and therefore their ability to make rational decisions independently. Uremia can cause a limited attention span and shortened memory. When uremia is present, adaptations must be made in communication style and the teaching approach. For example, short teaching sessions should include frequent episodes of repetition, followed by the request at critical points for the patient to provide feedback in relation to the material just presented. The uremic patient may also have a diminished response to stimuli, as well as an alteration in the ability to make decisions. This can occur because the patient's thought processes may be altered, such that the patient may have difficulty integrating ideas or concepts. In addition, the patient's perception of events can cause an unrealistic interpretation of the information presented or the sequence of events.

Diagnostic Tests

Several diagnostic tests may be performed to assist with the diagnosis of ARF. See Chapter 22 for a discussion of the following studies: kidney, ureter, and bladder radiography; retrograde pyelography; computed tomography; renal angiography; renal ultrasonography; and renal biopsy.

Intravenous Pyelography

This test provides visual assessment of the kidneys, kidney pelvis, ureters, and bladder, and it is useful in determining areas of dysfunction and in locating renal tumors and calculi. This procedure begins with an injection of radiopaque dye intravenously as a contrast medium. Complications can arise during this procedure as a result of the patient's reaction to the contrast medium, such as an allergic reaction. In addition, the dye acts as an osmotic agent causing diuresis that can precipitate a moderate to severe dehydration episode. The dye used during an IVP is also recognized as a nephrotoxic agent. Both the dehydration and the nephrotoxicity of the IVP can be prevented by the administration of a combination of a diuretic (i.e., mannitol, furosemide) and the prophylactic hydration of the patient, usually by a crystalloid (i.e., 5% dextrose in normal saline or 5% dextrose in half-normal saline) 24 hours before the procedure with as much as 1500 mL. Some protocols continue this hydration therapy during and even after the procedure. The administration of fluids causes a dilutional effect, thus minimizing the nephrotoxicity and the osmotic impact of the dye while at the same time hydrating the patient. The diuretic encourages the dye's rapid elimination through urinary excretion. However, the patient must have a urine output and must be able to tolerate the resulting increase in circulating extracellular volume, to be selected for this pretreatment approach.[11, 13–15]

Radionuclide Renal Scan

A renal scan begins with the administration of technetium compounds (Tc-99m) intravenously. Renal lesions are detected, as well as masses. This procedure is helpful in assisting with the diagnosis of ARF and chronic renal failure and in determining the status of a renal transplant. A renal scan is often used in place of an IVP when patients are allergic to contrast media.

Magnetic Resonance Imaging

This procedure provides direct imaging in several planes of the renal and urinary drainage system. With a better tissue characterization than offered by the computed tomography (CT) scan, magnetic resonance imaging (MRI) provides a method for detecting renal cystic disease, inflammatory processes, and renal cell carcinoma. In ARF and acute renal transplant rejection, MRI is especially helpful in detecting alterations in renal blood flow patterns.

Magnetic Resonance Urography

This form of magnetic imaging provides results similar to those of IVP but without the use of dye.

Nursing Diagnoses

During the course of acute renal failure, patients' physiologic problems vary according to the extent of the disease process. Some patients need support only for a short period of time until renal function resumes. The diversity of nursing diagnoses during acute renal failure reflects the multisystem involvement. In addition, the diagnoses also address loss of the kidney's ability to maintain homeostasis, including fluid, electrolyte, and acid-base balance. Throughout the disease process, the nursing diagnoses and etiologic factors may change as the patient moves toward recovery. Table 23–5 outlines many of the most common nursing diagnoses used in the care of the patient in ARF.

TABLE 23–5
Nursing Diagnoses

Problem Statement	Etiologic Factors
Alteration in urinary elimination	Oliguria
	Anuria
	Polyuria or nonoliguria
Fluid volume deficit	Increased urine output
	Body fluid loss without adequate replacement
Fluid volume excess	Oliguria
	Anuria
	Edema
Altered nutrition: less than body requirements	Increased catabolism
	Increased nutritional needs
Risk for impaired skin integrity	Uremia
	Malnutrition
	Immobility
Knowledge deficit	Lack of cognitive knowledge related to:
	Acute renal failure
	Dialysis or other treatments
Decreased cardiac output	Dehydration
	Overhydration
	Congestive heart failure
	Uremic pericarditis
	Uremia
Anxiety or fear	Lack of knowledge
	Uncertainty of prognosis
Activity intolerance	Uremia
	Anemia
	Hypocalcemia
Body image disturbance	Uremic changes
	Loss of ability to excrete urine
	Skin color changes
	Arteriovenous access
	Weight gain or loss
	Edema
	Uremic fetor
Altered thought processes	Uremia
	Shortened attention span
	Decreased memory
	Changes in perception
Risk for infection	Uremia
	Increased susceptibility to infection
Ineffective patient or family coping	Stress
	Inadequate or ineffective coping mechanisms
	Limited resources or support systems

Collaborative Management

Collaboration is essential for the physician, critical care nurse, and other health care team members managing the serious and complex issues confronting prevention and treatment of the critically ill patient at risk of ARF (Figure 23–1). The first step in managing ARF is prevention, and this can be accomplished by identifying patients who are at risk and eliminating or minimizing possible causes of ARF, such as unnecessary exposures to nephrotoxic agents or prolonged hypotensive episodes. By identifying the cause of the impending or actual case of ARF, the critical care practitioner can categorize the type of ARF: postrenal, prerenal, or intrarenal. Categorizing the ARF assists in understanding the underlying pathophysiologic features and the necessary medical or nursing interventions.

Another aspect of caring for the high-risk patient (Chart 23–1) is attempting to manage the primary critical care problem, for instance, cardiac failure or sepsis, because ARF usually occurs secondary to an exacerbation of the primary disease process.

Postrenal Management

Postrenal conditions can be ruled out early because these problems are easily diagnosed through the use of radiologic examination. If these conditions are present, a urology consultation may be necessary. The source of urinary obstruction must be removed, and any abnormality in the urinary collecting system must be corrected. Of course, the critically ill patient's ability to tolerate a urologic procedure to correct the postrenal condition must be seriously evaluated. Bladder neck or urethral obstruction often can be bypassed by the temporary placement of a transurethral or suprapubic catheter. Urethral obstructions may be initially treated by dilating the renal pelvis or ureter and performing percutaneous catherization. Obstructive lesions are

Text continued on page 559

CHART 23–1

Conditions That Put Patients at High Risk of Acute Renal Failure

- Hemodynamic instability
- Multisystem organ failure
- Trauma
- Intravenous hemolysis
- Rhabdomyolysis
- Use of nephrotoxic agents
- Complicated postoperative course

INTERDEPENDENT ACTIONS BASED UPON THE HUMAN RESPONSE TO ACTUAL OR POTENTIAL PROBLEMS

Hospital Day	Consults	Tests	Activity/Rest	Medical Interventions	Medications	Nutrition	Nurses' Signatures Date/Signature
Pre/post Admission Care Interval I	Social services Dietary Urology Vascular surgery Anesthesia Kidney center	CBC with differential Chem-20 Coagulation profile Urinalysis culture and sensitivity if indicated Urine osmolarity Urine electrolytes Serum uric acid Urine uric acid 24-hour creatinine clearance and protein collection Immune disease evaluation studies Renal biopsy if indicated Kidney, ureter, bladder radiographs IV pyelography Renal ultrasound	Bed rest with bathroom privileges with assistance	Renal dysfunction established Strict intake and output Daily weights Oxygen if indicated Fluid restriction Monitor FSBS if indicated Placement of vascular access for hemodialysis (Quinton, Perm cath) Placement of arteriovenous fistula Placement of peritoneal catheter for CAPD	Diuretics Anti-hypertensives Phosphate binders Kayexalate Multivitamin with folate Vitamin D analog Ferrous sulfate Sodium bicarbonate Diphen-hydramine Epogen Insulin therapy if indicated Antibiotics (IV, PO, IP) Stool softeners Others as needed Own (routine)	Low protein Low potassium Low sodium Low phosphorus Total parenteral nutrition if indicated Fluid restriction Diabetic diet if indicated	___ / ___ ___ / ___ ___ / ___ ___ / ___ ___ / ___ ___ / ___ ___ / ___ ___ / ___ ___ / ___ ___ / ___

Figure 23–1

Portion of a critical care pathway for acute and chronic renal failure. (Courtesy of the Tucson Medical Center, Division of Nursing, Tucson, AZ.)

INDEPENDENT ACTIONS BASED UPON THE HUMAN RESPONSE TO ACTUAL OR POTENTIAL PROBLEMS

Hospital Day	Assessment	Discharge Planning	Teaching	Psychosocial	Self Care	Nurses' Signatures Date/Signature
Pre/post Admission Care Interval I Date: _____	Weight on admission and daily	Contact care coordinator in utilization management	Assess learning needs of patient/significant other	Assess anxiety, fear, powerlessness, grieving, denial, non-compliance, depression, and alteration in relationship with significant other	Maintain optimum level of self-care	___ / ___
	Level of consciousness	Activities of daily living	Establish teaching plan			___ / ___
	Vital signs on admission and as ordered	Patient or significant others to know and understand disease process; if at home, care requirements and follow-up instructions	Evaluate progress/effectiveness of teaching	Assess coping strategies and interventions for stressors		___ / ___
	Skin color/integrity		Involve other staff to accomplish teaching/kidney center	Social worker to perform end-stage renal disease evaluation if chronic renal failure		___ / ___
	Depth/rate of respirations		equipment needs			___ / ___
	Lung sounds		Resource book, tapes while hospitalized (located in hemodialysis unit)			___ / ___
	Heart rate					___ / ___
	Temperature					___ / ___
	Bowel sounds					___ / ___
	Edema					___ / ___
	Signs and symptoms of infections					___ / ___
	If arteriovenous fistula present, check thrill/bruit		[Nurses: Patient may move to interval II once method of dialysis is established and uremia is stabilized]			___ / ___
	If CAPD catheter in place, check integrity at exit site/CAPD fluid					___ / ___
	Fluid balance					___ / ___

Hospital Day	Consults	Tests	Activity/Rest	Medical Interventions	Medications	Nutrition	Nurses' Signatures Date/Signature
Care Interval II		Predialysis laboratory tests as ordered (CBC, SMAC-20, HBSAG)	Bed rest with bathroom privileges with assistance	Renal dysfunction established Strict intake and output Daily weights Oxygen if indicated Fluid restriction Continue with hemodialysis 3 times weekly or CAPD exchanges QID or as ordered	Medications as ordered Note medications that are to be given every dialysis and those that are to be held before dialysis	Low protein Low potassium Low sodium Low phosphorus Total parenteral nutrition if indicated Fluid restriction Diabetic diet if indicated	___/___ ___/___ ___/___ ___/___ ___/___ ___/___ ___/___ ___/___ ___/___ ___/___ ___/___ ___/___

Figure 23–1 Continued

INDEPENDENT ACTIONS BASED UPON THE HUMAN RESPONSE TO ACTUAL OR POTENTIAL PROBLEMS

Hospital Day	Assessment	Discharge Planning	Teaching	Psychosocial	Self Care	Nurses' Signatures Date/Signature
Care Interval II Date: _____	Weight daily Level of consciousness Vital signs on admission and as ordered Skin color/integrity Depth/rate of respirations Lung sounds Heart rate Temperature Bowel sounds Edema Signs and symptoms of infections If arteriovenous fistula present, check thrill/bruit If CAPD catheter in place, check integrity at exit site/CAPD fluid Fluid balance	Contact care coordinator in utilization management Activities of daily living Individual needs identified Collaboration with renal center/social worker for continued outpatient therapy and home care requirements	Ongoing evaluation progression and effectiveness of teaching Initiate teaching form Resource book, tapes while hospitalized (located in hemodialysis unit) [Nurses: Patient may move to interval II once method of dialysis is established and uremia is stabilized]	Ongoing communication regarding continued medical management and needed support Social worker to perform end-stage renal disease evaluation if chronic renal failure	Maintain optimum level of self-care Encourage ongoing participation in care	_____ / _____ _____ / _____ _____ / _____ _____ / _____ _____ / _____ _____ / _____ _____ / _____ _____ / _____ _____ / _____ _____ / _____ _____ / _____

Figure 23-1 Continued

often removed percutaneously or are bypassed by insertion of a ureteric stent.

Most patients on removal of the source of obstruction experience a diuretic phase. The cause of this response is twofold. The diuresis occurs in an effort to correct the overhydration that resulted from the kidney's inability to excrete urine during the period of obstruction. The second reason is believed to be related to a temporary form of nephron damage that is the consequence of increased intrarenal pressure created by the presence of obstruction in the urinary collecting system. This damage remains for approximately 3 to 5 days, a period that correlates with the extent of the diuretic phase. The treatment during the diuresis is to replace two-thirds of the previous hour's urine with 5% dextrose in normal saline plus 30 mL. The additional 30 mL per hour represents the replacement of insensible fluid losses.

Prerenal and Intrarenal or Acute Tubular Necrosis Management

The reduced renal perfusion and other renal hemodynamic alterations associated with a prerenal condition and the early onset of ATN are treated alike, usually with fluid, diuretics, and vasopressors. In either prerenal or ATN, the diagnosis of dehydration must be made rapidly, and the appropriate replacement solution that reflects the type of losses (i.e., fluid, electrolyte, nutrient) needs to be administered. For example, blood loss needs to be replaced with the appropriate blood product, but in the interim, an extracellular volume expander may be used until the patient undergoes blood typing and crossmatching. However, even if dehydration is not present, the use of large boluses of intravenous fluid challenges has become part of the traditional therapy of ARF. Aggressive fluid administration by a volume expander, either a crystalloid or a colloid, after confirming that the patient's cardiovascular system can tolerate it, has proven to increase renal blood flow. Fluid therapy serves as a vehicle for prevention of prerenal ARF, and after the development of an ARF state, it has proven beneficial, particularly in oliguria to dislodge the tubular cells that slough off and obstruct the tubular space. The outcome is that more of the nephrons remain free of an obstructed source and allow the flow of urine. This effort promotes the formation of a nonoliguric rather than an oliguric state. Fluid is administered to prevent ATN, and once it is suspected of being present, the same fluid therapy may be continued to be administered, but with some caution if the patient has an oliguric ATN. The oliguric patient is prone to developing congestive heart failure secondary to the overhydration that results from the retention of fluids because the patient can no longer excrete the necessary urinary volumes to maintain body water balance (Table 23–6).

Diuretics are another mainstay of prevention and treatment of ARF. The two most commonly selected are furosemide and mannitol. Both agents are believed to improve renal blood flow, although this has not been substantiated consistently in medical research, and urinary flow through the tubules to assist in the removal of sloughed tubular cells. The use of diuretics must be managed carefully because the creation of a dehydrated state secondary to diuretic usage would only compound the impending or early-onset case of ARF. Measures must be planned and taken to prevent this complication. Furosemide can be administered as an intravenous bolus or a continuous low-dose infusion. The recommended bolus dose is 100 to 200 mg every 6 to 8 hours, whereas the continuous infusion dose usually begins low, at approximately 20 to 40 mg per hour. If the kidneys do not respond to this dose, then the amount of the infusion can be increased by increments of 20 mg every 2 hours. Maximal dosages of both forms of administration must be monitored because ototoxicity is a side effect of intravenous furosemide. The continuous low-dose infusion of furosemide has become preferable for several reasons. A higher incidence of renal responsiveness is noted, and a larger volume of urine output is observed. The incidence of diuretic intolerance is decreased; in fact, patients who may not respond to oral or intravenous furosemide may respond to the constant-infusion method because the tubule is exposed to a continuous, sustained level of the diuretic. In addition, a large bolus of intravenous furosemide may be more likely to stimulate a systemic vasoconstriction that could reduce renal blood flow; this effect is absent in a low-dose continuous approach.

Mannitol, another diuretic currently used, has not been proven to benefit the patient in ARF. This osmotic diuretic has the potential to increase plasma circulating volume and urinary flow through the tubules significantly. Although these effects seem beneficial, the increase in circulating volume must be able to be tolerated by the cardiovascular system, and research findings suggest that the tubules must respond to the increased workload resulting from the osmotic filtrate load by consuming more oxygen. This effect may actually contribute to the onset of ATN.

The most common vasopressor used in the prerenal and onset stage is dopamine at low-dose intravenous infusions. Despite its wide usage, the efficacy of this agent in ARF has not been substantiated. However, dopamine continues to be used in this situation. Administered in a dose range of 2 to 5 µg/kg per minute, with 3 µg/kg per minute as the best dosage for ARF, dopamine has been shown to improve renal blood flow. When dopamine is not able to prevent ARF, it may be able to contribute to the formation of the nonoliguric or less severe form of ARF. The goal of all the therapies described in this section is to implement

TABLE 23–6
Supportive Therapy in Ischemic and Nephrotoxic Acute Tubular Necrosis: General Guidelines

Patient Problems	Treatment
Extracellular Volume Overload	Restriction of salt (2–4 g/day) and water (usually <1 L per day) Diuretics, if responsive (usually loop and thiazide diuretics) Dialysis (daily or continuous)
Hyponatremia (Dilutional)	Restriction of oral water intake (<1 L/day) Restriction of hypotonic intravenous solutions (including dextrose-containing solutions)
Hyperkalemia	Restriction of dietary K^+ intake (20 to 50 mEq/day) Eliminate K^+ supplements and K^+-sparing diuretics Potassium-binding ion-exchange resins (e.g., sodium polystyrene sulphonate) Dialysis: consider low-K^+ dialysate Glucose (50 mL 50% dextrose) and insulin (10 U regular) Sodium bicarbonate (usually 50–100 nmol/L) Calcium gluconate (10 mL 10% solution over 5 min)
Metabolic Acidosis	Sodium bicarbonate (maintain serum bicarbonate >15 nmol/L, arterial pH > 7.2) Dialysis
Hyperphosphatemia	Restriction of dietary phosphate intake (<800 mg/day) Phosphate binding agents (calcium carbonate, aluminum hydroxide) Dialysis
Hypocalcemia	Calcium carbonate, PO (if symptomatic or if sodium bicarbonate to be administered) Calcium gluconate (10–20 mL 10% solution IV, consider whether emergency) Dialysis
Hypermagnesemia	Discontinue Mg-containing antacids Dialysis
Hyperuricemia	Treatment usually not necessary (if serum uric acid <15 mg/dL) Allopurinol and forced alkaline diuresis if >30 mg/dL
Nutrition	High dietary protein (35 to 50 kcal/kg of ideal body weight per day) Enteral and parenteral nutrition
Drug Dosage	Adjust doses for glomerular filtration rate (generally <10 mL/min) Avoid nonsteroidal anti-inflammatory agents, angiotensin-converting enzyme inhibitors, radiocontrast agents, and nephrotoxic antibiotics (unless absolute indication)

Data from Anderson, RJ: Prevention and management of acute renal failure. Hosp Pract 28:61–75, 1993.

them in a timely manner, to create a balance between cardiovascular function and renal blood and urinary flow.

Nutrition Management

The goals of nutritional therapy are to minimize uremic symptoms, to reduce the incidence of fluid, electrolyte, and acid–base imbalance, to produce an anabolic state, to decrease the patient's vulnerability to infections, and to minimize symptoms of anemia by providing adequate nutrition. In addition, research has shown that the administration of adequate protein intake actually promotes healing of the renal tubules and improves functioning of the immune system in the resistance to infection. Achieving these goals is a challenge because the patient in ARF usually maintains a catabolic state that increases protein requirements, as well as calories. The catabolic patient who does not receive adequate nutrition uses muscle protein for energy. The breakdown of significant amounts of muscle mass results in the further elevation of BUN and serum potassium levels; in addition, it exacerbates metabolic acidosis. The prescribed intervention is a high-calorie diet with a total of 30 to 35 kcal/kg per day of both lipids and carbohydrates, with a prescribed amount of glucose and triglycerides that is individualized for each patient. Amino acids, both essential and nonessential, are administered at 1.5 to 1.7 g/kg per day to minimize the catabolism. A combination of hyperalimentation (2 g/day of both essential and nonessential amino acids) and daily or continuous dialysis has been associated in isolated studies to increase the survival rate of the patient in ARF. One should consider the administration of water-soluble vitamins and iron supplements as additional nutritional support, as well to assist the patient in tolerating the effects of anemia.[16]

To determine the effectiveness of nutritional therapy, the nurse should monitor the patient's serum protein, albumin, hematocrit, and urea levels and should correlate the laboratory values to the patient's daily weight, level of mobility and other physical abilities, and personal sense of well-being, to ascertain the accomplishment of the nutritional outcomes.

Pharmacologic Management

The health care team must be aware that, during ARF, the dosages of pharmacologic agents that are primarily metabolized or excreted by the kidney must be adjusted. Extreme caution must be taken when a nephrotoxic agent is administered, such as radiologic contrast media and aminoglycoside antibiotics. Of course, whenever possible, a drug known to produce nephrotoxicity should be replaced by an equivalent agent or a close substitute. Collaborative interventions include the following: modifying the drug dosages to correlate with the degree of the renal failure, increasing the intervals between doses in an effort to maintain the appropriate blood levels, and monitoring serum drug levels to maintain them within therapeutic ranges.

Skin Care Management

The critical care nurse manages skin care primarily as an independent function. Uremic skin changes require frequent care and attention. The required plan is to initiate a regimen to keep the skin clean, dry, and intact, in addition to preventing bruising and minimizing itching. This goal can be accomplished by bathing the skin as necessary to remove uremic toxins, applying creams or lotions to treat dryness that may precipitate itching, developing a medication treatment plan with the physician for the prevention of itching, keeping bruised or open areas clean to prevent infection, monitoring the presence of edema, and avoiding tight shoes and clothing to eliminate the possibility of creating pressure points susceptible to skin breakdown. The desired outcome is the maintenance of intact skin, free of infection and itching.

Teaching Management

The patient in ARF and the family experience a knowledge deficit caused by the sudden onset of the renal disease. The patient, if alert and oriented, and the family need to be oriented to the ICU environment and the equipment. The prognosis needs to be explained, emphasizing the potential for renal recovery. Explanations of dietary and other restrictions assist the family in meeting the expectations of the health care providers.

Dialysis Selection and Management

The dialysis machine can be associated with many unusual perceptions by the patient and family, so a clear explanation of its purpose and function supports the patient and family in developing a realistic view of this procedure. Chart 23–2 gives indications for dialysis.

The management of ARF can be accomplished by the choice of any of three methods of dialysis. The critical care practitioner can select between the traditional two methods, hemodialysis and peritoneal dialysis, which are also available to patient in chronic renal failure, but the third choice is among a group of dialysis therapies specifically created for use in the critically ill patient in ARF. This group of therapies is called the continuous renal replacement therapies or CRRTs. The CRRTs offer a range of variations on hemodialysis. The forms of this dialysis procedure include continuous arteriovenous hemofiltration (CAVH), continuous arteriovenous hemodialysis (CAVHD), and the most recent adaptations, called continuous venovenous hemofiltration (CVVH) and continuous venovenous high-flux dialysis (CVVHD). The CRRTs have received much attention because of claims that their use is associated with decreased mortality and morbidity in the critically ill patient with ARF, although further study is necessary to substantiate these claims.

The basic principles of dialysis, diffusion, osmosis, and ultrafiltration or convection are the same whether the patient undergoing dialysis has ARF or chronic renal failure. However, specific aspects of selecting and managing the dialysis procedure are unique to the patient with ARF (Chart 23–3). These aspects follow, whereas detailed discussions of the types of dialysis,

---

CHART 23–2

Indications For Renal Dialysis

- Uremic syndrome (interfering with activities of daily living)
- Uremic pericarditis
- Volume overload
- Electrolyte imbalances
- Symptomatic metabolic acidosis
- Overdose (drug must be lipid free)

▶CHART 23–3
ETHICAL DILEMMA

Mr. S., age 84, has lived in a nursing home for the last 4 years. His only remaining relative is a sister who is 80 years old and lives independently at home. Even though Mr. S.'s sister is extremely devoted to him, she does not have the physical or financial means to care for him by herself. Mr. S. experienced a myocardial infarction and was taken to the local emergency department. Cardiac problems had begun in the patient more than 16 years ago, when he first suffered an anterior wall myocardial infarction. Since that episode, he has been treated for angina. A cardiac profile was completed, and the cardiac catherization revealed significant blockage in three vessels. As a result, a coronary artery bypass grafting was performed. The surgical procedure proved successful, but the first 3 postoperative days were complicated by respiratory distress as well as involvement of other organ systems. For example, several attempts to wean Mr. S. from the mechanical ventilator proved unsuccessful. He had few spontaneous respirations, and the blood gas values did not improve. Mr. S. also experienced dysrhythmias, and his cardiac output remained at 2.3 to 2.8. This low cardiac output proved compromising to his kidneys, and the blood urea nitrogen and serum creatinine had been climbing over the past 3

days. The risk of acute renal failure was growing when an episode of hypotension resulted in ischemic damage to the kidneys, commonly known as acute tubular necrosis (ATN). The onset of ATN greatly affects the patient mortality rate. On the third preoperative day, taking all these factors into consideration, Mr. S.'s sister was approached. She was asked to consider the possibility of initiating intra-aortic balloon pumping in conjunction with a form of continuous renal replacement therapy called continuous arteriovenous hemodialysis.

1. What is the number and duration of the organ systems that have failed? How would this affect your ethical decision making?
2. What are the quality of life factors before this admission that can be taken into consideration?
3. Considering that this is the third postoperative day, does this time factor influence your ethical decision making?
4. How would you present this case to Mr. S.'s sister?
5. If dialysis was initiated, at what point would you reevaluate the outcome of this procedure?

including indications, contraindications, and patient outcomes, appear in Chapter 24.

Hemodialysis has proven successful in the treatment of the critically ill patient. However, for this procedure to be successful, the patient must be able to tolerate certain situations unique to the implementation and management of this form of dialysis. For example, hemodialysis can be thought of as a hemodynamic procedure, especially in the critically ill patient. It requires approximately 1 U of blood or 250 to 350 mL to fill the dialysis circuitry, including the arteriovenous tubing and artificial kidney. A tolerance of this degree of acute blood loss is necessary to use hemodialysis, as well as the ability to be systemically anticoagulated. The inability of the patient to receive anticoagulation is an immediate contraindication for hemodialysis. To assist in the initial entry onto the machine, the priming solution composed of NS can be administered. If successful, this effort also assists in initially supporting the patient's blood pressure. A pump moves the patient's blood from the vascular system into and through the hemodialysis machine. Again, this "pulling" action on the cardiovascular system must be tolerated to continue

the procedure. The next hemodynamic insult occurs as a result of the rapid fluid and electrolyte shifts between the intracellular and extracellular compartments. Hemodialysis is known as an aggressive procedure; it rapidly depletes the extracellular space, consisting of both the vascular and interstitial space, of fluid and solute. This depletion occurs so quickly that the intracellular space does not have time to respond and therefore remains hyperosmotic in comparison with the extracellular space. An intracellular osmotic gradient further moves water from the extracellular space into the cell. The result, of course, is further loss of extracellular volume, especially in the vascular space. The clinical expression of this response is resistant hypotension, which may necessitate the administration of large amounts of a vascular volume expander (normal saline) in an already overhydrated patient as an attempt to raise the blood pressure. Within 30 to 60 minutes of initiating the hemodialysis procedure, the intracellular and extracellular compartments achieve equilibrium, and in response, the blood pressure should stabilize. However, intermittent periods of hypotension can occur throughout the entire procedure.

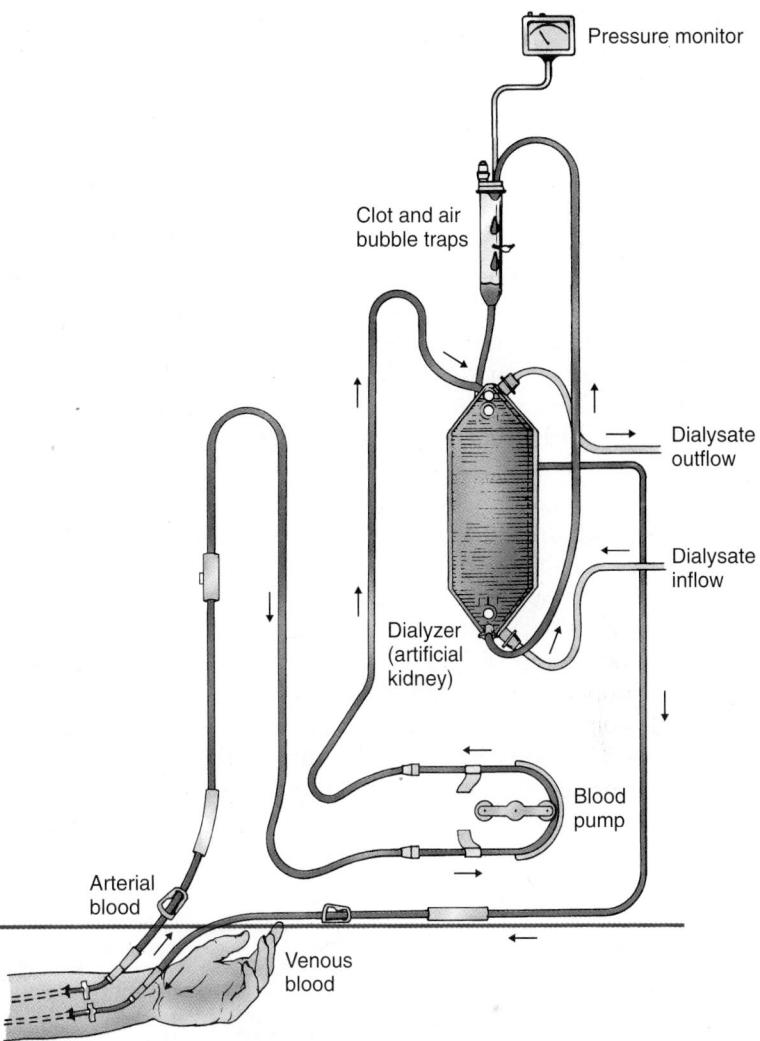

Pressure monitor

Clot and air
bubble traps

Dialysate
outflow

Dialysate
inflow

Dialyzer
(artificial
kidney)

Blood
pump

Arterial
blood

Venous
blood

Figure 23–2

Hemodialysis circuit. (From Ignatavicius DD, Workman
L, Mishler MA: Medical-Surgical Nursing, 3rd ed.
Philadelphia, W.B. Saunders, 1999.)

Dysrhythmias are another common problem in the first
30 to 60 minutes and are believed to be caused by the
cellular hyperosmolality and the rapid potassium shifts
synonymous within this time period. Stabilization of
the patient throughout these events allows continuation of the hemodialysis procedure until the last 30
minutes, when hypotension and dysrhythmia may
reappear as the result of true intracellular an extracellular compartment depletion. Any fluid that had been
removed earlier may need to be replaced at the final
stages of the hemodialysis procedure. When successful,
hemodialysis does provide the benefit of a rapid
method for the removal of excess fluid, electrolytes,
and wastes associated with uremia (Figure 23–2).

Peritoneal dialysis is usually used as a maintenance
procedure; therefore, it seems to have little benefit in
the critically ill patient who requires a means of rapid
correction of imbalances and the return to homeostasis. However, peritoneal dialysis has proven helpful
when hemodialysis is contraindicated or when it is
used in combination with hemodialysis. The hemodynamically unstable critically ill patient responds well

to the use of peritoneal dialysis for mild water removal
and then hemodialysis for the removal of solute (see
Figures 24–7 and 24–8).

The CRRTs were designed for the critically ill patient
and therefore offer several advantages not available in
either of the other traditional forms of dialysis. The
CRRTs use a hollow-fiber hemofilter that is more biocompatible in the critically ill patient than the hemodialysis membrane and is capable of a mild but
rapid form of fluid removal during hypotensive or
reduced blood flow states. This is possible because the
hemofilter has a low resistance that allows the patient's
own blood pressure, as low as 90/60 mm Hg, to drive
the blood flow through the dialyzer, although venovenous forms of CRRT use a blood pump to facilitate flow.
In addition, smaller volumes of blood are required to
fill the dialysis tubing and hemofilter, sometimes as
little as 40 mL. Because of these factors, the CRRTs have
proven beneficial as a dialysis method for the hemodynamically unstable patient. Another advantage is that
some forms of the CRRT use a minimal amount of anticoagulation. Finally, the continuous process of dialysis

provides a consistent means for reaching and maintaining homeostasis. The patient does not experience the rapid fluid and electrolyte shifts seen during hemodialysis, but rather the equal depletion of the intracellular and extracellular compartments. If the blood pressure drops, the critical care nurse can easily correct this hypotensive episode by replacing volume or by reducing the ultrafiltration rate.

CAVH is used primarily for the removal of fluid and some solute. It uses the patient's own blood pressure to facilitate the process of ultrafiltration or convection for water removal. CAVHD, also driven by the patient's blood pressure, incorporates the use of diffusion for efficient solute removal with its ultrafiltration processes. This is accomplished by the addition of peritoneal dialysis fluid, which is infused by a fluid administration pump into the hemofilter and established a diffusion gradient for solute removal. CVVH and CVVHD are more complex; these procedures use a special CRRT dialysis machine with a blood pump. As in hemodialysis, blood is pumped through venovenous tubing for both fluid and solute removal. The results are positive, despite the complexity of this technical procedure, which is usually performed by the critical care nurse (Figure 23–3).

Multidisciplinary Outcomes

The multidisciplinary outcomes for ARF focus on maintaining a homeostatic healing environment to promote renal repair, with the ultimate goal as the resumption of renal function (Chart 23–4). For prerenal failure, the outcome is to identify the causative factor, to promote resolution of renal hypoperfusion or nephrotoxicity, and to achieve the resumption of normal renal function. Postrenal failure outcomes involve the removal or resolution of the source of renal obstruction, followed by the resumption of normal urinary output. The outcomes for an intrarenal condition involve returning the patient to homeostasis for the promotion of renal healing, and ultimately, renal recovery, as exemplified by ability to concentrate urine. Other therapeutic outcomes that also promote homeostasis and renal healing are nutritional therapy and dialysis. For nutritional therapy, the goal is to minimize the uremic syndrome, to minimize or eliminate catabolic metabolism, and to promote a satisfactory nutritional state. The outcome for any form of dialysis is to control or minimize and prevent complications associated with uremia, including restoration of the fluid and electrolyte and acid–base balance (Table 23–7). Chart

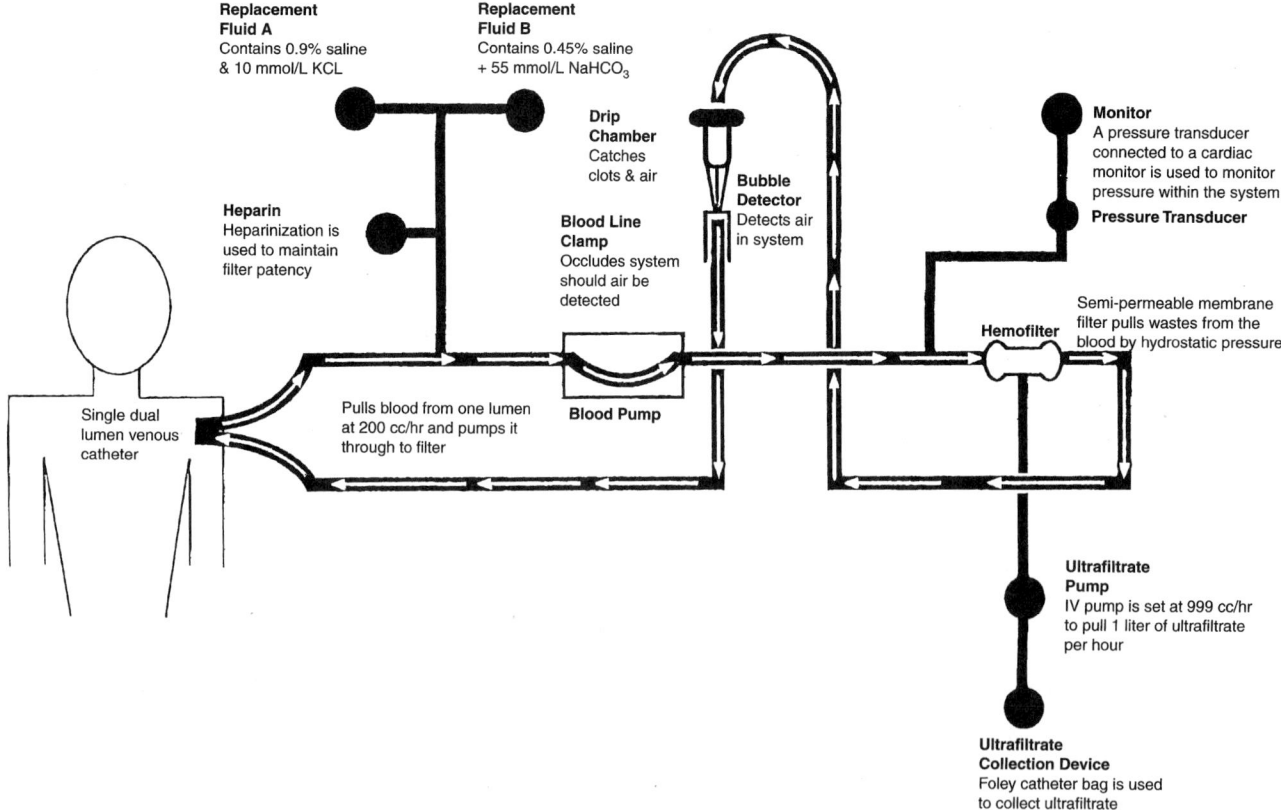

Figure 23–3

Schematic of continuous venovenous hemofiltration circuitry. (From Clevenger K: Setting up a continuous venovenous hemofiltration educational program: a case study in program development. Crit Care Nurs Clin North Am 10(2):235–244, 1998.)

23–5 provides further information regarding variables identified as predictors of morbidity and mortality in this patient population.

Critical Thinking Exercise

Mr. C., age 56, was involved in a motor vehicle accident in which he sustained lacerations to his head and face and broke his fibula and tibia of the right leg, which required surgical repair. Mr. C.'s accident occurred on a rural highway. Because of the location of the accident, critical time elapsed, approximately 2 hours, from the time of the accident to the time the patient arrived in the emergency room (ER). On entering the emergency room, Mr. C.'s vital signs and laboratory findings revealed the following: blood pressure, 98/60 mm Hg; heart rate, 118 beats per minute; respirations, 30 per minute; temperature, 37°C (98.6°F); blood urea nitrogen, 25; serum creatinine, 1.0 mg/dL; hemoglobin, 11; hematocrit, 33%; and red blood cells, 3.5.

An effort was made to begin to replace the blood loss experienced as a result of the accident. Because the type and crossmatch were being drawn, the ER clinicians ordered NS.

However, only a small volume was replaced before the patient was urgently moved to the operating room for the repair of the broken fibula and tibia. During the operative procedure, Mr. C. lost additional extracellular volume before the anesthesiologist had the time needed to replace the volume the patient required from the prior deficit. As a result, the patient had a hypotensive episode that was difficult to resolve and lasted more than 20 minutes. Extracellular volume replacement was finally accomplished by the rapid instillation of intravenous crystalloid fluid replacement and eventually blood replacement. Once the patient was stabilized, the procedure was completed, and Mr. C. was moved to the surgical ICU. On arrival in the ICU, the patient's vital signs and recent laboratory results were obtained. They were reported as follows: blood pressure, 116/82 mm Hg; heart rate, 124 beats per minute; respirations, 24 per minute; temperature, 37.1°C (98.8°F); blood urea nitrogen, 35; serum creatinine, 1.5 mg/dL; hemoglobin, 12; hematocrit, 35%; and red blood cells, 3.7. Mr. C.'s urine output was 47 mL the first hour after surgery and then decreased to approximately 30 mL per hour.

1. What do Mr. C.'s recent history, presenting signs and symptoms, vital signs, and laboratory findings suggest about his current renal status?

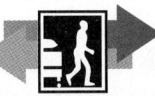

CHART 23–4

BEYOND THE ICU: LIFE AFTER ACUTE RENAL FAILURE

Many patients develop acute renal failure (ARF) as a complication of another event (e.g., trauma) or disease (e.g., congestive heart failure [CHF]). The majority of patients with ARF will experience an adequate return of kidney function, but the precipitating event will often influence the course of the patient's recovery. For example, patients recovering from traumatic events may require prolonged and complex care that includes dialysis. This care may be provided in a rehabilitation or transitional care unit. Nursing care that includes astute monitoring, emotional support, and education is necessary during this phase of the patient's recovery. Patients and their families need to understand that dialysis will be continued only until the patient's kidneys begin to resume functioning.

The patient recovering from ARF who returns home usually requires little to no further intervention. Follow-up care with the primary physician or nurse practitioner is recommended to monitor kidney function. If a primary disease such as CHF or hypertension triggered the episode of ARF, then the patient may benefit from follow-up care by a home health nurse. A concise teaching plan that not only educates the patient and family but also encourages

compliance with the medical regimen is developed and implemented by the nurse. Education regarding diet, exercise, weight control, fluid restrictions, and medications should be provided. Teaching strategies must be modified to meet individual patient learning needs (e.g., large print information sheets for patients with visual impairments). The goal for these patients is to assist them to achieve and maintain the best state of health so that their kidneys are not compromised again.

An additional resource that can be utilized by patients recovering from ARF and their families is the National Kidney Foundation. This organization provides timely information on a variety of topics related to kidney disease (e.g., diet, medications). The foundation can be reached at the following address:

National Kidney Foundation
30 East 33rd Street
New York, NY 10157
1-800-622-9010
Web Site: http://www.kidney.org

 **CHART 23-5**

RESEARCH UTILIZATION: PREDICTING OUTCOMES IN PATIENTS WITH ACUTE RENAL FAILURE

Abstract: A multicenter research study was conducted to address the outcomes of acute renal failure patients. Three specific areas were addressed: 1) hospital outcome; 2) analysis of prognostic factors using the variables of age, sex, preexisting chronic disease, previous health status, mechanism and type of acute renal failure, urine output, initial or delayed inclusion into the study, need for dialysis or mechanical ventilation, and three scoring systems computed at admission and at the conclusion of the study; 3) serum creatinine concentrations at ICU discharge and for survivors 6 months after the conclusion of the study. Three hundred and sixty patients were included in the study; 217 patients were admitted to the study at the same time they were admitted to ICU; 143 patients were admitted to the study after their ICU admission. The breakdown of types of acute renal failure occurred as follows: prerenal (N = 61), intrarenal (N = 282), postrenal (N = 17). The mechanism of acute renal failure was septic in 172 patients, hemodynamic in 115, toxic in 71 patients, and other in 105 patients. One hundred thirty-seven patients had at least 1 preexisting disease, including 39 with chronic renal insufficiency. Forty-one percent of the patients had been in good health 3 months before admission.

Critique: Two hundred ten (58%) of the patients died during the hospital stay, including 191 patients who died while still in the ICU. From the 210 patients who died during this study, 7 variables were identified as predictors of mortality: 1) advanced age, 2) altered previous health status, 3) hospitalization before ICU admission, 4) delayed occurrence of acute renal failure, 5) sepsis, 6) oliguria, and 7) severity of illness at the time of the study as assessed by the Simplified Acute Physiology Score, APACHE II, or organ system failure. Authors of the research study state that mortality rates remain high in acute renal failure (58%); an increasing incidence of multiorgan failure and sepsis is found in multicenter reports to account for the high rates. As a result of this study, the researchers suggested that therapeutic trials and new drugs or supportive therapies should be aimed at addressing these 7 variables, which are predictors of mortality in the patient with acute renal failure.

Nursing Considerations: One hundred forty-three of the foregoing subjects were admitted to the study after their ICU stay. This population could take advantage of the information learned from this study in the future. Possibly, we could identify high-risk groups of patients and begin early aggressive treatments to prevent permanent renal damage and to decrease morbidity and mortality rates. Nurses are the key to early identification of possible risk factors and the subsequent communication of this information to the physician.

Source: Brivet F, Kleinknecht D, Loirat P, et al: Acute renal failure in intensive care units—causes, outcome, and prognostic factors of hospital mortality: a prospective, multicenter study. Crit Care Med 24:192–198, 1996.

TABLE 23-7
Multidisciplinary Outcomes

Category	Outcome
Prerenal failure	Identification of causative factor and resolution of hypovolemic state
Postrenal failure	Identification of causative factor and resolution of the renal obstruction
Intrarenal failure or acute tubular necrosis	Restoration of renal perfusion and tubular obstruction and identification of and withdrawal of nephrotoxic agents or medications while minimizing of epithelial damage
Diet therapy	Minimizing of uremic toxicity, fluid and electrolyte imbalances, and prevention of catabolism
Dialysis	Control of the uremic state, restoration of fluid and electrolyte balance and acid–base balance, and provision of mechanism for waste removal

2. What preoperative measures could have been considered in Mr. C.'s case?
3. What relevance may the hypotensive episode have had in this case?
4. What nursing considerations exist for Mr. C.?

Key Concepts

➡ Many different etiologic factors are responsible for causing ARF. For diagnostic purposes, these causes are categorized into three groups: prerenal, renal, and postrenal. Each category has unique characteristics that differentiate it from the other groups. If the patient's problems are recognized before severe renal damage has occurred, ARF can be reversed. This is a differentiating factor between ARF and chronic renal failure.

➡ Postrenal failure is caused by an obstruction in the urinary tract. Obstructions can occur anywhere from the calyces to the urethral meatus. For the progression of ARF, it would be necessary for both kidneys to have developed an obstruction or a unilateral obstruction in a patient with only one kidney. In this situation, the patient presents in a uremic state with the BUN and serum creatinine at a 10:1 ratio.

➠ Prerenal failure is frequently the result of diminished renal perfusion. Because of decreased perfusion, the GFR decreases, which, in turn, decreases urine output. Many factors could cause this type of failure, including cardiogenic shock and certain medications (e.g., nonsteroidal anti-inflammatory drugs).

➠ Intrarenal or intrinsic renal failure results from actual damage to the kidney tissue, including parenchymal and nephron damage. Conditions that cause parenchymal damage are considered intrarenal. Intrarenal failure occurs most often after renal perfusion compromise or nephrotoxicity.

➠ ATN is the most common cause of ARF. The most frequent cause of ATN is a prolonged prerenal condition that has caused prolonged ischemia or hypovolemia. Exposure to classes of antibiotics and heavy metals has been discussed as a cause of tubular damage.

➠ Medications can be the cause of acute renal failure. Cisplatin, amphotericin B, pentamidine, tetracycline, and high-dose methotrexate or acyclovir are common nephrotoxic agents. Aminoglycosides, gentamicin, tobramycin, and amikacin bind to cells in the proximal tubules.

➠ Because of the vast functions of the kidneys, once they develop a crisis situation, such as in ARF, multiple systems are affected. Potential multisystem problems are electrolyte imbalances, pericarditis, pleural effusions and pulmonary edema, anorexia, nausea and vomiting, altered mental status, drowsiness, delirium, coma, psychosis, hypocalcemia, bleeding abnormalities, pruritus, and ecchymosis.

➠ ARF can be divided into four different stages. Each stage has a treatment focus along with specific patient concerns. The four stages associated with acute renal failure are: 1) onset, 2) oliguric or nonoliguric, 3) diuretic, and 4) recovery.

➠ For the patient in ARF, assessment information is crucial. ARF assessment should include information regarding 1) history of related renal symptoms, 2) systemic disease state, 3) family history of renal disease, 4) medication history, 5) physical assessment information, 6) vital signs, and 7) laboratory data analysis. A thorough assessment could be the key to finding the cause of ARF.

➠ IVP provides visual assessment of the kidneys, kidney pelvis, ureters, and bladder. It is used to determine areas of dysfunction and also to locate renal tumors and calculi.

➠ MRI provides direct imaging in several planes of the renal and urinary drainage system. In ARF and acute renal transplant rejection, it is especially helpful in detecting alterations of renal blood flow.

➠ CRRT is a form of hemodialysis. Types of CRRT include CVVH, CVVHD, CAVH, and CAVHD. These CRRTs allow replacement continuously instead of in large amounts at once, as in hemodialysis. This type of dialysis is used for the critically ill patient who is hemodynamically unstable.

References

1. Anderson RJ: Prevention and management of acute renal failure. Hosp Pract 28:61–75, 1993.
2. Baer CL: Acute renal failure. In: Hartshorn J, Lamborn M, Noll ML (eds): Introduction to Critical Care Nursing. Philadelphia, W.B. Saunders, 1993, pp 314–347.
3. Baer CL: Acute renal failure: recognizing and reversing its deadly course. Nursing 90 20:34–40, 1990.
4. Hullman P, Wolfson M: The patient with acute renal failure. Hosp Med 29:82–95, 1993.
5. Ulrich BT: Nephrology Nursing. Philadelphia, W.B. Saunders, 1989.
6. Brasfield K, Urden L: Renal disorders. In: Thelan L, Davie J, Urden L, et al (eds): Critical Care Nursing: Diagnosis and Management, 2nd ed. St. Louis, C.V. Mosby, 1994, pp 603–620.
7. Giordano B, Dossey B: Acute renal failure. In: Dossey BM, Guzzetta CE, Kenner CV (eds): Essentials of Critical Care Nursing: Body, Mind, Spirit. Philadelphia, J.B. Lippincott, 1990, pp 570–597.
8. Kernicki JG: Nursing management of the patient with acute renal failure. In: Ruppert S, Kernicki J, Dolan J (eds): Dolan's Critical Care Nursing: Clinical Management Through the Nursing Process. Philadelphia, F.A. Davis, 1996, pp 497–519.
9. King BA: Detecting acute renal failure. RN 57:34–40, 1994.
10. Whittaker AA: Patients with acute renal failure. In: Clochesy J, Breu C, Cardin S, et al (eds): Critical Care Nursing. Philadelphia, W.B. Saunders, 1993, pp 886–904.
11. Stark J: Acute tubular necrosis: differences between oliguria and nonoliguria. Crit Care Nurs Q 14:22–27, 1992.
12. Baer CL, Lancaster LF: Acute renal failure. Crit Care Nurs Q 14:1–21, 1992.
13. Alspach JG: Core Curriculum for Critical Care Nursing. Philadelphia, W.B. Saunders, 1991.
14. Melander S: Review of Critical Care Nursing: Case Studies and Applications. Philadelphia, W.B. Saunders, 1996.
15. Norris MK: Acute tubular necrosis: prevention of complications. Dimensions Crit Care Nurs 8:16–25, 1989.
16. Kierdorf HP: The nutritional management of ARF in the ICU. New Horizons 3:699–707, 1995.

24

Chronic Renal Failure and Renal Transplantation

Susan A. Pfettscher

Objectives

After completing this chapter, the student will be able to:

1. Differentiate the various causes of chronic renal failure (CRF).
2. Relate the pathophysiology of CRF to the diverse treatment strategies.
3. Interpret history, physical assessment, and diagnostic data for a patient presenting with CRF.
4. Plan appropriate interventions for the management of a patient with CRF.
5. Differentiate the care related to the renal replacement therapies for end-stage renal disease (ESRD): hemodialysis, peritoneal dialysis, and renal transplantation.
6. Evaluate outcome data relative to the current treatment strategies for patients with ESRD.

The term "chronic renal failure" describes a condition in which the kidneys are unable to eliminate metabolic waste products and excessive water from the body effectively. The cumulative signs and symptoms that develop in CRF are frequently referred to as uremia and include fluid overload, electrolyte imbalances, and coma. If the disorder is untreated, patients may experience pulmonary edema, cardiac dysrhythmias, and cerebral edema. Death may be a direct result of untreated hyperkalemia, massive pulmonary edema and cardiac failure, or respiratory arrest from cerebral edema and brain stem herniation. Although comfort measures and other medical treatments can be aggressively employed in the patient with renal failure, they are ineffective in maintaining life for an extended period.

Successful treatment of CRF has resulted from the development of replacement therapies that include hemodialysis, peritoneal dialysis, and the replacement of complete renal function with the transplantation of a human kidney.[1-5] The advent of hemodialysis and kidney transplantation to treat CRF required an entirely new approach to health care delivery. Initially, these treatments were not reimbursed by third-party payers because they were too expensive or were considered experimental. Selection committees, composed of health care professionals and lay persons, were formed at treatment facilities and determined which patients should receive treatment.[1,5,6] This system of treatment decision making generally excluded children, persons over age 50, those with other chronic diseases (e.g., diabetes, cardiovascular disease, primary hypertension), or those whose lifestyles were not socially acceptable based on criminal records, lack of family system or support, lack of employment or who were generally identified as not being contributing members of their communities.[1,5,6]

Public and political opinion regarding the discriminatory nature of patient selection for hemodialysis and renal transplantation led to the passage of PL 92-603 by the United States Congress in 1972.[7,8] This legislation guaranteed access to treatment for all patients with CRF without regard to social, economic, or other medical considerations. Payment for hemodialysis and transplantation was provided without discrimination through the Medicare program. Congress used the term "end-stage renal disease" to discriminate from other diagnoses. Using this definition, a patient with ESRD would be eligible for any form of dialysis or renal transplantation for irreversible kidney disease. This federal program remains unique in regard to access to and financial coverage of a disease entity.[2,9]

ETIOLOGY AND PATHOPHYSIOLOGY

The etiology of CRF is complex. The most common causes of CRF that are discussed can be categorized as 1) vascular, 2) glomerular, 3) interstitial, 4) congenital, and 5) genetic.[2, 10, 11]

The intact nephron theory explains the nature of the progression of renal failure. Because each nephron is an independently functioning structure within the kidney, it may or may not become diseased; nephrons lose function at different times within the kidney. As nephrons become diseased, others in close proximity functionally hypertrophy, thus compensating for lost function. Thus, more than 70% of functioning nephrons must be lost before one has a clinical indication by blood studies (elevations in blood urea nitrogen [BUN] and creatinine) that renal function has been compromised. ESRD becomes evident only when 90% of the nephrons are lost. This amount of loss is most frequently measured clinically using creatinine clearance values.[2, 11]

The etiology and epidemiology of ESRD have been and continue to be well described.[2, 12] Because of the federally funded ESRD program database requirements, a massive amount of clinical and sociodemographic data about patients with ESRD is available. However, some patients with ESRD may not be referred for ESRD treatment based on physician decision-making or patient choice. Few, if any, data are available to identify how many patients die of untreated ESRD in the United States, although this number is believed to be relatively small.

Vascular Renal Disease

Renal disease resulting from vascular lesions or disease correlates with cardiovascular disease as the leading cause of death in the United States. Hypertension (HTN), particularly untreated or poorly controlled HTN, results in sclerotic lesions that begin in the microvessels of the nephron and may extend to the larger vessels within the kidney. Thus, nephrosclerosis as the cause of ESRD occurs more frequently in the elderly and in ethnic groups with a higher incidence of primary HTN (e.g., blacks, Hispanics, and Asians).[2, 11, 13–16]

The sclerotic process in the kidney is the same as that in other small vessels including those of the peripheral, cerebral, and coronary systems. Antihypertensive therapy is directed at preventing disease in all of these vascular systems; the many drugs available to treat HTN allow the health care professional multiple alternatives for successful treatment while minimizing side effects.[17, 18]

Renal dysfunction improves or deteriorates with changes in blood pressure; the patient in a hypertensive crisis may have altered renal function that improves when the blood pressure is normalized. Similarly, patients whose blood pressure is not controlled with oral medications may show evidence of renal dysfunction that can be improved with adequate medication administration or may require other short-term interventions. Appropriate education by health care professionals may decrease the incidence of ESRD secondary to uncontrolled HTN. In addition, voluntary health care agencies play a significant role in public education. The National Kidney Foundation (NKF) sponsors programs for blood pressure and kidney disease screening for high-risk groups in many communities throughout the United States in an attempt to prevent the development and progression of renal disease.[19]

A major complication of all types of diabetes mellitus (DM) is the development of renal failure.[2, 11] A syndrome known as Kimmelstiel–Wilson syndrome can develop in patients who have had DM for several years. One component of this syndrome involves the development of atherosclerosis of the renal artery and glomerulosclerosis. Just as the microvessels in other organ systems of the body are sclerosed in diabetes, the macrovasculature and microvasculature of the kidney can be damaged, resulting in ESRD. Patients with DM and a coexisting diagnosis of HTN are at greatest risk for developing ESRD.[16]

Based on the findings of the Diabetes Complications and Control Trial (DCCT), the development of ESRD in diabetic patients may be slowed by the administration of angiotensin-converting enzyme (ACE) inhibitors. Because persons with all types of diabetes constitute the largest number of patients receiving ESRD treatment, pharmacotherapeutic management may have the potential to limit or prevent the development of this complication.[20]

Vascular lesions may also occur outside the kidney (prerenal or extrarenal) and can result in renal failure. In particular, renal artery stenosis secondary to a thrombus or sclerotic lesion may cause decreased renal function and progression to ESRD.[2] Careful physical assessment (sudden increase in blood pressure or presence of a renal bruit) and suspicion of such lesions may lead to early diagnosis and treatment, thus preventing the development of ESRD. Safer, noninvasive techniques of imaging for diagnosis and intervention rather than invasive surgery also assist in successful treatment. For example, angioplasty of a renal artery that is obstructed or stenosed by plaque formation can be performed to improve and preserve renal function. Similarly, when a thrombus obstructs the renal artery, an embolectomy can be performed to restore blood flow to a kidney.[2] Other lesions of the abdominal artery that occur above the renal artery junction may also alter blood flow to the kidneys. Sclerotic lesions or calcification in the aorta may decrease renal blood flow, resulting in HTN and renal disease. Because these types of lesions cannot be repaired surgically and because they may become progressively worse, renal dysfunction resulting in ESRD often occurs.[2]

The development of an abdominal aortic aneurysm often results in the impairment of renal blood flow and function. Although the surgical repair of this aneurysm may result in an episode of acute renal failure (ARF) (see Chapter 23), adequate renal function may not be restored, especially if the patient has underlying or preexisting renal disease from another cause. The additional loss of renal perfusion during the repair of the aneurysm may, in fact, precipitate ESRD.

The presence of cardiovascular disease may result in ESRD in some patients, especially those with other comorbidities. An example of these interacting pathophysiologic processes is a patient with type 2 DM, controlled HTN, and a history of myocardial infarction who presents with congestive heart failure (CHF). Although the signs and symptoms of renal disease in this patient may be similar to those of prerenal ARF, the renal failure in this patient cannot usually be reversed or improved significantly.[2, 11, 21–24] This renal failure exists secondary to decreased renal blood flow resulting from reduced cardiac output. The extent of renal dysfunction is increased by the coexistence of diabetic nephropathy and nephrosclerosis from HTN.

Glomerular Renal Disease

Glomerular renal disease is identified as those processes that affect the normal function of the glomerulus of the kidney resulting in decreased filtration of metabolic toxins or waste products, water, and electrolytes. In addition, lesions in the glomerular capillaries result in the inappropriate filtration of plasma proteins and red cells across this membrane.[2] Definitive diagnosis of the specific type of glomerulonephritis is made by pathologic examination of the kidney tissue. A renal biopsy must be performed to reach such a diagnosis.

In autoimmune glomerular disease, a person's own antibodies destroy the glomerular capillary structure. These antibodies may be formed as a result of an acute infection elsewhere in the body. The most classic example of this is a "strep throat" infection caused by beta streptococci that results in a secondary antibody response in the kidney. Because the antibody is the cause of the renal impairment, it cannot be treated with antibiotics. Consequently, autoimmune glomerular disease is considered a complication or sequela of another illness.[2, 25]

If the primary infection has not been treated or has been inadequately treated, the development of glomerular disease is more likely, but it is not always predictable. In addition, renal impairment may not become evident immediately; it may be diagnosed only years after the primary infection. Diagnosis is based on the patient's history or on kidney biopsy, if adequate tissue can be obtained. In these situations, it is assumed that renal dysfunction has been developing slowly through the destruction of individual nephrons.

Immunologic glomerular disease may develop aggressively, leading to accelerated renal failure, and is usually identified as rapidly progressive glomerulonephritis (RPGN). Along with the patient's history, if kidney function indicates the possibility of viable tissue available for pathologic analysis, a kidney biopsy will be done for specific diagnosis. Other autoimmune systemic diseases may also result in renal impairment. For example, patients diagnosed with systemic lupus erythematosus frequently develop some degree of renal impairment.[2]

Glomerulonephritis may or may not progress to ESRD; in particular, early diagnosis of this autoimmune process may allow specific treatment to halt its progression. Specific treatment with immunologic therapies including corticosteroids, cyclophosphamide (Cytoxan), azathioprine (Imuran), and cyclosporine (Neoral) may be ordered.[17] These treatments may not reverse the course of the renal disease, but they may delay loss of renal function. Consequently, the patient who begins treatment for ESRD may present with side effects of these drugs if they had been used in an attempt to prevent disease progression. In addition, if patients are not currently taking these medications, they may have knowledge of and experience with the effects, side effects, and complications. This experience may influence the use of such therapy and, in particular, may influence decision making regarding renal transplantation.[10, 13, 17, 26–30]

Before the onset of renal failure, glomerular disease may be diagnosed through blood studies showing increased serum levels of metabolic wastes (e.g., BUN and creatinine). The urinary excretion of protein (proteinuria) in the amount of several grams in 24 hours is more specific to glomerular disease. Systemic signs and symptoms of proteinuria include decreased serum protein, specifically serum albumin, with development of systemic edema secondary to decreased vascular oncotic pressure. Early morning edema of the eyelids and face may be particularly recognized by patients and others. The patient's urine output may be normal to increased. Because of this protein–fluid alteration, the patient does *not* generally develop significant hypertension. Protein loss may also result in diminished muscle mass, which may not be recognized as weight change because of its replacement with edema fluid.[2, 10, 11, 13]

Type 1 DM may also be classified as a cause of glomerular renal disease. The nephron lesion that develops (along with the vascular lesion previously described) involves the glomerular basement membrane; microalbuminuria develops early in the course of renal involvement and can be clinically measured in the person with type 1 DM. As mentioned earlier, pharmacologic management with ACE inhibitors may significantly slow or perhaps even prevent the development of ESRD in persons with type 1 DM.

Interstitial Renal Disease

Interstitial renal disease affects the dense tissue of the kidney that surrounds and supports the nephron structures in the kidneys. Damage to and scarring of this tissue prevents the multiple interactions of the vascular and tubular structures of the nephron. Pyelonephritis, an infection within the kidney, is a disease that affects the interstitium by scarring. Recurrent infections and the autoimmune process that often result from these infections have diminished as a cause of renal failure in the past 20 years. More aggressive diagnosis and more effective antibiotic therapy have been responsible for this improvement.[2]

Interstitial damage may also result from drugs and other toxic substances. The close monitoring of prescription drugs by the United States Food and Drug Administration (FDA) has minimized this problem. Historically, phenacetin, a drug administered as a pain reliever or added to pain relievers to aid effectiveness, caused irreversible interstitial renal disease. The withdrawal of this substance from the market by the FDA has decreased the number of patients developing ESRD from this drug.[2,10,11] Still, numerous drugs, including prescription drugs, have potential nephrotoxic effects.

Congenital Lesions

Congenital anomalies of the kidneys and urinary system may also lead to ESRD, although normal renal function may be maintained in some persons. Developmental anomalies resulting in misshapen kidneys (e.g., horseshoe kidney) may alter nephron structure and function.

Lower urinary tract anomalies may result in reflux and hydronephrosis, which destroys nephron mass and function. Careful newborn or pediatric assessment to determine the presence of such lesions allows early surgical correction that may prevent the development of renal disease. If surgical intervention is not indicated, close monitoring and management of the patient's condition may prevent or delay the onset of renal failure. No specific causes for the development of these congenital lesions have been identified.

Genetic Renal Disease

Genetic mutations leading to renal disease are relatively rare. The most significant genetic renal disease is polycystic renal disease, which is an autosomal dominant genetic disease. Thus, if one parent carries the gene, the disease can be expressed in 50% of offspring and equally between the sexes. Although cysts may develop by the second decade of life, renal dysfunction develops slowly. The patient usually experiences renal failure in the fourth to fifth decade of life. Families with this genetic mutation often report histories of loved ones dying of uremia over several generations. Current generations are now receiving dialysis or renal transplant therapy.

The pathophysiology of polycystic renal disease involves the presence of fluid-filled cysts within the kidney. As these cysts develop and increase in size, they destroy nephron function by the pressure they create in the kidney. Kidney size can increase as much as several times normal as these cysts grow. These large kidneys become space-occupying lesions in the abdominal cavity and may cause disturbances of the gastrointestinal (GI) tract. As these cysts increase in size, they may rupture, causing intense pain and bleeding resulting in hematuria. These cysts are also prone to infections. Removal of one or both kidneys may be considered once ESRD develops, especially if the patient has recurrent infections, multiple episodes of cyst rupture, or GI symptoms.[2,31]

Genetic counseling is offered to families and patients with a history of polycystic renal disease. Research on gene identification and mapping has resulted in the identification of the specific gene that causes polycystic renal disease. As with other genetic information now being identified, it is unclear how this knowledge will be integrated into the treatment plan. Other uncommon genetic syndromes may also lead to ESRD. It is beyond the scope of this chapter to explore these syndromes, and the reader is encouraged to consult texts on genetics for additional information.

Assessment

ESRD is chronic in two ways—progression of the disease usually occurs over a period of months to years, and, with the advent of treatment, the patient can usually live with this disease for many years. CRF can be described as "silent" during its progressive stage because it causes few or no symptoms. In addition, these symptoms may be so vague that they are either not reported or may be attributed to other illnesses. Patients who are not seeing a health care professional on a regular basis may seek medical attention only when fatigue, nausea and vomiting, or other symptoms persist and worsen.

The development of ESRD can be viewed as a continuum. Diminished renal reserve is the earliest stage of disease that can be clinically identified. During this stage, serum creatinine and BUN are slightly elevated above normal limits, and serum electrolytes are within normal limits. The patient has no evidence of fluid retention, and urine output is within normal range of 1 to 2 L per 24 hours. Red blood cell count and hematocrit remain in the normal range. Diminished renal reserve does not result in any symptoms. If renal disease is diagnosed at this stage, it is possible only through a comprehensive routine physical examination or another fortuitous circumstance (e.g., a visit to the emergency room for an unrelated problem).

Renal insufficiency reflects continued deterioration of kidney function to a level of 25% of normal. BUN and creatinine levels continue to rise, and, consequently, this stage is also described as the azotemic state. Electrolyte imbalance may be evident as serum levels of sodium, potassium, and chloride levels remain at high-normal levels while serum levels of calcium begin to lower and those of phosphorus begin to rise. Red blood cell count and hematocrit begin to fall as erythropoietin secretion diminishes. The patient may experience symptoms of fatigue from anemia, although it is not usually recognized as a debilitating problem requiring medical treatment. If the patient is not seeing a physician regularly, renal disease may not be diagnosed during this stage.

"Chronic renal disease" is a term that may be used to describe the period of functional loss preceding true ESRD. The patient is increasingly symptomatic with progressive fatigue, continued elevation of metabolic waste products, some electrolyte imbalance, and some fluid retention. These alterations are usually controlled with a regimen of antihypertensives, diuretics, phosphate-binding agents, erythropoietin replacement, and dietary restrictions. The patient may report a general sense of unwellness or may be unaware of the subtleties of these insidious metabolic changes.

Ultimately, the patient progresses to ESRD. As a medical diagnosis, ESRD is often used synonymously with uremia or CRF. During this stage, one sees significant elevations in serum creatinine and BUN resulting in symptoms of nausea, vomiting, headache, and altered sensorium. Urine output may be diminished, and the patient develops hypertension and edema from fluid retention. Significant anemia develops, creating a state of weakness and fatigue, and the patient often has a distinct gray pallor. Uremic fetor, a distinct sulfur-type odor, may be present and is often evident to persons in close proximity to the patient. Additionally, the patient may experience a metallic taste that negatively affects appetite. Patients report a fogginess in their thinking and concentration that interferes with normal cognition and short-term memory. These symptoms have been quantified through studies of brain function in patients with ESRD. If treatment with dialysis or transplantation is not initiated, patients with ESRD will die.[2, 10, 11, 13]

These terms describing the level of renal dysfunction and disease may be used indiscriminantly (e.g., renal failure rather than diminished reserve or even renal insufficiency when the BUN is 25, serum creatinine is 2.4, and the patient is asymptomatic). Recognizing the signs and symptoms of ESRD in addition to understanding the results of laboratory and diagnostic studies will assist the nurse to assess the current status of the patient correctly and to identify those risk factors that could further compromise the patient's renal function (e.g., nephrotoxic agents, fluid imbalance, and hypovolemia or hypotension). In addition, this knowledge allows the nurse to anticipate the treatments required for this patient as well as the patient's likely future.[11, 13, 18]

Physical Examination and Diagnostic Studies

The patient with ESRD may be exhibiting overt systemic signs and symptoms or may be at risk for complications that can develop in the uremic state. Although these complications can be dramatic, such as death from untreated uremia, they can be minimized or prevented with appropriate pre-ESRD treatment and the timely initiation of ESRD therapy. When patients with ESRD are adequately treated with replacement therapy, they should exhibit few of the complications of ESRD.

Subjective findings in the patient with ESRD may not have a direct correlation with objective findings from laboratory or other diagnostic studies. Patients develop signs and symptoms of uremia and systemic involvement in an individual manner. In addition, other health problems may exacerbate these signs and symptoms. For example, otherwise healthy patients may report few symptoms or may have coped with the symptoms related to ESRD in such a way that they describe the experience differently from patients who have had numerous complications of ESRD. In addition, many patients may not relate signs and symptoms to renal dysfunction because they are not knowledgeable of the complications.

Knowing the patient's history of onset of ESRD, previous management and treatment strategies, and the current replacement therapy regimen should assist the nurse in interpreting the relevant findings from a systemic assessment. The following sections briefly review the specific physical and diagnostic findings related to the assessment of a patient with ESRD.

Neurologic System
Neurologic symptoms include headache, sleep disturbances, cognitive process disturbances, lethargy, muscle irritability, and generalized irritability and fatigue.

These symptoms are thought to result from the elevated BUN, which causes cerebral edema (secondary to the osmotic load of BUN) in the cerebrovascular and cerebral spinal fluid compartments. Neurologic signs in an untreated or inadequately treated patient include projectile vomiting, seizures, and coma secondary to cerebral edema resulting in brain stem herniation and respiratory arrest.[2,4,11,13,32,33]

Cognitive process disturbances in patients with ESRD have been studied both qualitatively and quantitatively. Patients report alterations in short-term memory and concentration ability. They often report a "fuzziness" or "fogginess" in their thought processes. This dysfunction has been quantified by sophisticated neurologic testing. These disturbances are corrected with adequate replacement therapy. Recent research has also identified that these patients' cognitive abilities improve with correction of the anemic state.[33,34]

Assessment of these alterations may be difficult because patients may not recognize these subtle changes until they have improved with adequate treatment. Whenever possible, the family should be involved in the assessment of a patient's cognitive status. Because short-term memory changes are involved, patient teaching should be altered to provide short, frequent teaching sessions with reinforcement, and the family should be involved as much as possible.

Diagnostic studies may include electroencephalograms (EEGs) and computed tomography (CT) scans to rule out other causes of altered mental status. Evoked responses may also be used to measure cognitive function. Neurologic tests of short-term memory (such as serial sevens) and cognition may be performed by the primary physician or a consulting neurologist.[33,34]

Peripheral neuropathy may develop in the uremic patient and is exhibited as "restless leg syndrome" and by diminished nerve conduction times. These findings can involve both the upper and lower extremities and may result from the demyelination of both motor and sensory nerves. These findings may occur before treatment is begun or may develop secondary to inadequate treatment. If the cause is the uremic condition, it can be reversed with adequate dialytic treatment or successful renal transplantation. If components of peripheral vascular disease are present that may contribute to peripheral neuropathy or if the patient has diabetic neuropathy, this problem will not be adequately reversed with ESRD treatment.[2,35]

Assessment includes sensory testing by touch and sensation. The patient may not respond to any stimulation of the soles of the feet, and the lower and upper extremities may be described by the patient as numb or tingly. If the patient is awake and alert, the pattern of leg movement while in bed should be noted. Constant movement usually indicates and relieves restless leg syndrome. Often, the patient arises and walks during the night as a means to relieve peripheral neuropathy. Patient teaching should include prevention of injury to these extremities by heat or trauma.

Nerve conduction studies may be performed at the outset of ESRD diagnosis, but they are generally not particularly diagnostic at this time. These studies are more frequently performed at routine intervals after dialysis is begun to measure improvement or deterioration of neuropathy. The peripheral neuropathy associated with DM responds minimally to treatment.

Ocular changes, including papilledema, blurred vision, retinal hemorrhage, and sudden onset of blindness, may occur in the patient with ESRD. These complications may be related to the presence of uncontrolled HTN (primary or secondary to fluid overload) or to other primary illnesses resulting in renal failure (e.g., DM).[2,35]

Assessment may include observing whether the patient avoids reading documents (consent forms) or reports blurred or sudden changes in vision. Blood pressure measurement should be correlated with sudden changes in vision. Prior visual acuity and correction should be documented. Stabilization of or improvement in vision should be observed with adequate blood pressure control and ESRD treatment. Patients with coexisting DM may have more significant ocular changes and should receive care from an ophthalmologist.

Diagnostic studies should include regular eye examinations by an optometrist or ophthalmologist for all patients. Changes in prescriptions for corrective lenses are usually delayed until the patient's fluid volume status and blood pressure are well controlled with dialytic therapy. The patient with DM may have more significant changes related to diabetic retinopathy and may require laser therapy. Patients who have taken or are taking corticosteroids should be routinely monitored for the development of cataracts.

Cardiovascular System

Cardiovascular symptoms include chest pain, shortness of breath, dyspnea on exertion or at rest, and fatigue. Cardiovascular signs include peripheral edema, cardiac friction rub, elevated blood pressure and pulse alterations, pulmonary congestion seen on a radiograph, crackles, wheezes, and diminished breath sounds on auscultation, and cardiomegaly (on a radiograph or echocardiogram).

Hypertension, congestive heart failure (CHF), and pulmonary edema secondary to hypervolemia (fluid retention secondary to oliguria) are common findings in the patient with ESRD. These findings may be especially prominent in the uremic, untreated patient admitted to the critical care unit. For the patient with ESRD undergoing treatment, these findings may identify acute or chronic fluid overload from increased oral fluid intake or decreased residual renal function (increasing oliguria or anuria after ESRD treatment has been initiated).

Chest pain, shortness of breath or dyspnea, and increased fluid volume may be associated with worsening anemia. Myocardial ischemia can develop secondary to the anemic state even in the absence of coronary artery disease. Myocardial ischemia or infarction may cause typical and atypical symptoms, and these conditions should not be ruled out without appropriate diagnostic studies. Women and persons with DM are especially likely to report such symptoms related to myocardial insults.[2,13,21,22,35–37]

The patient with DM may be admitted with fluid overload secondary to increased thirst from hyperglycemia. The hyperosmolar glucose load not only creates additional thirst but also shifts interstitial and intracellular fluid into the extracellular (vascular) compartment. The cause of hyperglycemia should be identified in the patient with DM because it may reveal a more significant acute illness (e.g., infection) requiring treatment.

The cardiovascular changes associated with fluid overload may be corrected with adequate dialytic therapy and may not recur. Patients with primary HTN continue to have this condition and require antihypertensive drug therapy. In addition, patients who experience fluid overload between hemodialysis treatments may also require antihypertensive drugs to dilate the vascular compartment and to prevent complications of volume-overload HTN (e.g., strokes).

Patients who have concomitant cardiac disease (coronary artery disease, valvular disease, myocardial infarction, left ventricular hypertrophy, CHF) may continue to experience signs and symptoms of these conditions. Control of fluid balance and prevention of fluid overload through dialytic therapy and restricted fluid intake can minimize the signs, symptoms, and sequelae of these problems. Usual cardiovascular drug therapies are administered to these patients, although their dose and frequency may be changed because of altered renal function.[10,17,35]

For the patient admitted to the critical care unit, immediate dialysis may be required to treat fulminant pulmonary edema or CHF, although conservative treatment with oxygen therapy and body positioning may aid in relieving acute symptoms. Dialysis treatments may be performed daily until fluid removal is complete.

Occasionally, a patient may develop uremic pericarditis, a type of pericarditis in which straw-colored fluid accumulates in the inflamed pericardium resulting in the development of a pericardial friction rub and chest pain on inspiration. Pericarditis of this type is not the result of an infectious process, but it is due to inadequate dialytic treatment. Treatment includes aggressive dialysis therapy, usually daily, until symp-

toms resolve. The acutely ill patient with ESRD is also at risk of developing pericardial tamponade, a life-threatening emergency. If the patient develops recurrent pericarditis or if the pericardium becomes constrictive, surgical creation of a pericardial window or a pericardiectomy may be necessary.[2,38,39]

Proper assessment requires thorough auscultation of the heart sounds. Physical assessment of peripheral edema should include the severity and extent of edema. Changes in blood pressure, pulse, electrocardiographic (ECG) tracings, and radiographs should be monitored. Changes in patient status (improvement or deterioration) are critical nursing assessments. The nurse must distinguish the causes of fluid overload in the patient with ESRD. For example, myocardial decompensation resulting in pulmonary edema may not result from increased fluid intake but from worsening cardiac disease.

Diagnostic studies include routine ECGs for all patients. Specific cardiac diagnostic studies (e.g., echocardiogram, cardiac catheterization) are performed on patients who present with or develop new signs and symptoms of cardiac decompensation (e.g., angina).

Pulmonary System

Pulmonary symptoms in patients with ESRD may include shortness of breath, dyspnea on exertion or at rest, and a decreased level of consciousness.[2,10,13,35] Specific signs may include the presence of crackles and wheezes, decreased breath sounds, tachypnea, radiographic changes, and alterations in arterial blood gases.

The most frequent pulmonary complication of ESRD is the development of pulmonary edema secondary to fluid overload and CHF. Control of fluid intake and treatment of underlying cardiac dysfunction (if present) can prevent this problem. Other pulmonary diseases (e.g., chronic obstructive pulmonary disease, tuberculosis, emphysema) may also complicate the pulmonary status of the patient with ESRD.[36,40]

Assessment of the pulmonary system requires good auscultation and percussion skills in addition to the accurate interpretation of relevant diagnostic data. Determination of the improvement or deterioration in pulmonary function is an ongoing nursing priority. Discontinuation of dialysis treatment may result in pulmonary edema if fluid intake is not restricted. Because the hypoxia related to pulmonary edema precipitates patient discomfort, anxiety, and fear, edema should be prevented or treated with isolated fluid removal by dialysis.

Pulmonary diagnostic studies for the patient with ESRD include regular chest radiographs. Chest radiographs may be obtained to confirm fluid overload or pulmonary edema on an emergency basis. A chest radiograph may be performed for the dialysis patient to determine fluid volume status and to assist in establishing the patient's "dry weight."

Hematologic System

Hematologic symptoms in patients with ESRD may include easy or worsening fatigue, shortness of breath, dyspnea on exertion or at rest, decreased appetite, increased sleep, sensations of cold, decreased concentration, and bruising. Hematologic signs may include generalized pallor, pallor of conjunctival and mucous membranes, decreased body temperature, inattentiveness, inability to concentrate, weight loss, increased respiratory rate, decreased oxygen saturation, and tachycardia. Alterations in red blood cell indices indicate normochromic, normocytic anemia. Iron deficiency may also be present. Platelet deficiencies and red cell fragility are present and may alter bleeding times.[2, 41–43]

Significant anemia in the patient with ESRD need not exist at this time. The development of synthetic erythropoietin (Epogen) through recombinant biotechnology has provided most patients with replacement therapy and has significantly reduced many of the systemic complications.[44–48] Even as anemia is developing in the renal insufficiency stage, erythropoietin can be prescribed and administered to prevent symptomatic anemia. With erythropoietin therapy, patients' hemoglobin and hematocrit values are generally corrected to levels of 10 g/dL and 34%, respectively. In addition, iron may be administered either intravenously during dialysis treatment or orally.[42, 43]

Blood loss can be a problem for patients with ESRD. Blood loss from hemodialysis can be a treatment complication, and all efforts should be taken to prevent this complication. Acute blood loss that may develop from other causes (e.g., GI bleeding) should be treated appropriately and should not contribute to the patient's ongoing anemic state.

Platelet dysfunction has been identified as a complication of uremia that does not routinely cause clinical complications. Patients with ESRD are instructed to avoid routine over-the-counter use of aspirin products, although aspirin may be prescribed for other specific reasons.[2]

Assessment of the acutely ill patient with ESRD should be directed toward the patient's symptoms; correlation of these data with blood studies may lead to supportive therapies such as oxygen and transfusions. Blood loss should be minimized by the prudent selection of laboratory studies and the prevention of bleeding from venipuncture sites or other sites. Transfusion administration, if required, may be done during hemodialysis to minimize fluid overload. Conservation of energy for the anemic patient is paramount.

Diagnostic studies include the routine performance of complete blood counts (CBCs) to assess the progression of anemia or to assess for blood loss on an emergency basis. The patient receiving hemodialysis may have a weekly CBC (or hemoglobin or hematocrit) performed to measure the effectiveness or the proper dose of Epogen. Other studies may be performed to determine bleeding or clotting abnormalities.

Gastrointestinal System

GI symptoms reported by patients with ESRD may include indigestion, nausea, feeling of fullness, decreased appetite, and a metallic taste. Physical signs can include uremic fetor, vomiting, diarrhea, weight loss, and a positive Hematest on emesis and stool. As the uremic state develops, patients may experience severe anorexia, nausea, and vomiting. Development of these signs and symptoms generally indicates the need to initiate treatment. These symptoms improve and may be completely eliminated with adequate treatment.[2, 35]

Whether the incidence of GI ulcers or bleeding, diverticulitis, or hemorrhoids is increased in the ESRD patient population is unclear, although these problems are associated with significant morbidity. The prophylactic use of histamine (H_2) blockers may be considered to prevent GI bleeding or gastroesophageal reflux disease.

Assessment of the acutely ill patient with ESRD should include auscultating for the presence or absence of bowel sounds and the quality of bowel sounds and palpating the abdomen for pain or tenderness. Identification of the patient's usual dietary habits, including bowel patterns and recent changes, should be obtained. Hematesting emesis and feces may identify acute GI processes. Prevention and treatment of diarrhea or constipation may be required. Patients with ESRD are not usually given magnesium-containing cathartics because they are at risk for hypermagnesemia. In the controlled setting of the critical care unit, these agents may be administered if the situation is considered life-threatening.

Any GI alterations in the patient receiving peritoneal dialysis should be thoroughly assessed and may indicate the acute onset of peritonitis. In this situation, abdominal pain may be present, although it can be minimal or even absent.

Diagnostic studies include radiographic studies or direct visualization of the upper or lower GI tract. These studies are performed based on specific signs and symptoms and may reveal abnormalities that are only minimally related to the primary diagnosis of renal failure (e.g., gallstones, diverticula, hemorrhoids).

Fluid and Electrolyte Balance

For the patient with ESRD, symptoms of electrolyte imbalance are related to the electrolytes involved and may include weakness, muscle twitching, nausea, headache, fatigue, and heart palpitations. Similarly, signs of electrolyte imbalance may include edema, alterations in serum chemistry panels, ECG alterations, and positional blood pressure changes.

Diagnostic studies that assist in identifying the source of the fluid or electrolyte imbalance include the evaluation of blood chemistry studies and urine output (if the patient still produces urine). In the oliguric patient, edema may be present even when a fluid restriction order is followed. Assessment of edema requires an understanding of the patient's usual position (lying, standing, sitting) and oncotic pressure gradient (significant hypoalbuminemia, sodium balance). These factors result in fluid shifts from the vascular compartment. If the excess fluid remains in the vascular compartment, the patient may exhibit hypertension, which disappears when the excess fluid is removed with dialytic therapy. In addition to the physical assessment for edema, regular measurement of body weight identifies fluid increases and losses in the oliguric patient. In the patient with DM, the presence of hyperglycemia and its osmotic effects will result in or worsen fluid overload. The control of fluid intake and overload is achieved in these patients only if the hyperglycemic state (which causes uncontrollable thirst) is reversed or controlled.

Electrolyte imbalances of sodium, potassium, magnesium, chloride, and other ions usually depend on food intake, drug use, and intake of other dietary supplements. Generally, treated patients exhibit minimal increases in the levels of the electrolytes that normally are excreted by the functioning kidney (e.g., sodium and potassium). Dietary restriction of these electrolytes may keep these electrolytes within normal ranges. In addition, the vascular volume status of the patient must be considered, to assess the dilution versus the concentration of these ions in serum.[2, 10, 13, 35]

Drugs that contain electrolytes or other ions should not be administered to patients with ESRD. The use of over-the-counter medications, especially magnesium-containing medications (e.g., laxatives, antacids), herbal extracts, or dietary supplements may explain some electrolyte elevations in some patients. Instructions on avoiding these medications is a specific education need for patients with ESRD.

Electrolyte imbalances can be corrected by restrictions and dialysis. Most electrolyte imbalances are not life-threatening and respond to scheduled dialysis therapy. This is not the case, however, with potassium. For patients with ESRD, hyperkalemia and hypokalemia can be life-threatening. Hypokalemia occurs less frequently, but it is identified by signs and symptoms of cardiac dysrhythmias (flattened T waves), cramps, and generalized weakness. Once the imbalance is recognized and confirmed with serum measurement, administration of potassium by the intravenous or oral route quickly corrects this problem.

Even eating a single balanced meal (or a high-potassium food such as a banana) may be sufficient in the hypokalemic patient to relieve these symptoms.

Hyperkalemia is a more difficult problem to correct in this patient population. Because the functioning kidney is the organ that regulates potassium excretion and retention, loss of renal function creates a state of hyperkalemia. Although dietary intake is the most common cause of hyperkalemia, it is not the only source. Other sources must be considered, including occult bleeding with release of intracellular potassium, new drug therapies, ineffective dialysis therapy, and receipt of blood transfusions (stored blood has a greater potassium concentration because of red blood cell death during storage). If the serum level of potassium does not correlate with the ECG pattern or other patient signs and symptoms, the serum potassium should be rechecked.

Hyperkalemia causes specific cardiac dysrhythmias. In an untreated patient, the cardiac rhythm deteriorates from normal sinus rhythm with an elevated T wave to an ever-widening QRS complex and a bradycardia until a sine wave and cardiac standstill develops (Figure 24–1). Correlation of the severity of hyperkalemia with a serum potassium level is not always valid. Patients who have consistently higher serum potassium levels develop a physiologic refractiveness to this electrolyte, whereas patients who have had normal levels and who suddenly develop hyperkalemia are much more susceptible to cardiac dysrhythmias and cardiac arrest. Consequently, one patient may have a cardiac arrest at a potassium level of 8 mEq/L, while another may not have a cardiac arrest until the serum potassium is 11 mEq/L.

Treatment for hyperkalemia should be accomplished on an emergency basis. An intravenous "cocktail" is administered to shift potassium from the extracellular compartment back into the intracellular compartment, thus limiting its cardiotoxic effects. This is time-sensitive therapy because the excess potassium again leaves the intracellular space. However, it places the patient in a safer state while other treatments are initiated. Other treatment strategies that successfully remove potassium from the body are also described in Table 24–1.

Endocrine and Metabolic Systems

Signs and symptoms associated with dysfunction in the endocrine system in patients with ESRD follow the usual signs and symptoms for hypofunction of the endocrine glands (see Chapter 26). Essentially, all endocrine glands have been found to be affected by ESRD. Some of the alterations are subclinical and result in no specific signs and symptoms, nor do they require specific treatment. Diagnostic studies include blood studies of various hormone levels. Other studies specific to the endocrine system may be performed as

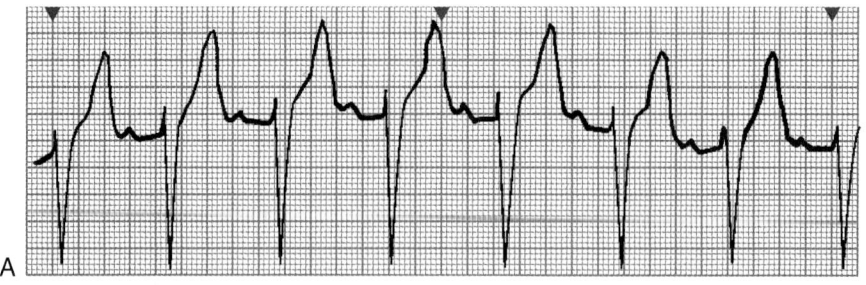

A

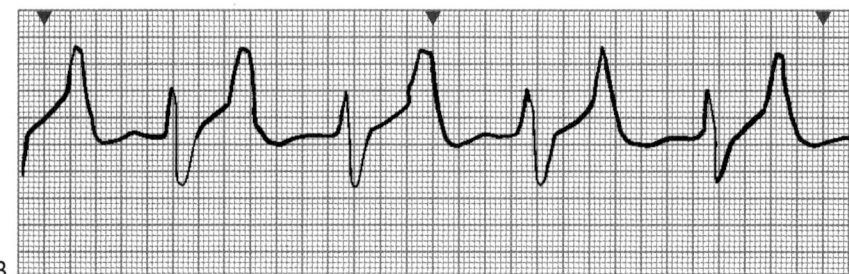

B

Figure 24–1

ECG tracings showing untreated hyperkalemia in a patient with end-stage renal disease leading to death, occurring over a period of 6 hours. *A,* Note the classic deterioration of the ECG beginning with elevated T waves. *B–D,* Progressive deterioration with widening and blunting of the QRS complex accompanied by decreasing rate. *E,* Development of a sine wave, which is incompatible with systemic perfusion and maintenance of life.

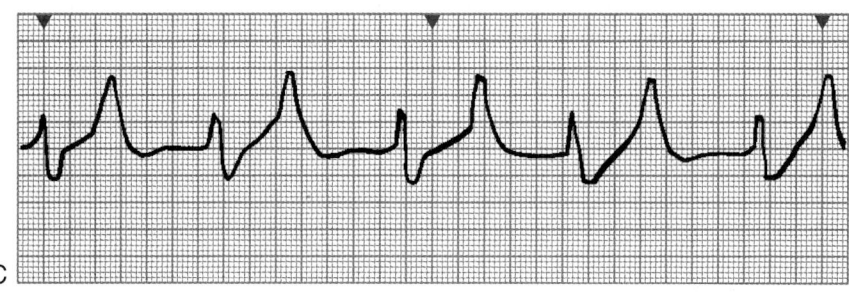

C

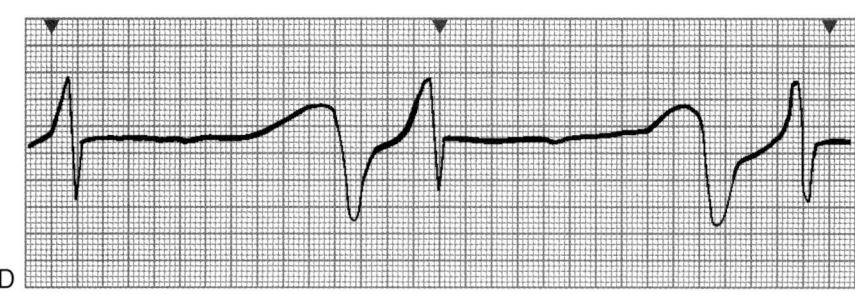

D

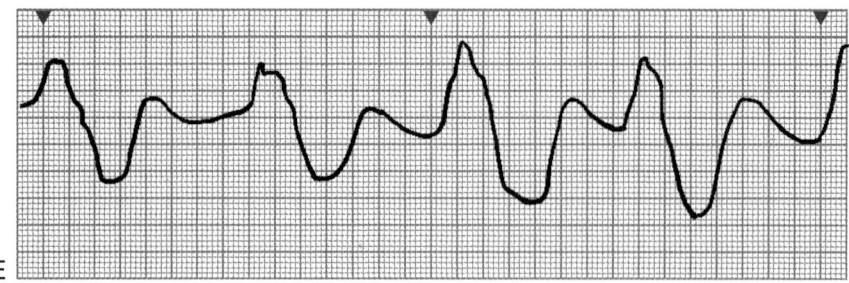

E

TABLE 24–1
Treatment of Hyperkalemia

Treatment Strategy	Mechanism of Action
Intravenous Therapy	
Calcium chloride	Stabilizes the irritability of cardiac muscle
Sodium bicarbonate	Improves metabolic acidosis, which alters cell wall potential (K+ moving out of cell is reversed)
50% glucose and regular insulin	Transports K+ from extracellular to intracellular compartment
Oral or Rectal Therapy	
Kayexalate (often mixed in liquid sorbitol)	Resin exchanges Na+ for K+ ion in the gastrointestinal tract; binds the K+ ion for excretion in the feces
	Sorbitol is an inert sugar that stimulates osmotic fluid shift into the gastrointestinal tract lumen; creates diarrhea, which enhances quick, efficient K+ loss
Extracorporeal Therapy	
Hemodialysis	Moves K+ from blood into dialysate by diffusion
Peritoneal dialysis	Removes K+ from body by diffusion

required by specific symptoms (e.g., radiographs, scans) (see Chapter 27).

The alteration in secretion of erythropoietin is discussed previously. The secretion of renin from the diseased kidneys may continue to cause HTN and can usually be adequately treated with antihypertensive drug therapy.

Altered carbohydrate metabolism has been observed in nondiabetic patients with ESRD, but it does not usually result in clinical signs and symptoms. The patient with ESRD who has coexisting DM may exhibit alterations in glucose control. Because the kidney is the organ that excretes insulin, the failing kidney is unable to perform this function. Thus, both endogenous and exogenous insulin will remain active in the body for a longer period. The result is the development of hypoglycemic episodes even when the patient is following the prescribed regimen. Adequate treatment is accomplished with reduction in insulin administration or oral hypoglycemic agents. Some patients with type 2 DM (who continue to produce insulin) may be able to discontinue their oral medications or insulin injections totally. These patients may believe and report that their DM is cured, although, unfortunately, this is not true, and the disease and its complications continue.[2,35]

Metabolic acidosis is the usual state of acid–base balance for the patient with ESRD secondary to the loss of renal function (see Chapter 22). This condition is usually corrected by adequate dialysis therapy and requires no other special treatment. However, the state of metabolic acidosis does contribute to other complications, including hyperkalemia and renal osteodystrophy.[2,10,35]

The calcium–phosphorus–vitamin D–parathormone interactions remain a major challenge in the management of patients with ESRD. This condition is frequently identified as the problem of renal osteoporosis or osteodystrophy. Because calcium and phosphorus

are filtered and reabsorbed or excreted by the functioning kidney to maintain normal serum levels, loss of renal function alters this balance. In addition, the kidney converts vitamin D to its most active form (dihydroxycholecalciferol), and this process allows for the absorption of calcium from the GI tract or through the skin from sunlight. Without renal function, calcium is not adequately absorbed from the GI tract. In addition, reabsorption may not be accomplished in the diseased kidney. Because of these disturbances, a state of hypocalcemia develops.[2,10,35]

In addition to this alteration, phosphorus, an end product of metabolism, is not excreted through the kidney, and serum levels rise. This imbalance of serum calcium and phosphorus in the circulation stimulates the secretion of parathormone, which is the hormone that maintains calcium levels in the blood. In an attempt to normalize serum calcium, parathormone stimulates calcium resorption from bone, resulting in the development of osteoporosis. When calcium and phosphorus are in the serum in such amounts that their mathematic product (serum calcium × serum phosphorus) exceeds 70, the complication of soft tissue calcification (calcium phosphate crystallization) develops. This complication may be identified as development of calcified blood vessels, bursitis in joints, skin lesions, and red eye syndrome from crystal deposition in the conjunctiva.[35,49,50]

Prevention and treatment of this endocrine complication of renal failure can be successful. Drug and diet therapies may be used to control both calcium and phosphorus levels. Controlling phosphate during the period of azotemia (before renal failure) is the best practice. Phosphate can be bound in the GI tract during digestion with the use of phosphate-binding agents. The most commonly used drugs to control hyperphosphatemia are calcium acetate (Phos-Ex) and calcium carbonate (Os-Cal).

If the phosphate level is controlled, the hypocalcemic state can be treated with the administration of activated vitamin D. The oral agents Rocaltrol and Calcijex can be given intravenously to improve absorption of dietary calcium. Because of improvements with these drug regimens, patients with renal failure rarely develop hypercalcemia. In addition, renal osteodystrophy can be prevented or minimized in most patients with ESRD.[51–53]

Altered sexual function and decreased reproductive hormone secretion may occur in the patient with ESRD. Adequate treatment may restore these hormones to normal levels, thus restoring and maintaining reproductive function. The role of anemia in reproductive function of the patient with ESRD has become more obvious with the use of erythropoietin (Epogen). Both males and females report improved sexual function, and pregnancy rates in women with ESRD have increased. In addition, improved antihypertensive therapies that do not suppress libido (in both men and women) or inhibit erection in males have contributed to improvement in the sexual and reproductive status of these patients.[54–56]

Assessment in the critical care setting should focus on changes that may affect the patient's current status. Physical assessment should include presence of bone deformities, surgical correction of fractures, or other signs and symptoms of renal bone disease. Systemic history taking, including a medication history, may reveal specific endocrine abnormalities in the patient with ESRD.

Integumentary System

Patients with ESRD may report constant itching, tingling, and dryness of the skin. Lesions caused by scratching may be open or healed, and patients may purposely cover the extremities to hide skin appearance. Petechiae may develop after scratching. Diagnostic studies include blood tests to determine specific hormonal abnormalities that may cause skin changes. Biopsies of skin lesions may be done if cellular changes (carcinomas) are suspected, although such lesions are not related to the diagnosis of ESRD. Lesions may be cultured if one suspects infection.

The primary alterations in integument that develop in patients with ESRD are dry skin and pruritus. Because treatment is readily available to these patients and is not usually delayed to the time of near death, uremic frost is rarely, if ever, seen. Uremic frost results from the crystallization of urea on areas of the skin and is a major irritant. It is unlikely that this would be the cause of integumentary disturbances in the treated patient.[2, 3, 10, 35]

Chronic fluid restriction may contribute to the dryness and itching of the skin. No other specific drugs and components of dialysis therapy have been shown to contribute to these complications.

Elevation of serum phosphorus and increased parathormone levels (discussed previously) that result from renal failure have been implicated in chronic pruritus. Deposition of calcium phosphate crystals in the epidermis can be observed in patients with ESRD. Often, patients scratch incessantly in an attempt to "remove" these crystals. It has been reported that subtotal parathyroidectomy to resolve tertiary hyperparathyroidism successfully relieves pruritus in about 50% of patients.[57]

As the nurse performs a systemic physical assessment or during other patient care activities, the patient's skin should be evaluated. The nurse should document the degree of dryness, the presence of healed or open lesions, and the condition of any open lesions. Orders for antipruritic drugs, antihistamines, sedatives, and topical agents should be requested, and the patient's response to these medications should be evaluated.

Nursing Diagnoses

The nursing assessment of the patient with ESRD should focus not only on those signs or symptoms arising from ESRD and the complications of ESRD, but also on those signs or symptoms that may result from other coexisting illnesses (e.g., cardiac disease, DM, systemic lupus erythematosus). This complex interaction of disease processes and clinical manifestations challenges the nurse to identify appropriate diagnoses, to monitor these patients for changes that may indicate improvement or deterioration of their condition. Table 24–2 provides a list of common diagnoses that relate to patients with ESRD.

Collaborative Management

Patients with ESRD can be treated with dialysis, and this procedure is generally performed on an outpatient basis or in the patients' own environment. The organization of health care delivery for patients with ESRD is based on a model of collaborative practice by a multidisciplinary health care team. Physicians, nurses, social workers, dietitians, and allied health professionals are all members of the team. When this team is effective, the patient receives quality care, usually outside the hospital setting.

Acute care nurses do not always have the luxury of seeing the healthy, rehabilitated patients with ESRD who are undergoing hemodialysis, or peritoneal dialysis or who have undergone successful renal transplant. Patients who are hospitalized are experiencing acute illnesses and are often the sickest of the ESRD population either from their primary disease, from complications of ESRD, or from coexisting morbidities (Chart 24–1). Nurses caring for patients with ESRD in the critical care or intermediate care setting should consult

TABLE 24–2
Nursing Diagnoses

Problem Statement	Etiologic Factors
Knowledge deficit (learning need)	New diagnosis of ESRD
	Decision about treatment modality
	Changes in therapeutic regimen
Activity intolerance, actual or potential	Untreated or inadequately treated anemia
	Acute or chronic blood loss
Fluid volume excess	Oliguria or anuria
	Excess intake related to thirst
	Excess sodium intake
	Hyperglycemia
	Edema secondary to decreased serum osmolality
Nutrition, less than body requirements	Dietary changes secondary to ESRD
	Gastroenteropathy
	Anorexia, nausea, and vomiting secondary to untreated uremia
	Development of other critical illnesses
Grieving, anticipatory	Loss of functioning body part (kidney)
	Loss of usual role and activities related to role
Anxiety, fear	Development of a new condition (ESRD)
	Development of a new complication
	Unknown prognosis
	Death
Family processes, altered	Interruption in usual roles related to severe illness of family member
	Increased dependence on family members
Thought processes, altered	Increasing retention of metabolic waste products resulting in uremia
	Untreated or inadequately treated anemia

with nephrology nurses and other members of the health team as needed.

The United States Renal Data System (USRDS) reports that younger patients with ESRD are less frequently hospitalized than older patients, and the length of stay for these patients is decreasing. However, the mean age of the ESRD population has been steadily rising.[16]

Hospitalization for patients with ESRD may begin with the initiation of treatment. If the patient presents in an acutely ill (uremic) state, immediate dialysis therapy is indicated. Temporary vascular access needs to be placed, and the patient may be discharged with a temporary access to continue treatment on an outpatient basis.

A major and, perhaps, the leading complication of ESRD in patients requiring hospitalization is loss of the vascular access. According to published data, clotting of vascular access is the leading cause of hospitalization.[16] Placement of a temporary access and surgical procedures either to salvage the clotted vascular access (embolectomy, angioplasty, or thrombolysis) or to create a new vascular access often requires hospitalization, especially if the patient's condition is unstable (presence of hyperkalemia). Inpatient dialysis is required to ensure the patient's safety and stability during this period.

The patient whose vascular access requires revision or replacement is a vulnerable patient who has lost his

or her "lifeline." Undoubtedly, the patient's greatest fear is that a new access cannot be created, and the patient is confronted with the prospect of death. The involvement of a competent surgeon who is dedicated to achieving vascular access is critical to solving these technical problems. During these stressful times, the nurse must provide emotional support to the patient and family.

Patients treated by peritoneal dialysis have had slightly higher rates of hospitalization than patients receiving hemodialysis, but this difference seems to be diminishing. The major causes of death in the ESRD population have been identified and provide an understanding of the reasons for hospitalization. In the ESRD population over age 20, 47.2% of the deaths in the years 1993 to 1995 were caused by cardiac events (cardiac arrest, acute myocardial infarction, or other cardiac). Cerebrovascular events caused another 6.7% of these deaths. It is clear from these data that cardiovascular disease in the ESRD population is common and contributes significantly to mortality. The second cause of death in this population was infection, accounting for 15.5% of all ESRD deaths in patients over age 20. This category included septicemia, acquired immunodeficiency syndrome (AIDS), and other infections.[16]

Decision making about ESRD treatment is a major event in the patient's life. Often, clinical pathways, care maps, or treatment algorithms are used to direct

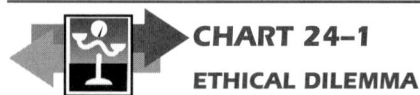

CHART 24–1

ETHICAL DILEMMA

Several authorities in the field of bioethics have suggested that the treatment of patients with end-stage renal disease (ESRD) was the catalyst for the development of this field. From the beginning, patients, families, physicians, nurses, other health care providers, and society have struggled with increasingly difficult issues surrounding the care of this patient population. The following case report represents some of these issues and the dilemmas they create.

Mrs. P. is a 65-year-old woman who developed ESRD approximately 12 years ago secondary to polycystic kidney disease. Married, with four adult children, she is a seamstress by occupation. She continued to work full-time after initiating hemodialysis and until she retired 3 years ago. Since that time, she and her husband have traveled throughout the United States. She has undergone dialysis in multiple facilities without incident. The arteriovenous fistula that was created at the beginning of her treatment has functioned without complication.

One week ago, Mrs. P. complained of a sudden severe headache and lost consciousness while preparing breakfast. Her husband immediately called 911, and she was transported to the hospital. On admission, she was comatose, with responses only to deep, painful stimuli. Although she was not apneic, Mrs. P. was intubated for respiratory support. A computed tomography scan of her brain revealed the presence of a large hemorrhage extending into the lateral ventricle. An electroencephalogram yesterday revealed generalized slowing of activity consistent with hypoxic encephalopathy. She has been removed from the ventilator and has adequate respiratory function. Her vital signs are now stable. Hemodialysis has been performed with minimal heparinization to prevent further bleeding. Total parenteral nutrition is being administered through a central venous catheter.

Mrs. P.'s family is at her bedside. Her children are overwhelmed by their mother's condition and have indicated that they are seeing improvement. Her husband has indicated that he sees no real improvement in her condition and knows that "some decisions" need to be made about her care. The physicians have indicated to him that she really does not require critical care at this time. Mrs. P. has not completed a durable power of attorney for health care, even though she had indicated frequently that she really should do that sometime. She has told her husband and children that she did not want to be maintained on "one of those breathing machines."

Mrs. P.'s nephrology team (physician, nurse, social worker, dietitian) have consulted with the neurologic and critical care staff. The staff and family are faced with questions and decisions about the following:

1. Should nutrition and fluid administration be continued? Should a feeding tube (e.g., percutaneous endoscopic gastrostomy) be placed for continued enteral nutrition?
2. Should hemodialysis treatment be continued for Mrs. P., who will most likely remain in a vegetative state? Defend your answer.
3. Should hemodialysis be continued without nutrition? Why or why not?
4. Should Mrs. P.'s comment about not wanting to be on a breathing machine be extended to include other life-sustaining treatment (enteral feeding, hemodialysis)?
5. Do all family members have to agree about these decisions? Who is the primary decision maker for this patient?
6. What is the nurse's role in this dilemma?

care. These guides should incorporate the patient's desires regarding treatment options. When used appropriately, these guides can document the patient's progress, changes in treatment modalities, and even end-of-life decisions (Figure 24–2).

Hemodialysis

When PL 92-603 was passed by Congress establishing the Medicare End-Stage Renal Disease Program, the collaborative team to care for patients receiving hemodialysis was formalized. These regulations required that ESRD facilities include a nephrologist, a registered nurse, a social worker, and a dietitian. Those team members, along with dialysis technicians and other ancillary patient care staff, remain the patient care providers in all Medicare-certified ESRD facilities (hemodialysis, peritoneal dialysis, and renal transplant centers).[7]

Today, most dialysis facilities are proprietary, for-profit facilities.[16] Patients come to the facility, undergo

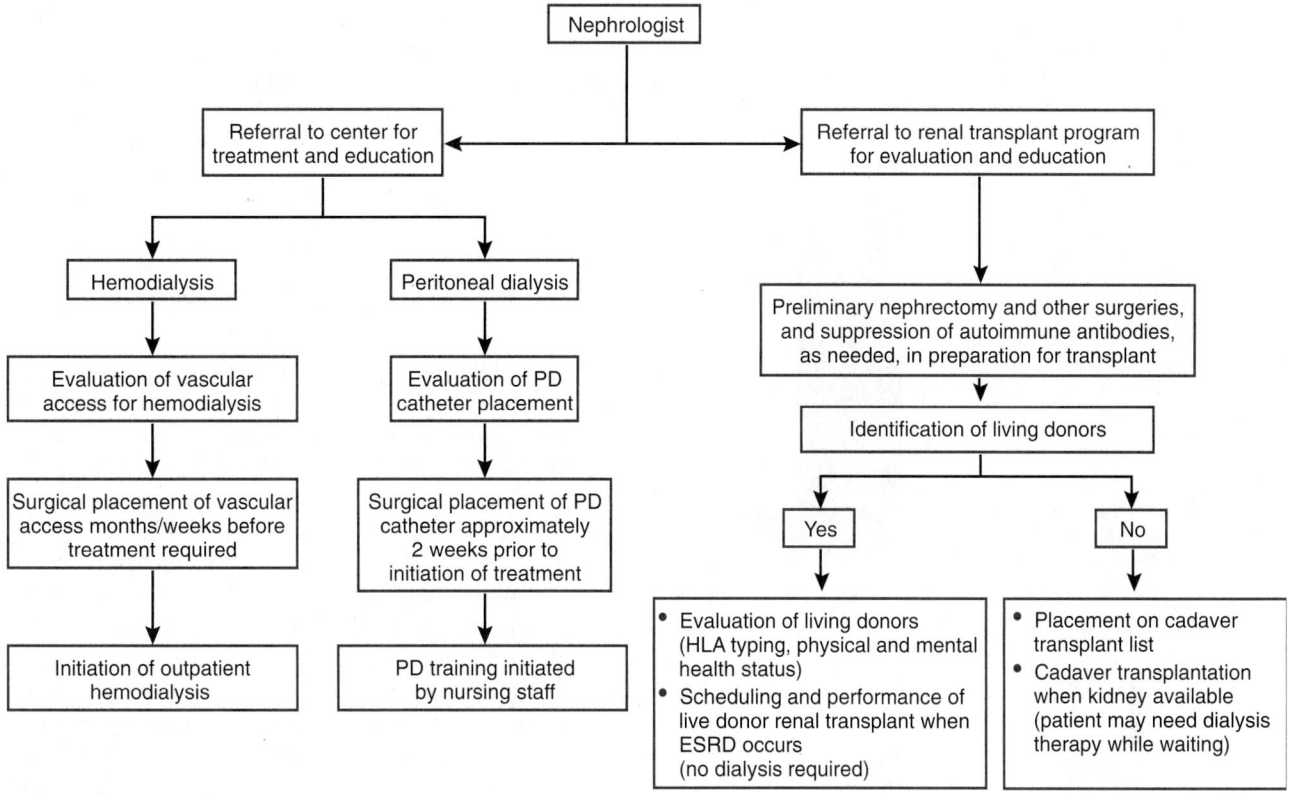

Figure 24–2

Treatment algorithm for a patient with end-stage renal disease. PD, peritoneal dialysis.

treatment, and return to their homes or workplaces. In 1996, data from the USRDS indicated that more than 200,000 patients underwent dialysis treatment in approximately 2000 facilities in the United States and its territories.[16]

Hemodialysis is a process that uses blood flow through an extracorporeal circuit to mimic the functions of the glomerulus of the human kidney. To perform this treatment, a dialyzer, dialysate solution (electrolytes and fluid compatible with blood), a circulatory, delivery, and monitoring system for the blood and dialysate, and vascular access are required[4,58] (Figure 24–3).

Dialyzer

The hemodialysis process removes small molecules (end products of metabolism and electrolytes) by an extracorporeal blood chamber (the dialyzer or "artificial kidney"). A semipermeable membrane forms the blood compartment of the dialyzer and is commonly designed as bundles of hollow fibers or as layers of membrane. These fibers are usually made of cellulose acetate, cuprophane, or other biocompatible materials. The blood is pumped from the patient into the top of the compartment and flows out the bottom to be returned to the patient. Because of the design of this device, the resistance to flow through the dialyzer is relatively low. The dialyzer and its tubing is a dispos-

able unit that can be resterilized and used again by the *same* patient (see Figure 24–3).[58–61]

The blood compartment of the dialyzer holds approximately 80 to 150 mL of blood, and the blood tubing holds another 50 mL. With approximately 200 mL of blood in the extracorporeal circuit, the patient undergoing treatment should experience minimal hemodynamic effects. The "phlebotomy" achieved at the initiation of treatment may actually slightly improve cardiopulmonary function in the patient with fluid overload, CHF, or pulmonary edema. Because the blood flow is in a closed circuit, the rate of flow can be controlled to maximize efficiency. A blood pump maintains blood flow at an average of 300 to 400 mL per minute. During a typical dialysis treatment of several hours, the patient's total blood volume flows through the dialyzer multiple times.

The vascular compartment also allows for the infusion of pharmacotherapeutic agents into the systemic circulation. Should the patient become hypovolemic secondary to rapid fluid removal during treatment, normal saline can be quickly infused into the vascular compartment. An almost immediate improvement in volume status should be achieved. Blood transfusions, plasma expanders, parenteral nutrition, and drugs can also be administered through this extracorporeal circuit. In addition, blood samples for testing can be withdrawn from this vascular circuit, rather than by venipuncture.

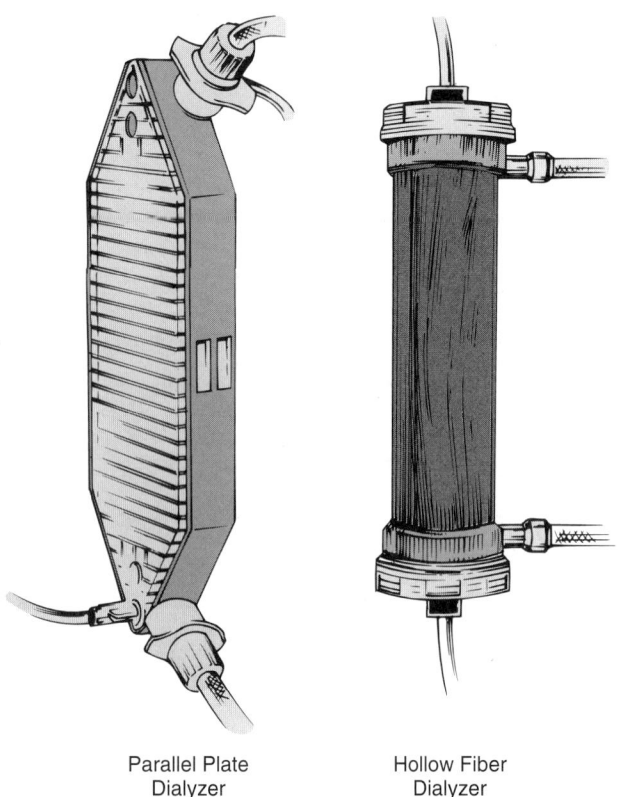

Parallel Plate
Dialyzer

Hollow Fiber
Dialyzer

Figure 24–3

Dialyzer disposable units. (From Ignatavicius DD, Workman ML, Mishler MA: Medical-Surgical Nursing Across the Healthcare Continuum, 3rd ed. Philadelphia, W.B. Saunders, 1999.)

Dialysate Solution

The space surrounding the blood compartment is the dialysate compartment, which contains a fluid (dialysate solution) that provides for equilibration of electrolytes and removal of waste products. During this process, excess electrolytes are removed, resulting in normal concentration in the blood. The movement of these particles is governed by the principles of diffusion and filtration. These are the same principles that explain the function of the glomerulus of the kidney. However, the selective reabsorption performed by the tubular system of the kidney cannot be replicated during hemodialysis.[61]

The dialysate solution used for hemodialysis is composed of a mixture of water and electrolytes. This mixture is isotonic and thus is compatible with human blood. Because the pores of the semipermeable membrane are micron size, bacteria and viruses that may be present in water cannot move from the dialysate into the blood compartment. Thus, the water supply used for dialysis does not need to be sterile. However, treatment of tap water can remove ions that can alter the electrolyte concentration of the final solution. Water treatment using deionization or reverse osmosis is used to provide a pure water supply.[4, 58–61]

The ions added to this water include sodium, calcium, magnesium, chloride, and bicarbon-

ate.[4, 58, 60, 62] Potassium is the electrolyte (ion) most frequently manipulated in dialysate solution. The concentration can range from 0 to 4 mEq/L, depending on the patient's serum level of potassium. This individual prescription allows for maximal correction of the patient's serum potassium during treatment with minimal development of significant hyperkalemia between dialysis treatments. Higher concentrations of potassium may be used in patients who are receiving digitalis preparations to prevent hypokalemia, which may exacerbate digitalis toxicity.[17]

Bicarbonate, which is mixed with the dialysate separately to prevent precipitation, is added to correct the metabolic acidosis that develops in renal failure. Glucose may also be added to the dialysate solution to remove additional fluid by the creation of an osmotic gradient across the semipermeable membrane. It may also be added to stabilize the blood glucose levels of patients with diabetes and thus to prevent hypoglycemia during hemodialysis.

End products of metabolism (e.g., BUN, creatinine) move efficiently across the semipermeable membrane depending on their molecular weight and size; none of these metabolites are present in fresh dialysate so a concentration gradient always exists between blood and dialysate. These molecules move from higher to lower areas of concentration. The movement of fluid (water) from the blood compartment to the dialysate is primarily controlled by a pressure gradient. Fluid removal is achieved by the creation of a pressure gradient between the blood compartment and the dialysate compartment. Fluid moves from an area of higher pressure to one of lower pressure. In the present dialysis systems, this pressure is actually a negative or vacuum pressure and thus allows the blood compartment to remain at relatively low positive pressures. The additional fluid (from the patient) added to the dialysate flow is measured, and this measurement is shown as a readout of total fluid removed during treatment.[36, 58, 63]

The semipermeable membrane also allows for the diffusion of particles back into the patient's blood from the dialysate solution if their concentration is lower in the blood than in the dialysate. Concentration gradients of ions and end products of metabolism decrease over time (within a few hours), and the hemodialysis process becomes less efficient. These principles of dialysis function are measured as clearance (just as creatinine clearance is measured) and are sometimes called dialysance.[36, 58, 59]

The prescription for hemodialysis is based on the performance characteristics of the dialysis equipment. The actual surface area of the semipermeable membrane determines the efficiency of the dialysis process. The more contact between blood and dialysate, the more dialysis is accomplished. In addition, the physical characteristics of the semipermeable membrane also influence dialysis efficiency.

Dialysis Monitoring

In addition to mixing and delivering the dialysate solution to the dialyzer, the dialysis machine also heats the dialysate solution to approximately 37°C to maximize patient comfort and solute movement. Although cooler dialysate solutions may be uncomfortable, they are not harmful to the patient. Overheated dialysate solutions can damage or destroy red blood cells.

Sensors monitor the electrical conductivity of the dialysate solution to ensure ion compatibility with blood. Hypertonic or hypotonic dialysate solutions can cause significant red cell damage and even death.

The pressure of blood flow through the dialyzer can be measured in both the arterial and venous blood lines, thus providing information about blood flow. These pressure monitors function to alert the nurse to decreased flow or increased resistance to flow in this extracorporeal chamber. A sensor also monitors for the presence of air in venous blood returning to the patient. Because of the high flow rates into the vascular access, an air embolus can be a life-threatening complication of hemodialysis.

Violation of any of the monitoring parameters performed by the dialysis equipment causes both audible and visible alarms that cannot be reset until the condition is corrected. Because all these monitoring systems and alarms are integrated within the dialysis hardware, the hemodialysis procedure (blood flow or dialysate flow) is halted when an unsafe condition exists. Although hemodialysis may appear to be a nearly fail-safe system, it cannot function in isolation. Careful monitoring of the patient during the procedure is a critical role of the nurse.[58,59]

Current dialysis equipment has incorporated several technologic advances. Some provide computer programs that allow the individual patient's prescription to be entered into the machine by diskette. Microprocessors provide constant readouts of dialysis parameters including time elapsed in treatment, fluid removed during treatment, and total volume of blood processed through the dialyzer during the treatment. Some machines also have noninvasive blood pressure monitoring capability.

Vascular Access for Hemodialysis

Central Venous Catheters. The use of central venous catheters has been successful in providing an access route for the emergency initiation of hemodialysis or for treatment while a permanent vascular access route is created and heals. Both double-lumen and triple-lumen catheters are placed and are used for hemodialysis. These catheters allow blood to be withdrawn from a shorter lumen and returned by a longer lumen back into the systemic circulation. Because of flow and pressure limitations within these catheters and the vessel in which they are placed, hemodialysis may not be most efficient or effective when this type of access is used (Figure 24–4).[64–66]

Central venous catheters may be placed in the right or left subclavian vein, the right or left jugular vein, and the right or left femoral vein. Placement in the femoral vein prevents mobility because the extremity needs to remain extended to prevent vascular injury, kinking, or displacement of the catheter. The patient can have fairly normal mobility when the catheter is placed in the subclavian or jugular vein. In the critical care setting, any of these routes may be accessed for hemodialysis. The patient's condition and placement of other vascular accesses may determine the site for these catheters.

When the catheter is not being used for hemodialysis, the lumen is flushed with a heparin solution according to the facility's policy. These catheters are generally not used for routine intravenous fluid administration, blood sampling, or medication delivery. Hemodialysis central catheters can be left in place for several weeks or even several months. General care of these catheters requires that they not be submersed in water (e.g., showering, deep tub bathing, swimming), to prevent infection at these sites.[67,68] Patients may or may not be taught how to change the dressings over these catheters. Although a suture is generally used to anchor these catheters in place, they have been known to be displaced. When this occurs, one usually sees no major sequelae. Although fatal complications are rare, they have been reported and are thought to be related to air emboli. The more common and critical complication of central catheters is the development of infection. Infections may be localized at the entry site or may result in septicemia. Infection continues to be one of the major complications of this access modality.[67–72]

Clotting of these catheters remains a major problem requiring emergency replacement. Even though heparin instillation is completed at the end of use, this

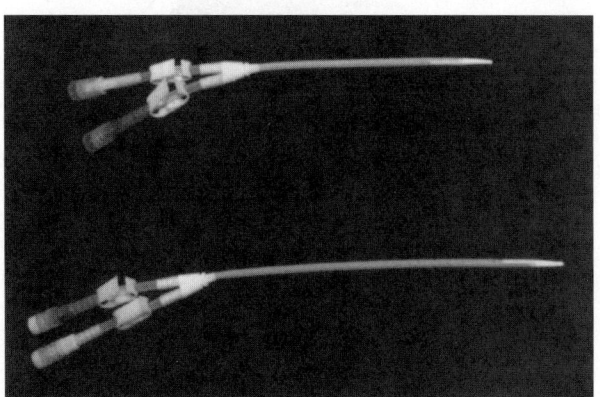

Figure 24–4

Subclavian dialysis catheters. (From Ignatavicius DD, Workman ML, Mishler MA: Medical-Surgical Nursing Across the Healthcare Continuum, 3rd ed. Philadelphia, W.B. Saunders, 1999.)

heparinized solution may be insufficient to maintain patency. Thrombolytics, such as streptokinase or urokinase, may be instilled in an attempt to dissolve a clot and to salvage the catheter.[73]

A permanent, surgically implanted double-lumen catheter may also be used for some patients (e.g., Hickman–Broviac catheter). These catheters are usually placed more centrally in the chest. They may or may not be routinely covered with a dressing.

Arteriovenous Fistulas. The arteriovenous (A-V) fistula for hemodialysis is surgically placed and is considered a permanent access. An A-V fistula is created by an anastomosis of a peripheral artery and vein. These anastomoses can be side to side, end to end, or end to side (Figure 24–5). An A-V fistula is usually created in the lower arm or, less frequently, in the upper arm. After creation of the fistula, the blood flow is redirected directly from the arterial to the venous system, thus bypassing the capillary bed between those vessels. The higher pressure and flow created in the venous system beyond the anastomosis create enlarged or engorged veins ("arterialization"). These enlarged veins with higher blood flow allow for cannulization with the large, usually 15-gauge needles needed to provide adequate blood flows for successful hemodialysis.

Nursing care of the patient with a new vascular access includes postoperative pain management, minimization of swelling through proper positioning (elevated at or above level of heart), assessment of blood flow to the extremity beyond the anastomosis (skin color and temperature, pulses, sensation, motor activity), and assessment of patency of the fistula. The assessment of blood flow through the anastomosis can be palpated, is described as a thrill, and feels like a constant vibratory, purring sensation. Auscultation at

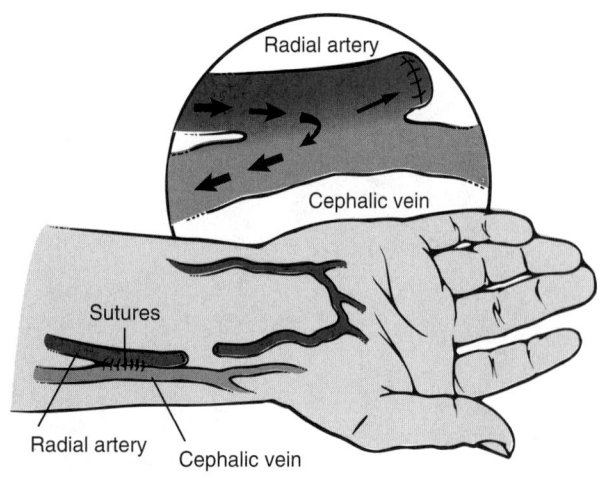

Figure 24–5

End to side arteriovenous fistula. (From Ignatavicius DD, Workman ML, Mishler MA: Medical-Surgical Nursing Across the Healthcare Continuum, 3rd ed. Philadelphia, W.B. Saunders, 1999.)

the site of anastomosis reveals a bruit, which is heard as a "whooshing" sound. If thick, extended dressings have been applied after the surgical procedure, this assessment may not be possible. The nurse should consult with the physician regarding changing the dressing to allow for assessment of function. If blood flow is strong through the A-V access, assessment of flow may be performed higher along the venous system. Absence of the thrill or bruit generally indicates absence of blood flow or clotting in the fistula and needs to be reported to the nephrologist or surgeon immediately.

After healing of the incision, the patient should be instructed to use this extremity normally and may even be instructed in physical exercises that assist to increase blood flow or engorgement of the venous system. In addition, the patient should be instructed to palpate the thrill in the fistula or to place the anastomosis to the ear to hear the bruit at least daily.

Complications associated with A-V fistulas may include the development of a steal syndrome, which diverts blood flow from the distal extremity and results in neurologic damage, ischemia, or necrosis of the extremity (often the fingers). High-output heart failure may also occur if the blood flow from the fistula to the right side of the heart is excessive relative to that patient's right heart function. Pseudoaneurysms may develop in these fistulas, particularly secondary to needle punctures, and can be surgically repaired. Infections in the fistula, which may result from needle punctures, may cause local abscesses, septicemia, or bacterial endocarditis. Finally, decreased blood flow resulting from various complications may cause a thrombosis in the A-V fistula resulting in its loss as the hemodialysis access.[4,74–76]

The physical appearance of enlarged, engorged veins along with "needle tracks" may be distressing and unsightly to the patient, who may hide them with long-sleeved clothing. The patient's concern about fistula appearance should be respected.

Ateriovenous Grafts. An A-V graft is created by placing a conduit between an artery and vein to allow some blood to flow between the artery and vein while not obliterating the flow of these native vessels. Several types of materials have been used to create these A-V grafts. Originally, the saphenous vein was used (not unlike their use in cardiac bypass surgery). Bovine grafts (processed, tanned, and sterilized carotid arteries of cows) have also been used. The most common material currently used is an artificial substance such as polyfluorotetraethylene, which allows for tissue ingrowth into its surface and thus reseals after needle puncture. A-V grafts are usually placed either in the lower or upper portion of the arm or in the upper thigh. However, these grafts can be placed between an artery and a vein in other places (e.g., across the abdomen, across the chest, or wherever an artery and vein may allow such a conduit to be placed). The graft itself is not as deep as the native vessels; tunneling allows for it to be placed through the subcutaneous tissue, thus allowing easy needle puncture (Figure 24–6).[9,71,77]

Assessment of this access and of the extremity in which it is placed is similar to that described for A-V fistulas. More swelling may occur immediately after surgical placement secondary to the subcutaneous tunneling required for placement. This swelling may also increase the patient's postoperative pain. A-V grafts are susceptible to clotting either at the anastomosis site or within the graft itself. They also are susceptible to infections resulting in cellulitis, septicemia, and bacterial endocarditis. In addition, stenotic lesions may develop, usually at the venous anastomosis of these grafts. Pseudoaneurysms may also develop in these conduits and may be able to be surgically repaired.[74,75,78–80]

Care of vascular access devices should be performed by nurses who are skilled in the use of these devices. Nephrology (dialysis) nurses should be consulted if one has any questions regarding a patient's dialysis access. Patients undergoing hemodialysis and their families are often well informed about their accesses and should also be consulted when there may be a change in the status of the access. Patients know that access complications mean additional surgery and pain. They are usually protective of their accesses and understand fully that their vascular access is their "lifeline."[12,60,81,82]

Peritoneal Dialysis

Peritoneal dialysis relies on the same principles of diffusion and filtration to achieve the removal of end products of metabolism, excess electrolytes, and water. The principle of osmosis is employed to promote fluid shifts from the peritoneal vasculature into the dialysis solution. This osmotic gradient is created by the concentration of glucose in the peritoneal dialysis solution.[4,60,83,84]

Peritoneal Dialysis Access

The development of a surgically placed, long-term catheter by Henry Tenckhoff allowed for exchanges to be performed without fluid leaking from the peritoneal cavity or without the constant risk of peritonitis from an open tunnel (fistula) from the peritoneum to the skin. The catheters used for peritoneal dialysis today are surgically implanted and are tunneled from the peritoneal cavity through the subcutaneous tissue and exit several inches away from the entry into the peritoneum. In addition, these catheters are "cuffed" with a velour material that allows tissue ingrowth into the cuff, thus sealing the tunnel at a location under the skin. If the peritoneal dialysis catheter has two cuffs, the second one lies in the tissue just outside the peritoneum (Figure 24–7).[85,86]

Although exit site infections and peritonitis remain major complications of peritoneal dialysis, their incidence has been reduced. When infections do occur, they may not result in catheter loss or treatment discontinuation. Treatment with intravenous and intraperitoneal antibiotics may be sufficient to eliminate the infection. When infections do not respond well to treatment, or if peritoneal dialysis becomes inadequate while treating an infection, the patient may be placed on hemodialysis. Peritoneal dialysis catheters may also become occluded with fibrin deposition (a type of incomplete clot). The addition of heparin to the peritoneal dialysis solution minimizes the formation of

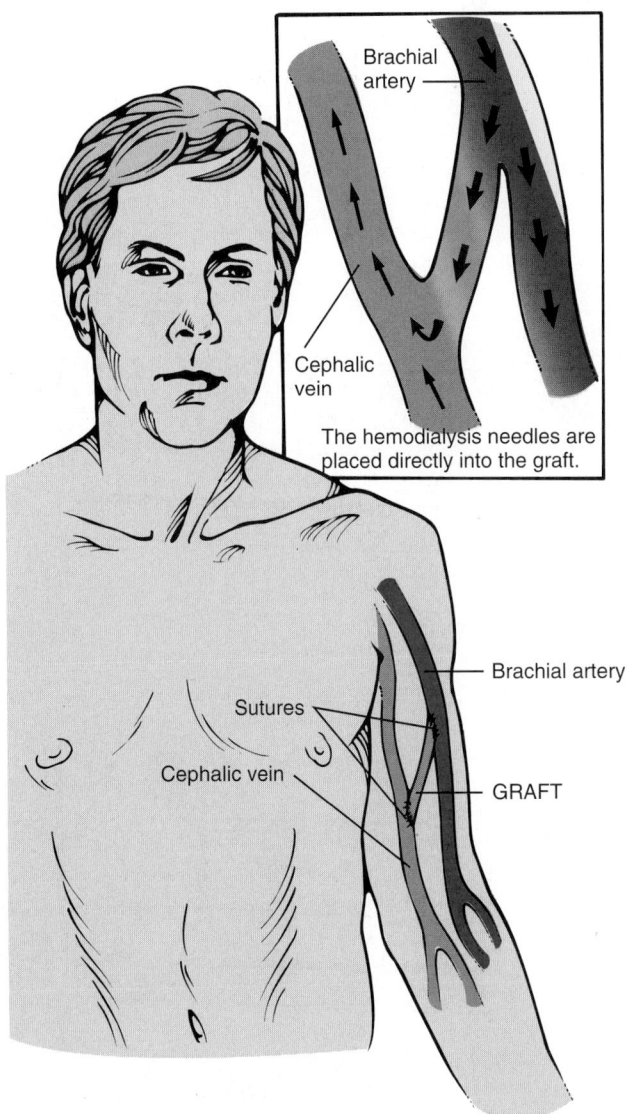

Brachial artery

Cephalic vein

The hemodialysis needles are placed directly into the graft.

Brachial artery

Sutures

Cephalic vein

GRAFT

Figure 24–6

Arteriovenous graft. (From Ignatavicius DD, Workman ML, Mishler MA: Medical-Surgical Nursing Across the Healthcare Continuum, 3rd ed. Philadelphia, W.B. Saunders, 1999.)

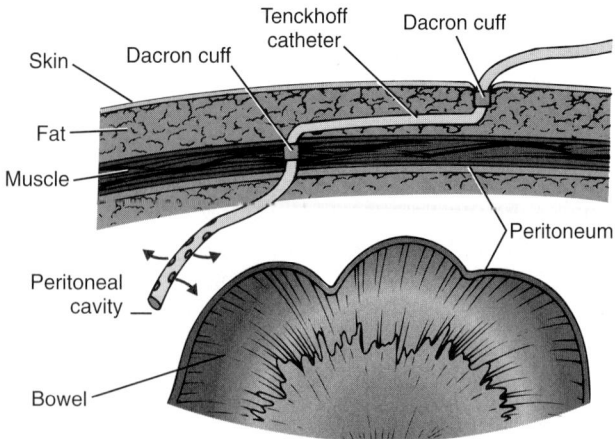

Figure 24–7

Tenckhoff catheter. (From Ignatavicius DD, Workman ML, Mishler MA: Medical-Surgical Nursing Across the Healthcare Continuum, 3rd ed. Philadelphia, W.B. Saunders, 1999.)

these fibrin aggregates, although the exact pharmacologic mechanism is unclear.[87]

After healing of the surgical and exit sites, care of the peritoneal catheter consists primarily of cleansing the exit site, usually while the patient showers. Institutional polices vary regarding the use of bacteriostatic agents around the exit site. Similarly, the patient may or may not prefer to place a dressing over the exit site. Such variations in care do not seem to have a significant impact on the incidence of catheter or exit site infection rates.[86,87]

Methods of Peritoneal Dialysis

Continuous ambulatory peritoneal dialysis (CAPD) is a manual method that involves multiple (usually four) exchanges a day. The peritoneal dialysis solution is packaged in plastic bags (similar to intravenous solutions) of varying volumes (1–3 L for adults per individual prescription). This sterile solution contains all essential electrolytes to ensure maintenance and correction of electrolyte balance. Acetate is added to correct metabolic acidosis through its conversion to bicarbonate by the liver. Generally, these solutions contain no potassium. Solutions are manufactured with concentrations of 1.5%, 2.5%, and 4.25% glucose, which is generally adequate to remove as much as several liters of fluid per day, depending on glucose concentration selected. Drugs can be added to these solutions as individually required. Regular insulin is often added to this solution, thus allowing the patient with DM freedom from subcutaneous injections.

An exchange in peritoneal dialysis consists of a fill, dwell, and drain cycle. The peritoneal dialysis solution flows by gravity into the peritoneal cavity (fill period), allowing for fluid (water), ions, and waste products to shift from the rich vasculature of the peritoneum into this cavity (Figure 24–8A). This fluid remains in the peritoneal cavity for several hours while dialysis occurs

(dwell period). Once the dwell cycle is completed, the fluid is drained out into a collection bag (drain period) (Figure 24–8B). New solution is instilled, marking the beginning of another exchange. The effluent (drainage) resembles urine output in color and clarity. One solution usually dwells in the peritoneal cavity overnight, allowing for shifts of larger molecules at slower rates and for patients to enjoy uninterrupted sleep.

The fill and drain periods each take approximately 20 to 30 minutes and can be performed in various physical locations. The exchange procedure is aseptic (sterile). The supplies required for an exchange are small enough that they can be carried in a tote bag, or briefcase.[60,84]

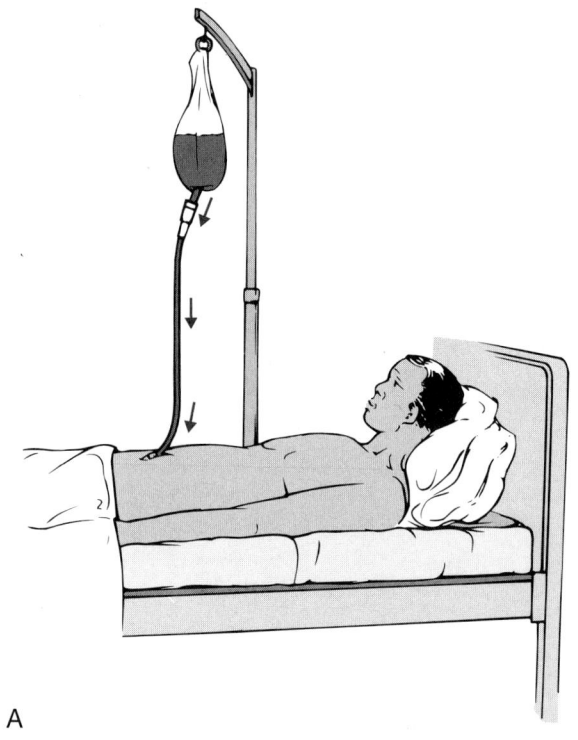

A

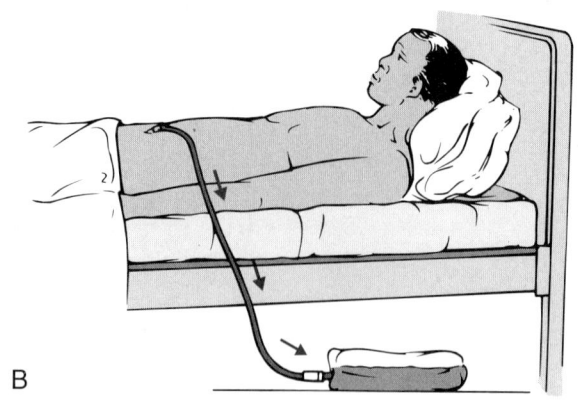

B

Figure 24–8

Manual peritoneal dialysis. A, Fill period. B, Drain period (follows a dwell cycle). (From Ignatavicius DD, Workman ML, Mishler MA: Medical-Surgical Nursing Across the Healthcare Continuum, 3rd ed. Philadelphia, W.B. Saunders, 1999.)

Automated peritoneal dialysis is performed using equipment that cycles specific volumes of solution in and out of the peritoneum at set intervals. Computerization of this equipment allows this information to be entered easily into the machine. The most recent peritoneal dialysis cyclers have been reduced to tabletop size, thus increasing the portability of this equipment and its integration into the patient's physical environment. Patients using the peritoneal dialysis cycler generally perform multiple overnight exchanges, with the final exchange remaining in the peritoneal cavity during the day (opposite of CAPD). This frees the patient from performing dialysis exchanges during the day. The cycler provides the patient with maximum freedom from a rigorous treatment regimen while achieving successful treatment of the patient's renal failure.

Both automated cyclers and a system of multiple bags attached to one set of tubing (octopus system) are used for the hospitalized patient to maintain the adequacy of peritoneal dialysis while minimizing disconnections in the system. The hospitalized patient receiving peritoneal dialysis is at high risk of nosocomial infection.[60,84]

In the critical care unit, the nurse performs standard system assessments, as previously described. Daily measurement of the patient's weight is important to ensure adequate fluid removal and balance. The patient's weight loss should correlate appropriately with the amount of fluid removed with each peritoneal dialysis exchange. Documentation of these exchanges is usually performed on flow sheets. Minimally, these flow sheets are used to document the volume of peritoneal dialysis fluid instilled and the volume of effluent. The difference between these two numbers is the volume of fluid removed through peritoneal dialysis.

Laboratory values for the patient receiving continuous peritoneal dialysis should reflect lower values for BUN and creatinine and normal electrolyte values. Abnormal values may indicate technical problems with the treatment or the presence of peritonitis, which adversely affects osmosis of fluid and filtration of solutes.

Patients who choose peritoneal dialysis as a treatment modality are taught by a specially trained dialysis nurse to perform this procedure independently. This teaching generally takes 1 week or less, with follow-up thereafter on a regular basis by the dialysis nurse or physician. Usually, stable patients return to the dialysis center every 4 to 6 weeks for assessment and are maximally involved in their care. When these patients are hospitalized, changes in procedures, schedules, or other parameters of treatment may create concern and anxiety.[88,89] Nurses must recognize this possibility and must provide an environment that supports the patient's sense of control whenever possible. For example, patients or significant others may wish to continue performing peritoneal dialysis ex-

changes, although this should not be assumed or expected. This involvement can provide the nurse with an excellent opportunity to assess the family's skills regarding the procedure and to provide education as needed (Chart 24–2).

Peritoneal dialysis allows the patient freedom from the 3 times weekly appointment for hemodialysis while providing adequate dialysis. It has special appeal for patients who find it difficult to sit for the 3 to 4 hours or for those who fear needle punctures. In addition, peritoneal dialysis allows greater freedom in dietary and fluid intake because treatment is constant rather than intermittent. Excess fluid, electrolytes, and waste products are removed shortly after their ingestion and absorption. This treatment does require daily therapy, however, and for some patients, this frequency and the rigorousness of the procedure are too great a burden.[90]

Continuous Renal Replacement Therapy

Continuous renal replacement therapy (CRRT) is an acute, hospital-based therapy similar to hemodialysis, although the mechanics of its delivery are different.[91–96] This therapy uses an extracorporeal circuit that removes plasma water and non–protein-bound solutes primarily through convection. Unlike hemodialysis, this treatment can be easily and successfully used for patients who have a significant fluid overload but who may not have renal failure.

The primary use of CRRT is for patients who are fluid overloaded and hemodynamically unstable and for whom hemodialysis may cause further instability and hypotension, thus preventing adequate fluid removal. These patients may have renal failure, heart failure that is diuretic resistant, or oliguria secondary to heart failure.[24] Patients who suffer from chronic fluid overload in the presence of renal failure, such as those with ascites or nephrotic edema, may also benefit from a course of CRRT.[24,91,97,98]

CRRT is also known as continuous A-V hemofiltration (CAVH) or continuous veno-venous hemofiltration (CVVH), depending on the vascular access route used to perform this treatment.[94,95] Catheters for these modalities can be placed in an artery and vein or in two veins. The blood flow through this extracorporeal circuit is relatively slow, at less than 200 mL per minute. If an arterial access is used, pressure gradients in the systems will be higher because of the patient's own mean arterial pressure. Venous blood flow into the system reduces the pressure in the system and decreases the amount of fluid removed. Although some practitioners use standard dialyzers for this treatment, a specially developed extracorporeal filter that is highly permeable to water and small to medium-sized solutes can be used. These filters have a low blood volume and low resistance to blood flow. If the patient's own blood

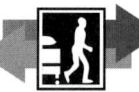

CHART 24–2

BEYOND THE ICU: PREVENTING COMPLICATIONS IN PATIENTS WITH ESRD

Patients with end-stage renal disease (ESRD) live in various settings in the community. Some patients may be living in their own homes and may perform all their life activities independently. Other patients may be living with family members who provide support and care for them by performing the activities they are unable to accomplish (e.g., errands, shopping, transportation) because of primary illnesses or complications. Other patients may be residing in other types of facilities that provide support based on disabilities or age (e.g., life-care communities, sheltered housing). Some patients reside in long-term facilities secondary to disabilities related to primary diseases or complications of their ESRD.

A primary goal of the ESRD health professional team is to prevent or minimize hospitalizations of patients receiving renal replacement therapy. Quality improvement and best practice programs in ESRD facilities are developed to address these issues. The design and organization of outpatient, freestanding dialysis facilities, however, require the use of hospital facilities to provide care that is beyond the scope of the facility's physical and human resources.

Frequent causes of hospitalization specific to the patient with ESRD include fluid overload resulting in congestive heart failure and pulmonary edema, vascular or peritoneal dialysis access occlusion, infections (signs and symptoms of sepsis) secondary to vascular or peritoneal dialysis access, and severe electrolyte imbalances. Patients who have had renal transplant may require hospitalization to treat episodes of rejection or infections.

Prevention of fluid overload for the patient undergoing hemodialysis or peritoneal dialysis is a primary objective of the nurse caring for these patients. Fluid intake and restriction are complex issues for the patient with ESRD and do not simply reflect an unwillingness to follow a prescribed regimen. Physiologic concepts of serum osmolality (particularly shifts in sodium and glucose) and shifts in serum osmolality caused by dietary and fluid intake and the composition of dialysate solutions should all be considered in the assessment of fluid overload in these patients.

Specific interventions to prevent fluid overload should include the following:

- Patient and family education regarding the content of fluid in foods, the relationship between sodium intake and thirst, and the interactions of glucose intake, blood glucose levels, and thirst.
- Exploration of the psychosocial variables that influence fluid intake such as boredom and social events.
- Assessment of the patient's dry weight at regular intervals to ensure that mass has not been lost and replaced by fluid; this requires expert physical assessment, review of the patient's history and treatment data, and diagnostic studies (e.g., chest radiograph).

Specific interventions to prevent vascular/peritoneal access failure should include the following:

- Initial and ongoing patient education regarding care of the access site.
- Prevention of infection through appropriate home care technique.
- Prevention of infection in the ESRD facility by use of appropriate infection-control procedures.
- Early diagnosis and treatment of access infections.
- Regular assessment of vascular access flow characteristics with attention to subtle changes in blood flow patterns.
- Expert surgical techniques in placement of vascular or peritoneal access, to maximize function and to minimize complications.

After discharge from an acute care facility (ICU), it is the general goal to return these patients to their previous environments. However, that arrangement may not be appropriate. Patients may require discharge to rehabilitation or long-term care facilities based on the outcome of their hospitalization and the ongoing care they require.

---

pressure does not support blood flow through the circuit or if controlled flow is desired, a roller pump may be used to maintain flow through the circuit.

Continuous ultrafiltration uses the principle of pressure gradients across a highly permeable membrane. The hydraulic pressure within the blood compartment is opposed by the hydrostatic pressure generated by the weight of the fluid column in the ultrafiltrate line. Oncotic pressure in the vascular compartment generated by plasma proteins also affects fluid removal by this system. These pressure gradients and the permeability of the membrane to water can result in the removal of as much as 10 to 15 L of water in 24 hours. If fluid replacement is necessary to maintain the hemodynamic status of the patient, normal saline can be administered into the venous line of the extracorporeal circuit.

The dialysate compartment of this ultrafilter must be filled with sterile fluid, and the dialysate usually used is a peritoneal dialysis solution with 1.5% glucose. Flow rates through the system are approximately 1 L per hour, and the solute content is compatible with blood, thus maintaining or correcting electrolyte and acid–base balance.

Solute removal with CRRT is comparable to that achieved with CAPD and can effectively treat ARF or CRF in the hospitalized patient. Heparinization of this extracorporeal circuit may be required because blood can easily clot at any point in the system. Some seriously ill patients with clotting dyscrasias may require little or no heparinization, whereas others may require large doses of anticoagulation. Both heparin and citrate have been used as anticoagulants for this procedure.[99] Patients may receive approximately 2000 units of heparin immediately before the initiation of treatment, and smaller amounts may be infused on a continual basis or given as bolus injections. The physician's orders should include the parameters for anticoagulation. If the extracorporeal circuit does clot, the entire system must be replaced. This can result in critical blood loss for the patient. When clots do develop, one usually sees a decrease in the volume of ultrafiltrate. Blood may also be lost if the fibers (semipermeable membrane) of the filter tear. The nurse must observe the ultrafiltrate as well as the filter carefully for the presence of blood because identifying this complication quickly can limit the loss of blood.

CRRT is usually performed by specially trained nurses. It is a labor-intensive therapy requiring a 1:1 ratio of patient to nurse. In some settings, hemodialysis nurses share responsibility for this treatment, particularly during the initiation of treatment and the changing of the hemofilter. The duration of this treatment is variable, depending on the patient's condition. It may be performed for less than 24 hours, or it may continue for as long as a week without interruption.[95,100]

Renal Transplantation

Renal transplantation is an alternative treatment option for patients with ESRD, although it is not considered a curative procedure.[101] The procedure involves using a kidney from one person to replace lost renal function in another person. The functioning kidney may be obtained from either a cadaveric organ donor or a live donor. Either of these donor sources can provide a successful transplant.

Live donor transplants have traditionally been accomplished with a genetically close family member serving as the organ donor. Based on genetic inheritance patterns, a sibling has a 25% chance of being human leukocyte antigen (HLA) identical to another sibling, a 50% chance of being half-identical, and a 25% chance of being totally dissimilar.[16,28,29,101] In the early experimental work in organ transplantation, this genetic and immunologic site that recognizes "nonself" was found on chromosome 6 and remains a factor in testing donor–recipient compatibility. Peripheral lymphocytes are used to perform HLA testing. Blood type is another measure of immunologic compatibility between donor and recipient. As in blood transfusions, blood type should be compatible, although Rh factor incompatibility is not a barrier to renal transplantation.[10,96]

Identical twins are immunologically privileged because they grew from the same ovum and sperm and share the same genetic tissue. Thus, a patient who receives a kidney from his or her identical twin does not experience rejection. Parents and offspring are half-alike because each parent contributes half of the offspring's genetic identity (Chart 24–3). More distant relatives or genetically unrelated individuals may also serve as kidney donors. With improvements in immunosuppressive therapy after renal transplantation, the role of HLA compatibility may no longer be the strongest variable in transplant success.

In the United States, the use of "emotionally related" donors (e.g., spouses, close friends) has been increasing. Blood type compatibility and acceptable

---

CHART 24–3

HLA Matching for Donor Compatibility

HLA identities here are represented as numbers to identify possible combinations

MOTHER	FATHER
1 2	3 4

OFFSPRING (CHILDREN)

Sibling 1	Sibling 2	Sibling 3	Sibling 4	Sibling 5
1 3	2 4	2 3	1 4	2 4

Siblings 2 and 5 are HLA identical; sibling 1 is totally dissimilar to siblings 2 and 5; sibling 3 is half-identical to siblings 1, 2, and 5.

Nonrelated donors may be identical, 50% match, 25% match, or totally dissimilar.

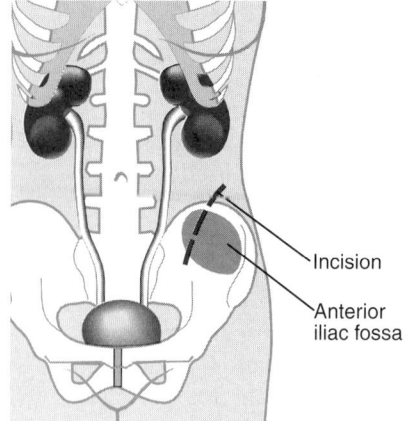

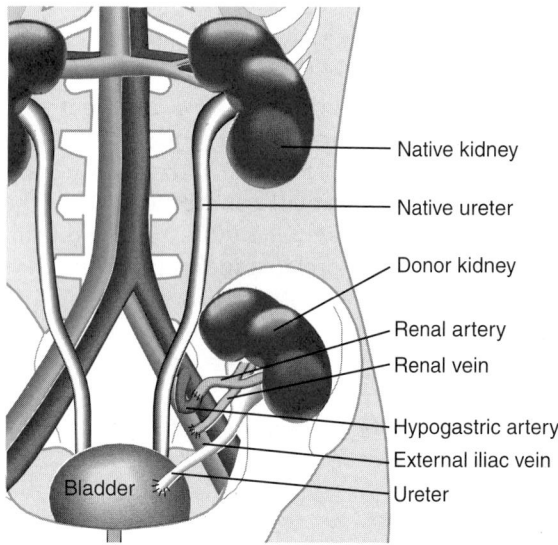

Figure 24–9

Kidney transplantation. (From Saunders Manual of Nursing Care. Philadelphia, W.B. Saunders, 1997.)

health status are primary criteria for acceptability of these donors.[16] After HLA testing identifies a compatible living donor, the donor undergoes a rigorous physical assessment to ensure that the surgical procedure and the removal of one kidney will not jeopardize the donor's health status. Although this operation provides no physical benefit for the donor, its continued performance has been justified as an act of altruism. Kidney donors have routinely reported that they derive much psychologic benefit from this act.[3, 101, 102]

Cadaver donors remain the primary source of kidneys for transplantation. These donors have suffered irreversible cessation of brain function, with maintenance of other vital organ functions. After declaration of death and consent for organ donation, kidneys (and usually other organs and tissues) are removed. Each cadaveric donor provides two patients

with renal transplants. The number of patients awaiting cadaveric kidney transplants continues to exceed the number of kidneys available from cadaver donors.[16, 103]

Before the actual kidney transplant is performed, final compatibility testing is performed between the donor (live or cadaver) and the recipient. This cross-match testing identifies cytotoxic antibodies that are directed toward the HLA antigens of the recipient and form secondary to exposure to blood transfusions or other foreign tissue. The cautious use of transfusions in patients with ESRD before renal transplant may limit the formation of such antibodies.

Transplant Surgical Procedure

The surgical procedure of kidney transplantation does not anatomically replace a native kidney. The kidney is usually left in place unless a specific disorder requires its removal. The transplanted kidney is placed in either the right or left iliac fossa. This placement allows for the anastomosis of the donor kidney's renal artery to the hypogastric artery and anastomosis of the renal vein to the iliac vein. The ureter is implanted into the bladder using a ureteroneocystostomy procedure. This surgical approach minimizes postoperative complications, enhances recovery, and allows for assessment of the transplanted kidney by more direct palpation and auscultation (Figure 24–9).[3, 28, 29, 102]

Postoperative Care of the Transplant Recipient

Care of the renal transplant recipient is directed to assessment of renal function as measured by urine formation and excretion of the end products of metabolism, maintenance or correction of fluid and electrolyte balance, assessment of urinary drainage related to the urologic surgical procedure, control of postoperative pain, and prevention of infection in an immunosuppressed patient.[13, 28, 29, 96] Renal transplant facilities usually have specialty nurses who are experts in the acute care of the transplant recipient and in the prompt recognition and treatment of transplant rejection. Patients who experience no complications after the renal transplant operation may be discharged from the hospital in approximately 7 days.[104]

Prevention and Treatment of Transplant Graft Rejection

In most cases of renal transplantation (with the exception of identical twins), the transplanted kidney is foreign tissue to the recipient. Because this organ is genetically dissimilar, the recipient's immunologic system recognizes this dissimilarity and begins to destroy this foreign tissue. This response has been defined as transplant rejection. Rejection events are commonly described as "acute" rejection or "chronic" rejection. A third type, known as "hyperacute" rejection, may occur at the time of the transplant surgery. This occurs when unidentified antibodies aggressively destroy the transplanted kidney when blood flow to the transplanted kidney is established. Fortunately, this type of rejection is rare because of pretransplant antigen–antibody testing.[13,28,29,96,105]

Because it is generally believed that the recipient's immune system always recognizes the donor kidney as foreign, the transplant recipient continues to receive immunosuppressive medications for the entire time the transplant is viable. Episodes of rejection are most likely to occur in the early months after a transplant. Although it is unclear whether a true state of physiologic tolerance to this foreign tissue develops, rejection episodes are less likely in the years after transplantation.

The acute (cellular) rejection response occurs when T cells are formed by the immune system and are released to directly attack and destroy the transplanted kidney. Signs and symptoms of this type of transplant rejection include decreased renal function and signs and symptoms of an inflammatory or immune response. This form of rejection can be controlled by immunosuppressive medications that work by suppressing the formation of T cells by the immune system.

Chronic (humoral) rejection forms B cells and is not as responsive to immunosuppressive medication. When B cells are formed as an immunologic response, this response stimulates the formation of memory cells that cannot be easily suppressed. Memory cells continue to recognize the transplanted kidney as foreign tissue and attempt to destroy it. Chronic rejection may continue over months to years and may result in failure of the transplanted kidney. Should renal failure occur, the patient returns to hemodialysis or peritoneal dialysis for renal replacement therapy. Some patients are able to receive subsequent transplants.

Current Immunosuppressive Drug Therapies

Protocols for the use of immunosuppressive drugs can vary among kidney transplant programs. Different combinations of these drugs may be used at different times during the patient's course of therapy. The use of immunosuppressive therapy is guided by the principle of balancing the therapeutic effects of these drugs against the side effects and complications. Dosages should provide maximum therapy while minimizing side effects and complications. Immunosuppressive therapy should be reduced or discontinued if the patient's kidney function does not improve with increased doses of medication or if the patient develops life-threatening complications (e.g., infection).[27,29,30,106] Table 24–3 is a summary of the major immunosuppressive drug therapies used to treat patients after renal transplantation.[12,26,96]

Survival after Renal Transplantation

Renal transplants have been performed since 1954. The clinical experience gained in these years has made it a safe and effective treatment for ESRD. In 1996, it was reported that more than 12,198 kidney transplants were performed; of this total, 3084 were from living related donors, and 619 were from living unrelated donors. Cadaver transplants were received by 8495 patients. In 1997, approximately 40,000 people were waiting for cadaveric renal transplants.[16]

According to the USRDS, patients who received renal transplants from living related donors between the years of 1985 and 1994 had a 96% survival rate; patients who received cadaveric transplants had a 92% survival rate at 1 year. One-year graft survival rates were 92.4% for kidneys from living related donors and 85.6% for cadaveric kidneys. At 5 years, it is calculated that at least 70% of transplants from living related donors will be functional, whereas 50 to 60% of cadaveric grafts will be functioning.[16,29,106]

The limited experience with kidney transplantation using emotionally related donors suggests that these recipients can anticipate survival rates closer to those achieved with genetically related donors. The number of patients in this group is small, so the data are tentative, although it seems clear that the outcome is better than that achieved for cadaveric kidney transplants. As noted previously, the rejection of a kidney transplant does not result in the patient's death. Rather, the patient may resume dialysis therapy. If a patient receives a successful transplant, all renal function returns. Although these patients require other medications, particularly immunosuppressives, they can expect to resume a normal life unencumbered by dialysis treatment.

Multidisciplinary Outcomes

Various health care professionals are directly and indirectly involved in the delivery and outcomes of care for the patient with renal failure. After the initial diagnosis of renal disease, the patient may continue to receive care from a primary physician. As renal function deteriorates, referral to a nephrologist is made for additional evaluation and discussion of treatment modalities. If dietary management of protein intake is needed or if other dietary interventions are indicated, referral to a dietitian is made. To manage issues of emotional adjustment as well as issues related to insurance coverage and ESRD Social Security benefits, the social worker may also be included in the patient's care. Ongoing, outpatient management is accomplished by the primary physician and, in some cases, by a nurse practitioner. For patients with comorbidities, this management may include other providers (e.g., cardiologists, diabetologists, ophthalmologists, pulmonologists) who also contribute to the patient's

TABLE 24–3
Immunosuppressive Drug Therapy After Kidney Transplantation*

Drug	Action	Nursing and Patient Implications
Azathioprine (Imuran)	Bone marrow suppression, specifically white blood cells; inhibits the early stages of cell differentiation and proliferation	Useful in preventing rejection but ineffective in treating acute rejection; may be administered intravenously and orally; major side effect: hepatotoxicity
Corticosteroids (Solu-Medrol, prednisone)	Immunosuppressive effects: interfere with gene transcription and alter cell function (RNA translation, protein synthesis, and secretion of cytokines and proteins); decrease number of circulating lymphocytes; inhibit events associated with T-cell activation; inhibit early proliferation of B cells Anti-inflammatory effects: inhibit accumulation of leukocytes at site of inflammation; inhibit macrophage function and decrease production of prostaglandins	Used in conjunction with other immunosuppressive drugs; short-term and long-term side effects such as Cushing's syndrome; adrenal crisis may develop if therapy is withdrawn abruptly (as may be the inadvertent case in patients whose transplanted kidneys have failed); may be given intravenously or orally
Cyclosporine (Sandimmune, Neoral)	Inhibits early activities of T-cell activation, sensitization, and proliferation	Used to prevent acute rejection; minimal effect on mature cytotoxic T cells, thus cannot reverse acute rejection; unclear effect on suppression of B cells and chronic rejection; can be administered intravenously and orally
Tacrolimus (Prograf)	Inhibits T-lymphocyte activation by binding to intracellular protein and forming a complex that prevents the generation of nuclear material for activated T cells	Effective as "rescue" or emergency therapy during an episode of acute or chronic rejection; may be reserved for the treatment of these events rather than used as a primary immunosuppressant
Antithymocyte Globulin (ATG, Atgam)	Antibody made from horse serum that binds to T- and B-cell lymphocytes as well as platelets and granulocytes thus depleting and lysing immunologically active cells and reversing acute rejection episodes	Usually reserved for prophylaxis or induction immediately before or at the time of transplant; also used for acute graft rejection that does not respond well to corticosteroids; side effects similar to those of serum sickness; in addition, patients may become sensitized to the horse serum and may be at risk of an anaphylactic reaction
Murine Monoclonal Antibody (OKT3)	Monoclonal antibody that suppresses T-cell–mediated rejection by binding to specific regions of the T cell, thus altering T-cell recognition of the antigen; blocks killer T cells that are attached to the transplanted kidney and renders them inactive	Used to suppress acute episodes of rejection; can only be given intravenously and may produce systemic reactions; may cause allergic reactions, including anaphylaxis
Mycophenolate (Cell Cept)	Suppresses T- and B-lymphocyte proliferation; inhibits the enzyme, inosine monophosphate dehydrogenase, which is required for protein synthesis	Often used in combination with cyclosporine and corticosteroids to prevent rejection

*Patients receiving immunosuppressive therapy are at higher risk of infection. The nurse should carefully investigate any (even subtle) changes in the patient's status because the usual signs and symptoms of infections may be masked. Use of invasive lines should be minimized, and adherence to aseptic technique must be absolute.

health care. Outcomes for patient care at this point are directed at restoring acid–base, fluid, and electrolyte balance, at achieving emotional balance, and at restoring nutritional status.

Once the patient begins treatment at an ESRD facility, the nurse manages the dialysis (hemodialysis and peritoneal dialysis) equipment, monitors patients for complications, and provides extensive patient education. Outcomes for patient care at this stage focus on maintaining fluid and electrolyte balance, avoiding infections, providing patient education, and preventing complications.[88,107,108]

In some situations, the patient with ESRD may be referred for renal transplant evaluation before dialysis is initiated. If it is medically possible, a kidney transplant (usually from a living donor) may be performed as the first treatment strategy. The renal transplant team is composed of staff similar to the staff at the dialysis facility. A successful renal transplant can only occur through collaboration between the dialysis team and the transplant team.

All these health care professionals work collaboratively to achieve the best quality of life for the patient for as long as possible. Patient care conferences are recommended to review the patient's status and to discuss treatment options and long-term plans. Patients and families should be included in these meetings whenever possible (Chart 24–4).

When patients with ESRD are hospitalized, collaboration between nurses from inpatient and outpatient settings is recommended. Dialysis and transplant nurses may have provided care for the patient for many years. Their knowledge of and relationship with the patient with ESRD should be respected and used to

---

CHART 24–4
RESEARCH UTILIZATION: PERCEPTIONS OF QUALITY OF LIFE

Abstract: Quality of life (QOL) is an increasingly important concept to both health care professionals and the general population. In this study, Molzahn and associates attempted to define the differences in ratings of QOL by patients with end-stage renal disease (ESRD), their physicians, and their nurses. In addition, these investigators identified sociodemographic variables that may explain any differences. This study used a cross-sectional, descriptive, comparative design. The sample included 215 patients, 42 nurses, and 7 physicians. The setting was one ESRD facility in a tertiary care hospital in Canada. The patient sample represented patients treated with all ESRD modalities.

Three established instruments were used to measure the patients' QOL. Physicians and nurses also measured QOL for those patients participating in the research. Statistical analyses were performed to measure the mean ratings of QOL by each of these three groups on each instrument. Correlations were calculated among the groups. Descriptive statistics were reported for four sociodemographic variables. Finally, an analysis of variables identified as significant predictors of the patient's perceptions of QOL was reported.

Findings included the following: patients with ESRD reported a QOL comparable to that of the general American population; kidney transplant recipients reported the highest QOL; nurses consistently rated patient QOL lower than patients did; and physicians rated patient QOL higher than both patients and nurses did.

Critique: The literature review is comprehensive and includes studies previously done in the ESRD community as well as in other settings of chronic illness or disability. The researchers clearly stated five research questions. The sample size is adequate for this study, but the setting is limited to a single dialysis unit in a tertiary care hospital in Canada. This sample size may limit both the findings and the generalizability to the ESRD population in the United States because of differences in the organization of ESRD treatment delivery. The researchers reported low stability reliability among some of the independent variables; they also acknowledged that data collection from the physicians was incomplete and could alter the findings. The mean age of the patient sample is much younger than that of the ESRD population in the United States and thus may also limit generalizability. Whether the physician and nursing samples are similar to their counterparts in the United States by demographics is unclear.

Nursing Considerations: These researchers have provided the health care community with information to consider seriously when caring for patients with ESRD. Nephrology nurses and physicians must be sensitive to the patients' perceptions of QOL and should engage in meaningful communication with these patients. In addition, physicians and nurses should communicate with each other regarding patients' reports of QOL. Because the tools used in these studies are brief and easy to administer, they could lend themselves to clinic use. The patients' perception of QOL could be documented at intervals during the course of treatment, especially when major medical events and decisions occur.

When patients with ESRD are hospitalized in the ICU, health care providers who are less familiar with these patients may be making judgments (both formal and informal) based on their own perceptions of patients' QOL. If treatment decisions are based on the health care professionals' perceptions of the patient's QOL, these decisions may be incongruent with the patient's perceptions.

Molzahn AE, Northcott HC, Dosseter JB: Quality of life of individuals with end stage renal disease: perceptions of patients, nurses, and physicians. J Am Nephrol Nurses' Assoc. 24:325–337, 1997.

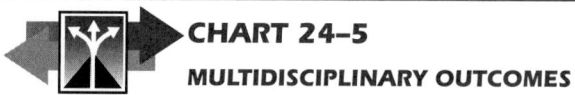

CHART 24–5
MULTIDISCIPLINARY OUTCOMES

Restoration and maintenance of fluid balance

Correction and maintenance of acid–base and electrolyte balance

Creation and maintenance of vascular or peritoneal access

Prevention of access infections

Restoration and maintenance of nutritional status

Prevention of renal osteodystrophy

Correction of anemia

Restoration and maintenance of role responsibilities

Performance and maintenance of successful renal transplant

provide expert care while the patient is hospitalized. Outcomes at this stage should involve resolution of the acute illness and restoration of renal replacement therapy. Chart 24–5 provides a summary of the multidisciplinary outcomes that can be anticipated for a patient with ESRD.

Critical Thinking Exercise

T.H. is a 36-year-old man who was diagnosed with type 1 DM when he was 9 years old. Complications of diabetes have been progressive, and he was diagnosed with renal failure 2 years ago. Dialysis treatment with CAPD was initiated approximately 6 months ago, but T.H. experienced several episodes of peritonitis during this time. CAPD was replaced with hemodialysis after placement of an A-V graft in his lower left arm. He recently underwent embolectomy (declotting) and revision of that graft. T.H. receives hemodialysis three times per week for 4 hours per treatment. He has continued to work for a local manufacturer, where he makes compact disks. Recently, T.H. developed dry gangrene of the third toe of his right foot. His current medications include: clonidine (Catapres), diltiazem (Cardizem), clonidine and minoxidil (Loniten), atenolol (Tenormin), bumetanide (Bumex), ranitidine (Zantac), clonazepam (Klonopin), cisapride (Propulsid), calcium acetate (Phoslo), Nephrocaps vitamins, Peri-Colace, and insulin (Humulin N). At 5:30 AM, T.H. went to the local emergency room with complaints of nausea and vomiting for 1 day and pain under his sternum, which was "tender to touch." He was scheduled for outpatient hemodialysis at 1500 (later this day).

The patient was alert and oriented to time and place; his respirations were rapid, at 26 per minute. His blood pressure was 150/84 mm Hg, and his heart rate was 64 beats per minute and regular. A right subclavian Permacath was in place; his left arm was red and swollen secondary to recent A-V graft surgery; and his left hand and nailbeds were cool and cyanotic.

The fingerstick glucose was too high to read. Arterial blood gases were as follows: pH 7.10, CO_2 23, PO_2 98, HCO_3^- 13. Laboratory results were as follows: potassium, 9.4; BUN 90; creatinine 12.9; glucose 664; and CBC: hemoglobin, 9.7, hematocrit, 38.6, and WBC 25,000. ECG tracing revealed widened QRS complexes.

An intravenous infusion of normal saline was placed in his lower right arm, and 600 mL was infused rapidly in the emergency room. 10 U regular Humulin insulin was given subcutaneously, and 10 U regular Humulin insulin was given by intravenous push, followed by a drip of regular Humulin insulin running at 5 U per hour; 1 ampule (50 mL) of sodium bicarbonate was given by intravenous push. He was admitted to the intensive care unit at 7:30 AM with orders for immediate hemodialysis. Hemodialysis treatment was initiated at 8:05 AM.

Hemodialysis treatment orders were as follows: 0 potassium dialysate solution; blood flow at 300 mL per minute by a right subclavian catheter; dialysis for 4 hours; fluid removal as tolerated (2200 mL of fluid were removed); administration of vancomycin 1 g intravenously at the end of treatment; serum potassium drawn at the beginning and end of treatment (results were 6.9 at 8:05 AM; 3.9 at 12:00 noon); blood cultures per protocol (preliminary report Gram-positive cocci; final report Staphylococcus aureus).

1. What are the most likely causes of T.H.'s hyperkalemia?
2. What treatments did he receive for hyperkalemia?
3. How could his fluid volume status be described based on history and assessment?
4. What has contributed to his nausea and vomiting and hyperglycemia?
5. What is the interpretation of his metabolic state, and what has contributed to this state?
6. T.H.'s CBC values reflect what conditions?
7. What is the interpretation of his uremic status?

Key Concepts

⟾ The cumulative signs and symptoms of CRF are often referred to as uremia and can include fluid overload, electrolyte imbalance, and coma.

⟾ Early diagnosis and management of diseases leading to renal failure may delay or even prevent the need for dialysis or renal transplantation.

⟾ Nursing care of acutely or critically ill patients with ESRD requires a solid understanding of pathophysiology of the disease and the interactions of the disease with other comorbidities.

⟾ The intact nephron theory describes the pathophysiologic process of CRF; as independently functioning nephrons become diseased, others hypertrophy and, compensate for the loss of function.

→ Cardiovascular disease and DM are the most common causes of CRF due to vascular disease.

→ Autoimmune glomerular disease results when the patient's own antibodies selectively destroy the glomerular apparatus of the kidney.

→ CRF from interstitial renal disease can result from pyelonephritis, an infectious process within the kidney, and from certain nephrotoxic drugs and substances.

→ Congenital anomalies (malformed kidneys, strictures in the lower urinary tract) can lead to CRF, although normal renal function may be maintained in some patients.

→ The most common genetic mutation leading to CRF is polycystic renal disease, an autosomal dominant genetic disease.

→ CRF can be viewed as a continuum, beginning with diminished renal reserve and progressing to renal insufficiency and, finally, the development of ESRD.

→ Patients are usually asymptomatic during the stage of diminished renal reserve, and often, this stage is not diagnosed.

→ Renal insufficiency results in increases in BUN and creatinine (azotemia), electrolyte imbalances, and decreases in red blood cells.

→ Patients with ESRD often present with significant elevations in BUN and creatinine, anemia, uremic fetor, and cognitive impairment.

→ Findings from a systemic assessment of a patient with ESRD should be correlated with data from laboratory and diagnostic studies.

→ Therapies for the treatment for hyperkalemia resulting from CRF can include intravenous drugs (e.g., calcium chloride, sodium bicarbonate, 50% glucose and insulin), oral or rectal drugs (e.g., sodium polystyrene sulfonate [Kayexalate]), or emergency dialysis.

→ Renal replacement therapies for the patient with ESRD include hemodialysis, peritoneal dialysis, and renal transplantation.

→ Patients undergoing dialysis treatment (hemodialysis, peritoneal dialysis) may achieve near-normal lifestyles and life expectancies with successful management.

→ Vascular access for hemodialysis can be through a centrally placed venous catheter or by a surgically constructed A-V fistula or graft.

→ Maintaining the vascular access (the patient's "lifeline") for the patient receiving hemodialysis is critical and involves diligent monitoring for complications (e.g., clotting, infection, steal syndrome).

→ Access for peritoneal dialysis involves the surgical placement of a catheter into the peritoneal cavity.

→ Both hemodialysis and peritoneal dialysis have advantages and disadvantages, and it is the patient, in collaboration with the dialysis team, who decides which method of renal replacement therapy is selected.

→ Patients and families, as members of the health care team, are taught to manage most of the care related to their dialysis and access devices.

→ CRRT is used for critically ill patients who have a significant fluid overload, but not necessarily from CRF.

→ Renal transplantation is a successful treatment for ESRD, providing patients with near-normal lifestyles.

→ Donors for kidney transplantation can be genetically related, emotionally related, or cadavers; donor–recipient compatibility is done using HLA testing.

→ The demand for donor kidneys far outweighs the supply.

→ Renal transplantation is the surgical implantation of a human kidney into the iliac fossa of a recipient. The procedure involves the anastomosis of the renal artery to the hypogastric artery, renal vein to external iliac vein, and implantation of the ureter into the recipient's bladder (native bladder) through a ureteroneocystotomy.

→ Patients who undergo renal transplantation need immunosuppressive therapy for the entire time the donor kidney remains viable.

→ Acute rejection of a transplanted kidney involves the formation of T cells by the immune system and usually responds well to immunosuppressive therapy.

→ Chronic rejection of a transplanted kidney may result in renal failure and the return of the patient to dialysis.

→ Continued research and development of new drug and biotechnologic therapies may result in the complete prevention of kidney transplant rejection.

→ Multidisciplinary health care teams (e.g., physicians, nurses, social workers, dietitians) work to provide the best quality of life for patients with ESRD.

References

1. Alexander S: They decide who lives, who dies: medical miracle puts a moral burden on a small committee. Life 53:102–110, 115–118, 123–125, 1962.
2. Brenner BM, Rector FC: The Kidney. Philadelphia, W.B. Saunders, 1991.
3. Danovitch GM (ed): Handbook of Kidney Transplantation. Boston, Little, Brown, 1992.
4. Daugirda JT, Ing TS (eds): Handbook of Dialysis, 2nd ed. Boston, Little, Brown, 1994.
5. Fox RC, Swazey JP: The Courage to Fail: A Social View of Organ Transplants and Dialysis, 2nd ed. Chicago, University of Chicago Press, 1979.

6. Institute of Medicine, Committee for the Study of the Medicare ESRD Program: Kidney Failure and the Federal Government. Washington DC, U.S. Government Printing Office, 1991.

7. Federal Register: Social Security Amendments of 1972, vol. 41. Washington, DC, Department of Health, Education, and Welfare, 1976.

8. Public Law 92-603. 92nd Congress. October, 1972.

9. Hartigan MF: Maintaining hemodialysis vascular access patency. Nephrol Nurs Today 3:1–8, 1993.

10. Pfettscher SA: Renal disorders. In: Holloway NM (ed): Nursing the Critically Ill Adult, 4th ed. Redwood City, CA, Addison-Wesley, 1993.

11. Richard CJ: Causes of renal failure. In: Lancaster L (ed): Core Curriculum for Nephrology Nursing, 3rd ed. Pitman, NJ, American Nephrology Nurses' Association, 1995.

12. Windus DW: Permanent vascular access: a nephrologist's view. Am J Kidney Dis 21:463, 1993.

13. Albee B, Beckman NJ, Shell HM: Patients with end-stage renal disease. In: Clocheys JM, Bleu C, Cardia S, et al (eds): Critical Care Nursing, 2nd ed. Philadelphia, W.B. Saunders, 1996.

14. Rimmer JM, Gennari FJ: Atherosclerotic renovascular disease and progressive renal failure. Ann Intern Med 118:712, 1993.

15. Qualheim RE, Rostand SG, Kirk KA, et al: Changing patterns of end-stage renal disease due to hypertension. Am J Kidney Dis 18:336–343, 1991.

16. US Renal Data System. 1996 Annual Data Report. [Online: http://www.med.umich.edu/usrds]. Washington, DC, Department of Health and Human Services, 1998.

17. Ateshkadi A, Johnson CA: Chronic renal failure. In: Young LY, Koda-Kimble MA (ed): Applied Therapeutics: The Clinical Use of Drugs. Vancouver, WA, Applied Therapeutics, 1995.

18. King B: Preserving renal function. RN 60:34–40, 1997.

19. National Kidney Foundation: Online: http://www.kidney.org

20. Diabetes Control and Complications Trial Research Group: The effect of intensive treatment of diabetes on the development and progress of long-term complication in insulin-dependent diabetes mellitus. N Engl J Med 329:977–986, 1993.

21. Held P, Levin N, Port F: Cardiac disease in chronic uremia: an overview. In: Parfrey PS, Harnett J (eds): Cardiac Dysfunction in Chronic Uremia. Boston, Kluwer Academic, 1992.

22. Ma K, Greene E, Ray L: Cardiovascular risk factors in chronic renal failure and hemodialysis populations. Am J Kidney Dis 19:505–513, 1992.

23. National Institutes of Health: NIH Consensus Statement: Morbidity and mortality of dialysis. November 1–3, 1993. Bethesda, MD, Department of Health and Human Services, National Institutes of Health, 1996.

24. Simpson IA, Simpson K, Rae AP, et al: Ultrafiltration in diuretic-resistant cardiac failure. Ren Fail 10:115–119, 1987.

25. Montseny J, Meyrier A, Kleinknecht D, et al: The current spectrum of infectious glomerulonephritis. Medicine 74:63–73, 1995.

26. Dupuis RE: Solid organ transplantation. In: Young LY, Koda-Kimble MA (eds): Applied Therapeutics: The Clinical Use of Drugs. Vancover, WA, Applied Therapeutics, 1995.

27. Payne JL: Immune modification and complications of immunosuppression. Crit Care Nurs Clin North Am 4:43–61, 1992.

28. Sigardson-Poor KM, Haggerty LM (eds): Nursing Care of the Transplant Recipient. Philadelphia, W.B. Saunders, 1990.

29. Smith SL: Tissue and Organ Transplantation: Implications for Professional Nursing Practice. St. Louis, Mosby–Year Book, 1990.

30. Young LY, Koda-Kimble MA (ed): Solid organ transplant. In: Applied Therapeutics: The Clinical Use of Drugs. Vancouver, WA, Applied Therapeutics, 1995.

31. McCarthy S, McMullen M: Autosomal dominant polycystic kidney disease: pathophysiology and treatment. J Am Nephrol Nurses' Assoc 24:45–57, 1997.

32. Marsh JT, Brown WS, Wolcott D, et al: RhuEPO treatment improves brain and cognitive function of anemic dialysis patients. Kidney Int 39:155–163, 1990.

33. Nissenson AR: Epoetin and cognitive function. Am J Kidney Dis 20(Suppl 1):21–24, 1992.

34. Pfettscher SA: Assessment of the learner: physiological readiness. Adv Ren Replace Ther 2:191–198, 1995.

35. Lancaster L: Systemic manifestations of renal failure. In: Lancaster L (ed): Core Curriculum for Nephrology Nursing. Pitman, NJ, American Nephrology Nurses' Association, 1995.

36. Gotch F, Keen M: Care of the patient on hemodialysis. In: Cogan MG, Schoenfeld PY (eds): Introduction to Dialysis, 2nd ed. New York, Churchill Livingstone, 1991.

37. Ritz E, Rambausek M, Mall G, et al: Cardiac changes in uraemia and their possible relationship to cardiovascular instability on dialysis. Nephrol Dial Transplant (Suppl 1):93–97, 1990.

38. Foley RN, Parfrey PS, Harnett JD: Left ventricular hypertrophy in dialysis patients Semin Dial 5:34–41, 1992.

39. Smith SH: Uremic pericarditis in chronic renal failure: nursing implications. J Am Nephrol Nurses' Assoc 20:432–439, 1993.

40. Kaupke C, Vaziri N: Pleural complications in end-stage renal disease. Semin Dial 4:189–197, 1991.

41. Eschbach JW, Abdulhodi MH, Brown JK, et al: Recombinant human erythropoietin in anemic patients with end-stage renal disease. Ann Intern Med 111:992–1000, 1989.

42. Fishbane S, Ungureanu V-D, Maesaka JK, et al: The safety of intravenous iron dextran in hemodialysis patients. Am J Kidney Dis 28:529–534, 1996.

43. Robbins KC, Sender JM, Kerhulas S, et al: Iron management in ESRD and the role of the nephrology nurse. J Am Nephrol Nurses' Assoc 24:265–272, 1997.

44. Evans RW, Rader B, Manninen DL, et al: The quality of life of hemodialysis recipients treated with recombinant human erythropoietin. JAMA 263:825–830, 1990.

45. Jensen SR, Eby SR, McMurray SD, et al: Clinical experience with erythropoietin in continuous ambulatory peritoneal dialysis. J Am Nephrol Nurses' Assoc 19:542–577, 1992.

46. Levin NW: Session II: The impact of epoetin alfa: quality of life and hematocrit level. Am J Kidney Dis 20(Suppl 1):16–20, 1992.

47. Lundin AP, Delano BG, Quinn-Cefaro R: Perspectives on the improvement of quality of life with epoetin alfa therapy. Pharmacotherapy 10:22S–26S, 1990.

48. Morris PJ: Kidney Transplantation: Principles and Practice. Philadelphia, W.B. Saunders, 1994.

49. Yucha CB: Renal control of calcium. ANNA J 20:440–446, 1993.

50. Yucha CB: Renal control of phosphorus and magnesium. J Am Nephrol Nurses' Assoc 20:447–453, 1993.

51. Emmett M, Simon MD, Kirkpatrick WG, et al: Calcium acetate control of serum phosphorus in hemodialysis patients. Am J Kidney Dis 17:544–550, 1991.

52. Mai ML, Emmett M, Sheikh MS, et al: Calcium acetate, an effective phosphorus binder in patients with renal failure. Kidney Int 36:690–695, 1989.

53. Nolan CR, Califano JR, Butzin CA: Influence of calcium acetate or calcium citrate on intestinal aluminum absorption. Kidney Int 38:937–941, 1990.

54. Bommer J, Kugel M, Schwobel B, et al: Improved sexual function during recombinant human erythropoietin therapy. Nephrol Dial Transplant 5:204–207, 1990.

55. Hou S, Orkowski J, Pahl M, et al: Pregnancy in women with end-stage renal disease: treatment of anemia and premature labor. Am J Kidney Dis 21:16–22, 1993.

56. Zarifian AA: Sexual dysfunction in the male end stage renal disease patient. J Am Nephrol Nurses' Assoc 19:527–532, 1992.

57. Shoop KL: Pruritus in end stage renal disease. J Am Nephrol Nurses' Assoc 21:147–153, 1994.

58. Keen ML, Lancaster LE, Binkley LS: Hemodialysis. In: Lancaster L (ed): Core Curriculum for Nephrology Nursing. Pitman, NJ, American Nephrology Nurses' Association, 1995.

59. Keen M, Gotch F: Dialyzers and delivery systems. In: Cogan MG, Schoenfeld PY (eds): Introduction to Dialysis, 2nd ed. New York, Churchill Livingstone, 1991.

60. Anonymous: Renal and urologic care. In: Nursing Procedures. Springhouse, PA, Springhouse Corporation, 1996.

61. Sargent J, Gotch F: Principles and biophysics of dialysis. In: Maher J (ed): Replacement of Renal Function by Dialysis, 2nd ed. Dordrecht, Kluwer Academic, 1989.

62. Almeida A, Van Stone JC: Dialysate sodium. Semin Dial 2:176–179, 1989.

63. Henrich WL: Hemodynamic instability during hemodialysis. Kidney Int 30:605–612, 1986.

64. Carbone V: Hemodialysis using the Permcath double lumen catheter. ANNA J 15:171–173, 1988.

65. Fan PY: Acute vascular access: new advances. Adv Ren Replace Ther 1:90–98, 1994.

66. Fan PY, Schwab SJ: Vascular access: concepts for the 1990s. J Am Soc Nephrol 3:1–11, 1992.

67. Levin A, Mason AJ, Kailash KJ, et al: Prevention of hemodialysis subclavian catheter infections by topical povidone-iodine. Kidney Int 40:934–938, 1991.

68. Maki DG, Ringer M, Alvarado CJ: Prospective randomised trial of povidone-iodine, alcohol, and chlorhexidine for prevention of infection association with central venous and arterial catheters. Lancet 338:339–343, 1991.

69. Bander SJ, Schwab SJ: Central venous angioaccess for hemodialysis and its complications. Semin Dial 5:121–128, 1992.

70. Goldstein MB: Prevention of sepsis from central vein dialysis catheters. Semin Dial 5:106–107, 1992.

71. Hartigan MF, Thomas-Hawkins C: Circulatory access for hemodialysis. In: Lancaster L (ed): Core Curriculum for Nephrology Nursing, 3rd ed. Pitman, NJ, American Nephrology Nurses' Association, 1995.

72. Ouwendyk M, Helferty M: Central venous catheter management: how to prevent the complications. J Am Nephrol Nurses' Assoc 23:572–583, 1996.

73. Northsea CL: Continuous quality improvement: improving catheter patency using urokinase. J Am Nephrol Nurses' Assoc 23:567–571, 1996.

74. Counts CS: Potential complications of the internal vascular access: implications for nursing care. Dial Transplant 22, 1993.

75. Feldman HI, Held PJ, Hutchinson JT, et al: Hemodialysis vascular access morbidity in the United States. Kidney Int 43:1091–1096, 1993.

76. Gaylord GM, Taber TE: Long-term hemodialysis access salvage: problems and challenges for nephrologists and interventional radiologists. J Vasc Interven Radiol 3:103–107, 1993.

77. Hartigan MF: Vascular access and nephrology nursing practice: existing views and rationales for change. Adv Ren Replace Ther 1:155–162, 1994.

78. Beathard GA: The treatment of vascular access dysfunction: a nephrologist's view and experience. Adv Ren Replace Ther 1:131–147, 1994.

79. Schwab SJ, Raymond JR, Saeed M, et al: Prevention of hemodialysis fistula thrombosis: early detection of venous stenosis. Kidney Int 36:707–711, 1989.

80. Stein P: Perioperative considerations of vascular access for dialysis. AORN J 60:947–958, 1994.

81. Kaufman JL: What is the duty of the surgeon in dialysis vascular access? Contemp Dial Nephrol 18:18–21, 1997.

82. Schwab S: What can be done to preserve vascular access for dialysis? Semin Dial 4:152–153, 1991.

83. Brunier GM: Calcium/phosphorus imbalances, aluminum toxicity, and renal osteodystrophy. ANNA J 21:171–177, 1994.

84. Prowant BF, Gallagher NM: Peritoneal dialysis. In: Lancaster L (ed): Core Curriculum for Nephrology Nursing, 3rd ed. Pitman, NJ, American Nephrology Nurses' Association, 1995.

85. Gokal R, Ash SR, Helfrich GB, et al: Peritoneal catheters and exit-site practices: toward optimum peritoneal access. Perit Dial Int 13:29–39, 1993.

86. Lewis SL, Prowant BF, Douglas C, et al: Nursing practice related to peritoneal catheter exit site care and infections. J Am Nephrol Nurses' Assoc 23:609–617, 1996.

87. Luzar MA: Exit-site infections in continuous ambulatory peritoneal dialysis: a review. Perit Dial Int 11:333–340, 1991.

88. Lowance DC: Factors and guidelines to be considered in offering treatment to patients with end-stage renal disease: a personal opinion. Am J Kidney Dis 21:679–683, 1993.

89. Pfettscher SA: Socioeconomic and Cultural Variables Influencing ESRD Treatment Decision-Making. Unpublished dissertation, 1991.

90. Wolfsson M, Strong C, Hamel K, et al: Difficulty accepting lifestyle limitations after the abrupt onset of end-stage renal disease, Adv Ren Replace Ther 2:246–254, 1995.

91. Chielewski C, Zellers L, Eyer J: Continuous arteriovenous hemofiltration in the patient with hepatorenal syndrome. Crit Care Nurs Clin North Am 2:115–121, 1990.

92. Highley RB: Continuous arteriovenous hemofiltration: a case study. Crit Care Nurse 16:37–40, 1996.

93. Merrill RH: The technique of slow continuous ultrafiltration. J Crit Illness 6:289–294, 1991.

94. Price C: Continuous renal replacement therapy, from a professional nursing perspective. Nephrol News Issues 3:31–36, 1989.

95. Price CA: Continuous arteriovenous ultrafiltration: a monitoring guide for ICU nurses. Crit Care Nurse 9:12–19, 1989.

96. Schanbacher BA, Lancaster L: Renal Transplantation. In: Lancaster L (ed): Core Curriculum for Nephrology Nursing, 3rd ed. Pitman, NJ, American Nephrology Nurses' Association, 1995.

97. Davenport A, Will E, Davidson A: Improved cardiovascular stability during continuous modes of renal replacement therapy in critically ill patients with acute hepatic and renal failure. Crit Care Med 21:328–338, 1993.

98. Lawyer LA, Velasco A: Continuous arteriovenous hemodialysis in the ICU. Crit Care Nurse 9:29–41, 1989.

99. Ashton D, Mehta R, Ward D, et al: Recent advances in continuous renal replacement therapy: citrate anticoagulated continuous arteriovenous hemodialysis. J Am Nephrol Nurses' Assoc 18:263–267, 1991.

100. Lievaart A, Voerman HJ: Nursing management of continuous arteriovenous hemodialysis. Heart Lung 20:152–158, 1991.

101. Hilton B, Starzonski R: Family decision making about living-related kidney donation. J Am Nephrol Nurses' Assoc 21:346–381, 1994.

102. Salvatierra O: Renal transplantation. In: Glenn J (ed): Urologic Surgery, 4th ed. Philadelphia, W.B. Saunders, 1991.

103. Evans RW, Orians CE, Ascher NL: The potential supply of organ donors. JAMA 267:239–246, 1992.

104. Hauser SP: Case management of the kidney transplant patient. J Am Nephrol Nurses' Assoc 22:369–375, 1995.

105. Rao KV: Mechanism, pathophysiology, diagnosis and management of renal transplant rejection. Med Clin North Am 74:1039–1057, 1990.

106. Rubin RH, Tolkoff-Rubin NE: The impact of infection on the outcome of transplantation. Transplant Proc 23:2068–2074, 1991.

107. Grumke J, King K: Missouri Kidney Program's patient-education program: a 10 year review. Dial Transplant 23:691–712, 1994.

108. Anonymous: Initiation or withdrawal of dialysis in end stage renal disease: guidelines for the health care team. New York, National Kidney Foundation, 1996.

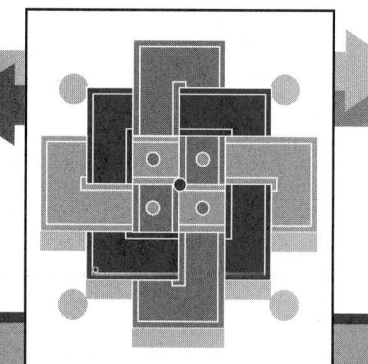

Endocrine Disorders

Taking Bold Steps to Improve Patient Care

In my position as a clinical nurse specialist (CNS), I frequently provide direct patient care to patients with complex cases. I first met T. on the Friday morning that she transferred to the intensive care unit (ICU) from the intermediate care unit. Her condition was diagnosed as deteriorating diabetic ketoacidosis (DKA). My associate and I began assessing T.'s condition as we settled her into the room. In my assessment of her, I decided that T. had something more than DKA. Our first concern was a pH of 7.0 that had persisted for about 8 hours in spite of hydration and insulin drip therapy. A Foley catheter was inserted, and her urine output was less than 10 mL over several hours. She complained of abdominal pain and was lethargic.

Once T. was settled and initial orders had been received and initiated, her husband arrived at the bedside. He was distraught because she had no chronic diseases and had been to her family physician just 2 days ago for "flu-like" symptoms. Her condition worsened, and she was admitted to the hospital. He was worried and shared that they were supposed to celebrate their twenty-fifth wedding anniversary in 2 weeks.

T.'s diagnosis puzzled me because she had no history of diabetes and had exhibited no symptoms that would indicate a new onset of the disease. I began to investigate her laboratory values and past medical history. We continued to adjust her insulin and fluids based on assessment and laboratory values. I spoke with the surgeon who was consulted for T.'s abdominal pain. He planned to observe her and felt that surgery was not indicated at this time. I ques-

tioned the diagnosis and asked the resident who was covering her case whether amylase and lipase had been drawn. I felt that the diagnosis of DKA was not appropriate. I kept checking the pH because it was not responding to fluid and insulin therapy. During the course of the day, we repeatedly asked for some orders for bicarbonate. The resident stated, "we don't treat pH 7.1 with bicarb, the fluids will take care of it." I was frustrated with that response. T.'s husband became more worried and needed reassurance and an explanation of what was happening to her. I continued to keep him informed and encouraged him to remain at her bedside.

Later in the early evening, the resident called a cardiologist to insert a pulmonary artery catheter for monitoring fluid status. The cardiologist ordered bicarbonate for the pH that still remained at 7.1. T.'s urine output remained minimal. Her level of consciousness had decreased as she became more lethargic. The fluid therapy and insulin drip continued to be titrated in an attempt to control her hyperglycemia and acidosis. T. was also given morphine for her severe abdominal pain.

I returned the next day to care for T. and learned that, during the night, a bicarbonate drip had been initiated. I also found that her amylase and lipase levels were elevated. I reported to the attending physician the changes in level of consciousness and requested renal and gastrointestinal consultations. The attending physician wanted to continue to observe the patient before ordering any consultations. The surgeon came in to check on T. and I updated him on her condition and again requested the consultations. He agreed and wrote the orders. I notified each specialist, and we soon confirmed a diagnosis of acute pancreatitis with secondary hyperglycemia. Fluids were adjusted, and the insulin drip was continued to try to regulate the hyperglycemia.

T. seemed to be trying to stabilize when I left. On my return the next day, I found her on the ventilator. During the night, she had developed some respiratory distress and required intubation to prevent cardiopulmonary arrest. During that day, she began to improve. The additional support to the respiratory system as well as the fluid management by nephrology and the management of pancreatitis by the gastrointestinal physicians enabled the healing process to begin.

One week after she arrived in the ICU, T. was sitting up in the chair and preparing to transfer back to the general floor. Within the next week, she was discharged home. We later received a letter from T. and her husband saying that she was doing well and that they would be going on a cruise to celebrate their anniversary.

I could not keep T. and her medical plan out of my mind and decided to bring the matter to the attention of the vice president of professional affairs. My concern was that this could happen again. We needed to address the issue of residents caring for ICU patients and DKA in particular. I was told that the directors of the residency program would take care of the problem. During the next 6 months, I was involved with or was made aware of five more patients with the diagnosis of DKA. They included problems similar to those I had encountered with T.'s case. Even though the other cases were not as severe as T.'s, they convinced me

that I must do something to guarantee better care for this patient population.

My first step was again to alert the vice president of professional affairs of the cases in question. Next I presented the cases to the Pharmacy and Therapeutics (P & T) Committee and enlisted the pharmacists' help to develop a protocol to be used in the treatment of DKA. I got together a task force consisting of myself, the diabetic educator, the CNS for surgical services, the director of the medical section for the residency program, an internal medicine physician, and a pharmacist from P & T Committee. Through collaboration and the use of national standards for the treatment of DKA, we developed a hospital protocol for treatment of the patient with DKA. The protocol was sent to the internal medicine section, the P & T Committee, and the College of Medicine residency program. All these areas endorsed the protocol. It is now available on all nursing units as a guide for residents and physicians to provide a quality plan of treatment for this patient population. Since the institution of this protocol, I have seen no new cases of DKA with the severe complications that occurred in T.'s case. We now have a baseline for assessment and a standardized plan for the care of these patients.

Georgiann Homuth, RN, MS, CCRN
Swedish American Health System
Machesney Park, Illinois

1998 AACN-3M Health Care Excellence in Clinical Practice Award Recipient

25

Endocrine Anatomy and Physiology

Karen L. Baker, Donna F. Hardwick, and Rubi Agana-Defensor

Objectives

After completing this chapter, the student will be able to:

1. Identify the anatomic structures of the basic endocrine glands.
2. Describe the physiologic functions of the basic endocrine glands.
3. Analyze the concept of negative feedback as a mechanism for hormonal regulation.
4. Contrast the endocrine system changes associated with the aging process.

Almost all the cells in the human body are influenced by the endocrine system. The overall purpose of the endocrine system is to maintain homeostasis despite constant changes in the external and internal environments. The endocrine system uses hormones to convey its information to nearly 50 billion target cells throughout the body.[1,2] Hormones are part of a communication chain linking the body systems with each other by specific hormonal receptors located on the surfaces of cells or within target cells to initiate their actions (Figure 25–1). The information transmitted results in the regulation of body functions and processes that govern our lives, such as growth and development, puberty and reproduction, metabolic functions, maintenance of internal homeostasis, and our response to stressors.

A hormone is typically defined as a chemical substance released by an endocrine gland that is transported through the blood to another tissue, where it acts to regulate the functions of the target tissue. The synthesis, rate, and degree of hormonal secretion are controlled by various regulatory mechanisms, such as the following: 1) spontaneous, basal, or direct hormone release; 2) endogenous rhythms of release (ultradian, circadian, monthly); 3) intervening influences such as stress, nutrition, illnesses, and other hormones; and 4) feedback control, in which the concentration of the hormone signals the need for more or less production. Negative feedback is the most common feedback control mechanism.

The body's goal is to maintain hormones in a homeostatic pattern, although endocrine glands have a natural tendency to oversecrete hormones. When too much hormonal function occurs, such as manifested by an elevated serum level or an excessive bodily function such as high blood pressure, a message *feeds back* to the endocrine gland. This *negative* feedback causes the gland to decrease its rate of secretion. This process is characteristic of the cyclic interaction of the anterior pituitary gland with the thyroid, adrenals, and gonads. Figure 25–2 illustrates this feedback mechanism.

Chemically, hormones are of three basic types: 1) steroids, 2) tyrosine (amino acid) derivatives, and 3) peptides or proteins (Table 25–1). Some hormones are secreted within seconds after the gland is stimulated and may develop full action within another few seconds to minutes, as in a trauma situation. The action of other hormones may require months for full effect, as in the example of the menstrual cycle. The quantity of hormones required to control most endocrine functions is incredibly minuscule, with concentrations in the blood ranging from as little as 1 picogram (pg) in each milliliter of blood up to a few micrograms per milliliter of blood.

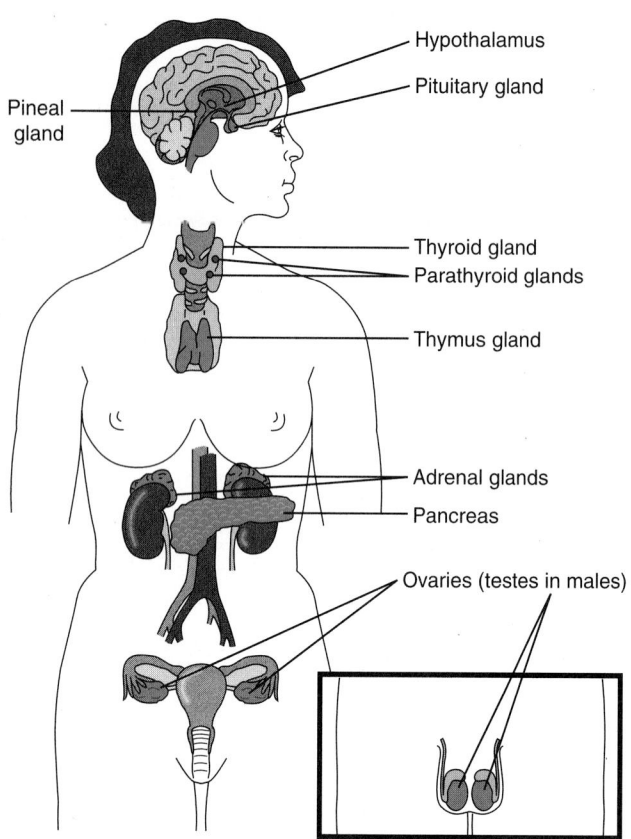

Figure 25–1

Anatomic location of the endocrine glands. (From Hansen M: Pathophysiology. Philadelphia, W.B. Saunders, 1998, p 798.)

STRUCTURE AND FUNCTION OF THE ENDOCRINE GLANDS

Hypothalamus

The hypothalamus is considered the "master controller" of most of the body's hormones. It acts as a link between the central nervous system and the endocrine system because it coordinates central nervous system input with hormone release. The hypothalamus contains hormone-producing cells, neurologic tissue, and neurotransmitters. The hypothalamus is in direct and indirect contact with all the sensory organs and is thereby involved in the control of behavior patterns that stem from basic biologic urges (i.e., feeding, drinking, body temperature regulation, sweating, pleasure and pain responses, activity and sleep, circulation, and respiration). In addition, the hypothalamus influences fluid and electrolyte balance and cell metabolism by the production and release of hypothalamic hormones, which directly stimulate the pituitary gland. These hormones are known as releasing hormones, such as corticotropin-releasing hormone (CRH), gonadotropin-releasing hormone (GnRH), growth hormone–releasing hormone (GHRH), and thyrotropin-releasing hormone (TRH), and inhibiting

hormones such as prolactin-inhibitory hormone (PIH), melanocyte-inhibitory hormone (MIH), and growth hormone–inhibitory hormone (somatostatin). The hypothalamus and the pituitary gland function as an integrated unit, with primary direction from the hypothalamus. The two parts of the pituitary gland are regulated differently by the hypothalamus. Each maintains separate linkages with the hypothalamus and secretes its own set of hormones. The posterior pituitary receives its signals from the hypothalamus through nerves; the anterior pituitary receives signals through blood vessels (Figure 25–3).

Pituitary Gland

The pituitary gland (or hypophysis) resides below the hypothalamus in a cartilage cover known as the sella turcica, which is just above the roof of the mouth (see Figure 25–1). The pituitary gland is really two distinct glands: the anterior pituitary gland and the posterior pituitary gland. It is approximately 1 cm in size and weighs 0.5 to 0.75 g.

Directly above the pituitary gland are the optic chiasm and the optic nerves. Other nearby vital tissues include the third ventricle, the sphenoidal and cavernous sinuses, the internal carotid arteries, and cranial nerves III to VI. Regulation of pituitary hormones is maintained by a continuous feedback system from target organs and direct hormone involvement.

Anterior Pituitary Gland

The anterior pituitary is the larger portion of the pituitary gland and produces seven hormones: growth hormone, thyrotropin or thyroid-stimulating hormone (TSH), adrenocorticotropin (ACTH), follicle-stimulating hormone (FSH), luteinizing hormone (LH), melanocyte-stimulating hormone (MSH), and prolactin (PRL). Growth hormone is an example of an anterior pituitary hormone that exerts its effect directly on tissue growth and protein synthesis. TSH stimulates the thyroid gland. ACTH stimulates the production of cortisol and aldosterone by the adrenal cortex (Figure 25–4).

Posterior Pituitary Gland

The posterior lobe of the pituitary gland comprises 25% of the gland. It secretes two hormones: oxytocin and antidiuretic hormone (ADH) or vasopressin. These hormones are produced by the hypothalamus, but they travel down nerve endings to the posterior lobe of the pituitary, where they are stored for future release. Oxytocin is mainly responsible for the milk letdown reflex and for contraction of the uterus. ADH maintains fluid balance by controlling the permeabil-

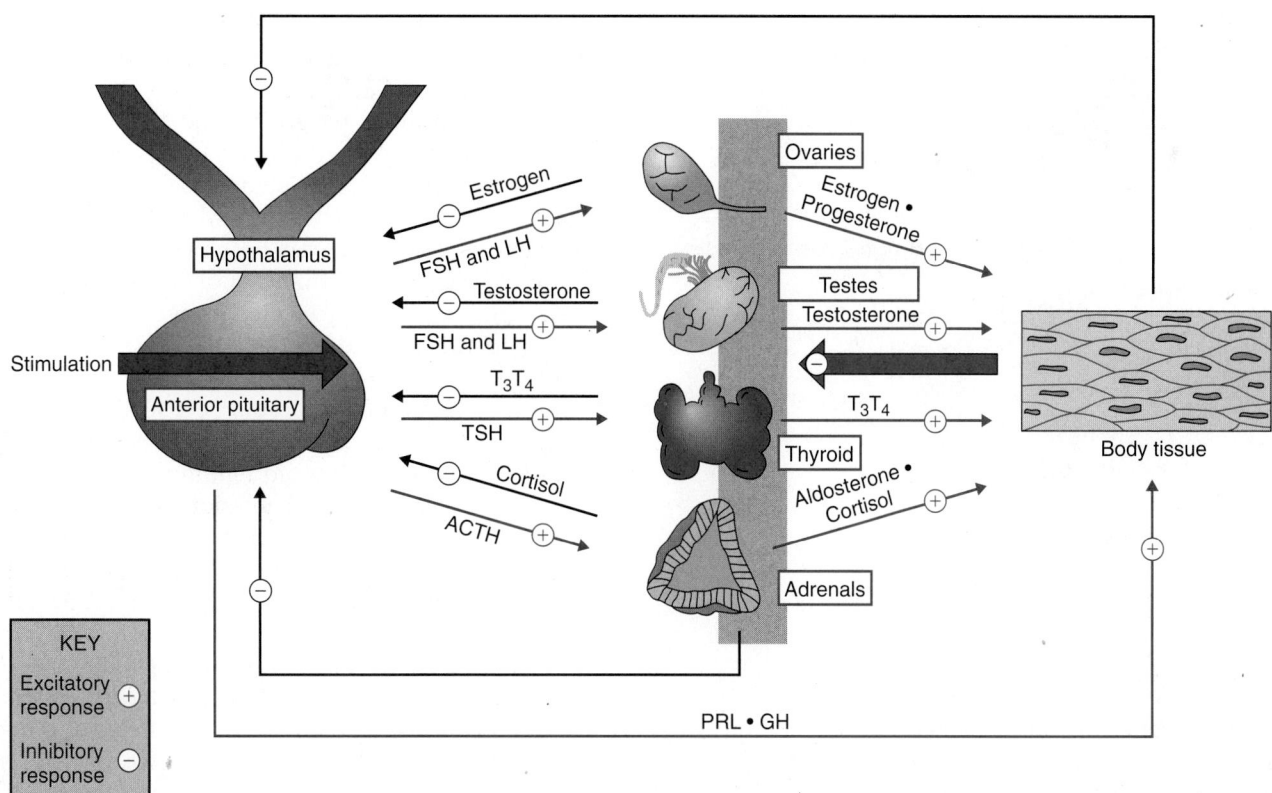

Figure 25–2

The feedback system of the hypothalamic–pituitary–target gland axis. ACTH, adrenocorticotropin; FSH, follicle-stimulating hormone; LH, luteinizing hormone; T₃, triiodothyronine; T₄, thyroxine. (From Ignatavicius D, Workman L, Mishler M: Medical-Surgical Nursing. Philadelphia, W.B. Saunders, 1999.)

TABLE 25–1
Chemical Makeup of Hormones

Steroids	Amino Acid Analogs	Peptides
(Product of Cholesterol Breakdown)	(Derivative of the Amino Acid Tyrosine)	(Large Proteins or Chains of Proteins)
Adrenal Cortex	**Thyroid**	**Anterior Pituitary**
Glucocorticoids (cortisol)	Thyroxine (T₄)	Adrenocorticotropin
Mineralocorticoids (aldosterone)	Triiodothyronine (T₃)	Growth hormone
Androgens		Follicle-stimulating hormone
	Adrenal Medulla	Luteinizing hormone
Ovaries	Epinephrine	Prolactin
Progesterone	Norepinephrine	Thyroid-stimulating hormone
Estrogen		Melanocyte-stimulating hormone
Testes		**Posterior Pituitary**
Testosterone		Antidiuretic hormone (Vasopressin)
		Oxytocin
Placenta		
Estrogen		**Pancreas**
Progesterone		Glucagon
		Insulin
		Parathyroid
		Parathyroid hormone
		Thyroid
		Calcitonin

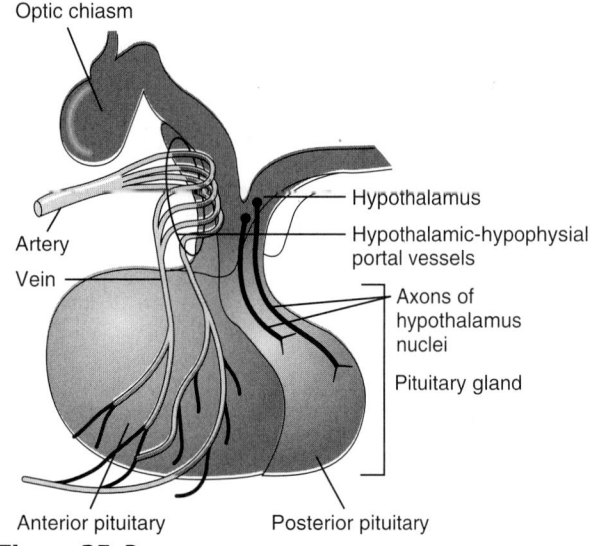

Figure 25–3

Anatomic relationship of the hypothalamus and the pituitary gland, with vascular and neurologic connections. (From Hansen M: Pathophysiology. Philadelphia, W.B. Saunders, 1998, p 800.)

ity of the collecting tubules and distal renal tubules, resulting in water reabsorption and decreasing plasma osmolality. Secretion of ADH into the circulation is controlled by the osmoreceptors in the hypothalamus. In the dehydrated patient, increased secretion of ADH occurs in an attempt to maintain appropriate osmolality and fluid balance. In the presence of high enough concentrations of ADH, vasoconstriction occurs, resulting in the elevation of blood pressure.

Thyroid Gland

The thyroid gland is located in the anterior aspect of the neck, just below the thyroid cartilage (see Figure 25–1). The gland is composed of two lateral lobes that wrap around the sides of the trachea and connect in front with a thin tissue called the isthmus. The thyroid centers vertically between the cricoid cartilage and the suprasternal notch. Each lobe is approximately 3 cm $\times$ 2 cm, and, in adults, it weighs around 15 g. The lobes are supported by the sternothyroid and cricothyroid muscles. The thyroid is a symmetric gland that is smooth and non-nodular. Thyroid enlargement or goiters frequently present in a posterior direction from the thyroid because of the relation to surrounding muscle groups. The recurrent laryngeal nerve lies proximal to each thyroid lobe, and the vagus nerve lies distal to each lobe. This close innervation is monitored during thyroid surgical procedures. The thyroid has an abundant blood supply with a blood flow rate of 5 mL/g per minute. The thyroid innominate mammary artery and the superior and inferior thyroid arteries stem from the carotid and subclavian arteries. Venous drainage flows from the superior, middle, and inferior thyroid veins into the internal jugular and subclavian veins.

The thyroid gland contains numerous follicles and parafollicular cells; each follicle is filled with colloid and has an epithelial membrane that secretes into the interior of the follicle. Thyroglobulin, a glycoprotein, is generated within the follicle and undergoes a process of iodination. Iodine, absorbed from the gastrointestinal tract and into the blood as iodide, is removed from the blood by the thyroid for this process. Thyroglobulin then biosynthesizes thyroxine (T_4) and triiodothyronine (T_3). The main structural component of the thyroid hormones T_4 and T_3 is the trace element iodine. Thyroglobulin can store or release T_4 or T_3 as needed by the body. The parafollicular cells of the thyroid gland secrete calcitonin, a hormone that functions to lower serum calcium levels.

When T_4 and T_3 are released from the thyroid gland and enter the blood, all but less than 1% immediately binds to thyroxine binding proteins. Consequently, the hormones are released to the tissue cells slowly. The

Figure 25–4

Interactive effects of the hypothalamic and anterior pituitary hormones. ACTH, adrenocorticotropin; CRH, corticotropin-releasing hormone; FSH, follicle-stimulating hormone; GH, growth hormone; GnRH, gonadotropin-releasing hormone; GRH, growth hormone–releasing hormone; LH, luteinizing hormone; MSH, melanocyte-stimulating hormone; PRH, prolactin-releasing hormone; T_3, triiodothyronine; T_4, thyroxine; TRH, thyrotropin-releasing hormone; TSH, thyroid-stimulating hormone.

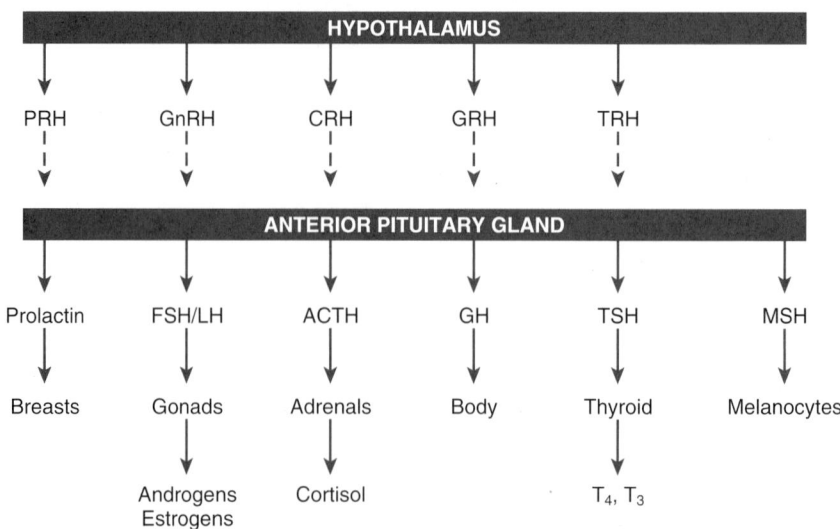

unbound hormones are the biologically active forms of the thyroid hormones. T_4 is secreted from the thyroid gland in much greater quantities than T_3. The majority of T_4 is deiodinated to T_3 within the tissue cells. T_3 is five times more potent than T_4. If unused, thyroid hormone is stored in the thyroid or is broken down by the liver and excreted into the stool. Similarly, dietary iodine not used by the thyroid is excreted through the renal system.

The thyroid hormones, specifically T_4 and T_3, stimulate sodium and potassium adenosine triphosphatase (ATPase) in most tissues. Consequently, the rate of sodium and potassium transport through cell membranes is increased. Because this process uses energy and produces heat, it is believed that this is one way in which the hormones increase the body's metabolic rate.

Additionally, the thyroid hormones improve muscle contractility and play a role in increasing diastolic contraction of the heart. Hypoxic and hypercapnic drive are affected by the thyroid hormones, as well as gastrointestinal motility, brain cerebration, and glucose availability. Other endocrine functions, mainly cortisol production, are also influenced by thyroid levels.

Thyroid gland function is modulated by hypothalamic and pituitary hormones. Hypothalamic TRH stimulates pituitary secretion of TSH, which follows a circadian rhythm in a pulsatile fashion with a peak level in the middle of the night. TSH, in turn, stimulates the thyroid gland to secrete T_4 and T_3 into the general circulation. Normal thyroid levels provide negative feedback to the pituitary gland and hypothalamus (Figure 25–5A). Feedback can be artificially altered by medications to stimulate or inhibit thyroid release.

Parathyroid Gland

The four parathyroid glands usually lie symmetrically superior and inferior to the thyroid gland (see Figure 25–1). They may also be found in the mediastinum, and some patients have a fifth gland. The glands consist primarily of chief cells that secrete parathyroid hormone (PTH). In conjunction with calcitonin and vitamin D, PTH aids in homeostasis of calcium regulation in the extracellular fluid, which is essential for life. PTH acts directly on the renal tubular lumen and on the bone osteoclasts to increase absorption of calcium into the extracellular fluid. Calcium circulates in the "free" or ionized state or it is bound to albumin. Ionized calcium, the active biologic form, serves as a readily available source of calcium if needed.

The PTH feedback system is stimulated by low ionized calcium blood levels. PTH can signal the decrease in renal excretion of calcium and the increase in intestinal absorption of calcium, assuming the pres-

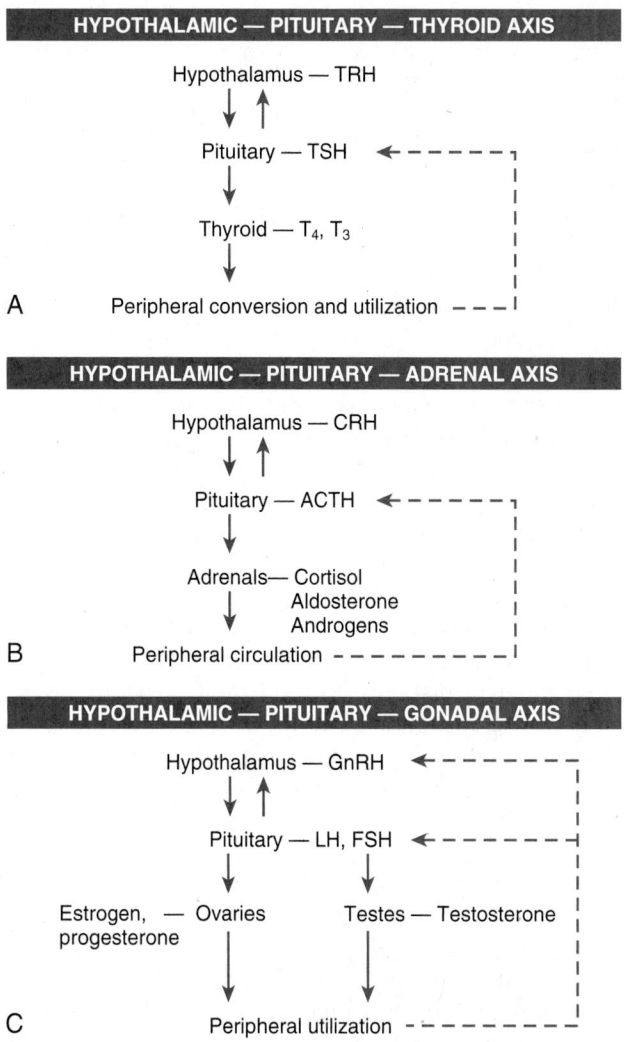

Figure 25–5

A, Hypothalamic–pituitary–thyroid axis. B, Hypothalamic–pituitary–adrenal axis. C, Hypothalamic–pituitary–gonadal axis. ACTH, adrenocorticotropin; CRH, corticotropin-releasing hormone; FSH, follicle-stimulating hormone; GnRH, gonadotropin-releasing hormone; LH, luteinizing hormone; T_3, triiodothyronine; T_4, thyroxine; TRH, thyrotropin-releasing hormone; TSH, thyroid-stimulating hormone.

ence of adequate vitamin D. Because the majority of calcium is stored in bones, PTH functions, further, to cause a rapid absorption of calcium from bones to meet extracellular needs. Calcitonin, a thyroid hormone, has an inverse relationship with PTH, in that it responds to elevated levels of serum calcium. It has limited ability, however, to reduce elevated serum calcium levels effectively in adults.

Pancreas

The pancreas weighs 60 g and is often described as having a head, a body, and a tail. It lies posterior to the stomach in a lateral position (see Figure 25–1). The main blood supply is from the mesenteric and celiac arteries. The pancreas is composed of two unique functions: exocrine and endocrine. The pancreas functions primarily as an exocrine gland, secreting enzymes for the digestion of food into the intestine. The islets of Langerhans, which comprise about 20% of the gland, serve the endocrine function of the gland. The islet cells consist of three types: 1) alpha cells, which secrete glucagon; 2) beta cells, which secrete insulin; and 3) delta cells, which secrete somatostatin.

Glucagon's principal activity is to increase the blood glucose level by accelerating the conversion of liver glycogen into glucose (gluconeogenesis). Insulin has an action opposite to that of glucagon. It decreases blood sugar level by promoting glucose entry from the blood into the cells. Blood glucose concentration is the major determinant of both insulin and glucagon secretion. An increase in serum glucose triggers insulin secretion and suppresses glucagon secretion.

Insulin is formed by the cleavage of proinsulin into active insulin and C peptide, a by-product. Fifty percent of insulin is secreted at a basal rate in pulsatile increments every 15 minutes. The other 50% is secreted in response to food intake. Insulin secretion has a circadian pattern, with greater amounts secreted in the morning and less in the afternoon and evening. The average secretion volume is 50 U per day for euglycemic adults. Insulin binds at the alpha subunit receptor sites of cell membranes, receiving glucose for transport into the cell. Insulin directs its effects on energy storage within the liver, muscle, and adipose tissue. Glycogen synthesis and storage occur in the liver in the presence of insulin. Insulin promotes protein and glycogen synthesis in muscle tissue. Insulin assists in triglyceride storage in adipocytes.

The absence of normal glucose levels triggers the processes of gluconeogenesis and glycogenolysis for carbohydrate generation. Type 1 diabetes mellitus is a state of beta cell destruction resulting in no available insulin for the cellular uptake of glucose. Impaired glucose tolerance (IGT) associated with hyperinsulinemia is a precursor to the development of type 2 diabetes mellitus. This disorder represents an index of insulin resistance or the inability of the cells to take up glucose in the presence of high circulating levels of insulin. Genetic susceptibility, obesity, and physical inactivity are contributing factors in the development of IGT and type 2 diabetes mellitus. Syndrome X comprises a potential central defect in which the consequences of insulin resistance and hyperinsulinemia affect lipid and blood pressure regulation.[3]

Adrenal Glands

An adrenal gland sits directly above the pole of each kidney (see Figure 25–1). Each gland weighs approximately 4 to 5 g and is structurally and functionally differentiated into two sections: cortex and medulla.

Adrenal Cortex

The outer portion, the adrenal cortex, comprises 90% of the gland by weight and is responsible for the production of glucocorticoids and mineralocorticoids. These hormones respond to physiologic stressors and modulate carbohydrate, fat, and protein metabolism as well as electrolyte balance. Androgens, responsible for the development of secondary sex characteristics, are also secreted by the adrenal cortex.

The adrenal cortex consists of three separate zones. The zone glomerulosa is the thin outer layer that secretes the mineralocorticoid aldosterone. Together, the zona fasciculata, the middle layer, and the zona reticularis, the inner layer, secrete the glucocorticoids (primarily cortisol) and the androgenic precursors. Synthesis of all adrenocortical hormones, which are steroid compounds, begins with the lipid cholesterol. Plasma lipoproteins are the major source of cholesterol for this process. A small amount of free cholesterol is present in the adrenal gland when rapid synthesis is required for hormonal production. Increased hydrolysis of stored cholesterol is necessary to replace the free cholesterol as it is used by the adrenal gland.

Aldosterone, the primary mineralocorticoid, influences extracellular fluid volume, blood pressure, and electrolyte balance by causing the kidneys to reabsorb sodium and, consequently, water and to excrete potassium. This complex process is influenced by several factors, such as serum levels of potassium, sodium, and ACTH and the activation of the renin–angiotensin system.

One of the primary mechanisms that controls the secretion of aldosterone is the potassium ion concentration in the extracellular fluid. Increased levels of potassium in the extracellular fluid stimulate the production of aldosterone by the adrenal cortex. Aldosterone increases the elimination of potassium by the kidneys in an attempt to maintain normal extracellular potassium levels. Decreased extracellular and intracellular potassium concentrations have the opposite effect. Low aldosterone production results in preservation of potassium by the kidneys. Changes in extracellular sodium may stimulate this same process of continuous intracellular and extracellular homeostasis. ACTH has only minor effects on the secretion of aldosterone. Complete absence of ACTH must be present to cause a deficiency of aldosterone.

A more complex process that controls aldosterone production is the renin–angiotensin pathway. This pathway is stimulated by a sudden change in blood pressure or a hypotensive episode. This change stimulates the juxtaglomerular cells of the kidney to secrete the enzyme renin. Renin and a plasma enzyme in the lung together convert angiotensinogen to angiotensin II. The presence of angiotensin II stimulates the adrenal cortex to increase its production of aldosterone, resulting in increased sodium reabsorption and water preservation. As a result, extracellular fluid volume is increased, with a resultant elevation in blood pressure. Angiotensin II is also a powerful vasoconstrictor that further assists in maintaining blood pressure.

Cortisol, the primary glucocorticoid, has many widespread effects on multiple body systems (Table 25–2). In times of physiologic or neurogenic stress, the anterior pituitary gland responds immediately by secreting ACTH. Within minutes, the adrenal gland responds by secreting cortisol. Cortisol promotes normal metabolism of carbohydrate, fat, and protein. During times of stress, cortisol production is exaggerated to support body systems in a "fight-or-flight" response. Stress would be a life-threatening event in the absence of cortisol.

During periods of stress, cortisol functions to maintain and raise serum blood sugar levels for energy use. To achieve this goal, cortisol depresses amino acid transport into muscle and other extrahepatic tissues and, consequently, protein synthesis. Further, cortisol

TABLE 25–2
Effects of Glucocorticoids

Target System	Consequences
Metabolism	Increase in gluconeogenesis Decrease in peripheral glucose uptake Insulin resistance Increase in glycogen synthesis Glycolysis, generally a catabolic process
Connective Tissue	Inhibition of fibroblasts causing loss of collagen and resulting in thinning of skin Easy bruising Poor wound healing
Bone and Calcium Metabolism	Inhibition of bone formation by decreasing cell proliferation Inhibition of RNA, protein, and collagen synthesis Stimulation of bone reabsorption leading to bone loss Stimulation of parathyroid hormone and vitamin D production and its effectiveness Reduction of gastrointestinal absorption of calcium
Growth and Development	Inhibition of growth in children secondary to decreased growth hormone
Hematologic and Immune System	Reduction in the number of mast cells Stabilization of lysosomal membranes, thus inhibiting release of histamine Decrease in capillary permeability Depression of phagocytosis Decrease of interleukin 1, which causes fever Atrophy of all lymphatic tissue
Cardiovascular System	Increase in cardiac output Increase in vascular tone Effects of catecholamines potentiated Regulation of adrenergic receptors Elevation of triglycerides and cholesterol because of an increase in lipolysis
Renal System	Increase in glomerular rate with electrolyte imbalances
Central Nervous System	Impairments in memory and concentration Insomnia with decreased REM sleep Increased stage II sleep Depression and acute "steroid psychosis"
Ophthalmologic System	Intraocular pressure thought to vary with cortisol level (paralleling the circadian rhythm of cortisol) Possible cataract formation
Other Hormones	Decrease in thyroid response to thyrotropin-releasing hormone Decrease in triiodothyronine because of a decrease in the conversion of thyroxine to triiodothyronine Decrease in the response of testes to luteinizing hormone leading to low testosterone levels Suppression of luteinizing hormone leading to low levels of estrogen and progesterone causing amenorrhea and anovulation

enhances protein catabolism, thereby mobilizing additional amino acids for transport to the liver for conversion into enzymes for several metabolic reactions. Amino acids may also be converted in the liver to glucose if reserves of glycogen and fat are low. This process is known as gluconeogenesis. Cortisol also promotes the mobilization of fatty acids from adipose tissue energy utilization.

The anti-inflammatory effects of cortisol have been a source of much research. The two primary effects include the ability of cortisol to block the initial stage of inflammation or to resolve inflammation rapidly if it has already begun. Because of this relationship, cortisol has been widely used as an effective anti-inflammatory agent in multiple disease processes.

The production of cortisol is regulated by the ACTH and the negative feedback mechanism. Low levels of cortisol stimulate the hypothalamus to produce CRH, which stimulates the pituitary to produce ACTH, which stimulates the adrenal cortex to produce cortisol. High levels of cortisol inhibit this process (see Figure 25–5B). The production of ACTH and of cortisol follows diurnal patterns. For example, cortisol peaks in the early morning shortly before awakening. Cortisol is also released in a pulsatile fashion throughout the day, with a gradual decline during the day reaching the lowest level during the initial stage of sleep. Individuals' light–dark cycles and feeding schedules dictate their own unique circadian rhythm. A disruption in this rhythm, such as a prolonged stay in the intensive care unit (ICU), may contribute to the phenomenon known as "ICU psychosis."[4]

Adrenal Medulla

The adrenal medulla, the inner portion of each adrenal gland, consists of chromaffin cells and accounts for 10% of the total adrenal weight. The sympathetic nervous system innervates the adrenal medulla. Stimulation by the adrenergic system causes the release of the catecholamines epinephrine and norepinephrine from the medulla. Catecholamines are both hormones and neurotransmitters. Neurotransmitters are chemical substances released from nerve endings that have local effects (see Chapter 38). The catecholamines are involved in the stress response and evoke adrenergic (elevated blood pressure, increased cardiac output), metabolic (increased rate of metabolism), and glycemic (glycogenolysis) responses. Thus, the adrenal medulla works in conjunction with the adrenal cortex to provide the body with extra resources to cope with stress.

Reproductive Glands

All sex hormones are controlled by a negative feedback system that stimulates the hypothalamus to secrete GnRH. GnRH then stimulates the anterior pituitary gland to release LH and FSH (see Figure 25–5C).

Ovaries

The female reproductive glands, the ovaries, are paired, oval organs. Each ovary is approximately 3 cm long, 2 cm wide, and 1 cm thick. These organs are usually located in the upper part of the pelvic cavity (see Figure 25–1). The two primary ovarian hormones are estrogen and progesterone. Estrogen is responsible for the development of the female secondary sex characteristics, such as increased growth of the uterus during puberty, and reestablishment of the endometrium after menstruation. Progesterone prepares the uterine endometrium for the reception and development of a fertilized ovum. The normal menstrual cycle pattern consists of the follicular phase, followed by the luteal phase (see Figure 25–5C).

Testes

The male reproductive organs, the testes, are oval and lie bilaterally in the scrotum. The scrotum serves as a protective shield and maintains a constant temperature, which is required for the sperm survival. Located in the pyramidal lobules of the testes are the seminiferous tubules. Embedded in the seminiferous tubules are Sertoli cells, which are responsible for spermatogenesis. Also embedded in the seminiferous tubules are Leydig cells, which secrete the androgens (testosterone).

Androgen production is controlled by the hypothalamic pituitary testicular axis (see Figure 25–5C) and is regulated by a negative feedback system. Low concentrations of testosterone stimulate GnRH release from the hypothalamus. In response, the pituitary releases LH. LH acts directly on the Leydig cells to release testosterone. A second negative feedback system, involving the pituitary and the Sertoli cells, controls spermatogenesis. FSH induces spermatogenesis. Once adequate spermatogenesis is established, the Sertoli cells produce a protein hormone called inhibin. Inhibin exerts an "inhibiting" action on the pituitary gland to halt the production of FSH.

Testosterone is perhaps the most important androgen of the male reproductive system. It is responsible for the development of the male external genitalia as well as changes in muscle bulk, skeletal growth, and male-pattern hair development. It is necessary for continued maintenance of these male characteristics, as well as for normal libido and functioning.

Cardiac and Renal Hormones

Any organ or tissue cell that produces hormones is part of the endocrine system. By this criterion, the kidneys and heart are members of the endocrine system.[5] Atrial natriuretic peptide (ANP) is a cardiac hormone released by the cardiac atrial muscle fibers in response to the overstretch of the atria (as seen in volume overload). ANP acts directly on the kidneys to cause a decrease in sodium reabsorption. This change results in an increased excretion of salt and, consequently, water, thereby reducing blood volume and blood pressure.

Erythropoietin, a glycoprotein, is produced primarily by the kidneys. It is unclear where exactly in the kidneys this hormone is produced. Erythropoietin stimulates red blood cell (RBC) production in the bone marrow and is released by the kidneys in proportion to the rate of RBC degradation. In addition, hypoxia causes a marked increase in the production of erythropoietin.

AGING INFLUENCE ON THE ENDOCRINE SYSTEM

Altered hormonal activity mirrors the theories of the aging process. The levels of most hormones and their responses to stimuli diminish by the age of 60 years. Changes in "self-regulation" are exemplified in autoimmune deficiencies such as type 2 diabetes and thyroid disorders. The "wear and tear" theory of aging may be reflected in the hypothalamus–pituitary–adrenal axis in the presence of stress. The "genetically programmed to stop" theory may be exhibited by the female reproductive hormones, estrogen and progesterone. The neuroendocrine system interacts extensively with the immune system; altered immune function may contribute to certain changes associated with aging. The quality of the endocrine feedback loop can then be affected, secondary to neurotransmitter changes.

Menopause occurs around the age of 50 years in women. There is a decline of estrogen and progesterone over several years before anovulation often referred to as a climacteric phase. Secondary effects of estrogen loss include changes in breast tissue, decreased bone density, and loss of the cardioprotective effects of this hormone. Women who have reached menopause have a marked increase in triglyceride and cholesterol levels, significantly raising their risk of coronary artery disease. The uterus and vagina decrease in size, elasticity, and lubrication, and the vaginal pH rises.

Male reproductive changes seen with aging include a decrease in spermatogenesis. Serum testosterone levels fall in older men, and this decrease can contribute to tissue changes in the prostate gland and loss of overall muscle mass. A compensating increase in serum LH may occur as a result of decreased testosterone.

Aging influences the way in which endocrine disease is manifested. A decrease in energy expenditure, lean body mass, basal metabolic rate, and physical activity is associated with aging. For example, a decrease in renal and liver clearance of cortisol and the loss of lean body mass contribute to decreased cortisol utilization. Injury and infection accentuate the lack of capacity of the metabolic response to stress.

Overall, hormone levels have a blunted amplitude, such as a lower peak level of cortisol, and peak concentrations occur earlier in the day and are not as high as in younger persons. Conversion of T_4 to T_3 is slowed in some persons after the age of 60 years. In addition, nocturnal surges of TSH diminish. Atrophy and fibrosis of the thyroid decrease levels of T_4, TSH, and T_3. Pancreatic changes result in increased glucose intolerance, peripheral insulin resistance, and hyperinsulinemia, which may be attributed to a sedentary lifestyle or obesity. Evidence indicates that growth hormone declines with age, specifically during the night.[6] With senescence, one also sees an increase in the sensitivity to ADH. Hormones that continue normal rates of secretion and receptor response are catecholamines and glucagon.

Key Concepts

➡ The endocrine system programs the body to maintain homeostasis of the metabolic processes as well as to promote growth and development.

➡ Most hormones are regulated by a negative feedback mechanism whereby sufficient levels of hormones signal the body to cease further production of more hormones.

➡ The target cells have specific receptor sites for hormones.

➡ Aging influences the endocrine system in various ways: circulating levels of some hormones are decreased, certain glands develop a diminished ability to respond to stimuli, and the stress response is reduced.

References

1. Kessler C: An overview of endocrine function and dysfunction. AACN Clin Issues Crit Care Nurs 3:289–299, 1992.
2. Kordon C, Bihoreau C: Integrated communication between the nervous, endocrine, and immune systems. Horm Res 31:100–104, 1989.
3. LeRoith D, Taylor S, Olefsky J: Diabetes Mellitus. Philadelphia, Lippincott–Raven, 1996, pp 509–577.
4. Robin N: Clinical Handbook of Endocrinology and Metabolic Disease. New York, Parthenon Publishing Group, 1996.
5. Ignatavicius D, Workman L, Mishler M: Medical-Surgical Nursing: A Nursing Process Approach. Philadelphia: W.B. Saunders, 1995.
6. Peterson A, Baker K: Endocrine Function in Gerontology Nursing. St. Louis, C.V. Mosby, 1996.

26

Endocrine Assessment

Karen L. Baker, Rubi Agana-Defensor, and Donna F. Hardwick

Objectives

After completing this chapter, the student will be able to:

1. Conduct a health history pertinent to the endocrine system.
2. Select key components of a physical examination of a patient with a suspected endocrine disorder.
3. Distinguish the normal variations in the physical examination of the endocrine system that are associated with aging.

The assessment of the endocrine system of a patient relies on findings from the triad of history, physical examination, and laboratory testing. The last item may involve measurements of hormone levels or their metabolites in plasma or urine either in the basal state or in response to provocative testing.

Some syndromes of hormonal excess or deficiency display overt problems in which the initial presentation may be life-threatening, such as diabetic ketoacidosis and severe thyrotoxicosis. In other syndromes, the clinical presentation is more often insidious, and the clinician must rely on laboratory testing and vague symptoms to establish a diagnosis. This is especially true in the early stages of most endocrine problems. For example, elderly patients with symptoms of hypothyroidism may be overlooked if their symptoms are attributed to the aging process. Thus, many manifestations of endocrine diseases should be considered in the differential diagnosis of many common complaints, such as weakness, fatigue, vague gastrointestinal discomfort, hypertension, and changes in weight. Patients with chronic endocrinopathies may cite these secondary complications as troublesome because they interfere with their quality of life.

HEALTH HISTORY

The health history often focuses on symptoms that are the patient's chief complaint. Individual presentation may vary, yet asking specific questions may help to illustrate the clinical picture and to establish a diagnosis. Most endocrinopathies have a subtle presentation until reserves have been reached, so numerous combinations of symptoms may appear along the continuum of the disease process (Table 26–1).

Medical and Family History

For every patient, the nurse should elicit information regarding endocrine problems or associated conditions such as autoimmune disease, tuberculosis, or fungal disease. Common autoimmune disorders or autoantibodies are related to Hashimoto's thyroiditis, Addison's disease, and diabetes mellitus. Does the patient have a history of head and neck radiation in childhood that may have induced thyroid changes? The nurse should identify all the medications the patient is currently taking or has recently taken, for example, a recent history of steroid use for acute or chronic diseases. The nurse should ask the patient whether he or she has used over-the-counter cortisone cream or taken any body-building drugs? Does the patient smoke or chew tobacco, and what is his or her estimation of alcohol and recreational drug use? These social behaviors may exacerbate endocrine symptoms. Family history taking is beneficial, specifically with first-degree relatives.

Review of Systems

The nurse should query patients regarding changes in shoe, hat, or ring size and the fit of their clothes.

TABLE 26–1
Hormonal Activity Suggested by Clinical Findings

Clinical Findings	Hormonal Influence
Hemodynamic Regulation	
Hypertension	↑ Catecholamines; ↑ aldosterone; ↑ ACTH/cortisol; ↑ GH
Tachycardia	↑ Catecholamines; ↑ FT$_4$; ↑ GH; ↑ aldosterone; ↑ cortisol; ↓ PTH
Body temperature	↑ Cortisol; ↑ FT$_4$ (heat intolerance); ↓ FT$_4$, ↑ rT$_3$ (cold intolerance)
Hypotension	↓ ACTH/cortisol; ↑ catecholamines (orthostatic); ↓ aldosterone
Electrocardiographic changes	↑/↓ PTH; ↑ catecholamines (dysrhythmias); ↑/↓ ACTH/cortisol
Gastrointestinal Disturbances	
Nausea and vomiting	↑ PTH; ↓ ACTH/cortisol; ↓ insulin; ↑ catecholamines
Constipation	↑ Catecholamines; ↑ GH; ↓ ADH; ↑ PTH
Anorexia	↓ ACTH/cortisol; ↑ PTH
Diarrhea	↓ ACTH/cortisol; ↓ insulin (gastroparesis)
Abdominal pain	↓ ACTH/cortisol; ↑ PTH; ↑ thyroid
Polyphagia	↓ Insulin
Polydipsia	↓ Insulin
Weight loss	↑ Catecholamines; ↑ FT$_4$; ↓ ACTH/cortisol; ↓ insulin; ↓ AVP (diabetes insipidus)
Weight gain	↑ ACTH/cortisol; ↑ aldosterone (fluid retention); ↓ insulin (↑ glucose); ↑ ADH (fluid retention); ↓ FT$_4$, ↑ rT$_3$
Fluid and Electrolyte Imbalances	↑/↓ ACTH/cortisol; ↑/↓ ADH; ↑/↓ aldosterone; ↑/↓ PTH; ↑/↓ insulin
Genitourinary Disturbances	
Polyuria	↓ Insulin; ↑ PTH; ↓ ADH (diabetes insipidus)
Kidney stones	↑ PTH (↑ calcium); ↑ GH
Weakness and Fatigue	↑ Catecholamines; ↓ FT$_4$, ↑ rT$_3$; ↑/↓ PTH; ↓ insulin; ↑/↓ Aldosterone; ↑/↓ GH; ↑/↓ ACTH/cortisol
Infection	↓ Insulin; ↑/↓ ACTH/cortisol; ↑ GH
Mobility	↑/↓ ACTH/cortisol; ↑ GH
Tetany	↓ PTH (severe)
Pain and Discomfort	↑/↓ ACTH/cortisol; ↑ GH
Bone	↑ PTH; ↑ cortisol (fractures due to wasting of bone matrix); ↑ TSH, ↓ FT$_4$
Joint	↑ GH; ↓ FT$_4$, ↑ rT$_3$
Headache	↑ catecholamines (pheochromocytoma); ↑/↓ ACTH/cortisol; ↑ GH, ↑ AVP
Neuropathy	↓ Insulin
Paresthesia	↓ PTH (low calcium)
Visual Disturbances	
Visual field defects	↓ Insulin (retinopathy); ↑ ACTH/cortisol; ↑ FT$_4$
Exophthalmos	↑ FT$_4$ (Graves' disease)
Behavioral and Cognitive Disorders	
Lethargy	↑ PTH; ↓ thyroid; ↓ insulin; ↓ ACTH/cortisol
Anxiety and nervousness	↑ Catecholamines; ↓ PTH; ↑ ACTH/cortisol
Confusion	↓ FT$_4$, ↑ rT$_3$ (thyrotoxicosis); ↑ insulin (hypoglycemia); ↑ PTH
Body Image Disturbances	↑ ACTH/cortisol
Thick, oily skin	↑ GH
Dry skin	↓ FT$_4$, ↑ rT$_3$; ↓ insulin; ↑ GH; ↓ ACTH/cortisol
Hirsutism	↑ ACTH/cortisol; ↑ androgens
Diaphoresis	↑ Catecholamines (profuse in pheochromocytoma); ↑ insulin (hypoglycemia); ↓ PTH; ↑ ACTH/cortisol
Hyperpigmentation	↓ ACTH/cortisol (pituitary stimulated to produce ACTH and MSH)
Goiter	↓ FT$_4$, ↑ rT$_3$
Fat distribution	↑ ACTH/cortisol
Striae	↑ ACTH/cortisol

ACTH, adrenocorticotropin; ADH, antidiuretic hormone; FT$_4$, free thyroxine; GH, growth hormone; MSH, melanocyte-stimulating hormone; PTH, parathyroid hormone; rT$_3$, reverse triiodothyronine.

Changes in facial features should also be assessed. It is important to assess for a change in skin conditions such as dryness, edema, bruising, or sores that heal slowly. Has there been a change in hair growth patterns, such as facial hair appearing on women? Does the patient have purplish stretch marks (striae) on the abdominal, inner thighs, and arms? These signs are often a part of the complex clinical manifestations associated with hyperadrenal function (Figure 26–1). Prolonged hoarseness may be caused by hypothyroidism. The nurse asks patients to recall their weight from several years ago, 1 year ago, and 6 months past, to review fluctuations. Weight changes and fat redistribution may be due to disorders of the pancreas, thyroid, or adrenal glands. In addition, because many endocrine disorders are exacerbated by stress, any

recent emotional and physical stressors must be ascertained. It is important to evaluate any changes in thirst or fluid intake because these signs may indicate pituitary dysfunction, specifically, the inappropriate secretion of antidiuretic hormone (ADH) from the pituitary.

Fatigue is a common symptom of several endocrine disorders, specifically diabetes mellitus, hypothyroidism, adrenal insufficiency, and panhypopituitarism. Complaints of blurry vision may be related to hyperglycemia. The hallmark symptoms of polydipsia, polyuria, and polyphagia should precipitate further investigation for the presence of diabetes mellitus. Increased urination, nocturia, and nocturnal falls from osmotic diuresis may be clinical features of hyperglycemia in elderly people. A history of recurrent infections or poor wound healing is also more common in the elderly. A history of hyperlipidemia can be a key preliminary finding in patients with type 2 diabetes mellitus.

For all patients, a history of hypertension should be ascertained. Secondary hypertension from an endocrine source can accompany such disorders as primary aldosteronism, Cushing's syndrome, and pheochromocytoma and can be drug induced (oral contraceptives, sympathomimetics, thyroid hormone excess, and steroids). The effects of the adrenal medulla hormones, the catecholamines, increase blood pressure by increasing cardiac output, increasing peripheral resistance by vasoconstrictive action on the arterioles, and increasing renin release from the kidneys.[1] Episodes of hypertensive crisis indicate pheochromocytoma, a tumor of the adrenal medulla. This presentation includes a diastolic blood pressure of more than or equal to 120 mm Hg with evidence of end-organ damage, especially liver and cardiac failure. The presence of concurrent disease states, particularly diabetes mellitus and any adrenal involvement, precludes the use of certain classes of antihypertensives. Tachycardia, diarrhea, restlessness, sweating, fever, tremors, palpitations, anxiety, and hyperactivity are some of the signs that can accompany hyperthyroidism.

The history of the female reproductive system generally begins with an emphasis on assessing the patient's menstrual cycle. Specifics such as age at onset of menstruation, duration, flow, dysmenorrhea, dyspareunia, and changes in libido are all pertinent areas to explore. Normal reproductive changes associated with aging include "hot flashes," insomnia, irritability, irregular menstrual cycle patterns, and fatigue. These symptoms often accompany menopause or complete cessation of menses. Questions regarding the practice of breast self-examination, use of contraceptives, pregnancy, last menstrual cycle, sexually transmitted diseases, and Pap smear results should be incorporated into a comprehensive gynecologic history.

The health history of the male reproductive system includes assessment of the development of secondary

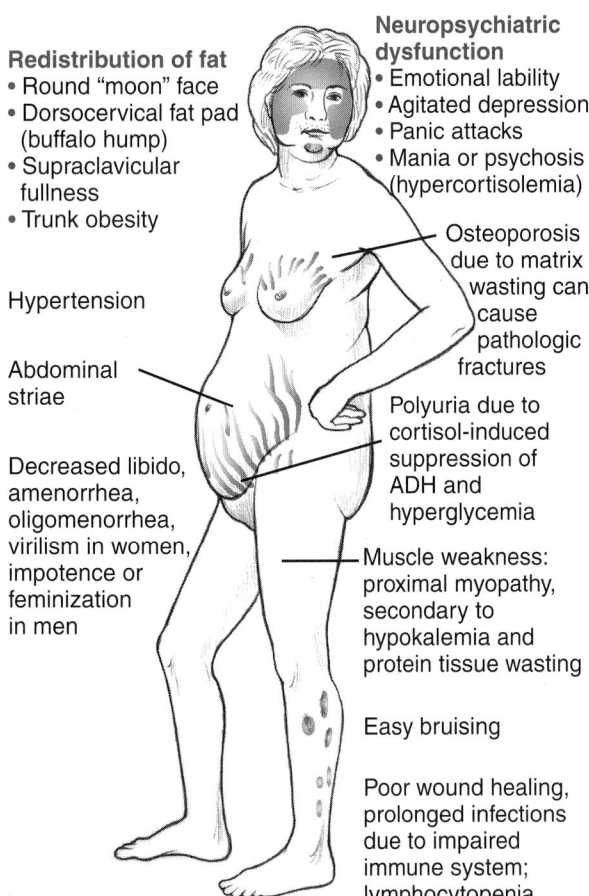

Redistribution of fat
• Round "moon" face
• Dorsocervical fat pad (buffalo hump)
• Supraclavicular fullness
• Trunk obesity

Hypertension

Abdominal striae

Decreased libido, amenorrhea, oligomenorrhea, virilism in women, impotence or feminization in men

Neuropsychiatric dysfunction
• Emotional lability
• Agitated depression
• Panic attacks
• Mania or psychosis (hypercortisolemia)

Osteoporosis due to matrix wasting can cause pathologic fractures

Polyuria due to cortisol-induced suppression of ADH and hyperglycemia

Muscle weakness: proximal myopathy, secondary to hypokalemia and protein tissue wasting

Easy bruising

Poor wound healing, prolonged infections due to impaired immune system; lymphocytopenia

Complications
Cardiovascular complications are the major causes of morbidity and mortality. Other complications:
• Congestive heart failure
• Hypertension
• Dependent edema
• Left ventricular hypertrophy
• Pathologic fractures
• Masked infections

Figure 26–1

Common clinical manifestations of hyperadrenal function (Cushing's syndrome). (From Saunders Manual of Nursing Care. Philadelphia, W.B. Saunders, 1996, p 1404.)

sexual characteristics. Questions should address penis, testes, and scrotum size, lack of muscle mass development, deepening of voice, and absence of hair development on face, axillary, and pubic areas. Furthermore, the following areas should be explored: presence of penile discharge, erectile dysfunction, urinary difficulties, testicular pain or swelling, and libido changes. As with female patients, it is also important to obtain information regarding the onset of puberty and the presence of secondary sexual characteristics. Failure of penis and testes enlargement with lack of muscle mass development usually indicates inadequate testosterone or androgen levels.

PHYSICAL EXAMINATION

Thyroid Gland

The thyroid gland is one of the few palpable endocrine glands in the human body. To inspect the thyroid, the patient should be seated with the neck flexed slightly forward and to the right. The patient should be instructed to swallow, and the nurse should observe for noticeable masses or enlargement.

To palpate the thyroid, the nurse should stand behind the patient and press fingertips on the left side of the patient's trachea and displace it to the right. The nurse's right fingers should retract the sternocleidomastoid muscle. The nurse then should palpate the

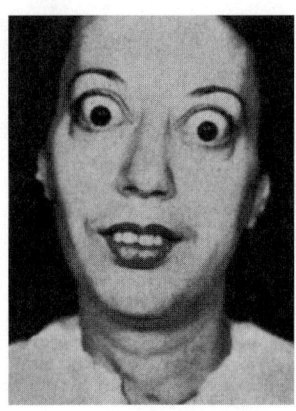

Figure 26–3
Exophthalmos. (From Wilson JD, Foster DW: Williams Textbook of Endocrinology, 8th ed. Philadelphia, W.B. Saunders, 1992, p 1330.)

gland with the right fingertips and then reverse this process for the opposite side (Figure 26–2). The gland is assessed for size, consistency, such as firmness and hardness, and tenderness. A normal thyroid gland usually has a smooth contour, is nontender, and is not easily palpable.[2]

The lymph nodes in the neck should be palpated in a gentle circular motion; normal nodes are movable and discrete. Auscultation of the thyroid can help to detect any bruits resulting from a marked increase in blood flow through the lobes indicating potential hyperthyroid function.

The ankle reflex, induced by striking the Achilles tendon, has a slow relaxation phase in hypothyroid patients. Cardiac muscle contractility testing can measure the peripheral effects of thyroid hormone function by assessing the preejection period or the left ventricular ejection time. Exophthalmos in hyperthyroidism causes a classic startled look because of increased orbital fat and fluid in the extraocular muscles (Figure 26–3). This condition may be accompanied by lid lag. If observed, the nurse should further assess the eye for potential infections or abrasions resulting from the lack of full protective covering of the eye.

Parathyroid Glands

Examination of the parathyroid glands is done indirectly by observing the patient for signs of hypercalcemia or hypocalcemia. Hypercalcemia is manifested in patients by nausea, vomiting, muscle weakness, tremors, fatigue, muscle hypotonicity, and dysrhythmias.

Neuromuscular excitability can be due to the effects of hypocalcemia. An early symptom is paresthesia, whereas tetany is a late symptom. Prolonged low calcium levels can cause organic brain syndrome. Chvostek's and Trousseau's signs are physical tests that can assess for hypocalcemia in patients.

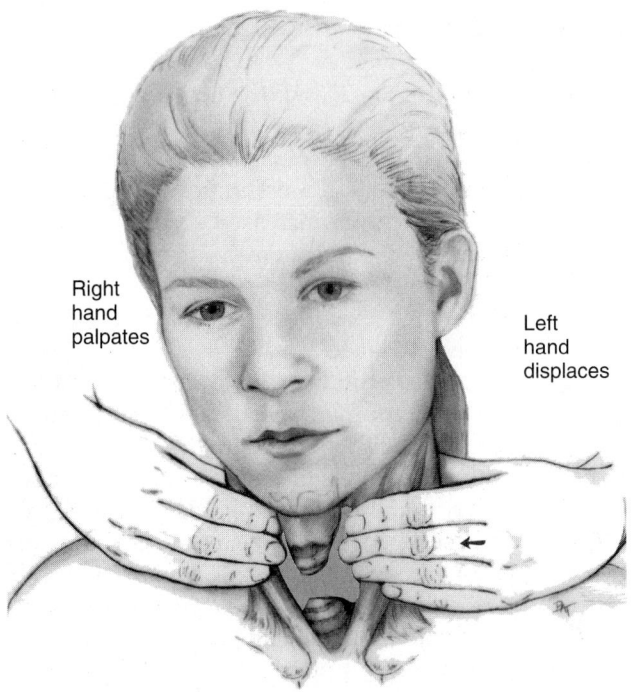

Right hand palpates

Left hand displaces

Figure 26–2
Palpation of the thyroid gland. (From Jarvis C: Physical Examination and Health Assessment, 2nd ed. Philadelphia, W.B. Saunders, 1992, p 283.)

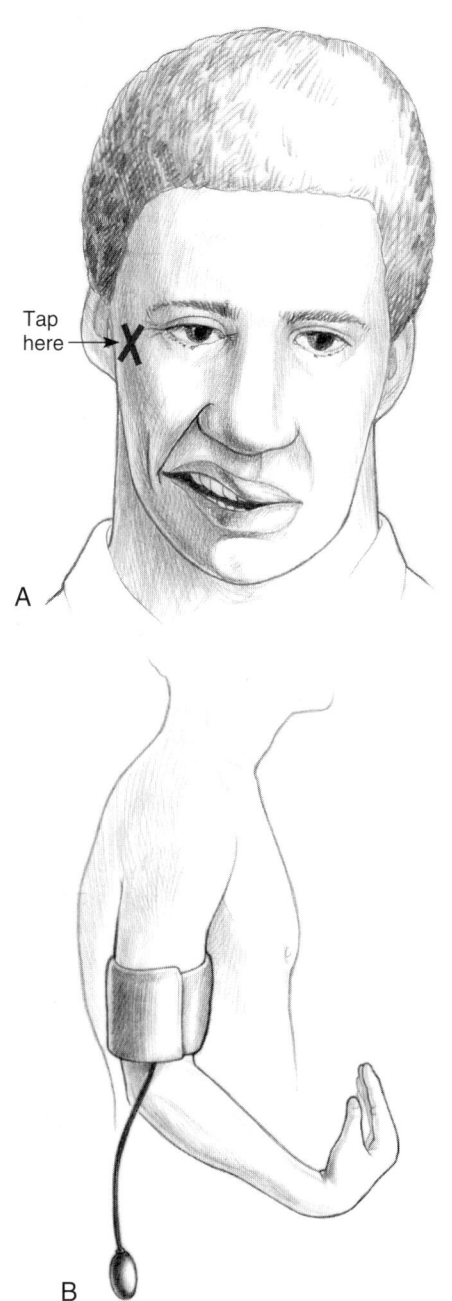

Tap
here →

A

B

Figure 26–4

Physical tests for hypocalcemia. A, Positive Chvostek's sign. B, Positive Trousseau's sign. (From Saunders Manual of Nursing Care. Philadelphia, W.B. Saunders, 1996, p 272.)

Chvostek's sign is evoked by taping the cheek anterior to the ear lobe (Figure 26–4*A*). This test induces a positive response of a hemifacial contraction (nerve twitch of the mouth) in hypocalcemic patients. Trousseau's sign is elicited by inflating the blood pressure cuff to 20 mm Hg above the patient's systolic pressure for 3 minutes. Regional ischemia to the ulnar nerve causes a carpal spasm or the twitching of the fingers or hand (see Figure 26–4*B*). Baseline assessment of both tests is encouraged because a positive response can occur in some eucalcemic persons. Both Chvostek's and

Trousseau's signs can be incorporated into scheduled vital sign times. Other physical findings in the hypocalcemic patient include paresthesias of the hands and feet, muscle cramps, nausea, vomiting, depression, and irritability. Tetany in hypocalcemia patients may be masked by uremia, hypokalemia, or hypermagnesemia.

Pituitary Gland

Impairment of pituitary function can be indirectly assessed by checking cranial nerves III for pupillary reactions, III, IV, and VI for extraocular movements, and V for corneal reflexes, facial sensation, and jaw movements (mastication) (see Chapter 39). This assessment provides information on the impact of pressure, size, or enervation resulting from possible tumor growth on the pituitary gland.

Care after a transsphenodial hypophysectomy (pituitary resection) should include an assessment for cerebrospinal fluid leakage. This complication is best noted from the presence of clear drainage from the nose, which is often felt by the patient or seen on the mustache dressing. The drainage appears as a "halo"; the center is serosanguineous, and the outer circle is clear or yellowish. This finding may suggest a cerebrospinal fluid leak that requires more investigation. Initial interventions include increasing the head of the bed briefly to verify a cerebrospinal fluid leak.[3]

Adrenal Glands

Similar to the pituitary gland, the adrenal glands are assessed by their effectiveness or the absence of expected actions. The body's management of physical and emotional stressors is most indicative of adrenal function. The demand for increased cortisol availability accompanies such conditions as trauma, surgery, fever, burns, and dehydration.[4] In the absence of normal cortisol, for example, an infection may be masked, with no evidence of fever.

Signs of overproduction of adrenal cortex hormones include hyperglycemia, increased fat distribution in the face and abnormally on the shoulders and trunk, hypernatremia, hypokalemia, hypertension, menstrual irregularity, and decreased libido. The overproduction of these hormones also influences skin integrity, leading to easy bruising and discoloration, and results in muscle wasting with a decrease in the muscle strength of limbs (see Figure 26–1).

Clinical signs and symptoms that may present in a patient with a hypofunctioning adrenal cortex include hyponatremia, hyperkalemia, hypoglycemia, decreased cortisol levels, increased skin pigmentation, particularly in the skin folds and around scar tissue, and muscular weakness. Weakness of lower extremity muscles can be assessed by asking the patient to rise from a squatting position without the use of other accessory muscles or assistance. Patients with any degree of muscular weakness are challenged by this directive.

Clinical signs and symptoms that may present in a patient with a hyperfunctioning adrenal medulla include severe headache, excessive perspiration, palpitations, pallor, nausea, vomiting, paroxysmal or sustained hypertension, and postural hypotension and tachycardia. Tests of baseline and postural blood pressures and heart rate are invaluable in patients with a suspected adrenal tumor.

Pancreas

The examination of the pancreas focuses on the symptoms related to diabetes mellitus. Two fasting blood sugars greater than 126 mg/dL are supportive of a diagnosis of diabetes. However, the patient usually presents with complaints of increased urination, thirst, and weight loss. The nurse should also inspect the patient's feet, skin, and lower limbs for signs of ischemia and the presence of ulcers and abrasions. These secondary findings, associated with complications of peripheral vascular disease, may also be indicative of hyperglycemia. The nurse should test sensory loss in the patient's feet for pain and temperature with an alternating pattern using dull–sharp, warm–cold. A diminished sensation of vibration with the tuning fork placed on the finger and toe may indicate peripheral neuropathy. Cranial nerves III, IV, VI, and VII may also reveal secondary complications of diabetic neuropathy (see Chapter 39). Obesity, as measured by a body mass index of more than 25 kg/m^2 and, more selectively, an enlarged abdominal girth shaping a pear figure, are noted risk factors for type 2 diabetes in older persons.[5] Finally, women presenting with persistent vaginal yeast infections should also be suspected of having hyperglycemia.

Male and Female Reproductive Glands

The breasts of both male and female patients should be examined for enlargement, asymmetry, induration, and breast discharge. In males with breast enlargement, gynecomastia, the nurse should perform a concurrent assessment of the testes because breast enlargement can indicate the presence of testicular cancer. Any complaints of breast or lower abdominal pain should be thoroughly explored for endocrinopathies. For females, a complete internal pelvic and bimanual examination is necessary for ruling out lesions and masses and for localizing tenderness.

Finally, the nurse should check for the presence of secondary sexual characteristics and gender habitus, such as fat distribution and hair pattern, in all patients suspected of having an endocrine disorder.

NORMAL VARIATIONS ASSOCIATED WITH AGING

As persons age, the levels of most endocrine hormones diminish. In addition, the physiologic response to these hormones also decreases. These changes can be manifested in several ways and are related to the specific hormones and target organs. The most common endocrine manifestations associated with aging are the changes seen with menopause. In addition to the cessation of menses, secondary effects associated with the loss of estrogen include changes in breast tissue, decreases in bone density, and increases in triglycerides and cholesterol. Finally, the uterus and vagina decrease in size, elasticity, and lubrication, possibly contributing to changes in sexual functioning.

Changes in aging also result in a reduced response in the hypothalamus–pituitary–adrenal axis. This can be manifested by a diminished stress response in times of physiologic (hypoxia, trauma, pain) and/or psychological (anxiety) stress. Consequences include a decrease in the secretion of cortisol and aldosterone. These hormonal decreases are demonstrated by a decreased ability to maintain sodium and fluid volume balance. Compensatory responses to postural changes in vital signs and volume depletion are diminished.[6]

Similarly, the hypothalamus–pituitary–thyroid axis demonstrates a slowed response as one ages. Changes in thyroid function include atrophy and fibrosis. Whether these changes are a result of the aging process or of disease remains unclear. However, hypothyroidism is seen frequently in the elderly. Early signs of hypothyroidism (e.g., skin and hair changes, neurologic changes) often go unnoticed by health care providers or are considered normal changes associated with aging.[6]

Pancreatic changes seen in the elderly result in increased glucose tolerance, peripheral insulin resistance, and hyperinsulinemia. The development of type 2 diabetes mellitus is common in the elderly and can be attributed to a sedentary lifestyle and/or obesity.

With aging, sensitivity to ADH is increased. However, there is also a decrease in renal function associated with aging that diminishes the ability to concentrate urine.[6] Consequently, as persons age, nocturia is frequently reported.

In summary, management of patient care begins with a thorough health assessment and physical examination. Plans of care should account for the patient's level of independence, knowledge, living arrangements, lifestyle, and concurrent illnesses. The nurse needs to discern and integrate the patient's reported history, current laboratory data, vital signs, results of diagnostic testing, such as electrocardiogram or bedside blood glucose monitoring, with the presenting signs and symptoms. Clearly defining what the patient perceives as his or her baseline of activity and health can be a starting point from which to negotiate health goals. The next step is for the nurse to identify appropriate nursing diagnoses from the comprehensive assessment and physical examination. This step enables the nurse to formulate a plan of care that has measurable and meaningful outcomes.

Key Concepts

➡ Symptoms of endocrine disease result from the cumulative effects of the oversecretion or undersecretion of hormones on the target organ or system.

➡ Endocrine disorders are often manifested by chronic problems and are not diagnosed until an acute crisis occurs.

➡ A thorough history may assist the nurse in recognizing the slow trend of changes often associated with endocrine problems. For example, asking the patient about a difference in hair growth or weight over the past 6 months may reveal more insightful information.

➡ Diagnosis and treatment of endocrine disorders depend on information from a combination of laboratory values and patient symptoms.

➡ In the elderly population, it is important not to assume that physical or mental changes are due to the effects of aging.

References

1. Gumowski J, Loughran M: Adrenal gland. Nurs Clin North Am 9:747–769, 1996.
2. United States Preventive Services Task Force: Clinical guidelines, adult screening for cancer protection: thyroid examination. Nurse Prac 30:65–67, 1995.
3. Barker E: Cranial surgery. In: Neuroscience Nursing. St. Louis, C.V. Mosby, 1994, p 275.
4. Felig P, Baxter J, Froham L: Endocrinology and Metabolism, 3rd ed. New York, McGraw-Hill, 1995.
5. Finucane P, Sinclair A: Epidemiology. In: Diabetes in Old Age. New York, John Wiley & Sons, 1995.
6. Blevins DR, Cassmeyer VL: Assessment of the endocrine system. In: Phipps WJ, Cassmeyer VL, Sands JK, et al (eds): Medical-Surgical Nursing: Concepts and Clinical Practice, 5th ed. Philadelphia, C.V. Mosby, 1995, pp 1189–1190.

27

Endocrine Laboratory and Diagnostic Tests

Julie A. Jamison

Objectives

After completing this chapter, the student will able to:

1. Identify the target tissues of the endocrine hormones.
2. Discuss commonly ordered tests used to identify concerns regarding the endocrine glands.
3. Identify factors that may produce inaccuracies in endocrine test results.
4. Identify acceptable parameters for home diagnostic test methods used in the care of patients with diabetes mellitus.
5. Develop patient teaching plans related to endocrine testing.

The endocrine system coordinates with the nervous system to regulate major functions of the body. The hormones secreted by the endocrine glands influence metabolism and growth, regulate fluid and electrolyte balance, respond to stressors, and promote the development of sexual characteristics. Glands of the endocrine system include the hypothalamus, pituitary, thyroid, parathyroid, pancreas, adrenals, ovaries, and testes. When hormones produced by these glands are secreted to the target tissues in amounts above or below physiologic requirements, a multitude of conditions can occur that require medical intervention and nursing care in the critical care setting.

This chapter provides information about laboratory and diagnostic methods and patient teaching for conditions resulting from endocrine dysfunction. Discussions of growth hormone and hormone disorders that affect the ovaries, testes, or mammary glands are not included in this chapter. Table 27–1 provides an overview of alterations in endocrine hormone secretions and the conditions that result from variations in those hormone levels.

HYPOTHALAMUS AND PITUITARY

The hypothalamus coordinates the neuroendocrine response with the pituitary gland. Secretion from the posterior pituitary is controlled by nerve impulses that originate in the hypothalamus and terminate in the posterior pituitary. Inhibiting and releasing factors secreted in the hypothalamus act on the cells in the anterior pituitary. The anterior pituitary releases hormones that act on target tissues in other parts of the body.[1] The hypothalamus receives feedback from all areas of the nervous system. The feedback increases or inhibits endocrine hormone secretion from the pituitary.

Antidiuretic hormone (ADH), also known as arginine vasopressin, regulates fluid balance in the body based on this feedback system. ADH from the posterior pituitary acts on the distal tubules and collecting ducts of the kidney to reabsorb water and to reduce the urine volume without changing the rate of solute excretion. Osmolality of the extracellular compartment is maintained by the kidneys as urine is concentrated. Failure of the negative feedback system results in secretion of a greater than normal amount of ADH by the posterior pituitary. This change promotes additional reabsorption of water by the renal tubules, thus increasing the volume of the extracellular compartment. This condition leads to water overload and dilutional hyponatremia and is known as the syndrome of inappropriate antidiuretic hormone (SIADH). Patients with SIADH produce a small volume of highly concentrated urine.

A deficit in secretion of ADH by the posterior pituitary (central diabetes insipidus [DI]) or an inability of

TABLE 27–1
Conditions Resulting From Alterations in Endocrine Hormones

Hormones	Target Tissue/Organ	Hormone Level	Effects	Condition
Hypothalamic and Pituitary Hormones				
Antidiuretic hormone	Kidney	Increased	Water retention	SIADH
		Decreased	Water excretion	Diabetes insipidus
Thyrotropin-releasing factor	Thyroid	Increased	Impaired intracellular chemical reactions	Hyperthyroidism (Graves' disease, thyroid crisis)
		Decreased		Hypothyroidism (myxedema)
Adrenocorticotropin	Adrenal cortex	Increased	Metabolism, fluid and electrolyte changes	Cushing's disease
		Decreased		Adrenal insufficiency (Addison's disease)
Thyroid and Parathyroid Hormones				
Calcitonin	Bone	Increased	Changes in bone and calcium metabolism	Hypocalcemia
		Decreased		Hypercalcemia
Parathyroid hormone	Bone	Increased	Changes in bone and calcium metabolism	Hypercalcemia
		Decreased		Hypocalcemia
Pancreatic Hormone				
Insulin	Muscle, body cells	Increased	Metabolism, fluid and electrolyte changes	Hypoglycemia
		Decreased		Hyperglycemia (diabetic ketoacidosis, hyperglycemic hyperosmolar nonketotic coma)

SIADH, syndrome of inappropriate antidiuretic hormone.

the kidney tubules to respond to ADH (nephrogenic) results in DI. This condition causes excessive amounts of dilute urine to be excreted. To compensate for the volume loss, patients with DI drink large quantities of fluid.[2] A thorough discussion of the pathophysiology and management of patients with SIADH and DI is presented in Chapter 29.

Laboratory Testing for Diabetes Insipidus and the Syndrome of Inappropriate Antidiuretic Hormone

Clinical signs and symptoms, physical assessment, medications, and health history are reviewed with the laboratory data. Laboratory tests indirectly assess the function of the hypothalamus and pituitary glands. Blood, plasma, serum, and urine tests are used to evaluate alteration in endocrine function. Additional tests evaluate the function of the gland by suppressing or stimulating secretion of the hormone. Standard pre-

cautions must be followed when obtaining or testing any blood or body fluids. A comparison of the laboratory findings for DI and SIADH is found in Table 27–2.

Electrolytes

Electrolytes are tested to obtain baseline values. Serum electrolytes affected by changes in ADH secretion are chloride, sodium, and magnesium. In SIADH, all these electrolytes are decreased by osmotic dilution. Chloride values less than 80 mEq/L, sodium values less than 120 mEq/L, and magnesium values less than 1.0 mEq/L are in critical ranges.

Serum Osmolality

Serum osmolality measures the concentration of particles in solution. Nonfasting serum osmolality normal values are 275 to 295 mOsm/kg H_2O; values less than 265 mOsm/kg H_2O or greater than 320 mOsm/kg H_2O are critical. Drug interferences contributing to

TABLE 27–2

Comparison of Laboratory Findings in Diabetes Insipidus and Syndrome of Inappropriate Antidiuretic Hormone

Laboratory Tests	Diabetes Insipidus		Syndrome of Inappropriate Antidiuretic Hormone
	Central	Nephrogenic	
Serum			
Antidiuretic hormone (ADH)	Decreased	Normal or increased	Increased
Osmolality	Increased	Increased	Decreased
Electrolytes			
Sodium	Increased	Increased	Decreased
Chloride	Increased	Increased	Decreased
Magnesium	Normal or increased	Normal or increased	Decreased
Urine			
Output	Increased	Increased	Decreased
Specific gravity	Decreased	Decreased	Increased
Osmolality	Decreased	Decreased	Increased
Water Deprivation ADH Stimulation Test	Diagnostic	Diagnostic	—
Water Loading ADH Suppression Test	—	—	Diagnostic

low values are chlorthalidone, cyclophosphamide, and thiazide. Random urine osmolality values can range from 50 to 1200 mOsm/kg H_2O, but with average fluid intake, they are usually 300 to 900 mOsm/kg H_2O. Urine osmolality values in SIADH are elevated in relation to the low serum osmolality values; specific gravity is increased because of water reabsorption.

High serum osmolality values and low urine osmolality values are common in DI. Drugs that produce increases in serum osmolality are corticosteroids, glycerin, lorcainide, mannitol, urea, methoxyflurane postoperatively, and extremely large doses of insulin.

In DI, serum chloride and sodium levels are elevated because of output of 5 to 15 L of dilute urine per day.[3] A critical range for chloride is greater than 115 mEq/L. Sodium concentrations greater than 155 mEq/L can result in renal and cardiovascular complications when combined with volume depletion from dehydration. Serum magnesium levels may remain unchanged. Magnesium levels appear normal by laboratory testing, even though magnesium body stores are depleted by 20%.[4] This is because most magnesium in the body is intracellular, and serum levels reflect less than 1% of the total body magnesium.

ADH Levels

Elevated plasma levels of ADH are found with SIADH or nephrogenic DI. Levels are decreased in central DI. Normal plasma ADH values are 1 to 5 pg/mL.[4] The ADH reference value increases or decreases as the os-

molality and blood volume changes in the blood sample. In preparation for this test, patients may not exercise or have food for 8 to 10 hours before the blood is obtained, but they should be well hydrated. ADH secretion is higher during the night, in conditions of pain, stress, or exercise, and when the patient is in an erect position. Lower secretion of ADH occurs with hypertension, recumbent position, and hypo-osmolality. These factors need to be evaluated in relation to the time and results of the test.

Many drugs increase ADH levels and should be withheld before testing, if possible for 8 to 10 hours. Narcotic analgesics, thiazides, tricyclic antidepressants, antineoplastics, antipsychotics, barbiturates, carbamazepine, chlorpropamide, clofibrate, cyclophosphamide, nicotine, and rarely furosemide interfere with the test.[4] Drug interference from demeclocycline, ethanol, lithium carbonate, and phenytoin lowers values of ADH.

Usual procedures for obtaining blood specimens are followed. The sample is obtained in a plastic rather than a glass tube to prevent degradation of ADH. Significant deterioration of ADH occurs at room temperature or with prolonged storage, so blood samples must be processed quickly according to laboratory guidelines.

Water Loading ADH Suppression Test

In persons with normal secretion of ADH from the posterior pituitary, as fluid intake and water volume increase, ADH is suppressed, urine output increases, and urine osmolality decreases. In patients with SIADH, values from the water load test reflect abnormalities in serum osmolality, increased ADH levels, and urine output of less than half the water loading dose.[5]

In preparation for the test, the patient takes nothing by mouth after midnight. The patient begins the test by voiding and discarding the urine. A tap water loading dose of 1000 mL is administered to the patient to drink in 15 to 30 minutes. Tietz[4] suggests that the water loading dose may be 20 mL/kg of body weight. Intravenous fluid may be used. Urine and blood specimens are collected hourly for 4 to 5 hours. Urine is evaluated for volume, specific gravity, and osmolality. Serum osmolality and ADH values are obtained at hourly intervals. Specimen collection procedures and laboratory guidelines must be followed for ADH serum testing. Poor nutritional status, stress, and drug therapy can interfere with interpretation of endocrine test results.[6] Drugs that interfere with test results include demeclocycline, lithium carbonate, methoxyflurane, chlorpropamide, clofibrate, cyclophosphamide, diuretics, and diazoxide, and these agents should be withheld for 12 hours if possible.

Patients with a history of congestive heart failure risk potential fluid volume overload. Seizures and fatal hyponatremia can occur in patients with SIADH because of impaired fluid and electrolyte balance. The nurse should observe the patient for signs of nausea, vomiting, abdominal fullness, fatigue, or rales and assess for symptoms of hyponatremia, which include anxiety, muscle weakness, altered level of consciousness, and a rapid, thready pulse.

Water Deprivation ADH Stimulation Test

This test, used to establish the diagnosis for DI, evaluates the body's ability to balance water and electrolytes. In persons with normal ADH secretion, fluid restriction should stimulate the release of ADH to conserve urine and to maintain serum osmolality. Reference ranges after fluid restriction are urine osmolality more than 500 mOsm/kg, serum osmolality less than 300 mOsm/kg, and plasma ADH in an appropriate range for the serum osmolality, with weight loss less than 3% from the baseline weight. In central DI, urine osmolality or urine specific gravity does not change in response to water deprivation. If the kidney responds to the administration of ADH by concentrating urine, then the diagnosis of central DI can be established. A 10% increase in urine osmolality occurs after aqueous ADH is administered. In nephrogenic DI, water deprivation or the administration of ADH does not affect urine osmolality.[4]

Drugs that affect the water loading ADH suppression test also interfere with the water deprivation test

and should be withheld for 8 to 10 hours. Fluid restriction begins at 6:00 AM. The patient voids and is weighed. Serum osmolality is collected for a baseline measure. Urine samples are tested hourly for specific gravity and osmolality. When two consecutive urine samples have less than a 30 mOsm/kg change, serum osmolality and ADH values are obtained. The patient is again weighed, and 5 U of aqueous ADH is administered subcutaneously. After 1 hour, urine osmolality is measured. Patients remain at rest and are observed closely for signs of fluid volume deficit. Hourly assessments of blood pressure and weight loss are essential. Serum sodium levels are monitored for increased values. Specimen collection guidelines are followed for obtaining blood and urine samples. Specific guidelines must be followed in handling ADH samples.

THYROID AND PARATHYROID

Thyroid function is controlled by the hypothalamus and pituitary glands and is regulated by a negative feedback system. The thyroid secretes three hormones: calcitonin, important for calcium metabolism and phosphorus regulation; triiodothyronine (T_3); and thyroxine (T_4). T_4 comprises approximately 93% of the hormones secreted, and T_3 comprises 7%; T_3 has the stronger metabolic effect.[1] Release of T_3 and T_4 is controlled by thyrotropin-releasing hormone (TRH) from the hypothalamus, which regulates thyrotropin or thyroid-stimulating hormone (TSH) from the anterior pituitary.

Excessive secretion of TSH is associated with primary hypothyroidism. Primary hypothyroidism is characterized by increased serum TSH, reduced metabolic processes, and symptoms of mental dullness, lethargy, weight gain, constipation, and dry skin.[1]

The four parathyroid glands secrete parathyroid hormone (PTH), which maintains blood calcium levels, neuromuscular activity, blood clotting, and cell membrane permeability.[2] Hyperparathyroidism with resultant hypercalcemia causes dysfunction of many body systems. Hypoparathyroidism reduces osteoclastic activity of the bones. When the parathyroids are surgically removed, tetany rapidly develops.

Laboratory Testing for Hyperthyroidism and Hypothyroidism

Hyperthyroidism results in an increase in serum sodium values, but the condition decreases triglyceride and total cholesterol values. Hypothyroidism increases magnesium, triglyceride, and total cholesterol levels and lowers serum sodium.

Thyroid Hormone Levels

Circulating thyroid hormone is measured by radio immunoassay of T_3, T_4, free T_3 (FT$_3$), and free T_4 (FT$_4$). Assessment of the pituitary–thyroid axis is measured by TSH and the thyroid response to the administration of TRH.[7] FT$_4$ and TSH levels are often used as screening tests for thyroid disease and for evaluating thyroid function in hospitalized adults. These two tests have a sensitivity of 99.5% and a specificity of 98%.[8]

T_4, with a normal value of 5 to 12 μg/dL, varies because serum binding protein levels fluctuate. The unbound T_4 or FT$_4$ is physiologically active, with adult values of 0.8 to 2.3 ng/dL. FT$_4$ levels increase with hyperthyroidism and decrease with hypothyroidism. FT$_4$ is also used to evaluate levothyroxine for thyroid replacement therapy. No special patient preparation is required for drawing venous blood for this test. Total T_4 reference values must be correlated with the patient's age for accurate evaluation of results. Drugs increasing FT$_4$ results include amiodarone, aspirin, propranolol, and danazol. Total T_4 values are increased by estrogens, heroin, amphetamines, methadone, thyroid preparations, oral contraceptives, propranolol, amiodarone, and iopanoic acid. FT$_4$ results are lowered by anticonvulsants, especially phenytoin, and methadone. Decreases are seen in T_4 levels with androgens, asparaginase, aspirin, corticosteroids, large doses of furosemide, isotretinoin, lithium, penicillin, reserpine, sulfonamides, somatotropin, and T_3.[4]

Normal serum values of FT$_3$ are 260 to 480 pg/dL for adults; 99% of T_3 is bound to thyroxine-binding globulin (TBG). FT$_3$ is responsible for the physiologic activity of T_3. FT$_3$ and total T_3 values (normal adult 80–100 ng/dL) are elevated in hyperthyroidism and are decreased in hypothyroidism. Drug interferences that raise FT$_3$ and T_3 values include dextrothyroxine, estrogens, heroin, methadone, oral contraceptives, terbutaline, dinoprost tromethamine, and, rarely, amiodarone. High altitude also increases values.[4] Drugs decreasing FT$_3$ and T_3 results are phenytoin, cimetidine, dexamethasone, iodides, lithium, large doses of salicylates, amiodarone, androgens, asparaginase, propylthiouracil, and oral cholecystographic agents.[9]

Thyroid Panel

A thyroid panel typically includes FT$_4$, total T_4, total T_3, T_3 uptake, T_7 or FT$_4$ index, and the TSH assay. T_3 uptake is a ratio between unsaturated TBG in the patient's specimen and a laboratory control sample. The T_7 or FT$_4$ index is a mathematic calculation used to correct the T_4 for the amount of TBG in the patient's blood sample.

TSH Assay

The TSH assay uses two TSH-specific monoclonal antibodies to distinguish euthyroid from hyperthyroid patients. Using a venous blood sample, the test is able to detect serum TSH as low as 0.1 μU/mL, with adult norms up to 5.4 μU/mL. The TSH assay is the single most sensitive test for primary hypothyroidism. TSH is high in primary hypothyroidism and low in hyperthyroidism.[8] TSH secretion has an early morning peak and an evening low. When using immunoassay methods, lithium, radiographic dyes, morphine, and metoclopramide increase values, whereas heparin, dopamine, L-dopa, corticosteroids, carbamazepine, aspirin, and T_3 decrease values.[4,9] Table 27–3 summarizes the laboratory tests used to evaluate abnormal thyroid function.

The parathyroid glands regulate calcium and phosphorus levels. A decrease in one mineral results in an increase in the other.[1] Critical ranges for calcium are less than 6 mg/dL or greater than 14 mg/dL. Less than 1 mg/dL is considered critical for phosphorus.[5]

The PTH level is obtained from a fasting venous blood sample. PTH has a short half-life, so the specimen must be placed on ice and processed according to laboratory guidelines. Drug interferences that increase values include anticonvulsants, corticosteroids, isoniazid, lithium, phosphates, and rifampin. Cimetidine, pindolol, and propranolol decrease test results.[4] Normal values vary according to the test method used, whether serum or plasma is tested, and the time the specimen was obtained. Baseline PTH values can be obtained in the morning, whereas the highest secretion of PTH is in the evening.[4,5] Serum calcium and phosphorus levels should be obtained at the same time, to

TABLE 27–3

Comparison of Laboratory Findings in Primary Hypothyroidism and Hyperthyroidism

Laboratory Test	Hypothyroidism	Hyperthyroidism
Serum TSH	>7 μU/mL	<0.1 μU/mL
Serum FT$_4$	<0.5 ng/dL	>4 ng/dL
FT$_4$ index	Low	High
Thyroid autoantibodies	Indicates autoimmune disease	
Thyroxine-binding globin	Used when FT$_4$ is low but TSH is normal	

FT$_4$, free thyroxine; TSH, thyroid-stimulating hormone.

compare ratio values. Frequent assessments of calcium, phosphorus, potassium, and magnesium levels are important for the patient with parathyroid dysfunction.[2]

PANCREAS

The endocrine functions of the pancreas are carried out by the alpha, beta, and delta cells in the islets of Langerhans. Insulin is an important anabolic hormone produced by the beta cells and is essential in regulating blood glucose concentrations. Amylin, a beta cell hormone discovered in 1987, is cosecreted with insulin in response to rising glucose concentrations. Amylin affects glucose and glycogen metabolism and may delay gastric emptying.[10] Other endocrine hormones produced are glucagon from the alpha cells and somatostatin from the delta cells.

Patients with pancreatic endocrine dysfunction experience hyperglycemia associated with diabetes mellitus, diabetic ketoacidosis, hyperglycemic hyperosmolar nonketotic syndrome (HHNK), or hypoglycemia that occurs as a complication of therapy.

Laboratory Testing for Hyperglycemia and Hypoglycemia

Because of insufficient levels of insulin in the person with diabetes mellitus, plasma glucose concentrations increase, producing osmotic diuresis and changes in fluid and electrolyte balance. Movement of electrolytes from intracellular to extracellular compartments results in fluctuations in sodium and potassium levels. Serum creatinine, osmolality, and blood urea nitrogen increase in response to dehydration. Serum pH becomes acidotic. *Ketones* are produced from fat metabolism and can be tested in the urine or blood. Patients taking levodopa, paraldehyde, isoniazid, phenazopyridine, and phthalein compounds may have false-positive results when testing for ketonuria.[11] Ketones are not normally present in the urine. To test for ketones, a ketone reagent strip is dipped in urine, timed according to directions, and compared with a color chart from the manufacturer.

Fasting Glucose

Normal fasting glucose is 70 to 110 mg/dL. Two-hour postprandial values are 70 to 140 mg/dL. Patients with insufficient insulin risk diabetic ketoacidosis or HHNK at glucose values of 300 mg/dL or higher. Drug interferences contributing to elevated values are corticosteroids, diuretics, estrogens, antidepressants,

glucagon, isoniazid, lithium, phenytoin, salicylates, beta blockers, theophylline, and rifampin.[4] Lowered values are caused by alcohol, anabolic steroids, marijuana, monoamine oxidase inhibitors, oral antidiabetic agents, insulin, acetaminophen and aspirin in large doses, antihistamines, and gemfibrozil. Glucose levels less than 60 mg/dL are considered hypoglycemic. The nurse must provide immediate and appropriate treatment for hypoglycemia. Glucose testing reflects the current glycemic level and is subject to rapid change by other counterregulatory hormones, stress, food, and exercise.

Blood for glucose testing may be obtained from a venous sample or a fingerstick for frequent blood glucose monitoring at the bedside. Blood glucose monitoring is a key component for patients in the intensive care unit as well as when they return home. In the hospital or home health care setting, blood glucose monitoring must comply with national clinical laboratory standards. Normal blood glucose ranges are applicable with blood glucose meters. Many brands of meters are available for hospital and home use. Directions for use must be followed to obtain accurate blood glucose values.

Glycosylated Hemoglobin

The glycosylated hemoglobin (HbA_{1c}) test reflects the average blood glucose concentration over the previous 2 to 3 months. Glucose irreversibly attaches to the hemoglobin molecule of the red blood cell. The amount of glucose bound to the red blood cell over its 120-day life span provides the HbA_{1c} value. This test is not affected by numerous drug interferences or patients' efforts at short-term compliance, as is the glucose test. Patients with elevated hemoglobin levels or those receiving heparin therapy may have increased values. Hemolytic anemia and high levels of immature erythrocytes contribute to low results. Random venous samples are used for this test. Normal ranges are from 4 to 7%, but they vary with the laboratory method used.

Insulin levels, C-peptide, glycosylated serum protein, fructosamine, amylin, and the glucose tolerance test are important tools for the diagnosis and treatment of pancreatic hormone dysfunction, but they are not routinely used within the intensive care setting for care related to the patient with diabetes mellitus.

ADRENAL GLANDS

The adrenal glands consist of two distinct parts: the adrenal medulla and the adrenal cortex. The primary hormones produced by the adrenal cortex are aldosterone (mineralocorticoid), cortisol (glucocorticoid), and androgens. Primary adrenal insufficiency (Addison's disease) results when secretion of both aldosterone and cortisol are inadequate. Secondary adrenal insufficiency results from failure of the anterior pituitary to synthesize and secrete adrenocorticotropin (ACTH). In adrenal hypersecretion (Cushing's disease), excess cortisol is secreted, or a pituitary tumor may produce too much ACTH.6

Laboratory Testing for Adrenal Insufficiency or Hypersecretion

Adrenocortical insufficiency produces many electrolyte imbalances. Serum sodium, glucose, and chloride values are low, whereas serum magnesium, potassium, blood urea nitrogen, creatinine, and urine sodium are increased.[4] Glucose and electrolyte values should be obtained every 2 to 4 hours for the patient with acute adrenal insufficiency. ACTH fasting plasma levels are determined using venous blood. ACTH levels are increased in primary and are decreased in secondary adrenal insufficiency. Normal values vary according to the time of day and increased stress on the patient. Morning values are 15 to 100 pg/mL, whereas evening values are less than 50 pg/mL. ACTH is unstable in blood. The specimen must be drawn in a plastic tube, placed on ice, and processed according to laboratory guidelines. Test values are increased in hypoglycemia and with insulin, levodopa, and ADH. Dexamethasone and other corticosteroids lower tests results.

Cortisol Levels

In primary adrenal insufficiency, cortisol values are decreased. As with ACTH, these values are affected by time of day, patient stress levels, drug interferences, and age. The patient may have food and fluids. Venous blood is drawn at 8:00 AM and 4:00 PM. Morning normal values are 6 to 28 μg/dL, evening values are 2 to 12 μg/dL.[4,5] Urine cortisol levels mimic serum levels, with free cortisol increasing urine values when plasma values are high.

ACTH Stimulation Test

The ACTH stimulation test evaluates adrenal function. When ACTH is given, plasma cortisol levels should increase. An exaggerated response to ACTH indicates cushingoid symptoms. With administration of ACTH, the nurse should observe the patient for bronchospasm, seizures, hyperglycemia, hypokalemia, elevated blood pressure, sodium and fluid retention, or mood swings. A low response indicates adrenal insuf-

ficiency. Test methods include a rapid screen, a 24-hour test, or a 3-day test. The patient takes nothing by mouth (is NPO) after midnight. At 8:00 AM, plasma cortisol levels are drawn. In the rapid test, an intramuscular injection of a synthetic ACTH drug is given, followed by plasma cortisol levels in 30 and 60 minutes. With normal test results, cortisol levels should increase more than 7 μg/dL above baseline.[6]

Aldosterone

Aldosterone can be measured in serum or urine. The 24-hour urine tests avoid the diurnal variations and are more reliable. Normal values are 6 to 25 μg per 24 hours.[5] Other urine tests are for 17-hydroxycorticosteroids (17-OHCS) and 17-ketosteroids (17-KS). Both tests require urine to be collected over 24 hours. Normal values vary with age, gender, and drug interferences. 17-OHCS values are increased by stress, licorice, and drugs including cefoxitin, chloral hydrate, erythromycin, hydroxyzine, methicillin, paraldehyde, phenothiazine, spironolactone, and quinine. Drugs decreasing 17-OHCS levels include estrogens, oral contraceptives, phenytoin, meperidine, and morphine.[4] Twenty-four-hour urine collection procedures should be followed. The 17-OHCS are a group of steroids, cortisone and hydrocortisone, in the urine. Elevated test results indicate adrenal hyperfunction, and low results indicate hypofunction.

The 17-KS are male hormone metabolites secreted from the adrenal cortex and testes. Elevated test results indicate hyperfunction, whereas decreased values are seen with adrenal hypofunction. Normal values vary with age and gender and are affected by stress and drug interferences.[5]

DIAGNOSTIC TESTING FOR ENDOCRINE FUNCTION

Diagnostic test methods are also used to evaluate the patient with endocrine dysfunction. Basic principles for patient care must be followed with any diagnostic procedure. The patient is informed about the purpose and general procedure for the test. Signed consent forms are obtained according to the institution's policy. Assessments, health history, and contraindications for the test such as pregnancy, allergies, or prior responses to test procedures are completed. Guidelines for test preparation and aftercare must be followed. The nurse should allow the patient time to ask questions or express concerns, and the discussion should include family members. Care provided to the patient before and after the test is documented.[12] The nurse should ask the patient about specific allergies to iodine or contrast media and be alert to signs and symptoms of allergic reaction when contrast dyes are used in testing.

Radiologic Examinations

Radiologic examinations (x-ray studies) may be used as a preliminary step in assessing abdominal endocrine glands and in visualizing bony structures of the skull. The sella turcica surrounds and protects the pituitary gland. Skull fractures, tumors, and tissue swelling can cause changes detectable by x-ray studies. Patients receiving skull radiographs must remove glasses, dentures, hair clips, and other objects above the neck. Multiple views of the skull are obtained.

Angiography is a radiographic study of vascular structures after introduction of a radiopaque contrast dye. Angiographies are used to evaluate patency of vessels or to identify abnormal vascularization resulting from tumors. Sites used to introduce the dye through a catheter include the carotid, brachial, and femoral arteries. Before the test, the patient is NPO after midnight. Policies and procedures for diagnostic testing are followed; information about hypersensitivity to iodine or contrast dyes must be obtained, as well as the anticoagulant status of the patient. The test takes 1 to 2 hours to complete. After the test, the patient lies flat, with sandbags placed over the catheter insertion site to maintain pressure for hemostasis. The site is assessed frequently for hemorrhage or hematoma formation; peripheral pulses are evaluated with vital signs and are compared with the preprocedure assessment.

Nuclear Scans

Nuclear scans are used to detect an intracranial mass, abscess, cancer, metastasis, or trauma to the head. In the thyroid, a scan detects a thyroid mass, determines the size, structure, and position of the gland, or evaluates thyroid function.[5] The radionuclide (isotope) is administered orally or intravenously. Procedures and instructions for nuclear scans vary with the organ tested and the radionuclides used.

Radionuclides for brain scans are administered intravenously, with the waiting time after the injection and before the scan ranging from 45 minutes to 3 hours, depending on the isotope used. Food or fluids are not restricted. Lugol's solution or potassium perchlorate is given before the scan to block uptake of the isotope by the salivary glands, thyroid, and choroid plexus. The patient needs to remain still during the procedure, which lasts half an hour to 1 hour.

Three days before a thyroid scan, thyroid hormones, iodine compounds, seafood, iodized salt, corticosteroids, aspirin, phenothiazines, sodium nitroprusside, multivitamins, and cough syrups containing iodide are discontinued with physician approval.[5] Food and fluids are restricted for 8 hours before testing if oral iodine radionuclide is used. Waiting times after receiving the isotope until scanning vary from 30 minutes to 24 hours. The scan takes 30 minutes to complete.

The dose of radionuclide is low and does not affect other people coming in contact with the patient. The substance is excreted in the urine in 6 to 24 hours. Nuclear scans are contraindicated for patients who are pregnant or are breast-feeding.[12]

Computed Tomography

Computed Tomography (CT) scans produce an x-ray beam that examines body sections from many angles.[5] Structures in the head, neck, pancreas, and adrenal glands are examined. Scans may be done with or without contrast dye. The patient is strapped to a special table in the CT scanner and must lie still. Many patients express fears of claustrophobia; analgesics and sedatives may be ordered. Patients may take medications, food, and fluids. If contrast dye is used, they may be NPO 2 to 4 hours before the procedure. For a total-body CT scan, the test may take 30 to 60 minutes.

Magnetic Resonance Imaging

Magnetic resonance imaging (MRI) produces cross-sectional images using magnetic energy sources. The patient is not exposed to radiation. Contrast dyes are occasionally used with this imaging test. There are no food or fluid restrictions. Safety issues are a major concern with MRI. Because of the strong magnetic field, absolute contraindications exist for any implanted device including pacemakers, drug infusion pumps, cochlear implants, intrauterine contraceptive devices, neurostimulators, and other prosthetic devices. Patients with metallic fragments, surgical clips, pins, screws, plates, wire sutures, or mesh cannot be scanned. Contraindications exist for the patient who has epilepsy or is pregnant. Hearing aids, dentures, wigs or other items must be removed. Conscious sedation may be used for patients during the 45- to 90-minute procedure.[12]

Ultrasonography

Ultrasonography is used to evaluate the thyroid, parathyroids, pancreas, and adrenal glands. High-frequency sound waves are used to produce an image of the structure examined. Gel, lotion, or oil is applied to the skin to enhance contact with the transducer and to permit easy movement across the skin. Ultrasound is a noninvasive procedure that is without radiation risk, requires little patient preparation, and takes 20 to 45 minutes to complete.

Key Concepts

⟶ The patient's clinical signs and symptoms, physical assessment, health history, and current medications must be correlated with endocrine laboratory data.

⟶ Medications, activity, gender, and patient stress levels are factors that affect endocrine hormone test levels.

⟶ Some endocrine secretions have diurnal variations. Laboratory reference ranges must be correlated with the time of day the specimen was obtained.

⟶ Because of the rapid degradation of many endocrine hormones, laboratory specimen collection guidelines are followed precisely to obtain accurate results.

⟶ Blood glucose values change rapidly because of effects of food, stress, exercise, and the influences of counterregulatory hormones.

⟶ HbA$_{1c}$ provides an indication of the average blood glucose values over the past 3 to 4 months.

⟶ Diagnostic tests use radiographic images, contrast dyes, radionuclides, magnetic fields, and sound waves to elicit information about the endocrine glands.

References

1. Guyton AC, Hall JE: Textbook of Medical Physiology, 9th ed. Philadelphia: W.B. Saunders, 1996.
2. Anderson K (ed): Mosby's Medical, Nursing and Allied Health Dictionary, 4th ed. St. Louis, C.V. Mosby, 1994.
3. Bianco CM: Diabetes insipidus. Am J Nurs 96:30–31, 1996.
4. Tietz N (ed): Clinical Guide to Laboratory Tests, 3rd ed. Philadelphia, W.B. Saunders, 1995.
5. Kee JL: Laboratory and Diagnostic Tests With Nursing Implications, 4th ed. East Norwalk, CT, Appleton & Lange, 1995.
6. Toto KH: Endocrine physiology: a comprehensive review. In: Toto KH (ed): Crit Care Nurs Clin North Am 6: 637–659, 1994.
7. Miller M: Endocrine disorders: new technology allows quick, accurate diagnosis. Geriatrics 51:52–55, 1996.
8. Behnia M, Gharib H: Primary care diagnosis of thyroid disease. Hosp Pract 31:121–126, 131–134, 1996.
9. Surks MI, Sievert R: Drugs and thyroid function. N Engl J Med 333:1688–1694, 1995.
10. Kolterman O (ed): Beta Cell Dysfunction in Diabetes: The Role of Amylin and Insulin [brochure]. San Diego, Oxford Clinical Communications, 1996.
11. Watson J, Jaffe MS: Nurses Manual of Laboratory and Diagnostic Tests, 2nd ed. Philadelphia, F.A. Davis, 1995.
12. Fischbach F (ed): A Manual of Laboratory and Diagnostic Tests, 5th ed. Philadelphia, W.B. Saunders, 1996.

28

Diabetic Ketoacidosis and Hyperglycemic Hyperosmolar Nonketotic Coma

Debbie Hinnen and Belinda Childs

Objectives

After completing this chapter, the student will be able to:

1. Differentiate the etiology and pathophysiology of diabetic ketoacidosis (DKA) and hyperglycemic hyperosmolar nonketotic coma (HHNK).
2. Identify the presenting signs and symptoms and diagnostic tests related to the patient in DKA or HHNK.
3. Differentiate the treatment strategies for DKA and HHNK.
4. Identify appropriate nursing diagnoses for the patient experiencing DKA or HHNK.
5. Evaluate the outcomes of the collaborative management of the patient with DKA or HHNK.

ETIOLOGY AND PATHOPHYSIOLOGY

Diabetes is a complex disease characterized by disturbances in carbohydrate, fat, and protein metabolism caused by hormone imbalances, primarily insulin and glucagon. Type 1 diabetes is an autoimmune disease of familial predisposition. Type 2 diabetes is a disease of insulin resistance with obesity as a classic hallmark. Whether a disease of insulin deficiency or of insulin resistance, the common denominator is the presence of hyperglycemia.

Type 1 Diabetes

Type 1 diabetes occurs in fewer than 10% of the people with diabetes. It is an autoimmune disease in which it is thought that a viral trigger initiates a cascade of destruction. Islet cell antibodies are present in a subclinical level for years before symptoms occur. A viral illness such as chickenpox or influenza occurs, and massive autoimmune activity destroys the beta cells. This process precipitates an absolute insulin deficiency, potentially leading to diabetic ketoacidosis (DKA). Peak

times for diagnosis are preadolescence, school age, ages 5 to 6 years, and young adulthood. However, Type 1 diabetes can occur at any age. DKA is characterized by uncontrolled hyperglycemia (>300 mg/dL), metabolic acidosis (pH < 7.30), and the unique diagnostic feature of increased plasma ketone bodies.[1]

Type 2 Diabetes

Type 2 diabetes occurs in 80 to 90% of people with diabetes. Usually, it occurs after age 45, with the highest incidence over the age of 65 years. An increasing incidence of maturity onset of diabetes in youth (MODY) is occurring in children and adolescents.

Type 2 diabetes is a disease of insulin resistance. However, both type 1 and type 2 diabetes have a familial predisposition with strong genetic links. The precipitating trigger in type 2 diabetes is usually obesity. Endogenous insulin production is still occurring, but insulin resistance is present. This condition has various causes including insulin receptor defects, hepatic glycogen release, poor glucose utilization and uptake by the muscle, glucose transporter defects, and other cellular defects. All these problems result in hyperglycemia. Because the person with type 2 diabetes is still producing insulin, this prevents the ketogenesis cycle and thus DKA. However, persons with type 2 diabetes are more susceptible to hyperosmolar nonketotic coma (HHNK). In HHNK, patients tend to be more hyperglycemic (>600–800 mg/dL) and less ketotic (ketones < 5 mmol). Considerable overlap exists between the two disorders and, consequently, their treatment.

Incidence of Diabetes

The incidence of diabetes is increasing at about 6% per year.[2] Sixteen million Americans have diabetes and half of them are undiagnosed. About 7 to 7.5 million Americans have type 2 diabetes. Only about 700,000 have type 1 diabetes. Most people have type 2 diabetes and are not ketosis prone and therefore are more likely to develop HHNK. DKA, on the other hand, contributes to a significant percentage of emergencies in any general hospital. The National Diabetes Data Group[2] estimates an annual incidence of DKA at 3 to 8 episodes per 1000 patients with diabetes. New patients with diabetes present with ketoacidosis about 20 to 30% of the time. Mortality from DKA remains at about 8 to 14% and increases with age, severity of underlying precipitating factors, and degree of metabolic derangements.[3]

Infection is the most common precipitating cause of DKA and is responsible for about 30 to 40% of all DKA admissions.[1] Other causes of DKA are related to omission of insulin injections, especially in adolescents, and underlying illness such as cerebrovascular accidents in the elderly (Chart 28–1). Patient education with early triage and sick day insulin management may allow hyperglycemia to be treated at home.

In some cases when home management is not done by the patient, critical care intervention is initiated by emergency rooms and is followed up by home health care facilities. This venue of care delivery will continue to increase in frequency as managed care gains influence in the United States. This represents a vast opportunity for patient and professional education. Self-management training for people with diabetes empowers patients to initiate and resolve mild DKA at home with telephone support from the health professional. With the patient as the central focus, collaborative practice with many health professionals is occurring in today's integrated health care system.

Pathophysiology

The absolute (type 1) or relative (type 2) insulin deficiency seen in diabetes is responsible for hyperglycemia. The resultant effect of counterregulatory hormones, primarily glucagon, leads to a catabolic action that causes hyperglycemia, ketosis, and ultimately ketoacidosis. In normal fuel metabolism, energy is provided through carbohydrate, fat, and protein. Fuel substrates are absorbed as glucose, free fatty acids, glycerol, and amino acids. If glucose is not immediately needed for energy, it is stored as glycogen in the liver and muscles, or it is stored as triglycerides in the adipose tissue.

Insulin and glucagon are the primary hormones that control fuel metabolism. Insulin functions primarily in the fed state to stimulate nutrient utilization and storage when glucagon secretion is suppressed. Glucagon functions primarily in the fasting state to supply the body's energy needs by releasing glycogen.

Diabetic Ketoacidosis

In type 1 diabetes, severe insulin deficiency results in the inability of muscle and adipose tissue to use glucose. Without the counterregulatory effects of insulin, glucagon triggers an accelerated rate of hepatic glucose production by glycogenolysis and gluconeogenesis. Poor peripheral glucose utilization and excessive hepatic glucose production combine to create hyperglycemia. To compensate for the starvation of peripheral muscle tissues, lipolysis (fat breakdown) is stimulated, and ketones (beta-hydroxybutyrate and acetoacetic acid) are produced as a by-product of free fatty acid metabolism in the liver. This exacerbates an insulin-resistant state, which decreases insulin binding to its receptors and alters glucose uptake through operation of the glucose–fatty acid cycle.

Glucose and ketones are osmotically active. Their excretion in the urine leads to osmotic diuresis and dehydration. Volume depletion secondary to hyperglycemia-induced osmotic diuresis is also a factor. Severe depletion may lead to decreased urine output. Improving fluid volume with rehydration alone may vastly lower plasma glucose levels. Without the administration of insulin, severe dehydration, electrolyte imbalance, metabolic acidosis, coma, and even death may occur (Figure 28–1).

Primary precipitating factors for DKA include undiagnosed type 1 diabetes, uncontrolled diabetes, severe illness, infection, and psychosocial causes such as poor access to health care, insulin, blood glucose testing supplies, and stress.

Signs and symptoms of DKA can easily be confused with other conditions. The nonspecific fatigue and frequent urination (polyuria) of early ketosis may suggest a urinary tract infection. As the condition deteriorates, weight loss, abdominal tenderness, and electrolyte imbalance from nausea and vomiting may seem like the flu. These symptoms are also confused

CHART 28-1

RESEARCH UTILIZATION: PRECIPITATING FACTORS OF DKA

Abstract: The objective of this study was to identify the causes of diabetic ketoacidosis (DKA) in a large urban hospital. Over a 3-month period, all African-Americans who were 18 years old or older who were admitted in moderate to severe DKA, as defined by a serum glucose greater than 250 mg/dL, bicarbonate less than 15 mmol/L, and pH less than 7.35, were studied. Diabetes nurse educators reviewed medical records and interviewed patients. Information obtained included precipitating causes of DKA, content of previous diabetes education, frequency of home blood glucose monitoring, recognition of symptoms of metabolic decompensation, and types of medical assistance obtained after the patient became ill.

In the 3-month study period, there were 56 admissions. Seventy-five percent of these patients had known diabetes. The other 25% were persons with newly diagnosed diabetes. In the patients with known diabetes, the most common cause of DKA was stopping of insulin therapy. This occurred in 67% of the cases. Lack of funds or inability to reach the hospital to obtain insulin was reported as the cause for stopping the insulin in 50% of the patients. Twenty-one percent stopped their insulin because of lack of appetite, and 14% stopped their insulin because they did not know how to manage their diabetes on sick days. Eighty percent of the patients with known diabetes remembered being instructed on glucose testing and acute and chronic complications, but only 28% recalled being instructed on dose adjustment, and 35% remembered instruction on sick day management. Over half (55%) of those patients with known diabetes recognized the symptoms of decompensation, but only 5% contacted the diabetes center. The majority went to the emergency room.

The authors concluded that, in the urban African-American population, two-thirds of the episodes of DKA could be prevented with improved access to care and patient education. Good glycemic control reduces complications. The Diabetes Control and Complications Trial (DCCT) was a 10-year, prospective study conducted by the National Institutes of Health. The study demonstrated that retinopathy could be reduced by up to 75% by reducing hemoglobin A_{1c} to 7%, and the risk of the other associated complications, such as neuropathy and nephropathy, could be reduced. The DCCT confirmed that intensive diabetes management and medical support facilitated those improvements. Access to care and patients empowered for self-management produced extremely positive outcomes.

Critique: The authors identified a significant problem that is costly and potentially has devastating consequences for the patient. The problem was identified in a health care facility in which diabetes care is provided by a multidisciplinary team. Success had been achieved in the early years of the program (1974–1986), but cases of DKA had failed to decline since that time. An important translation of this study is that even though the patient population was urban African-American the difficulty in financing and accessing supplies is relevant for many persons with diabetes.

A standard structured patient interview was used. The question format was a structured yes–no response format. Interviewing as a method can be influenced by interviewer bias, but combining the interview with the chart audit increases the validity.

Fifty-six patients were evaluated. Data were examined by analysis of variance and χ^2. Considering the relatively small sample size, these were appropriate tests to use for statistical analysis.

Nursing Implications: This study highlights the tragedy of the costliness of diabetes to the patient who has difficulty in obtaining insulin and glucose testing supplies. The nurse is often the primary referral source and coordinator of care. Home health nurses should be utilized for teaching, follow-up, and care whenever possible. The social services in the community and other community resources should be made available to patients suspected of being in need of financial support.

Sick day education is necessary for all patients with diabetes. Retention of information used so seldom is likely low, so the more important nursing implication is providing phone numbers, pager access, and clear information on accessing the health care triage system in emergencies. Telephone triage for the educated person with diabetes can prevent most emergency room visits and admissions for DKA.

Source: Musey V, Klatka M, Lee J, et al: Diabetes in urban African-Americans. I. Cessation of insulin therapy is the major precipitating cause of diabetic ketoacidosis. Diabetes Care 18:483–489, 1995.

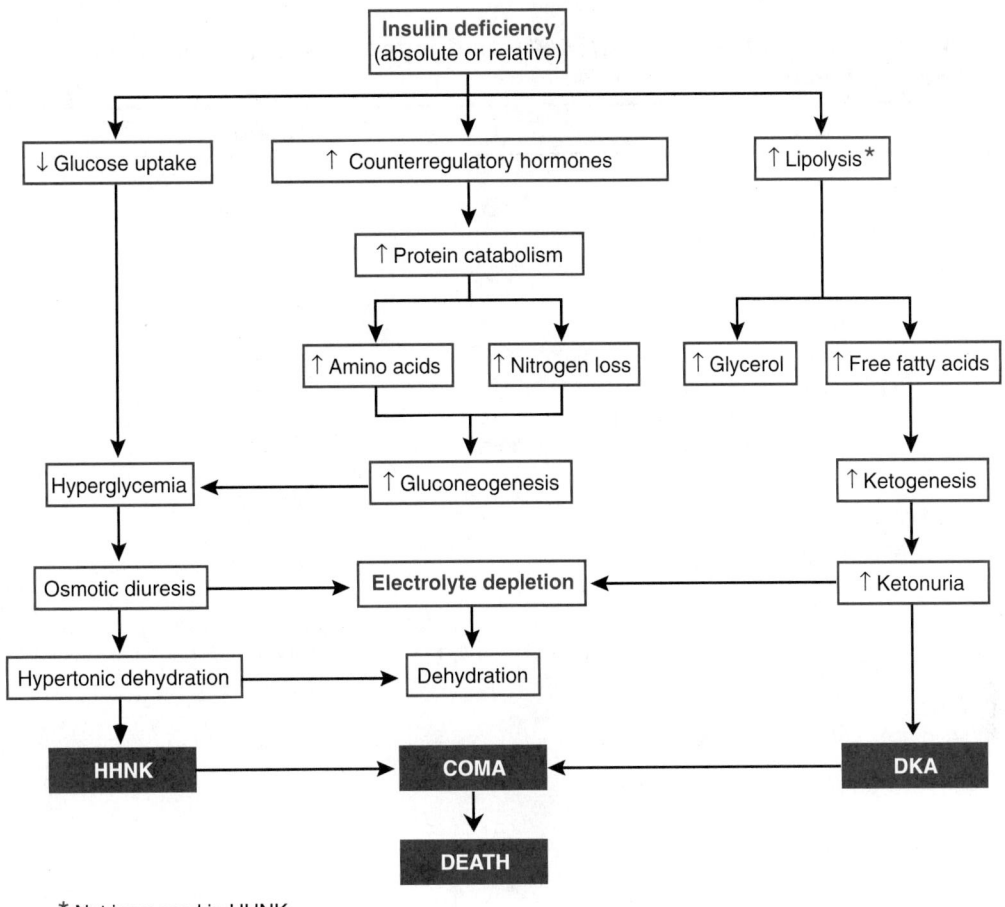

* Not increased in HHNK

Figure 28–1

Pathophysiologic pathways for diabetic ketoacidosis (DKA) and hyperglycemic hyperosmolar nonketotic coma (HHNK).

with alcohol consumption, especially the ketotic (acetone) breath. This factor further reinforces the need for all persons with diabetes to wear medical identification. When severe DKA occurs, classic Kussmaul's respiration, a deep and labored breathing, is present. The features of DKA and HHNK are summarized in Table 28–1.

Hyperglycemic Hyperosmolar Nonketotic Syndrome

The pathophysiology of HHNK is similar to that of DKA, with the notable absence of overproduction of ketone bodies. Thus, ketoacidosis does not occur. The extreme hyperglycemia that characterizes this syndrome results from the decrease in urine output. The escape route for glucose is diminished or absent. At the same time, hepatic glucose production continues unabated, and glucose is released into a steadily shrinking plasma–extracellular space. The result is an extremely high concentration of glucose. With the lack of ketosis, the obvious severity of the illness is not

evident, and the patient in HHNK may not be diagnosed until the dehydration is so severe that consciousness is altered (see Figure 28–1).

HHNK usually occurs in elderly patients with type 2 diabetes. Some endogenous (internal) insulin production prevents significant lipolysis and ketosis. This is the primary differentiation between DKA and HHNK. Further distinctions in HHNK include the presence of extremely high plasma glucose (600–1000 mg/dL) and osmolality (>350 mOsm). The resulting osmotic diuresis can cause severe dehydration and a decrease in glomerular filtration rate. In the face of decreasing renal function, glucose cannot be effectively excreted in the urine, and blood glucose continues to rise, causing intracellular dehydration and hyperosmolarity. Nursing assessment should include monitoring for severe dehydration and neurologic manifestations such as stupor that may progress to coma.[4]

The mortality rate in HHNK is sometimes reported as high as 50%, depending on the underlying illness. The high osmolality leads to poor perfusion and dehydration that may predispose patients to vascular occlusion. Extreme levels of measured serum osmolality

TABLE 28–1

Comparison of Diabetic Ketoacidosis (DKA) and Hyperglycemic Hyperosmolar Nonketotic Coma (HHNK)

Feature	DKA	HHNK
Age of patient	Usually <40 years	Usually >60 years
Duration of symptoms	Usually <2 days	Usually >5 days
Glucose level	Usually <600 mg/dL	Usually >800 mg/dL
Sodium concentration	Likely normal or low	Likely normal or high
Potassium concentration	High, normal, or low	High, normal, or low
Bicarbonate concentrate	Low	Normal
Ketone bodies	Present	Usually absent
pH	Low, <7.3	Normal
Serum osmolality	Usually <350 mOsm/kg	Usually >350 mOsm/kg
Cerebral edema	Often subclinical, occasionally clinical	Rarely occurs
Assessment		
Skin	Flushed; dry, warm	Pallor: moist, cool
Breath	Fruity, acetone	Normal
Vital signs	Blood pressure decreased	Blood pressure decreased
	Pulse increased	Pulse increased
	Kussmaul's respirations	Respiration normal
Gastrointestinal	Severe abdominal pain, nausea, vomiting	Mild abdominal pain, nausea, vomiting
Mental status	Lethargic	Lethargic
Level of consciousness	Decreasing	Decreasing
Urine output/fluid intake	Increased initially, decreased with dehydration	Increased initially, decreased with dehydration
Prognosis	8–14% mortality	10–20% mortality
Subsequent course	Insulin therapy required in nearly all cases	Insulin therapy not required in many cases

have been associated with the development of coma and an increased mortality. One formula for calculating effective osmolality is[5]

$$2(Na) + \frac{Glucose}{18} + \frac{BUN}{2.8}$$

HHNK is insidious. Patients typically come to seek medical attention later and are much sicker. Precipitating factors are usually dehydration, medications such as steroids and thiazide diuretics, acute illness, cerebral vascular accident, and advanced age. Any elderly person with or without diabetes who has deteriorated central nervous system function and is severely dehydrated should be evaluated for HHNK.

Assessment

Signs and Symptoms of Ketoacidosis and Hyperglycemic Hyperosmolar Nonketotic Coma

DKA has no specific signs and symptoms, but it has rather a constellation of signs and symptoms that should alert the clinician to the possibility of the diagnosis. Symptoms may mimic those of other diseases or conditions. Any person presenting with coma, shock, dehydration, respiratory distress, or any other evidence of major illness should have an immediate screening of blood or urine glucose and urine ketones. Any person with known diabetes who has nausea, vomiting, abdominal pain, central nervous system depression, shortness of breath, fever, localized signs of infection, or unexplained glucose levels of greater than 250 mg/dL should be screened for DKA.

Unlike DKA, which usually occurs in patients with type 1 diabetes, HHNK is commonly found in the elderly patient with mild or undiagnosed type 2 diabetes. Often, the patient is taking oral agents and is not monitored well. Someone who lives alone or anyone unable to communicate his or her needs may potentially become dehydrated from lack of fluids. The absence of significant ketosis is what differentiates HHNK from DKA. The signs and symptoms of HHNK are similar to those of DKA, with several exceptions (see Table 28–1).

The assessment process includes establishment of a previous history of diabetes. If diabetes has been previously diagnosed, then events leading to the current status must be obtained, including other diabetes complications, diabetes medication history, previous episodes of DKA, or severe hypoglycemia. A physical assessment should be conducted. An evaluation of laboratory values is necessary.

The typical manifestations of hyperglycemia are polyuria, polydipsia, polyphagia, and blurred vision.

Nonspecific symptoms include weakness, lethargy, malaise, and headache. The most profound symptoms of HHNK are related to the significant hyperglycemia, which is often greater than 800 mg/dL (normal 60–150 mg/dL), and the marked elevation in serum osmolality.

Gastrointestinal System
In DKA, gastrointestinal symptoms include nausea, vomiting, and abdominal pain. It is not clear what leads to the gastrointestinal symptoms, but the acidotic state is thought to be a factor. Abdominal tenderness is common and often is mistaken for an "acute abdomen." Signs include tenderness to palpation, diminished bowel sounds, and some muscle guarding, especially in children.[4] The gastrointestinal symptoms of HHNK are generally mild compared with those of DKA.

Respiratory System
Respiratory symptoms of DKA include Kussmaul's respiration, which is described as an "inability to catch one's breath." Kussmaul's respirations are very deep, labored respirations and represent an attempt by the body to correct metabolic acidosis. Acetone breath may be present. Acetoacetate, one of the ketone bodies, is converted to acetone, which is excreted by the lungs. Acetone is described as having a fruity odor and can often be detected on the patient's breath. Kussmaul's respirations rarely occur in HHNK.

Vascular System
In both DKA and HHNK, symptoms of dehydration (intravascular volume depletion) are likely, including hypotension, tachycardia, dry mucous membranes, decreased skin turgor, and decreased eyeball pressure. Dehydration can also be assessed by observing for decreased neck vein filling from below when the patient is lying flat and by obtaining postural vital signs. Body fluid losses can be estimated by subtracting the admission weight from a recent known dry weight. Hypotension usually occurs with at least 10% dehydration. Severe dehydration is a clinical hallmark of HHNK.

Cardiovascular System
Cardiac dysrhythmias are common with alteration in the potassium level, with flattened or inverted T waves and the appearance of U waves that indicate hypokalemia. Tall symmetric T waves, a widened QRS complex, and loss of P waves indicate hyperkalemia. Asystole may occur with either imbalance, if it is severe enough.

Neurologic System
Mentation changes may be present in both DKA and HHNK. Patients in DKA may be alert, obtunded, stu-

porous, or in frank coma. The level of consciousness is best correlated with serum osmolality, less well with glucose concentrations, and least well with serum pH.[4] Hyporeflexia or decreased reflexes may occur with decreasing potassium levels. Although hypothermia is often found, fever suggests the presence of an underlying infection.

Lethargy and confusion are common with HHNK, but frank coma is unusual. Mentation correlates best with serum osmolality. Focal neurologic deficits may be present, including hemisensory deficits, hemiparesis, aphasia, myoclonic jerking, and seizures. A positive Babinski sign may be present. Hypothermia or hyperthermia may be found in HHNK.

Renal System
In these emergencies, the patient is usually anuric on admission and remains oliguric until rehydrated. The creatinine and blood urea nitrogen are likely elevated because of the reduced glomerular filtration rate and dehydration.

Medication History
All medications ingested by the patient, including all prescriptions and over-the-counter medications, should be reviewed. Special consideration should be given to the insulin doses taken, including type, species, and units given. Any missed doses in the previous 48 hours should be noted. For the patient in HHNK, special consideration should be given to all oral diabetes medications and thiazide diuretics.

Laboratory and Diagnostic Tests

An initial diagnosis of DKA can be made by clinical impression and bedside testing, including a capillary blood glucose determination and a blood or urine ketone test. Additional laboratory tests should be obtained to guide treatment.

Blood Glucose and Blood or Urine Ketone Tests
In DKA, the glucose level is usually greater than 300 mg/dL, with an average of 600 mg/dL.[1] Normal plasma glucose levels are between 60 and 150 mg/dL. The glucose level may be less than 250 mg/dL, especially if the patient with diabetes has ingested large amounts of alcohol. The value may also be greater than 600 mg/dL if the patient has had long-standing poor glucose control. In contrast to DKA, the blood glucose level in HHNK is often greater than 800 mg/dL and can be as high as 2000 mg/dL. Because of the profound dehydration, the serum sodium is usually higher in HHNK than in DKA. The patient with HHNK also has a higher osmolality than the patient in DKA. The serum osmolality reflects the degree of intracellular dehydration. Testing for blood

or urine ketones should be initiated when blood glucose levels are greater than 250 mg/dL.

Electrolyte and pH Tests

The potassium level may be high, low, or normal. The plasma potassium averages 5.2 mEq/L, but it can be less than 3.5 or more than 6 mEq/L on admission.[1] Plasma blood urea nitrogen and creatinine usually are slightly elevated because of reduced renal blood flow and dehydration.

The pH can range from 6.8 to 7.3 in DKA. The pH may be higher than expected or even normal if the patient has concurrent metabolic alkalosis from diuretic ingestion or mineralocorticoid action. In DKA, the carbon dioxide (CO_2) value is usually less than 20 mEq/L. A CO_2 of less than 20 mEq/L but greater than 15 mEq/L signifies DKA, whereas a CO_2 of <15 mEq/L signifies acidosis.[6] The plasma anion gap is usually between 16 and 30.

Other Diagnostic Tests

Infection should not be excluded as a precipitating factor because of a normal or subnormal temperature. Leukocytosis is present in nearly all cases of DKA.[6] Meningeal signs call for computed tomography or magnetic resonance imaging of the head, followed by a lumbar puncture. Blood cultures may be warranted in patients with fever of unknown origin. A urinalysis should be evaluated for bacteria and nitrites. If leukocytes or nitrites are present, a sterile urine specimen should be obtained. A pulmonary infection should be ruled out if any respiratory disease is noted on physical assessment.

Rectal and pelvic examinations should not be deferred if the abdominal pain and nausea and vomiting do not resolve with initial treatment because appendicitis, pelvic inflammatory disease, diverticulitis, and cholecystitis may be the source of the pain.

As suggested with the patient with DKA, underlying causes for HHNK must be evaluated, including testing for stroke, myocardial infarction, or underlying infection if the presenting symptoms warrant such testing. An electrocardiogram (ECG) should be evaluated for an acute silent myocardial infarction in older adults and in patients with type 1 diabetes for longer than 15 years.

Nursing Diagnoses

The care of patients presenting with DKA and HHNK requires astute observational and assessment skills. This care is provided by nurses as well as by other members of the health care team across various settings within the acute care facility and extending into the community. This collaborative approach to the care of patients with DKA or HHNK can be guided by nursing diagnoses (Table 28–2). These diagnoses rarely involve nursing alone, but instead, draw on the expertise of the multidisciplinary team to deliver holistic care.

Collaborative Management

The management of patients experiencing DKA and HHNK requires an interdisciplinary approach and usually begins in the emergency room (Chart 28–2). Physicians, critical care nurses, diabetes educators including nurses, dietitians, social workers, and behaviorists, pharmacists, and clergy may all be part of the team. Others who may play a role before and after discharge are exercise specialists, case managers, and home health nurses. Patients with diabetes require ongoing support, and the critical care nurse begins the return to the home environment and initiates the process of preventing future admissions for DKA or HHNK.

The goals of treatment for DKA and HHNK are to correct the fluid and electrolyte disturbances, to provide adequate insulin to restore and maintain normal glucose metabolism and to correct acidosis in DKA, to prevent complications resulting from the treatment of DKA and HHNK, and to provide the patient and family with education and follow-up.

TABLE 28–2
Nursing Diagnoses

Problem Statement	Etiologic Factors
Fluid volume deficit	Osmotic diuresis
Decreased cardiac output	Hypovolemia, increased osmolality, dehydration, electrolyte disturbances
Altered nutrition, less than body requirements	Insulin deficiency
Risk for altered tissue perfusion, cerebral	Cerebral edema secondary to rehydration and rapid glycemic shifts
Knowledge deficit, learning need	Disease process, prognosis, treatment, and self-management techniques
Anxiety	Sudden hospitalization; new diagnosis; realization that diabetes is a chronic disease, requiring lifelong self-management, lifestyle changes, and follow-up for prevention of long-term complications
Anticipatory or dysfunctional grieving	Loss of previous level of health and lifestyle

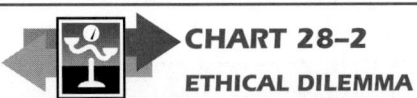

CHART 28-2

ETHICAL DILEMMA

Diabetes educators reported that the majority of ethical conflicts (75%) concerned disagreements with the physician regarding the quality of medical care the patient was receiving.[7] The registered nurse is often caught between personal responsibility for the welfare of the patient and professional responsibility to support the medical doctors.

Mrs. S., age 38, presents to the emergency department on New Year's Eve at 11:30 PM with vomiting and labored breathing. She has a strong odor of rotten fruit on her breath. She and her husband had been at a New Year's Eve party. The resident physician orders a chemistry 24 profile and does a brief history and physical examination.

The patient has not been feeling well for about 1 week. She thought she had a urinary tract infection because of frequent urination. The family medical history is unremarkable except for a maternal grandmother who had diabetes. The patient's blood sugar is found to be 350 mg/dL.

The resident diagnoses acute alcohol intoxication and prepares to discharge the patient.

1. What is of immediate concern in this case?
2. What additional data are needed to confirm or rule out the diagnosis?
3. What ethical principles are involved in this situation?
4. What is the nurse's role in the decision-making process regarding the treatment of this patient?

Patients with moderate to severe DKA and HHNK require immediate emergency attention. Severe DKA and HHNK should be monitored and treated in an intensive care unit (ICU). Chart 28–3 depicts an example of standing orders used to direct the care of these patients while in the ICU. Patients with moderate DKA are defined as those who cannot retain oral fluids, who have a CO_2 of less than 20 mEq/L but greater than 15 mEq/dL, and who have alterations in mental status. Many times, these patients, as well as patients with early HHNK, can be managed in alternative settings (Chart 28–4).

In the rare situation in which cardiac or respiratory arrest has occurred, an adequate airway must be established and respiratory function must be maintained. Management includes oxygen administration as necessary.

The largest possible intravenous line for rapid administration of saline must be started and its patency maintained. Fluid and electrolyte replacement is based on individual needs. Adequate fluid replacement is critical for lowering blood glucose levels. Hyperglycemia persists even with insulin therapy if fluid replacement is inadequate.

Consideration should include maintenance needs, replacement requirements, and ongoing fluid and electrolyte losses. Monitoring of blood pressure, pulse, and intake and output is necessary to determine whether adequate hydration is occurring. Bladder catheterization may be necessary but it is not recommended if the patient is able to void.

Initial fluid replacement for DKA should be made with one-half normal saline (0.45%) or normal (0.9%) saline. For adults, the initial replacement depends on the degree of dehydration and the patient's cardiovascular status. In general, 1 to 2 L should be delivered in the first 1 to 2 hours for adults.

When the serum glucose is decreased to approximately 250 mg/dL, intravenous fluids should be changed to include glucose. Even though the blood glucose level may be decreased, the acidosis is likely not resolved. Adequate amounts of insulin must continue to be given and glucose must be administered until the acidosis is adequately resolved.

As in DKA, fluid replacement in HHNK depends on the patient's state of hydration and cardiovascular status. Elderly patients should always have continuous cardiac monitoring. The patient with HHNK probably will be in the ICU.

The first 2 L of fluids are usually 0.9% normal saline to raise the circulating volume, but then the infusion is switched to hypotonic solutions. Up to 12 L of fluids may be infused in a 24- to 36-hour period. The rate of administration must be guided by body weight, urine output, kidney function, and the presence or absence of congestive heart failure. In patients with prior congestive heart failure or renal failure, central venous pressure monitoring is indicated. Failure to show improvement may mean inadequate rehydration.[1] Fluid requirements are higher in HHNK because of the extreme dehydration and hyperosmolarity.

Hypokalemia, if not treated properly, can lead to death. Potassium should be given immediately if hypokalemia is present, as noted by the ECG or laboratory findings. All patients with DKA, once urine flow has been established, require potassium replacement. Potassium may be added in the second to fourth hour of treatment or sooner, depending on the T-wave changes and confirmed by laboratory values. Potassium is usually replaced at concentrations of 20 to 40 mEq/L. Sometimes, half is given as potassium chloride and half as potassium phosphate. If the initial

CHART 28–3

Orders for Patients Admitted to the ICU With a Diagnosis of Diabetic Ketoacidosis or Hyperglycemic Hyperosmolar Nonketotic Coma

1. Blood sugar by Accu-Check and test urine ketones on admission.
2. Stat CBC, Chem-7, UA. Call results. CO_2 <10 Requires critical care bed.
3. Repeat Chem-7 every 2 hr ×2, then in 4 hr, and then in 8 hr. Call results.
4. Check urine each void until negative for ketones.
5. NPO. Sips of sugar-containing clear liquids when blood sugar and electrolytes become stabilized and patient is without GI distress.
6. Vital signs q2h × 8 hr.
7. Telemetry.
8. Oxygen at 2–3 L PRN at nurses' discretion.
9. Foley catheter PRN.
10. A. Start IV of 1000 NS at _____ hr. KCL _____ mEq/KPO_4 _____ mmL added to above solution (10–20 mL/kg IBW for first liter).
    B. Second liter _____ at _____ hr. KCL _____ mEq/KPO_4 _____ mmL added to above solution.
    C. When BS falls approximately to 250 or 1/2 of admitting BS, 1000 D_5 1/2 NS or D_{10} 1/2 NS at _____ hr. Add KCL _____ mEq/KPO_4 _____ mmL to above solution.
11. If BS > 500 _____ U (human regular) insulin IV push (0.1 U/kg IBW) one time only (NTE 10 U). Recheck in 15–30 min.
12. Human regular insulin, 50 U in 50 NS syringe pump IV piggyback, below filter, run at _____ hr (0.1U/kg).
13. BS hourly. BS goal 120–200 mg/dL.
14. BS falls by 50–100 hourly, and insulin titrated by nurses to maintain that rate of fall per No. 15, 16, and 17.
15. If BS does not fall by 50 mg/dL/hr, increase insulin infusion by 1 U greater per hr.
16. If BS falls greater than 100 per hr, decrease insulin infusion by 1–2 U less per hr.
17. When BS is less than 120 mg/dL; shut syringe pump off. Call attending physician. Recheck blood sugar in 1/2 hr. If blood sugar is above 120 mg/dL, restart syringe pump at 1–2 U less per hr. Do not keep insulin pump off >30 min.
18. If BS remains less than 120 mg/dL for >30 min, D_5 1/2 NS with K^+ (per No. 10C) will be changed to D_{10} 1/2 NS with K^+.
19. Routine hypoglycemia orders.
20. When starting subcutaneous insulin, give first dose 30 min before discontinuing syringe pump IV insulin.
21. Insulin protocol 0.25–2.0 U/kg human regular insulin = total daily dose.
    35% total daily dose before breakfast.
    22% total daily dose before lunch.
    28% total daily dose before supper.
    15% total daily dose at midnight.
22. Discontinue telemetry when syringe pump is discontinued if cardiac condition is stable.

Adapted with permission from Via Christi Health System, Wichita, KS.

phosphate (PO_4) is high, then potassium chloride only is given.

Potassium concentrations can drop rapidly from those obtained initially because of the intravascular volume expansion and increased renal excretion resulting from increased renal perfusion of the kidneys, both conditions secondary to rehydration. Insulin administration also causes an increase in intracellular potassium. Continuous monitoring of the potassium concentration and ECG findings are guides to therapy. Clinically significant signs of hypokalemia include skeletal weakness progressing to paralysis, rapid diminution or absence of deep tendon reflexes, and

dysrhythmias, including flattened or inverted T waves. The development of shallow, gasping respirations, in contrast to Kussmaul's respirations, may also be noted. Symptoms of hyperkalemia include tall symmetric T waves, loss of the P wave, and widening of the QRS complex. Deep tendon reflexes are hyperactive. Monitoring of the serum electrolytes every 2 to 4 hours is likely necessary the first 12 to 24 hours of treatment in severe DKA.

Potassium replacement is also necessary in HHNK. Potassium loss is less in HHNK than in DKA, probably as a result of milder acidosis and lack of vomiting associated with HHNK. Because the patient is usually

CHART 28–4
Beyond the ICU: Managing DKA and HHNK

Many cases of mild to moderate diabetic ketoacidosis (DKA) and some cases of early hyperglycemic hyperosmolar nonketotic coma are likely to be managed in a partial day care setting, in emergency rooms, clinics, and even at home. The nurse is challenged to use astute nursing assessment skills to monitor when the patient is too critically ill to be managed outside the intensive care setting. The risk of electrolyte imbalance, including hypokalemia and hyperkalemia, cerebral edema, and other complications, must be monitored carefully.

Fluid replacement is likely to be initiated in the Emergency Department. Initial laboratory data, especially the carbon dioxide values, determine the acuity of the patient. What previously could have been an admission may now be an observation (23-hour) or partial day (outpatient) treatment. Six to 8 hours of fluids and low-dose insulin infusion may circumvent the need for inpatient admission. Home health nurses are accepting referrals of patients with DKA who are discharged from the emergency department. Continuing fluid replacement and insulin by infusion or injection will require hourly glucose monitoring. The capability for quick laboratory data

turnaround for electrolytes is also necessary. In a collaborative practice model, a nurse with preapproved protocols for DKA may resolve this emergency situation and may thus avert the need for a hospital admission.

Many outpatient clinics including family practice settings are providing rehydration as a clinic service. The nurse plays an integral role in this collaborative practice setting through assessment, intervention, evaluation, and education.

In the home setting, the patient and family require self-management education, including an understanding of signs and symptoms indicating that the patient's condition is deteriorating. These signs and symptoms could include Kussmaul's respiration, persistent vomiting, decreasing mental alertness, positive urine ketones, and failure of the blood glucose level to decline. Important components of the home health plan are identification of the health care practitioner to notify for management and the means of notifying the practitioner. The nurse and physician must be able to monitor the patient's electrolyte status even in the home environment.

---

oliguric, potassium likely needs to be added as the patient becomes better hydrated and produces and excretes more urine.

Treatment with sodium bicarbonate is controversial and is not recommended by most diabetes specialists. The acidosis of DKA is corrected in time by insulin inhibition of ketogenesis. Bicarbonate also increases the risk of hypokalemia. If used, bicarbonate should be given by slow intravenous infusion over several hours. It should not be given as a bolus injection, except in cardiac arrest. Doses of 50 to 100 mEq bicarbonate in 250 to 1000 mL of 0.45% normal saline can be administered over 30 to 60 minutes. The arterial pH should be checked after 50 to 100 mEq is administered, and monitoring should be continued until the pH reaches 7.10. Potassium levels must be monitored frequently, and additional potassium may need to be administered.[1]

In HHNK, bicarbonate is not needed unless the patient has severe lactic acidosis. However, with the increased use of the biquinides such as metformin in the treatment of type 2 diabetes, lactic acidosis is a consideration.

Although phosphate and magnesium levels are usually normal or elevated on admission, body stores of both are often depleted in DKA. Occasionally, they are depleted in HHNK. Insulin administration frequently produces hypophosphatemia and a less dramatic fall in magnesium. Some physicians use potassium phosphate to correct or attenuate the hypophosphatemia. If rhabdomyolysis, central nervous system deterioration, cardiac dysfunction, or hemolysis parallels the initial fall in plasma phosphate, then replacement is definitely needed.

Insulin treatment protocols vary from institution to institution. All patients in DKA need insulin. Regular or lispro insulin should be used. Lispro insulin's time action is like that of regular insulin when given intravenously: onset in 5 minutes, peak in 10 to 15 minutes, and clearance in 20 to 30 minutes. Intravenous low-dose concentrations are the most widely used method of insulin administration. The benefits of low-dose insulin infusion include the reduced risk of hypoglycemia and hypokalemia because the glucose and potassium decreases are more predictable. Typically, 0.1 to 0.2 U/kg is given per hour up to 10 to 12 U per hour. An intravenous or intramuscular bolus of regular insulin may be given before the initiation of the continuous insulin infusion.[6]

The insulin is administered through a piggyback intravenous line inserted below the filter: 1 U of insulin per 1 mL intravenous fluid is the common dilution in a 50-mL syringe, to decrease adherence to the tubing and to allow accurate titration of the dose. The blood glucose level should drop between 75 and 100 mg/dL per hour with proper insulin therapy and rehydration. In many institutions, nurses are provided standing orders with which to adjust the insulin infusion to obtain a 75- to 100-mg/dL decrease in glucose per hour (see Chart 28–3). Subcutaneous insulin may be

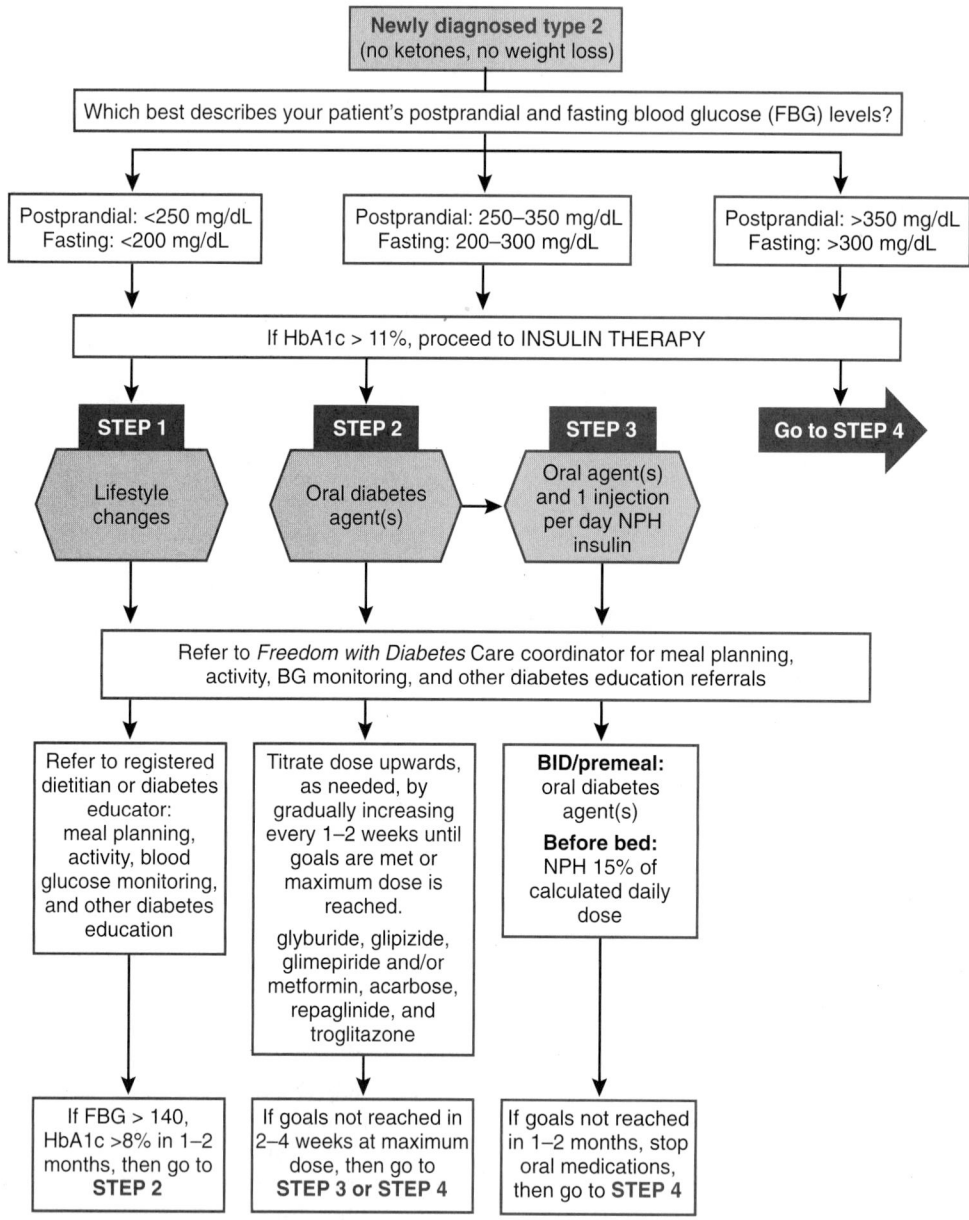

Figure 28–2

An example of diabetes management protocol. (With permission from Via Christi Health System, Wichita, KS.)

given when the patient is able to eat. Subcutaneous regular insulin should be given 30 minutes before discontinuing intravenous insulin to provide adequate insulin coverage.

Frequent nursing assessments, including hourly bedside blood glucose monitoring, are required by patients receiving intravenous insulin. Urinary ketone bodies may take several days to clear and are not useful in management decisions. Urine glucose monitoring is not useful in the management of DKA. Glucose spills into the urine normally when the blood glucose level is greater than 160 to 180 mg/dL. However, the urine glucose threshold is often elevated with age and the complications of diabetes.

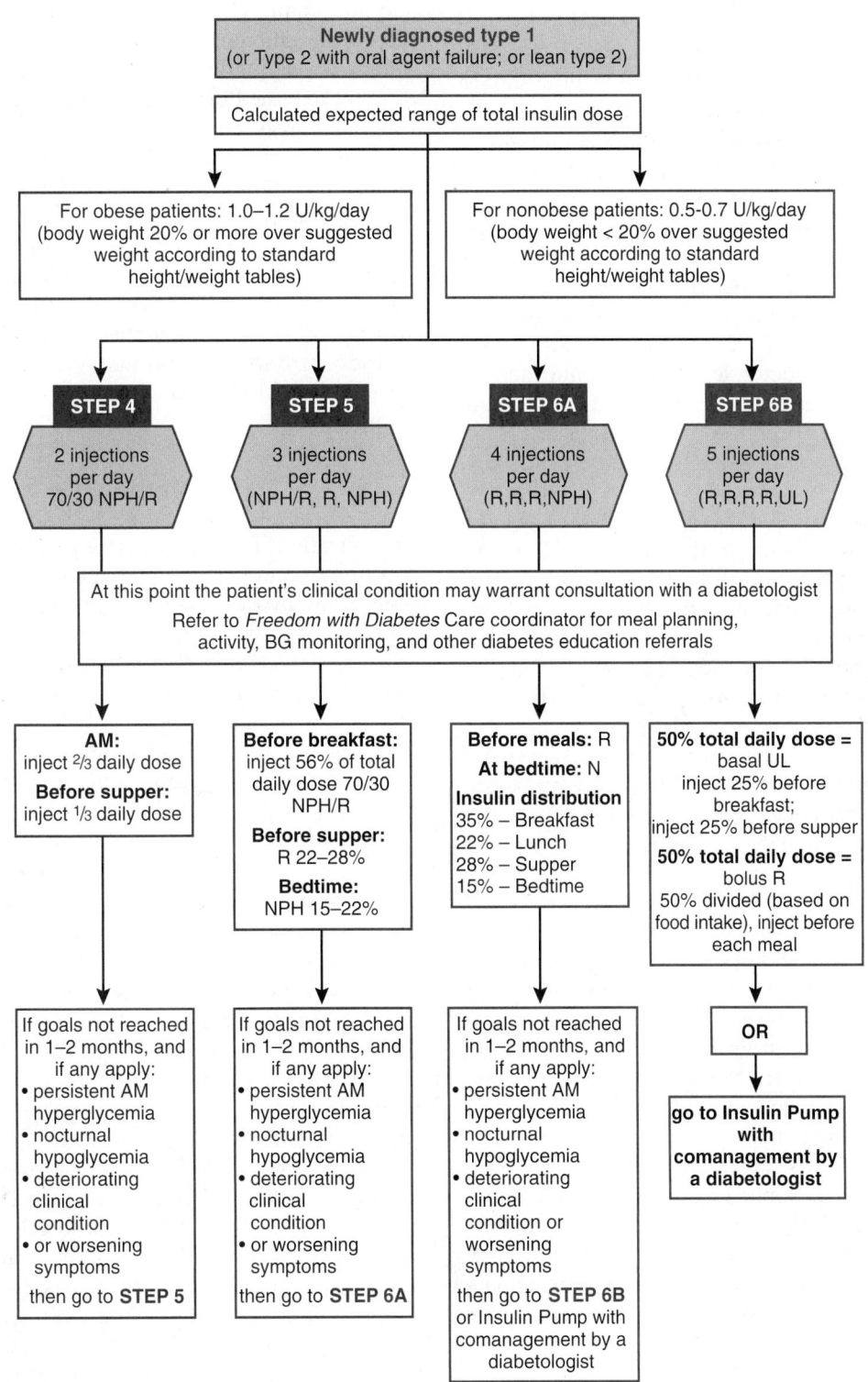

Figure 28–2 Continued

For mild DKA, low-dose intramuscular regular insulin or subcutaneous lispro insulin may be given sometimes as frequently as hourly. Intramuscular insulin has a faster onset than subcutaneous insulin and in patients with dehydration is absorbed more consistently. Dose calculations are the same as for intravenous administration. Intravenous or oral fluids are used to rehydrate.

Admission to a partial stay unit for intravenous fluids is common for the treatment of mild to moderate DKA. Small sips of sodium-containing fluids should be given at frequent intervals. It is important to prevent and treat the dehydration. Some programs advocate using glucose-containing liquids and additional insulin to correct the metabolic imbalance.[6]

In HHNK, insulin initiation may be instituted, as described for DKA treatment. Less insulin is typically required because the patient is not ketotic. Fluid replacement has a major impact on the hyperglycemia, but insulin is still required even in patients taking oral antihyperglycemic agents. If the patient is newly diagnosed with type 2 diabetes, long-term insulin therapy likely will not be needed, but oral agents and a diet and exercise regimen will need to be established.

The nurse should also assess the patient's skin. It is always important to assess the skin integrity of the patient with diabetes. Underlying cellulitis may be the precipitating factor leading to the DKA or HHNK. An egg crate or an air mattress should be used for the stuporous or comatose patient. Frequent turning is required. Frequent oral hygiene is appropriate, especially for the patient taking nothing by mouth (NPO).

The patient's ability to learn at the time of the hospitalization and knowledge level related to diabetes need to be assessed by the nurse. Initial assessment and teaching can begin with the family. The nurse can also initiate a plan of care for ongoing education and self-management while the patient is hospitalized and after discharge.

Self-management training is a critical part of the treatment plan for patients with diabetes. Meal planning, exercise, medications, stress management, sick day management, self blood glucose monitoring, and the interaction of all these components are elements of the content to be taught. Problem solving and blood glucose record review are the skills necessary for intensive insulin management. Figure 28–2 is an example of a diabetes management protocol used to coordinate the efforts of the health care team to achieve these goals. Sophisticated patients do independent insulin, calorie, and exercise adjustment. Sick day supplements of regular or lispro insulin may require support from the diabetes team to calculate dosages. Patients taking oral antihyperglycemic agents often learn similar skills and develop competence in self-management.

Nutritional Considerations

The average adult needs a minimum of 100 to 125 g of glucose per day for protein sparing and ketosis prevention.[8] This represents 400 to 500 calories of sugar-containing liquids such as 36 ounces of carbonated beverage, sugared gelatin, or juice in a 24-hour period. One liter of 5% dextrose has 50 g of glucose.

If the patient has nausea and vomiting, the patient should remain NPO until the nausea and vomiting are resolved. Antiemetics are not recommended because one of the side effects is drowsiness, which makes it difficult to assess the level of consciousness. The resolution of nausea and vomiting is one way to determine whether the acidosis of DKA is resolving. Ice chips or sips of clear liquids may be given until the nausea and vomiting subside.

A return to the normal meal plan should occur when the patient's DKA or HHNK has resolved and bowel sounds have returned. Subcutaneous insulin or an oral antihyperglycemic agent should be resumed on the return to a normal meal plan. Additional calories may need to be provided after DKA to replace the diminished glycogen stores.

Monitoring for Complications

Complications from the treatment of DKA and HHNK contribute significantly to patient mortality. Careful monitoring by the nurse is essential. Potential complications and specific causes and treatment strategies are noted in Table 28–3. Additionally, vitals signs, serum electrolytes, capillary blood glucose levels, and urine ketones are monitored every 1 to 2 hours initially (see Chart 28–3). Cardiac monitoring is continuous. Neurologic evaluation including reflexes, muscle tone, and sensorium should be evaluated by the nurse every 1 to 2 hours until the patient's condition is stable.

Multidisciplinary Outcome

The care of patients with DKA or HHNK is challenging. Rapid identification and appropriate treatment of these conditions are integral to patient outcomes. A multidisciplinary and collaborative approach is required to ensure quality patient outcomes. Chart 28–5 summarizes the expected outcomes for patients experiencing DKA or HHNK.

Priority outcomes for patients with DKA or HHNK are both physiologic and psychosocial. Normalization of electrolytes and acid–base balance and cessation of any nausea or vomiting are necessary to restore the patient's fluid and electrolyte status. Fluid replacement to correct hypovolemia and to increase systemic perfusion is aimed at maintaining cardiac output and

TABLE 28–3
Complications of Diabetic Ketoacidosis and Hyperglycemic Hyperosmolar Nonketotic Coma

Complication	Etiology	Treatment
Cardiac dysrhythmias	Electrolyte abnormalities	Correction with alterations in intravenous fluids
Hyperkalemia	Acidosis, insulin deficiency, decreased renal tubular secretion, iatrogenic	Insulin/glucose, sodium bicarbonate
Hypokalemia	Potassium loss	Addition of potassium chloride or phosphate
Cerebral edema	Hyperosmolar consequences	Mannitol, intubation, ventilation
Pulmonary edema	Neurogenic, increased capillary permeability	Supplemental oxygen, diuresis
Hypoglycemia	Osmotic physiologic changes	Decrease in insulin infusion, increase in glucose infusion
Acute kidney failure	Severe volume depletion or papillary necrosis	Temporary dialysis

stabilizing vital signs. Careful monitoring for early signs of neurologic (e.g., cerebral edema) and cardiopulmonary (e.g., congestive heart failure) changes is paramount in preventing and rapidly treating complications related to rehydration and glycemic shifts. Nutritional deficiencies are corrected by providing intravenous glucose and, ultimately, by progressing the patient to a normal oral caloric intake.

Identifying the causes of DKA or HHNK is essential to long-term outcomes. Knowing whether DKA or HHNK was precipitated by new-onset diabetes, infection, or missed medication can guide the nurse and other team members in planning for discharge teaching. Preparation of the patient for return to the community involves an in-depth assessment of the patient's ability to self-manage the diabetes. This assessment often generates referrals to the dietitian, diabetes educator, case manager, or home health nurse. This multidisciplinary approach is needed to address the holistic needs of the patient and the family both before and after discharge from the acute care setting.

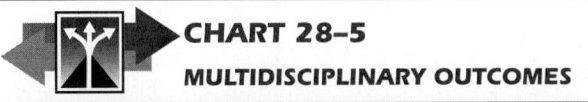

CHART 28–5

MULTIDISCIPLINARY OUTCOMES

Restoration of fluid, electrolyte, and acid–base balance
Maintenance of adequate cardiac output
Correction of nutritional deficiencies
Identification of causative factors
Prevention of complications related to treatment
Preparation of the patient and family for management of the treatment regimen after discharge

Critical Thinking Exercise

Mr. R. is a 35-year-old white man who is known to have type 1 diabetes mellitus. He was found by a neighbor to be stuporous but responsive to vigorous shaking. Emergency medical services were contacted, and Mr. R. was transported to the emergency department of a local hospital.

The neighbor, who accompanied Mr. R., reported that the patient lived alone and had not been eating or taking his insulin as he should for several days. He also stated that when Mr. R. did take his insulin, he was reusing his needles and syringes. The neighbor requested that social services be consulted to review the patient's living situation. Mr. R.'s clothing was soaked in urine and appeared to have been worn for several days.

Physical examination revealed poor skin turgor, hot, dry, flushed skin, dry mucous membranes, fruity breath odor, and deep, rapid respirations. In addition, the patient had a right below-the-knee amputation. A large, malodorous wound with copious, thick, brown drainage was present on the left foot on the heel. The skin near the wound was dark purplish, and the lower leg was edematous.

During the examination, the patient would rouse, moan, complain of abdominal pain, and beg for water. Vital signs were as follows: blood pressure, 84/48 mm Hg; pulse, 136; respirations, 46; and rectal temperature, 97.2°F. Arterial blood gases were as follows: pH, 7.15; bicarbonate, 13; and P_{CO_2}, 34.2. Electrolytes were as follows: sodium, 129 mEq/L; potassium, 5.6 mEq/L; CO_2, 12 mEq/L; glucose, 693 mg/dL; creatinine, 1.6 mg/dL; and blood urea nitrogen, 40 mg/dL. Blood count was as follows: hemoglobin, 15 g/dL; hematocrit, 49.5%; white blood count, 34,000/mm³. Urine ketones were 4+, and serum ketones were 4+. Mr. R.'s urine output was limited. He voided 60 mL in the first 2 hours while he was in the emergency room.

An intravenous infusion of normal saline was started immediately in the emergency room. On arrival in the ICU, cardiac monitoring was initiated. Blood cultures were ordered times two. Urine and wound cultures were obtained. Intravenous insulin was initiated by continuous infusion, and the insulin was titrated by protocol to lower the blood glucose by 50 to 100 mg/dL per hour. A Foley catheter was inserted.

1. Discuss the clinical signs and symptoms that contribute to the diagnosis of DKA in this patient.
2. Consider the interventions ordered up to this point and provide rationales for each.
3. The nursing diagnoses of decreased cardiac output, alterations in fluid volume, and alterations in tissue perfusion, cerebral, have been made. What nursing interventions would you anticipate relative to these diagnoses?
4. Considering Mr. R.'s social situation, what nursing interventions should occur?

Key Concepts

➠ DKA and HHNK are two conditions that can generally be prevented with early intervention and with patient and health professional education.

➠ Recognition of signs and symptoms and of common precursors to DKA and HHNK is the responsibility of all health care providers.

➠ Aggressive treatment and careful monitoring are required to prevent the mortality and morbidity of DKA and HHNK.

➠ The initial treatment of both DKA and HHNK is rehydration and management of the fluid and electrolyte imbalance. Insulin in low-dose continuous infusion is the next treatment consideration.

➠ Careful monitoring and appropriate intervention prevent complications of treatment, such as hypokalemia.

➠ Patient and family self-management education is essential, including sick day management.

➠ Case management and home follow-up with the involvement of a multidisciplinary team facilitate the prevention of recurrence and improve the quality of life for the patient with diabetes.

References

1. DeFronzo R, Matsuda M, Barrett E: Diabetic ketoacidosis. Diabetes Rev 2:209–238, 1994.
2. National Institutes of Diabetes, Digestive, and Kidney Disease: Diabetes Statistics. NIH Publication No. 95–1468. Bethesda, MD, National Institutes of Health, 1995.
3. Fishbein H, Palumbo P: Acute metabolic complications in diabetes. In: Diabetes in America, 2nd ed. Bethesda, MD, National Institutes of Health, 1995, pp 283–287.
4. Davidson M: Hyperglycemia. In: Peragallo-Dittko V, Godley K, Meyer J (eds): A Core Curriculum for Diabetes Education, 2nd ed. Chicago, American Association of Diabetes Educators, 1993, pp 303–332.
5. Miller LR: Patients with fluid and electrolyte disturbances. In: Clochesy C, Breu S, Cardin AA, et al (eds): Critical Care Nursing, 2nd ed. Philadelphia, W.B. Saunders, 1996.
6. Guthrie DW, Guthrie RA: Acute complications. In: Nursing Management of Diabetes Mellitus, 4th ed. New York, Springer, 1998.
7. Redman B, Fry S: Ethical conflicts reported by registered nurse/certified diabetes educators. Diabet Educator 22:219–224, 1996.
8. Childs B: Perioperative issues. In: Peragallo-Dittko V, Godley K, Meyer J (eds): A Core Curriculum for Diabetes Education, 2nd ed. Chicago, American Association of Diabetes Educators, 1993, pp 382–385.

29

Diabetes Insipidus and Syndrome of Inappropriate Antidiuretic Hormone

Joanne Konick-McMahan

Objectives

After completing this chapter, the student will be able to:

1. Relate the pathophysiology of diabetes insipidus (DI) and syndrome of inappropriate antidiuretic hormone (SIADH) to plan of care and collaborative management.
2. Identify physical examination and laboratory findings specific to the patient with DI and SIADH.
3. Compare and contrast the diagnostic workups for DI and SIADH.
4. Develop a collaborative plan of care for the patient with DI and SIADH.
5. Evaluate achievement of multidisciplinary outcomes for patients with DI and SIADH.

DI and SIADH are endocrine problems resulting from the fluid regulating activity of antidiuretic hormone (ADH). Both pathophysiologic states lead to fluid and electrolyte abnormalities as well as accompanying neurologic complications.

This chapter addresses the etiology and pathophysiology of DI and SIADH, along with assessment of these critically ill patients, including health history, physical examination, and diagnostic workup. Nursing and collaborative diagnoses are followed by collaborative management, including fluid and electrolyte management and pharmacologic interventions. Multidisciplinary outcomes specific to DI and SIADH are followed by a case study.

ETIOLOGY AND PATHOPHYSIOLOGY

Diabetes Insipidus

DI is a problem of impaired conservation of water by the kidney. Neurogenic DI occurs as a result of a lack of ADH, whereas nephrogenic DI is secondary to inability of the kidney to respond to ADH. The result of

excess water excretion in the critically ill patient with DI, whether neurogenic or nephrogenic, is polyuria, low urine specific gravity, hypernatremia, and fluid deficit.

Neurogenic or central DI develops because of a lack of ADH from the hypothalamus or posterior pituitary gland in spite of plasma osmolality that would normally cause release of ADH. This condition may be related to a disruption of the neural pathways leading to release of the ADH, or it may result from structural damage to the hypothalmus or the posterior pituitary gland.

Causes include an idiopathic variety that may be autoimmune, in which the ADH-producing cells are destroyed by one's own immune system. Neurogenic or central DI may also be caused by head trauma, hypoxic or ischemic encephalopathy such as after cardiopulmonary arrest, or surgery such as pituitary or hypophysectomy procedures.

Neurogenic DI is the most common complication in the patient who has had a hypophysectomy; up to 40% of these patients develop DI, which may last for up to 3 months.[1] This condition is usually transient secondary to swelling, but it may be permanent if more than 80% of the supraoptic and paraventricular nuclei or the proximal end of the pituitary stalk is destroyed.[2]

The pathophysiologic feature in neurogenic DI is lack of the hormone with resultant polyuria as the kidney tubules lose their stimulus to conserve water. Usually, the thirst center stimulates the individual to drink and thus maintain fluid balance. However, in the critically ill patient, the thirst mechanism may not be functional, or the patient may not be able to obtain water. Examples include the very young, patients with a decreased level of consciousness, or those with damage to the thirst center in the hypothalamus. Hypovolemia and dehydration occur along with hypernatremia (sodium level greater than 145 mEq/L).

Nephrogenic DI is caused by decreased ability of the kidney tubule to respond appropriately to ADH. Elevated levels of ADH are present because of overstimulation of the posterior pituitary, but the kidney does not respond. The most common reasons for this type of DI are use of the drug lithium, hypercalcemia (>10 mg/dL), and hypokalemia (<3.5 mEq/L). Other causes include osmotic agents such as glucose or mannitol, Sjögren's syndrome, amyloidosis, and renal failure.

The pathophysiology of nephrogenic DI may be of several types. The first potential cause is reduced ADH action on the collecting tubule of the kidney. Therefore, ADH is present, but the tubule does not respond to it. Hypercalcemia, hypokalemia, and the use of lithium, demeclocycline, and amphotericin B lead to DI in this way.

A second cause of nephrogenic DI is a decreased osmotic pressure gradient between the cortex and medulla of the kidney as a result of osmotic diuresis. Osmotic diuresis occurs when heavy substances are filtered through the kidney and pull water with them to be excreted. Substances leading to this include glucose, urea, mannitol, and the loop diuretics such as furosemide (Lasix). Protein malnutrition and renal failure also have this effect.

A third form of nephrogenic DI occurs in the second half of pregnancy. The cause here is thought to be rapid breakdown of ADH by a substance produced by the placenta. This leads to the polydipsia and polyuria of DI.

Unknown mechanisms lead to nephrogenic DI in the case of exposure to or ingestion of methoxylflurane, ifosfamide, and propoxyphene. The primary pathophysiologic feature of nephrogenic DI is decreased response to ADH by the collecting tubules of the kidney. This leads to polyuria, dilute urine with low osmolality, hypernatremia, and high plasma osmolality.

Syndrome of Inappropriate Antidiuretic Hormone (SIADH)

SIADH, by comparison with DI, is caused by too much ADH release, stimulating the kidney to retain water and resulting in water intoxication. This overproduction occurs in the setting of low serum osmolality and hyponatremia. These two triggers normally inhibit ADH release, but in SIADH, this feedback mechanism is ineffective.

SIADH can be caused by many situations. Malignant diseases are the most frequent causes of SIADH, especially oat cell carcinoma of the lung. Malignant tumors of the pancreas, duodenum, lymph, prostate, or thymus may also lead to SIADH because these cells produce a hormone identical to ADH.

Central nervous system problems lead to ongoing production of ADH despite normal feedback parameters. These conditions include meningitis, brain abscess and tumors, head trauma, subarachnoid hemorrhage, and Guillain–Barré syndrome.

Pulmonary problems such as tuberculosis, pneumonia, lung abscess, and positive-pressure ventilation have been associated with SIADH. Tuberculosis consolidations may produce and release ADH just as malignant tumors do. Positive-pressure ventilation causes the release of ADH by its effect of decreasing venous return to the right side of the heart. This stimulates the baroreceptors to cause the release of ADH to retain water at the kidney.

Certain drugs have been associated with SIADH. Drugs enhancing ADH release include chlorpropamide, carbamazepine, cyclophosphamide, vincristine, antidepressants, and narcotics. Diuretics, especially the thiazide diuretics, act on the distal nephron to slow free water excretion and cause the euvolemic hyponatremia associated with SIADH.[3, 4]

SIADH produces clinical symptoms related to the effect of free water retention by the kidney. Increased amounts of free water in the blood lead to hypotonic or dilute body fluids. Glomerular filtration by the kidney increases, leading to sodium excretion. The clinical picture produced by this overproduction or increased response to ADH is water retention with hyponatremia (serum sodium < 135 mEq/L).

Table 29–1 provides a summary of the pathophysiology, etiology, clinical presentation, and treatment objectives of a patient with DI and SIADH. A detailed discussion of the assessment, diagnosis, and collaborative management of a patient with DI and SIADH follows.

Assessment

Health History

Diabetes Insipidus

The patient with DI most commonly presents in the clinical setting with a history of head trauma, surgery, disease, or ischemia of the hypothalmus or pituitary areas. If the DI is nephrogenic, the history may include renal disease or exposure to drugs such as lithium or

TABLE 29-1

Comparison of Diabetes Insipidus (DI) and Syndrome of Inappropriate Antidiuretic Hormone (SIADH)

	DI	SIADH
Pathophysiology	Neurogenic: lack of ADH Nephrogenic: lack of kidney response to ADH	Oversecretion of ADH by tumor or overstimulation
Etiology	Neurogenic: idiopathic, brain injury, pituitary or hypothalmic surgery Nephrogenic: lithium, hypercalcemia, hypokalemia	Malignancies, especially lung, brain injury or surgery, pulmonary disease or mechanical ventilation, drugs
Signs and Symptoms	Polyuria, polydipsia, dehydration if free water not given Neurologic signs of hypernatremia related to brain cell dehydration	Weight gain without edema Neurologic signs of hyponatremia related to cerebral edema
Laboratory Data		
Plasma osmolality	High, > than 295 mOsm/kg	Low, < than 280 mOsm/kg
Serum sodium	Normal or >145 mEq/L	Low, <135 mEq/L
Urine osmolality	Low, <250 mOsm/kg	Normal or high, >100 mOsm/kg
Urine sodium	Normal or low	>20 mmol/L
Treatment Objectives	Correction of underlying cause Free water replacement Neurogenic: ADH replacement Nephrogenic: thiazide diuretics	Correction of underlying cause Fluid restriction Hyponatremia: saline, hypertonic if symptomatic with sodium less than 120 mEq/L

demeclocycline. The onset of symptoms, primarily polyuria, may be acute, such as after head trauma, or chronic, related to situations such as tumor. These primary situations are reasons to be alert for the signs of fluid deficit. Early intervention with adequate fluid replacement is needed to avoid hypovolemia.

Syndrome of Inappropriate Antidiuretic Hormone

The patient with SIADH may have a health history of a central nervous system problem such as head trauma or stroke. SIADH may also be seen along with a pulmonary problem including pneumonia, positive-pressure ventilation, or cancer of the lung. Other malignancies such as duodenal or pancreatic tumors or lymphoma may produce this syndrome. These diagnoses should alert a health care provider to the potential for the neurologic complications related to hyponatremia of SIADH.

Clinical Presentation

Diabetes Insipidus

Polyuria is the usual presenting symptom that attracts the clinician's attention in DI. Polyuria, defined as a urine output greater than 3 L per day, should be considered whenever a patient with the appropriate clinical history has a urine output of more than 200 mL per hour for 2 consecutive hours. This finding should be reported to the physician, and the patient should continue to be monitored.

If the patient is awake, excessive thirst and polydipsia may be a clinical finding as well. If free water intake, either orally or intravenously, is not sufficient to maintain intravascular volume, hypernatremia and dehydration may result.

Hypernatremia in DI occurs because of ongoing loss of free water resulting from lack of or ineffective ADH at the kidney tubule. Clinical signs of hypernatremia are predominantly found in the neuromuscular system and range from lethargy and confusion to seizure and coma at high levels (160–170 mEq/L) of sodium.

Dehydration or volume depletion results if free water is not replaced adequately in DI. Clinical signs include tachycardia, orthostatic hypotension, poor skin turgor, sunken eyes, thick secretions, and dry mucous membranes. Hypotension because of hemodynamic compromise can result if ongoing free water loss is not adequately replaced. With sufficient nursing intervention to ensure free water replacement and adequate therapy of the cause of DI, hypotension should not occur.

The clinical presentation of the patient with DI includes polyuria, thirst and polydipsia (if these systems are intact), and dehydration if free water replacement is not adequate. The physical examination findings include urine output of 200 mL per hour or greater, neurologic findings related to hypernatremia, and cardiovascular findings related to dehydration or volume depletion because of free water loss.

Syndrome of Inappropriate Antidiuretic Hormone

The physical examination and clinical findings of SIADH depend on the rate of development and level of the dilutional hyponatremia.[3] Sodium levels of less than 120 mEq/L that develop in less than 48 hours are associated with increased neurologic signs as well as with higher mortality.

Neurologic findings are thought to be the result of cerebral edema occuring because of water intoxication or excess free water in the vascular system. This free water leads to a low serum osmolality or a dilute serum. The brain, with a higher osmolality, attracts water from the serum. The movement of water into the brain creates cerebral edema. The neurologic findings of hyponatremia include change in level of consciousness, confusion, headache, and lethargy. As hyponatremia progresses, if not detected or treated, neurologic findings can include decreased deep tendon reflexes, seizures, coma, and even death. Careful attention to sodium levels in those critically ill patients with the potential to develop SIADH becomes extremely important.

Assessment findings of SIADH can also include those related to increased extracellular fluid volume including weight gain without edema, increased blood pressure, and crackles on lung auscultation. Decreased urine output may also be a finding related to the effect of ADH on the kidney to conserve water. Changes in gastrointestinal function related to hyponatremia present as anorexia, nausea, and vomiting.

Triphasic Pattern

A three-part combination of DI and SIADH can occur in patients who have a clinical history of neurologic injury or surgery (Figure 29–1). The first phase occurs in hours or days after surgery or injury and presents as polyuria resulting from impairment of ADH release. The second phase is the SIADH phase and lasts 2 to 14 days. This phase presents as oliguria, water saving, and hyponatremia. The third phase occurs as ADH stores are depleted and DI with polyuria reappears. This DI may be transient, resolving in days, or chronic.

Laboratory and Diagnostic Tests

Diabetes Insipidus

Polyuria in critically ill patients may have many causes. Those causes need to be considered before a diagnostic workup for DI. Hyperglycemia, diabetes mellitus, drugs such as mannitol, and excessive intravenous fluid replacement may all lead to polyuria. Ruling out these situations is important before a DI workup.

Laboratory tests to diagnose DI include plasma osmolality, urine osmolality, urine specific gravity, serum sodium, and plasma ADH levels. A water deprivation

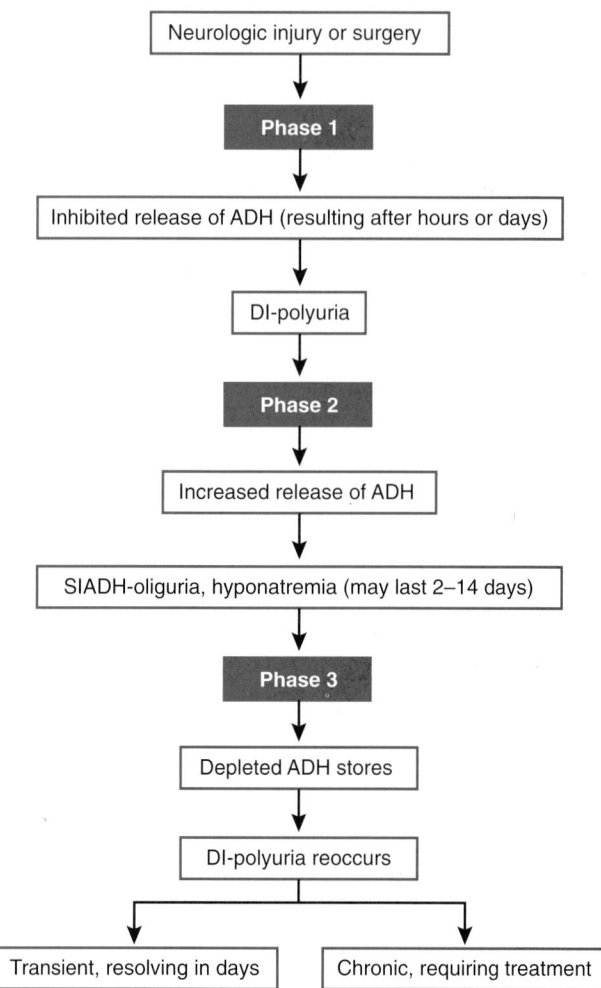

Figure 29–1

Triphasic pattern of diabetes insipidus (DI) and syndrome of inappropriate antidiuretic hormone (SIADH).

test is rarely done in the critically ill patient because of the risk of hypovolemia. If the patient is hypernatremic with dilute urine, DI is confirmed, and further testing is not warranted.[5]

Plasma osmolality is usually greater than 295 mOsm/kg H_2O because of free water loss in DI. Urine osmolality and urine specific gravity are low because of increased free water in the urine. Serum sodium is elevated (>145 mEq/L) when free water intake does not meet urine output. ADH serum levels are not usually measured unless there is a question of partial lack of secretion or action.

When the diagnosis of DI has been confirmed by the foregoing data, administration of ADH is used to determine whether the DI is neurogenic or nephrogenic. Subcutaneous injection of 5 U of vasopressin or intranasal use of 10 μg of 1-desamino-8-D-arginine vasopressin (desmopressin acetate [DDAVP]) is used. Patients with neurogenic DI do respond with decreased urine output and increased urine concentration and osmolality. The response to ADH administration by patients with nephrogenic DI is unchanged urine volume and concentration.

The water deprivation test, used to diagnose DI when it can be safely carried out, consists of two parts. The first part involves water restriction until 3 to 5% of body weight is lost or two to three consecutive hourly urine samples have osmolalities that vary by less than 10%. The aim is to increase serum osmolality to above 295 mOsm/kg H_2O or sodium to more than 145 mmol/L. When those values have been reached, ADH is administered subcutaneously or by nasal spray. A urine sample is collected 1 hour after ADH is given. If neurogenic or central DI is present, the urine sample will show increased concentration and decreased volume. Patients with nephrogenic DI have no response. The obvious risk of hypovolemic shock in the critically ill patient limits the water deprivation test to rare occasions.

Syndrome of Inappropriate Antidiuretic Hormone

The diagnostic workup for SIADH includes ruling out disease associated with renal, liver, or adrenal disorders. Therefore, the patient should have no orthostatic blood pressure changes or tachycardia, no hypokalemia, and no rise in blood urea nitrogen to indicate prerenal disease.

The laboratory tests used to determine the presence of SIADH are similar to those used for DI. The values, however, reflect the effect of ADH causing water retention in the presence of a fluid status that would normally inhibit ADH release. Serum osmolality is below 280 mOsm/kg H_2O because of the extra water the kidney is saving as a result of excess ADH. Serum sodium is below 135 mEq/L because of dilution. Urine osmolality is inappropriately concentrated, usually greater than 100 mOsm/kg H_2O, when compared with diluted serum. Urine sodium is greater than 20 mmol/L because of increased glomerular filtration as a result of hypotonic volume expansion.

When comparing and contrasting the diagnostic workup for DI and SIADH, it is evident these clinical syndromes are at opposite ends of the spectrum. DI, because of lack of hormone or response to that hormone, produces a concentrated serum and large amounts of dilute urine. This condition may result in hypernatremia if free water is lost and is not repleted in the critically ill patient. SIADH, in comparison, produces dilute serum, hyponatremia, and concentrated urine because of water conservation by the kidney.

Nursing Diagnoses

The care of patients with DI or SIADH may occur in the emergency room, in the intensive care unit (ICU) during stabilization or in the postinjury or surgical phase, and in the intermediate care unit. Length of stay and stabilization depend on the underlying cause and the type of intervention needed.

As members of a multidisciplinary team in these settings, nurses use nursing and collaborative diagnoses to plan care. Throughout the patient's hospitalization for DI or SIADH, the priority diagnoses relate to the consequences of alterations in fluid and electrolyte balance. Altered thought processes are an associated diagnosis during acute treatment of hypernatremia in DI and hyponatremia in SIADH. Patient safety is an additional diagnosis that relates to the neurologic findings associated with the sodium imbalance in DI and SIADH. Anxiety and knowledge deficit are important nursing diagnoses during the workup and follow-up management of the cause of DI and SIADH. Sleep pattern disturbance, related to polydipsia and polyuria, is a pertinent nursing diagnosis for the patient with DI who is alert, ambulatory, and without a urinary catheter until treatment is initiated.

The patient's clinical history, presenting symptoms, and cause of DI and SIADH guide the selection of pertinent nursing diagnoses to drive management during the critical care phase (Table 29–2).

Collaborative Management

The many potential primary diagnoses that can lead to DI or SIADH set the stage for a multidisciplinary team that includes physicians, acute care nurses, community nurses, dietitians, social workers, and clergy. Oncology nurses and hospice nurses may also be a part of the team if appropriate. The settings for care include the emergency room, ICU, intermediate care unit, medical–surgical unit, home, and hospice.

Diabetes Insipidus

Identification of the underlying cause is important in the collaborative management of the patient with DI. Brain tumors that are causing the problem need to be removed. In the case of a pituitary tumor, the DI may continue and may be a chronic problem. If the cause is not treatable, such as postresuscitation ischemia, support with fluid and pharmacotherapeutics is necessary until the edema of the hypothalamus–pituitary area resolves.

Rehydration
Preventing hypovolemic shock by adequate oral or intravenous intake is the primary goal or outcome for the patient with DI. If the patient is able, oral fluids of sufficient quantity are the therapy of choice. If the patient is not able to drink or to respond to thirst stimulus, then intravenous fluids are given.

The intravenous fluid of choice is free water, that is, hypotonic dextrose and water at a rate to equal to the output of the previous hour or several hours. This is

TABLE 29–2
Nursing Diagnoses

Diabetes Insipidus

Problem Statement	Etiologic Factors
Fluid volume deficit	Impaired conservation of water by the kidney
Altered thought processes	Hypernatremia secondary to excess water loss
Risk for injury	Central nervous system alteration secondary to hypernatremia; thromboembolism secondary to hemoconcentration
Decreased cardiac output	Excess volume loss
Anxiety	Sudden change in health status, hospitalization, unknown prognosis
Knowledge deficit (learning need)	Diagnosis, treatment plan, follow-up care
Fatigue	Hypernatremia, hypovolemia, disrupted sleep
Sleep pattern disturbance	Polydipsia, polyuria
Risk for impaired skin integrity	Loss of water from interstitial spaces

Syndrome of Inappropriate Antidiuretic Hormone

Problem Statement	Etiologic Factors
Fluid volume excess	Compromised regulatory mechanism secondary to excessive secretion of antidiuretic hormone
Altered thought processes	Water intoxication, hyponatremia, cerebral edema
Risk for injury	Seizure activity secondary to hyponatremia
Anxiety	Sudden change in health status, hospitalization, unknown prognosis
Risk for impaired skin integrity	Immobility
Knowledge deficit (learning need)	Diagnosis, treatment plan, follow-up care

the therapy of choice for hypernatremia in this case. Accurate intake and output records as well as ongoing daily weight assessments become vitally important. Frequent monitoring of plasma sodium and evaluations of osmolality are important indicators of therapeutic effectiveness. Ongoing monitoring for signs of hypovolemic shock is also essential.

If systolic blood pressure falls to less than 90 mm Hg, that is an indicator of circulatory failure, and the patient requires more aggressive fluid repletion with isotonic saline. When intravascular volume and hemodynamic stability are achieved, then hypotonic fluid replacement should resume. When the polyuria subsides, the serum sodium and osmolality levels should return to normal.

Pharmacotherapeutics

Neurogenic or central DI is effectively treated with ADH medications during the acute phase of illness. This is replacement therapy for the ADH not being produced and released by the hypothalamus and pituitary, respectively. The types of ADH preparations used include vasopressin, desmopressin, and lypressin (Table 29–3).

Synthetic vasopressin or Pitressin Synthetic is structurally identical to natural vasopressin. Available as an aqueous solution with 20 U/mL, synthetic vasopressin can be given subcutaneously, intramuscularly, or by intranasal inhalation. It is useful as a rapid-acting, short-duration (2–8 hours) treatment for DI during the initial acute management or postoperatively in the

TABLE 29–3
Drug Therapy for Diabetes Insipidus

Drug	Indication	Route of Administration
Vasopressin (Pitressin)	Acute	Subcutaneous Intramuscular Intranasal
Desmopressin acetate (DDAVP)	Acute/chronic	Intravenous Subcutaneous Intranasal
Lypressin	Acute/chronic	Intranasal

cranial surgical patient. From 5 to 10 U subcutaneously would be utilized every 8 to 12 hours, with dose titration depending on decreased urine response.

Side effects of vasopressin or Pitressin Synthetic are related to its pressor effect. Pitressin can lead to anginal attacks in patients with coronary artery disease, and intravenous nitroglycerin may be used to counteract this effect. Patients may also develop resistance to ADH preparations.[5]

DDAVP can be administered intravenously, subcutaneously, or intranasally. Intravenous DDAVP has an antidiuretic effect 10 times that of intranasal form. The intranasal form is the most common form; however, the intravenous or subcutaneous forms may be more reliable as well as more appropriate in the critically ill patient with an impaired cognitive state. The nasal approach for transsphenoidal hypophysectomy with resultant packing makes intravenous or subcutaneous DDAVP more reliable for those requiring this operation for removal of a pituitary tumor.

DDAVP lasts for 8 to 24 hours with 10 to 40 μg intranasally or 2 to 4 μg intravenously or subcutaneously. Because it is longer acting than vasopressin, DDAVP is usually given in two divided doses or is individualized to patient response. DDAVP has no vasopressor action compared with vasopressin. DDAVP is comparatively more expensive.

The third ADH preparation used to treat neurogenic or central DI is lypressin. It is in nasal spray form with 50 USP pressor Units/mL. The disadvantage of lypressin is its short duration of action (2–6 hours), which requires administration four times per day. It is used for patients who are unresponsive to the other forms of ADH or who are allergic to the systemic varieties of ADH.[6]

With any of the foregoing ADH replacements, overtreatment can occur, leading to excess free water and hyponatremia. This potential adverse effect necessitates careful calculation of hourly intake and output and frequent monitoring of serum osmolality and sodium levels during ADH replacement therapy for DI.

Other drugs may be used in partial central DI to increase ADH release by the neurohypophysis or to increase the action of ADH in the kidney. These drugs include clofibrate, chlorpropamide, and carbamazepine. Clofibrate (used to treat hyperlipidemia), at doses of 500 mg orally three to four times per day, may have side effects of gastrointestinal problems and gallstones (cholelithiasis). Clofibrate may increase ADH release.

Chlorpropamide (an oral hypoglycemic), given one to two times per day in doses of 125 to 250 mg, increases the action of ADH, but hypoglycemia limits its dose effect. Carbamazepine, 100 to 300 mg two times per day, increases the action of ADH, but it can be toxic to liver and bone marrow. These drugs, used cau-

tiously because of side effects, may decrease polyuria by 50%.[7]

Nephrogenic DI is characterized by polyuria occurring because the tubule is unable to respond to ADH. Most frequent causes are hypercalcemia and long-term lithium use. The hypercalcemic patient quickly reverses the polyuria as soon as the serum calcium is decreased to more normal values. The patient with lithium-induced nephrogenic DI may have permanent tubular injury or may respond to drug therapy.

Nephrogenic DI may respond to the administration of thiazide diuretics such as hydrochlorothiazide, 25 mg one to two times per day, in combination with a low-sodium diet. This combination has been effective in decreasing polyuria, theoretically by creating a mild fluid volume deficit and increasing sodium and water reabsorption in the proximal tubule of the kidney. Less water then flows by the collecting tubules that are ADH sensitive.

The challenge in both neurogenic and nephrogenic DI is to provide adequate fluid replacement while medication doses are being adjusted to decrease water output by the kidney. Avoiding water overload as a result of too much medication is part of that challenge to the multidisciplinary critical care team.

Nutrition

Parenteral hyperalimentation is an important part of the needs of the critically ill patient with DI to ensure healing. However, hyperalimentation may contribute to water loss if blood sugar levels are not controlled. Hyperglycemia, an osmotic load, causes increased water loss by the kidney as the glucose is filtered. This change may lead to water deficit in the patient with DI if it is not tightly controlled. Frequent monitoring of serum glucose with sliding-scale insulin dosing is important to prevent additional fluid loss because of hyperglycemia.

Enteral tube feedings can pull water into the gastrointestinal tract and may lead to diarrhea. The loss of water can lead to hypovolemia in the critically ill patient with DI when it is added to the urinary losses. Nursing actions to decrease the diarrhea related to tube feeding include controlling volume to avoid too large a load in the gastrointestinal tract and the addition of water to a hypertonic tube feeding solution to decrease its concentration or osmolality.

For critically ill patients with DI who are able to eat, a diet low in sodium and protein is important to decrease the solute load. This diet decreases the amount of water necessary to filter protein through the kidney and helps to decrease water loss.

Skin Care

As water is lost from the interstitial areas, the skin becomes vulnerable to breakdown. Frequent turning, repositioning, padding of bony prominences, and massage of those areas are important preventive nursing actions to avoid skin breakdown.

Elimination

Polyuria in the critically ill patient with DI is best managed with a urinary catheter in the acute stages. Careful catheter care is required to avoid urinary tract infections, and the catheter should be removed as soon as possible.

The bowels may become constipated if water deficit occurs. Lack of stool should be noted and managed by a suppository or enema before impaction occurs.

Syndrome of Inappropriate Antidiuretic Hormone

Treatment of the primary problem causing SIADH is as important as the measures to treat the SIADH itself. If the problem is a drug, such as the thiazides or chlor-propamide, then stopping those drugs is primary treatment. This may be all that is needed to return the patient to a baseline state. Some primary problems such as cancer may require surgery or long-term treatment to decrease the effect of the SIADH (Chart 29–1). Along with the primary treatment, fluid restriction, management of hyponatremia, and blocking ADH action are necessary therapies in SIADH.

Fluid Restriction

The primary problem in SIADH is too much free water in the serum that dilutes sodium and causes hyponatremia. Fluid restriction is first-line therapy to decrease the amount of free water available. The restriction is usually to 1000 mL per day and includes oral and intravenous free water. All intravenous medications should be mixed in normal saline, not dextrose in water, and in minimal volumes. The result of this fluid restriction should be a steady rise in serum sodium and a decrease in body weight. Patients with asymptomatic SIADH may have spontaneous remission in 1 to 2 weeks with fluid restriction alone.

Electrolyte Replacement

Acute life-threatening hyponatremia exists if sodium levels are lower than 120 mEq/L occurring in less than 24 to 48 hours of time. Neurologic manifestations, including seizures and coma, are the most severe symptoms in this case because of cerebral edema. Cerebral edema is caused as water is pulled into the brain's circulation because of higher sodium levels than serum. In this situation, the use of hypertonic saline, 3 or 5%, is necessary to bring the sodium to 120 mEq/L, the minimum serum sodium to avoid severe, life-threatening neurologic symptoms.

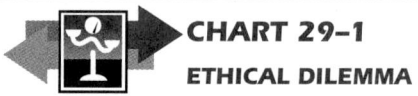 **CHART 29–1**

ETHICAL DILEMMA

Mr. V. is a 59-year-old man admitted because of mental confusion. His family has noted a 35-pound weight loss over 6 months with increasing fatigue and a nonproductive cough. Mr. V. has smoked 2 packs of cigarettes per day (ppd) for 25 years, as well as drinking a 6-pack of beer per day for 15 years.

Physical examination reveals a temperature of 98°F, a heart rate 95 and regular with a normal electrocardiogram, and a respiratory rate of 18. Blood pressure is 140/80 mm Hg without orthostasis. Neurologic examination reveals confusion with long- and short-term memory loss, as well as decreased deep tendon reflexes. The chest radiograph shows a left lower lobe mass, whereas a computed tomography scan of the head is normal. Laboratory values are as follows: sodium, of 115 mEq/L; potassium, 3.8 mEq/L; chloride, 80 mEq/L; blood urea nitrogen, 8; creatinine, 0.9; glucose, 90 mg/dL; and serum osmolality, 234 mOsm/L.

Mr. V. is admitted to the ICU with hyponatremia, syndrome of inappropriate antidiuretic hormone,

and possible lung cancer. He is fluid restricted with initial treatment with 3% (hypertonic) saline for 6 hours. After his sodium reaches 120 mEq/L, the intravenous solution is changed to normal saline at an hourly rate of 20 mL. Mr. V.'s confusion clears as his sodium rises to 128 mEq/L by the second hospital day. He is treated with oxazepam to prevent symptoms of alcohol withdrawal.

Bronchoscopy on the third hospital day reveals small cell carcinoma of the left lung. Mr. V.'s wife and daughters do not want the patient to know his diagnosis because "He'll be depressed and just give up."

1. What information is necessary for the family to have to address fully the decision to withhold information?
2. Who should be part of the team addressing these issues?
3. Would you support the family in this decision?
4. How would you support Mr. V.?

CHART 29-2

RESEARCH UTILIZATION: NURSING INTERVENTIONS FOR EDUCATION OF PATIENTS DISCHARGED AFTER TRANSSPHENOIDAL SURGERY

Abstract: Hyponatremia related to the syndrome of inappropriate antidiuretic hormone (SIADH) has been thought to be an infrequent occurrence after transphenoidal surgery for pituitary adenoma. This retrospective study of 2297 patients of a single surgeon from 1971 to 1993 found 42 patients (1.8%) who presented 4 to 13 days postoperatively with nausea and vomiting, headache, malaise, dizziness, confusion, anorexia, and seizures as clinical signs of hyponatremia. The number of patients found makes hyponatremia more common in this population after discharge than previously thought. The average decrease in sodium was from 138.7 mEq/L before discharge from the hospital to 121.6 mEq/L on readmission. All patients were treated with fluid restriction or fluid restriction and salt replacement, with resolution in 1 to 6 days.

Two patients had ADH levels measured on presentation and were found to be low normal. Based on these two results, the authors pose the theory that SIADH is not the cause of the hyponatremia seen postoperatively in these patients.

Critique: A large sample of one surgeon's population, this retrospective study accomplishes its goal of clarifying the frequency, presentation, and outcome of this group with hyponatremia postoperatively. A prospective study with consistent data of ADH measurement would increase the scientific worth of the study.

The authors did not make a convincing case for hyponatremia in these patients as being unrelated to SIADH. A study with consistent ADH measurement would give a more accurate picture of the role of the hormone in hyponatremia in this population. The study does delineate symptoms as well as the need for saline replacement along with fluid restriction to correct the hyponatremia in this population.

Nursing Considerations: Acute care nurses and other health care providers must be aware of the signs and symptoms presented in this study population. Monitoring and timely intervention are necessary to prevent complications of hyponatremia during hospitalization.

Patients in this population, as well as their care givers, must be educated regarding the signs and symptoms of hyponatremia and the importance of early feedback to their health care providers. The chance that these symptoms of potentially life-threatening electrolyte imbalance will happen at home is likely, given earlier discharge at present than in the 1970s and 1980s when some of these patients were hospitalized. Quick response to patients and care givers who call with the signs and symptoms found in this study may prevent more serious sequelae of hyponatremia. Home health care nurses, caring for an increasingly acutely ill population such as these patients, must be aware of the presentation, to ensure early detection and intervention.

Source: Taylor SL, Tyrrell JB, Wilson CB: Delayed onset of hyponatremia after transsphenoidal surgery for pituitary adenomas. Neurosurgery 37(4):649–654, 1995.

Hypertonic saline requires a pump for infusion and must be administered at a cautious rate to avoid too rapid correction of sodium levels; 3% saline is administered at a rate of 1 to 2 mL/kg per hour to raise the serum sodium no faster than 1 to 2 mEq/L per hour for the first 3 to 4 hours.[7] The goal is a target of 120 to 125 mEq/L over 24 to 48 hours.

The reason for caution in sodium replacement is the rare complication of osmotic demyelination. This demyelinating process in the brain has been found especially in the pons and leads to delayed neurologic changes such as flaccid quadriplegia, pseudobulbar palsy, and alterations in mental state.[5] Avoiding too rapid correction of sodium in all situations is prudent.

The nurse must monitor for signs of intravascular fluid overload during hypertonic saline administra-

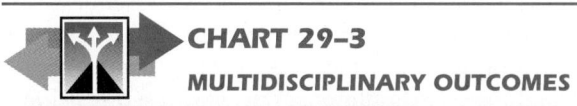

CHART 29-3

MULTIDISCIPLINARY OUTCOMES

Restoration of fluid and electrolyte balance
Prevention of complications related to treatment strategies
Preservation of cerebral functioning
Prevention of injury
Restoration of psychosocial balance
Achievement of self-management of therapeutic regimen

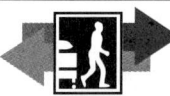

CHART 29–4
BEYOND THE ICU: HOME MANAGEMENT OF PATIENTS WITH DI OR SIADH

Caring for patients recovering from diabetes insipidus (DI) or syndrome of inappropriate antidiuretic hormone (SIADH) often extends beyond the ICU to the home setting. Careful evaluation of the patient's needs on discharge guides the nurse in determining whether or not the patient would benefit from follow-up by the home health nurse. Discharge planning should begin on admission, to maintain the continuity of care after discharge.

The home health nurse evaluating a patient recovering from DI or SIADH needs excellent assessment and teaching skills. Monitoring for early manifestations of alterations in fluid and electrolyte balance is a priority. For patients with DI, this includes signs and symptoms of hypernatremia and hypovolemia (lethargy, fatigue, hypotension, tachycardia, poor skin turgor, thirst, weight loss, polyuria). For patients with SIADH, this includes signs and symptoms of hyponatremia and fluid overload (headache, confusion, irritability, restlessness, nausea or vomiting, weight gain, tachycardia, decreased urine output). Patients and their families must also receive instructions on how to monitor for these signs and symptoms. For patients and families, teaching the importance of taking daily weights as an indicator of fluid status is equally important. In addition, they need to know the significance of contacting the physician if any of these signs and symptoms develop and of keeping all scheduled appointments.

Instructions on medications, including the purpose, dose, route of administration, frequency, and side effects, are an important component of patient and family teaching. The nurse should provide verbal and written information that is easily understood. In the case of medications with unusual routes of administration (e.g., intranasal desmopressin for patients with DI), the nurse should observe the patient administering the medication whenever possible. In this way, any needed corrections to the patient's technique can be made. For patients with SIADH, and especially those treated with diuretic therapy, the nurse needs to provide specific diet instructions. Information on maintaining a diet that provides adequate salt and potassium is important to avoid complications related to electrolyte imbalances (hyponatremia, hypokalemia) secondary to the drug therapy. The nurse should also emphasize the importance of maintaining the medication regimen and the consequences of interrupting or discontinuing medications. Finally, all patients should be encouraged to obtain and wear a Medic-Alert identification device.

Caring for patients recovering from DI or SIADH and their families in the home setting can be challenging and rewarding. Most often, these patients have experienced a life-threatening health crisis. Emotional support, in addition to the necessary patient education, is also provided by the home health nurse as needed. By doing so, the patient and family fully benefit from the continuity of care and from a holistic approach to their needs.

---

tion. This complication can occur as fluid volume expands. Signs and symptoms include tachycardia, tachypnea, increased blood pressure, shortness of breath, lung crackles, increased central venous pressure, and increased pulmonary artery pressure. A loop diuretic may be used in severely symptomatic patients with SIADH to cause free water loss during hypertonic saline use.

Diuretic Therapy
A loop diuretic, such as furosemide, may be used as mentioned earlier to help with the correction of water excess. Low doses (20 mg furosemide twice daily) may be utilized along with saline to correct the dilutional hyponatremia. Electrolytes should be closely followed in such cases to manage additional losses related to the diuretic.

Skin Care
The critically ill patient with symptomatic acute hyponatremia as a result of SIADH is frequently immobile, perhaps comatose. This patient requires frequent turning, massage, and padding of bony prominences. If the patient has seizures, siderails should be padded to avoid injury.

Long-Term Management
Chronic hyponatremia is a fall in or persistence of hyponatremia for longer than 48 hours. These patients are usually asymptomatic because the body and brain have time to adjust to the hypo-osmolar serum. This situation is best managed with fluid restriction and a diet high in salt. Drug therapy may be an adjunct.

Drugs used to treat the chronic form of SIADH include demeclocycline and lithium carbonate. Demeclocycline is an antibiotic that blocks the kidney's response to ADH, thus allowing for free water loss. This drug's onset of action is several days, so it is not used acutely. Lithium has a similar mechanism of action in SIADH, but it has increased toxicity as well as a variety of responses. Therefore, demeclocycline is more commonly used to treat chronic SIADH.

Chart 29–2 describes the need for patient education concerning signs and symptoms of hyponatremia after transsphenoidal hypophysectomy. Of these patients, 1.8% presented with neurologic changes of hyponatremia 4 to 13 days after surgery. Patients discharged after this surgery must be made aware of the signs of hyponatremia as well as how to contact the health care team.

Multidisciplinary Outcomes

DI and SIADH have similarities in the goals that health care providers wish to achieve during critical illness (Chart 29–3). *Restoration of fluid and electrolyte balance* is a primary goal in DI to restore volume and to treat hypernatremia and, in SIADH, to cause volume loss and to increase sodium. *Prevention of complications* of undertreatment, overtreatment, or too rapid correction is common to both DI and SIADH. Dehydration, fluid overload, and neurologic effects of rapid sodium correction are the complications specific to DI, whereas neurologic complications and volume overload are specific to SIADH.

Preservation of cerebral functioning is an outcome pertinent to patients with both DI and SIADH during diagnosis and treatment of the primary problem. *Prevention of injury* in both DI and SIADH revolves around the neurologic symptoms along with cardiovascular and skin effects of these two problems in critical care.

Restoration of psychosocial balance is an outcome for critically ill patients with DI and SIADH and their families as they deal with searching for a cause and then dealing with that cause of the DI and SIADH. *Self-management of the therapeutic regimen* is an outcome for patients with both DI and SIADH who develop chronic disease and require medication or diet teaching (Chart 29–4). These multidisciplinary outcomes are appropriate in the various settings in which care of the patient with DI or SIADH takes place.

Critical Thinking Exercise

Mr. S. is a 45-year-old man with a brain tumor. After resection of the tumor, he requires a tracheostomy for airway protection and to facilitate ventilator weaning. After weaning, he is transferred to a medical–surgical unit. He suffers a cardiopulmonary arrest with about 5 minutes of unwitnessed time between being observed and being found apneic.

Mr. S. is resuscitated and is transferred to the ICU. His heart rhythm is normal sinus without electrocardiographic changes. Initially, he requires dopamine for blood pressure support, but he is weaned from dopamine after 16 hours with blood pressures of 120/70 to 80 mm Hg. He is ventilated on assist/control mode with normalized blood gases and 40% FiO_2. Mr. S. is unresponsive and is found to have seizure activity on an electroencephalogram (EEG). He is treated with phenytoin (Dilantin), with resolution of seizure by EEG, but he remains unresponsive, with pupils equal and reactive to light. A computed tomography scan of his head shows no changes from before the cardiac arrest.

On day 2 of his ICU stay, Mr. S. has urine outputs of 400 mL from 9 AM to 10 AM and 500 mL from 10 AM to 11 AM.

1. Discuss additional data you would obtain before conferring with the physician.
2. What potential complications would you be anticipating? How would you monitor for those complications?

Mr. S. continues to make 400 to 600 mL urine per hour. The urine specific gravity was 1.005, with an osmolality of 180 mOsm/kg. Mr. S.'s serum sodium, which was 136 mEq/L on ICU admission, rose to 150 mEq/L, with a rise in plasma osmolality to 300 mOsm/kg. His urine output is replaced with intravenous fluid to replace the previous hour's output.

3. Provide a rationale for the type of intravenous fluid you would expect to be utilized.
4. Given the laboratory results, what intervention would you anticipate to control the urine volumes?

Mr. S. is given 5 U subcutaneous aqueous vasopressin (Pitressin), with a decrease in urine volume to 200 mL over the next 2 hours. Five hours later, Mr. S. receives another dose of subcutaneous Pitressin and every 6 hours thereafter.

5. How would you monitor the effectiveness of this therapy other than urine volume?
6. Mrs. S. asks you how long Mr. S. will need to be on the Pitressin. What answer would you give?

Key Concepts

➡ Neurogenic DI is the result of the lack of ADH, whereas nephrogenic DI is the result of the kidney's inability to respond to ADH.
➡ The result of both types of DI is excess water excretion by the kidney, thus causing polyuria.
➡ Neurogenic DI can be the result of an idiopathic condition, a brain injury, or surgery of the pituitary or hypothalamus.
➡ The critically ill patient is at risk for dehydration and hypernatremia with DI because of the inability to respond to thirst. Clinical signs of hypernatremia include lethargy, seizures, and coma.

➡ Nephrogenic DI is commonly seen because of the drug lithium, hypercalcemia, or hypokalemia.

➡ SIADH is the result of excess ADH, which causes the kidney to retain free water in excess of solute. SIADH can be the result of malignant diseases that produce their own ADH, central nervous system diseases, pulmonary problems, or drugs.

➡ Hyponatremia is the clinical problem produced by SIADH because of free water dilution of the serum sodium. Sodium levels of less than 120 mEq/L are life-threatening, especially if the change occurs over 48 hours or less. Cerebral edema occurs, leading to change in level of consciousness to coma and seizures.

➡ Laboratory studies diagnostic of DI include plasma osmolality greater than 295 mOsm/kg H_2O, serum sodium greater than 145 mEq/L, and urine osmolality less than 250 mOsm/kg H_2O. Response to ADH replacement therapy differentiates neurogenic from nephrogenic DI. Patients with nephrogenic DI have no decreased urine response to ADH therapy.

➡ Water deprivation testing is not commonly used in critically ill patients because of the danger of hypovolemia in an already compromised individual.

➡ Laboratory studies diagnostic of SIADH include serum osmolality less than 280 mOsm/kg H_2O, serum sodium less than 135 mEq/L, urine osmolality greater than 100 mOsm/kg H_2O, and urine sodium greater than 20 mmol/L.

➡ Collaborative management of the critically ill patient with neurogenic DI includes rehydration with free water and use of ADH replacement therapy.

➡ Three forms of ADH replacement are available: vasopressin, desmopressin, and lypressin.

➡ Other drugs may be used to increase ADH release or to increase ADH action in the kidney. They are clofibrate, chlorpropamide, and carbamazepine. All have potential side effects.

➡ Patients with nephrogenic DI respond to correction of underlying problems such as hypercalcemia or removal of lithium. Thiazide diuretics may also be used in low doses.

➡ Fluid loss as a result of hyperglycemia induced by parenteral hyperalimentation must be minimized by control of blood sugar levels. Diarrhea because of hypertonic tube feeding must also be controlled.

➡ Fluid restriction, usually to 1 L of oral and intravenous intake per day, may be enough to correct the dilutional hyponatremia of SIADH.

➡ Hypertonic saline is used if the patient with SIADH is symptomatic with a serum sodium less than 120 mEq/L. Correction of serum sodium must occur slowly, to avoid the osmotic demyelination syndrome.

➡ Loop diuretics may be used along with hypertonic saline to correct the water excess and hyponatremia.

➡ Chronic forms of SIADH may be treated with fluid restriction, a high-salt diet, and demeclocycline or lithium. These two medications block the actions of ADH on the kidney tubule leading to free water loss.

➡ Outcomes for patients with DI and SIADH include restoring fluid and electrolyte balance along with preventing complications, preventing injury and preserving cerebral tissue perfusion, restoring psychological balance, and enabling the patient to manage care outside the acute hospital setting.

References

1. Loriaux TC, Drass JA: Endocrine and diabetic disorders. In: Kinney MR, Packa DR, Dunbar SB (eds): AACN's Clinical Reference for Critical Care Nursing, 3rd ed. St Louis, Mosby–Year Book, 1993.
2. Bell TN: Diabetes insipidus. Crit Care Nurs Clin North Am 6:675–685, 1994.
3. Batcheller J: Syndrome of inappropriate antidiuretic hormone secretion. Crit Care Nurs Clin North Am 6:687–692, 1994.
4. Freedland MJ, Kruse JA: Hyponatremia and hypernatremia. In: Kruse JA, Parker MM, Carlson RW, et al (eds): Pocket Companion to Principles and Practice of Medical Intensive Care. Philadelphia, W.B. Saunders, 1996.
5. Freedland MJ: Diabetes insipidus. In: Kruse JA, Parker MM, Carlson RW, et al (eds): Pocket Companion to Principles and Practice of Medical Intensive Care. Philadelphia, W.B. Saunders, 1996.
6. Malseed RT, Goldstein FJ, Balkon N: Pharmacology, Drug Therapy and Nursing Considerations. Philadelphia, J.B. Lippincott, 1995.
7. Black RM: Disorders of plasma sodium and plasma potassium. In: Rippe JM, Irwin RS, Fink MP, et al (eds): Intensive Care Medicine. New York, Little, Brown and Company, 1996.

30

Thyroid Crisis and Myxedema Coma

Danni Brown

Objectives

After completing this chapter, the student will be able to:

1. Compare and contrast the underlying pathophysiology of thyroid crisis and myxedema coma.
2. Select appropriate nursing diagnoses for a patient experiencing thyroid crisis or myxedema coma.
3. Differentiate the emergency treatment for the patient presenting with thyroid crisis versus myxedema coma.
4. Plan appropriate interventions for the prevention and early treatment of patients experiencing thyroid dysfunction.

Thyroid crisis, also called thyroid storm, and myxedema coma are extreme conditions that occur in hyperthyroid and hypothyroid states, respectively. Although both these states are extremely rare, both are serious, life-threatening medical conditions that require rapid diagnosis and aggressive treatment to achieve successful outcomes. To understand the manifestations of severe dysfunctions of the thyroid gland, the nurse must first have a firm grasp on normal hormonal function.

Thyroid hormones, thyroxine (T_4) and triiodothyronine (T_3), are iodine-based compounds produced in the thyroid gland. Most of the hormones travel through the body bound to proteins and are inactive in the bound state. T_4, the physiologically inactive hormone, is converted to T_3 by the enzymatic removal of an iodine molecule. T_3 is the physiologically active hormone. It affects most cells in the body and controls metabolism, oxygen consumption, heat production, and therefore temperature regulation.

ETIOLOGY AND PATHOPHYSIOLOGY

Thyroid crisis is a rare but life-threatening condition occurring in patients with hyperthyroidism. The exact pathophysiology is not fully understood. Thyroid crisis occurs most often in women and during times of stress in patients with hyperthyroidism (e.g., infection, trauma, or surgery).[1] Several theories have been postulated on the exact mechanism, but none has been proven. One theory suggests an increase in circulating thyroid hormone.[2] Several studies, however, have shown no difference in the circulating levels of thyroid hormone between patients with uncomplicated hyperthyroidism and patients with thyroid storm. The actual level of hormone in the blood may not be as important as the rate at which levels increase.[2]

Other theories include a change in tissue response to thyroid hormone and activation of the sympathetic nervous system. Sympathetic nervous system stimulation is responsible for most of the signs and symptoms associated with thyroid storm. Thyroid hormone is known to have an effect on the adrenergic receptors in certain tissues, thereby increasing the sensitivity to circulating catecholamines.

Apathetic thyroidism is a condition often seen in the elderly. Patients with apathetic thyroidism are at high risk of thyroid storm. These patients do not develop the usual signs and symptoms of hyperthyroidism and often have only a single symptom, such as tachycardia, muscle weakness, or depression.[3] The diagnosis of hyperthyroidism is often not made until thyroid storm develops.

In contrast, myxedema coma is an extreme and life-threatening form of decompensated hypothyroidism. It is almost always precipitated by a stress state, such as an illness, infection, or trauma.[4] Although most patients do not present with true coma, a classic sign of advanced hypothyroidism is an alteration in central nervous system (CNS) functioning. This change may be manifested as lethargy, confusion, disorientation, or obtundation.

In addition to the CNS abnormalities, low circulating levels of T_3 and T_4 result in lowered metabolism and loss of heat generation. The body attempts to compensate with peripheral vasoconstriction, decreasing blood flow to the extremities. This change allows blood to be shunted toward the center of the body, or core, thus preserving central body temperature and vital organ function. However, this higher central blood volume increases circulation to and fluid loss from the kidneys. The elderly are more strongly affected by a hypothyroid state. It is more difficult for the elderly patient to maintain a normal body temperature because heat generation decreases with age, independent of thyroid state.[5] A hypothyroid condition makes it even more difficult to maintain core temperature. The elderly must peripherally vasoconstrict maximally to maintain core temperature. This process can cause moderate to severe dehydration over time.

Patients with chronic hypothyroidism have an interstitial accumulation of a mucopolysaccharide and water causing a nonpitting edema, hence the term "myxedema." This edema can be in the skin, giving a swollen appearance to the face and extremities; the vocal cords, causing hoarseness; the heart, causing pericardial effusions; and the lungs causing pleural effusions.

It is important in the critically ill patient to differentiate sick euthyroid syndrome from hypothyroidism. In the person with a nonthyroidal illness, T_4 has an alternative degradation pathway. Rather than the usual conversion of T_4 to T_3, an energy-saving pathway is used, and T_4 is degraded to reverse T_3 (rT_3). Because rT_3 is not physiologically active, metabolism is decreased and oxygen consumption is decreased during the healing phase. This mechanism is adaptive, not pathologic. Sick euthyroid syndrome is differentiated from hypothyroidism by a normal thyroid-stimulating hormone (TSH) and elevated rT_3.

Assessment

There are no specific clinical or laboratory findings to diagnose either thyroid storm or myxedema states, but rather a constellation of signs and symptoms that, when considered together, makes up the clinical picture.

Health History

Both thyroid storm and myxedema states are associated with a preexisting disruption of normal thyroid physiology—hyperthyroidism and hypothyroidism, respectively. The patient and family should be questioned carefully to elicit any past history of thyroid disorder or symptoms consistent with thyroid disorders not previously diagnosed. This includes any incidence of dizziness, lightheadedness, weakness, or palpitations. The nurse should also ask questions specific to disturbances in thought process, activity level, or tolerance to heat or cold. Information should include the intensity and duration of any symptoms, as well as the identification of any precipitating factors related to the current health crisis.

Physical Examination

The patient in thyroid crisis manifests intensification of the effects of thyroid hormone. All body systems can be affected by high circulating levels of T_3. In addition, the effect of catecholamines is heightened. Often, the patient also presents with goiter (an enlargement of the thyroid gland) and exophthalmos (a protrusion of the eyeballs). These two symptoms are seen in the condition known as Graves' disease. The patient appears anxious, disoriented, or even obtunded. He or she is tachycardic, with heart rates frequently as high as 150 to 180 beats per minute and often irregular. In addition to the tachycardia, the patient has hyperpyrexia, with a body temperatures as high as 40 to 41°C (Chart 30–1). The patient's skin is warm and diaphoretic. The patient also has hypertension, with a widened pulse pressure early in the development of thyroid storm. As the cardiovascular system decompensates in progressive thyroid storm, the patient develops hypotension.

Myxedema coma, in contrast, is the most severe form of hypothyroidism. These patients present with diminution of effects of thyroid hormone. They have cool, pale skin and body temperatures as low as 31 to 32°C. Although few patients present in a coma, all patients have moderate to severe alteration in mental status. They may be disorientated, lethargic, or even psychotic. Edema is also a common characteristic of hypothyroidism, and patients with myxedema often have nonpitting edema of the extremities. Respiratory failure is a classic finding in hypothyroidism. Patients with slow, shallow respirations resulting in hypercapnia may require emergency intubation and mechanical support to maintain respiratory function. The cardiovascular changes associated with hypothyroidism include bradycardia and hypotension.

In both thyroid storm and myxedema coma, all attempts must be made to identify the precipitating factors to the decompensated state. Interventions need

CHART 30–1

RESEARCH UTILIZATION: DETERMINING THE OPTIMAL SITE FOR ASSESSING BODY TEMPERATURE

Abstract: Many studies have compared temperature readings from different sites in hypothermic and normothermic patients, but none has compared methods in febrile patients. In this study, oral, axillary, rectal, tympanic, and pulmonary artery temperature readings were obtained in rapid sequence from 13 patients with temperatures higher than or equal to 37.8°C. A total of 113 sets of temperature measurements was collected. Results indicated that rectal temperature correlated most closely with pulmonary artery temperature, followed by oral, tympanic, and axillary temperatures. Rectal and tympanic methods were most sensitive in detecting temperatures higher than 38.3°C. The researchers concluded that rectal temperatures should be considered when assessing temperature in febrile patients. When the rectal site is contraindicated, then either the tympanic or the oral route can be used. Axillary temperature did not correlate well with core (pulmonary artery) temperature. The researchers recommended that this method should not be used clinically to assess for fever.

Critique: This study had several limitations. The sample size was small, and the researchers failed to test the thermometers and pulmonary artery catheters for accuracy. In addition, only one brand of thermometer was used for each site. Finally, the researchers did not establish interrater reliability among the data collectors.

Nursing Implications: Nurses caring for febrile patients need to measure temperature accurately to provide appropriate interventions. A falsely low temperature may delay needed treatment, and a falsely elevated temperature may initiate unnecessary treatments (e.g., administration of antibiotics, collection of specimens for cultures). Although this study did not include patients experiencing fever from thyroid crisis, the information has clinical importance. The approach to the measurement of temperature in febrile patients must, minimally, be consistent. This implies that the nurse or technician must use the same site to obtain temperature measurements, to document the site used, and to communicate this information to others caring for the patient. Further research is needed to determine fully whether or not the rectal site has definitive advantages over other sites. Based on findings from this study, however, it is recommended that nurses avoid the use of the axillary site to assess for the presence or absence of fever.

Source: Schmitz T, Bair N, Falk M, et al: A comparison of five methods of temperature measurement in febrile intensive care patients. Am J Crit Care, 4:286–292, 1995.

to be aimed at both the treatment of the thyroid disorder and the treatment of the precipitating event (e.g., the initiation of antibiotics for infection).

Laboratory and Diagnostic Tests

History and clinical presentation are important in the diagnosis of either thyroid storm or myxedema coma. Thyroid function testing should be done in any patient suspected of having any disruption in normal thyroid physiology. These tests include serum T_4, T_3, TSH, free T_4 (FT_4), and free thyroxine index (FTI). T_3 level is not usually helpful in diagnosing hypothyroid states because it is expected to be low in a patient with a critical illness, as mentioned in the discussion of sick euthyroid syndrome. A radioiodine uptake study, either the standard 24-hour test or an abbreviated 2-hour test, is helpful in diagnosing hyperthyroid states. Other blood tests helpful in completing the clinical picture are serum glucose, electrolytes, and complete blood counts, including a white cell count with differential. The patient with hyperthyroid state has elevated total and free serum levels of T_4 and T_3. TSH is depressed in primary thyroid disorders, but it may be elevated in secondary hyperthyroidism. A radioiodine uptake study is also elevated. Other abnormal laboratory findings include hyperglycemia, elevated white blood cell count, often with a shift to the left, hypercalcemia, and elevated transaminases, creatine kinase, and alkaline phosphatase. Chest radiographic findings may show pulmonary edema.[2]

The patient with hypothyroid state has depressed levels of T_4, FT_4, and FTI. TSH is elevated in primary hypothyroidism and is depressed in secondary hypothyroidism. Other abnormal laboratory findings include hypoglycemia, hyponatremia, a low white blood cell count with a mild shift to the right, and arterial blood gases with a low partial pressure of oxygen (PO_2) and an elevated partial pressure of carbon dioxide (PCO_2). Chest radiography reveals an enlarged heart that may be due to a pericardial effusion or a dilated myocardium.[6]

The diagnosis of thyroid storm and of myxedema coma is difficult to make and often can be missed. If the index of suspicion is high enough, treatment should be started even before all laboratory results have been received. Prompt treatment of these life-threatening conditions is critical for the patient's survival. Table 30–1 provides a comparison of the pathophysiology and physical assessment and laboratory findings found in patients experiencing thyroid crisis or myxedema coma.

Nursing Diagnoses

Patients with severe forms of thyroid dysfunction, thyroid crisis, and myxedema states require rapid assessment, diagnosis, and management of the physio-

logic sequelae. The plan of care established by the health care team needs to be comprehensive. Nurses need to identify individualized nursing diagnoses to direct the plan of care (Table 30–2). The immediate priorities of care in the intensive care unit (ICU) are the achievement or maintenance of cardiovascular and neurologic stability as well as the restoration of normothermia. Patient education, although initiated in the ICU, is a major focus during the patient's recovery beyond the ICU and after discharge (Chart 30–2).

Collaborative Management

The ultimate goal of treatment for patients experiencing either thyroid crisis or myxedema coma is correction of the abnormal thyroid state. In addition, these patients require rapid stabilization of altered cardiopulmonary and thermoregulatory systems. Con-

TABLE 30–1
Comparison of Thyroid Crisis (Storm) and Myxedema Coma (State)

Thyroid Crisis	Myxedema Coma
Pathophysiology	
Excessive circulating thyroid hormone	Inadequate circulating thyroid hormone
Precipitating event: trauma, surgery, infection, emotional stress, medication overdose	Precipitating event: infection, trauma, emotional stress, exposure to cold, interruption of medications
Physical Assessment Findings	
Cardiovascular: tachycardia, atrial and/or ventricular dysrhythmias, systolic hypertension	Cardiovascular: bradycardia, pericardial effusion, hypotension
Nutrition: weight loss	Nutrition: weight gain
Respiratory: dyspnea, tachypnea	Respiratory: hypoventilation, respiratory failure
Thermoregulation: fever	Thermoregulation: hypothermia
Neuromuscular: agitation, restlessness, emotional lability, wakefulness	Neuromuscular: decreased level of consciousness, psychosis, coma
Gastrointestinal: nausea, vomiting, diarrhea	Gastrointestinal: ileus
Laboratory Findings	
Elevated T_4, FT_4, and FTI	Decreased T_4, FT_4, and FTI
Decreased TSH	Elevated TSH
Hypernatremia; hypercalcemia; elevated transaminases, creatine kinase and alkaline phosphatase; hyperglycemia	Hypokalemia, elevated cholesterol and triglycerides, hypoglycemia
Treatment Strategies	
Medications: drugs that block synthesis (e.g., PTU), release (e.g., iodides) and/or peripheral conversion (e.g., glucocorticoids) of thyroid hormone; beta blockers; antibiotics (if infection present); antipyretics	Medications: thyroid hormone replacement (e.g., L-T_4), glucocorticoids, antibiotics (if infection present)
T_4 removal: plasmapheresis, dialysis; ablative therapies (e.g., surgery)	
Supplemental oxygen as needed	Ventilatory support as needed
Intravenous glucose and vitamins	Fluid replacement to maintain blood volume
Active cooling: blankets (taper once patient's temperature = 38°C), ice packs, fans	Passive rewarming
Identification and treatment of precipitating event	Identification and treatment of precipitating event

FT_4, free thyroxine; FTI, free thyroxine index; PTU, propylthiouracil; TSH, thyroid-stimulating hormone.

TABLE 30-2
Nursing Diagnoses

Problem Statement	Etiologic Factors
Thyroid Storm	
Hyperthermia	Increased heat generation secondary to hypermetabolic state
Altered nutrition, less than body requirements	Increased need for nutrition secondary to hypermetabolic state
Impaired gas exchange	Increased oxygen demand secondary to hypermetabolic state
Sleep pattern disturbance	Interruption in sleep–rest patterns secondary to hypermetabolic state
Altered thought processes	Change in cerebral metabolism
Anxiety	Uncertainty regarding illness; hospitalization
Risk for fluid volume deficit	Excessive water losses secondary to vomiting, diarrhea, sweating
Myxedema Coma	
Decreased cardiac output	Myocardial depression secondary to insufficient thyroid hormone
Hypothermia	Lack of heat generation from decreased metabolism
Impaired gas exchange	Depressed respirations secondary to muscular weakness
Altered thought processes	Psychosis, coma
Fluid volume deficit (intravascular)	Shifting of intravascular fluids secondary to the accumulation of mucopolysaccharides and, consequently, water in the interstitial space
Constipation	Decreased gastrointestinal motility

sideration must also be given to identification and treatment of the precipitating condition (see Table 30–1). The nurse must monitor the patient's response to treatment carefully, to ensure the achievement of this goal.

Thyroid Crisis

The treatment of high circulating levels of thyroid hormones is aimed at blocking the synthesis, secretion, and peripheral conversion of the hormones. Propylthiouracil (PTU) is a drug that blocks the synthesis of the hormones in the thyroid gland and inhibits conversion of T_4 to T_3 in the periphery. Methimazole (Tapazole) is another drug that blocks the synthesis of the hormones, but it has no effect peripherally. Beta-blocking agents, such as propranolol (Inderal), inhibit the conversion of T_4 to T_3, as well as block the cardiovascular effects of hyperthyroidism. Glucocorticoids also

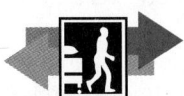

CHART 30-2

BEYOND THE ICU: MANAGING PATIENTS WITH THYROID DYSFUNCTION AFTER DISCHARGE

The patient with severe thyroid dysfunction usually has a chronic but stable thyroid condition that has been disrupted by a physiologic or emotional stressor (e.g., trauma, surgery, infection, crisis). This stressor usually precipitates an abrupt decompensation in the condition that requires emergency management in an ICU. After recovery from the acute event, the patient requires specific nursing interventions to ensure maintenance of a normal state. The nurse should assess the family dynamics and home care situation to determine whether resources are adequate. It may be appropriate to consult social services for assistance with the patient's discharge needs. Because many patients are discharged sooner and sicker than previously, home care nurses may be needed to follow the patient and family in the community to continue or evaluate the education process.

Long-term and adequate control of the hypothyroid or hyperthyroid state is essential. The patient and family must understand the medication regimen and the potential side effects of the medications. The patient may also need to have blood levels checked periodically to ensure proper dosing of the medication and a euthyroid state. In addition, the patient and family must have a solid understanding of the effects of stressors on thyroid function. The patient and family should also be knowledgeable about early signs and symptoms of decompensation and should know when to seek medical care. Prevention or early intervention is the primary mechanism for avoiding a health crisis in these patients. Finally, patients should be encouraged to obtain and carry MedicAlert identification.

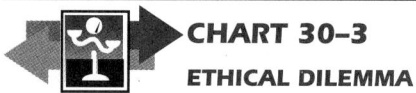

CHART 30-3

ETHICAL DILEMMA

Mrs. H. is a 75-year-old woman who was admitted to the intensive care unit this morning after being found unresponsive in her apartment. She has been treated for the past 10 years with synthetic thyroid replacement for idiopathic hypothyroidism. Eight months ago, she was diagnosed with ovarian cancer and received chemotherapy. She is currently in remission. She has also been under the care of a psychiatrist for treatment of clinical depression that became debilitating after the death of her husband 3 years ago. During her a visit with her primary care provider last week, she expressed a desire to discontinue all her medications and "get this over with." Her admitting diagnosis is severe hypothyroidism (myxedema state), secondary to discontinuance of replacement therapy and superimposed infection. At present, she is unconscious and is receiving thyroid replacement, intravenous fluids, and mechanical ventilation to maintain her respiratory status. An abdominal ultrasound has revealed a probable abscess. She has been started on antibiotics. Her only living relative, a niece from out of town, arrived this afternoon. Mrs. H.'s niece is requesting that all treatment be stopped and the patient be allowed to die. The niece believes that this is her aunt's wish but does not have any written documentation, such as a living will, to substantiate this belief.

Mrs. H. lives alone in an apartment complex for the elderly. Her husband died 3 years ago after 53 years of marriage. They had no children. Her only sister died 5 years ago after a long struggle with cancer. She has only the one niece, who appears extremely concerned about her aunt.

1. What are the ethical issues related to care decisions for Mrs. H. at this time?
2. What are the legal issues related to care decisions for Mrs. H. at this time?
3. Is Mrs. H.'s niece acting in the patient's best interest? Defend your response.
4. What is the nurse's role in the decision-making process for this patient?
5. What resources could be accessed to resolve this dilemma?

inhibit the conversion of T_4 to T_3 as well as treat any adrenal insufficiency that may occur. Iodine administration and lithium carbonate block the secretion of synthesized hormones from the thyroid gland. Neither should be given until synthesis of the hormones has been stopped with either PTU or methimazole. In extreme cases, plasmapheresis, peritoneal dialysis, and plasma exchange have been used to help lower circulating hormone levels when other measures fail.

The hyperthermia seen with thyroid storm is the result of excessive heat production unregulated by the hypothalamus. The high body temperatures can be treated with the antipyretic acetaminophen (Tylenol). Aspirin should never be used because it can cause the unbinding of thyroid hormones in circulation and may increase free hormone levels. Antipyretics alone may not lower body temperature. Cooling blankets and ice packs may also be required to help lower extremely high body temperatures.

Other supportive therapies for the patient in thyroid storm include adequate hydration and the correction of any electrolyte imbalances. Supplemental oxygen, antidysrhythmics, and sedation, as indicated, should be employed. Adequate nutrition, including vitamins, is also important to supply substrate for the hypermetabolic state.

Clinical improvement can be expected within 24 to 48 hours after the initiation of therapy. The best gauge of response is the patient's mental status. Decrease in body temperature and resolution of tachycardia are also signs of improvement. Once the thyroid storm has been treated, it is important to discuss definitive treatment options with the patient, to prevent the likelihood of another event. Ablation therapy, either surgical or chemical with radioactive iodine, has been successful in treating hyperthyroidism.

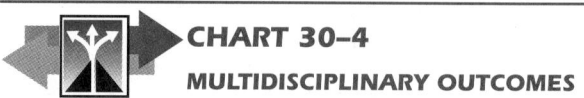

CHART 30-4

MULTIDISCIPLINARY OUTCOMES

Restoration of thermoregulation
Restoration of adequate nutrition
Restoration of fluid and electrolyte balance
Restoration of cerebral functioning
Restoration of elimination pattern
Patient education regarding health maintenance
Prevention of complications of treatments

Myxedema Coma

Myxedema coma requires prompt thyroid replacement. Levothyroxine (Synthroid) should be given intravenously. All patients must be monitored closely during the administration of the drug and for some time afterward. Hormone replacement increases the patient's metabolic rate, oxygen consumption, and cardiac workload. This sudden increase in demand can precipitate an acute myocardial infarction, especially in patients with a history of coronary artery disease. Patients should receive intravenous thyroid replacement for 2 to 10 days, after which oral replacement therapy can be initiated.

Other important supportive therapies for the patient with myxedema state include fluid resuscitation, respiratory support, and temperature control. A pulmonary artery catheter may be necessary to assess fluid status adequately and to guide resuscitation efforts. The patient's response to fluid resuscitation must be carefully monitored, and electrolytes must be checked to prevent an exacerbation of the dilutional hyponatremia that is common in severe hypothyroidism.[3] An intravenous solution of both saline and dextrose is recommended if hypoglycemia is present. A solution of 10% dextrose may be necessary if severe hypoglycemia is present. Intubation and mechanical ventilation are often necessary to treat respiratory failure. Rewarming the patient must be done with care. Passive rewarming, using blankets to cover the patient, is usually sufficient. A warming blanket should never be used to raise the patient's body temperature. This type of active rewarming can cause peripheral vasodilation. In the dehydrated patient, this condition could lead to profound hypotension.

Care of patients presenting with severe hypothyroid or hyperthyroid states poses many challenges to the health team. With prompt diagnosis and treatment, these patients usually respond quickly, and remaining interventions are focused on recovery and prevention of future thyroid crises (Chart 30–3).

Multidisciplinary Outcomes

The goal for both the patient with thyroid storm and the patient with myxedema coma is the return to and maintenance of a euthyroid state (Chart 30–4). Achievement of this goal is evidenced by a normal body temperature, vital signs within normal limits, and normal or baseline cognitive ability. Patient education is essential because the patient must understand the need for continuous therapy and must know the signs and symptoms of an alteration in thyroid function. Prevention and early intervention are the best approaches to treating patients with thyroid dysfunction.

Critical Thinking Exercise

Mrs. S. is a 68-year-old woman admitted to the intermediate care unit from the emergency department (ED), where she presented with an elevated temperature. She has a past medical history of coronary artery disease (for 9 years), breast cancer (treated with surgery and chemotherapy 5 years ago), and dental surgery for a tooth abscess 2 days before admission. In addition, she described a history of increasing tremors, weight loss (10 lb), increased appetite, and restlessness developing over the past 2 weeks. Her chest radiograph (done in the ED) was normal, and her initial laboratory results and vital signs were as follows:

		(Normal Range)
Sodium	151	*(135–145 mEq/L)*
Potassium	4.0	*(3.5–5.0 mEq/L)*
Chloride	99	*(100–106 mEq/L)*
CO_2	22	*(24–30 mEq/L)*
Blood urea		
* nitrogen*	29	*(8–25 mg/dL)*
Creatinine	1.0	*(0.6–1.5 mg/dL)*
Hematocrit	37.8	*(37–48%)*
Hemoglobin	13.3	*(12–16 g/dL)*
White blood		
* count*	13.6	*(4.3–10.8 × 10^3*
		cells/μL)
pH	7.44	*(7.35–7.45)*
PO_2	90	*(80–100 mm Hg)*
PCO_2	33	*(35–45 mm Hg)*
HCO_3^-	23	*(24–28 mEq/L)*
Heart rate	*119 beats/min*	
Blood pressure	*166/62 mm Hg*	
Temperature	*40.3°C*	
Respiratory		
* rate*	*26/min*	

Specimens (urine and blood) were collected and sent for culture. Mrs. S.'s temperature remained elevated (>39°C) despite repeated doses of acetaminophen. She developed nausea, vomiting, and diarrhea. An obstructive series was ordered and was negative. She developed atrial fibrillation with a rapid ventricular response and complained of palpitations. She was transferred to the ICU for further evaluation and treatment. The results of her endocrine panel were as follows:

		(Normal Range)
T_3	203	*(40–185 ng/dL)*
FT_4	3.9	*(0.8–2.3 ng/dL)*
Total T_4	14	*(5.0–11.0 μg/dL)*
TSH	0.2	*(0.5–8.9 μU/mL)*
Total cortisol	6	*(5–25 μg/dL at 8:00*
		AM)

It was determined that Mrs. S. was experiencing thyroid storm. PTU and esmolol (Brevibloc) were ordered, as well as a cooling blanket.

1. What do you believe were the precipitating events that led to Mrs. S.'s thyroid crisis?

2. Identify three priority nursing diagnoses (with interventions) for Mrs. S. at this point and provide rationales for your choices.
3. Provide rationales for the medications ordered for Mrs. S. What additional medications could also be ordered for this patient and why?
4. What key elements need to be included in the discharge education for this patient?

Key Concepts

➡ Thyroid crisis and myxedema coma usually occur when a precipitating and stressful event moves a patient from a controlled hyperthyroid or hypothyroid state to an uncontrolled hyperthyroid or hypothyroid state, respectively.

➡ The primary symptoms seen in thyroid crisis include hyperthermia, tachycardia, and hypertension.

➡ A patient in myxedema coma is hypothermic, obtunded, and often in respiratory distress.

➡ Patients in thyroid crisis have elevated levels of T_4 and T_3 and a decreased level of TSH, if the hyperthyroidism is a primary disorder.

➡ Patients in myxedema coma have depressed levels of T_4 and T_3 and an elevated level of TSH, if the hypothyroidism is a primary disorder.

➡ The goal of treatment for both thyroid crisis and myxedema coma is the correction of the abnormal thyroid state.

➡ Treatment of patients experiencing thyroid crisis includes medications that block the synthesis, release, and peripheral conversion of thyroid hormones.

➡ Treatment of patients experiencing myxedema coma includes the prompt replacement of thyroid hormones.

➡ Treatment of patients with either thyroid crisis or myxedema coma includes attention to restoration of normothermia, adequate nutrition, and fluid balance.

➡ Patient education is critical to helping patients prevent further episodes of thyroid dysfunction.

References

1. Lammon CA, Hart G: Recognizing thyroid crisis. Nursing 23:33, 1993.
2. Tietgens ST, Leinung MC: Thyroid storm. Med Clin North Am 79:169–184, 1995.
3. Spittle L: Diagnoses in opposition: thyroid storm and myxedema coma. Clin Issues Crit Care Nurs 3:300–308, 1992.
4. McMorrow ME: Myxedema coma. Am J Nurs 96:55, 1996.
5. Nicoloff JT, LoPresti JS: Myxedema coma: a form of decompensated hypothyroidism. Endocrinol Metab Clin North Am 22:279–290, 1993.
6. Tsitouras PD: Myxedema coma. Clin Geriatr Med 11:251–258, 1995.

31

Adrenal Crisis (Addison's Disease)

Lisa Ann Bove

Objectives

After completing this chapter, the student will be able to:

1. Relate the pathophysiology of adrenal insufficiency or crisis to the anticipated plan of care.
2. Identify assessment parameters and diagnostic studies used to identify adrenal insufficiency or crisis.
3. Plan collaborative care that extends across the health care continuum for patients experiencing adrenal insufficiency or crisis.
4. Select appropriate interventions for patients experiencing adrenal crisis.
5. Evaluate the effects of the collaborative care on anticipated outcomes for a patient experiencing adrenal crisis.

Nurses care for patients with various disease processes. Perhaps one of the most challenging is the patient in adrenal crisis. These patients are often admitted for unrelated problems, such as gastrointestinal surgery, infectious diseases, or respiratory problems. Adrenal crisis can occur as a complication of these problems. A firm understanding of the etiology and pathophysiology of adrenal insufficiency and crisis is important to developing an appropriate plan of care and, ultimately, to the patient's outcome.

ETIOLOGY AND PATHOPHYSIOLOGY

Primary adrenal insufficiency (Addison's disease) is also known as hypoadrenalism and hypocorticism and strikes about 1 in 100,000 people.[1,2] It is a rare endocrine disorder that afflicts men and women equally. First identified by Dr. Thomas Addison in 1849, primary adrenal insufficiency was initially associated with tuberculosis (TB) because 70 to 90% of his patients also had TB on autopsy. As the treatment of TB improved and fewer patients contracted TB, fewer patients demonstrated signs of adrenal insufficiency and crisis. Today, adrenal insufficiency is separated into two types, primary and secondary, with each having its own causes and treatments.[3]

Each person has two adrenal glands, one located at the upper portion of each kidney. Each adrenal gland has two components, the adrenal medulla and the adrenal cortex. The center of the adrenal gland, the medulla, is part of the autonomic nervous system and secretes catecholamines (Table 31–1). Around 90% of the secretion from the medulla is epinephrine, and the rest is norepinephrine. Catecholamines regulate metabolic pathways commonly known as the "fight-or-flight" syndrome. Epinephrine causes vasoconstriction, resulting in decreased blood flow to the nonessential organs, such as the gastrointestinal tract and skin, while increasing venous return, thus increasing cardiac output. It also increases heart rate and contractility, to ready the body for increases in metabolic demands. Finally, epinephrine acts to relax the smooth muscles of the bronchioles, thereby increasing vital capacity and tidal volume.

The adrenal cortex, the outer portion of the adrenal gland, secretes three kinds of adrenocorticosteroid hormones: glucocorticoids (cortisol), mineralocorticoids (aldosterone), and sex hormones (androgens). These hormones affect glucose and electrolyte metabolism and exert effects similar to those of testosterone,

TABLE 31-1
Structures and Functions of the Adrenal Gland

Structure	Hormone	Function
Adrenal Cortex	Corticosteroids	
	Mineralocorticoids (aldosterone)	Causes the reabsorption of sodium and the elimination of potassium
	Glucocorticoids (cortisol)	Responsible for the metabolism of carbohydrates, proteins, and fats; assists in the stress and the anti-inflammatory responses
	Sex hormones (androgens)	Thought to be partly responsible for the preadolescent growth spurt
Adrenal Medulla	Catecholamines	
	Epinephrine	Causes actions similar to the stimulation of the sympathetic nervous system: vasoconstriction, cardiac stimulation, and bronchiole relaxation; participates in the "fight or flight" syndrome
	Norepinephrine	Increases peripheral resistance (vasoconstriction)

respectively. Adrenal regulation of glucocorticoids is maintained by hormone release from the hypothalamus and pituitary glands (Figure 31–1). Not until more than 90% of the adrenal cortex is lost does adrenal insufficiency develop.

Adrenal insufficiency is caused by lack of sufficient adrenocorticosteroids. This deficiency is the result of a failure of the adrenal gland to produce adequate levels of cortisol. Insufficient cortisol production can result from a disorder of the adrenal glands themselves (primary adrenal insufficiency) or from a failure to produce adequate adrenocorticotropin (ACTH) (secondary adrenal insufficiency). Adrenal crisis is an acute adrenal insufficiency and can be life-threatening.

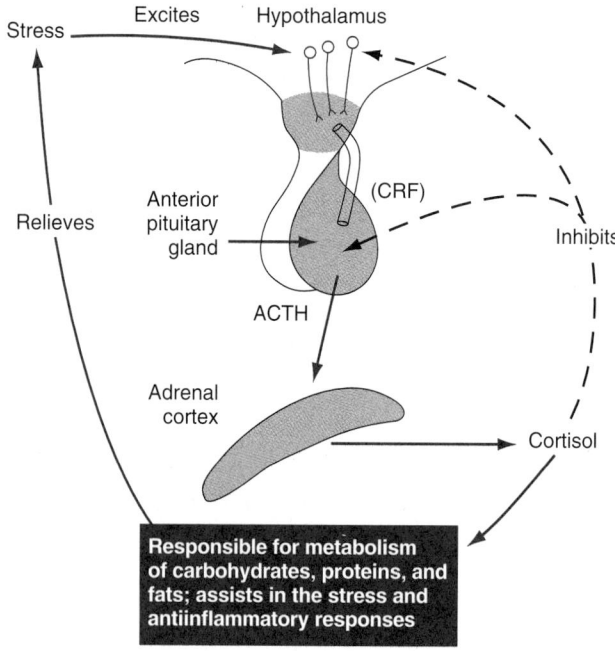

Figure 31-1
Feedback mechanisms controlling the release of glucocorticoid (cortisol) from the adrenal gland. (Modified from Guyton AC, Hall JE: Textbook of Medical Physiology, 9th ed. Philadelphia, W.B. Saunders, 1996, p 966.)

Primary Adrenal Insufficiency (Addison's Disease)

Most cases of primary adrenal insufficiency are caused by a gradual loss of functioning adrenal cortex resulting from the creation of antibodies to the adrenal gland.[4] The destruction of the adrenal gland by the autoimmune response is 25% more common in women than in men. TB of the adrenals, formally the most common cause, has decreased because of an overall decrease in the incidence of TB.[5] Other causes include sepsis, acquired immunodeficiency syndrome (AIDS), fungal infections such as histoplasmosis, and surgical removal of the adrenal gland secondary to metastatic disease. In these cases, the adrenal cortex tissue slowly atrophies and eventually requires removal.

Secondary Adrenal Insufficiency

Secondary adrenal insufficiency is caused by inadequate secretion of ACTH from the pituitary gland or by abrupt withdrawal of exogenous adrenocortical hormone (e.g., cortisone) therapy. Inadequate ACTH secretion results from either altered hypothalamic function, which is responsible for pituitary hormone regulation, or primary disorders of the pituitary; both conditions decrease production of ACTH. Exogenous adrenocortical hormone administration suppresses the body's normal secretion of adrenal hormones and interferes with normal feedback mechanisms regulating the hormones. Abrupt withdrawal of exogenous adrenocortical hormones precipitates an acute state of adrenal insufficiency.

Adrenal Crisis

Adrenal crisis is caused by the body's inability to continue to maintain homeostasis because of insufficient cortisol. It is usually precipitated by a stressful event such as surgery or infection or other illnesses (Chart 31–1). Adrenal crisis affects both glucocorticoids and mineralcorticoids. Glucose metabolism is impaired, and inadequate circulating blood glucose levels lead to poor healing, decreased cerebral perfusion, and cardiac irregularities. Inadequate aldosterone levels lead to sodium and water loss and potassium retention. These conditions cause severe dehydration, and, eventually, circulatory collapse and shock. Lack of circulating blood volume also contributes to inadequate cerebral blood flow and cardiac dysrhythmias.

Pathophysiology

Whether primary or secondary, adrenal insufficiency leads to decreased hepatic glucose output and hypo-glycemia resulting from altered hormone control. Insufficient cortisol also reduces the levels of digestive enzymes in the stomach and can cause nausea, vomiting, and diarrhea, as well as fluid and electrolyte imbalances. Insufficient aldosterone leads to increased sodium and water loss and to potassium retention. The resultant hyperkalemia also contributes to dysrhythmias and decreased cardiac output, leading to further hypovolemia and hypotension. As hypotension and hypovolemia develop, the patient moves into life-threatening adrenal crisis and can experience shock, coma, and death, if the condition is not treated rapidly.

Finally, in primary adrenal insufficiency, increased levels of circulating ACTH (in response to the decrease in adrenal hormones) can contribute to abnormal deposits of melanin pigment in the skin and mucous membranes. It is thought that the changes in pigmen-

---

CHART 31–1

RESEARCH UTILIZATION: EXPLORING THE PATIENT'S NEED FOR STEROIDS DURING SURGERY

Abstract: Patients taking long-term replacement hormones for the treatment of secondary adrenal insufficiency (AI) are routinely ordered additional steroids to prevent hypotension in the perioperative period. The rationale for this approach is based on the belief that the acute stress of surgery precipitates a need for greater doses of steroids. This study was a randomized, double-blind study to determine whether or not patients with secondary AI actually required an increase in steroids during the perioperative period.

Patients who were taking prednisone for secondary AI were randomly assigned to receive preoperative and postoperative injections of cortisol (N = 6) or saline (N = 12) in addition to their regularly scheduled doses of prednisone. Subjects underwent various major operations that included joint replacements and abdominal operations. Results demonstrated that two patients, one from each study group, experienced transient hypotension that resolved with fluid replacement. No significant differences were found between the groups' average pulse rates or blood pressures during the perioperative period. The researchers concluded that patients with secondary AI do not experience hypotension caused by an increased need for cortisol during surgery when given only their regularly scheduled dose of steroids.

Critique: The strength of this study was the strong design. Randomized, double-blind clinical studies are the hallmark of solid, clinical research. Unfortunately, the sample size was small, and the study should be duplicated using larger numbers of patients to confirm the results.

Nursing Implications: In periods of acute stress such as major surgery, the body initiates several physiologic responses, including the increased production of cortisol. This response is thought to be necessary to maintain hemodynamic stability during the period of stress. Patients taking exogenous steroids for secondary AI have an absent or blunted cortisol response to stress. Although it remains unclear whether surgical patients with secondary AI require supplemental doses of steroids during the perioperative period, regularly scheduled doses of replacement steroids must be maintained. The nurse caring for these patients must ensure that these medications are ordered and administered in a timely manner. Further, the nurse must be equally attentive to signs and symptoms of adrenal crisis (hypotension, tachycardia, tachypnea, changes in level of consciousness) that could be precipitated by this stressful event.

Source: Glowniak JV, Loriaux DL: A double-blind study of perioperative steroid requirements in secondary adrenal insufficiency. Surgery 121:123–129, 1997.

tation are as much a result of the increased levels of ACTH as of the concurrent increases in circulating melanocyte-stimulating hormone (MSH).

Assessment

Symptoms of adrenal insufficiency usually progress slowly in patients with all causes of the disorder except surgical removal of the adrenal or pituitary glands and abrupt withdrawal of exogenous adrenocortical hormones. Nurses can contribute to the care of these patients with thorough assessment. Because many of these patients are admitted to the critical care unit for reasons other than adrenal crisis, prompt identification of symptoms is imperative. Nonspecific signs of hemodynamic instability can point to many types of shock. Patients in adrenal crisis may have, in addition to the signs of shock, muscular discomfort and weakness, weight loss, and skin and mucosal hyperpigmentation.[6]

Signs and Symptoms Associated with Adrenal Insufficiency

Patients with adrenal insufficiency may present with chronic worsening fatigue, muscle weakness, and weight loss. Patients may report craving for salty foods because of inadequate salt levels. Women may report irregular menstrual periods or cessation of menses. In addition, they may also report a decrease or loss of body, axillary, and pubic hair resulting from diminished production of sex hormones. They may also present in adrenal crisis with severe hypotension and the other classic signs of shock. The patient's health history is especially important for gathering information that points to the appropriate place in the continuum of adrenal insufficiency. Questions should focus not only on presenting symptoms but also on previous surgeries, other hormonal irregularities, and original symptoms. Many symptoms are ignored until a stressful event such as an infection causes a patient to become severely ill, precipitating a crisis. The health history should also focus on the use of current and past medications. Patients may neglect to list medications such as cortisol that they may have stopped taking (Chart 31–2). In addition, a report that the patient recently was taking antibiotics or cold and flu medications should prompt the care giver to investigate a recent illness that may have precipitated this event.

Clinical Presentation

Patients with adrenal insufficiency may present with anorexia, nausea and vomiting, diarrhea, abdominal pain, weakness, fever, and orthostatic hypotension. Skin changes are also common with areas of hyperpigmentation, most visible on scars, skin folds, and pressure points. Irritability and depression are often seen in these patients. Symptoms of hypoglycemia may also exist.

Patients in adrenal crisis may present with the following: severe, sudden onset, and penetrating back or

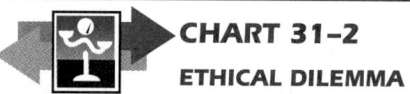

CHART 31–2

ETHICAL DILEMMA

Mrs. T. is a 64-year-old woman with a history of adrenal insufficiency (AI) for which she has been taking dexamethasone (Decadron). The cause of her AI is a pituitary tumor for which Mrs. T. refused surgery. Her past medical history includes insulin-dependent diabetes, angina, and crippling arthritis. She has been confined to her house for the past year. This morning, Mrs. T.'s caretaker was unable to awaken her. Paramedics were called, and Mrs. T. was taken to the emergency department.

On arrival to the hospital, Mrs. T. was unresponsive, hypotensive, tachycardic, tachypneic, febrile, and hyperglycemic. A diagnosis of adrenal crisis and diabetic ketoacidosis was made. Aggressive therapy was initiated and included fluids, insulin, electrolyte replacement, and hydrocortisone. Over the next 48 hours, Mrs. T. responded well. When she was able to communicate, she admitted to you that she purposely withheld her medications, including her dexamethasone and insulin. She tells you that she is "ready to die" and that she will plan her "suicide" better next time.

1. As the nurse caring for this patient, how would you respond to Mrs. T.'s admissions (withholding medications and planning to commit suicide)?
2. How would your personal feelings influence your response to Mrs. T.?
3. What is the dilemma in this situation?
4. What ethical principles are involved in this dilemma?
5. What resources to help resolve this dilemma are available to the nurse? The patient?

abdominal pain; fever; severe hypotension; cardiac dysrhythmias, including tachycardias; increased respiratory rate; changes in level of consciousness; or even coma. In addition, these patients often have many electrolyte imbalances and may exhibit signs of dehydration.

Laboratory and Diagnostic Tests

The diagnosis of adrenal insufficiency may be difficult in the early stages because symptoms are often vague and mild. If patients are hemodynamically stable, x-ray studies and computed tomography scans of the pituitary and adrenal glands are completed to determine the overall state of the glands. Suggestive laboratory findings include hypoglycemia, hyponatremia, hyperkalemia, hypercalcemia, decreased serum osmolality, and an increased blood urea nitrogen/creatinine ratio (Table 31–2). Definitive diagnosis of primary adrenal insufficiency is confirmed by high levels of serum ACTH, whereas the reverse is true for secondary adrenal insufficiency, in which serum ACTH levels are normal or decreased. In both conditions, low levels of ACTH in the urine and low levels of cortisol in the serum are found.[7]

To determine the cause of inadequate cortisol levels, two diagnostic laboratory tests can be done. The ACTH stimulation test, also called the cosyntropin (Cortrosyn) test, confirms adrenal cortex destruction if repeated ACTH injections fail to cause a rise in plasma cortisol and urinary 17-hydroxycorticosteroids. A normal response is an increase in the serum cortisol level of at least 5 μg/dL over baseline and a peak serum cortisol level of at least 20 μg/dL.[8] Patients with secondary adrenal insufficiency respond to these injec-

tions within 48 to 72 hours with a delayed but normal rise in plasma cortisol and urinary 17-hydroxycorticosteroids. If the adrenal gland is functioning, but not adequately stimulated by pituitary release of ACTH, repeated doses of exogenous ACTH increase plasma cortisol and urinary 17-hydroxycorticosteroids.

Secondary adrenal insufficiency can further be confirmed with the use of the metyrapone (Metopirone) stimulation test. Metyrapone is a drug that reduces cortisol secretion from the adrenal gland. Normally, a compensatory increase in ACTH is anticipated. In secondary adrenal insufficiency, an impaired response or no response confirms the diagnosis.[3]

Nursing Diagnoses

Patients exhibiting signs and symptoms of adrenal crisis are in need of rapid and accurate diagnoses. Once these diagnoses are made, the combined efforts of the health care team are needed to initiate the appropriate treatment plan. This team can include the physician, nurse, discharge planner, dietitian, social worker, and home health nurse. Priority nursing diagnoses for patients in adrenal crisis are found in Table 31–3.

Collaborative Management

The immediate goals of therapy are to administer replacement hormones and to restore fluid and electrolyte balance. Initial treatment focuses on treating the

TABLE 31–2
Laboratory and Diagnostic Findings in Adrenal Insufficiency

Definitive Laboratory Findings	Suggestive Laboratory Findings
Primary Adrenal Insufficiency	**Primary or Secondary Adrenal Insufficiency**
Increased serum ACTH	Hypoglycemia
Decreased urine ACTH	Hyponatremia
Decreased serum cortisol	Hyperkalemia
Abnormal ACTH stimulation test	Hypercalcemia
	Decreased serum osmolality
	Increased blood urea nitrogen blood urea nitrogen/ creatinine ratio
Secondary Adrenal Insufficiency	
Decreased or normal serum ACTH	
Decreased urine ACTH	
Decreased serum cortisol	
Normal ACTH stimulation test	
Abnormal metyrapone stimulation test	

ACTH, adrenocorticotropin.

TABLE 31–3
Nursing Diagnoses

Problem Statement	Etiologic Factors
Fluid volume deficit	Excessive sodium and water losses secondary to inadequate circulating adrenal mineralocorticoids (aldosterone)
Decreased cardiac output	Hypovolemia, secondary to abnormal sodium and water losses, dysrhythmias, secondary to hyperkalemia
Altered thought processes	Hypovolemia, secondary to abnormal sodium and water losses; hyponatremia, hyperkalemia, and hypoglycemia secondary to inadequate circulating glucocorticoids and mineralocorticoids
Altered nutrition, less than body requirements	Reduced glucocorticoid hormone levels
Anxiety or fear	Acute onset of life-threatening disease process, subsequent hospitalization, and treatment modalities
Activity intolerance	Hypotension, muscular weakness, cerebral changes
Risk for body image disturbance	Body changes (hyperpigmentation, loss of body hair) from reduced adrenocorticosteroid levels
Risk for infection	Compromised immune response or corticosteroid replacement therapy

hypovolemia and cardiac dysrhythmias. Fluid resuscitation is begun immediately with a saline and glucose solution. The amount of replacement fluids depends on the depth of the hypovolemic state.[9] Electrolytes are also replaced based on laboratory results. Table 31–4 presents an example of standards of care for a patient in adrenal crisis that can be used to guide the health care team in the collaborative management of the patient.

Hemodynamic monitoring may be necessary to assess fluid status accurately and to monitor the effectiveness of fluid replacement. Pulmonary artery pressure readings should continue every 1 to 2 hours depending on the patient's response to fluid replacement. Cardiac index should remain at 2.5 to 4.0 L/m^2 per minute, and mean arterial pressure should be maintained between 60 and 100 mm Hg. Efforts to maintain adequate tissue perfusion include fluid volume replacement and, if necessary, positive inotropic support with medications such as dobutamine or renal-dose dopamine.[10, 11]

In addition, patients should be placed on continuous electrocardiographic monitoring and watched for signs and symptoms of hyperkalemia including premature ventricular contractions, tall peaked T waves, and ventricular tachycardia. Glucose-insulin or ion-exchange resins such as sodium polystyrene sulfonate (Kayexalate) to treat the hyperkalemia are used cautiously because they may predispose the patient to rebound hypokalemia once steroid replacement is begun.[7]

Once baseline blood studies are obtained, treatment focuses on cortisol replacement. Cortisol replacement does not wait for laboratory confirmation.[12] Replacement helps to stabilize blood pressure and cardiac function. If hypotension is severe and retractable, a 10-mg bolus of dexamethasone can be given intravenously.[12] Otherwise, the patient is started on 100 mg

hydrocortisone intravenously every 6 hours for 24 hours, then 50 mg every 6 hours for the next 24 hours.

Response should be rapid, with an improvement of symptoms within 12 hours. As improvement continues, intravenous hydrocortisone is tapered, and oral steroids are initiated and are gradually tapered to less than 30 mg per day by about the fifth day.[4] After the crisis has passed, further evaluation is completed to pinpoint the underlying condition, and a maintenance treatment regimen is begun.

A quiet, stable environment and emotional support for the patient and family are necessary during the acute stage of the illness. Patients have often only had vague, poorly defined symptoms before this crisis and are usually taken by surprise at the seriousness of the disease. They may have additional diagnostic studies to undergo, and they may also have to consider the possibility of accepting a chronic illness. Patient and family education during the acute phase as well as the chronic phase of the disease is important. Patients must maintain their hormone-replacement regimen and must rapidly report any stressors, such as infections, to their physicians, to prevent future incidences of adrenal crisis (Chart 31–3).

Multidisciplinary Outcomes

Care of patients experiencing adrenal insufficiency involves a team effort. Close communication among the nurse, physician, discharge planner, and other appropriate team members should facilitate a rapid recovery for the patient. Chart 31–4 summarizes the anticipated outcomes of the collaborative management of patients in adrenal crisis.

TABLE 31–4
Adrenal Crisis: Standards of Care

Problem	Patient Outcomes	Collaborative Interventions
Fluid Volume Deficit	Hemodynamics will return to or remain within normal limits (CI, 2.5–4.0 L/min/m^2; MAP > 60 mm Hg; PAD, 5–15 mm Hg; HR, 60–100 beats/min).	Monitor vital signs hourly including CVP and PA pressure readings; assess intake and output and daily weights. Monitor ECG continuously for dysrhythmias related to fluid and electrolyte imbalances. Monitor hemodynamic parameters (CO, CI, PAOP, SVR) every 2 hours. Administer D$_5$NS to restore volume while monitoring for signs of shock versus volume overload. Encourage sodium-rich fluids once patient can tolerate oral fluids.
	Patient will be alert and oriented to person, place, and time.	Check neurologic signs hourly. Reorient patient as needed.
Electrolyte Imbalances		
Hyperkalemia	Serum potassium levels will return to and remain at normal levels (3.5–5.5 mEq/L).	Monitor serum potassium q4h. Assess patient for muscle weakness and hyperreflexia.
	Patient will not experience life-threatening cardiac dysrhythmias related to hyperkalemia (e.g., ventricular tachycardia).	Monitor ECG for ventricular ectopy (premature beats), tall peaked T waves, and prolonged QRS interval. Prevent iatrogenic increase in potassium by providing low potassium hyperalimentation (if needed) and IV solutions free of potassium, i.e., saline and dextrose in place of Ringer's solutions. In cases of severe hyperkalemia, serum potassium-reducing agents such as kayexalate (for potassium = 5.5 − 6.5 mEq/L) can be ordered rectally, orally, or by nasogastric tube. Monitor patient for potassium-rich diarrhea, indicating the removal of potassium. Hypertonic glucose and insulin infusions (for potassium > 6.5 mEq/L), IV calcium gluconate (for potassium > 7.5 mEq/L), or sodium bicarbonate infusions may also be considered. (These treatments temporarily shift potassium into the cells and not out of the body. Patients need to be monitored for signs of over-treatment [hypokalemia], as well as for returning turning signs of hyperkalemia.)
Hyponatremia	Serum sodium levels will return to and remain at normal levels (135–145 mEq/L).	Monitor serum sodium levels q4h. Assess patient for nausea, abdominal cramps, fatigue, confusion, irritability, and signs of dehydration. Replace fluid volume with 0.45 or 0.9 NS solutions.
Glucocorticoid Deficit	Glucocorticoids will be replaced, and serum levels will remain adequate.	Administer hydrocortisone as ordered (100 mg IV, q6h initially) then taper the dose (as the patient's condition permits) while initiating an oral maintenance dose
	Serum glucose levels will return to and remain at normal levels (80–120 mg/dL).	Monitor blood glucose q2–4h. Administer fluids containing dextrose until oral intake is tolerated.
Education Need	Patient and family will verbalize drug regimen and potential factors requiring an adjustment of drug dosage.	Discuss disease process with patient and family. Explain possibility of long-term treatment with steroid-replacement drug therapy and the dangers of abruptly stopping replacement drug. Encourage patient to obtain and wear a medic alert bracelet. Discuss factors that can precipitate an increase in replacement drug therapy, such as infections, stress, and other disease processes.

CI, cardiac index; CO, cardiac output; CVP, central venous pressure; D$_5$NS, 5% dextrose in normal saline; ECG, electrocardiogram; HR, heart rate; IV, intravenous; MAP, mean arterial pressure; NS, normal saline; PA, pulmonary artery; PAD, PA diastolic; PAOP, pulmonary artery occlusive pressure; SVR, systemic vascular resistance.

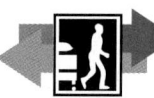

CHART 31–3

BEYOND THE ICU: MONITORING PATIENTS WITH ADRENAL CRISIS ACROSS HEALTHCARE SETTINGS

The care of patients experiencing adrenal crisis may occur in various health care settings. The importance of rapid assessment and initiation of treatment cannot be understated. Adrenal crisis represents an acute, life-threatening situation.

Emergency Department: Many times, patients report to an emergency department because of the abrupt change in their health status. In this setting, a rapid and thorough assessment by the triage nurse is critical to facilitate an accurate diagnosis. Initiation of intravenous lines, administration of supplemental oxygen, electrocardiographic monitoring, and the collection of baseline laboratory values are usually performed by the nurse with or without the assistance of ancillary care providers. Patients are usually stabilized and are transferred to the ICU as soon as possible.

Intensive Care Unit: Patients usually respond to treatment within 24 hours. During this time, the nurse must diligently assess the patient for complications and evaluate the effectiveness of treatment strategies. Discharge planning should begin at admission. Depending on the patient's situation, a case manager may be assigned to follow the patient. In addition, discharge planning for follow-up in the home or for placement in a new environment should be considered.

Equally important, the nurse in the acute care setting must be aware of the possibility of adrenal crisis in patients admitted with trauma, sepsis, or other serious illnesses. In these situations, the body may not be able to produce sufficient levels of cortisol needed to maintain homeostasis. Consequently, the nurse must monitor for symptoms of adrenal crisis in any patient with an unexplained hemodynamic instability.

Surgical Units: Patients can be admitted to outpatient or inpatient surgical units for various surgical procedures. The nurse in these settings must be equally attentive to the possibility of adrenal crisis precipitated by the trauma of surgery as well as the fluid and electrolyte imbalances that may occur in the postoperative patient. Signs and symptoms of impending shock, such as hypotension, diminished pulses, cool and pale skin, tachycardia, and reduced urine output, should be noted immediately. Prompt interventions contribute to a positive patient outcome.

Home Care Considerations: As the nurse prepares the patient recovering from adrenal crisis for discharge, it may be appropriate to initiate follow-up care in the home. In this setting, the nurse should recommend that the patient obtain and carry a medical alert bracelet and emergency medication, especially when traveling. In addition, detailed information regarding drug administration, drug interactions, and side effects should be provided.

Diet, exercise, and lifelong hormonal replacement need to be incorporated into most patients' lifestyles. Patients need to know that, in stressful situations, such as infection, fever, routine dental care, and positive or negative changes in lifestyle, they may need an adjustment in their hormone replacement dosage. Occasionally, female patients may also need additional education and support related to administering intramuscular injections of testosterone (synthetic androgen).[13]

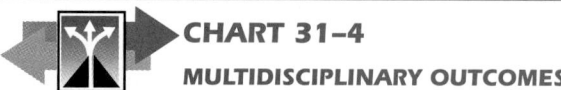

CHART 31–4

MULTIDISCIPLINARY OUTCOMES

Restoration and maintenance of the cardiac functioning
Restoration of fluid and electrolyte balance
Improvement in nutritional status
Preservation of cerebral functioning
Self-management of the therapeutic regimen

Critical Thinking Exercise

Mrs. N., a 68-year-old white woman, was admitted to the intensive care unit (ICU) after being discovered in her home by her niece. According to her niece Christine, Mrs. N. had not been feeling well for several days. When Christine checked on her aunt this morning, she found her confused and difficult to arouse. On admission, Mrs. N. was hypotensive, disoriented, lethargic, and tachycardic. She was given 2 L of 5% dextrose in normal saline and started on dobutamine at 5 μg/kg per minute. She was placed on continuous cardiac monitoring and a 50% face mask. A pulmonary artery catheter was placed 24 hours later, when she still did not respond to therapy. Initial central venous pressure was 2 mm Hg, pulmonary artery diastolic pressure was 5 mm Hg, and cardiac index was 2.8 L/m² per minute. Her systolic blood pressure continued to remain in the low 90s in spite of increases in dopamine.

When questioned about Mrs. N.'s health history, Christine reported that Mrs. N. had a history of rheumatoid arthritis and had taken 30 mg prednisone daily for the last 6 months. For the past 2 days, Mrs. N. had a gastrointestinal disorder with severe nausea and vomiting. During this time, she had not been able to keep any food or fluids down. She had no other concurrent health problems.

Once this information was passed on to the attending physician, Mrs. N. was given an immediate dose of 100 mg hydrocortisone intravenously. Additional doses were ordered every 6 hours. Within 24 hours, Mrs. N.'s vital signs were improving, and she was alert and oriented.

1. What precipitated Mrs. N.'s adrenal crisis?
2. What diagnostic test would confirm adrenal crisis? Why or why not would this test be ordered for Mrs. N.?
3. What aspects of patient education would be important for the nurse to include when preparing this patient for discharge?

Key Concepts

➠ Addison's disease (primary adrenal insufficiency) strikes about 1 in 100,000 people. In this situation, one sees a gradual loss of functioning adrenal cortex that is usually due to an autoimmune response.

➠ Symptoms of adrenal insufficiency usually progress slowly in patients with all causes of the disorder except surgical removal of the adrenal or pituitary glands and abrupt withdrawal of exogenous adrenocortical hormones.

➠ Adrenal crisis is an acute adrenal insufficiency that is life-threatening.

➠ Definitive diagnosis of primary adrenal insufficiency is confirmed by increased levels of ACTH in the blood, decreased levels of ACTH in the urine, and low levels of cortisol in the serum.

➠ The ACTH stimulation test, also called the cosyntropin (Cortrosyn) test, confirms adrenal cortex destruction if repeated ACTH injections fail to cause an increase in plasma cortisol and urinary 17-hydroxycorticosteroids.

➠ If the adrenal gland is functioning but not adequately stimulated by pituitary release of ACTH (secondary adrenal insufficiency), repeated doses of exogenous ACTH increase plasma cortisol and urinary 17-hydroxycorticosteroids, but administration of metyrapone, which stimulates endogenous ACTH production, causes no response.

➠ The immediate goals of therapy for adrenal crisis are to administer replacement hormones and to restore fluid and electrolyte balance.

References

1. Corrigan E: Adrenal Crisis. NIH Publication No. 90–2054. Bethesda, MD, National Institutes of Medicine, 1989.
2. Epstein CD: Adrenal cortical insufficiency in the critically ill patient. AACN Clin Issues Crit Care Nurs 3:705–713, 1992.
3. Zelissen P, Bast E, Croughs R: Associated autoimmunity in Addison's disease. J Autoimmun 8:121–130, 1995.
4. Longcope C: Hypoadrenal crisis. In: Rippe JM, et al (eds): Intensive Care Medicine, 3rd ed. Philadelphia, Lippincott-Raven, 1996, pp 1319–1323.
5. Salem M, Guarino AH, Chernow B: Adrenal dysfunction in the intensive care unit. In: Shoemaker WC, Ayres SM, Grenvik A, et al (eds): Textbook of Critical Care, 3rd ed. Philadelphia, W.B. Saunders, 1996, pp 1096–1100.
6. Kong M, Jeffcoate W: Eighty-six cases of Addison's disease. Clin Endocrinol 41:757–761, 1994.
7. O'Donnell M: Addisonian crisis. Am J Nurs 97:41, 1997.
8. Tietz NW (ed): Clinical Guide to Laboratory Tests, 3rd ed. Philadelphia, W.B. Saunders, 1995.
9. Russell S: Hypovolemic shock. Nursing 94 24:34–51, 1994.
10. Loriaux DL, McDonald WJ: Adrenal insufficiency. In: DeGroot LJ (ed): Endocrinology, 3rd ed. Philadelphia, W.B. Saunders, 1995.
11. Fallo F, Fanelli G, Cipolla A, et al: Twenty-four hour blood pressure profile in Addison's disease. Am J Hypertens 7:1105–1109, 1994.
12. Marino P: Adrenal and thyroid disorders in the ICU. In: Marino P (ed.): The ICU book. Philadelphia, Lea & Febiger, 1991, pp 557–568.
13. Tucker S, Canobbio M, Paquette E, Wells M: Adrenal cortical insufficiency. In: Tucker S, Canobbio M, Paquette E, Wells M (eds.): Patient Care Standards: Collaborative Practice Planning Guides. St Louis, Mosby–Year Book, 1996, pp 459–462.

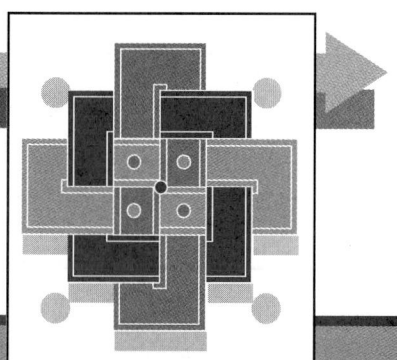

Gastrointestinal Disorders

Knowing What the Right Things Are for the Patient and the Family

Eleanor was 73 years old. Her admission history revealed a woman who had passed her 5-year survival rates on first lung, then breast, and finally throat cancers, all requiring surgical resections. When she and her family were informed that she had esophageal cancer, they thought they were dealing with "just another one." Surgery would be done, she'd recuperate, get some chemotherapy if needed, and life would go on.

I was assigned to take care of Eleanor, postoperative day 2 from an esophagectomy. After report, I introduced myself to Eleanor. She was a frail elderly woman sitting up in a chair at her bedside, using every ounce of her energy to breathe. She was on a non-rebreather mask, her oxygen saturation was uncomfortably low, the chest tube exit sites were saturated with drainage, and yet she smiled at me and said, "Hello." I did a quick assessment, and put Eleanor back to bed. In consideration of her past lobectomy, the surgeons were adamant about not wanting to reintubate Eleanor. We gingerly performed nasal-tracheal suctioning and chest physiotherapy, and decreased her oxygen demands in every possible way. Five hours into my shift, she spiked a temperature, was reintubated, and her blood pressure decreased. Approximately 6 hours into the shift, I allowed Eleanor's family to come in.

Eleanor was very sick for a very long time. She was dependent on vasopressors, inotropes, sedatives, and pain medication for 6 weeks; the ventilator for much longer. During Eleanor's sickest phases, I was a facilitator for the children—Susan, Pete, Ann, Julia, and Jim. They wanted to be told what was wrong with their mother and exactly what we did for treatment. They wanted simple answers in terminology that they could understand. They wanted the best care for their mother that modern technology could offer. I tried to give them both. They wanted their mom back. We allowed them to keep 24-hour vigilance at her bedside. They held her hand and talked to her while we worked around the bed. They weren't obtrusive or bothersome. They were just there and we allowed them to be there.

While I took care of Eleanor, her children talked about how they couldn't give up on this wonderful lady. She was an Army Air Corps nurse who served in World War II,

married a pilot, and found herself with four children all under the age of 8, as well as a step-daughter, when her husband died. She worked at this hospital until raising a family required her full-time attention. All of her previous cancer surgeries had been done at this hospital. She had recuperated from all those surgeries here and the children were determined that she'd recuperate from this one—here.

We held family conferences during which we addressed Eleanor's treatment plan and discharge planning with the surgeon and social workers. However, the lymph nodes that were resected from the present surgery revealed metastasis. The family would not consider a "do not resuscitate" status. They wanted everything done to save their mom. The nursing staff was frustrated with the situation. I gave my colleagues encouragement by complimenting them on the high quality of care they gave Eleanor and her family.

Finally, we began to see a change for the better. Eleanor was slowly weaned off the pressors, then the sedatives, and finally the pain medication. It took her at least 10 days to exhibit signs of her former personality. Oh, what a delightful woman!

Discharge planners pressured her family to make plans for moving Eleanor to a long-term care facility that could accommodate ventilator weaning. The family was firm in their decision not to move their mother. Eleanor wanted to stay with us, and the children wanted her to stay with us. The entire family was even more determined to get Eleanor off the ventilator. Every day we would see a little improvement. Eleanor was a strong person. She joked with us, using gestures, mouthing her words, and writing notes. She signed her notes "E." She was determined to get well.

About a week into her third month in the unit, Eleanor had been off the ventilator for 2 days. The surgeons transferred her to an acute care ward, but the move lasted less than 24 hours. Eleanor was rushed back, unresponsive and blue. The family was devastated. They felt we had been too hasty in transferring their mother out of the unit. I listened to them and nodded sympathetically. Within 3 days, Eleanor was back to her laughing, joking self, but she was also on the ventilator. She would have bleak days when she saw no end in sight. I encouraged her children to do everything possible to give her hope. One evening I arranged for Jim to bring her old deaf cocker spaniel, Holly, in for pet visitation. The dog won her over. She finally smiled and told us we were crazy.

Shortly thereafter we had another family conference. This time the surgeons told the children that their mother needed to be transferred to a ventilator rehabilitation center. The discharge planner gave them several places to visit and asked them to pick where they would like to place their mom. I had given Julia my home telephone number some time before when she was troubled, and told her to call if she ever needed to talk. She called me after the discharge planner asked them to start looking for a placement facility. We talked for a long time. I offered to go with them to the site visits.

Our nursing staff tried to prepare Eleanor for the move. We told her about ventilatory rehabilitation facilities and what wonderful places they were. We encouraged her to give the move a try. We answered her questions and listened to her concerns. Finally, she consented to the move. I had the family bring in a home permanent for Eleanor's hair, and Julia, Ann, Jim, Susan, and I permed Eleanor's hair. It was all she needed to get herself and the children motivated to find a rehabilitation facility. The following week, we went to visit another one of the facilities. It met all their criteria. It had aggressive pulmonary, speech therapy, dietary, and physical rehabilitative departments. The children went back to Eleanor with glowing reports. They were excited that they had the ideal place for their mom. Eleanor was discharged from our facility shortly thereafter, waved "good-bye," and mouthed that she'd see us later.

Julia kept me posted on Eleanor's progress at the new facility. They anticipated her discharge home within 10 days. I was so happy for everyone. Two days later, Julia called very upset and said, "They say Mom is in a coma. She had another one of those events last night. I can't believe this is happening. I hate that place." For 3 days, Julia and I held lengthy telephone conversations. Julia said that the physicians at the facility were telling them that Eleanor was in a persistent vegetative state, that she'd never get better. The rehabilitation facility asked the family to find a long-term care facility for Eleanor. Julia asked me whether I thought the doctors where I work would accept Eleanor back for a second opinion.

Our ICU director would not approve the transfer unless we had a family meeting and formulated an evaluation, treatment, and discharge plan. The oncology surgeon and I

decided we needed group support for this move to be a positive experience for everyone involved. We convened an ethics committee meeting and the surgeon presented the case at the meeting. The next day, the family met with the ethics committee, the nurse managers of the units, a legal representative, discharge planning personnel, the surgeon, a neurologist, and myself. The family made it clear that they wanted a second opinion from our medical staff, and if Eleanor was truly in a persistent vegetative state they wanted to have her taken off the ventilator and be allowed to breathe on her own. They were firm in their decision that Eleanor would never want to live on a ventilator the rest of her life.

Two days later, Eleanor was transferred back to our facility. The needed testing was done. Our physicians concurred with the diagnosis of persistent vegetative state. Three days were allowed for family members to arrive and say their good-byes. As the time grew closer to taking Eleanor off the ventilator, the children had questions about dying, funerals, and grieving. We answered them. At 4:20 PM Eleanor was placed on nebulized room air via a trach collar. All of the children, sisters, and spouses were there. The chaplain was there to give spiritual support. The oncology surgeon sat at the bedside and held Eleanor's hand. She was pronounced dead 1 hour later. There wasn't a dry eye in the room. Five months of suffering and fighting were over. Eleanor died peacefully. As we were all walking out of the room, Julia and Jim handed me the guardian angel pin that had faithfully hung above Eleanor's bed for months. They said, "Here, you need to have this. You have truly been our guardian angel through all this. You will never know how much you mean to all of us."

The oncology surgeon and I attended the funeral later that week. The children were the pallbearers. I know in my heart that we did right things for this family and their mother. Eleanor was truly a delightful lady. May she rest in peace.

Christine L. Nelson, RN, BSN, CCRN
Surgical ICU
David Grant Medical Center
Travis Air Force Base
California

1998 AACN-Siemens Excellence in Caring Practices Nominee

32

Gastrointestinal Anatomy and Physiology

Donna W. Markey

Objectives

After completing this chapter, the student will be able to:

1. List the organs of the gastrointestinal (GI) tract.
2. Describe the mucosal structure and function of the GI tract (gut) wall and peritoneum.
3. Describe the functional anatomy of the organs of the GI tract.
4. Identify the structure and function of the accessory organs: liver, gallbladder, and pancreas.
5. Explain the neurologic and hormonal control mechanisms of the GI tract.
6. List the factors influencing blood supply to the GI tract.
7. Define the immune and nonimmune defense mechanisms of the GI tract.
8. Differentiate the digestive and absorptive properties of the GI tract.
9. List the structural and functional changes in the GI tract associated with aging.

The GI system provides the mechanisms for the digestion and absorption of nutrients essential for sustaining the body's structure and functions. It breaks down ingested food, prepares it for uptake by cells, and eliminates any end products. The integrity of the GI system is one of the body's basic defense mechanisms against bacteria and other pathogens. The GI tract extends as a hollow lumen from the mouth to the anus. The organs of the GI tract are the mouth and pharynx, esophagus, stomach, and the small and large intestine. Additionally, the processes of digestion and absorption depend upon the contributions of the accessory organs: the liver, gallbladder, and pancreas (Figure 32–1).

ANATOMY

Understanding the anatomy of the GI tract is essential to the critical care nurse in any setting. Acute and critically ill patients experience primary GI diseases, such as Crohn's disease or ulcerative colitis, and secondary GI diseases, such as mesenteric ischemia secondary to cardiogenic shock. These illustrate the need for the critical care nurse to have a strong foundation of knowledge in GI anatomy and physiology upon which to base a patient's treatment plan and the nurse's clinical decision making. First in this discussion of the GI anatomy, the composition of the wall of GI tract and its overlying serous membrane, the peritoneum, are considered. The mucosal structures of the gut wall, as it is commonly called, are consistent throughout the length of the GI tract and abdomen. Second, the anatomy of the organs of the GI tract is discussed.

Gut Wall

There are four major layers that comprise the gut wall from the esophagus to the anal canal. These four layers from the inside out are the mucosa, submucosa, muscularis, and serosa (Figure 32–2).

Mucosa

The mucosa is the innermost layer of the GI tract. This layer is exposed to the nutrient components of food eaten and absorbs both nutrients and fluids. The thickness and function of the mucosa varies with the

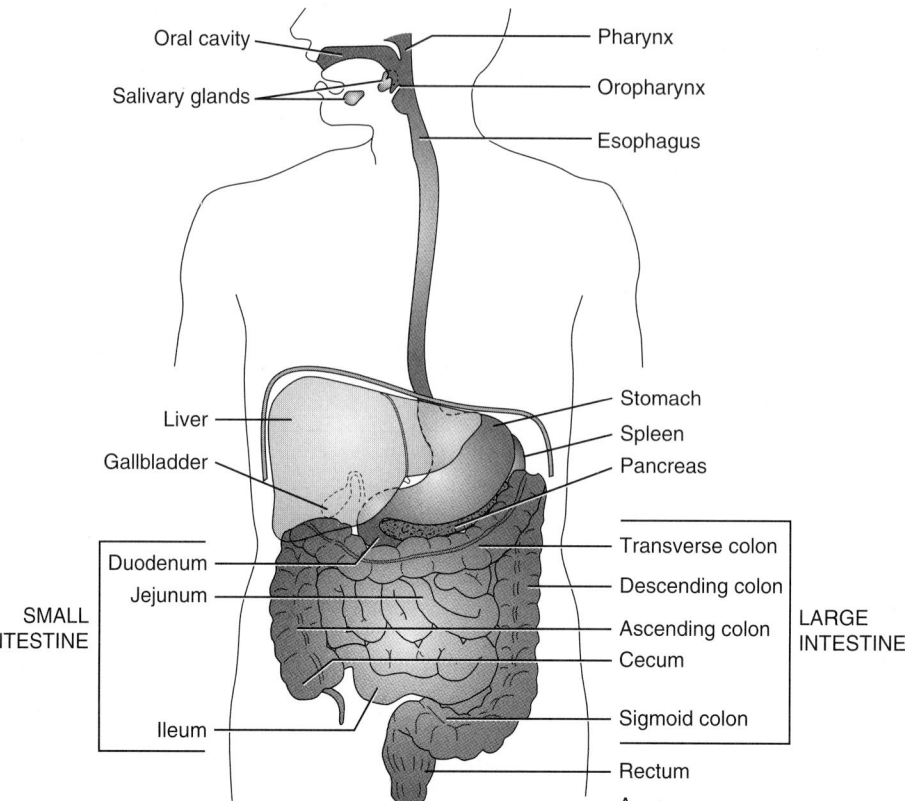

Figure 32–1

The gastrointestinal tract. (Redrawn from Black JM, Matassarin-Jacobs E: Medical-Surgical Nursing: Clinical Management for Continuity of Care, 5th ed. Philadelphia, WB Saunders, 1997, p 1686.)

anatomic location along the tract. Epithelial cells comprise the mucosal layer. Squamous epithelial cells line the esophagus, whereas columnar epithelium lines the stomach. The tight mesh of epithelial cells forms junctions that serve as an effective barrier against the passage of large molecular substances and bacteria. The mucosa contains specialized cells throughout the length of the GI tract. The cell type and function varies depending on the anatomic location. Many of these cells are secretory, releasing substances such as mucus or digestive enzymes to aid in the passage or digestion of food.[1–3]

In critical illness, the integrity of the mucosa can break down as a result of trauma, stress, medications, or surgery. The result of the impaired mucosal integrity can be bleeding, inflammation, and infection.

Submucosa

The submucosa connects the mucous and muscular layers. This highly vascular layer supports the blood vessels leading to the inner mucous layer. The submu-

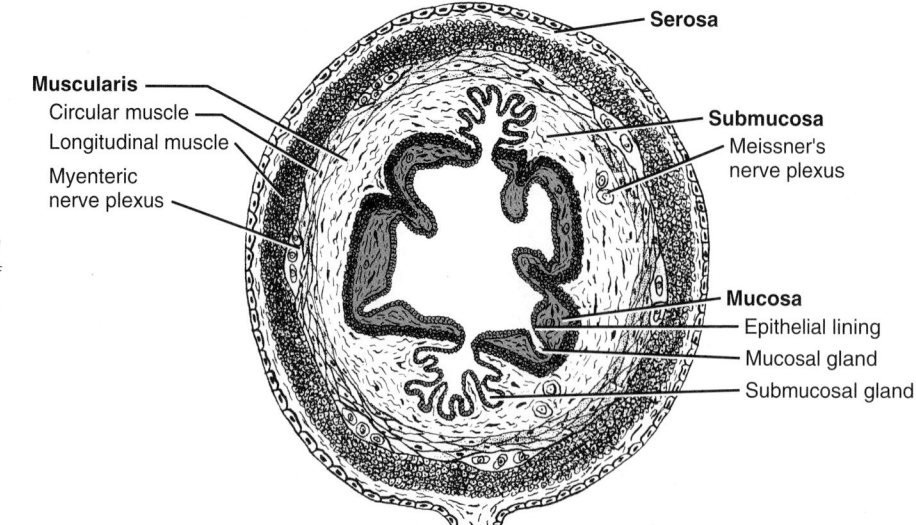

Figure 32–2

Cross section of the gut wall. (Modified from Guyton AC, Hall JE: Textbook of Medical Physiology, 9th ed. Philadelphia, WB Saunders, 1996, p 512.)

cosa also contains one plexus of the enteric nervous system, the submucosal plexus (Meissner's nerve plexus). This is a part of the autonomic nerve supply to the muscularis mucosa.[1-3]

Muscularis

The mouth, pharynx, and esophagus consist, in part, of skeletal muscle that produces voluntary swallowing. The rest of the GI tract muscularis consists of smooth muscle. The smooth muscle layer is generally found in two sheets: an inner ring of circular fibers and an outer ring of longitudinal fibers. In the stomach, there is an additional ring of oblique fibers. These fibers combine in their efforts to rhythmically contract to mechanically break down food, mix it with digestive enzymes, and propel it through the tract. The muscularis also contains the second nerve plexus, the myenteric plexus, which lies between the longitudinal and circular fibers.[1-3]

Serosa

The outermost layer, the serosa, is derived from the peritoneum. It covers the entire surface of the gut. It is composed of connective tissue and epithelium. This is known as the visceral peritoneum as it adheres to the visceral organs of the abdomen.[1-3]

Peritoneum

The peritoneum is the largest serous membrane of the body. Other serous membranes are the pericardium and the pleura, surrounding the heart and lungs, respectively. Serous membranes consist of a layer of simple squamous epithelium and a layer of connective tissue. The parietal peritoneum lines the wall of the abdominal cavity. The visceral peritoneum covers some of the abdominal organs and constitutes their serosa. The potential space between the parietal and visceral peritoneum is called the peritoneal cavity. This space is generally fluid filled. This fluid lubricates the two layers and prevents friction during organ movement.[1,3]

Inflammation of the peritoneum (peritonitis) is a serious condition that can rapidly spread throughout the abdominal cavity because of the continuous nature of the peritoneum. Peritonitis may occur with intestinal perforation or sometimes may follow abdominal surgery. As the inflammatory process resolves, adhesions may form and cause future bowel obstruction.

The peritoneum contains large folds that weave in and out of the viscera. These folds bind the organs to each other and contain the blood and lymph vessels and the nerves that supply the abdominal organs. One large fold of the peritoneum is the mesentery. This is an outward fold of the serous coat of the intestines. The mesentery binds the small intestine to the posterior abdominal wall. The mesentery facilitates intestinal motility and supports blood vessels, nerves, and lymphatics. The mesocolon is a peritoneal fold that binds the large intestine to the posterior abdominal wall. Impaired blood flow through the mesentery can result in intestinal ischemia. This can occur as a consequence of cardiogenic or hypovolemic shock in critically ill persons.

Other important peritoneal folds are the falciform ligament, the lesser omentum, and the greater omentum. The falciform ligament attaches the liver to the anterior abdominal wall and diaphragm. The lesser omentum arises from the serosa of the stomach and duodenum, suspending the stomach and duodenum from the liver. The greater omentum is a large fold in the serosa of the stomach overlying the intestines, wrapping around the transverse colon and attaching to the posterior abdominal wall.[1,3]

Organs of the GI Tract

Mouth and Pharynx

The chewing of food in the mouth initiates the processes of digestion. The preparation of the food bolus for digestion results from the coordinated activities of the teeth, cheeks, tongue, gums, and palate. The mechanical process of chewing (mastication) breaks food down into smaller particles. This process creates more surface area for exposure to digestive enzymes and GI mucosa. The stimulation caused by mastication signals the salivary glands to produce the first enzyme, amylase, to come in contact with the food ingested.

Saliva is necessary for comfort, hygiene, and digestion. Saliva is produced and released by the parotid, submaxillary, and sublingual glands. Together they secrete about 1 L of saliva per day. Mucin, the salivary secretion released primarily by the sublingual and submaxillary glands, reduces friction between food particles and the oropharyngeal and esophageal mucosa. It aids chewing and swallowing. Ptyalin, secreted by the parotid gland, initiates carbohydrate digestion by converting starches to disaccharides.

The pharynx lies behind the nose, mouth, and larynx and is continuous with the esophagus. The three sections of the pharynx are the oropharynx, nasopharynx, and laryngeal pharynx. There are seven openings into the pharynx: the two posterior nares, the two eustachian tubes, the mouth, the larynx, and the esophagus.

The pharynx plays an important role in the act of swallowing (Figure 32–3). The swallowing response is

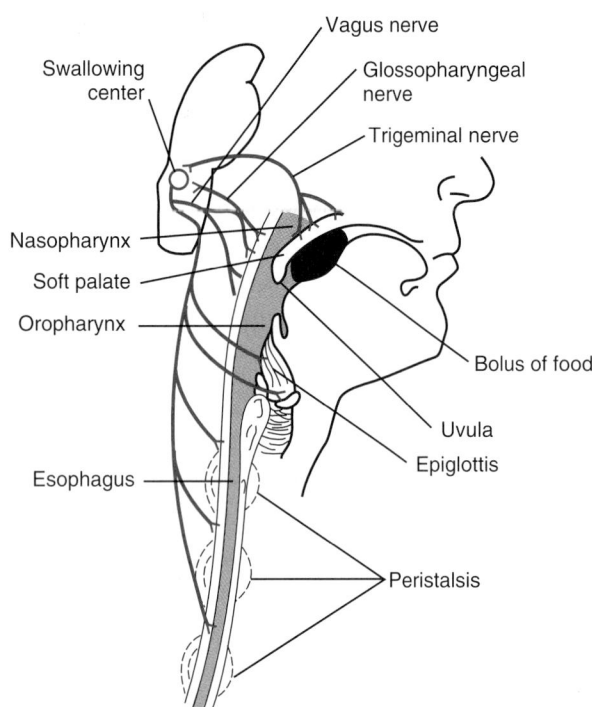

Figure 32–3

Swallowing mechanism and involved structures. (Modified from Guyton AC, Hall JE: Human Physiology and Mechanisms of Disease, 6th ed. Philadelphia, WB Saunders, 1997, p 515.)

initiated by the brain stem. Afferent nerve endings from the back of the throat, stimulated by the presence of food and chewing, travel via the vagus, glossopharyngeal, and trigeminal nerves to the brain stem. Neural fibers from the brain stem travel in the trigeminal, hypoglossal, and vagus nerves to innervate muscles of the mouth and throat. The jaw shuts and soft palate rises during swallowing. The nasopharynx and oropharynx close to prevent the movement of oral contents into the nose or trachea. For a brief moment, breathing ceases and the food bolus passes from the mouth to the esophagus.[1,2,4]

Esophagus

The esophagus is a hollow tube that allows the passage of ingested food from the pharynx to the stomach (see Figure 32–1). It is approximately 9 inches in length, running posterior to the trachea as it descends the posterior mediastinum and crosses the diaphragm.

The entrance and exit of a food bolus is regulated at each end of the esophagus by spincters. The upper esophageal sphincter consists of skeletal striated muscle fibers. Contraction of the upper esophageal sphincter relaxes the esophageal opening and allows for passage of a food bolus into the esophagus. Relaxation of the sphincter facilitates peristalsis and movement of the bolus downward to the stomach.

Primary and secondary peristalsis are responsible for the movement of the food bolus through the esophagus. Primary peristalsis is a continuation of the wave that initiates within the pharynx with swallowing (Figure 32–3). This wave passes from the pharynx to the stomach within 8 to 10 seconds. If all the food fails to move forward to the stomach with primary peristalsis, secondary peristalsis occurs. Secondary peristalsis is initiated in response to the stretch of the esophagus by the remaining food bolus.

The lower esophageal sphincter functions to allow the forward passage of food into the stomach. It also prevents the reflux of gastric contents into the esophagus. This sphincter is not anatomically distinct from the esophagus. It is a thickening of the esophageal circular muscle in the lowest aspect of the esophagus at its union with the stomach. It normally remains tonically constricted until peristaltic waves signal it to relax to allow the passage of food. A functioning lower esophageal sphincter allows the esophagus to maintain its normally alkaline environment. The esophagus does not tolerate the presence of gastric secretions. The high acidity of gastric secretions can cause mucosal damage and pain. Mucus is secreted by glands within the esophageal wall to provide lubrication for the smooth passage of the food bolus into the stomach. These glands are most prevalent at the lower aspect of the esophagus.[1–3]

Stomach

The stomach is the most dilated part of the GI tract. Located between the esophagus and the small intestine, it lies in the upper abdomen, behind the anterior wall of the abdomen and beneath the diaphragm. The stomach is described in four parts: the cardia, the fundus, the body, and the antrum or pylorus (Figure 32–4).

The cardia surrounds the lower esophageal sphincter. The fundus is the rounded portion above and to the left of the cardia. The large central portion is the body. Physiologically, there is no difference in function between the fundus and the body, thus some authors do not distinguish an anatomic difference between these areas. The body tapers down inferiorly to the antrum or pylorus as it joins the duodenum. A thick ring of circular fibers forms the pyloric sphincter between the stomach and the small intestine.

The stomach serves three primary functions:

1. To store large quantities of food until it can be accommodated in the duodenum
2. To mix ingested food with gastric secretions until a semifluid mixture, chyme, is formed
3. To regulate the rate of emptying food from the stomach into the small intestine to enable appropriate digestion and absorption by the small intestine

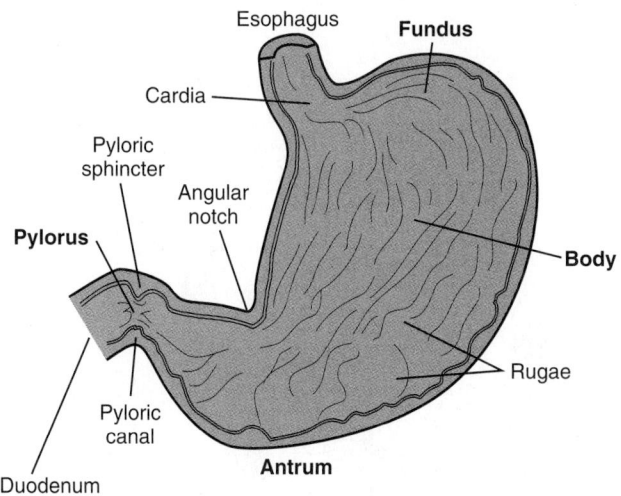

Figure 32-4

Anatomy of the stomach. (Modified from Guyton AC, Hall JE: Human Physiology and Mechanisms of Disease, 6th ed. Philadelphia, WB Saunders, 1997, p 516.)

The rate of stomach emptying is normally dependent on characteristics of the diet. Calorie-rich, high-fat foods empty more slowly than less dense foods. The hormone gastrin has a stimulatory effect on the pyloric pump. Gastrin levels increase in response to high-protein meals, resulting in more rapid emptying. Gastrin is secreted by specialized cells within the stomach and duodenal walls.[1-3]

Small Intestine

The small intestine consists of the duodenum, the jejunum, and the ileum (see Figure 32–1). It is here that the bulk of digestion and absorption occurs. The mucosa throughout the small intestine is modified to allow the small intestine to complete the processes of digestion and absorption (Figure 32–5). The mucosal layer contains many pits lined with glandular epithelium. These intestinal glands or pits secrete the intestinal digestive enzymes. The submucosa of the duodenum is equipped with mucus-secreting glands, Brunner's glands, to protect the walls of the small intestine from the action of the digestive enzymes.[1,2]

Mucosal folds (plica) within the small intestine slow the passage of chyme. This allows more time for digestion and absorption to occur. The folds are most numerous in the jejunum and proximal ileum. Absorption occurs from villi, which cover the mucosal folds (Figure 32–6). The villi secrete digestive enzymes and absorb nutrients. A villus is composed of absorptive columnar cells and mucus-secreting goblet cells. Closely adherent columnar cells form tight junctions. These intercellular spaces are the site for water and electrolyte absorption. Microvilli form tiny projections on the surface of each columnar epithelial cell. These

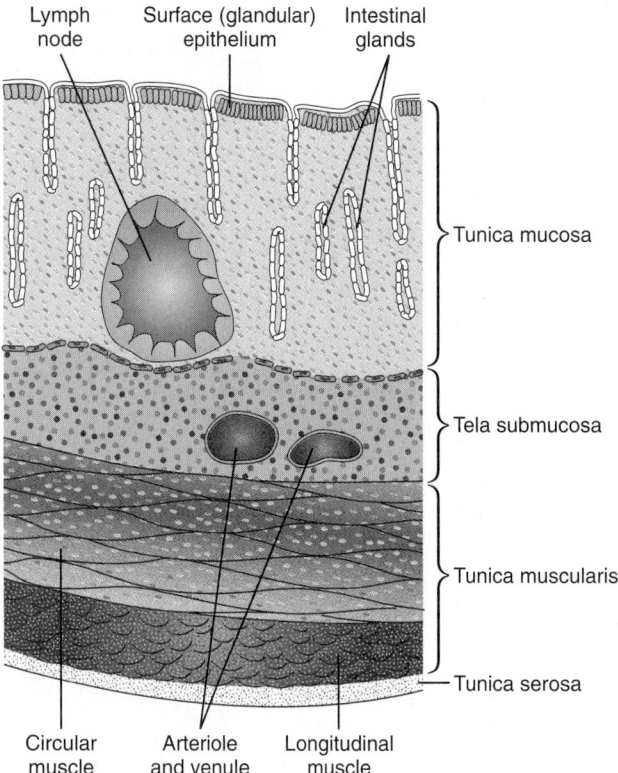

Figure 32-5

Cross section of the small intestine wall. (Redrawn and modified from Black JM, Matassarin-Jacobs E: Medical-Surgical Nursing: Clinical Management for Continuity of Care, 5th ed. Philadelphia, WB Saunders, 1997, p 1693.)

fingerlike projections collectively create a mucosal surface known as the brush border (Figure 32–7). The plica, villi, and microvilli greatly increase the absorptive surface area of the intestinal membrane.[1-3]

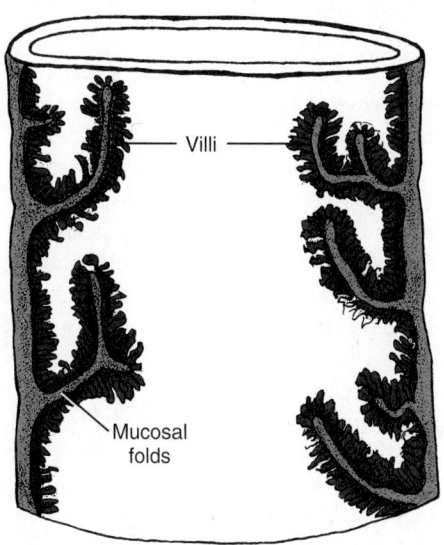

Figure 32-6

Longitudinal section of the small intestine showing villi that cover the mucosal folds. (Modified from Guyton AC, Hall JE: Human Physiology and Mechanisms of Disease, 6th ed. Philadelphia, WB Saunders, 1997, p 539.)

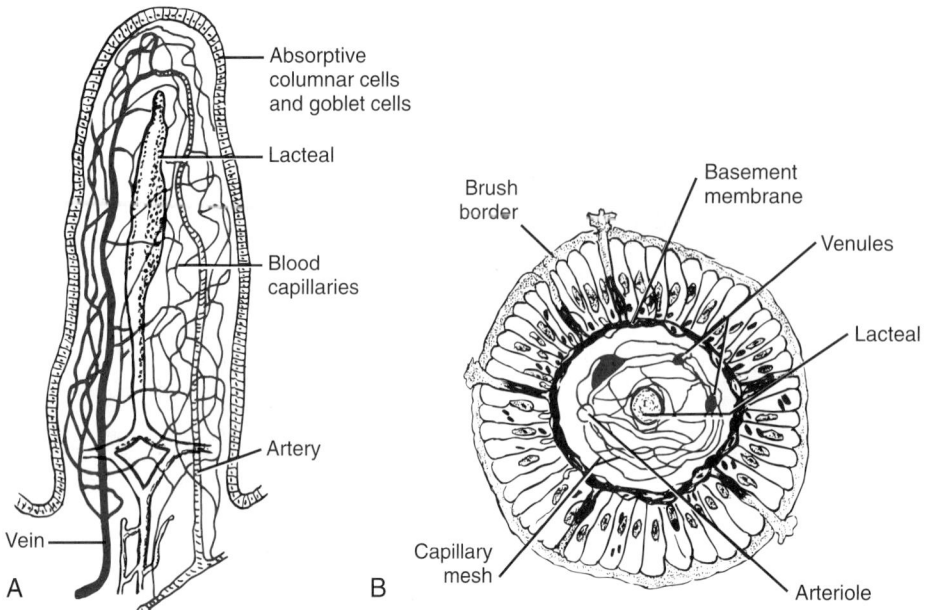

Figure 32–7

A, Longitudinal section of villus showing the blood supply. B, Cross section showing epithelial cells and basement membrane. (Modified from Guyton AC, Hall JE: Human Physiology and Mechanisms of Disease, 6th ed. Philadelphia, WB Saunders, 1997, p 540.)

The villi are contained within a connective tissue core of the lamina propria. A network of vessels, an arteriole, a venule, capillary mesh, and a lacteal (lymphatic vessel) are within this core (see Figure 32–7). In addition, the lamina propria contains lymphocytes; plasma cells, which produce immunoglobulins; and macrophages.[4] The lacteal (lymphatic channel) is important for the absorption and transport of fat molecules.

Lacteal contents flow to regional lymph nodes and channels that ultimately drain into the thoracic duct. There is an abundance of lymphatic tissue in the walls of the small intestine. Single lymph nodules, called solitary lymph nodules, are most numerous in the lower ileum. Peyer's patches are aggregated lymph nodes found predominantly in the ileum.[1, 3, 4]

The crypts of Lieberkühn are located at the base of the villi (Figure 32–8). They contain undifferentiated and secretory cells. The undifferentiated cells are the precursor to columnar epithelial cells that form the villi. The cells arise from the crypt and move to the tip of the villus, maturing in shape and function as they progress. After becoming columnar cells and reaching their destination, they function for a few days and then are sloughed into the intestinal lumen to be digested. Sloughed cells are an important source of endogenous protein. The entire epithelial population is replaced approximately every 4 to 7 days. Factors negatively influencing this process of cell proliferation include starvation, vitamin B_{12} deficiency, cytotoxic drugs, and irradiation. This results in decreased absorption, diarrhea, and malnutrition. Nutrient intake stimulates cell production.[1–4]

The duodenum, the broadest part of the small intestine, is approximately 25 cm (10 inches) long. The passage of chyme into the duodenum is regulated by the pyloric sphincter and antral contractions. The pyloric sphincter prevents reflux (retrograde flow) of duodenal contents back into the stomach. Like stomach contents to the esophagus, duodenal contents are caustic to the stomach. The duodenum lies in close communication with the liver, the gallbladder, and the pancreas. Three to 4 inches below the pylorus, both the

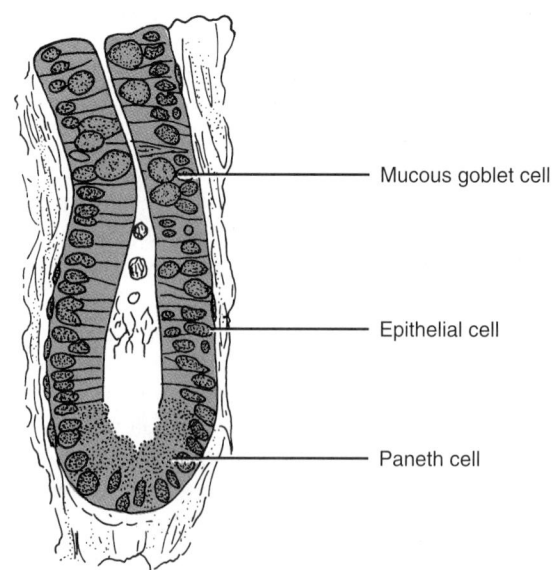

Figure 32–8

Crypts of Lieberkühn, located in all parts of the small intestine, between villi. (From Guyton AC, Hall JE: Human Physiology and Mechanisms of Disease, 6th ed. Philadelphia, WB Saunders, 1997, p 534.)

common bile duct and the pancreatic duct enter the duodenum.[1]

The transition from the duodenum to the jejunum is marked by a suspensory ligament, the ligament of Treitz. The jejunum is approximately 2.5 m (8 feet) long and extends to the ileum. It is thicker, wider, and more vascular than the ileum. The villi within the jejunum are also larger than those within the ileum. Brunner's glands, found throughout the duodenum, are only present in the upper segment of the jejunum.

The ileum is approximately 3.6 (12 feet) long and joins the large intestine at the ileocecal valve. It occupies the umbilical, hypogastric, right iliac, and pelvic regions of the abdomen.[1,4]

Large Intestine

The overall functions of the large intestine are the completion of absorption, the manufacture of certain vitamins, the formation of feces, and the expulsion of feces from the body. The large intestine is about 1.5 m (5 feet) long and averages 6.5 cm (2.5 inches) in diameter. It extends from the ileum to the anus. The large intestine is divided into four regions: cecum, colon, rectum, and anal canal (see Figure 32–1).

The ileocecal valve guards the opening from the ileum to the cecum of the large intestine (Figure 32–9). The valve allows the passage of luminal contents from small intestine to large intestine. The cecum lies below the ileocecal valve as a blind pouch or cul-de-sac, about 6 cm (2 to 3 inches) long. The vermiform appendix is a twisted, coiled tube extending off the cecum, and its length is approximately 8 cm (3 inches). The opposite open end of the cecum joins with the colon.

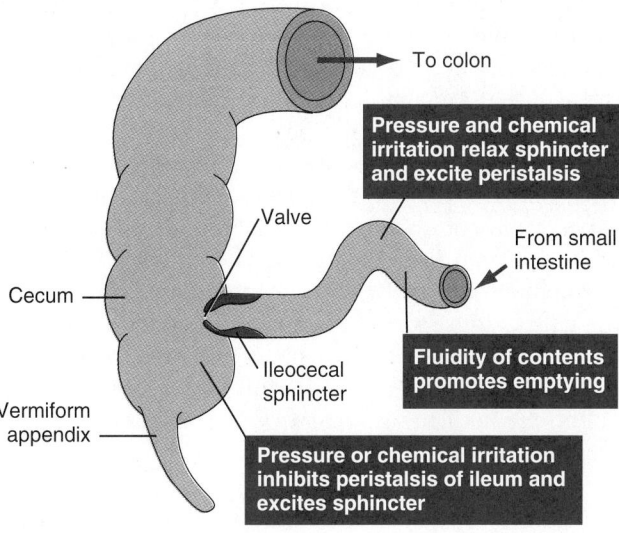

Figure 32–9

Emptying at the ileocecal valve. (Modified from Guyton AC, Hall JE: Human Physiology and Mechanisms of Disease, 6th ed. Philadelphia, WB Saunders, 1997, p 519.)

The colon is divided into four portions: ascending, transverse, descending, and sigmoid (see Figure 32–1). The ascending portion rises along the right side of the abdomen, reaches the undersurface of the liver, and turns abruptly left. This area is known as the right colic flexure or hepatic flexure. Here the transverse colon travels across the upper abdomen to the spleen, where it again makes a sharp turn and forms the left colic or splenic flexure. Below the splenic flexure, the colon moves downward as the descending colon to the area overlying the iliac crest. The sigmoid colon begins at the left iliac crest, moves inward to the midline, and terminates as the rectum. The rectum is the last 20 cm (7 to 8 inches) of the GI tract. It lies anterior to the sacrum and coccyx. The terminal 2 to 3 cm (1 inch) of the rectum is called the anal canal. The anus is the external opening from the anal canal. The anus is guarded by an internal sphincter of smooth muscle and an external sphincter of skeletal muscle.[1,3]

The wall of the large intestine differs from the wall of the small intestine in the following ways. No villi or permanent circular folds (plicae circulares) are found in the mucosa. The mucosa does contain columnar epithelium with numerous goblet cells. Goblet cells secrete the mucus that aids in the passage of colonic contents through the colon. Solitary lymph nodes are found in the mucosa. The longitudinal muscles of the mucosa do not form a continuous sheet as they do elsewhere in the GI tract. Here they are broken up into three flat bands called taenia coli. Each band runs the length of the large intestine. Tonic contractions of the bands gather the colon into a series of pouches called haustra. This gives the colon its puckered appearance.

Accessory Organs

Liver

The liver is the largest gland in the body. It is situated in the upper right part of the abdominal cavity (see Figure 32–1). Vertically, it measures 6 to 7 inches in height. It lies just below the right diaphragm. Liver consistency is that of a soft solid. It is quite friable and easily lacerated. This is commonly seen in traumatic injuries, such as are sustained by unrestrained drivers in motor vehicle accidents and fall victims.

The liver is lobulated, having two main lobes, the right and the left. The right lobe appears greater than the left, yet they are almost equal in size.[5] These lobes are further broken down into subsegments. The lobes of the liver are made up of numerous lobules. The lobules are the functional units of the liver. A lobule consists of cords of hepatic cells (hepatocytes) arranged in a radial pattern around a central vein (Figure 32–10). Sinusoids, the endothelial lined spaces between the cords, convey blood. The sinusoids are

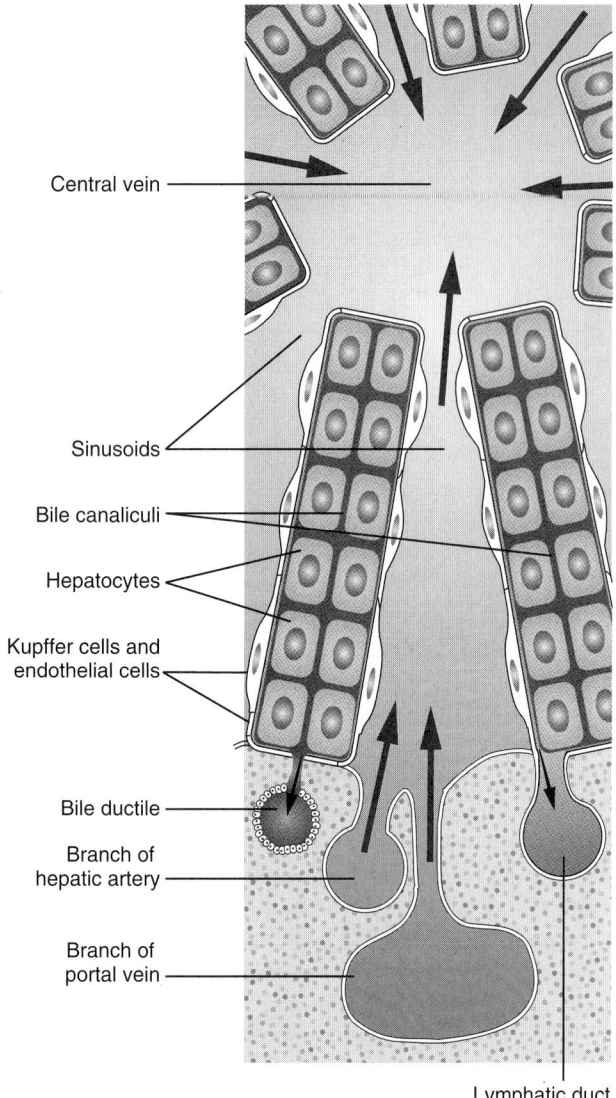

Central vein

Sinusoids

Bile canaliculi

Hepatocytes

Kupffer cells and
endothelial cells

Bile ductile

Branch of
hepatic artery

Branch of
portal vein

Lymphatic duct

Figure 32–10

Schematic drawing of a liver lobule. (Redrawn from Black JM, Matassarin-Jacobs E: Luckman and Sorensen's Medical-Surgical Nursing: A Physiologic Approach, 4th ed. Philadelphia, WB Saunders, 1993, p 1680.)

also partly lined with Kupffer cells. The Kupffer cells destroy worn-out white and red blood cells and bacteria. The major functions of the liver are listed in Chart 32–1.

The blood supply of the liver comes from two sources. The hepatic artery carries oxygenated blood to the liver. The hepatic portal vein carries nutrient-rich, deoxygenated blood from the intestines. Both the hepatic artery and the hepatic portal vein carry blood into the sinusoids of the lobules, where oxygen, most of the nutrients, and certain toxins are extracted by the hepatic cells. The nutrients are stored or used to make new materials. The toxins are either stored or detoxified. Products manufactured by the hepatic cells and nutrients needed by other cells are returned to the blood. The blood then drains into the central vein and

CHART 32–1
MAJOR FUNCTIONS OF THE LIVER

Bile formation
Metabolism of drugs and hormones
Substrate metabolism
Protein synthesis, including those associated with coagulation
Detoxification of noxious substances
Phagocytosis via Kupffer cells

passes into a hepatic vein on its way to the inferior vena cava.[4]

Under normal conditions, bile is not secreted into the blood. Bile is manufactured by the hepatic cells and secreted into bile capillaries or canaliculi that empty into small ducts (see Figure 32–10). The network of small ducts eventually merge to form the right and left hepatic ducts. These ducts leave the liver united together as the common hepatic duct. The common hepatic duct joins with the cystic duct of the gallbladder to form the common bile duct. The common bile duct empties into the duodenum via the ampulla of Vater. The passage of bile is regulated by a valve in the common bile duct, the sphincter of Oddi. When the small intestine is empty, the sphincter is closed and bile backs up via the cystic duct to the gallbladder, where it is stored (Figure 32–11).[1,3,6]

Gallbladder

The gallbladder is a sac located along the underside of the liver (see Figure 32–11). Its inner wall consists of a mucous membrane arranged in rugae resembling those of the stomach. A bile-filled gallbladder expands to the size and shape of a pear. The middle muscular coat of the wall consists of smooth muscle fibers. Like elsewhere in the GI tract, these muscle fibers are capable of contraction. Contraction of these fibers ejects bile into the cystic duct. The gallbladder holds approximately 30 mL of bile. As mentioned previously, the gallbladder stores bile until it is needed for digestion. The release mechanism is initiated through a signal that the duodenum is full or receiving a food bolus, chyme. The sphincter of Oddi relaxes and bile is secreted into the duodenum.[1,3,6]

Pancreas

The pancreas is a long and irregularly shaped soft gland, comparable in its structure to the salivary

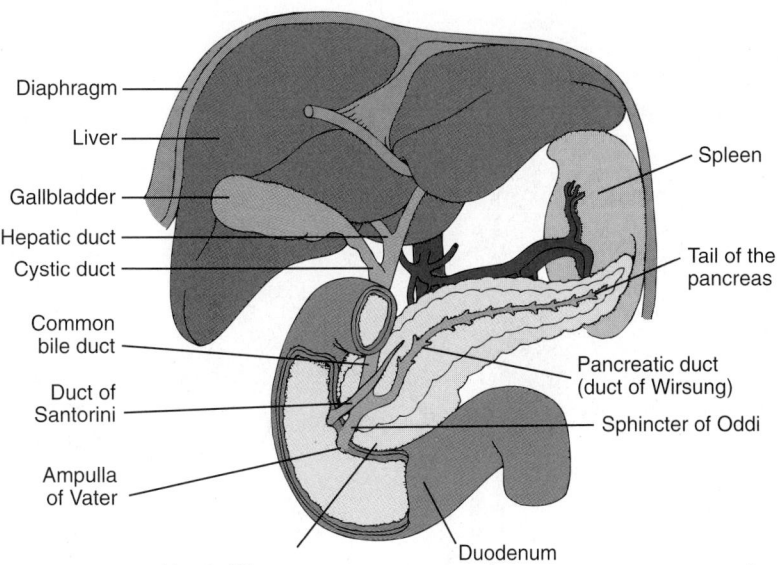

Figure 32–11

Gallbladder and pancreas with connections to the liver and duodenum. (From Ignatavicius DD, Workman LL, Mishler MA: Medical-Surgical Nursing: A Nursing Process Approach, 3rd ed. Philadelphia, WB Saunders, 1999.)

glands. It lies transversely across the posterior wall of the abdomen. It varies in length from 5 to 6 inches (12.5 cm). It is anatomically described as having a head, body, and tail. The head is the widest portion at the far right of the gland. It conforms to the concave shape of the descending portion of the duodenum. Its relationship to the duodenum is similarly important as that of the liver and gallbladder (see Figure 32–11).

The pancreas is made up of small clusters of glandular epithelial cells. Some clusters, islets of Langerhans, form the endocrine portions of the pancreas. The islets of Langerhans consist of alpha and beta cells that secrete glucagon and insulin. The acini are the exocrine portion of the pancreas. Secreting cells of the acini release a mixture of digestive enzymes called pancreatic juice, which is dumped into small ducts attached to the acini. Pancreatic enzymes leave the pancreas through its principal excretory duct, the pancreatic duct or duct of Wirsung.

In most people, the pancreatic duct joins with the common bile duct and enters the duodenum via the ampulla of Vater. An accessory duct, the duct of Santorini, may also lead from the pancreas and empty into the duodenum about 2.5 cm (1 inch) above the ampulla of Vater (see Figure 32–11).[1,3,6]

Lesions obstructing the ampulla of Vater or common bile duct are not uncommon conditions in acute and critically ill patients. Gallstones obstructing the ampulla of Vater may result in gallstone pancreatitis. Obstructive jaundice (yellowing of the skin, mucous membranes, and sclera) resulting from the retrograde flow of bile into the liver, backing up into the blood, and epigastric pain may be the hallmark symptoms of this life-threatening condition. This condition is described further in Chapter 37.

PHYSIOLOGY

Blood Supply of the Gastrointestinal System

Splanchnic circulation is the system responsible for the blood supply of the GI system (Figure 32–12). It includes blood flow through the entire GI tract and the accessory organs, the liver, gallbladder, pancreas, and spleen. All of the blood flowing through the gut, spleen, and pancreas enters the liver via the portal vein. This blood passes through the millions of liver sinusoids and leaves the liver via the hepatic veins that empty into the vena cava of the general circulation. Reticuloendothelial cells lining the liver sinusoids remove bacteria and other particulate matter that may enter the circulation from the GI tract (see Figure 32–10). This prevents the direct access of potentially harmful agents into the body.

Nutrients absorbed from the gut are also transported in the portal venous blood to the liver sinusoids. Here, the reticuloendothelial and hepatic cells absorb and temporarily store one-half to three-fourths of all the absorbed nutrients.

The walls of the stomach and the small and large intestine receive their blood supply via the celiac and the inferior and superior mesenteric arteries. On entering the gut wall, the arteries branch into smaller arteries that encircle the gut wall. These further branch into yet smaller arteries that penetrate the wall and spread along the muscle bundles, into the villi, and into the submucosal network beneath the epithelium. This microvasculature performs the secretory and absorptive functions of the gut. Circulation through the villus is shown in Figure 32–7.

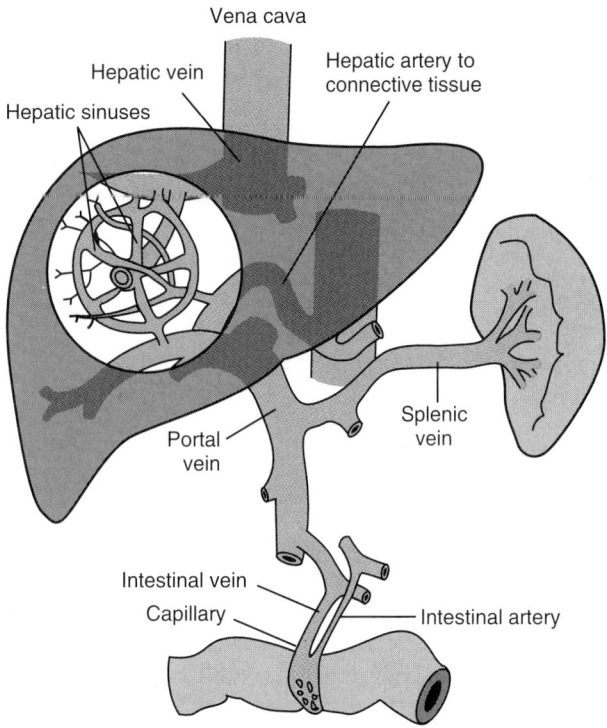

Figure 32–12

Splanchnic circulation. (From Guyton AC, Hall JE: Human Physiology and Mechanisms of Disease, 6th ed. Philadelphia, WB Saunders, 1997, p 522.)

Factors Affecting Gastrointestinal Blood Flow

Blood flow to each area of the gut and each layer of the gut wall depends on the level of local activity. Increased motor activity (peristalsis) in the gut increases blood flow in the muscle layers of the intestinal wall. Active absorption through the submucosa layer increases blood supply to the villi and surrounding tissue. Following a meal, the blood flow increases as high as 100% to 150%, usually lasting for 3 to 6 hours.[2,6]

Theories to explain the increased blood flow are not well established. However, there are some facts that help to explain this phenomenon. First, several of the intestinal hormones secreted during digestion do have a vasodilatory effect. Those known to have this effect are cholecystokinin, vasoactive intestinal peptide, gastrin, and secretin. Second, some of the intestinal glands secrete two kinins into the gut wall, kallidin and bradykinin, at the same time they release their secretions into the gut lumen. These kinins are powerful vasodilators. Third, decreased oxygen concentration in the gut wall can increase intestinal blood flow by up to 50%. The increased metabolic rate during gut activity most likely lowers the oxygen concentration enough to cause vasodilatation. It is also possible that the release of adenosine, another vasodilator, in response to low

oxygen levels may increase blood flow. It is most likely that the combination of these factors results in increased intestinal blood flow in response to digestion, absorption, and increased activity.[2]

Parasympathetic innervation to the stomach and intestines may also play a role in increasing local blood flow, while it is simultaneously increasing glandular secretion. However, the sequence of this stimulation is not yet clear. It is possible that it is actually the increased glandular secretions that stimulate the parasympathetic nerves to cause increased blood flow (circulation).

Sympathetic stimulation directly affects circulation to all of the GI tract by causing intense vasoconstriction of the arterioles within the gut wall. This vasoconstriction greatly decreases blood flow. Prolonged vasoconstriction, as occurs in patients in a shock state, leads to ischemia and ulceration of the luminal surfaces of the stomach and intestines. The breakdown in the integrity of the intestinal walls results in an inability to serve as a barrier against bacteria and foreign toxins. Gram-negative bacteria from within the intestines can translocate via the damaged mucosal wall to invade the blood. Ulceration also increases the incidence of stress ulcers and precipitates GI bleeding as discussed in Chapter 35.[2,6,7]

Hormonal Control

The hormones of the GI system have both stimulatory and inhibitory effects on the processes of secretion, digestion, motility, and absorption. The stomach and small intestine are chiefly responsible for the secretion of these hormones. The hormones and their actions are described in Table 32–1.

Neurologic Control of the Gastrointestinal Tract

Intrinsic Control

The enteric nervous system is the nervous system of the GI tract. It lies within the wall of the gut. It is comprised of roughly 100,000,000 neurons, a number equal to the number of neurons in the entire spinal cord. The enteric nervous system controls GI movements and secretions. Two plexi are the main components of the enteric system: an outer plexus lying between the longitudinal and circular muscular layers, called the myenteric plexus, and an inner plexus, called the submucosal plexus, that lies in the submucosa (Figure 32–13).

The myenteric plexus controls the GI movements (motility) and the submucosal plexus controls GI secretions and local blood flow. The myenteric plexus is a linear plexus extending down the intestinal wall.

TABLE 32–1
Hormones of Digestion

Hormone	Origin	Actions
Gastrin	Antrum of stomach in response to acetylcholine stimulation of antral cells	▪ Stimulates secretion of hydrochloric acid by the parietal cells ▪ Stimulates secretion of pepsin by the chief cells ▪ Promotes stomach emptying ▪ Stimulates pancreatic secretion (acinar cells)
Secretin	Duodenal and jejunal secretion in response to acidic gastric juice emptied from the stomach to the pylorus	▪ Augments the action of cholecystokinin ▪ Stimulates pancreatic and hepatic bicarbonate and water secretion ▪ Mild inhibition of gastrointestinal motility to facilitate digestion
Cholecystokinin (CCK)	Jejunal secretion in response to fatty substances in the intestinal contents	▪ Increases contractility of the gallbladder ▪ Moderates inhibition of the stomach ▪ Stimulates pancreatic enzyme secretion (amylase, lipase, trypsin)
Gastric inhibitory peptide (GIP)	Mucosal secretion of the small intestine in response to fat and carbohydrate in the chyme	▪ Decreases motor activity of the stomach ▪ Slows gastric emptying ▪ Stimulates secretion of insulin by the pancreas
Vasoactive intestinal peptide (VIP)	Small intestine secretion in response to the acidic gastric juice emptied into the duodenum	▪ Main effects are similar to secretin ▪ Stimulates intestinal secretions to decrease the acidity of chyme ▪ Inhibits gastric secretin

Adapted from Alspach J: Core Curriculum for Critical Care Nursing, 4th ed. Philadelphia, WB Saunders, 1991.

Because of its location between the longitudinal and circular fibers of smooth muscle, it controls motor activity along the length of the gut. Neurons of the myenteric plexus are of both the excitatory and inhibitory type. Excitatory effects are:

- Increased tone (contraction) of the gut wall
- Increased intensity of contractions
- Increased rate of the rhythm of contractions
- Increased velocity of conduction of excitatory waves along the gut wall, causing more rapid movement of the peristaltic waves

Inhibitory effects result from the secretion of an inhibitory transmitter from the fiber endings. The resulting inhibitory signals repress the contraction of intesti-

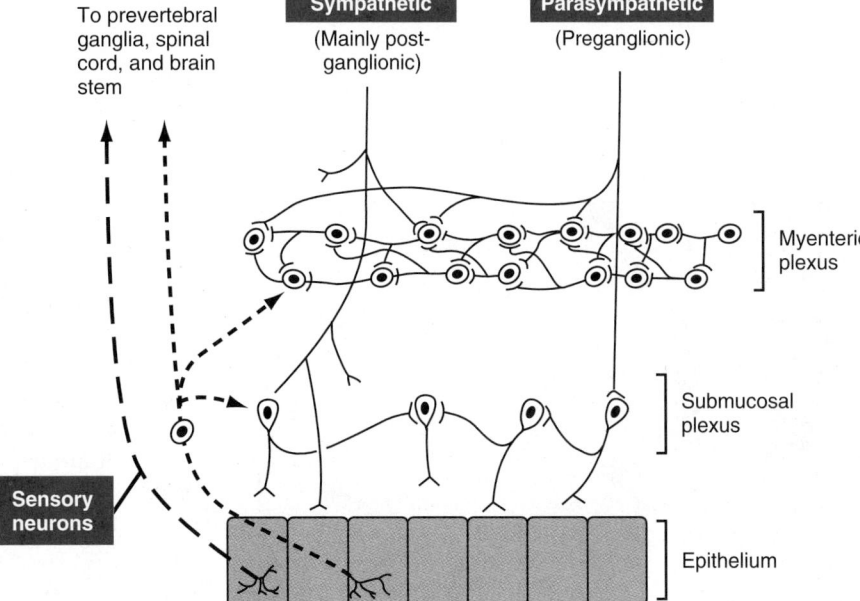

Figure 32–13

Diagram showing neural control of the gut wall. (From Guyton AC, Hall JE: Human Physiology and Mechanisms of Disease, 6th ed. Philadelphia, WB Saunders, 1997, p 513.)

nal sphincter muscles. The release of sphincter muscle tone promotes the movement of food between segments of the GI tract. In contrast, the submucosal plexus is responsible for a much finer level of control. It is mainly concerned with controlling function within the inner wall of each minute segment of the intestine. Many sensory signals originate from the GI epithelium and are integrated in the submucosal plexus to control local intestinal secretion, local absorption, and local contraction of the submucosal muscle that causes various degrees of infolding of the stomach mucosa. Neurotransmitters secreted by the enteric neurons are listed in Chart 32–2. The specific function of all of these is not yet known. The two most familiar are acetylcholine and norepinephrine. Acetylcholine excites GI activity; norepinephrine almost always inhibits GI activity. This is also true of epinephrine, which reaches the GI tract via the blood after its release from the adrenal medulla.[2,6]

Extrinsic Control

Despite its ability for fully independent function, the enteric nervous system also connects with the sympathetic and parasympathetic systems. These extrinsic nerves can further activate or inhibit GI functions. Sensory nerve endings present in the gut wall send afferent fibers to both plexi of the enteric system and to the prevertebral ganglia of the sympathetic nervous system. These sympathetic nerve transmissions travel to the spinal cord and the brain stem (see Figure 32–13).

Parasympathetic Innervation
Cranial and sacral divisions comprise the parasympathetic supply to the gut. The cranial parasympathetics are transmitted almost extensively via the vagus nerves. These fibers provide innervation to the esophagus, stomach, pancreas, and first half of the large in-

testine. A few fibers also innervate the mouth and pharynx. The sacral parasympathetics originate in the second, third, and fourth sacral vertebrae and pass through the pelvic nerves to the distal half of the large intestine. The sigmoid, rectum, and anal regions are better supplied than other areas of the large intestine. These fibers function in the defecation reflexes.

The postganglionic neurons of the parasympathetic system are located in the myenteric and submucosal plexi. Stimulation of the parasympathetic system causes a general increase in the activity of the enteric nervous system.

Sympathetic Innervation
The sympathetic fibers to the GI tract originate in the spinal cord between the segments T5 and L2. The sympathetics innervate all portions of the GI tract. The sympathetic nerve endings secrete norepinephrine. As a result, these have an inhibitory effect on GI activity. Norepinephrine has a direct effect on smooth muscle to inhibit activity and a major inhibitory effect directly on the neurons of the enteric nervous system. Strong stimulation of the sympathetic system can totally block movement of food through the GI tract, as can occur in a critically ill patient in a shock state.

Reflexes of the Gastrointestinal Tract

Three different types of GI reflexes are supported through the mechanisms of the enteric nervous system in combination with the sympathetic and parasympathetic systems. These are described in Table 32–2.

Defense Mechanisms of the Gastrointestinal Barrier: Lymphatic and Immune Function

The immunologic structure and function of the GI tract plays a major role in the body's defense against bacteria, parasites, and other toxic pathogens. The GI system has two major mechanisms of defense: nonimmunologic and immunologic.

Nonimmunologic Defense

Nonimmunologic defenses are those provided by salivary secretions, gastric acidity, bile salts, peristalsis, intestinal microflora, and the mechanical barrier formed by intestinal epithelial cells and the mucous coat overlying the epithelial cells. Antibacterial agents within the saliva are active against foreign antigens and microorganisms ingested with food. Pathogens that survive the mouth then confront gastric acidity and intestinal bile salts in the stomach and small intestine. Gastric pH and bile salts combine effects to create a microenvironment that is highly unfavorable for growth. After surviving these conditions, an offending

---

CHART 32–2

NEUROTRANSMITTERS SECRETED BY THE ENTERIC NEURONS

Acetylcholine
Adenosine triphosphate
Dopamine
Substance P
Somatostatin
Met-enkephalin
Norepinephrine
Serotonin
Cholecystokinin
Vasoactive intestinal polypeptide
Leu-enkephalin
Bombesin

TABLE 32–2
Gastrointestinal Reflexes

Reflex Type	Reflex Name	Description/Effect
Enteric nervous system based		Control: gastrointestinal (GI) secretion, peristalsis, mixing contractions, local inhibitory effects
Gut to prevertebral sympathetic ganglia and back to GI tract	Gastrocolic reflex	Signals from stomach to cause evacuation of the colon
	Enterogastric reflex	Signals from the colon and small intestine to inhibit stomach motility and secretion
	Colonoileal reflex	Signals from the colon to inhibit ileal emptying
Gut to spinal cord or brain stem and back to GI tract		Reflexes from stomach and duodenum to brain stem, then back to stomach to control gastric motor and secretory activity
		Pain reflexes to cause general inhibition of entire GI tract
	Defecation reflex	Defecation signals travel to spinal cord and back to produce colonic, rectal, and abdominal contractions

organism must then adhere to an epithelial surface to initiate colonization and invasion across the epithelium. Peristaltic action of the mucosal surfaces dislodges microorganisms and prevents stagnation of chyme through its continuous motion.

Indigenous bacterial flora resident in the GI tract limit proliferation and adherence of potentially pathogenic bacteria. The large number of anaerobes normally present prevents the overgrowth of other gram-negative and gram-positive bacteria. *Bacteroides fragilis* is the main anaerobic bacterium, and *Escherichia coli* is the main aerobic bacterium considered normal bowel flora.[8,9] These bacteria effectively inhibit the adherence of pathogenic bacteria through the secretion of short-chain fatty acids in the epithelial mucous layer.

Further mechanical resistance to offending luminal substances is provided by the intestinal epithelial cells and its overlying mucous coat. Goblet cells, as discussed earlier, secrete mucus over the microvillus surface of the intestine. This provides an extensive physical barrier to the passage of potential pathogens and may actually contribute to their removal.

Immunologic Defense

The immunologic defenses of the GI tract are provided by gut associated lymphoid tissue (GALT). Roughly 25% of the intestinal mucosa is lymphoid tissue and approximately 70% to 80% of all immunologic secreting cells are reported to be within the intestine. This makes the GI tract one of the largest immune organs within the body.[9]

The GALT is composed of organized and nonorganized lymphoid tissue. The nonorganized lymphoid tissue consists of both lymphoid cells within the lamina propria and intraepithelial lymphocytes. The lymphoid cells within the lamina propria include T-helper cells (of the CD4 type), B cells, plasma cells, mucosal mast cells, and macrophages. The intraepithelial lymphocytes consist mainly of T-suppressor cells.

The organized lymphoid tissue consists of lymphoid follicles, such as Peyer's patches of the small intestine, and lymphoid nodules of the small and large intestine. Peyer's patches are an important site for antigen penetration and the expression of mucosal immunity. Peyer's patches are said to "sample and transport" microorganisms and antigens in the intestinal lumen to lymphoid tissue within the patch. Stimulated lymphocytes then leave the Peyer's patch, travel through the lymphatic system, and return to take up residence in the mucosal membranes (lamina propria) as immunoglobulin A (IgA)-producing cells. IgA functions as an antimicrobial defense molecule in the intestine. This pathway protects the entire GI tract by routing the antigen-specific immune cells into the systemic circulation and back to the length of the intestine where it defends against the offending pathogen.

Optimal mucosal defense depends on the coordinated efforts of the nonimmunologic and immunologic processes. Traumatic injuries, burns, hemorrhagic shock, radiation injury, intestinal obstruction, protein malnutrition, and parenteral nutrition can all interfere with the integrity of the intestinal mucosa. In the case of parenteral nutrition, it has been observed that the lack of enteral stimulation results in mucosal atrophy and bacterial overgrowth. Mucosal barrier breakdown accompanying each of the aforementioned conditions allows the translocation of intestinal pathogens to the systemic circulation. Intestinal bacteria have been observed to cause systemic disease in immunodeficient patients, such as the critically ill.[9,10]

Digestive and Absorptive Properties

Digestion

Minor aspects of digestion do begin in the upper GI tract. In the mouth, secretions of amylase mix with saliva to begin the breakdown of starch. Amylase is quickly inactivated upon reaching the stomach and therefore does not contribute to carbohydrate digestion. No further digestion occurs between the mouth and stomach.

Hydrochloric acid (HCl) and pepsin are the initiators of digestion in the stomach. HCl is secreted by the parietal cells, primarily located in the body and fundus. At an intragastric pH of 2 to 4, the rate of HCl secretion is approximately 2 to 3 mEq per hour. This rate can be increased up to 10-fold by factors such as vagal stimulation, hormonal stimulation, and chemical properties of the chyme. The antral hormone gastrin and neurotransmitter acetylcholine directly stimulate parietal cells to release HCl. Histamine, present throughout the GI tract, is also a HCl stimulant. Current drug therapy for peptic ulcer disease targets histamine receptors. Histamine (H_2) receptor blockers effectively decrease HCl release.[6]

The acid environment of the stomach promotes the conversion of pepsinogen to pepsin. Pepsinogen is a proteolytic enzyme released by gastric chief cells. Pepsin begins the breakdown of protein, although it may not be essential for normal protein breakdown and absorption.

Parietal cells of the stomach also secrete intrinsic factor. Intrinsic factor binds to vitamin B_{12} and is essential for transport and absorption of this vitamin in the terminal ileum. Vitamin B_{12} plays an essential role in the formation of red blood cells. An intrinsic factor or vitamin B_{12} deficiency can result in anemia. Surgical removal of the stomach or atrophy of the gastric mucosa would result in an intrinsic factor deficiency, as would resection of the terminal ileum.

The stomach also secretes fluids rich in electrolytes including sodium and potassium. Loss of these fluids through vomiting or gastric suction (common in the ICU) can lead to fluid and electrolyte imbalances and acid–base disturbances.

Endocrine cells, located among the gastric epithelial cells of the antrum, produce and secrete gastrin. Gastrin is a peptide hormone produced by specialized cells in the gastric and duodenal mucosa. Its release is regulated by neural stimulation, chemical properties of the diet, and distention of the stomach wall. Gastrin stimulates the release of HCl, pepsinogen, and pancreatic enzymes.

The small intestine is the primary site of both digestion and absorption. The functional unit of the small intestine is the villus. The structure of the villus has been described previously (see Figure 32–7). Enzymes within the brush border are responsible for the breakdown of disaccharides and peptides. The digestion of proteins, fats, and carbohydrates is initiated by duodenal pancreatic enzymes. Additional enzymes located along the mucosal brush border complete the digestive processing of proteins and carbohydrates.[6]

Protein. Protein digestion begins in the stomach with pepsin and continues to a much greater extent as the chyme passes into the duodenum. Proteolytic enzymes synthesized in the pancreas enter the duode-

num, in their inactive form, via the pancreatic duct. The pancreatic duct often joins with the common bile duct and enters the duodenum via the ampulla of Vater. On entering the small intestine, these enzymes are activated by enterokinase. Within the small intestine lumen, pancreatic proteolytic enzymes break down proteins to peptides. Enzymes of the microvilli within the brush border are responsible for the final breakdown of peptides to amino acids.[6]

Carbohydrates. As mentioned previously, carbohydrate digestion is initiated via salivary amylase in the mouth. Starches and simple sugars are then hydrolyzed by exposure to HCl in the stomach. The small intestine is the site of carbohydrate exposure to pancreatic amylase. Pancreatic amylase breaks down starches to disaccharides. The mucosal brush border then cleaves disaccharides to monosaccharides, which are absorbed through the intestinal lumen.[6]

Fat. Triglycerides are dietary fat composed of glycerol and fatty acids. Dietary fat is emulsified by bile salts in the small intestine. As described earlier, bile salts are formed in the liver, stored in the gallbladder, and secreted into the duodenum. Fats emulsified by these bile salts are further broken down by pancreatic lipase. The fat molecules break down to monoglycerides and fatty acids. They are then surrounded by a water-soluble barrier and transported to the absorptive surface. These fat products enter the mucosal epithelial cells, releasing the bile salts to diffuse back into the lumen for recycling or reabsorption, via the ileum, to the liver. Digestion is totally completed in the small intestine.[6]

Absorption

As with digestion, absorption occurs chiefly in the small intestine. The stomach absorbs limited substances; for example, alcohol and aspirin are chiefly absorbed from the stomach.

TABLE 32–3

Sites of Absorption for Digested Nutrients

Site	Nutrient Absorbed
Small Intestine	
Duodenum	Iron
	Calcium
	Fat
	Sugars
	Amino acids
Jejunum	Sugars
	Amino acids
Ileum	Bile salts
	Vitamin B_{12}
Large Intestine	Water
	Electrolytes

Data from Heitkemper M, Westfall U: Gastrointestinal physiology. In Clochesy J, Breu C, Cardin S, Rudy E, Whittaker A, eds. Critical Care Nursing. Philadelphia, WB Saunders, 1996.

Nutrients are absorbed via active and passive transport and facilitated diffusion. Carbohydrates are absorbed as monosaccharides, and proteins are absorbed as amino acids. These substances then move into the circulation. Fats are absorbed as fatty acids and glycerol. They are then reconstituted to triglycerides, cholesterol, and phospholipids to form chylomicrons. Chylomicrons are absorbed into the lymph system, and then travel to the venous circulation. Table 32–3 lists the expected absorptive locations for digested nutrients. The small intestine is also the site for absorption of fluids and electrolytes arising from food, and gastric and intestinal secretions.

Even though the colon absorbs some drugs, it is chiefly responsible for the absorption of fluid and electrolytes. The large intestine absorbs roughly 85% of its total fluid content. The remaining 15% is excreted in the feces. The absorptive function of the colon is not

TABLE 32–4
Structural and Functional Changes Associated With Aging

Structure	Functional Changes
Mouth	▪ Drooping of lower face and lips is caused by reduced circumoral muscle tone; older persons have difficulty keeping their mouth closed during sleep and eating, decreased production of saliva, and excessive dryness.
	▪ There is increased incidence of oral carcinoma in persons older than age 50 years, especially squamous cell: lower lip, tongue, gingiva, floor of mouth. Painless lesions appear as ulceration, induration, fungal lesion, or elevation.
	▪ Receding gums lead to exposed roots of teeth and loosening. Elderly persons are four times more likely to have root caries.
	▪ Inflammation appears as gingivitis resulting from plaque on neck of teeth. Halitosis, bad taste, bleeding result.
	▪ There is increased tooth decay from wear on enamel and dentin. Removal of teeth results in bone loss and atrophy. Dentures loosen and can cause mucosal trauma.
	▪ Reduced number of taste buds result in decreased sense of taste. Eating becomes less pleasurable, appetite diminishes.
Esophagus	▪ Decreased peristalsis is caused by neurologic changes. The gag reflex becomes weak. Dysphagia and chest pain are common signs of esophageal disorders. Diffuse esophageal spasm mimics chest pain of myocardial infarction.
	▪ Incompetence of lower esophageal sphincter resulting from neurologic changes increase esophageal reflux. Resulting mucosal damage leads to inflammation, ulceration, bleeding, or strictures. Symptoms include heartburn or retrosternal burning that increases with bending or lying down; regurgitation.
Stomach	▪ Decreased gastric blood flow reduces absorptive surface and delays gastric emptying. Diminished absorption of carbohydrates, fats, vitamin D, and calcium results.
	▪ Decreased stomach volume and gastric acid content further alter digestive processes.
	▪ Acute onset of burning epigastric pain beginning 1 to 4 hours after meals that is relieved by food or antacids is a classic scenario for a gastric ulcer. Elderly persons may also be pain free or have an unusual pain pattern.
Gallbladder	▪ There is slight dilation of common bile duct. Size of gallbladder is generally unchanged; emptying is not affected.
	▪ Incidence of gallstones increases with each decade of life; indigestion, belching, and flatulence are sometimes associated with gallbladder disease. Acute cholecystitis may result from gallstones and usually includes obstruction of common bile duct, producing biliary colic and jaundice.
Liver	▪ Number of hepatocytes, and weight and size of liver generally decrease, but liver function parameters are usually unchanged.
	▪ Hepatitis is more likely to be drug induced.
	▪ Cirrhosis, as the end stage of chronic hepatitis, occurs among elderly alcoholics and sometimes diabetics.
Small intestine	▪ Absorption, motility, and blood flow decrease, resulting in impaired nutrient absorption.
Large intestine	▪ Diverticuli incidence increases from roughly 5% at 50 years of age to 50% at 80 years of age. Primary complications of diverticuli are infection and inflammation that can cause fever and abdominal pain, especially in the left lower quadrant.
	▪ Increased frequency of colon polyps necessitates their removal and routine screening.
	▪ There is increased frequency of colon cancer. Persons age 60 years and older are at greatest risk. Signs include change in bowel habits, bleeding, weight loss, mucoid stools, and iron-deficiency anemia. Right colon tumors are associated with anemia; left colon tumors more commonly present with constipation, rectal bleeding, and abdominal pain.
	▪ Decreased intestinal peristalsis leads to constipation, defined in terms of frequency and hardness of stool.

considered vital to life. However, a disruption in this function caused by surgical resection of the colon can result in significant fluid and electrolyte disturbances, especially in the immediate postoperative period or during times of illness typically associated with fluid imbalance, such as infection, high fever with dehydration, vomiting, or diarrhea.[6]

NORMAL STRUCTURAL AND FUNCTIONAL CHANGES ASSOCIATED WITH AGING

Physiologic changes in every body system accompany aging. These changes generally begin in the fifth decade of life. Table 32–4 describes the most common changes found in the GI tract as people age. These changes pose important considerations for the critical care nurse preparing to care for the acute and critically ill elderly.[4,11,12]

Key Concepts

⇒ The GI system provides the mechanisms for the digestion and absorption of nutrients essential for sustaining the body's structure and function.

⇒ The gut wall is composed of four layers: the mucosa, the submucosa, the muscularis, and the serosa.

⇒ The mucosa is responsible for the absorption of nutrients and fluids.

⇒ The muscularis contains longitudinal and circular fibers responsible for the rhythmic contraction that mechanically breaks down food and propels it through the GI tract.

⇒ The serosa is derived from the peritoneum and covers the entire gut surface. It provides a layer of protection and contains the network of blood and lymph vessels and the nerves that supply the abdominal organs.

⇒ Oral secretions—saliva, mucin, ptyalin—aid chewing and swallowing, and initiate carbohydrate digestion in the mouth.

⇒ The vagus, glossopharyngeal, and trigeminal nerves in communication with the brain stem are responsible for the act of swallowing.

⇒ The lower esophageal sphincter is responsible for maintaining an alkaline environment within the esophagus by preventing reflux of gastric contents.

⇒ The stomach serves three primary functions: 1) the storage of large quantities of food; 2) the mixing of ingested food with gastric secretions to form chyme; and 3) the regulation of the rate of emptying chyme into the duodenum.

⇒ The small intestine consists of the duodenum, the jejunum, and the ileum. It is the principal location for the digestion and absorption of nutrients.

⇒ Brunner's glands, within the submucosa of the small intestine, secrete mucus to protect the walls from the action of digestive enzymes.

⇒ Mucosal folds (plica), villi, and microvilli are the functional units of the small intestine. They are responsible for increasing the mucosal surface area for both digestion and absorption.

⇒ The villi contain a network of blood and lymphatic vessels. They secrete digestive enzymes and absorb nutrients. The lymphatic vessels, within the villi, absorb and transport fat molecules.

⇒ The primary functions of the large intestine are the completion of absorption, the manufacture of certain vitamins, and the formation and expulsion of feces from the body.

⇒ The ileocecal valve guards the opening from the ileum to the cecum of the large intestine.

⇒ Longitudinal muscles of the mucosa of the colon run in three flat bands called taenia coli. Tonic contractions of these bands gather the colon into a series of pouches called haustra. This causes puckering of the colon as feces pass through it.

⇒ Functions of the liver include 1) bile formation; 2) drug and hormone metabolism; 3) substrate metabolism; 4) protein synthesis, especially those associated with blood coagulation; 5) detoxification of noxious substances; and 6) phagocytosis via Kupffer cells.

⇒ Bile formed in the liver travels via the common hepatic duct to the cystic duct for storage in the gallbladder.

⇒ A signal from the duodenum stimulates the release of bile. Bile travels via the cystic duct to the common bile duct and enters the duodenum via the ampulla of Vater.

⇒ The gallbladder is located under the right lobe of the liver. It holds approximately 30 mL of bile.

⇒ The exocrine pancreas cells, or acini, secrete pancreatic enzymes that enter the duodenum to aid in digestion.

⇒ The stomach and the small and large intestine receive their blood supply from the celiac and the inferior and superior mesenteric arteries.

⇒ GI blood flow is affected by the level of local activity, the vasodilatory effects of intestinal hormones, the effects of the kinins—kallidin and bradykinin, and the oxygen levels within the gut wall.

⇒ Hormones of the GI system stimulate and inhibit secretion, digestion, motility, and absorption. The stomach and small intestine are the chief suppliers of these hormones.

⇒ The enteric nervous system is composed of two nerve plexi: the submucosal and the myenteric. These nerve plexi interface with the sympathetic and parasympathetic nerve pathways to innervate and regulate the GI system. Together they control motility, secretions, blood flow, digestion, and absorption.

→ The GI tract plays a major role in the body's defense against bacteria, parasites, and other toxic pathogens. It has two mechanisms of defense: immunologic and nonimmunologic. Nonimmunologic defenses include salivary secretions, gastric acid, bile salts, peristalsis, normal bowel flora, and the mucous coat lining the gut lumen. Immunologic defenses include lymphoid cells within the lamina propria of the mucosal layer containing T-helper cells, B cells, plasma cells, mucosal mast cells, and macrophages. Intraepithelial lymphocytes contain T-suppressor cells.

→ Lymphoid tissue is organized as Peyer's patches in the small intestine and as solitary lymphoid nodules throughout the small and large intestine.

→ HCl and pepsin initiate digestion in the stomach. Gastrin, acetylcholine, and histamine all stimulate HCl production and secretion. HCl and pepsin initiate protein breakdown.

→ Parietal cells of the stomach secrete intrinsic factor. Intrinsic factor binds to vitamin B_{12} and is essential for transport and absorption of this vitamin in the terminal ileum. Vitamin B_{12} is a factor in the formation of red blood cells.

→ The small intestine is the primary site of both digestion and absorption. Brush border enzymes break down disaccharides and peptides. Duodenal pancreatic enzymes digest proteins, fats, and carbohydrates.

→ The colon is chiefly responsible for the absorption of fluid and electrolytes. Roughly 85% of its daily fluid content is absorbed and the remaining 15% is excreted in feces.

→ Many structural and functional changes in the GI system accompany aging. This should be considered carefully when caring for the critically ill elderly.

References

1. Gray H: Gray's Anatomy: The Anatomical Basis of Medicine and Surgery, 38th ed. New York, Churchill, 1995.
2. Guyton A, Hall J: Textbook of Medical Physiology, 9th ed. Philadelphia, WB Saunders, 1996.
3. Tortora G, Anagnostakos N: The digestive system. In Principles of Anatomy and Physiology. New York, Harper and Row, 1990, pp 733–783.
4. Huether S: Structure and function of the digestive system. In McCance K, Huether S, eds. Pathophysiology: The Biologic Basis for Disease in Adults and Children. St. Louis, CV Mosby, 1990, pp 1174–1211.
5. Smith S: Patients with liver dysfunction. In Clochesy J, Breu C, Cardin S, Rudy E, Whittaker A, eds. Critical Care Nursing, Philadelphia, WB Saunders, 1993, pp 970–1008.
6. Heitkemper M, Westfall U: Gastrointestinal physiology. In Clochesy J, Breu C, Cardin S, Rudy E, Whittaker A, eds. Critical Care Nursing. Philadelphia, WB Saunders, 1993, pp 929–944.
7. Rice V: Shock, a clinical syndrome: an update. Part 2. The stages of shock. Crit Care Nurse 11(5):74–79, 1991.
8. Briones TL: The gastrointestinal system. In Alspach JG, ed. Core Curriculum for Critical Care Nursing, 4th ed. Philadelphia, WB Saunders, 1991, pp 748–765.
9. Langkamp-Henken B, Glezer J, Kudsk K: Immunologic structure and function of the gastrointestinal tract. Nutr Clin Pract 7(3):100–108, 1992.
10. Cuff PA: Acquired immunodeficiency syndrome and malnutrition: role of gastrointestinal pathology. Nutr Clin Pract 5:43–53, 1990.
11. Esberger K: Guide to gastrointestinal problems of elders. Geriatr Nurs 12(2):74–75, 1991.
12. Shad M: Gastrointestinal issues in older adults. In Schmidt Lagen A, ed. Core Curriculum for Gerontological Nursing. St. Louis, CV Mosby, 1996, pp 553–563.

33

Gastrointestinal Assessment

Una Elizabeth Westfall

Objectives

After completing this chapter, the student will be able to:

1. Collect a thorough health history of the gastrointestinal (GI) system.
2. Perform an abdominal physical examination.
3. Describe why referred pain patterns are important when doing an abdominal assessment.
4. Differentiate the gastrointestinal organs in the abdominal and retroperitoneal spaces.
5. Determine elements to use when characterizing gastrointestinal symptoms.
6. Link the importance of the GI assessment with aging differences.
7. Determine the most helpful components of a dietary assessment for selected intensive care unit (ICU) patients.
8. Highlight nutritional beliefs for at least five different ethnic or religious groups.

Gastrointestinal (GI) system assessment by the critical care nurse is needed to achieve multiple goals. Among these goals are to aid in 1) detecting system/organ/tissue changes in structural integrity; 2) detecting system/organ/tissue changes in functional integrity; 3) diagnosing GI and extragastrointestinal causes of illness when GI signs or symptoms are present; 4) determining system components that are intact, functional, and healthy; 5) identifying components for symptom management by nurses; 6) formulating a comprehensive nursing care approach for the intensive care patient; or 7) monitoring treatment effectiveness.

By collecting focused, timely data using an organized approach, a more comprehensive picture of the GI system can be obtained. In an intensive care situation, when and how completely components are assessed is often dictated, in part, by the dynamic status of the patient. For example, on admission, gathering a complete nutritional history is often not appropriate. However, the patient's hypermetabolic state and nutritional status can directly contribute to multiple health outcomes, including length of stay, morbidity, and, in some cases, mortality.[1] Thus, the sensitivity of the nurse in deciding not only what information to solicit but also when to solicit information is a major contribution to the patient's well-being.

Throughout the course of a patient's intensive care stay, the nurse is continually challenged to construct an accurate comprehensive picture of the patient in a dynamic situation. Integrating presenting signs and symptoms is one of the many tasks accepted by the critical care nurse. Some GI signs or symptoms may need to be handled both as isolated entities and as part of a larger composite. For example, actions may be needed to control a symptom, such as vomiting or abdominal pain. At the same time, the symptom may be part of a larger picture and, as such, provides valuable information for identifying and correcting the underlying cause.

Many GI signs and symptoms may result from non-GI sources. Projectile vomiting, for example, often originates from a central nervous system condition. Thus, the nurse is faced with gathering data which may or may not have as its origin the GI tract. The context of the data is critical in providing the most accurate representation and, subsequently, in making decisions for medical and nursing diagnoses and treatment.

Reasons for GI assessment can change over the illness trajectory or intensive care stay. The importance of selected history and physical components also vary. Initially, necessary data may focus primarily on obtaining, refining, ruling in, or ruling out medical diagnoses. The dynamic status of the intensive care patient challenges the nurse to maintain a current database as well as to solicit additional information helpful in individualizing nursing care consistent with the patient's current status. With a more protracted illness, the nutritional status increases in importance.

A GI assessment encompasses the entire GI tract from mouth to anus and includes accessory organs of the liver, gallbladder, and pancreas. Organs and tissues comprising the system pass through several regions of the body, that is, oral cavity, neck, thorax, and abdomen. Thus, disruptions within the regions have the potential to adversely alter structural or functional capacity of the GI system.

CHART 33–1

ELEMENTS OF GASTROINTESTINAL HISTORY

Personal Health History

Any preexisting gastrointestinal (GI) condition
GI surgeries or injuries: oral, pharyngeal, esophagus, stomach, small bowel, colon, liver, gallbladder, pancreas
Abdominal surgeries or injuries
GI disorders or diseases including peptic ulcer, polyps, gallstones
Past GI examinations (e.g., colonoscopy)
Prior GI bleeding
Past hospitalizations
Blood transfusions
Major illness such as diabetes or cancer
Pancreatitis
Drugs—prescription; over-the-counter drugs; recreational drug use
Alcohol use—types, quantity, patterns, consequences
Smoking or chewing tobacco
Recent travel history
Hepatitis or cirrhosis of the liver
Hepatitis vaccine

Family Medical History

Malabsorption syndrome
Familial Mediterranean fever (periodic peritonitis)
Gallbladder disease
Hirschsprung disease, aganglionic megacolon
Polyposis
Colon cancer

Description of GI Symptoms

Type
Onset
Location
Intensity
Duration
Frequency, if appropriate
Character (e.g., if pain—sharp, dull, burning; if diarrhea—watery, copious, explosive, undigested food)
Aggravating and alleviating factors

Relationship to other symptoms, events, or activities (e.g., food intake)

Regional Elements: Mouth and Throat

Dental status—toothache or tooth abscess, pattern of dental care, dental appliances and fit
Gingiva—bleeding gums, sore gums
Mucous membranes—sores or lesions and location in mouth
Tongue—altered taste
Voice—hoarseness, changes in voice
Throat/swallowing—difficulty swallowing, sore throat

Regional Element: Thorax and Abdomen

Heartburn
Dysphagia
Indigestion
Nausea
Eructations
Vomiting—character (color, consistency, quality, duration, frequency); relationship to other symptoms, events, or activities; medications
Hematemesis
Abdominal pain (characterize)
Jaundice
Dark urine
Fever and chills

Regional Element: Lower Abdomen

Rectal condition
Hemorrhoids
Flatulence
Stools—patterns, aids; color, frequency, consistency, changes in stool shape, odor
Bowel regularity; use of laxatives, stool softeners
Change in bowel habits—diarrhea, constipation, fecal impaction
Blood in stools

HEALTH HISTORY

Completing a focused GI history and physical examination is dependent on many factors, including purpose, constellation of symptoms, and patient stamina. Chart 33–1 highlights the elements of a GI history. Initially, history information may be obtained more quickly and easily from family members, significant others, or friends. Personal health, including preexisting GI conditions, previous GI or abdominal surgeries or injuries, and hospitalizations, as well as family history are fixed. Thus, this information needs to be completed only once. However, if obtained from someone other than the patient, there may be selected aspects to verify with the patient. An advantage of this approach is that it can conserve patient energy.

Data about regional aspects, or GI signs or symptoms, may need to be updated throughout the current hospital course; many GI symptoms are nonspecific.

PHYSICAL EXAMINATION

Oral and Throat

The GI system physical examination includes structures along the full length of the alimentary canal. The clinical physical examination should begin with the

TABLE 33–1
Oral Assessment Tool

Category	Tools for Assessment	Methods of Measurement	Numerical and Descriptive Ratings*		
			1	2	3
Voice	Auditory	Converse with patient	Normal	Deeper or raspy	Difficulty talking or painful
Swallow	Observation and tongue blade	Ask patient to swallow. To test gag reflex, gently place blade on back of tongue and depress	Normal swallow	Some pain on swallow	Unable to swallow
Lips	Visual/palpatory	Observe and feel tissue	Smooth, pink, and moist	Dry or cracked	Ulcerated or bleeding
Tongue	Visual/palpatory	Feel and observe appearance of tissue	Pink and moist and papillae present	Coated or loss of papillae with a shiny appearance with or without redness	Blistered or cracked
Saliva	Tongue blade and visual	Insert blade into mouth, touching the center of the tongue and the floor of the mouth	Watery	Thick or ropy	Absent
Mucous membranes	Visual	Observe appearance of tissue	Pink and moist	Reddened or coated (increased whiteness) without ulcerations	Ulcerations with or without bleeding
Gingiva	Tongue blade and visual	Gently press tissue with tip of blade	Pink and stippled and firm	Edematous with or without redness	Spontaneous bleeding or bleeding with pressure
Teeth or dentures (or denture-bearing area)	Visual	Observe appearance of teeth or denture-bearing area	Clean and no debris	Plaque or debris in localized areas (between teeth if present)	Plaque or debris generalized along gum line or denture-bearing area

*Each category is assigned a numerical rating. Total ratings can range from 8 to 24. The higher the rating, the greater the risk of oral breakdown.

(Reprinted with permission of June Eilers, RN, MSN, CS, University of Nebraska Medical Center, Omaha, NE.)

oral cavity (Table 33–1). This is especially important for intubated patients. Although the mouth can easily be examined, it may be inadvertently neglected. Additionally, the condition of the mouth may change rapidly in the critically ill patient. Thus, establishing an initial oral assessment and conducting a periodic oral assessment (e.g., at least daily) can aid in keeping structures intact or in beginning treatment as soon as disruptions start.

Any secretions, oral odor, or odor changes should be investigated. Findings suggest that there may well be a relationship between pneumonia and mouth colonizations in intubated patients.[2] Additionally, an oral tube can be a source of noxious fluid if it leaks. Such fluid can be corrosive to oral structures. Even soft tubes may compress structures in the mouth, as well as hinder vision when inspecting oral structures.

The presence of bilateral gag reflexes should be noted. A coordinated swallow is the best protection against aspiration. With suppression of the reflex, the patient is at increased risk for complications, including aspiration.

The presence of a nasal or oral tube in the stomach or small intestine prevents the lower esophageal sphincter from closing completely. Gastric reflux may result, with caustic effects to esophageal tissues, and, on occasion, up to the oropharyngeal region. If delayed gastric emptying is present, such reflux and subsequent damage to structures may intensify.

Abdomen

A traditional abdominal assessment encompasses intra-GI and extra-GI structures. Additionally, GI structures are found both in the peritoneal and retroperitoneal areas.[3–6] Figure 33–1 shows two com-

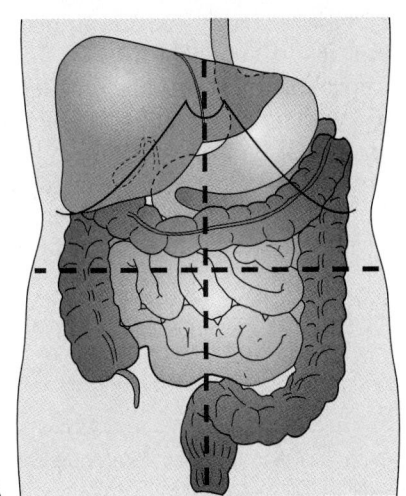

A

Right upper quadrant (RUQ)	Left upper quadrant (LUQ)
Liver and gallbladder	Left liver lobe
Pylorus	Stomach
Duodenum	Body of pancreas
Head of pancreas	Splenic flexure of colon
Hepatic flexure of colon	Portions of transverse and descending colon
Portions of ascending and transverse colon	Spleen
Kidney	Kidney
Adrenal gland	Adrenal gland

Right lower quadrant (RLQ)	Left lower quadrant (LLQ)
Cecum and appendix	Sigmoid colon
Portion of ascending colon	Portion of descending colon

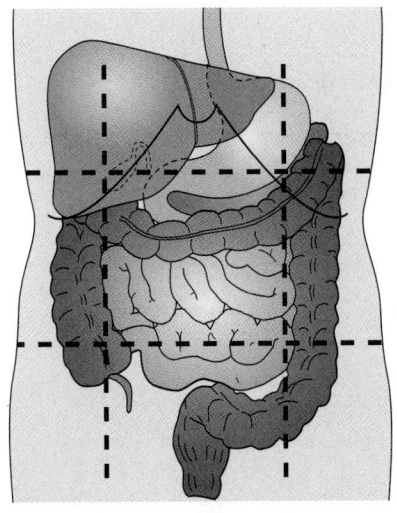

B

Right hypochondriac	Epigastric	Left hypochondriac
Right liver lobe	Pyloric end of stomach	Stomach
Gallbladder	Duodenum	Tail of pancreas
Upper pole of kidney	Pancreas	Splenic flexure of colon
	Portion of liver	Spleen
		Upper pole of kidney

Right lumbar	Umbilical	Left lumbar
Ascending colon	Omentum	Descending colon
Portion of duodenum and jejunum	Mesentery	Tail of pancreas
Lower pole of kidney	Lower part of duodenum	Portions of jejunum and ileum
	Jejunum and ileum	Lower pole of kidney

Right inguinal	Suprapubic or hypogastric	Left inguinal
Cecum	Ileum	Sigmoid colon
Appendix	Bladder	
Lower end of ileum		

Figure 33–1

Abdominal mapping approaches and underlying organs. A, Division of the abdomen into four quadrants. B, Division of the abdomen into nine areas.

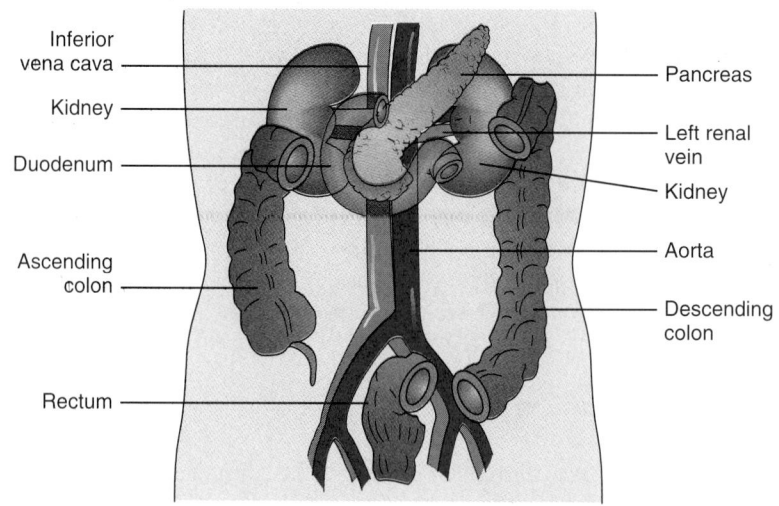

Figure 33–2

Retroperitoneal structures and their alignment in the adult patient.

monly used abdominal mapping approaches and structures found in each division. Figure 33–2 displays structures and their alignment behind the posterior parietal peritoneal membrane, that is, retroperitoneum. Chart 33–2 presents the physical examination procedure for abdominal assessment of the GI system. Common abnormal signs are found in Table 33–2. To minimize bowel sound disruption, the examination sequence is as follows: 1) inspection; 2) auscultation; 3) percussion; and 4) palpation—both light and deep.

Abdominal inspection includes examination of any openings, tubes, drains, or fluids leading to the skin surface. Gut regions have specific functions in the digestion and absorption of nutrients. To accommodate these, normal fluid volumes, pH levels, and properties vary widely throughout the system. Table 33–3 lists normal GI volumes and pH levels by gut section. Large volume losses can occur rapidly and may require timely replacement of individually formulated fluids. The pH variability within the

TABLE 33–2
Abnormal Abdominal Signs

Sign	Features	Conditions
Blumberg	Rebound tenderness	Peritoneal irritation; inflamed or perforated appendix
Cullen	Periumbilical ecchymosis	Intraabdominal bleeding; pancreatitis; ectopic pregnancy
Grey Turner	Flank ecchymosis	Intraabdominal bleeding; pancreatitis
Iliopsoas muscle	Right lower quadrant pain when right leg elevated against tension	Inflamed or perforated appendix (inflamed iliopsoas muscle)
Murphy	Sharp pain and abruptly stops inspiration when palpating under liver border	Cholecystitis
Obturator muscle	Abdominal pain when right leg rotated at hip (internal and external)	Inflamed or perforated appendix

TABLE 33–3
Gastrointestinal Fluid

Location	Daily Volume	Contents	pH
Oral	1000–2000 mL	Mucus, water, ions, H_2O, amylase, immunoglobulins	6.0–7.0
Esophagus	300–800 mL	Mucus	
Stomach	1500–2000 mL	Mucus, HCl, H_2O, ions, intrinsic factor, pepsinogen	1.0–3.5
Liver (bile)	500–1000 mL	Bile salts, H_2O, ions, bilirubin	7.8
Pancreas	1000–1800 mL	H_2O, ions, enzymes	8.0–8.3
Small intestine	1200–3000 mL	H_2O, ions, mucus, enzymes, peptides	7.5–8.9
Colon	Variable	Mucus	7.5–8.0

Modified from Westfall U, Heitkemper M: Gastrointestinal physiology. In Clochesy I, Breu C, Cardin S, Whittaker A, Rudy E, eds. *Critical Care Nursing,* 2nd ed. Philadelphia, WB Saunders, 1996, p 988.

CHART 33–2

ELEMENTS OF ADULT GASTROINTESTINAL PHYSICAL EXAMINATION

Oral and Oropharynx (Inspection and Palpation)

See Table 33–2 for oral assessment tool.
Gag reflex—presence bilaterally

Abdomen (Gastrointestinal System Focus)

Sequence: Inspection, auscultation, percussion, palpation

Approach: Four quadrants or nine sections (see Figure 33–1)

1. Inspection—surface characteristics using consistent approach
   Skin color—moles, lesions (particularly nodules), scars (location, configuration, relative size), spider angiomas
   Contour—may need to measure circumference
   Movement—respiration, peristalsis, pulsations
   Symmetry
   Venous return pattern
   Hair distribution
   Presence of tubes or openings (e.g., colostomy or ileostomy); note locations, output consistency, and pH
2. Auscultation—bowel sounds using consistent approach (diaphram of stethoscope)
   Frequency—normally 5–35 per minute
   Pitch—small bowel normally high pitch; colon normally low pitch
   Character—clicks, gurgles, rumbling

   Vascular sounds (bell of stethoscope)

   Location
   Pitch
   Timing—bruits over aortic, renal, and femoral arteries; venous hums in epigastric area and around umbilicus

   Friction rubs (diaphragm of stethoscope)

   Pitch
   Location
   Relationship to respiration—normally not audible; if present, often over liver or spleen

3. Percussion—presence of air, fluid, or solid masses using consistent approach
   Tones and tone changes
   Location—normally tympany predominant sound when there is air in stomach and intestine; normally dullness over organs and solid masses, including distended bladder
   Fluid wave of shifting dullness (may not be detected if less than 500 mL)

   Liver border

   Location upper right quadrant and lower right chest
   Size—normal liver span approximately 6 to 12 cm (2½ to 4½ inches) at midclavicular line
4. Palpation—feel for areas of tenderness, muscle spasms, masses, fluid with light palpation (approximately 1 cm depth) using consistent approach with pillow under knees if possible
   Muscle resistance or guarding
   Rigidity
   Tenderness
   Large masses (if detected, not surface location)

   Feel for organs in abdomen with deep palpation (approximately 5 to 8 cm or 2 to 3 inches)

   Liver edge—location, size, mobility, consistency or border smoothness
   Gallbladder—normally not palpable, below liver margin
   Masses—location, size, shape, tenderness, consistency, mobility, surfaces, pulsation, movement with respiration
   Rebound tenderness—normally not present, location
   Fluid wave—normally not present

Specific Abnormal Signs: See Table 33–4 for common abnormal signs.

Rectal Area (Inspection and Palpation): Surface characteristics:
   Condition of anus and surrounding skin
   Presence of hemorrhoids
   Presence of tubes
   Presence of large bowel contents—consistency, quantity
   Palpable fecal mass above internal sphincter

system can lead to damage of surrounding structures if secretions leak out. If these caustic secretions are on the skin, they quickly can lead to skin breakdown. Additionally, when secretions exceed their normal pH range, ionic shifts may lead to fluid and electrolyte imbalances. Thus, checking the pH of fluids reaching the skin surface may direct early actions to maintain or achieve fluid and electrolyte balance. Contents or fluids may also be tested for unanticipated contents such as blood. As blood moves through the tract, its normal character is changed by actions of digestion.

Bowel sounds, resulting from air or fluid movement through the gut lumen, may radiate within the abdomen. Thus, the actual location of such sounds may be misleading at the surface. Normally, bowel sounds occur from 5 to 35 per minute. Characteristics to note include frequency, pitch, and loudness. Altered bowel sounds may occur in many conditions, such as those listed in Table 33–4.

Auscultation for friction rubs and vascular sounds should be pursued before percussion or palpation. When present, friction rubs are most often associated with abnormal contact between the peritoneal membrane and abdominal organs, especially the liver or the spleen. For example, an epigastric, sustained venous hum may be audible in the presence of compromising portal hypertension. Bruits occur from turbulent blood flow through arteries. Their presence may reflect partially disrupted flow in the vessel.

Percussion in the critically ill patient may be deferred, particularly if there is conspicuous abdominal

TABLE 33–4
Abnormal Bowel Sounds

State	Bowel Sound Frequency
Diarrhea	Hyperactive
Early mechanical bowel obstruction	Hyperactive
Esophageal bleeding	Hyperactive
Gastroenteritis	Hyperactive
Hyperkalemia	Hyperactive
Resolving paralytic ileus	Hyperactive
Gastric bleeding	Hypoactive
Hypokalemia	Hypoactive
Inflammation	Hypoactive
Intraabdominal bleeding	Hypoactive
Late bowel obstruction	Hypoactive (may be high–pitched tingling at obstruction)
Paralytic ileus	Hypoactive or absent
Peritonitis	Hypoactive or absent
Pneumonia	Hypoactive
Mechanical obstruction	Mixed hypoactive and hyperactive

guarding. Only after nonpainful areas have been tested should painful areas be examined. Fluid in the abdomen or pleural space produces a dull sound on percussion. Conversely, air either contained in an organ (e.g., stomach and intestines) or within the abdomen can produce a tympanic sound. Most often, suspect findings lead to more complete assessment activities.

Palpation includes both light and deep touch. Light touch can be used to determine location and character of some somatic abdominal pain as well as to detect surface abnormalities. Attention to abdominal guarding can alert the nurse to the appropriateness of using deep palpation. Deep palpation is used to assess for organ megaly. Rupture or tissue disruption associated with an underlying pathologic condition, such as a pancreatic pseudocyst, grossly distended stomach, or hepatic inflammation, may occur from too much pressure. Other techniques for deep palpation of GI organs, such as the liver and retroperitoneal structures, are presented in physical assessment texts (e.g., Jarvis[4]).

When present, abdominal pain is often a nonspecific symptom.[7, 8] As viscera, abdominal organs contain limited pain receptors. Those present characteristically produce diffuse, more dull responses. Referred pain of organs and pathologic conditions within the abdomen are depicted in Figure 33–3. Pain from encapsulated abdominal organs, such as the liver or the spleen, originates from capsule receptors.

Inflammation of the internal peritoneal membrane pressing against an organ results in rebound tenderness. It is only with finger release from palpation that a sharp, localized pain is reported. This inflammation may be in response to multiple conditions such as GI organ inflammation, infection, abscess formation, or release of bowel contents into the abdomen.

Lower Gastrointestinal Tract

The GI system terminates at the anus. Examination of the anus includes inspection for the presence of stool or leaking colon contents, visible fissures, as well as any tissue normally found above the external or internal sphincters. Disease or treatment options for the critically ill often influence GI motility, resulting in either diarrhea or constipation. Some treatment conditions, such as the supine position, limited or no GI intake, and opioids, decrease intestinal peristalsis. Initially, bowel status may be deferred, because there are more immediate care priorities. However, if left unattended, constipation and its more severe form, fecal impaction, will likely occur.

Besides inspection, palpation may be used to assess for anal sphincter tone. Such assessment may give some clues of GI incontinence problems.

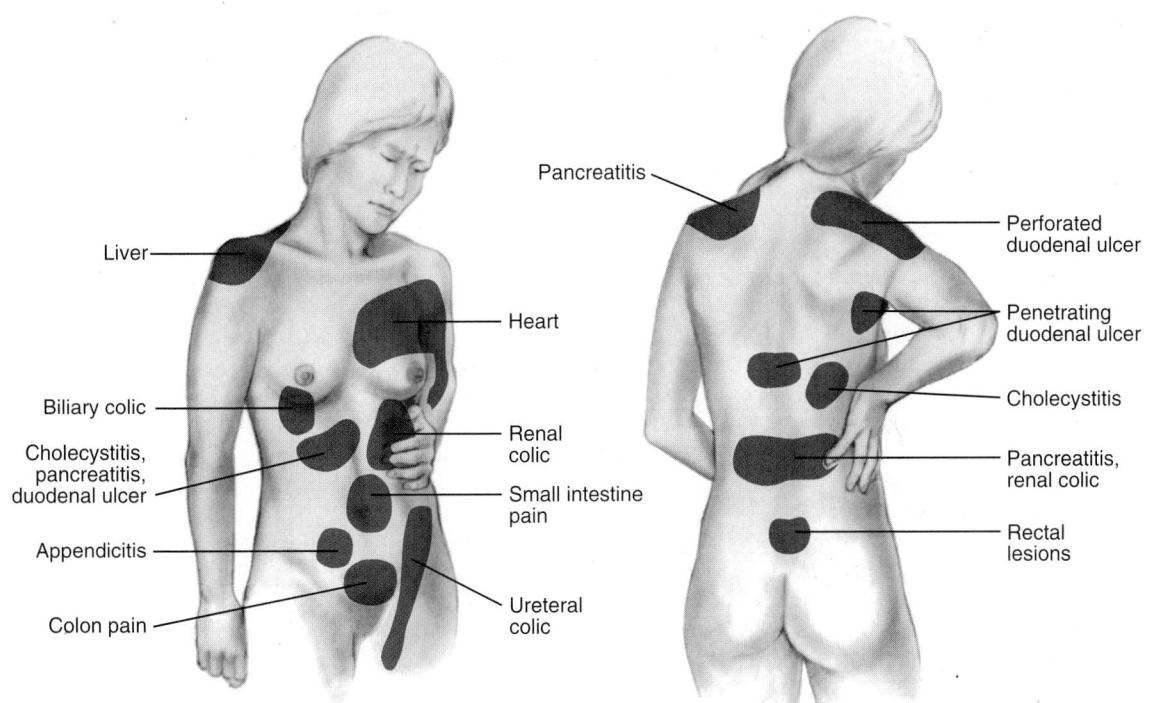

Figure 33–3

Referred pain locations and organs for abdominal contents. (From Jarvis C: *Physical Examination and Health Assessment*, 2nd ed. Philadelphia, WB Saunders, 1992, p 636.)

Nutritional Assessment

A nutritional assessment contains history, physical, and biochemical elements, and is directed toward macronutrient and micronutrient status. Macronutrients are proteins, carbohydrates, and fats. Micronutrients include fat and water-soluble vitamins, minerals, electrolytes, and trace elements. Over the illness trajectory, circulating and storage nutrient pools shift such that multiple macronutrient or micronutrient disequilibrium states can result. Stores may be depleted to provide the body with needed elements. Many measurements may only detect circulating levels of nutrients, thereby leading to an incomplete or misleading nutritional picture.

The nutritional status of the critically ill patient is dynamic. Data gathering often begins with a screening assessment. Later, a more comprehensive, as well as an ongoing approach, is needed. Traditional components of a nutritional assessment include historical and physical examination data, including anthropometric measurements, and biochemical analysis. Biochemical analysis contains measures of visceral and circulating proteins, total lymphocyte count, and cell-mediated immunity.

None of these measures, by itself, is nutritionally specific. The critically ill patient may have undergone medical management that interferes with accuracy of one or more of these measurements. Obtaining an accurate weight on admission may be precluded by such aspects as health status, treatments, and limited mobility. Fluid resuscitation can dilute serum, resulting in lower levels of circulating substances. Conversely, albumin may be used in treatment, resulting in an artificially high serum albumin level. Both albumin and prealbumin levels may be influenced by disease or treatment factors, as well as by nutritional status.

A clinical assessment of nutritional status that encompasses history, symptoms, and physical features is shown in Figure 33–4. This subjective global assessment focuses on five history elements and one physical status area.[9, 10] Within the physical status component are anthropometric measures of triceps skin fold thickness (TSF) and mid-arm muscle circumference (MAMC) to estimate subcutaneous fat reserves and protein reserves, respectively.

In addition to the current hypermetabolic state, a critically ill or injured patient already may have short- or long-term nutritional deficiencies. A nutritional health screen for nutritional problems has been developed[11, 12] and is presented in Figure 33–5. Calculations to guide nutritional management decisions need to take into consideration the person's nutritional status before the current physiologically unstable state. Thus, information about appetite, diet, intake patterns, attitudes toward food and eating, food intolerance, allergies, patterns of alcohol use, and food avoidances before hospitalization can be helpful in planning care.[13–16] Consideration of relevant cultural or religious beliefs about food may enhance oral intake for

(Select appropriate category with a checkmark, or enter numerical value where indicated by "#.")

A. **History**
   1. Weight change
      Overall loss in past 6 months: amount = #_____ kg; % loss = #_____
      Change in past 2 weeks _____ increase,
                             _____ no change,
                             _____ decrease.
   2. Dietary intake change (relative to normal)
      _____ No change
      _____ Change _____ duration = #_____ weeks.
                    _____ type: _____ suboptimal solid diet, _____ full liquid diet,
                             _____ hypocaloric liquids, _____ starvation.
   3. Gastrointestinal symptoms (that persisted for > 2 weeks)
      _____ none, _____ nausea, _____ vomiting, _____ diarrhea, _____ anorexia.
   4. Functional capacity
      _____ No dysfunction (e.g., full capacity)
      _____ Dysfunction _____ duration = #_____ weeks.
                    _____ type: _____ working suboptimally,
                             _____ ambulatory,
                             _____ bedridden.
   5. Disease and its relation to nutritional requirements
      Primary diagnosis (specify) _____

      _____
      Metabolic demand (stress): _____ no stress, _____ low stress,
                             _____ moderate stress, _____ high stress.
B. **Physical** (for each trait specify: 0 = normal, 1+ = mild, 2+ = moderate, 3+ = severe)
   # _____ loss of subcutaneous fat (triceps, chest)
   # _____ muscle wasting (quadriceps, deltoids)
   # _____ ankle edema
   # _____ sacral edema
   # _____ ascites
C. **SGA rating** (select one)
   _____ A = Well-nourished
   _____ B = Moderately (or suspected of being) malnourished
   _____ C = Severely malnourished

Figure 33–4

Features of subjective global assessment (SGA) for nutritional status. The final SGA rating is determined on the basis of clinical judgment of the features, rather than by an explicit numeric scheme. (From Detsky A, McLaughlin J, Baker J, et al: What is the subjective global assessment of nutritional status? JPEN J Parenter Enteral Nutr 11:8–13, 1987.)

the critically ill patient.[5, 17] Table 33–5 highlights nutritional beliefs for several such groups. Although most groups exclude persons who are ill from dietary restrictions, the patient may still cherish such practices.

As the patient moves through the illness trajectory, nutritional modifications are needed. Thus, periodic nutritional assessment updates are necessary. With a protracted condition, body stores of macronutrients and micronutrients may decline to dangerously low levels. Thus, selected nutritional supplements are needed for current body functioning as well as to replenish these stores.

NORMAL VARIATIONS ASSOCIATED WITH AGING

Physical changes occur throughout the GI system with aging.[18–20] Beginning with the oral cavity, there is a decrease in salivary flow. The buccal mucosa is less vascular and thinner. The tongue may be more fissured, and thus more difficult to clean. Some or all of an aging patient's teeth may be lost. Thus, the nurse must check for the presence of oral prosthetics, the condition of the underlying mucous membranes, and appliance fit.

Gut motility is decreased in the elderly patient. There is also some decrease in digestive enzymes secretion and protective mucus. Intestinal bacterial flora can undergo changes, either in number or ability. Often the end result is that the bacteria present are less able to participate in digestion. Additionally, there is some increase in epithelial atrophy. The ability of the small intestine to complete digestion and absorption for certain substances is diminished with age. The micronutrient calcium is an example of one such substance.

The size of the liver begins to decrease around the age of 50 years. With decreasing cardiac output that accompanies aging, hepatic blood flow decreases. With this reduction, drugs, hormones, and other substances normally metabolized by the liver remain active

DETERMINE YOUR NUTRITIONAL HEALTH

The Warning Signs of poor nutritional health are often overlooked. Use this checklist to find out if you or someone you know is at nutritional risk.

Read the statements below. Circle the number in the yes column for those that apply to you or someone you know. For each yes answer, add the number in the box. Total your nutritional score.

	YES
I have an illness or condition that made me change the kind and/or amount of food I eat.	2
I eat fewer than 2 meals per day.	3
I eat few fruit or vegetables, or milk products.	2
I have 3 or more drinks of beer, liquor or wine almost every day.	2
I have tooth or mouth problems that make it hard for me to eat.	2
I don't always have enough money to buy the food I need .	4
I eat alone most of the time.	1
I take 3 or more different prescribed or over-the-counter drugs a day.	1
Without wanting to, I have lost or gained 10 pounds in the last 6 months.	2
I am not always physically able to shop, cook and/or feed myself.	2
TOTAL	

Total Your Nutritional Score. If it's —

0–2 **Good!** Recheck your nutritional score in 6 months

3–5 **You are at moderate nutritional risk.** See what can be done to improve your eating habits and lifestyle. Your office on aging, senior nutrition program, senior citizens center or health department can help. Recheck your nutritional score in 3 months.

6 or more **You are at high nutritional risk.** Bring this checklist the next time you see your doctor, dietitian or other qualified health or social services professional. Talk with them about any problems you may have. Ask for help to improve your nutritional health.

DETERMINE

The nutrition checklist is based on the following warning signs. Use the word DETERMINE to help you remember them.

D – Disease
E – Eating Poorly
T – Tooth Loss/Mouth Pain
E – Economic Hardship
R – Reduced Social Contact
M – Multiple Medicines
I – Involuntary Weight Loss/Gain
N – Needs Assistance in Self Care
E – Elder Years Above Age 80

Remember that warning signs suggest risk, but do not represent diagnosis of any condition.

Figure 33–5

Nutritional health screen. (Reprinted with permission by the Nutrition Screening Initiative, a project of the American Academy of Family Physicians, and the American Dietetic Association and the National Council on the Aging, Inc., and funded in part by a grant from Ross Products Division, Abbott Laboratories.)

longer in the body. There may be an increase in biliary lipids with aging. Lipids of particular interest are phospholipids and cholesterol. With their increase, gallstone formation may be enhanced.

With age, often there is increased subcutaneous fat deposits around the abdomen and hips. Abdominal muscle tone may decrease and the abdominal musculature normally thins. If obesity is not present in the aged patient, abdominal organs may be easier to palpate.

Finally, pain in the elderly patient may be a less reliable symptom. The intensity and quality may be diminished. Additionally, if confusion is present, historical information and current reports about GI symptoms may be misleading or inaccurate.

Key Concepts

⇒ The dynamic situation of the critically ill patient requires ongoing assessment of the GI system to construct an accurate, comprehensive patient picture.

⇒ Many GI signs and symptoms may originate from non-GI sources.

⇒ GI assessment includes the entire GI tract and accessory organs.

⇒ History information may be obtained more quickly and easily from family members, significant others, or friends.

⇒ In the abdomen, there are GI structures in the peritoneal and retroperitoneal spaces.

⇒ The sequence to follow in an abdominal examination is inspection, auscultation, percussion, and palpation.

⇒ Abdominal inspection includes examining any openings, tubes, drains, or fluids leading to the skin surface.

⇒ The surface location of bowel sounds may be misleading because such sounds may radiate within the abdomen.

⇒ Abdominal pain is often a nonspecific symptom.

⇒ Abdominal pain that is reported is often referred pain.

TABLE 33–5
Beliefs Relating to Nutrition

Group	Nutritional Beliefs
Adventist (Seventh Day Adventist; Church of God)	Meat prohibited in some groups Lacto-ovo vegetarian diet common Pork, some seafood, some spices, alcohol, caffeine, coffee, or tea discouraged
African-American	May seek help from others, including Root Doctor who uses herbs, oils, and so on
Baptist (multiple groups)	Discourage caffeine and alcohol (some groups)
Black Muslim	Prohibit alcohol, pork, and meat of dead animals or foods common among American blacks (e.g., cornbread, collard greens)
Buddhist Churches of America	Varies with culture Vegetarian diet common Alcohol discouraged
Chinese	Folk healers include herbalists Wide use of medicinal herbs Meals sometimes planned to balance hot and cold Milk intolerance relatively common Spices (e.g., monosodium glutamate and soy sauce) may impede some diet prescriptions
Church of Christian Science	Caffeine and alcohol beverages discouraged
Church of Jesus Christ (Mormon)	Prohibit caffeine (e.g., some teas, coffee, colas, and selected carbonated soft drinks), alcohol Moderation in all things encouraged Fasting for 24 hours on first Sunday of each month (from after evening meal Saturday to evening meal Sunday) Elderly, ill, pregnant persons exempt from fasting
Cuban-American	Nutrition important Traditional Cuban diet rich in meat and starch
Episcopal	Old tradition not often practiced to maintain fast day with no meat
Four-square	Moderation in all things
Friends (Quakers)	Most practice moderation Alcohol discouraged
Greek Orthodox	Church-designated fast periods—usually on all Wednesdays and Fridays, 40 days before Christmas, during Lent, and August 1 to 14 Usually avoid meat, dairy products (for some), and olive oil Shellfish and fish sometimes allowed
Haitian	Foods possess characteristics: hot/cold; light/heavy Work to be in harmony with one's life cycle and bodily states
Hindu	Many dietary restrictions Beef and veal not eaten; some are strict vegetarian
Islam (Muslim/Moslem)	Prohibit all pork and pork products Shellfish possibly prohibited Animals to be slaughtered in proscribed manner (halal) Daylight food and drink fasting during ninth month of Mohammedan year (Ramadan) Exemptions for young children, those ill, traveling, elderly, pregnant, or lactating Other fast days encouraged in Islamic year No alcohol
Japanese	Older persons avoid some food combinations (e.g., milk and cherries; watermelon and crab) May believe pickled plums have special properties
Jehovah's Witness	Eat nothing that has had blood added Can eat animal flesh if meat bled properly
Judaism (Orthodox and Conservative)	Numerous dietary kosher laws that may be influenced by local practices, family, and cultural tradition No pork or shellfish Meat allowed from animals that are vegetable eaters, have cloven hoofs, chew their cud, and are ritually slaughtered, or fish with scales and fins Prohibit any combination of meat and milk; milk products can be served first, with meat following in a few minutes; milk may not be swallowed for several hours after eating meat

TABLE 33-5
Beliefs Relating to Nutrition Continued

Group	Nutritional Beliefs
Judaism (Orthodox and Conservative)	24-hour fasting part of Yom Kippur and other holiday observances
	Matzo replaces leavened bread or grain products during Passover week
	Not required to fast if adverse to health, elderly, pregnant, or persons younger than 13 years old
Mexican American	May adhere to "hot" and "cold" food prescriptions
Middle Eastern	Some lactose intolerance
	Seasonal fresh fruits and vegetables encouraged
	Diet uses many foods of plant origin
	Meal times tend to be later than in United States; middle meal often followed by nap
Native Americans (many tribes)	Specialists use herbs
Nazarene	Alcohol prohibited
Puerto Rican	Folk healers often use herbs
Roman Catholic	Fasting or abstaining from meat mandatory on Ash Wednesday and Good Friday; fasting optional during Lent
	Traditionally no meat on Fridays during Lent
	Exempt from fasting if detrimental to health or in children, elderly
	Some may adhere to rule of eating fish on Friday
Russian Orthodox	No meat or dairy products on Wednesdays, Fridays, period before Christmas, during Lent, period between Pentecost and July, and 2 weeks in August
	Fish or shellfish are acceptable; wine and oil may be prohibited during fast
	Two fasting levels: (1) no meat or dairy (fish acceptable); (2) no meat, dairy, fish, shellfish, wine, or oil
Vietnamese	May use special diets to prevent illness
	Lactose intolerance common

Data from Seidel H, Ball J, Dains J, Benedict G: Mosby's Guide to Physical Examination. St. Louis, Mosby, 1996, pp 40–48, and Packard D, McWilliams M: Cultural foods heritage of Middle Eastern immigrants. Nutrition Today 28(3):6–12, 1993.

⟱ Rebound tenderness is identifiable only with release of pressure.

⟱ Several treatments of the critically ill can depress intestinal peristalsis, making these patients at increased risk for constipation or fecal impaction; yet, other conditions or treatments, including medications, can cause diarrhea.

⟱ A nutritional assessment includes attention to macronutrients and micronutrients.

⟱ The critically ill patient is in a hypermetabolic state, and the nutritional status in the critically ill patient is dynamic.

⟱ Periodic nutritional assessment updates are needed to maintain a current plan and treatments.

⟱ Several changes with aging can make the oral cavity more fragile.

⟱ Gut motility decreases with age.

⟱ With the reduced hepatic blood flow seen with aging, substances normally metabolized or detoxified by the liver remain active longer in the body.

⟱ Pain in the elderly may not be a reliable indicator of underlying problems.

References

1. American Society of Parenteral and Enteral Nutrition: Nutrition Assessment Anthology. Silver Spring, MD, Author, 1991.

2. Treloar DM, Stechmiller JK. Use of a clinical assessment tool for orally intubated patients. Am J Crit Care 4(5):355–360, 1995.

3. Goins W, Rodriguez A: Retroperitoneal injuries. In Maull K, Rodriguez A, Wiles C III, eds. Complications in Trauma and Critical Care. Philadelphia, WB Saunders, pp 442–452.

4. Jarvis C: Physical Examination and Health Assessment. Philadelphia, WB Saunders, 1996.

5. Seidel H, Ball J, Dains J, Benedict G: Mosby's Guide to Physical Examination. St. Louis: Mosby, 1996.

6. Sosa J, Reines H: Evaluating the acute abdomen. In Civetta J, Taylor R, Kirby R, eds., Critical Care, 3rd ed. Philadelphia, Lippincott-Raven, 1099–1108.

7. Bonica J: The Management of Pain, 2nd ed. Vol. 1. Philadelphia, Lea & Febiger, 1990.

8. Burkhart C: Guidelines for rapid assessment of abdominal pain indicative of acute surgical abdomen. Nurse Practitioner 17(6):39,43–44,46,49, 1992.

9. Detsky A, McLaughlin J, Baker J, Johnston N, Whittaker S, Mendelson R, Jeejeebhoy K: What is subjective global assessment of nutritional status? JPEN J Parenter Enteral Nutr 11:8–13, 1987.

10. Jeejeebhoy K, Detsky A, Baker J: Assessment of nutritional status. JPEN J Parenter Enteral Nutr 14:193S–198S, 1990.

11. Dwyer J: Nutrition Screening I: Toward a Common View. Washington, DC, Nutrition Screening Initiative, 1991.

12. Posner B, Jette A, Smith K, Miller D: Nutrition and health risks in the elderly: the nutrition screening initiative. Am J Public Health 83:972–978, 1993.

13. DeHoog S: The assessment of nutritional status. In Mahan L, Escott-Stump S, eds. Krause's Food, Nutrition, & Diet Therapy, 9th ed. Philadelphia, WB Saunders, 1996, pp 361–386.

14. Ham R: The signs and symptoms of poor nutritional status. Prim Care 21(1):33–54, 1994.

15. Nikolaus T, Bach M, Siezen S, Volkert D, Oster P, Schlierf G: Assessment of nutritional risk in the elderly. Ann Nutr Metab 39:340–345, 1995.

16. Stack J, Babineau T, Bistrian B: Assessment of nutritional status in clinical practice. Gastroenterologist 4(Suppl I):S8–S15, 1996.

17. Packard D, McWilliams M: Cultural foods heritage of Middle Eastern immigrants. Nutrition Today 28(3):6–12, 1993.

18. Luggen A, ed. *NGNA Core Curriculum for Gerontological Nursing.* St. Louis: Mosby, 1996.

19. Reuben D, Greendale G, Harrison G: Nutrition screening in older persons. J Am Geriatr Soc 43:415–425, 1995.

20. Worthington-Roberts B, Williams S, eds. Nutrition Throughout the Life Cycle, 3rd ed. St. Louis, Mosby–Yeark Book, 1996.

34

Gastrointestinal Laboratory and Diagnostic Tests

Una Elizabeth Westfall

Objectives

After completing this chapter, the student will be able to:

1. Differentiate between liver and pancreatic function tests.
2. Link liver diagnostic tests with specific liver functions.
3. Specify strengths and shortcomings for using an albumin level to determine the nutritional status of a patient in intensive care.
4. Compare and contrast the diagnostic procedures of abdominal computed tomography (CT), ultrasonography, and magnetic resonance imaging regarding purpose, indications, contraindications, and nursing care.
5. Describe three types of gastrointestinal (GI) endoscopies including purpose, location viewed, nursing preparation, and nursing follow-up.

Multiple laboratory and diagnostic tests are used to isolate GI disorders. Generally, multiple abdominal findings are used to confirm the presence of a particular disorder. Even with history and physical examination data, there are large portions of the GI tract that remain hidden. The oral cavity is the only portion of the GI system visible to the eye. Thus, laboratory and diagnostic test findings, coupled with history and physical data, contribute to accurate diagnosis of GI problems.

LABORATORY TESTS

Liver

Tests for structural and functional integrity of the liver include several blood tests that focus on the hepatocyte (i.e., liver cell) as well as on different liver functions.[1, 2] Major liver functions include metabolism of carbohydrates, proteins, and fats; formation and excretion of bile; synthesis of certain circulating proteins such as albumin and several coagulation factors; synthesis of cholesterol; detoxification of substances such as ammonia, an end product of protein metabolism,

and many pharmacologic agents; steroid metabolism; and storage of fat-soluble vitamins and selected minerals such as copper and iron. Testing hepatocyte integrity often includes measuring cellular enzymes, selected proteins manufactured in the liver, clotting ability and factors, and end products such as ammonia or drug levels. Common laboratory tests for the hepatobiliary system focus on bilirubin, cholesterol, and other lipids. It follows that patterns of abnormalities are more useful than any single laboratory test of liver function.[3, 4]

With hepatocyte damage or destruction, intracellular enzymes are released into the blood. Many of the enzymes are found in other body tissues as well. Thus, recent work identifying isoenzymes has been helpful in isolating enzymatic components from the liver. Common enzyme tests used to evaluate the liver are listed in Table 34–1.

Alkaline phosphatase has an isoenzyme, AP-1, alpha2, that originates in the liver, and an isoenzyme AP-3,beta2, that arises in the intestine. Two isoenzymes of lactate dehydrogenase (LD or LDH) are of interest in suspected liver pathology. LD4 and LD5 are the major LD isoenzymes from the liver and skeletal muscle.

TABLE 34–1
Common Liver Enzyme Blood Tests

Enzyme (Serum)	Reference Values	Comments
Alkaline phosphatase (ALP) and isoenzyme	Norms: Adult: 20–90 U/L at 30°C (SI units) 25–97 U/L at 37°C (SI units), 4–13 U/dL (King-Armstrong) ALP₁ 20–130 U/L	ALP is found mainly in bone and liver and also in intestine, kidney, and placenta. Since ALP is produced by several systems and cells in the body, its activity is classified as nonspecific; therefore other liver function tests should be performed to confirm the diagnosis. In severe liver damage (e.g., cancer of liver, hepato-cellular problems) serum ALP is greatly increased. ALP isoenzymes assist in identifying the origin of the problem. ALP_1 is of liver origin, and ALP_2 is of bone origin.
5'Nucleotidase (5'NT or 5'N)	Norms: <17 U/L	5'NT is specific to liver cells. ALP and 5'NT are measured at the same time, since both enzymes are found in liver cells and are elevated in hepatocellular disease. However, serum ALP will be elevated in bone disease, but 5'NT will not be increased.
Leucine aminopeptidase (LAP)	Norms: 8–22 mU/mL, 12–33 IU/L, 75–200 U/mL, 20–50 U/L at 37°C (SI units)	LAP enzyme is found mainly in liver tissue. Serum LAP is elevated in liver disease (e.g., cancer of the liver, viral hepatitis, acute necrosis of the liver, and extrahepatic biliary obstruction). LAP, 5'NT, and ALP tests are frequently ordered together to confirm liver disease. If only ALP is elevated and the other two enzymes are not, bone disease would be probable.
Alanine aminotransferase (ALT or SGPT)	Norms: Adult: 5–35 U/mL (Frankel) 5–25 mU/mL (Wroblewski) 4–35 U/L at 37°C (SI units)	ALT/SGPT is found primarily in liver cells and is effective in diagnosing hepatocellular obstruction. AST is found in liver cells; however, it is more specific to cardiac muscle and skeletal muscle. Serum ALT is slightly to moderately increased in cancer of the liver and cirrhosis. It is highly increased during viral hepatitis and drug hepatotoxicity.
Lactic dehydrogenase (LD/LDH) Isoenzymes	Norms: Adult: 100–190 IU/L Isoenzyme LDH₅ 6%–16%	LDH is elevated in heart, lung, liver, and renal disease. To determine if the increased LDH is due to liver disease, LDH isoenzymes are measured. LDH_5 rises before jaundice occurs and falls before bilirubin level does.
Gamma-glutamyl transferase/ transpeptidase (GGT/GGTP)	Norms: Adult: Male: 4–23 IU/L Female: 3–13 IU/L Average: 0–45 U/L	GGT/GGTP is found mostly in the liver and kidney and small amounts in heart muscle, spleen, and prostate gland. It is a more sensitive indicator for liver disease than other liver enzymes (e.g., ALP and AST/SGOT). Elevated GGT/GGTP occurs in cirrhosis of the liver, alcoholism, cancer of the liver, viral hepatitis, and acute pancreatitis.

AST, aspartate aminotransferase.
From Kee J: Laboratory and Diagnostic Tests with Nursing Implications, 4th ed. Stamford, CT, Appleton & Lange, 1995, pp 543–546.

Measurements of two types of transaminase intracellular enzymes, alanine aminotransaminase (ALT) and aspartate aminotransaminase (AST), are often requested when liver injury is suspected. AST is distributed in multiple body tissues, such as the heart and muscle, as well as the liver. ALT is primarily found in the liver and kidneys. The circulating half-life of ALT is more than twice that of AST, that is, 47 and 17 hours, respectively.[2] Elevated levels may be markers of liver injury or necrosis. However, in a situation in which most liver tissue has been destroyed, such as chronic cirrhosis, the enzyme levels may be low or normal because little functional tissue remains.

Normal values for liver function tests are listed in Table 34–2. Forms of serum bilirubin include total,

conjugated (direct), and unconjugated (indirect). Additionally, the urinary end product, urobilinogen, can be measured when liver or biliary disorders are suspected. The breakdown of red blood cells gives rise to bilirubin. The unconjugated form is bound to albumin; the conjugated form circulates freely in the blood. Normally, bilirubin is converted to a water-soluble form in the liver. If the amount of bilirubin entering the liver exceeds its capacity, the unconjugated bilirubin level is elevated. If the liver transformation occurred but there is difficulty in excreting the conjugated form, the conjugated bilirubin level is elevated.

In the duodenum, conjugated bilirubin is converted to urobilinogen. Decreased levels of urobilinogen can occur with severe liver damage, inflammatory disease,

TABLE 34–2
Common Liver Function Laboratory Tests

Liver Function Tests (Blood or Urine)	Reference Values	Comments
Bilirubin, total (blood)	Adult: 0.1–1.2 mg/dL	Serum sample
Indirect/unconjugated	0.1–1.0 mg/dL	Form bound to albumin
Direct/conjugated	0.1–0.3 mg/dL	Water-soluble form
Urobilinogen (urine)	0–0.02 mg/dL	Conjugated form likely because unconjugated form not water soluble
Proteins, total (blood)	Adult: 5.0–8.0 g/dL	Several proteins make up total value
Albumin	3.5–5.0 g/dL	Electrophoresis enables amount and type of protein in sample to be identified
Globulin	0.8–3.0 g/dL	
Prothrombin time (blood)	Adult: 12–14 seconds	Interinstitutional level variations
Factor II	100% normal activity	Requires vitamin K
Fibrinogen (blood)	Adult: 200–400 mg/dL	Synthesized by liver
Factor I		Converted to fibrin by thrombin
Activated plasma (blood) thromboplastin time (APPT)	21–35 seconds	Screens for coagulation disorders; often used to monitor heparin therapy
		Prolonged in liver disease or vitamin K deficiency
Cholesterol (blood)	Adult: <200mg/dL	Synthesized cholesterol transported as low-density or high-density lipoproteins
		Liver esterifies ~70% circulating cholesterol
High-density lipoproteins (HDL)	Men: 35–70 mg/dL	HDLs carry excess cholesterol back to liver
	Women: 35–85 mg/dL	High levels protective
Low-density lipoproteins (LDL)	<130 mg/dL desirable	Carry most of cholesterol from liver to tissues; high levels atherogenic
	>159 mg/dL high risk	
Very-low-density lipoproteins (VLDL)	25%–50%	VLDL degradation is major source of LDL
Ammonia (blood)	Adult: 15–45 μg/dL	End product of protein metabolism; converted to urea in liver
	11–35 μmol/L (SI units)	

or obstruction in the biliary system. Elevated levels may occur in early cirrhosis or hepatitis.

Many serum proteins are synthesized by the liver. Protein electrophoresis can be used to identify types and amounts of protein present. The protein albumin is decreased in liver cell damage, as well as in conditions such as malnutrition and renal disease. The circulating half-life of albumin is approximately 20 days. Thus, by itself, it may give a falsely optimistic picture in a dynamic situation. Additionally, with administration of albumin, the serum level reflects therapeutic contributions as well as amounts produced by the liver during the prior 2- to 3-week period. To more accurately measure nutritional status, a prealbumin level may be sought. Prealbumin levels are not affected by albumin infusion. Furthermore, the half-life of prealbumin is considerably shorter.[5] Comparison of common serum proteins often used in nutritional assessment is shown in Table 34–3.

Coagulation factors and anticlotting factors are adversely affected by liver disease. The liver stores vitamin K and uses it in synthesizing several necessary clotting factors. Studies of clotting factors such as fibrinogen, prothrombin time (PT), and activated partial thromboplastin time (APTT) or partial thromboplastin time (PTT) can aid in determining the functional status

of these elements. The PTT and APTT test for the same liver functions. Extensive damage and hepatocyte necrosis can delay coagulation. Some clotting-related values have been reported to manifest a circadian cycle, or sleep-wake difference.[6–8] Such variability can influence interpretation of levels, as well as affect anticoagulant therapy adjustments.

Cholesterol is a lipid that can be synthesized in the liver. Derangement in lipoprotein metabolism can occur with hepatic disorders. With prolonged liver damage and poor nutrition, the circulating cholesterol level can be low. When there is obstruction of flow from the biliary tract, serum levels of cholesterol may be elevated. Elevated triglycerides with hepatocyte injury are often found in the low-density lipoprotein (LDL) fraction or in the phospholipids in very-low-density lipoprotein (VLDL). Furthermore, there may be a decrease in the high-density lipoproteins (HDL).[2]

Multiple substances are detoxified by the liver. Ammonia, an end product of amino acid metabolism, is detoxified in the liver to urea. When the liver ceases to function, ammonia builds up in the circulation. Also, if intrahepatic portal shunting occurs, circulating ammonia bypasses the liver, thereby leading to an elevated serum level.

TABLE 34–3

Common Serum Proteins and Nutritional Status

Serum Protein	Half-life	Degree of Reduction		
		Mild	Moderate	Severe
Albumin (g/dL)	20 days	2.8–3.4	2.1–2.7	<2.1
Transferrin (mg/dL)	4–8 days	150–200	100–149	<100
Prealbumin (mg/dL)	2 days	10–15	5–9	<5

Data from Gibson R: Principles of Nutritional Assessment. New York, Oxford University Press, 1990, pp 547–549.

If pharmacologic agents are metabolized or excreted by the liver and liver function is compromised, systemic levels may exceed the therapeutic range, or drug effects may be prolonged. Drug peak and trough levels may be requested to determine how effectively pharmacologic substances are being cleared by the liver.

Pancreas

Pancreatic blood studies commonly include levels of amylase, lipase, glucose, triglycerides, and calcium, both total and ionized. These studies are outlined in Table 34–4. Serum amylase is found in multiple body tissues, including the pancreas (P-form), parotid glands (S-form), intestine, liver, and fallopian tubes. In contrast, the major and primary source of lipase is the pancreas. Not only the level, but the duration of elevation, can be important in diagnostic patterns. For example, in acute pancreatitis, the level of serum amylase can read four to six times the normal limit. Levels return to normal within 3 to 4 days. However, serum amylase levels often remain elevated when a pancreatic pseudocyst is present.

Several therapeutic conditions can influence the level of serum amylase. For example, intravenous glucose can lead to a decrease in amylase. Several drugs that are often used with critically ill patients, such as meperidine, morphine, and codeine, can elevate amylase levels.

In addition to digestive enzymes, cells within the pancreas contribute to blood glucose levels through the hormones of insulin and glucagon. With pancreatic disruption, their production or secretion can be altered. Thus, blood glucose levels may need to be monitored frequently.

Often, the critically ill patient receives glucose intravenously. During their hypermetabolic state, patients

TABLE 34–4

Common Laboratory Tests for the Pancreas

Pancreatic Tests (Blood or Urine)	Reference Values	Comments
Amylase (blood)	Adult: 25–125 U/L	Interinstitutional variations
		Levels increase in acute pancreatitis; return to base in <5 days
Amylase (urine)	2-hr 2–34 units	Levels low—pancreatic insufficiency
	24-hr 24–408 units	Urine values 6–10 hr behind blood changes
		Refrigerate specimen
Lipase (blood)	Adult: 10–140 U/L	Pancreas major source
		In blood with organ damage
		Remains elevated after amylase returns to baseline
Fasting glucose (blood)	Adult: 65–110 mg/dL	Intravenous glucose may prevent "fasting" level
		Multiple intensive care factors cause increase (e.g., physical stress)
		Multiple factors cause decrease (e.g., liver damage, starvation)
Triglycerides (blood)	Male: 30–100 mg/dL	Measure body's ability to metabolize fat
	Female: 35–110 mg/dL	Elevation with liver disease, alcohol use, pancreatitis, among other conditions
Serum calcium (blood)		
Total	Adult: 8.6–10.0 mg/dL	Circulating Ca^{++} ionized (50%); protein bound (50%)
	2.15–2.5 mmol/L	Hypoalbuminemia common cause of low total calcium
		High total calcium levels in cancer of liver, pancreas, and other organs
Ionized	Adult: 4.65–5.28 mg/dL	Used to track disorders including cancer, acute pancreatitis
	1.16–1.32 mmol/L	

may temporarily become insulin resistant or glucose intolerant. If the glucose level exceeds the ability of the body to maintain blood glucose within the normal range, multiple mechanisms are activated. When glucose exceeds the renal threshold, it is excreted in the urine and acts as an osmotic diuretic. Furthermore, elevated blood glucose levels can exert a depressant effect on the central nervous system.

DIAGNOSTIC TESTS

Diagnostic tests often used to examine selected portions of the GI system are identified in Table 34–5 and diagnostic tests for gastrointestinal disorders are identified in Table 34–6. Common noninvasive abdominal diagnostic tests include x-ray studies and fluoroscopy, forms of CT, ultrasonography, and magnetic resonance imaging. Invasive diagnostic tests often used to investigate GI conditions include nuclear scans, peritoneal lavage, endoscopies, biopsies, and angiography.

The nurse is often the person who is in the position to listen to concerns of the patient or family when diagnostic tests are scheduled. From this information, preparation can be tailored for the critically ill patient, family, or significant other. In part because these people often have limited reserves, diagnostic test preparation is often streamlined. Thus, knowing institutional policies for test preparation, including the need for informed consent authorization, as well as any precautions to take during or following the test, can help the critically ill patient and family prepare for the diagnostic procedure. Explanations that are brief, but informative and complete, may be most helpful in this environment that is already stressful. The element of time may assume unanticipated dimensions for the patient or family. If there are delays, the nurse can

keep the family or patient informed of the progress, thereby reducing unnecessary speculation.

X-ray Studies and Fluoroscopy

X-rays are used to inspect soft and bony tissues within the body. In part because of their short wavelength, these rays can penetrate dense tissues and the absorbed rays result in images that can be recorded on photographic film. Different body tissue densities result in distinct shades on the developed film. By convention, x-ray images have air appearing as black, bone (tissue high in density) appearing white, and soft tissues in shades of gray. Because the stomach and intestines normally contain some air, these structures appear darker on the x-ray than does a solid organ such as the liver.

X-ray studies may be obtained of structures such as the esophagus, stomach, small bowel, or colon, as well as regions such as the peritoneal and retroperitoneal spaces. Such diagnostic tests may be conducted without introduction of a contrast substance, with a radiopaque substance, or with a gas such as oxygen, carbon dioxide, nitrous oxide, or nitrogen. When contrast media are used to visualize part of the GI tract, these substances can be given orally, rectally, or by injection.

X-rays permit visualization of body tissues along a flat plane. If a structure overlays the area to be viewed, the desired image may be obstructed. An often-ordered x-ray study is the abdominal plain film or "flat plate." The patient is most often supine, upright, or positioned on the left side (left lateral decubitus position). The latter positions can be used especially when there is a suspicion of free air in the abdomen, such as from a perforated bowel. Air is evident just below the diaphragm in Figure 34–1.

TABLE 34–5
Diagnostic Tests for Gastrointestinal System

Test	Description/Purpose
Angiography	X-ray studies of selected vascular beds and flow
Biopsy	Invasive procedure resulting in collection of tissue from organ or structure
Computed tomography (CT)	X-ray study producing cross-sectional images of underlying structures and tissues
Endoscopy (see Table 34–7)	Uses fiberoptic instrument to visually inspect internal organs or tissues; may also be used for certain procedures or treatments
Fluoroscopy	Series of rapid x-ray beams that provide data about movement and location of organs within gastrointestinal (GI) tract
Magnetic resonance imaging	Uses magnetic energy sources that result in coronal, axial, or sagittal images without radiation
Nuclear scan	Visual inspection of organ or organ portion; nonuniform radioactive uptake in tissues often indicates disease; also used to detect motility within GI tract
Radiography	Beams of short wavelength x-rays penetrate tissues; the amount of x-ray absorbed dependent on tissue density. Results transfer to photographic film. Density can be altered with air or contrast media
Spiral computed tomography	Conventional CT technique modification resulting in three-dimensional data composite
Ultrasonography (sonogram)	Visual inspection of soft tissue structures through use of high-frequency sound waves

TABLE 34–6
Diagnostic Tests for Gastrointestinal Disorders

Diagnostic Test	Indications	Contraindications	Nursing Actions
X-ray examination, flat plate Abdomen	Aid in diagnosis of intraabdominal conditions (e.g., intestinal obstruction, organ rupture, masses, foreign bodies, abnormal fluid or air)	Known early pregnancy	Protect patient gonads with shield.
X-ray examination, contrast Upper gastrointestinal (GI) tract	Visualize esophagus, stomach, duodenum, into jejunum, and pathologic conditions (e.g., hiatal hernia, tumors, peptic ulcer, foreign bodies)	Allergy to contrast medium; inability to tolerate contrast medium or positions	Solicit allergy history for contrast media. If needed, schedule other tests before barium use. Obtain pretest and posttest vital signs. Assist with needed positioning. Check on limiting oral or enteral intake before test. Take actions to help patient expel contrast medium. Record stool color, amount, consistency.
Small intestine	Visualize jejunum, ileum, cecum, pathologic conditions (e.g., Meckel's diverticulum, tumors, Crohn's disease, visceral hernia)	Allergy to contrast medium; inability to tolerate contrast medium or positions	Solicit allergy history for contrast media. If needed, schedule other test before barium use. Obtain pretest and posttest vital signs. Assist with needed positioning. Check on limiting oral or enteral intake before test. Take actions to help patient expel contrast medium. Record stool color, amount, consistency.
Colon (barium enema)	Visualize colon structure and filling pathologic conditions (e.g., obstructions, fistulae, tumors, diverticulae, polyps, stenosis)	Allergy to contrast medium; inability to tolerate needed pretest cleansing of bowel, contrast medium, or positions	Solicit allergy history for contrast media. If needed, schedule other tests before barium use. Obtain pretest and posttest vital signs. Assist with needed positioning. Check on colon preparation to use with patient. Take actions to help patient expel contrast medium. Record stool color, amount, consistency
Computed tomography scan	Visualize abdomen, retroperitoneal structures, tumors, cysts, abscess, fluid pocket, or air in cavity	Avoid barium if perforation in GI tract suspected, allergy to contrast media, claustrophobia, physiologically unstable	Solicit history for possible allergy to contrast materials. If needed, schedule other tests before barium use. Obtain pretest and posttest vital signs. Assist patient to lie still. Give sedative. Assess patient for allergic reaction, passing of contrast media.

TABLE 34–6
Diagnostic Tests for Gastrointestinal Disorders *Continued*

Diagnostic Test	Indications	Contraindications	Nursing Actions
Ultrasound sonography	Characterize abdomen and retroperitoneal soft tissues, fluid pocket or air in cavity, abscess; observe movement	Scar tissue over area to be studied distorts signal. Dressings preclude access to skin above site of interest. Fatty tissue can alter wave (obese patient may not be candidate). Barium and air distort echo. Open wounds limit lubricant use.	Limit patient's enteral or oral intake. Inform patient that gel will be applied to skin over examination area. Help patient lie quietly in supine decubitus position; often some controlled breathing is needed. Pressure may be applied with transducer.
Magnetic resonance imaging	Evaluate abdomen, retroperitoneal structures, abdominal neoplasms, abscesses, cysts, ascites, fluid pocket, air in cavity	Internal metallic devices; attached external metal objects; claustrophobia; obesity; physiologic instability; inability to maintain still position	Remove external metal objects, dental appliances. Obtain accurate history regarding internal metal/metallic implants. Assist patient to lie still.
Radionuclide scanning	Visualize organs; elements of GI motility; detect location of lower GI bleeding	Pregnant or breast-feeding; some recent nuclear dynamic instability	Solicit history of allergy, pregnancy, breast feeding, recent nuclear exposure history. Obtain weight and age to use in calculating dose. Note drainage tubes. Remove metal. Report whether patient recently received barium, which may not have cleared tract. After test, monitor injection site. Have visitors and pregnant staff avoid prolonged contact until nuclide is cleared from patient's body.
Peritoneal lavage	Abdominal blunt and penetrating trauma	Medical judgment regarding usefulness	Assemble sterile catheter, equipment for insertion, sterile normal saline. Observe insertion site for bleeding, leakage, infection. Obtain vital signs before and after procedure.
Biopsy: organ specific Liver (percutaneous)	Tissue needed for examination	Bleeding disorder; major ascites; infection at site	Obtain baseline and follow-up vital signs. Obtain signed permission Ensure sterile procedure. Turn patient to right side after biopsy. Observe for pneumothorax, bleeding. Provide pain control measures.
Liver (transvenous)		Bleeding disorder; biliary obstruction	Obtain baseline and follow-up vital signs. Obtain signed permission Ensure sterile procedure.

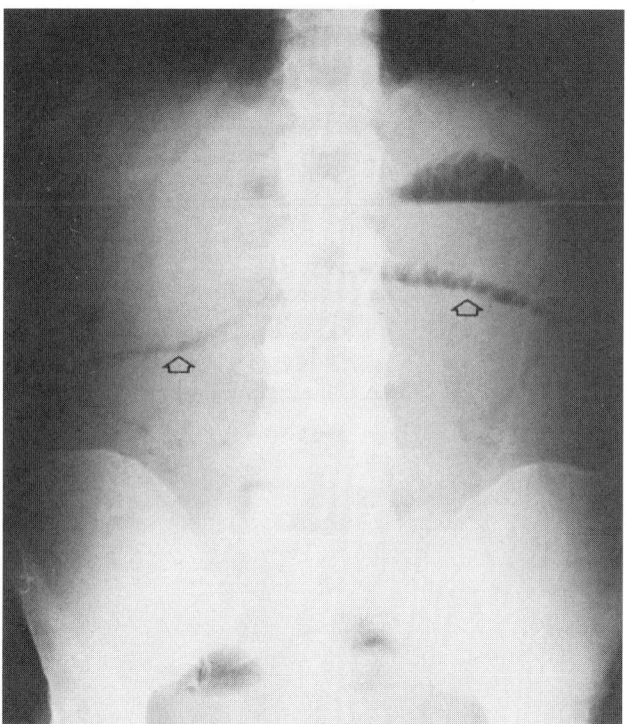

Figure 34–1

Flat plate upright abdominal radiograph showing small bowel obstruction with a string of beads sign. Small amounts of air are trapped between valvulae in the superior portion of fluid-distended loops (*arrows*). (From Putman C, Ravin C: Textbook of Diagnostic Imaging, vol. 1, 2nd ed. Philadelphia, WB Saunders, 1994, p 784.)

Most often, a plain film uses only natural contrasts of tissues, and can be helpful in detecting such GI conditions as intestinal obstruction, ruptured organs, foreign bodies, and abnormal fluids such as ascites. Such a film gives information about the size, position, and shape of the GI organs as well as the spleen and kidneys.

With introduction of contrast media into the GI system, more details can be added to the tissues and structures visible on x-ray film. To prevent nonsoluble radiopaque contrast media from moving out of the GI tract, barium sulfate should not be used unless the GI tract is known to be intact. A water-soluble substance such as diatrizoate meglumine (Gastrografin) can be used in place of barium sulfate. Figure 34–2 shows the use of water-soluble contrast media, in this case when detecting a perforation in the esophagus.

Because radiopaque substances conceal structures behind them, diagnostic tests not requiring contrast substances should be completed first. Additionally, contrast media given to improve visualization in the upper GI tract can obscure findings in the lower tract until the substance has been expelled. On the other hand, absorbable gases may be used to enhance the contrast between tissues of interest. Figure 34–3 is an example of air contrast used to visualize a hiatus hernia.

Depending on the area to be visualized, during the test, the patient may be asked to change positions and

to breathe at specific times. If possible, metal materials should be removed from the patient before the radiograph is obtained.

When a contrast medium is used to visualize the upper GI tract, food and fluid may need to be withheld from the patient before the study. The patient may be asked to swallow the substance or it may be administered through an enteral tube. The study is most often performed in a special diagnostic department. A critically ill or debilitated patient may be unable to participate in such studies.

Following the test, the contrast solution needs to be expelled. Laxatives may be ordered. For the critically ill patient already at risk for constipation because of medications and limited mobility, evacuation of barium or diatrizoate meglumine may be particularly challenging. The nurse needs to observe and record stools for amount, color, and consistency. If not removed from the tract, contrast substances can harden and lead to problems such as fecal impaction. Preexisting conditions, such as an ileostomy or colostomy, can alter the care needed following contrast medium administration.

If only the colon is to be assessed, actions are often needed to ensure the large bowel is clean. However,

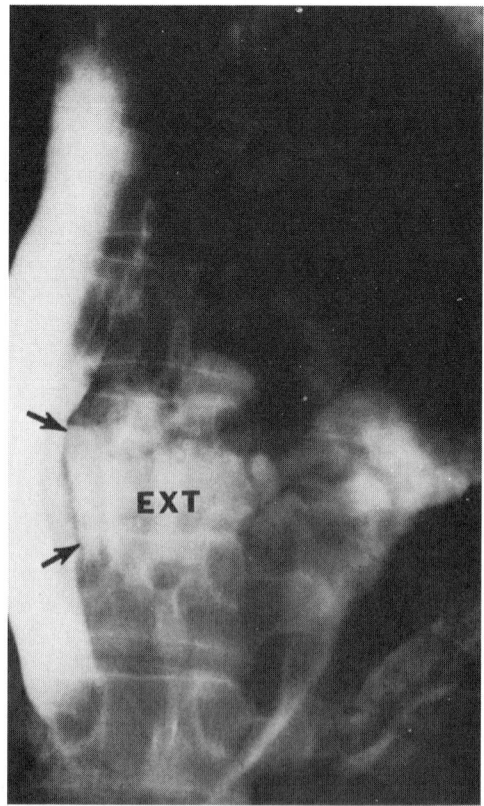

Figure 34–2

Use of water-soluble contrast with radiography showing esophageal perforation (*arrows*) resulting from endoscopic trauma. Extravasation (EXT) of water-soluble contrast into the mediastinum and pleural space is visible. (From Putman C, Ravin C: Textbook of Diagnostic Imaging, vol. 1, 2nd ed. Philadelphia, WB Saunders, 1994, p 697.)

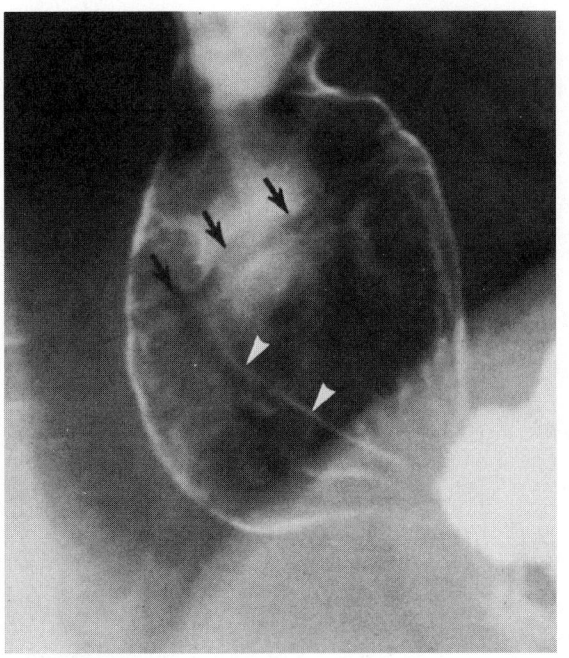

Figure 34–3

Use of air as contrast in a radiograph of the distal esophagus and stomach showing a hiatus hernia above the diaphragm. Distal to the thin mucosal web *(arrows)* are gastric folds *(arrowheads)*. (From Putman C, Ravin C: Textbook of Diagnostic Imaging, vol. 1, 2nd ed. Philadelphia, WB Saunders, 1994, p 679.)

the rigor required for complete visualization may be poorly tolerated by a person who is critically ill. Preparation traditionally includes actions to minimize new substances entering from the upper GI tract as well as actions to clean the large bowel with laxatives and enemas. The nurse should consult with radiology personnel and the medical team to ensure patient safety in this pretest period. Inadequate colon preparation is illustrated in Figure 34–4.

A fluoroscopy study is a series of rapid sequential radiographs. This technique records tract activity as it takes place inside the body. Such activities can include movement, filling, and placement of a radiopaque substance throughout any region of the GI tract. The patient must be able to assume and maintain a position that allows multiple pictures of the desired area. Exposure to x-rays is greater with this test than from a conventional x-ray study. Actions identified previously to assist with passing contrast from the body also apply for contrast media introduced into the GI tract.

Computed Tomography

CT or computed axial tomography (CAT) is a noninvasive technique that produces detailed cross-sectional

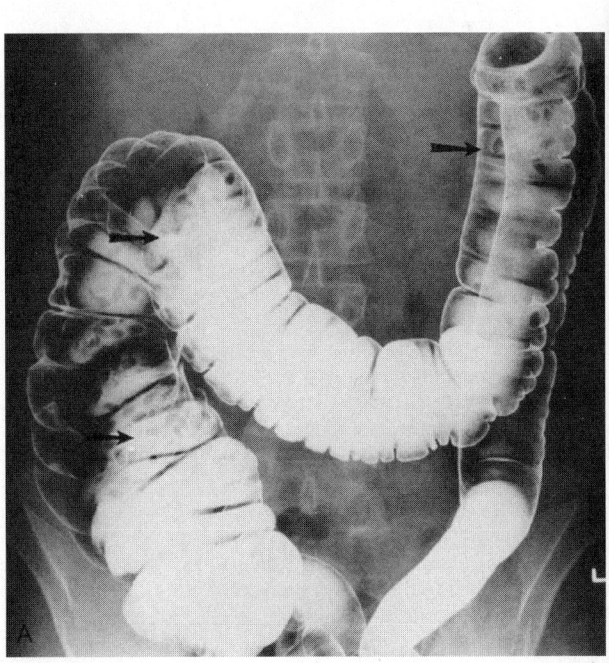

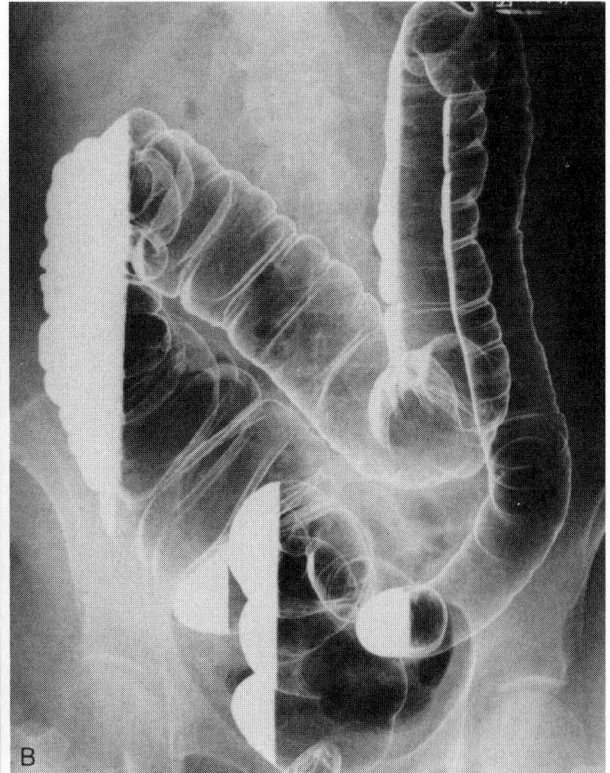

Figure 34–4

Radiograph showing evidence of inadequate bowel preparation. *A,* Film from a double-contrast barium enema shows multiple nodular filling defects *(arrows)* that could be mistaken for polyps. *B,* Decubitus film is helpful because the filling defects are no longer present as a result of having fallen into the barium pool, a finding indicating that they represent nonadherent fecal residue. (From Putman C, Ravin C: Textbook of Diagnostic Imaging, vol. 1, 2nd ed. Philadelphia, WB Saunders, 1994, p 823.)

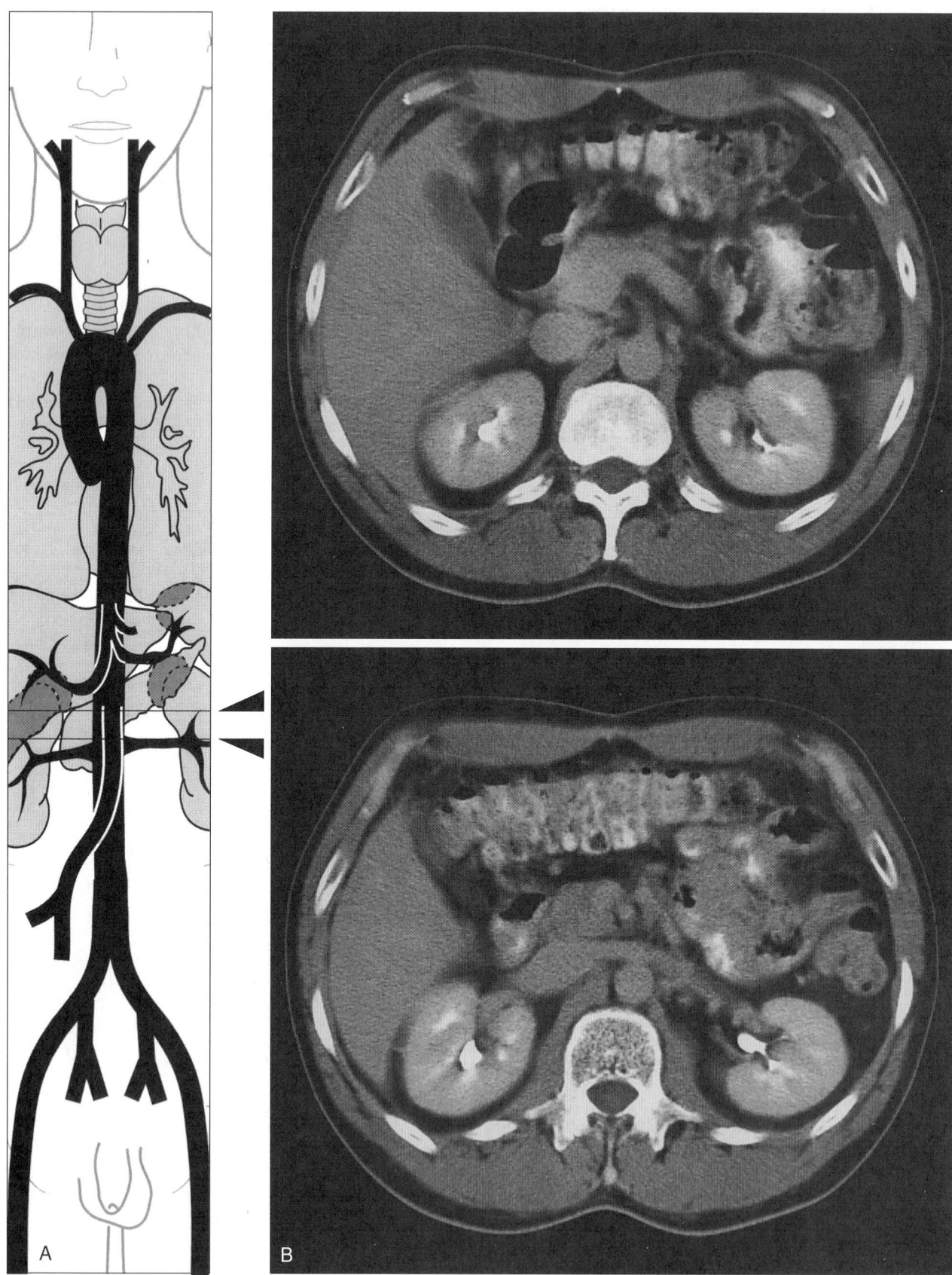

Figure 34–5

Computed tomography (CT) of an abdominal slice. *A,* Vertical schematic identifying location of transverse abdominal image. *B,* CT image showing anatomic structures at this transverse level. (From Wegener O: Whole Body Computed Tomography. Boston, Blackwell Scientific Publications, 1993, pp 46–47.)

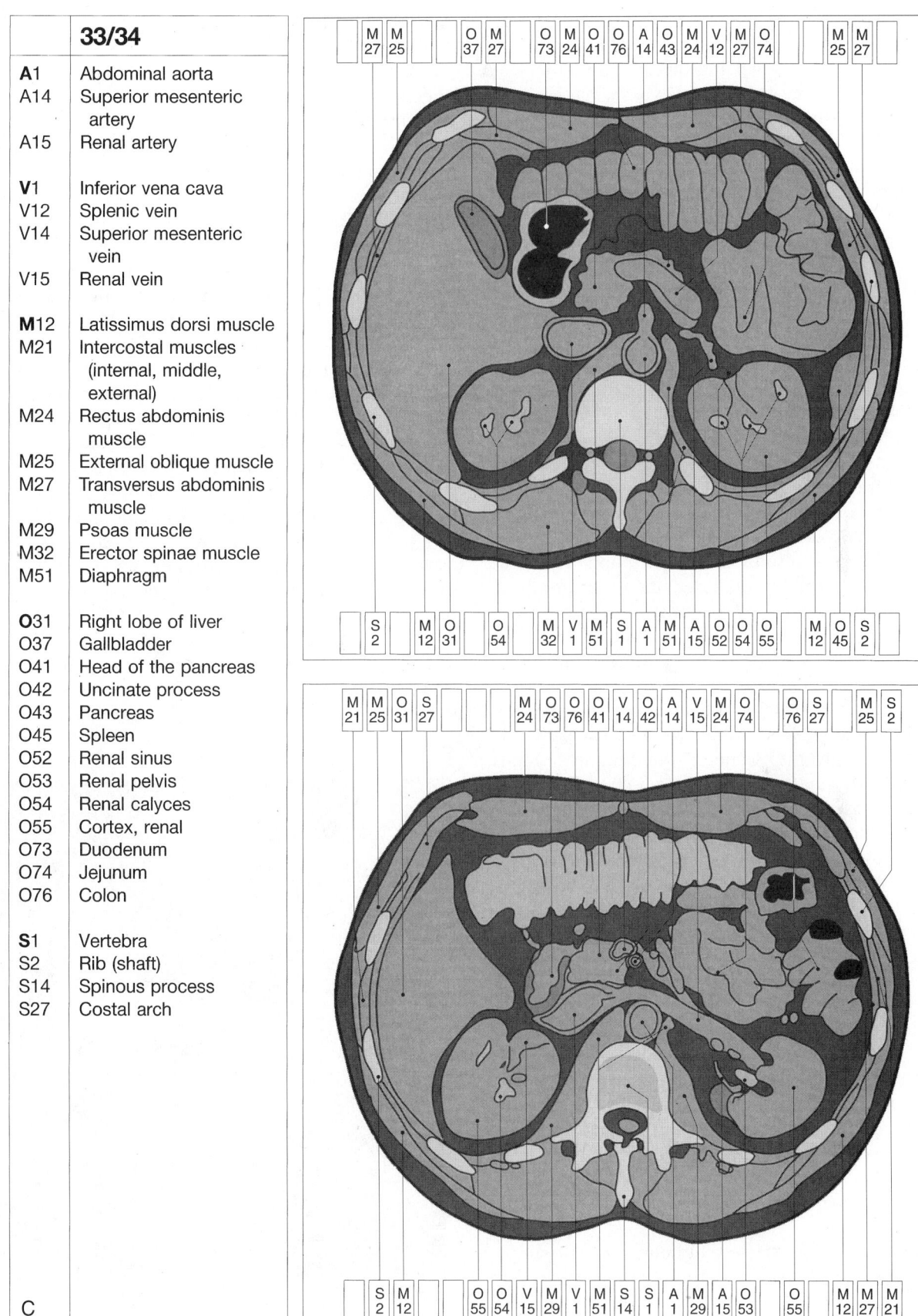

33/34

A1	Abdominal aorta
A14	Superior mesenteric artery
A15	Renal artery
V1	Inferior vena cava
V12	Splenic vein
V14	Superior mesenteric vein
V15	Renal vein
M12	Latissimus dorsi muscle
M21	Intercostal muscles (internal, middle, external)
M24	Rectus abdominis muscle
M25	External oblique muscle
M27	Transversus abdominis muscle
M29	Psoas muscle
M32	Erector spinae muscle
M51	Diaphragm
O31	Right lobe of liver
O37	Gallbladder
O41	Head of the pancreas
O42	Uncinate process
O43	Pancreas
O45	Spleen
O52	Renal sinus
O53	Renal pelvis
O54	Renal calyces
O55	Cortex, renal
O73	Duodenum
O74	Jejunum
O76	Colon
S1	Vertebra
S2	Rib (shaft)
S14	Spinous process
S27	Costal arch

C

Figure 34–5 Continued

C, Transverse schematic identifying anatomic structures visible in the corresponding CT image. (From Wegener O: *Whole Body Computed To-mography.* Boston, Blackwell Scientific Publications, 1993, pp 46–47.)

x-ray images of body tissues.[9] The CT "slice" originates from the gathering of many angles of a fan-shaped x-ray beam revolving around the patient. A computer transforms the multiple views, synthesizing them into a single image. Figure 34–5 contains a schematic of the abdominal area being viewed, the image, and a drawing with structures identified from this upper abdominal CT scan. Tissue absorbance of the x-ray beams permits visual construction of organs as well as parts of their internal structure within the cross-sectional slice. As with x-ray images, air appears black, bone (tissue high in density) appears white, and soft tissues, shades of gray.

To better visualize the gut, a radiopaque contrast material may be given by mouth or through a gastric tube before the CT scan. Commonly, barium sulfate or diatrizoate meglumine and organic iodides are used for gut visualization and injection, respectively. If there is any suspicion of a break in structural integrity in the GI tract, barium should not be used. It can seep through an opening into the cavity. If barium is to be used, other x-ray examinations should be completed before it is introduced. Visualization of abdominal structures can be occluded by a barium-filled bowel. An intravenous (IV) contrast substance may be used to assess blood flow and vascularity in given body locations as well as to better outline questionable areas.

The patient needs to be able to lie supine and quiet on a motorized stretcher during the test. The patient is moved through the scanner; the scanner rotates around the patient to produce cross-sectional views of underlying tissues. Patients may be asked to hold their breath to enhance the images. However, unrequested patient movement adversely affects picture clarity. The presence of treatment equipment or patient instability can prohibit use of this diagnostic test.

It is important to determine whether the patient has an allergy to potential contrast materials that may be used. Allergic reactions may range from mild to severe, including death. Baseline vital signs should be recorded before the injection of contrast material. Iodine contrast material can elicit adverse respiratory and cardiovascular effects. Iodine often causes patients to experience flushing, a feeling of warmth, taste changes, or nausea and vomiting. Delayed allergic reactions to contrast media may occur. Often these occur as hives or other skin reactions. Antihistamines may be ordered to control the more bothersome effects.

Sedation may be ordered, although patient status and current treatments may limit the type or amount that may be used. Claustrophobia may be experienced during the test.

A recent innovation is the spiral CT scanner. This technique uses continuous inspection that results in even more realistic three-dimensional images.

Ultrasonography

Ultrasonography, or sonography, of the abdomen is a simple noninvasive diagnostic technique that uses high-frequency sound waves. In an ultrasound study, a transducer is in contact with the skin over the area to be examined. The transducer acts to both deliver sound waves that penetrate the body and receive echoes that bounce off underlying tissues and structures. The echo, or reflection, pattern varies with tissue density. Thus, tissue location, size, shape, and texture can be detected in the resulting computer image.[10] A subhepatic abscess is visible in Figure 34–6.

Although one of the easiest diagnostic tests to perform, conditions of the critically ill may prevent an ultrasound study from being used. An open abdominal wound or abdominal dressings can preclude use of the needed skin surface lubricant. Abdominal guarding may limit the contact needed between the transducer and the skin surface to obtain an accurate depiction of underlying structures. Prior abdominal disease and treatment, including scarring or adhesions, may distort the sound signal, resulting in a less than accurate image. Furthermore, fatty tissue can interfere with the sound wave signal.

The patient is asked to lie quietly, usually in a supine or decubitus position. There is no pain with the procedure. However, abdominal tenderness may contribute to discomfort. If rebound tenderness is present

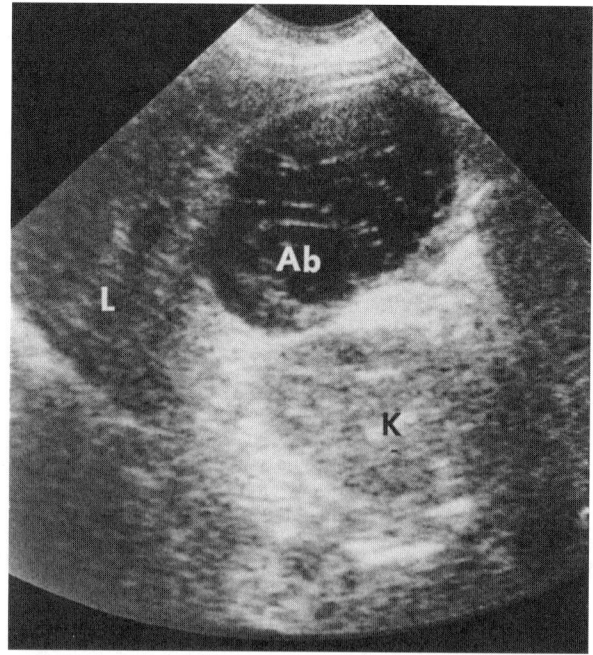

Figure 34–6

Sonogram (ultrasound) image showing a subhepatic abscess. The abscess (Ab) is detected by sonography as a rounded cystic mass with internal echoes, debris, and septations. L, liver; K, kidney. (From Putman C, Ravin C: Textbook of Diagnostic Imaging, vol. 1, 2nd ed. Philadelphia, WB Saunders, 1994, p 851.)

over the area being examined, pain is reported when pressure is released. Patients may be asked to control their breathing in certain ways or at certain times to improve the image.

Food or liquid in the GI tract can interfere with the ultrasound image. If the critically ill patient is receiving enteral or oral feedings, the nurse should verify what actions need to be taken, or for what length of time, before the ultrasound test. Because large amounts of air or contrast media can interfere with sound wave reflections, scheduling of other diagnostic or treatment procedures may need to be orchestrated to obtain the best sonographic results.

Magnetic Resonance Imaging

Magnetic resonance imaging includes sophisticated, noninvasive diagnostic methods that provide detailed coronal, axial (i.e., transverse), or sagittal plane images of the body with unique soft tissue contrast without the use of x-rays. Figure 34–7 shows examples of coronal and axial abdominal views. The procedure involves placing the patient inside a specialized scanner. Powerful electromagnets in the scanner create a strong but uniform magnetic field. Normally, randomly oriented tissue nuclei become aligned in the direction of the field's poles. Properly timed radio frequencies momentarily disrupt this alignment. As nuclei spin back into alignment, they give off faint signals of their own. These signals are captured, measured, and transformed by a computer. The resulting image displays varying tissue densities in a measured body section.[11]

Magnetic reasonance imaging of the abdomen can be particularly helpful in visualizing abdominal and retroperitoneal tissues and organs, including the liver, pancreas, stomach, small intestine, and large intestine, as well as abnormalities such as neoplasms, abscesses, or cysts. This test is motion sensitive. Some critically ill patients may be unable to control movement for the time needed to complete the test.

The magnetic field may be as much as 60,000 times as strong as that of the Earth's. It would follow that external or internal metal within the magnetic field needs to be evaluated for safety. Any external metal objects worn by a patient are to be removed. Additionally, internal metal objects that are magnetic are contraindications for this test. Such metal objects may include implanted devices such as cardiac pacemakers, heart valves, implanted drug infusion pumps or similar devices, catheters with metal hubs, some intrauterine contraceptive and prosthetic devices, as well as metal objects such as bullets, shrapnel, surgical clips, plates, screws, rods, pins, or wire mesh or sutures. The presence of nonmagnetic stainless steel shows as an artifact, but does not automatically eliminate the person from having a magnetic resonance

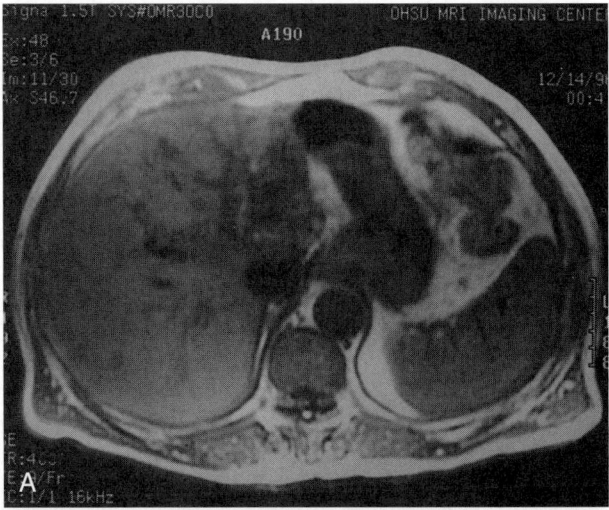

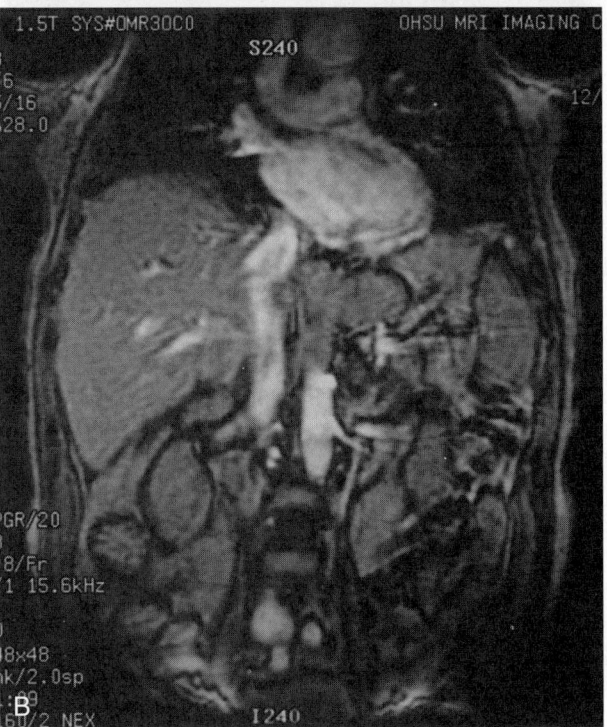

Figure 34–7

Magnetic resonance imaging of the abdomen with (A) coronal and (B) axial views.

imaging study. Hazards related to the magnetic field can include displacement of metal objects, internal heating of the metal or tissues, damage to electromechanical implants, or twisting of metal objects such as wire mesh or surgical clips. When this test is being considered for a given patient, information is needed about internal metal objects. The nurse should check with the institution's laboratory personnel to verify what implanted devices are contraindications for an MRI and to verify any institutional policy to ensure proper permission has been secured.

The patient needs to lie supine and still while inside the magnetic chamber. Respiratory movements can interfere with accurate images, especially in the upper abdominal region. Many critically ill patients may be unable to maintain this position, or they may have equipment attached that would prevent the test being performed. Additionally, the scan room has been arranged to eliminate metal objects. Specialized non-ferrous metal equipment can be used in the test room Such equipment may include cardiac and respiratory monitoring systems. Patient resuscitation may pose special challenges if only magnetic metal equipment is available. Should resuscitation of a patient be needed, equipment such as oxygen tanks, monitors, or IV poles may not be available in the immediate proximity.

Placement in the chamber may cause some patients to experience claustrophobia. Patient preparation includes explaining about the chamber size, the noise level and possible knocking sounds, as well as the need to remain still. Sedation may be used for an adult who may experience claustrophobia if not contraindicated by present status or treatments.

Nuclear Scans

Radionuclide imaging, or scans, are diagnostic approaches that can be used to view organs or organ subsections not visible by simple x-ray images. They also can provide data about organ functional ability. In radionuclide imaging, small doses of the administered radioactive material are distributed in the tissues of interest. The dose is adjusted by body weight and patient age. The output from a radionuclide scan following GI bleeding is shown in Figure 34–8.

These studies are usually performed in a nuclear medicine department. Under emergency conditions, a scan may be conducted at the bedside. The critically ill patient must be able to be safely transported to and from the location.

Gamma electromagnetic radiation is most commonly used in these diagnostic procedures. Imaging can be either static, when the gamma camera and patient are stationary, or dynamic, when a series of images correspond to the radionuclide moving through the tissue of interest. A radionuclide can be given intravenously or orally. Technetium (^{99m}Tc) is a commonly used tracer for GI studies. It clears the body in 24 hours. However, each tracer substance, such as iodine and thallium, has its own half-life, body clearance route, and time. Thus, the length of time that care providers need to exercise precautions is dictated by the tracer substance used. In some circumstances, other drugs may be ordered to amplify the effects of the diagnostic substance.

GI radionuclide scans may be used to evaluate structures such as salivary glands, liver, gallbladder, and biliary tract. Regional motility can be assessed by

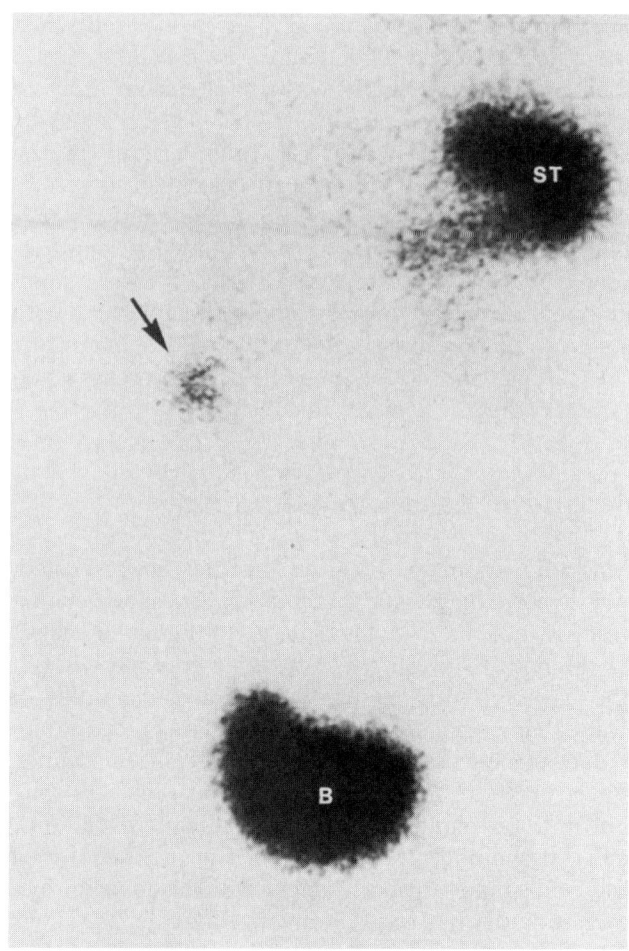

Figure 34–8

Radionuclide scan in a child after gastrointestinal bleeding and showing Meckel's diverticulum. The diverticulum is demonstrated by focal uptake of technetium-99m pertechnetate (arrow). Normal radiotracer accumulation is seen within the stomach (ST) and urinary bladder (B). (From Putman C, Ravin C: Textbook of Diagnostic Imaging, vol. 1, 2nd ed. Philadelphia, WB Saunders, 1994, p 783.)

a gastroesophageal reflux scan or a gastric emptying scan. After the tracer substance is introduced, a timed series of images is taken. Furthermore, lower GI blood loss can be sought with a blood loss scan. For active bleeding, ^{99m}Tc sulfur colloid may be used because extravasation of the tracer into the bowel can be detected. For intermittent or smaller bleeding, ^{99m}Tc-tagged red blood cells may be more useful if bleeding occurs within 24 hours of red blood cell tagging. However, for patients who are hemodynamically unstable, this scan is contraindicated.

The presence of barium can interfere with scan results. Thus, a radionuclide scan should be scheduled before a barium contrast study. When testing for gastroesophageal reflux, graded pressures are applied to the abdomen with images obtained before and after pressures are increased. Scans to characterize gastric emptying include a solid and a liquid phase. The speed of such emptying has been shown to vary over the course of a day.[12]

After receiving the diagnostic radioactive material, pregnant staff and visitors should limit contact with the patient until the tracer has been degraded or eliminated from the body. Usual precautions with body fluids and bowel contents provide safety for the small diagnostic doses.

Peritoneal Lavage

Following abdominal trauma, peritoneal lavage may be used to aid in determining the extent of injury through detecting the presence of GI secretions, contents, or free blood in the peritoneum. This invasive procedure requires sterile insertion of a catheter into the abdominal cavity, usually below the umbilicus. After placement of the lavage cannula, 1 L of warmed solution, usually normal saline, is infused by gravity. The solution is then drained by gravity, with study of the drained fluid. Positive findings can include blood, red blood cells, white blood cells, or the presence of bacteria from the gut, bile, or food particles. Peritoneal lavage is used with both blunt and penetrating trauma.[13] However, rather than being definitive, it is often one of a test series following abdominal trauma as illustrated by the algorithms in Figures 34–9 and 34–10.

Endoscopies

A series of diagnostic tests for the GI system called endoscopies use fiberoptic light and a lens system. This light enables inspection of internal surfaces of organs. If blood vessels are engorged, they can be visible when examining the luminal surfaces. Removal of tissue for further testing (e.g., sampling such as biopsy), as well as some treatments (e.g., suction, cauterizing bleeding vessels, or laser surgery), may be performed during endoscopic procedures visualizing tissues of the upper or lower GI tract. Prophylactic antibiotics are often given for GI endoscopies if the patient has an implanted artificial valve or metal such as shrapnel or a hip replacement.

Endoscopic examination of the upper GI tract can include inspection of structures from the oral cavity to the ligament of Treitz, found at the junction of the duodenum and the jejunum. Structures to be examined are often included in the endoscopic name. Common endoscopic tests are outlined in Table 34–7.

For the critically ill patient, the procedure is most often performed at the bedside or the operating room. To ease equipment passage through the mouth for an upper GI endoscopy, a spray anesthetic is often used for the throat. Sedation may be administered intravenously. To protect the patient and equipment, a mouthpiece is inserted. The endoscope is inserted

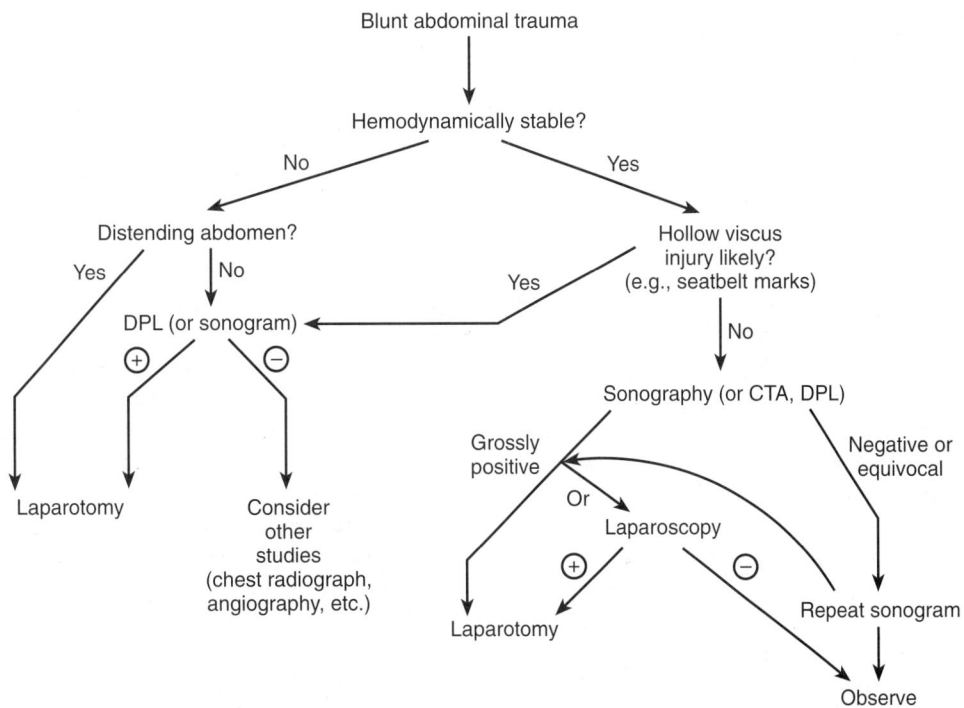

Figure 34–9

Suggested diagnostic algorithm for use with blunt abdominal trauma. CTA, computed tomography of the abdomen; DPL, diagnostic peritoneal lavage. (Modified from Elliott D, Militello P: Pitfalls in the diagnosis of abdominal trauma. In: Maull K, Rodriquez A, Wiles C III [eds]: Complications in Trauma and Critical Care. Philadelphia, WB Saunders, 1996, p 146.)

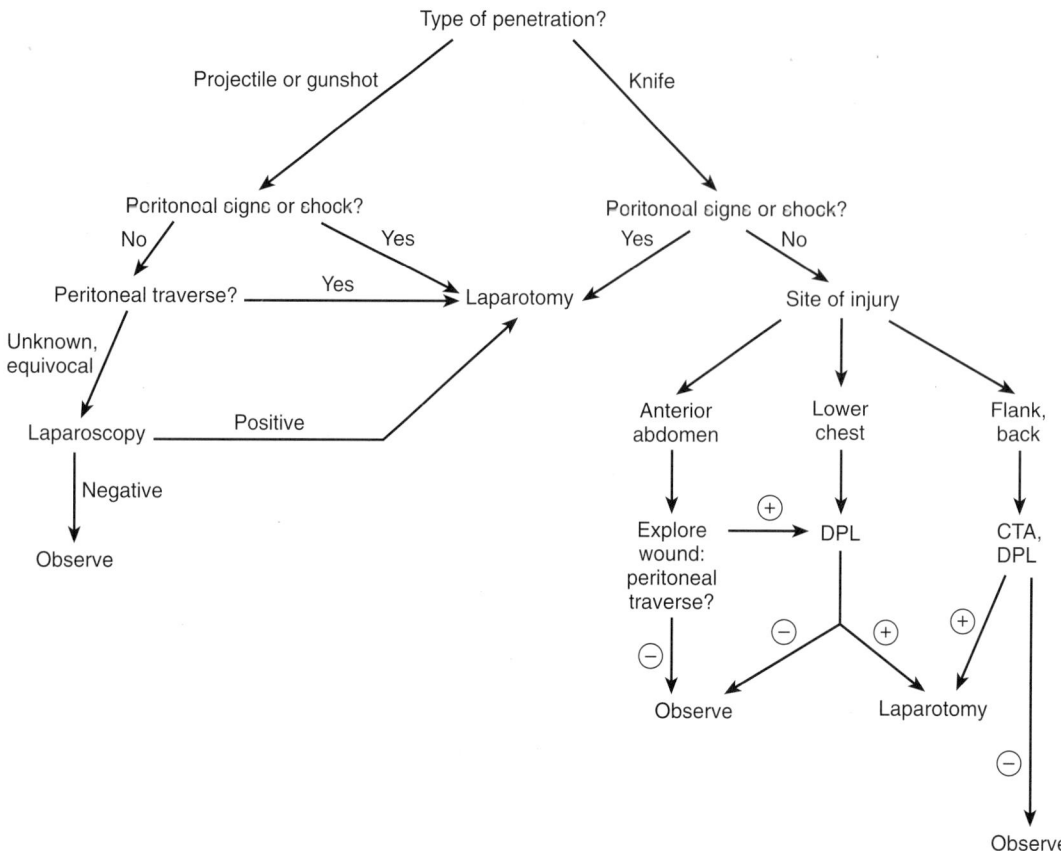

Figure 34–10

Suggested diagnostic algorithm for use in penetrating abdominal trauma. CTA, computed tomography of the abdomen; DPL, diagnostic peritoneal lavage. (Modified from Elliott D, Militello P: Pitfalls in the diagnosis of abdominal trauma. In: Maull K, Rodriquez A, Wiles C III [eds]: Complications in Trauma and Critical Care. Philadelphia, WB Saunders, 1996, p 147.)

through the mouthpiece and slowly advanced to the desired location. Air can be injected just ahead of the scope to distend the lumen, thereby minimizing mucosal trauma.

Although infrequent, complications involve perforation, bleeding, local irritation, sore throat, or drug reactions. Posttest care includes periodically measuring vital signs as well as positioning the patient to prevent injury or aspiration until the gag reflex returns and sedative effects subside.

A colonoscopy is an endoscopic test to examine the large intestinal mucosa as far up as the ileocecal valve. If the rigorous preparation required for visualizing the large intestine cannot safely be tolerated by the critically ill patient, this test should not be performed. Preparation most often includes a clear liquid diet for 2 to 3 days and laxatives 1 to 3 days before the test; a purgative to produce diarrhea; enemas until return is clear; or an oral washout solution. Combinations of sedatives may be given to assist the patient to relax, as well as to reduce bowel spasms. For best visibility, the preferred patient position is the left lateral or Sim's position. However, prone positioning may be needed in certain situations. A better view of tissues occurs during instrument withdrawal rather than during insertion.

Because of potential bleeding problems or infection from colon bacteria, clotting studies and prophylactic antibiotics are often requested as part of the test preparation. Following the study, stools should be observed for blood. Abdominal pain should be noted and thoroughly characterized. Large amounts of flatus may be expelled after the procedure to remove air injected during insertion of the endoscope.

Examining the sigmoid colon and rectal mucosa and the anal canal can be achieved by endoscopy. The flexible scope is seldom passed more than 40 cm into the bowel from the anus. For the critically ill patient, bowel preparation is often minimal or waived. The patient must be able to assume a position that permits endoscope insertion and visualization of the lumen. As with the more invasive colonoscopy, perforation and bleeding are serious but unusual complications.

An additional endoscopic test that enables examination of the hepatobiliary or pancreatic system is a retrograde cholangiopancreatography (ERCP). In this test, a flexible endoscope is passed into the duodenum until the ampulla of Vader is visible. The tip of the endoscope is positioned at the ampulla so a contrast medium can be injected to visualize the biliary or pancreatic system. There are many treatment

TABLE 34–7
Endoscopies of the Gastrointestinal System

Endoscopy Test	Indications	Contraindications	Nursing Actions
Esophagogastro-duodenoscopy	Visualization of upper gastrointestinal (GI) mucosal structures for diagnostic or treatment plans; may locate source of upper GI bleeding	Serious cardiovascular or respiratory compromise	Obtain baseline and ongoing vital signs. Safely administer intravenous (IV) sedation. Ensure airway is correctly placed. Position patient to aid breathing. Perform oral care before and after procedure. Check for return of gag reflex. Hold patient's oral intake until gag reflex returns. Assist patient to attain side-lying position after test until alert. Obtain signed permission form; sedation may be used.
Colonoscopy	Visualization of large intestine structures for diagnostic or treatment plans; may locate source of lower GI bleed	Preparation exceeds patient's tolerance; perforating diseases of the colon; peritonitis; recent bowel surgery; serious cardiovascular or respiratory compromise	Obtain baseline and ongoing vital signs. If patient is on oral intake, give clear liquids, then nothing by mouth; clarifying bowel prep is needed. Anticholinergics may be given. Position patient in Sim's or left lateral position. Check for clotting before test. For fragile patients, antibiotics may be given before and after test. Observe patient stools after test. Obtain signed permission form; sedation may be used.
Proctoscopy/ sigmoidoscopy/ Proctosigmoid-oscopy	Visualization of sigmoid colon and rectal mucosal structures for diagnostic or treatment plans; may locate source of sigmoid or rectal bleeding		Obtain baseline and ongoing vital signs. Laxative or enema may be ordered before test. If symptoms are acute, prep is likely to be waived; obtain signed permission form.
Endoscopic retrograde chol-angiopancrea-tography (ERCP)	Evaluate biliary/pancreatic systems using contrast medium	Allergy to contrast substance; inability to tolerate position	Solicit history for contrast medium allergies and recent barium use. Obtain signed permission form; conscious sedation is used. Restrict patient's intake before test. Assist patient into left lateral position. Topic anesthetic into oropharynx. Ensure mouthpiece is in place. Give anticholinergics IV to relax duodenum and papilla. Obtain baseline vital signs and ongoing assessment. Position patient to aid breathing. Provide oral care before and after procedure. Check for return of gag reflex. Patient may experience abdominal discomfort, sore throat. After test, observe for cholangitis or pancreatitis.

options that can be done with ERCP, such as stone removal, stints, or drain placement. Pretest and posttest care include those highlighted for an upper GI endoscope and when contrast is used. Positioning, monitoring, and safety precautions until the gag reflex returns and vital signs are stable are important in posttest care. Complications can include cholangitis or pancreatitis; nurses should obtain periodic vital signs as well as report nausea or vomiting or posttest sharp abdominal pain. As with other studies using contrast medium, attention to patient response and clearing of the substance is a consideration in this posttest care.

Angiography

Contrast media injected into selected arteries or veins of the GI tract can be used to visualize blood flow,

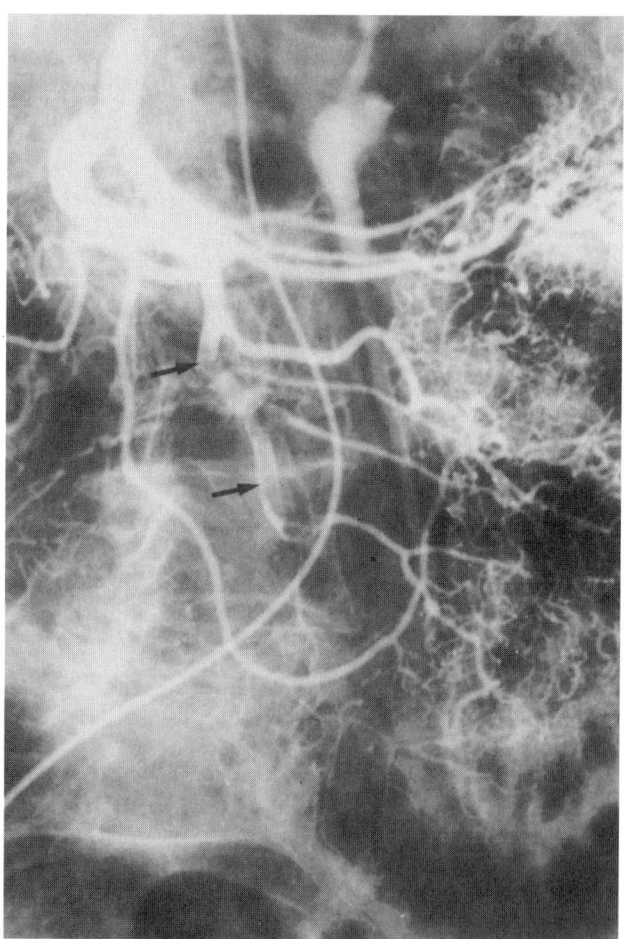

Figure 34–11

Arteriogram of the superior mesenteric vasculature demonstrating an embolic occlusion (arrows) of the jejunal branch vessels and a corresponding lack of mural blood flow to the midjejunal loops. (From Putman C, Ravin C: Textbook of Diagnostic Imaging, vol. 1, 2nd ed. Philadelphia, WB Saunders, 1994, p 804.)

vessels, and flow disruptions. Nursing care before and following an angiography is detailed in the cardiovascular section, Chapter 8. A selective superior mesenteric arteriogram demonstrates an occlusion of the jejunal branch vessels (Figure 34–11).

Biopsy

A small sample of tissue may be removed from various GI organs for pathologic study. A frequent biopsy site is the liver. Such a biopsy can be done at the bedside, and may be performed through the skin, percutaneously, or transvenously. Sterile technique is necessary to prevent infection in an already compromised patient. The patient may receive a sedative and pretest and posttest antibiotic therapy. If the biopsy route is percutaneous, a local anesthetic is injected at the biopsy site. Following removal of the tissue, the patient is turned to the right side, in an effort to apply pressure to the site. Vital signs should be obtained on a regular basis, often for 24 hours. Because of the liver location, the biopsy route traverses the pleura and diaphragm. Thus, after biopsy, the patient should be observed for signs of a right-sided pneumothorax or hemorrhage.

Laboratory, as well as noninvasive and invasive diagnostic, tests take on added importance for the clinician seeking to confirm GI-related diagnoses.[14] Nursing actions can ease the patient and family through tests that can aid in diagnosis and treatment of GI symptoms and diseases.

Key Concepts

⟹ Because large portions of the GI tract are hidden from view, constellations of laboratory and diagnostic tests, in combination with history and physical examination data, contribute to accurate diagnosis of GI problems.

⟹ Liver laboratory tests include tests for the hepatocyte as well as liver functions.

⟹ Testing hepatocyte integrity often includes cellular enzymes, selected proteins, clotting ability, and detoxified end products.

⟹ With hepatocyte damage, intracellular enzymes are released into the circulation.

⟹ ALT is primarily found in the liver and kidneys. Elevated levels may be markers for liver injury or necrosis.

⟹ Serum bilirubin forms are conjugated (direct) or unconjugated (indirect).

⟹ Conjugated bilirubin is converted to urobilinogen in the duodenum.

⟹ Urobilinogen is excreted and can be measured in the urine.

➡ If bilirubin is conjugated in the liver but there is an obstruction in the biliary tract, conjugated bilirubin level in the blood increases.

➡ Protein electrophoresis can be used to identify types and quantities of proteins in the blood.

➡ Albumin levels are reduced in liver cell damage.

➡ The long half-life of albumin (approximately 20 days), makes it an unreliable measure of nutritional status in the dynamic, critically ill patient.

➡ Coagulation factors and anticlotting factors manufactured in the liver are adversely affected by liver disease.

➡ Derangement in lipoprotein metabolism can occur with hepatic disorders.

➡ Ammonia, an end product of protein metabolism, is detoxified in the liver to urea.

➡ Drug peak and trough levels may be requested to determine how well pharmacologic substances normally metabolized by the liver are being cleared.

➡ Pancreatic blood studies often include both total and ionized levels of amylase, lipase, glucose, triglycerides, and calcium.

➡ Whereas amylase is found in several body tissues, the major source of lipase is the pancreas.

➡ Abdominal diagnostic tests include noninvasive and invasive approaches.

➡ Diagnostic test preparation is often streamlined for the critically ill.

➡ Upright or left lateral decubitus position x-ray examinations are used when there is suspicion of free air in the abdomen.

➡ It is important to solicit information from the patient about possible allergy to planned contrast materials.

➡ Barium sulfate should not be used as contrast medium unless the GI tract is known to be intact.

➡ Water-soluble contrast medium may be used in place of barium sulfate.

➡ During some abdominal x-ray studies, patients may be asked to change positions or follow breathing instructions.

➡ Contrast solution needs to be expelled because it can harden and lead to constipation or fecal impaction.

➡ Patient movement, physiologic instability, or equipment can prohibit use of CT as a diagnostic test.

➡ Conditions of the critically ill, such as open abdominal wounds, abdominal dressing, or abdominal guarding, may prevent an ultrasound examination from being used.

➡ Powerful electromagnets in the scanner create a strong but uniform magnetic field for magnetic resonance imaging.

➡ Magnetic resonance imaging is motion sensitive.

➡ External or internal metal within the magnetic field is a contraindication for magnetic resonance imaging.

➡ In radionuclide imaging, small doses of the administered radioactive material are distributed in the tissues of interest.

➡ The length of time that care providers and family members need to use precautions with patients having nuclear scans is dictated by the tracer substance used.

➡ Following abdominal trauma, peritoneal lavage may be used to determine whether there are GI secretions, contents, or free blood in the peritoneum.

➡ Endoscopies are diagnostic tests that use fiberoptic light and a lens system to inspect the internal surfaces of structures in the GI tract.

➡ Posttest care for an upper GI endoscopy includes positioning the patient to prevent injury or aspiration until the gag reflex returns and the sedative wears off.

➡ Perforation and bleeding are serious but unusual complications for GI endoscopies.

➡ In a percutaneous liver biopsy, the biopsy route transverses the pleura and diaphragm. Postbiopsy care includes placing the patient on the right side, obtaining frequent vital signs, and observing the patient for signs of a pneumothorax or hemorrhage.

References

1. Brockmoller J, Roots I: Assessment of liver metabolic function: Clinical implications. Clin Pharmacokin 27:216–248, 1994.
2. Pincus M, Shaffner J: Assessment of liver function. In: Henry J (ed): Clinical Diagnosis and Management by Laboratory Methods, 19th ed. Philadelphia, WB Saunders, 1996, pp 253–267.
3. Theal R, Scott K: Evaluating symptomatic patients with abnormal liver function test results. Am Fam Physician 53:2111–2119, 1996.
4. Wallah J: Interpretation of Diagnostic Tests, 6th ed. Boston, Little, Brown and Company, 1996.
5. Gibson R: Principles of nutritional assessment. New York, Oxford University Press, 1990.
6. Decousus H, Croze M, Jaubert J, et al: Circadian changes in anticoagulant effect of heparin infused at a constant rate. BMJ 290:341–344, 1985.
7. Decousus H, Boissier C, Perpoint B, et al: Circadian dynamics of coagulation and chronopathology of cardiovascular and cerebrovascular events. Ann NY Acad Sci 618:159–165, 1991.
8. Schved J, Gris J, Eledjam J: Circadian changes in anticoagulant effect of heparin infused at a constant rate (Letter). BMJ 290:1286, 1985.
9. Wegener O: Whole Body Computed Tomography. Boston, Blakwell Scientific Publications, 1993.
10. Rosenthal T, Siepel T, Zubler J, et al: The use of ultrasonography to scan the abdomen of patients presenting for routine physical examinations. J Fam Pract 38:380–385, 1994.

11. Edelman R, Hesselink J, Zlatkin M: Clinical magnetic resonance imaging, 2nd ed. Vol. 1. Philadelphia, WB Saunders, 1996.
12. Goo R, More J, Greenberg E, et al: Circadian variation in gastric emptying of meals in humans. Gastroenterology 93:515–518, 1987.
13. Elliott D, Militello P: Pitfalls in the diagnosis of abdominal trauma. In Maull K, Rodriguez A, Willes C III (eds): Complica-tions in Trauma and Critical Care. Philadelphia, WB Saunders, 1996, pp 145–158.
14. Sosa J, Reines H: Evaluating the acute abdomen. In: Civetta J, Taylor R, Kirby R (eds): Critical Care, 3rd ed. Philadelphia, Lip-pincott-Raven, 1997, pp 1099–1108.

35

Acute Gastrointestinal Bleed

Carolyn J. Driscoll

Objectives

After completing this chapter, the student will be able to:

1. Relate the pathophysiology associated with gastrointestinal (GI) bleeding to the assessment findings.
2. Differentiate between upper and lower GI bleeding.
3. Describe patients at risk for the development of GI bleeding.
4. Identify patients at greater risk for the development of complications associated with GI bleeding.
5. Select collaborative interventions appropriate for the care of the patient with GI bleeding.
6. Evaluate effects of collaborative care on anticipated outcomes for a patient with GI bleeding.

GI bleeding is a common critical care problem. The blood supply to the GI tract is extensive and close to the surface so that bleeding from multiple causes can easily occur. GI bleeding can range in severity from very mild, slow occult blood loss to sudden massive hemorrhage. There is a larger arterial blood supply to the upper GI tract near the stomach and esophagus because digestion requires a massive blood supply. For this reason, upper GI bleeds are more likely to produce arterial hemorrhage. Bleeding in the lower GI tract is more commonly of venous origin. Although this is less threatening, it can be evasive to diagnose.[1]

Upper GI tract hemorrhage, which can be serious and life threatening, is defined as bleeding proximal to the ligament of Treitz.[2] The vasculature in the upper GI tract predisposes this area to arterial hemorrhage.[1] The annual incidence of upper GI bleeding is 150 per 100,000 population,[3] with a mortality rate of 5% to 10%.[4] In patients with acute upper GI hemorrhage, comorbid disease is the cause of death approximately 70% of the time.[5] The most frequent cause of upper GI bleeding is peptic ulcers (Table 35–1). Men are more likely than women to have an upper GI bleed, although women are more likely to bleed from gastric ulcers. The risk of development of a GI bleed increases significantly between the third and ninth decade of life.[4]

Lower GI bleeding is defined as hemorrhage below the ligament of Treitz.[6] Patients with acute lower GI bleeding tend to be older than those with upper GI bleeding, have more concomitant medical problems, and therefore have increased morbidity. Mortality rate from acute lower GI bleeding also ranges between 5% and 10%.[6]

ETIOLOGY AND PATHOPHYSIOLOGY

Upper Gastrointestinal Bleeding

Esophageal Bleeding

Esophageal varices are large dilated veins in the submucosa of the stomach and lower esophagus.[7] These veins become dilated when blood is unable to flow through the liver normally. Cirrhosis, schistosomiasis, and noncirrhotic portal hypertension are the most common causes of increased portal pressure (portal hypertension). As a result of the increased portal pressure, collateral channels develop to decompress the splanchnic circulation. The esophagogastric junction, perianal and periumbilical regions, and retroperitoneum are common locations for collateral channel formation. Even though one might expect that the development of collateral circulation would be sufficient to decrease portal hypertension, this does not occur in the splanchnic system. Instead, the increased inflow of blood to the splanchnic circulation, when coupled

TABLE 35–1

Diagnosis in Patients with Upper GI Hemorrhage

Finding	Occurrence
Peptic ulcers	45%
Duodenal 23%	
Gastric 22%	
Gastric erosions	30%
Varices	15%
Esophagitis	13%
Mallory-Weiss tears	8%
Tumors	4%
Esophageal ulcers	2%
Angiodysplasia	0.5%
Other lesions	6%

Total more than 100% because patients may have had more than one lesion

Adapted from Silverstein FE, Gilbert DA, Tedesco FJ, et al: The National ASGE Survey on Upper Gastrointestinal Bleeding: I study design and baseline data. Gastrointest Endosc 27:73–79, 1981.

with resistance through the liver, maintains the portal hypertension.[8]

Approximately 10% of upper GI hemorrhage in the United States is caused by varices.[1,9] One-third of patients with cirrhosis bleed from varices, with an overall mortality rate for those patients of about 30%.[10] The incidence of bleeding increases with the severity of liver disease. The risk of death and rebleeding is highest immediately after a variceal bleed.[8,11]

Factors that precipitate bleeding from esophageal varices in individuals are not fully understood. Several endoscopic grading systems have been devised to predict the risk of bleeding. Large varices are more likely to bleed than small varices.[12] As varices increase in size, the wall thickness decreases, leading to increased risk of rupture. Neurohumoral responses in the gut may also be involved in variceal bleeding. Food in the gut increases splanchnic flow, which increases portal hypertension.[8] Circadian rhythms may also be a factor in the timing of variceal bleeding. One study has shown that the peak incidence of variceal bleeding occurred at 8:00 AM and 8:00 PM.[13] Even though the aforementioned factors may contribute to variceal bleeding, the degree of liver dysfunction is the most important factor in determining prognosis.[12]

Although it is difficult to evaluate the hemodynamics of the splanchnic circulatory system during acute variceal bleeding, several studies have been performed. These studies suggest that portal venous pressure is increased around the time of a variceal bleed and that the peak of portal venous pressure during a bleeding episode is an important risk factor for rebleeding and mortality.[12]

Inflammation of the esophagus, or esophagitis, is another cause of bleeding in the upper GI tract.

Esophagitis may occur as the result of reflux of gastric or duodenal contents into the esophagus. Normally, the lower esophageal sphincter prevents the reflux of gastric contents into the esophagus. These contents are often highly acidic and irritating to the lining of the esophagus. With frequent exposure over time, the esophagus can become inflamed. Certain individuals with lower sphincter tone at the esophagus may be more prone to the development of esophageal inflammation, but a combination of different factors may also contribute to an inflammatory response. Reflux esophagitis is the most common cause of esophageal inflammation (Table 35–2). Other causes may include infection, acquired immunodeficiency syndrome (AIDS), and medication-induced injury.[14,15]

Delayed gastric emptying also contributes to the development of reflux esophagitis by lengthening the period of time that gastric contents may come in contact with the esophagus, as well as contributing to increased acidity of those contents. Hyperemia, increased capillary permeability, edema, tissue fragility, and erosion, which may develop as a result of reflux esophagitis, contribute to the potential for bleeding. Fibrosis and thickening of the esophageal wall may also develop.[3] Reflux esophagitis is commonly associated with iron deficiency rather than overt bleeding. Severe esophagitis is usually clinically evident.[16]

Although the inflammation associated with esophageal reflux most often is confined to the superficial layer of the esophagus, it may sometimes erode deeper into the submucosa, resulting in an ulcer.[17] Serious hemorrhage from such ulcers is responsible for

TABLE 35–2

Causes of Esophagitis

Common Causes

Reflux esophagitis
Infectious esophagitis
   Candida esophagitis
   Herpetic esophagitis
   Cytomegalovirus
Acquired immunodeficiency syndrome
Caustic esophagitis
Radiation esophagitis
Medication-induced injury

Rare Causes

Crohn's disease
Ulcerative colitis
Graft-versus-host disease
Zollinger-Ellison syndrome
Thermal injury
Trauma

From Ott DJ: Radiology of the oropharynx and esophagus. In: Castell DO (ed): The Esophagus. Boston, Little, Brown, 1995, pp 673–689.

approximately 2% of upper GI bleeding.[3] Ulcers associated with reflux esophagitis may penetrate deeper into a nearby organ or blood vessel, such as the aorta, although this is uncommon. This type of deep esophageal ulceration occurs more frequently with Barrett's esophagus.[17]

Barrett's esophagus is the condition in which abnormal mucosa (Barrett's mucosa) replaces the normal squamous epithelium of the distal esophagus, as a result of gastroesophageal reflux disease (GERD). It is believed that esophageal epithelium, which has been injured and exposed to reflux contents during healing, results in the development of Barrett's mucosa.[17] Complications associated with Barrett's esophagus include esophageal ulceration, hemorrhage, stricture, and cancer.[18]

Even though Barrett's esophagus is most often implicated in the development of esophageal ulcers, other causes may be responsible. Infection with cytomegalovirus or herpes simplex virus, especially in the immunocompromised host, may result in the development of esophageal ulcers.[15] Inflammatory changes associated with Crohn's disease may also progress to ulcer formation.[19] Finally, the use of nonsteroidal anti-inflammatory drugs (NSAIDs) has also been associated with the development of esophageal ulcers.[20]

Bleeding from esophageal tumors accounts for approximately 4% of upper GI bleeds.[3] Most esophageal tumors are malignant, with squamous cell carcinoma and adenocarcinoma being seen most often.[21] The presence of Barrett's esophagus increases an individual's risk of development of cancer and, in some reports, adenocarcinoma developed in as many as 50% of patients with Barrett's esophagus.[17] There are approximately 10,000 new cases of esophageal cancer diagnosed each year. The symptoms of esophageal cancer are typically nonspecific, with dysphagia most often being the presenting symptom. Bleeding from esophageal cancers is uncommon, but may occur because of ulcer formation or erosion of the tumor into a vessel such as the aorta.[21]

Mallory-Weiss tears are lacerations of the cardia of the stomach and the gastroesophageal junction caused by vomiting or retching. Although they are usually superficial, deep tears and even perforations are possible. The most common presenting symptom is hematemesis (85% of cases). Approximately 10% of patients are seen only with melena, and abdominal pain is extremely rare.[22] The use of endoscopy has increased the knowledge about Mallory-Weiss tears, and it is more common and less fatal than initially believed. There is a strong association with chronic alcoholism and recent binge drinking as well as a history of prior vomiting, retching, or violent coughing. Hiatal hernias are often present, and men younger than 50 years of age are most often affected.[20]

Gastric Bleeding

Peptic Ulcer Disease. Peptic ulcer disease, which includes gastric and duodenal ulcers, is a common, serious medical problem. Mortality as a result of peptic ulcer disease is low, although patients endure substantial pain and suffering as a result of this disease. The two most important factors associated with peptic ulcer disease are infection with the *Helicobacter pylori* bacteria and the use of NSAIDs. Cigarette smoking has also been linked to an increased incidence of ulcer disease, slower healing rates, and higher rates of ulcer recurrence.[23]

H. pylori is a common infection, yet peptic ulcer disease develops in only a small proportion of infected individuals. Conversely, approximately 90% to 100% of patients with duodenal ulcers and 70% to 90% of patients with gastric ulcers have *H. pylori* present in their stomach. Treatment of the *H. pylori* infection has been shown to increase the rate of healing in duodenal ulcers when compared to standard H_2-blocker therapy. More importantly, it has been shown that treatment of *H. pylori* infection decreases subsequent recurrences and therefore becomes a cure for what would otherwise become a chronic, relapsing disease.[23] Current *H. pylori* eradication therapy includes antibiotics in combination with other medications such as proton-pump inhibitors or bismuth preparations.

One of the most common side effects associated with the use of NSAIDs is ulcer formation. It is estimated that gastric or duodenal ulcers develop in approximately 25% of patients taking NSAIDs, including salicylates such as aspirin, on a regular basis (Chart 35–1). Inhibition of prostaglandins is believed to be the most important mechanism associated with the formation of ulcers. Prostaglandins increase mucous secretion, bicarbonate secretion, and mucosal blood flow as well as inhibit gastric acid secretion. With the use of NSAIDs, these actions are decreased and may contribute to the formation of gastroduodenal ulcers.[23] Because most NSAID users derive benefit from taking these agents and complications do not develop, it is important to identify factors that predispose patients to the development of complications associated with the use of these medications (Chart 35–2).

Smoking tobacco is an additional risk factor for the development of ulcer disease. Ulcers are approximately two times more likely to develop in smokers than in nonsmokers, and there is a direct relationship between the amount of smoking and the incidence of ulcer formation. The presence of *H. pylori* infection in smokers increases the risk of ulcer formation even further. Cigarette smoking may provide a more favorable environment for, or increase the susceptibility to, *H. pylori* infection.[24]

Bleeding from gastric ulcers occurs when the ulcer erodes into the wall of a blood vessel. Ulcers that are

CHART 35–1

BEYOND THE ICU: LIMITING GI COMPLICATIONS FROM COMMONLY ADMINISTERED MEDICATIONS

GI complications of treatment with NSAIDs are a major cause of morbidity and mortality. The use of NSAIDs for the management of pain has become commonplace and is seen in the outpatient as well as acute and critical care setting.

Several studies have evaluated the relationship between the use of NSAIDs and the development of GI bleeding. In one meta-analysis, 12 studies evaluating the relationship between the use of NSAIDs in the community and the development of serious peptic ulcer complications, which required admission to a hospital, were compared. This meta-analysis has suggested that ibuprofen was associated with the lowest risk of development of severe GI toxicity, which may be related to the fairly low dose used in clinical practice. Ketoprofen, which is also available over the counter, and piroxicam had the highest risk of development of GI bleeding. Middle rankings for the development of GI bleeding were given to aspirin, sulindac, naproxen, and indomethacin.

Another study investigated the relationship between the presence and location of ulcers, *H. pylori* infection, NSAID use, and GI tract bleeding. Patients with duodenal and benign gastric ulcers were evaluated. Whereas greater than 90% of each group had *H. pylori* detected, all those who were *H. pylori* negative were using NSAIDs. Additionally, the frequency of NSAID use was very high in those patients with GI bleeding. Eighty-four percent of patients with gastric ulcers and 62% of patients with duodenal ulcers reported the use of NSAIDs. One conclusion was that NSAID use may be responsible for most bleeding complications of ulcer disease, regardless of *H. pylori* status.

What these studies show is that the use of NSAIDs, which has become common in most households, can have very serious side effects. Because many of these medications are available over the counter, patients feel safe in using them for the relief of pain. Dosage guidelines are outlined on the box, yet patients can take higher doses, which can approach, and even surpass, doses that were previously only available by prescription. Many pa-

tients with liver disease believe they should avoid acetaminophen for analgesia and use NSAIDs instead. For those patients with portal hypertension as a result of cirrhosis, this choice can further increase their risk of bleeding.

It is important to question patients carefully about their medication use. It is not uncommon for patients to provide a list of medications that relate specifically to the problem for which they are being evaluated, while not including medications they may be taking for other medical conditions. Also, it may be necessary to specifically ask about the use of over-the-counter medications, because many people believe that these do not really "count" as medications.

Because NSAID use has become so commonplace, GI complications related to their use can be seen in many practice settings. In addition to the outpatient setting, NSAIDs have gained popularity in the management of postsurgical pain in the acute care setting. Even though it is believed that the use of medications such as ketorolac provide adequate pain relief, without some of the side effects associated with narcotic use, they are not without their own potential complications. In one case, the use of ketorolac for as few as 4 days to manage breakthrough abdominal pain was associated with the development of a bleeding ulcer, which ultimately increased the patient's hospital stay.

But, NSAID use is not the only medication that may increase the risk of development of GI bleeding. Calcium antagonists such as diltiazem, nifedipine, and verapamil have also been associated with the development of GI bleeding. This may be related to the inhibition of platelet aggregation and vasodilation associated with the use of this class of medication.

It is important for nurses in all practice settings to be aware of the potential side effects of the multitude of medications that are in use. Careful assessment of medication use, including dosage and pattern of use, as well as evaluation of GI complaints is important. This may allow for the early identification and perhaps prevention of GI complications.

Data from Henry D, Lim LLY, Garcia-Rodriguez LA, et al: Variability in risk of gastrointestinal complications with individual nonsteroidal anti-inflammatory drugs: results of a collaborative meta-analysis. BMJ 312:1563–1566, 1996; Al-Assi MT, Genta RM, Karttunen TJ, et al: Ulcer site and complications: relation to Helicobacter pylori infection and NSAID use. Endoscopy 28:229–233, 1996; Lilly LL, Guanci R: Med errors: adverse effects of NSAIDs. Am J Nurs 95:17, 1995; and Pahor M, Guralnik JM, Fryberg CD, et al: Risk of gastrointestinal haemorrhage with calcium antagonists in hypertensive persons over 67 years old. Lancet 347:1061–1065, 1996.

CHART 35–2

> **Risk Factors for Complications Associated with NSAID Use**
>
> Prior history of peptic ulcer disease
> Prior history of GI bleeding
> Age older than 60 years
> Use of higher doses
> Concomitant use of corticosteroids
> Tobacco use
> Alcohol use
>
> From Isenberg JI, McQuaid KR, Laine L, et al: Acid-peptic disorders. In: Yamada T, Alpers DH, et al (eds): Textbook of Gastroenterology. Philadelphia, JB Lippincott, 1995, 1347–1430.

located high on the lesser curve of the stomach are at high risk of eroding into the left gastric artery, leading to significant bleeding.[25] The consumption of alcohol or the use of NSAIDs has been associated with the development of gastric ulcers.[2,26,27] Another major contributing factor is the *H. pylori* bacteria. First identified in 1984, the *H. pylori* bacteria is the most common cause of peptic ulcer disease and is the major cause of 80% of gastric ulcers.[28,29]

Bleeding associated with gastritis comes from diffuse, superficial lesions in the gastric mucosa. Local irritants, such as alcohol, NSAIDs, or corticosteroids may contribute to the development of these lesions.[26,27] Major physiologic stressors such as burns, trauma, sepsis, and even long-distance running are also often associated with gastritis. Endoscopic studies have shown that gastroduodenal damage occurs in 52% to 100% of patients within 18 to 24 hours of admission to an intensive care unit (ICU). Hepatic failure, renal failure, and respiratory insufficiency also increase a patient's susceptibility to stress ulceration.[30] Decreased splanchnic blood flow during times of severe stress may contribute to the breakdown in normal mucosal defenses.[2] Congestive gastropathy, congestion, and stasis of the gastric mucosa associated with portal hypertension are also associated with the development of gastritis.[30]

Cancer. Although the incidence is low in the United States, carcinoma of the stomach is the second most common cause of cancer in the world (second only to lung cancer), accounting for almost 10% of cancers worldwide.[31] Stomach cancer appears to have a complex, multifactorial origin. Whereas dietary factors have traditionally been given the greatest emphasis, the role of *H. pylori* is receiving increasing attention. Dietary factors have been implicated in the development of gastric carcinoma because of the striking re-

gional variation worldwide. However, one single dietary item, or combination of items has not been identified. The intake of nitrates and nitrites has also been implicated in the development of gastric cancer. It has been noted that the incidence of gastric cancer is lower in more developed countries.[32] Additional factors include chronic inflammation and gastric atrophy because they are frequent precursors to gastric cancer. *H. pylori,* the most common known cause of chronic gastritis, is also suspected of playing a role in the development of gastric cancer.[28,33]

Diagnosis of gastric cancer is difficult because symptoms are typically vague and nonspecific. For this reason, gastric cancers are often advanced at the time of diagnosis. Gastric cancers may cause acute GI bleeding or may result in anemia secondary to chronic GI blood loss. Metastatic tumors to the stomach, although unusual, may also result in significant bleeding in approximately 20% of the cases.[32]

Angiodysplasia. Angiodysplasia and arteriovenous malformations occur throughout the GI tract and may account for as much as 4.4% of GI bleeding. Bleeding and anemia may be the only symptoms of angiodysplasia, which are also known as vascular ectasias or angiomas.[34] For patients with lesions located in the upper GI tract, hematemesis is a frequent occurrence, although it is not usually life threatening. In fact, spontaneous cessation of bleeding usually occurs.[35]

Small Intestine

Angiodysplasias are the most common cause of small intestinal bleeding, accounting for 70% to 80% of cases. Bleeding from angiodysplasias can range from brisk to occult. However, the reason these lesions bleed is unclear. It has been suggested that high pressures cause thin-walled capillaries to bleed or that food erodes the mucosa. Localized ischemia may cause thinning and ulceration of the mucosa, which leads to bleeding. The natural history of these lesions is also not well known. Angiodysplasia of the small intestine is usually seen in elderly patients (mean age of 60 years) with equal frequency in men and women.[22]

Thirty percent of patients with *Crohn's disease* have distribution of their disease localized to the small intestine. Gross bleeding is unusual in Crohn's disease, occurring in 4% to 11% of patients with ileitis. This may result from the inflammation associated with Crohn's disease eroding into blood vessels. These episodes are usually self-limited and do not recur.[36] Bleeding, however, does not usually occur alone, and most patients also have the more common symptoms of Crohn's disease, such as diarrhea and abdominal pain.[37]

Meckel's diverticulum is a congenital diverticulum of the small intestine. This anomaly is present in 2% of the population and is more common in men than in women.[38] The most common clinical presentation of a Meckel's diverticulum is GI bleeding. This occurs in 25% to 50% of patients who are seen with a complication.[39] The bleeding can present as melena, or bright red blood per rectum, and is classically described as appearing as "currant jelly."[40] The source of bleeding is usually an ileal ulcer with ectopic gastric mucosa in the diverticulum.[39] Bleeding is typically more common in children than adults.[40]

Lower Gastrointestinal Bleeding

In the United States, four diseases account for the majority of lower GI bleeding: diverticulosis, angiodysplasia, internal hemorrhoids, and malignant tumors. Diverticulosis and angiodysplasia are the leading causes of acute bleeding, whereas hemorrhoids and colonic neoplasia are the most common causes of chronic blood loss from the lower GI tract. Other causes of lower GI bleeding include polyps, ulcerative colitis, Crohn's disease, and rectal fissures (Table 35–3). Eighty percent of bleeding episodes resolve spontaneously, with a risk of recurrence in 25% of the patients. Most lower GI bleeding, unlike upper GI bleeding, is slow and intermittent and does not require hospitalization.[41]

Diverticular Bleeding

Diverticular bleeding occurs in only 3% of patients with diverticulosis, yet it is the most common cause of major lower GI hemorrhage. Diverticular bleeding presumably occurs when a colonic artery penetrates into the diverticulum. The artery ruptures into the sac of the diverticulum causing extensive bleeding. Diverticulitis, or inflammation, is not usually present and the vessel rupture is thought to be the result of pressure erosion.[42]

TABLE 35–3
Diagnosis in Patients with Lower Gastrointestinal Bleeding

Finding	Occurrence
Diverticulosis	43%
Angiodysplasia	20%
Undetermined	12%
Neoplasia	9%
Colitis	9%
Radiation 6%	
Ischemic 2%	
Ulcerative 1%	
Other	7%

Adapted from Boley SJ, DiBiase A, Brandt LJ, et al: Lower intestinal bleeding in the elderly. Am J Surg 137:57–64, 1979.

Diverticular bleeding usually presents with acute, painless, maroon to bright red hematochezia, although melena may also occur. Bleeding diverticula often result in significant blood loss, which may be poorly tolerated by the elderly patient. Bleeding stops spontaneously in approximately 80% of cases and no further intervention is necessary. Among this group of patients, only 25% have repeated episodes of diverticular bleeding.[43]

Angiodysplasia

Angiodysplasia is another common cause for acute lower GI bleeding. The clinical presentation of lower GI bleeding from angiodysplasia is different from diverticular bleeding. Patients present with weakness, fatigue, dyspnea on exertion, and heme-positive stools. Although bleeding can occasionally be massive, most often it is slow, chronic, and occult. Angiodysplastic lesions are small, typically less than 5 mm, multiple, and most often located in the colon and cecum. The cause of angiodysplastic lesions is unclear, although they are thought to be acquired with aging. It is thought that bleeding is a result of tension in the blood vessels in the colon surrounding these lesions. This leads to dilation of the blood vessels in the angiodysplastic lesions and results in friable areas.[6]

Hemorrhoids

Hemorrhoids, one of the most common causes of intermittent lower GI bleeding, are estimated to occur in 50% to 80% of the U.S. population. It is rare that the amount of bleeding is large enough to cause iron deficiency anemia or to warrant transfusion. Typically, the patient notes bright red blood on the toilet tissue or around the stool, but not mixed in with the stool. However, massive bleeding from hemorrhoids can occur, most typically in patients with rectal varices as a result of portal hypertension. Anal fissures can cause symptoms similar to hemorrhoids, but they are usually associated with pain.[6]

Tumors and Polyps

Benign and malignant tumors and polyps are fairly common, especially in elderly persons. Ten percent to 20% of these patients have bleeding from these lesions, although it is usually slow, chronic, and self-limiting. More advanced lesions usually have other symptoms of obstruction, such as weight loss or change in the caliber of the stools.[6] Colorectal cancer is the most common malignant lesion to cause occult GI bleeding in the Western countries.[44] Colonoscopy is indicated for further evaluation of these lesions.[6]

Inflammatory Bowel Disease

Diarrhea is the most common symptom of ulcerative colitis and is often associated with blood in the stool. The degree of bleeding from inflammatory bowel disease is usually small to moderate, although, rarely, it can be massive. And, although it is not uncommon for an iron deficiency anemia to develop, transfusions are not usually required. Bleeding associated with Crohn's disease is also usually small to moderate in amount, and is thought to be related to thrombocytosis. In very rare instances, life-threatening hemorrhage can result when the underlying inflammation ulcerates into adjacent arteries.[6] The treatment of bleeding associated with inflammatory bowel disease is management of the underlying disorder.[42]

Ongoing Bleeding

Although most lower GI bleeding in adults is usually mild and self-limited, a small percentage of patients have ongoing bleeding, which may result in shock or hypotension, requiring ICU observation. Frequently, these patients are elderly and have other concomitant medical or surgical problems. Identification of the source of bleeding is important, and colonoscopy or anoscopy is performed. If a bleeding site is not identified, further interventions, including upper endoscopy, red blood cell scanning, and angiography, should be performed. The most common bleeding lesions resulting in massive lower GI bleeding are colonic angiomas (angiodysplasia) and diverticula.[45]

Assessment

Hematemesis, or bloody vomitus, can be either a bright red color or resemble coffee grounds. Bright red blood occurs when the bleeding is rapid, or it does not come in contact with gastric acid.[1] The presence of hematemesis confirms an upper GI source of bleeding in approximately 90% of the cases. Melena, which is black, tarry, foul-smelling stool, occurs when bleeding is slower. This is the result of degradation of the blood in the small intestine. Sense of smell is an excellent way to assess blood. When blood is passed with stool it has a characteristic foul odor. Although the presence of melena is most often an indication of an upper GI source of bleeding, it may also occur as a result of bleeding in the colon.[42] As little as 50 to 100 mL of blood in the upper GI tract can cause melena. Larger amounts of bleeding (1000 to 2000 mL) can produce melena for up to 5 days and heme-positive stools for up to 12 days. Whereas black stools can occur while taking some medications, such as iron, they are not tarry.[2] Hematochezia is bright red blood from the rectum. It may be mixed with stool and usually indicates a lower GI source of bleeding. If hematochezia is present with an upper GI bleed, there is massive hemorrhage (Table 35–4).[42]

Blood Loss

It is important to quickly assess the patient to determine the urgency of the situation. Initial assessment should include the patency of the patient's airway, breathing, circulation, and vital signs. It is important to know the correlation between the volume of blood lost and the clinical findings. If the volume of blood lost is small, there may be little or no clinical assessment findings. As the volume of blood loss increases, the variety of physical findings also increases.

Blood loss of 500 mL or less typically has no clinical findings. With blood loss of 750 to 1250 mL, slight tachycardia (less than 110 bpm), slight decrease in blood pressure, as well as cool hands and feet may correlate to mild shock. As blood loss increases, up to 1750 mL, the tachycardia worsens (100–120 bpm), pulse pressure decreases, and systolic blood pressure decreases to 90 to 100 mm Hg. The patient may exhibit pallor, diaphoresis, restlessness, and oliguria.[46] As blood loss continues, the patient may exhibit shortness of breath, decreased oxygen saturation, and even chest pain. A patient who is already "dry" or dehydrated demonstrates signs and symptoms of blood loss with the loss of a smaller volume of blood. Postural hypotension of 10 mm Hg or higher usually indicates at least a 20% reduction in blood volume. Shock occurs when blood loss approaches 40% of total blood volume.[42] With massive blood loss, greater than 2500 mL, tachycardia is severe (greater than 120 bpm) and the systolic blood pressure drops below 90 mm Hg.[46] With massive blood loss, bradycardia, rather than tachycardia, may be present because of vagal slowing of the heart.[42] The extremities become cold, pallor is extreme, mental stupor is present, and the patient becomes anuric.[46]

The initial hematocrit obtained from a patient who is acutely bleeding does not always accurately reflect

TABLE 35–4
Sources of Bleeding

Assessment Finding	Source of Bleeding
Hematemesis	
Bright red blood	Upper GI
Coffee ground material	Upper GI
Melena	Upper GI, rarely
Black, tarry, foul-smelling stool	lower GI
Hematochezia	Lower GI, rarely
Bright red blood mixed with stool	upper GI

Adapted from Elta GH: Approach to the patient with gross gastrointestinal bleeding. In: Yamada T, Alpers DH, et al (eds): Textbook of Gastroenterology. Philadelphia, JB Lippincott, 1995, pp 671–698.

the amount of blood loss. The hematocrit is a measure of the erythrocyte (red blood cell) volume as a percentage of the total blood volume. As blood is lost, extravascular fluid begins to move intravascularly. However, while this process begins almost immediately, it can take 24 to 48 hours for equilibration to occur. As external fluid, such as normal saline, is given to the patient, the hematocrit value may appear to precipitously decrease. For this reason, it is important to not rely only on laboratory values as a means of assessing blood volume loss. Instead, clinical assessment of the patient's blood pressure and pulse, as well as any evidence of continued bleeding is a more sensitive evaluation. In patients with anemia from chronic blood loss, however, the hematocrit is an accurate representation of the degree of anemia. Despite all this, it is still important to send blood samples to the laboratory for serial assessment of hematocrit, platelets, coagulation factors, and blood typing and crossmatch.[46]

Nursing Diagnoses

The care of patients with GI bleeding is complex and requires keen assessment skills. Diagnoses that are appropriate for patients diagnosed with GI bleeding are listed in Table 35–5.

Collaborative Management

It is crucial that one of the first interventions in the care of the patient with acute GI bleeding is fluid replacement. Many of the complications of GI bleeding, such as the development of shock, are the result of acute volume loss (see Chapter 47). Large-bore intravenous (IV) access (14- or 16-gauge), should be established.

However, blood has been safely transfused through IV catheters as small as 20 or 22 gauge, if it is first diluted with 100 to 250 mL of normal saline. For the hemodynamically unstable patient, it is preferable that at least two IV lines be started. While IV access is being established, oxygen therapy should be started, with pulse oximetry for continual monitoring. Also during this time, continuous cardiac monitoring should be initiated.

Fluid replacement should begin immediately with 250 to 1000 mL of crystalloid (normal saline or lactated Ringer's) to maintain a systolic blood pressure of greater than 90 mm Hg. Vital signs should be monitored after every bolus, and breath sounds should be monitored frequently to assess for fluid overload. If the patient has not responded to the infusion of 2 to 3 L of crystalloid, then infusion of blood products should be considered. A Foley catheter should be placed to assist with monitoring the fluid replacement therapy. Urine output should be maintained at 30 to 50 mL per hour. In patients with underlying cardiac, pulmonary, renal, or hepatic disease, a central venous or pulmonary artery catheter may be inserted to further monitor fluid replacement.[47]

In addition to patients who remain unstable after infusion of 2 to 3 L of crystalloid, patients who experience angina or ischemic changes on electrocardiogram may also need blood product administration. Whole blood transfusions should be considered for exsanguinating patients because it provides increased colloid osmotic pressure and decreases the total fluid requirements of the patient. Infusion of O-negative blood can be initiated until the patient's blood has been typed and crossmatched. It is safe to infuse type-specific blood as well as type O blood. Packed red blood cells are typically infused because this decreases the patient's exposure to plasma antibodies and de-

TABLE 35–5
Nursing Diagnoses

Problem Statement	Etiologic Factors
Fluid volume deficit, risk for	Hypovolemia secondary to blood loss
Tissue perfusion, altered: cerebral, cardiac, respiratory, renal, peripheral	Hypovolemia and decreased oxygenation secondary to anemia
Gas exchange, impaired	Hypovolemia, anemia
Anxiety	Fear of bleeding, threat of death
Aspiration, risk for	Hematemesis and potential changes in level of consciousness
Nutrition, less than body requirements, altered	Decreased appetite secondary to bowel irritability
Pain	Bleeding and discomfort
Diarrhea	Decrease in intestinal transit time secondary to effects of blood in GI tract
Thought processes, altered	Decreased oxygen to the brain secondary to anemia
Infection, risk for	Suppressed immunity
Fatigue	Anemia, decreased oxygenation
Knowledge deficit	Precipitating factors, hospital procedures, therapeutic interventions, discharge information

creases the likelihood of fluid overload when compared with whole blood transfusions. Blood and blood products should be infused through a filter and warmed before infusion. If rapid infusion is necessary, a blood warmer should be used. Each unit of packed cells should elevate a patient's hematocrit by 3 points. As additional blood work is obtained, this allows for evaluation of whether the bleeding has stopped.

Serial hemoglobin values are obtained to assess for cessation of bleeding; they are not usually done to evaluate the effect of packed cell administration. The initial hematocrit may represent the patient's prehemorrhage baseline, because blood loss involves the loss of plasma as well as red blood cells. There may be a decrease of 6 points in the hematocrit after the infusion of 2 L of crystalloid, because this replaces the plasma volume, without supplying additional red blood cells. The optimal time to check the hematocrit is 10 to 20 minutes after the completion of a crystalloid infusion.[2]

Fresh frozen plasma (FFP) may be used for patients who have a coagulopathy or have been receiving warfarin (Coumadin) therapy. Although FFP is not crossmatched like packed red blood cells, it is still necessary to know the blood type of the patient. As with packed red blood cells, type O-negative FFP can be infused until the blood type is available. A blood type can be determined in approximately 30 minutes. FFP has also been used in massive transfusions when coagulation studies are not available. For this use, 1 unit of FFP may be given for every 5 to 6 units of packed red blood cells.

Platelet transfusions may be necessary for patients who have thrombocytopenia, perhaps associated with portal hypertension, or because of platelet consumption. The goal is maintenance of the platelet count above $50,000/mm^3$. Platelets can be ordered as "random donor," which is a compilation of units from many donors, or single donor, which, as the name implies, is from one donor. In random donor platelets, 5 to 10 units are usually ordered at a time. This is equivalent to 1 unit of single donor platelets. Single donor platelets offer the advantage of not exposing the patient to many different donor antibodies, thereby potentially decreasing the possibility of a transfusion reaction. Whereas some literature states that each unit of random donor platelets given should elevate the platelet count by 5000 to $10,000/mm^3$, this can be difficult to predict and is dependent on the individual patient's ability to accept the platelets (Table 35–6).[2, 48]

Therapeutic Interventions

Nonvariceal bleeding from the upper GI tract stops spontaneously approximately 80% of the time, whereas in variceal bleeding, only approximately 60% of bleeding stops spontaneously.[2] In lower GI tract bleeding, spontaneous cessation of bleeding occurs in approximately 80% of cases, although approximately 25% of these patients rebleed.[26] For patients in whom bleeding does not stop, some type of therapeutic intervention is necessary. This can include pharmacotherapy, mechanical tamponade, transjugular intrahepatic portosystemic shunt, endoscopic therapy, or surgery.

Pharmacotherapy

Antacids

Antacids are indicated for the relief of symptoms associated with hyperacidity related to the diagnosis of conditions such as peptic ulcer disease and gastritis. Antacids control gastric pH by binding with and neutralizing hydrogen ions. Antacid therapy has been a standard method of managing stress ulcers since the late 1970s, although it is not currently first-line therapy for the control of peptic ulcer disease.[23] To control gastric pH, antacids must be administered frequently, occasionally as often as hourly. Measurement of gastric pH must be done frequently to evaluate effectiveness and titrate doses. Accurate measurement of gastric pH can be difficult because the aspirate of gastric contents is drawn through the same nasogastric tube by which the antacids are administered. Nasogastric tubes must

TABLE 35–6
Blood Products and Laboratory Work

Blood Products	Necessary Laboratory Work	Comments
Red blood cells	Crossmatch	Raises hematacrit 3 points per unit
Fresh frozen plasma	Blood type	In massive transfusions, may give 1 unit for every 5–6 units of packed red blood cells
Platelets	Blood type	6–8 units random = 1 unit single; goal is platelet count >50,000/mm³
Cryoprecipitate	Blood type	Most commonly administered source of exogenous von Willebrand's factor (carrier protein for factor VIII)

Data from McGuirk TD, Coyle WJ: Upper gastrointestinal tract bleeding in emergency medicine, Part 1. Emerg Med Clin North Am 14:523–543, 1994; Longstreth GF: Epidemiology of hospitalization for acute upper gastrointestinal hemorrhage: a population based study. Am J Gastroenterol 90:206–210, 1995.

be frequently clamped and released between doses, which is a time-consuming procedure.[49]

Side effects associated with antacid administration include constipation and diarrhea. Aluminum and calcium products form insoluble salts, which precipitate out in the intestines, causing constipation. Magnesium products attract and retain water, causing an osmotic effect, leading to diarrhea. Aluminum antacids bind with phosphate in the GI tract, which can lead to decreased phosphate levels. Even though that may be the intended use in patients with renal failure, it bears watching in other patients so that appropriate replacement therapy can be instituted.

Digitalis preparations can also be adversely affected by antacid administration. There is the potential for levels to be either higher or lower than normal. Additionally, many drugs can be adversely affected by the administration of antacids as a result of the change in the gastric pH. For this reason, it is important to not administer any oral drug within 1 to 2 hours before or after an antacid. This can present a particular problem if the administration of the antacids is frequent.[50]

Histamine Receptor Antagonist

Because of the problems associated with the administration of antacids, histamine (or H_2) receptor antagonists have become a more desirable option for the control of gastric pH. These agents block the histamine stimulation of acid-secreting cells, thereby influencing gastric pH. The four H_2 receptor antagonists that have been approved by the Food and Drug Administration (FDA) are cimetidine, ranitidine, famotidine, and nizatidine (Table 35–7). All of these agents are used in oral form for the management of ulcer disease. However, in the management of acute GI bleeding, continuous IV infusion, which eliminates the use of nizatidine, is preferred. Bolus infusion over 15 to 30 minutes is also acceptable. Continuous IV administration of H_2 receptor antagonists can be used in hyperalimentation solutions or maintenance IV lines.[49,51]

H_2 receptor antagonists have been well tolerated with an overall low rate of reported side effects. Common side effects include headache, dizziness, diarrhea, and constipation. Because these drugs alter the acidic environment in the stomach, there may be alterations in the absorption, metabolism, or excretion of certain drugs. With the exception of ketoconazole, changes in the absorption of drugs is rarely clinically significant.[52]

Cimetidine, and to a lesser extent ranitidine, decrease hepatic blood flow and inhibit cytochrome P-450, which can result in potential drug interactions as a result of altered metabolism. In most cases, this altered metabolism is not clinically significant. However, additional attention is warranted when medications with narrow therapeutic-to-toxic-level ratios, such as theophylline, phenytoin, lidocaine, quinidine, and warfarin, are given. Additional medications metabolized by the P-450 cytochrome that may be affected include some beta-blockers (propranolol, metoprolol), calcium channel blockers (except diltiazem), tricyclic antidepressants, and benzodiazepines.[53]

Ranitidine binds five to 10 times less avidly to cytochrome P-450 than cimetidine and has far less potential for significant drug interactions. Famotidine and nizatidine do not exhibit any significant alteration of the cytochrome P-450 and are virtually devoid of any significant related drug interactions.[54] For this reason, these medications are more commonly recommended in patients with liver disease. It is important to remember that H_2 receptor antagonists and antacids should be given 1 hour apart.[49]

Sucralfate

Sucralfate is another medication used in the management of ulcers. Sucralfate is given orally, either in pill form or slurry. It forms a thick, viscous paste in the stomach, which protects the ulcer. It is hypothesized that this protective barrier may absorb substances, such as pepsin and bile salts, thereby protecting the ulcer from further erosion, and allowing healing to begin.

Sucralfate has minimal (3%–5%) systemic absorption and so has very few side effects associated with its use. Constipation may occur in 3% of patients. Sucralfate should be administered on an empty stomach. It has been shown to bind to several drugs, such as quinolone antibiotics, phenytoin, and warfarin, decreasing their absorption. Significant interactions are rare and can be avoided by giving sucralfate separately from other medications.[55]

Sucralfate should not be administered with tube feedings because of the potential for the development

TABLE 35–7

Histamine Receptor Antagonists

	Cimetidine	Ranitidine	Famotidine	Nizatidine
Brand names	Tagamet	Zantac	Pepcid	Axid
Equivalent dosage (orally)	1600 mg	300 mg	40 mg	300 mg
Intravenous infusion	Yes	Yes	Yes	No
Serum half-life	1.5–2.5 hr	2–3 hr	2.5–4 hr	1–2 hr

Data from Feldman M, Burton ME: Histamine$_2$-receptor antagonists. N Engl J Med 323:1749, 1990.

of nonabsorbable compounds.[49] For this same reason, if a patient only has a flexible feeding tube through which to administer sucralfate, it is of vital importance that thorough flushing of this medication is completed before restarting any tube feedings. If this is not done, the feeding tube may become irreparably blocked, necessitating replacement. Additionally, sucralfate should not be administered within 30 minutes of antacids.[49]

H$^+$,K$^+$-ATPase Inhibitors (Proton Pump Inhibitors)

H$^+$,K$^+$-ATPase inhibitors, also known as proton pump inhibitors, inhibit the acid secretory pump, which is the final step in the acid secretory process. Omeprazole inhibits basal and stimulated acid secretion. After 1 week of therapy, basal acid secretion is inhibited by almost 100%, and stimulated acid secretion is inhibited by 98%.

Because omeprazole degrades rapidly in the acidic environment of the stomach, it is administered as enteric-coated capsules containing granules that dissolve in the small intestines. While it was previously thought that this would limit the use of omeprazole in the critically ill patient, recent studies have shown otherwise. One study demonstrated that a simplified omeprazole suspension consisting of omeprazole, 20 mg/10 mL of 8.4% sodium bicarbonate solution, administered via a nasogastric tube, prevented clinically significant gastrointestinal bleeding and maintained gastric pH greater than 5.5 in mechanically ventilated patients without negative side effects. This method of delivery may be a safe and effective option for administering omeprazole to critically ill patients who are at risk for stress ulceration.[56]

Side effects associated with the use of omeprazole have been few, although nausea and abdominal pain have been rarely seen. As with H$_2$ receptor antagonists, omeprazole may inhibit the absorption of drugs, such as ketoconazole, which require an acidic environment. A dose-related inhibition of the P-450 cytochrome has been noted. Partial inhibition of diazepam, phenytoin, and warfarin has been noted, although in most situations, this has been clinically insignificant.[23]

Prostaglandins

Natural prostaglandins in the GI tract have a multitude of biologic effects, which include inhibition of gastric acid production, promotion of mucous production, and promotion of water and electrolyte absorption.[49] The half-life of natural prostaglandins is short, approximately several minutes, so synthetic prostaglandins have been developed for clinical use. The only FDA-approved synthetic prostaglandin is misoprostol. Misoprostol is readily absorbed from the GI tract, is excreted in the urine, although dose reduction for chronic renal failure is not necessary, and does not affect hepatic cytochrome P-450 drug metabolism.[23]

It has been demonstrated that misoprostol inhibits gastric acid secretion and stimulation of mucosal defense mechanisms. Although the gastric acid secretion inhibition is not as potent as the H$_2$ receptor antagonists are, it is believed that the ulcer healing effect of misoprostol is a result of a constellation of actions. Stimulation of mucous and bicarbonate secretion is believed to enhance the pH mucous barrier and mucosal blood flow. Misoprostol has been well tolerated, with the most common side effect being diarrhea (10%–30%), although this may be self-limited.[23] Because misoprostol can stimulate uterine contractions, leading to bleeding and miscarriage, its use is contraindicated for pregnant women.[49]

Vasopressin

The IV infusion of vasopressin, used for the temporary management of GI bleeding, is often started as soon as the diagnosis is certain. Vasopressin decreases portal pressure by vasoconstricting the splanchnic arteries, thereby reducing blood flow. Bleeding is usually controlled soon after the vasopressin infusion is started. However, the infusion should be maintained at least 6 hours after the bleeding has stopped, although 24 hours is preferred.[57]

Complications of vasopressin therapy are a result of the vasoconstrictive properties of the medication.[57] Vasopressin reduces coronary blood flow and increases blood pressure. This increases oxygen demand while decreasing myocardial oxygen supply.[58] Coronary artery vasoconstriction can result in bradydysrhythmias, ventricular dysrhythmias, angina, myocardial infarction, and decreased cardiac output.[57,59] For this reason, cardiac monitoring during vasopressin infusion is essential. Abdominal cramps and bowel ischemia may also develop.[57]

In addition to cardiac vasoconstriction, blood flow to the splanchnic system, via the mesenteric artery, is also decreased. This places the patient at risk for bowel ischemia. Ischemic bowel causes third space extracellular fluid loss, resulting in fluid and electrolyte imbalance, acid-base imbalance, and symptoms of bowel ischemia, which include abdominal pain and distention, paralytic ileus, nausea, and diarrhea. Assessment for these conditions should be included in the nursing care of patients receiving this therapy.[57–59]

Concurrent administration of nitroglycerin can minimize some of the undesirable side effects of vasopressin. Nitroglycerin, which decreases preload and systemic vascular resistance, improves blood flow to the coronary arteries, decreasing the workload of the heart. A reduction of portal pressure also contributes to control of bleeding.[58]

Additional parameters that should be included in the nursing assessment include peripheral pulses, capillary refill, and skin temperature and color, which may be decreased as a result of the vasoconstrictive effects of vasopressin. The skin over the extremities may appear mottled. Urinary output should also be monitored. Vasopressin can cause water retention, resulting in water intoxication. Symptoms of water intoxication include change in mental status and low serum sodium concentration. Hourly intake and output, daily body weight, daily serum sodium levels, and frequent evaluation of neurologic status should also be included in the nursing assessment of these patients.[58] Arterial blood gas may be monitored to assess for metabolic acidosis caused by lactic acid buildup.

Somatostatin

Somatostatin, a naturally occurring polypeptide, lowers portal venous pressure by vasoconstriction of the splanchnic circulation. Whereas somatostatin causes vasoconstriction, it has fewer systemic side effects than vasopressin. Because of its very short plasma half-life, continuous IV administration is necessary.[60] In comparison to vasopressin, somatostatin results in superior control of bleeding and it has been shown to be as effective as sclerotherapy in controlling bleeding.[61]

Octreotide

Octreotide is a synthetic analog of somatostatin that has similar hemodynamic properties but a longer duration of action.[62] Although it is usually given IV in the management of acute GI bleeding, it may also be administered subcutaneously. Octreotide has been shown to control bleeding better than vasopressin with decreased incidence of side effects such as headache, chest pain, and abdominal pain. However, mortality rate related to bleeding esophageal varices was no different between the two groups. Octreotide has also been shown to be as effective as emergency sclerotherapy in the control of variceal hemorrhage.[61]

Mechanical Tamponade

Esophageal or gastric balloon tamponade tubes have been used effectively for the temporary control of active esophageal and gastric variceal bleeding that cannot be controlled with pharmacotherapy or sclerotherapy. The basic esophagogastric tube has two balloons, one for the stomach and one for the esophagus, and a distal port to drain the gastric contents. The Sengstaken-Blakemore tube is the most widely known (Figure 35–1). A nasogastric tube should also be inserted to aspirate esophageal and pharyngeal secretions. Some tubes, such as the Minnesota tube, already have a fourth port as part of the tube for drainage of these secretions. When the balloons are inflated, pressure is applied in the esophagus and at the cardioesophageal junction. For the tube to function

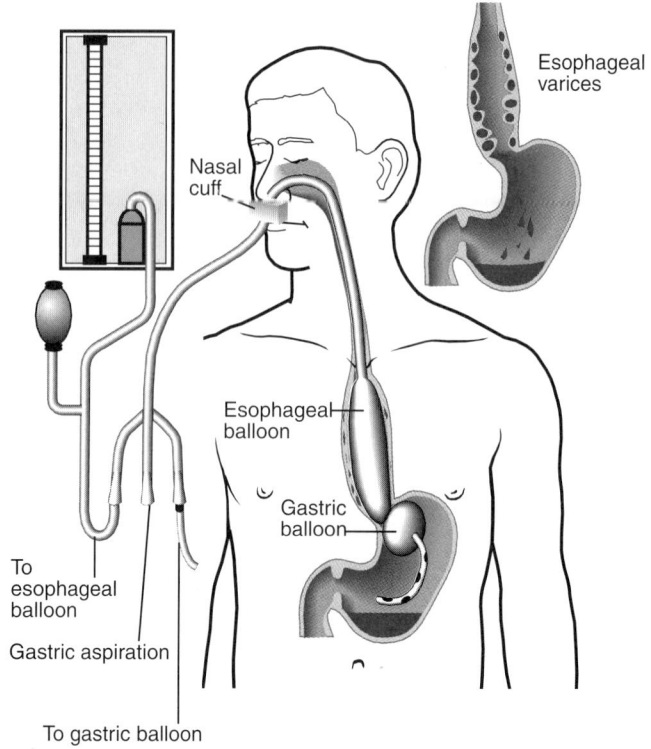

Figure 35–1

Sengstaken–Blakemore tube. (Modified from Saunders Manual of Nursing Care. Philadelphia, W.B. Saunders, 1996, p 1325.)

properly, tension must be applied so that the gastric balloon is held firmly in place at the cardioesophageal junction.[59] Even though balloon tamponade tubes control bleeding in up to 90% of patients initially, long-term control by other methods is still required.[2]

Before insertion, each balloon should be inflated to assess for leaks. The balloons are then deflated and clamped to ensure they remain deflated during insertion. Once the tube has been inserted, through the mouth or nose, a radiograph is required to verify placement before inflation of the balloon. Upon confirmation of placement, the gastric balloon is inflated using a specified amount of air, as per manufacturer recommendations. It is then pulled back until resistance is felt and secured according to hospital protocol, which may involve the use of a football helmet, traction, or another method. This ensures that the balloon is applying pressure to the gastroesophageal junction. If bleeding continues once the gastric balloon is inflated, then the esophageal balloon is also inflated. The esophageal balloon is inflated until a desired pressure (usually between 25 and 40 mm Hg) is obtained. This is measured with a mercury manometer.[59]

Normal capillary pressure ranges between 10 and 15 mm Hg, whereas arterial pressure is between 30 and 40 mm Hg. The goal is to keep the pressure in the esophageal balloon at the lowest level to prevent bleeding. Pressures above 45 mm Hg place the patient at risk for necrosis or rupture. For this reason, it is important that the pressure in the esophageal balloon be measured frequently and that the balloon be deflated periodically.[59] The frequency and procedure for this may vary based on the tube used or the policy of the institution.

The major complications associated with the use of balloon tamponade include necrosis, rupture or erosion of the esophagus, occlusion of the airway by the balloon, or pulmonary aspiration. Careful monitoring of the esophageal balloon pressure to prevent pressures above 45 mm Hg assists in the minimization of this complication. Inflation of the esophagogastric balloon should be limited to 24 to 36 hours. Upward migration of the esophageal balloon may cause occlusion of the airway. This can occur with sudden or gradual deflation of the gastric balloon. For this reason the gastric balloon should never be deflated while the esophageal balloon remains inflated. Scissors should be kept at the bedside to cut the esophageal balloon in case of an emergency. However, the most frequent complication associated with the use of the esophagogastric balloon tamponade tube is aspiration pneumonia. To protect the airway and minimize the development of this complication, endotracheal intubation is recommended before insertion of the balloon tube. Low, intermittent aspiration of gastric and esophageal contents reduces the risk for pulmonary aspiration. And, unless the patient is hemodynamically compromised, the head of the bed should be elevated at 30° to 45°.[59]

Transjugular Intrahepatic Portosystemic Shunt

The transjugular intrahepatic portosystemic shunt (TIPS) is a nonsurgical method of creating a portosystemic shunt. This shunt is created by the insertion of a metal stent, via a transjugular approach, that connects the portal vein to the hepatic vein (Figure 35–2). This results in the diversion of approximately 70% of the blood flow, which comes from the portal vein, through the liver to the hepatic vein, which drains the blood from the liver. TIPS should not be considered a first-line intervention for the management of acute variceal bleeding. Rather, it should be used in patients who have had repeated episodes of variceal bleeding that have been unresponsive to other therapies. This may mean that they have not responded to medical treatment, including sclerotherapy, at their first acute variceal bleed, or it may mean that they have had multiple hospital admissions for variceal bleeding (Chart 35–3).

The use of the TIPS is not without risks. Serious life-threatening complications occur in 1% to 2% of cases. These include hemoperitoneum, hemobilia, hepatic ischemia, sepsis, and death. Minor complications, which occur in approximately 8% of cases, include hematoma, stent migration, hemolysis, and fever.

Chronic complications associated with TIPS include portal or splenic vein thrombosis (1%–15%), chronic hemolysis (1%–3%), worsening hepatic function (1%–5%), shunt stenosis (33%–66%), and hepatic encephalopathy (15%–30%).[63]

An absolute contraindication to the placement of a TIPS is right-sided heart failure. The shunt that is created increases the blood flow back to the right side of the heart, further compromising the patient. Polycystic liver disease, which increases the risk of complications during insertion, and hepatic failure are also absolute contraindications. Relative contraindications to TIPS insertion include active intrahepatic or systemic infection, severe hepatic encephalopathy that is poorly controlled by medical therapy, portal vein thrombosis, and severe coagulopathy.[63]

Nursing responsibilities when caring for a patient after a TIPS procedure include assessing for complications associated with a TIPS insertion. Assessment should include evaluation for right-sided heart failure, including close monitoring of intake, output, and daily weights, the development or worsening of hepatic encephalopathy, and recurrence of bleeding. Additionally, patient and family teaching should be instituted regarding potential complications and any necessary follow-up.

Endoscopic Therapy

Endoscopy has become accepted as the diagnostic study of choice in upper GI hemorrhage, and can be valuable in locating the source of a lower GI bleed. Endoscopy, which is the insertion of a flexible, lighted endoscope into the GI tract, either from above or below, provides a mechanism for a variety of therapeutic interventions. These may include injection of a sclerosing agent, variceal band ligation, use of a heater probe, or combination therapy.

Injection Sclerotherapy

Endoscopic injection sclerotherapy can be performed emergently at the time of the initial endoscopy, or it can be delayed until the variceal bleeding has been controlled by other methods. This therapy involves the injection of a sclerosing agent into the varices, resulting in decreased bleeding. The mechanism of action is not yet fully understood. A variety of sclerosing agents are used and selection of which one to use is dependent on the personal choice of the physician performing the procedure. Sclerosants commonly seen in the United States include ethanolamine, sodium morrhuate, and sodium tetradecyl sulfate. A newer agent, cyanoacrylate, although not currently approved by the FDA, is gaining popularity. This agent is slightly different than the standard sclerosants because it acts as a liquid tissue adhesive, which increases its efficacy in the treatment of gastric varices.[64]

Normal anatomy

Hepatic vein

Portal vein

Inferior vena cava

Splenic vein

Renal vein

Mesenteric vein

A

Splenorenal shunt

B

Portacaval shunt

C

Mesocaval shunt

D

Transjugular Intrahepatic Portosystemic Shunt

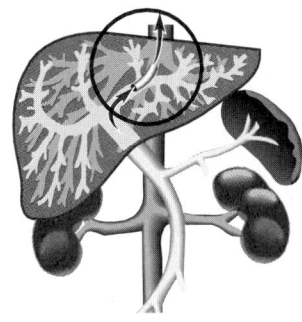

E

Figure 35–2

A, Normal anatomy. *B,* Splenorenal shunt: splenectomy with anastomosis of the splenic vein to the left renal vein. *C,* Portacaval shunt: surgical shunting of the blood from the portal system (portal vein) to the venous system (inferior vena cava). *D,* Mesocaval shunt: side anastomosis of the superior mesenteric vein to the proximal end of the inferior vena cava. *E,* Transjugular intrahepatic portosystemic shunt: radiologic surgical procedure that uses the normal vascular anatomy of the liver to create a shunt with the use of a metallic stent; the shunt is between the portal and systemic venous systems within the liver and is aimed at relieving hypertension. (Modified from Saunders Manual of Nursing Care. Philadelphia, W.B. Saunders, 1996, p 1327.)

Emergency sclerotherapy is performed during acute bleeding to stop active variceal hemorrhage. This has been shown to improve hemostasis and decrease transfusion requirements as well as rebleeding. After acute hemostasis, elective sclerotherapy is performed at 1- to 3-week intervals to obliterate remaining varices to prevent recurrent bleeding.

There are few contraindications to the performance of sclerotherapy. Perforation of the GI tract is one. The presence of deep ulcerations at previous sclerotherapy injection sites is another. After healing, repeat injection is possible. Coagulopathy, however, is not necessarily considered a contraindication because many patients with portal hypertension have some degree of coagulopathy.[64]

Sclerotherapy is a safe procedure, although complications can occur. To minimize patient discomfort, sedation is given. The most common complications asso-

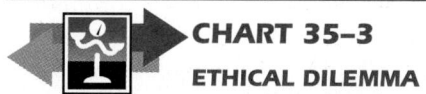

CHART 35–3

ETHICAL DILEMMA

Mr. H. is a 42-year-old homeless man who was admitted to the ICU with acute variceal bleeding. This is his third admission in 3 months. Mr. H. is an alcoholic who drinks as much as he can get his hands on, which, on average, is about a quart of whiskey a day. He has been evaluated by the addictions consult team and has refused all help. Mr. H. has stated that he does not want to stop drinking and that he does not care if it kills him.

In the ICU, Mr. H. is combative and confused, striking out at hospital personnel. He has advanced liver disease as a result of his alcohol use and has portosystemic encephalopathy. Mr. H. initially refuses all treatment. He is argumentative, cursing frequently, and attempts to pull out all his IV lines and remove his oxygen. His initial laboratory work reveals an Hgb of 7.0 and Hct of 22. His ammonia level is elevated at 60 (normal, 11–35). It is decided that a blood transfusion is necessary, as well as an upper endoscopy to identify and treat the source of bleeding.

Mr. H. refuses to sign consent for the endoscopy and does not want the blood transfusion. The nasogastric tube, which Mr. H. has not yet pulled out, continues to drain copious amounts of bright red blood. A follow-up complete blood count reveals an Hgb of 5 and Hct of 18. At this point, Mr. H. is sedated, the endoscopy is performed, and transfusions started.

Mr. H.'s next of kin, his wife, is contacted. However, Mrs. H., although still legally married to Mr. H., has had little or no contact with him for the past 3 years. She states that she left him because of his drinking and does not want to be involved with his care now.

Mr. H.'s bleeding is controlled. He was intubated during the upper endoscopy and cannot speak. To prevent him from harming himself, he is in restraints and is receiving IV sedatives. Because Mr. H. has had several episodes of variceal bleeding in the past 3 months, additional therapeutic options to control his varices are discussed. These options include the insertion of a TIPS, as well as liver transplantation.

1. Mr. H. has stated that he does not want any interventions performed. Why is the decision made to proceed with emergency treatment?
2. What role should Mrs. H. play in making additional decisions regarding Mr. H.'s care?
3. What impact does Mr. H.'s refusal to stop drinking have on treatment options and use of resources, such as blood transfusions?
4. What factors should be evaluated when considering additional therapeutic interventions.
5. Should Mr. H. be considered as a candidate to receive a liver transplant? Defend your response.

---

ciated with this procedure are transient and self-limiting (Table 35–8). Sore throat, low-grade fever, dysphagia, and retrosternal pain may occur in more than half of patients. More serious complications, which may be

TABLE 35–8
Common Complications of Sclerotherapy

Area Affected	Complication
Esophageal	Ulcer formation
	Bleeding ulcers
	Perforation
	Strictures
	Dysphagia
Pulmonary and thoracic	Aspiration pneumonia
	Pleural effusions
Systemic	Low-grade fever
	Transient bacteremia

Adapted from Young HS, Matsui Suzanne M, Gregory PB: Endoscopic control of upper gastrointestinal variceal bleeding. In: Yamada T, Alpers DH, et al (eds): Textbook of Gastroenterology. Philadelphia, JB Lippincott, 1995, pp 2969–2991.

systemic or limited to the esophagus or lungs and thoracic cavity may develop in 10% to 15% of these patients.[65] Bleeding is always a risk because sclerotherapy may start a variceal bleed.

All sclerosants cause the formation of ulcers at the site of injection in almost every patient within 2 to 4 days. Deep ulcerations may delay additional sclerotherapy sessions. Significant bleeding from these ulcers may occur in 2% to 13% of patients. Acute esophageal perforation usually occurs shortly after a sclerotherapy session and is seen more frequently with the use of a rigid scope or an overtube. Delayed esophageal perforation from necrosis of ulcers may be fatal. Esophageal strictures, which appear to correlate with the number of sclerotherapy sessions, and dysphagia may also occur.[65]

Aspiration pneumonia develops in approximately 5% of patients, with those undergoing emergency sclerotherapy being at greater risk. Pleural effusions may occur in up to half of all patients who have received sclerotherapy, and even though most are clinically insignificant, some patients require thoracentesis. Adult respiratory distress syndrome, pneumothorax, and subcutaneous emphysema are less common complications of sclerotherapy.[65]

Development of a low-grade fever is a common complication of sclerotherapy. However, prolonged fever, for more than 2 days, requires additional evaluation for an infectious source. Transient bacteremia has also been reported, although the incidence of clinical significance varies. Death from acute complications of sclerotherapy is infrequent, occurring in about 1% to 2% of cases.[65]

Variceal Band Ligation

Variceal band ligation, an alternative to sclerotherapy, involves the application of a rubber band around the base of a varix, similar to hemorrhoid banding. Once the band has been placed on the base of the varix, blood supply is cut off and thrombosis occurs. The bands fall off within 1 to 2 weeks, are nonabsorbable, and are therefore passed spontaneously in the stool. The advantages of variceal band ligation over sclerotherapy include fewer local and systemic complications, lower rebleeding rates, and fewer endoscopic sessions to obliterate varices. Esophageal strictures are less common with band ligation, although no significant differences were noted with pulmonary infections or bacterial peritonitis.[66]

Drawbacks associated with variceal band ligation include limited field of view, blood pooling within the banding mechanism during active bleeding, and misfiring of the bands. Also, many banding devices are single shot, which requires removal of the device for reloading after each firing. An overtube is placed to facilitate removal and reintroduction of the banding device. The overtube has been associated with several complications including esophageal perforation, laceration, and hematoma. As the use of multishot banding devices becomes more common, complications associated with the overtube may decrease as will the length of time necessary for the procedure.[66]

Endoscopic Electrocoagulation

Endoscopic electrocoagulation has been used successfully for the emergency control of nonvariceal upper GI bleeding as well as for hemorrhoidal bleeding. Electrocoagulation involves the application of direct electric current to the hemorrhoid or bleeding lesion, resulting in submucosal fibrosis. Excess electrical current is grounded through the patient's body, although occasionally discharges occur that cause injury at sites distant from the area of intended tissue destruction. Electrocoagulation is also used for the palliative management of esophageal tumors.

Monopolar and bipolar electrocoagulation probes are available. Monopolar electrocoagulation involves the use of high-frequency alternating electric current. Heat is generated at the site of the probe, causing he-

mostasis. Serious complications such as perforation, postcoagulation syndrome, and delayed hemorrhage have occurred.[67] Bipolar probes use two electrodes for the administration of the electric current. Complications may include hemorrhage, fistula formation, and strictures.[68]

Laser Therapy

Another method of applying heat or thermal energy to coagulate or vaporize tissue is with the use of a laser. The site of bleeding must be clearly seen so that the laser can be targeted effectively. No delayed bleeding or postcoagulation syndromes were reported with this technique.[67] However, one disadvantage of laser therapy is that it is expensive and not easily portable, so that transport to the ICU for emergency treatment is difficult.[69] It is also important to remember that eye shields are essential when laser therapy is in use.

Heater Probe

A heater probe is a metal-tipped catheter through which electric current can be applied to heat tissue, causing coagulation. Even though monopolar, bipolar, and multipolar probes have been developed, the monopolar probes have fallen out of favor because of difficulty in controlling the depth of penetration from the heat, increasing the risk of complications. This therapy is portable and effective, so that most emergency endoscopy carts are equipped with an electrocautery device, such as the heater probe, as well as sclerosants.[69]

Photocoagulation

Photocoagulation, using infrared light or lasers, stimulates fibrosis of the submucosal tissue, resulting in eradication of hemorrhoids. This is a relatively safe procedure and can be performed in the outpatient setting. Unlike electrocoagulation, no electric current is applied to the patient, so there is decreased likelihood of complications. Typically, one hemorrhoid cushion is photocoagulated per session, so, on average, 3 to 5 sessions are necessary.[70]

The nurse caring for the patient undergoing an endoscopic procedure has several responsibilities. Before the procedure, the nurse is responsible for adequate patient preparation, which includes food and medication restriction. This is often less of a priority in an acute bleeding episode. Attending to the psychological needs of the patient or family should include reassurance and an explanation of the procedure. A brief history, focusing on any pertinent medical or surgical history, as well as a brief physical assessment, including baseline vital signs should be obtained.

During the endoscopic procedure, the responsibility of the critical care nurse may vary. In some institutions, a nurse from the endoscopic unit may be present during a bedside procedure. However, the overall focus of nursing responsibility during the procedure is to ensure the patient's safety and well-being. The emphasis is on monitoring and assessing the patient. The nurse may assist with technical aspects as well. In this case, it is important to have a thorough knowledge of the procedure. Throughout the procedure, it is important to continually assess the patient and his or her response to sedation.

At the completion of the procedure, it is important to monitor the patient's response to the procedure and any medications giving during the procedure. An assessment should be performed to identify any potential or actual complications associated with the procedure.[71]

Surgical Procedures

Surgical intervention may be required for the management of GI bleeding that is unresponsive to other therapeutic interventions. Patients who continue to bleed for more than 24 hours, require more than a 6- to 8-unit transfusion, or have recurrent bleeding despite endoscopic treatment require surgery.

Surgical Shunts

For patients with bleeding esophageal or gastric varices who are unresponsive to pharmacologic, endoscopic, or mechanical intervention, surgical options are explored. The creation of a portal-systemic shunt to divert blood away from the liver decreases the portal pressure and decompresses the esophageal and gastric varices. Several portal systemic shunt procedures can be performed (Figure 35–2). In selective shunt procedures, varices are decompressed while preserving portal vein flow. In nonselective shunt procedures, all portal blood flow is diverted to the systemic circulation.

The distal splenorenal shunt is the most widely recommended selective shunt procedure. In this procedure, the venous blood supply from the left upper quadrant of the abdomen is shunted away from the portal circulation, which decompresses the blood supply to the esophagus and upper stomach. Superior mesenteric blood flow to the liver is maintained, which decreases the incidence of portal systemic encephalopathy. Because this operation is more time-consuming than nonselective shunts, it is not often performed in emergency situations.[59]

The most commonly used emergency surgical shunt procedure is the end-to-side portacaval shunt. This involves the ligation of the hepatic end of the portal vein and anastomosis of the portal vein to the vena cava. The incidence of portal-systemic encephalopathy after this procedure is 50%.[59]

The side-to-side portacaval shunt, which involves the anastomosis of a side of the portal vein to the side of the vena cava, results in better control of ascites. The mesocaval shunt, which involves the positioning of a prosthetic graft to divert portal blood flow from the liver to the vena cava, has similar outcomes to the portocaval shunt in regard to morbidity and portal systemic encephalopathy.[59]

Gastric Surgical Interventions

The decision to electively operate in patients with intractable peptic ulcer disease is based on severity and duration of symptoms, response to medication, patient compliance, frequency of recurrence, and past complications. Which surgical procedure to perform remains controversial.

One approach is to decrease the production of stomach acid. This can be accomplished by severing the nerves that stimulate acid production or by removing the acid-secreting portion of the stomach. A vagotomy, which is severing of the vagus nerve, eliminates the stimulation to the gastric cells, resulting in decreased acid production. Several vagotomy procedures are possible and include a truncal vagotomy or selective gastric vagotomy. Because gastric motility is also stimulated by the vagus nerve, a gastroenterostomy or pyloroplasty must also be performed to provide for gastric emptying. This is not necessary with the highly selective vagotomy because gastric motility is preserved.

Surgical removal of the acid-producing portion of the stomach is another option for the treatment of gastric ulcer. This is accomplished by performing a Bilroth I or II procedure. In the Bilroth I procedure, the distal portion of the stomach is removed with an anastomosis to the proximal portion of the duodenum. In the Bilroth II procedure, the distal portion of the stomach is removed and anastomosed to the jejunum. The stump of the duodenum is surgically closed.[72]

Multidisciplinary Outcomes

Multidisciplinary outcomes identified for patients with GI bleeding are summarized in Chart 35–4.

Critical Thinking Exercise

Mrs. J. is an 80-year-old woman with rheumatoid arthritis who was seen at the emergency department with complaints of dizziness, shortness of breath, and chest pain. She is a poor historian, but relates that this has been occurring with increasing frequency over the past 2 weeks. Initial evaluation reveals a heart rate of 110, respiratory rate of 28, and peripheral oxygen saturation of 92%. Continuous cardiac monitoring and 4 L of oxygen supplementation are initiated. A 12-lead electrocardiogram (ECG) is performed.

Additional questioning reveals that Mrs. J. has smoked two packs of cigarettes a day for the past 60 years, has a

> ## CHART 35–4
>
> **MULTIDISCIPLINARY OUTCOMES**
>
> Identification and stabilization of GI bleeding
> Restoration and maintenance of fluid volume
> Restoration and maintenance of electrolyte and acid-base balance
> Normalization and maintenance of cardiac output and tissue perfusion
> Normalization of ventilation and gas exchange
> Prevention of complications associated with acute illness
>
> Restoration and maintenance of adequate nutrition and patterns of elimination
> Identification of risk factors related to GI bleeding
> Self-management of therapeutic regimen, including discontinuation of use of alcohol, if appropriate
> Achievement of optimal level of functioning

history of coronary artery disease, and has been taking corticosteroids and NSAIDs for the management of her rheumatoid arthritis.

On physical examination Mrs. J.'s lungs were clear, no dysrhythmias were noted, and EKG was normal, although her pulse was weak. Nailbeds were pale and capillary refill was sluggish. During this time, Mrs. J. also stated that she had been having black tarry stools for several weeks, which she thought started after she began taking iron supplements. Blood work revealed the following:

Complete blood count: white blood cell count—4.6; Hgb—8.4; Hct—26.5; platelets—279.

Arterial blood gas: pH—7.36; P_{O_2}—70; P_{CO_2}—44; O_2 sat—92%.

Blood type: O positive.

The decision was made to transfer Mrs. J. to the ICU for further evaluation and management. While in the ICU, an upper endoscopy was performed and a diagnosis of upper GI bleeding was made.

1. What presenting symptoms influenced the decision to admit Mrs. J. to the ICU?
2. What was the cause of Mrs. J.'s chest pain?
3. What assessment findings were clues that Mrs. J.'s chest pain was not of cardiac origin?
4. Mrs. J.'s hematocrit was 26.5. Discuss whether this is an accurate measurement and what factors affect the hematocrit value in the presence of bleeding.
5. What factors increase Mrs. J.'s risk for the development of peptic ulcer disease?
6. Describe the rationale for performing the upper endoscopy.
7. What interventions would be expected for Mrs J. based on her clinical presentation and diagnosis?

Key Concepts

➤ GI bleeding is a common critical care problem.
➤ Upper GI bleeding has a mortality rate of 5% to 10%.

➤ Esophageal varices account for one of 10 upper GI bleeds.
➤ Peptic ulcer disease is a common, serious medical problem, associated with a high incidence of GI bleeding.
➤ Two common causes of peptic ulcer disease are infection with the *H. pylori* bacteria and use of NSAIDs.
➤ Lower GI bleeding has a mortality rate of 5% to 10%.
➤ Diverticulosis and angiodysplasia are the leading causes of lower GI.
➤ The initial hematocrit may not be an accurate assessment of blood loss.
➤ Fluid replacement is a crucial first step in caring for the patient with acute GI bleeding.
➤ Blood product administration may be necessary depending on the severity of blood loss.
➤ A variety of pharmaceutical options exist for the control of gastric pH. These include antacids, H_2 blockers, sucralfate, and proton pump inhibitors.
➤ IV vasopressin, somatostatin, and octreotide can be used for the temporary management of GI bleeding. The use of vasopressin alone for the control of GI bleeding has been associated with many side effects. These have been improved with the concomitant administration of nitroglycerin.
➤ Mechanical balloon tamponade is another temporary measure to control active bleeding.
➤ TIPS is a nonsurgical method of creating portosystemic shunting as a mechanism to control GI bleeding.
➤ Endoscopic therapy has become the treatment of choice for the management of GI bleeding by many practitioners.
➤ Injection sclerotherapy can be performed emergently. Follow-up sessions are necessary to obliterate remaining varices and prevent recurrent bleeding.
➤ The use of variceal band ligation is gaining in popularity, although its use for emergent control of GI bleeding remains under investigation.

⟹ Surgical intervention is indicated for the control of GI bleeding that is unresponsive to other therapeutic interventions. The most common surgical shunt created for the control of emergent GI bleeding is the end-to-side portacaval shunt. The distal splenorenal shunt is the most widely recommended selective shunt procedure, but because of the lengthy operative time required, this procedure is not often performed in emergency situations.

⟹ The decision to perform surgical intervention, such as a vagotomy, to control intractable peptic ulcer disease is based on severity and duration of symptoms, response to medication, patient compliance, frequency of recurrence, and past complications.

References

1. Labovich TM: Selected complications in the patient with cancer: spinal cord compression, malignant bowel obstruction, malignant ascites and gastrointestinal bleeding. Semin Oncol Nursing 10:189–197, 1994.
2. McGuirk TD, Coyle WJ: Upper gastrointestinal tract bleeding in emergency medicine, Part 1. Emerg Med Clin North Am 14:523–543, 1994.
3. Huether SE, McCance KL, Tarmina MS: Alterations of digestive function. In: McCance KL, Huether SE, (eds): Pathophysiology: The Biologic Basis for Disease in Adults and Children. St. Louis, CV Mosby, 1994, pp 1212–1266.
4. Longstreth GF: Epidemiology of hospitalization for acute upper gastrointestinal hemorrhage: a population-based study. Am J Gastroenterol 90:206–210, 1995.
5. Gilbert DA: Epidemiology of upper gastrointestinal bleeding. Gastrointest Endosc 36(Suppl):S8–S13, 1990.
6. Bono MJ: Lower gastrointestinal tract bleeding, Part 1. Emerg Med Clin North Am Gastrointest Emerg 14:547–556, 1996.
7. Huston CJ: Ruptured esophageal varices. Am J Nursing 4:43, 1996.
8. McCormick PA: Pathophysiology and prognosis of oesophageal Varices. Scand J Gastroenterol 207(Suppl):1–5, 1994.
9. Silverstein FE, Gilbert DA, Tedesco FJ, et al: The National ASGE Survey on Upper Gastrointestinal Bleeding: I study design and baseline data. Gastrointest Endosc 27:73–79, 1981.
10. Sanyal AJ, Purdum PP, Luketic VA, et al: Bleeding gastroesophageal varices. Semin Liver Dis 13:328–341, 1993.
11. Sanyal AJ, Feedman AM, Shiffman ML, et al: Transjugular intrahepatic portosystemic shunt (TIPS) for uncontrolled variceal hemorrhage in advanced cirrhotics at high risk for surgery: a prospective study (Abstract). Gastroenterology 104:A985, 1993.
12. McCormick PA, Jenkins SA, McIntyre N, et al: Why portal hypertensive varices bleed and bleed: a hypothesis. Gut 36:100–103, 1995.
13. Merican I, Sprengers D, McCormick PA, et al: Diurnal pattern of variceal bleeding in cirrhotic patients J Hepatol 19:15–22, 1993.
14. Ott DJ: Radiology of the oropharynx and esophagus. In: Castell DO (ed): The Esophagus. Boston, Little, Brown, 1995, pp 41–91.
15. Pegram PS: Esophagitis in the immunocompromised host. In: Castell DO (ed): The Esophagus. Boston, Little, Brown, 1995, pp 635–657.
16. Richter JM: Occult gastrointestinal bleeding. Gastroenterol Clin North Am 1:53–66, 1994.
17. Spechler SJ: Complications of gastroesophageal reflux disease. In: Castell DO (ed): The Esophagus. Boston, Little, Brown, 1995, pp 533–545.
18. DeMeester TR, Peters JH: Surgical treatment of gastroesophageal reflux disease. In: Castell DO (ed): The Esophagus. Boston, Little, Brown, 1995, pp 577–617.
19. Johnson D: Esophageal involvement in other inflammatory conditions. In: Castell DO (ed): The Esophagus. Boston, Little, Brown, 1995, pp 673–689.
20. Semble EL: Nonsteroidal anti-inflammatory drugs and esophageal damage. In: Castell DO (ed): The Esophagus. Boston, Little, Brown, 1995, pp 691–698.
21. Haddad NG, Fleicher DE: Neoplasms of the esophagus. In: Castell DO (ed): The Esophagus. Boston, Little, Brown, 1995, pp 269–291.
22. Katz PO, Salas L: Less frequent causes of upper gastrointestinal bleeding. Gastroenterol Clin North Am 22:875–889, 1993.
23. Isenberg JI, McQuaid KR, Laine L, et al: Acid-peptic disorders. In: Yamada T, Alpers DH, et al (eds): Textbook of Gastroenterology. Philadelphia, JB Lippincott, 1995, 1347–1430.
24. Raskin JB, Chong J: NSAID induced ulcerations. In: Bayless TM (ed): Current Therapy in Gastroenterology and Liver Disease. St. Louis, Mosby.
25. Swain CP: Pathophysiology of bleeding lesions. Gastrointest Endosc 36:S21–S22, 1990.
26. Gabriel SE, Jaakkimainen L, Bombardier C: Risks for serious gastrointestinal complications related to the use of nonsteroidal anti-inflammatory drugs. Ann Intern Med 115:787–796, 1991.
27. Kelly JP, Kaufman DW, Koff RS, et al: Alcohol consumption and the risk of major upper gastrointestinal bleeding. Am J Gastroenterol 90:1058–1064, 1995.
28. Marshall BJ: *Helicobacter pylori.* Am J Gastroenterol 89(Suppl): S116–S128, 1994.
29. NIH Consensus Conference: *Helicobacter pylori* in peptic ulcer disease. JAMA 272:65–69, 1994.
30. Chamberlain CE: Acute hemorrhagic gastritis. Gastroenterol Clin North Am 22:843–873, 1993.
31. Pisani P, Parkin DM, Ferlay J: Estimates of the worldwide incidence of eighteen major cancers in 1985. Int J Cancer 55:891–903, 1993.
32. Boland CR, Scheiman JM: Tumors of the stomach. In: Yamada T, Alpers DH, et al (eds): Textbook of Gastroenterology. Philadelphia, JB Lippincott Co, 1995, pp 1494–1523.
33. Parsonnet J, Friedman GD, Vandersteen DP, et al: *Helicobacter pylori* infection and the risk of gastric carcinoma. N Engl J Med 325:1170–1171, 1991.
34. Steger A: Acute gastrointestinal bleeding. In: Bouchier IAD, Allan RN, Hodgson HJF, Keighley MRB (eds): Gastroenterology: Clinical Science and Practice. London, WB Saunders Company Ltd, 1994, pp 957–974.
35. Clouse RE: Vascular lesions: ectasias, tumors, and malformations. In: Yamada T, Alpers DH, et al (eds): Textbook of Gastroenterology. Philadelphia, JB Lippincott, 1995, pp 2471–2489.
36. Thompson H: Crohns disease. In: Bouchier IAD, Allan RN, Hodgson HJF, Keighley MRB (eds): Gastroenterology: Clinical Science and Practice. London, WB Saunders Company Ltd, 1994, pp 1128–1134.
37. Farmer R, Hawk W, Turnbull R: Clinical patterns in Crohn's disease: a statistical study of 615 cases. Gastroenterology 68:627–635, 1975.
38. Lewis BS: Small intestinal bleeding. Gastroenterol Clin North Am 23:67–91, 1994.
39. Cullen JJ, Kelly KA. Current Management of Meckel's Diverticulum. Adv Surg 29:207–214, 1996.
40. Kusumoto H, Yoshida M, Takahashi I, et al: Complications and diagnosis of Meckel's diverticulum in 776 patients. Am J Surg 164:382–383.
41. Boley SJ, DiBiase A, Brandt LJ, et al: Lower intestinal bleeding in the elderly. Am J Surg 137:57–64, 1979.

42. Elta GH: Approach to the patient with gross gastrointestinal bleeding. In: Yamada T, Alpers DH, et al (eds): Textbook of Gastroenterology. Philadelphia, JB Lippincott, 1995, pp 671–698.

43. Spencer J: Lower gastrointestinal bleeding. In: Bouchier IAD, Allan RN, Hodgson HJF, Keighley MRB, (eds): Gastroenterology: Clinical Science and Practice. London, WB Saunders Company Ltd, 1994, pp 975–988.

44. Cook IJ, Pavlli P, Riley JW, et al: Gastrointestinal investigation of iron deficiency anemia. BMJ 292:1380–1382, 1986.

45. Savides TJ, Jensen DM: Severe lower gastrointestinal bleeding. In: Bayless TM (ed): Current Therapy in Gastroenterology and Liver Disease. St. Louis, Mosby, 1994, pp 465–469.

46. Englert DA, Rupert SD: Patients with gastrointestinal bleeding. In: Clochesy J, Breu C, Cardin S et al (eds): In Critical Care Nursing. Philadelphia, WB Saunders, 1993, pp 945–969.

47. Kankaria AG, Fleischer DE: The critical care management of nonvariceal upper gastrointestinal bleeding. Crit Care Clin 11:347–368, 1995.

48. Lundberg GD: Practice parameter for the use of fresh-frozen plasma, cryoprecipitate and platelets. JAMA 271:777–781, 1994.

49. Prevost SS, Oberle A: Stress ulceration in the critically ill patient. Crit Care Nurs Clin North Am 5:163–169, 1993.

50. Kuhn MA: Pharmacotherapeutics: a nursing process approach. In: Kuhn MA, (ed): Philadelphia, FA Davis, 1994, pp 1082–1105.

51. Feldman M, Burton ME: Histamine$_2$-receptor antagonists. Standard therapy for acid-peptic diseases—Part 2. N Engl J Med 323:1749–1755, 1990.

52. Hansten PD: Drug interactions with antisecretory agents. Aliment Pharmacol Ther 5(Suppl 1):121, 1991.

53. Levitt MD: Lack of clinical significance of the interaction between H$_2$ receptor antagonists and ethanol. Aliment Pharmacol Ther 7:131–138, 1993.

54. Shamburek RD, Schubert ML: Control of gastric acid secretion. Histamine H$_2$ receptor antagonists and H$^+$K$^+$-ATPase inhibitors. Gastroenterol Clin North Am 21:527–550, 1992.

55. McCarthy DM: Sucralfate. N Engl J Med 325:965, 1991.

56. Phillips JO, Metzler MH, Palmieri TL, et al: A prospective study of simplified omeprazole suspension for the prophylaxis of stress-related mucosal damage. Crit Care Med 24:1793–1799, 1996.

57. Czaja A: Bleeding esophageal varices. In: Rakel RE (ed): Conn's Current Therapy. (ed): Philadelphia, WB Saunders, 1996, pp 451–461.

58. Burns SM, Martin MJ: VP/NTG therapy in the patient with variceal bleeding. Crit Care Nurse 10:42–49, 1990.

59. Kerber K: The adult with bleeding esophageal varices. Crit Care Nurs Clin North Am 5:153–162, 1993.

60. Hanisch E, Doertenbach J, Usadel KH: Somatostatin in acute bleeding oesophageal varices: pharmacology and rationale for use. Drugs 44(Suppl 2):24–35, 1992.

61. Jutabha R, Jensen DM: Management of upper gastrointestinal bleeding in the patient with chronic liver disease. Med Clin North Am 80:1035–1068.

62. Burroughs AK: Acute management of bleeding oesophageal varices. Drugs 44(Suppl 2):14–23, 1992.

63. Shiffman ML, Jeffers L, Hoofnagle JH, et al: The role of transjugular intrahepatic portosystemic shunt for the treatment of portal hypertension and its complications: a conference sponsored by the National Digestive Diseases Advisory Board. Hepatology 22:1591–1597, 1995.

64. Young HS, Matsui Suzanne M, Gregory PB: Endoscopic control of upper gastrointestinal variceal bleeding. In: Yamada T, Alpers DH, et al (eds): Textbook of Gastroenterology. Philadelphia, JB Lippincott, 1995, pp 2969–2991.

65. Schuman BM, Beckman JW, Tedesco FJ, et al: Complication of endoscopic injection sclerotherapy: a review. Am J Gastroenterol 82:823–830, 1987.

66. Laine L, Cook D. Endoscopic ligation compared with sclerotherapy for treatment of esophageal variceal bleeding: a meta-analysis. Ann Intern Med 123:280–287, 1995.

67. Jensen DM: Acute lower GI bleeding—emergency colonoscopy for whom? Postgraduate Course, Integrating Visual, Technical and Cognitive Skills in Endoscopy, 1996.

68. Heier SK: Laser use and photodynamic therapy for gastrointestinal cancer. In: Bayless TM (ed): Current Therapy in Gastroenterology and Liver Disease. St. Louis, Mosby, 1994, pp 89–96.

69. Baillie J: Upper gastrointestinal bleeding. In: Bayless TM (ed): Current Therapy in Gastroenterology and Liver Disease. St. Louis, Mosby, 1994, pp 132–138.

70. Barnett JL, Raper SE: Anorectal diseases. In: Yamada T, Alpers DH, et al (eds): Textbook of Gastroenterology. Philadelphia, JB Lippincott, 1995, pp 2027–2050.

71. Society of Gastroenterology Nurses and Associates: Gastroenterology Nursing: A Core Curriculum. St. Louis, Mosby–Year Book, 1993, pp 6–7.

72. Debas HT, Orloff SL: Surgery for peptic ulcer disease and postgastrectomy syndromes. In: Yamada T, Alpers DH, et al (eds): Textbook of Gastroenterology. Philadelphia, JB Lippincott, 1995, pp 1523–1543.

36

Hepatic Disorders

Marian S. Altman

Objectives

After completing this chapter, the student will be able to:

1. List the causes of liver failure.
2. Relate the pathophysiology of liver disease to the clinical manifestations.
3. Differentiate the four stages of hepatic encephalopathy.
4. Discuss assessment findings of patients with liver disease.
5. Select appropriate nursing interventions used to care for patients with liver disease.
6. Discuss the current treatment modalities for liver disease.
7. Review future therapies for the treatment of liver disease.

The liver is one of the most vital organs in the body, performing over 400 functions that affect each body system. When the liver cannot perform its many functions, failure ensues. Loss of liver function can lead to secondary organ failures. Virtually every organ system in the body is affected by liver failure (Table 36–1).

Hepatic failure is a clinical syndrome characterized by massive necrosis resulting in the clinical manifestations of liver disease. Hepatic failure can occur suddenly in the event of acute liver disease, or it can have an insidious onset, chronic liver disease. Hepatic failure is defined as a loss of 60% of the hepatocytes. Symptoms of hepatic failure are usually noted after 75% of hepatocyte function is lost.

ETIOLOGY

Acute hepatic failure may be the result of viral, chemical, metabolic, or ischemic factors (Chart 36–1). The most common causes of acute liver failure are viral hepatitis and drug-induced liver injury.[1] Causes of chronic liver disease include cirrhosis, chronic cholestatic disease, chronic viral hepatitis, excessive alcohol consumption, malnutrition, diabetes mellitus, alpha$_1$-antitrypsin deficiency, Wilson's disease, hemochromatosis, repeated toxin exposure, and malignant diseases such as hepatocellular carcinoma and cholangiocarcinoma.

Viral Causes

Hepatitis is widespread inflammation of the liver in response to a virus, drugs, or an autoimmune disease. As the disease progresses, inflammation and edema of the liver cells occur. Hepatocellular necrosis develops, resulting in liver enlargement. Five different types of viral hepatitis are recognized. Hepatitis A, B, C, D, and E can all cause acute hepatocellular necrosis. Hepatitis B is the most common causative agent[2] (Table 36–2). Hepatitis may be acute or chronic.

Acute hepatitis is a condition lasting less than 6 months with either resolution of liver damage or rapid progression of necrosis, which may be fatal. Chronic hepatitis is a result of a sustained inflammatory process lasting longer than 6 months. Hepatitis may result from viral infection, toxic exposure, long-term alcohol intake, or bacterial infection.

Other viral causes of liver disease include Epstein–Barr virus, cytomegalovirus, and herpes viruses 1, 2, and 6. Acute liver failure caused by herpes virus is usually associated with immunosuppression and can be treated with an antiviral agent. Varicella-zoster, Coxsackie B, adenoviruses, rubella, rubeola, mumps, and yellow fever virus may also cause liver disease.

Chronic hepatitis leads to inflammation, necrosis, and fibrosis. Cirrhosis may result. Chemical agents, viral agents, and alcohol abuse may cause this form of hepatitis.

TABLE 36–1
Clinical Findings of Liver Failure

Body System	Pathophysiology	Signs and Symptoms
General	Ineffective metabolism of carbohydrate, fat, and protein	Decreased weight Muscle wasting Malnourishment
	Inability to store vitamins and iron	Malaise and fatigue
Cardiovascular	Hyperkinetic circulation	Increased cardiac output and heart rate Systolic ejection murmur Bounding pulses
	Hypotension related to third spacing Fluid and electrolyte imbalances	Decreased blood pressure and renal blood flow Dysrhythmias Peripheral edema
Immune	Splenomegaly	Leukopenia Increased infection risk
	Decreased Kupffer cell function	Increased infection risk
Skin	Inability to conjugate bilirubin Inability to detoxify hormones	Jaundice Palmar erythema Hair loss
	Elevated bile salts Decreased synthesis of clotting factors Portal hypertension	Pruritus and dry skin Bruising, purpura, and ecchymosis Caput medusae Spider angiomas
	Hyperlipidemia	Xanthomas
Endocrine	Inability to detoxify or inactivate hormones	Peripheral edema Increased weight Moon face and striae Testicular atrophy Gynecomastia Decreased libido Impotence Menstrual abnormalities
	Decreased glycogen related to decreased carbohydrate metabolism	Hypoglycemia
Gastrointestinal	Elevated methylmercaptan levels Decreased fat metabolism	Fetor hepaticus, anorexia, nausea, and vomiting Steatorrhea and malnutrition Hyperlipidemia
	Portal hypertension Inability to conjugate bilirubin Decreased synthesis of clotting factors	Hematemesis, melena, and hematochezia Clay-colored stools Epistaxis and gingival bleeding Heme-positive stools
Hematologic	Splenomegaly Inability to synthesize clotting factors	Red blood cell destruction and anemia Nosebleeds, gum bleeds, disseminated intravascular coagulation, thrombocytopenia, and ecchymosis
Neurologic	Inability to absorb fat-soluble vitamins	Sensory disturbances, peripheral degeneration, paresthesia, foot drop, nystagmus, and ptosis
	Inability to conjugate ammonia	Personality changes and asterixis Change in level of consciousness
Renal	Decreased circulating volume	Decreased renal blood flow, glomerular filtration rate, and urine output Elevated blood urea nitrogen and creatinine
	Inability to conjugate bilirubin Inability to detoxify hormones	Dark, foamy urine (tea colored) Increased urine osmolality
Pulmonary	Ascites	Diaphragm elevation, shortness of breath, decreased lung expansion, and pulmonary edema or effusion
	Increased 2,3,-diphosphoglycerate levels	Decreased oxygen saturation and partial pressure of oxygen

Data from Covington H: Nursing care of patients with alcoholic liver disease. Crit Care Nurse 13:51, 1993; and Reishtein J: Liver failure: case study of a complex problem. Crit Care Nurse 13:38, 1993.

CHART 36–1

Causes of Acute Hepatic Failure

Viral
Viral hepatitis: A, B, C, D, E
Acute alcoholic hepatitis

Viral Associated with Immunosuppression
Cytomegalovirus
Herpes simplex
Epstein–Barr
Yellow fever
Adenovirus
Varicella-zoster

Chemical
Hepatotoxic drugs
   Isoniazid (INH)
   Rifampin
   Cancer chemotherapy
   Acetaminophen (Tylenol)
   Tetracycline
   Valproate sodium (Depakene)
   Phosphorus
   Monoamine oxidase inhibitors
   Alpha-methyldopa (Aldomet)
   NSAIDs (Nonsteroidal anti-inflammatory drugs: ibuprofen [Advil])

Drug overdose: acetaminophen
Anesthetic agents—halothane
Industrial toxins
   Carbon tetrachloride
   Herbicides
Mushroom poisoning:
   Amanita phalloides species

Pregnancy-Related
Fatty liver of pregnancy
Eclampsia

Medical
Wilson's disease
Budd–Chiari syndrome
Acute leukemia and lymphoreticular malignancies
Graft-versus-host disease
Reye's syndrome
Gram-negative septicemia
Ischemia, hypoxic injury, or shock
Veno-occlusive disease after bone marrow transplantation

Data from Smith S: Patients with hepatic disorders. In: Clochesy J, Breu C, Cardin S, et al (eds): Critical Care Nursing. Philadelphia, W.B. Saunders, 1993, p 980; and Sussman N, Lake J: Treatment of hepatic failure, 1996: current concepts and progress toward live dialysis. Am J Kidney Dis 27:621, 1996.

Chemical Causes

Liver disease may result after exposure to certain substances such as drugs or chemicals. A major function of the liver is drug metabolism, by converting lipid-soluble drugs to a water-soluble compound, which the kidney excretes. Drugs may cause liver failure predictably, when taken in excess doses, or idiosyncratically.

Acetaminophen (Tylenol) is an example of a drug, that when taken in doses larger than recommended, predictably causes liver damage. Ingestion of as little as 10 g (30 regular-strength tablets) of acetaminophen can cause significant damage. An overdose occurs with more than 15 g of acetaminophen ingested by an adult. Acetaminophen toxicity may occur if the drug is taken as directed on a regular basis in some persons.

Acetaminophen toxicity is dose dependant, but the effect is exaggerated by alcohol, starvation, and drugs that induce the cytochrome P450 pathway in the liver

for metabolism. Approximately 97% of acetaminophen is metabolized through conjugation and is excreted in the urine. The other 2 to 3% is metabolized by the P450 pathway, which converts acetaminophen to a potentially toxic metabolite. Conjugation of the metabolite renders it harmless. When excessive amounts of the drug are ingested, the P450 pathway becomes the primary route of metabolism. The result is production of an increased amount of hepatotoxic metabolite. As glutathione is depleted, liver necrosis occurs. Massive necrosis may lead to fulminant hepatic failure and death. The extent of liver damage may be predicted by acetaminophen blood levels within 4 to 12 hours after ingestion. High acetaminophen levels in a patient with a partial thromboplastin time (PTT) of more than 100, pH of less than 7.3, and serum creatinine of more than 3.0 mg/dL are associated with a poor prognosis.[3]

An idiosyncratic drug or chemical reaction is one that may not be predicted and occurs for unknown reasons in susceptible persons. An idiosyncratic reac-

TABLE 36–2
Types of Viral Hepatitis

Virus	Risk Factors	Risk of Liver Failure	Modes of Transmission	Miscellaneous
Hepatitis A (HAV)	Poor personal hygiene Poor sanitation Household contact Sexual contact Employment or attendance at a day care center International travel	Low	Fecal–oral transmission by person-to-person contact Ingestion of contaminated food (e.g., raw shell-fish or frozen foods) or water Parenteral transmission (rare)	Acute, not chronic Enterovirus Usually self-limiting Good prognosis Occurs in children more than in adults
Hepatitis B (HBV)	Homosexual contact Heterosexual contact Intravenous drug abuse Work in health care environment Transfusion of blood products Dialysis Tattooing or body piercing 40% of those infected have no known risk factors	High	Exposure to infected blood or other body fluids Perinatal transmission (rare)	Most common cause of fulminant hepatic failure Chronic carriers suffer no liver damage, but can transmit virus Can be asymptomatic DNA virus
Hepatitis C (HCV)	Same as HBV	Moderate	Exposure to infected blood or other body fluids Fecal–oral transmission (rare) Perinatal transmission (rare)	RNA virus
Hepatitis D (HDV)	Same as HBV HBV infection	High	Exposure to infected blood or other body fluids Perinatal transmission (rare)	Seen with hepatitis B as a co-infection
Hepatitis E (HEV)	Same as HAV (in endemic regions)	High, especially in pregnant women	Fecal–oral transmission Ingestion of contaminated drinking water	Enteric non-A, non-B Affects young and middle-aged adults Underdeveloped countries with contaminated water supplies Rare in the United States

Adapted from Hansen M: Pathophysiology. Philadelphia, W.B. Saunders, 1998, p 784.

tion occurs as toxic metabolites are produced through hepatic drug metabolism. It is believed that hypersensitivity plays a part in the liver damage. Examples of these agents include isoniazid (INH), allopurinol (Zyloprim), methyldopa (Aldomet), sulfonamides, halothane, and phenytoin (Dilantin). Damage may also occur as a result of exposure to chemicals such as industrial cleaning solvents, fluorinated hydrocarbons, and tetrachloroethane or by sniffing glue. Liver damage can occur either from short-term or prolonged exposure.

The mushroom species, *Amanita phalloides*, may cause hepatic failure when ingested. The *Amanita* mushroom is found in temperate forests in the late summer and fall. One to three mushrooms can cause fulminant hepatic failure. Symptoms are noticed 6 to 12 hours after eating the mushrooms and persist for 1 to 4 days. Fulminant hepatic failure may occur in 4 to 8 days after ingestion. Hepatic failure is preceded by profuse sweating, severe abdominal pain, vomiting, and watery diarrhea.[4]

Metabolic Causes

Lipid infiltration of the liver is the most common metabolic cause of liver disease. Fatty liver is a result of the accumulation of excess lipids in the intact liver cells. This is a result of either increased synthesis or release of lipoproteins by the liver.

Triglycerides, cholesterol, and phospholipids are all involved. If the fatty deposits encroach on normal liver cells, alteration in liver function is observed. Some of the clinical conditions associated with fatty liver include starvation, obesity, diabetes, pregnancy, total parenteral nutrition, chronic alcoholism, and Reye's syndrome. Treatment is symptomatic.

Acute fatty liver of pregnancy occurs in the third trimester and is characterized by the sudden onset of jaundice, hypoglycemia, altered mental status, and possibly preeclampsia. Rapid delivery of the infant is the treatment of choice.

Another metabolic cause of liver failure is hemochromatosis, which is the result of excess of iron deposits in lysosomes that cause enzymes to spill into the liver. These enzymes damage the hepatocytes and cause fibrosis in the sinusoids and bile ducts, leading to portal hypertension. Hemochromatosis, a familial disease, is relatively rare and occurs in men more often than in women. Treatment consists of phlebotomy and support.

Ischemic Causes

Liver disease is also caused by ischemia, as the result of cardiac insufficiency or failure. Factors affecting the oxygenated blood supply to the liver include systemic shock, cardiac arrest, myocardial infarction, cardiomyopathy, pulmonary embolism, and damage to the liver that prevents oxygenated blood from reaching it. Occlusion of hepatic venous outflow, as occurs in Budd–Chiari syndrome, may also cause liver failure. Veno-occlusive disease, which occurs as a result of cancer chemotherapy or bone marrow transplantation, is another cause of hepatic failure.

PATHOPHYSIOLOGY

Acute hepatic failure is the result of sudden, massive necrosis of liver cells, commonly from viral infection or exposure to hepatotoxins. Acute hepatic failure is a life-threatening form of liver disease associated with signs and symptoms of encephalopathy and coagulopathy. Acute hepatic failure can develop in less than 8 weeks from the onset of illness in a patient without preexisting liver disease. The diagnosis is based on the symptoms of acute liver disease, hepatic encephalopathy, and liver failure. The prognosis is poor, and death may occur. Treatment is symptomatic and supportive. The hepatocytes can regenerate in 4 to 5 weeks if the function of the liver can be supported and if no further damage occurs.

Cirrhosis

Cirrhosis is the fourth leading cause of death in adults older than 40 years of age in the United States.[2] Cirrhosis is described as fibrous tissue changes secondary to chronic injury. Liver tissue is usually able to regenerate after injury. However, with chronic injury, there is irreversible fibrous scarring, and regeneration nodules form and cause irreparable functional damage. Fibrous scarring and nodules distort the vascular bed, leading to portal hypertension and shunting. Hepatocyte function is disturbed.[5] Any chronic disease of the liver may result in cirrhosis.

Several types of cirrhosis are recognized (Table 36–3). Primary cirrhosis is thought to be an autoimmune disease in which cytotoxic lymphocytes attack the biliary epithelium and cause bile duct destruction. Laennec's cirrhosis, or alcoholic cirrhosis, which usually develops after years of daily alcohol consumption, accounts for more than 50% of all cases of cirrhosis.[2] The pathophysiologic process in alcoholic cirrhosis is the oxidation of alcohol to aldehyde by the liver, a change that causes permanent hepatocellular damage. Excessive alcohol intake causes proliferation of smooth endoplasmic reticulum in the hepatocytes. This increases cholesterol production and accumulation in the liver. Mitochondria swell, leading to inflammation, necrosis, and fibrosis of liver cells. Cardiac cirrhosis is associated with right-sided heart failure, which causes liver cell anoxia and subsequent necrosis.

Cholestatic disease may also cause cirrhosis. Primary biliary cirrhosis is a chronic disorder of the bile duct. It occurs in women more often than in men, and generally it occurs in the fourth or fifth decade. An

TABLE 36–3
Types of Cirrhosis

Type	Cause	Treatment
Primary	Autoimmune bile duct destruction	Supportive and symptomatic
Secondary or obstructive	Prolonged bile duct obstruction	Relief of obstruction
Laennec's	Alcohol intake	Symptomatic and abstinence
Cardiac	Right-sided heart failure	Reversal of cause
Postnecrotic	Liver cell necrosis secondary to infection, metabolism, and toxicities	Symptomatic
Cryptogenic	Unknown	Symptomatic and transplantation

autoimmune mechanism is thought to cause this type of liver disease.[5]

Sclerosing cholangitis is a result of chronic, fibrosing inflammation in all parts of the biliary tract that results in obliteration of the biliary tree. The cause is unknown. One theory is that bacteria or toxic bile acids reach the liver by the portal system and cause an autoimmune response in the biliary tree. There is no specific treatment other than liver transplantation.

Portal Hypertension

The major sequelae of cirrhosis are portal hypertension, liver failure, ascites, hepatorenal syndrome, and encephalopathy. The normal liver offers little resistance to blood flow and is known as a low-pressure system. As the liver fails, the blood flow is reduced secondary to vasoconstriction, resulting in portal hypertension. Cirrhosis also impedes blood flow and thus increases pressure in the portal system. This change results in significant congestion and dilatation of the veins in the portal system and shunting of blood away from the liver. A backward flow is created away from the liver, to the spleen, stomach, and esophagus in an effort to maintain venous return to the heart. Collateral channels may develop in the gastric fundus, esophagus, abdominal wall, and rectum. These collateral channels shunt blood away from the high-pressure portal system to an area of lower pressure in the gastrointestinal (GI) tract.

As these low-pressure veins become distended with blood, the vessels enlarge, and varices develop. The dilated, thin-walled veins of the esophagus and GI tract are easily traumatized and therefore may rupture and bleed easily. The risk of bleeding increases as portal pressure increases.

The collateral system that is a result of portal hypertension also causes skin changes. Spider angiomas or nevi are vascular lesions that appear as a central red body with radiating branches. Spider angiomas appear primarily on the upper anterior thorax, arms, and face. These lesions are arterial, blanche when touched, and can bleed profusely. Abdominal veins radiating from the umbilicus also dilate secondary to portal hypertension, causing caput medusae.

Immunologic Alterations

Patients with liver failure may have difficulty mounting a response to infection. The Kupffer cells of the liver normally filter blood arriving by removing bacteria, antigens, by-products of coagulation, and other harmful substances. Portal hypertension decreases blood flow to the liver. Because the blood flow through the liver is decreased or stagnant, the Kupffer cells do not function. GI tract organisms are not filtered in the liver and may enter the systemic circulation. Portal hypertension also causes blood to become sequestered in the spleen, with resulting splenomegaly, which causes destruction of white blood cells, red blood cells, and platelets. Many functions of the leukocytes such as fighting infection are impaired. All these malfunctions contribute to the high risk of infection and bacteremia in these patients.[6]

Fluid Alterations

Portal hypertension causes increased hydrostatic pressure, which forces fluid out of the vessels and into the peritoneal cavity. Fluid dynamics are altered, with decreased synthesis of albumin as a result of liver failure. Albumin is responsible for oncotic pressure; therefore, decreased levels cause fluid to move into the peritoneal cavity. As this protein-rich fluid shifts, peripheral edema in dependent areas and ascites occur. As fluid moves from the vascular space, circulating volume decreases, and renal perfusion is lowered.

Ascites

Ascites, excess fluid in the peritoneal cavity, is seen in patients with acute and chronic liver failure. It is usually milder and more persistent in patients with chronic liver failure. Ascites may occur early or late in hepatic failure. Causes of ascites are altered plasma oncotic pressure related to decreased albumin synthesis and increased portal venous pressure. As ascites develops, fluid is drawn from the intravascular space to the peritoneal cavity, thus causing a decrease in circulating volume. Aldosterone and antidiuretic hormone (ADH) are stimulated and cause sodium and water to be reabsorbed in the renal tubules in an effort to increase intravascular volume (Figure 36–1).

An increase in aldosterone and in ADH results in increased sodium and water retention, and dilutional hyponatremia occurs. Although the body is actually fluid overloaded secondary to hyperaldosteronism, the fluid is shifted into the potential spaces, thereby decreasing circulating volume. The lymph system attempts to remove the excess fluid volume, but the fluid continues to accumulate. Finally, the lymph system is overwhelmed, and lymph leaks into the peritoneal cavity through the thoracic and hepatic ducts. Lymph pulls intravascular fluid with it, also causing ascites. On examination of the patient, the clinician finds a distended abdomen, shifting dullness in the abdomen, and a fluid wave. There is no tenderness to palpation. Jugular vein distention and elevated right atrial pressures are noted. Ultrasonography is used to confirm the presence of ascites.

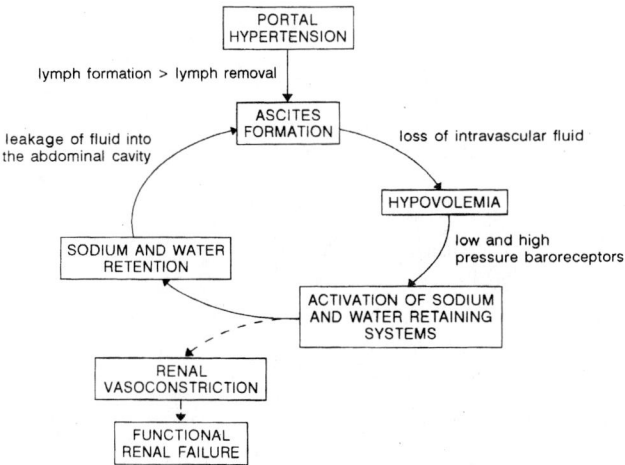

Figure 36–1

Pathogenesis of ascites and renal abnormalities in liver failure. (From Gitlin N: In: Zakim D, Boyer T [eds]: Hepatology: A Textbook of Liver Disease, 3rd ed. Philadelphia, W.B. Saunders, 1996.)

Alterations in Hormone Metabolism

As blood is shunted away from the liver, substances normally detoxified and metabolized by the liver such as hormones, chemicals, and drugs fail to reach their destination. Glucocorticoids such as cortisol, mineralocorticoids such as aldosterone, and ADH are not inactivated by the liver. Circulating aldosterone and ADH cause the kidneys to reabsorb free water and sodium. This process increases the circulating volume and may contribute to ascites. Ascites decreases circulating volume, a change that causes ADH and aldosterone to be released, again to increase the circulating volume. When endocrine hormones are not deactivated by the diseased liver, weight gain, a rounded, edematous face, scant body hair, gynecomastia, and impotence may occur.

Alterations in Fat Metabolism

Bile, which consists of bile salts, bile pigments, and cholesterol, decreases the surface tension of fat in the gut by agitating it and making fatty acids more soluble. This process allows fat and fat-soluble vitamins (A, D, E, and K) to be absorbed. Bile salts are produced by the hepatocytes from cholesterol in a 1:1 relationship. However, not all the cholesterol is used when making bile salts.

As the liver fails, fat metabolism becomes ineffective. The production of bile salts is decreased, causing up to 40% of lipids to be lost in the stool. This condition causes steatorrhea, characterized by fatty, greasy stools that are foul smelling. Serum levels of cholesterol rise and may cause gallstones.

Malnutrition may result from decreased absorption of fat, fat-soluble vitamins, and minerals. Decreased absorption of fat-soluble vitamins may have many side effects. Vitamin A deficiency may lead to night blindness after an extended period of deficiency. Vitamin D deficiency causes decreased serum calcium absorption in the gut that results in calcium resorption from the bone to increase serum calcium levels. Bone demineralization occurs and may lead to osteomalacia, kyphosis, and fractures. Vitamin K deficiency may result in coagulopathies. Vitamin B deficiency leads to decreased folic acid levels, causing macrocytic anemia. Decreased niacin may cause sensory disturbances. Decreased levels of Vitamin B_6 cause peripheral nerve degeneration and palsy of cranial nerve VI.

Alterations in Bilirubin Metabolism

Hepatic failure leads to a decreased ability to conjugate bilirubin. Bilirubin is the end product of red blood cell destruction and provides the bile with pigment. As the red blood cell is destroyed, the heme molecule attaches to the albumin and creates unconjugated or indirect bilirubin. This type of bilirubin is not soluble and cannot be excreted. Bilirubin is made soluble or is conjugated by the liver and is excreted in the bile, urine, and feces, a process that gives them their characteristic color.

As unconjugated bilirubin levels increase, bilirubin is deposited in the skin, mucous membranes, sclera, and elastic tissues. This results in a jaundiced appearance. Unconjugated bilirubin also crosses the blood–brain barrier and deposits in the brain tissue.

Metabolic Alterations

Metabolic functions of the liver include the metabolism of carbohydrates, fats, and proteins. Carbohydrates arrive in the liver as simple sugars. The liver metabolizes the carbohydrates to energy for immediate use. Any extra carbohydrate in the liver is stored as glycogen (glycogenesis) and can be released when glucose is needed by the body but is unavailable (glycogenolysis).

Excess carbohydrates are converted by the liver to triglycerides, which are then stored. Triglycerides are metabolized to glycerol and fatty acids when needed for energy production. Fatty acids are broken down further into ketones, which are converted to meet cellular energy needs. If glycogen stores are depleted, the liver is able to convert amino acids and fatty acids to glucose. This process is called gluconeogenesis. Thus, through the liver, the body is able to maintain glucose homeostasis.

The liver can usually continue to store and make glucose during liver disease. If the liver is unable to do so, the kidneys can assume gluconeogenesis. Patients may develop an elevated glucose level related to the inability to store glycogen. Hypoglycemia may occur as a result of impaired liver function secondary to altered glucose release, gluconeogenesis, or altered levels of insulin.[7] Hypoglycemia is noted more frequently in patients with acute liver disease than in patients with chronic liver disease.

Alterations in Protein Metabolism

The liver synthesizes 90% of all plasma proteins. The major proteins metabolized by the liver are albumin, globulin, and fibrinogen. As the liver fails, protein synthesis is decreased, and less fibrinogen and fewer clotting factors are made. Coagulation factors II, V, VII, IX, and X, those of the extrinsic clotting cascade, are deficient. All the factors listed except factor V are vitamin K dependent. Vitamin K is lipid soluble and therefore depends on bile salts for intestinal absorption. Failure of bile salt secretion leads to a deficiency of vitamin K–dependent clotting factors. An elevated prothrombin time (PT) and PTT result, putting the patient at risk for bleeding because of a deficiency of clotting factors.

The liver is also unable to remove activated clotting factors, and this limitation leads to the formation of microthrombi and consumption of platelets and fibrinogen. As these clots break down, fibrin split products are released that are anticoagulants. The liver is unable to synthesize more clotting factors, and bleeding results. This process may lead to disseminated intravascular coagulation (DIC). Potential bleeding sites are the nasopharynx, lungs, kidneys, retroperitoneum, and breaks in skin integrity, such as phlebotomy or catheter sites. GI bleeding is related to the development of gastric erosions and or the rupture of esophageal varices.

Hepatorenal Syndrome

An association between liver failure and renal failure was first described in patients with cirrhosis. Renal failure without an obvious cause that develops concurrently in a patient with hepatic failure is termed "hepatorenal syndrome." The kidneys are structurally normal, with no evidence of primary renal disease, but renal hypoperfusion occurs as the circulating volume of blood decreases. This condition leads to a decrease in the glomerular filtration rate and a subsequent decrease in urine output.[8]

The clinical presentation of hepatorenal syndrome is listed in Chart 36–2. Hepatorenal syndrome is usually irreversible; therefore, the prognosis is poor. Diagnosis is by exclusion of other causes of acute renal failure such as decreased circulating volume to the kidney, acute tubular necrosis, or postrenal obstruction.

Treatment focuses on identifying patients at risk, avoiding nephrotoxic drugs, maintaining circulating volume, and preventing an accumulation of substances normally inactivated by the liver. Hemodialy-

---

CHART 36–2

Hepatorenal Syndrome: Clinical Presentation

Concentrated urine
Urinary sodium <10 mmol/L
Elevated blood urea nitrogen and serum creatinine
Oliguria
Hyponatremia often found
Urinalysis: mild proteinuria, granular casts, hematuria
Nausea and vomiting
Thirst

---

sis or other renal replacement therapies may be indicated. Renal perfusion may be maintained by vasodilator effects of low-dose dopamine.

Hepatic Encephalopathy

Encephalopathy has been defined as a complex neuropsychiatric syndrome characterized by a global depression of central nervous system (CNS) function that may progress to impaired consciousness and coma.[6] Toxic substances in the portal blood enter the systemic circulation and reach the brain without first being metabolized by the liver. Hepatic encephalopathy occurs in patients with acute and chronic liver failure and may be either acute or chronic. Increased intracranial pressure, cerebral edema, and coma are commonly seen with acute hepatic encephalopathy, and mortality is high. Chronic hepatic encephalopathy manifests with subtle neurologic changes in a more persistent form and is typically associated with portosystemic shunting of blood. Clinical findings of hepatic encephalopathy range from subtle neurologic defects to coma. Causes are numerous and varied. Encephalopathy is divided into four stages (Table 36–4).

The underlying pathogenesis of encephalopathy is an increase in the level of nitrogenous wastes in the blood resulting from liver failure. The liver metabolizes amino acids for immediate energy or storage. During this process, carbon dioxide and ammonia are released as by-products. Ammonia can also be formed from the degradation of protein or from the metabolism of blood by the natural flora of the gut. As blood is shunted away from the diseased liver, ammonia is not converted to water-soluble urea, which is excreted by the kidneys. Ammonia levels rise. Ammonia crosses the blood–brain barrier and causes a deterioration of brain function. The stage of encephalopathy does not correlate with the ammonia level. A normal ammonia

TABLE 36-4
Stages of Encephalopathy

Stage*	Mental State	Neuromuscular Changes	Electroencephalographic Changes
1	Subtle behavior and personality changes; irritability; mood swings; mild confusion; decreased attention span; slow mentation; slurred speech; lack of cooperation but rational; disordered sleep	Slight asterixis; normal tone and reflexes	None
2	Accentuation of 1; drowsiness; inappropriate behavior; marked slowed mentation; confusion and disorientation	Asterixis; reflexes brisk; increased muscle tone; impaired fine motor skills	Generalized slowing; abnormal
3	Sleeping most of time but can be aroused; marked confusion; may be disruptive or violent; incoherent speech	Asterixis; local or flexion response to pain; signature unrecognizable	Abnormal
4	Possible response to pain only; coma possible	Asterixis absent; extends to pain; positive Babinski test; hyperreactive reflexes	Abnormal

*Prognosis for stages 1 to 2 is good. Stages 3 to 4 have a much worse prognosis. Once stage 3 or 4 develops, the patient is at risk for the development of multiorgan complications in addition to hepatic failure, and the mortality rate is high. Cerebral edema is estimated to occur in 75 to 80% of patients in stage 4 and is the leading cause of death.
  Data from Lee W: Acute liver failure. N Engl J Med 329:1862–1872, 1993; Sherlock S: Fulminant hepatic failure. Adv Intern Med 38:245–267, 1993; and Sussman N: Fulminant hepatic failure. In: Zakin D, Boyer T (eds): Hepatology: A Textbook of Liver Disease, 3rd ed. Philadelphia, W.B. Saunders, 1996.

level may be noted in a few patients with hepatic encephalopathy. Patients with high ammonia levels may demonstrate stage I signs and symptoms of encephalopathy. Other mechanisms thought to contribute to the encephalopathy are reduced neural excitation and decreased transmission and certain amino acid reductions.[6,9] Encephalopathy is associated with an increased protein intake or GI bleeding, hypoxia, infection, electrolyte abnormalities, drugs such as sedatives and alcohol, and a decreased circulating volume.

Patients with hepatic encephalopathy develop a distinctive breath odor called fetor hepaticus. The sweet fecal breath is a result of the excretion of mercaptan, a metabolite formed from sulfur-containing amino acids, through respirations instead of through liver detoxification. Mercaptans are neurotoxic and can potentiate ammonia toxicity.

Assessment

The clinical manifestations of hepatic failure are directly related to a lack of the normal physiologic functions performed exclusively by the liver. The clinical findings of liver failure, the pathophysiologic features, and the body systems affected are listed in Table 36–1. Problems that can develop include coagulopathy, ascites, cerebral edema, portal hypertension with the potential for bleeding, and mental status changes.

Clinical findings of acute liver failure differ from those of chronic hepatic insufficiency. Patients with chronic hepatic failure develop nonspecific signs and symptoms of malaise and nausea, followed by jaundice, and the rapid onset of altered mental status. Clinical findings vary in relation to timing of the physical examination and the progression of the disease process. Clinical findings associated with acute hepatic failure may occur in less than 2 weeks. Examination of the patient reveals a tender, enlarged liver and decreased hepatic dullness to percussion. Hypoglycemia and elevated PTT and liver function tests are noted. Hemodynamic changes include elevated cardiac output, decreased systemic vascular resistance, and hypotension.

The clinical findings of liver disease have been categorized into a classification system known as Child's classification (Table 36–5). Studies have documented that the life expectancy dramatically decreases from years to months as the patient's Child's classification progresses from A to B to C. Patients in class C have a median survival rate of 2 to 8 months. Patients in class A or B have a survival rate of 12 to 54 months.[10] Surgical risk also increases as the patient approaches class C. Patients with Child's class C have progressed to stage 3 or 4 encephalopathy.

Cerebral edema occurs in three-fourths of patients who progress to grade IV encephalopathy.[1] Cerebral edema may progress to decerebrate rigidity, posturing, and then brain stem respiratory patterns and apnea if

TABLE 36–5
Child's Classification of Patients With Liver Disease

Parameter	Class		
	A	B	C
Serum bilirubin (mg/dL)	<2.0	2–3	>3
Serum albumin (g/dL)	>3.5	3–3.5	<3.0
Ascites	Absent	Moderate	Tense
Encephalopathy	Absent	Grade I–II	Grade III–IV
Prothrombin time (sec > nL)	<4	4–6	>6
Operative mortality	<1%	10%	>50%

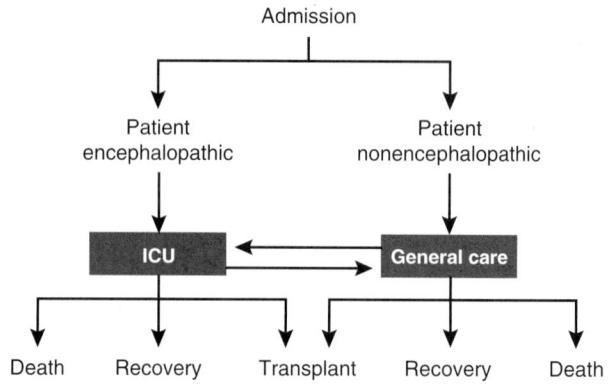

Figure 36–2
Course of hospitalization for patient with liver failure.

left untreated. These changes occur rapidly. Signs of increased intracranial pressure (dilated pupils, brisk deep tendon reflexes, and clonus) occur late and thus are an unreliable guide for timing of treatment.

Nursing Diagnoses

Nursing care of the patient with acute hepatic failure focuses on continuous assessment of the patient, supportive care while the hepatocytes regenerate, evaluation of interventions, and treatment of complications. The patient with hepatic failure is admitted to an acute care facility, possibly the intensive care unit (ICU), as the patient becomes more encephalopathic and as hepatic function declines (Figure 36–2). Many nursing diagnoses are applicable to a patient experiencing hepatic failure (Table 36–6).

Collaborative Management

A collaborative, multidisciplinary approach to patient management is essential to a favorable outcome. The management of liver failure focuses on supporting liver function until it can regenerate while protecting other body systems from failure. Priorities include maintaining circulating volume, stabilizing hemodynamics, providing nutritional support, and controlling ammonia levels to prevent the progression of encephalopathy and its complications. Treatment is also focused on relief of symptoms. Alcohol and other liver toxins must be avoided. Patients with acute liver failure are critically ill and need management in the ICU.

Intensive Care Management

Patients who progress to grade III or IV hepatic encephalopathy need ICU monitoring. Patients who are

TABLE 36–6
Nursing Diagnoses

Problem Statement	Etiologic Factors
Risk for fluid volume deficit	Hemorrhage secondary to decreased clotting ability
Impaired gas exchange	Anemia, hypoxemia, ascites
Alteration in thought process	Elevated ammonia levels, electrolyte imbalances
Alteration in nutrition: less than body requirements	Decreased metabolism of fats, protein, carbohydrates, anorexia, malabsorption
Impaired skin integrity	Ascites, increased bile salts, edema, decreased mobility
Fluid volume deficit	Ascites, third spacing, decreased albumin
Risk for infection	Decreased Kupffer cell function, leukopenia, splenomegaly
Risk for injury	Hepatic encephalopathy
Risk for altered sexual function	Inability to detoxify hormones
Sleep pattern disturbance	Hospital environment, encephalopathy
Diarrhea	Lactulose administration
Risk for activity intolerance	Deconditioning, electrolyte imbalances
Self-care deficit	Deconditioning, encephalopathy
Ineffective airway clearance	Encephalopathy, gastrointestinal bleeding, intubation
Body image disturbance	Jaundice, ascites

cared for in the ICU have been shown to have an improved survival rate.[1] Patients need frequent assessment for signs and symptoms of cerebral edema, bleeding, infection, changes in hemodynamics, oxygenation, and neurologic function. Patients in acute hepatic failure require pulmonary artery pressure monitoring to help manage intravascular volume and to optimize oxygenation. Intubation may be indicated for fatigue or respiratory depression or to protect the airway of an encephalopathic patient. Positive end-expiratory pressure (PEEP) may be required to achieve an adequate partial pressure of oxygen (PO_2). However, PEEP may also decrease cardiac output. Frequent assessment of breath sounds, respiratory rate and pattern, arterial blood gases, and serial chest radiographs is essential. Pulmonary hygiene, turning, coughing, deep breathing, incentive spirometer usage, and suctioning as needed are a focus of patient care.

Cerebral edema develops in 75 to 80% of patients with fulminant hepatic failure in stage 4 encephalopathy and is a major cause of death.[11] Patients who develop cerebral edema require intracranial pressure monitoring. A monitoring device is also inserted in patients who progress to encephalopathy stage 3 or 4. Stimuli that increase intracranial pressure should be avoided. Cerebral perfusion pressure (mean arterial pressure − intracranial pressure) must be kept above 50 mm Hg. Hypotension, hypoxia, and hypercapnia should be avoided. Patients are positioned with the head of the bed elevated. Mannitol, 0.3 to 0.4 g/kg in a 20% solution, may also be given by rapid intravenous infusion for treatment of cerebral edema. The dose may be repeated.

Medical Management of Gastrointestinal Bleeding

All patients with upper GI bleeding should be admitted to the ICU for treatment of the hemorrhage and for close monitoring to minimize complications. Treatment of upper GI bleeding includes immediate intravascular volume repletion with a large-bore catheter. Packed red blood cells are indicated for patients with active bleeding or a hematocrit less than 30.[10] Assessment of blood volume and restoration of blood volume should precede a diagnostic workup. Correction of underlying coagulopathy with fresh frozen plasma is important before endoscopy or other invasive procedures.

Patients with variceal bleeding should take nothing by mouth (NPO), and a nasogastric tube may be inserted to allow gastric decompression of nitrogenous substances and administration of medications. The nasogastric tube can also allow the practitioner to test the patient's gastric contents for blood. Temporizing measures to slow or to stop variceal bleeding include mechanical balloon tamponade and administration of pharmacologic agents such as vasopressin. These therapies are usually instituted after endoscopy confirms variceal bleeding.

GI bleeding necessitates a gastroenterology consultation. Panendoscopy is indicated for the diagnosis in patients with upper GI bleeding. Sclerotherapy is used to treat active bleeding and is performed using an endoscope equipped with a needle filled with a sclerosing agent such as sodium morrhuate. The bleeding vessel is located, the needle is inserted into it, and then the sclerosing agent is injected. The sclerosing agent causes a thrombus to form in the vein and stops the bleeding. Numerous studies have confirmed the long-term efficacy and safety of sclerotherapy. Definitive hemostasis can be achieved.[10] Potential complications include esophageal ulceration, bleeding, stricture, fever, substernal chest pain secondary to esophageal spasms, and perforation.

Pharmacologic agents such as vasopressin, somatostatin, and octreotide may be used to decrease portal pressure by vasoconstriction of the splanchnic vasculature. These agents are not usually administered until diagnosis of bleeding with endoscopy and treatment with sclerotherapy have been completed. One meta-analysis found somatostatin to be more efficacious than vasopressin in controlling acute bleeding. Studies have also concluded that octreotide and somatostatin are as efficacious as sclerotherapy in controlling active bleeding.[10]

Pitressin (synthetic vasopressin) causes vasoconstriction of arterioles in the gut that decreases portal flow and pressure. Pitressin may be administered intra-arterially or intravenously with a loading dose of 20 U in 50 mL of 5% dextrose in water (D_5W) and given over 30 minutes. A maintenance dose of 0.1 to 0.5 U per minute with a maximum dose of 0.9 U per minute follows the bolus. This drug is discontinued with a taper over 24 hours. Side effects include coronary vasoconstriction, dysrhythmias, myocardial infarction, bradycardia, decreased cardiac output, hypertension, and abdominal cramps. Continuous electrocardiographic (ECG) monitoring is advised.

Somatostatin is a polypeptide that causes vasoconstriction, thus decreasing gastric esophageal collateral blood flow while increasing resistance to blood flow. The drug's effects are limited to the splanchnic circulation, so it has fewer side effects. Octreotide is a synthetic analog of somatostatin and has a much longer half-life. Propranolol, a beta blocker, may also be used.

Balloon tamponade may be used to control esophageal bleeding by placing pressure on the bleeding varices. Three types of tubes are used to control esophageal bleeding. The Sengstaken–Blakemore tube (see Figure 35–1) has three lumina: a gastric balloon, an esophageal balloon, and a lumen to aspirate gastric contents. The Minnesota tube is similar to the Blakemore tube; however, it has a larger gastric balloon and a fourth lumen to aspirate the esophagus. The Linton tube has a single gastric balloon, which is larger than the other tubes, and lumina to aspirate the stomach and esophagus. The balloons may be inflated to tamponade bleeding. Mechanical tamponade has been shown to stop bleeding more effectively than pharmacologic interventions. However, a Sengstaken–Blakemore tube inserted before sclerotherapy increases transfusion requirement and complications. Potential complications of tamponade are ulceration, necrosis, perforation, aspiration, and bleeding.[10]

Surgical Management of Gastrointestinal Bleeding

Medical management with sclerotherapy and pharmacologic agents is implemented initially to treat bleeding varices. If the bleeding is uncontrolled, surgical intervention may be necessary. Portal pressure and complications of esophageal varices can be addressed with a portosystemic shunt. Shunts divert blood flow from the portal to the systemic circulation, which bypasses the liver and decreases portal hypertension. Shunts decrease the risk of recurrence of upper GI hemorrhage from varices, but they may increase disease and mortality.[12] Shunts are only palliative (Table 36–7).

Transjugular Intrahepatic Portosystemic Shunt

An alternative treatment for portal hypertension and bleeding esophageal varices is transjugular intrahepatic portosystemic shunt (TIPS). TIPS is a nonsurgical, invasive radiologic procedure. The portal vein is accessed through the right internal jugular vein. The portal and hepatic veins are then connected by punching a hole and inserting an expandable metal stent (see Figure 35–2). The goal is to decrease the portal to hepatic vein gradient to 10 mm Hg or less. TIPS is associated with a decrease in the incidence of morbidity and mortality associated with surgery in patients with acute hemorrhage or severe liver dysfunction. Complications include intraperitoneal hemorrhage, hematoma, fever, encephalopathy, transient oliguric renal failure, bacteremia, subendocardial myocardial infarction, shunt stenosis, shunt occlusion, laceration, contrast complications, and bile duct trauma. The morbidity and mortality related to this procedure are influenced by patient demographics and technical expertise. Patients with

Child's class A typically have a lower mortality than those with Child's class C cirrhosis.[12, 13]

Acetaminophen Overdose Management

Acetaminophen overdose causes depletion of glutathione, which binds the drug and causes liver failure. The goal of initial management of acetaminophen overdose is to prevent continued drug absorption. Interventions include evacuating the stomach and absorbing acetaminophen with activated charcoal. N-Acetylcysteine (Mucomyst) is given, and it replenishes the glutathione and limits hepatic damage. This agent is available as an oral preparation given by nasogastric tube and is most effective when given within 24 hours of ingestion of acetaminophen. A loading dose of 140 mg/kg is given and is followed by seven doses of 70 mg/kg at 4-hour intervals. Treatment may be discontinued after 24 hours if clotting times and renal function remain within normal limits.[4]

Nonintensive Care Management

Depending upon a patient's physiologic condition and other hepatic factors, the following management techniques may or may not be performed in the ICU.

Encephalopathy Management

Encephalopathy is treated by identifying and correcting precipitating factors. Frequently, one must monitor a patient's neurologic status, reorient the patient as needed, protect the patient from injury, and treat any changes. Encephalopathy may be caused by azotemia, sedation, GI bleeding, infection, increased protein intake, hypoxia, drugs such as sedatives or anesthetics, alcohol, constipation, and aggressive diuresis that leads to intravascular volume depletion. The exact pathogenesis of hepatic encephalopathy is uncertain; however, a decrease of nitrogenous products from the gut and circulation is accompanied by clinical improvement. In early encephalopathy, withdrawal of dietary protein and administration of lactulose is beneficial. At a more advanced stage of encephalopathy, there is little evidence that these measure are advantageous.[11]

TABLE 36–7
Types of Shunts Used to Treat Portal Hypertension

Shunt	Selective	Indication	Anastomosis	Other
Portacaval	No	Most common	Portal vein to inferior vena cava	End to end or side to side
Splenorenal	Yes	Hypersplenism	Splenic vein to left renal vein	Decreased chance of variceal re-bleed
				Possible shunt thrombosis
Mesocaval	Yes	Portal vein thrombosis Previous splenectomy Ascites	Superior mesenteric to inferior vena cava	Increased graft occlusion

It is important to rule out any concurrent process that could cause mental status changes and to begin treatment of encephalopathy while other causes of mental status changes are being excluded.[10] Avoidance of hepatotoxic drugs and sedatives is essential. Treatment is aimed at decreased absorption of nitrogenous products from the gut, withdrawal of oral protein, and administration of lactulose and, if needed, nonabsorbable neomycin.[14]

Ammonia levels must be monitored. Treatment of high ammonia levels includes bowel cleansing with neomycin and lactulose. Neomycin, a nonabsorbable antibiotic, destroys the flora in the GI tract that breaks down protein and results in ammonia production. Neomycin can be administered by mouth or by enema. However, an enema may not be recommended because it may cause rectal bleeding in patients with coagulopathies. The dose is generally 500 mg to 1 g every 6 hours or a 200-mL enema of 1% solution. Neomycin can cause ototoxicity and nephrotoxicity; therefore, lactulose is usually the drug of choice.

Lactulose is a nonabsorbable disaccharide that is converted in the bowel to lactate and other acids. Lactulose acidifies the bowel environment and binds the ammonia. The laxative effect of this treatment causes the ammonia to be excreted in the stool. Side effects of this therapy may be bloating, cramping, nausea, or vomiting. Severe diarrhea may result. The dose is 15 to 30 g given three to four times a day, or until the patient has two to four stools. An enema of 300 mL of 50% lactulose and 700 mL of water three times daily can also be used.

Nutrition Management

A patient's nutritional status must be assessed within a few days. Adequate calories are needed to prevent muscle breakdown for gluconeogenesis. A dietary consultation is indicated to assess a patient's caloric intake and dietary needs. Dietary supplements, tube feedings, or total parenteral nutrition may be indicated.

The oral or enteral route is preferred, to maintain intestinal mucosal integrity and to decrease bacterial translocation. Salt intake should be restricted to less than 2 g per day to prevent fluid alterations. Many patients with hepatic failure feel nauseated and may vomit. Metoclopramide (Reglan) and hydroxyzine (Vistaril) may be indicated. Frequent small feedings may also be indicated. Mouth care before eating may promote a patient's appetite. It is also important to assess the patient's food preferences.

Protein intake may be restricted to 40 g per day or 0.5 to 1.0 g/kg per day to decrease the body's nitrogen load. Patients in severe stress or fulminant hepatic failure may need more protein. Patients in coma should receive no protein.[15] The use of branched-chain amino acids to meet the caloric requirement of patients with hepatic failure is controversial. Researchers have reported that patients with cirrhosis and hepatic encephalopathy who receive branched-chain amino acids have less protein catabolism and enhanced protein synthesis.[14] However, other investigators have reported no good evidence to support the branched-chain amino acid formulation in providing nutritional support.[4] Glycogen stores are diminished and insulin levels are high in liver disease. Patients with acute hepatic failure may become hypoglycemic and may need intravenous infusions of 10 to 20% dextrose. Fingersticks every 1 to 2 hours and as needed to determine a patient's glucose level are essential. Boluses of 50 mL of 50% glucose or continuous infusions of 10% dextrose for glucose levels of less than 70 mg/dL may also be administered for patients who are hypoglycemic.

Ascites Management

Ascites is managed by treating the cause. Medical treatment focuses on salt restriction of 2 to 3 g per day, fluid restriction of 0.75 to 1.5 L per day, daily weights, strict intake and output (I & O), and the prudent use of diuretics. Medications such as antacids or antibiotics that may be sodium rich should also be restricted. Serum and urine electrolytes must be monitored regularly. Diuretics such as spironolactone (Aldactone), a potassium-sparing diuretic, thiazide diuretics, or loop diuretics may be used. Potassium-sparing diuretics decrease aldosterone and thereby reverse the secondary hyperaldosteronism. The dose of spironolactone is 25 mg three times daily and can be increased slowly to 300 mg per day. It is important to monitor the patient's fluid and electrolyte status regularly and to avoid overdiuresis. The goal is to decrease body weight by 0.5 kg per day. Patients with urinary sodium levels greater than 20 mmol per day and fractional sodium excretion greater than 0.2% tend to respond to lower doses of 100 to 150 mg per day. Careful monitoring for signs and symptoms of hypovolemia, azotemia, and sodium and potassium imbalance is needed. Potassium levels should be determined frequently, and patients should be observed for signs and symptoms of hypokalemia from excessive diuretics and signs and symptoms of hyperkalemia from too much potassium replacement.[16] Loop diuretics may be added if the patient is unresponsive to spironolactone alone.

Paracentesis. Paracentesis, puncture of the abdominal cavity to remove ascitic fluid, is a procedure once abandoned because of its association with frequent complications, but it has been reintroduced. Paracentesis provides only temporary relief and is usually performed to relieve pressure on the diaphragm and to prevent respiratory complications. Ascitic fluid that is withdrawn may be replaced with intravenous colloids such as salt-poor albumin. Diuretics should be administered to prevent reaccumulation of ascites. Repeated paracentesis for large amounts of fluid removal may be needed. It is important to analyze all ascitic fluid withdrawn for infection. Peritonitis may occur at any time, in the absence of an identifiable intra-abdominal source, and must be treated with antibiotics. Nurses should observe the patient for signs and symptoms of fluid depletion and sepsis after the procedure.

Shunts. A peritoneal venous shunt (LeVeen shunt) may be used for patients refractory to medical treatment of ascites. A collecting cannula is surgically inserted in the peritoneal cavity and is tunneled under the skin to the superior vena cava. Ascitic fluid is then drained from the abdomen and is reinfused into venous circulation (Figure 36–3). The shunt must be clamped or removed before any abdominal surgery to prevent air embolism.[6] If the patient is a candidate for liver transplantation treatment of ascites should not include the surgical placement of shunts, which may lead to increased complications during the transplant procedure.[17] The LeVeen shunt is contraindicated in patients with encephalopathy, recent abdominal surgery, congestive heart failure, DIC, or decompensated liver disease.[2] These shunts are associated with high rates of infection, occlusion, and coagulopathy. No evidence suggests that treatment with a peritoneal venous shunt significantly increases long-term survival.[18]

Fluid and Electrolyte Management
A patient's fluid and electrolyte status may be affected by liver disease and also by interventions used to treat the disease. The nurse must monitor and prevent hy-

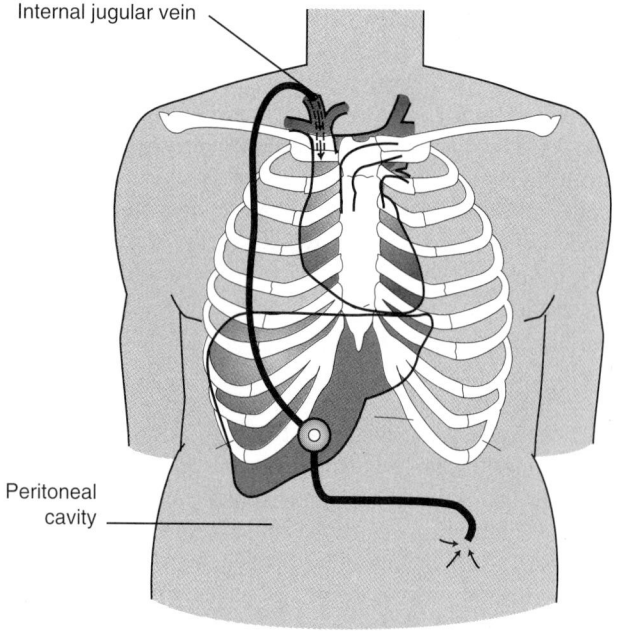

Figure 36–3
Peritoneal venous shunt.

Internal jugular vein

Peritoneal cavity

perkalemia and intravascular volume depletion. Frequent vital signs, strict I & O, and daily weights are essential. The following laboratory values should be monitored daily: potassium, glucose, urinary sodium, blood urea nitrogen (BUN), and creatinine. Urine output should be monitored hourly and maintained at more than 30 mL per hour. A patient's volume status is carefully monitored by frequent vital signs and hemodynamic monitoring of pulmonary artery pressures and cardiac output. If signs and symptoms of volume depletion occur, intravenous fluid volume replacement is indicated, and diuretics should be discontinued. Volume is usually replaced with blood if the patient's hemoglobin is low; otherwise, a combination of colloids and crystalloids is used. Ringer's lactate should be avoided because lactate is chiefly metabolized by the liver. It is important to assess the patient for orthostatic blood pressure changes.

Coagulopathy Management
Liver failure is associated with an abnormal clotting cascade. This association is due to a decrease in the synthesis of clotting factors, a consumptive coagulopathy state, activation of the fibrolytic pathway, and platelet abnormalities. Coagulopathy is usually not treated, but treatment may include administration of vitamin K, fresh frozen plasma, and platelets.[8] Vitamin K, 10 mg subcutaneously, may be given every day for 3 days. Patients are then given 10 mg by mouth every day. Fresh frozen plasma may be administered for uncontrolled bleeding or in anticipation of procedures. Administration of fresh frozen plasma in the absence of bleeding has not been shown to be valuable.[11] Platelets may be given as needed to keep the platelet count greater than 50,000 mm^3.[1] It is also essential to discontinue any aspirin-containing products. Frequent monitoring of PT, PTT, and fibrinogen is needed. Histamine (H$_2$) blockers are given to prevent stress ulcers and hemorrhage.

Infection Management
Infection is managed by prevention and early detection. Careful hand washing, avoidance of invasive procedures and lines when possible, frequent line changes, venipuncture and wound site assessment, regular pulmonary hygiene, and strict aseptic technique help to prevent infection in patients with hepatic failure. Regular microbial surveillance and aggressive treatment of presumed infections are essential because prophylactic regimens have been shown to be of little benefit.[1] Antibiotics are given as indicated by culture sensitivities. Bacterial and fungal infections are common in patients with acute liver failure and are related to the immunologic defects of the disease as well as to iatrogenic causes such as catheters and endotracheal tubes. Gram-positive organisms such as streptococci and *Staphylococcus aureus* usually enter the

skin through indwelling catheters. All catheter tips should be cultured on removal. *Candida* species are usually responsible for the fungal infections. Fungal infections always accompany a bacterial infection.[4] Fungal infections typically occur later in the hospital stay.

Hepatitis Treatment

No specific treatment has been identified for viral hepatitis infections. Treatment of these patients is supportive. Patients need rest until the liver is no longer tender and their serum bilirubin levels are within normal limits. A low-fat, high-carbohydrate diet is recommended to assist in the maintenance of adequate nutrition. If a patient is unable to ingest food orally or is unable to keep food in the stomach because of nausea or vomiting, intravenous feedings may be initiated. Corticosteroids may be used to slow the disease progression and to alleviate symptoms. Exposure to all types of hepatitis carries danger, but hepatitis B poses the greatest risk. An immunization exists for those exposed to hepatitis B. After exposure, passive immunoprophylaxis can be obtained through use of high anti-HBs titer hepatitis B immune globulin. There is also a vaccine for active immunization against hepatitis B, Recombivax-HB, and Engerix-B. This vaccine is administered over a 6-month period prophylactically and provides active immunity against hepatitis B. This vaccine is recommended for all health care personnel who may have contact with patients infected with hepatitis B or for personnel who are at risk of needle-sticks. Standard precautions should also be followed.[2]

Liver Transplantation

Liver transplantation has revolutionized the treatment of advanced liver disease. Transplantation is a highly successful procedure for patients with advanced and untreatable liver disease. The types of liver disease for which patients undergo liver transplantation include fulminant hepatic failure, cirrhosis, sclerosing cholangitis, biliary atresia, and metabolic disorders in children. Indications for liver transplantation include encephalopathy, severe ascites, coagulopathy, hepatorenal syndrome, recurrent variceal hemorrhage, severe bone disease with fractures, recurrent cholangitis, and severe progressive hepatic insufficiency.[6]

Contraindications include malignant disease outside the hepatobiliary system, sepsis and infection outside the hepatobiliary system, human immunodeficiency virus (HIV)-positive status, and severe cardiorespiratory compromise.[18] Advances in procurement techniques, preservation solutions, surgical techniques, and immunosuppression have all contributed to encouraging results. Both short-term and long-term survival rates have improved in recent years. However, outcome still remains a function of the degree of illness at the time of surgery.[18] Unfortu-

nately, there are not enough organ donors to meet the demand of organ recipients (Chart 36–3). Alternative treatments such as hepatocyte transplantation and partial liver graft transplantation from living related donors are being used.

Future Management

The liver is a dynamic organ performing greater than 400 functions. An artificial liver has been difficult to develop, and its development lags behind that of mechanical devices used for other vital organs. Extracorporeal liver assist devices (ELADs) and bioartificial livers have been developed and are now being tested in clinical trials. An ELAD consists of a mass of liver cells housed in a hollow fiber bioreactor.

Treatment is performed using modified dialysis equipment. A patient's plasma is perfused through a filter cartridge containing hepatocytes. One type uses a charcoal filter and porcine hepatocytes grown on hollow fiber supports. A second type of device contains human hepatoma cells grown on hollow fibers. The goal is to remove toxic metabolites until the patient's own liver can regenerate and function. These devices only contain hepatocytes and therefore can only correct imbalances attributable to hepatocellular injury, not those originating from nonparenchymal cells. ELADs should allow patients to recover from acute liver failure or to be supported until a liver transplant can be performed.[8,19]

Multidisciplinary Outcomes

Caring for a patient with acute or chronic liver disease requires early assessment, identification, and prompt treatment by a collaborative health care team. Patients with acute liver failure and those with advanced chronic liver failure must be managed appropriately in the ICU. It is important that critical care nurses understand the pathophysiology, clinical presentation, and treatment of patients with liver disease so that the most favorable patient outcomes can be achieved (Table 36–8 and Chart 36–4).

Critical Thinking Exercise

Mr. C. W. is 56 years old with a history of cirrhosis. He was admitted to the medical intensive care unit accompanied by his wife. His wife stated that he had been complaining of nausea and vomiting the night before admission. On awakening this morning, she found him lethargic and confused. Because of the seriousness of his condition, a pulmonary artery catheter and a Foley catheter were inserted. The patient was also placed on a cardiac monitor, and admission laboratory samples were sent. Laboratory results were as

> **CHART 36–3**
>
> **ETHICAL DILEMMA**
>
> Ms. Y. is a 40-year-old woman who presented to the emergency room vomiting bright red blood and with an altered mental status. The patient reported a history of alcohol abuse since the age of 16 years, cirrhosis, esophageal varices, thrombocytopenia, and hemolytic anemia. Her hemoglobin was 6.6 g/100 mL, and the patient was transfused with 2 U packed red blood cells. Her liver function tests, prothrombin time, and partial thromboplastin time were all abnormally elevated.
>
> Ms. Y. denied that alcohol is a problem. She became tearful and angry when the topic of substance abuse was discussed. The patient had never been a patient in a substance abuse program. She was separated from her husband and had no other family.
>
> On discharge from the acute care setting, Ms. Y. entered an inpatient substance abuse program, which she completed. As an outpatient, she completed the 12 steps of Alcoholics Anonymous (AA) and regularly attended support group meetings. Six months later, the patient remains alcohol free and continues to attend AA meetings three times per week.
>
> Ms. Y.'s liver disease has progressed. She now presents to her local transplant program to be worked up as a possible liver transplant recipient.
>
> 1. Liver transplantation has revolutionized the treatment of advanced liver disease. Unfortunately, there are not enough donor organs to meet the demand of organ recipients. Who shall receive a transplant when not all patients can? Is the goal of transplantation to save patients regardless of length of survival or to transplant organs in patients with the greatest life expectancy?
>
> 2. Allocation of scarce resources has both ethical and moral implications. How should the decision-making process of recipient selection be defined? Should it be defined by medical criteria alone, by medical criteria with an ethical focus, by medical criteria with a psychosocial focus, or by all factors that may influence the outcome of the procedure? Should selection criteria be standardized nationally?
>
> 3. Can medical factors be considered without unintentional personal bias and values affecting the decision?
>
> 4. Organ donors are in short supply, and organs are rationed among transplant centers. Rationing is in conflict with the United States Constitution, which supports the tenet that all Americans are equal. Some end-stage disease is the result of self-infliction. Should patients who never had a normal liver because of a medical condition such as primary biliary cirrhosis be given priority over patients with self-induced end-stage liver disease through an overdose or alcohol abuse?
>
> Data from Kelso L: Alcohol-related end-stage liver disease and transplantation: the debate continues. AACV Clin Issues Crit Care Nurs 5:501–506, 1994; Killeen T: Alcoholism and liver transplantation: ethical and nursing implications. Perspect Psychiatr Care 29:7–12, 1993; Murray B: The lottery of life: should organ transplants be used to even the odds? Dimensions Crit Care Nurs 14:266–272, 1995; and Thomas D: Organ transplantation in people with unhealthy lifestyles. AACN Clin Issues Crit Care Nurs 4:665–668, 1993.

follows: sodium, 137; chloride, 101; BUN, 22; aspartate aminotransferase, 68; total bilirubin, 3.7; potassium, 3.4; carbon dioxide, 23; serum creatinine, 1.2; alanine aminotransferase, 124; lactate dehydrogenase, 356; ammonia, 174; albumin, 2.8; globulin, 2.0; PT, 28; PTT, 46; white blood cells, 12,500; hemoglobin, 10.7; hematocrit, 34; and red blood cells, 3.6.

The patient's vital signs on admission were as follows: blood pressure, 86/42 mm Hg; heart rate, 132; respiratory rate, 26; temperature, 101.2° F; right atrial pressure, 3; pulmonary artery systolic, 12; pulmonary artery diastolic, 6; pulmonary artery occlusive pressure, 6; and cardiac output, 3.5.

Blood gases on room air were as follows: PaO_2, 58; $PaCO_2$, 23; pH, 7.43; HCO_3^-, 24; and SaO_2, 78%.

The patient's physical examination revealed the following:

Neurologic: Confused; localizes to pain; uncooperative; asterixis noted; pupils 2 mm that react to light; extraocular eye movements intact; moderate weakness noted in both upper and lower extremities

Cardiovascular: ECG showing sinus tachycardia with occasional premature ventricular contractions; capillary refill prolonged; skin cool to touch; heart tones diminished

Respiratory: Breath sounds clear and decreased on the right; chest expansion decreased on the right; patient dyspneic with exertion; nonproductive cough noted

GI: Abdomen firm and distended; bowel sounds hypoactive; nasogastric tube in place draining dark brown liquid

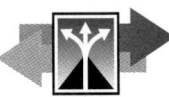

TABLE 36–8
Multidisciplinary Outcomes

Phase	Outcome
Primary care	Identification of patients at risk for liver failure
	Identification of precipitating factors
Acute care	Identification of precipitating factors
	Treatment or elimination of cause
	Minimization of hepatic toxicity
	Support of hepatic function
Intensive care	Maintenance of hemodynamic stability and adequate oxygenation
	Support of hepatic and other body system function
	Treatment or elimination of cause
	Maintenance of fluid and electrolyte balance
	Prevention of renal failure, gastrointestinal bleeding, and cerebral edema
	Prevention or detection of complications
Intermediate care	Maintenance of fluid and electrolyte balance
	Prevention or detection of complications
	Initiation of patient education
	Discharge preparation of patient and family
Community	Home health as indicated
	Patient education
	Return to previous or improved level of health and function

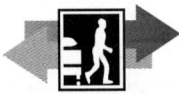

CHART 36–4

BEYOND THE ICU: MANAGING PATIENTS WITH LIVER FAILURE FROM ALCOHOL ABUSE

Patients at risk for liver failure may be identified in the primary care setting. Liver failure has many causes, as discussed throughout this chapter, but the leading cause is alcohol abuse. Alcohol abuse is also the leading cause of cirrhosis. Follow-up care in the community for the patient with acute liver failure can be facilitated by home health agencies. Home health nurses may provide medical interventions, patient education, and assessments of patient compliance. Patients are routinely followed on discharge by both their primary care physician and a hepatologist.

If the acute liver failure is due to alcoholism, the issues of substance abuse and addiction must be addressed with the patient. Community referrals can be suggested and appointments made; however, the patient must decide to access this care to prevent further liver damage. Community support groups and inpatient admission to rehabilitation facilities are additional options to assist in recovery from alcoholism.

If initial recommendations to decrease alcohol intake are not followed, further damage will be done to the liver. These patients then progress to the more chronic stage in which irreversible damage has been done to their liver. Once the patient has reached this stage, few options are available. Patients with acute liver disease or advanced stages of chronic liver disease need critical care nursing. If the prognosis is grave for the patient in hepatic failure on discharge from the hospital, hospice care needs to be considered. The use of this agency allows the patient to stay at home with loved ones for support. If families choose this option, hospice can assist with meeting the patient's needs such as obtaining necessary pain relief. Hospice can also prevent unnecessary hospitalizations by providing needed care within the patient's home. Hospice can also serve as an important resource for family members experiencing the loss of a loved one.

that is heme positive and has a pH of 4.5; formed clay-colored stool noted

Genitourinary: Foley catheter in place draining dark brown, foamy fluid with a foul odor

Skin: Turgor poor, yellow tinged, spider angiomas on thorax; mucous membranes yellow tinged and dry; patient's wife stating patient's gums bleed on brushing teeth

Psychosocial: Irritable and angry when awake; frequent napping noted

1. List the abnormal laboratory values and physical assessment signs and symptoms that are indicative of hepatic disease, and discuss their causes.
2. Mr. W.'s precipitating cause of hepatic disease is cirrhosis. What other precipitating factors are associated with acute and chronic hepatic failure?
3. Describe the major physiologic functions of the liver.
4. Why does Mr. W. have an increased risk of infection?
5. List the appropriate nursing diagnoses that apply to patients with hepatic failure.

Key Concepts

➡ Hepatic failure is a clinical syndrome characterized by presence of liver disease or functional impairment resulting from massive necrosis. Hepatic failure can occur suddenly, as in the event of acute liver disease, or it may present with an insidious onset. The most common causes are viral hepatitis and drug-induced liver injury.

➡ Acute hepatic failure results from a sudden massive necrosis of liver cells. This is due most often to viral infection or exposure to hepatic toxins. This condition lasts longer than 6 months and either resolves or is followed by progression of necrosis, which can be fatal.

➡ Any chronic disease of the liver may result in cirrhosis. Cirrhosis is any fibrous tissue change secondary to a chronic injury. Fibrous scarring and nodules distort the liver's vascular bed and lead to portal hypertension and shunting.

➡ Portal hypertension is the end result of cirrhosis of the liver. It is defined as an elevated pressure (>12 mm Hg) within the portal system that results in shunting of systemic circulation away from the liver.

➡ Portal hypertension creates a backflow of pressure to the spleen, stomach, and esophagus in an effort to maintain venous return to the heart. As low-pressure veins become distended, thin-walled vessels become at risk for trauma and hemorrhage.

➡ Gluconeogenesis is the ability of the liver to convert amino acids and fatty acids to glucose. If the liver is damaged, patients may exhibit elevated glucose levels related to their inability to store glucose.

➡ Hepatorenal syndrome is an association between liver failure and renal failure. Renal hypoperfusion leads to decreased glomerular filtration and decreased urine output. Vasodilators may be needed, or hemodialysis or other renal replacement modes may be required.

➡ Encephalopathy is a result of toxic substances in the systemic circulation that have advanced to the CNS. This condition usually causes impaired consciousness or coma.

➡ Encephalopathy can occur in acute and chronic liver failure and can also be acute or chronic. Patients should be assessed for subtle neurologic signs that suggest this development.

➡ Abnormal clotting cascades are associated with liver failure because of the decrease in the synthesis of clotting factors and the activation of the fibrolytic pathway.

➡ Coagulopathies are sometimes treated and other times not, depending on the stage of liver failure. It is important to assess PT, PTT, and fibrinogen levels as needed.

➡ Patients with liver failure also need to discontinue any form of aspirin and may be taking H_2 blockers to prevent stress ulcers and hemorrhage.

References

1. Lee W: Acute liver failure. N Engl J Med 329:1862–1872, 1993.
2. Smith S: Patients with hepatic disorders. In: Clochesy J, Breu C, Cardin S, et al (eds): Critical Care Nursing. Philadelphia, W.B. Saunders, 1993, pp 970–1008.
3. Smith S: Liver transplantation for acute hepatic failure: a review of clinical experience and management. Am J Crit Care 2:137–144, 1993.
4. Sussman N: Fulminant hepatic failure. In: Zakin D, Boyer T (eds): Hepatology: A Textbook of Liver Disease, 3rd ed. Philadelphia, W.B. Saunders, 1996.
5. Butler R: Managing the complications of cirrhosis. Am J Nurs 94:46–49, 1994.
6. Reishtein J: Liver failure: case study of a complex problem. Crit Care Nurse 13:36–45, 47, 1993.
7. Fingerote R, Bain V: Fulminant hepatic failure. Am J Gastroenterol 88:1000–1010, 1993.
8. Sussman N, Lake J: Treatment of hepatic failure, 1996: current concepts and progress toward liver dialysis. Am J Kidney Dis 27:605–621, 1996.
9. Zaloga G: Nutrition in Critical Care. St. Louis, C.V. Mosby, 1994.
10. Jutabha R, Jensen D: Management of upper GI bleeding in patients with chronic liver disease. Med Clin North Am 80:1035–1068, 1996.
11. Williams R, Gimson A: Intensive liver care and management of acute hepatic failure. Dig Dis Sci 36:820–826, 1991.
12. Bouley G, Grimshaw G, Lindewall K, et al: Transjugular intrahepatic portosystemic shunt: an alternative. Crit Care Nurse 16:23–28, 1996.
13. Pagliaro L, D'Amico G, Luca A, et al: Portal hypertension: diagnosis and treatment. J Hepatol 23 (Suppl 1):36–44, 1995.
14. Gitlin N: Hepatic encephalopathy. In: Zakin D, Boyer T (eds): Hepatology: A Textbook of Liver Disease, 3rd ed. Philadelphia, W.B. Saunders, 1996.

15. Gecelter G, Comer G: Nutritional support during liver failure. Crit Care Clin 11:675–683, 1995.

16. Chiou S, Changchien C: Management of end-stage liver disease. Transplant Proc 25:2948–2952, 1993.

17. Kelso L: Fluid and electrolyte disturbances in hepatic failure. AACN Clin Issues Crit Care Nurs 3:681–687, 1992.

18. Jaffe D, Chung R, Friedman L: Management of portal hypertension and its complications. Med Clin North Am 80:1021–1034, 1996.

19. Conlin C: Extracorporeal liver assist device: hope for the future. Crit Care Nurs Q 17:73–78, 1995.

37

Acute Pancreatitis

Karen K. Giuliano and Susan S. Scott

Objectives

After completing this chapter, the student will be able to:

1. Identify the most common causes of pancreatitis.
2. Relate the pathophysiology of pancreatitis to the presenting signs and symptoms.
3. Identify the nursing diagnoses associated with pancreatitis.
4. Plan the collaborative management of a patient with pancreatitis.
5. Select interventions to manage the most common complications of pancreatitis.

Pancreatitis is an inflammatory disease process in which proteolytic and lipolytic enzymes are activated and released within the pancreas, resulting in autodigestion of the organ. It is divided into acute and chronic forms. Chronic pancreatitis results in permanent tissue damage in which pancreatic cells are progressively replaced by fibrotic, nonfunctioning tissue. The result is progressive impairment of function by the organ. Patients with chronic pancreatitis experience repeated outbreaks of the disease and painful periods that may alternate with pain-free periods.

Acute pancreatitis is an acute attack to a previously normal pancreas in which permanent damage to the organ does not usually occur. It may be seen as a single episode or as recurrent attacks. The organ usually heals and returns to normal after the acute episode, unless complications result in scarring of the pancreatic tissue. The severity of the disease ranges from the mild edematous form that resolves spontaneously to the most severe form that results in necrosis and hemorrhage of the organ; the latter is associated with multiorgan failure and death. The mortality rate for pancreatitis is about 10% unless complications develop. About 25% of patients with acute pancreatitis have complications, in which case, the mortality rate jumps to 50% or more.[1] Pain relief for the patient with pancreatitis is a primary nursing focus, regardless of the severity of the disease, and patients with the more severe form require the most comprehensive critical nursing and medical interventions.

ETIOLOGY AND PATHOPHYSIOLOGY

The precise cause of pancreatitis is unclear, but under a variety of circumstances, pancreatic enzymes are activated within the pancreas and digest the pancreatic tissue itself. This process is termed *autodigestion*. In the normal pancreas, protective mechanisms prevent autodigestion. Pancreatic enzymes are in their inactive form, and this state of inactivity prevents damage to the pancreas by these enzymes. Other protective mechanisms in the pancreas that prevent autodigestion are localized and systemic protease inhibitors and specialized storage systems within the (pancreatic) acinar cells. In pancreatitis, there is a disruption of the protective mechanisms, and these enzymes digest both the pancreas itself and tissues and vessels surrounding the pancreas.

The severity of acute pancreatitis ranges from the mild form, which resolves spontaneously, to the severe form, in which shock, organ failure, and death can occur. The most common type of pancreatitis is the mild form, termed *edematous pancreatitis*.[1] With edematous pancreatitis, there is interstitial edema and mild necrosis of the fat surrounding the pancreas.

Necrotizing pancreatitis is the term used for the severe form of the disease. Necrotizing pancreatitis may begin as the edematous form and may become more severe, or it may present initially in the necrotizing form. This severe form of acute pancreatitis results in necrosis of the pancreatic tissue. When proteolytic enzymes damage tissue and blood vessels surrounding the pancreas, hemorrhage within and around the pancreas occurs. This is termed *hemorrhagic pancreatitis*. For the pathophysiologic progression of pancreatitis, see Figure 37–1.

The causes of acute pancreatitis include biliary tract disease, chronic alcoholism, drug ingestion, trauma, and idiopathic, with the most common causes being biliary tract disease and alcoholism (Chart 37–1.)

Biliary Tract Disease

Biliary tract disease is the most common cause of acute pancreatitis in the nonalcoholic population.[2] When biliary tract disease occurs, a gallstone or edema and inflammation from passage of a stone obstruct the flow of enzymes through the pancreatic duct, and it is

CHART 37–1

Causes of Pancreatitis

Biliary tract disease
Alcohol
Trauma
Hypertriglyceridemia
Hypercalcemia
Idiopathic
Infection
Shock
Medications
   Diuretics
   Steroids
   Transplant medications

hypothesized that the obstruction of the duct is what triggers the acute pancreatitis. Ordinarily, the enzymes in the pancreatic duct are not activated and so do not result in autodigestion. Research suggests, however, that after the pancreatic duct is obstructed, digestive enzymes are activated within the pancreatic cells, resulting in the cellular damage that is seen with pancreatitis. Although there are several other theories as to why biliary tract stones result in the onset of acute pancreatitis, most researchers agree that the aforementioned situation is the most likely cause.[3]

Chronic Alcoholism

Alcoholism is the most common cause of pancreatitis in men. It is unclear how ethanol ingestion results in pancreatitis, but possibilities include the induction of ischemia due to secondary hypertriglyceridemia or a toxic effect to pancreatic cells. It is thought that elevated triglycerides lead to injury to pancreatic blood vessels.[2] Usually, the first attack of alcohol-induced pancreatitis does not occur until the patient has undergone years of alcohol consumption, although there have been some cases of the disease after as little as one exposure to alcohol.

Drugs

Exposure to drugs is another cause of acute pancreatitis. The most common culprits are thiazide diuretics, furosemide, and ethycrinic acid. Pentamidine and dideoxyinosine, which are medications used to treat acquired immunodeficiency syndrome or acquired immunodeficiency syndrome–related complex, are also associated with pancreatitis. Immunosuppressive

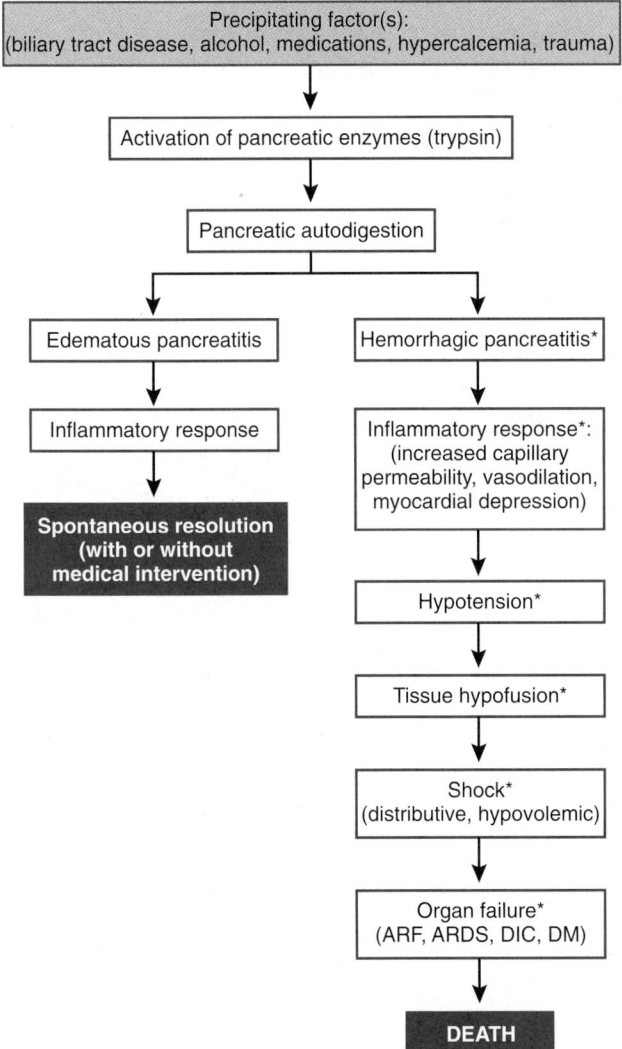

Figure 37–1

Pathophysiologic progression of pancreatitis. The asterisk indicates that the disease may respond to treatment and resolve at any point in the disease process. ARF, acute renal failure; ARD, acute respiratory distress syndrome; DIC, disseminated intravascular coagulation; DM, diabetes mellitus.

agents, such as those used with organ transplantation, also put patients at risk for developing acute pancreatitis. Miscellaneous drugs also associated with pancreatitis include steroids, tetracycline, and estrogens.[3]

Trauma

Damage to the pancreas as the result of trauma is another cause of this disease. Penetrating trauma to the organ itself can occur with a knife or a gunshot wound or with surgery on the pancreas and can result in leakage of pancreatic enzymes and autodigestion of the pancreas. Blunt abdominal trauma, as occurs with motor vehicle crashes and falls, can damage the pancreas, causing leakage of enzymes into the pancreas and to the surrounding tissues.

Idiopathic pancreatitis was thought to account for 10 to 20% of cases, although some research suggests that many patients whose pancreatitis seems to have no identifiable cause in fact have biliary sludge and biliary tract disease.[4] Pancreatic duct obstruction or conditions that interfere with drainage from the pancreatic duct can also cause pancreatitis and include tumors, cysts, inflammatory lesions, and hypercalcemic disorders. Surgery to the areas immediately surrounding the pancreas can result in localized inflammation, which can interfere with the drainage of secretions. Hypercalcemia can lead to stone formation in the pancreatic duct, thereby obstructing the flow of pancreatic secretions from the pancreas. Hypercalcemia is also associated with increased secretion of pancreatic enzymes; this increase magnifies the inflammatory process associated with pancreatitis.

Assessment

Signs and Symptoms of Acute Pancreatitis

The clinical presentation of acute pancreatitis may range from a patient who is asymptomatic to someone who appears acutely ill, vomiting, and writhing in pain.

Abdominal

Abdominal pain is the most common symptom of pancreatitis, although it may be difficult to assess for its severity, quality, and location in the critical care population, where patients often have a decreased level of consciousness. Patients who have undergone abdominal surgery or who have sustained abdominal trauma may have abdominal pain from causes other than pancreatitis, and so the pancreatitis may go undetected. The pain that occurs is thought to be the result of peritoneal inflammation caused by leakage of pancreatic secretions.

The character of the abdominal pain is usually described as constant and is often severe, with the patient either frequently changing position, or if peritonitis is present, assuming a fetal position in the attempt to diminish the pain. It may be located over the entire abdomen or may be limited to the epigastric region. The patient's abdomen is often distended, and if there is peritoneal involvement, the abdomen is rigid, there are no bowel sounds, and rebound tenderness is present. Nausea and vomiting are common, and unlike nausea from other causes, the nausea associated with pancreatitis is not relieved by vomiting. The vomiting is usually frequent and in small amounts and is gastric in origin. In addition to vomiting, there may be loose, foul-smelling stools.

The clinician should continuously assess the patient for hemorrhage. If the pancreatitis is associated with hemorrhage and bleeding around the pancreas, the bleeding can extend into the tissues. This may be seen as ecchymosis in the flank region, termed *Grey Turner's sign,* and ecchymosis in the periumbilical area, termed *Cullen's sign.*

Hemodynamic

One of the effects of pancreatic autodigestion and damage to surrounding tissues by the activated pancreatic enzymes is inflammation. With tissue damage, there is inflammation, and along with tissue damage, there is a release of chemicals that cause the capillaries to increase their permeability to fluids. When this occurs, fluid in the capillaries leaks into the interstitial space around the pancreas and particularly into the abdominal cavity and retroperitoneal space. The volume of fluid that leaks into the tissues is often so great that it can result in hypovolemia. In fact, even a mild case of acute pancreatitis can result in the shift of 6 L of fluid into the third space, and in more severe cases of the disease, there is a shift of even greater amounts of fluid. This fluid volume deficit (hypovolemia) may manifest as increased thirst, dry mucous membranes, poor skin turgor, flat neck veins, low blood pressure, tachycardia, and decreased urine output. Under normal circumstances, when hypovolemia occurs, the body attempts to maintain circulation by narrowing the blood vessels and increasing the cardiac output. This is an attempt to maintain circulating volume within the blood vessels in order to deliver adequate oxygen and nutrients to the cells. With pancreatitis, the activated enzymes cause pancreatic cellular and local vascular damage, leading to an inflammatory response. This response results in the release of agents (including myocardial depressant factor, histamine, and prostaglandin) that interfere with the body's ability to respond and lead to shock and circulatory collapse. The release of these agents (referred to as chemical mediators and vasoactive substances) results in vasodilation, myocardial depression, and increased capillary permeability. The patient experiences a fluid volume deficit as fluid leaks from the vascular compartment into the tissues. An alteration in cardiac output occurs as myocardial contractility is decreased because of the myocardial depressant factor. This is compounded by the vasodilation, which interferes with the normal vasoconstrictive response that ordinarily occurs when the sympathetic nervous system is stimulated by hypovolemia. Vasodilation, myocardial depression, and hypovolemia all interfere with the ability to deliver oxygen to the cells. When the amount of oxygen available to the cells is insufficient (e.g., shock), tissue ischemia and cellular death occur. Tachycardia occurs as the body attempts to increase cardiac output to maintain tissue perfusion. Impaired tissue perfusion is often manifested as decreased level of consciousness, delayed capillary refill (>3 seconds), cool extremities, clammy skin, and various degrees of organ failure. If circulating blood volume is not adequately replaced, circulation to the kidneys decreases, leading to decreased urine output. Decreased perfusion to the kidneys eventually results in acute renal failure if left untreated.

Respiratory
Respiratory failure is one of the leading causes of death in acute pancreatitis.[2] The alterations in gas exchange associated with pancreatitis are complex and are related to a number of factors. Pleural effusions occur in up to 15% of patients, particularly on the left side, because this is more proximal to the pancreas, although they may develop bilaterally. Pleural effusions are fluid collections that occur as pancreatic secretions leak into the pleural space and cause an increased production of pleural fluid.[5] If the effusion is large enough, it can reduce lung volume and produce difficulty breathing. A pleural effusion may be discovered because of the presence of decreased breath sounds and dullness to percussion over the affected area.

Shallow respirations and a weak cough can occur because abdominal pain causes the patient to splint. This, in turn, results in atelectasis, which causes a decrease in the amount of oxygen reaching the alveolar-capillary membrane. This reduces the amount of oxygen entering the blood, making less available for cellular metabolism.

Other changes in respiratory status are caused by impaired gas exchange across the alveolar-capillary membrane as a result of noncardiogenic pulmonary edema or acute respiratory distress syndrome. If circulating chemicals associated with the inflammatory response involve the lung, the capillaries become more permeable to fluids. When this increased capillary permeability occurs, protein-rich fluids leak into the lung tissue. This interferes with the ability of oxygen and carbon dioxide to cross the alveolar-capillary membrane. In addition to the fluid leakage into the lungs, there is damage to type II pneumocytes in the alveoli, which are responsible for surfactant production. Surfactant is a substance found in the alveoli that maintains the surface tension within the alveoli. Without surfactant, alveolar collapse occurs more easily. Initially, in an attempt to improve oxygenation, tachypnea and hyperventilation occur and can compensate for some degree of respiratory compromise. However, respiratory failure eventually occurs as the patient fatigues, warranting mechanical ventilation because the patient can no longer continue to sustain adequate ventilation and oxygenation.

Laboratory and Diagnostic Tests

Laboratory Tests
Some laboratory values suggest pancreatitis. Amylase level is usually elevated. It increases 2 to 12 hours after the onset of the disease and may be greater than 1000 IU/L. It returns to normal levels within 3 to 6 days. Lipase levels rise with pancreatitis as well and remain elevated longer than the amylase levels, so that finding may suggest that pancreatitis is present, despite a normal amylase level. Triglyceride levels are increased in some patients, particularly the alcoholic population.[3] Hypokalemia and hypomagnesemia are common and occur as the result of vomiting, nasogastric suction, and fluid and electrolyte shifts. Hypomagnesemia can contribute to hypocalcemia by disrupting the function of the parathyroid gland, which is responsible for the release of calcium from bone and for total body calcium balance. Both hypokalemia and hypomagnesemia contribute to the hypotension that already exists.

Hypocalcemia is a common abnormality in patients with pancreatitis, although the exact cause of hypocalcemia is not completely understood. It is known that serum calcium levels drop in the presence of a low serum albumin level. When the albumin level is low, the total serum calcium is low because 50% of total body calcium is bound to serum proteins, such as albumin. When the serum albumin level is low, the total amount of serum calcium is low. The total amount of serum calcium includes the protein-bound and ionized calcium. This low level does not reflect the amount of ionized calcium in the body. Ionized calcium makes up 50% of the total serum calcium. It is the ionized calcium that is involved in biologic activities, such as muscle and nerve cell function. Therefore, a patient with a low total serum calcium level may not exhibit any signs of hypocalcemia, because the biologically active portion of the total serum calcium (ionized) is not reduced. One can calculate the corrected calcium level for a patient with a low albumin level by adding 0.8 to the total calcium calculation for every factor of 1 that the albumin level is less than 4 (e.g., if the serum calcium level is 6.0 and the albumin level is 2, one would add 1.6 to the calcium level, to reach a corrected calcium level of 7.6, which brings the calcium level to within normal limits).

Although the low serum albumin level explains the asymptomatic hypocalcemia, it does not explain why patients experience symptomatic hypocalcemia. It is thought that the symptomatic hypocalcemia is due to calcium ion deposition in areas of fat necrosis around the pancreas; this phenomenon occurs with pancreatitis. Patients who have a reduced amount of available ionized calcium have symptomatic hypocalcemia. The signs of hypocalcemia include bronchospasm, neuromuscular irritability, decreased cardiac output, tetany, cardiac dysrhythmias, and congestive heart failure. Also seen are a positive Chvostek's sign and positive Trousseau's sign.

Diagnostic Tests

Computed tomography is used to identify acute pancreatitis, but as many as 21% of patients with this disease have negative results.[5] Abdominal ultrasounds may be used initially to identify biliary tract problems, such as stones and bile duct dilation. Later in the course of the disease, ultrasound studies may be performed to detect and monitor pancreatic inflammatory masses and pseudocysts.[3]

Severity of Illness

Because pancreatitis has such a broad range of severity, numerous scoring systems have been developed in an attempt to predict the severity of the disease. Some scoring systems look at the complications of the disease. The Ranson criteria are commonly used for patients with pancreatitis. This system considers patient age, white blood count, blood glucose level, and other laboratory values (Chart 37–2). The number of positive prognostic signs that are present in the patient is linked to the patient's mortality rate. The greater number of positive signs a patient has, the greater the patient's mortality rate. A score of 7 or greater is associated with a 100% mortality rate.[6] Although the patient's mortality rate does not alter the nursing care requirements, it does allow the nurse to help the patient's significant others prepare for a less than positive patient outcome (Chart 37–3). Other systems are those based on the appearance of the pancreas on computed tomographic scan, the presence of comorbid illnesses, or the systemic release of pancreatic enzymes.[1]

Nursing Diagnoses

Several nursing diagnoses reflect the problems encountered by patients who are diagnosed with acute pancreatitis. Many of the diagnoses are discussed and

CHART 37–2

> ### *Ranson's Criteria*
>
> On admission (or diagnosis):
> Age >55 years
> White blood count >16,000/mm^3
> Blood glucose level >200 mg/dL
> Serum lactic dehydrogenase level >350 IU/L
> Aspartate transaminase >250 Sigma-Frankel
>   U%
> During the initial 48 hours:
> Fall in hematocrit >10%
> Blood urea nitrogen level increase >5 mg/dL
> Partial pressure of arterial oxygen <60 mm
>   Hg
> Base deficit >4 mEq/L
> Estimated fluid sequestration >6L
> Serum calcium level <8 mg/dL

presented in the case study. The predominant nursing diagnoses for the patient diagnosed with acute pancreatitis are outlined in Table 37–1.

Collaborative Management

Because the acuity of pancreatitis ranges from mild to severe, the treatment of individual patients varies according to the severity of the disease. Because the basic pathophysiology of pancreatitis leads to widespread alterations in all organ systems, comprehensive and ongoing assessment is important for all patients with pancreatitis, regardless of the severity of their disease. The nursing care of these complex patients can sometimes seem overwhelming, and a multidisciplinary approach to assessment, intervention, and evaluation based on the patient's needs is imperative.[7]

Cardiac Output

It is widely believed that early and aggressive fluid resuscitation is the single most important intervention in decreasing the morbidity and mortality related to acute pancreatitis. If fluid resuscitation is not initiated aggressively enough, the severe hypovolemia associated with acute pancreatitis causes inadequate tissue perfusion, which then progresses to multiorgan failure. As much as one-third of the circulating volume can be lost into the interstitial space,[8] and that amount is even greater if the patient has additional fluid losses from open wounds, bleeding, excessive vomiting, or gastrointestinal suctioning.

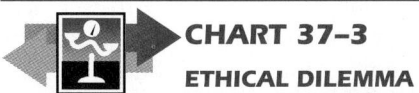

CHART 37–3

ETHICAL DILEMMA

B. D. is a 60-year-old man admitted to the intensive care unit (ICU) with hemorrhagic pancreatitis. The patient admits to drinking a case of beer every day for the past several years. He also says that he is unemployed and has no health insurance. He denies any medical problems but says that he has not seen a doctor because of lack of insurance. On arriving into the ICU, he tells his nurse that he would not want any heroic measures to keep him alive. The following day, he becomes restless, he is in obvious respiratory distress, and his oxygen saturation drops to 60%. His temperature is 38.5°C, his blood pressure is 80/40 mm Hg, his pulse is 130, and his skin is cool and clammy.

Significant laboratory values are as follows:

White blood count	18,000/mm^3
Amylase level	1000 U/L
Glucose level	350 mg/dL
Total calcium level	6.9 mg/dL
Albumin level	2.0 mg/dL
Aspartate transaminase level	300 Sigma-Frankel U%
Lactate dehydrogenase level	500 IU/L

B. D. experiences respiratory failure and is subsequently intubated and placed on mechanical ventilation. His estranged wife arrives and is shocked at what she sees. She tells you that she has not seen B. D. for 3 years since making him leave the house because of his drinking problem. She says that this is all her fault and that it never would have happened if she had not kicked him out. When the physician arrives, he describes the severity of the illness to B. D.'s wife and asks her how aggressive she wants his treatment to be. B. D.'s wife replies that she wants "everything done."

1. What are the ethical issues in this case?
2. How can you advocate for B. D.?
3. What do you think B. D.'s wife needs to know in order to make informed decisions about his care?
4. What options are available to a clinician in the event that treatment does not coincide with a patient's expressed wishes?

The interventions and monitoring that may be necessary for managing the volume replacement in a patient with acute pancreatitis depend primarily on the severity of the disease. Urine output is one indication of the patient's vascular volume status and should be maintained at a rate of at least 0.5 to 1.0 mL/kg per hour.[9] Thirty milliliters of urine per hour is not adequate for every patient. It is important to individualize urine output goals for each patient based on his or her weight because intravascular volume varies according to a patient's body size. Daily weights are another way to assess fluid balance. However, daily weights simply reflect overall fluid balance—they do not give information about the loca-

TABLE 37–1
Nursing Diagnoses

Problem Statement	Etiologic Factors
Pain	Pancreatic infiltration, sepsis, systemic immune response
Tissue perfusion, altered	Sepsis, systemic immune response
Gas exchange, impaired	Changes in pulmonary blood flow, pulmonary edema, ventilation-perfusion mismatches, pleural effusion
Decreased cardiac output	Loss of intravascular volume, sepsis
Fluid volume deficit	Loss of intravascular volume, interstitial fluid accumulation
Skin integrity, risk for impaired	Poor nutrition, interstitial fluid accumulation, vasoconstriction, immobility
Infection, risk for	Generalized immunosuppression due to critical illness, numerous invasive procedures, pancreatic necrosis
Nutrition, less than body requirements: altered	Lack of gastrointestinal route for feeding, increased metabolic needs
Knowledge deficit	Disease process, diagnostic workup, treatment strategies, prognosis

tion of the body fluids. Because it is vascular fluid volume, not overall fluid volume, that is important to assess in the patient with acute pancreatitis, daily weights are often of limited value for guiding fluid replacement.

Hemodynamic parameters can be especially helpful in guiding the fluid resuscitation for patients with acute pancreatitis, and maximizing cardiac output is particularly important.[2] Because the body's first compensatory response to hypovolemia is tachycardia (based on the formula that cardiac output = heart rate × stroke volume), some assessment of cardiac output can be made, even in the absence of a pulmonary artery catheter. However, for many patients with acute pancreatitis, central monitoring by use of either a central venous catheter or a pulmonary artery catheter is needed to adequately measure the patient's response to fluid replacement. Some patients may require as much as 18 to 25 L of fluid replacement in the first few days of their acute pancreatitis to maintain their pulmonary artery occlusive pressures in the range of 16 to 20 cm H_2O.[2] Although this pressure may seem high in the face of the large pulmonary capillary leaks associated with pancreatitis, it is necessary for overall organ and tissue perfusion. More conservative fluid replacement may directly benefit the lungs by decreasing capillary leakage and lung water, but it indirectly leads to more organ hypoperfusion and ischemic damage by further contributing to an already inadequate circulating volume. In addition, because patients with acute pancreatitis are often receiving significant levels of positive end-expiratory pressure (PEEP), some amount of that PEEP level would be reflected in the pulmonary artery occlusive pressure (PAOP) measurement, so actual vascular volume would not be as high as a PAOP of 16 to 20 cm H_2O might indicate.

Because myocardial depressant factor is thought to be released from the injured pancreas, other interventions to improve cardiac output often include inotropic support. The specific choice of inotropic agent depends on the patient's overall status, especially systemic vascular resistance. If systemic vascular resistance were low, an agent with both inotropic and vasoconstrictive properties, such as dopamine, epinephrine, and norepinephrine, might be used. If systemic vascular resistance were high, agents with primarily inotropic properties, such as dobutamine, amrinone, and milrinone, would probably be better choices. In many cases, combinations of different agents are used and can be titrated specifically to the patient's individual response. Figure 37–2 summarizes the considerations in cardiac output management for a patient with acute pancreatitis.

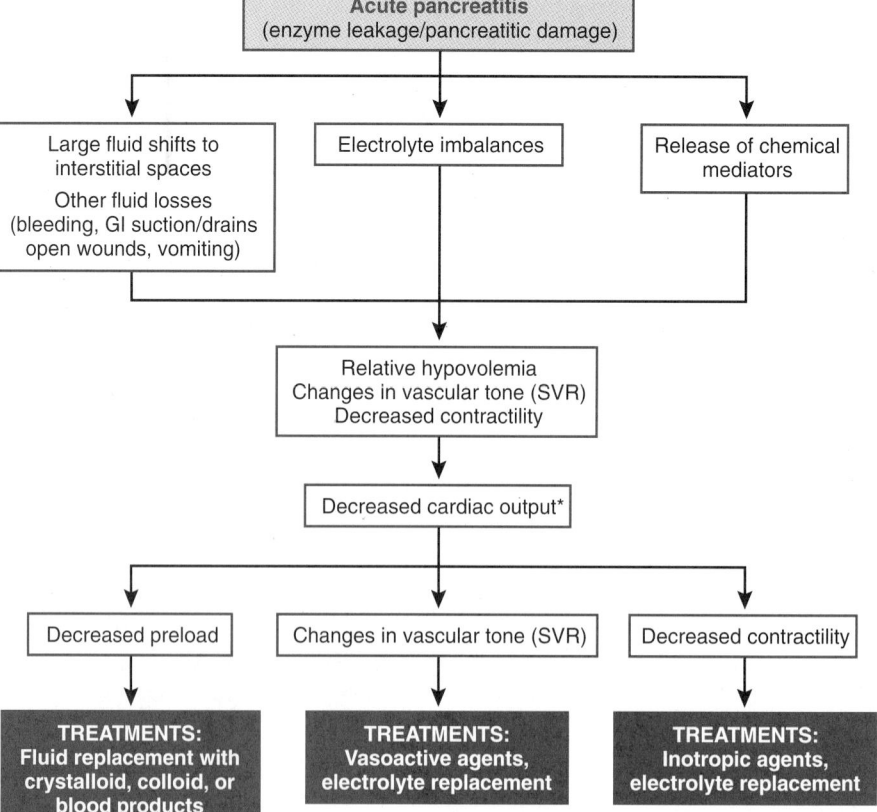

Figure 37–2

Pathophysiology and hemodynamic management in the patient with acute pancreatitis. The asterisk indicates that heart rate will change in response to catecholamines (stress response) and to the interventions used to optimize stroke volume. If measures to improve cardiac output fail, decreased tissue perfusion, cellular ischemia, and organ failure may occur. SVR, systemic vascular resistance.

Oxygenation

Respiratory insufficiency is the most common complication of acute pancreatitis.[2] Not all of the mechanisms that contribute to the respiratory failure so commonly seen with acute pancreatitis are well understood. However, several pathologic changes occur specifically as a manifestation of the acute pancreatitis that are known to contribute to respiratory compromise. These are listed in Chart 37–4.

Treatment of the patient with acute pancreatitis who is experiencing respiratory insufficiency should be directed at minimizing respiratory complications and supporting respiratory function. Humidified oxygen is usually indicated for all patients, even those who do

---

CHART 37–4

Factors Associated with Respiratory Failure in the Patient with Pancreatitis

Abdominal pain leading to guarding and decreased respiratory excursion.

Pancreatic enzymes entering the pleural cavity either via the lymph circulation or through direct seepage and leading to pleural effusions.

Increased serum levels of phospholipase A (an enzyme that catalyzes the breakdown of lecithin, a major component of surfactant), which decreases the amount of surfactant and leads to atelectasis and alveolar edema.

Release of trypsin from the damaged pancreas causes widespread clotting abnormalities, particularly disseminated intravascular coagulation, which leads to microemboli in the lung and consequently causes ventilation/perfusion mismatches.

Abdominal pressure from either paralytic ileus and/or retroperitoneal edema places pressure directly on the diaphram and compromises its ability to flatten during inspiration.

Pulmonary hypertension secondary to pulmonary vasoconstriction.

Complement-induced neutrophil aggregation, which increases capillary wall permeability and increases alveolar edema.

Hypertriglyceridemia, which is often secondary to ethyl alcohol abuse, leads to the release of free fatty acids, which cause injury to lung tissues.

Vigorous fluid resuscitation, although necessary, contributes to increases in lung water.

---

not require intubation and mechanical support. Pleural taps may be performed for large effusions; however, this intervention may provide only temporary relief because the underlying reasons for the pleural effusions continue to be present until the pancreatitis resolves. Intubation and mechanical ventilation are indicated if the partial pressure of oxygen falls below 60 mm Hg and tachypnea is present.[2]

Positive end-expiratory pressure is an important intervention for patients with respiratory failure resulting from acute pancreatitis. PEEP improves oxygenation by preventing alveolar collapse during expiration. The use of PEEP recruits more alveoli to participate in gas exchange, thus decreasing ventilation/perfusion mismatches. In some cases, it may be necessary to apply high levels of PEEP (15–20 cm H_2O) in order to have any appreciable increase in partial pressure of arterial oxygen. Careful management while the patient is receiving PEEP is extremely important. Although PEEP is often successful at improving oxygenation, it can compromise cardiovascular function by putting direct pressure on the ventricles and reducing preload and cardiac output. This is particularly important in a patient with acute pancreatitis, whose cardiovascular function is already compromised. "Optimal PEEP" is the amount of PEEP it takes to maximize oxygenation while minimizing barotrauma and decreases in cardiac output. Nursing care should be directed at carefully balancing both the respiratory and the cardiovascular effects of PEEP to best meet the patient's overall needs. This can be accomplished by carefully assessing the patient's response to incremental changes in the level of PEEP.

Another negative consequence of PEEP is barotrauma. Peak inspiratory pressures should be monitored because a sudden increase can indicate barotrauma and pneumothorax. Other signs and symptoms associated with pneumothorax include dyspnea, hypotension, decreased breath sounds, and limited chest wall excursion. Patients should also be monitored for the presence of subcutaneous emphysema, another possible indication of barotrauma. Additionally, the possibility of autoPEEP always exists, and patients should be carefully monitored for its presence. AutoPEEP is air trapping that can result in overinflation of alveoli and barotrauma. Respiratory waveform monitoring can be a particularly useful tool for detecting autoPEEP.[10] Any time mechanical ventilation with PEEP is being used, methods for reducing the risk of barotrauma should be implemented, including using appropriate ventilator settings, controlling respiratory rate, using sedation, and using neuromuscular blockade. In addition, modes of ventilation that improve inspiratory/expiratory flow patterns should be considered.[11]

Pain is another important factor to consider in pulmonary care, especially because nursing is responsible for the ongoing assessment of pain and the administration of pain medication. Pancreatitis is usually very painful for most patients. Inadequate pain control leads to guarding and decreased respiratory excursion and contributes to an overall decrease in pulmonary function for patients with pancreatitis. Keeping the patient as pain-free as possible encourages the patient to take deeper breaths without the fear of increased pain.

Other factors that contribute to a decrease in pulmonary function include the effects of pancreatic enzyme release, microthrombi from disseminated intravascular coagulation, and a distended abdomen. Interventions directed at controlling these problems are subsequently beneficial for overall pulmonary function.

Electrolyte and Acid–base Balance

The electrolyte imbalances associated with pancreatitis are many and have widespread effects throughout most organ systems. One of the most common electrolyte imbalances associated with pancreatitis is hypocalcemia. A normal serum calcium is between 9.0 and 10.0 mg/dL; this measurement includes both protein-bound and ionized calcium.[12] Ionized calcium accounts for about 50% of the total calcium level. A decrease in serum calcium level for patients with pancreatitis is largely a reflection of hypoalbuminemia, and in many cases, the ionized calcium level is at normal or near-normal levels.[2] However, in more severe cases of pancreatitis, the level of ionized calcium, which is the calcium important for various cellular functions, is also decreased. Therefore, intravenous replacement of calcium should be guided by measurements of ionized as well as total calcium levels. Because calcium is important for the proper functioning of the neuromuscular and cardiovascular systems, the patient with pancreatitis should be assessed for both neuromuscular irritability and cardiovascular abnormalities. The patient's clinical presentation should then determine the specific needs for calcium replacement.

Two of the major cations in the pancreatic juice are sodium and potassium. Therefore, the leakage of pancreatic enzymes, as well as other factors, such as fluid shifts and gastrointestinal losses, contributes to both hyponatremia and hypokalemia. The serum levels of both of these electrolytes should be monitored in patients with pancreatitis, and a combination of serum levels and clinical presentation should guide electrolyte replacement. The major effects of hyponatremia are on the central nervous system and are manifested by changes in level of consciousness. The major effects of hypokalemia are muscle weakness and changes in cardiovascular function. Although clinical presentation is perhaps the best guide for replacement, its use is often difficult because the pathophysiologic changes

associated with pancreatitis are so widespread. Therefore, careful monitoring of serum levels and replacement of electrolytes are especially important.

Hyperglycemia is another common manifestation of pancreatitis. Hyperglycemia results from both an increase in glucagon release and islet cell destruction from the injured pancreas.[2] Although administration of insulin should be used to control serum glucose levels, it should be used carefully in order to avoid rebound hypoglycemia as the glucagonemia resolves.

Pain Control

Most patients with pancreatitis experience severe abdominal pain. It is often deep and piercing, may be present anywhere in the abdomen, and may radiate to the back. The initial step in pain control is a detailed assessment of pain. Because pain is a subjective experience, the most important part of the pain assessment is patient self-report.[13] Although self-reports of pain can be difficult to get from critically ill patients, various tools are available that can be used to assist bedside nurses in the assessment of pain (Figure 4–5). If possible, your pain assessment should include the patient's descriptive words regarding his or her pain, the location and severity of his or her pain, both aggravating and relieving factors associated with the pain, cognitive and physiologic responses to the pain, and the patient's goals for pain management.[14]

Many pharmacologic treatment options are available for pain. Acetaminophen and nonsteroidal anti-inflammatory agents can be used either for mild pain or as an adjunct to opioids. In patients with severe pancreatitis, opioids are usually necessary for adequate pain relief. Various agents, doses, and routes can be used for effective pain management in patients with pancreatitis who experience severe pain.

Many nonpharmacologic interventions can also assist in pain relief. Repositioning patients into a position in which they are most comfortable is one of the simplest. Application of heat, touch, or massage may be helpful for some patients. Relaxation exercises include slow, rhythmic breathing; guided imagery; and music.[13] The benefit of the nonpharmacologic interventions is that they are easy to do, are essentially without risk, and can involve participation by family or significant others as well.

Care of the Gastrointestinal Tract

Because the underlying cause of all the pathophysiologic alterations associated with pancreatitis stems from release of pancreatic enzymes into the pancreas and subsequent pancreatic autodigestion, minimizing pancreatic activity is of paramount importance in the treatment of a patient with pancreatitis. This is of utmost importance for decreasing the likelihood that the pancreatitis will deteriorate and cause the patient to have severe complications, such as shock, hemorrhage, and sepsis. By minimizing pancreatic activity and halting the disease process, further tissue damage is prevented, and tissue healing can occur.[15] For this reason, it is important to give the patient nothing by mouth (NPO) because oral intake is a natural stimulant for pancreatic enzyme secretion. Because the patient may require NPO status for an extended period of time, nutritional support is extremely important. In the face of sepsis resulting from pancreatitis, the body's nutritional needs are greatly increased,[16] making the need for adequate nutritional support even more important.

Although there is no dispute regarding the need for adequate nutritional support for the patient with pancreatitis, there is some disagreement as to the preferred route. Most experts suggest the use of parenteral nutrition.[15] However, parenteral administration of nutrition is associated with numerous risk factors, including sepsis, pneumothorax, air embolism, subclavian artery laceration, subclavian vein thrombosis, and metabolic complications.[17] As a general rule in patient care, the enteral route is the preferred route of administration of nutrition, but the patient with pancreatitis presents a special challenge because enteral administration of feedings stimulates pancreatic enzyme secretion. The enteral route may not be appropriate for patients with pancreatitis, because gastrointestinal tract functioning may be decreased or excessive diarrhea may be occurring. In addition, the risk of pulmonary aspiration should always be a consideration, especially in the face of the marked pulmonary pathology already associated with pancreatitis. Although adequate nutrition is of utmost importance for patients with pancreatitis to prevent the undernutrition commonly associated with this disease process, the most appropriate method varies from patient to patient.[16]

Gastrointestinal suctioning is a common clinical intervention for gastric decompression; however, its true therapeutic role in altering the course of pancreatitis is unknown. However, if patients are experiencing the nausea and vomiting, gastrointestinal suctioning is usually indicated.

The prevention of gastric and duodenal ulcers should be facilitated by the use of prophylactic therapy. Therapy may include intravenous administration of histamine$_2$ blockers, antacid therapy, or both. Gastric pH levels should be maintained at 5 or above, and histamine$_2$ blocker doses should be increased if the pH drops below 5.[2]

Pharmacologic Therapy

The pharmacologic therapy required by patients with pancreatitis can be complex and widespread. Therapy should be guided by the severity of the disease as well as by the specific pathologic derangements that occur with each patient. As previously discussed, elec-

trolytes should be replaced as necessary, insulin should be used conservatively for the control of hyperglycemia, pain medication should be administered in amounts great enough to relieve the patient's pain, and medications for the prevention and treatment of ulcers should be administered.

Antibiotics, including antifungals, are commonly used as a treatment for patients with pancreatitis; however, there are many things to consider related to their use. First, not all patients with pancreatitis have the same risk factors for infection. The group at highest risk are patients who experience pancreatic necrosis. Major pancreatic necrosis involving greater than 10% of the pancreas occurs in approximately 10% of patients with acute pancreatitis, and about one-half of these patients will become infected.[18] Infected pancreatic necrosis is the most common cause of fatal outcome in patients with pancreatitis.[19, 20] Therefore, this is the group that is most likely to benefit from appropriate antibiotic therapy. However, even within this group,[2] Frey and Araida raised many unanswered questions related to the use of antibiotic therapy.

Are all patients with necrotizing pancreatitis at the same risk for infection?
Should prophylaxis be used, and if so, what is the proper timing?
Should all infections, even those with late onset, be treated aggressively?
What are the most effective antibiotic agents and course of therapy for patients with necrotizing pancreatitis?

These questions are important because prolonged use of antibiotics increases the likelihood of the development of resistant organisms and secondary infections.

Considering all the evidence to date and weighing the risks and benefits,[2] Frey and Araida recommended a 14- to 28-day course of prophylactic antibiotic therapy for all patients with necrotizing pancreatitis confirmed by a computed tomographic scan. The ideal agent should penetrate pancreatic tissues in levels great enough to be effective for treating infection. Buchler and colleagues[19] measured antibiotic levels in pancreatic tissue, juice, and cyst fluid 30 minutes after intravenous administration. Results indicated that imipenem, ofloxacin, ciprofloxacin, and cefotaxime are the agents of choice. Results also indicated that the aminoglycosides, which are often widely used in patients with pancreatitis, did not reach levels therapeutic enough to treat the infections and therefore would not likely be effective.[19]

Surgical Intervention

Although not all patients with pancreatitis require surgical intervention, it is necessary for some patients. In particular, all patients with infected necrotic areas of the pancreas or peripancreatic tissue require operative removal of the necrotic tissue.[2] The pancreatic necrotic tissue becomes a site for abscess formation, which is one of the most serious complications of pancreatitis. In most cases, undrained abscesses are fatal.[21]

Options for surgical treatment for draining pancreatic abscesses include a closed-drainage procedure and/or an open-drainage procedure. Closed drainage is usually used in patients with less necrosis for which only one operative procedure is expected to be sufficient for complete removal of all necrotic tissue. Intraoperative insertion of drains is necessary to clear the operative area of active pancreatic enzymes that continue to be secreted in the postoperative phase.[22]

Open packing and drainage is another technique for the removal of necrotic pancreatic tissue. This type of procedure is usually necessary for patients who have a large degree of pancreatic necrosis. In the open procedure, the abdominal wound is packed and left open underneath the dressing. The patient then returns to the operating room every few days for débridement until all the necrotic tissue is finally removed. Another variation is using an open procedure with a continuous irrigation of antibiotic solution to control infection while the wound is open. This irrigation continues using a system of drains once all the necrotic tissue is removed. The constant infusion of antibiotic solution also helps control uremia in patients with impaired renal function because it functions in a way similar to peritoneal dialysis.[2] Although these types of procedures are the most common for infected pancreatic necrosis that are reported in the literature, the emergence of new techniques of closed procedures for these patients is beginning.[23] Also, regardless of the specific type of surgical procedure used, decreasing pancreatic exocrine function in the postoperative phase is important in healing and in prevention of postoperative complications. There is increasing evidence that octreotide may have a therapeutic role in decreasing pancreatitic exocrine function.[24, 25]

Pancreas transplantation is not indicated as a treatment for pancreatitis. The only indication for a pancreas transplant is insulin-dependent diabetes mellitus. However, a patient who has chronic pancreatitis may eventually become a candidate if the chronic nature of the pancreatitis damages the insulin-producing islet cells and subsequently causes the patient to become insulin dependent.

Pancreatic pseudocyst occurs in about 10% of patients with pancreatitis, making it the most common complication of pancreatitis.[21] If the main pancreatic duct becomes blocked as a result of pancreatitis, duct rupture occurs, and pancreatic secretions are released. This fluid then forms a pseudocyst, which can be located in various areas around the pancreas.

Small pseudocysts may resolve spontaneously, but larger ones usually require surgical intervention. Surgical intervention is important to prevent the occurrence of complications of pancreatic pseudocysts, which may include rupture, hemorrhage, infection, and obstruction. Surgical procedures for the treatment of pseudocysts include excision, internal drainage, and external drainage. The choice for the appropriate surgical procedure depends on the size of the pseudocyst, the maturity of the fibrous lining, the presence or absence of infection in the pseudocyst fluid, and the complications associated with each procedure (Table 37–2).

Multidisciplinary Outcomes

The care of the patient with pancreatitis is complex and requires a collaborative working relationship between the physician, the nurse, and the entire team caring for the patient. This is especially important with pancreatitis because the acuity of the patient's illness has such a broad range. In the mild stage, pain, fluid and electrolyte balance, infection, and the underlying cause of the disease must be carefully managed to halt the disease process and to prevent the development of complications (Chart 37–5). In the more severe stages, the team approach to management is even more imperative. Quick and appropriate treatment increases the likelihood that the patient will be able to recover from the many pathophysiologic changes that occur with

TABLE 37–2

Surgical Interventions for the Treatment of Pancreatic Pseudocyst

Surgical Intervention	Pseudocyst Characteristics	Complications
Excision	Small pseudocysts; easiest for pseudocysts located in the tail of the pancreas	Bleeding
External drainage	Used if fibrous lining of pseudocyst has not matured; used with infected pseudocysts	Fistula formation; skin excoriation; fluid and electrolyte imbalances; further infection; pseudocyst recurrence
Internal drainage	Mature pseudocyst; non-infected	Bleeding

Data from Butler RW, Smith SL: Acute Pancreatitis. Part II: Complications and Surgical Management. Aliso Viejo, CA, American Association of Critical Care Nurses, 1993, pp 13–25.

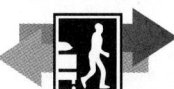

CHART 37–5

BEYOND THE ICU: NEEDS OF PATIENTS RECOVERING FROM PANCREATITIS

There are many related factors to consider in the care of the patient with pancreatitis across a variety of settings. Although the patient's care in the critical care area is focused on treatment of the pathology associated with severe pancreatitis, the patient's need for care is just as acute in other settings. Care in settings outside of the critical care area should focus on two major areas: (1) the factors known to contribute to pancreatitis and (2) the continued care needs of a patient who is recovering from an episode of pancreatitis.

Because alcoholism is one of the major causes of pancreatitis, anyone whose pancreatitis is a result of alcohol abuse requires aggressive counseling and treatment in order to prevent further pancreatitis episodes. This care should begin in the acute care area, but it is even more necessary in the community setting so that once patients begin to feel better and have access to alcohol, they will have developed the internal and external resources to facilitate continued abstinence. Alcoholism is associated with numerous comorbid conditions in addition to pancreatitis, so treatment of alcoholism is of utmost importance for the patient's overall health. Ideally, treatment should include the patient's family as well.

Patients with abnormally high serum triglyceride levels are also at risk for pancreatitis as well as various cardiovascular complications. Patients with high serum triglyceride levels should be managed carefully in both the acute care and the community settings. Dietary counseling and pharmacologic interventions are usually necessary to maintain serum triglyceride levels at more normal levels. The participation of the patient's family and/or significant others is important for the success of the long-term management of this risk factor.

Patients who are recovering from a recent episode of pancreatitis may have a variety of health care needs, such as the treatment of wounds or the management of blood sugar. If wound healing is not complete by the time a patient is discharged from a hospital setting, appropriate arrangements must be made to continue the patient's care after discharge. Use of subacute settings, home care assistance, and/or participation by the patient and family are all options to be considered and used as appropriate. The most effective and feasible options vary with each patient. A complete and thorough nursing assessment of the patient's resources and abilities is important in helping determine the best way to meet the overall goal of promoting wound healing for each patient.

Diabetes is another complication that may develop and need continued treatment after discharge from a hospital. If the pancreatic islet cells are damaged from the pancreatitis, insulin may be required temporarily or permanently, depending on the level of islet cell damage. The new onset of diabetes requires comprehensive management of the patient in both the acute care and the outpatient settings in order to teach patients how to care for themselves and keep their glucose levels within a normal range. Teaching regarding diet, exercise, blood glucose testing, administration of insulin, and signs and symptoms of changes in blood glucose level are all necessary for both the patient and the family.

Finally, patients who have chronic pancreatitis should be aware of the signs and symptoms associated with the onset of an episode of pancreatitis. Because the most successful outcomes of pancreatitis depend primarily on early detection and treatment, the long-term effects of chronic pancreatitis can be minimized if patients are treated promptly with each episode.

severe pancreatitis and prevent the progression of the disease to the point of coma and death. See Table 37–3 for a list of outcomes according to phases of the illness.

Critical Thinking Exercise

A. P. is a 37-year-old female who presents in the emergency department complaining of severe abdominal pain and vomiting for 3 days. She has a history of gallbladder disease but states that the pain is much more severe than her usual gallbladder pain. She has no other significant medical history. Her physical assessment is significant for rapid shallow respirations, dry mucous membranes, poor skin turgor, and midepigastric pain that is rebound in character. A. P. states that she is very thirsty. With further assessment, you note that A. P. is confused.

Her vital signs are as follows: blood pressure, 88/50 mm Hg; temperature, 38.2°C; heart rate, 140 and regular; and respiratory rate, 35.

Laboratory values were as follows: serum amylase, 500 U/L; lipase, 100 U/L; calcium, 6.4 mg/dL; and albumin, 2.5 g/dL.

Arterial blood gases reveal a metabolic acidosis. Arterial oxygen saturation is 90% on 100% oxygen via a nonrebreather mask. Urine output has consisted of 10 mL of con-

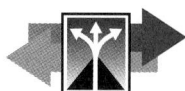

TABLE 37–3
Multidisciplinary Outcomes

Phase	Outcome
Emergency department	Establishment of diagnosis
	Volume resuscitation
	Stabilization of vital signs
Intensive care unit	Determination of cause
	Pancreatic rest
	Nutritional support
	Pulmonary support
	Cardiovascular support
	Fluid and electrolyte management
	Skin/wound care
	Blood glucose management
	Patient/family support
	Preparation of patient for a coordinated transfer to the intermediate care unit
Intermediate care unit	Nutritional support
	Skin/wound care
	Blood glucose management
	Patient and family teaching
Community	Avoidance of ethyl alcohol
	Adequate nutrition
	Continued skin/wound care
	Maintenance of normal serum triglyceride level
	Blood glucose management
	Patient and family teaching
	Psychological support for patient and family

centrated urine in the past half hour. Two large-bore intravenous lines are inserted, and 0.9% saline is started at 300 mL per hour. She is admitted to the intensive care unit with a diagnosis of acute pancreatitis.

1. Why is pain control so important for A. P.?
2. What does the character of A. P.'s respirations and her arterial oxygen saturation suggest?
3. What is the significance of A. P.'s thirst, poor skin turgor, low blood pressure, tachycardia, and dry mucous membranes?
4. Which laboratory values are consistent with a diagnosis of pancreatitis?
5. Which additional laboratory values do you anticipate will be ordered in order to obtain a Ranson score for A. P.?

Key Concepts

➡ Acute pancreatitis is the result of the activation of pancreatic enzymes in the pancreas, resulting in autodigestion of the organ.

➡ Acute pancreatitis is divided into the mild form, which resolves spontaneously, and the hemor-

rhagic form, which may result in multiorgan system failure and death.

➡ The most common causes of pancreatitis are alcoholism and biliary tract disease.

➡ Most patients have varying degrees of abdominal pain, and because pain can exacerbate the attack and contribute to respiratory problems, its control is critical. Both pharmacologic and nonpharmacologic methods are available for pain control.

➡ Release of activated enzymes results in the inflammatory response, which causes large fluid shifts. Patients with pancreatitis require large volumes of fluid. Inadequate fluid resuscitation can lead to organ failure.

➡ Electrolyte imbalances occur as a result of actual loss and/or shifting of electrolytes from compartments. Calcium, magnesium, sodium, and potassium are particularly affected.

➡ Pulmonary problems develop as a result of pleural effusions, acute respiratory distress syndrome, and atelectasis, and respiratory failure is the most common complication of pancreatitis.

➡ Nutritional support must be maintained via parenteral nutrition in patients with an ileus to avoid malnutrition. Nutritional balance is very important in the healing process for patients with pancreatitis.

➡ Infected pancreatic necrosis is the leading cause of death in patients with pancreatitis.

➡ Decreasing pancreatic exocrine function is one of the most important aspects of the care of the patient with pancreatitis.

➡ Appropriate antibiotic and antifungal treatment is necessary for all patients with infectious complications.

➡ A variety of surgical interventions are available to treat the complications associated with acute pancreatitis.

References

1. Forsmark CE, Toskes PP: Acute pancreatitis: medical management. Crit Care Clin 11:295–309, 1995.
2. Frey CF, Araida T: Acute pancreatitis. In: Sivak ED, Higgins TL, Seiver A (eds): The High Risk Patient Management of the Critically Ill. Baltimore, Williams & Wilkins, 1995, pp 1015–1045.
3. Steer ML: Acute pancreatitis. In: Rippe J, Irwin RS, Fink MP, Cerra FB (eds): Intensive Care Medicine, 3rd ed. Boston, Little, Brown, 1996, pp 1744–1764.
4. Balinger AB: Is intervention necessary after a first episode of acute idiopathic pancreatitis? Gut 38:293–295, 1996.
5. Wright JE, Shelton BK: Desk Reference for Critical Care Nursing. Boston, Jones & Bartlett, 1993, pp 905–913.
6. Ranson JH, Rifkind KM, Roses DF, et al: Prognostic signs and the role of operative management in acute pancreatitis. Surg Gynecol Obstet 139:69–81, 1974.
7. Noone J: Acute pancreatitis: An Orem approach to nursing assessment and care. Crit Care Nurse 15:27–37, 1995.
8. Hennesey K: Patients with acute pancreatitis. In: Clochesky JM, Breu C, Cardin S (eds): Critical Care Nursing, Philadelphia, WB Saunders, 1993, pp 1009–1025.

9. Potts JR: Acute pancreatitis. Surg Clin North Am 68:281–299, 1988.

10. Aloi A, Burns SM: Continuous airway pressure monitoring in the critical care setting. Crit Care Nurse 15:66–74, 1995.

11. Geisman LK, Ahrens T: Auto-PEEP: An impediment to weaning in the chronically ventilated patient. AACN Clin Issues Crit Care Nurs 2:391–397, 1991.

12. Guyton AC: Textbook of Medical Physiology, 8th ed. Philadelphia, WB Saunders, 1991.

13. Agency for Health Care Policy and Research: Management of Cancer Pain, Clinical Practice Guidelines. Rockville, MD, U.S. Dept. of Health and Human Services, publication #94-0592, 1994.

14. Agency for Health Care Policy and Research: Management of Cancer Pain, Quick Reference Guide for Clinicians. Rockville, MD, U.S. Dept. of Health and Human Services, publication #94-0592, 1994.

15. Smith SL, Butler RW: Acute Pancreatitis: An Overview. Aliso Viejo, CA, American Association of Critical Care Nurses, 1993, pp 1–11.

16. Marulendra S, Kirby DF: Nutritional support in pancreatitis. Nutr Clin Pract 10:45–53, 1993.

17. Matarese LE, Steiger E, Jewett BE: Nutritional support in the management of the critically ill. In: Sivak ED, Higgins TL, Seiver A (eds): The High Risk Patient Management of the Critically Ill. Baltimore, Williams & Wilkins, 1995, pp 1249–1277.

18. Bradley EL, Allen K: A prospective longitudinal study of observation versus surgical intervention in the management of necrotizing pancreatitis. Am J Surg 161:19–24, 1991.

19. Buchler M, Malfertheiner P, Freiss H, et al: Human pancreatic tissue concentration of bactericidal antibiotics. Gastroenterology 103:1902–1908, 1992.

20. Stanton R, Frey CF: Comprehensive management of acute necrotizing pancreatitis and pancreatic abscess. Arch Surg 125:1269–1275, 1990.

21. Ranson J: Acute pancreatitis. In: Schwartz S, Ellis H (eds): Maingot's Abdominal Operations, 8th ed. Norwalk, CT, Appleton-Century-Crofts, 1985, pp 2061–2076.

22. Butler RW, Smith SL: Acute Pancreatitis: Complications and Surgical Management. Aliso Viejo, CA, American Association of Critical Care Nurses, 1993, pp 13–28.

23. Farkas G, Marton J, Mandi Y, Szederkenyi E: Surgical strategy and management of infected pancreatic necrosis. Br J Surg 83:930–933, 1996.

24. Buchler M, Freiss H, Klempa I, et al: Role of octreotide in the prevention of postoperative complications following pancreatic resection. Am J Surg 163:125–131, 1992.

25. Buchler M, Freiss H: Inhibition of pancreatic secretion to prevent postoperative complication following pancreatic resection. Acta Gastroenterol Belg 56:271–278, 1993.

26. Allardyce DB: Incidence of necrotizing pancreatitis and factors related to mortality. Am J Surg 154:295–299, 1987.

27. Peterson KJ, Solie CJ: Interpreting lab values in pancreatitis. Am J Nurs 94:56A-B–56-F, 1994.

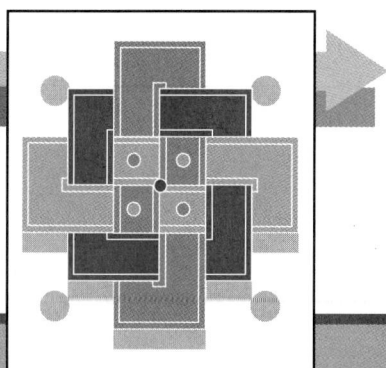

Neurologic Problems

Hope Gives Patient the Will to Live

There seemed to be nothing unusual about that night in April 1996. The 11 to 7 shift started the same as every other—report on 10 patients, all of whom had suffered traumatic injuries caused by senseless accidents or complications of disease. Working in the high observation unit of a rehabilitation hospital, we see many patients who still need critical care nursing but who are ready to start the long, arduous process of physical rehabilitation.

I listened carefully as the tape went on to describe the individual patients and their needs. "In 301W is a new admission, Mrs. S., a 56-year-old female with a brain stem infarct. She is completely paralyzed but can blink her eyes. She stares blankly and is slow to respond. Even though she can blink appropriately to simple questions of orientation, it doesn't seem like there is anyone at home upstairs. I guess that's a blessing. She has a new trach and is on 40% O_2. There is no swallow reflex, so she is fed through a PEG tube. Her family was here earlier. They are very supportive but emotional. There's not really much we can do at this point except to continue anticoagulant therapy and monitor her cardiac and respiratory status. The prognosis given to her husband is poor."

I don't know why I was so eager to take her as my patient. Maybe it was because she was the same age as my mother or because I fear being in a similar situation myself someday. In any case, as a critical care nurse for 15 years, I knew that there was more to be done for her than was mentioned in report.

I distinctly remember the first time I saw Mrs. S. Her room was dimly lit and quiet, except for the occasional alarms of the cardiac monitor and pulse oximeter and the steady gurgling of the oxygen humidifier. She lay still on her back. Her chest was rising and falling quite rhythmically. I walked up to her and said "Good evening Mrs. S. My name is Holly, and I will be your nurse tonight. We are all terribly sorry for your circumstances, but we're delighted that you are here. Our job is to work like crazy to get you out of this mess and get you back home with your family, where you belong." Mrs. S. looked up at me. Her eyes were smiling and I began to feel her spirit.

During my assessment, she started coughing violently. The respiratory therapist, another nurse, and I tried to help her through it. She looked terrified. As we bagged her and helped to remove the secretions, I was close to her ear telling her everything that we were doing and trying to calm her fears. Just when the worst was over, she looked at me and mouthed a few words I thought I understood. But this couldn't be, not from a person with such a severe brain stem stroke, or from someone who is questionably "not at home upstairs." "What?" I asked. "Can you say that again for me, only a little slower?" Again her lips started moving, enunciating each syllable. "What is my ox-y-gen sat-u-ra-tion?" Tears filled my eyes as I realized that not only was someone "at home," but a very intelligent someone as well. "Yes, yes!" I said with both relief and delight. "It's 98% and you're doing fine."

I wondered why no one reported that she could mouth words. Did we miss something? Maybe this was new! As I continued with my assessment, I explained everything to her. I told her about rehabilitation. The team would work with her and her family on goals that they could help set. I'm not sure she believed me. She knew she was still very ill and that there was a high risk she would have another stroke and die.

By this time, Mrs. S. had been in the hospital for 2 weeks. I asked her if she had had a good bath and shampoo since her stroke. Somewhat embarrassed, she said she hadn't. I thought that a nice shower might help her to feel better. I explained that if she was willing, I'd put her on a stretcher and take her to the shower room for some "girl time." Her eyes opened wide. "But how can you move me with all the tubes and equipment?" she asked. I assured her that I had experience in both critical care and rehabilitation nursing and promised that I would monitor her every step of the way.

My position at the time was a dual role of staff nurse and nursing supervisor, so I had to ask if she could wait until I made rounds on the other units and complete a few other necessary tasks first. She smiled and blinked softly.

When I returned to the unit, the other staff members told me that Mrs. S. couldn't sleep. She had decided to wait up for the shower. So I went into her room and started gathering all of the supplies we would need. I could see that she was anxious but that it wasn't going to stop her. It took four of us to get her on the stretcher and connect all of the portable equipment. We looked like a parade going to the shower room at 2 AM!

The shower was a wonderful experience for both of us. I remember the smell of the raspberry soap her daughter had brought. We talked a little as I bathed her, but mostly there was a reflective silence. Mrs. S. seemed to have something on her mind. I watched as her tension faded and a new woman emerged. She started dozing while I shampooed her hair. After we put her back in bed, she immediately fell asleep. She slept quietly the rest of the night.

The next evening I went in to find a completely different woman! Surrounded by her family, she was alive! I was introduced to her husband, son, daughter, son-in-law, and daughter-in-law. They were the most attentive family I'd ever seen, and they were delighted at how much better she seemed to be. They rejoiced in telling me about Barbara, as we were now asked to call her, and what a remarkable person she is. Their stories were filled with love and laughter.

Barbara was in charge of the family. It wasn't always easy, but she made it work. She took care of everything and everyone. She was active with her children, in her church, and with her husband in a car collectors' club. She found tranquillity in painting and could complete several pieces in an evening. And she wrote with all the style and humor of Erma Bombeck. No doubt it was difficult for them to see her this way and even more difficult for Barbara, for the first time in her life, to be dependent on them.

Our staff fell in love with Barbara and her family. Her stay at our hospital lasted about 4 months. Rehabilitation was slow, but it was her inner strength and the never-ending support of her family and our staff that kept her going. We learned so much about life from Barbara. She was truly an inspiration to everyone who met her.

One day, during the third month of her stay, she told me something that explained a lot of my unanswered questions from that first night. We often shared special stories, but this one I would never have expected. She told me that in the acute care hospital, shortly after her stroke, she overheard some staff members talking. They said that it was a "tragedy" that she survived because she would more than likely be a "vegetable" for life. They went on to comment about what a burden she would be to her family. Someone said that it would be best if she passed away so that it would be easier on everyone.

Barbara had understood completely, and being the caring, independent person she was, she felt they were probably right. She loved her family but, based on what she had heard, thought she would no longer be able to do anything for them. Not wanting to be a negative force in her

family members' lives, she thought it best to help get this over as quickly as possible. But how? She had virtually no control over anything. She was completely paralyzed and could do nothing for herself except breathe. Barbara also knew that she was having cardiac dysrhythmias, and they seemed to be related to her breathing. So she thought if she could hold her breath long enough, the dysrhythmias would become aggravated and solve her problem for her.

Barbara waited for her family to leave, then said a prayer and held her breath. "I held my breath so long and kept thinking any minute now I should begin to die." She kept holding and holding, but nothing happened. "I must have held my breath for a good 5 minutes. I didn't even feel the need to start breathing again. What was going on? That's when I remembered I had a trach and I couldn't even kill myself." Barbara laughed and cried at the same time while she told me this. I held her and cried too.

"I just knew that rehabilitation for me was impossible. I was too far gone already." That's why she seemed so despondent when she was first admitted. She had almost given up. Barbara went on to say that the reason she told me this was because her life was changed that first night. "You treated me like I had worth. And even though I thought you were nuts, you kept talking about the future, saying that anything is possible. You weren't afraid to touch me or talk to me. You took the time to try to understand me. The shower washed away many of my fears and I began to feel human again. Now I wanted more than anything to live."

I think about Barbara and her family almost every day. And I am proud and honored to have made a difference in their lives. One year later, she continues to progress at home. She can feed herself and perform some simple activities of daily living independently. For about 10 minutes, four times a day, she stands out of her wheelchair. She remains a very important part of her family and a symbol of strength and courage to many others. It's obvious that the "tragedy" was not in her survival but most assuredly would have been in her death.

Holly L. Cirlin, RN, BSN, CCRN, CRRN, CNA
HEALTHSOUTH Rehabilitation Institute of San Antonio
San Antonio, Texas

1998 AACN-Siemens Excellence in Caring Practices Award Recipient
© 1998 by the American Association of Critical Care Nurses

38

Neurologic Anatomy and Physiology

Phyllis Dubendorf

Objectives

After completing this chapter, the student will be able to:

1. Describe the microanatomy and physiology of the nervous system.
2. Identify the structural components of the nervous system, including the brain, spinal cord, and peripheral nervous system.
3. List the functions of localized areas of the central nervous system.
4. Discuss the basic concepts of intracranial dynamics.
5. State the normal neurologic structural and functional changes associated with aging.

ANATOMY AND PHYSIOLOGY

The brain, spinal cord, and their supportive structures comprise the elements of one of the most complex systems of the body, the nervous system. This system receives, transmits, organizes, processes, and integrates all of the information from the environment and allows the individual to perform a motor or behavioral response to it, such as kicking a ball and calculating a math problem. The nervous system shapes our ability to learn, contemplate, and perform. Despite the complexity of skills and behaviors based in the nervous system, there remain only two types of cells on which the nervous system is based, the *neurons* and the *neuroglia*. Neurons are cells active in the transmission of impulses; neuroglia are supportive cells that hold the neurons together (neural glue).

Microanatomy of the Nervous System

Neurons

The neuron is an excitable cell whose functions are to receive stimuli, conduct impulses, and transmit messages to surrounding neurons. There are three basic components to all neurons, the *cell body* or perikaryon, *dendrite*, and *axon* (Figure 38–1). The cell is surrounded by a *plasma membrane*, which is made up of proteins and lipids.

The short processes of the cell are called *dendrites*. Dendrites are responsible for receiving information and conducting it toward the cell body. Many small branches of the dendrites, called *dendritic spines*, increase the surface receptive area of the cell.

Axons tend to be the longest processes of the cell, with lengths ranging from several micrometers to longer than a meter in extreme cases, as seen in the cells of peripheral skin receptors carrying impulses to the spinal cord. Axons carry impulses away from the cell body and communicate with other neurons (see Figure 38–1).

Synapse

A *synapse* is present wherever two or more neurons communicate with each other.[1] A synapse can be (1) *axodendritic,* communicating with a body of dendrites; (2) *axosomatic,* communicating with a cell body; or (3) *axoaxonic,* communicating with another axon. Communication at any synapse results in either inhibition or excitation and takes place by either chemical or electrical stimulation.

Most communication in the nervous system is chemical. A *neurotransmitter* is released from *synaptic vesicles* located at the distal end of the axon (Figure 38–2). These neurotransmitters flow across the synapse and affect the action potential of the receiving neuron, either

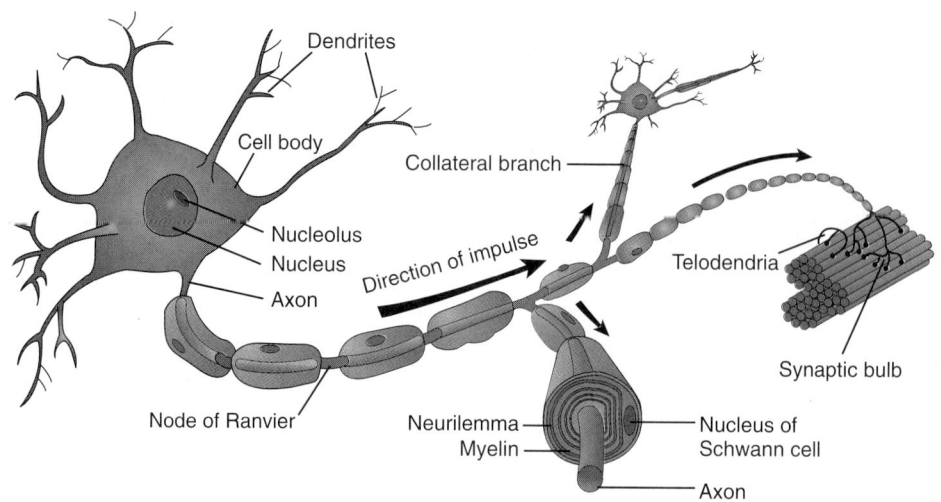

Figure 38–1

Structure of a typical neuron. (Redrawn from Applegate E: The Anatomy and Physiology Learning System. Philadelphia, WB Saunders, 1995, p 158.)

raising or lowering it, thereby inhibiting or exciting the neuron (Table 38–1). The neurotransmitter is then degraded by enzymes located in the *synaptic cleft* or it is taken up by the presynaptic axon terminal. There are many known neurotransmitters, such as *acetylcholine, norepinephrine, epinephrine, dopamine, glycine, serotonin, gamma-aminobutyric acid, enkephalins, substance P,* and *glutamic acid.* Most neurons produce and release only one type of neurotransmitter. Certain neurotransmitters may be produced and released in specific areas of the nervous system. For example, dopamine is primarily released in the *substantia nigra,* whereas acetylcholine is produced and released in the central and peripheral nervous systems.

Impulse Transmission. The neuron at rest is considered to be a "charged" cell. The difference between the intracellular and extracellular charge is called the *resting potential* of the cell. Like other cells of the body,

the neuron's resting potential lies in the sodium, chloride, calcium, and potassium concentrations within and outside of the cell. When enough stimulation has occurred to change the permeability of the cell membrane, *depolarization* occurs. Depolarization of the cell results in release of excitatory or inhibitory neurotransmitters at the synapses. As the neurotransmitter affects the action potential of the next neuron, an impulse is generated and is carried through the neuron and down the axon. The speed of this transmission is affected by the presence or absence of a *myelin sheath,* which is formed by *oligodendrocytes* in the central nervous system, and *neurolemmocytes (Schwann cells)* in the peripheral nervous system (see Figure 38–1). Oligodendrocytes are able to myelinate multiple axons, whereas each Schwann cell is able to myelinate only one nerve fiber. These cells wrap themselves around the cell axons, forming a kind of insulation. The number of

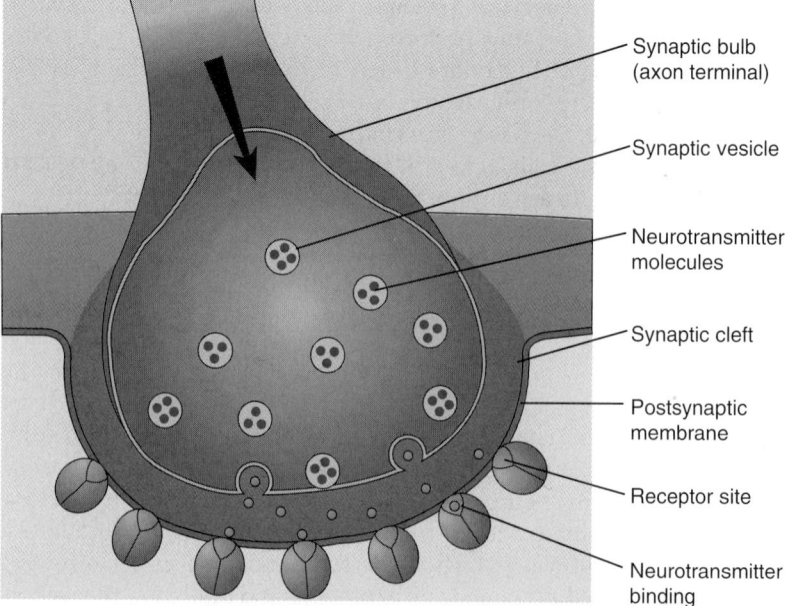

Figure 38–2

Components of a synapse. (Redrawn from Applegate E: The Anatomy and Physiology Learning System. Philadelphia, WB Saunders, 1995, p 163.)

TABLE 38–1
Neurotransmitters and Their Actions

Neurotransmitter	Action
Acetylcholine	Excitatory
Dopamine	Inhibitory
Endorphin	Excitatory
Enkephalin	Excitatory
Gamma-aminobutyric acid	Inhibitory
Glutamate	Excitatory
Glycine	Inhibitory
Histamine	Excitatory/inhibitory
Norepinephrine	Excitatory
Serotonin	Inhibitory
Substance P	Excitatory

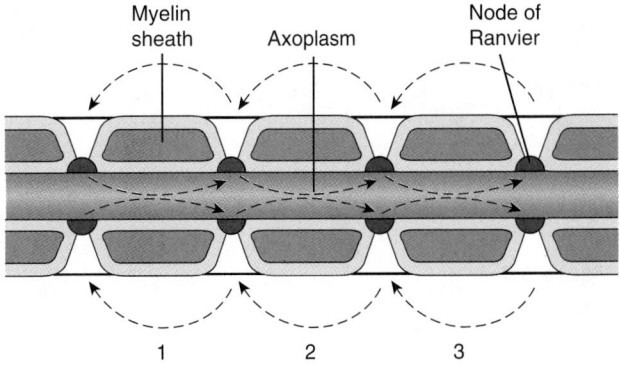

Figure 38–3

Saltatory conduction. (Redrawn from Guyton A: Basic Neuroscience Anatomy and Physiology. Philadelphia, WB Saunders, 1991, p 78.)

layers wrapped determines the thickness of the myelin sheath. Unlike their cousins in the central nervous system, Schwann cells lay down a basement membrane, forming an architecture that enables regeneration of myelin in the periphery, a property that does not exist in the central nervous system.

Myelin is a discontinuous layer, interrupted at specific intervals to create *nodes of Ranvier,* breaks in the insulation that allow ions to cross, continuing the action potential. Impulses traveling down myelinated axons jump from node to node, a phenomenon called *saltatory conduction* (Figure 38–3). This unique quality of the neuron allows impulses to travel in an extremely rapid fashion.

Nonmyelinated fibers are also present in both the central and the peripheral nervous systems. Nonmyelinated fibers conduct impulses at a slower speed.

Neuroglia

The *neuroglia* are specialized nonexcitable cells found in the nervous system that act as the glue that holds the neurons together. These cells are smaller and more abundant than neurons. In fact, there are five to 10 times more glial cells than neurons (Table 38–2). There are four types of neuroglia: astroglia, oligodendrocytes, microglia, and ependyma.

Astroglia, or *astrocytes,* are small, star-shaped cells that have many processes branching out from the cell body. These small cells form a network around neurons and nerve fibers and absorb certain neurotransmitters in addition to exerting phagocytic properties. These cells proliferate and fill in space at the death and degeneration of neurons, resulting in a scarring or *gliosis* of the tissue. Processes of astroglia extend out from the cell body and attach to capillary surfaces,

TABLE 38–2
Neuroglial Cell Types

Cell Type	Location	Description	Special Function
Astrocytes	CNS	Star shaped; numerous radiating processes with bulbous ends for attachment	Bind blood vessels to nerves; regulate the composition of fluid around neurons
Ependymal cells	CNS (line the ventricles of the brain and central canal of spinal cord)	Columnar cells with cilia	Active role in formation and circulation of cerebrospinal fluid
Microglia	CNS	Small cells with long processes; modified macrophages	Protection; become mobile and phagocytic in response to inflammation
Oligodendrocytes	CNS	Small cells with few, but long, processes that wrap around axons	Form myelin sheaths around axons in the CNS
Schwann cells*	PNS	Flat cells with a long, flat process that wraps around an axon in the PNS	Form myelin sheaths around axons in PNS; active role in nerve fiber regeneration

*Some authorities do not consider these to be neuroglia because they are in the PNS.
CNS, central nervous system; PNS, peripheral nervous system.
Modified from Applegate EJ: The Anatomy and Physiology Learning System Textbook. Philadelphia, WB Saunders, 1995.

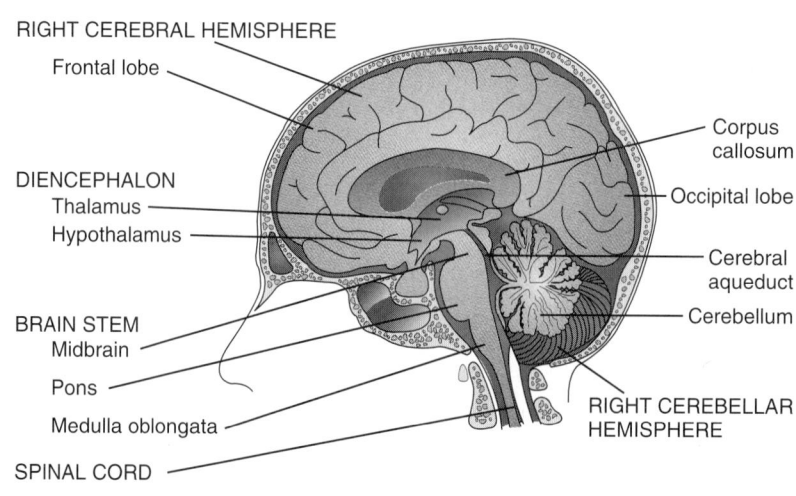

Figure 38–4

Lobes and functional areas of the cerebrum. (Redrawn and modified from Applegate E: The Anatomy and Physiology Learning System. Philadelphia, WB Saunders, 1995, p 167.)

suggesting that these cells may be part of the complex system called the *blood–brain barrier.*

Oligodendrocytes are small cells responsible for the myelination of the central nervous system. Oligodendrocytes have many processes enabling them to attach to and myelinate multiple nerve fibers. Although found only in the peripheral nervous system, Schwann cells perform a function similar to oligodendrocytes in the central nervous system, that of myelination.

Microglia appear to be dormant in the brain and spinal cord until an inflammatory or destructive process occurs. These cells then migrate to the area of injury, where they act as phagocytes.

Cells that line the ventricles and the central canal of the spinal cord are called *ependymal cells.* These cells possess *microvilli* and *cilia* that facilitate the flow of cerebrospinal fluid (CSF). Ependyma may also be involved in the production of CSF; however, this func-

tion is mainly accomplished by the *choroid plexus,* specialized cells found mainly in the ventricles of the brain.

Neurons bundle together to form nerve fibers and, ultimately, nerve tracts. These fibers and tracts are held together by neuroglia, or nerve glue, and form the functional complement of the most complex system in the body, the nervous system.

The Brain

The central nervous system consists of the brain and spinal cord. The specific functions of the brain and spinal cord can be localized into discrete areas. The brain is divided generally into areas known as the *cerebrum, diencephalon, brain stem,* and *cerebellum* (Figures 38–4 and 38–5).

Figure 38–5

The diencephalon, brain stem, and cerebellum. (Redrawn and modified from Applegate E: The Anatomy and Physiology Learning System. Philadelphia, WB Saunders, 1995, p 168.)

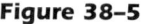

Cerebrum

The cerebrum consists of the left and right hemispheres, which are separated by the *deep longitudinal fissure*. The cortical surface area is increased by the presence of *gyri*, which are folds of cortical tissue, and *sulci*, the fissures created by the folds. Within each hemisphere are *frontal, parietal, temporal,* and *occipital* lobes, named for the bones of the skull under which they lie. The lobes are separated by specific sulci. The outermost covering of the cerebrum is gray matter, known as the *cerebral cortex*. This 2- to 5-mm layer is made up of cell bodies, unmyelinated axons, dendrites, and synapses of billions of cells.[2] Beneath the outer gray area is a layer of myelinated cells and neuroglia known as the *white matter*. This area serves as fiber pathways that facilitate communication between various parts of the brain. The lobes of the cortex can also be mapped into specific functions, either primary or associative. Primary cortical areas have a specific function with regard to their stimulation. Associative areas assist with the integration and processing of an impulse and may ascribe a certain significance to an experience. The cerebrum consists of

TABLE 38–3
Cerebral Cortex: Structures, Functions, and Results of Injury

Structure	Function	Injury May Result in
Frontal Lobe		
Motor cortex	Voluntary motor activity. Coordinates sequences of individual muscle movements or combines muscle movements.	Weakness/paralysis on the side opposite the injury.
Premotor cortex	"Practice-makes-perfect" area.	Difficulty with sequenced or skilled movements.
Prefrontal cortex	Concentration, organization, and higher intellectual functions.	Disorders of concentration, calculation, impulsivity, insight, and memory.
Broca's speech area	Controls and coordinates larynx and mouth to produce words.	"Expressive" or motor aphasia.
Parietal Lobe	Receives and integrates sensations, e.g., touch, pinprick, temperature, vibration, and proprioception.	Sensory perception disorders.
Temporal Lobe		
Auditory area	Receives and integrates tone, loudness, spoken words, and music.	Difficulty interpreting or understanding sound.
Wernicke's area (usually left dominant)	Interprets all kinds of language (written, spoken, felt, or generated within the brain). Connects to Broca's area via the arcuate fasciculus.	"Receptive" aphasia
Occipital Lobe	Receives and integrates visual stimuli.	Visual dissociation/cortical blindness/field cuts.
Commissural Fibers		
Corpus callosum	Connects frontal, parietal, and occipital lobes.	Impaired communication between the cerebral hemispheres.
Anterior commissure	Connects the temporal lobes.	
Basal Ganglia Caudate nucleus Globus pallidus Putamen	Exerts coordinative effect on finer motor movements initiated in the frontal lobe, resulting in smooth, controlled muscle contraction.	Discoordinate motor movements.
Reticular Formation	Network of nerve cells modulating motor and sensory systems and influencing level of wakefulness.	Loss of consciousness and coma.
Limbic System	Communicates with the hypothalamus, autonomic nervous system, and endocrine system to influence aspects of emotional behavior, particularly fear, anger, emotions associated with sexual behaviors and visceral responses to emotions.	Disorders of emotional responses.
Hippocampus	Recent memory	Disorders of recent memory

the following structures: frontal lobe, parietal lobe, temporal lobe, occipital lobe, commissural fibers, basal ganglia, reticular formation, limbic system, and hippocampus. See Table 38–3 for specific cerebral structures, functions, and examples of deficits caused by injury.

Diencephalon

The term *diencephalon* means the "between brain." In primitive animals, this area connects the cerebrum with the highest area of the brain stem, the midbrain. The diencephalon provides a similar function in humans; however, the connection between the diencephalon and the cerebrum is not easily demarcated. Its structures refer to the those around the third ventricle (discussed later) and include the *thalamus* and the *hypothalamus* (see Figure 38–5; Table 38–4).

The *pituitary* is a small gland that is primarily involved in regulating the hormonal activity of the body. The pituitary releases regulatory hormones, including growth hormone, adrenal-stimulating hormone, thyroid-stimulating hormone, prolactin, follicle-stimulating hormone, and luteinizing hormone. The pituitary also stores and releases oxytocin and vasopressin. The specific functions of the pituitary and its hormones are discussed in Chapter 25.

The *internal capsule* arises from the motor cortex and travels down through the basal ganglia in order to be further organized into tracts connecting to lower portions of the brain. The internal capsule connects the frontal cortex to many other areas of the brain, including the pons, the cranial nerve nuclei, and the spinal cord. Lesions in the internal capsule may result in contralateral weakness or hemiparesis.

Brain Stem

The *brain stem* is located beneath the cerebrum and the diencephalon. It is located in front of the cerebellum and serves many important functions. Primarily, it is the connection between the higher centers of the brain, the cerebellum, and the spinal cord. It serves as the passage for all ascending sensory input and descending motor impulses. Many important regulatory functions are governed here, such as heart rate and respiration. Almost all cranial nerve nuclei originate within some component of the brain stem. The brain stem is subdivided into three parts, the *midbrain*, the *pons*, and the *medulla* (see Figure 38–5 and Table 38–5). Disorders of the brain stem can result in severe neurologic deficits, such as paralysis, respiratory failure, cardiovascular decompensation, and cranial nerve deficits.

Cerebellum

The *cerebellum* is located behind the brain stem and has fiber connections to the three components of the brainstem: the midbrain, the pons, and the medulla (see Figure 38–5). These fiber connections are called the *inferior, middle,* and *superior cerebellar peduncles.* The cerebellum's main functions are coordination, balance, and regulation of muscle tone. These functions are affected by elaborate communication networks of neurons that send sensory information from vestibular nuclei and muscle spindle fibers directly to the cerebellum or via brain stem nuclei with connections to the cerebellum. These networks convey information regarding balance, skeletal muscle contraction, and muscle tension to the cerebellum, which in turn exerts its influence on motor fiber activities of the cerebral cortex. Although

TABLE 38–4

Diencephalon: Structures, Functions, and Results of Injury

Structure	Function	Injury May Result in
Thalamus	A major relay station of the brain. Processes all sensory and motor information. Coordinates and regulates all functional activity of the cerebral cortex.	Loss of consciousness, loss of sensory function, and loss of motor function.
Hypothalamus	Regulatory center for • Autonomic nervous system • Body temperature • Endocrine activities • Thirst • Satiety • Emotional expressions Synthesizes releasing and inhibiting factors affecting the release of hormones from the pituitary. Synthesizes oxytocin and vasopressin, which are then stored and released from the pituitary.	Severe obesity or wasting, sexual disorders, hyperthermia, hypothermia, diabetes insipidus, sleep disturbances, and emotional disorders.

TABLE 38–5
Brain Stem: Structures, Functions, and Results of Injury

Structure	Function	Injury May Result in
Midbrain	Contains many connections to higher and lower centers of the brain. Involved with reflex movements of the head, eye, and neck in response to visual stimuli.	A variety of motor and sensory disturbances, including paralysis, anesthesias, and cranial nerve deficits, particularly involving the eye.
Cranial nerves	Cranial nerves III (oculomotor) and IV (trochlear) nuclei are located here.	Cranial nerve dysfunction—extraocular movements and pupil constriction.
Substantia nigra	Concerned with muscle tone.	Discoordination (Parkinson's disease).
Cerebral aquaduct	Cerebrospinal fluid pathway.	Hydrocephalus.
Pons	Has many connections to the higher and lower centers of the nervous system and to the cerebellum.	A variety of motor and sensory disturbances.
Pneumotaxic and apneustic centers	Control rate and length of respiration.	Respiratory failure.
Cranial nerves	Houses nuclei for cranial nerves V (trigeminal), VI (abducens), VII (facial), and VIII (acoustic).	Cranial nerve dysfunction: motor and sensory to face, extraocular movements, and hearing.
Cerebral aquaduct	Cerebrospinal fluid pathway.	Hydrocephalus.
Medulla	Governs many basic functions of the body, including rhythm of respiration, rate and strength of heartbeat, and cardiovascular tone. Mediates swallowing, coughing, vomiting, and sneezing reflexes.	A variety of motor and sensory disturbances, including paralysis, anesthesias, loss of consciousness, respiratory and cardiac decompensation.
Pyramids	A bundle of fibers that are part of the voluntary motor or corticospinal tract. These tracts cross or decussate in the medulla.	Paralysis.
Fourth ventricle	Cerebrospinal fluid chamber.	Hydrocephalus.
Cranial nerves	Cranial nerves IX (glossopharyngeal), X (vagus), XI (accessory), and XII (hypoglossal) nuclei.	Cranial nerve dysfunction: tongue, swallowing, and gag, neck weakness

voluntary motor impulses are initiated in the cortex, it is the cerebellum that coordinates the fluidity and control of the movement via feedback loops, which are initiated only when sensory information has been evaluated. Disorders of the cerebellum result in ataxia, incoordination, and loss of muscle tone.

Supportive Structures and Mechanisms of the Brain

Skull

The skull is a rigid, bony structure composed of eight cranial bones and 14 facial bones. The part of the skull that encloses the brain is called the *cranium* and is composed of the frontal, occipital, sphenoid, and ethmoid bones in addition to the two parietal and temporal bones. These bones are like plates, attached together at areas called *sutures* (Figure 38–6).

The two bones not seen from an external view of the cranium are the *sphenoid* and ethmoid bones (see Figure 38–6). These two bones make up the anterior portion of the *basilar skull*. The ethmoid bone is projected upward between the two orbits. The sphenoid

bone is shaped like a butterfly. The occipital-sphenoid junction is known as the *basilar suture*. The sphenoid has many ridges curving up to hold the structures of the underside of the brain. One such formation, the *sella turcica*, encloses the descending lobes of the pituitary. Many openings, or *foramina*, are also located within the sphenoid bone. These openings allow for the passage of arteries and cranial nerves. Understanding the relationship between the basilar skull and its overlying structures is imperative in understanding the pathophysiology of many brain injuries.

Meninges

The *meninges* are located between the skull and the brain and form a protective supportive covering around the brain and spinal cord. The meninges are composed of three layers: the dura, the arachnoid, and the pia (Figure 38–7). The dura is a tough, fibrous outermost layer that covers and compartmentalizes the intracranial cavity. The dura creates compartments by folding over on itself and forms the *falx cerebri*, which separates the left and right hemispheres, and the *tentorium cerebelli*, which separates the cerebrum from the

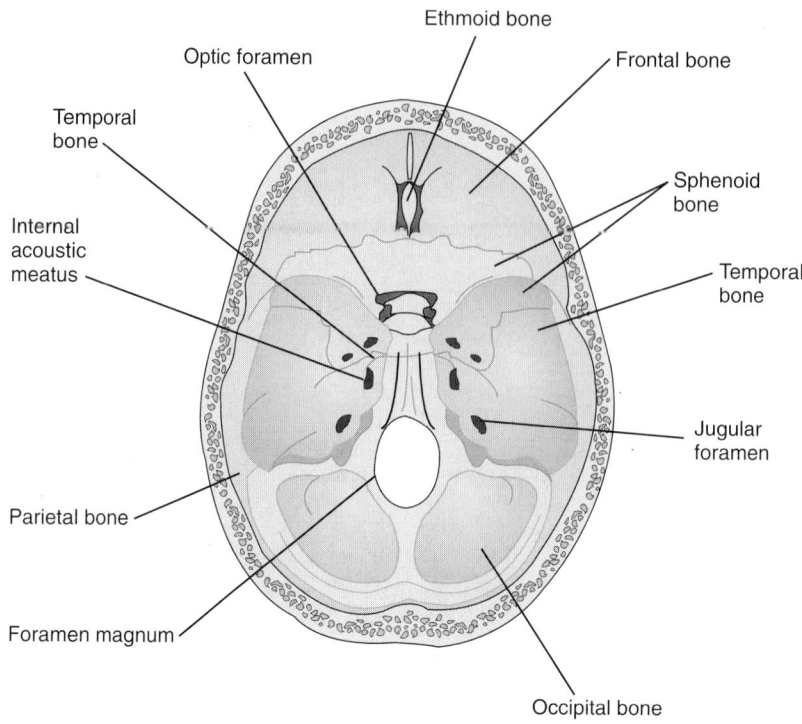

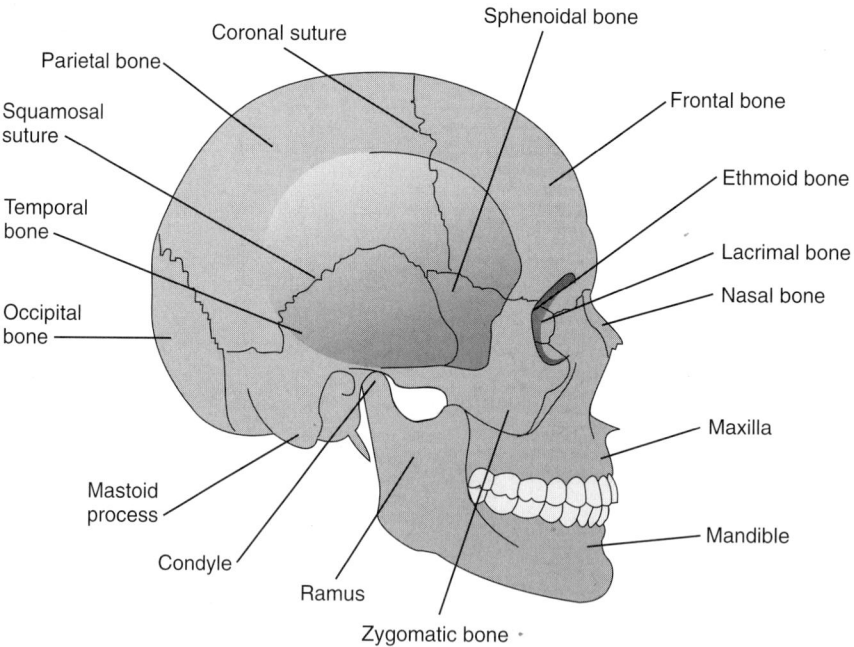

Figure 38–6

Skull. A, Internal view of the skull floor. B, Lateral view of the skull.

A

B

cerebellum. The *arachnoid* is a thin, delicate layer loosely adhering to its underlying structures. The *pia* is a vascular membrane lying closest to the brain, covering arteries as they enter the substance of the brain.[1]

Between these layers of meninges are spaces, one actual and two potential spaces, that must be identified. Above and below the dura are the potential *epidural space*

and the *subdural space.* Typically, these areas are involved when there has been trauma or infection to the cranium, and both are spaces where blood, fluid, or pus can accumulate, causing increased pressure on the brain.

Beneath the arachnoid layer lies the *subarachnoid space,* a real space in which cerebrospinal fluid freely circulates. It contains large blood vessels and is formed

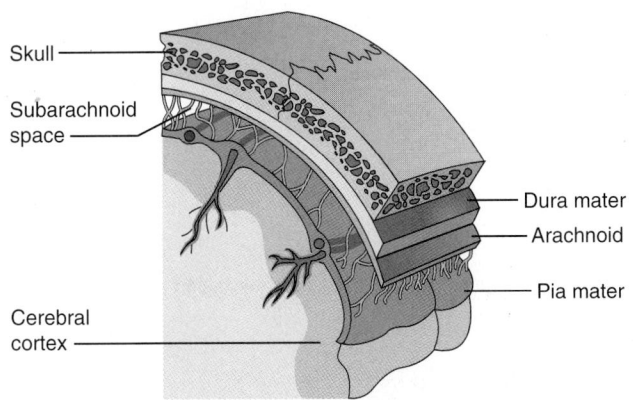

Figure 38–7

Meninges. (Redrawn from Applegate E: The Anatomy and Physiology Learning System. Philadelphia, WB Saunders, 1995, p 166.)

by delicate connective tissue. Pockets of cerebrospinal fluid are formed in areas where the arachnoid and pia are separated by wide gaps. Two of these areas are notable, the *cisterna magnum*, located inferior to the cerebellum, and the *lumbar cistern*, located below the second or third lumbar vertebrae. Both of these areas are used for sampling cerebrospinal fluid, by either a C1-2 puncture or a lumbar puncture.

Ventricles

The ventricular system synthesizes and facilitates the flow of CSF. CSF is formed primarily in the lateral ventricles by specialized cells called choroid plexus. Lateral ventricles are found in both cerebral hemispheres and consist of anterior, inferior, and posterior horns. The CSF flows from the lateral ventricles through the *interventricular foramina* to the *third ventricle*, which is located in the center of the brain. From here, CSF flows through the *aqueduct of Sylvius* on its way to the *fourth ventricle*, which is located in the pons. The *foramina of Luschka* and *Magendie* open from the fourth ventricle and allow CSF to flow into the subarachnoid space around the brain and the spinal cord (Figure 38–8).

Cerebrospinal Fluid

Cerebrospinal fluid is generally a clear, colorless or light straw-colored fluid. Its makeup is remarkably like that of serum plasma; however, there is about one-half the glucose content and only a trace of protein. Concentrations of sodium, calcium, and magnesium also differ. CSF is thought to act as a cushion between the delicate nervous tissue and its overlying support-ive structures. It is likely to play a part in the nourish-ing neural cells and removing metabolites from the nervous tissue.

Cerebrospinal fluid is generally free of cells, with the exception of lymphocytes. CSF pressure, measured in a lateral recumbent position, measures 60 to 150 mm

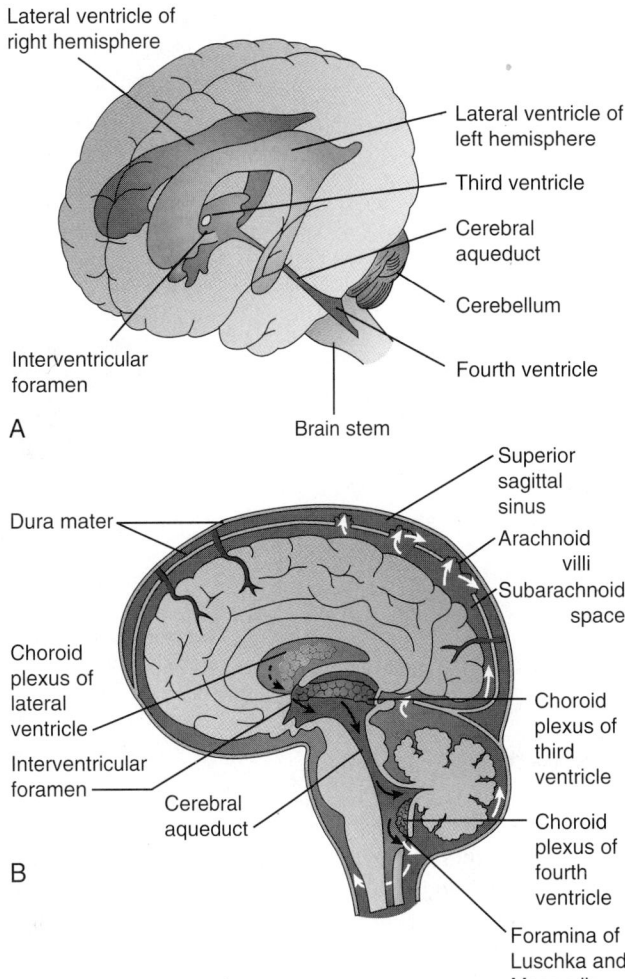

Figure 38–8

A, Ventricular system. B, Flow of cerebrospinal fluid. (Redrawn and modified from Applegate E: The Anatomy and Physiology Learning System. Philadelphia, WB Saunders, 1995, p 172.)

H_2O. The total volume of the CSF found at any one time in the ventricles, subarachnoid space, and cis-terns is 130 mL; however, approximately 500 mL of CSF is produced daily (Table 38–6). CSF is reabsorbed into the venous system through *arachnoid villi* located in the subarachnoid space (see Figure 38–8).

TABLE 38–6
Normal Components of Cerebrospinal Fluid

Components	Normal Value
Color	Clear
Red blood cells	0
White blood cells	0–5 mm³
Glucose	50–75 mg/100 mL
Protein	15–45 mg/100 mL
Chloride	700–750 mg/100 mL
Lactate	1.6 mg/100 mL

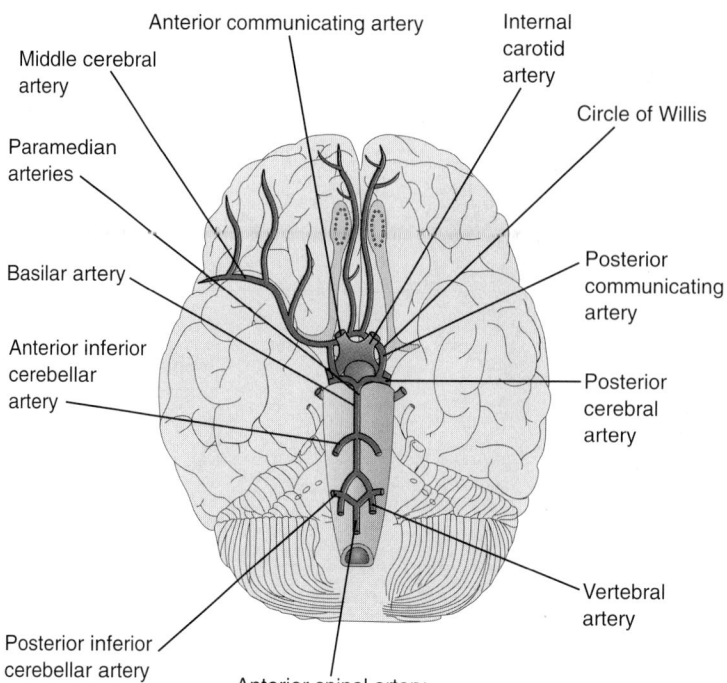

Figure 38–9

Cerebral circulation.

Circulation

The blood flow to and from the brain is dynamic and vital to the function of the neurons. If blood flow to the brain is impaired, ischemia and tissue injury occur. For this reason, blood flow to the brain is a complex process with built-in physiologic fail-safe mechanisms, namely the blood–brain barrier and autoregulation, to be discussed later in this section.

The brain is supplied by two distinct circulatory regions, an anterior supply arising from the two *carotid arteries* and a posterior supply arising from the two *vertebral arteries*. These circulations come together at

the base of the brain in an area known as the *circle of Willis* (Figure 38–9). Cerebral arteries arise from the anterior and posterior circulations to feed specific cerebral structures (Table 38–7).

The circle of Willis lies at the base of the brain and forms the anastomosis between the anterior and posterior circulations. The circle of Willis is formed from the anterior communicating, anterior cerebral, internal carotid, posterior communicating, posterior cerebral, and basilar arteries. Because of these connections, a malformation impairing blood supply to a localized area of the brain may be overcome by retrograde filling from the other side. However,

TABLE 38–7
Cerebral Circulation

Circulation	Supplies Blood to the
Anterior	
External carotid	Face and neck
Internal carotid	
Ophthalmic artery	Structures of the orbit
Middle cerebral artery	Lateral surfaces of both cerebral hemispheres—frontal, parietal, and temporal lobes
Anterior cerebral artery	Medial frontal cortex and central structures of the brain
Posterior	
Vertebral artery	
Anterior/posterior spinal arteries	Upper portions of the spinal cord
Posterior inferior cerebellar artery	Brain stem and cerebellum
Basilar artery	
Anterior inferior cerebellar artery	Cerebellum, pons, and medulla
Superior cerebellar arteries	Cerebellum, pons, and medulla
Posterior cerebral arteries	Occipital and temporal lobes

because of the increased number of arterial anastomoses in the circle, defects in the arterial vessel wall leading to aneurysms are common. Aneurysms may develop anywhere in the intracranial circulation.

Venous Drainage

The *venous sinuses* and veins of the brain differ from venous systems found in other parts of the body. They have no muscular tissue in their walls, and they have no valves. The veins lie in the subarachnoid space and ultimately pierce the dura to drain into the venous sinuses in the dural folds. Sinuses provide a low pressure channel for the flow of venous blood back to the general circulation ultimately via the *jugular veins*. Major sinus complexes include the superior sagittal sinus, the inferior sagittal sinus, the straight sinus, the transverse sinus, the sigmoid sinuses, and the jugular bulbs (see Figure 38–8; Figure 38–10).

Blood–Brain Barrier

The *blood–brain barrier* is a discriminative property exclusively found in the capillary structure of the brain and spinal cord. This barrier is a function of a network of cells involving tight junctions between the endothelial cells in the capillary wall, a continuous basement membrane surrounding these endothelial cells, and astrocytic processes called *perivascular feet* that attach to the capillary wall. This architecture prevents the entry of certain molecules into the neuron. The permeability of the blood–brain barrier is inversely related to the size of the molecules and is directly related to their lipid solubility. Small molecules pass readily, whereas medium-sized molecules, such as glucose and electrolytes, pass more slowly. The blood–brain barrier is largely impermeable to proteins and other large organic molecules.[1] The blood–brain barrier protects the brain from toxic substances but also prevents the admission of many therapeutic agents, a factor that impedes systemic treatment of some neurologic diseases and infections.

Autoregulation

Autoregulation is a property of the cerebral blood vessels that enables them to vasodilate or vasoconstrict to maintain a constant cerebral blood flow despite fluctuations in the systemic blood pressure. This property has likely resulted from the fact that the brain is highly dependent on two specific substrates: oxygen and glucose. Because there are no mechanisms to store these substrates in the brain, it is necessary for the brain to accurately regulate the flow of blood to deliver them. The brain uses glucose and oxygen in the process of energy production to maintain transmembrane activities and also to synthesize neurotransmitters.[2] Autoregulation operates most effectively within certain physiologic parameters, namely, a mean arterial blood pressure of between 60 and 130 mm Hg, and also within normal parameters of intracranial pressure.

Basic Concepts of Intracranial Dynamics

The brain and its surrounding supportive structures create a dynamic environment that responds uniquely to the needs of the neurons. The three major components of this environment are the brain, the cerebrospinal fluid, and the cerebral circulation. The skull forms a fixed, rigid space around these components.

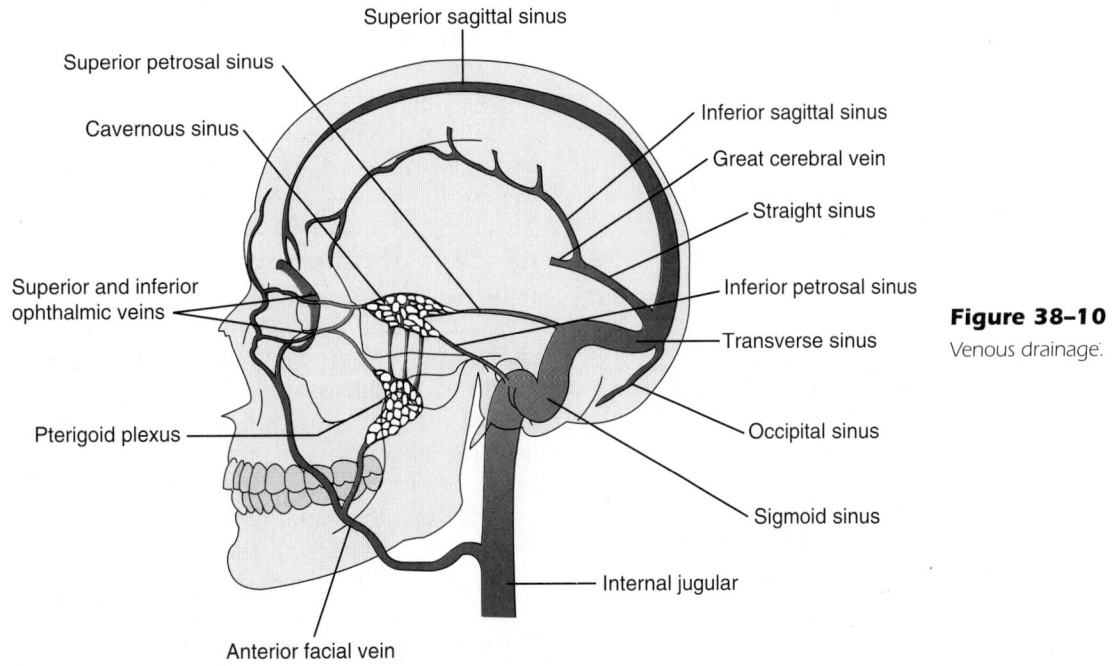

Figure 38–10

Venous drainage.

The relationship between the brain, CSF, and blood within this bony structure can be measured, in part, by the *intracranial pressure* (ICP). This pressure is usually between zero and 15 mm Hg in adults when measured at the level of the foramen of Monro (externally at the level of the tragus of the ear).

Intracranial Pressure

An understanding of the *modified Monro-Kellie hypothesis* is necessary to comprehend further pathophysiologic changes related to ICP. This hypothesis states that the rigid skull is filled to capacity with its three components: brain matter, CSF, and blood. To maintain a steady intracranial pressure, if one of these components increases in ratio, another must decrease. Many normal physiologic changes in ICP are easily compensated for, such as coughing, sneezing, changes in position, and Valsalva maneuver. Such compensatory mechanisms include shunting of CSF down the spinal cord to large cisterns, compression of the low pressure venous system, decreased production of CSF, and vasoconstriction of the cerebral vessels to accommodate increases in pressure. Compensatory mechanisms allow the brain to be responsive to relatively small changes in volume without a change in ICP.

Another property of the brain is *compliance,* or the ability to add volume without a resultant change in pressure. Such a concept can be explained by a *volume–pressure curve*[2] (Figure 38–11). At the lowest point of the curve, both volume and pressure are at their lowest levels. As volume is increased, the pressure rises slightly, until compliance maximizes. Larger

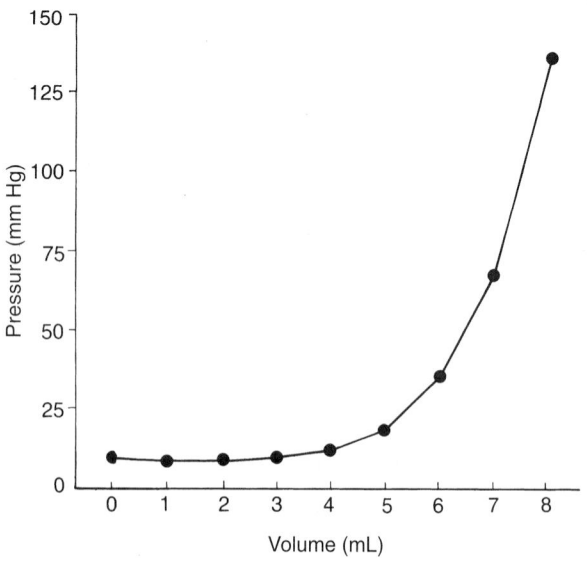

Figure 38–11

Volume–pressure curve: the relationship between volume and pressure within the intracranial space. As the volume reaches the point at which pressure begins to rise, small increases in volume cause large rises in intracranial pressure. (From Marshall SB, Marshall LF, Vos HR, et al: Neuroscience Critical Care: Pathophysiology and Patient Management. Philadelphia, WB Saunders, 1990.)

TABLE 38–8
Conditions Influencing Intracranial Pressure

Category	Example
Increased intrathoracic pressure	Sneezing
	Vomiting
	Coughing
	Valsalva maneuver
	Suctioning
	Positive end-expiratory pressure
Increased activity	Changes in position
	Range of motion
	Isometric exercises
	Neck flexion
Psychological stress	Emotional upset
Ventilation deficits	Decreased PaO_2
	Increased $PaCO_2$
Temperature	Hyperthermia
Metabolic	Seizures

Modified from Barker E: Anatomy and physiology of the nervous system. In Barker E (ed): Neuroscience Nursing. St. Louis, Mosby, 1994, pp 295–323.
PaO_2, partial pressure of arterial oxygen; $PaCO_2$, partial pressure of arterial carbon dioxide.

changes in volume, such as those caused by brain tumors, hydrocephalus, and intracranial hematomas, rapidly deplete compensatory mechanisms. Each additional volume forces the intracranial pressure to rise exponentially. In the critically ill patient, normal activity may result in a critical rise in ICP (Table 38–8).

In an environment of increased intracranial pressure, blood flow is reduced, and the neuron risks ischemia and hypoxia. If hypoxic, the neuron loses its basic protective mechanism, autoregulation, or the ability of the cerebral vessels to dilate or constrict depending on the metabolic needs of the neuron. Once autoregulation is lost, there in unrestricted blood flow to some parts of the brain, resulting in further increases in volume and pressure.

With any increase in volume and pressure, the brain expands within the cranial vault and presses against the compartments created by the folds of the dura. This expansion and pressure results in dysfunction of the affected neurons demonstrated by neurologic deficits. These deficits may be manifested by a decrease in level of consciousness, weakness, pupillary changes, confusion, or other symptoms.

Intracranial pressure can be measured many ways. One of the most common ways is to insert a catheter into the subarachnoid space surrounding the cerebrum or directly into one of the lateral ventricles, usually on the nondominant side. A fluid-filled column in contact with the CSF transmits fluid pressure waves, which are then digitized and measured by electronic means. There are also means to measure the ICP via an epidural electrode method, which is less accurate but also less invasive than other methods that breech the dura. The most recent means of measuring ICP is fiberoptically. A fiber optic sensor can be placed either within fluid or within the brain matter itself and can transmit information regarding the pressure of the brain. Any of these readings reflect the local pressure of the brain; for example, if brain swelling occurs on the side of the monitoring device, the pressure readings may be higher than if the device were on the opposite side, and vice versa.

Cerebral Perfusion Pressure

The measurement of intracranial pressure is only one parameter that is useful in evaluating cerebral dynamics. *Cerebral perfusion pressure* (CPP) is a reflection of the global circulatory status of the brain. CPP is derived from subtracting the ICP from the mean arterial pressure (MAP): CPP = MAP − ICP. This measurement of CPP goes a step beyond the measurement of ICP. For example, if two patients have an ICP of 15 mm Hg, the patient with the higher MAP would have a higher perfusion pressure. CPP is an *estimate* of the perfusion to the brain. Optimally, the CPP is maintained at greater than 60 to 70 mm Hg in order to maintain neuronal function. Alternately, CPP values greater than 100 mm Hg represent hyperperfusion, or too much blood flow to the brain.[2] Irreversible brain ischemia occurs if the CPP falls to or below 40 mm Hg.

Cerebral Oxygen Delivery

Intracranial pressure and cerebral perfusion pressure are two important parameters, but they are indirect measurements of cerebral circulation at best. Most importantly, are the neurons receiving the required substrates of oxygen and glucose, and if they are, are they using these substrates? It has become possible to measure the use of oxygen by the neuron. This is accomplished by insertion of a monitoring catheter into the jugular bulb, which transmits the oxygen saturation of the venous blood. This oxygen value is compared to the simultaneous oxygen value of the arterial blood system. The difference is calculated, and a determination of the cerebral oxygen extraction can be made. Because the brain is the only organ draining blood into the proximal jugular system, it is a more direct reflection of the metabolism of the neurons. By use of these values, certain variables may be manipulated. For example, if the brain is extracting too much oxygen from the arterial blood, efforts to maximize oxygen content and also to slow the metabolism of the brain are made.

The Spinal Cord

Contiguous with the brainstem is the *spinal cord,* an elongated, cylindric organ. The spinal cord acts as the "highway" for information. It is the structure through which information from the periphery enters and is organized before going to the higher centers of the brain for processing, and it carries impulses from those higher centers to end-organs, such as the muscles, heart, lungs, gut, and bladder.

The spinal cord extends from the level of the foramen magnum to approximately the level of the second lumbar vertebrae. The areas of the spinal cord are grouped by function and include the cervical, thoracic, lumbar, and sacral segments (Figure 38–12). The terminal end of the spinal cord is made of a tapered area called the *conus medullaris.*

The cross-section of the spinal cord reveals many discrete areas. The center contains a butterfly-shaped area made up of gray matter containing cell bodies, dendrites, synapses, and unmyelinated axons. It is here that specific nuclei are located that have specialized functions and target structures. This gray matter is surrounded by a corresponding component of white matter. These areas are myelinated axons organized as tracts to transport messages up and down the spinal cord. These tracts are addressed later in this chapter under nervous system pathways.

The spinal cord is made of the same delicate tissue as the brain and is therefore enclosed in a similar protective environment, including the vertebral column and the meninges.

Supportive Structures of the Spinal Cord

Vertebral Column

The *vertebral column,* or the spine, is a series of bones with two functions: (1) it is a protective covering for the spinal cord, and (2) it provides structure and support to the trunk. The vertebral column is composed of 33 vertebrae: seven cervical, 12 thoracic, five lumbar, five sacral (fused), and four coccygeal (fused) (Figure 38–13). The most flexible areas of the spine are the cervical and lumbar segments, posing these areas at greatest risk for injury.

There are two parts to each vertebrae, the anterior (*body*) and posterior (*arch*) segments. The opening in the middle of the vertebrae is the vertebral foramen, which encloses the spinal cord (Figure 38–14). The body is the largest part of the vertebrae and has a large, two-sided flattened surface to which fibrocartilages attach. Spinal nerves, arteries, and veins exit from the body via openings.

The arch is composed of two pedicles and two laminae. There are a number of processes off the arch that provide sites for articulation and attachments for muscles and ligaments. This ensures structural stability in the spine. The spinous process is a posterior projection off the laminae on which muscles and ligaments also attach.

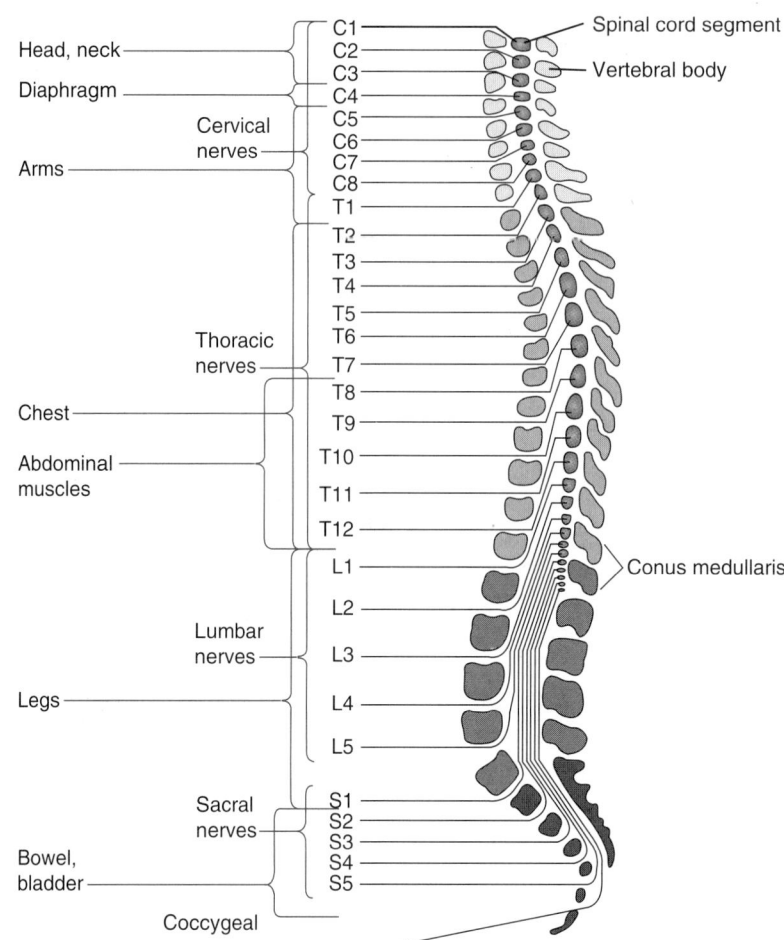

Figure 38–12

Segments of the spinal cord.

The stability of the spinal column is ensured by the intervertebral disk and muscle connections, but most notably by ligamentous support. The *anterior* and *posterior longitudinal ligaments* and the *ligamenta flava* secure the anterior and posterior elements of the spine and prevent excessive flexion and extension.

The first two cervical vertebrae are called the *atlas* (C1) and the axis (C2). The first cervical vertebra is like a ring, which articulates with the base of the skull. The second cervical vertebra has the usual components of the structure but also has a vertical projection called the *odontoid process* on which C1 is situated. These are specialized vertebrae that allow for rotation of the head (Figure 38–15).

Each vertebra from the second cervical vertebrae to the sacrum is cushioned by an *intervertebral disk*. These disks differ in shape, size, and thickness, depending on their location within the spine. The two basic components of the disk are the *nucleus pulposis,* the central gelatinous substance, and the *annulus fibrosis,* a fibrous capsule surrounding the nucleus pulposis.

Spinal Cord Circulation

Like the brain, the spinal cord is extremely dependent on blood supply to provide spinal neurons with the necessary substrates of oxygen and glucose. Major blood supply to the spinal cord is provided by the posterior spinal arteries, the anterior spinal artery, the segmental arteries, and the great anterior medullary artery of Adamkiewicz. Injury to these vessels results in dysfunction of the spinal cord.

Peripheral Nervous System

The peripheral nervous system (PNS) essentially contains the neurons outside of the brain and spinal cord. The peripheral nervous system is the final portion of the pathway for the motor impulse. Muscles are innervated via these fibers. Alternately, the PNS is the beginning pathway for sensory impulses since sensations are collected, organized, and transmitted from the peripheral fibers. Cranial nerves, spinal nerves, peripheral nerves, and their connecting fibers are all considered part of the peripheral nervous system.

Cranial Nerves

There are 12 pairs of cranial nerves exiting from the brain, primarily from the brain stem. Cranial nerves have numerous functions. They can innervate striated

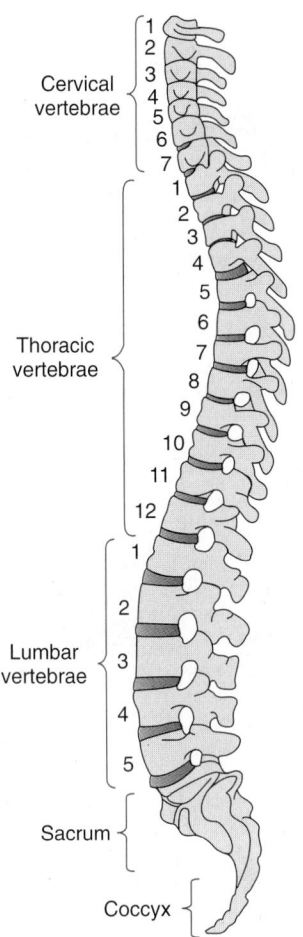

Figure 38–13

Spine.

where the medial fibers of the optic nerve cross, which allows the information from each optic nerve fiber to communicate with both sides of the occipital cortex. The fibers continue posteriorly and separate into optic tracts. The optic tracts synapse in an area of the thalamus and the midbrain. From the thalamus, the fibers continue to the visual cortex, where primary vision and visual association are appreciated. The role of the midbrain is reflexive. The head automatically turns toward any object within the visual field in order to determine whether to continue looking at it. The optic nerve and optic tracts are relatively long pathways that must travel through many areas of the brain. For this reason, a lesion occurring at any point in this pathway can result in visual problems, including blindness, loss of visual acuity, visual field defects, and visual agnosias (inability to recognize an object).

Oculomotor Nerve (Cranial Nerve III). The *oculomotor nerve* arises from the brain stem and innervates the muscles of the eyes that allow the eye to look upward, medially, downward, and up and outward. The oculomotor nerve also innervates the muscle that raises the eyelid and muscles that control the constriction of the pupil and the thickness of the lens. Lesions affecting this nerve result in *ptosis,* drooping of the lid, pupillary dilation, and limited extraocular movements.

Trochlear Nerve (Cranial Nerve IV). The *trochlear nerve* arises from the midbrain and is responsible for one extraocular movement, the simultaneous movement of the eye downward and inward.

Trigeminal Nerve (Cranial Nerve V). The *trigeminal nerve* arises from the superior aspect of the pons and is responsible for facial and corneal sensation and for the muscles of mastication. The trigeminal nerve is the largest of the cranial nerves and trifurcates into the

muscle *(motor nerves),* or they can synapse in the sensory nuclei *(sensory nerves).* Some cranial nerves serve both functions (Figure 38–16).

Olfactory Nerve (Cranial Nerve I). The *olfactory nerve* is concerned only with the sense of smell and is one of the few cranial nerves that does not exit from the brain stem. It consists of nerve cells that are located in the mucosa of the nasal cavity which then travel through the ethmoid bone and enter the olfactory bulb on the underside of the frontal lobe bilaterally. These bulbs then transition to olfactory tracts, which carry messages to specific olfactory areas located in the cerebral cortex. These areas send nerve fibers to many other areas of the brain, such as the temporal and frontal cortexes, the limbic system, and the hypothalamus. Although the olfactory nerves only serve to perceive odors, connections to higher centers allow for emotional and autonomic responses to these stimuli.

Optic Nerve (Cranial Nerve II). The *optic nerve* is primarily responsible for transmitting information regarding vision. The fibers of the optic nerve originate in a layer of the retina and exit from the posterior aspect of the eyes as the optic nerve. These nerves travel posteriorly and join to become the *optic chiasm,*

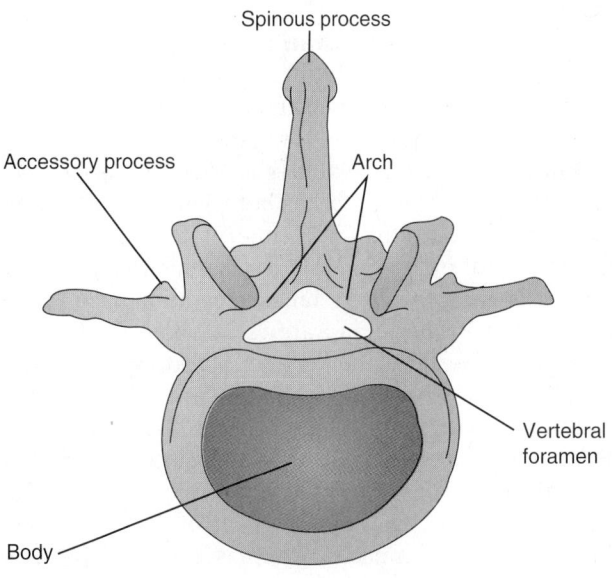

Figure 38–14

Vertebral body.

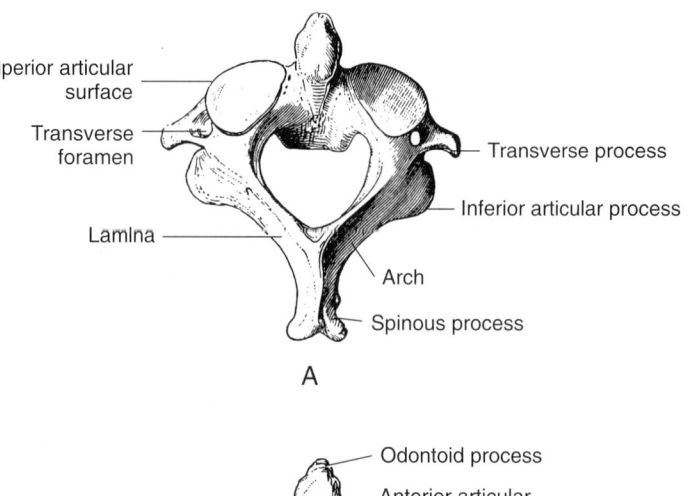

A

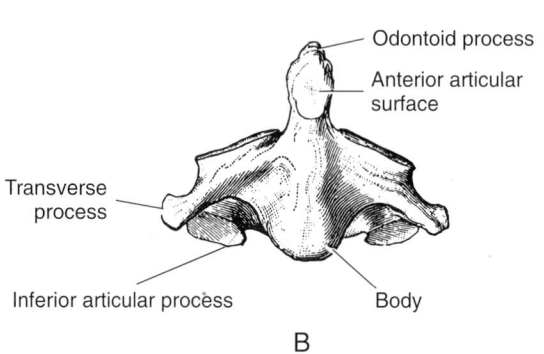

B

Figure 38–15

Specialized vertebrae. *A,* Atlas (C1). *B,* Axis (C2). (From Marshall SB, Marshall LF, Vos HR, et al: Neuroscience Critical Care: Pathophysiology and Patient Management. Philadelphia, WB Saunders, 1990, p 55.)

ophthalmic, maxillary, and *mandibular* branches. The ophthalmic division carries sensory information from the skin of the forehead, the upper face, the bridge of the nose, the cornea, and the eyelid. The maxillary component carries information from the upper jaw, the cheek, the upper teeth, and the mucous membranes of the palate and nasal and sinus cavities. The mandibular division transmits information from the skin of the lower face, the lower teeth, and the mucous membranes of the oral cavity. Motor fibers to the muscles of mastication also travel along the mandibular division.

Abducens Nerve (Cranial Nerve VI). The *abducens nerve* originates in the pons and is responsible for lateral extraocular movement. Cranial nerves III, IV, and VI are usually tested together.

Facial Nerve (Cranial Nerve VII). The *facial nerve* arises from the pons and has both sensory and motor functions. The motor fibers innervate the muscles of the face and are responsible for symmetry of expression. The sensory fibers innervate the anterior two-thirds of the tongue and are responsible for taste in that area. The facial nerve nuclei also synapse with facial motor fibers of both cerebral hemispheres, forming a facial motor pathway. Like other long pathways of the nervous system, lesions along any part of the pathway result in dysfunction. Lesions of the facial nerve specifically result in drooping of the same-sided (ipsilateral) facial muscles, whereas lesions of the cerebral motor cortex result in opposite-sided (contralateral) motor dysfunction. The nucleus of each facial nerve travels in close proximity to the nucleus of cranial nerve VIII, the acoustic nerve. Occasionally, lesions of the eighth cranial nerve affect the function of the facial nerve as well.

Acoustic Nerve (Cranial Nerve VIII). The *acoustic nerve* is the lowest cranial nerve related to the pons, and is responsible for hearing and balance. The *cochlear* division is involved in hearing. Vibrations of the *tympanic membrane* are transmitted via fibers from the hearing apparatus located in the inner ear. These transmissions travel along the eighth nerve until they arrive at the pontine nuclei, which convey them to areas of the midbrain concerned with auditory reflexes and to areas of the temporal cortex.

The *vestibular* division collects information from the *semicircular canals, saccule,* and *utricle,* which enables the brain to detect positions and movements of the head. This information is transmitted via the vestibular nerve to the pontine nuclei, and then directly to the inferior cerebellar peduncle to connect to the cerebellum. This process of information transmission allows any corrections in body position or muscle tension to be made via descending fibers through the spinal cord. Extraocular movements also allow for visual fixation on an object while the head is moving.

Glossopharyngeal Nerve (Cranial Nerve IX). The *glossopharyngeal nerve* originates in the medulla. It is a motor and sensory nerve responsible for movement and sensation of the pharynx, innervation of the parotid gland, and taste of the posterior one-third of the tongue. Sensory information from the *carotid sinus,*

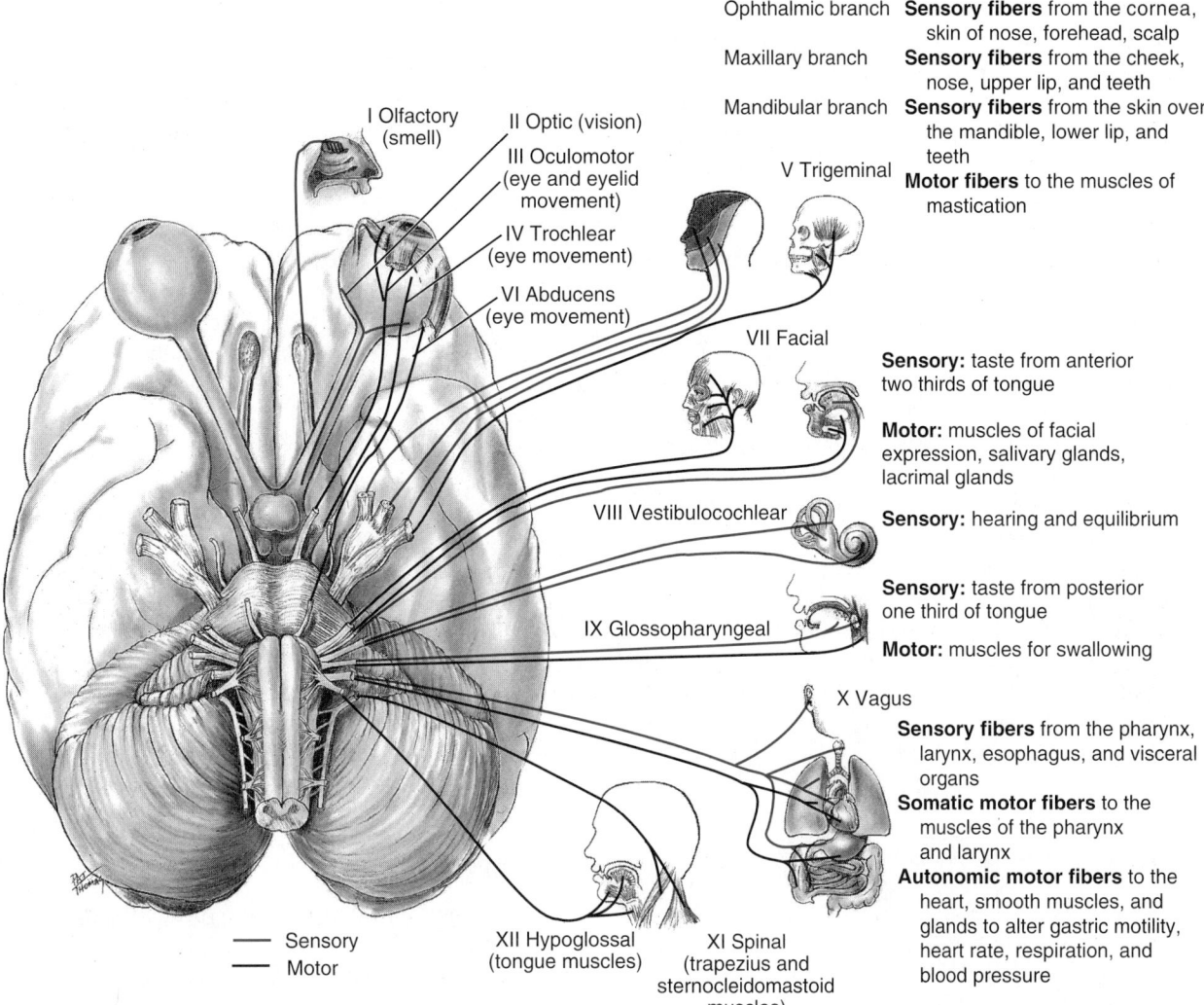

Figure 38–16

Cranial nerves. (From Polaski A, Tatro S: Luckmann's Core Principles and Practice of Medical-Surgical Nursing. Philadelphia, WB Saunders, 1995, p 248.)

a baroreceptor located at the bifurcation of the carotid artery, also travels with the glossopharyngeal and vagus nerves. This association results in the *carotid sinus reflex,* assisting in the regulation of the arterial blood pressure. Lesions of the glossopharyngeal nerve result in loss of the *gag reflex.*

Vagus Nerve (Cranial Nerve X). The *vagus nerve* is also a mixed motor/sensory nerve; however, it has more complex functions than other cranial nerves because of its role in the parasympathetic nervous system. The vagus nerve exits from the medulla, traveling in close approximation with the glossopharyngeal nerve and jugular veins. The motor portion of the vagus nerve innervates portions of the pharynx and the larynx. In addition, the motor portion of the nerve descends to parasympathetic motor fibers that innervate the involuntary muscles of the bronchi, heart, esophagus, stomach, small intestine, and large intestine (to the transverse colon). These fibers are explained further later in this chapter.

Sensory fibers of the vagus nerve carry information from the skin around the ear, internal viscera, and pharynx. Lesions affecting the vagus nerve result in vocal cord paralysis and swallowing/gag dysfunction.

Spinal Accessory Nerve (Cranial Nerve XI). The *spinal accessory nerve* exits from the medulla and is solely a motor nerve. It innervates the *trapezius* and the *sternocleidomastoid muscles,* which are responsible for shoulder shrugging and head turning.

Hypoglossal Nerve (Cranial Nerve XII). The *hypoglossal nerve* is a motor nerve that originates in the medulla and provides innervation to the tongue. Lesions of the hypoglossal nerve result in tongue deviation toward the injured side.

Spinal Nerves

Thirty-one pairs of spinal nerves emanate from the spinal cord. These nerves form the pathway for sensory information to be retrieved from the periphery and for motor information to be dispersed to the appropriate end muscle or structure. Each spinal segment consists of a pair of spinal nerves and the corresponding portion of the spinal cord. Cervical nerves are named against the cervical vertebrae over which they pass. The first cervical nerve exits above the first cervical vertebrae; therefore, the second cervical nerve is located between the 1st and 2nd cervical vertebrae. Despite the fact that there are only seven cervical vertebrae, there is an eighth cervical nerve (C8), which exits between the seventh cervical vertebrae and the first thoracic vertebrae. All other distal spinal nerves are named for the vertebrae under which they pass. For example, the fourth thoracic nerve (T4) exits between the 4th and 5th thoracic vertebrae. All spinal nerves are named in relation to their corresponding vertebrae. The spinal roots at the distal end of the spinal cord are known as the *cauda equina,* or "horse's tail," and are composed of lumbar, sacral, and coccygeal nerve roots (Figure 38–17).

The spinal nerve carries both motor and sensory information; therefore, there are two specific places in the spinal cord that this information must be synapsed in order to be integrated: (1) the sensory *dorsal root* and (2) the motor *anterior root.*

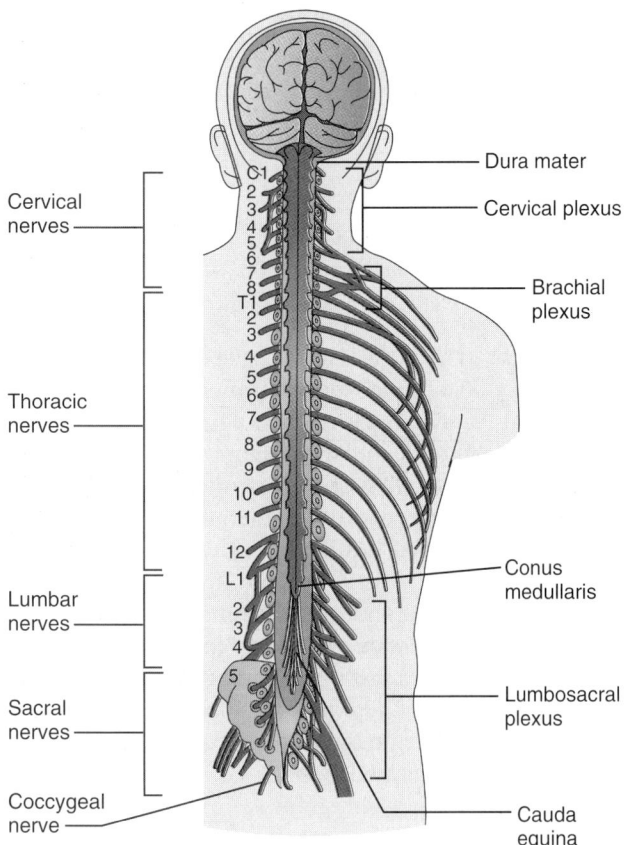

Figure 38–17

Peripheral nerves and plexuses. (Redrawn and modified from Applegate E: The Anatomy and Physiology Learning System. Philadelphia, WB Saunders, 1995, p 173.)

Dorsal (Posterior) Nerve Root. The *dorsal root* transmits sensory information from each nerve root to a specific cutaneous area on the body. These discrete areas are called *dermatomes* (Figure 38–18). Information regarding touch, temperature, pain, vibration, and proprioception is transmitted via the nerve fiber, synapsed in the *dorsal root ganglion,* and transferred to sensory tracts in the spinal cord.

Anterior Nerve Root. The *anterior roots* convey motor information from the brain and spinal cord to their associated spinal nerve. The spinal nerves innervate striated muscle for the performance of motor activities. They also innervate smooth and cardiac muscle.

Nerve Plexuses

A *nerve plexus* is formed from a grouping of individual spinal nerves that have branched and then joined other adjacent spinal nerves to form a network of fibers. This enables the nerve fibers to redistribute through the peripheral nervous system. There are four major nerve plexuses: cervical, brachial, lumbar, and sacral (see Figure 38–17; Table 38–9). Lesions of a specific plexus or part of a plexus result in motor weakness and sensory dysfunction distal to the lesion.

Peripheral Nerves

Once the nerve plexuses have branched and then joined together, this complex may give rise to a peripheral nerve (see Table 38–9). Peripheral nerves innervate specific body areas whose distributions are similar to the groupings of cutaneous dermatomes. Peripheral nerve injury may result from trauma or disease and usually results in loss of sensory and motor function in the distribution of that nerve.

Reflexes

Reflexes are involuntary motor activity in response to a sensory stimulus.[2] The simplest type of reflex is known as a *reflex arc.* A reflexive response is elicited if a sensory stimulus transmitted via the posterior root synapses with an interneuron, which then synapses with the corresponding anterior root, finally effecting a response from the responding target. Muscle stretch reflexes reflect the balance between inhibitory and excitatory fibers governing a specific muscle. A simple example of this is a muscle stretch reflex, or *deep tendon reflex,* in which a tendon is stimulated and causes an involuntary muscle contraction (Table 38–10).

Cutaneous stimulation may also produce a reflexive response known as *superficial reflexes.* Some of these reflexes can be considered protective, such as the blink and the gag reflexes.

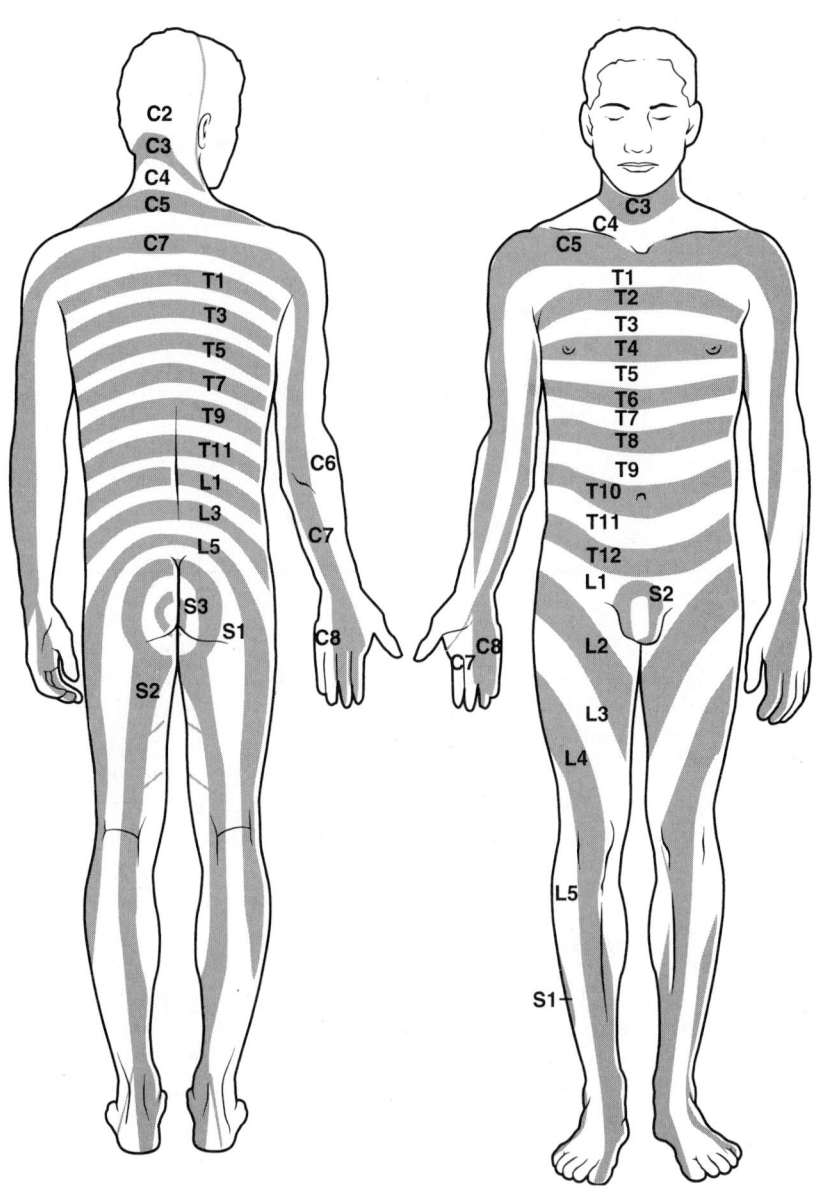

Figure 38–18

Dermatomes. (From Saunders Manual of Nursing Care. Philadelphia, WB Saunders, 1996, p 657.)

Other specialized reflexes of the body are elicited with different kinds of sensory stimuli. For example, the auditory reflex is elicited if a loud or sudden noise occurs, resulting in an automatic turning of the head toward the noise. A similar visual reflex is elicited if an object is within peripheral vision, again causing head turning toward the object. Other common reflexes include sneezing, coughing, and vomiting.

Nervous System Pathways

Sensory Pathways

The sensory pathways of the body are complex networks of nerve fibers transmitting information from skin or visceral receptors and conveying them through the peripheral nerves, nerve plexuses, spinal roots, and ultimately, to the tracts of the spinal cord in order to be relayed through and to higher centers of the brain (Figure 38–19). As the impulses ascend through this complex system, they become more modulated. Sensations perceived in the periphery include pain, temperature, crude touch (nondiscriminative), proprioception, vibration, and discriminative touch. These sensations are transmitted through two different pathways of the spinal cord: (1) the *spinothalamic tract*, and (2) the *posterior columns*.

Spinothalamic Tract. Located in the anterior aspect of the spinal cord, the *spinothalamic tract* conveys information regarding pain, temperature, and crude touch. Crude touch involves the ability to identify a touch or pressure sensation; however, there is no discriminative quality to the sensation (i.e., sharp

TABLE 38-9
Spinal Nerve Plexuses and Involved Structures

Plexus	Location	Spinal Nerves Involved	Region Supplied	Major Nerves Leaving Plexus
Cervical	Deep in the neck, under the sternocleidomastoid muscle	C1-C4	Skin and muscles of neck and shoulder; diaphragm	Phrenic
Brachial	Deep to the clavicle, between the neck and axilla	C5-C8, T1	Skin and muscles of upper extremity	Musculocutaneous Ulnar Median Radial Axillary
Lumbosacral	Lumbar region of the back	T12, L1-L5, S1-S4	Skin and muscles of lower abdominal wall, lower extremity, buttocks, external genitalia	Obturator Femoral Sciatic Pudendal

From Applegate EJ: The Anatomy and Physiology Learning System Textbook. Philadelphia, WB Saunders, 1995.

versus dull cannot be perceived). Pain pathways involve connections to effect reflex responses in addition to connections to the thalamus and the sensory cortex in the parietal lobe. Pain impulses start in the nerve endings and travel through specialized pain fibers to the dorsal (sensory) root fibers of the spinal cord, which in turn synapse with fibers of the spinothalamic tract. This tract then ascends, sending the information to the thalamus, where it is routed to the appropriate area of the sensory cortex. The spinothalamic tract carries pain information only from all parts of the body except for the face. Painful stimuli from the face are conveyed through cranial nerve V (trigeminal).

Posterior Columns. Proprioception, vibration, and discriminative touch are stimuli carried by the tracts of the *posterior columns.* Proprioception is the ability to perceive the position of a body part in space. Discriminative touch is the ability to identify two distinct points on the skin if two stimuli are simultaneously applied. This information is perceived by several specialized kinds of nerve endings, including those responsible for tactile stimulation, muscle stretch stimulation, and fibers conveying information from muscles, joints, and tendons regarding their position and activity. These impulses travel through the periph-

eral system to the spinal cord, where some fibers are involved in reflex pathways and others conduct information up the long fibers of the spinal cord. These axons extend their way through the same side of the spinal cord and cross in the medullary area. Once crossed, this impulse travels to thalamic areas, and then finally to the sensory cortex in the parietal lobe.

Motor Pathways

Motor fibers of the nervous system exert their influence on skeletal muscle to affect reflexive and voluntary motor activity. Motor impulses typically start in the motor strip of the cerebral cortex, travel via fibers in the central nervous system, and synapse to fibers in the peripheral nervous system to reach their target muscle (Figure 38–20). Fibers in the brain and spinal cord are associated with the central nervous system and are known as *upper motor neurons.* Fibers in the spinal nerves, nerve plexuses, and peripheral nerves are associated with the peripheral nervous system and are called *lower motor neurons.*

Upper Motor Neurons. Motor pathways originating in the higher centers of the cerebral cortex and the brainstem are known as *upper motor neuron* pathways. These include all motor pathway fibers in the brain and the spinal cord down to, but not including, the anterior horn of the spinal cord. The most important upper motor neuron pathway is the *corticospinal tract,* whose fibers carry voluntary motor impulse information through the spinal cord. Motor impulses start in the motor strip of the cerebral cortex, then descend through the cerebrum, where they are organized into bundles. These bundles continue to the area of the brain stem, and then cross, or decussate, in the medulla (see Figure 38–20). From here, fibers continue down the spinal cord and finally end in the anterior

TABLE 38-10
Muscle Stretch Reflexes

Muscle Stimulated	Nerve Root Involved
Biceps	C5,6
Brachioradialis	C5,6
Triceps	C6,7
Quadriceps (patellar)	L2,3,4
Gastrocnemius (ankle)	S1

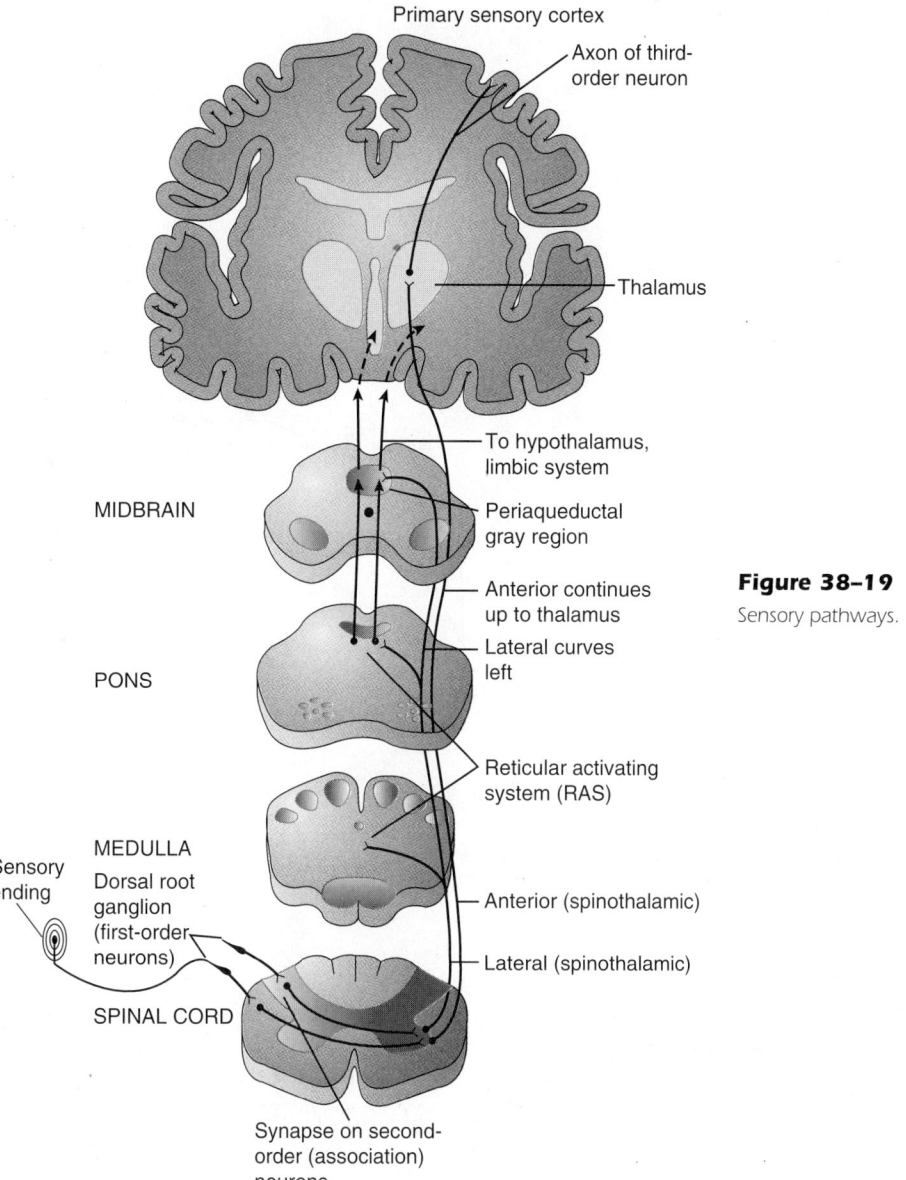

Primary sensory cortex

Axon of third-order neuron

Thalamus

To hypothalamus, limbic system

MIDBRAIN

Periaqueductal gray region

Anterior continues up to thalamus

Lateral curves left

PONS

Reticular activating system (RAS)

MEDULLA

Sensory ending

Dorsal root ganglion (first-order neurons)

Anterior (spinothalamic)

Lateral (spinothalamic)

SPINAL CORD

Synapse on second-order (association) neurons

Figure 38–19
Sensory pathways.

horn cell, where motor impulses synapse from the fibers of the upper motor neuron pathway to fibers of the lower motor neuron pathway.

Motor pathways for cranial nerve motor activity follow the *corticobulbar* tract, which starts in the motor cortex and ends in the motor nuclei of the specific cranial nerve. Lesions affecting upper motor neuron pathways result in exaggerated reflexes and spastic paralysis of the involved muscles. Typically, these involve injury to the brain and spinal cord.

Lower Motor Neurons. The *lower motor neuron* pathway begins in the anterior horn cell of the spinal cord and consists of the spinal roots, the nerve plexuses, and the peripheral nerves. Cranial nerves are also considered to be lower motor neuron pathways. Lower motor neurons play a large role in the innervation of the skeletal muscle, completing the pathway from the motor strip to the muscle, allowing for gross and fine motor activity.

Lower motor neuron lesions are usually peripheral, such as lesions to the spinal roots from a herniated disc and traumatic injuries resulting in damage to nerve plexuses. Lower motor neuron injuries result in characteristic flaccid muscle paralysis and a loss of reflexes distal to the lesion.

Autonomic Pathways

The *autonomic nervous system* governs the body's visceral responses under normal circumstances and also in times of stress. These peripheral pathways are not typically under conscious control, and their activity results in control of cardiac muscle, smooth muscle of the gastrointestinal tract, and glandular secretion.

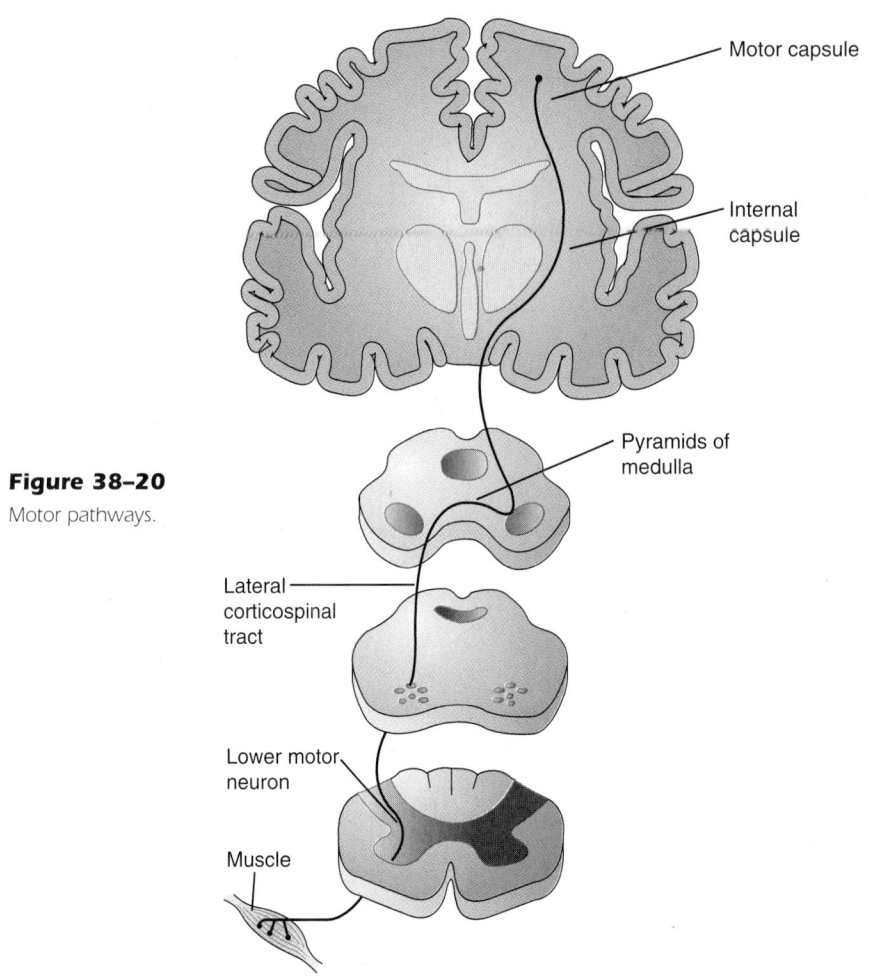

Figure 38–20

Motor pathways.

Autonomic pathways are divided into two branches: (1) the *sympathetic nervous system* and (2) the *parasympathetic nervous system*. These two systems work synergistically with each other to balance the body's responses to varied circumstances (Figure 38–21 and Table 38–11).

Sympathetic Nervous System. The *sympathetic nervous system* responds when the body is under stress.

TABLE 38–11

Characteristics of the Sympathetic and Parasympathetic Divisions of the Autonomic Nervous System

Affected Structure	Parasympathetic Stimulation	Sympathetic Stimulation
Pupil	Constricts	Dilates
Heart rate	Decreases	Increases
Cardiac contractility	Decreases	Increases
Bronchi	Constricts	Dilates
Sweat glands	—	Increases secretion
Lacrimal glands	Increases secretion	Decreases secretion
Salivary glands	Increases secretion	Decreases secretion
Peripheral arteries	—	Vasoconstricts
Coronary arteries	Dilates	Constricts
Skeletal muscle	—	Constricts, increased strength
Gastrointestinal motility	Increases	Decreases
Gastrointestinal sphincters	Relaxes	Contracts
Gallbladder	Relaxes	Contracts
Urinary bladder	Contracts	Relaxes
Adrenal medulla	—	Stimulates

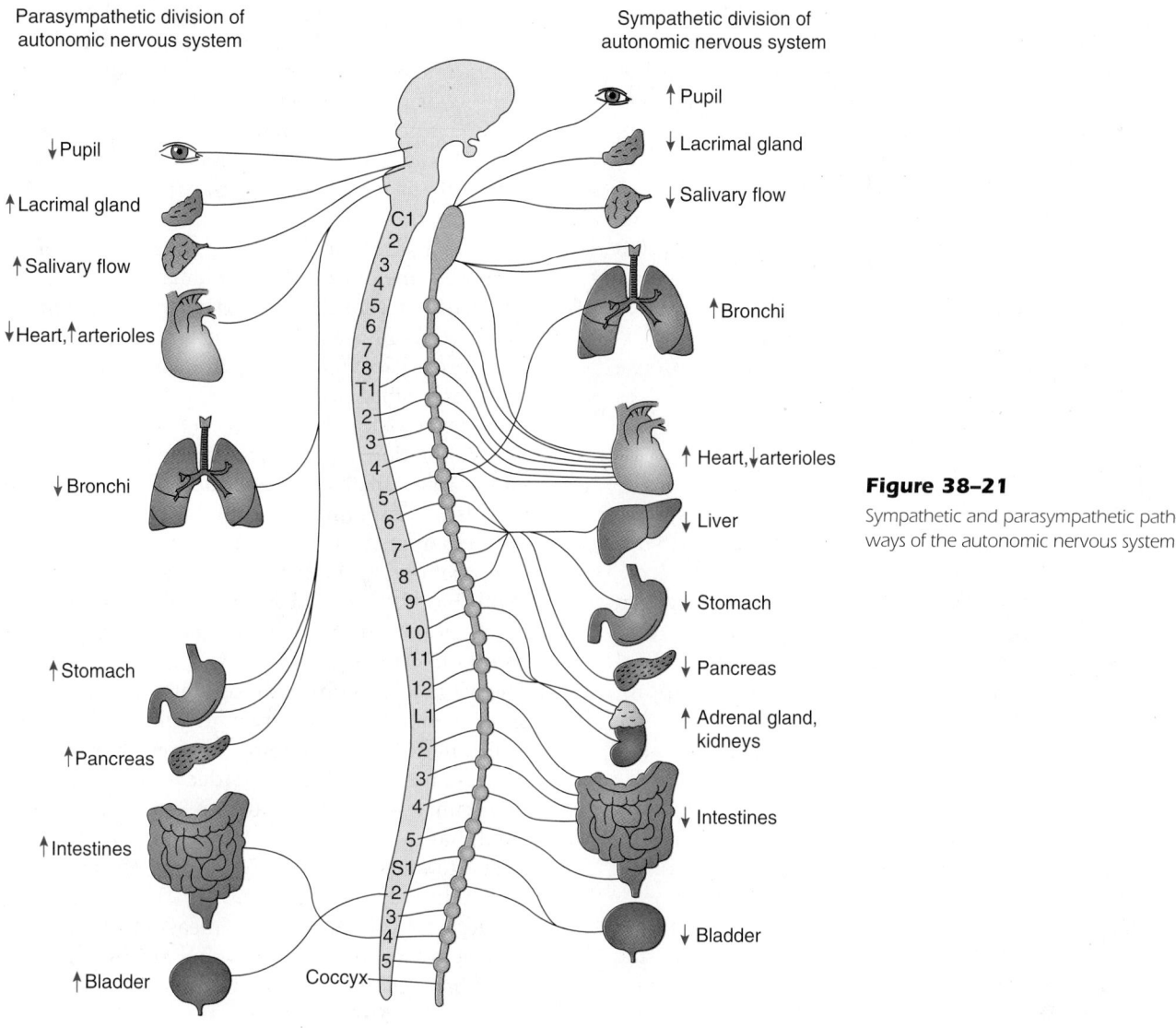

Parasympathetic division of
autonomic nervous system

↓Pupil

↑Lacrimal gland

↑Salivary flow

↓Heart,↑arterioles

↓Bronchi

↑Stomach

↑Pancreas

↑Intestines

↑Bladder

Sympathetic division of
autonomic nervous system

↑Pupil

↓Lacrimal gland

↓Salivary flow

↑Bronchi

↑Heart,↓arterioles

↓Liver

↓Stomach

↓Pancreas

↑Adrenal gland,
kidneys

↓Intestines

↓Bladder

Coccyx

Figure 38–21

Sympathetic and parasympathetic pathways of the autonomic nervous system.

This is part of the "fight or flight" mechanism. Under stress, the heart rate increases, the blood pressure increases, the pupils dilate, and the circulation is shunted to the muscles, heart, and respiratory tree, while blood is shunted away from the digestive tract.

Sympathetic fibers originate from the thoracolumbar areas of the spinal cord. Even sympathetic fibers to the head, such as those used to dilate the pupil, are mediated by upper thoracic fibers.

Parasympathetic Nervous System. The *parasympathetic nervous system* governs the body's homeostatic responses under normal circumstances. This system innervates almost all of the same organs as the sympathetic system, but it effects an entirely different response. The parasympathetic system causes the cardiac and breathing muscles to slow, the blood pressure to decrease, the pupil to constrict, and blood to be shunted to the digestive system.

Parasympathetic fibers originate from cranial and sacral nerve fibers. Cranial nerve fibers innervate the parasympathetic responses of the eye, the secretory glands, and the viscera (via the vagus nerve). Sacral fibers govern responses of the bowel and bladder.

NORMAL STRUCTURAL AND FUNCTIONAL CHANGES ASSOCIATED WITH AGING

Numerous anatomic changes occur as the body ages, and the neurologic system is no exception. Changes in the neurologic system do not necessarily mean loss of intelligence and function, however. Aging affects the nervous system in three basic ways: changes in the brain, the neurons, and the peripheral nerves.

Age-related changes in the brain are frequently manifested by cerebral atrophy and, with that, enlargement of the ventricles. There may also be an alteration in the synthesis, transmission, and metabolism of neurotransmitters. For these reasons, an elderly person may demonstrate an atypical response to increases in intracranial volume. Because of decreased brain mass, neurologic symptoms may not be exhibited until a large volume of one of the intracranial components has accumulated. Cortical deficits may impair pain perception. Neurons diminish in size, and axons degenerate as the body ages. Conduction of nerve impulses is also affected, and myelinated nerve fibers decrease with age. Supportive structures of the spine are also affected. Osteoporosis and intervertebral disc disease may result in pain and localized neurologic deficits. The sympathetic nervous system is also slowed, impairing the elderly person's response in times of stress.[2]

Key Concepts

⟹ The major structures of the nervous system include the brain, the spinal cord, and their supportive structures.

⟹ The primary functions of the nervous system include receiving, transmitting, organizing, processing, and integrating internal and external stimuli such that an individual can respond appropriately to it.

⟹ The basic elements of the nervous system consist primarily of two types of specialized cells: (1) neurons and (2) neuroglia. Neurons are involved in the transmission of nerve impulses, and the neuroglia are supportive cells that hold neurons together.

⟹ Depolarization refers to the change in the membrane potential of a neuron and results in the release of excitatory or inhibitory neurotransmitters at the synapse.

⟹ The central nervous system consists of the brain and the spinal cord. The brain is divided into the cerebrum, the diencephalon, the brain stem and the cerebellum.

⟹ The cerebrum consists of a right and a left hemisphere. Frontal, parietal, temporal, and occipital lobes are located within each hemisphere.

⟹ The diencephalon connects the cerebrum with the highest area of the brain stem, the midbrain.

⟹ The brain stem connects the higher centers of the brain with the spinal cord and is divided into the midbrain, the pons, and the medulla.

⟹ The major functions of the cerebellum include coordination, balance, and regulation of muscle tone.

⟹ The part of the skull that encloses the brain is called the cranium and consists of eight cranial bones.

⟹ The meninges, located between the skull and the brain and extending down the spinal cord, are a protective covering. The meninges are composed of the dura, the arachnoid, and the pia.

⟹ There are two potential spaces (epidural and subdural) and one actual space (subarachnoid) between the layers of the meninges. Cerebrospinal fluid (CSF), which is synthesized in the ventricles of the brain, circulates freely in the subarachnoid space.

⟹ Cerebrospinal fluid is thought to provide nourishment for the neural cells, removal of metabolites from neural tissue, and a cushion between the nervous tissue and overlying structures. CSF is generally free of cells and contains approximately 50 mg of glucose/100 mL and a trace of protein.

⟹ The blood–brain barrier is a discriminative property located exclusively in the capillaries of the brain and spinal cord that serves to protect the brain from toxic substances.

⟹ Autoregulation is a property of the cerebral circulation that dilates or constricts cerebral blood vessels to maintain a constant blood flow in spite of fluctuations in systemic blood pressure.

⟹ The relationship between the components of the skull (blood, CSF, and brain matter) can be measured, in part, by the ICP. Normal ICP in adults is zero to 15 mm Hg.

⟹ The Monro-Kellie hypothesis states that the rigid skull is filled to capacity with blood, CSF, and brain matter. If any one of these components increases, then another must decrease in order to maintain a steady intracranial pressure.

⟹ Compliance refers to the ability of the brain to adjust to small increases in volume without a resultant increase in pressure.

⟹ Intracranial pressure can be measured invasively by placing a catheter into the subarachnoid space or a fiberoptic sensor into brain matter or the subarachnoid space. Noninvasively, ICP can be measured by use of an epidural electrode.

⟹ Cerebral perfusion pressure reflects the global status of the cerebral circulatory system. CCP = MAP − ICP. CCP should be maintained at greater than 60 to 70 mm Hg.

⟹ The spinal cord is contiguous with the brain stem and acts as a highway for information from the periphery traveling to the higher centers of the brain and for information traveling from the brain to target organs, such as heart and lungs.

⟹ The vertebral column, or spine, provides protection for the spinal cord and support for the trunk of the body. The vertebral column consists of 33 vertebrae: seven cervical, 12 thoracic, five lumbar, five sacral (fused), and four coccygeal (fused).

⟹ The peripheral nervous system consists of neurons outside the brain and spinal cord and includes the cranial nerves, the spinal roots, the nerve plexuses, the peripheral nerves, and the reflexes.

⟹ The 12 pairs of cranial nerves exit primarily from the brain stem and have either motor or sensory

➡ functions. Some cranial nerves serve both functions.

➡ There are 31 pairs of spinal nerves leaving the spinal cord. These nerves retrieve sensory information from the periphery and disperse motor information to the end muscles.

➡ Dermatomes are discrete areas that transmit sensory information to the dorsal root of the spinal cord.

➡ There are four major nerve plexuses: (1) cervical, (2) brachial, (3) lumbar, and (4) sacral. These groupings of spinal nerves form networks of nerve fibers.

➡ Reflexes are involuntary motor responses to a stimulus. The deep tendon reflexes are an example of the simplest type of reflex, known as the reflex arc.

➡ The sensory nervous system pathways consist of the spinothalamic tract and the posterior columns.

➡ The spinothalamic tract is located in the anterior aspect of the spinal cord and is responsible for conveying information about pain, temperature, and touch.

➡ Sensory stimuli related to proprioception, vibration, and discriminative touch are carried by the posterior columns of the spinal cord.

➡ Upper motor neurons are located in the central nervous system. The corticospinal tract carries voluntary motor impulses through the spinal cord.

➡ The autonomic nervous system governs the body's visceral responses during normal circumstances and in times of stress. The autonomic system consists of the sympathetic and parasympathetic nervous systems.

➡ The sympathetic nervous response ("fight") includes an increase in heart rate and blood pressure, dilation of pupils, and shunting of blood to vital organs and away from nonvital organs, such as the gastrointestinal tract.

➡ The parasympathetic nervous response ("flight") includes a decrease in heart and respiratory rate, pupillary constriction, and shunting of blood to the gastrointestinal tract.

➡ Age-related changes in the brain include cerebral atrophy and ventricular enlargement. Consequently, elderly persons may demonstrate an atypical response to increases in intracranial volume; that is neurologic symptoms may not appear until a large volume of one of the intracranial components has accumulated.

➡ The response of the sympathetic nervous system slows with age and may impair the elderly person's ability to respond in times of stress.

➡ Loss of intelligence is not an expected age-related change.

References

1. Snell RS: Clinical Neuroanatomy for Medical Students, 3rd ed. Boston, Little, Brown, 1992.
2. DePace, D: Anatomy and physiology of the nervous system. In Barker, E (ed): Neuroscience Nursing. St. Louis, CV Mosby, 1994, pp 3–48.

39

Neurologic Assessment

Diane Schwenker

Objectives

After completing this chapter, the student will be able to:

1. Collect a pertinent health history from a patient or a family of a patient to identify or eliminate the possibility of a neurologic problem.
2. Differentiate the physiology of arousal and wakefulness.
3. Outline the components of a complete mental status examination for an adult.
4. Accurately use the Glasgow Coma Scale for assessing level of consciousness and central nervous system integrity.
5. Apply appropriate assessment techniques to evaluate the functioning of the 12 pairs of cranial nerves.
6. Demonstrate the evaluation and interpretation of muscle strength testing.
7. Differentiate the techniques for evaluating sensory and motor pathways in the critically ill adult.
8. Describe the impact of normal aging on neurologic function.

Neurologic assessment requires a basic understanding of the multiple neurologic pathways in the body. Components of the neurologic system include the brain, spinal cord, and peripheral nervous system. Within these components are pathways for voluntary, autonomic, and reflex activity. Observations of behavior, affect, speech patterns, memory, performance of motor tasks, response to sensory stimuli, and interpretation of sensory input indicate the integrity of the neurologic pathways. Absent or abnormal responses provide information that aids in determining which neurologic structure or pathway may be impaired. This chapter describes methods for performing a neurologic examination as well as interpreting the data from the neurologic examination. Information on conducting a neurologic examination on a conscious patient who may be acutely ill is presented first. Special considerations for conducting the examination on the unconscious patient are presented next. Neurologic tests that may be considered as the patient's condition permits are also described. Finally, the impact of aging on the neurologic system and, ultimately, on the neurologic examination is discussed.

HEALTH HISTORY

Neurologic problems can be evidenced in various body systems, with subjective symptoms originating in different locations. Review of past medical records may be helpful in providing baseline health information before the interview begins. Assistance from family, significant others, and health records may be essential in order to obtain a health history from a patient who is neurologically impaired or critically ill. Therefore, it is beneficial for the nurse to develop a systematic process for obtaining the health history. The following is an example of a process to assist the nurse in conducting a comprehensive interview.

First, the nurse should identify the patient's chief complaint. Obtaining this information in the form of a subjective statement is best. Using the acronym OLD CART as a guide, the nurse should fully explore the patient's chief complaint. Chart 39–1 gives an example of the categories and questions that should be explored.

Next, the patient's general health should be assessed with regard to any recent infections or illnesses, injuries, immunizations, or medical treatments. After

CHART 39-1

Using the OLD CART to Explore the Chief Complaint

Onset—When did the symptom(s) first begin?

Location—Where do the symptoms occur? Have the patient point to or describe the anatomic boundaries of the location of the symptoms.

Duration—How long do the symptoms last? minutes? hours? days? weeks?

Characteristics—What do the symptoms feel like? May suggest that the patient rate any pain or discomfort on a rating scale of 1–10 with 1 = minimal pain/discomfort and 10 = the worst pain the patient can imagine. Is there a pattern to the symptoms? Do the symptoms move to other locations?

Associated symptoms—What, if anything, precedes, accompanies, or follows the onset of the symptoms?

Relieving and/or exacerbating factors—Can you describe those things that relieve the symptoms? What, if anything, makes the symptoms worse?

Treatments and effects—What treatments/remedies have been tried (especially any over-the-counter medications)? Which of these have worked, and how effective have they been?

this, the nurse should explore specific symptoms or events that might suggest or rule out a neurologic problem. This line of inquiry is called a review of systems. Questions should be organized in a head-to-toe review of body systems. Table 39–1 presents areas for exploration during the review of systems that are specific for symptoms that might suggest a possible neurologic dysfunction.[1,2]

PHYSICAL EXAMINATION

Level of consciousness and mental status indicate the integrity of the cerebral hemispheres (see Chapter 38). Assessment of mental status can be divided into categories of consciousness and thought content. Consciousness is dependent on normal function of the reticular activating system, the arousal and wakefulness system in the brain. The reticular activating system is an integration of the brain stem and cerebral hemispheres that supports eye opening and attention in the awake state. Normal arousal and wakefulness are evidenced by the ability to accurately interpret and respond to en-

TABLE 39-1
Review of Systems for Neurologic Screening

System	Screening Topics
Head	Dizziness
	Headaches
	Pain
	Fainting
	Head injury
	History of stroke
Eyes	Last vision check, use of eyeglasses or contact lenses
	Changes in vision (e.g., blurred or double vision, "floaters")
	History of glaucoma, cataracts, infections
	Pain
	Redness
	Discharge
	Excessive tearing
	Sensitivity to light
	Injury
Ears	Any hearing impairment, use of hearing aid
	Discharge, blood, fluid, pus
	Pain
	Ringing, any unusual sounds
	Infections
Nose	Nosebleeds
	Infections, sinus infection
	Discharge
	Frequency of colds
	Nasal obstruction
	Injury
	Hay fever
	Changes in sense of smell
Mouth and throat	Changes in sense of taste
	Difficulty swallowing
	Last dental check, condition of teeth and gums
	Changes in voice, hoarseness
	Changes in speech, word finding, slurring
	Postnasal drip
Musculoskeletal	Weakness (paresis)
	Paralysis
	Muscle stiffness
	Limited range of motion
	Joint pain
	Arthritis
	Gout
	Back/neck problems
	Muscle cramps
	Deformities, congenital or acquired
Neurologic	Fainting
	Dizziness
	Blackouts
	Loss of memory
	Loss of consciousness
	Speech disorders

Table continued on following page

TABLE 39–1
Review of Systems for Neurologic Screening *Continued*

System	Screening Topics
Neurologic (continued)	Disorientation
	Numbness
	Tingling
	Burning
	Stroke
	Tremors
	Unsteadiness of gait
Psychiatric	Psychiatric disorders (e.g., depression, suicidal ideation, mania)
	Mood swings
	Nervousness
	Hallucinations
	General behavioral change
Social	Drug and alcohol use
	Drug reactions or allergies

vironmental stimuli; these are functions of the cerebral hemispheres. Thought content is measured by evaluation of the function of several specific areas of the cerebral hemispheres and other supratentorial structures. The use of thought content testing in combination with level of consciousness (LOC) examination results in a comprehensive evaluation of a patient's most complex levels of brain function (Chart 39–2).

The acutely ill patient may not have the energy or the LOC needed for the extensive questioning related to a full mental status examination. Tests for orientation, short-term and long-term memory, affect, posture, calculations, and general information can help the nurse formulate a general statement regarding a patient's mental status. Family interviews and review of the patient's chart for previous neurologic examinations, cognitive testing, occupational therapy assessments, or neuropsychiatric evaluations may provide valuable information for deter-mining a patient's baseline capabilities and level of function until more extensive testing can be performed.

Pupillary Reflex

Normal pupils are equal and round and constrict in response to light (reactive) or near stimulus (accommodation). The words "pupils equal, round, and reactive to light and accommodation" define the acronym PERRLA. This acronym is commonly used to document normally functioning pupils. The constrictive pupillary response involves the integration of a complete circuit of afferent sensory fibers to the cerebral cortex of the occipital lobe and brain stem, then efferent motor fibers back to the ciliary muscles of the eyeball (see Chapter 38).

The procedure for evaluating pupillary function involves several steps. In normal lighting, the nurse should make several observations of the pupils. First, the size of each pupil should be estimated by use of a visual reference for estimating pupil size. Figure 39–1 is an example of a neurologic assessment flow sheet used to document findings from neurologic checks. Eye medications, barbiturates, and age can affect pupillary size. The shape of pupil should also be

CHART 39–2

Mental Status Examination for the Conscious Patient

I. Level of consciousness: orientation to person, place, time, and events
II. Thought content
   A. Short-term memory—Ask the patient to remember 5–7 unrelated words (e.g., tunnel, basket, cat, hamburger, rain, tree, lamp) at the beginning of your evaluation. Test the patient's recall of this list later during the evaluation. Ask the patient to name the content of his or her most recent meal.
   B. Long-term memory—Long-term memory can be evaluated by asking questions about the patient's date of birth and address.
   C. Judgment—Ask the patient what he or she would you do if he or she found a checkbook with a name and address inside the front cover.
   D. Calculations—Have the patient count backward by threes, starting from a hundred.
   E. Abstract thought—Ask the patient what "a stitch in time saves nine" means?
   F. Attention—Does the patient keep pace with the interview or do you have to repeat questions or regain his or her attention?
   G. Posture—Is the patient sitting upright and midline? If not, what observations can you make about the patient's posture?
   H. Affect—Note and describe the patient's facial expression.
   I. General information—Give clues as to a current event and attempt to elicit the actual event from the patient (e.g., outcome of a recent election, an upcoming holiday).

HUP
Hospital of the
University of Pennsylvania

**NEUROLOGICAL ASSESSMENT
FLOW SHEET**

Signature / Title	Init.	Signature / Title	Init.

Dates		
Times		
Initials		

GLASGOW
- Eye Opening
- Verbal Response
- Motor Response
- Total Score

EYES
- Visual Blurring (+ or -) — R / L
- Visual Diplopia (+ or -) — R / L
- Size (See Scale) R — Size / Reaction
- Reaction L — Size / Reaction

EOM'S
- R (+ or -) — L U M D
- L (+ or -) — L U M D

Facial Droop (+ or -) — R / L

Limb Movement (See Scale)
- R — Arm / Leg
- L — Arm / Leg

OTHER

GLASGOW COMA SCALE

EYE OPENING
4 Spontaneously
3 To voice
2 To painful stimuli
   i.e., nailbed pressure,
   sternal rub, procedures
1 None

VERBAL RESPONSE
5 Oriented times three
4 Confused
3 Inappropriate words
2 Incomprehensible sounds
   i.e., moan, grumble
1 None

MOTOR RESPONSE
6 Obeys commands
   i.e., holds up 2 fingers
5 Localizing to pain
   i.e., identifies and
   attempts to remove painful
   stimulus
4 Withdrawals (pain)
3 Abnormal flexion (pain)
2 Extension (pain)
1 None

PUPIL SIZE
1 2 3 4 5 6 7 8

EXTRAOCULAR MOVEMENT

U=UP   M=Medial
D=Down   L=Lateral

LIMB MOVEMENT
5. Limb movement normal
4. Active movement against
   gravity and resistance
3. Active movement
   against gravity
2. Active movement with
   gravity eliminated
1. Minimal movement
O. No response, total paralysis
U. Unable to test strength
   of extremity

132988 6/94

Figure 39–1

Neurologic assessment flow sheet. (Courtesy of the Hospital of the University of Pennsylvania, Philadelphia.)

noted. Although normally round, one or both pupils may be oval, irregular, or keyhole in shape from eye surgery or increased intracranial pressure (ICP). Finally, the nurse should note the position of the pupil, either midline or deviated.

Next, the nurse should move a bright and focused light beam from the side of the patient's head toward the nose. The pupillary response (constriction) in that eye should be noted. Darkening the room may be helpful if pupillary constriction is difficult to see. The nurse should retest the same eye and note the pupillary response (consensual) in the unstimulated or opposite eye. Both pupils should constrict in response to stimulus in one eye. Each eye should be tested for direct and consensual responses. During this testing, the nurse should note the rate and the quality of pupillary constriction. Pupils should constrict briskly. Slow, "bouncing" (hippus), or absent pupillary reactions are abnormal findings. To test for accommodation, the nurse should move an object from arm's length toward the patient's nose. The patient's eyes should move toward the nose, and the pupils should constrict (accommodate) as the object comes closer. Abnormal pupillary reactions can be the result of injury to the eyeball itself or to any part of the sensory and motor fibers in the brain or brain stem. Damage to specific cerebral structures can be related to the type of pupillary abnormality observed (Figure 39–2).

Motor Function

Motor function should be evaluated in all four extremities as well as the neck, assuming the absence of a spinal injury. Motor strength scoring should be reviewed before the examination is performed. Figure 39–1 is an example of a neurologic assessment flow sheet used to monitor a patient's neurologic status. In the critically ill patient, limitations on mobility imposed by physician order must be respected during the examination. Proximal and distal motor strength should be evaluated. If deficits are identified in tests of proximal or distal strength, a full evaluation of each muscle group should follow. Figure 39–3 is a list of extensive muscle function tests.

The nurse evaluates neck strength by asking the patient to lift his or her head from the bed. The arms should be tested for proximal strength first at the shoulder. The nurse asks the patient to extend his or her arms as though holding a tray. The nurse, using only one arm, should apply downward pressure while asking the patient to resist. Distal strength can be tested by evaluating strength of grasp. It is advisable to offer the patient only two crossed fingers to squeeze to avoid causing discomfort to the nurse. A simple but revealing examination for upper extremity weakness is the pronator drift. The patient is requested to close the eyes and extend the arms at the level of the shoulder with palms facing up. The arms are observed for

Figure 39–2

Abnormal pupillary responses due to injury to selected cranial structures. A, Ipsilateral pupil is fixed and dilated. B, Pupils are small, equal, and reactive. C, Unilateral Horner's syndrome (small pupil with partial ptosis). D, Pupils are midposition and nonreactive. E, Pupils are small and nonreactive (pinpoint). F, Pupils are fixed and dilated.

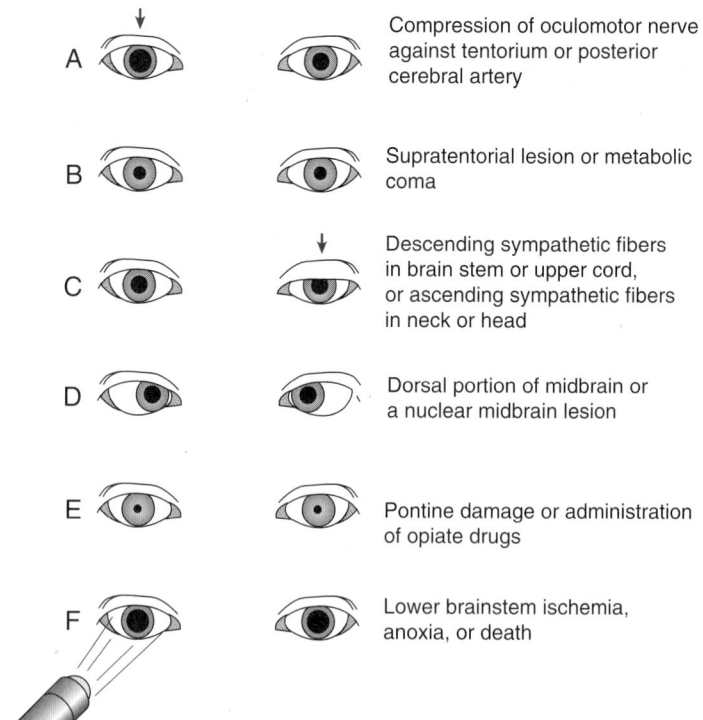

A Compression of oculomotor nerve against tentorium or posterior cerebral artery

B Supratentorial lesion or metabolic coma

C Descending sympathetic fibers in brain stem or upper cord, or ascending sympathetic fibers in neck or head

D Dorsal portion of midbrain or a nuclear midbrain lesion

E Pontine damage or administration of opiate drugs

F Lower brainstem ischemia, anoxia, or death

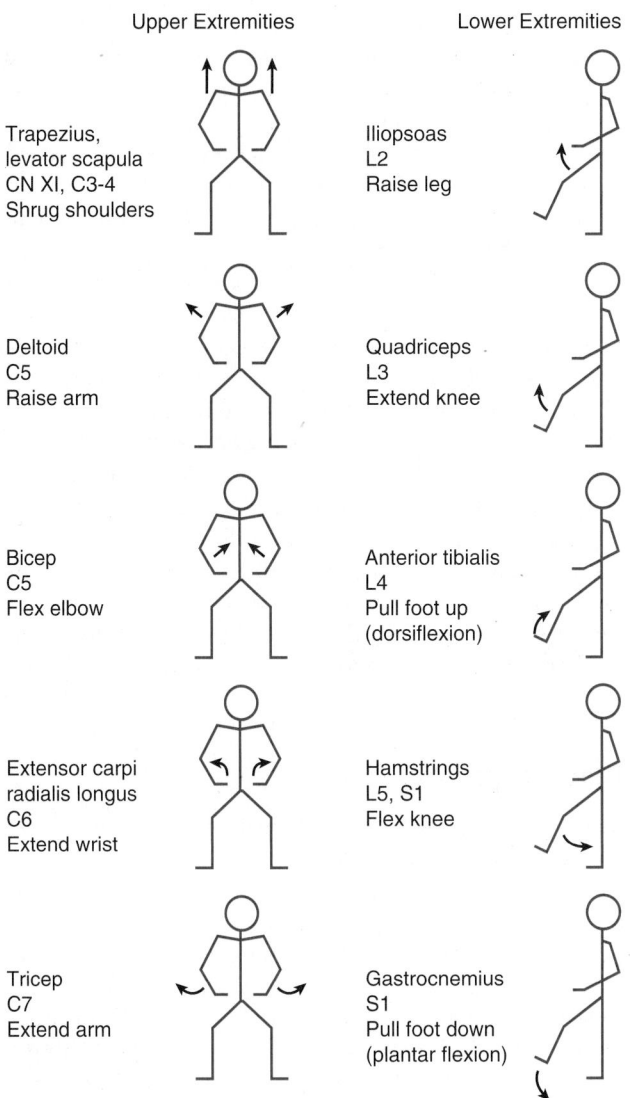

Upper Extremities

Lower Extremities

Trapezius,
levator scapula
CN XI, C3-4
Shrug shoulders

Iliopsoas
L2
Raise leg

Deltoid
C5
Raise arm

Quadriceps
L3
Extend knee

Bicep
C5
Flex elbow

Anterior tibialis
L4
Pull foot up
(dorsiflexion)

Extensor carpi
radialis longus
C6
Extend wrist

Hamstrings
L5, S1
Flex knee

Tricep
C7
Extend arm

Gastrocnemius
S1
Pull foot down
(plantar flexion)

Figure 39–3

Extensive evaluation of muscle function testing. A, Upper extremities (C3–T1). B, Lower extremities (L2–S1). (Courtesy of Phyllis Dubendorf, Drexel Hill, PA.)

drifting from the original position and for pronation of the wrists.

The legs can be tested proximally by evaluation of hip flexion, lifting the knee from a sitting position or raising the leg from a supine position. Leg raises can be difficult for patients with back or abdominal pain. Distal strength in the leg is tested by evaluating dorsiflexion and plantar flexion of the foot.

Results of strength tests should be documented by use of the same five-point objective scale each time to ensure consistent and comparable results (see Figure 39–1, Chart 39–3). The nurse should first permit the patient to independently extend and flex the muscle or muscles being tested to evaluate range of motion and ability to oppose gravity. Then, resistance is offered by the nurse to determine scores of 3, 4, and 5. To identify small versus absent movement, the muscle group being tested should be exposed. Palpation may be necessary in order to note slight movements that would receive a score of 1.

Sensory Function

In the acutely ill patient, it is possible to gain general information about the sensory function of the cerebral cortex, spinal tracts, and peripheral nerves in a simple examination of tactile sensation. After instructing the patient to close his or her eyes, the nurse should touch each side of the patient's body in corresponding locations and should ask the patient to identify the site and the quality of the stimulation. Questions such as, "Where did I touch you? Did it feel the same on each side or different?" are useful in obtaining data on sensory function. The nurse should ask the patient to further describe any unusual or painful sensations associated with the stimulus. Similar to motor strength scoring, pain assessments should use a consistent and objective rating scale. A full examination of sensory function in a medically stable patient is discussed in the section on additional neurologic tests.

Vital Signs

Ongoing assessment of the patient's vital signs can provide the nurse with important information regarding the stability of the patient's neurologic status. Changes in vital signs in the conscious patient may be

---

CHART 39–3

Motor Strength Scoring

The following scale is often used as an objective measure of motor strength:

5—normal strength, resists equally opposing force

4—offers resistance but is able to be overcome by examiner

3—able to overcome gravity, e.g., moves in a vertical plane but no resistance to examiner

2—cannot oppose gravity, moves only in horizontal plane

1—flicker of muscle movement, visible or palpable

0—no movement

Note: Range of motion measures joint mobility, and some adaptation in technique may be required in assessment of muscle strength.

the result of neuromuscular weakness, decreasing LOC, or sympathetic nervous system dysfunction. In the unconscious patient, vital sign changes may signal serious declines in neurologic function. Vital sign changes always warrant increased observation and monitoring by the nurse. Attention to the individual components of vital sign assessment is necessary in order to monitor the patient for early changes in status, to initiate appropriate interventions, and to evaluate the patient for expected outcomes.

Respiratory Patterns

In the conscious patient, abnormal respiratory patterns may indicate the need for pulmonary suctioning, repositioning, or increased monitoring. Noisy or snoring respirations should alert the nurse to a partially obstructed airway. Partial airway obstruction may be caused by a relaxation of the jaw, neck, or pharyngeal structures or may indicate an increase in respiratory muscle weakness, a decrease in LOC, and/or a decrease in the ability to maintain a clear airway. A partially obstructed airway caused by unmanageable secretions or weakness can often be corrected by coughing, suctioning, or repositioning (neck in neutral position or extension, side lying, or both). The patient at risk for airway obstruction should be observed closely for any signs of respiratory distress. For further monitoring for early signs of obstruction, continuous pulse oximetry (to measure oxygen saturation) is recommended. Arterial blood gas evaluations may be indicated if symptoms of partial airway obstruction develop or persist. Relief of partial airway obstruction is imperative to prevent hypoxia and/or hypercapnia.

Another change in respiratory pattern that may be observed in the conscious patient is apnea, or the cessation of regular breathing for some period of time. The nurse should observe the patient's respirations for a full minute, noting the movement of the chest wall and the pattern of breathing. The nurse should document respiratory rate and pattern, length of apneic periods, and any impact on vital signs or oxygen saturation. Periods of apnea may remain stable or may progress to levels that require oxygen therapy and/or airway support.

Heart Rate

Neurologically mediated irregularities in heart rate can occur as a result of increasing ICP, brain stem dysfunction, interrupted or malfunctioning sympathetic pathways, and events that increase amounts of circulating catecholamines. Increased ICP may initially cause episodes of tachycardia, and as pressure increases further, bradycardia may develop. Bradycardia is one of the three components of Cushing's triad, a late and ominous sign of neurologic injury. Stroke-related or hemorrhage-related ischemia or any injury to the brain stem may result in fluctuating heart rates or atrial dysrhythmias.

Spinal shock, caused by injury to the spinal cord above the level of T6, results in diminished or absent sympathetic activity below the level of the injury. The effect on heart rate is bradycardia. As long as blood pressure remains adequate for perfusion, treatment is often not required.

Autonomic dysfunction may occur in such neurologic diseases as Guillain-Barré syndrome. Malfunctioning sympathetic nervous system pathways often cause tachydysrhythmias (see Chapter 8). Increased amounts of catecholamines in the bloodstream may occur as a result of neurologic trauma and disease (e.g., tumor of the adrenal medulla). Increased heart rate, premature atrial contractions, and, less commonly, premature ventricular contractions may occur. Monitoring the effects of tachydysrhythmias on cardiac output and blood pressure should guide interventions.

Blood Pressure

Blood pressure is largely controlled by the medulla, the vasomotor center in the brain stem. Disruptions in blood pressure control occur whenever ischemia or injury to the vasomotor center occurs. Hypertension can occur in patients with increasing ICP. This results from the downward pressure exerted on the brain stem by the increasing intracranial volume. Continued increases in ICP may result in the classic Cushing's triad. This triad includes bradycardia in the presence of hypertension, widening pulse pressure (the difference between the systolic and the diastolic blood pressures), and irregular respirations. Usual pulse pressures do not exceed 50 mm Hg. Even in a hypertensive crisis, in which the systolic pressure may exceed 200 mm Hg, the diastolic pressure rises as well, maintaining a near-normal pulse pressure. In Cushing's triad, systolic pressure rises while diastolic pressure remains normal or low. An example might be a blood pressure of 220/70 mm Hg with a pulse pressure of 150 mm Hg. Cushing's triad is a late or preterminal sign in the patient with increasing ICP. A complete discussion of increasing ICP can be found in Chapter 41.

Autonomic dysfunction occurring in some neurologic disease states may cause hypotension if vasoconstrictive reflexes are impaired and vasodilation results. Episodes may be brief and resolve seemingly spontaneously. Persistent or recurrent hypotension may require intervention (see Chapter 47). Other causes of blood pressure instability may need to be ruled out before a neurologic cause is assumed. Continuous assessment of the perfusion of the brain and kidneys is used to guide interventions.

Temperature

Mechanisms in the central nervous system for temperature control involve central regulation from the hypothalamus and peripheral vasoconstriction and dilation. Injury to the hypothalamus may result in central nervous system fever. Central fevers may be dramatically high and resistant to antipyretic therapy.

Injury to the spinal cord resulting in decreased response to sympathetic stimulation disrupts the normal vasoconstriction needed for heat conservation; this results in indiscriminate vasodilation and subsequent heat loss. When this situation occurs, a condition known as poikilothermia, or taking on the temperature of the surrounding environment, develops.

EXAMINATION OF THE PATIENT WITH AN ALTERED LEVEL OF CONSCIOUSNESS

The neurologic examination of patients with altered LOCs presents several challenges to the nurse. Modifications in assessment techniques are necessary for accurate data regarding the neurologic status of these patients to be obtained. Figure 39–1 is an example of a flow sheet that is used to monitor the neurologic status of a patient with a real or potential altered LOC.

Level of Consciousness

Level of consciousness is the most sensitive indicator of cerebral function. Therefore, measures of LOC are important parameters in neurologic evaluation. Objective measures of LOC assist the nurse in effectively communicating the patient's condition. The Glasgow Coma Scale (GCS) is a commonly used measure of LOC (see Figure 39–1) in both conscious and unconscious patients. The scale has been found to accurately measure changes in LOC, is universally known and therefore aids in the consistent communication of a patient's condition, can easily be taught and, over time, has some value in predicting outcomes of coma.[3,4] The GCS does not critically evaluate brain stem function. Other tests, such as oculocephalic and oculovestibular reflexes, apnea tests, and perfusion studies, are necessary for evaluation of patients at very low LOCs (GCS = 3). The GCS is limited in evaluating the LOC of patients who are intubated or have swollen eyes or wired jaws. Continued research is needed to find tools that best measure changes in LOC in midranges of the GCS.[4]

If there is a risk for changing LOC, such as in stroke or head injury, and after brain surgery, accurate measurement of LOC may be critical to the patient's outcome. The LOC, rather than a change in vital signs,

is the first indicator of a developing neurologic problem. At lower LOCs (GCS < 11), it is more difficult to arouse and maintain wakefulness in a patient. Even lower LOCs (GCS < 6) are primarily mediated by the brain stem and involve less integration with the complex and refined functions of the cerebral hemispheres.

The GCS measures LOC by assigning a score to patient responses to various stimuli. Categories of responses are eye opening, verbal response, and motor response. Scores range from a low of 3 to a high of 15. The score is derived from the most complex response attainable or, differently stated, the patient's very best response. The total score reflects the level of integrity of the reticular activating system and the cerebral hemispheres. GCS scores may vary one or two points from one evaluation to another as a result of normal sleep-wake cycles. In this case, a change in scores may reflect a normal variation. Conversely, a change in score of only one point may also indicate a serious change in LOC. As with most assessment parameters, knowledge of the patient's baseline scores and pattern of responses is important in evaluating the responses subsequently observed. Additional documentation regarding the details of the patient's responses can be an important adjunct to the numeric score.

Sometimes, conditions exist that prohibit an accurate examination in one of the three categories. That category is then considered untestable. Such untestable situations are documented as "U" and are not assigned a numeric value.

Eye Opening

Eye opening is a function of arousability or wakefulness that is mediated by the reticular activating system. Impaired wakefulness, reflected by delayed or absent eye opening, is indicative of dysfunction in the reticular activating system. Dysfunctions in this system may be caused by injuries to brain tissue that result in structural disruption, ischemia, and changes in the biochemical environment. Alert and attentive behavior is a function of the cerebral hemispheres; therefore sleepiness or decreased attention may indicate impaired LOC.

A GCS of 4 (spontaneous eye opening) in this category is a sign of an intact arousal system. The patient is observed with eyes open in the presence of the nurse and with no apparent or required stimulus. A score of 3 is assigned when a verbal stimulus is required to effect eye opening. The verbal stimulus delivered should progress from a normal voice to one as loud as necessary before the next level of stimuli is assessed. Patients who are sedated or hearing impaired may require elevated tones of voice. It is important to note the level of verbal stimulus and the duration of stimulus required to wake the patient. Increased observation is indicated if the patient requires loud stimuli after previously responding to normal voice because this indicates a change in the level of stimulus required for a patient response. Such a subtle change may be an early warning of decreasing LOC. The examination should be repeated to confirm the finding, and then the finding should be reported. It is important to avoid tactile stimulation in the evaluation of response to verbal stimulus because the use of touch is another level of stimulus and may confuse scoring.

A GCS of 2 implies that a painful stimulus is required to effect eye opening. The nurse may deliver a painful stimulus in several ways. Infraorbital pressure is applied by putting a thumbtip into the notch felt at the medial aspect of the superior orbit. A sternal rub is delivered by applying the knuckles of a closed fist to the midsternum. A trapezius squeeze is delivered by compressing the belly of the trapezius muscle between the nurse's thumb and fingers. Nail bed pressure is applied with a firm instrument, such as a pencil and a pen. The instrument is placed on the fingernail at the base or where it exits the skin. Care should be taken to avoid compressing the skin of the finger because this action may cause a bruise. However, any of these tests may result in some visible bruising. The nurse should provide the patient's family with an explanation of the purpose of these tests and of the origin of any bruising that may result from these tests.

Response to painful stimuli may depend on maintaining the stimulus for 20 to 30 seconds before a patient with impaired LOC can react. Some nurses have difficulty inflicting painful stimuli. It may be helpful to remember that the purpose of this examination is to identify the earliest indication of changing LOC. Decreasing LOC usually indicates worsening of the patient's condition. Often, rapid intervention is required to protect brain tissue and to preserve the patient's level of function.

A GCS of 1 indicates the absence of eye opening, even in the presence of painful stimuli. Untestable conditions for this category may include extensive periorbital edema or eyelids that are sutured closed for corneal protection.

Verbal Response

Normal speech and orientation require a high level of cerebral integration. Changes in this category may be the first indication of deterioration. Nonverbal patients (e.g., intubated patients) may be able to be tested by use of handwritten responses, picture boards, or simple nodding of their heads or blinking of their eyes in response to questions asked by the nurse.

A GCS of 5 in this category indicates that the patient is oriented. Normal orientation consists of knowing one's name; where one is; the day, date, and time; and what one is doing in the hospital. Environment, med-

ication, and metabolic sequelae of a critical illness can affect a patient's ability to track the date and the time of day. If, on questioning, a patient is unable to recall this information completely and accurately he or she should be reoriented with the correct information. Retesting should result in recall of the correct data. Memorization of responses to orientation questions is possible, and altering the questions to require the name of the hospital one time and the name of the city or state another may help determine the difference.

A GSC of 4 is assigned to patients who are confused. For some patients, this score represents a baseline. If a patient cannot answer orientation questions accurately, a score of 4 should be conferred. Patients with a change in LOC may exhibit subtle changes in orientation.

Some patients may be able to articulate responses but the content is inappropriate as a result of impaired cognition. For these patients, a GCS of 3, indicating an inappropriate response, is assigned. Perseveration, the repetitive use of a single response, and profanity are common responses that would support a rating at this level.

A GCS of 2 is assigned to patients whose responses are incomprehensible. Grunting, mumbling, moaning, and utterances of any kind that are not able to be understood are possible responses at this level and indicate an impaired LOC.

For patients who are unable to iterate any verbal responses, a GCS of 1 is assigned. Untestable conditions for this category may include intubation or wired jaws. As mentioned previously, however, alternate forms of communication should be attempted before a U is recorded for this category.

Motor Response

Injury to a cerebral hemisphere, a spinal cord tract, a peripheral nerve, a muscle, or a bone may impair the movement of an extremity. All four extremities should be tested for motor strength to ensure that the patient's best response is observed. GCS scores describe characteristic patterns or postures indicative of levels of function in the brain. Decorticate posturing (abnormal flexion) occurs when the cortex of the cerebral hemispheres is not engaged. Decerebrate posturing (abnormal extension) indicates loss of integration with the cerebral hemispheres.

A GCS of 6 indicates that the patient follows commands. The nurse should ask the patient to hold up one finger or to wiggle the toes. This is a reliable approach to the initial examination in this category. Nurses often ask patients to "squeeze my fingers." In altered states of consciousness, patients can effect a grasp response that reflects a primitive frontal lobe reflex and not the ability to follow commands. If the patient can follow a one-step or simple command, then the nurse should follow this with a complex command (e.g., "Lift your right arm; now put it down."). The ability to follow complex commands indicates a higher level of function. Following complex commands is not reflected in GCS scoring but should be noted in the nurse's documentation.

Localization is the identification of an uncomfortable stimulus and an attempt to remove it. A GCS of 5 is assigned to this patient response. This response is dependent on observation of spontaneous movement or use of noxious stimuli to elicit a response (see the discussion of types of painful stimuli under GCS of 2 for eye opening). For example, a patient's response to a sternal rub may involve moving his or her hand to the sternal area and attempting to grasp the nurse's hand. A spontaneous movement may also qualify as localization (e.g., the purposeful removal of an endotracheal tube).

A GCS of 4 indicates withdrawal from a painful stimulus. The best test for the presence of withdrawal is nail bed pressure. Responses can be observed in each extremity. Normal withdrawal must be differentiated from flexion withdrawal.

Flexion withdrawal, or decorticate posturing, is an abnormal patient response and is assigned a GCS of 3. Flexion and internal rotation are observed at the wrist and shoulder. Lower extremities internally rotate. In the extreme situation, flexed wrists may be brought up over the chest to the chin.

Abnormal extension, or decerebrate posturing, is characterized by extension and internal rotation in the upper and the lower extremities. Extreme extension of the arms may cause the tricep muscles to bulge, even if they are not well developed. Patients demonstrating this response receive a GCS of 2.

A GCS of 1 indicates no response to painful stimuli. Untestable situations may include therapeutic immobilization of an extremity, high-level spinal cord injury, therapeutic paralysis (e.g., during mechanical ventilation), or paralysis resulting from neurologic disease in which little or no motor ability exists in the extremities (e.g., Guillain-Barré syndrome).

Pupillary Response. Patients with decreased LOC may not cooperate during an eye examination. Furthermore, it is possible, particularly with patients with encephalitis, subarachnoid hemorrhage, or increased ICP, that the patient is photophobic and that the eye examination is uncomfortable. It is important to optimize the examination conditions to ensure that the examination is completed accurately and quickly. The nurse should limit the direct lighting in the room that may cause reflections or interfere with the examination light. Dim, tangential lighting is best. The nurse should use a small beam light source for pupillary stimulation.

- Oculocephalic (doll's eye) reflex. Doll's eyes reflex is present in the comatose patient with intact brain stem function. It is imperative that the stability of the cervical spine is ensured before this examination is performed. The reflex is elicited by briskly rotating the patient's head side to side while holding the eyes open. A normal response involves the eyes initially moving in the direction opposite to the head rotation and then moving back toward midline. An absent response indicates significant brain stem injury and is demonstrated by the patient's eyes remaining in line with the position of the head (Figure 39–4).[5]

- Oculovestibular (iced water caloric) reflex. This reflex is also used to test brain stem function and may be considered for use in the patient whose cervical spine has not been fully assessed or has been determined to be unstable. The determination of an intact tympanic membrane, by use of an otoscope, is a prerequisite for this test.

  The patient is positioned supine with the neck flexed 30°. Twenty to 30 mL of ice water is expressed from a large syringe into the external auditory canal. The normal response is the slow, conjugate movement of the eyes toward the stimulated ear canal with a rapid return to midposition (Figure 39–5).[5]

Cranial Nerves. Examination of the cranial nerves (CNs) provides additional information regarding the integrity of the brain stem. Not all the CNs, however, can be tested in patients who are critically ill. The nurse must decide which CN tests are appropriate for each patient.

Cranial nerve III innervates the eyelid muscles that allow the eyes to look upward, medially, downward, and up and out. Part of the evaluation of LOC involves the identification of the stimulus that results in eye opening. When the eyes are open, the nurse should evaluate the function of the muscles operating the lid by comparing the exposed portion of the upper lid. If the lids appear unequal, there may be damage to the motor function of CN III. Whenever possible, extraocular eye movements should be assessed to further evaluate CN III, as well as CNs IV and VI (Figure 39–6).

Pupillary constriction in response to light is also under the control of CN III. See Figure 39–2 for abnormal pupillary responses caused by CN III damage.

Cranial nerve VII innervates the muscles of the face and is responsible for facial symmetry. This nerve can be evaluated in the unconscious patient during spontaneous yawning or during evaluation of a patient's response to pain when a grimace is likely to be observed. During spontaneous facial movements, it is possible to observe for asymmetry of the facial features by looking at the corners of the patient's mouth and the nasolabial folds (the facial crease extending from the side of the nose to the corner of the mouth).

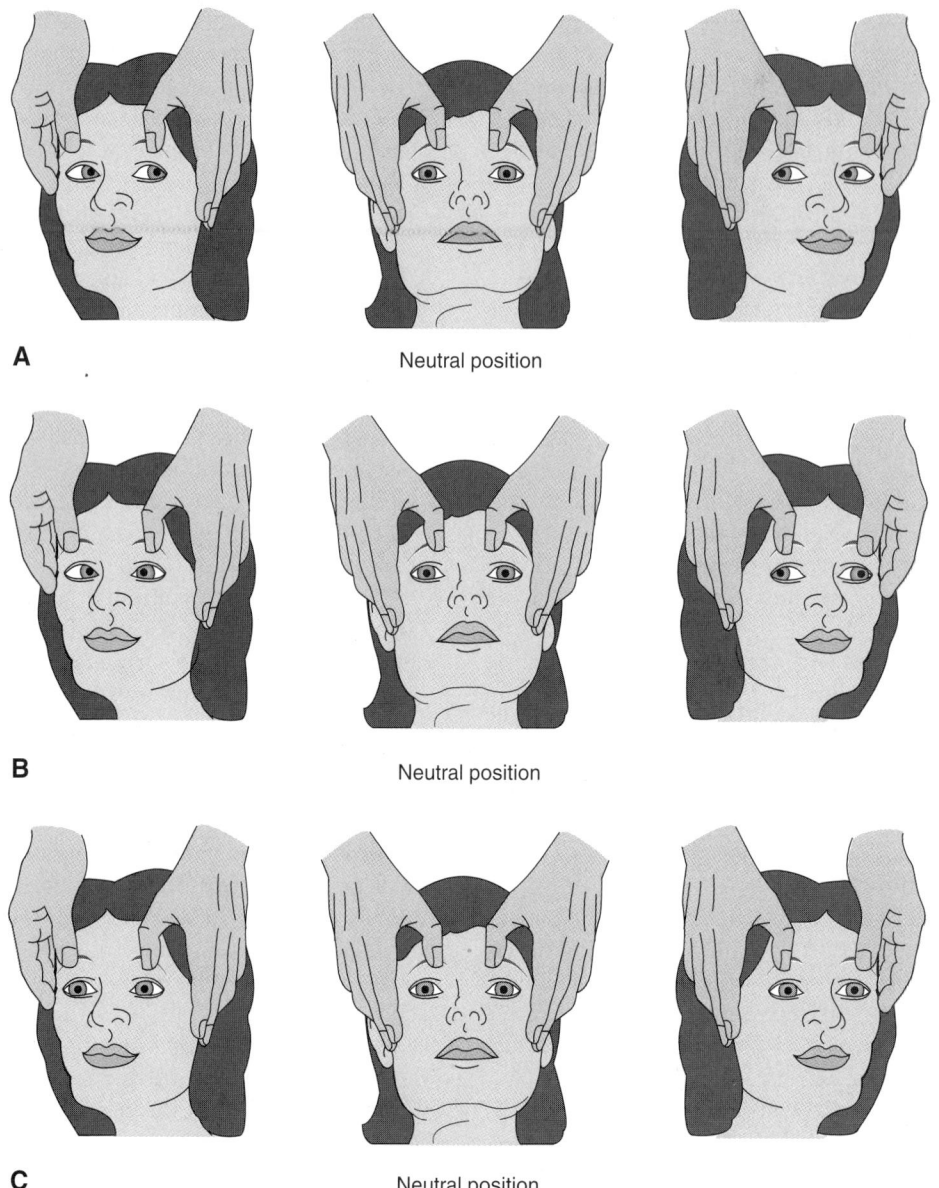

Figure 39–4

Oculocephalic (doll's eye) reflex. A, Normal response. B, Abnormal response indicating some degree of brain stem injury. C, Absent response.

On the affected side of the patient's face, the corner of the mouth droops, and there is flattening or less definition of the nasolabial fold. The normally functioning side of the face may appear abnormal when compared with the serene appearance of the impaired side (see Figure 39–1).

Protective Reflexes. The corneal, cough, and gag reflexes are described as protective reflexes because they serve to guard the patient from certain physiologic dangers.

- *Corneal reflex.* CNs V and VII are responsible for the corneal reflex. This reflex protects the eye by closing the eyelid in the presence of a stimulus. To test for this reflex, the nurse should stimulate the patient's cornea with a wisp of sterile cotton or a sterile eye drop. This should result in the simultaneous and complete closure of the eyelids. The stimulus reception for this reflex is mediated by the afferent fibers of CN V and the response by CN VII. Absence of this reflex indicates the need for protection of the cornea on the affected side.

- *Cough and gag reflexes.* These reflexes are primarily responsible for protecting the patient's airway and are under the control of CNs V, IX, and X. The gag reflex should occur in response to the stimulation of the patient's posterior pharynx or posterior one-third of the tongue. The cough reflex should occur with stimulation of the trachea during suctioning or during movement of a tracheal airway device. Absence of these reflexes indicates profound decreased LOC and potential for aspiration. Observa-

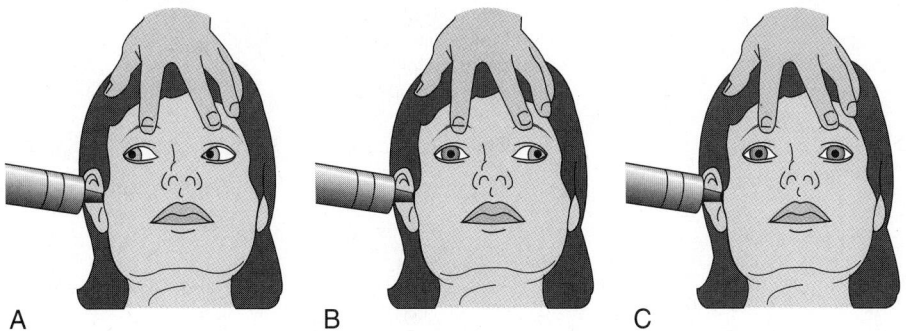

Figure 39–5

Oculovestibular (iced water caloric) reflex. *A,* Normal response. *B,* Abnormal response (dysconjugate eye movement) indicating brain stem injury. *C,* Absent response, indicating significant brain stem injury.

tion for these reflexes can be made whenever these anatomic regions are stimulated (e.g., oral care with a swab, tracheal suctioning, placement of an endotracheal or nasotracheal tube, placement of an orogastric or nasogastric tube).

Evaluation of Vital Signs

As with the conscious patient, the frequent assessment of the vital signs of the unconscious patient can provide the nurse with critical data regarding changes in neurologic status. For any patient with an altered LOC, it is extremely important for the nurse to assess the patient's pattern of respirations for a full minute. Any change in the unconscious patient's respiratory pattern should prompt the nurse to initiate a full neurologic assessment. Abnormal respiratory patterns in the unconscious patient may provide information about specific locations of lesions or injured areas of the brain (Figure 39–7).

Fluctuations in heart rate and development of atrial dysrhythmias may indicate vasomotor instability secondary to increasing ICP in the unconscious patient. These observations should also alert the nurse to increase the frequency and the depth of neurologic evaluations.

Cushing's Triad

As mentioned earlier, irregular respirations are one of the components of Cushing's triad—a syndrome seen only in unconscious patients. This syndrome consists of bradycardia with systolic hypertension, a widening pulse pressure, and irregular respirations. Cushing's triad reflects increasing brain stem ischemia and is possibly a terminal sign of increased ICP.

ADDITIONAL NEUROLOGIC TESTS

The neurologic examination discussed here requires more wakefulness, strength, and mobility than may be available in the critically ill patient. For the patient who is able to perform the following tests, critical information about specific areas of the nervous system can be obtained.

Mental Status Examination

This examination provides valuable information about attention, memory, and cognition. It is important to tailor this examination to the patient's language and

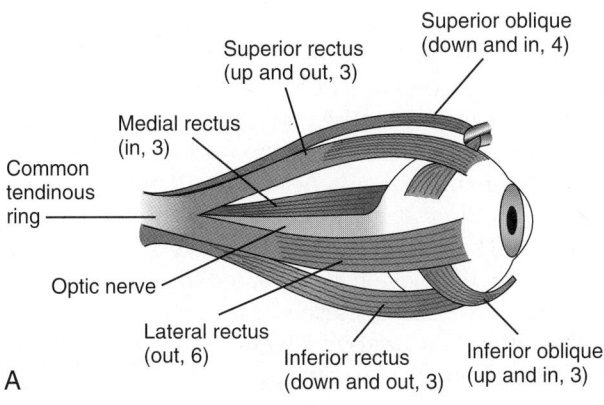

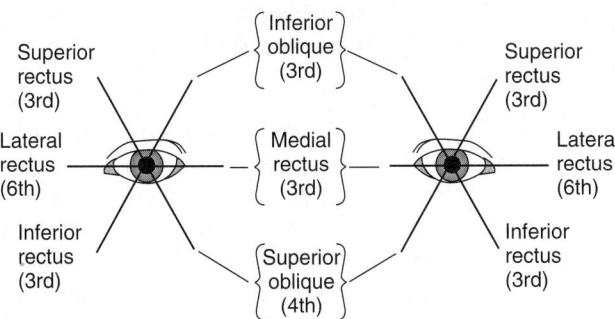

Figure 39–6

Cranial nerve function relative to eye movement. *A,* Extraocular muscles and associated cranial nerve supply. *B,* Six cardinal fields of vision.

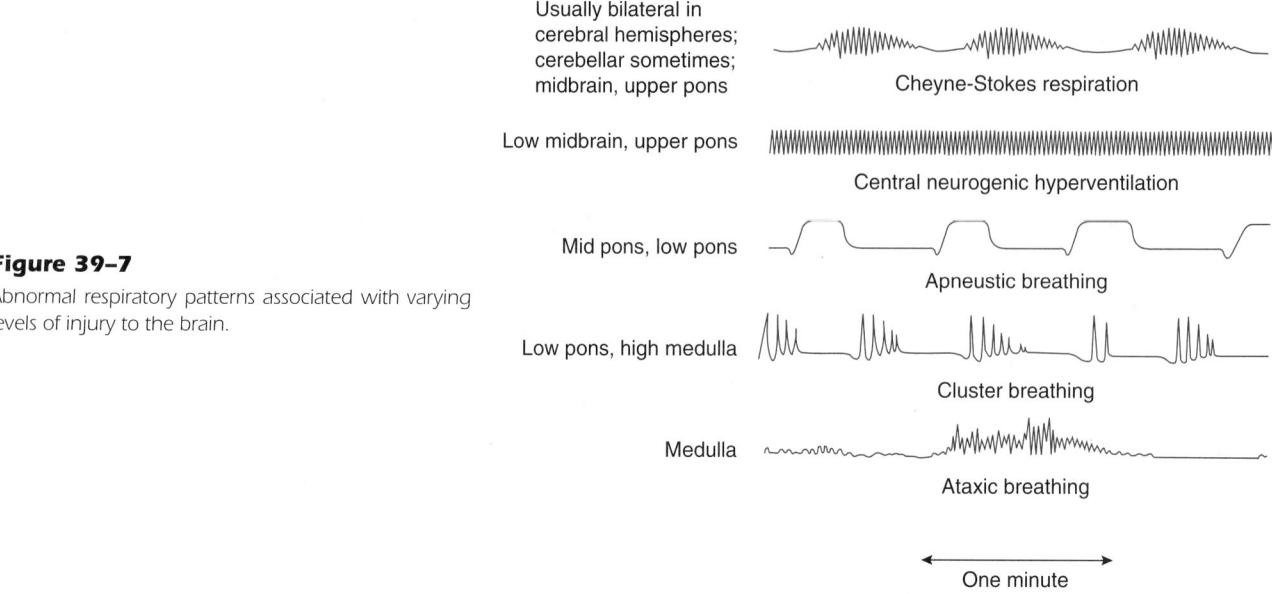

Figure 39-7

Abnormal respiratory patterns associated with varying levels of injury to the brain.

Usually bilateral in cerebral hemispheres; cerebellar sometimes; midbrain, upper pons — Cheyne-Stokes respiration

Low midbrain, upper pons — Central neurogenic hyperventilation

Mid pons, low pons — Apneustic breathing

Low pons, high medulla — Cluster breathing

Medulla — Ataxic breathing

One minute

education level to gain the best information and to avoid discomfort for the patient (see earlier discussion and Chart 39-2).

Cranial Nerve Testing

All cranial nerves should be tested in the conscious patient for a full assessment of brain stem and cerebral function.[6] Some aspects of cranial nerve function are not routinely tested, but these are mentioned here as a matter of information.

Olfactory (Cranial Nerve I)

Cranial nerve I is assessed by stimulating each nostril with a potent scent, such as coffee, vanilla extract, cinnamon, and scented soap. These substances can be carried in sealed tubes or canisters. Volatile substances or small particles should not be used so that eye irritation or inhalation of the sample is avoided. A decreased or altered sense of smell may indicate a lesion in the base of the anterior skull, where nasal receptors are located; a lesion along the olfactory tract to the brain stem; or a lesion from a generalized head injury.

Optic: (Cranial Nerve II)

Cranial nerve II is assessed by evaluation of visual acuity and visual fields. The nurse should have the patient hold normal-sized printed material at a bent arm's length (approximately 14 inches), and the patient should be able to be read with any usual corrections (e.g., glasses and contact lenses). Each eye is assessed independently. A full evaluation using a Snellen chart results in the quantification of visual acuity with the familiar 20/20 to 5/200 scale. Severely diminished vision is assessed by holding fingers up in the patient's line of vision and asking for a count, or, in the worst case, asking the patient to identify the presence or absence of a light source. Visual acuity changes, such as blurring and diplopia, can occur with trauma, tumors, and vascular abnormalities as a result of optic nerve involvement and should be monitored (see Figure 39-1).

Visual fields are tested by confrontation, one eye at a time. The nurse covers his or her eye opposite to the patient's covered eye. From a distance of 3 feet, the nurse moves one or two fingers on each hand from each side of the patient's head toward the face. The fingers should be seen simultaneously by the patient and nurse. The patient is asked to report the number of fingers seen, thus vision is evaluated in each half of an upper or lower field. Various optic nerve–mediated abnormalities can exist and include blindness, hemianopsia, and quadrantic defects (Figure 39-8).

Oculomotor (Cranial Nerve III), Trochlear (Cranial Nerve IV), and Abducens (Cranial Nerve VI)

These three CNs are evaluated together because they control extraocular movements of the eyes. The eyes are evaluated for conjugate movement in each of the six cardinal fields of gaze. Eyes are also tested individually in the six cardinal fields of vision: lateral, out and up, in and up, medial, down and in, and down and out (see Figures 39-1 and 39-6).

Cranial nerve III also controls pupillary constriction and eyelid elevation. See earlier discussion for complete testing of the pupillary reflex and eyelid movement.

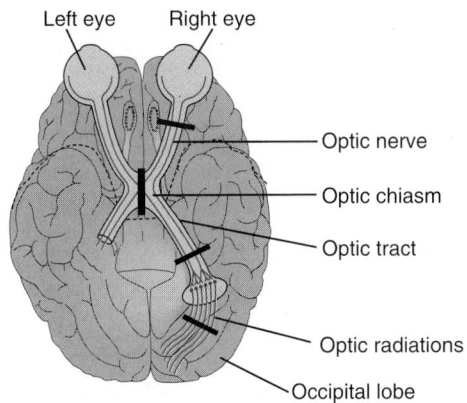

Left eye   Right eye

Optic nerve

Optic chiasm

Optic tract

Optic radiations

Occipital lobe

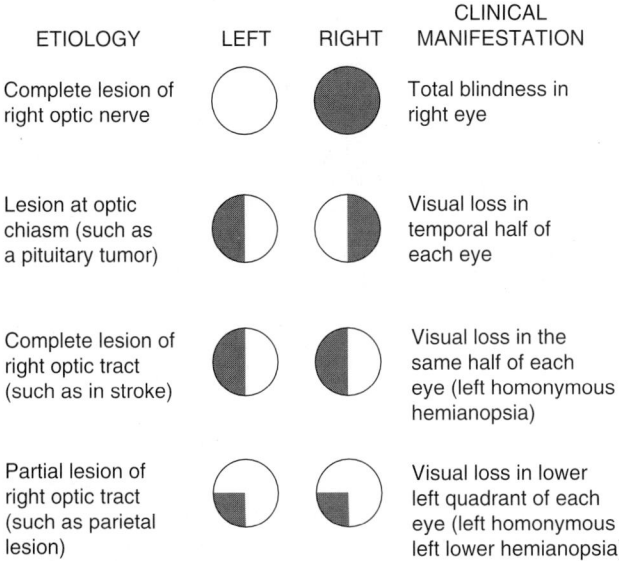

ETIOLOGY	LEFT	RIGHT	CLINICAL MANIFESTATION
Complete lesion of right optic nerve			Total blindness in right eye
Lesion at optic chiasm (such as a pituitary tumor)			Visual loss in temporal half of each eye
Complete lesion of right optic tract (such as in stroke)			Visual loss in the same half of each eye (left homonymous hemianopsia)
Partial lesion of right optic tract (such as parietal lesion)			Visual loss in lower left quadrant of each eye (left homonymous left lower hemianopsia)

Figure 39–8

Visual field defects produced by selected lesions in the visual pathways.

Trigeminal (Cranial Nerve V)

Cranial nerve V is assessed by evaluating the patient's facial sensation, corneal reflex, and ability to chew food. Sensation is tested along three branches of the nerve. With the patient's eyes closed, the nurse should run a wisp of cotton across the most anterior aspect of the nose to the eyebrow and forehead; the upper lip, the lateral aspect of the nose to cheek, and the temporal area of the face; and the lower lip, the chin, and the area of face anterior to the ear. The patient is asked to identify touch and compare sensations on each side of the face. Muscles used for chewing can be evaluated one side at a time by having the patient clench his or her teeth on a tongue blade and then attempting to remove the blade from each side.

Facial (Cranial Nerve VII)

Cranial nerve VII is evaluated by observing for symmetry in expressions and testing strength of muscles on each side of the face. The nurse should observe the patient wrinkle his or her forehead and exaggerate a smile. Resistance testing should be performed on each side by having the patient puff out his or her cheeks while the nurse applies mild pressure.

Cranial nerve VII also provides for taste on the anterior two-thirds of the tongue. This function can be tested by applying small amounts of salt or sugar grains to this portion of the patient's tongue and asking him or her to identify the taste.

Acoustic (Cranial Nerve VIII)

Cranial nerve VIII is assessed by evaluating the patient's hearing acuity in each ear. To evaluate gross hearing, the nurse should whisper into a cupped hand, testing one ear at a time. The Weber and Rinne tests are performed to evaluate air and bone conduction capabilities. CN VIII is also responsible for balance and position sense.

Glossopharyngeal (Cranial Nerve IX) and Vagus (Cranial Nerve X)

Assessment of these CNs involves stimulating the posterior tongue or the posterior pharynx on each side with a tongue blade to elicit a gag reflex or observing symmetric elevation of the soft palate on utterance of and "ahh."

The vagus nerve also supplies parasympathetic nerve fibers to the organs of the thorax and abdomen and provides motor functions for speech and swallowing and most of the sensory functions in the external ear canal.

Spinal Accessory (Cranial Nerve XI)

Cranial nerve XI is evaluated by requesting the patient to turn his or her head to the side against the resistance of the nurse's hand. This tests the motor function of the sternocleidomastoid muscle.

Hypoglossal (Cranial Nerve XII)

Tongue strength is evaluated by observing for deviation from the midline position when the patient protrudes his or her tongue. Deviations occur toward the weak side and may also indicate problems with swallowing or speech.

Evaluation of Sensation

Sensory function is determined by intact tracts of the spinal cord and peripheral nerves and accurate interpretation of transmitted information primarily in the temporal and parietal lobes of the brain. As previously discussed, sensory function is tested during the examination of the cranial nerves. Peripheral nerve stimulation tests complete the sensory examination. Peripheral sites are tested for pain, temperature, touch, position, and vibration.

All sensation is tested in corresponding locations on each side of the body in a head-to-toe direction. The characteristics and patterns of sensory changes help define the structures involved. Parietal and temporal lobe dysfunctions are characterized by altered perceptions in two-point discrimination, tactile localization, stereognosis, and graphesthesia.[2]

Spinal nerves have well-delineated anatomic boundaries illustrated in the dermatome figure (see Figure 38–18). Sensory changes along those boundaries imply injury to specific nerve roots. Deficits in sensing pain, temperature, or light touch involve the corticospinal tracts of the spinal cord. Deep pressure, proprioception, and vibration are communicated via the dorsal column. Injury to a peripheral nerve results in sensory or motor deficits or pain specific to the distribution of the nerve. The following tests are commonly used to assess sensation in patients.

Light Touch

The nurse assesses light touch by first asking the patient to close his or her eyes. The nurse, using a wisp of cotton, tissue, or gauze, lightly touches the patient's exposed skin. The patient is instructed to report when the stimulus is sensed.

Discrimination

Discrimination relates to the patient's ability to distinguish between sharp and dull. Using a cotton applicator or a broken tongue blade, the nurse randomly applies the sharp or dull end of the instrument, asking the patient to identify the sensation. Discrimination between hot and cold can also be tested by use of specimen cups or tubes filled with warm and cold water.

Proprioception

Proprioception is tested by asking the patient to report the position of a finger or toe. With the patient's eyes closed, the nurse should take the patient's hand and move the index finger up or down. The patient is asked to report the position of the finger. The same examination is performed on the opposite hand and on the feet, using the great toe.

Vibration

Vibration is tested by holding a vibrating tuning fork on a bony prominence and asking patient to report when vibration is sensed.

Tactile Localization

Tactile localization is tested with the patient's eyes closed. A peripheral site is stroked in different locations on each side of the body. The nurse then asks the patient to identify each site.

Stereognosis

Stereognosis refers to the ability of the patient to identify an object by touch. Items that are commonly used are keys and paper clips. With the patient's eyes closed, the nurse places the object selected in the patient's palm and asks him or her to identify the object. The opposite hand should be tested with a different object.

Graphesthesia

Similar to stereognosis, graphesthesia is the ability of the patient to identify a number drawn in the palm. With the patient's eyes closed, the nurse draws a single digit number in the patient's palm and asks him or her to identify the number. Both palms should be tested, with a different number in each palm.

Evaluation of Motor Function

When you ask a patient to perform a voluntary motor action you are testing the integrity of the somatic nervous system. To perform a complete motor assessment, it is helpful to have the patient sitting upright and facing the nurse. With many of the limitations of acute illness, it is often difficult to have a patient accurately demonstrate muscle strength (see Figure 39–3 and Chart 39–3).

The functions of the autonomic nervous system include peripheral vasoconstriction, pilomotor function, sphincter control, glandular secretion, and peristalsis. Certain neurologic diseases and spinal nerve injuries can alter function of the autonomic functions.

Fine motor function and balance are coordinated by the cerebellum. To assess these, the following examinations are performed on each side of the body and evaluate accuracy, rapidity, and fluidity of movement.

Finger-to-Nose Test

The nurse should hold a finger up at arm's length from patient. The patient is instructed alternately touch the nurse's finger and then his or her own nose. The patient should be able to repeat this sequence several times.

Heel-to-Knee Test

With the patient in a supine or sitting position, the nurse should instruct him or her to move the heel of one foot to the knee of the opposite foot and slide the heel down the anterior aspect of the opposite leg. The patient should be asked to perform this movement bilaterally.

Rapid Alternating Movement

The nurse should place the patient in a sitting position. The patient should be instructed to rapidly pronate and supinate his or her hand, tapping the thigh on the same side with each movement. This should be repeated several times and as quickly as possible. The nurse should compare one side with the other. The patient's movements should be quick and fluid.

Romberg Test

The patient should be instructed to stand with his or her eyes closed and arms extended from the sides. Without touching the patient, the nurse should place his or her arms under the patient's to prevent the patient from falling. The patient may demonstrate a slight sway but should be able to maintain this position without falling.

Gait Evaluation

A normal gait is a rolling movement from heel to toe with a fluid shifting of weight from one foot to the other. This is accompanied by a smooth swing of the arms from the shoulder with the forward arm and leg opposite to each other. Gait disturbances may be indications of central or peripheral nerve injury. Further evaluation should be performed if an abnormal gait is observed. In addition, the patient should be observed using any assistive devices, such as a walker and a cane.

Reflexes

Peripheral deep tendon reflex testing elicits information about the integrity of nerve pathways to the spinal cord and back to the stimulated area. A reflex hammer is used to stimulate the biceps, brachioradialis, patellar, and Achilles tendons bilaterally. Reflexes are graded from 0 (absent) to +4 (hyperactive). Normal reflexes are graded +2 (Figure 39–9).[7]

In order to elicit the biceps reflex, the biceps tendon is palpated at the medial aspect of the arm. The nurse should support the patient's arm and stimulate the tendon while observing for bicep contraction and the resultant elbow flexion.

The brachioradialis reflex is tested by first locating the brachioradialis tendon, which is proximal to the styloid process (lateral aspect) of the wrist. The nurse should observe for supination of the hand when this tendon is stimulated.

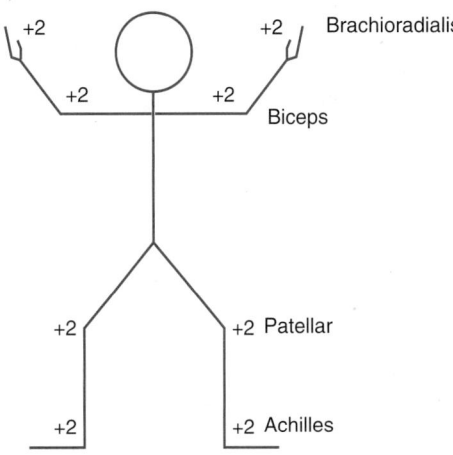

Figure 39–9
Deep tendon reflexes.

The patellar tendon is located just under the patella. The patient should be seated with his or her lower legs swinging freely or supported under the knee. Stimulation of this tendon results in contraction of the quadricep muscle and extension of the knee. While the patient is still in this position, the nurse should locate the patient's Achilles tendon, which is just above the heel at the ankle. Stimulation of this tendon results in plantar flexion.

The Babinski reflex is a pathologic reflex; that is, it is always abnormal when it occurs in an adult. To check for a Babinski reflex, the nurse should stimulate the lateral aspect of the patient's foot from the heel to the ball of the foot by use of a firm instrument, such as the handle of a reflex hammer. Normally, plantar flexion of the great toe is observed, and the Babinski reflex is negative. If dorsiflexion of the great toe and fanning of the remaining toes occur, the patient is said to have a positive Babinski reflex.

EFFECTS OF AGING ON THE NERVOUS SYSTEM

Some decline in sensory and motor function is expected with age, but this expectation may mask conditions that require treatment. Sensory deficits may exist as a result of diminishing number of cells or as a result of pathologic processes that are more common in the aged. It is important to differentiate between effects of aging and a treatable pathology. Screening for vision and hearing problems during the physical examination may help to identify treatable problems.

Age-associated changes in the neurologic system bring an increased risk for Parkinson's disease, stroke, and dementia.[8] It is more likely that the nurse can associate dementia with a cause if careful questioning about the nature and the progression of symptoms occurs during the taking of the patient's history. Many causes of dementia are amenable to treatment.

TABLE 39-2

Normal Aging: Effects on the Nervous System

System	Effects of Aging
General	Decreased brain size causing traction on bridging veins and increasing risk for subdural hemorrhage secondary to trauma
	Decreased number of functional neurons
	Decreased vibratory and position sense in lower extremities
	Decreased two-point discrimination
	Decreased reflexes and reaction times
	Increased sleep disturbances, decreasing rapid eye movement and stage 4 sleep
	Degenerative connective tissue and bone may increase risk for spinal compression
	Significant risk for depression
	Increased risk for stroke, Parkinson's disease, and dementia
Vision	Presbyopia (decreased near vision)
	Arcus senilus (opaque white ring around the periphery of the cornea)
	Cataracts
	Smaller, less reactive pupils
	Slower adaptation to darkness
	Decreased color discrimination (especially between blue and green)
	Decreased upward and downward gaze
Hearing	Presbycusis
	Deterioration of hair and bone
	Loss of "f," "s," "th," "ch," "sh" sounds
Taste	Decreased number of taste buds
	Xerostomia (decreased saliva production by one-third)
	Atrophy of the oral mucosa
Motor function	Overall strength decreases by 10–45% as a result of loss of motor cortex and spinal cord tracts for motor function
	Decreased velocity of peripheral nerve conduction
	Loss of total number of muscle cells
	Decreased number and bulk of muscle fibers
	Stooped posture related to degeneration of intervertebral discs
	Short, shuffling gait with loss of arm swing on walking
	Decreased dorsiflexion of foot

Depression and alcoholism are occurring with increasing frequency in the elderly population, and therefore screening questions for these problems should also be included in the history. Table 39–2 gives additional information about the physiologic changes that are associated with the normal aging process.[9]

Key Concepts

⟹ Arousal is a function of the reticular activating system and is a component of consciousness that allows all sensory systems to be "on alert."

⟹ The Glasgow Coma Scale (GCS) is used to measure arousal by evaluating eye opening. Arousal becomes impaired when level of consciousness (LOC) is decreased.

⟹ The cranial nerves are a set of 12 nerves that control a combination of sensory and motor functions in the head and neck. Brain or brain stem injury can temporarily or permanently affect the function of these nerves.

⟹ Normal LOC, or awareness, integrates the function of the peripheral nervous system with the brain stem and the cerebral hemispheres. The functional assessment of this integration relates to the ability of the patient to interpret sensory input and to formulate an appropriate response.

⟹ The assessment of mental status reflects the integrity of all brain functions. Tools that evaluate orientation, mood or affect, attention and concentration, thought content for judgment and abstract reasoning, ability to calculate, and memory test the functions that comprise mental status.

⟹ In the assessment of a patient for sensory and motor functions, it is important that all extremities are tested. Comparisons are made between right and left sides and upper and lower extremities. Assessment of the sensory and motor functions of the face should also be performed bilaterally.

⟹ Wakefulness is determined by an intact and integrated central nervous system. "Awake and alert" or "wakes easily" are terms commonly used to describe a normal LOC.

➡ Aging does involve a decline in sensory and motor functions. It is important that this expectation not mask underlying conditions that could require treatment.

References

1. Bates B: A Pocket Guide to Physical Exam and History Taking, 2nd ed. Philadelphia, JB Lippincott, 1995, pp 6–8.
2. Swartz MH: Textbook of Physical Diagnosis: History and Examination. Philadelphia, WB Saunders, 1989, pp 22–23.
3. Juarez VJ, Lyons M: Interrater reliability of the Glasgow coma scale. J Neurosci Nurs 25:283–286, 1995.
4. Segatore M, Way C: The Glasgow coma scale: time for a change. Heart Lung 21:548–557, 1992.
5. Hickey JV (ed): Neurological and Neurosurgical Nursing, 4th ed. Philadelphia, JB Lippincott, 1997.
6. Geary S: Nursing management of cranial nerve dysfunction. J Neurosci Nurs 27:102–108, 1995.
7. Jarvis C: Physical Examination and Health Assessment. Philadelphia, WB Saunders, 1992.
8. Cassel C (ed): Geriatric Medicine. New York, Springer-Verlag, 1997.
9. Barclay L, Wolfson L (eds): Clinical Geriatric Neurology. Philadelphia, Lea & Febiger, 1993.

40

Neurodiagnostic Tests and Procedures

Jane C. Van Tatenhove and Carleen B. Kelley

Objectives

After completing this chapter, the student will be able to:

1. Compare the preprocedure and postprocedure nursing care for common radiologic procedures used to diagnose neurologic problems.
2. Describe the purpose and the significance of Doppler and electrophysiologic studies for the patient with neurologic problems.
3. Formulate appropriate patient teaching plans for patients undergoing various neurologic tests.
4. Differentiate the purpose and the physiologic principles of intracranial pressure monitoring.
5. Identify indications and contraindications for intracranial pressure monitoring.
6. Compare and contrast the various methods used to measure intracranial pressure.
7. Select appropriate troubleshooting interventions for intracranial pressure monitoring systems.

Historically, in order to study the central nervous system, indirect techniques were developed to overcome the brain's complexity and inaccessibility. Early techniques, such as lumbar puncture (LP), plain radiography, pneumoencephalography, and electroencephalography (EEG), have been replaced by more direct visualization and measurement methods, such as computed tomography (CT), angiography, magnetic resonance imaging (MRI), and intracranial pressure (ICP) monitoring. These methods are so impressive that there may be a temptation to substitute them for a careful, detailed history and physical assessment. However, a thorough clinical assessment along with an understanding of the neurodiagnostic procedures is essential to a complete assessment.

RADIOLOGIC PROCEDURES

Skull Radiographs

In the past, plain films of the skull were considered a routine part of the study of the neurologic patient. CT and MRI have increased the ability to visualize pathol-

ogy and have greatly eliminated the need for skull x-ray studies.[1]

Although limited in general use, skull x-ray studies may still be used to identify the following: tumors of the skull, foreign bodies (especially metal objects before MRI), calcified brain lesions, skull fractures, and bone erosion.[2]

Skull films usually include anteroposterior and lateral views (Figure 40–1). Certain landmarks are identified to determine the presence of a pathologic condition. For example, fractures greater than 0.5 cm are often associated with cerebral contusions, and most depressed skull fractures require surgical débridement. Many fractures of the skull and face may result in pneumocephalus. In addition, the pineal body, which is normally calcified in the adult, is a midline structure. If it appears to be skewed to one side, pressure from a space-occupying lesion may be responsible for the deviation.[3] Figure 40–1 shows a bullet wound to the head with fragments throughout the cerebrum.

Skull x-ray studies are relatively painless. Other than ensuring that the patient lie still for the brief time necessary to take the films, there is no preparation or postprocedure care required.

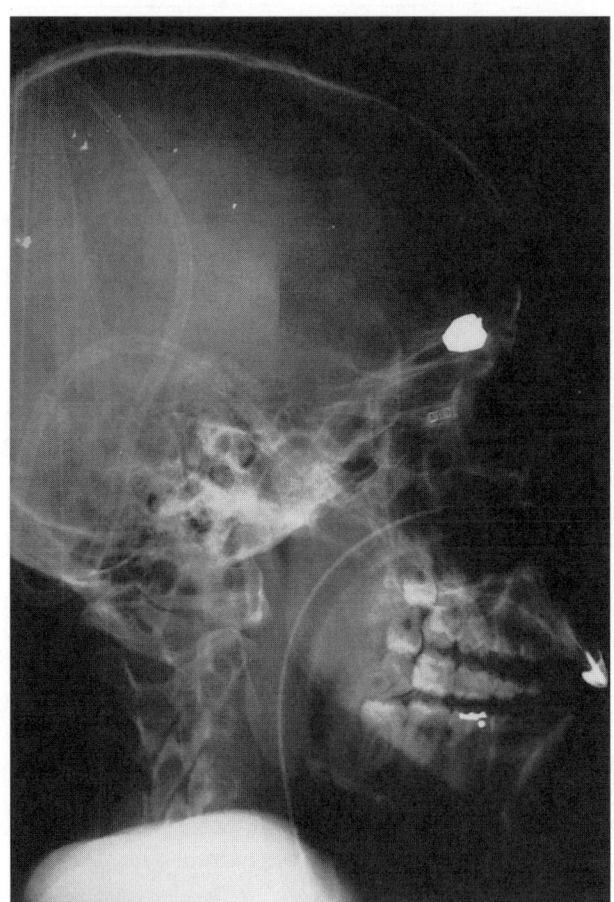

Figure 40–1

Lateral skull radiograph with bullets and brain fragments.

Spinal Radiographs

Spinal films, which are obtained extensively in emergency departments and trauma units, are simple x-ray studies of various regions of the spine: cervical, thoracic, lumbar, and sacral (see Chapter 38). Indications for spinal films include the following: known or presumed trauma to the back or vertebral column (e.g., from motor vehicle accidents, falls), pain, and motor and/or sensory impairment.

Vertebrae are highly irregular anatomic structures that require anterior, posterior, and lateral views to rule out the possibility of fracture.[3] These views are usually sufficient to identify a fracture in the thoracic and lumbar regions of the spine. Cervical spine clearance, however, is frequently not accomplished with these films because a clear view of C1–2 and C6–7 is difficult to obtain. An improved view of C1–2 is obtained by taking an odontoid, or "Waters' view," x-ray study through the patient's open mouth. For C6–7 views, adequate visualization often requires the nurse or technician to pull down firmly on the patient's arms while the lateral film is being taken. Even so, a "swimmers view" to drop the scapula may still be needed. This lateral film is taken with the opposite arm raised over the head.[4] On some occasions, the simple x-ray studies are still not adequate to visualize the spine, and further films and studies, such as CT and MRI, may be necessary. In the critically ill patient, it is often difficult to obtain an assessment of neck pain and motor and sensory impairment because of loss of consciousness or use of sedation. In such cases, the cervical spine evaluation may be delayed, and the patient may be admitted to the critical care unit with spinal precautions and a rigid collar. Flexion and extension films may then be obtained, although this practice is controversial. In the sedated or comatose patient who cannot communicate neck pain, this manipulation may cause new or additional spinal cord damage.[5]

In general, before spinal radiography is performed, the patient should be cooperative and able to communicate neck pain and tenderness. Critically ill or injured patients who are unconscious or sedated may not be able to communicate and, therefore, may be admitted to the intensive care unit with a cervical collar and spinal precaution orders in place. When the patient is cooperative and able to communicate clearly, further films may be obtained.

Nursing care involves positioning the patient to obtain adequate films while maintaining cervical alignment and immobilization. Patients who require transfer to a stretcher usually require three to four persons with a draw sheet, slide board, and/or total body lift to maintain cervical precautions. Most important, the cervical spine should be treated as unstable until proved otherwise. A rigid cervical collar, bed rest with the head of bed less than 30°, and log rolling of the patient are required until additional films can be obtained.

Computed Tomography

Since its development in the 1960s, CT has become the primary tool for demonstrating the presence of any of the following: abnormal calcifications, brain edema, hydrocephalus, tumors, cysts, hemorrhages, clots, intracranial shifts, and herniation. It falls short, however, in detecting some vascular lesions.[6] CT is fast, noninvasive, and safe. The care of patients with head injury has been revolutionized by CT because an accurate diagnosis can be made in minutes, allowing rapid initiation of therapy. Consequently, mortality from epidural, subdural, and intracerebral hematoma has been significantly reduced.

Computed tomography provides a mathematically reconstructed view of multiple "slices" of the head. This is accomplished by passage of intersecting x-ray beams and measurement of the density of substances through which the x-ray beam passes (Figure 40–2). The denser the substance through which the x-ray beam passes, the whiter it appears on the finished film.

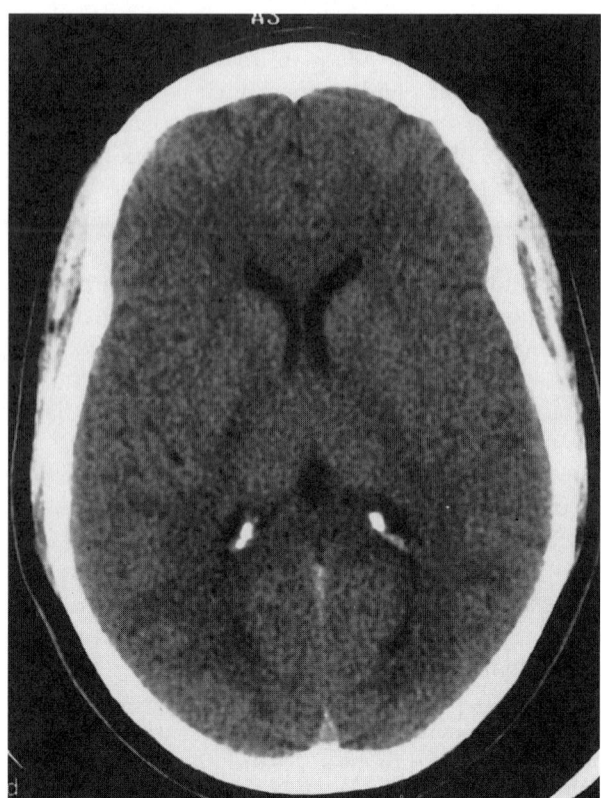

Figure 40–2

Normal computed tomography scan, horizontal slice.

The less dense a substance, the blacker it appears (Table 40–1).

Tissue density changes with pathology. For example, freshly clotted hemorrhage appears more dense; edematous tissue appears less dense. The diagnostic sensitivity of CT can be increased by the intravenous injection of an iodinated contrast agent. When there are abnormalities, these agents often pass into the abnormal tissue through defects in the blood–brain barrier. Iodine in the contrast agent absorbs a large quantity of the x-rays, making the lesion white.[2]

Computed tomography is indicated in a diagnostic workup for headache, head trauma with associated loss of consciousness, seizures, hydrocephalus, suspicion of space-occupying lesions, hemorrhage, or vascular lesions and edema. Serial CT scans are indicated to detect developing hematomas, increased swelling, or new lesions in the severely head-injured patient and

TABLE 40–1
Computed Tomographic (CT) Color of Various Substances

Substance	Color on CT Film
Bone	White
Blood	Off white
Tissue	Shaded gray
Cerebrospinal fluid	Off black
Air	Black

the patient who has undergone surgery. CT has several advantages over MRI: more rapid results, few contraindications, up to 50% less expensive, and ability to scan other body parts simultaneously.

Before the procedure, the patient should be clean and free of hairpins, jewelry, and metal objects. No dietary restrictions are necessary unless contrast agents are used. If so, clear liquids or nothing by mouth (NPO) for 6 to 8 hours before the procedure may be ordered in nonemergency situations. The patient's renal status should be assessed before the contrast agent is administered because the agent is cleared from the body through the kidneys.

When contrast agents are used, a skin test may be performed to check for an allergic reaction to iodine. Patients should be told that they may experience flushing, transient headache, nausea, or vomiting when the contrast is injected.

The need for the patient to remain perfectly still should be emphasized. Some patients may require sedation to prevent motion. There is no special postprocedure care unless the patient has received contrast media. If so, the patient should be monitored for signs and symptoms of reaction, including hives, skin rash, itching, headache, and nausea. If symptoms are severe, an antihistamine may be administered. After the procedure, the patient should be hydrated to help clear the dye from the body.[3]

Magnetic Resonance Imaging

Magnetic resonance imaging is like CT in that MRI provides "slice" imaging of the brain. MRI is better than CT in the respect that it uses nonionizing energy (radiation) and the slice images can be visualized in any plane, versus the horizontal plane of CT scan.

Magnetic resonance imaging is accomplished by placing the patient in a powerful magnetic field, which causes the hydrogen protons of the neuronal tissues and cerebrospinal fluid (CSF) to align themselves in the orientation of the magnetic field. Different types of neuronal tissue (gray versus white) emit energy at different frequencies. In MRI, the application of a radiofrequency pulse into the field causes the protons to resonate or "gyrate," and change their axis of alignment. When the radiofrequency pulse is removed, the protons return to their original alignment. The radiofrequency energy that was absorbed and then emitted is subjected to computer analysis, and an image of the different frequencies is constructed.[1] The images are truly remarkable, differentiating gray matter from white matter, a characteristic that allows the clinician to identify all discrete nuclear structures and lesions within them (Figure 40–3).

Magnetic resonance imaging is superior to CT in identifying several abnormalities: extraaxial hemorrhages, brain stem injuries, posterior fossa injuries,

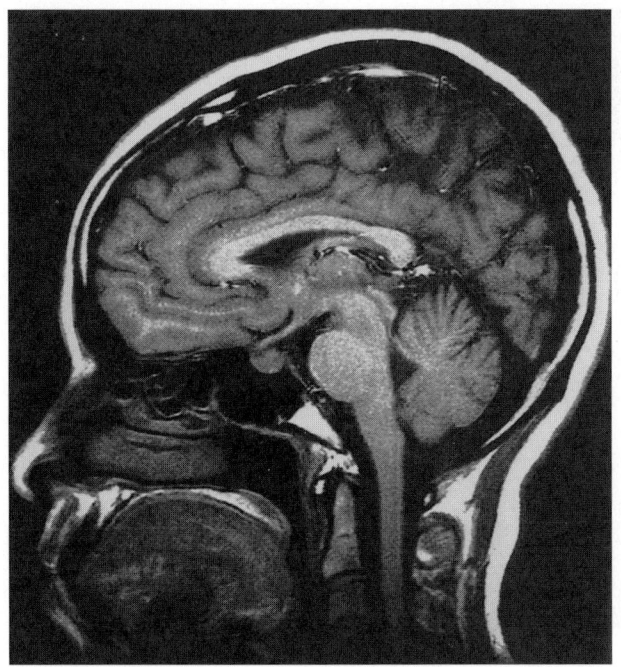

Figure 40-3

Normal magnetic resonance imaging scan, vertical slice.

and nonhemorrhagic lesions. The sharpness and detail of the images produced allow MRI to serve as a "knifeless biopsy" for diagnostic purposes and to identify abnormalities even before structural changes have occurred.[3]

Unfortunately, MRI's magnetic field, radiofrequency interference, and limited size make equipment such as artificial pacemakers, prosthetic devices (e.g., metallic heart valves, orthopedic replacements), artificial limbs, respirators, hemodynamic monitoring equipment, and ICP monitoring equipment a contraindication to the imaging. Technical problems can be overcome by the use of special monitoring and ventilator equipment that is not sensitive to the magnetic field or radiofrequency interference. MRI has been known to move intracranial clips and metal bullet fragments in the brain. Therefore, MRI personnel should be contacted before performing the procedure on anyone with implanted ferrous metal objects. If patients are not sedated or comatose, they should be informed that the procedure is lengthy (45–60 minutes) and requires the patient to lie motionless in a tight, enclosed space. Some patients are severely claustrophobic and may require an "open" MRI. These are spacious MRI scanners located in most metropolitan areas and major medical centers that accommodate obese and claustrophobic patients.

Positron Emission Tomography

Positron emission tomography (PET) differs from CT and MRI in its ability to detect brain function rather than brain anatomy. PET detects the emission of

photons from a previously injected biochemical compound labeled with an isotope that traces a specific biologic process (in the case of head-injured patients, the distribution and utilization of glucose in the various regions of the brain). Decay of these isotopes results in the emission of a subatomic particle called a positron. Each positron decay sends a two-directional signal that is picked up by tomograph detectors. The data are analyzed by a computer, and an image is reconstructed.

Positron emission tomography is not yet a common diagnostic tool because it is still in an early stage of development. It is primarily available at major research centers that have the on-line cyclotron necessary for its use. PET holds promise for understanding the complex physiologic process of epilepsy, dementia (e.g., Alzheimer's disease), cerebrovascular disease, trauma, and mental illness. Patient preparation is similar to that for the patient undergoing a brain scan.

Cerebral Angiography

Cerebral angiography has been nearly supplanted by CT and MRI, yet it remains the definitive diagnostic test for delineating lesions of the cerebral vasculature, such as arteriovenous malformations and cerebral aneurysms. It is the only study that can demonstrate cerebrovascular stenosis, occlusions, thrombus, and ulcerated plaques (Figure 40–4).[7] Most recently, cerebral angiography with balloon angioplasty or coiling of aneurysm has become the treatment of choice for a number of cerebral vasculature abnormalities.

Cerebral angiography involves the injection of radiopaque contrast medium into the intracranial or extracranial vasculature. A catheter is placed in the femoral artery and is threaded up to the aorta and into the cerebral circulation. Other less common injection sites include the brachial, axillary, and subclavian arteries. Contrast medium is injected, and a succession of radiographs are taken as the contrast medium progresses from the arterial circulation to the capillary bed to the venous circulation. Four-vessel angiography involves injections into the right and left internal carotid arteries and the right and left external carotid arteries. One-vessel angiography is performed if the area of disease has already been identified by other means or as a follow-up to evaluate vascular surgery.

Overall morbidity and mortality from angiography is reported to be 0.1 to 2.5%. Although complications are rare, they can be severe: cerebral embolus, hemorrhage, clot formation, vasospasm, thrombus of the distal extremity, and allergic reaction to the contrast medium. Contraindications to the procedure include allergy to radiopaque dye, anticoagulant therapy, bleeding disorders, recent embolic or thromboembolic events, and severe liver, thyroid, or kidney disease. The patient is generally NPO for at least 4 hours before

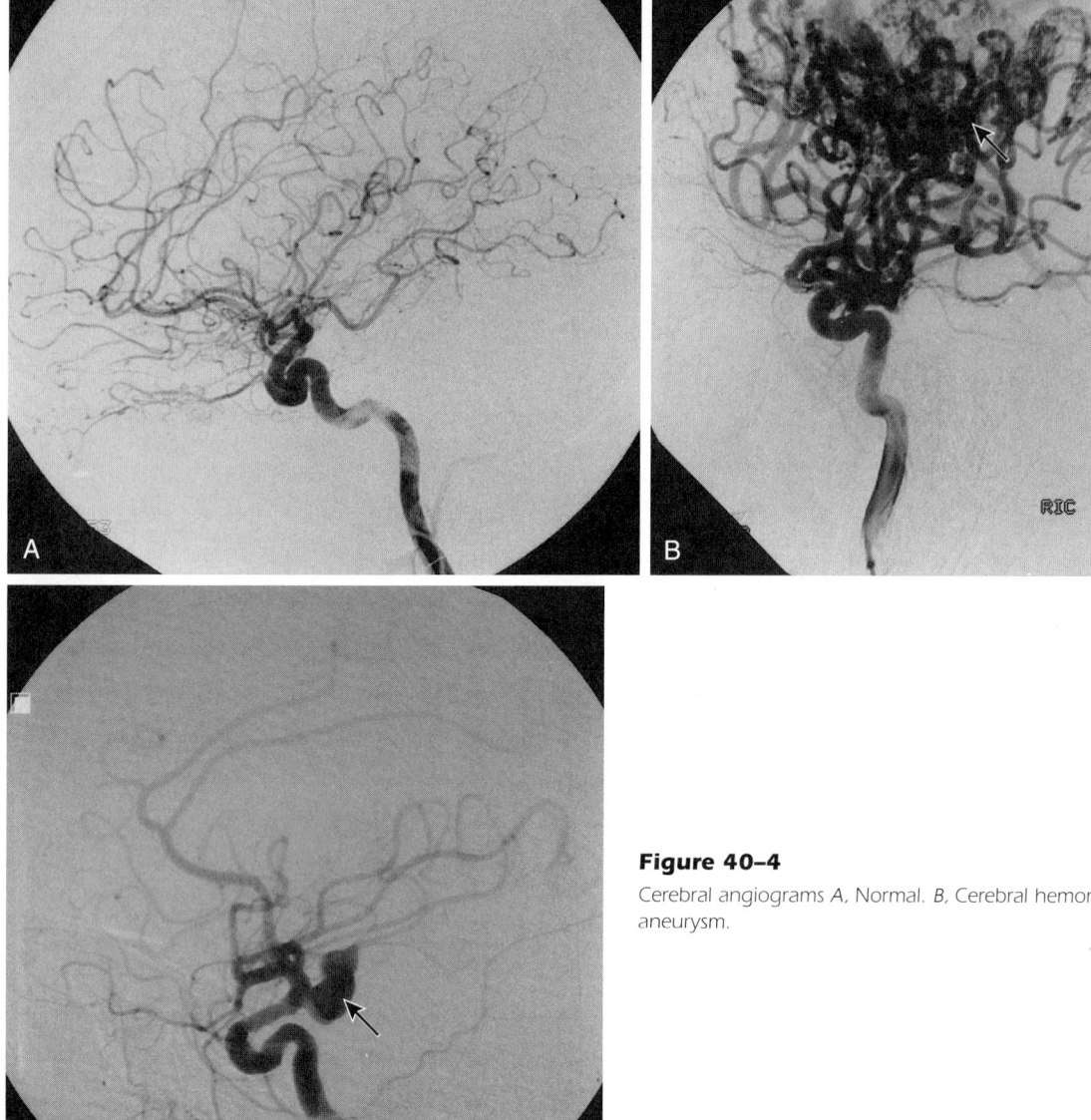

Figure 40–4

Cerebral angiograms *A*, Normal. *B*, Cerebral hemorrhage. *C*, Cerebral aneurysm.

the procedure, and an intravenous line is inserted to maintain hydration. After the procedure, bed rest is maintained for several hours, and the catheterized extremity is kept straight. Vital signs, catheter insertion site, distal extremity perfusion (color, temperature, sensation, and peripheral pulses), and neurologic status should be assessed and documented every 15 minutes for the first hour and at least every hour thereafter for 4 to 6 hours.

The nurse should explain the purpose and general procedure for the test and should emphasize the contrast medium's side effects of burning, headache, and/or pressure. After the procedure, the nurse reviews the need for frequent monitoring, for bed rest with the leg straight, and for an increased fluid intake to eliminate the dye.

Digital Subtraction Angiography

Digital subtraction angiography is a computer-assisted radiographic procedure used to visualize the carotid arteries and cerebral vessels. Like angiography, radiographic dye is injected into either the venous or the arterial circulation, but significantly less dye is necessary than that required for angiography. The image produced is made more distinct by the elimination (subtraction) of surrounding and interfering anatomic structures. Films taken before and after dye injection are superimposed on each other, and all matching images are subtracted. Shadows and distortions of bone or other material are eliminated. Thus, only the dye-enhanced cerebral vessels are left for evaluation.

Digital subtraction angiography is similar to angiography except that the patient is required to be perfectly motionless. The patient must hold his or her breath and refrain from swallowing while the films are being taken. Patient management and teaching are also similar to that with cerebral angiography.

Myelography

Myelography allows visualization of the lumbar, thoracic, cervical, or entire spinal column. A lumbar or cisternal (base of the skull) puncture into the subarachnoid space is performed, and approximately 10 mL of CSF is removed. Contrast medium is then injected, and films are taken of the spinal cord and vertebral column (Figure 40–5). Indications for myelography include herniated intervertebral disks, tumors, congenital anomalies, and bony fragments or growths. Either water-based or oil-based contrast media may be used.

Nursing care of the patient undergoing a myelogram varies, depending on the type of contrast medium used.

Oil-Based Media

Iophendylate (Pantopaque) is an iodine compound suspended in an oil base. Oil-based media are heavier than CSF and therefore must be maneuvered into position with a tilt table. The oil-based medium is removed at the end of the procedure by aspirating with a syringe. As much medium as possible is removed to prevent irritation of neural tissue. The oil-based medium and possible side effects of neural tissue irritation should be explained to patients before the procedure, and patients should be NPO for at least 4 hours before the procedure. Sedative, analgesic, or anticholinergic medications may also be given before the procedure. After the procedure, the patient's neurologic status and vital signs should be monitored frequently while the patient lies flat in bed for 6 to 24 hours. Fluids are encouraged to help eliminate the contrast, and intake and output data are carefully recorded. Analgesics may be prescribed for the most common side effect, which is headache. Lying flat is the recommended position for managing headache. The nurse should observe the patient for complications from the myelography: severe back pain, spasms, nuchal rigidity, neurovascular changes, fever, nausea, and vomiting.

Water-Based Media

Water-based media diffuse upward toward the cranial vault, regardless of patient positioning. The patient's head is kept elevated at all times, and the patient is kept quiet to avoid rapid upward diffusion of the

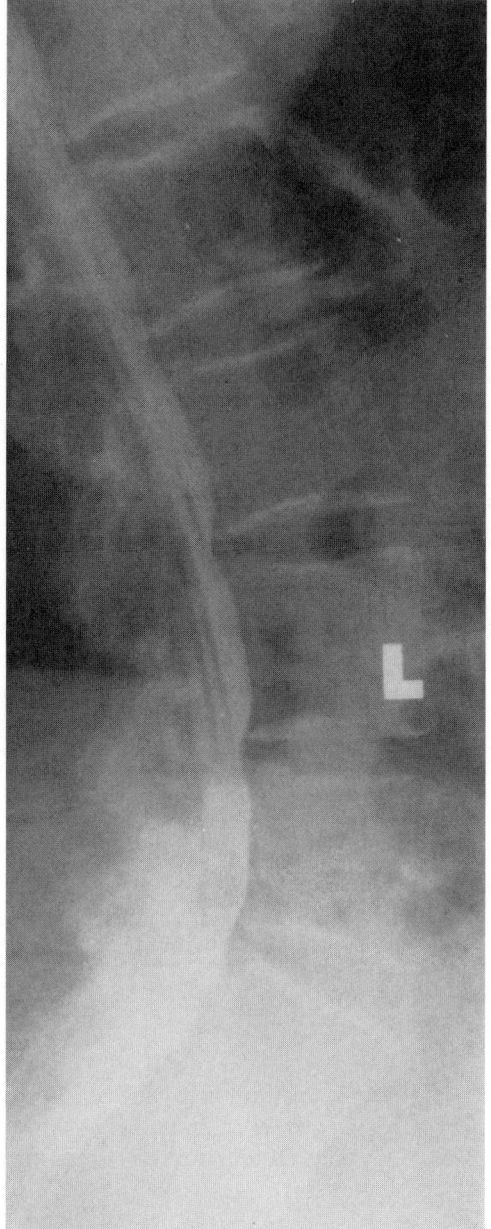

Figure 40–5
Lumbar myelogram.

medium. If contrast medium enters the cranial vault, seizures could result. Patients should be NPO 4 hours before the procedure except for fluids. Sedatives or analgesics may be given before the procedure. Major tranquilizers, monoamine oxidase inhibitors, and stimulants should be discontinued 48 hours before the procedure. After the procedure, nursing care is focused primarily on the prevention of seizures. All patient transfers, transport, and postprocedure care should ensure that the patient's head is elevated 30 to 45°. Frequent vital sign and neurologic assessments should be performed for 12 to 24 hours after the procedure. Patients should be kept quiet and as motionless as possible during this time. Fluid consumption should be encouraged to eliminate the contrast medium, and intake and output should be recorded. Medications may be ordered for headache, backache, and neck stiffness, which are side effects of the procedure.

ELECTROENCEPHALOGRAPHY

An EEG is a diagnostic tool to detect and localize abnormal electrical activity of the brain. The EEG measures cerebral function, much like the electrocardiogram of the heart. EEG benefits patient care in three broad areas: (1) identification and characterization of seizures, (2) assessment of coma, and (3) confirmation of brain death. The EEG may also determine cerebral injury or infarct and some head injuries, but it is most commonly employed if cerebral dysfunction cannot be visualized by CT, MRI, or radiography.[8] The procedure consists of affixing 21 electrodes to the scalp and ears with a jelly or paste. Electrical activity of the brain, brain waves, are recorded at rest, after hyperventilation, with photic stimulation, and during sleep. The electrical activity is amplified one million times and is recorded on graph paper. An EEG consists of more than 300 pages of recorded cerebral electrical activity. Brain waves are classified based on the number of cycles per second (Table 40–2).

Abnormal Electroencephalographic Findings

The most pathologic finding is a "flat" or electrocerebral silent EEG. Causes of a flat EEG include brain death, central nervous system depressant (barbiturate)

ingestion, and hypothermia. Slow wave findings may be either focal or diffuse. Focal slow waves may be related to dysfunction in a localized area secondary to tumor, hemorrhage, or clot. Diffuse slow waves are usually seen with toxic, metabolic, degenerative, or infectious conditions.

Spikes and sharp waves occur either as part of seizure discharges or in patients with epilepsy. These EEG abnormalities can be either diffuse or focal (Figure 40–6).

Continuous Electroencephalographic Monitoring

Continuous EEG monitoring in the intensive care unit is receiving increasing attention. Many experts believe that continuous EEG should become an integral part of monitoring of all neurologic intensive care patients. Typically, a patient's neurologic status is monitored by clinical observation or "neuro checks" at assigned intervals. Even under the best circumstances, these assessments are often subjective and detect functional deterioration after it has occurred.[9] The goal of continuous EEG monitoring is to detect subclinical seizures or nonconvulsive seizures, which may indicate inadequate vascular supply before functional deterioration. This is especially useful in the critically ill patient who requires sedation and/or paralysis. Automated digital EEG hardware with color display monitors is a convenient way to trend EEG events (percentage of alpha waves) in the intensive care unit; however, obstacles such as dealing with cumbersome amounts of data and training nurses to interpret the data have until now prevented widespread implementation in intensive care units.

Preparation of the patient for EEG requires that the scalp and hair be free of creams, clips, or other items. Depending on the indication for the EEG, it may be important that any stimulants or sedatives be withheld. In addition, the patient may be required to stay awake the night before the procedure; however, these preparations are often not possible in the critically ill patient. If the EEG is being performed to confirm brain death, family counseling and teaching should be performed to clarify misconceptions and to lend support.

ELECTROMYOGRAPHY

Electromyography evaluates the electrical activity of muscles. A concentric needle, usually a 24-gauge by 3 to 4 cm long or a solid steel needle coated with an insulating plastic is inserted into a muscle and is advanced by steps to several depths. Variations in electri-

TABLE 40–2
Electroencephalographic Wave Classification

Wave	Cycles per Second	Findings
Delta	1–4	Seen in sleep
		Not normal in awake adult
Theta	4–8	Originates from temporal and parietal lobes
		Normal in drowsiness
Alpha	8–13	Most prominent in occipital leads
		Considered normal in adult
		Can be blocked by beta waves
Beta	13–35	Most prominent in frontal and central areas
		Opening of eyes, mental activity, anxiety, or apprehension

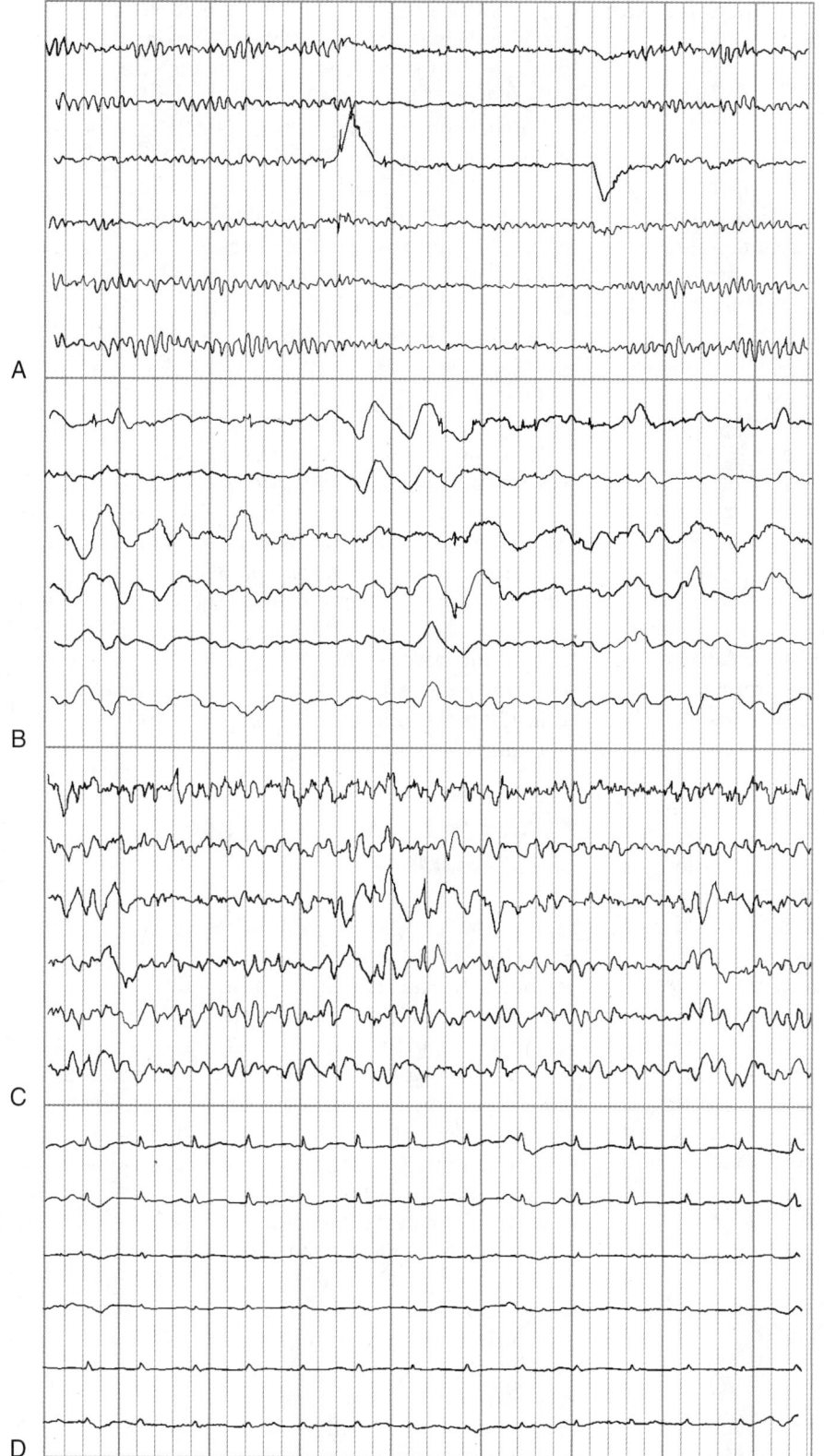

Figure 40–6

Electroencephalograms. *A,* Normal. *B,* Generalized slowing. *C,* Temporal spikes (seizures). *D,* Electrocerebral silence.

cal activity between the needle and a skin electrode are displayed on an oscilloscope and/or loudspeaker. The electrical activity is recorded during the insertion of the needle and the contraction of the muscle. Two types of activity observed by electromyography have particular significance: fibrillations and fasciculations.

These electrical patterns may signal denervated muscle and lower motor neuron disease, respectively. Nerve conduction studies are often performed in conjunction with electromyography.

Patient management and teaching involve informing the patient of the procedure and the expected discomfort. Patient cooperation is also important. No special postprocedure care is necessary.

EVOKED POTENTIALS

An evoked potential is an electrical manifestation of the brain's response to an external stimulus. In clinical neurophysiology, evoked potentials are a noninvasive means of applying repetitive sensory stimuli and recording the impulse generated as it travels through the brain stem and into the cerebral cortex. Evoked potentials are conducted if a diagnosis is not confirmed by clinical or other diagnostic testing. Three types of evoked potentials are used in the clinical setting: (1) visual evoked potentials/response, which use light stimulus; (2) somatosensory evoked potentials/response, which use electrical shock; and (3) brain stem auditory evoked potentials/response, which use click or sound stimulus.

The auditory stimulus (brain stem auditory evoked response) is used most often in the critically head-injured patient because it is easily performed at the bedside. The procedure involves applying earphones to the patient and delivering a series of click stimuli. The impulse then travels up the auditory regions of the brain stem to the cortex. Normally, the recorded response is a series of five to six positive voltage waves. The most common abnormal responses are absence of all waves (brain death), prolonged waves (brain stem dysfunction/conduction), and absence of a wave or waves (brain stem dysfunction at a specific region).

Preparation and postprocedure care involve teaching awake patients about the test and possible sensations from the electrical shock. The brain stem auditory evoked response is not affected by central nervous system depressants; therefore, this test is easily used in the critical care area for the head-injured patient. If the procedure is being performed to confirm brain death, family teaching and counseling should be conducted to facilitate an understanding of the test results and to support the family.

BRAIN SCANNING (CEREBRAL BLOOD FLOW STUDIES)

Cerebral blood flow (CBF) studies, often referred to as a brain scan, measure the amount of blood flow throughout the brain or in a single region of the brain. The goal of CBF studies is to detect areas of increased or decreased cerebral circulation during cerebral vasospasm; during operative procedures, such as aneurysm clipping; for arteriovenous malformation; or after carotid endarterectomy. CBF studies have also been used to confirm brain death. The application of

CBF measurements has been limited to clinical research because of a lack of evidence regarding CBF in the head-injured patient as well as the effect of metabolic state on CBF.

Cerebral blood flow averages 50 to 55 mL per 100 g of cerebral tissue per minute, or about 15 to 20% of the cardiac output.[7] Overall, flow in gray matter is normally three to four times higher than that in white matter. The most common method of CBF measurement involves inhalation of the isotope xenon-133 via a ventilator circuit for 3 to 5 minutes. Sixteen to 32 electrodes are placed around the skull, and clearance of xenon is calculated by a computer. Other methods involve injecting a radioisotope or inhaling nitrous oxide.

This noninvasive procedure requires minimal patient management outside of encouraging the awake patient to increase fluid intake and verifying the patient's allergies before administering the isotope. If an isotope is injected, the patient is informed that some mild burning may be felt. The awake patient is reassured that the radioactive material is excreted rapidly and poses no health hazard. If the scan is being performed to confirm brain death, family teaching and counseling should be conducted for support and explanation of the test results.

TRANSCRANIAL DOPPLER ULTRASOUND

The use of Doppler ultrasound as a screening technique for carotid artery occlusion (extracranial) is well established. Transcranial Doppler ultrasound is the newest diagnostic tool used to detect vasospasm after aneurysm clipping. There is great interest in the use of transcranial Doppler ultrasound for the head-injured patient. A probe over the temporal bone usually allows for flow information from the anterior, posterior, and middle cerebral arteries. An ultrasonic signal that is reflected from the moving red blood cells is transmitted back to a computerized spectral analysis machine. Generally, the higher the flow, the narrower the vessel.[9a] Figure 40–7 depicts bedside Doppler ultrasound studies of a cerebral artery with and without spasm. Use of serial (daily) Doppler studies reduces the need for angiography and provides verification and evolving information about flow through the cerebral vessels. Doppler ultrasound is a noninvasive, easy to perform bedside test that requires no patient preparation or postprocedure care.

LUMBAR PUNCTURE

Lumbar puncture involves entering the subarachnoid space of the spinal column with a needle and a stylet.

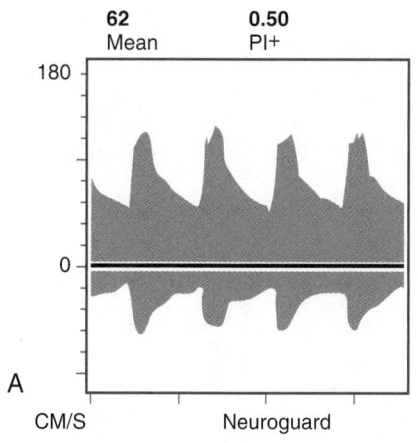

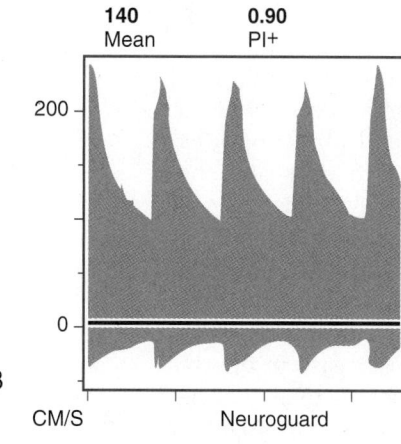

Figure 40–7

Transcranial Doppler waveforms. A, Normal waveform. B, Vasospasm.

Indications for a LP are measurement of CSF and pressure, removal of bloody or infected CSF, injection of medications to achieve spinal anesthesia, analgesia, and treatment of infection (administration of antibiotics). Contraindications for LP include increased ICP and CSF infection. An LP should not be preformed on any patient suspected of having increased ICP—brain stem herniation could occur if lumbar puncture is preformed in this setting. Occasionally, an intracranial monitor is placed before the LP to assess the patient's ICP.

Lumbar puncture with drainage and pressure monitoring has been introduced to critical care units for patients who have undergone aortic aneurysm repair. Studies have shown that LP drainage after aortic cross-clamp may relieve spinal cord swelling and ischemia.

Using aseptic technique, an 18- to 22-gauge hollow needle is introduced into the subarachnoid space at L4–5, which is usually below the end of the spinal cord. Flexion of the lumbar spine is necessary for safe insertion of the needle. The patient can be placed in either the lateral recumbent position with the knees and head tucked toward each other or sitting (leaning) over a bedside table. After the needle is successfully in the subarachnoid space, the stylet is removed, and a pressure monitoring system may be connected in order to measure entrance CSF pressure. Once this measurement is obtained, samples of CSF are collected for laboratory analysis.

Before the procedure, patients should empty their bladder and be informed about the importance of positioning during the procedure. After the procedure, patient care involves monitoring neurologic and vital signs frequently, encouraging fluids, administering analgesics for headache, and maintaining the patient in supine position. Complications of LP are related to CSF leak or subarachnoid trauma. Patients may experience severe headache, lower back and leg spasms, nuchal rigidity, difficulty voiding, and fever. Treatment of a CSF leak may require the injection of blood into the dura, known as a "blood patch," in an attempt to stop CSF leakage.

INTRACRANIAL PRESSURE MONITORING

Since 1960, when Lundberg determined that ICP monitoring could be performed safely, ICP monitoring has been used as a standard method of neurologic evaluation in the brain-injured patient.[10] ICP monitoring allows the clinician to manage the brain-injured patient through continuous objective data and not just neurologic assessment alone; it provides prompt recognition of elevated pressure in the brain, facilitating early diagnosis of a developing mass lesion; it guides therapy by proving the effectiveness of medical and nursing interventions; and it can assist in predicting patient outcome and prognosis. ICP monitoring, along with its subsequent medical and nursing interventions, can prevent uncontrolled intracranial pressure and cerebral herniation. Several research studies have shown that the presence of the ICP monitor to guide therapy in the brain-injured patient actually improves patient outcome by reducing mortality rates from 50% to 28 to 36%.[10–12]

Principles

Three principles govern the pathophysiology of increased intracranial pressure and its secondary effects on brain injury. The *Monro-Kellie hypothesis*, the *volume–pressure curve* and *cerebral perfusion pressure* (CPP) are essential principles to understand in order to interpret ICP values.

Monro-Kellie Hypothesis

In 1783, Alexander Monro introduced the concept that there are compartments in the intracranial space that have the potential to change volumes. This was supported by observations of Kellie some 40 years later. This Monro-Kellie hypothesis was tested repeatedly and today is one of the main principles underlying cerebral pathophysiology.

Fundamental to this hypothesis is that the intracranial space is composed of three components: (1) brain substance (80%), (2) blood (10%) and (3) CSF (10%). These components are housed in a fixed space, the skull, that does not readily expand. Normal ICP is derived from the pressure these components place on each other with an average value of 3 to 15 mm Hg. The modified Monro-Kellie hypothesis states that an increase in volume of one of the intracranial components must be compensated by a decrease in one or more of the other components so that the total volume remains fixed; if not, the ICP increases (Figure 40–8).

Volume–Pressure Curve

As stated earlier, the three intracranial components are brain tissue, blood, and CSF. The relationship between the volume of these three components and their pressure on each other is best described by the volume–pressure curve shown in Figure 40–9. As the intracranial volume begins to increase, the ICP remains within the normal range as a result of compensatory mechanisms. The intracranial components compensate by displacing CSF down the spinal canal or through the arachnoid villa into the venous system to keep the ICP within normal range (see Figure 40–9, point A on the graph). As the volume in the cerebrum continues to increase, other buffering mechanisms, such as autoregulation, are used to keep the ICP within normal limits (see Figure 40–9, point B on the graph). Autoregulation is the automatic vasodilation and vasoconstriction of the cerebral blood vessels to maintain CBF at nearly normal levels despite marked changes in arterial pressure, ICP, and CPP. As the volume increases further (see Figure 40–9, point C on the graph), autoregulation is no longer able to com-

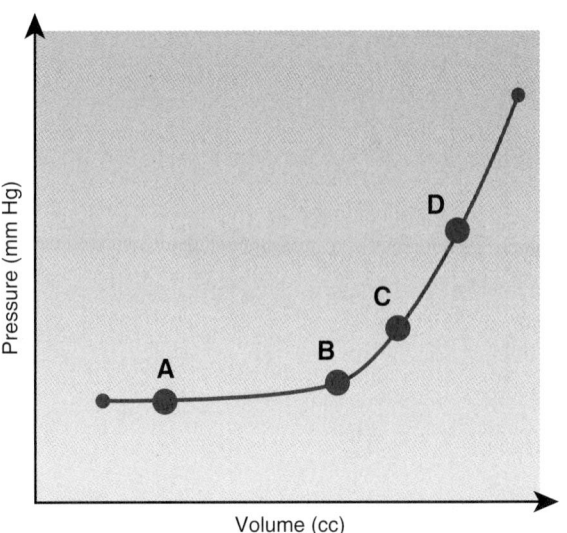

Figure 40–9

Volume–pressure curve.

pensate for the increased pressure, and the intracranial space becomes less compliant or less able to tolerate an increase in volume, and the ICP increases. Finally, the intracranial space becomes noncompliant, and any additional increase in volume leads to a dramatic increase in ICP (see Figure 40–9, point D on the graph). The shape of the volume–pressure curve is also dependent on the rate of the increase of the volume. Slow rates of increased volume, like those caused by slow-growing tumors, can be accommodated with minimal changes in ICP. Conversely, the brain does not have time to compensate for rapidly developing hematomas, and ICP can rise quickly.

Cerebral Perfusion Pressure

Cerebral blood flow must be maintained at an adequate level to provide a continuous supply of oxygen and glucose to the brain cells. It is difficult to measure CBF; therefore, an estimated pressure, CPP, is used. CPP is the difference between the mean arterial pressure (MAP) and the opposing force of the ICP on the cerebral arteries.[13]

$$CPP = MAP - ICP$$

The average CPP is 80 to 100 mm Hg, with a range of 60 to 150 mm Hg. A CPP below 60 mm Hg may lead to cerebral ischemia, and a sustained CPP of 30 mm Hg results in neuronal cell death. Therefore, a dangerously low CPP may have two results: a high ICP or a low MAP. For example, Patient A had an increased ICP of 30 mm Hg and a normal MAP of 80 mm Hg. The nurse would immediately begin interventions to decrease his ICP because his CPP was 50 mm Hg (80–30 mm Hg), a value that leads to cerebral ischemia and

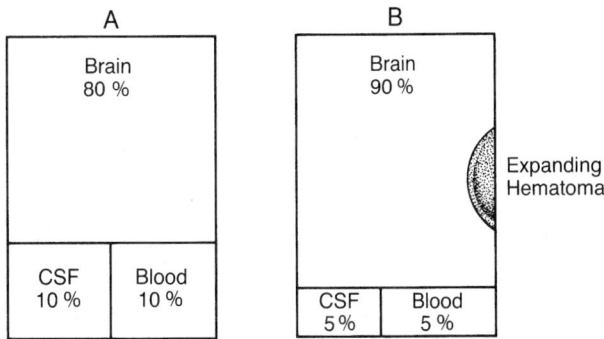

Figure 40–8

The Monro-Kellie hypothesis. *A,* Schematic representation of the three intracranial components. *B,* Schematic representation of intracranial compensation when brain volume is increased. *CSF,* cerebrospinal fluid. (From Cardona VD, et al: Trauma Nursing. Philadelphia, WB Saunders, 1994, p 393.)

neuronal cell death. However, Patient B has an ICP of 12 mm Hg, not high enough to start ICP interventions, but his MAP is 62 mm Hg also leaving him with a CPP of 50 mm Hg. Interventions in the second example would stress increasing the blood pressure to increase cerebral perfusion to the brain.

Indications for Intracranial Pressure Monitoring

The criteria for ICP monitoring depend on the patient, but in general, head-injured patients who are comatose with a Glasgow Coma Score of 8 or less should be monitored. ICP monitors can also be used in patients with nontraumatic neurologic disorders, such as subarachnoid hemorrhage, hydrocephalus, brain tumors, and intracerebral hemorrhage. The main objective for intensive monitoring of the ICP is to help the brain-injured patient maintain adequate cerebral perfusion and oxygenation while the brain recovers.[14] Whereas earlier severe head-injury studies concen-

trated on the importance of preventing ICP elevations, current evidence emphasizes the importance of maintaining the CPP at an adequate level.[13–15] The only reliable way to measure CPP is to continuously measure blood pressure and ICP.

There is no agreement among neurosurgeons about which ICP monitoring device is optimal. Certain ICP monitoring devices, placed within the cerebral ventricles, can contribute directly to decreasing the elevated ICP by draining CSF out of the catheter. Other devices, placed in the intraparenchymal or epidural space, are thought to provide more accurate readings and are easier to place and maintain (Table 40–3).

Contraindications to Intracranial Pressure Monitoring

Contradictions to ICP monitoring are few. Although ICP monitoring has been shown not to be necessary in mildly to moderately head-injured patients, it is not contraindicated.[16]

TABLE 40–3
A Comparison of Intracranial Pressure (ICP) Monitoring Devices

ICP Monitoring Devices	Catheter Placement	Advantages	Disadvantages
Intraventricular catheter	Anterior horn of the lateral ventricle	Drains CSF Most accurate and reliable measure of ICP	Most difficult to place Highest risk of infection Need for transducer leveling and repositioning of head Unable to obtain accurate ICP reading when draining CSF
Subarachnoid	Subarachnoid space	No penetration of the parenchyma, less risk of infection or hemorrhage Easier to place than intraventricular catheter Useful when unable to place intraventricular catheter because of edema	Accuracy and reliability over time are poor May be unable to drain CSF Can become clotted with blood clot or brain tissue Requires intact skull for accurate ICP readings Need for transducer leveling and repositioning of head
Epidural	Epidural space	No penetration of dura layer Easiest to place Low infection risk Can be used for longer periods of time No adjustment of transducer with head movement needed	Indirect measurement of ICP/questionable accuracy Unable to drain CSF Unable to recalibrate or rezero after placement
Fiberoptic	Epidural, subarachnoid, or parenchymal space	Accurate and reliable Easier to place Can be used longer term No adjustment of transducer with head movement needed	Unable to drain CSF Unable to recalibrate or rezero after placement Requires large investment in equipment/hardware for fiberoptics Fiberoptics can be broken if cable is kinked

CSF, cerebrospinal fluid.

Methods of Intracranial Pressure Monitoring

Intraventricular Catheters

Intraventricular devices (ventriculostomies), placed in the anterior horn of the lateral ventricle, are fluid-filled catheters connected to an external strain gauge or a catheter tip pressure transducer (Figure 40–10). If possible, the nondominant hemisphere of the patient's brain is chosen for placement (the right side for 90% of patients). The ICP value obtained is from deep within the brain and is therefore considered most reflective of the whole brain pressure.[17] However, these devices must be maintained with utmost accuracy. Leveling of the pressure transducer at the foramen of Monro (outer hypocanthus of the eye or top of the ear) and maintaining the fluid-filled system free of air bubbles, leaks, clots, and artifact are essential (Figure 40–11).

Subarachnoid Catheters

This type of device is a bolt or a screw placed in the subarachnoid space. This device may or may not be capable of draining CSF. However, the insertion is easier than that of a intraventricular catheter (see Figure 40–10).

Epidural Catheters

Epidural devices are usually a fiberoptic catheter tip pressure transducer with no CSF draining capabilities (see Figure 40–10). The dura is not penetrated with this method, and it is considered a relatively noninvasive and indirect measurement of ICP. The epidural device is the least common and has the least risk for infection.

Fiberoptic Catheters

The fiberoptic ICP device may be placed in the epidural, subdural, or parenchymal space to obtain ICP measurement (see Figure 40–10). This monitoring system is connected to a transducer or a pressure-sensing device located at the distal tip of the intracranial catheter. It is very accurate, and waveforms are comparable to those obtained with intraventricular catheters. No CSF can be withdrawn with this system (Figure 40–12).

The various methods for ICP monitoring have distinct advantages and disadvantages (see Table 40–3). The newest technology being developed combines the fluid-filled intraventricular catheter drainage system with a fiberoptic transducer for the most advantages and the most accurate results.

Intracranial Pressure Waves

Pulse Waveform

The ICP pulse waveform is observed on a real-time pressure display and corresponds to the patient's heartbeat. The normal pulse waveform has three defined peaks. These three peaks, P1, P2, and P3, descend in a sawtooth pattern (Figure 40–13). The P2 portion of the pulse waveform increases as cerebral compliance decreases. If P2 is larger than or equal to P1, a state of decreased cerebral compliance exists

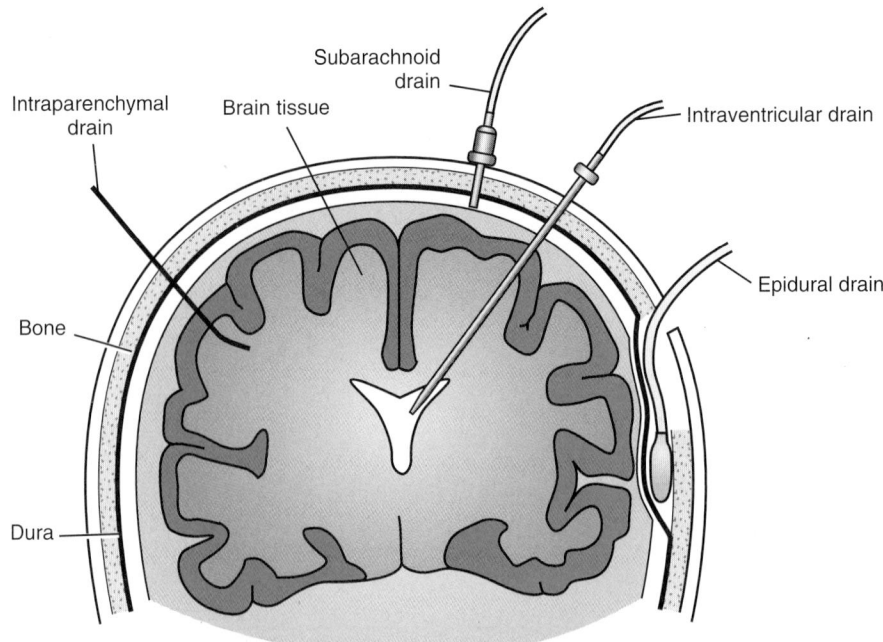

Figure 40–10
Location of intracranial pressure monitors.

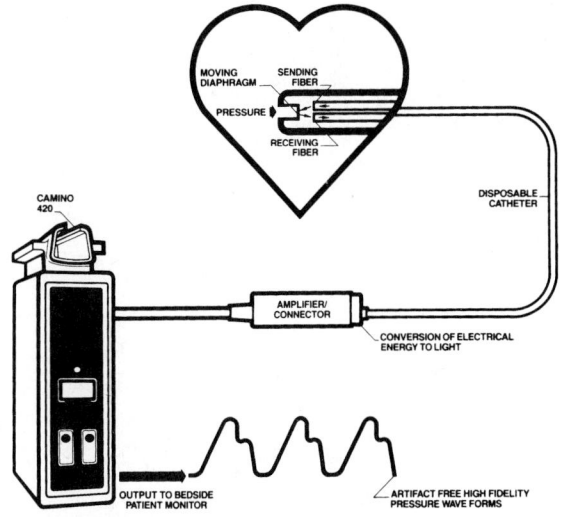

Figure 40-12

Intraparenchymal fiberoptic intracranial pressure monitoring. (From Cardona VD, et al: Trauma Nursing. Philadelphia, WB Saunders, 1994, p 416.)

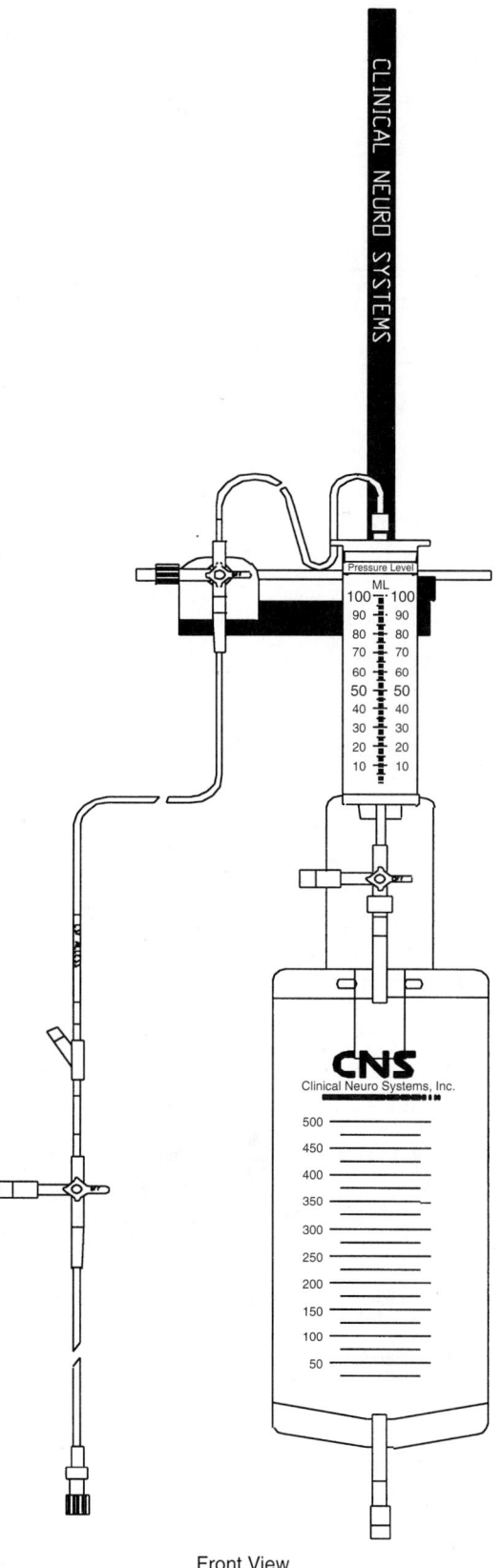

Front View

Figure 40-11

Central nervous system intraventricular drainage system. (From Connell Neurosurgical, Exton, PA.)

(Figure 40–14). One must consider clotting of the ICP monitor if the P1, P2, or P3 pulse waveforms are not visible or are flat.

A,B,C, Trend Waveforms

In 1960, Lundberg identified three types of abnormal ICP trend waveforms and labeled them A, B, and C.[11] These pressure waves are graphically displayed data that reflect spontaneous alterations in ICP associated with respiration, systemic blood pressure, and deteriorating neurologic status over minutes to hours.

A waves, also called plateau waves, are the most clinically significant waves. A waves have a baseline ICP of greater than 20 mm Hg and often plateau for 15 to 20 minutes at ICPs of 30 to 70 mm Hg (Figure 40–15A). These waveforms are produced by changes in the cerebral blood volume. They indicate a noncompliant brain if small fluctuations in volume of any of the three components in the brain lead to dramatic increases in ICP. Because of early interventions, A waves are rarely seen; however, a blunted version of them can be seen in severely injured patients. Treatment of these waveforms is focused on decreasing the ICP and preventing the CPP from falling to a critical level.

B waves are sharp sawtooth waveforms that occur approximately every 0.5 to 2 minutes and can raise the ICP from 5 to 70 mm Hg (see Figure 40–15B). These waveforms indicate an injured brain that is beginning to lose its compensatory mechanisms for fluctuations in ICP. B waves may progress to A waves.

C waves are small, rhythmic waves that occur at normal levels of ICP (see Figure 40–15C). They are related to normal fluctuations in respirations and blood pressure. Their significance is unknown.

Figure 40–13

Normal intracranial pressure waveform.

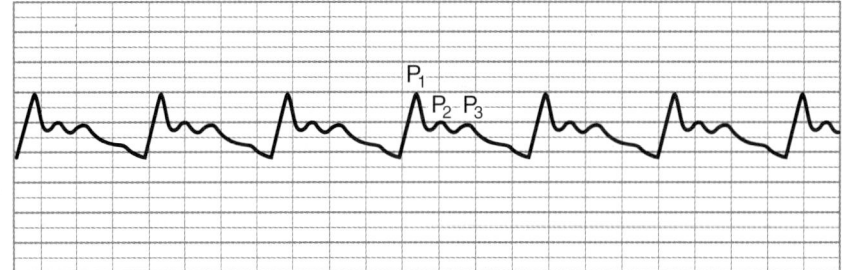

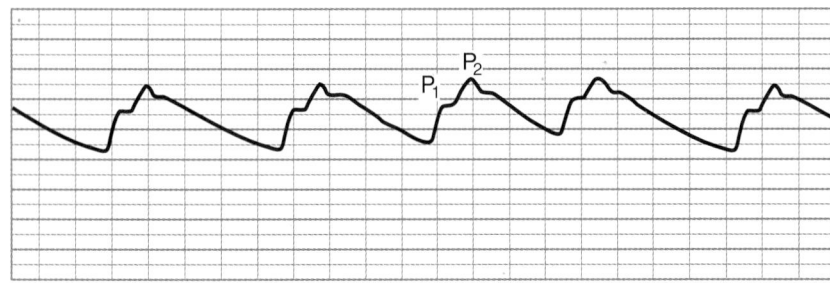

Figure 40–14

Increased intracranial pressure waveform with decreased compliance. Note that P_2 is greater than P_1.

Figure 40–15

Brain waves. *A*, A waves. *B*, B waves. *C*, C waves. (From Cardona VD, et al: Trauma Nursing. Philadelphia, WB Saunders, 1994, p 419.)

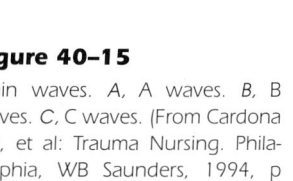

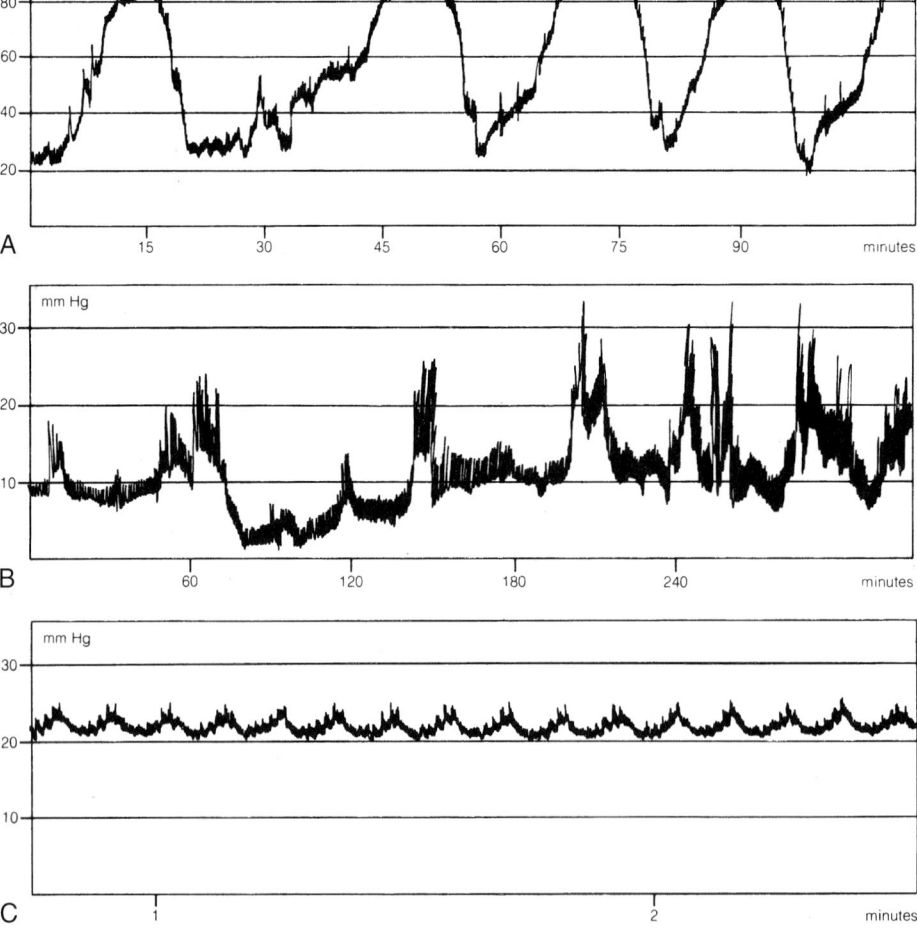

TABLE 40-4
Nursing Considerations During Intracranial Pressure (ICP) Monitoring

Nursing Considerations	Rationale
Maintain knowledge of the indications for ICP monitoring	Timely assembling of equipment is required because of the critical condition of the patient.
Assemble equipment accurately	It is important to be familiar with the type of ICP monitor to be used. For accurate ICP readings: 　The intraventricular catheter needs to be leveled, with zero being the outer canthus of the eye or the foramen of Monro; a physician's order must be obtained for the level of the drainage system above that zero point. 　For other ICP monitoring devices, the transducers may be at the level of the outer canthus of the eye and zeroed appropriately. 　Fiberoptic monitors are calibrated before insertion and level of the device is not a factor. Use strict sterile technique when setting up the ICP monitor. Do not connect the transducer of any ICP monitor to a flush system.
Keep patient free from infection	Maintain aseptic technique with all dressing changes and troubleshooting of devices. Keep all stopcocks in closed position and sterile. Monitor insertion site for redness, swelling, warmth, or drainage. Administer antibiotics as prescribed.
Monitor vital signs and neurologic status frequently	Record ICP readings with the patient in the same position according to the physician's order or the nursing standards of care. Record ICP readings more frequently if unstable. Record high and mode ICP if the monitor is continuous. Begin medical and nursing interventions as prescribed for ICP > 20 mm Hg or CPP < 60–70 mm Hg.
Monitor the effect of nursing interventions on the patient's ICP	Space out nursing interventions: ICP has been shown to increase with turning of the patient and with endotracheal suctioning. Bathing may or may not increase ICP. Noise has been associated with increases in ICP. ICP should return to baseline in no more than 4–5 minutes after stimulation or a nursing care activity.
Document thoroughly	Document ICP/CPP values, waveforms, neurologic assessments, type of ICP monitoring device, location and condition of insertion site, dressing changes, amount and color of CSF drainage. This will provide the necessary information for evaluating patient trends and effectiveness of medical and nursing therapies.
Troubleshoot the ICP monitoring system as needed	For dampened waveform: 　Compare waveform with outgoing registered nurse. 　Change scales on monitor if appropriate. 　Check all stopcocks/connections. 　Check level of monitor if appropriate. 　Rezero monitor/transducer. 　Look for evidence of pulsatile fluid in catheter if appropriate. 　Try to drain system if physician's order is in place. 　Manually flush transducer only. 　Call neurosurgeon/physician to flush monitoring system if appropriate. For absent waveform: 　Check all stopcocks/connections. 　Check level of monitor if appropriate. 　Rezero monitor/transducer. 　Look for evidence of pulsatile fluid in catheter if appropriate. 　Try to drain system if physician's order is in place. 　Manually flush transducer only. 　Call neurosurgeon/physician to flush/replace monitoring system.

Monitoring for Complications

Intracranial pressure monitoring complications include infection, hemorrhage, malfunction, obstruction, and malposition. Although these complications rarely produce long-term morbidity, they can produce inaccurate ICP readings and can increase costs by requiring replacement of the device.

Although infection is the most commonly noted complication, there have been no reports in large prospective studies of clinically significant intracranial infections associated with ICP monitoring devices.[18]

Catheters in place greater than 5 days have been shown to be associated with an increase in infection rates.[19]

The overall incidence of hemorrhage and hematomas with all ICP devices is 1.4%, and, specifically, 1.1% with intraventricular catheters.[20, 21] Parenchymal fiberoptic catheter tip devices are associated with a 2.8% hematoma rate.[22, 23]

The incidence of malfunction and obstruction in fluid-coupled catheters is 6 to 16% and 9 to 40%, respectively, in the fiberoptic devices.[23, 24] There are no reported studies on malposition of the catheter or drainage system.

TABLE 40–5
Nursing Considerations for Transport of the Patient With a Neurologic Deficit

Nursing Actions	Rationale
Confirm precise time and location of test with department.	Excessive waiting outside the ICU can place the patient at risk for deterioration.
Notify ancillary departments who will need to accompany patient: respiratory therapy, nursing assistants/technicians.	Give other personnel as much time as possible to prepare for patient's needs, e.g., transport ventilator, pressure transducers, and pulse oximeter.
Gather transport supplies: Emergency medications/pack. Sedatives if needed. Transport monitor. Routine medications needed during lengthy procedure (diuretics, antihypertensives). Emergency intubation equipment.	Ensure appropriate patient monitoring to maintain standards of care while at the test. Emergency preparedness while the patient is off the unit in a remote location is required.
Attach patient to transport monitor and transport ventilator/Ambu bag as required.	Minimally, ECG, BP, and pulse oximetry should be monitored. ICP monitoring is vital for the patient requiring ICP assessment or therapy.
Ensure that all equipment (e.g., IVs, monitors, blankets, beds, oxygen) is unplugged. Check the status of all equipment's battery power at this time.	Ensures a smooth transport out of the room and enough battery power to provide uninterrupted delivery of therapy.
Transport to the procedure department.	If the patient is traveling with a ventilator and other equipment, ensure that passageways and elevators are accessible in order to avoid delays.
Assist with transferring patient to the diagnostic table.	Three to four people may be needed to transfer the patient safely.
Position monitoring equipment and other devices so that they can be observed easily during the test.	Allows the nurse to continually assess the patient during the test.
Perform neurologic and hemodynamic assessment before test.	Establishes patient stability after transport and obtains baseline data before the start of the test.
Monitor and record patient parameters (ECG, BP, pulse oximetry, and ICP) during examination.	Provides documentation of the patient's physiologic responses during test.
Transfer patient and equipment back to stretcher or bed and then transport patient to ICU.	Three to four people may be needed to transfer the patient safely and to transport the patient to the ICU.

ICU, intensive care unit; IV, intravenous line; ECG, electrocardiogram; BP, blood pressure; ICP, intracranial pressure.

Nursing Care Considerations

Accurate monitoring of the neurologic status and ICP measurement is essential for the neurologically impaired patient. The nurse must be knowledgeable about the indications for ICP monitoring in order to anticipate the need to assemble the equipment. ICP devices are most commonly placed by a neurosurgeon in the emergency department and trauma resuscitation settings or in the operating room. Nurses in intensive care units and neurosurgical units also may assist the neurosurgeon in the placement of the monitoring system. Nurses in intermediate care units may see intraventricular catheters for continued drainage of CSF in preparation for a more permanent shunt system.

Nursing care considerations include assembling the equipment, accurate set-up and calibration of the equipment, assessment of the patient during insertion of the monitor, and observation for complications that could lead to neurologic deterioration and inaccurate ICP readings (Table 40–4). Nurses are also responsible for continuous monitoring of the patient and the equipment, for troubleshooting for the ICP monitoring system, and for rapid response to emergency situations involving the ICP monitoring system.

Patient and family teaching should include the purpose and benefit of the ICP monitoring device, the causes of increased ICP, and the reinforcement of the physician's explanation of medical management.

TRANSPORTING THE PATIENT WITH A NEUROLOGIC DEFICIT

Standards for neurodiagnostic testing have resulted in more frequent brain imaging and testing. Nurses caring for critically ill patients are accompanying patients to these tests more routinely and emergently. The process of transporting a patient and obtaining the needed image or test may cause significant stress to an already injured brain. To avoid further injury or deterioration, the nurse must ensure that all preparations for transport are complete and that necessary supplies are present before taking a patient out of the intensive care unit. Table 40–5 identifies the nursing actions required to safely transport a critically ill patient.

It is particularly important to provide critically ill patients on a ventilator with a transport ventilator if they require more than 50% fraction of inspired oxygen (FIO_2) or positive end-expiratory pressure of greater than 5. The transport ventilator prevents any increases in ICP because the patient is not ventilated with an Ambu bag. Ventilation with an Ambu bag may cause endotracheal motion, fluctuations in oxygenation, and subsequent increases in ICP. In addition, it is important to monitor the patient's electrocardiogram, blood pressure, and pulse oximetry during transport. For the brain-injured patient who is receiving therapy for increased ICP, it is vital that the patient's ICP be monitored closely and that the necessary therapy or agents to treat the increased ICP are accessible during the test.

Key Concepts

⇒ Earlier neurodiagnostic tests, such as lumbar puncture, skull radiography, and electroencephalography, have been mostly replaced by newer techniques that allow more direct visualization and measurement, such as computed tomography (CT), angiography, magnetic resonance imaging, (MRI), and intracranial pressure (ICP) monitoring.

⇒ The spine is considered unstable until spinal radiographs rule out injury. Consequently, full precautions are required (e.g., cervical alignment and immobilization) until the results are available.

⇒ A CT scan is indicated for severe headache, head trauma, seizures, hydrocephalus, hemorrhage, or suspicion of lesions. This diagnostic test is quick, less expensive than the MRI, and has few contraindications.

⇒ A complete history of the patient's allergies should be explored for all tests that require the use of a contrast medium. Patients should also be informed that they may experience flushing, transient headache, and nausea/vomiting when the contrast medium is injected.

⇒ Magnetic resonance imaging is superior to CT in attempting to identify extraaxial hemorrhage, brain stem and posterior fossa injuries, and nonhemorrhagic lesions.

⇒ Position emission tomography is still in the early stage of development and holds promise for understanding such disorders as epilepsy, dementia, trauma, and mental illness.

⇒ Patient care after angiography includes monitoring of vital signs, catheter insertion site, and neurologic status. If the femoral artery is used, the patient must remain in bed with the extremity kept straight, and the nurse must assess the distal extremity for signs of adequate perfusion.

⇒ Patient care after myelography is dependent on the type of contrast medium used. The most common side effect with oil-based media is headache; with water-based media, the nursing care is focused on the prevention of seizures.

⇒ Electroencephalography is most commonly ordered if cerebral dysfunction cannot be visualized by CT scan, MRI, or radiography.

⇒ Evoked potentials are a noninvasive technique that involves applying repetitive sensory stimuli and recording the impulse generated as it travels through the brain stem and the cerebral cortex. The auditory stimulus (brain stem auditory evoked response) is easily performed at the bedside.

➡ The use of transcranial Doppler ultrasound in patients with head injuries is gaining interest. Generally, the higher the flow, as measured by the computerized spectral analysis machine, the narrower the vessel.

➡ Patient teaching regarding neurodiagnostic testing should include the critical information needed to ensure patient safety and cooperation before and after the test or tests.

➡ The three principles governing ICP include the Monro-Kellie hypothesis, the volume–pressure curve, and cerebral perfusion pressure (CPP).

➡ The average CCP is 80 to 100 mm Hg. Pressures below 60 mm Hg predispose the patient to cerebral ischemia, and sustained pressures below 30 mm Hg result in brain death.

➡ In general, patients with head injuries who are comatose and have Glasgow Coma Scores of 8 should have ICP monitoring.

➡ There are many advantages and disadvantages to each of the different types of ICP monitoring catheters. Regardless of which catheter is selected, the main objective of ICP monitoring is to maintain cerebral perfusion and oxygenation while the injured brain recovers.

➡ The ICP waveform has three peaks that descend in a sawtooth pattern. When the P2 portion of the pulse waveform is larger than or equal to P1, a state of decreased cerebral compliance exists.

➡ There are three types of abnormal ICP trend waveforms: A, B, and C. A waves, or plateau waves, indicate a highly noncompliant brain, and treatment is focused on decreasing ICP and preventing the CCP from falling to critical levels.

➡ Complications of ICP monitoring include infection, hemorrhage, malfunction, obstruction, and malposition. Diligent nursing care can prevent many of these complications and can provide early detection and intervention of others.

➡ Transporting patients with a neurologic deficit can be challenging. Nurses must adequately plan for the care the patient will require while off the unit in order to limit any additional stress to the patient's already injured brain.

References

1. Adams RD, Victor M (eds): Principles of Neurology, 5th ed. New York, McGraw-Hill, 1993, pp 11–34.
2. Waxman SG, de Groot J: Imaging the brain. In: Waxman SG: Correlative Neuroanatomy. Norwalk, CT, Appleton & Lange, 1994, pp 291–303.
3. Hickey JV: The Clinical Practice of Neurological and Neurosurgical Nursing, 3rd ed. Philadelphia, JB Lippincott, 1992.
4. Thelan LA, Davie JA, Urden LD, Lough ME: Critical Care Nursing: Diagnosis and Management, 2nd ed. St. Louis, CV Mosby, 1993, pp 515–521.
5. Montgomery JL, Montgomery ML: Radiographic evaluation of cervical spine trauma: procedures to avoid catastrophe. Postgrad Med 95:173–196, 1994.
6. Cardona VD, Hurn PD, Mason PJ, et al.: Trauma Nursing. Philadelphia, WB Saunders, 1994.
7. Marshall SB, Marshall LF, Vos HR, Chestnut RM: Neuroscience Critical Care. Philadelphia, WB Saunders, 1997.
8. Nuwer MR: Electroencephalograms and evoked potentials: monitoring cerebral function in the neurosurgical intensive care unit. Neurosurg Clin North Am 5:647–659, 1994.
9. Jordan KG: Continuous EEG and evoked potential monitoring in the neuroscience intensive care unit. J Clin Neurophysiol 10:445–475, 1993.
9a. Manno EM: Transcranial Doppler ultrasonography in the neurocritical care unit. Crit Care Clin 13(1):79–93, 1997.
10. Marshall LF, Gautille T, Klauber MR, et al.: The outcome of severe closed head injury. J Neurosurg 75:528–536, 1991.
11. Marmarou A, Tabaddor K: Intracranial pressure: physiology and pathophysiology. In: Cooper PR (ed): Head Injury, 2nd ed. Baltimore, Williams & Wilkins, 1991, pp 56–72.
12. Ghajar JB, Hariri R: Survey of critical care management of comatose head injured patients in the United States. Crit Care Med 23:560–567, 1996.
13. Rosner MJ, Daughton S: Cerebral perfusion pressure management in head injury. J Trauma 30:933–941, 1990.
14. Rosner MJ, Rosner SD, Johnson AH: Cerebral perfusion pressure: management protocol and clinical results. J Neurosurg 83:949–962, 1995.
15. Prendergast V: Current trends in research and treatment of intracranial hypertension. Crit Care Nurs Q 17:1–8, 1994.
16. Chestnut RM, Marshall LF: Management of head injury: treatment of abnormal intracranial pressure. Neurosurg Clin North Am 2:267, 1991.
17. Schickner DJ, Young RF: Intracranial pressure monitoring: fiberoptic monitor compared with ventricular catheter. Surg Neurol 37:251–254, 1992.
18. Shapiro S, Bowman R, Callahan J, Wolfla C: The fiberoptic intraparenchymal cerebral pressure monitor in 244 patients. Surg Neurol, 45:278–282, 1996.
19. Bader MK, Littlejohns L, Palmer S: Ventriculostomy and intracranial pressure monitoring: in search of a 0% infection rate. Heart Lung 24:166–172, 1995.
20. Piper IR, Miller JD: The evaluation of the wave-form analysis capability of a new strain-gauge intracranial pressure microsensor. Neurosurgery 36:1142–1145, 1995.
21. Paramore CG, Turner DA: Relative risks of ventriculostomy infection and morbidity. Acta Neurochir (Wien) 127:79–84, 1994.
22. Artu F, Terrier A, Gibert I, et al.: Monitoring of intracranial pressure with intraparenchymal fiberoptic transducer: technical aspects and clinical reliability. Ann Fr Anesth Reanim 11:424–429, 1992.
23. Yablon JS, Lantner HJ, McCormack TM, et al.: Clinical experience with a fiberoptic intracranial pressure monitor. J Clin Monit 9:171–175, 1993.
24. Chambers IR, Kane PJ, Choksey MS, et al.: An evaluation of the Camino ventricular bolt system in clinical practice. Neurosurgery 33:866–868, 1993.

41

Acute Head Injury

Karen March

Objectives

After completing this chapter, the student will be able to:

1. Describe the mechanisms of injury for acute brain injury.
2. Differentiate primary versus secondary brain injury.
3. Identify the principal attributes of each type of primary brain injury.
4. Relate the major factors contributing to secondary brain injury to the pathophysiologic consequences.
5. Apply appropriate primary and secondary assessment techniques to a patient with an acute brain injury.
6. Relate the diagnostic workup of the brain-injured patient to the management plan.
7. Develop a plan for the collaborative management of the brain-injured patient.
8. Evaluate the effectiveness of the collaborative management of increased intracranial pressure.

There are different terminologies used in discussions of trauma to the structures associated with the brain; acute head injury, brain injury, traumatic brain injury (TBI), closed head injury, and penetrating head injury. Acute head injury is a generic term used in discussions about an injury to the head and its structures, whereas brain injury refers only to injuries to the brain itself. A TBI is one that results from a traumatic event and may result from a blunt or a penetrating injury. The term closed head injury refers to a blunt injury to the brain that does not result in an open skull fracture. A penetrating injury results from a missile, such as a knife, gun, hammer, and baseball bat. Traumatic brain injury is the preferred terminology.

Trauma is the leading cause of death for persons younger than 45 years.[1] Between one-third and one-half of all trauma deaths are the result of a TBI. Hundreds of thousands of people seek medical care for a TBI each year, and 60 to 80% of these are a mild or a minor injury. There are probably many more injuries that are never seen by health care personnel.[2,3]

Traumatic brain injury is most common between the ages of 15 and 25 years, with peaks seen in infants and in the elderly. Males are twice as likely to sustain a TBI as females. Lower socioeconomic groups also appear to be at a greater risk.

The major cause of TBI is motor vehicle crashes. Falls are the second leading cause in all age groups and are the leading cause in the elderly and in preschoolers. Interpersonal violence is fast approaching the leading cause of brain injury in the urban setting. For the infant, child abuse is the number one cause of TBI. Other mechanisms of TBI include motorcycle crashes, motor vehicles hitting pedestrians and cyclists, cyclist crashes, and sport-related injuries.[4]

Trauma specialists believe that traumatic injury is the result of preventable events that are rarely an "accident." Therefore, the best way to treat an injury is to prevent it from occurring. Injury prevention strategies are aimed at legislation to protect the individual and to educate the public on how to protect themselves from situations that put them at risk. Some of the legislative efforts are drinking and driving laws, cyclist and motorcycle helmet laws, seatbelt and car seat laws, driver's side air bags, and firearm legislation. Programs such as "Think First" and "Trauma Nurses Talk Tough," are education programs that focus on teaching youths the consequences of their behaviors.

ETIOLOGY AND PATHOPHYSIOLOGY

Mechanism

The pathology of TBI can be divided into two stages: primary and secondary injury. The primary injury occurs at the time of injury or impact. The secondary injury results from the events that follow the injury that affect oxygenation and perfusion of brain tissue.

Primary injury occurs when kinetic force is applied to the cranium and brain. These forces are acceleration, deceleration, acceleration-deceleration, and coup-contrecoup. Acceleration force occurs when a moving object (baseball, fist, hammer) hits a stationary head. A deceleration force occurs when a moving head hits a stationary object (windshield, wall, the ground). Acceleration-deceleration forces occur during high-speed motor vehicle crashes and car versus pedestrian crashes. Coup-contrecoup is the result of movement of the intracranial contents within the cranium. The brain first hits the wall of the cranium underlying the initial impact (coup), then bounces in the opposite direction and hits the cranium directly opposite the initial impact (contrecoup). These forces produce shear, tensile, and compressive strains on the cranium and brain, tearing tissue, vessels, and axons and fracturing bone.[5, 6]

Primary Injury

Injuries may be divided into focal or diffuse injuries. A focal injury is one that produces a macroscopic lesion: scalp lacerations, skull fractures, lacerations and contusions of the brain, epidural hematomas, subdural hematomas, and intracerebral hematomas. Diffuse brain injury is microscopic or neuronal: concussion and diffuse axonal injury.[7]

Skull Fractures. Scalp lacerations are disruptions of the outermost protective layer of the brain that is very vascular and may bleed profusely. Gentle pressure and a sterile dressing should be applied to stop the bleeding. All wounds should be gently inspected for evidence of an underlying skull fracture. A brain injury may or may not accompany a scalp laceration.

Skull fractures may be divided into linear, depressed, or basilar. A linear fracture is a crack in the skull. The severity of the fracture depends on the location of the fracture and the damage to the underlying tissues. Usually, linear fractures require no surgical intervention; however, in the pediatric population a growing linear fracture may develop into a leptomeningeal cyst. A leptomeningeal cyst is a widening of the fracture created by the intrusion of the arachnoid membrane into the fracture. Surgical treatment may be required to remove the cyst and to repair the dura and cranium.[8–10] A depressed skull fracture is a fracture that displaces the bone with or without lacera-

tion of the dura and brain tissue. Surgical elevation of the fracture, débridement of the brain tissue, and repair of the dura may be performed, followed by antibiotic administration.[11, 12]

Basilar skull fractures are linear fractures at the base of the skull. Basilar fractures in the anterior fossa may result in periorbital ecchymosis (raccoon or panda eyes) and blood or cerebral spinal fluid (CSF) drainage from the nose (rhinorrhea). Basilar skull fractures in the middle or posterior fossa result in bruising over the mastoid process (Battle sign) and blood and CSF drainage from the ear (otorrhea). Figure 41–1 illustrates locations of fractures. Any drainage from the nose or ear should be assessed for the presence of CSF either by dipping the fluid for glucose with a Dextrostix or, if blood is present, performing a halo ring test (dropping a few drops of CSF on a pillowcase or a paper towel; blood congeals in the center and the CSF forms a ring around it). The nose or ear should never be packed when a CSF leak is present; obstructing the flow of CSF may increase the risk of infections. Patients with rhinorrhea or otorrhea are treated with antibiotics. Most CSF leaks seal themselves after several days of bed rest with the head of the bed elevated; if not, a lumbar or ventricular drain is inserted to lower the CSF pressure against the tear. Surgery is reserved for larger defects or those that do not heal. Basilar fractures involving the petrous bone may also result in seventh and eighth cranial nerve injury, producing facial droop, dizziness, tinnitus, or hearing loss.[11]

Lacerations and Contusions. Lacerations and contusions of brain tissue are usually found in the frontal and temporal lobes. Often these are related to the impact of the tissues on the rough bony surface of the basal cranium. A laceration is the tearing of the brain that can also occur beneath a depressed skull fracture. A contusion is the bruising of the cortical surfaces of the brain. Patients may be restless and agitated and may have poor short-term memory, speech and motor dysfunction, or coma. Surgical débridement of necrotic tissue is performed if ICP is difficult to control medically.

Hematomas. A linear fracture across the temporal bone may lacerate the middle meningeal artery, producing an epidural hematoma, shown in Figure 41–2A. Epidural hematomas account for about 0.2 to 6% of head injuries and occur more frequently in children and young adults. An epidural hematoma is called the "talk and die syndrome" because the patient may have a lucid period, rapidly deteriorate, and die. The morbidity and mortality arise from the rapid expansion of the hematoma from the arterial bleeder, causing uncal herniation, not direct brain injury. The hematoma lies outside the dura between the dura and cranium, displacing the brain. The patient classically has ipsilateral pupillary changes that progress from a sluggish and elliptical pupil to a dilated and fixed one.

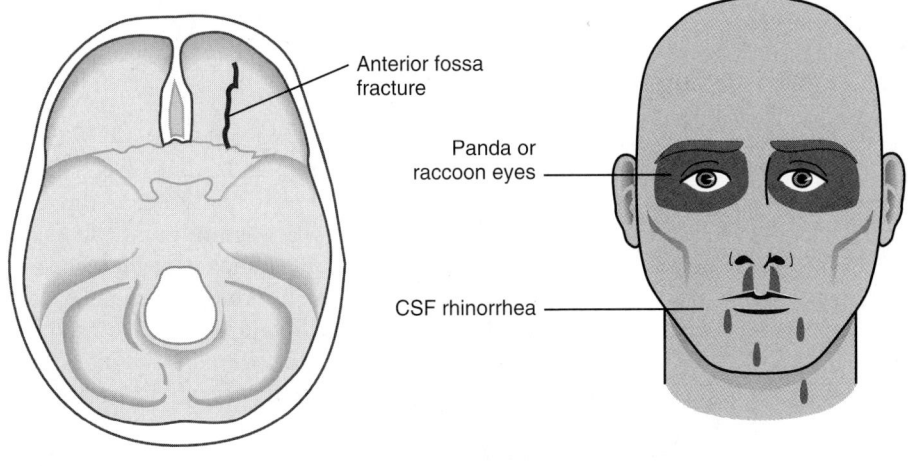

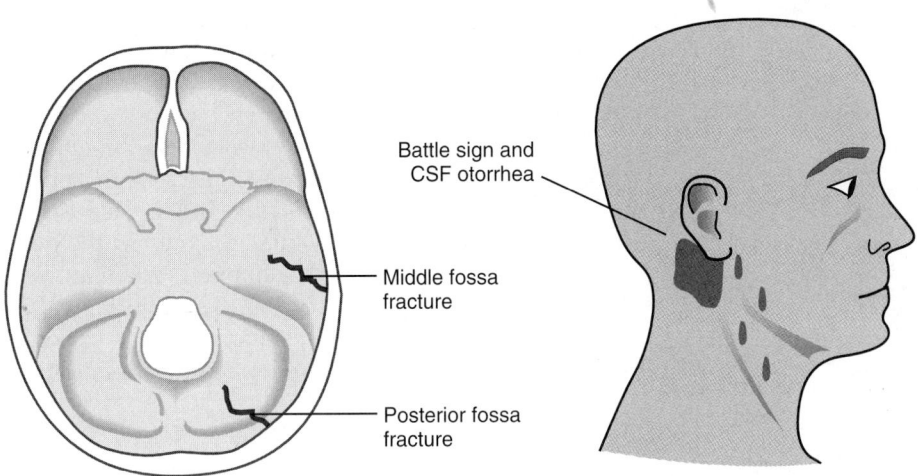

Figure 41–1

Location of and symptoms associated with basilar skull fractures.

There are simultaneous contralateral motor changes that progress from a mild hemiparesis to decortication, decerebration, or flaccid paralysis. Epidural hematoma may also be caused by lacerated veins and may occur subfrontally and in the posterior fossa. Treatment is usually surgical removal of the clot. With early treatment, the prognosis is usually good.

Subdural hematomas (SDH) carry the second highest morbidity and mortality. The hematoma originates from venous bleeding from the cortex or bridging veins between the surface of the brain and the dura, as shown in Figure 41–2*B*, making the progression slower than with an epidural hematoma. SDH is associated with direct injury to the brain. There are three types of SDH. An acute SDH is symptomatic within the first 24 to 72 hours after injury and usually requires immediate surgical evacuation. A subacute SDH is symptomatic 72 hours to 2 weeks after injury and requires close observation for symptoms of increased intracranial pressure (ICP) and herniation. Surgical evacuation depends on the consistency and the size of the clot. Chronic SDH usually produces delayed symptoms, 2 weeks or more after the trauma, and mimics dementia. Chronic SDHs are most often

seen in the elderly or chronic substance abusers with brain atrophy. Bleeding is slow and there is more space in the cranium for the clot to expand before the patient experiences neurologic compromise. Treatment consists of burr holes, irrigation, and insertion of drainage catheters to slowly drain the clot. Patients are nursed in the supine position to promote drainage and to avoid reaccumulation of the clot. Placing the head in the supine position allows the brain tissue to expand and take up the space in the cranium where the clot previously was. If the clot is too viscous, a craniotomy is performed. Mortality rates range from 30 to 63%. Preoperative neurologic status, age, timing of surgery, ICP, size of hematoma, and extracranial factors affect outcome.[5, 12, 13]

An intracerebral hematoma is a well-circumscribed area of bleeding into the parenchyma tissue of about 2 cm or more. Motor vehicle crashes and falls are the most common causes of intracerebral hematoma. Intracerebral hematomas produce focal neurologic deficits related to their locations. Surgical removal of the clot is performed if the clot is large, well circumscribed, and easily accessible. Others are left to reabsorb on their own. Mortality rates range from 25 to

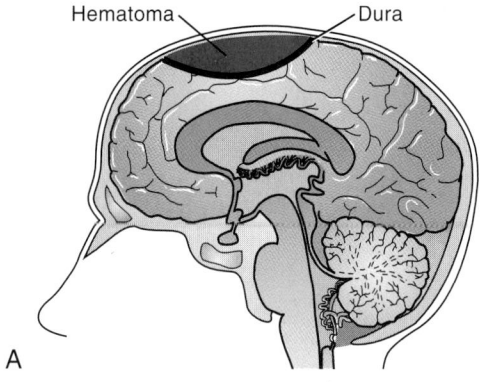

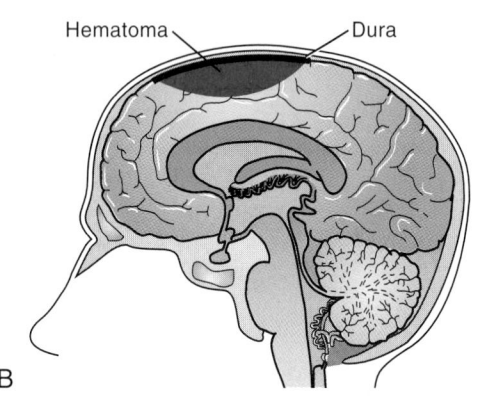

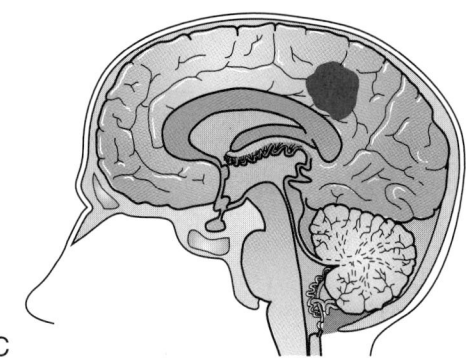

Figure 41–2

Types of hematomas. *A.* Epidural hematoma. *B.* Subdural hematoma. *C.* Intracerebral hematoma.

60%. The poor outcome is related to the severity of the injury required to produce these injuries.[12, 14] Figure 41–2C shows an intracerebral hematoma.

Penetrating Injuries. With the increase in violence in our society, there has been an increase in penetrating injury from gunshots. The morbidity and mortality from these injuries depend on the type of weapon, the shape and trajectory of the bullet, the structures hit by the bullet, and whether the bullet crosses the midline. Generally, transventricular gunshot wounds are fatal, and overall, 50 to 60% of these patients die. Controversy exists about aggressive surgical débridement of the wounds and vigorous removal of the bullet and bone fragments. Routine use of antibiotics has decreased the incidence of meningitis, but brain abscesses occur at a rate of 5 to 10%.[12, 15, 16]

Other causes of penetrating injuries are knives, arrows, scissors, spears, nails, and other objects. Stab wounds are less common and usually occur through the thinner tables of bone, like the orbit and the zygomatic area. Injury to cerebral tissues is more localized and may result in little or no neurologic deficits unless an intracerebral hematoma develops or vital structures are hit.[12] Surgery may be performed to explore and clean the wound and to repair lacerated vessels and dura.

Diffuse Injuries. Cerebral concussion is the temporary loss of consciousness, and amnesia usually lasts less than 6 hours with little or no long-term neurologic sequelae. Computed tomography shows no macroscopic lesions and is read as normal. This may also be referred to as a mild diffuse injury.[6]

High-speed motor vehicle crashes result in angular deceleration forces that shear the interface between the gray and the white matter of the brain. This causes tearing and fraying of myelinated axons in the deep white matter, much like what happens when an electric cord is stretched (Figure 41–3). This injury is called diffuse axonal injury (DAI), shearing injury, or Strich injury. Computed tomographic scans often appear

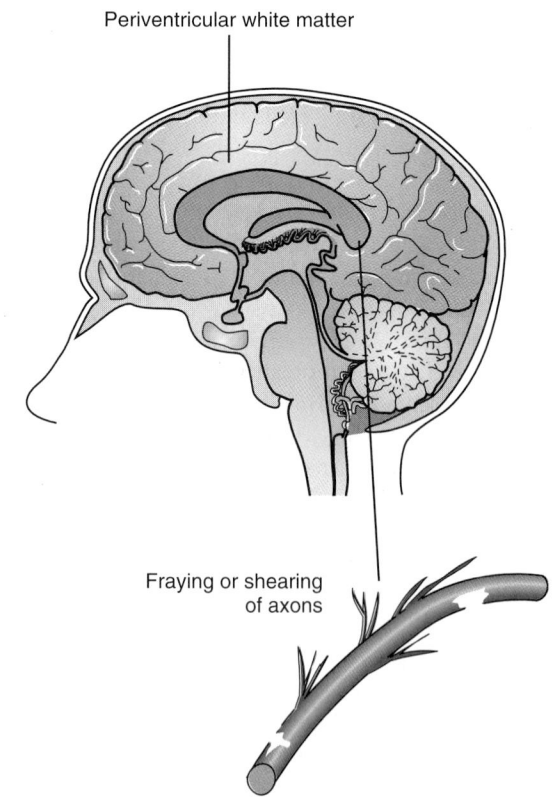

Figure 41–3

Schematic of diffuse axonal injury.

normal or show punctate hemorrhages in the corpus callosum, the periventricular area, or the brain stem. Molecular and biochemical changes produce further destruction of neurons and worsening of the neurologic condition.[17] DAI carries high morbidity and mortality directly related to the severity of the injury: mild, moderate, or severe. Mild DAI results in a loss of consciousness for 6 to 24 hours. Patients with moderate DAI have prolonged coma and a 20% mortality. Those with severe DAI also have prolonged coma as well as brain stem dysfunction, leading to hemodynamic and cardiac instability. Mortality increases to 60 to 70%.[7] Autonomic dysfunction, or "storming," is often seen after DAI, producing increased ICP, dilated pupils, diaphoresis, hypertension, tachycardia, and abnormal flexion or extensor posturing. These symptoms diminish with time and may be moderated with propranolol, morphine sulfate, and bromocriptine.[18, 19] No treatment studies have been reported to date.

Traumatic Subarachnoid Hemorrhages. Traumatic subarachnoid hemorrhage, bleeding into the subarchnoid space resulting in vasospasm, occurs in 25 to 40% of TBI.[20–22] A study by Greene and colleagues[21] found that patients with subarachnoid hemorrhage spent more time in the intensive care unit and in the hospital and had a worse outcome. Blood in the subarachnoid space puts the patient at risk to develop cerebral vasospasm, which is narrowing of the vessel lumen, that may result in a delayed ischemic event. The risk for developing vasospasm is greatest 3 to 7 days after the bleeding and subsides about 10 days after the bleeding. Administering nimodipine, a calcium channel blocker, has been shown to improve outcome in patients with traumatic cerebral vasospasm.[23]

Mild Traumatic Brain Injuries. Patients who sustain a mild or subtle TBI often go unrecognized, even when they require hospitalization for other injury. The computed tomographic scan is normal, there may or may not be a loss of consciousness, and the Glasgow Coma Scale (GCS) score is 13 to 15. It is only after patients try to resume their normal activities that the deficits become apparent. Symptoms can be somatic, cognitive, and emotional-behavioral, as shown in Chart 41–1. Sequelae from a mild TBI, if left untreated, may result in loss of employment and disruption of the family. Educating the patient and the family on coping strategies and acknowledging that the symptoms are real can help the patient get through this limited disability.[24, 25]

Secondary Injury

After TBI, biophysical and biochemical changes occur that alter perfusion, leading to neuronal dysfunction and death. The severity and the significance of these changes can be moderated if we have an understanding of the processes. In the past, management after brain injury has been focused on treating increased ICP. Now, treatment focuses on promoting adequate perfusion. Figure 41–4 illustrates systemic and intracranial events that affect cerebral perfusion.[26]

When caring for patients after TBI, the nurse should understand what happens to cerebral blood flow (CBF). CBF is a function of influx pressures, systemic arterial blood pressure (SABP), efflux pressure, venous outflow, vascular radius, and blood viscosity. Normally, CBF remains constant over a wide range of mean SABP, 50 to 150 mm Hg. As mean SABP falls, vessels dilate; as mean SABP rises, vessels constrict. As these mechanisms fail, the brain injury can worsen: (1) hypotension decreases cerebral perfusion, leading to ischemia; (2) unmediated hypertension leads to vasogenic edema and further increased ICP.[5, 27]

CHART 41–1

Symptoms of Mild Traumatic Brain Injury

SOMATIC
- Headache
- Dizziness
- Nausea and vomiting
- Blurred vision
- Tinnitus and hearing difficulties
- Drowsiness
- Seizures (rare)

COGNITIVE
- Amnesia of event
- Impaired attention and concentration
- Impaired short-term memory
- Disorientation and/or confusion
- Slow thinking and information processing
- Poor judgment
- Mental fatigue

EMOTIONAL-BEHAVIORAL
- Agitation
- Irritability
- Apathy
- Depression
- Emotional instability
- Sleep disturbance
- Lower tolerance for frustration
- Loss of sexual drive
- Intolerance to ethyl alcohol

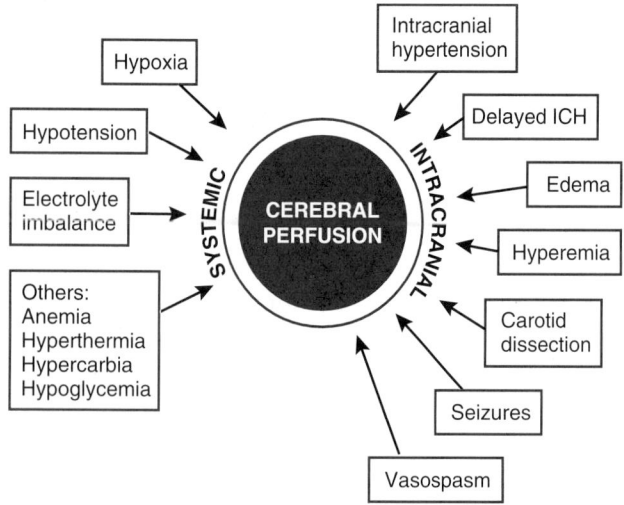

Figure 41-4

Systemic and intracranial events that affect cerebral perfusion.

Compensatory mechanisms that control CBF are called cerebral autoregulation. These mechanisms can be divided into metabolic, myogenic, and chemical. Table 41–1 demonstrates cerebrovascular effect of each mechanism. Metabolic regulation is the coupling or matching of CBF to metabolic demand. When demand decreases, as occurs during sleeping, CBF also decreases. Myogenic regulation, also referred to as adrenergic or sympathetic, is the vascular tone that adjusts to changes in transmural pressure. The chemical regulation that is called metabolic by some authors refers to the effect of extravascular pH on vascular diameter. When carbon dioxide levels rise or oxygen levels fall (hypoxia), the patient becomes acidotic, and cerebral vessels dilate. If carbon dioxide levels decrease or the patient is hyperoxygenated, the patient becomes alkalotic and vessels constrict. Impaired autoregulation, which may be regional or global, may affect the patient's responsiveness to treatment. Vasomotor paralysis (loss of autoregulation) usually results in death.[28,29]

For the first several hours after a TBI, CBF studies have shown that CBF drops as much as half and, in 30% of patients with TBI, to 18 mL/100 g of brain per minute. Normal CBF is about 50 mL/100 g of brain per minute. Ischemia occurs when CBF drops below 20 mL/100 g of brain per minute, and neuronal death occurs when CBF drops to 10 to 15 mL/100 g of brain per minute. Figure 41–5 represents the pathophysiologic changes of decreased cerebral blood flow. The presence of ischemia in the first hours is correlated with poor outcome. Prior studies at 18 and 24 hours failed to show significant ischemia. This acute response of CBF appears to be related to the impact and not to hypotension; however, hypotension can compound the effects of low CBF.[28]

After the initial event, patients may remain ischemic, referred to as oligemic cerebral hypoxia, or patients may become hyperemic. Hyperemia is an increase in CBF in relationship to demand and often also an increase in cerebral blood volume. Hyperemia may be relative or absolute. When cerebral metabolism is normal and CBF is increased beyond the tissue needs, absolute hyperemia occurs. During coma, cerebral metabolic demand normally decreases; therefore, CBF should decrease. If demand decreases but CBF remains at normal levels, the patient has a relative hyperemia. As brain tissue dies, patients may become progressively more hyperemic.[30] In the past, children were thought to have hyperemia more frequently, referred to as malignant brain edema; however, some investigators suggest that this is not true.[31]

One way we can monitor if we are meeting the demand of the brain tissue is to calculate the patient's cerebral perfusion pressure (CPP). CPP is the sum of the mean SABP minus the ICP (mean SABP − mean ICP = CPP). Normal CPP is 80 to 100 mm Hg. Studies suggest that in the patient with a brain injury, CPP should be maintained at greater than or equal to 70 mm Hg. A CPP of less than 40 mm Hg results in ischemia.[27,32]

Ischemic and hypoxic events trigger a chain of biochemical responses and neurotoxic processes. These

TABLE 41-1
Mechanisms of Autoregulation

Mechanism	Vasoconstriction	Vasodilation
Metabolic		
↑ demand		X
↓ demand	X	
Myogenic		
↑ SABP	X	
↓ SABP		X
Chemical		
↑ PaO_2, ↓ $PaCO_2$, ↑ pH	X	
↓ PaO_2, ↑ $PaCO_2$, ↓ pH		X

PaO_2, partial pressure of arterial oxygen; $PaCO_2$, partial pressure of arterial carbon dioxide; SABP, systemic arterial blood pressure.

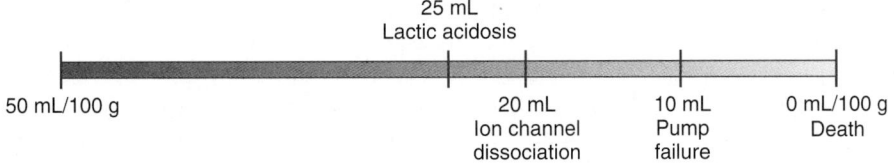

Figure 41–5

Effects of altered cerebral blood flow on cellular function.

include regulation of calcium, sodium, and potassium ion channels, release of excitotoxic amino acids, production of superoxides and free radicals, peroxidation of lipid, and release of inflammatory mediator, all of which result in cellular damage (Figure 41–6). As cellular damage progresses, edema and neuronal death ensue, leading to increased ICP, further ischemia, and cell damage. If this process is not abated, brain death occurs.[33-36]

Increased ICP is a result of uncompensated increases in intracranial volume: blood, brain (hematoma, tumor, edema), or CSF. Cerebral edema is defined as an increase in brain tissue water. It is thought that five types of edema exist: (1) cytotoxic, (2) vasogenic, (3) interstitial, (4) hydrostatic, and (5) hypo-osmotic. Cytotoxic edema is caused by the failed ion channels of the cell membrane, allowing sodium and water to enter the cell. Vasogenic edema results from a disruption in the blood-brain barrier, increasing capillary permeability, transmural pressure, retention of extravasated fluids and proteins in the interstitial space. Interstitial edema is caused by high-pressure obstructive hydrocephalus in which CSF infiltrates the periventricular tissues. An increase in transmural vascular pressure results in hydrostatic edema, an increase in extracellular fluid. Lastly, hypo-osmotic edema is a shift in fluid resulting in a critically low serum sodium level or osmolarity. Women may be more susceptible to this because of higher levels of estrogen.[5]

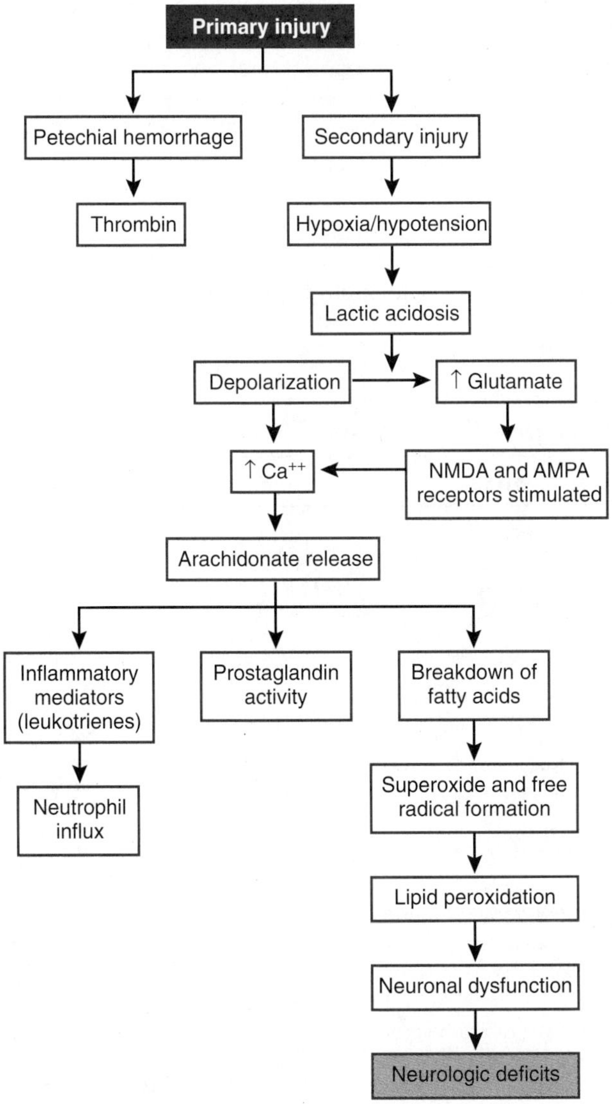

Systemic Impact of Acute Brain Injury

Acute brain injury affects not only the central nervous system but also all body systems. When the brain is injured, the sympathetic nervous system is stimulated; that, in turn, stimulates the adrenal cortex and medulla, increasing the circulating corticoid and catecholamine levels. Glucocorticoids increase the metabolism of carbohydrates, fats, and proteins. Mineral corticoids stimulate the retention of water and sodium. Antidiuretic hormone is also released from the posterior pituitary, influencing the retention of water. If antidiuretic hormone is not secreted, excessive diuresis and diabetes insipidus result.

Increases in serum catecholamine levels stimulate the cardiovascular system, producing hypertension, electrocardiographic changes, and cardiac dysrhythmias. Common electrocardiographic changes include peaked P waves, prolonged QT intervals, depressed ST segments, inverted T waves, and large U waves. It is difficult to distinguish some of these electrocardiographic changes from myocardial ischemic changes. Cardiac dysrhythmias that most commonly occur are bradycardia, nodal rhythms, and sinus tachycardia; less common are sinus dysrhythmias, atrial fibrillation, premature ventricular contractions, heart block, and ventricular tachycardia.[37,38]

Pulmonary dysfunction may be neurogenic. Inadequate ventilation may be the result of abnormal respiratory patterns or reduced functional residual capacity, causing the retention of partial pressure of arterial

Figure 41–6

Ischemia cascade in brain injury.

carbon dioxide, vasodilation, and increased ICP. Abnormal respiratory patterns include Cheyne-Stokes, central neurogenic hyperventilation, apneusis, and ataxia. Pulmonary edema may be neurogenic rather than cardiopulmonary. It is theorized that the sympathetic stimulation increases pulmonary capillary permeability, thus increasing pulmonary alveolar fluid and impeding ventilation.[37,39,40]

During the stress response, patients may become hyperglycemic. Increased epinephrine and cortisol levels inhibit the release of insulin; promote glyconeogenesis, gluconeogenesis, and lipolysis; and decrease glucose utilization by muscle and adipose tissue. Insulin is not recommended in the first 72 hours unless the glucose level increases to greater than 200 mg/dL.

Vascular occlusion, disseminated intravascular coagulopathy, or anemia may develop after brain injury. Catecholamines and thromboplastin released from the injured brain stem increase platelet and plasma fibrinogen levels, shortening clotting and prothrombin times. Thromboplastin activates the clotting cascade and converts to free thrombin, causing platelets to aggregate and fibrin to form. This can cause either a consumption coagulopathy or vascular occlusion. Anemia results from a decrease in red cell mass.

Secondary infection, such as pneumonia, is common after brain injury and may be partly due to the immunosuppression that results from the effects of the catecholamine-induced disturbance in phagocytosis. Catecholamines depress neutrophil and lymphocyte function.

The gastrointestinal system is also affected. Gastric motility is often decreased and acidity increased. The acidity is influenced by the increase in catecholamines and glucocorticoids. This increase in acidity may result in the development of a gastritis or a gastric ulcer.[6,37,41,42]

Assessment

Recognition and management of TBI begin with the prehospital providers. Mortality statistics vary among regions in part as a result of access to health care in different areas. Studies show that hypotension (<90 mm Hg systolic) and hypoxia (partial pressure of arterial oxygen < 60 mm Hg) increase morbidity and mortality.[43,44] Assessment and management of the patient's airway, breathing, and circulation (ABCs) diminish the secondary effects of the brain injury. Recognition and management of an acute brain injury and transport to definitive care optimize the patient outcome.

Signs and Symptoms of Traumatic Head Injury

During the primary survey, the neurologic assessment consists of evaluating pupillary reactivity and equality and level of consciousness. The acronym AVPU (alert, verbal, pain, unresponsive) signifies the level of consciousness. During the secondary survey, a brief history of the events and mechanism is taken, vital signs are assessed, and a more extensive neurologic evaluation is performed with the GCS shown in Table 41–2. The GCS ranges from 3 to 15. At this time, the examiner assesses for decreased consciousness, GCS of 13 or less (no eye opening to verbal or noxious stimuli, confusion, abnormal vocalization or no vocalization, and localization or abnormal motor movements), pupillary changes (inequality, nonreactivity, or pontine), and symmetry of neurologic findings.[45]

When the patient reaches the hospital, a more comprehensive neurologic evaluation is performed and is repeated at regular intervals to monitor the patient's progress. The initial evaluation includes (1) level of consciousness; (2) pupillary assessment; (3) brain stem reflexes; (4) identification of focal or localizing signs; (5) survey for external signs of head trauma; (6) vital signs, which may include ICP monitoring; (7) concurrent injuries, such as craniofacial and spinal injuries; and (8) assessment of preexisting conditions that may confound the patient's condition. Table 41–3 highlights components of the assessment. Agreement between examiners is important to determining when the patient has a change in neurologic status. Performing an examination together is one way to ensure that the examination is interpreted consistently. A deteriora-

TABLE 41–2
Glasgow Coma Scale

Response	Rating
Eye opening (1–4)	
▪ Opens eyes spontaneously	4
▪ Opens eyes to verbal stimuli	3
▪ Opens eyes to pain	2
▪ No eye opening	1
Best verbal (1–5)	
▪ Oriented	5
▪ Confused (disoriented)	4
▪ Inappropriate (swearing, yelling)	3
▪ Incomprehensible sounds (moans)	2
▪ None	1
▪ Intubate	1T
Motor (6–1)	
▪ Follows commands	6
▪ Localizes to pain (purposeful)	5*
▪ Normal flexion (withdrawal)	4*
▪ Abnormal flexion (decortication)	3*
▪ Extension (decerebration)	2*
▪ None	1*

*Noxious stimuli testing is best performed with a central stimuli to avoid eliciting a spinal reflex or not eliciting a response if a spinal cord injury is present.

TABLE 41–3
Comprehensive Neurologic Assessment

Component	Possible Findings
Level of consciousness	Orientation Hypoarousal: lethargy, obtunded, stupor Hyperarousal: restlessness, agitation Language—dysphasia, dysarthria Mentation—memory, attention
Pupillary assessment	Examination—size, shape, response to light, consensual Abnormal pupils—unilateral fixed and dilated, bilateral fixed and dilated, pinpoint
Brain stem reflexes	Corneals Extraocular movements—doll's eyes (oculocephalic reflex), caloric (oculovestibular reflex), gaze, tracking Cough Gag
Focal/localizing signs	Glasgow Coma Scale—motor 6 Follows commands 5 Localizes to pain (purposeful) 4 Normal flexion (withdrawal) 3 Abnormal flexion (decortication) 2 Extension (decerebration) 1 None Pronator drift Muscle strength 5 Normal power 4 Moves against gravity with some resistance 3 Moves against gravity without resistance 2 Moves without gravity 1 Flicker of movement 0 No movement Facial droop
External signs of head injury	Bruises, lacerations, abrasions
Vital signs	Respirations—Cheyne-Stokes, central neurogenic hyperventilation, apneustic, ataxic Heart rate—sinus tachycardia, bradycardia Blood pressure—hypertension, hypotension
Preexisting conditions	Head injury, stroke, peripheral nerve injury, spinal cord injury, Parkinson's disease, cardiac disease, pulmonary disease, other

tion in two parameters indicates a worsening of the patient's neurologic condition and necessitates physician notification. Strict attention must be paid to patterns of neurologic deterioration that signify herniation.[5,46]

The GCS is used not only to monitor the patient's progress but also to guide additional neurologic assessment and to predict outcome. The severity of the injury dictates the focus of the neurologic examination. The GCS is used to categorize the severity of the injury; a GCS of 13 to 15 indicates a mild injury; a GCS of 9 to 12, a moderate injury; and a GCS of 3 to 8, a severe injury. A mild head injury requires assessment of higher cognitive functions and subtle neurologic focal deficits. The patient with a moderate or severe head injury will have impaired consciousness and often focal neurologic deficits.

Laboratory and Diagnostic Tests

After the patient is hemodynamically and medically stabilized in the emergency department, diagnostic studies are performed to assess the cause of the injury. Anterior-posterior and lateral radiographs of the skull are used primarily to look for skull fractures or to assess penetrating objects. Computed tomography is commonly performed to assess for mass lesions, edema, swelling, infarcts, fractures, penetrating objects, and herniation. Magnetic resonance imaging is usually reserved for further evaluation of DAI, brain stem injury, chronic SDH, and neurologic deficits that are not well explained. Arteriography is used to assess cerebrovascular injury.[5,47]

Other diagnostics that may help determine the extent of the brain injury include auditory, visual and somatosensory brain stem evoke potentials, cerebral

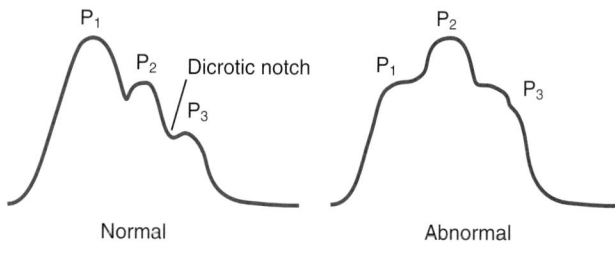

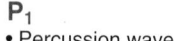

P_1
- Percussion wave
- Reflects the ejection of blood from the heart transmitted through the choroid plexus in ventricles

P_2
- Tidal wave
- Reflective of brain bulk or compliance, vasoparalysis, swelling, and edema
- Reflects venous compartment
- $P_2 = 80\% P_1$

P_3
- Dicrotic notch

Figure 41–7

Intracranial pressure waveforms, normal and abnormal.

blood flow studies, cerebral metabolic studies, nuclear medicine scans, transcranial Doppler monitoring,[22] and monitoring of saturation of jugular venous oxygen, lactate, and glucose. Retrograde jugular catheters or saturation of jugular venous oxygen catheters are diagnostic tools managed by the nurse at the bedside. These catheters assess the balance between CBF and the demand of the tissues. Data may be obtained by use of intermittent blood samples or continuously with a fiberoptic oximetric catheter. Information obtained from these catheters allows the caregivers to adjust their treatment to optimize perfusion.[5,48,49]

Another emerging bedside tool for the nurse is ICP waveform analysis. The focus of ICP monitoring has been on the level of the ICP and the frequency of the pressure fluctuations.[50] Figure 41–7 illustrates the components of normal and abnormal ICP waveforms. Studies suggest that the ICP waveform is predictive for the development of disproportionate increases in ICP. Normally, P1 is greater than P2; however, as compliance decreases, P2 increases to equal to or greater than P1. This change in the waveform can alert the nurse to the changing status of the intracranial compartment and can allow for adjustments in care to minimize the impact.[51,52]

Nursing Diagnoses

Using the nursing process, the nurse performs an assessment and formulates a list of nursing diagnoses appropriate to the patient. Table 41–4 lists appropriate diagnoses for these patients.

Collaborative Management

Management of increased ICP is designed to reestablish equilibrium of the intracranial contents (blood, brain, and CSF) that are housed in a rigid container, the skull. Normally as one or more of the contents increase, there is a reciprocal decrease in the other contents. This concept is known as the Monro-Kellie doctrine. Some investigators describe these relationships

TABLE 41–4
Nursing Diagnoses

Problem Statement	Etiologic Factors
Altered tissue perfusion, cerebral	Cerebral edema or intracranial bleeding secondary to TBI
Decreased adaptive capacity, intracranial	Cerebral edema or intracranial bleeding secondary to TBI
Altered thought processes	Cerebral trauma or sedation
Impaired gas exchange	Hypoventilation or neurogenic pulmonary edema secondary to TBI
Ineffective airway clearance	CNS depression, poor cough effort secondary to TBI
High risk for aspiration	CNS depression, reduced gag reflex
Impaired verbal communication	Frontal or temporal lesions secondary to TBI
Fluid volume deficit	Diuretic therapy or diabetes insipidus secondary to pituitary dysfunction
Impaired physical mobility	Altered LOC, paralysis, or activity restrictions secondary to increased ICP
Pain	Headache secondary to TBI
Altered nutrition, less than body requirements	Altered LOC, dysphagia
Ineffective family coping	Sudden and traumatic injury of a family member
Risk for impaired skin integrity	Immobility, paralysis
Risk for disuse syndrome	Immobility, paralysis
Risk for injury	Thromboembolism secondary to immobility
Self-care deficit (ADLs)	Physical limitations resulting from TBI
Altered urinary elimination	Altered LOC
Constipation	Altered LOC
Body image disturbance	Physical limitations resulting from TBI
Knowledge deficit, learning needs	Treatment strategies, prognosis, rehabilitation process

ADL, activity of daily living; TBI, traumatic brain injury; CNS, central nervous system; LOC, level of consciousness; ICP, intracranial pressure.

Figure 41-8

PHYSICAL Protocol

PATIENT NEEDS	Current Level of Functioning & Short-term Goal for Severe Impairment (4-6 Weeks)	Short-term Goal for Moderate Impairment (4-6 Weeks)	Short-term Goal for Mild Impairment (4-6 Weeks)	Current Level of Functioning at Patient's Optimal Discharge Status
PHYSICAL (as they affect mobility, self-care, and communication) --↓ROM --Abnormal tone --↓Strength --↓Balance/Coordination --Altered Mobility --Altered Self-care --Motor Speech/Voice Impairments (PT, OT, KT, RN, SP)	**Current Functioning** Patient is dependent in bed mobility and all transfers. FIM-1 Patient is completely dependent in ambulation (w/c or walking). FIM-1 Patient is total care in ADLs. FIM-1 Patient is intelligible less than 25% of the time, and requires feedback to be understandable at all or to use a communication device. FIM-1 **Patient/Family Goals** Patient demonstrates baseline abilities in bed mobility and tolerates upright positioning in w/c for up to two hours. Performs bed ↔ w/c transfers with 50 to 75% assist. FIM-2 Tolerates upright positioning in w/c for up to two hours. Performs w/c mobility 50 - 100 feet with assist 25% to 50% of the time. FIM-2 Performs sit ↔ stand with maximum assist. Patient participates in basic self-care with maximal assistance. FIM-1 Patient is intelligible 25% of the time; enunciates or uses a communication device with feedback. FIM-1	**Patient/Family Goals** Patient repositions self in bed 25% of the time. Performs bed ↔ w/c transfers with 25 to 50% assist. FIM-3 Performs tub/toilet transfers with 50 to 75% assist. FIM-2 Performs w/c mobility independently for 50 feet/household distances. FIM-5 Walks with assistive device 150+ feet and with moderate to minimal assist. FIM-3/4 Patient participates in self-care with moderate physical assistance. FIM-3 Patient is intelligible 50% of the time; enunciates with feedback. FIM-2	**Patient/Family Goals** Patient will reposition self in bed with less than 10% assist. Performs bed ↔ w/c transfers with less than 10% assist. FIM-4 Performs tub/toilet transfers with less than 25% assist. FIM-4 Performs w/c mobility independently on the ward and to and from therapies 150+ feet. FIM-6 Walks with assistive device (if necessary) and contact guard to standby supervision for 150+ feet. FIM-4/5 Patient performs self-care activities with set-up. FIM-5 Patient is intelligible 75% of the time; enunciates with only occasional feedback. FIM-4	**Current Functioning** Patient is independent in bed mobility and all transfers with adaptive equipment as needed. FIM-6 Independently ambulates (w/c or walking) a minimum of 150 feet with or without assistive device on even or uneven terrain. FIM-6/7 Patient is independent in self-care with or without adaptive equipment. FIM-6 Patient is intelligible more than 90% of the time, and enunciates with only occasional feedback to speak clearly. FIM-6

ORIENTATION & MEMORY Protocol

PATIENT NEEDS	Current Level of Functioning & Short-term Goal for Severe Impairment (4-6 Weeks)	Short-term Goal for Moderate Impairment (4-6 Weeks)	Short-term Goal for Mild Impairment (4-6 Weeks)	Current Level of Functioning at Patient's Optimal Discharge Status
ORIENTATION & MEMORY (as they affect ward behavior, mobility, and communication) --Confused, Disoriented, and Wandering Behaviors --Confabulation --Learning and Retention Problems --Prospective Memory Deficits (SP, RN, NP, Entire Team)	**Current Functioning** Patient is disoriented to person, place, and time. Unable to use environmental cues or written material for orientation even with maximum assistance. Patient does not recognize or know their treatment staff or ward environment. FIM-1 Requires maximum assist to remember previous day events. FIM-2 **Patient/Family Goals** Patient is inconsistently oriented to person, place, and time. Utilizes environmental cues and/or written material for orientation with maximum assistance. Patient is aware of staff and the ward environment. Patient remembers previous day events with moderate assist. FIM-3 Patient returns with verbal cues, if and when he occasionally wanders off. Patient stops confabulating when given verbal redirection.	**Patient/Family Goals** Patient is oriented X 3 using external memory aids or other technique with moderate cues. Patient is aware of staff and familiar surroundings within the hospital; he/she does not wander off. Patient exhibits day-to-day recall with minimal cues and can state circumstances of his/her injury. FIM-4 Patient knows his/her schedule and attends therapy independently using external device as needed.	**Patient/Family Goals** Patient functionally utilizes external memory aids to manage scheduled and unexpected activities within the hospital environment with pm cues. Patient independently finds his/her way to activities by using environment cues; may require minimal assistance in unfamiliar settings. Patient exhibits day-to-day recall but may have occasional gaps. FIM-6	**Current Functioning** Patient consistently utilizes external memory aides (pm) to orient self and manage activities within the hospital environment. Patient orients self independently to environmental surroundings. Patient orients self to environmental surroundings, but requires minimal assistance in unfamiliar settings. Patient exhibits day-to-day recall but may have occasional gaps. FIM-6

Sample of a clinical protocol used for patients with traumatic brain injury. (With permission from U.S. Department of Veterans Affairs and the University Healthcare Consortium: *Drug and Disease Treatment Guidelines Source Book*, pp 242–244.)

Illustration continued on following page

PATIENT NEEDS — ATTENTION (as it affects self-care, mobility, communication, & leisure activities)

PATIENT NEEDS	Current Level of Functioning & Short-term Goal for Severe Impairment (4-6 Weeks)	Short-term Goal for Moderate Impairment (4-6 Weeks)	Short-term Goal for Mild Impairment (4-6 Weeks)	Current Level of Functioning at Patient's Optimal Discharge Status
ATTENTION (as it affects self-care, mobility, communication, & leisure activities)	Current Functioning			Current Functioning
--Inattention to safety issues in transfers and gait	Patient has difficulty following simple directions even in quiet environment. FIM-1			Patient is aware of safety issues and remains injury free.
--Inattention to toileting, bathing, feeding, or ADL tasks	Patient interrupts and shifts topic in conversation 75% of the time. FIM-1			
--Inattention to posture and position				
--↓ toleration of environmental stimuli		Patient/Family Goals	Patient/Family Goals	
--Altered perception and body neglect	Patient remains injury free through staff and significant other intervention	Patient shows beginning awareness of safety issues but requires minimal to moderate supervision to remain injury free.	Patient is aware of safety issues but requires occasional cueing to remain injury free.	
--↓ pragmatic communication skills (e.g., active listening)	Patient/Family Goals	Patient is able to attend to environmental stimuli, but requires cueing 25-50% of the time.	Patient is able to attend to environmental stimuli, but requires cueing <25% of the time.	Patient is able to attend to environmental stimuli consistently.
	Patient demonstrates ability to attend to important environmental stimuli with cueing. Patient begins to focus on staff/tasks.			
(SP, RN, NP, Entire Team)	Patient begins to become aware of his body position and posture, but requires cueing 80-90% of the time.	Patient begins to self-monitor and correct posture & position; requires cueing 25-50% of the time.	Patient self-monitors and corrects posture & position; requires cueing less than 25% of the time.	Patient self-monitors and corrects posture & position.
	Patient can follow simple directions in structured environment. FIM-2	Patient can follow complex directions in a clinic environment with minimal distractions. FIM-3	Patient can follow complex directions in a clinic environment with moderate distractions. FIM-5	Patient can follow complex directions, even in distracting environments. FIM-7
	Patient listens (does not interrupt) and stays on topic with maximal cues. FIM-2	Patient listens (does not interrupt) and stays on topic with moderate cues. FIM-3	Patient listens (does not interrupt) and stay on topic with minimal cues. FIM-4	Patient listens (does not interrupt) and stay on topic with occasional cues. FIM-6

PATIENT NEEDS — EXECUTIVE FUNCTIONS (as it affects self-care, mobility, communication, & community re-entry)

PATIENT NEEDS	Current Level of Functioning & Short-term Goal for Severe Impairment (4-6 Weeks)	Short-term Goal for Moderate Impairment (4-6 Weeks)	Short-term Goal for Mild Impairment (4-6 Weeks)	Current Level of Functioning at Patient's Optimal Discharge Status
EXECUTIVE FUNCTIONS (as it affects self-care, mobility, communication, & community re-entry)	Current Functioning	Current Functioning	Current Functioning	Current Functioning
--↓ initiation	Patient is unable to initiate or follow-through with ADLs. Requires total assistance. FIM-1			Patient independently initiates all activities. FIM-7
--impulsivity	Patient does not monitor his/her conversations, shifts topics, is verbose, and makes inappropriate comments. FIM-1			Patient modifies interactions in new environments with occasional cues. FIM-5
--↓ awareness of deficits				
--Refusal of therapies	Patient does not initiate use of memory notebook, does not keep track of time, and is not accepting of feedback.			Patient keeps track of time, but may require occasional assistance; independently uses external cueing devices.
--↓ judgment				
--Poor self-monitoring/ correction	Patient is not aware of deficits, demonstrates poor judgment, and does not understand reason(s) for treatment/hospitalization. FIM-1			Patient becomes aware of errors and corrects them; may require occasional cues. FIM-5
--Sequencing problems				
--↓ problem-solving			Patient/Family Goals	Patient participates in therapy with only occasional cues; verbalizes his/her need for follow-up treatment, if necessary.
--Poor pragmatic communication	Patient/Family Goals	Patient/Family Goals		
--Prospective memory deficit	Patient initiates simple activities 25% of the time; requires external direction 75% of the time. FIM-2	Patient initiates simple activities (e.g., basic ADLs) 75% of the time, requires external direction 25% of the time. FIM-4	Patient initiates all activities 75% of the time; requires external direction less than 10% of the time. FIM-5	Patient plans and participates in community re-entry activities with minimal assist from staff/significant other. FIM-4
(SP, RN, NP, Entire Team)	Patient successfully modifies his/her interactions 25% of the time after feedback. FIM-2	Patient successfully modifies his/her interactions 50% of the time after feedback. FIM-3	Patient successfully modifies his/her interactions 75% of the time after feedback. FIM-4	Patient successfully compensates for changes in routine in most situations. FIM-6
	Patient keeps track of time for schedule and therapy assignments with maximal assist.	Patient keeps track of time for schedule and therapy assignments with moderate assist.	Patient keeps track of time for schedule and therapy assignments with minimal assist.	
	Patient begins to show awareness of deficits by correcting some errors. FIM-2	Patient becomes aware of errors and corrects them with moderate cues. FIM-3	Patient becomes aware of errors and corrects them with minimal cues. FIM-4	
	Patient participates in therapy with maximal cues.	Patient participates in therapy with moderate cues.	Patient participates in therapy with only occasional cues; verbalizes his/her need for treatment.	
	Patient begins to utilize staff and significant other input in self-care and therapeutic activities. FIM-2	Patient begins to participate in community re-entry activities with moderate assist from staff/others. FIM-3	Patient plans and participates in community re-entry activities with minimal assist from staff/others. FIM-4	
	Patient accepts changes in routine 25% of the time without inappropriate emotional response. FIM-2	Patient accepts changes in routine 50% of the time without inappropriate emotional response. FIM-3	Patient accepts changes in routine 75% of the time without inappropriate emotional response. FIM-4	

Figure 41-8 Continued

PSYCHOSOCIAL

PATIENT NEEDS	Short-term Goal for Severe Impairment (4-6 Weeks) Patient/Family Goals	Short-term Goal for Moderate Impairment (4-6 Weeks) Patient/Family Goals	Short-term Goal for Mild Impairment (4-6 Weeks) Patient/Family Goals	Current Level of Functioning at Patient's Optimal Discharge Status — Current Functioning
PSYCHOSOCIAL --adjustment --sexuality --family/significant other support --alcohol/drug use --psychiatric disorder --spiritual (RC, CM, SW, NP, RT, RN, Entire Team)	Family/significant others participate in interview to assess psychosocial needs. Family/significant others verbalize awareness of support groups/services and attend/participate as needed.	Family/significant others utilize family support group for education, support, and adjustment. If geographically unrealistic, family/significant others utilize telephone contacts for support and education.	Family/significant others utilize family support group for education, support, and adjustment. If geographically unrealistic, family/significant others utilize telephone contacts for support and education.	Family/significant others utilize family support group for education, support, and adjustment. If geographically unrealistic, family/significant others utilize telephone contacts for support and education.
	Patient/significant others verbalize awareness of patient/family counselor and his/her role, and participate in individual counseling (prn).	Patient participates in individual counseling as indicated by their individual needs.	Patient participates in individual and/or group counseling	Patient utilizes individual therapy and/or support groups for guidance with problem-solving and assistance with overall emotional adjustment to disability. Patient provides peer support to other TBI patients.
	Patient interacts with others in the patient support group.	Patient interacts with others in the patient support group. Patient verbalizes beginning awareness of deficits and their impact.	Patient provides peer support to other TBI patients. Patient utilizes support groups for guidance with problem-solving and assistance with overall emotional adjustment to disability.	
	Patient respond to re-direction for inappropriate behavior 25-50% of the time. Family significant other verbalizes understanding of re-direction techniques. FIM-2	Patient responds to re-direction for inappropriate behavior but requires re-direction 50-75% of the time. Family significant other verbalizes understanding of re-direction techniques. FIM-3	Patient responds to re-direction for inappropriate behavior and requires re-direction less than 25% of the time. Family significant other verbalize understanding of re-direction techniques. FIM-4	Patient responds to re-direction for inappropriate behavior and requires re-direction less than 10% of the time. Family significant other verbalize understanding of re-direction techniques. FIM-5
	Patient and significant other verbalize awareness of purpose and possible safety risks involved in future therapeutic passes.	Patient and significant other verbalize awareness of purpose and possible safety risks involved in therapeutic passes. Successfully complete therapeutic day passes.	Patient and significant other verbalize awareness of purpose and possible safety risks involved in therapeutic passes. Successfully complete therapeutic over-night passes.	Patient and significant other successfully complete therapeutic over-night passes.
	Patient participates in 1:1 recreational and/or leisure activities.	Patient interacts with others in recreational/ leisure activities in hospital.	Patient interacts with others in recreational/ leisure activities both in and out of the hospital.	Patient interacts with others in recreational/ leisure activities both in and out of the hospital.

EDUCATION

PATIENT NEEDS	Short-term Goal for Severe Impairment (4-6 Weeks) Patient/Family Goals	Short-term Goal for Moderate Impairment (4-6 Weeks) Patient/Family Goals	Short-term Goal for Mild Impairment (4-6 Weeks) Patient/Family Goals	Current Level of Functioning at Patient's Optimal Discharge Status — Current Functioning
EDUCATION Knowledge deficits regarding: --Program/goals/treatment --Medical status --Diet & medication --Physical condition --Cognitive problems --Safety issues --Psychosocial issues --Drinking/driving risks --Benefits and follow-up service (CM, Entire Team)	Family/significant others receive Head Injury educational materials. Family/significant other recognize patient's needs and the roles of TBI team members.	Patient/significant others begin to identify roles of staff members. Family/significant others verbalize general knowledge of rehabilitation expectations and goals.	Patient and family/significant others demonstrate understanding of TBI risk factors through successful weekend passes.	Family/significant others demonstrate understanding of TBI risk factors through successful weekend passes or community re-entry trips. Patient & significant others verbalize knowledge of community resources for continued quality of life.
	Patient and/or significant others meet with doctor to discuss medical needs.	Patient and/or significant others meet with doctor to discuss medical needs.	Patient and/or significant others meet with doctor to discuss medical needs.	
	Patient and/or significant others meet with TBI team to review evaluation findings, treatment plan, and discharge goals and date.	Patient and/or significant others communicate with TBI team to review evaluation findings, treatment plan, and discharge goals and date.	Patient and/or significant others communicate with TBI team to review evaluation findings, treatment plan, and discharge goals and date.	

DISCHARGE NEEDS / OTHER NEEDS

PATIENT NEEDS	Short-term Goal for Severe Impairment (4-6 Weeks) Patient/Family Goals	Short-term Goal for Moderate Impairment (4-6 Weeks) Patient/Family Goals	Short-term Goal for Mild Impairment (4-6 Weeks) Patient/Family Goals	Current Level of Functioning at Patient's Optimal Discharge Status — Current Functioning
DISCHARGE NEEDS --Placement --Equipment needs --Vocational/avocational issues --Follow-up needs (SW, CM, VRT, RC, Entire Team)	Patient & significant other verbalize awareness of tentative length of stay; make decisions regarding disposition based on team's recommendations.	Patient & significant other verbalize awareness of tentative length of stay; make decisions regarding disposition based on team's recommendations.	Patient & significant other verbalize awareness of tentative length of stay; make decisions regarding disposition based on team's recommendations.	Patient & significant other have made decisions regarding disposition based on team's recommendations.
	Patient & significant other verbalize awareness of rehabilitation goals and expectations, and discuss alternatives for treatment follow-up with team.	Patient & significant other verbalize awareness of rehabilitation goals and expectations, and discuss alternatives for treatment follow-up with team.	Patient & significant other verbalize awareness of rehabilitation goals and expectations, and discuss alternatives for treatment follow-up with team.	Patient & significant other verbalize awareness of continuing rehabilitation/medical needs and follow-up plans.
	Patient is involved in continuing ADL assessment to determine equipment needs; necessary equipment ordered and education provided in its use.	Patient is involved in continuing ADL assessment to determine equipment needs; necessary equipment ordered and education provided in its use.	Patient is involved in continuing ADL assessment to determine equipment needs; necessary equipment ordered and education provided in its use.	Patient has completed ADL. Patient/family/significant other demonstrate safe use of adaptive equipment 100% of the time; necessary equipment ordered.
	Patient/family/referral source provide vocational/avocational history. If appropriate, patient completes vocational evaluation.	Patient/family/referral source provide vocational/avocational history. If appropriate, patient completes vocational evaluation.	Patient/family/referral source provide vocational/avocational history. If appropriate, patient completes vocational evaluation.	Patient/family/significant other begin to follow-up on recommendations for independent living or vocational services.
	Patient/family/significant other participate in exploration of available independent living or vocational services with the vocational counselor; make application for community-based services and Veterans Benefits	Patient/family/significant other participate in exploration of available independent living or vocational services with the vocational counselor; make application for community-based services and Veterans Benefits	Patient/family/significant other participate in exploration of available independent living or vocational services with the vocational counselor; make application for community-based services and Veterans Benefits	
OTHER NEEDS				

Figure 41-8 Continued

as the volume–pressure relationship: initially, as volume increases, there is little or no increase in ICP because of the compensatory mechanisms previously discussed. As these compensatory mechanisms become exhausted, there is a linear increase in pressure with increases in volume. These concepts are integral to the physiology of ICP treatment.[53] See Figure 41–8 for an example of a clinical protocol for TBI.

Surgical Management of Increased Intracranial Pressure

Studies show patients with mass (hematomas) lesions do better if the lesion is removed. The size and accessibility of the lesion are determining factors to whether surgery is performed. Speed is of the essence to decrease the extent of the neurologic damage from increased ICP. Depressed skull fractures that lacerate the dura and brain tissue, as well as penetrating injuries, require débridement and repair. In some institutions, when ICP is refractive to treatment, a craniectomy, or removal of the bone, may be performed to relieve pressure. In these patients, the dura remains intact or is augmented, limiting the protrusion of the intracranial contents. The bone is reimplanted weeks or months later when the patient is more clinically stable. Craniofacial injuries that involve the sinuses and vascular injuries may also require surgical repair.[1,13]

Nonsurgical Management of Increased Intracranial Pressure

In the past 2 decades, our understanding of brain injury has increased remarkably. We know that secondary injury plays a considerable part of the consequences of TBI; therefore, we must focus our management not only on ICP in order to improve outcome but also on all factors affecting perfusion. In 1995, a hallmark document was introduced, "Guidelines for the Management of the Severe Head Injury."[54] These guidelines were compiled to assist practitioners to improve outcomes in their patients. This section highlights these recommendations for management as well as others. Table 41–5 summarizes the guidelines for the management of severe head injury.

Airway Management
Managing the acute head injury starts with managing ABCs. Assessment and management of the airway in the patient with TBI with an uncleared cervical spine begin with opening the airway by use of a jaw thrust or chin lift, followed by clearing the airway of debris by a finger sweep or gentle oropharyngeal suctioning. Patients who are unable to maintain an adequate airway should be intubated. Strict attention is given during intubation to maintain cervical spine precau-

tions and to minimize increased ICP. Recommendations include oral intubation with manual inline traction and rapid sequence intubation with a combination of a sedative and short-acting paralytic or nasal intubation if the patient has spontaneous respirations. Aggressive management of the airway averts hypoxemia. Patients with an adequate airway should initially be placed on 100% nonrebreather mask, assessed frequently for airway patency and adequacy of ventilation, and receive regular pulmonary hygiene (see Chart 41–2).[45,46,55]

Hyperventilation
Patients who require intubation for airway management should maintain adequate oxygenation with a partial pressure of arterial oxygen of about 100 mm Hg and a partial pressure of arterial carbon dioxide of about 35 mm Hg. Hypercapnia results in cerebral vasodilatation, increased cerebral blood volume, and increased ICP. Hyperventilation should be avoided unless signs of herniation are exhibited and then should be used judiciously. Hyperventilation reduces ICP by causing cerebral vasoconstriction and by reducing CBF. CBF is reduced to half during the first 24 hours; therefore, hyperventilation may worsen the ischemia. For every millimeter change in partial pressure of carbon dioxide, there is a 3% reduction in CBF. Studies show that patients who were aggressively hyperventilated had a worse outcome then those who were not. During acute deterioration, gentle hyperventilation using an Ambu or anesthesia bag may be used at a rate of 12 to 20 breaths per minute. If chronic prophylactic hyperventilation with a partial pressure of arterial carbon dioxide of less than 30 mm Hg is required to treat refractory increased ICP, jugular oxygen saturation monitoring is recommended to help avoid cerebral ischemia. Patients who are aggressively hyperventilated should be hyperemic.[56,57]

Hemodynamics and Fluid Resuscitation
Initial management of cerebral circulation begins with the pulse and the blood pressure. The pulse may be tachycardic or bradycardic, depending on the systemic hemodynamics and the ICP. Tachycardia occurs when the patient is in hypovolemic shock or early increased ICP. Bradycardia is a sign of late increased ICP and herniation. The brain is rarely the cause of hypotension—an extracranial source of bleeding should be sought, such as the chest, abdomen, pelvis, long bone fractures, and scalp lacerations. Hypotension from a brain injury indicates a brain stem injury and is usually terminal. Hypotension should be aggressively treated with intravenous fluids using isotonic solutions, such as normal saline and lactated Ringer's solution. Euvolemia is the goal. Concerns about increasing cerebral edema during fluid resuscitation appear to be unwarranted. Hypotonic solutions may increase cere-

TABLE 41–5
Summary of Guidelines for the Management of Severe Head Injury

Standard	Guideline	Option
Chronic prophylactic hyperventilation should be avoided in absence of increased ICP during first 5 days.	All areas of the United States should have an organized trauma system.	Neurosurgeons should have an organized plan to care for neurotrauma.
Barbiturate therapy should be considered for refractory increased ICP if hemodynamically stable.	Avoid hypotension and hypoxia.	Priority of treatment—complete fluid resuscitation. No treatment for increased ICP unless signs of herniation present.
Glucocorticoids are not recommended in severe head injury.	ICP monitoring appropriate for GCS 3–8, with abnormal CT scan or with 2 or more of the following: age >40 yr, motor posturing, BP ≤90 mm Hg.	Mean SABP should be maintained >90 mm Hg.
Prophylactic anticonvulsants (phenytoin, carbamazepine, phenobarbital) are not recommended for preventing late posttraumatic seizures.	ICP treatment threshold 20–25 mm Hg. Treatment for ICP should be corroborated by clinical examination.	CPP should be maintained at a minimum of 70 mm Hg.
	Prophylactic hyperventilation should be avoided during the first 24 hours.	Brief hyperventilation may be necessary to treat acute neurologic deterioration or longer for refractory increased ICP.
	Mannitol is effective to treat increased ICP. Bolus better than continuous infusion.	Use of mannitol without ICP monitoring is indicated with signs of herniation or neurologic deterioration. Maintain euvolemia, serum osmolarity < 320 mOsm
	Nutritional replacement: 140% resting metabolism expenditure (RME) if nonparalyzed, 100% if paralyzed.	Preferable feeding method: gastrojejunostomy.
		Early posttraumatic seizures may be treated with phenytoin or carbamezepine, or no treatment may be given. Does not appear to affect outcome.

Modified from Brain Trauma Foundation and the Joint Section on Neurotrauma and Critical Care of the American Association of Neurological Surgeons and the Congress of Neurological Surgeons: Guidelines for the Management of Severe Head Injury. Park Ridge, IL, The Brain Trauma Foundation, 1995.

ICP, intracranial pressure; GCS, Glasgow Coma Scale; CT, computed tomography; BP, blood pressure; SABP, systemic arterial blood pressure; CPP, cerebral perfusion pressure.

bral edema secondarily to decreases in osmolarity and sodium level. Glucose solutions have been shown to increase morbidity and should be avoided. Hypertonic saline (3%) and colloid solutions may be useful in fluid resuscitation while simultaneously decreasing cerebral edema. These fluids cause a shifting of fluids from the extravascular spaces to the intravascular space by increasing intravascular sodium and oncotic pressures and also help to keep fluids intravascularly.[46,58]

Aggressive management of hypertension should be avoided unless the mean SABP exceeds 130 to 140 mm Hg. An increase in systemic pressure is a compensatory mechanism to maintain adequate perfusion during increased ICP. If treatment of hypertension should be necessary, extreme caution should be used to avoid excessive decreases in blood pressure and CPP.

Some clinicians advocate improving CPP by use of fluids and vasoactive drugs in patients with increased ICP. Some studies suggest that patients have a better outcome if CPP is maintained above 70 to 80 mm Hg. Keeping the patient euvolemic or slightly hypervolemic instead of dehydrated helps to maintain CPP.[27,28]

Managing the ABCs is important not only in the initial management but also throughout the hospitalization. Studies suggest that hypotension (systolic blood pressure <90 mm Hg) and/or hypoxia (partial pressure of arterial oxygen <60 mm Hg) anytime during the acute phase after injury increases the mor-

CHART 41-2

RESEARCH UTILIZATION: LIMITING THE EFFECTS OF AIRWAY SUCTIONING

Abstract: A quasiexperimental, within-subject design study was conducted in two university-affiliated intensive care units to determine the effect of suction catheter insertion and tracheal stimulation on the cerebrovascular and systemic vascular systems of adults with severe brain injury. Thirty intubated and mechanically ventilated patients aged 31 ± 15 years participated in the study. The patients' response to insertion of the suction catheter and tracheal stimulation was compared to the response to suctioning. Mean intracranial pressure (MICP), mean arterial pressure (MAP), cerebral perfusion pressure (CPP), and heart rate (HR) were measured immediately before catheter insertion, during insertion, and during application of negative pressure of suctioning as measures of cerebrovascular and systemic vascular status. Descriptive statistics were applied to data by use of either independent t-test or Mann-Whitney U test, and the data were graphed. Each hypothesis was examined with a dependent t-test with a $P <0.025$. Catheter insertion and tracheal stimulation independently increased MICP, CPP, and MAP. During application of negative pressure for suctioning, MICP and HR increased, but MAP and CPP did not significantly increase. Investigators concluded that the greatest effects on the cerebrovascular and systemic vascular systems occurred during the insertion of the catheter for suctioning rather than the application of suction for removal of secretions. They concluded that interventions to minimize airway stimulation during suctioning are needed.

Critique: Each day, intubated patients require suctioning of their airway to maintain patency. The patients with intracranial lesions present with the unique issue of preserving cerebrovascular integrity. Numerous studies have examined the endotracheal suctioning procedure in adults with and without brain injury. These studies have focused on hyperoxygenation; hyperventilation/hyperinflation procedures before, during, and after suctioning; number of catheter passes; and blunting the cough response that has been attributed to the increase in ICP. This study focused on determining at which point in the suctioning procedure systemic and cerebrovascular parameters were most affected. The study clearly identified the independent (catheter insertion, tracheal stimulation, and negative pressure for suctioning) and dependent variables (MAP, CPP, MICP, and HR) and outlined the procedure, making this study easily replicated. The authors discussed the current body of knowledge and research that exists on suctioning and the special consideration of the patient with brain injury, as well as outlined the deficits of the research in this area: (1) the mechanism by which endotracheal suctioning increases ICP is unknown, and (2) there is a lack of interventions to prevent or minimize the deleterious effects of suctioning. The data showed a significant increase in MICP from 19 to 22 mm Hg and in HR from 99 beats per minute to 113 beats per minute and no significant change in CPP (97 to 94 mm Hg) or MAP (no change) between insertion of the suction catheter and application of suction. The authors concluded that a well-designed study to examine interventions such as lidocaine administration to diminish the adverse effects of endotracheal suctioning are needed.

Nursing Implications: Endotracheal suctioning has an adverse effect on ICP, but the pathophysiology is unclear, and how these effects can be controlled is less clear. The use of lidocaine during suctioning may be useful. Other techniques suggested are measuring the length of the endotracheal tube, limiting the insertion of the catheter to slightly more than the tube length to minimize irritation of the trachea, and using a smaller suction catheter. Hyperoxygenation and hyperinflation should clearly be performed to minimize the effects of apnea and airway closure that occur with suctioning and are best achieved with the ventilator.

Source: Brucia J, Rudy E: The effect of suction catheter insertion and tracheal stimulation in adults with severe brain injury. Heart Lung 25:295–303, 1996.

---

bidity and mortality; therefore, maintaining adequate oxygenation and perfusion is imperative.[43,59]

Positioning

There are two aspects of positioning that must be kept in mind: (1) maintaining a neutral head position and (2) maintaining a backrest or head of bed position.

Lipe and Mitchell[60] demonstrated that lateral head rotation, flexion, or extension alters venous outflow. Careful attention to maintaining a neutral head alignment promotes venous drainage. There has been much debate in the literature over the optimal backrest position. Rosner and Coley[61] and others advocated that patients be in the supine position to promote CPP. Others

TABLE 41-6
Summary of Pharmacologic Management of Increased Intracranial Pressure

Drug	Dose Range	Mechanism of Action	Special Considerations
Sedatives:			
Midazolam	0.01–0.1 mg/kg IV	Sedative, hypnotic, anxiolytic, amnesic, skeletal muscle relaxant, anticonvulsant	Respiratory and cardiac depression
Lorazepam	0.01–0.06 mg/kg IM/IV		
Diazepam	1–10 mg IV		
Propofol	5–50 µg/kg/min or greater	Sedative, hypnotic	May produce hemodynamic instability and respiratory depression
			Tubing and solution should be changed every 12 hours
			Rapid onset and elimination, allowing assessment
			Slowly wean continuous infusions
			Expensive
Haloperidol	0.03–0.07 mg/kg IM/IV	Central antidopaminergic, weak anticholinergic	Extrapyramidal symptoms—rigidity
Morphine sulfate	1–10 mg IV	Analgesic	Respiratory depression
Short-acting paralytics:			
Pancuronium	0.1 mg/kg IV	Neuromuscular blocking agents	Patient must be intubated
Vecuronium	0.1 mg/kg		May be given in intermittent bolus or infusion
Atracurium	0.4–0.5 mg/kg		Will affect neurologic examination
Lidocaine	1–1.5 mg/kg IV or intratracheally	Stabilizes cell membrane Blunts cough	Monitor cardiac rhythm
Mannitol	0.25–1 G/kg IV	Osmotic diuretic, decreases CSF production, changes rheology of RBCs	Best response with bolus administration
			Avoid dehydration—keep serum osmolarity less than 315–320 mOsm
Furosemide	0.5–1 mg/kg IV	Loop diuretic, decreases CSF production	Avoid dehydration
	0.15–0.3 mg/kg if given with mannitol		
Barbiturates:			
Pentobarbital	10 mg/kg over 30 min	Suppresses neuronal activity Stabilizes cell membranes	Suppresses cardiovascular and immune systems
	5 mg/kg × 3 hr, followed by 1–2 mg/kg/hr	Decreases CBF, CMRO$_2$, and glucose utilization	Keep hydrated
			Support with vasopressors
			Consider PA catheter
			Monitor levels (3–4 mg/dL)
Thiopental	5–11 mg/kg over 15–30 min		
	4–8 mg/kg/hr		

IV, intravenously; IM, intramuscularly; CBF, cerebral blood flow; CMRO$_2$, cerebral metabolic rate of oxygen; CSF, cerebrospinal fluid; RBC, red blood cell; PA, pulmonary artery.

advocated elevating the head of the bed 30 to 60° to promote venous outflow and CSF drainage into the spinal canal.[62,63] It is best to consider all options and to evaluate the best position for each patient, observing the ICP and CPP in each position.[64,65]

Pharmacologic Management
Pharmacologic management of patients with acute head injury can be divided into those drugs that treat increased ICP and those that treat pathologic changes in brain injury. Table 41-6 summarizes the medications

commonly used to treat these patients. Agitation and excessive movement may occur after head injury and can contribute to increased ICP. Agitation after a head injury may be the result of biochemical imbalances from excessive levels of catecholamines and cortisol or may be a sign of pain, hypoxia, and the possibility of alcohol withdrawal.[66] Treatment for agitation should be aimed at the underlying cause. A patient in pain should be given analgesics. Hypoxia is treated with oxygen and/or increased ventilation. Alcohol withdrawal is treated with benzodiazepines. The biochemical imbalance seen after head injury is difficult to treat and has had limited study.

Excessive movement can occur when a patient resists the ventilator, coughs, and pulls against restraints, as well as during posturing and abnormal motor movements. Sedation alone or with paralytic agents is used to treat these excessive movements that result in increased ICP. Benzodiazepines are commonly used and vary in their length of action. Morphine sulfate can be used and is easily reversed. Propofol has gained popularity in the intensive care unit setting and, when used for brief periods, is useful and is short acting. Short-acting paralytics, such as pancuronium bromide, vecuronium, and atracurium, can be used to control excessive movements but must be accompanied by hypnotic agents and analgesics. These agents are given in intermittent doses when agitation causes increased ICP or as a constant infusion in severe cases. The latter results in an inability to perform a neurologic assessment except for pupillary assessment.[67–70]

Sedation and blunting of the cough reflex help control sustained increased ICP during suctioning. Short-acting barbiturates, like thiopental and morphine sulfate, are often used. Lidocaine intratracheally has long been used by anesthesiologists to blunt the cough reflex during intubation. Studies suggest intravenous lidocaine may also help by lowering the baseline ICP and blunting increases.[71–74]

Mannitol, an osmotic diuretic, is a treatment for patients with increased ICP and cerebral edema. Mannitol decreases ICP by increasing the intravascular-to-extravascular osmotic gradient, causing a shift in fluid from the brain tissues to the intravascular space, and by improving CBF by decreasing blood viscosity. There is also a decrease in CSF production. Intermittent boluses appear to be more effective than continuous infusion. Careful attention must be paid in order to avoid systemic dehydration. Serum osmolarity should be maintained below 320 mOsm because excessive hyperosmolarity can result in acute renal tubular necrosis. Other osmotic diuretics have been used in the past; however, mannitol is most effective.[75, 76]

There is some evidence that loop diuretics, such as furosemide, lower increased ICP. Its effects include shifting of extravascular fluid into the intravascular space and suppressing CSF production as much as 70%. Advocates of using furosemide suggest using it alone and in conjunction with mannitol to enhance the effects of mannitol. Again, dehydration must be avoided.[75]

Corticosteroids have not been shown to be effective in treating increased ICP or in improving outcome from head injury and may result in gastrointestinal bleeding and hyperglycemia. It has been shown to be effective in treating vasogenic edema seen with brain tumors. Corticosteroids should not be given after head injury.[77]

Seizures

Late posttraumatic seizures should not be treated prophylactically with anticonvulsants. Treatment of early posttraumatic seizures, within the first 7 days after TBI, is recommended. Control of seizures in the immediate postinjury period decreases secondary injury resulting from increased oxygen consumption and release of neurotransmitters. Long-term use of anticonvulsants may result in neurobehavioral and other side effects. If patients experience late posttraumatic seizures, they should be treated with the same approach as used with any patient with new onset of seizures.[78]

Approximately 10 to 15% of severe head injury is refractory to medical and surgical management for increased ICP. Patients in this group who are hemodynamically stable should be considered for treatment with high-dose barbiturates. Barbiturates appear to work by several mechanisms: improving vasomotor tone, suppressing metabolism, and inhibiting free radical–mediated lipid peroxidation. The most commonly used barbiturate is pentobarbital, although thiopental and phenobarbital have been used. Barbiturate coma not only suppresses the central nervous system but also suppresses the myocardium, resulting in decreased cardiac output and hypotension, often requiring cardiac support. Additional fluid resuscitation using crystalloids and colloids and the addition of an inotropic agent and vasoactive drugs may be needed to counteract these complications. Drug levels are monitored, with the goal of 3 to 4 mg/dL; for pentobarbital however, some patients may require a higher level to obtain therapeutic benefit. Electroencephalographic monitoring may require a higher level for a therapeutic benefit to be obtained. Electroencephalographic monitoring to a pattern of burst suppression appears to be more reliable. The neurologic examination is unable to be elicited except for the ability for the pupils to become fixed and dilated.[79–81]

Neuroprotectants

A new category of investigational drugs is emerging called "neuroprotectants." These drugs do not treat increased ICP but are aimed at treating or altering some of the pathologic pathways that occur in ischemia. Classifications of drugs include lipid peroxidase inhibitors, free radical scavengers, excitatory amino acid antagonists, receptor antagonists, endogenous opioid peptide antagonists, calcium channel blockers, specific and nonspecific inhibitors of the arachidonic acid metabolic pathway, and gangliosides. Many of these drugs need to be given within a short time after injury to be effective.[5, 72]

Temperature Regulation and Hypothermia

Body temperature has a direct effect on cerebral metabolism. For every degree centigrade change in body temperature, there is a 5.4% change in cerebral metabolism.

A fever in a brain-injured patient may result in worsening ischemia; therefore, close attention and management of hyperthermia are imperative. Hypothermia reduces cerebral metabolism and CBF and cerebral blood volume and therefore decreases ICP. Complications associated with severe hypothermia may outweigh the benefits. Experimental studies have suggested that mild-to-moderate hypothermia decreases neuronal injury possibly by reducing the release of excitatory amino acids. Clinical trials are underway.[82-84]

Cerebrospinal Fluid

Drainage of CSF with a ventricular catheter is an effective treatment for increased ICP. Lumbar puncture and lumbar drainage catheters to drain CSF should not be used in acute TBI, because of the risk of central herniation. In the presence of cerebral edema, removal of small volumes of CSF may produce dramatic decreases in ICP. Care must be taken not to overdrain and collapse the ventricles[72] (see Chapter 40 for care of a patient requiring ICP monitoring).

Consequences of Intracranial Hypertension

At times, despite the best efforts to control increased ICP, the patient's brain herniates, and the patient dies.

Herniation is the displacement of brain tissue from compressing and displacing adjacent structures. There are four types of herniation: (1) cingulate, (2) transtentorial, (3) central or rostral caudal, and (4) infratentorial. Table 41–7 describes the signs and symptoms of each syndrome. When compression of the cardiopulmonary regulatory centers occurs, death is imminent. Figure 41–9 illustrates anatomic landmarks associated with deteriorating neurologic status.

Ethical Considerations

In the care of the patient with a severe head injury, several ethical dilemmas may arise: withdrawal of life support, including nutrition, water, and ventilatory support; treatment of pain; and organ donation. How the health care team perceives these situations influences their ability to care for the patient and the family. Chart 41–3 illustrates an ethical dilemma faced by the health care team caring for the severely brain-injured patient.

Ten percent of patients with severe head injury are refractory to treatment of increased ICP, leading to death or prolonged coma.[85] Survival in a persistent vegetative state may be worse than death. Patients are unaware of themselves or their environment, depending totally on the care of others. Patients exist in this

TABLE 41–7
Signs and Symptoms of Herniation

Cingulate	Uncal	Central	Infratentorial
Lateral displacement of the cingulate gyrus under falx cerebri	Lateral and downward displacement of the temporal lobe through the tentorium incisura	Downward displacement of the cerebrum and diencephalon onto the brain stem	Downward displacement of the brain stem through the foramen magnum
Decreased LOC	Early: altered LOC, ipsilateral pupil dilation, disconjugate doll's eyes, contralateral motor weakness	Early: altered LOC, Cheyne-Stokes respiration, small pupils, localization to noxious stimuli, intact doll's eyes	Precipitous increase in SABP, small pupils, disconjugate gaze, ataxic respirations, quadraparesis
	Late: central neurogenic hyperventilation or Cheyne-Stokes respiration, ipsilateral fixed and dilated pupil, disconjugate doll's eyes, contralateral decortication or decerebration	Late diencephalon: altered LOC, Cheyne-Stokes respiration, small pupils, decortication, intact doll's eyes	
		Midbrain, upper pons: coma, central neurogenic hyperventilation, fixed mid-position, irregular pupils, disconjugate doll's eyes, decerebrate posturing	
		Pons, upper medulla: coma, ataxic respiration, dilated fixed pupils, flaccid, lower extremities—triple flexion	

LOC, level of consciousness; SABP, systemic arterial blood pressure.

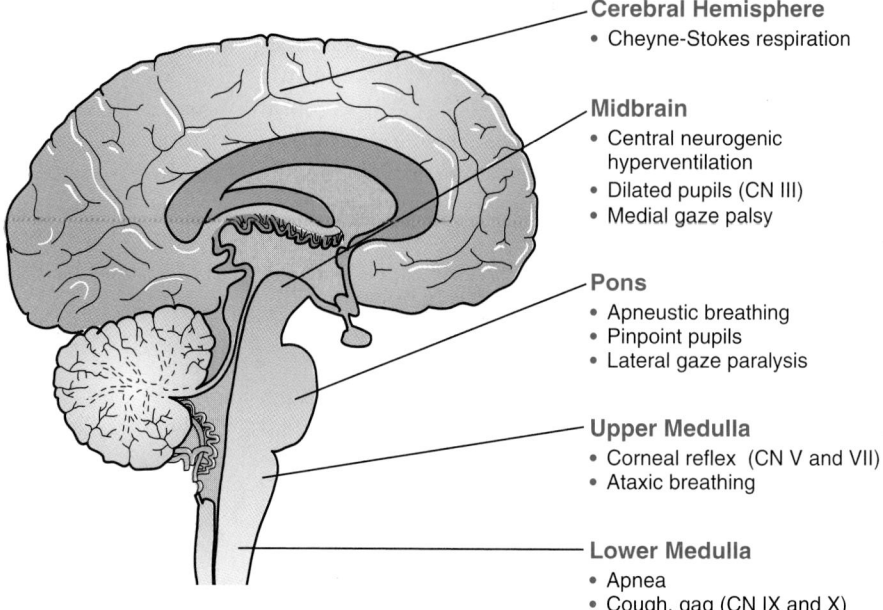

Figure 41–9

Progression of signs and symptoms with herniation.

Cerebral Hemisphere
- Cheyne-Stokes respiration

Midbrain
- Central neurogenic hyperventilation
- Dilated pupils (CN III)
- Medial gaze palsy

Pons
- Apneustic breathing
- Pinpoint pupils
- Lateral gaze paralysis

Upper Medulla
- Corneal reflex (CN V and VII)
- Ataxic breathing

Lower Medulla
- Apnea
- Cough, gag (CN IX and X)

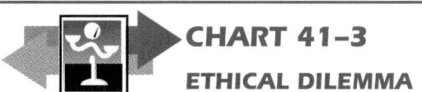

CHART 41–3

ETHICAL DILEMMA

Mr. J. is a 17-year-old patient who was in a motor vehicle crash. The driver in the crash died, a companion is also hospitalized in grave condition, and a fourth person was discharged with minor injuries. Mr. J. has a large right subdural hematoma and intracranial hemorrhage. Other injuries include a tension pneumothorax treated with a chest tube and an aortic dissection. He undergoes evacuation of the subdural hematoma and right hemicraniectomy with massive extrusion of the brain from the defect. The postoperative computed tomographic scan demonstrates an intracerebral hematoma occupying two-thirds of the right hemisphere and massive herniation of the brain through the craniectomy. You are told that this is the worst computed tomographic scan the physician has ever seen. Intracranial pressures are 30 to 50 mm Hg. The Glasgow Coma Scale score is 4T (decerebrate posturing), pupils are fixed at 6 bilaterally, and no brain stem reflexes are present except that the patient is initiating respirations. The decision by the general surgeon is to manage the aortic injury conservatively.

The family is approached about the gravity of the situation. The physicians explain the patient's injuries and the treatment options, including the recommendation to treat the aortic injury conservatively, and if the patient survives, surgery could be per-formed at a later date. The family is told that if the patient survives, he will probably never wake up. The family wishes everything to be done.

The next day, the patient continues as he was the previous day, with intracranial pressures of 30 to 50 mm Hg, and is taken to the operating room for an aortic stent. Mr. J.'s neurologic examination is unchanged.

On day three, Mr. J.'s intracranial pressure increases to 70 to 80 mm Hg, his mean arterial blood pressure is 160 mm Hg, and his heart rate drops to 30 to 40 beats per minute. The patient now has a Glasgow Coma Scale score of 3T but still initiates respirations. The family still wants to continue everything. As the nurse, you are frustrated because this patient is a full code. The patient dies 6 days after admission.

1. What ethical dilemma arises during the first encounter with the family?
2. Should the surgery for repairing the aortic injury have been performed?
3. Was there a better way to approach the family about the patient's injuries and whether or not he should be treated?
4. Should the health care team have taken the decision to treat out of the hands of the family? Was treatment futile? Defend your responses.

state for days, months, and even years. When the patient's prognosis is such, a decision regarding discontinuation of life-sustaining treatments arises. If family members have discussed their desires about life support measures, the decision to withdraw support is easier, especially when decision makers are in agreement. It is when health care matters have not been discussed that dilemmas arise.

In 1986, the American Medical Association published a paper on withholding or withdrawing life support. It stated that there was no difference in withholding or withdrawing life support in the presence of a terminal illness or irreversible coma.[86] In 1988, the American Nurses Association stated that the nurse has the duty to prevent pain and suffering. When it is decided to allow a patient to die, the ventilator is removed, and nurses often support the patient by alleviating their suffering with morphine sulfate.[87] We say that we want to make them more comfortable. Does a comatose patient feel pain? How do we determine pain? It can be argued that patients who respond to noxious stimuli still feel pain, but the patient who is unresponsive may not. Are we treating the patient or ourselves? How much morphine is all right? 2 mg, 5 mg, 20 mg, 200 mg? When does this treatment become euthanasia?

Why is it easier to not give a treatment than to withdraw treatment? In the eyes of the law, there is no difference. Discussion revolves around whether it is more humane to never start an intervention or to give a trial treatment and withdraw it. The idea of taking something away gives rise to feelings of active assistance, whereas withholding is more passive.

Brain Death

Before 1968, death was defined as the cessation of bodily functions—no circulatory or respiratory function.[53] In 1968, Harvard Medical School defined guidelines for brain death that opened the doors for organ donation for transplantation. Brain death is the cessation of CBF and of all vital brain stem functions, including pupillary reflexes, extraocular reflexes, corneal reflex, cough, gag, and breathing. Brain death is different from clinical death because the patient's heart is still beating. Each state legislates the requirements for the diagnosis of brain death. Guidelines for the determination of death were established in 1981.[88] Besides a clinical examination that demonstrates the absence of brain stem function, diagnostic tools, such as transcranial Doppler, electroencephalography, angiography, nuclear medicine scanning, and blood flow studies, may be used to corroborate brain death. Other requirements outlined are establishment of a cause of coma be established and the fact that two separate examinations can be carried out separated by a designated period of time. Once brain death is established, life support measures can be withdrawn and organ donation can be considered.

TABLE 41–8
Multidisciplinary Outcomes

Outcome	Prehospital/ Emergency Department	Critical Care	Acute Care	Subacute/ Acute Rehab	Community
Maintenance of adequate cerebral tissue perfusion	X	X	X	X	X
Effective airway clearance	X	X	X	X	X
Effective respiratory pattern	X	X	X	X	X
Maintenance of adequate oxygenation	X	X	X	X	X
Improvement in nutritional status		X	X	X	X
Prevention of complications	X	X	X	X	X
Restoration of fluid and electrolyte balance	X	X			
Self-management of therapeutic regimen			X	X	X
Improvement in responsiveness	X	X	X	X	X
Improvement in self-care activities			X	X	X
Improvement in communication		X	X	X	X
Improvement in mobility		X	X	X	X
Maintenance of bowel function		X	X	X	X
Maintenance of bladder function	X	X	X	X	X
Maintenance of comfort	X	X	X	X	X
Prevention of skin breakdown	X	X	X	X	X
Improvement in thought processes		X	X	X	X
Improvement in activity tolerance			X	X	X

For many of the lay population, the concept of irreversible brain damage and brain death is difficult to comprehend. The patient's heart is still beating, but the medical team says that the individual is dead because the brain is no longer functioning. How can this be? How nurses and other health care providers perceive death and dying is influenced by many factors, such as education, exposure to death, religion, and cultural beliefs. All health care providers must respect and understand what contributes to an individual's belief about death in order to help them make the necessary life and death decisions.

The Mandatory Donation Request Act was established in 1987 and requires health care providers to approach the next of kin about organ donation in the event of a patient's death.[88] Organ donation can be hindered by religious and cultural beliefs about the body and afterlife as well as by misconceptions about what happens when another person's organs are inside a person. Families who do consent to donate organs often feel that their loved one's death was not in vain, that that patient lives on by helping another to live. It is usually best for the request to be made by someone other than the direct care givers to avoid an appearance of conflict of interest. Bereavement counseling should also be provided to assist families and friends to deal with their loss. This counseling can be provided by a trained nurse, social worker, chaplain, or other designee.[88]

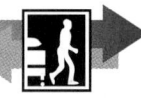

CHART 41–4
BEYOND THE ICU: CARING FOR PATIENTS WITH TBI ACROSS SETTINGS

Despite the advances in treatment for traumatic brain injury, once the injury occurs, the patient will never be the same. Outcomes vary widely, from patients who are independent with subtle yet often devastating cognitive dysfunction to patients who are gravely disabled or comatose and require assistance with activities of daily living or total care.

The best cure for a brain injury is to never have one. Injury prevention initiatives include legislation and safety regulations that alter the kinetic forces that injure persons and educational programs that instruct the public on how injuries occur. These programs are offered in the schools, at public events, and through the media. Nurses are often involved in these community-focused programs as a function of their positions in a health care agency or as a part of the activities of their professional organization. The exposure of nurses to the consequences of trauma provides them with the necessary credibility to appeal to the various program audiences.

Patients who survive a traumatic brain injury require high levels of physical care and intensive rehabilitation. In the intensive care unit, the nurse begins the rehabilitation process concurrent with stabilization of the patient's physiologic needs. Basic nursing care, such as the prevention of skin breakdown and the maintenance of joint mobility (range-of-motion exercises, proper positioning of limbs, and splinting as needed), is provided and sets the stage for the rehabilitation process. Once the patient's intracranial pressure and cerebral perfusion pressure are stable, more aggressive rehabilitation begins, and the focus shifts from prevention of secondary injury to maintenance and promotion of function.

As soon as possible, the patient is moved out of the intensive care unit, and if the patient progresses, therapy that promotes independence in self-care is initiated. Some patients transfer from the intensive care unit to either an intermediate care unit or an acute care unit and then to a rehabilitation unit. This process may take days, weeks, or months. In each of these settings, nurses with well-developed assessment and technical skills are needed to provide the high level of physical and emotional care required by these patients. Others patients make slower or no progress and require placement in a transitional facility until they are ready for rehabilitation or long-term care.

For the patient who is comatose after a brain injury, a sensory stimulation program may be started in the intensive care unit to elicit the patient's interaction with the environment. Patients who remain comatose or who have limited recovery are transferred to a skilled nursing facility or a subacute rehabilitation unit to continue their recovery. The comatose patient requires intensive physical care. Attention to maintaining a patent airway and adequate ventilation is imperative to avoid a return to the intensive care unit for a respiratory complication. Meticulous care of the skin, bowel and bladder, nutrition and hydration, and prevention of deep vein thrombosis may continue indefinitely. The systemic effects of the head injury leave these patients vulnerable for repeated complications, including pulmonary emboli and sepsis. Nurses with critical care skills are needed to care for these patients because early identification of potentially lethal complications is imperative to patient outcomes.

Multidisciplinary Outcomes

Multidisciplinary outcomes for the patient with TBI can be prioritized according to the phase of the care. Some outcomes carry throughout the continuum of care (Table 41–8). The role of the nurse in these patient outcomes spans more than the emergency department and the intensive care unit. Chart 41–4 more fully describes the continuum of care beyond the intensive care unit and the role of the nurse across these settings.

Critical Thinking Exercise

Mr. J. is a 25-year-old man who had a TBI in a high-speed motor vehicle crash. Medics found him unrestrained, unresponsive to verbal stimuli, with a right pupil fixed and dilated and a left pupil sluggishly reactive, decerebrate on the left, and decorticate on the right to noxious stimuli. His SABP was 160/75 mm Hg, his heart rate was 110, his pulse was thready, and his respirations were 30/min. He was placed in a cervical collar, orally intubated, and bagged on 100% oxygen, and an intravenous of lactated Ringer's solution was started. There are no other injuries.

In the emergency department, the patient is noted to have bilateral fixed and dilated pupils and bilateral decerebrate posturing. Mannitol 100 g is administered intravenously, a Foley catheter is inserted, and the patient undergoes computed tomography. The scan reveals a large right fronto-temporal SDH. The patient is taken to the operating room, where the hematoma is removed and a Camino ICP monitor is inserted.

After surgery, the patient is taken to the neurosurgical intensive care unit. Mr. J. is placed on a ventilator, and his partial pressure of arterial oxygen is 104 mm Hg and his partial pressure of arterial carbon dioxide is 35 mm Hg. His pH is 7.34. Several hours after arriving at the intensive care unit, Mr. J.'s ICP spikes to 35 mm Hg. He is given 100 g of mannitol intravenously. His ICP returns to a baseline of 15–18 mm Hg. During the next several hours, his ICP spikes two more times, and he is given mannitol, 100 g, each time with good results.

1. Discuss the implications of the clinical signs and symptoms observed by the medics.
2. What should the nurse be concerned about when giving mannitol?
3. What other treatments might be considered and why?

Mr. J. continues to have increased ICP, spiking to 30 to 40 mm Hg. The neurosurgeon hyperventilates him to a partial pressure of carbon dioxide of 30 mm Hg, but his ICP continues to spike. Neurologically, Mr. J.'s right pupil is greater than the left, and they are sluggish; he is bilaterally decerebrate; he has disconjugate gaze; and he has positive corneal, cough, and gag reflexes. CPP is 56 to 74 mm Hg. Serum osmolarity is 312 mOsm.

4. What treatment might be tried now and why?

Mr. J. continues to have increased ICP, despite aggressive management. His neurologic status has deteriorated to fixed and dilated pupils, flaccid and absent corneal reflexes, and a weak cough. The neurosurgeon talks to the family.

5. What are the family's options for care?

Key Concepts

→ The primary injury occurs at the time of the impact and is the result of the kinetic forces applied to the brain tissues. Prevention strategies are aimed at educating the public to minimize the occurrence of these events.

→ Secondary injury results from the events that affect the perfusion after the primary injury. Treatment strategies are aimed at minimizing secondary injury.

→ Injury to the brain has many systemic effects: pulmonary, cardiac, fluid and electrolyte, gastrointestinal and nutrition, coagulation, and immune.

→ Assessment of the neurologic injury requires an integration of a comprehensive neurologic examination with current diagnostic technology.

→ The treatment of patients with intracranial hypertension (increased intracranial pressure) is guided by evidence-based "Guidelines for the Management of Severe Head Injury." These guidelines as well as other treatments are focused on the collaborative management of secondary injury.

References

1. National Center for Health Statistics: Births, marriages, divorces, and deaths for 1990. vol. 39, no. 12, Hyattsville, MD, 1991.
2. Kraus J, Nourjah P: The epidemiology of mild head injury. In: Levin H, Eisenberg H, Benton A (eds): Mild Head Injury. New York, Oxford Press, 1989, pp 8–22.
3. Evans R: The post-concussion syndrome and the sequelae of mild head injury. Neurol Clin 10:815–847, 1992.
4. Leroux P, Grady M: Epidemiology of head injury. In: Lam A (ed): Anesthetic Management of Acute Head Injury. New York, McGraw-Hill, 1995, pp 1–9.
5. Avellino A, Lam A, Winn R: Management of acute head injury. In: Ablin M (ed): Textbook of Neuroanesthesia with Neurosurgical and Neuroscience Perspectives. New York, McGraw-Hill, 1996, pp 1137–1175.
6. Spielman-McGinnis J: Central nervous system I: head injuries. In: Cardon V, et al. (eds): Trauma Nursing: From Resuscitation Through Rehabilitation. Philadelphia, WB Saunders, 1988, pp 365–418.
7. Gennarelli TA: Head injury in man and experimental animals: clinical aspects. Acta Neurochirur, Suppl (Wien) 32:1–13, 1983.
8. Johnson D: Head injury. In: Echekberger M, Pratsch G (eds): Pediatric Trauma Care. Rockville, Aspen Publishing, 1988.

9. Vernon-Levett P: Head injuries in children. Crit Care Nurs Clin North Am 3:411–421, 1991.

10. Ward J: Pediatric issues in head trauma. New Horiz 3:539–545, 1995.

11. Wilberger J, Chen D: The skull and meninges. Neurosurg Clin North Am 2:341–350, 1991.

12. Leroux P, Winn HR: Surgical management of acute head injury. In: Lam A (ed): Anesthetic Management of Acute Head Injury. New York, McGraw-Hill, 1995, pp 101–141.

13. Obana W, Pitts L: Extracranial lesions. Neurosurg Clin North Am 2:351–372, 1991.

14. Aldrich EF: Surgical management of traumatic intracerebral hematomas. Neurosurg Clin North Am 2:373–386, 1991.

15. Kauffman H: Treatment of civilian gunshot wounds to the head. Neurosurg Clin North Am 2:387–398, 1991.

16. Kennedy F, Gonzalez P, Dang C: The Glasgow Coma Scale and prognosis in gunshot wounds to the brain. J Trauma 35:75–77, 1993.

17. Adams J, Graham D, Gennarelli TA: Head injury in man and experimental animals: neuropathology. Acta Neurochir Suppl (Wien) 32:15–30, 1983.

18. Bullard D: Diencephalic seizure: responsiveness to bromocriptine and morphine sulfate. Ann Neuro 21:609–611, 1985.

19. Rossitch E, Bullard D: The autonomic dysfunction syndrome: etiology and treatment. Br J Neurosurg 2:471–487, 1988.

20. Martin N, Doberstein C, Zane C, et al.: Post-traumatic cerebral arterial spasm: transcranial Doppler ultrasound, cerebral blood flow, and angiographic findings. J Neurosurg 77:575–583, 1992.

21. Greene K, Jacobowitz R, Marciano F, et al.: Impact of traumatic subarachnoid hemorrhage on outcome in non-penetrating head injury. Part II: relationship to clinical course and outcome variables during acute hospitalization. J Trauma 41:964–971, 1996.

22. Weber M, Grolimund P, Seiler RW: Evaluation of post-traumatic cerebral blood flow velocities by transcranial Doppler ultrasound. Neurosurgery 27:106–112, 1990.

23. Bailey I, Bell B, Gray J, et al.: The effect of nimodipine on outcome after head injury: a prospective randomized controlled trial. In: Scriabine A, Teasdale G, Tettenborn D, Young W (eds): Nimodipine: Pharmacological and Clinical Results in Cerebral Ischemia. New York, Springer-Verlag, 1990, pp 263–265.

24. Rutherford W: Post-concussion symptoms: relationship to acute neurological indices, individual differences and circumstances of injury. In: Levin H, Eisenberg H, Benton A (eds): Mild Head Injury. New York, Oxford Press, 1989, pp 217–228.

25. Zasler N: Mild traumatic brain injury: medical assessment and intervention. J Head Trauma Rehabil 8:13–29, 1993.

26. Doberstein C, Hovda D, Becker D: Clinical considerations in the reduction of secondary brain injury. Ann Emerg Med 22:993–997, 1993.

27. Lang E, Chestnut R: Intracranial pressure and cerebral perfusion pressure in severe head injury. New Horiz 3:400–409, 1995.

28. Bouma G, Muizelaars J: Cerebral blood flow in severe clinical head injury. New Horiz 3:384–394, 1995.

29. Kontos HA: Regulation of cerebral circulation. Annu Rev Physiol 43:393–407, 1981.

30. Obrist WD, Langfitt TW, Jaggi JL, et al.: Cerebral blood flow and in comatose patients with acute head injury. J Neurosurg 61:241–253, 1984.

31. Muizelaar JP: Cerebral blood flow, cerebral blood volume and cerebral metabolism after severe head injury. In: Becker D, Gudemann S (eds): Textbook of Head Injuries. Philadelphia, WB Saunders, 1989, pp 221–240.

32. Rosner M, Daughton S: Cerebral perfusion management in head injury. J Trauma 30:933–941, 1990.

33. Grady M, Shapira Y: Pathophysiology of head injury: central nervous system effects. In: Lam A (ed): Anesthetic Management of Acute Head Injury. New York, McGraw-Hill, 1995, pp 11–24.

34. Hayes R, Jenkins L, Lyeth B: Neurochemical aspects of head injury: role of excitatory neurotransmission. J Head Trauma Rehabil 7:16–28, 1992.

35. Siesjo B: Basic mechanisms of traumatic brain damage. Ann Emerg Med 22:959–969, 1993.

36. Vink R: Magnesium and brain trauma. Magnes Trace Elem 10:1–10, 1991.

37. Domino K: Pathophysiology of head injury: secondary systemic effects. In: Lam A (ed): Anesthetic Management of Acute Head Injury. New York, McGraw-Hill, 1995, pp 25–58.

38. Clifton G, Robertson C, Kyper K, et al.: Cardiovascular response to severe head injury. J Neurosurg 59:447–454, 1983.

39. Eggleston C: Clinical correlation of neurogenic pulmonary edema to increased intracranial pressure. J Neurosurg Nurs 14:245–254, 1982.

40. Rogers F, Shackford S, Trevisani G, et al: Neurogenic pulmonary edema in fatal and non-fatal head injury. J Trauma 39:860–868, 1995.

41. Clifton G, Ziegler M, Grossman R: Circulating catecholamines and sympathetic activity after head injury. Neurosurgery 8:10–13, 1981.

42. Muwaswes M: Increase intracranial pressure and its systemic effects. J Neurosci Nurs 17:238–243, 1985.

43. Chestnut R, Marshall S, Piek J, et al.: Early and late systemic hypotension as a frequent and fundamental source of ischemia following severe brain injury in Traumatic Coma Bank. Acta Neurochir Suppl (Wien) 59:121–125, 1993.

44. Marmarou A, Holdaway R, Ward J, et al.: Traumatic brain tissue acidosis: experimental and clinical studies. Acta Neurochir (Wien) 57:160–164, 1993.

45. Emergency Nurses Association: Initial assessment. In: Jacobs BB, Baker P (eds): Trauma Nursing Core Course Manual. Chicago, Emergency Nurses Association, 1995, pp 43–72.

46. Grady M, Lam A: Management of acute head injury: initial resuscitation. In: Lam A (ed): Anesthetic Management of Acute Head Injury. New York, McGraw-Hill, 1995, pp 87–100.

47. Gean A, Kates R, Lee S: Neuroimaging in head injury. New Horiz 3:549–561, 1995.

48. Robertson C, Cormio M: Cerebral metabolic management. New Horiz 3:410–422, 1995.

49. Sheinberg M, Kanter MJ, Robertson CS, et al.: Continuous monitoring of jugular venous oxygen saturation in head injured patients. J Neurosurg 76:212–217, 1992.

50. Cardosa E, Rowan J, Galbraith S: Analysis of cerebrospinal fluid pulse wave in intracranial pressure. J Neurosurg 59:817–821, 1983.

51. Willis M: Interpretation of intracranial pressure waveforms: the predictive value of P2 elevation in the diagnosis of decreased adaptive intracranial capacity. Masters Thesis, University of Washington, 1991.

52. Mitchell P, Kirkness C, March K, et al.: Intracranial pressure and transcranial Doppler waveform analysis, 1997, unpublished data.

53. Newell D: Brain death. In: Lam A (ed): Anesthetic Management of Acute Head Injury. New York, McGraw-Hill, 1995, pp 271–284.

54. Brain Trauma Foundation and the Joint Section on Neurotrauma and Critical Care of the American Association of Neurological Surgeons and the Congress of Neurological Surgeons: Guidelines for the Management of Severe Head Injury. Park Ridge, IL, The Brain Trauma Foundation, 1995.

55. Abram K: Airway management and mechanical ventilation. New Horiz 3:474–487, 1995.

56. Marion D, Obrist W, Carlier P, et al.: The use of moderate therapeutic hypothermia for patients with severe head injury: a preliminary report. J Neurosurg 79:354–362, 1993.

57. Muizelaar J, Marmarou A, Ward J, et al.: Adverse effects of prolonged hyperventilation in patients with severe head injury: a randomized trial. J Neurosurg 75:731–739, 1991.

58. Zornow M, Prough D: Fluid management in patients with traumatic brain injury. New Horiz 3:488–498, 1995.

59. Winchell R, Simons R, Hoyt D: Transient systolic hypotension: a serious problem in the management of head injury. Arch Surg 131:533–539, 1996.

60. Lipe H, Mitchell P: Positioning the patient with intracranial hypertension: how turning and head rotation affect the internal jugular vein. Heart Lung 9:1031–1037, 1980.

61. Rosner M, Coley I: Cerebral perfusion pressure, intracranial pressure and head elevation. J Neurosurg 65:636–641, 1986.

62. Durward Q, Amacher A, DelMaestro R, Sibbald W: Cerebral and cardiovascular responses to changes in head elevation in patients with intracranial hypertension. J Neurosurg 59:938–944, 1983.

63. Kenning J, Toutant S, Saunders R: Upright patient positioning in the management of intracranial hypertension. Surg Neuro 15:148–152, 1981.

64. Feldman Z, Kanter M, Robertson C, et al.: Effect of head elevation on intracranial pressure, cerebral perfusion pressure and cerebral blood flow in head injury patients. J Neurosurg 76:207–211, 1992.

65. March K, Mitchell P, Grady M, Winn R: Effect of backrest position on intracranial and cerebral perfusion pressures. J Neurosci Nurs 22:375–381, 1990.

66. Jackson R, Mysiw J: Abnormal cortisol dynamics after traumatic brain injury. Am J Phys Med Rehabil 68:18–23, 1985.

67. Brooke M, Patterson D, Questad K, Basak K: Agitation and restlessness after closed head injury: a prospective study of 100 consecutive admissions. Arch Phys Med Rehabil 73:320–323, 1992.

68. Fowler S, Hertzog J, Wagner B: Pharmacological interventions for agitation in head injury: patients in the acute care setting. J Neurosci Nurs 27:119–125, 1995.

69. Prielipp R, Coursin D: Sedative and neuromuscular blocking drug use in critically ill patients with head injury. New Horiz 3:456–468, 1995.

70. Rao N, Jellinek H, Woolston D: Agitation in closed head injury: haloperidol effects on rehabilitation outcomes. Arch Phys Med Rehabil 66:30–34, 1985.

71. Brucia J, Owens D, Rudy E: The effects of lidocaine on intracranial hypertension. J Neurosci Nurs 24:205–214, 1992.

72. Eisenhart K: New perspectives in management of adults with severe head injury. Crit Care Nurs Q 17:1–12, 1994.

73. Hamill J, Bedford R, Weaver D, Colohan A: Lidocaine before endotracheal intubation: intravenous or laryngotracheal. Anesthesiology 55:578–581, 1981.

74. Kerr M, Rudy E, Brucia J, Stone K: Head injured adults: recommendations for endotracheal suctioning. J Neurosci Nurs 25:86–91, 1993.

75. Bullock R: Mannitol and other diuretics in severe neurotrauma. New Horiz 3:448–452, 1995.

76. Davis M, Lucatorto M: Mannitol revisited. J Neurosci Nurs 26:170–174, 1994.

77. Kelly D: Steroids in head injury. New Horiz 3:453–455, 1995.

78. Temkin N, Haglund M, Winn H: Causes, prevention and treatment of post-traumatic epilepsy. New Horiz 3:518–522, 1995.

79. Eisenberg H, Frankowski R, Constant C: High-dose barbiturate control of elevated intracranial pressure in patients with severe head injury. J Neurosurg 69:15–23, 1988.

80. Lowenstein D, Aminoff M, Simon R: Barbiturate anesthesia in the treatment of status epilepticus: clinical experience with 14 patients. Neurology 38:395–400, 1988.

81. Miller J, Piper I, Chan K: Control of intracranial pressure in patients with severe head injury. J Neurotrauma 9:S317–S326, 1992.

82. Clifton G, Allen S, Barrodale P, et al.: A phase II study of moderate hypothermia in severe brain injury. J Neurotrauma 10:263–271, 1993.

83. Metz C, Holzshuh M, Bein T, et al.: Moderate hypothermia in patients with sever head injury: cerebral and extracerebral effects. J Neurosurg 85:533–541, 1996.

84. Shiozaki T, Sugimoto H, Taneda M, et al.: Effects of mild hypothermia on uncontrollable hypertension after severe head injury. J Neurosurg 79:363–368, 1993.

85. Wilberger J, Cantell D: High dose barbiturates for intracranial pressure control. New Horiz 3:469–473, 1995.

86. Fry S: New ANA guidelines on withdrawing or withholding food and fluid from patients. Nurs Outlook 36:122–123, 148–150, 1988.

87. Wurzbach ME: The dilemma of withholding or withdrawing nutrition. Image: J Nurs Scholarship 22:226–230, 1990.

88. Black P: Conceptual and practical issues in the declaration of death by brain death criteria. Neurosurg Clin North Am 2:493–501, 1991.

42

Spinal Cord Injury

Connie A. Jastremski

Objectives

After completing this chapter, the student will be able to:

1. Describe the mechanisms of spinal cord injury (SCI).
2. Discuss the implications of a stable injury versus an unstable injury.
3. Differentiate the symptoms seen in a patient with anterior cord syndrome, Brown–Séquard syndrome, central cord syndrome, and a complete injury.
4. Compare the clinical picture of a patient with spinal shock with that of a patient with neurogenic (distributive) shock.
5. Provide a rationale for the use of various pharmacologic agents in the treatment of the patient with acute SCI.
6. Perform a spinal cord assessment.
7. Plan appropriate nursing strategies for the patient with SCI who requires a surgical intervention.
8. Develop collaborative care plans for the acute phase of care for the patient with SCI.
9. Select appropriate interventions aimed at preventing or managing the complications related to SCI.
10. Analyze some of the ethical dilemmas faced by the health care team in caring for the patient with SCI.

SCI with neurologic deficit is considered one of the most devastating traumatic injuries one can suffer. Approximately 7600 to 10,000 new cases of SCI occur each year in the United States; the frequency is similar in other developed countries.[1, 2] The number of persons with SCI living in the United States at any one time ranges from 183,000 to 203,000.[3] Eighty percent of these injuries affect young men between the ages of 20 and 24 years. This injury, which effects every physiologic system in the body, had an 80% acute mortality rate in 1946 and now has a 6% mortality rate.[4] This significant decrease in mortality is related to better emergency medical services and increased knowledge regarding the mechanisms of injury that have resulted in better interventions directed at treating the injury. In addition, public education regarding the use of seat belts and helmets, the addition of airbags to automobiles, and the increased legal consequences of drinking under the influence of alcohol have significantly contributed to a decrease in the severity of SCI seen in the late 1990s.

Of all SCIs, cervical SCI is the most challenging, and the patient generally requires critical care interventions immediately after the injury. These patients are the focus of this chapter, although many of the concepts discussed in terms of types of injury, assessment, diagnostic workup, and management apply to all patients with SCI. In 1992, the American Spinal Injury Association recommended that the term "quadriplegia" be dropped in favor of "tetraplegia," which is more contemporary.[5] Throughout this chapter, the term tetraplegia is used to describe the patient with high cervical SCI and loss of motor power to all four extremities.

The care of the patient with SCI is complex and demanding. It is critical that the nurses who care for these patients understand the pathophysiology of SCI, the rationale for the interventions to treat these patients, and the actual and potential problems these patients experience, to provide the highest quality care to these severely injured patients.

ETIOLOGY AND PATHOPHYSIOLOGY

The spinal cord is one of the most intricate and delicate components of the central nervous system. Unfortunately, when the spinal cord is injured, the entire physiologic system of the body is disrupted, and the injury produces numerous long-term consequences for the patients. The cost of SCI is high. The average yearly health care costs vary according to the severity of the injury and the resulting disability.[2] The average cost of care for the person with a high cervical SCI in the first year, including initial hospitalization, is approximately $415,000, whereas the person with paraplegia incurs costs up to $152,000 during the first year. Total aggregate costs for 1 year were estimated to be $5.6 billion for all patients with SCI, including those newly injured patients and the approximately 200,000 postinjury patients.[6] These figures represent only the beginning for these patients; annual costs in subsequent years are as high as $75,000 for the tetraplegic patient.[2, 4]

SCI occurs most frequently in young people, with the highest incidence in adolescent males between the ages of 15 and 20 years, with a male-to-female ratio of 4:1.[5] Table 42–1 describes the usual causes of SCI in the United States. Causes also vary by geographic region. Although penetrating injury to the spinal cord accounts for only 15% of all SCI, children under the age of 15 years show a disproportionately higher incidence. One study, reported by the Regional Spinal Cord Injury Care System of Southern California, found that preinjury factors, cause (blunt versus penetrating), and ethnicity did not contribute significantly to individual patient outcomes; only severity of the injury affected the outcome.[7]

Although the incidence of SCI is relatively low in comparison with that of other trauma, the morbidity and mortality remain high in this patient group. These patients require lifetime care for the multiple systems affected by the injury, and they have an overall readmission rate of 57%.[4] Improvement in the acute care of SCI has been credited with the decreased mortality and the prevention of life-threatening complications frequently associated with early death in these patients. Factors that affect survival include the level of injury, the extent of paralysis, the numbers and types of associated injuries, and the age of the patient at the time of injury. The elderly do less well than typical young, otherwise healthy, patients. Patients who do survive the acute phase of the injury tend to have a near-normal life expectancy.

In the past decade, a much better understanding of the pathophysiology of the SCI and of the mechanisms of secondary damage has developed. SCI is multiphasic, involving morphologic damage to the spinal cord. The mechanical trauma to the spinal cord results in tissue necrosis and loss of function. Many axons are damaged directly by the physical deformation of the spinal cord, the primary injury.[3] Secondary injuries continue to cause axonal damage and further neurologic deficit. These secondary injuries include petechial hemorrhages progressing to hemorrhagic necrosis, enzymatic lipid hydrolysis with lipid peroxidation, loss of calcium from the extracellular space and other electrolyte changes compatible with tissue and vascular damage, ischemia of the tissue with a resultant decrease in available oxygen and lactic acidosis, free radical release into the tissue, structural changes in the gray and white matter, and inflammation with neuronophagia.[3, 8] The hemodynamic changes that occur after SCI are major contributors to the resultant damage to the spinal cord. Autoregulation, the ability of the spinal cord tissues to maintain a constant blood flow despite changes in arterial blood pressure, is lost during the acute phase (the first 24 hours) of injury, thus profoundly decreasing the blood supply to the spinal cord.

Much remains to be learned about the pathophysiology of acute SCI, but with the current characteristics that have been identified, many new treatments have been introduced to minimize progressive damage. Drug therapy is now directed at the acute secondary response (neuroprotective agents), membrane stabilization (neuroregenerative therapy), and sustained function (restorative agents that enhance neural elements).[8]

Mechanism of Injury

SCI results from compression, contusion, or transection of the spinal cord. The major mechanisms of injury are flexion, flexion–rotation, hyperextension, and compression (axial loading). Flexion injury, with tearing of the posterior ligaments and dislocations of the vertebral body, is the most unstable injury. This injury is often associated with neurologic deficits. Hyperextension injury is the most common mechanism of SCI.

TABLE 42–1
Spinal Cord Injury

Cause of Injuries	Percentage (%)
Motor vehicle crashes	50
Falls	18
Sports injuries	15
Penetrating injuries	15
Industrial accidents	2

Types of Injury

There are many ways to classify SCI: by level (cervical, thoracic, lumbar, sacral), by degree (complete, partial or incomplete), and by mechanism (flexion, hyperextension, compression, or rotation). Fractures can occur in any part of the vertebra. The actual shape of the vertebrae makes them easy to fracture. Vertebral fractures may be caused by direct or indirect trauma and may be stable or unstable. Stability is maintained if all the anterior ligaments and posterior ligaments, plus one ad-

ditional structure, such as the lamina or spinous process, are intact.[9, 10] If a fracture is determined to be unstable, consideration should be given to immediate surgical intervention, to allow the patient mobility.

Many different types of fractures can occur, and these fractures can be seen with or without associated SCI. It is important to understand the various types of fractures and their potential to cause associated SCI. The fractures can be classified as simple, compression, comminuted, teardrop, or special involving the atlas (C1) or axis (C2). Injuries to the vertebra can also be

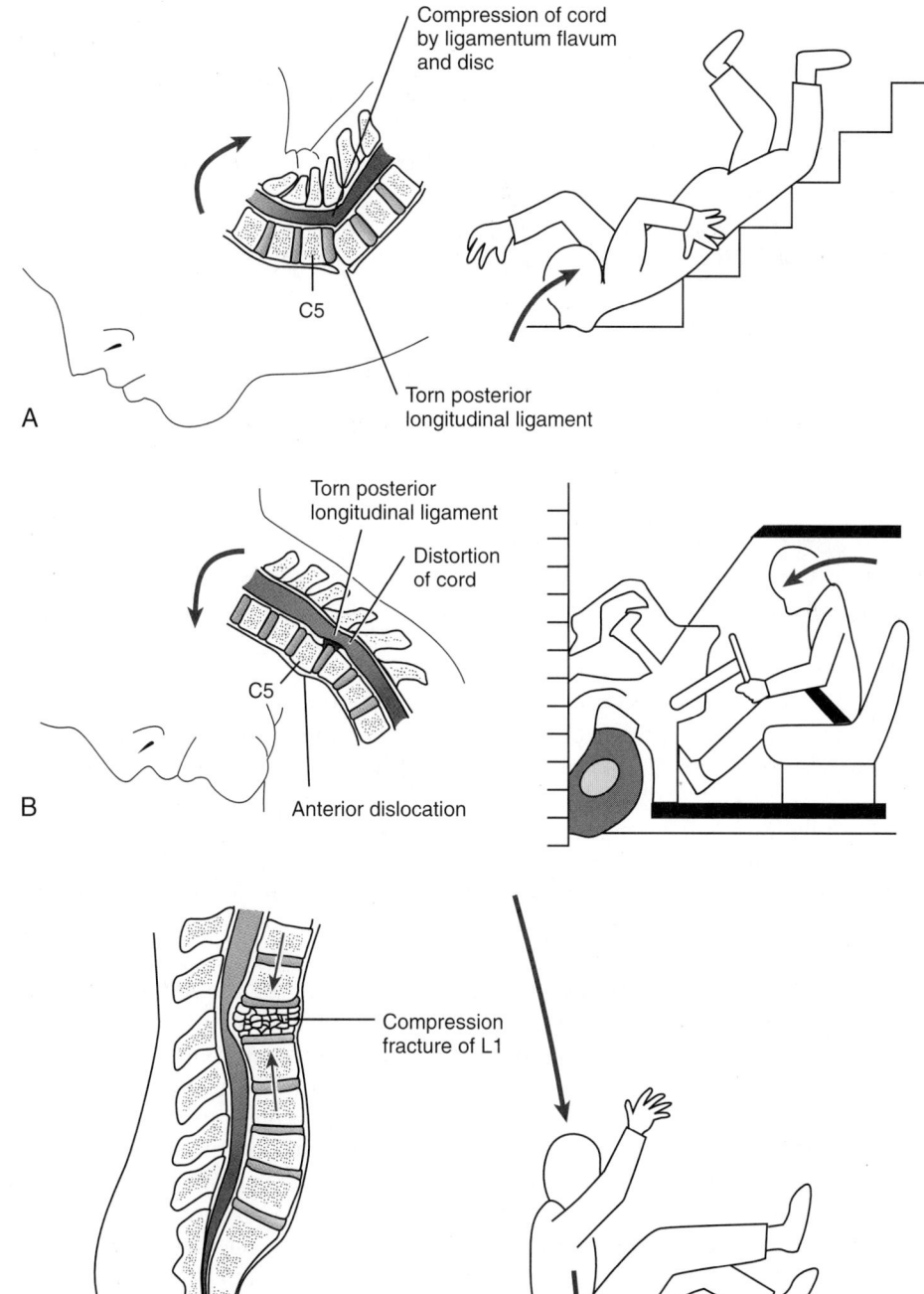

Figure 42–1

Examples of closed spinal cord injury mechanisms. *A,* Hyperextension injury resulting from a fall on steps. *B,* Hyperflexion injury resulting from a head-on collision. *C,* Compression fracture associated with an axial loading injury resulting from a fall.

classified as follows: dislocations, in which one vertebra overrides another with unilateral or bilateral facet dislocation; subluxation, which is a partial or incomplete dislocation of one vertebra over another; or fracture–dislocation, characterized by bone dislodgment and movement of one vertebra over another.

A simple fracture can occur along smooth surfaces of the bones such as the transverse process, facets, lamina, or pedicles. Alignment remains intact, and these fractures are usually without neural involvement.

A wedge fracture is a compression fracture involving the vertebral body and is generally seen in axial loading injuries or severe hyperextension or hyperflexion injuries (Figure 42–1A,B). A teardrop fracture, involving a piece of bone that actually breaks off, may also occur. Neural compression may or may not be present. This type of bony injury may also be seen in conjunction with a fracture–dislocation injury.

A comminuted or burst fracture is always associated with an axial loading-type injury that causes the vertebral body to shatter (see Figure 42–1C). The axial loading may be caused by something falling on a person's head, landing on one's head, such as in a diving accident, or trying to land on one's feet when jumping from a high place. In this serious bony injury, bone fragments are driven into the spinal cord and may cause complete transection of the cord at the level of the injury.

Special fractures include a bursting of the C1 ring as a result of axial loading on the head (see Figure 42–2A). This injury is called a Jefferson fracture and causes pain in the area, but it is not usually associated with neurologic deficit. If the fractured bone is displaced, the injury is fatal.

Atlanto-occipital dislocations are produced by an avulsion of the atlas from the occipital bone attachment. Death is usually immediate. If there is no neurologic involvement at the time of injury, recovery is complete.

The odontoid process (dens) of C2 can be fractured in many ways. If the dens fractures forward into the spinal canal, death occurs instantly. If the dens fractures and does not displace or if it displaces laterally, usually no neurologic deficit is seen and recovery is complete. A hangman's fracture occurs when the arch of the C2 vertebra is fractured (see Figure 42–2B). This patient is usually asymptomatic but does need to be immobilized to prevent neurologic damage.

Spinal levels include the cervical, thoracic, lumbar, and sacral areas. The cervical and lumbar areas are more prone to injury because they have a great deal of movement and are flexible. A cervical injury with spinal cord tissue damage is likely to result in loss of motor function in all extremities, known as tetraplegia. This injury is the most devastating and has the highest mortality rate (Table 42–2).

The classification of injury by degree is stated in terms of loss of neurologic function. The patient may have a

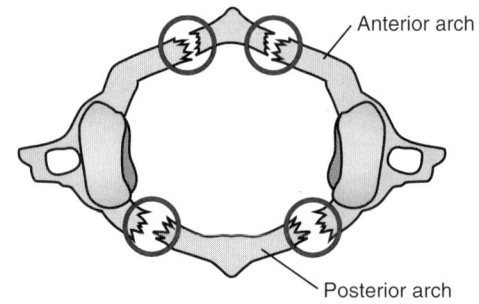

A   C1 (Atlas) Superior view

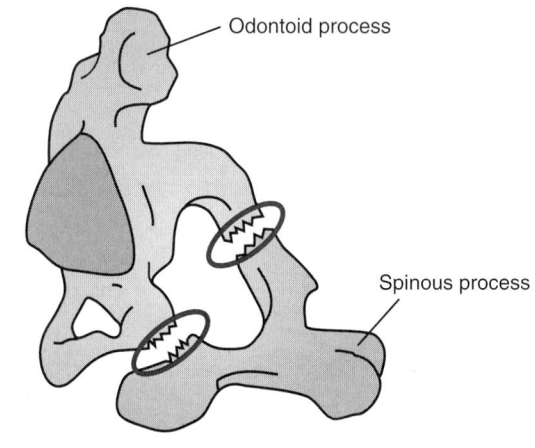

B   C2 (Axis) Lateral view

Figure 42–2

Examples of spinal fractures. A, Jefferson's fracture. B, Hangman's fracture.

complete injury with total loss of motor and sensory function below the level of the injury immediately after the injury. If the injury is complete, function will not return, as a result of irreversible spinal cord damage. A partial or incomplete injury results in a varying picture of neurologic deficit that depends on the area of the spinal cord that has been damaged. This injury results in a mixed loss of motor and sensory function.

Partial injuries can further be classified into syndromes that reflect the areas of the spinal cord involved in the injury. The central cord syndrome is one example of an incomplete or partial injury. This syndrome usually follows a hyperextension injury in patients who have a narrowed spinal canal. Central cord syndrome results in a motor weakness of the extremities that is greater in the upper extremities and worse in the distal areas. These symptoms are related to microscopic hemorrhages and edema that occur in the central area of the gray matter (Figure 42–3A). Recovery depends on the extent of the hemorrhaging and the ability to relieve the pressure on the spinal cord.

The anterior cord syndrome is the most common of the incomplete injuries. Compression of the anterior

TABLE 42–2
Levels of Injury and Expected Functional Ability

Cervical Level of Injury	Normal Function	Expected Function
C1–C2	Head and neck control Respiratory muscle control Shoulder shrug	Limited movement of the head and neck Ventilator dependent Electric wheelchair with breath or head control Dependent in all ADLs Use of mouthstick to type, write, or turn pages
C3–C4	Mouth control Shoulder or scapular movement Diaphragm movement	Good head and neck control May or may not be ventilator dependent, but needs ventilator support acutely Dependent in all ADLs Electric wheelchair with breath, head, or shoulder controls
C5	Shoulder flexion Elbow flexion Increased scapular function	Full head, neck, shoulder, and diaphragm control Can assist in ADLs, but still requires major assistance Can feed self with special assistive devices Able to move wheelchair for short distances, but does better with an electric wheelchair
C6	Good wrist flexion Wrist extension Shoulder rotation and abduction	Independent in feeding and some grooming with assistive devices Can roll over in bed Requires minor assistance in transfer Can drive a car with hand controls
C7	Elbow extension Strong wrist extension Shoulder full movement Some finger control	Transfers independently Independent in most ADLs Excellent bed mobility
C8–T1	Normal hand strength	Bed and wheelchair independent

ADLs, activities of daily living.

spinal artery by the displacement of the vertebral body backward with a flexion injury, thrombosis of the artery, or a herniated intervertebral disc causes ischemia (see Figure 42–3B). Because this artery supplies the anterior two-thirds of the spinal cord, symptoms include loss of motor function below the level of injury and a varying loss of sensation. Posterior functions are generally preserved, so the patient retains some touch sensation, along with position sense (proprioception) and vibratory sensation. If the syndrome is caused by bony compression of the artery, surgical decompression is necessary.

A rare syndrome associated with an incomplete injury caused by hemisection of the spinal cord is the Brown–Séquard syndrome (see Figure 42–3C). This syndrome results in an ipsilateral loss of motor function and a contralateral loss of pain and temperature sensation. Penetrating injuries more often cause this syndrome than does blunt trauma; however, each patient should be tested bilaterally for motor and sensation after any trauma because the syndrome can be found with blunt trauma, hemorrhage, or herniated intervertebral disc.

Additional Issues

Spinal shock is a physiologic disruption of the function of the spinal cord that occurs with SCI. This temporary suspension of function is caused by the loss of input to the spinal cord from the higher cerebral centers. Symptoms include flaccid paralysis, absence of muscle contractions, and loss of sensation below the level of injury. All reflexes are lost, and the patient has bowel and bladder dysfunction. The body's ability to control its temperature is also lost, so the patient becomes poikilothermic, meaning that the body temperature reflects the ambient room temperature and the patient is unable to shiver to warm up or perspire to cool down.

Spinal shock usually appears immediately after the injury, but it can take several hours to manifest itself fully.[11] Clinically, spinal shock can persist for days or weeks, and it can be prolonged by infection or other complications.[9, 11] There is no treatment. This phase of spinal injury ends when the elicitable reflexes such as the cutaneospinal and muscle spindle reflex arcs return. The skeletal muscles become spastic. The patient exhibits signs of an upper motor neuron

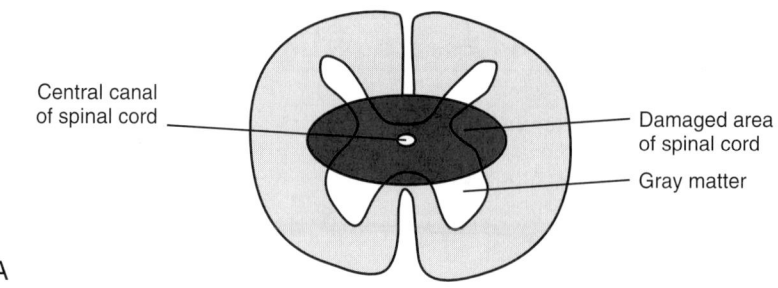

A

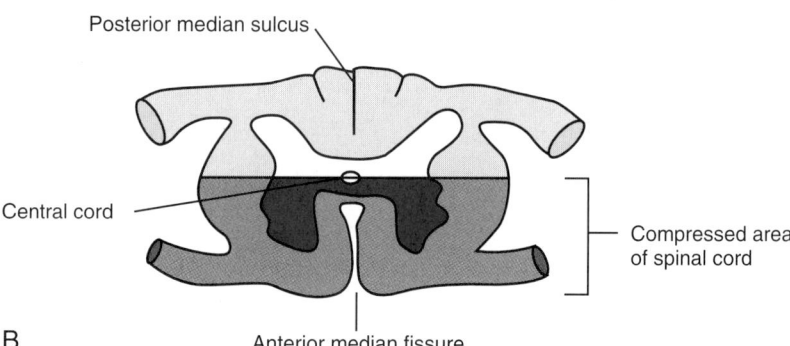

B

Figure 42–3

Three syndromes associated with incomplete (partial) spinal cord injury lesions. *A,* Central cord syndrome. *B,* Anterior cord syndrome. *C,* Brown–Séquard syndrome. (From Barker E: *Neuroscience Nursing.* St. Louis, C.V. Mosby, 1994, p 356.)

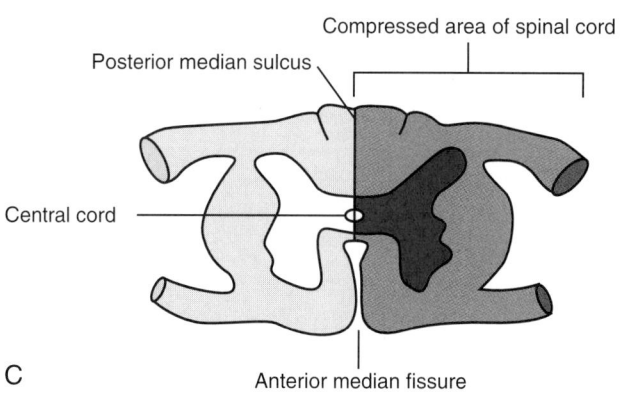

C

problem at this time, with the muscle becoming spastic with increased muscle tone, heightened stretch reflexes, and exaggerated flexor muscle movement.

In patients with a cervical or upper thoracic SCI, neurogenic shock, a form of distributive shock, is also a problem. This shock state is caused specifically by the loss of brain stem and high center control of the sympathetic nervous system. The loss of sympathetic outflow allows the parasympathetic system to be engaged unopposed. The overwhelming parasympathetic influence results in hypotension from peripheral vasodilatation, severe bradycardia, loss of the cardiac accelerator reflex, and loss of the ability to sweat below the level of the lesion. One must consider other reasons for hypotension before labeling the patient as having neurogenic shock. For example, severe hemorrhage may be precipitating the hypotension. Chapter 47 gives greater detail about distributive shock and its sequelae.

Assessment

At the Scene

Assessment of the patient with SCI begins at the scene of the trauma. It is most important to determine whether SCI is present or could be present as soon as possible. As with all victims of traumatic injury, the focus is on the ABCs: airway, breathing, and circulation. The airway should be checked for any obstructions that would impair breathing. If the airway is closed or if the patient is not breathing, the airway should be opened gently using a jaw thrust maneuver. The patient's neck should be maintained in a neutral position because movement may worsen the patient's condition and may even create a neurologic deficit. A patient with a cervical fracture or cervical compression at C4 or above stops breathing and needs to be intubated in the field. The patient's blood pressure and heart rate should be measured and recorded. If the patient is hypotensive or bradycardic, the patient may be in neurogenic shock. Care should be taken not to overload the patient with fluids at the scene of the accident because this may cause pulmonary edema in a patient who has normovolemia and is experiencing a fluid shift from peripheral vasodilatation. In many instances, it is difficult to determine whether the patient is in hemorrhagic shock before arrival at the hospital, so fluids need to be given to try to increase the blood pressure. Rescuers at the scene must perform a motor and sensory assessment and must note the exact time of the onset of any neurologic symptoms. The time of onset is used to determine the type of therapy the patient can receive in the definitive care center. The assessment focuses on motor and sensory function. It should include the ability to move any muscle or muscle groups voluntarily, the presence of any painful areas in the neck, thorax, back, or other areas of the body, and the assessment of proprioception. One must note the circumstances of the accident that caused the spinal cord injury—type of accident, position of the patient when found, location of patient when found, whether the patient had voluntary movement at any time after the accident and subsequently lost that movement, and any complaints at the time of the accident.

Emergency Department

After the patient is stabilized and is brought to the emergency department, a more thorough assessment is done. At this point, information obtained by the rescuers should be given to the staff, including the report of the accident scene, the stability of the patient, and the results of the neurologic assessment. This assessment should be recorded because it serves as the baseline for all future assessments.

Attention during this phase of care remains focused on the ABCs and the motor, sensory, and reflex examination. There is always the danger of losing the airway and breathing ability in the patient with cervical SCI, even if the primary injury is below the C4 level. The injured cervical spinal cord becomes edematous after the injury, and the edema spreads upward, causing an ascension of the initial level of injury. Respiratory insufficiency is a serious threat to the patient after SCI. Respiratory failure remains the leading cause of death in patients with tetraplegia. Frequent assessments of the patient's respiratory status include observations of chest wall movement, measurements of vital capacity, forced expiratory volume, arterial blood gases, and continuous oxygen saturation, and examinations of chest radiographs. Hypoxemia is to be avoided because it only contributes to the neurologic damage. An arterial oxygen pressure (PaO_2) of at least 80 mm Hg and a normal arterial pressure of carbon dioxide ($PaCO_2$) are the respiratory outcome parameters that should be established for these patients.[9, 10]

Monitoring the vital signs, including cardiac rate and rhythm, is important throughout the initial management phase and the critical care phase. An arterial line, pulmonary artery catheter, and cardiac monitoring assist the care team in the continual assessment of the patient's cardiovascular status during the time of spinal shock and neurogenic shock. If an arterial line is not used, then a noninvasive blood pressure cuff should be applied, and the blood pressure should be monitored at least every 15 minutes for the first few hours after admission. In addition to hypotension from decreased systemic vascular resistance, cardiac preload is also decreased. The use of the information derived from the pulmonary artery catheter allows for the appropriate management of the hypotension and the prevention of fluid overload in these patients.

Heart rate is closely monitored for bradycardia. Atropine should be given to the patient who is symptomatic from the slowed heart rate. If repeated doses of atropine are needed to improve the patient's heart rate, consideration should be given to the use of a transcutaneous or transvenous pacemaker during the acute phase of the illness. Left ventricular function is usually depressed secondary to the lack of sympathetic outflow, and it can lead to cardiac dysrhythmias including heart block.[9, 10] If the patient is in type II, second-degree heart block or third-degree heart block and is symptomatic, a pacemaker is indicated. Monitoring of the cardiac rhythm during the initial phase of injury is critical to detect any life-threatening dysrhythmias.

Neurologic Assessment

The neurologic assessment of the patient initially includes the testing of the patient's level of consciousness, using the Glasgow Coma Scale or similar tool, and motor and sensory examination. Other injuries can occur concurrently with SCI, especially closed head injuries, but the focus of this assessment is on the spinal cord.

Precise and reliable neurologic assessment is a necessary tool for determining the extent and pattern of injury and recovery after SCI.[12] Detailed assessment over the first 72 hours can be useful in establishing the patient's potential for walking after recovery from the initial injury. In 1992, the Standard Neurological Classification of Spinal Cord Injury was adopted and revised in 1996 (Figure 42–4). This international scale unified the American Spinal Injury Association (ASIA) and the National Acute Spinal Cord Injury Study (NASCIS) scoring approaches, defined spinal cord

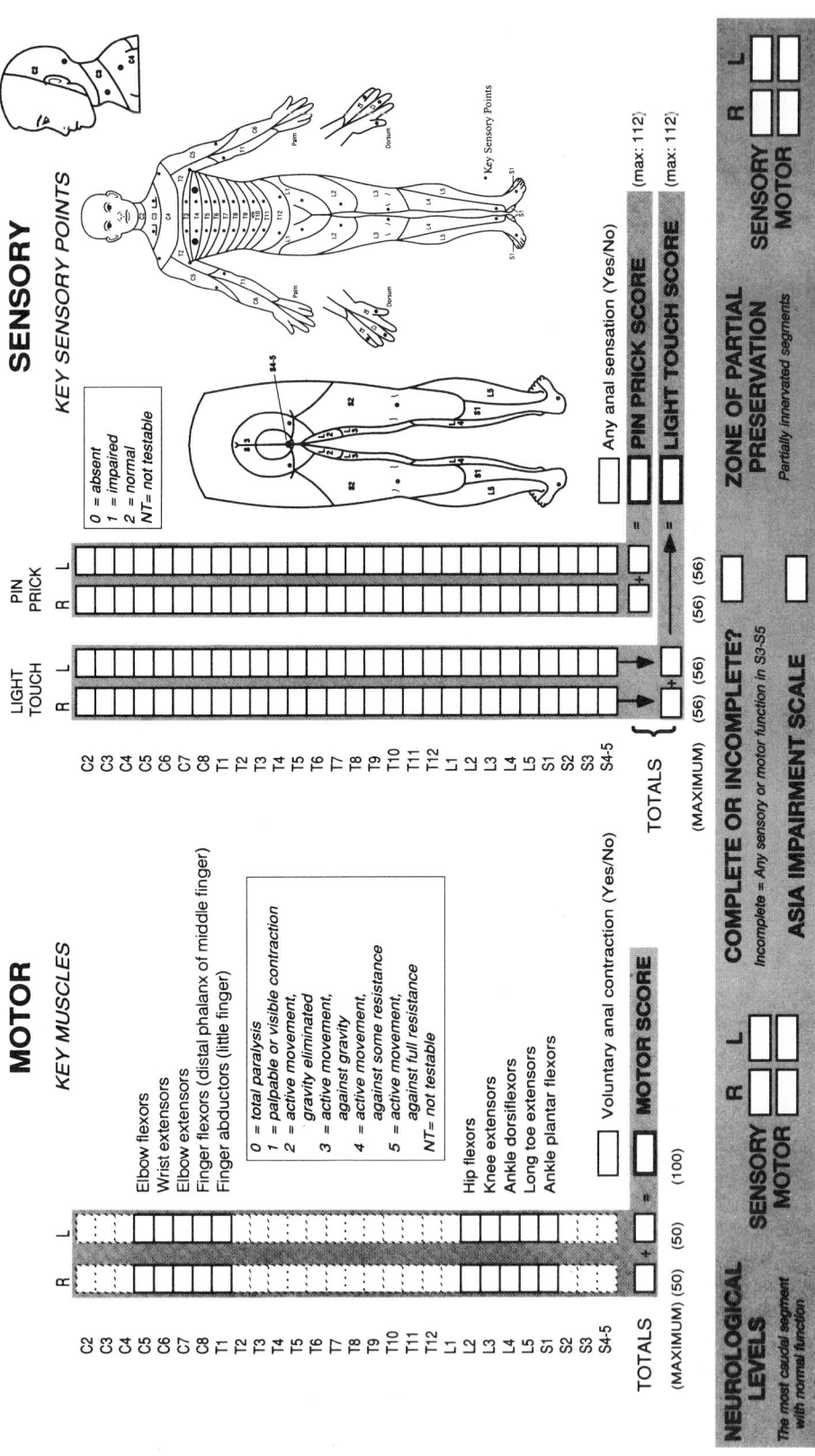

Figure 42–4

1996 Standard Neurological Classification of Spinal Cord Injury. A, Motor: key muscles. B, Sensory: key sensation points. (With permission from the American Spinal Injury Association, Atlanta, GA, 1996.)

injury levels and syndromes, specified an objective impairment scale, and recommended a functional assessment instrument (Figure 42–5).[13] The motor assessment focuses on 10 major muscle groups, 5 in the arms and hands and 5 in the hips, legs, and feet. Each group is tested bilaterally and is assigned a score ranging from 0, meaning complete paralysis, to 5, indicating active movement against full resistance. Scores of 1 to 4 indicate varying degrees of strength in movement. The muscle function scores are added together, and the most points a person can attain is 100[13,14] (see Figure 42–4*A*). Other motor groups may be tested if desired, and the tool allows for testing of all major muscle groups, but only the 10 identified are scored for the purposes of scoring the patient.

LEVELS		
	7 Complete independence (timely, safely) 6 Modified independence (device)	No helper
	Modified Dependence 5 Supervision 4 Minimal assist (subject = 75%+) 3 Moderate assist (subject = 50%+) **Complete Dependence** 2 Maximal assist (subject = 25%+) 1 Total assist (subject = 0%+)	Helper

Self-Care	**Admit**	**Discharge**
A. Eating	☐	☐
B. Grooming	☐	☐
C. Bathing	☐	☐
D. Dressing, upper body	☐	☐
E. Dressing, lower body	☐	☐
F. Toileting	☐	☐
Sphincter Control		
G. Bladder management	☐	☐
H. Bowel management	☐	☐
Mobility		
Transfer:		
I. Bed, chair, wheelchair	☐	☐
J. Toilet	☐	☐
K. Tub, shower	☐	☐
Locomotion	W☐	W☐
L. Walk/wheelchair	C☐ ☐	C☐ ☐
M. Stairs	☐	☐
Communication	A☐	A☐
N. Comprehension	V☐ ☐	V☐ ☐
O. Expression	V☐ ☐	V☐ ☐
	N☐	N☐
Social Cognition		
P. Social interaction	☐	☐
Q. Problem solving	☐	☐
R. Memory	☐	☐
Total FIM	☐	☐

NOTE: Leave no blanks; enter 1 if patient not testable due to risk

Figure 42–5

Functional independence measures. (With permission from the Research Foundation of the State University of New York, New York, NY.)

The sensory scale requires testing of the dermatomes. Using pinprick and light touch as the two sensations, each major dermatome is tested bilaterally. In the case of sensation, the patient can be scored as 0, indicating absent sensation, 1, representing impaired sensation, or 2, which is normal sensation to pinprick and light touch (see Figure 42–4*B*). The total score for the patient who is normal neurologically is 112 for pinprick and 112 for light touch. It is important to test both pinprick and light touch because they are carried to the higher centers in different areas of the spinothalamic tracts of the spinal cord and may indicate the area of injury more precisely for the health care team. When testing sensation, the patient should be asked to close his or her eyes, so the visual input is taken away. The tester should begin on the patient's face, where it is presumed sensation is normal. This maneuver allows the patient to know what the pinprick and light touch feel like on a neurologically normal area of the body. This technique helps the patient to describe abnormalities of sensations, as well as areas of total loss of sensation. The patient describes what he or she is feeling and where on the body the sensation is felt as the examination progresses. The assessment tool also asks for the tester to identify, based on the examination, whether the injury is complete or incomplete using the ASIA Impairment Scale (Figure 42–6).

Proprioception should be assessed as well. An injury to the posterior spinal cord results in a significant loss of proprioception. The patient is asked to close his or her eyes and to identify whether the great toe or the thumb is in the up or down position (moved away or toward the head).

A major problem with using these assessment tools is that the patient must be awake and able to follow commands and to indicate the presence of sensation. If the patient is unconscious from a closed head injury or is sedated because of mechanical ventilation, these assessment tools will not be helpful to the clinician.

For the first 72 hours, the patient's motor and sensory function should be assessed frequently (every 1–2 hours), along with vital sign measurements, to determine any changes from baseline. Careful documentation of all assessment data is critical to detect neurologic deterioration and the need for intervention.

Diagnostic Workup

After initial stabilization of the injured spine and the patient, diagnostic testing should be done to determine the nature of the injury.[15] The golden rule in caring for the patient with SCI is to prevent further injury, so it is critical to determine the extent of the original injury and the appropriate therapeutic intervention, that is, surgical versus nonsurgical treatment, as soon as possible after admission.

A cervical spine radiograph is obtained immediately after admission to establish the level of injury

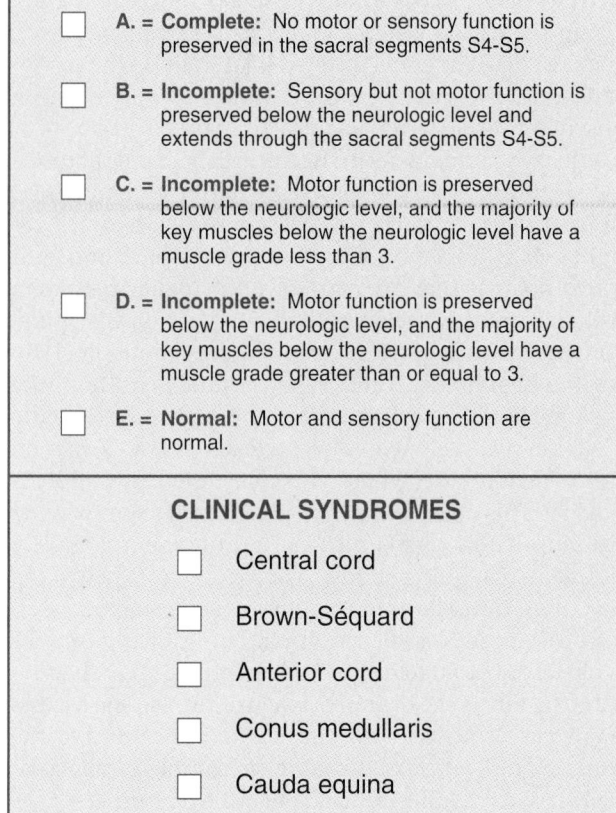

A. = Complete: No motor or sensory function is preserved in the sacral segments S4-S5.

B. = Incomplete: Sensory but not motor function is preserved below the neurologic level and extends through the sacral segments S4-S5.

C. = Incomplete: Motor function is preserved below the neurologic level, and the majority of key muscles below the neurologic level have a muscle grade less than 3.

D. = Incomplete: Motor function is preserved below the neurologic level, and the majority of key muscles below the neurologic level have a muscle grade greater than or equal to 3.

E. = Normal: Motor and sensory function are normal.

CLINICAL SYNDROMES

☐ Central cord

☐ Brown-Séquard

☐ Anterior cord

☐ Conus medullaris

☐ Cauda equina

Figure 42–6

American Spinal Injury Association Impairment Scale. (With permission from the Research Foundation of the State University of New York, New York, NY.)

and the extent of bony injury. At this time, thoracic and lumbosacral films should also be obtained if the patient is hemodynamically stable enough to tolerate the procedures to ensure that no other spinal damage has occurred. The radiographs are taken with the patient in a neutral position, on a backboard, and with neck protection to prevent any movement. All seven cervical vertebrae must be visualized to the top of T1 in the anterioposterior and lateral views of the neck. This may be difficult because C7 can easily be obstructed by the shoulders or muscles that are in spasm after the injury. An open-mouth view may be needed to view the odontoid process (dens) of C2.

Computed tomography (CT) scanning is generally helpful to delineate the type of bony injury and to determine the presence of spinal cord compression. It can be done in combination with a myelogram to enhance visualization of the spinal canal. Indications for CT with myelogram include neurologic deficit in the presence of a normal radiograph, thoracic spine injury with deficit, determination of the presence of bone in the spinal canal, and after reduction of the spinal column in patients with neurologic deficit to ensure adequate spinal cord decompression.

Magnetic resonance imaging (MRI) is the newest diagnostic tool to be used to determine the extent of the SCI. This test may be difficult to perform in the critically ill patient because no ferrous metal can come in contact with the patient during the examination.[9] This test will be much easier to obtain in the future because more products, such as cervical tongs, are being made with titanium. MRI should be done if the patient has an incomplete spinal cord syndrome or neurologic deficit without obvious fracture identified by plain radiograph or CT scan.[16] This test enables one to diagnose spinal cord contusion, edema, and hemorrhage. The images from MRI correlate with the neurologic status of the patient better than the other diagnostic tools and are better predictors of outcome.[16]

The best diagnostic tool for determining the extent of the SCI and establishing a prognosis is the somatosensory evoked potential (SEP). The evoked potential from the stimulation of a peripheral nerve in the arm or leg below the level of injury reflects the sensory function of the spinal cord in carrying messages along the neural pathway to the higher centers of the brain. In a patient with a complete injury, SEPs are absent because no information is able to pass the area of damage. In patients with an incomplete injury, altered responses are noted, but the pathway may be able to carry the messages, a good prognostic sign. In early injury, when the patient is still experiencing spinal shock and the clinical examination may demonstrate a complete injury, the SEP can indicate that the injury is partial. This information may change the interventions for the patient to a more aggressive therapeutic regimen.[17] The combination of clinical examination, CT or MRI, and SEP can give the clinician the information needed to plan the medical therapies that will produce the best possible outcomes (see Table 42–2).

Nursing Diagnoses

The nursing management of the patient with SCI is extremely complex because of the effects of this injury on all body systems. This patient requires the care of a multidisciplinary team from the outset. The management of this patient actually begins in the field, before arrival in the emergency department. The assurance of an adequate airway, of breathing, and of circulation is critical. Of major concern also during this phase of care is the acute immobilization of the cervical spine before transport. Once the patient has been stabilized and transported to the definitive care center, the diagnosis can be made and the therapeutic plan can be initiated. The goals of care are to prevent secondary injury and complications and to prepare the patient for reintegration to home. Many high-risk diagnoses are present in these patients and persist from the acute phase of care

TABLE 42–3
Nursing Diagnoses

Phase of Hospitalization	Problem Statement	Etiologic Factors
Emergency Department	Decreased cardiac output	Peripheral vasodilation
	Impaired gas exchange	Muscle paralysis
	Ineffective airway clearance	Muscle paralysis
	Ineffective breathing pattern	Muscle paralysis
	Impaired mobility	Muscle paralysis
	Risk for injury	Unstable spinal cord injury
	Ineffective temperature regulation	Disruption of hypothalamic control
	Constipation	Muscle paralysis and spinal shock
	Urinary retention	Muscle paralysis and spinal shock
Intensive Care Unit	In addition to above:	
	Risk for injury	Cardiovascular problems and venostasis
	Altered nutrition, less than body requirements	Inability to access nutrients, gastrointestinal inactivity, and increased metabolic demand
	Impaired gas exchange	Respiratory insufficiency
	Fear	Psychological impact of the injury
Intermediate Care Unit	In addition to above:	
	Risk for injury	Autonomic dysreflexia
	Risk for impaired skin integrity	Injury and paralysis
	Sexual dysfunction	Paralysis and loss of higher center control
	Ineffective individual coping	Psychological distress, body image disturbances, feelings of powerlessness, and unknown future
	Ineffective family coping	Change in family roles

to rehabilitation. A priority list of nursing diagnoses associated with the various phases of care is contained in Table 42–3.

Collaborative Management

The patient with cervical SCI and neurologic deficit is a challenge to any nurse. A multidisciplinary team approach, including physicians representing many specialties, nurses, respiratory therapists, rehabilitative specialists, clergy, social workers, and counselors, is needed to ensure that the patient's holistic needs are met. Because this injury affects every body system, multiple medical specialists may be involved in the patient's care. It is important to have one coordinator of the patient's care. Coordination ensures that all actual and potential patient problems are addressed in a timely manner. A pathway or multidisciplinary care plan can be used to assist in the coordination and documentation of care. Figure 42–7 provides an example of a critical pathway to guide the acute care of the patient with SCI.

Emergency Department

On arrival to the emergency department, a complete history, including a history of the accident, is obtained, and the primary trauma survey is done. Once the patient has been stabilized, and if it is within 8 hours of the injury, the patient should be started on high-dose methylprednisolone (Solu-Medrol). The dosing regimen has been precisely determined, based on the results of the second National Acute Spinal Cord Injury Study.[1, 18–26] This multicenter study found that patients given high-dose methylprednisolone within 8 hours of the injury (onset of symptoms) had improved neurologic recovery.[18] The patient is given an intravenous loading dose of 30 mg/kg of body weight over 15 minutes. After 45 minutes, an infusion of 5.4 mg/kg per hour of methylprednisolone is delivered over the next 23 hours.[13, 18, 23, 27] Despite controversies and unresolved issues surrounding the use of high-dose methylprednisolone, it is the recommended initial therapy.[13, 19, 26] If the injury is more than 8 hours old, high-dose methylprednisolone is contraindicated.[18, 27] In addition, a study examining the impact of high-dose methylprednisolone on penetrating SCIs showed no significant improvement in functional outcome for this patient population.[28]

The National Acute Spinal Cord Injury group that conducted the original methylprednisolone study furthered their work and published the results of another study with high-dose methylprednisolone and tirilazad (Freedox) (a 21-aminosteroid agent).[27] The

Text continued on page 884

R Adams Cowley Shock Trauma Center

Inclusion Criteria: Bony, ligamentous and/or neurologic
injury to the spine at or above T5 level with neurologic deficit

Team Physician: _____
Critical Care Physician: _____
Orthopedic Surgeon/Neuro Surgeon: _____

OR Procedures _____

Date _____ 01/96

Date/ Hospital Day	first 6 hours	6 - 24 hours	Day 2	Day 3	Day 4	Day 5
NEUROLOGIC Maintain or improve Neurologic function R/O other SCI Normothermia	Consult ___ Neurosurgery ___ Orthopedics SC assessment (on admission, level check with VS) CT ___ MRI ___ Steroids † ___ Study: ___ Sedation: ___ C/T/L Spine X R ___ Temp Q1-2°	SC evaluation (check sc level with VS check) Analgesia/Sedation: Antianxiety Med:	SC evaluation QD + prn Analgesia/Sedation: Antianxiety Med:	SC evaluation QD + prn Analgesia/Sedation: Evaluate need for speech/lang. cognitive screen Y/N Evaluate need for augmentative communication Y/N Antianxiety Med:	SC evaluation QD + prn Assess and establish sleep pattern Weaning analgesia/sedation	SC evaluation QD + prn Evaluate pain/ dysesthesia mgt.
RESPIRATORY Maintain Adequate Gas Exchange Maintain $Pa0_2$ ___ $Sp0_2$ ___ $PaC0_2$ ___ $ETC0_2$ ___	Airway intubated Y/N 0_2 apparatus: $Sp0_2$ monitored Monitor for Respiratory failure PT consult CXR:	Monitor for respiratory failure $Sp0_2$ monitored CPTq ___ ISq ___ vol ___ Assist cough Abdominal binder ___	Assess for weaning Implement weaning protocol $Sp0_2$ monitored Consider L.T. airway mgt (i.e. trach?) ISq ___ vol ___ CPTq ___ CXR:	$Sp0_2$ monitored ISq ___ vol ___ CPTq ___ CXR:	$Sp0_2$ monitored ISq ___ vol ___ CPTq ___ CXR:	$Sp0_2$ monitored ISq ___ vol ___ CPTq ___ CXR:
CV Maintain adequate tissue perfusion Maintain Hgb ___	VS Q1° Maintain MAP > 80-90mmHgx4D DVT prophylaxis: ___ Arterial line ___	VSq ___ Labs S/U calf/thigh girth qd	VSq ___ Labs S/U calf/thigh girth qd	VSq ___ Labs S/U calf/thigh girth qd Change Peripheral IV	Labs S/U calf/thigh girth q 12° Change AL/Central Line	VSq ___ Labs: calf/thigh q 12° Initiate fluid restriction ___ cc/day
GI/NUTRITION R/O intra-abdominal injury Maintain nutritional intake to meet metabolic needs Maintain bowel elimination	NPO except meds GI prophylaxis: ___ R/O Intra-abdominal injury Y/N	Nutrition consult ___ prealbumin ___ Diet: ___ Bowel regimen:	Diet: TF/TPN	Diet: Receiving rec'd goal TF/TPN Y/N Check BM	Diet:	Diet: Check BM

This pathway represents the course of care for the majority of patients in this casetype. Including resource utilization and outcomes. Each patient will have variations from this pathway almost every day.

Figure 42-7

Sample critical pathway for care of the spinal cord injured patient. (With permission from the University of Maryland Medical System, Baltimore, MD.)

	1st 6 Hours	6-24 Hours	Day 2	Day 3	Day 4	Day 5
GU Maintain adequate u/o	Insert Foley I + O	I + O	Assess for bladder training I + O	I + O	I + O	I + O
ID Remain infection free			Fever pack protocol	Fever pack protocol	Fever pack protocol	Fever pack protocol
SKIN Skin remains intact	Off Backboard in 2° with MD assistance Implement skin prevention protocols	If on regular bed use dynamic sleep surface Waffle cushion on Stryker frame				
MUSCULOSKELETAL Stabilize and maintain alignment of fractures and dislocation	Initial spinal alignment Initial stabilization plan: traction type: _____ wt: _____ bed: _____ Bedrest Use Sulkoff board for patient transports	Clarify plan for stabilization/mobilization PT evaluation _____	OT consult: Brace: 90° film with Brace	Splints: Evaluate for progressive sitting (high back wheelchair with cushion) OT tx plan:	Splints: OOBq _____ for _____ minutes Assistance required _____ chair _____ cushion _____ Dependent weight shifts position _____ pressure relief _____ Ace/Teds Y/N	Splints: OOBq _____ for _____ minutes ? F/U X-ray:
PSYCHOSOCIAL/ TEACHING Patient/family state understanding of injury and treatment	Initial patient/family contact - nurse - prognosis discussed/documented by neuro/ortho _____ Social work consult _____ Family contact with patient _____ ASAP _____ Evaluate family desire for clergy Y/N	Provide initial Neurotrauma Booklet Plan Family Conference Substance Abuse _____	Determine teaching plan Evaluate need for psych consult	Initial Skin Care teaching (provide preventing pressure ulcer brochure) Establish Mutual Schedule with patient	Implement teaching plan	Evaluate patient/family understanding of injury/implications Educate on Autonomic Dysreflexia Guidelines for functional outcomes (PT/OT/Nsg) Education Review Nutrition Education
DISCHARGE Patient discharge to appropriate setting with necessary supports		Refer to Rehab Network _____ D/C Coordinator _____	Insurance status verified _____ Financial Counselor consult _____ Rehab Network contact patient/family _____ Apply for MA _____	Multi-disciplinary family Conference Referral to SCI hotline		Rehab Family Conference
Variance						

Date/ Hospital Day	Day 6	Day 7	Day 8	Day 9	Day 10	CLINIC
NEUROLOGIC Maintain or improve Neurologic function	SC evaluation QD + prn	SC evaluation QD + prn	SC evaluation QD + prn	Forward D/C SCI evaluation to Clinic		Study protocol requirements: SCI evaluation Assess pain mgt. and spasm mgt.
RESPIRATORY Maintain Adequate Gas Exchange Maintain $Pa0_2$ ___ $Sp0_2$ ___ $PaC0_2$ ___ $ETC0_2$ ___	Exubation Y/N Assess for trach monitor $Sp0_2$ ___ ISq ___ vol ___ CPTq ___ Assist cough	monitor $Sp0_2$ ___ ISq ___ vol ___ CPTq ___ Assist cough	monitor $Sp0_2$ ___ ISq ___ vol ___ CPTq ___ Assist cough	monitor $Sp0_2$ ___ ISq ___ vol ___ CPTq ___ Assist cough		Assess for complications including hoarseness
CV Maintain adequate tissue perfusion Maintain Hgb ___	VSq ___ Labs: calf/thigh girth qd. 12°	VSq ___ Labs: calf/thigh girth 12°	VSq ___ Labs: calf/thigh girth 12°			Labs: Assess for DVT Continue DVT prophylaxis Y/N
GI/NUTRITION Maintain nutrition intake to meet metabolic needs Maintain bowel elimination	Hold TF for exubation Once exubated evaluate start po diet ? Swallow evaluation Y/N Diet:	Weight ___ Diet:	 Diet:	Nutrition D/C summary in chart Diet:		Evaluation for constipation Weight ___ Weight change from D/C ___

	Day 6	Day 7	Day 8	Day 9	Day 10	CLINIC
GU Maintain adequate u/o Establish urine elimination pattern	D/C Foley Initiate q 4° intermittent caths I + O	Cathq ____ I + O	Cathq ____ I + O	Cathq ____ I + O		Assess bladder training: Self cath capability:
ID Remain Infection free	Fever pack protocol	Fever pack protocol	Fever pack protocol	Fever pack protocol		
SKIN Skin remains intact						Assess skin integrity: wound check: pin site check:
MUSCULOSKELETAL Stabilize and maintain alignment of fractures/dislocation. Optimize patient mobility	Splints: OOBq ____ for ____ minutes Lateral transfer/total lift	Splints: OOBq ____ for ____ minutes Evaluation for spasms Initiate antispasmodic:	Splints: OOBq ____ for ____ minutes Lateral transfer/total lift	Splints: OOBq ____ for ____ minutes		Films at 2wks, 6wks, 3mos, 6mos, 1yr, 2yrs post fixation A/P: Y/N Lateral: Y/N Others: Evaluate PT care Evaluate mobility progress
PSYCHOSOCIAL/ TEACHING Patient/family state understanding of injury and treatment	Educate about rehab					Assess mental health Assess family and support systems Assess drug dependency Assess sexual fx Referrals: Education provided on:
DISCHARGE Patient discharge to appropriate setting with necessary supports		F/U on rehab plan	Evaluate patient's condition for D/C Prepare and copy D/C summaries Copy physician consult sheets Call report to rehab in PM	Plan F/U Clinic visit Films required for Clinic visit: D/C to rehab facility		MA obtained: Establish primary care MD: Home referrals: Vocational rehab: Next clinic appt.:
Variance						

Figure 42-7 Continued

883

results continued to demonstrate that patients who receive high-dose methylprednisolone do the best neurologically. All patients in the study received the bolus dose of methylprednisolone and then were randomly assigned to the 24-hour group (5.4 mg/kg per hour for 24 hours); the 48-hour group (5.4 mg/kg per hour for 48 hours); or the tirilazad group. This group received 25 mg/kg bolus infusions every 6 hours for 48 hours. Motor changes and functional independence measures (FIM) were assessed at 6 weeks and at 6 months. This study demonstrated that all patients who received methylprednisolone within 3 hours of the injury showed the most improvement on the 24-hour regimen. Patients treated within 3 to 8 hours improved more on the 48-hour dosing. Finally, those patients who received tirilazad for 48 hours showed motor recovery rates equivalent to those of the patients receiving methylprednisolone for 24 hours.[27] The researchers recommended that patients treated within 3 hours of the injury should be maintained on the current regimen of 24 hours of methylprednisolone, whereas those receiving treatment within 3 to 8 hours of injury should be given the new 48-hour tirilazad therapy for the best outcomes.[27] These recommendations have not become standard at this time. The group also suggests further study into the dosing of tirilazad.[27]

Respiratory Support

The respiratory status of the patient must be assessed frequently to ensure a patent airway and adequate respiratory effort. A continuous pulse oximeter to monitor oxygen saturation should be placed immediately on admission to the emergency department. A baseline arterial blood gas determination should also be made to assess the patient's respiratory status on admission. A respiratory therapist or anesthesiologist should be available to intubate the patient should the patient have difficulty with respiratory effort, suffer hypoxia, or develop clinical signs of respiratory arrest. The intubation should be done using the jaw thrust maneuver to prevent any flexion or extension of the neck. Edema after SCI causes the spinal cord to swell upward so respiratory compromise is a likely problem in the patient with a high cervical injury, especially at C5 and above. Many physicians believe that elective intubation is best in cervical injuries that are likely to cause respiratory compromise. The endotracheal tube should be removed as soon as the patient has stabilized neurologically and is no longer in danger of respiratory arrest.

Spinal Shock

The patient will most likely be brought to the emergency department in spinal shock. The clinical presentation of the patient with spinal shock is flaccid paralysis, loss of sensation below the level of injury, loss of bowel and bladder control, usually resulting in fecal and urinary retention, and poikilothermia. The patient should have a Foley catheter inserted as quickly as possible to prevent severe overdistention of the bladder, especially if a great deal of fluid had been administered during resuscitation and stabilization in the field. Bladder training is started after spinal shock is over in most instances.

A nasogastric tube is inserted into the stomach and is connected to low suction to drain the stomach and to prevent vomiting and aspiration. Abdominal distention can occur quickly, and this condition lifts the diaphragm and interferes with respiratory effort, which may already be compromised.

The loss of sensation prevents the patient from feeling any pain below the level of injury. A thorough secondary assessment is absolutely necessary to discover other possible injuries such as fractured bones or intra-abdominal bleeding.

Cardiovascular Support

Monitoring of heart rate and rhythm should be done routinely in these patients. As described earlier, these patients experience a loss of sympathetic outflow causing bradycardia. Left ventricular function is also depressed, and the poor ventricular function is exacerbated by the release of beta-endorphin in response to the injury. It may be prudent to have an external pacemaker on standby for these patients. In addition to cardiac monitoring, cardiac enzymes should be monitored in the presence of electrocardiographic changes that indicate ischemia to the heart muscle. Left ventricular dysfunction can lead to significant cardiac dysrhythmias and severe heart block.

The lack of sympathetic outflow leads to hypotension, which needs to be treated with drugs to raise the blood pressure and to increase the cardiac output to 1.5 times normal. A pulmonary artery catheter may be inserted in the emergency department to gather data to determine further medical interventions and to monitor fluid balance. Fluids should be administered cautiously to avoid risking pulmonary edema.

Precautions should be taken during this time to keep the patient normothermic. These patients tend to take on the ambient temperature of the environment because of the loss of temperature regulation by the hypothalamus. Blankets may be necessary to keep the patient warm at this time.

Conservative Versus Surgical Treatment

Once the diagnosis has been confirmed, decisions must be made regarding the best way to manage the patient. Conservative management consists of immobilization of the patient in Gardner–Wells or Vinke tongs (Figure 42–8) or a halo vest or brace (Figure 42–9) with or without traction. The goal of this approach is not only to immobilize the patient to prevent

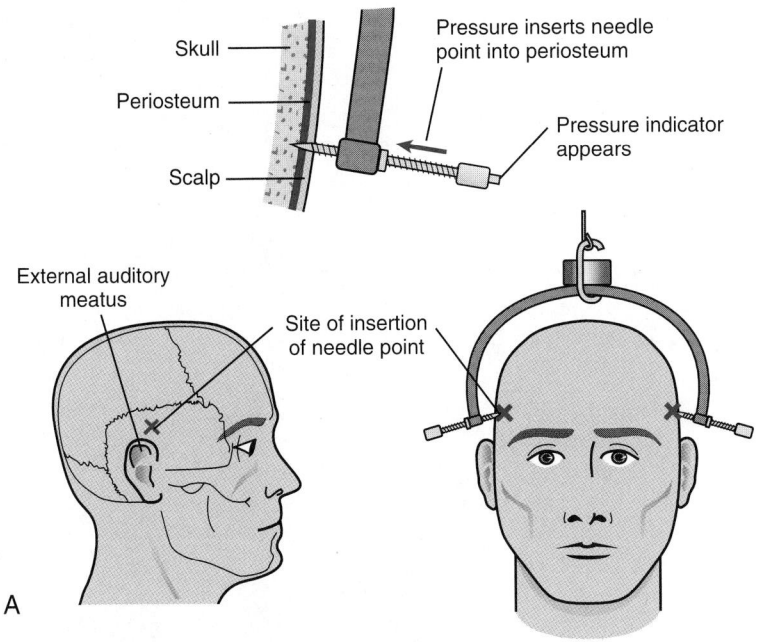

Skull

Periosteum

Scalp

Pressure inserts needle point into periosteum

Pressure indicator appears

External auditory meatus

Site of insertion of needle point

A

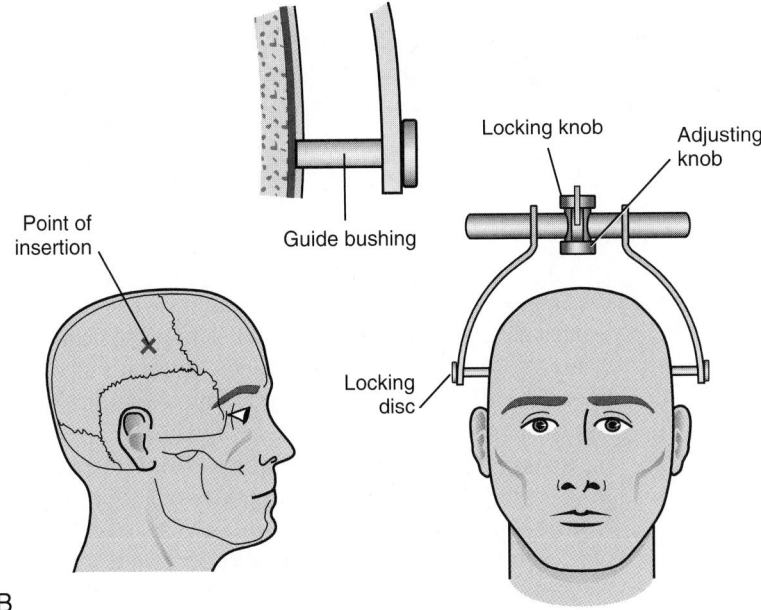

Point of insertion

Guide bushing

Locking knob

Adjusting knob

Locking disc

B

Figure 42–8

Cervicals immobilization device. A, Gardner-Wells tongs with traction. B, Vinke tongs. (Redrawn from Rothman RH, Simeone FA (eds): The Spine, 2nd ed. Philadelphia, W.B. Saunders, 1992, p 1642.)

further injury, but also to reduce the bony deformity and realign the vertebrae. Patients can be placed in a regular bed and cared for adequately with this type of traction. Sometimes a specialty bed is needed, such as a kinetic treatment table, if the patient needs additional turning to prevent or treat atelectasis.

Surgical intervention should be done as soon as possible after the injury to preserve and perhaps improve spinal cord function. Early surgery (within the first 24 hours) is generally done if the patient has radiologic evidence of spinal cord compression, a progressive neurological deficit, a comminuted fracture with a chance that the bone will dislodge and penetrate the spinal cord, penetrating injuries, or evidence of bone frag-

ments in the spinal canal.[29] The surgical procedure chosen is determined by the surgeon. The type of procedure to be done depends on the degree of bony injury and instability and the location of the injury. The procedures performed include spinal cord and nerve root decompression by spinal cord realignment and, when necessary, removal of bone, soft tissue, or foreign bodies from the spinal canal. Depending on the degree of vertebral instability, these procedures are combined with a spinal stabilization or fusion procedure to prevent further injury and to allow patient mobility. The approach to the surgical procedure is posterior if the laminar or spinous process is involved. Posterior instrumentation, placing wires, pins, or screws into the

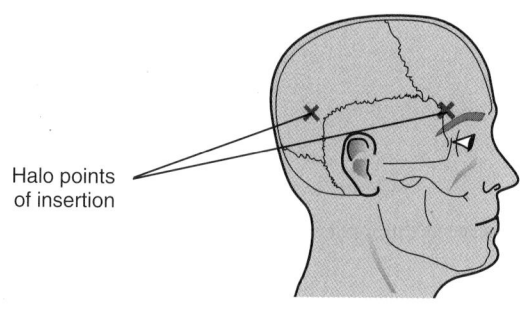

Halo points
of insertion

Figure 42–9

The halo provides four-point skeletal fixation through a circumferential steel ring placed above the ears and eyebrows. The raised portion of the ring is located over the occiput. The halo can be attached to free weights, or it may be fixed directly to a body vest with steel uprights between the ring and the vest. (Redrawn from Rothman RH, Simeone FA (eds): The Spine, 2nd ed. Philadelphia, W.B. Saunders, 1992, pp 1641, 1643.)

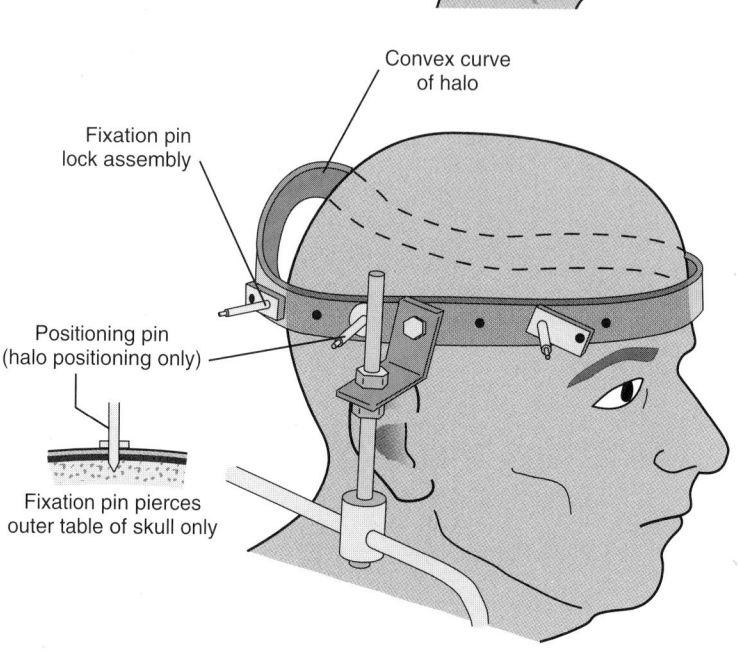

Convex curve
of halo

Fixation pin
lock assembly

Positioning pin
(halo positioning only)

Fixation pin pierces
outer table of skull only

spinous process, is done to stabilize the bones and to prevent bony movement. An anterior approach is done if the vertebral body itself or the ligaments that surround the body have been damaged. When an anterior approach is used, the surgeon must fuse the vertebral bodies together for stability. With the anterior approach in the cervical area, the major postoperative concern is a compromised airway resulting from swelling in the operative area.[10] The overall goals of operating on the patient are to provide stability in the injured area, to permit early mobility, and to minimize the risks of secondary neurologic injury as well as the systemic complications associated with immobility.

Once physiologic and neurologic stabilization measures have been accomplished by nonoperative or operative means, the patient is transferred to the intensive care unit (ICU) for continued monitoring, management, and nursing care. A holistic approach to care is critical because every body system is affected by SCI.

Critical Care

Cardiovascular Care

The major cardiovascular problems are related to the loss of sympathetic outflow. The patient experiences a profound peripheral vasodilation that, in turn, affects cardiac output, cardiac index, systemic vascular resistance, and tissue perfusion. The tissue perfusion of the spinal cord is also altered by the inflammatory responses after the injury, thereby creating tissue hypoxia.

Several therapeutic interventions are focused on improving the cardiovascular status of the patient. Continuous monitoring of the hemodynamics and cardiac function of the patient is important to direct interventions to support the cardiac output and systemic perfusion. Hypotension and low cardiac output respond to the use of inotropic agents, as opposed to fluid resuscitation. Dopamine (Intropin) (3–5 µg/kg per minute) is the drug of choice to treat the loss of sympathetic outflow during neurogenic shock. The goals of using an inotropic agent are to keep the mean systemic arterial pressure at 80 to 90 mm Hg and to maintain a cardiac output at 1.5 times normal.[10] Dobutamine (Dobutrex) may be added to support cardiac function because left ventricular function is often depressed in these patients. This augmentation of cardiovascular function should be maintained for a minimum of 72 hours, to counter the effects of neurogenic shock and to improve spinal cord perfusion during the initial injury phase.[24] The patient should have a pulmonary artery catheter placed to ensure appropriate monitoring of the hemodynamic parameters and to assess the effectiveness of the therapeutic interventions.

Bradycardia also occurs in these patients, but it is usually well tolerated by patients with adequate fluid volume and cardiac index. Atropine should be available at the bedside of the patient with bradycardia. If the patient is asymptomatic and does not have type II second-degree heart block or third-degree heart block, continued observation is all that is necessary. If the patient is symptomatic with hemodynamic changes, shortness of breath, and decreased level of consciousness, then atropine, 1 mg, should be administered. If symptoms persist, consideration should be given to transcutaneous or transvenous pacing of the patient. Vasovagal responses to turning and suctioning may also need to be treated to prevent deterioration in cardiovascular functioning. Continuous cardiac monitoring is necessary to identify significant bradycardic episodes and other dysrhythmias, especially ventricular dysfunction.

As neurogenic shock resolves, the cardiovascular status generally stabilizes. The patient may remain with a low blood pressure and bradycardia, but systemic vascular resistance and cardiac parameters are generally improved.

Respiratory Care

Altered respiratory function is a serious threat to the patient with cervical SCI. Some degree of respiratory insufficiency should be suspected in all patients with tetraplegia, even if the injury is below C5. Insufficiency may result from airway obstruction, intercostal or diaphragmatic muscle paralysis, associated thoracic or tracheal trauma, or aspiration.[10] Gastric dilatation and ileus may contribute to respiratory problems by limiting diaphragmatic excursion. A past history of respiratory problems such as asthma or chronic obstructive pulmonary disease also adds to the potential for the development of severe respiratory insufficiency. When the diaphragm is the only active muscle of respiration, fatigue can also contribute to ineffective breathing patterns.

Respiratory complications continue to be a major cause of morbidity and mortality after cervical SCI, with a reported incidence of 38 to 83%.[30] Atelectasis and pneumonia are frequent complications in patients with SCI. An impaired cough reflex leads to the accumulation of secretions that can lead to pneumonia. If the secretions cannot be cleared, recombinant human DNAse, which is similar to surfactant, can be administered to resolve the atelectasis.[31]

Pulmonary embolus is another complication that can interfere with the pulmonary function of the patient with SCI. It can occur anytime from the time of injury, with a peak incidence at about 78 days.[32] Thirteen percent of all patients with SCI suffer pulmonary emboli at some time after their injury. The usual cause of the pulmonary emboli is deep venous thrombosis (DVT), which occurs as a result of paralysis and immobilization and is associated with hypercoagulability and decreased vascular tone. The incidence of DVT has been reported to vary from 14 to 100%.[33] During the acute phase of care, several things need to be done to prevent DVT. Nurses should perform passive range-of-motion exercises to the lower extremities to decrease venous stasis, turn patients at least every 2 hours, elevate the patient legs above the level of the head once the spine is stabilized, and use graduated compression stockings or a pneumatic compression device to decrease the risk of DVT.[34] Low-molecular-weight heparin (e.g., Lovenox) has emerged as an extremely effective method for DVT prophylaxis in other high-risk patient populations, such as patients who have had hip and knee operations, but little has been published on the safety and efficacy in patients with SCI. The use of this form of prophylaxis is gaining wider acceptance, and in some centers, patients are started on low-dose anticoagulation on admission.

Physical assessment of the chest, including observation, inspection, palpation, percussion, and auscultation, should be done with assessment of the patient's vital signs for the first 72 hours. Chest expansion and abdominal movement should be observed to determine whether the accessory muscles are being used for respiration. Bedside pulmonary function studies can be done to determine the patient's work of breathing and to ascertain whether support is needed. Tidal volume, minute volume, inspiratory and expiratory volumes, vital capacity, and residual capacity should all be measured on a routine basis during the first few days after the injury. Continuous pulse oximetry can be useful in assessing changes in oxygen saturation. Chest radiographs can be used to assess for any respiratory complications, as well as for the resolution of complications.

In patients with ineffective breathing patterns from muscle paralysis and weakness of the chest wall, aggressive chest physical therapy is necessary to mobilize and clear secretions to prevent atelectasis. Use of Trendelenburg's position, when this position is not contraindicated, may be necessary to move the secretions from the lower lobes to the upper areas of the lung. Care must be taken when the patient is head down because this position may cause a vasovagal response and increased bradycardia.

The use of a "quad-assist" cough augments the abdominal muscles during the expiratory phase of ventilation to help the patient clear secretions from the airway. As in the Heimlich maneuver, the nurse places a fist or heel of the hand between the umbilicus and the diaphragm and presses down on the abdomen and pushes up (toward the head) when the patient coughs.[9] The patient is instructed to take the deepest breath possible and repeat it three times. At the end of the third breath, the patient is told to attempt to cough, and the nurse assists at that point. This intervention may need to be performed hourly, or even more frequently, if the patient has a large amount of secretions. Standard nursing interventions of turning and adequate hydration aid in helping to mobilize the secretions.

If the patient has an endotracheal tube or tracheostomy, suctioning is done to clear the secretions. Close monitoring of the patient is necessary during suctioning because a vasovagal response occurs, especially in patients with high cervical SCI. This response can result in severe bradycardia, even to asystole.[9]

Immobilization and Mobility
The primary goal of management remains to prevent further deterioration in function and to maximize the patient's functional outcome. Continued neurologic assessment of the patient's motor and sensory function is essential. Neurologic deterioration during the acute phase of care may indicate a delayed response to the injury, a lack of stability in the area of injury, swelling of the spinal cord, failure of the immobilization or operative intervention to stabilize the injury, or a secondary injury related to continued impairment of tissue perfusion to the spinal cord. During the first 72 hours of care, neurologic assessments should be done every hour, and the results should be recorded.

The rationale for surgical intervention is described earlier in the chapter. Whether the patient has had an operative procedure or not, the patient needs to remain in traction or a halo vest until healing occurs. The patient is immobilized to prevent new injury to the spinal cord. Traction may be applied to the tongs or halo ring to keep the vertebrae in proper alignment or to decompress the bony impingement on the spinal cord. A specialty bed, such as a kinetic therapy bed or a Stryker-type frame, may or may not be needed for these patients, depending on the stability of the injury.

The patient depends on the nursing and physical therapy staff for any mobility at this time. The paralysis caused by the injury, the spinal shock, and the forced immobility of bed rest and traction require that the staff do range-of-motion exercises to maintain the patient's joint mobility. Passive range of motion should be done at least every 4 hours to all joints including those of the hands and feet. This maneuver prevents contractures, which can start quickly after the injury. Range-of-motion exercises also improve the venous return from the lower extremities, to help prevent the formation of DVT. All joints should be in a neutral position when the patient is lying at rest. Supportive devices such as antidrop foot splints, antirotational booties, trochanter rolls, high-top tennis shoes, and wrist and forearm splints can all be used in the ICU to assist in maintaining the joints in proper alignment.[9]

Immobilizing the patient is important to prevent further injury, but it has a detrimental effect on most other body systems, including the respiratory system, the gastrointestinal system, and the integumentary system, as well as the patient's psychological well-being. As soon as spinal shock is over and the patient has attained hemodynamic stability, efforts should be made to mobilize the patient. Of course, spinal stability must be achieved before mobilization can be considered.

Skin Integrity
The changes in the patient's skin integrity are related not only to immobility, but also to the poor tissue perfusion after the injury. The patient may have been made to lie on a hard backboard for many hours during the initial assessment and diagnostic periods. This prolonged lying in one position in the presence of poor tissue perfusion can precipitate a disruption in skin integrity. Meticulous skin assessment and preventive skin care are initially the responsibility of the nursing staff, but ultimately they are the responsibility of every member of the team, including the patient. Certain risk factors can make the patient more prone to pressure ulcer in addition to the restriction in activity. These factors are degree of immobility, complete SCI, impaired cognitive function, urinary disease, diabetes, cigarette smoking, hypoalbuminemia, and anemia.[35] These risk factors should be noted in the patient's medical record, and increased diligence should be applied to the skin of the patient with the additional risk factors. While the patient is confined to bed, turning every 1 to 2 hours is mandatory to prevent pressure on any one area of the skin. If turning is prohibited because of instability of the injury, a specialty bed that turns the patient should be considered. Skin breakdown should be avoided at all costs in these patients. Once a decubitus ulcer develops, the patient's rehabilitation is delayed until healing starts; the wound has a high risk of infection that could delay wound healing, and the ulcer has a poor chance of healing completely because of poor blood perfusion to paralyzed areas of the body. Prevention of disruption of the skin integrity is paramount.

Gastrointestinal Function
Alterations in the gastrointestinal functioning accompany SCI. These dysfunctions include gastric dilatation, paralytic ileus, and gastrointestinal bleeding. As previously mentioned, a nasogastric tube should be placed in the emergency department to decompress the stomach. Patients are generally well nourished before the traumatic event, with an adequate nutritional store of proteins and fats.[10] The gastrointestinal system is usually in shock after the injury, so feeding the patient is not possible. If the spinal shock resolves within 3 days, enteral feeding should be started to

prevent starvation and to decrease negative nitrogen balance. Postpyloric feedings are generally better tolerated in these patients, especially if the ileus persists.[10] If the ileus is prolonged, total parenteral nutrition may be necessary until enteral feedings can be tolerated.

Elimination

A bowel program for the patient should begin within 2 days of admission. Patients with cervical SCI lose the sensation and the urge to defecate, but they may retain some reflex defecation ability. Administering glycerin suppositories, followed by digital stimulation of the internal sphincter every other day, may be all that is necessary to stimulate the rectum to empty. If this does not work, adding a laxative to the regimen, along with a stool softener, can enhance the bowel program. The goal is for the patient eventually to have a routine for defecation that can be planned for, thus preventing any accidental emptying of the bowel. Caution must be used when digital stimulation is done because this activity can cause an autonomic dysreflexic episode after spinal shock has resolved.

While the patient is in the acute phase of neurogenic shock and is receiving hemodynamic support, an indwelling Foley catheter should be in place. This catheter is removed as soon as possible because it can contribute to bladder atonicity, making later reflex emptying of the bladder more difficult.[9, 36] The goals of urologic management of the patient are to maintain a low-pressure bladder reservoir and to render the patient as free of bladder symptoms as possible.[36]

Clean intermittent catheterization (CIC) has changed the urologic management of the patient with SCI dramatically.[37] Criteria for using CIC include negative urine cultures after removal of the indwelling catheter, the patient's tolerance of a fluid restriction of 1800 to 2200 mL of fluid in a 24-hour period, and the need not to use diuretics.[9] The goal of the program is to stimulate the reflex emptying of a full bladder. The need for catheterization is based on the amount of urine obtained from each catheterization, usually done every 4 hours initially. Frequency of catheterization decreases as the bladder gains automaticity. Pharmacologic manipulation may be used as an adjunct to decrease bladder hyperactivity (anticholinergic agents) or to decrease bladder residual volume (cholinergic agents), although these drugs are used infrequently.[36] Some controversy remains over the frequency of urinary complications after the use of CIC (Chart 42–1).

Psychosocial Needs

Patients with SCI suffer a profound sense of loss. They have a real loss of physical control over themselves and their world. They have also lost the ability to be independent. Their sense of powerlessness is reinforced by their total dependence on others to care for

them and to provide for their every need. All these issues can lead to depression in the patient with SCI. During the critical care phase of the illness, little can be done to change the dependent state. A few interventions can be done to give these patients some control, even in the ICU. Care givers can include patients in planning of care and goal setting. The cognitive ability of these patients is usually unimpaired; therefore, they can participate in the cognitive decisions that need to be made. With increased understanding of the SCI and the ramifications of the injury, patients can help in designing a plan of care that will be best suited to their individual needs and desires. Contracting with these patients for goal attainment also gives them control over what will be done.

One tangible source of control for the patient is the ability to control the immediate environment, such as telephone, lights, television, and bed movement, with environmental control units.[37] These specially designed bed units are costly, but they can be important in raising the self-esteem of a patient and in providing a sense of control. These units are primarily used outside the ICU, but they may have a place in the unit as well.

Depression is another problem seen in patients with SCI. This depression can prevent the patient from becoming actively engaged in his or her care. Depression reduces the patient's energy and creates negative expectations and social withdrawal for the patient.[38] The depression may be related to forced dependency, or it may be a normal coping strategy. The nurse must be careful to individualize patient care, be consistent in approach, and be realistic in goal setting. Each patient adapts to this stressor differently.[39] The nurse should begin to work with the patient and the support systems in the ICU to enhance the adaptation process.[10] Patients are less likely to become depressed if their independence is fostered and if they are encouraged to develop new sources of self-esteem.[38]

Pain is little understood in the patient with a SCI.[8] Certain pain syndromes are associated with SCI based on the nature of the lesion, the structures damaged, and the secondary pathophysiologic changes created by the injury. Some links have been made by researchers between pain and depression in these patients. One study reported that the relationship between pain and depression is real and develops over time, and reducing the pain has a greater effect on reducing the depression more than reducing the depression has on reducing the pain.[40] Of course, in the critical care unit, the patient may be so hemodynamically unstable that treating pain with drugs that could lower respirations and blood pressure may not be possible. This creates a dilemma for the critical care nurse caring for the patient.

SCI affects not only the patient's psychological well-being, but also the patient's entire social support

Abstract: Since its introduction in the early 1970s, clean intermittent catheterization (CIC) has dramatically changed the urologic management of the neurogenic bladder. CIC is used during the acute period of spinal cord injury (SCI) to drain the bladder; it is also used during bladder retraining to determine the residual urine in the bladder, and it can be used for long-term bladder drainage. The objectives of a SCI population of 159 patients were to evaluate the overall incidence of complications of CIC and to study patients who had performed CIC for more than 2 years before discontinuance (group 1) and patients who had used CIC for more than 5 years (group 2). The reasons for the long-term CIC, the frequency of urinary tract infections, and the rates of urethral strictures were evaluated. The analysis of group 1 showed a rate of lower urinary tract infection of 28% and of asymptomatic cytobacteriologic infection of 60%. Chronic pyelonephritis was not observed, and infection was always confined to the lower urinary tract, a finding consistent with other studies. The rates of epididymitis and urethral stricture were 10 and 5.3%, respectively. Sixty-two percent of the group of patients who had performed CIC for 2 years remained incontinent of urine, and 89% of the group who had used CIC for more than 5 years showed a satisfactory degree of continence. The factors related to the acceptance of the use of long-term CIC by these patients were continence and the ability to perform the CIC independently. In the group that used CIC the longest, urethral stricture was reported 19% of the time and epididymitis, 28.5%. These two complications (urethral tolerance and urethroprostatic infection) increased with the number of years CIC was used. The authors concluded that CIC was an excellent technique to minimize urinary complications in the patient with SCI. The occurrence of the complications of urethral stricture and urethroprostatic infections remained high with long-term use of CIC. These investigators recommended finding a better technique to prevent these complications and proposed a long-term study using two groups of patients performing CIC, one group using currently available catheters and another using nonreusable hydrophilic catheters.

Critique: Although this study was done in France, a replication in the United States probably would produce similar results. Unfortunately, small subgroups of patients were used in the second part of the study (N = 8 for the group using CIC for 2 years, and N = 21 for the group using CIC > 5 years). All patients studied were male; therefore, the findings cannot be generalized to female patients with SCI. The findings do suggest, however, that despite its effectiveness, CIC poses some long-term risks, and perhaps new catheters or even new techniques are needed to prevent these complications.

Nursing Considerations: It was surprising to find little nursing research in the area of SCI. This study examined patient acceptance and the long-term effects of CIC and therefore does have an impact on nursing practice, particularly in the acute phase of care, when CIC is usually started. The study suggests that the patient's acceptance of the procedure is related to the degree of continence achieved with CIC. The group that used CIC the longest reported an 89% continence rate. The earlier CIC is started, the better the chance that the patient will be able to attain some degree of continence by using CIC. The second factor in continued use of CIC is the ability of the patient to perform the catheterization. Tetraplegics can perform CIC and should be taught early because this helps to foster early independence and acceptance of the procedure.

Because the study did not include women, it is harder to predict whether the same findings would hold true for women with SCI. Women can be taught CIC, although the techniques for women are slightly different. Continence would seem to be a motivator for women as well as for men in continuing to use CIC for a long period.

Nurses should be familiar with the CIC technique and the methods for teaching patients to perform the procedure independently. In the hospital setting, a sterile technique is used, but generally, at home, the patient uses a clean technique. This may predispose the patient to lower urinary tract infections, which can cause the patient permanent harm. As suggested by the researchers, studies should be conducted using newer catheters that may cause less harm to the patients. This area of research should be explored by nurses in both acute and rehabilitation phases of care.

CIC is used by almost all tetraplegic patients to control urinary output. Nurses need to remain abreast of all research on the use of CIC, including patient motivators related to performance and long-term use of CIC.

Source: Perrouin-Verbe B, Labat JJ, Richard I, et al: Clean intermittent catheterization from the acute period in spinal cord injury patients: long-term evaluation of urethral and genital tolerance. Paraplegia 33:619–624, 1995.

system. The family and significant others may develop an understanding of the implications of the injury at different stages than the patient. This difference disrupts normal relationships between the patient and these support systems. The family and the patient may need to find new support systems to cope effectively with this crisis. For family members to be able to assist the patient in moving toward adaptation, they must understand the problems, mobilize their social support network, and cope effectively. Only when family members have been able to adapt to the new situation will they be able to help the patient to cope effectively. The family and the patient must go through the grieving process so that adaptation can begin.

Sexual Dysfunction

The critically ill patient with a SCI is not generally focused on the sexual dysfunction that accompanies the injury, but this important aspect of care should not be ignored. Sexuality is a multifaceted health concept that integrates psychological components, personal value systems, interpersonal relationships, and personal presentation, as well as the physiologic components of sexual activities.[41] The sexuality needs of the patient should be assessed in the early phases of care. The patient will need counseling by professionals to avoid becoming an asexual being. The nurse should be aware that the patient may be worried about sexual function and should address issues that the patient may bring to the nurse's attention. Sexual counseling is usually started in the intermediate or rehabilitation phase of care.

The nurse should create a climate for honest, open communication. One model for addressing the issues of sexuality is the P–LI–SS–IT model. This model offers an interventional approach that facilitates breaking down the barriers of knowledge deficit, value conflict, and general discomfort[41] (Table 42–4). P or level I is the permission-giving level that allows the nurse to give the patient permission to voice sexual concerns. This also gives the nurse permission to refer the patient's questions to another professional. This level is usually the only part of the model approached in the ICU. LI represents level II, the limited information level. SS is the specific suggestion level (level III), and level IV is the intensive therapy level or IT.[41] The last three levels are important to the patient once rehabilitation begins.

Prevention of Complications

The patient with SCI has the potential for many complications. One major goal of the acute care of these patients is to prevent such complications. The average length of stay for the patient with SCI in the ICU is 4 days, a period that limits the nurse's contact with these patients.[42] Patients who have complicated injuries or who require more critical care may stay as long as 2.5 months.[42] The latter groups of patients are more likely to experience complications and need to be monitored closely.

Autonomic Dysreflexia

Autonomic dysreflexia, also known as autonomic hyperreflexia, is a potentially life-threatening complication of SCI. It occurs in 83 to 85% of tetraplegic patients within a few weeks or months after the injury. It accompanies any injury that interferes with the splanchnic outflow (at T5 to T8).[43] The injury interrupts the normal pathway for information from the lower part of the body to the brain. The presence of a noxious stimulus is transmitted from the periphery to the spinal cord and activates a sympathetic response. This

TABLE 42–4
P–LI–SS–IT Model for Sexual Counseling

Level		Interpretation
I	P	Permission giving: nurse allows patient to voice sexual concerns
Nurse: *You seem anxious when your girlfriend is here. Do you have concerns we have not addressed for you? Do you have questions about your future relationship?*		
II	LI	Limited information given to patient
Nurse: *You will be able to have a sexual relationship, but the way in which you engage in sexual acts will change.*		
III	SS	Specific suggestions given to patient and significant other or partner regarding sexual options
Nurse to patient and significant other: *Remember to touch your partner where he still has feeling, like stroking the face and shoulders gently and lovingly. This stroking can be stimulating to the tetraplegic patient because sensitivity to touch is heightened now.*		
IV	IT	Intensive sexual counseling (therapy) for patient and partner
Nurse: *You are both ready to discuss how the actual sexual act can be carried out. We have some films for you to watch. These films are of a tetraplegic and his partner preparing to and having sexual intercourse. I will be here and we can discuss what you see, what your feelings are, and how this will apply to you.*		

dysreflexia is not seen until after spinal shock and neurogenic shock have resolved. Although this problem is manageable, serious consequences can result if it is not handled quickly or correctly.[43, 44]

Autonomic dysreflexia may result from various stimuli, including an overdistended bladder, a distended bowel, skin breakdown, excess skin stimulation or pressure, sudden changes in the environmental temperature, infection, and pain. The exaggerated sympathetic response causes a peripheral vasoconstriction, which elevates the patient's blood pressure to extremely high levels. The blood pressure increase causes a response in the carotid baroreceptors, which triggers a vagal response in the brain stem that lowers the pulse, but has no effect on the blood pressure.[43] The patient generally complains of a sudden onset of severe headache. The nurse notes diaphoresis and flushing above the level of the lesion and coolness and pallor below the level. The hypertension may be so severe that it causes a hemorrhagic stroke.[10] The symptoms are relieved when the noxious stimulus is removed.

The key element of management of autonomic dysreflexia is prevention. The patient at risk should be placed on a bowel and bladder program as soon as possible. Skin should be protected from pressure and breakdown. Special pressure pads should be placed on the patient's chairs. Adequate nutrition should be maintained.

If the patient develops the signs and symptoms of autonomic dysreflexia, interventions are aimed at removing the triggers and avoiding serious complications.[44] The patient should be placed in the sitting position immediately to help to lower the blood pressure. The physician should be notified promptly. The nurse then begins the assessment to determine the source of the noxious stimulus and remove it if possible. If the blood pressure does not respond, the patient may require ganglionic blocking agents to disrupt the hyperreflexic state.[10] Hydralazine (Apresoline), trimethaphan (Arfonad), atropine, and diazoxide (Hyperstat) are some of the recommended agents.[44] Nifedipine (Procardia) may also be used to treat the symptoms or as a prophylactic measure.[43]

Because the patient with a SCI is managed by a multidisciplinary team, the entire team needs to be educated regarding this complication and its treatment. In addition, the patient, family members, and other care givers must also know what autonomic dysreflexia is, what triggers it, and how it is treated should it occur.

Respiratory Complications

Even after the acute phase of care, respiratory complications are common in the patient with cervical SCI. Pneumonia, atelectasis, and aspiration occur frequently in these patients. The best way to prevent these complications is to keep the patient mobilized and to limit the time spent lying or sitting in bed. When eating or being fed, the patient should be sitting up at a 90° angle. Deep breathing and incentive spirometry should also be used to prevent collapse of the alveoli.

Some patients remain ventilator dependent because of the level of the injury (C4 or above). These patients are more prone to respiratory complications than those who can breathe on their own. The incidence of continued respiratory complication is reported to be between 36 and 83% in these patients.[30] Diligent respiratory care is important to prevent pneumonia and atelectasis. For some of these patients, removal from the ventilator for periods of time may decrease the number of complications. In one study, patients with a diaphragmatic pacemaker reported a better ability to move in an electric wheelchair and better phonation. This device decreased the patients' dependency and improved their outlook as well as their satisfaction with their care.[45] Although the true incidence of respiratory complications was not reported in this study, greater mobility would appear to contribute to reduced complications.

Another respiratory complication is pulmonary embolus. Prophylactic measures, such as sequential compression devices and low-dose heparin, are moderately effective in reducing the risk of DVT. In addition to mobilizing the patient and performing range-of-motion maneuvers, some physicians are recommending the prophylactic insertion of a vena cava filter in this high-risk population.[32] This is a reasonable measure to prevent the occurrence of a potentially lethal pulmonary embolus (see Chapter 19).

Musculoskeletal Complications

Spasticity from excessive muscle tone and exaggerated reflexes occurs in all patients with SCI. The spasticity may become severe and may interfere with the rehabilitation of the patient. Spasticity occurs in a predominant pattern of flexion or extension.[22] Extensor spasticity occurs in two-thirds of these patients. It is important to control spasticity so a patient can be mobile. Pain can also occur with severe spasms, so control of spasms is important to control pain. Factors known to trigger spasm include cold temperatures, anxiety, fatigue, emotional distress, infections, fecal impaction, and decubitus ulcers.[22]

The management of spasticity involves various physical therapy techniques, such as passive range of motion, stretching exercises, the application of cold or heat to the muscles in spasm, and electrical stimulation of the muscle group. Alcohol and phenol injections have been used with some success. The use of pharmacologic agents is reserved for severe spasticity unrelieved by other therapies. Antispasmodics such as baclofen (Lioresal) and dantrolene (Dantrium) can be administered alone or in combination with the other therapeutic interventions listed earlier.

In addition to spasms, which usually diminish in magnitude after 2 years, the patient will also have muscle atrophy, fibrous changes, and muscle contractures. These changes in the muscle will inhibit mobility and may prevent bracing in a patient. The only way to limit these natural changes in a muscle that is not being used is to keep the patient as mobile as possible and to continue exercising the muscles frequently.

Heterotopic ossification (HO) represents a frequent complication of the skeletal system of the patient with SCI. This complication is seen in patients with tetraplegia and in those with paraplegia. HO is newly formed bone, which has a high rate of turnover, as seen in growing bone.[46] In SCI, the incidence of HO is 20 to 25%, with the predominate areas below the level of the injury, especially in the hips, thighs, and knees.[47] HO can begin as soon as 2 to 3 weeks after the injury. The physical findings, however, may not be present for 10 weeks after the injury. HO causes significant morbidity to the patient with SCI who is in rehabilitation. The patient is generally placed on bed rest when HO is diagnosed. This approach not only delays further rehabilitation, but it may cause other complications for the patient. The clinical diagnosis may be difficult because HO can mimic DVT, hematoma, ruptured Baker's cyst, or cellulitis.[47] At this time, little evidence suggests that any treatment is effective for HO. Keeping the patient as mobile as possible in hopes of preventing the onset of HO is the best treatment.

Gastrointestinal Complications

The patient with SCI is prone to gastrointestinal bleeding during the acute phase of the injury. One explanation for this complication is the unopposed parasympathetic influence on gastric secretions. The stimulation of the parasympathetic system increases the release of hydrogen ions and an increase in hydrochloric acid in the stomach with delayed emptying of the stomach. The use of a nasogastric tube early to drain the stomach and the addition of histamine (H_2) blockers and proton pump inhibitors can prevent the bleeding.

These are the major complications of SCI. The nurse must be attentive to the development of any complications because they will delay the patient's rehabilitation and reintegration to home. Because all body systems are affected by SCI, complications can arise in any body system in addition to those highlighted here.

Psychological Response

As the patient attempts to adapt to the loss he or she is experiencing, ongoing psychological support is needed. The SCI is truly a catastrophic event, and usual coping strategies may be ineffective or unable to be used by the patient. Constant attention is needed to the psychological needs of the patient throughout hospitalization and even after rehabilitation. Some variables that have been associated with low quality of life and unsatisfactory coping in the patient with SCI are the presence of severe, unrelieved pain, age older than 35 years at the time of the trauma, and being held blameless for the accident.[48] Support groups have been used, and, for some patients, they provide the necessary psychological outlet for the grief and anger. Other patients need individualized attention to their needs.

The family members or significant others of the patient also need support. The entire world is changing for these people, including role changes and new, unfamiliar roles. Again, support groups may be of some help. The entire process of adjustment can take many years.[22] Many families do not survive this crisis as a whole; separation and divorce are common after SCI.

The patient with SCI with complete loss of all motor and sensation can create ethical dilemmas for the health care team. How do team members uphold the ethical principles of beneficence and nonmaleficence, when they know that the patient, particularly the ventilator-dependent patient, will face a lifetime of complications from the injury? The struggles to get through the day and to become an integrated member of society may be extremely difficult physically and psychologically for the patient. How can the patient's autonomy be maintained when the patient is totally dependent on others for all care activities? These issues are indeed ethically challenging for the patient and the care giver (Chart 42–2).

Future Trends

Considerable research is being directed at better pharmacologic treatment for SCI, based on a better understanding of the pathophysiologic responses to the injury. The success of high-dose methylprednisolone in treating complete and incomplete SCI has inspired even more research into better drugs to improve the outcome from these injuries.[1, 18, 27, 49, 50] Several agents are designed to help to reduce the extent of secondary neuronal injury in animal models, and some are in human trials as well.[26]

One agent being studied for its ability to improve outcome after SCI is ganglioside GM_1 (Syngen). Gangliosides are complex acidic glycolipids present in high concentrations in the cells of the central nervous system with neuroprotective and neurofunctional restoration potential.[26]

Other agents undergoing trial in the treatment of SCI include opiate antagonists, free radical acid scavengers, calcium channel blockers, and 4-aminopyridine. Preliminary studies with animal models have been favorable for all these agents, but large clinical trials are needed to determine their effectiveness in improving patient outcomes.

> **CHART 42–2**
>
> **ETHICAL DILEMMA**

Tom was a 42-year-old executive vice president for a large manufacturing firm. He lived in New York City and was visiting the shore for the weekend. He was body surfing and suddenly hit his head on a rock. The lifeguard pulled him from the water and began cardiopulmonary resuscitation because he was not breathing. The rescue helicopter was called, and 2 hours after Tom took his first dip in the ocean, he was admitted to the level I trauma center with the tentative diagnosis of complete cervical spine injury at the level of C2. He was intubated by the paramedics at the scene and was manually ventilated until his arrival at the trauma center. On admission, he was awake and tracking with his eyes. He was blinking to questions (double blink for yes; one blink for no). He was on a backboard with cervical immobilization in place. He was placed on a ventilator immediately and had a Foley catheter inserted. Primary and secondary surveys revealed no other injuries. The patient underwent cervical spine radiographs. The films showed a complete fracture dislocation of C3 with bone visible in the spinal canal. C2 had a fracture of the odontoid process, which was also protruding into the spinal canal. Both these injuries had done tremendous damage to the spinal cord. The patient was taken to the operating room to remove the bone in the spinal canal.

Five hours after the injury, the patient was admitted to the neurotrauma ICU. The patient was unconscious from sedation and anesthesia, on a ventilator with controlled respirations, and receiving dopamine and dobutamine to be titrated to a mean systemic blood pressure of 90 mm Hg. A pulmonary artery catheter was in place, and the patient was in a halo vest. He required one-to-one nursing for the first 8 hours postoperatively.

By day 3, the patient was awake and appeared to be alert. He always tracked with his eyes and appeared to blink appropriately to yes-and-no questions. He had atelectasis thought to be caused by the aspiration of ocean water and was on a triple-antibiotic regimen. Even though his mother and eldest brother had been contacted, no family members had arrived at the trauma unit as yet. One of his significant others did come on day 2, but she stated that she could only stay a few days.

On day 3, the speech pathologist who had been working with Tom stated that he had hooked him up to a blink computer so the staff could better interact with Tom. Tom would blink at a letter, and the computer would type that letter. Tom's first typed message was surprising: "Please stop. I want to die. Don't do any more to me." The staff members were shocked at the message. They tried to talk to Tom to calm him down, but, instead, he became angry and agitated. The physician called for a psychiatric consultation, although he believed that this reaction was not necessarily inappropriate.

The psychiatrist arrived on day 4 and interviewed Tom. In his opinion, Tom was not situationally depressed, and the request was a legitimate one on Tom's behalf. It was simply that Tom did not want to be a ventilator-dependent tetraplegic. Despite the psychiatrist's comments, the staff members were still unable to grasp what Tom really meant. "He couldn't want to die."

After several more days had passed, Tom's request was becoming more adamant. He was frustrated by the medical and nursing staffs' perceived lack of compassion for him and was becoming more angry. A request was made for his brother and mother to come to the center. Tom did not have an advanced directive, so the staff would need to deal with the closest family members.

The decision was made to comply with Tom's wishes and to stop all treatment, including the ventilator. To ease his suffering, he was started on a morphine drip, which would be increased as needed to keep him comfortable. The nursing staff was divided on this issue. The nurse manager had multiple meetings to assist the staff in dealing with this ethical dilemma.

1. What are the major ethical principles that apply to this case?
2. How should the nurse manager handle the staff members' feelings?
3. Is removal from the ventilator an act of active euthanasia? Defend your answer.
4. What were the nurses' responsibilities in caring for Tom after his wishes were known?
5. Do you feel this patient was truly able to decide for himself about withdrawal of treatment? Why or why not?

In addition to new pharmacologic agents, technologies are being applied to improve the functional outcome and the quality of life for the tetraplegic patient. With the paraplegic patient, some success has been found with functional neuromuscular stimulation. The application of this therapeutic support has allowed some paraplegic patients to walk on crutches. This technology has now been applied to a group of tetraplegic patients, with exciting results.[51] In the tetraplegic patient, functional neuromuscular stimulation can provide the ability to exercise, stand, and transfer, even in the presence of medical complications and upper extremity impairment.[51] More research is needed into other technologies that can be applied to improve the quality of life of all patients with SCI.

Multidisciplinary Outcomes

The multidisciplinary team sets outcomes for the patient with SCI throughout the care continuum. These outcomes can be determined for the various phases of care (Table 42–5). The overall outcome is to reintegrate the patient to society. This goal implies that the patient will be as independent as possible and recognizes that the patient will require lifelong follow-up care.

Some studies have looked at the outcomes of patients after acute hospitalization for SCI. In one study, patients cared for at an acute SCI unit had significantly decreased lengths of stay and significant improvements in neurologic recovery compared with patients cared for in a general hospital unit.[25] The strength of an acute SCI unit is that the focus is on caring for the patients with SCI from the time of stabilization until rehabilitation. The unit uses a multidisciplinary approach from the initial assessment of the patient and during all phases of care.[25] More attention should be given to creating centers of excellence for the delivery of care to patients with SCI. Centers where physiologic, psychological, and psychosocial needs can be dealt with on a consistent basis will enhance patient outcomes.

SCI affects every physiologic system in the body, and, because of this, many patients require hospital-

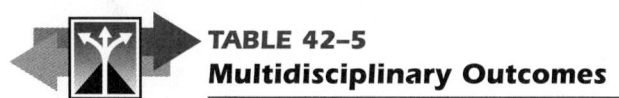

TABLE 42–5
Multidisciplinary Outcomes

Phase of Recovery	Outcome
Emergency Department	Stabilization of the vertebral column Diagnosis of injury Initiation of high-dose methylprednisolone therapy if appropriate (within 8 hours of onset of symptoms) Initiation of appropriate ventilatory support Insertion of indwelling Foley catheter Insertion of nasogastric tube Stabilization of patient for transfer to the ICU
Intensive Care Unit	Restoration of hemodynamic stability including blood pressure and fluid balance Stabilization of cardiac rate and rhythm Maintenance of normothermia Maintenance of adequate oxygenation with or without ventilatory support Initiation of active rehabilitation protocols Increased mobility Initial psychological interventions Preparation of patient for transfer to a step-down unit or rehabilitation center
Intermediate Care Unit and Rehabilitation	Prevention of deep venous thrombosis and heterotropic ossification Increased independence in activities of daily living Stable respiratory function Improvement in psychosocial functioning Education of patient, family, or significant other regarding care of patient Bladder control by intermittent catheterization Alternate-day bowel movements at a predictable time Ability to detect and treat autonomic dysreflexia Preparation for reintegration to society
Community	Prevention of complications Maintenance of adequate respiratory function and oxygenation Psychological adaptation to disability

Nurses are familiar with the acute care of the patient with spinal cord injury (SCI). However, the nurse may not be as prepared to receive and care for the patient with chronic SCI who develops an acute problem several months to several years after the acute injury. The patient with SCI can develop some unique sequelae of the SCI anytime during his or her lifetime and may require hospitalization.

Cardiovascular Sequelae: The patient with an SCI has many changes in the cardiovascular system that are seen throughout the patient's lifespan. Autonomic dysreflexia and orthostatic hypotension are two major problems these patients experience that may be significant enough to cause an admission to the ICU.

Autonomic dysreflexia or hyperreflexia, as it is also known, is an uninhibited sympathetic response to a noxious stimulus. Severely elevated blood pressure caused by the response can be life-threatening and can lead to hemorrhagic stroke or myocardial infarction. Additionally, seizures have also been documented with the onset of hypertension from autonomic dysreflexia. Because the tetraplegic patient usually is hypotensive, blood pressure of 130/80 mm Hg can be considered hypertensive.[2] The nurse should suspect autonomic dysreflexia if the systolic blood pressure is greater than 20 mm Hg above the patient's baseline.[2] According to the guidelines for autonomic dysreflexia of the American Association of Spinal Cord Injury Nurses, the first line of treatment for the high blood pressure (systolic pressure >140 mm Hg) should be to elevate the patient's head to 90° and to place the patient's legs in a dependent position if possible. In addition, 1 inch of 2% nitroglycerin above the level of injury should be applied. Pharmacologic intervention is started if the systolic blood pressure is greater than 160 mm Hg. Nifedipine (Procardia), 10 mg, should be administered every 20 to 30 minutes until blood pressure is controlled. The patient needs to be watched closely for any rebound hypotension because this can occur rapidly after any intervention for blood pressure elevation. The most important elements for the nurse to remember are that the noxious stimuli must be removed to treat the hyperreflexia appropriately and that pharmacologic interventions are only administered if the patient remains symptomatic after the problem is corrected or if the noxious stimuli cannot be controlled quickly.

A second major concern with the patient with SCI is orthostatic hypotension. This problem develops early in the patient's postinjury course and especially during mobilization. Symptomatic low blood pressure can cause syncope and loss of consciousness. Some interventions that can be used to support the blood pressure include antiembolism stockings and abdominal binders to promote the return of blood to the heart and brain, leg elevation when the patient is in bed, and adequate hydration. In addition, the patient should be monitored for anemia.

Respiratory Sequelae: The patient with a thoracic or cervical SCI is always at risk of pulmonary complications. Pulmonary deterioration can occur more rapidly in these patients, so they require vigilant monitoring of the respiratory system. Along with the patient's subjective reports of increased work of breathing, the patient should be observed for increased use of accessory neck muscles, difficulty or inability to expectorate secretions, generalized fatigue, rapid, shallow breathing with exaggerated abdominal movements, diminished or absent breath sounds, and pale or dusky color.[2] These signs indicate impending respiratory failure due to fatigue, and interventions focused on ventilation, oxygenation, and mobilization of secretions must be started quickly.

The patient with severe respiratory failure may require intubation and ventilation for a short while. The goal should be to return the patient to his or her previous respiratory status as soon as possible to prevent long-term ventilation or need for other assistive devices.

Genitourinary System Sequelae: Patients with SCI have neurogenic bladder. These patients are more likely to develop urinary tract infections (UTIs). The symptoms of fever, chills, and perhaps a change in urine color and odor should alert the nurse to a possible UTI. Additionally, the patient may demonstrate an increased spasticity in the muscles and the onset of autonomic dysreflexia in the presence of an infection. The UTI must be treated aggressively in these patients to prevent septicemia. Knowing the patient's routines for bladder care and close attention during hospitalization to those routines can prevent problems.

Musculoskeletal System Sequelae: Spasticity can occur at any time after the resolution of spinal shock. The spasm can become severe and may interfere with the patient's ability to maintain a level of independence and mobility. A spasticity manage-

CHART 42–3

BEYOND THE ICU: MANAGING THE SEQUELAE OF SPINAL CORD INJURY (CONTINUED)

ment plan that focuses on preventing or controlling the stimuli that cause the spasticity is usually initiated. At times, the spasticity requires more treatment, especially if the patient has developed a resistance to oral pharmacologic therapy with agents such as baclofen (Lioresal). An alternative invasive method for controlling refractory spasticity has been approved by the United States Food and Drug Administration.[2] This involves the continuous infusion of intrathecal baclofen through an implantable delivery system. With the pump in place, the patient should be free of spasm. The nurse must monitor the patient for signs and symptoms of drug over-

dose such as extreme drowsiness, confusion, and respiratory depression.

The most important aspect of care for the patient with SCI who is admitted to the hospital is to know the status of that patient before the hospitalization. All attempts should be made to maintain previous patterns of care, especially with regard to nutrition, bowel care, bladder care, and skin care. Illness, whether related to the SCI or caused by other problems, is extremely stressful for the patient. The goal should be to minimize the stress and to have the patient return to his or her normal patterns as quickly as possible.

---

ization for acute problems that may develop over their lifetime. Chart 42–3 discusses some of the sequelae that occur in patients with SCI and that the nurse may encounter.

Critical Thinking Exercise

A 28-year-old white man was involved in a motor vehicle crash. He is brought to the emergency room on a backboard with a neck brace in place. The vehicle had been involved in a head-on crash with a telephone pole, and the speedometer was stuck on 65 miles per hour. The driver was wearing a seat belt, and his airbag had deployed. He had only minor injuries and was taken to another local emergency department.

The passenger did not have a seat belt on and was thrown out of the car on impact when the passenger door flew open. He did have a brief (<5 minutes) loss of consciousness, but he was awake, alert, and oriented when the ambulance arrived at the scene. The patient stated that as soon as he woke up he realized that he could not move anything except his head. He complained of severe pain in his neck at the level of C5. Two intravenous lines were started at the scene, and the patient received 3 L of fluid before arrival in the emergency department. It has been less than 2 hours since the patient was injured. Significant findings on your assessment are that the patient is alert, but sleepy. He is complaining of headache and neck pain at the level of C5. His pupils are equal and react equally to light. The patient is unable to move his extremities or to shrug his shoulders. He can feel pain and pressure applied to his face and upper neck, but nothing below that. You note that his abdomen is moving up and down with each breath and he is working hard to breathe. He has no discernible chest wall movement. His temperature is 36°C, and his extremities feel cold. His blood

pressure is 84/50 mm Hg, his pulse is 42, and his respirations are 28 and labored. A pulse oximeter is applied, and the oxygen saturation is 92% on a 40% face mask. The patient is placed on a cardiac monitor, and cervical spine films and blood work, including arterial blood gases, have been ordered. Intravenous fluids have been decreased to 50 mL per hour in each intravenous line (total, 100 mL per hour). The patient remains on the backboard with the cervical collar in place.

1. At this point in the care of this patient, what is your most important concern?
2. Discuss the rationale for the interventions that have been ordered to this point, including the cardiac monitor, arterial blood gas, and the decrease in intravenous fluids.
3. It is less than 2 hours since the injury and loss of function, so high-dose methylprednisolone is ordered to be started in the emergency department. What dose would the nurse plan to administer?

The patient is transferred to the CT scanner for a CT myelogram, which shows a fracture dislocation of the C5 vertebrae, a pedicle fracture of C6, and a laminar fracture of C7. With that amount of damage to the vertebral column, this injury is determined to be unstable, and surgery is performed, including an anterior cervical fusion from C3 to T1. After surgery, the patient is transferred to the ICU for management and care.

On admission, the patient's vital signs are as follows: blood pressure, 90/50; heart rate, 40; and respirations, 24. The patient is awake and looks anxious. You are to start a dobutamine drip to maintain a mean arterial pressure of 85 mm Hg.

4. What dose of methylprednisolone are you maintaining at this point and why? When will you discontinue the methylprednisolone?

5. Describe your assessment strategy for monitoring the respiratory status of this patient. Provide rationales.
6. What drugs would you have at the bedside to treat symptomatic bradycardia in this patient?
7. Three of the major nursing diagnoses during the emergency and ICU phases of care are alteration in temperature regulation related to disruption of hypothalamic control, potential for injury related to unstable spinal cord injury and venostasis, and alteration in bowel and bladder function related to muscle paralysis and spinal shock. What are the nursing interventions related to these diagnoses during this phase of care?
8. How will the psychological concerns of this patient be handled during the critical care phase of care?

Key Concepts

⟹ SCI is the result of a trauma that causes the vertebrae to compromise the spinal cord by compression, contusion, or physiologic transection.

⟹ Secondary injuries occur after the primary injury and include petechial hemorrhages progressing to hemorrhagic necrosis, enzymatic lipid hydrolysis with lipid peroxidation, loss of calcium for the extracellular space and other electrolyte changes compatible with tissue and vascular damage, ischemia of the tissue with resultant decrease in available oxygen and a lactic acidosis, free radical release into the tissue, structural changes in the gray and white matter, and inflammation with neuronophagia.

⟹ The major mechanisms of injury are flexion (most unstable injury), flexion–rotation (usually unstable), hyperextension (most common and most stable), and axial loading (stable with burst fractures of the vertebral body).

⟹ Spinal cord syndromes occur with an incomplete or partial SCI. Central cord syndrome follows hyperextension injury and is manifested by weakness in the extremities that is greater in the upper extremities than the lower. Anterior cord syndrome is caused by compression of the anterior spinal artery and results in loss of the motor response below the level of injury with varying loss of sensation. Brown–Séquard syndrome is caused by a hemisection of the spinal cord, thus producing an ipsilateral loss of motor function and a contralateral loss of sensation.

⟹ Spinal shock occurs immediately or shortly after SCI, and the signs are a temporary loss of all function (motor, sensory, and reflexive) below the level of the injury. This includes a flaccid paralysis of the extremities and loss of bowel and bladder control.

⟹ Neurogenic shock, which occurs in patients with injury at T6 or above, is caused by a lack of sympathetic nervous system outflow. The loss of sympathetic input results in severe bradycardia, hypotension from peripheral vasodilation, loss of cardiac accelerator reflex, and loss of the ability to sweat above the level of the lesion. Neurogenic shock is a self-limiting problem and resolves within 3 to 5 days of the injury.

⟹ A history of the traumatic event helps the care givers to understand the type and extent of the injury.

⟹ Patients brought to the emergency department within 8 hours of the injury are candidates for high-dose methylprednisolone therapy. If patients present within 3 hours of the injury, the loading dose of 30 mg/kg is given in a bolus over 15 minutes followed by 23 hours of 5.4 mg/kg methylprednisolone per hour in an intravenous infusion.

⟹ If the patient presents between 3 hours and 8 hours of the onset of symptoms, the loading dose is given as above, followed by 5.4 mg/kg per hour for 48 hours.

⟹ The important components of the neurologic assessment in SCI are the motor and sensory evaluations done hourly and compared with previous assessments.

⟹ Patients with SCI must be kept immobile until spinal cord stability is established.

⟹ All body systems are affected by SCI, so all body functions must be supported when caring for these patients.

⟹ Cardiovascular support consists of cardiac and hemodynamic monitoring for the first 72 hours after the injury, inotropic drug support for the hypotension and low pulmonary artery occlusion pressures, treatment of symptomatic bradycardia, monitoring for cardiac dysrhythmia and left ventricular function, and prevention of pulmonary emboli from DVT.

⟹ Respiratory support includes frequent assessment of the work of breathing and oxygenation and intubation, if necessary, to support respiratory status.

⟹ Gastrointestinal support includes placement of a nasogastric tube to prevent vomiting, gastric distention, aspiration, and early nutrition.

⟹ Indwelling catheterization of the bladder for the time of inotropic support is critical, followed by the removal of the catheter and CIC to retrain the bladder for automatic emptying.

⟹ Support of bowel emptying should start on day 1 of hospitalization, to prevent distention of the bowel. Stool softeners, laxatives, and suppositories with rectal stimulation should be given on a routine, consistent schedule to assist the patient in gaining control of rectal emptying.

One model for addressing sexuality issues for the patient with SCI is the P–LI–SS–IT model. P is the permission-giving level for permission for the patient to voice concerns about sexuality and sexual activity. This is usually the only part of the model addressed in the ICU. LI is the limited information level. SS is the specific suggestion level, and IT represents the intensive therapy level.

Autonomic dysreflexia (hyperreflexia) is a complication of SCI that occurs in patients with injury above T6. This syndrome is potentially life-threatening and is triggered by noxious stimuli including an overdistended bladder, a distended bowel, skin breakdown and infection, excessive skin stimulation, sudden changes in environmental temperatures, and pain.

Hyperreflexia is manifested by extreme hypertension (systolic blood pressure > 20 mm Hg above baseline), severe headache, and diaphoresis and flushing above the level of the injury and pallor below. The treatment is focused on removing the stimulus causing the event and treating the blood pressure if it remains elevated despite removal of the stimulus.

Pain in the patient with SCI presents a challenge to care givers. Certain pain syndromes are seen in patients with SCI. The method chosen to treat the pain can have secondary consequences in these patients.

Patients with SCI suffer a profound sense of loss and body image disturbance. These psychological responses can lead to severe depression in these patients. Fostering independence is one therapeutic intervention that appears to minimize depression.

All aspects of the tetraplegic patient's life are affected by the SCI, as are the lives of his or her family and significant others.

Future therapies are aimed at stopping the spinal cord tissue damage after injury, inducing axonal regeneration, and improving motor outcome.

References

1. Bracken MB: Pharmacological treatment of acute spinal cord injury: Current status and future projects. J Emerg Med 11:43–48, 1993.
2. Wirtz KM, LaFavor KM, Ang R: Managing chronic spinal cord injury: issues in critical care. Crit Care Nurse 16:24–35, 1996.
3. Anderson DK, Hall ED: Pathophysiology of spinal cord injury. Ann Emerg Med 22:48–53, 1993.
4. Runge JW: The cost of injury. Emerg Med Clin North Am 11:241–253, 1993.
5. Spoltore TA, O'Brien AM: Rehabilitation of the spinal cord injured patient. Orthop Nurs 14:7–14, 1995.
6. Berkowitz M: Assessing the socioeconomic impact of improved treatment of head and spinal cord injuries. J Emerg Med 11:63–67, 1993.
7. Waters RL, Adkins RH: Firearm versus motor vehicle related spinal cord injury: preinjury factors, injury characteristics, and initial outcome comparison among ethnically diverse groups. Arch Phys Med Rehabil 78:150–155, 1997.
8. Yezierski RP: Pain following spinal cord injury: the clinical problem and experimental studies. Pain 68:85–94, 1996.
9. Walleck Jastremski C: Patients with spinal cord injury. In: Clochesy JM, Breu C, Cardin S, et al (eds): Critical Care Nursing, 2nd ed. Philadelphia, W.B. Saunders, 1996, pp 812–830.
10. Walleck C: Neurotrauma: spinal cord injury. In: Barker E (ed): Neuroscience Nursing. Philadelphia, C.V. Mosby, 1994, pp 352–375.
11. Atkinson PP, Atkinson JLD: Spinal shock. Mayo Clin Proc 71:384–390, 1996.
12. Ditunno JF Jr, Graziani V, Tessler A: Neurological assessment in spinal cord injury. Adv Neurol 72:325–333, 1997.
13. Young W: Secondary injury mechanisms in acute spinal cord injury. J Emerg Med 11:13–22, 1993.
14. El Masry WS, Tsubo M, Katoh S, et al: Validation of the American Spinal Injury Association (ASIA) motor score and the National Acute Spinal Cord Injury Study (NASCIS) motor score. Spine 21:614–619, 1996.
15. Fehlings MG, Lounm D: Initial stabilization and medical management of acute spinal cord injury. Am Fam Physician 54:155–162, 1996.
16. Davis SJ, Khangure MS: A review of magnetic resonance imaging in spinal trauma. Australas Radiol 38:241–253, 1994.
17. Curt A, Dietz V: Ambulatory capacity in spinal cord injury: significance of somatosensory evoked potentials and ASIA protocol in predicting outcome. Arch Phys Med Rehabil 78:39–43, 1997.
18. Bracken MB, Shepard MJ, Collins WF, et al: A randomized controlled trial of methylprednisolone or naloxone in the treatment of acute spinal cord injury: results of the second national acute spinal cord injury study. N Engl J Med 322:1405–1411, 1990.
19. Ducker TB, Zeidman SM: Spinal cord injury; role of steroid therapy. Spine 19:2281–2287, 1994.
20. Faden AI: Pharmacological treatment of central nervous system trauma. Pharmacol Toxicol 78:12–17, 1996.
21. Faden AI: Therapeutic approaches to spinal cord injury. Adv Neurol 72:377–386, 1997.
22. Hickey JV: The Clinical Practice of Neurological and Neurosurgical Nursing, 4th ed. Philadelphia, Lippincott–Raven, 1997, pp 419–465.
23. Hilton G, Frei J: High-dose methylprednisolone in the treatment of spinal cord injuries. Heart Lung 20:675–680, 1991.
24. McBride DQ, Rodts GE: Intensive care of patients with spinal trauma. Neurosurg Clin North Am 5:755–766, 1995.
25. Tator CH, Duncan EG, Edmonds VE, et al: Neurological recovery, mortality, and length of stay after acute spinal cord injury associated with changes in management. Paraplegia 33:254–263, 1995.
26. Zeidman SM, Ling GS-F, Ducker TB, et al: Clinical applications of pharmacologic therapies for spinal cord injury. J Spinal Disord 9:367–380, 1996.
27. Bracken MB, Shepard MJ, Holford TR, et al: Administration of methylprednisolone for 24 or 48 hours or tirilazad mesylate for 48 hours in the treatment of acute spinal cord injury: results of the third National Acute Spinal Cord Injury randomized controlled trial. JAMA 277:1575–1604, 1997.
28. Levy ML, Gans W, Wijesinghe HS, et al: Use of methylprednisolone as an adjunct in the management of patients with penetrating spinal cord injury: outcomes analysis. Neurosurgery 39:1141–1149, 1996.
29. Schnee CL, Ansell LV: Selection criteria and outcome of operative approaches for thoracolumbar burst fractures with and without neurologic deficit. J Neurosurg 86:48–55, 1997.
30. Lemons VR, Wagner FC Jr: Respiratory complications after cervical spinal cord injury. Spine 19:2315–2320, 1994.
31. Voelker KG, Chetty KG, Mahutte CK: Resolution of recurrent atelectasis in spinal cord injury patients with administration of re-

combinant human DNAse. Intensive Care Med 22:582–584, 1996.

32. Wilson JT, Rogers FB, Wald SL, et al: Prophylactic vena cava filter insertion in patients with traumatic spinal cord injury: preliminary results. Neurosurgery 35:234–239, 1994.

33. Kim SW, Charallel JT, Park LW, et al: Prevalence of deep vein thrombosis in patients with chronic spinal cord injury. Arch Phys Med Rehabil 75:965–968, 1994.

34. Bright LD, Georgi S: How to protect your patient from DVT. Am J Nurs 94:28–32, 1994.

35. Salzberg CA, Byrne DW, Cayten CG, et al: A new pressure ulcer risk assessment scale for individuals with spinal cord injury. Am J Phys Med Rehabil 75:96–104, 1996.

36. Nygaard IE, Kreder KJ: Spine update: urological management in patients with spinal cord injury. Spine 21:128–132, 1996.

37. Holme SA, Kanny EM, Guthrie MR, et al: The use of environmental control units by occupational therapists in spinal cord injury and disease services. Am J Occup Ther 51:42–48, 1997.

38. Boekamp JR, Overholser JC, Schubert DS: Depression following spinal cord injury. Int J Psychiatry Med 26:329–349, 1996.

39. Rintala DH, Young ME, Spencer JC, et al: Family relationships and adaptation to spinal cord injury: a qualitative study. Rehabil Nurs 21:67–74, 1996.

40. Carins DM, Adkins RH, Scott MD: Pain and depression in acute traumatic spinal cord injury: origins of chronic problematic pain? Arch Phys Med Rehabil 77:329–335, 1996.

41. Hodge AL: Addressing issues of sexuality with spinal cord injured persons. Orthop Nurs 14:21–24, 1995.

42. Richmond TS, Metcalf J, Daly M: Requirements for nursing care services and associated costs in acute spinal cord injury. J Neurosci Nurs 27:47–52, 1995.

43. Adsit PA, Bishop C: Autonomic dysreflexia: don't let it be a surprise. Orthop Nurs 14:17–20, 1995.

44. Pinder PM: Protocols constructed around the nursing process. 3. Autonomic dysreflexia. College Health 43:229–230, 1995.

45. Esclarin A, Bravo A, Arroya D, et al: Tracheostomy ventilation versus diaphragmatic pacemaker ventilation in high spinal cord injury. Paraplegia 32:687–693, 1994.

46. Chantraine A, Nusgens B, Lapiere CM: Biochemical analysis of heterotopic ossification in spinal cord injury patients. Paraplegia 33:398–401, 1995.

47. Mysiw WJ, Tan J, Jackson RD: Heterotopic ossification: the utility of osteocalcin in diagnosis and management. Am J Phys Med Rehabil 72:184–187, 1993.

48. Stensman R: Adjustment to traumatic spinal cord injury: a longitudinal study of self-reported quality of life. Paraplegia 32:416–422, 1994.

49. Katoh S, El Masry WS, Jaffrey D, et al: Neurologic outcome in conservatively treated patients with incomplete closed traumatic cervical spinal cord injuries. Spine 21:345–351, 1996.

50. Merry WH, Cogbill TH, Annis BL, et al: Functional outcome after incomplete spinal cord injuries due to blunt injury. Injury 27:17–20, 1996.

51. Triolo RJ, Biari C, Uhlir J, et al: Implantable functional neuromuscular stimulation systems for individuals with cervical spinal cord injuries: clinical case reports. Arch Phys Med Rehabil 77:1119–1128, 1996.

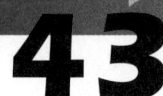

Guillain–Barré Syndrome

Lisa Plowfield

Objectives

After completing this chapter, the student will be able to:

1. Understand the pathophysiology of Guillain–Barré syndrome (GBS).
2. Describe the presenting signs and symptoms of GBS.
3. Identify the diagnostic evaluation of the patient with GBS.
4. Select nursing interventions appropriate for the patient and family during the acute phase of GBS.
5. Compare and contrast current modalities used to treat GBS.
6. Evaluate the effectiveness of the prescribed plan of care for the patient with GBS.

GBS is considered an autoimmune disease that affects 3000 to 4000 Americans a year, with a worldwide incidence of 1.0 to 1.5 cases per 100,000 persons a year.[1, 2] Not all mechanisms of the disease are known; the syndrome, however, has a classic presentation and progression and is self-limiting. Synonyms for GBS include acute inflammatory polyneuropathy and acute inflammatory demyelinating polyradiculoneuropathy.

ETIOLOGY AND PATHOPHYSIOLOGY

GBS usually presents as a bilateral ascending flaccid paralysis accompanied by areflexia and hypotonia. Some persons report sensory impairment and pain as well. The pattern of symmetric flaccid paralysis that appears in a toe-to-head progression is a result of an inflammatory demyelination of the peripheral nerves. The demyelination is thought to result from an autoimmune response to peripheral nerve antigens.[3] The immune mechanisms involved include humoral and cell-mediated responses, but the triggering mechanism has not been identified.[1]

The axons of the peripheral nervous system are covered with myelin, which is interrupted by nodes of Ranvier. The myelin insulation and the nodes of Ranvier allow for rapid impulse conduction. In GBS, the immune system identifies the myelin as non-self and attempts to destroy it. Demyelination results in impaired nerve impulse conduction. This process slows, distorts, and may stop impulse transmission. The immune attack on the myelin causes inflammation and edema, which further impair nerve conduction.

Once the ascending progression ends, demyelination stops. The process of demyelination may end at any point, or it may extend to involve all extremities, the autonomic nervous system, and the cranial nerves. After demyelination, remyelination and recovery occur slowly. If the axon has been damaged during the period of demyelination, permanent deficits may result. Symptoms usually progress for up to 2 weeks after the onset; this progression is usually followed by a plateau phase of 1 to 4 weeks.[4] Return of function usually begins after the plateau phase.

GBS may be preceded by a nonspecific viral infection, often respiratory or gastrointestinal. This syndrome has also been associated with *Campylobacter jejuni* and *Mycoplasma pneumoniae* infections, cytomegalovirus, the Epstein–Barr virus, and the human immunodeficiency virus (HIV). Some cases of GBS have also been identified after administration of vaccines, surgery, streptokinase therapy, herpes zoster and herpes simplex infections, and hepatitis B and during pregnancy.[3,5]

Assessment

The assessment process includes a health history specific to the known preceding factors. The assessment should involve a health history, which includes identification of any progression of symptoms. The nurse should also assess the patient's respiratory and neuromuscular function and sensation. A complete assessment can help to distinguish GBS from various neurologic diseases and variants of GBS.

Health History

Significant history related to GBS includes a recent viral infection and any significant history of immune dysfunction. If HIV serostatus is unknown, the nurse should assess the patient for HIV risk factors. Recent life stressors that may affect immune function also need to be investigated. The history of present illness should include a detailed description of the onset and progression of symptoms. If these elements are not noted by the patient, the nurse should question symmetry of symptoms, sensory symptoms, and respiratory function.

Signs and Symptoms

GBS usually presents with neuromuscular symptoms of weakness and tingling sensations and reports of having difficulty in accomplishing tasks that require physical activity. Some patients, however, may overlook symptoms until the respiratory system has become involved.

Clinical Presentation

The physical assessment should include an evaluation of neurologic function, noting the pattern of motor function and any sensory involvement. Cranial nerve assessment should help to identify impairment of motor and sensory functions as well. The motor functions of the cranial nerves are affected in GBS; most commonly affected are CN IX (glossopharyngeal), CN X (vagus), CN VII (facial), CN III (oculomotor), CN VI (abducens), and CN IV (trochlear) (Table 43–1). Gait should be assessed, noting any ataxia. Assessment of respiratory function includes noting any use of accessory muscles and the presence of shallow, tachypneic respirations. The ability to cough and a positive gag reflex should be assessed.

As GBS progresses, involvement of the autonomic nervous system may result in tachydysrhythmias, blood pressure instability, gastrointestinal dysfunction, sweating, and flushing.[3] Vital signs should be assessed for abnormalities of heart rate and blood pressure. Postural blood pressure should be assessed. If the patient is unable to stand, a two-position (seated and lying) assessment may be done.

If the patient first presents with an acute onset that has already affected respiratory function, ability to cough, or swallowing, respiratory monitoring needs to occur during the assessment to avoid respiratory arrest. When the patient is unable to answer assessment questions, the family should be asked to provide the health history and to detail the onset and progression of symptoms.

Laboratory and Diagnostic Tests

The diagnosis of GBS is usually determined by ruling out other neurologic, psychologic, and immunologic causes of impairment. The diagnostic evaluation specific to GBS includes a lumbar puncture with cerebrospinal fluid (CSF) examination, nerve conduction studies, and pulmonary function tests.

Lumbar Puncture

A lumbar puncture is performed to examine the CSF. After the first week of symptoms, an elevated concentration of protein in the absence of few or no cells is highly characteristic of GBS.[1] CSF may also be examined for lymphocyte counts. The presence of lymphocytes in the CSF is not characteristic of GBS, but it is common in clients with HIV infection.

Nerve Conduction Studies

Electromyography is used to record the electrical activity of skeletal muscles. Nerve conduction velocities document the excitability of motor and sensory nerves. Needle electrodes are used to deliver an electrical impulse and to innervate a muscle. The conduction of the impulse can be timed to determine any delay or absence of nerve impulse transmission.[6] These studies are used to determine the presence of demyelination and its severity.

Pulmonary Function Tests

With disease progression, pulmonary function may be affected. Vital capacity, tidal volumes, and inspiratory effort are monitored frequently to determine the patient's need for mechanical ventilation. When vital capacity falls below 15 to 20 mL/kg or the inspiratory effort is less than −25 cm H_2O, the patient is at great risk of respiratory failure.[1]

TABLE 43–1
Cranial Nerves Commonly Affected in Guillain–Barré Syndrome

Cranial Nerve	Motor Function
CN III Oculomotor	Elevation of eyelids
	Extraocular movement
CN IV Trochlear	Extraocular movement (downward and inward)
CN VI Abducens	Extraocular movement (outward)
CN VII Facial	Facial expressions
CN IX Glossopharyngeal	Swallowing
CN X Vagus	Swallowing, gag reflex

TABLE 43–2
Nursing Diagnoses

Problem Statement	Etiologic Factors
Ineffective airway clearance	Respiratory muscle impairment secondary to demyelination
Ineffective breathing patterns	Respiratory muscle impairment secondary to demyelination
Impaired physical mobility	Demyelination process
High risk for decreased cardiac output	Autonomic dysfunction
Sensory perceptual alterations (varies for each person)	Demyelination
Altered nutrition, less than body requirements	Swallowing dysfunction, autonomic dysfunction
High risk for aspiration	Loss of gag and swallowing reflexes
Pain (varies for each person)	Demyelination
Anxiety or fear	Sudden hospitalization, rare disease, unpredictable course
Powerlessness	Immobility, autonomic dysfunction
Knowledge deficit, learning need	Disease and recovery process, treatment strategies
Risk for ineffective family coping	Sudden and critical illness of a family member, change in family roles
High risk for impaired skin integrity	Immobility

Nursing Diagnoses

Once a patient has a tentative diagnosis of GBS with continued progression, respiratory function is imperative to monitor. Monitoring may initially occur in a medical–surgical unit. As soon as respiratory compromise is detected, the patient is usually transferred to the intensive care unit (ICU) for care. The care of patients with GBS presents a challenge and requires rigorous management to avoid complications and permanent disability. Some of the common nursing diagnoses appropriate for the patient with GBS who requires critical care hospitalization are presented in Table 43–2. Other diagnoses may be used, based on the individual patient's and family's experience with GBS.

Collaborative Management

Because the patient with an acute onset and severe case of GBS may have quadriplegia with autonomic dysfunction while remaining alert and oriented but unable to communicate, the management of the patient with GBS requires multidisciplinary care. The patient's management extends across the continuum of care from the critical care unit to medical–surgical units to rehabilitation centers and on into home care. The overall goal of care is to provide support during the acute phase of illness, so that the patient remains in the best possible condition for remyelination to occur.[7] In addition to supportive care, some immunologic therapies may be instituted to lessen the severity and to attempt to halt any further progression of GBS. Figure 43–1 is an example of a care map that guides the collaborative care of patients with GBS while in the ICU.

Respiratory Management

As noted previously, the GBS patient who is hospitalized in the ICU has a particularly severe case of GBS and requires mechanical ventilation for respiratory support. Fewer than thirty percent of patients with GBS require mechanical ventilation.[8] Intubation and mechanical ventilation should be initiated when respiratory monitoring indicates that the patient is at great risk of respiratory failure (Chart 43–1). Proactive support helps to eliminate complications that may arise from instituting support after the crisis of respiratory arrest.[1] If the need for mechanical ventilation persists beyond 7 to 10 days, a tracheostomy is indicated for long-term support. Arterial blood gases are used to monitor respiratory function while the patient is receiving ventilatory support.

Some patients with GBS have reported sensations of drowning in their secretions; frequent suctioning may help to alleviate some of these sensations. Suctioning may also result in a vasovagal response that can result in profound bradycardia.[4] Oxygenation with 100% before and immediately after all suctioning may help to alleviate some of this response[9] (Chart 43–2). Patients with severe cases of bradycardia may, however, require insertion of a temporary pacemaker.[1,4] Pulmonary hygiene is a function of a team of health care providers including the nurse, respiratory and physical therapists, and physicians. Usually, the nurse who is at the bedside most consistently is able to coordinate the respiratory care of the critically ill patient.

Once the patient's symptoms have reached a plateau and the patient begins to support his or her own respiratory function, weaning from the ventilator may begin. Weaning usually occurs in the critical care unit or the intermediate care unit. When a patient's vital capacity is greater than 15 mL/kg, weaning should be considered. Additional factors are involved in the decision to wean the patient from the ventilator; these include

Text continued on page 908

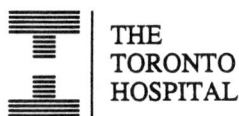

THE
TORONTO
HOSPITAL

CARE MAP

Care Map No.: NS053
Case Type: GUILLAIN-BARRE SYNDROME (ICU) PLATEAU PHASE
Physician: Length of Stay: 4 weeks
Page 1 of 8   Nursing Unit:

Date Admitted:
Date Developed: December 18, 1991
Revision Date: March 17, 1992
Developed By: Dr. V. Brill, Dr. P. Houstan,
B. Reid, I. Hart, A. Leavens, K. Davison, V. Boyer, R. Batson,
A. Potts, B. Thomas, T. Kelleher, S. Bisaillon, M. Hall, L. Roy,
A. Saliba, E. Green, R. Lascelle, B.A. Sjaarda, A. Hall, N.
Neary, E. Shaul, P. Mann, J. Marr

Patient Problem	Day 1	Day 2	Day 3	Day 4	Day 5	Day 6	Day 7
Date:							
1. Respiratory insufficiency R/T ascending paralysis	Patient weaned from ventilator and able to maintain adequate respiratory function spontaneously	>	>	>	>	>	>
2. Fear/anxiety R/T ascending weakness and loss of control	Communicates awareness of progress	>	>	>	>	>	>
	Communicates decreased feelings of fear and anxiety	>	>	>	>	>	>
3. (a) Impaired mobility R/T decreased strength and function (b) Activity intolerance R/T decreased strength and function	Patient communicates some understanding of disease progression	>	>	>	>	>	>
4. Impaired communication	Patient communicates via more extensive system or is extubated	>	>	>	>	>	>
5. Cardiac arrhythmias and altered BP R/T autonomic instability	Patient maintains adequate BP-no episodes of syncope	>	>	>	>	>	>
	Pulse rate & rhythm WNL for patient	>	>	>	>	>	>
6. (a) Alteration in comfort (pain, paresthesias) (b) Sensory deficit uncompensated (paresthesias)	Patient reports any increase in discomfort	>	>	>	>	>	>
7. Alterations in skin/nerve integrity	Skin/nerves (ulnar, peroneal) free from pressure damage	>	>	>	>	>	>
8. Potential for malnutrition and dehydration	Patient's intake remains WNL for height and weight	>	>	>	>	>	>
9. Depression R/T progression of disease and slow recovery rate	Understands nature of phases of disease and recovery period						
10. Emotional lability R/T body image disturbance, progression of disease and length of recovery							
Signature N							
/Position D							
E							

Figure 43–1

An example of a care map for a patient with Guillain–Barré syndrome in the intensive care unit. Please note that pages 5 to 8 (covering days 15 through 28) repeat the information shown on pages 3 and 4 and are not included here. (Courtesy of the Toronto Hospital, Toronto, Canada.)

Case Type: GUILLAIN-BARRE SYNDROME (ICU) PLATEAU PHASE
Page 2 of 8

Critical Path	Day 1	Day 2	Day 3	Day 4	Day 5	Day 6	Day 7
Date:							
1. Consults	Neurology (on admin)	>					
	Physio	>					
	O.T.	>					
	Dietician as indicated	>	>	>	>	>	>
	Speech as indicated	>	>	>	>	>	>
	Social Work as indicated	>	>	>	>	>	>
	Chaplaincy prn	>	>	>	>	>	>
	Pain Clinic (optional)	>	>	>	>	>	>
	E.N.T. (optional)	>	>	>	>	>	>
	Swallowing Team (1 week post trach. & before enteral feeds)	>	>	>	>	>	>
2. Tests	Weight Q Wed.	>	>	>	>	>	>
	V.C./N.I.F.	>	>	>	>	>	>
	EMG, NCS, L.P	>	>	>	>	>	>
	Blood Work - CBC, ESR, LYTES, ABG's, PT/PTT, mono spot, LFT'S, Renal F'n, as ordered.	>	>	>	>	>	>
	Immunoelectrophoresis	>	>	>	>	>	>
	HIV with verbal consent of Pt/Family	>	>	>	>	>	>
	GBS Neuro Assessment weekly	>	>	>	>	>	>
3. Treatments	Plasmapheresis or gammaglobulin (TG)	>	>	>	>	>	>
	Physio-(Resp. & mobility program)	>	>	>	>	>	>
	Splints, Velfoam for skin & nerves	>	>	>	>	>	>
	AES for ↓BP	>	>	>	>	>	>
	Mechanical Ventilation	>	>	>	>	>	>
	Turning & neutral body alignment, skin care, eye care, & mouth care	>	>	>	>	>	>
	Foam/air mattress on admission, heel cups, bed cradle	>	>	>	>	>	>
4. Medications	Heparin/Coumadin as ordered	>	>	>	>	>	>
	Analgesic as ordered	>	>	>	>	>	>
	Antihyper/hypotensives as ordered	>	>	>	>	>	>
	Bowel routine	>	>	>	>	>	>
5. Diet	D/C enteral feeds per Silastic tube Clear fluids to soft DAT when trached after swallowing assessment	>	>	>	>	>	>
6. Activity	Sit in bed, up in tilt chair, walking as tolerated	>	>	>	>	>	>
	Written, posted schedule of care (by nursing) to include all services	>	>	>	>	>	>
7. Teaching	Start to discuss plans to transfer to unit	>	>	>	>	>	>
	Patient/Family teaching re: course of disease & treatment modalities as indicated (see GBS pamphlet & booklet)	>	>	>	>	>	>
	Inform family of GBS Society (see GBS pamphlet)	>	>	>	>	>	>
8. Discharge Planning	Patient/Family conference as required	>	>	>	>	>	>
Signature N							
/Position D							
E							

Figure 43–1 *Continued*

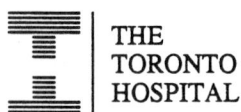

THE
TORONTO
HOSPITAL

CARE MAP

Care Map No.: NS053
Case Type: GUILLAIN-BARRE SYNDROME (ICU) PLATEAU PHASE
Physician: Length of Stay: 4 weeks
Page 3 of 8   Nursing Unit:

Date Admitted:
Date Developed: December 18, 1991
Revision Date: March 17, 1992

Patient Problem	Day 8	Day 9	Day 10	Day 11	Day 12	Day 13	Day 14
Date:							
1. Respiratory insufficiency R/T ascending paralysis	Patient weaned from ventilator and able to maintain adequate respiratory function spontaneously	>	>	>	>	>	>
2. Fear/anxiety R/T ascending weakness and loss of control	Communicates awareness of progress	>	>	>	>	>	>
	Communicates decreased feelings of fear and anxiety	>	>	>	>	>	>
3. (a) Impaired mobility R/T decreased strength and function (b) Activity intolerance R/T decreased strength and function	Patient communicates some understanding of disease progression	>	>	>	>	>	>
4. Impaired communication	Patient communicates via more extensive system or is extubated	>	>	>	>	>	>
5. Cardiac arrhythmias and altered BP R/T autonomic instability	Patient maintains adequate BP- no episodes of syncope	>	>	>	>	>	>
	Pulse rate & rhythm WNL for patient	>	>	>	>	>	>
6. (a) Alteration in comfort (pain, parethesias) (b) Sensory deficit uncompensated (parethesias)	Patient reports any increase in discomfort	>	>	>	>	>	>
7. Alterations in skin/nerve integrity	Skin/nerves (ulnar, peroneal) free from pressure damage	>	>	>	>	>	>
8. Potential for malnutrition and dehydration	Patient's intake remains WNL for height and weight	>	>	>	>	>	>
9. Depression R/T progression of disease and slow recovery rate	Understands nature of phases of disease and recovery period						
10. Emotional lability R/T body image disturbance, progression of disease and length of recovery							
Signature N							
/Position D							
E							

Figure 43–1 *Continued*

Case Type: GUILLAIN-BARRE SYNDROME (ICU) PLATEAU PHASE
Page 4 of 8

Critical Path	Day 8	Day 9	Day 10	Day 11	Day 12	Day 13	Day 14
Date:							
1. Consults	Neurology (on·admin)	>					
	Physio	>					
	O.T.	>					
	Dietician as indicated	>	>	>	>	>	>
	Speech as indicated	>	>	>	>	>	>
	Social Work as indicated	>	>	>	>	>	>
	Chaplaincy prn	>	>	>	>	>	>
	Pain Clinic (optional)	>	>	>	>	>	>
	E.N.T. (optional)	>	>	>	>	>	>
	Swallowing Team (1week post trach. & before enteral feeds)	>	>	>	>	>	>
2. Tests	Weight Q Wed.	>	>	>	>	>	>
	V.C./N.I.F.	>	>	>	>	>	>
	EMG, NCS, L.P	>	>	>	>	>	>
	Blood Work - CBC, ESR, LYTES, ABG's, PT/PTT,	>	>	>	>	>	>
	mono spot, LFT'S, Renal F'n, as ordered.	>	>	>	>	>	>
	Immunoelectrophoresis	>	>	>	>	>	>
	HIV with verbal consent of Pt/Family	>	>	>	>	>	>
	GBS Neuro Assessment weekly	>	>	>	>	>	>
3. Treatments	Plasmapheresis or gammaglobulin (TG)	>	>	>	>	>	>
	Physio-(Resp. & mobility program)	>	>	>	>	>	>
	Splints, Velfoam for skin & nerves	>	>	>	>	>	>
	AES for ↓BP	>	>	>	>	>	>
	Mechanical Ventilation	>	>	>	>	>	>
	Turning & neutral body alignment, skin care, eye care, & mouth care	>	>	>	>	>	>
	Foam/air mattress on admission, heel cups, bed cradle	>	>	>	>	>	>
4. Medications	Heparin/Coumadin as ordered	>	>	>	>	>	>
	Analgesic as ordered	>	>	>	>	>	>
	Antihyper/hypotensives as ordered	>	>	>	>	>	>
	Bowel routine	>	>	>	>	>	>
5. Diet	Clear fluids to soft DAT when trached after swallowing assessment	>	>	>	>	>	>
6. Activity	Sit in bed, up in tilt chair, walking as tolerated	>	>	>	>	>	>
	Written, posted schedule of care (by nursing) to include all services	>	>	>	>	>	>
7. Teaching	Start to discuss plans to transfer to unit	>	>	>	>	>	>
	Patient/Family teaching re: course of disease & treatment modalities as indicated (see GBS pamphlet & booklet)	>	>	>	>		>
	Inform family of GBS Society (see GBS pamphlet)	>	>	>	>	>	>
8. Discharge Planning	Patient/Family conference as required	>	>	>	>	>	>
Signature N							
/Position D							
E							

Figure 43–1 *Continued*

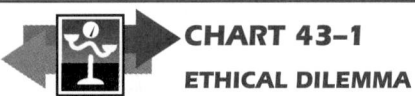

CHART 43–1

ETHICAL DILEMMA

Mr. J. is a 46-year-old dentist who has been HIV positive for 8 years. A year ago, he had his first case of Pneumocystis carinii pneumonia. After the onset of AIDS, he wrote and signed an advance directive that states his desire to not be placed on mechanical ventilation for life support. He presented to the emergency department with numbness, tingling, and decreased strength and reflexes of the lower extremities. Within 2 hours of his admission, he was unable to move his legs. His lumbar puncture was significant for increased protein in the cerebrospinal fluid. On neurologic consultation, a tentative diagnosis of Guillain–Barré syndrome was made. As his vital capacity begins to decrease, it becomes evident that he will require mechanical ventilation for respiratory support during the acute onset of Guillain–Barré syndrome.

1. Knowing that some cases of Guillain–Barré syndrome are brief and require only temporary ventilatory support, what is your role as a nurse in discussing with Mr. J. his need for mechanical ventilation?
2. How does the patient's positive HIV status influence the decision-making process?
3. Who should be involved in the decision to place Mr. J. on a ventilator?
4. What beliefs do you, the nurse for Mr. J., have that could influence your desire to have him placed on the ventilator? Or not placed on the ventilator?

infection, anemia, electrolyte disturbances, fatigue, and past history of chronic lung disease.

Autonomic Nervous System Management

Two-thirds to three-quarters of patients with GBS have autonomic nervous system involvement.[1, 2] Common symptoms of autonomic dysfunction are listed in Table 43–3. Continuous cardiac monitoring and frequent blood pressure monitoring are used to detect autonomic nervous system involvement of the cardiac system. Tachydysrhythmias have been noted in patients with GBS. Ventricular ectopy and atrioventricular conduction blocks have also been reported, but they are less common.[10] Cardiovascular autonomic dysfunction is difficult to manage and requires continuous monitoring because changes can occur within

seconds, and patients may be labile as a result of the demyelination.[1]

Labile blood pressure is common over short periods. If hypotension persists, volume expanders are usually the treatment of choice because the patient's response to vasopressors tends to be unpredictable as a result of the autonomic neuropathy.[8] Volume expansion, however, must be monitored closely because the patient with autonomic dysfunction may not be able to adjust cardiac output appropriately.[1] As noted earlier, bradycardia may require temporary pacing. Atropine, which is used effectively in many patients, may not be therapeutic because some patients with GBS fluctuate between bradycardia and tachycardia.[1] The cardiac response to medications may be unpredictable and potentially life-threatening. For patients who are highly unstable, use of a pulmonary artery catheter is usually indicated for hemodynamic monitoring. Death from GBS is commonly associated with cardiac arrest during the progression phase as a result of demyelination within the autonomic nervous system.[2]

The patient with GBS may also have gastrointestinal, genitourinary, and integumentary autonomic dysfunction. All these systems must be assessed frequently, so that their functions (or dysfunctions) may be used to complete the full assessment of the patient's status. For example, ileus may prevent nutrient absorption, or excessive sweating may require additional fluid replacement.

Nutritional Support

Nutritional support is required when the patient is mechanically ventilated. Gastrostomy tubes are preferred by some clinicians to limit the risk of aspiration, repeat placement, and obstruction of narrow-lumen nasogastric tubes.

Prevention of Complications of Immobility

Additional care that needs to be planned and implemented is meticulous support to prevent the complica-

TABLE 43–3

Signs of Autonomic System Involvement in Guillain–Barré Syndrome

System	Signs and Symptoms
Cardiac	Dysrhythmias, particularly tachydysrhythmias
	Labile blood pressure
	Hypertension
	Hypotension
	Abnormal hemodynamic response to drugs
Neurologic	Pupillary dysfunction
Gastrointestinal	Constipation
Genitourinary	Retention
Integumentary	Flushing and sweating

CHART 43–2
RESEARCH UTILIZATION: ENDOTRACHEAL SUCTIONING

Abstract: Two methods of hyperoxygenation delivery were compared to determine which method preserved physiologic respiratory parameters more effectively. The methods of hyperoxygenation included use of a manual resuscitation bag (MRB) versus the ventilator. Twenty-nine patients in an ICU who required mechanical ventilation participated in this study. Each subject received both suctioning methods. Physiologic parameters monitored and recorded before and after each suctioning episode included partial pressures of oxygen and carbon dioxide (PaO_2 and $PaCO_2$), oxygen saturation (SaO_2), pH, heart rate, mean arterial pressure (MAP), and peak airway pressure. Significantly higher PaO_2 and SaO_2 levels were found with the ventilator hyperoxygenation method. No differences were found in $PaCO_2$, pH, or heart rate. Peak inspiratory pressure was greater with the MRB hyperoxygenation technique. In both techniques, MAP increased after suctioning, but it returned to baseline within 2 minutes after suctioning. The findings support the current closed system of ventilator hyperoxygenation.

Critique: The delivery of differing fraction of inspired oxygen (FIO_2) levels by each method limits a true comparison of these techniques. The study, however, supports current practice of ventilator hyperoxygenation. The researchers provide an excellent discussion of their findings with practical application.

Nursing Considerations: The patient with GBS who requires mechanical ventilation also requires suctioning. Because of the frequency with which some patients need suctioning, this study has some practical implications that the nurse should consider when caring for the patient with GBS. This study supports the use of ventilator hyperoxygenation, which is a closed system of oxygen delivery and subsequent suctioning. The immobile, ventilator-dependent patient is prone to developing pneumonia. Using the closed system may help to decrease the risk of pneumonia.

Patients with GBS may have autonomic dysfunction. The alteration in MAP indicates a need to monitor closely the patient's blood pressure and ability to adapt to hemodynamic altering situations. The patient with GBS may not have a return to baseline MAP within 2 minutes of the suctioning episode. This study highlights the need to monitor hemodynamic changes during the common ICU practice of suctioning.

In addition, this study supports the use of ventilator hyperoxygenation in patients who have a vasovagal response. Some patients' vasovagal response may be so severe that temporary pacing is indicated. Clinicians using the ventilator hyperoxygenation deliver higher FIO_2 levels and maintain higher PaO_2 and SaO_2 levels; this heightened oxygenation may help to reduce the severity of the vasovagal response.

Source: Grap MJ, Glass C, Corley M, Parks T: Endotracheal suctioning: ventilator vs manual delivery of hyperoxygenation breaths. Am J Crit Care 5:192–197, 1996.

tions of immobility, which can prolong acute care hospitalization and may increase residual disabilities. Pneumatic compression boots or supportive hosiery may be used to limit thrombosis; for patients at high risk of thrombosis, heparin therapy may be used. The health care team needs to provide range of motion to limit contractures and shortening of tendons. High-top sneakers can be used to prevent footdrop. (Families often feel helpless; purchasing high-top sneakers is often a therapeutic activity for family members.)

Patients with GBS are frequently unable to communicate many of their needs. When the cranial nerves are involved, communication becomes particularly challenging. Referral to a speech therapist may be helpful in developing creative strategies to maintain communication with the patient.

Sensory impairment may heighten patients' responses to stimuli or may mask feelings of pressure and the need to be repositioned. Sensations of burning and being "on fire" have been reported; some patients report comfort with use of ice packs and having their hands touching the cool metal side rails. Pain is extremely variable. Nurses need to assess and intervene for the comfort of the patient with GBS.

Psychological and Family Care

GBS is a frightening disease for patients and their family members. Information and education about the disease process and prognosis need to be provided on admission. Because the patient's cognitive awareness is preserved in spite of quadriplegia and facial immobility, all team members and family members should speak to the patient directly and should not discuss the patient as if he or she were not present. The inability to communicate can be frustrating as well as depressing. Family members may be able to assist the staff with communication and the patient's preferences.

Because some patients with GBS may spend weeks in an ICU, families and the patient need to be reminded of the temporary paralysis, excellent prognosis, and potential for full recovery with GBS. Education about recovery and rehabilitation needs after GBS should be provided as soon as the diagnosis is made, so that families may begin to plan for discharge with the multidisciplinary team. Referrals to social workers facilitate the family's management of the extended hospitalization and the discharge planning process (Chart 43–3). Active discharge planning to a rehabilitation center or to the home should begin as soon as the patient begins to demonstrate a return of function.[11] Families should also be linked to community resources that address GBS or neurologic disease. The GBS Foundation is available to provide families with information and support and to have former patients with GBS visit families and patients.

Immunologic Care

The immunologic treatment of GBS is directed at decreasing the severity and limiting the progression of autoimmune symptoms. Two therapies are used: plasmapheresis and intravenous immunoglobulin (IVIG). The use of corticosteroids had been common, but it is no longer considered therapeutic.

Plasmapheresis

Plasmapheresis is an exchange of plasma products performed to lessen the concentration of circulating antibodies that are causing demyelination of the peripheral nerves. Plasma is removed and is replaced with either albumin or fresh frozen plasma (FFP). This treatment is recommended for use in severe cases and during the first week of symptoms for its greatest effect; plasmapheresis instituted after 14 days has not demonstrated any significant improvement.[7, 8] The exact amount of plasma exchanged and the timing remain varied; some sources document four to six plasma exchange treatments of 40 to 50 mL/kg administered every 2 days[10] to four or five exchanges of 200 to 250 mL/kg every day[11] to 12 exchanges of more than 95% of the patient's estimated plasma level beginning with the first two or three exchanges on a daily basis.[12] Studying a large randomized group of patients, the French Cooperative Group on Plasma Exchange in GBS recommends two plasma exchanges for patients with mild GBS and four plasma exchanges for patients with moderate and severe GBS with plasma

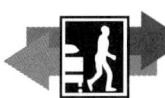

CHART 43–3

BEYOND THE ICU: CARE ISSUES OF THE PATIENT WITH GBS

Patients with Guillain–Barré syndrome (GBS) usually remain in the ICU until they are medically stable and extubated. Once they are transferred from the ICU, care is primarily focused on rehabilitation and recovery. The extent of rehabilitation and home care required depends on the patient's level of physical mobility and the presence of complications from prolonged immobility at discharge. Discharge planning begins as soon as the diagnosis of GBS is made. A multidisciplinary approach is required to address the complex needs of these patients and can include social service, home health care, physical therapy, and other community agencies, such as the GBS Foundation. Some patients are discharged to rehabilitation centers for weeks of therapy; others are discharged to their homes and are followed up with home-based nursing care and physical therapy. The impact of this disease can be emotionally and financially overwhelming to the family. All the necessary support services should be identified and initiated before discharge.

In some instances, extubation of patients with GBS may be compromised by other comorbidities such as a history of emphysema. When this occurs, patients may be transferred from the hospital, before weaning from the ventilator, to a subacute or transitional care unit. These units may be found within the hospital setting, or they may be freestanding facilities. A high level of skilled nursing is required in these settings. Patients require astute nursing care that focuses on maintaining an adequate airway and effective breathing patterns. Meticulous attention to sterile technique during suctioning is paramount to prevent pulmonary infections that could delay weaning and recovery. Aggressive physical therapy is also initiated during this time, to restore and maintain the patient's optimal level of mobility. Once weaning is accomplished, patients may still require further rehabilitation. This may be accomplished in the home setting or in a rehabilitation facility.

exchange volumes of 40 mL/kg.[13] Complications associated with plasmapheresis include infection, hypotension, hypocalcemia, bleeding, electrolyte imbalances, and allergic responses; these complications, however, are rare.[4]

TABLE 43–4
Multidisciplinary Outcomes

Phase of Illness	Outcome
Progression Phase	Stabilization of the symptoms by instituting plasmapheresis or intravenous immunoglobulin therapy Maintenance of adequate respiratory function by monitoring progression of symptoms and instituting ventilatory support before respiratory arrest occurs Stabilization of autonomic dysfunctions Development of a communication method Prevention or detection of complications of immobility
Plateau Phase	Maintenance of respiratory support Maintenance of hemodynamic stability Prevention or detection of complications of immobility Preparation for discharge from the ICU
Remyelination Phase	Restoration of respiratory function Preparation for discharge to rehabilitation unit or home Return to previous level of health Return to home and previous role functions

Plasmapheresis was demonstrated as an effective treatment for GBS in two large randomized studies.[14, 15] The documented effects of treatment include reduced ventilator dependency, shortened acute care hospitalizations, an earlier return of physical function and strength, and an improved outcome at 1 year.[4, 11]

Intravenous Immunoglobulin

IVIG is another immunologic treatment for GBS that is demonstrating promising results of earlier recovery.[16] IVIG is a blood product derived from the pooled plasma of a large group of individuals; the major component is IgG with a trace of IgA.[17] IVIG is recommended for patients with GBS in whom plasmapheresis is contraindicated. The recommended dose of IVIG is 0.4 g/kg daily for 5 days.[1, 17] The action of IVIG in GBS remains unclear. Although rare, complications of IVIG therapy include allergic reactions, tachycardia, and hypotension.[4, 17]

Corticosteroids

As noted earlier, corticosteroids have been used frequently and in high doses to help limit the inflammatory response of the autoimmune dysfunction. This approach, however, is no longer considered therapeutic.[1, 4] Randomized controlled studies failed to demonstrate therapeutic value. Controversial reports of relapse and prolonged disability add to the current recommendation that corticosteroids not be used to treat GBS.[7]

Multidisciplinary Outcomes

Multidisciplinary outcomes for the patient with GBS should be identified by the specific phase of illness and across the continuum of care. The ultimate goal of care should be to support the patient until function returns (Table 43–4). Disease progression in GBS is highly variable. Some patients present with weakness and some autonomic dysfunction and may require short-term ICU monitoring, with a return to health in a few weeks. For patients with a severe and acute onset of GBS, the ICU hospitalization may be of several weeks' duration; these patients require close monitoring and case management to regain the highest level of function possible after GBS.[18] The coordination of high-level care results in the fastest recovery with the least residual impairment.

Critical Thinking Exercise

Ms. S. is a 39-year-old mother of four; she does not work outside the home in order to raise her family. Her children range in age from 10 years to 9 months. Her husband is employed full time as a delivery person for a local small business; he works as many hours of overtime as possible to support his wife and children.

Ten days ago, Ms. S. reported having had a gastrointestinal "bug" with vomiting and diarrhea. About 4 days ago, Ms. S. began to feel tired; she reported having difficulty in climbing the stairs and feeling as if she just could not move another step. Her legs felt as if they were weighted down. Ms. S. was diagnosed with GBS 2 days ago; in the last 24 hours, she was intubated. Her motor paralysis symptoms continue to progress with involvement of the cranial nerves. Ms. S. is unable to swallow without choking and has little ability to make facial expressions. She is unable to wrinkle her forehead or to smile. Ms. S. is also beginning to have some ptosis.

In addition to the progression of her motor paralysis, her blood pressure readings are beginning to fluctuate, and her heart monitor displays occasional bursts of tachycardia and supraventricular beats.

1. What events led to the diagnosis of GBS?
2. What is the most likely cause of her labile blood pressure and tachydysrhythmias?
3. Which cranial nerves are affected?
4. What interventions could you use to continue to communicate with Ms. S.?
5. What therapies are available to help limit this acute phase of GBS?
6. What is Ms. S.'s prognosis?

Key Concepts

➡ GBS is an autoimmune and self-limiting disease characterized by demyelination of peripheral nerves.

➡ GBS presents as a classic picture of bilateral ascending weakness and paralysis that may be associated with sensory symptoms.

➡ Diagnosis of GBS is made by ruling out other neurologic, immunologic, and psychologic origins of disease and by the clinical presentation of symptoms.

➡ Because of the progressive nature and onset of GBS, the patient's respiratory function must be monitored, and ventilatory support must be provided when respiratory failure is imminent.

➡ Autonomic dysfunction may also result from the demyelination of peripheral nerves.

➡ The primary goal of care is to support the patient until remyelination and recovery occur.

➡ Supportive care of the patient includes respiratory management, hemodynamic and cardiac monitoring, nutritional support, psychologic care, and the prevention and detection of complications of immobility.

➡ Plasmapheresis, the treatment of choice, may help to limit symptom progression and may hasten recovery.

➡ Complications of plasmapheresis are rare but include bleeding, allergic responses, hemodynamic instability, and hypocalcemia.

➡ When the patient is hospitalized in the ICU for an extended length of time, psychologic support to the patient and family should include emphasizing the temporary nature of this disease and the high likelihood of full recovery.

➡ Outcomes of care focus on returning the patient to his or her previous level of health and functioning because full recovery is common with GBS.

References

1. Hund EF, Schuchardt V, Ropper AH: Acute inflammatory polyneuropathy (Guillain–Barré syndrome). In: Hacke W, Hanley DF, Einhaupl KM, et al (eds): Neurocritical Care. New York, Springer, 1994.
2. The Italian Guillain–Barré Study Group: The prognosis and main prognostic indicators of Guillain–Barré syndrome. Brain 119:2053–2061, 1996.
3. McCombe PA: The Guillain–Barré syndrome and acute dysautonomia. In: Pender MP, McCombe PA (eds): Autoimmune Neurological Disease. London, Cambridge University Press, 1995.
4. Sommer N, Winer JB: Inflammatory and infectious polyneuropathy. In: Brandt T, Caplan LR, Dichgans J, et al (eds): Neurological Disorders: Course and Treatment. New York, Academic Press, 1996.
5. Awong IE, Dandurand KR, Keeys CA, et al: Drugs associated with Guillain–Barré syndrome: a literature review. Ann Pharmacother 30:173–180, 1996.
6. Brumback RA: Neurology and Clinical Neuroscience, 2nd ed. New York, Springer, 1996.
7. Hickey JV: The Clinical Practice of Neurological and Neurosurgical Nursing, 4th ed. Philadelphia, Lippincott–Raven, 1997.
8. Adams RD, Victor M, Ropper AH: Principles of Neurology, 6th ed. New York, McGraw-Hill, 1997.
9. Dam V, Wild MC, Baum MM: Effect of oxygen insufflation during endotracheal suctioning on arterial pressure and oxygenation in coronary artery bypass graft patients. Am J Crit Care 3:191–197, 1994.
10. Parry GJ: Guillain–Barré Syndrome. New York, Thieme, 1993.
11. Donohoe KM: Autoimmune disorders. In: Barker E (ed): Neuroscience Nursing. Philadelphia, CV Mosby, 1994.
12. Petajan JH: Acute inflammatory polyneuropathy. In: McKendall RR, Stroop WG (eds): Handbook of Neurovirology. New York, Marcel Dekker, 1994.
13. French Cooperative Group on Plasma Exchange in Guillain–Barré Syndrome: Appropriate number of plasma exchanges in Guillain–Barré syndrome. Ann Neurol 41:298–306, 1997.
14. French Cooperative Group on Plasma Exchange in Guillain–Barré Syndrome: Efficiency of plasma exchange in Guillain–Barré syndrome: role of replacement fluids. Ann Neurol 22:743–761, 1987.
15. The Guillain–Barré Syndrome Study Group: Plasmapheresis and acute Guillain–Barré syndrome. Neurology 35:1096–1104, 1985.
16. van der Meche FGA, Schmitz PIM, the Dutch Guillain–Barré Study Group: A randomized trial comparing intravenous immune globulin and plasma exchange in Guillain–Barré syndrome. N Engl J Med 326:1123–1129, 1992.
17. Chipps E, Skinner C: Intravenous immunoglobulin: implications for use in the neurological patient. J Neurosci Nurs 26:8–17, 1994.
18. Marr JA, Reid B: Implementing managed care and case management: the neuroscience experience. J Neurosci Nurs 24:281–285, 1992.

44

Neurovascular Disorders

Anne W. Wojner

Objectives

After completing this chapter, the student will be able to:

1. Relate the pathophysiologic origins of specific neurovascular disorders resulting in stroke to the clinical presentation and unique multidisciplinary needs of these patients.
2. Identify the key components of the assessment of a patient experiencing a stroke.
3. Apply the nursing process to design an individualized plan of care for ischemic and hemorrhagic stroke victims.
4. Use the nursing process to plan total care in preparation for a dignified death in the patient with neurologic dysfunction.
5. Evaluate the effectiveness of a multidisciplinary care regimen aimed at optimizing functional outcomes in the patient with neurologic dysfunction.

The term "stroke" originated in the sixteenth century when the outcomes of this neurologic disease were believed to be caused by a "stroke" of God's hand in response to wrongful living.[1] The term "cerebral vascular accident" (CVA) evolved in the 1900s, but it has recently been replaced by the original term "stroke," both because of the disease's nonaccidental nature and because of the multiple mechanisms for stroke production.[2]

In the United States, stroke is the number 1 cause of disability among adults and the third leading cause of death. The annual incidence of stroke in the United States totals approximately 400,000; of this number, 150,000 strokes result in death.[3] Mortality related to stroke varies according to the type of stroke incurred. In ischemic stroke, 30-day mortality has been reported at 15%, whereas in subarachnoid hemorrhage (SAH), a 30-day mortality of 46% has been reported. The highest 30-day mortality in stroke occurs among the hemorrhagic group suffering from intraparenchymal brain hemorrhage (IPBH), with a mortality rate reported at 83%.[4] Chart 44–1 lists significant risk factors for the development of stroke.

The National Stroke Association's (NSA) screening program revealed that the public is unaware of stroke warning signs and confuses these important indicators with well-publicized cardiac symptoms such as chest pain and shortness of breath. Additionally, the study

also revealed that only two of five participants screened indicated that they viewed stroke as a medical emergency necessitating a call to 911. Forty-five percent stated that they would first call their physician before seeking emergency treatment, and an alarming 3% revealed that they would not seek treatment, but instead would "wait and see" whether symptoms worsened.[5]

Functional disability after stroke has been described by stroke survivors as their most significant and terrifying life experience.[6] A state of unconsciousness may result secondary to stroke, fostering the need for both psychosocial and physiologic care of both patient and family. Chart 44–2 describes outcomes after a period of unconsciousness identified through research that the nurse should know about when caring for stroke patients. The nurse is challenged to orchestrate interdisciplinary therapies that reduce the incidence of disability and enhance functional independence to improve quality of life for stroke patients and their family.[7]

ETIOLOGY AND PATHOPHYSIOLOGY

Ischemic Penumbra

Stroke results from loss of brain tissue perfusion, regardless of whether the triggering event is ischemic or hemorrhagic. After loss of arterial blood flow, a zone

CHART 44-1

Risk Factors Associated With the Development of Stroke

Hypertension
Smoking
Obesity
Drug and alcohol abuse
Sedentary lifestyle
Hyperlipidemia
Atrial fibrillation
Left ventricular hypertrophy
Heart failure
Ischemic heart disease
History of transient ischemic attacks
Diabetes
Elevated hematocrit levels

of ischemia develops, referred to as the "ischemic penumbra." The penumbra is made up of severely ischemic core tissue surrounded by tissue that may be potentially viable. The central core of the penumbra dies rapidly, but the fate of the tissue lying between the junction of the viable and infarction zones depends on local perfusion conditions.[8] Viability thresholds for individual cells and neuronal networks vary, driving the duration of the penumbra from mere hours to days, as the stroke process evolves and is completed.[9, 10] Early intervention aimed at restoring cellular perfusion may produce complete recovery without neurologic deficit because of these thresholds.

The stroke process begins with a fall in cellular perfusion. Autoregulatory responses produce immediate local vasodilation aimed at restoring perfusion. A continued fall in perfusion pressure despite vasodilation is referred to as "misery perfusion," indicating a state of cellular oxygenation delivery and consumption mismatch. Misery perfusion triggers an increase in oxygen extraction by brain tissues to ensure aerobic cellular metabolism.[11] Failed compensatory mechanisms results in cellular ischemia, which leads to metabolic dysfunction, neuronal electrical failure, and, ultimately, cellular death.[7]

Ischemic Metabolic Cascade

The sequence of events at the onset of cellular ischemia has important implications for new and future stroke treatments. Researchers are now focusing on the metabolic response to ischemic brain injury, to determine the timing of intracellular and extracellular reactions and the critical physiologic links in the chain of untoward events.[7]

The metabolic cascade that leads to cell death begins with the massive release and impaired uptake of glutamate, an excitatory neurotransmitter that causes a cellular influx of calcium ions and the migration of intracellular potassium to outside the cell. Once calcium is inside the cell, an increase in intracellular glycolysis is triggered to enhance generation of adenosine triphosphate (ATP). ATP is used by the cell to operate cellular pumps aimed at maintaining proper intracellular ionic gradients. The increased focus on glycolysis slows intracellular protein synthesis, which is essential in maintaining integrity of the cell wall and internal cellular structures.[12, 13] The cell's poor state of perfusion forces anaerobic metabolism of intracellular glucose, which increases the intracellular lactic acid load. As illustrated in Figure 44–1, this combination of a lack of protein synthesis and increased intracellular lactic acid produces deadly results: cellular destruction from the inside out.[7, 12]

Types of Stroke

Ischemic Stroke

Ischemic stroke is the most common type of stroke, accounting for approximately 70% of all strokes. Patho-

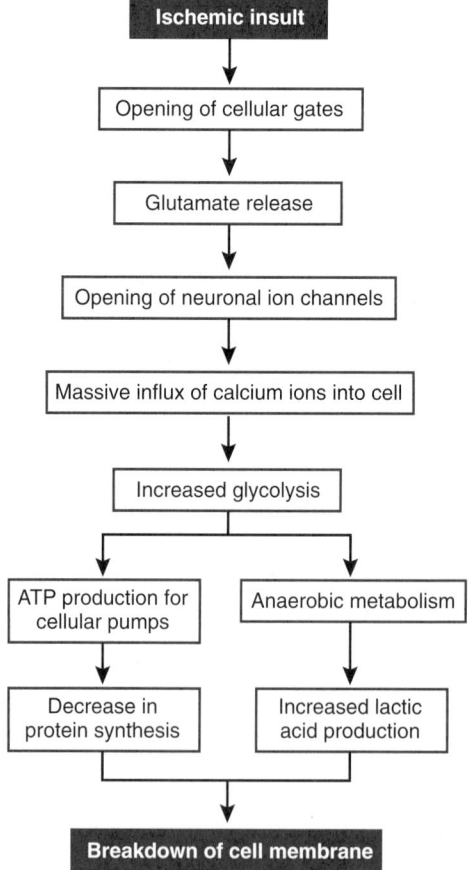

Figure 44–1

The metabolic cascade that leads to cell death.

CHART 44-2

RESEARCH UTILIZATION: THE UNCONSCIOUS EXPERIENCE

Abstract: Little is known about the patient's perspective of unconsciousness or coma. This study sought to describe the experiences of patients with a documented history of unconsciousness. Phenomenologic interviews of 100 formerly hospitalized patients with a documented unconsciousness event were conducted. Patients were found to experience one or more of five discrete states. Unconsciousness, defined as a total absence of awareness of self and environment even when externally stimulated, was experienced by 27% of the sample. Inner consciousness, or lack of awareness of the external environment, but presence of an awareness of the inner self, was experienced in 9% of patients. Perceived unconsciousness, or the ability to hear, understand, and respond emotionally, coupled with an inability to respond physically was experienced in 27% of patients. Distorted consciousness, defined as unreal perceptual, memory, or personality distortions occurred in 14% of patients. Finally, paranormal experiences, including near-death experiences (NDE), out-of-body experiences not associated with NDE, visits by a deceased significant other, and visits by the "Grim Reaper," occurred in 23% of patients. Patients consistently reported hesitancy related to discussing these occurrences with significant others for fear of being perceived as mentally disturbed.

Critique: This study describes the patient's perspective of unconsciousness as a multifaceted phenomenon. Traditional approaches to nursing care of the unconscious or perceived unconscious states are generally incorporated into nursing education. However, nursing approaches to the unconscious patient experiencing active perceptual distortions or hallucinations, NDE or other paranormal phenomena, or the presence of solely an inner consciousness state are lacking.

Nursing Considerations: Unconscious patients require vigilant nursing care. The nurse must cautiously assess for clinical signs suggestive of perceived unconsciousness, perceptual distortions or hallucinations, or the occurrence of a paranormal experience. Acting as a patient advocate, the nurse should facilitate creation of a healing, safe environment, including one-way or, when possible, two-way communication techniques. Patients, when able, should be invited to have a therapeutic dialog about their unconsciousness experience. The nurse should use open-ended statements such as, "Tell me what you remember about your time in the intensive care unit." Probing questions should follow, to open the conversation further. Patients should be reassured that their experiences are not unusual. The family should be included in the discussion once a trusting relationship has been established and the patient feels well supported and comfortable.

The domain of unconsciousness from the patient's perspective is relatively unexplored. Nurses must commit themselves to learning from their patients' shared experiences and contributing their knowledge to the profession, to enhance both nursing science and patient outcomes.

Source: Lawrence M: The unconscious experience. Am J Crit Care 4:227–232, 1995.

genic mechanisms responsible for this type of stroke include local vessel thrombosis and embolism.[3, 9]

Thrombotic Stroke. Thrombotic or atherosclerotic strokes have a pathogenic mechanism similar to that of occlusive coronary artery disease. Intracranial collateral circulation develops in this type of stroke as vessel diameter slowly decreases over time. Transient ischemic attacks (TIAs) are a common precursor to thrombotic stroke as vessel lumens become dangerously narrow.[8] Thrombotic strokes occur most commonly during sleep or sedentary periods, when lowered resting arterial pressures produce inadequate perfusion through narrowed vessel lumens.[14]

Lacunar Stroke. Lacunar strokes occur in small, penetrating arteries in the deep gray or white matter, when a thrombus develops secondary to lipohyalinosis, which coats arterial vessel walls with a hyaline–lipid material. The infarcted brain tissue sloughs, producing a small cavity or lake. This type of ischemic infarct occurs commonly in patients with chronic hypertension.[14]

Embolic Stroke. Approximately 20% of ischemic strokes are the result of intravascular emboli.[3] The origin of the emboli producing the stroke may include the heart (secondary to atrial fibrillation, diseased heart valves, infectious endocarditis, and cardiac myopathy), the carotid vessels, and the venous circulation in patients with patent foramen ovale.[2, 8] Embolic strokes usually occur during periods of activity.[14]

Perioperative ischemic stroke in patients undergoing cardiopulmonary bypass (CPB) for cardiac surgery has been documented since 1954.[15] The development of this type of stroke is thought to be related to comorbid factors as well as to CPB and surgical technique, gas emboli, valvular emboli, or plaque that breaks loose during clamping or subsequent unclamping of a brittle aorta.[8] A mean of 62 emboli has been recorded by transcranial Doppler (TCD) during coronary artery bypass, whereas a mean of 1339 emboli has been recorded by TCD during heart valve replacement. During cardiac valve replacement, 70 to 100% of patients studied with TCD experienced brain embolism.[16]

Hemorrhagic Stroke

Hemorrhagic stroke is part of a general category sometimes referred to as nontraumatic, intracranial hemorrhage (ICH). The incidence of hemorrhagic stroke differs widely by racial groups, with the highest incidence occurring in Asians (specifically the Japanese), an intermediate incidence found in African-Americans, and the lowest incidence found in Caucasians. Still unexplained by science, cold weather months are most commonly associated with ICH.[17] Hemorrhagic stroke has three pathologic origins: IPBH; aneurysmal SAH; and hemorrhage sustained from rupture of a vascular malformation.

Primary Intraparenchymal Brain Hemorrhage. IPBH occurs much more infrequently than ischemic strokes. This type of stroke afflicts approximately 40,000 Americans annually.[18] Causes of IPBH include severe hypertension, arteriosclerosis, tumors, blood dyscrasia, substance abuse, and other degenerative diseases affecting the brain's vascular system.[19, 20]

In IPBH, high arteriolar pressure results in the direct release of blood into the brain tissues. Adjacent arterioles and capillaries rupture secondary to high local pressures and cause the hematoma to enlarge at its periphery like a rolling snowball, collecting blood along its pathway.[21] Mortality rates for patients with IPBH vary widely, but the presence of coma in the early hours after the bleeding carries a mortality rate that is virtually 100%.[19]

Aneurysmal Subarachnoid Hemorrhage. Each year in the United States, approximately 28,000 new cases of aneurysmal SAH are documented.[22] SAH is the accumulation of blood in the subarachnoid space, most often at the base of the brain. The most common cause of SAH is a ruptured intracranial aneurysm, but head trauma, coagulopathies, tumors, and rupture of an arteriovenous malformation (AVM) may also result in SAH.[8] The mean age of SAH occurrence is approximately 50 years; women have a higher incidence of SAH than men.[23, 24]

Comorbid conditions associated with aneurysm formation include hypertension, cerebral atherosclerosis, vascular asymmetry at the circle of Willis and pregnancy-induced hypertension (PIH).[25] De novo or "new" aneurysm growth has been documented by angiographic study in high-risk persons with previously negative angiograms for aneurysm.[26] Incidental intracranial aneurysms occur in approximately 1% of the general population and carry an associated rate of rupture of 1%.[27] An estimated 3 to 24% of patients with aneurysms demonstrate the presence of multiple intracranial aneurysms on angiography.[20, 23] Rupture of more than one intracranial aneurysm at a time is considered unusual.

Approximately 7% of intracranial aneurysms are classified as familial aneurysms.[28] The mechanism for inheritance is autosomal dominance with variable penetrance and expression. Familial aneurysms rupture at an earlier age and smaller size than do sporadically occurring aneurysms.[29] This finding has caused practitioners to advocate regular screening of directly related family members when a relative has been diagnosed with familial aneurysms.[28]

Most aneurysms occur within the anterior circulation fed by the internal carotid artery (ICA). Aneurysms are classified by size as minute, small (less than 10 mm), large (10–20 mm), or giant (>20 mm).[20] Table 44–1 lists the reported incidence of intracranial aneurysms by arterial site.

Three leading hypotheses are related to the development of intracranial aneurysms. Although much remains unclear, environmental contributors, stress, and congenital factors may play a role in the genesis of intracranial aneurysms. The congenital hypothesis suggests that an inherent weakness in the wall of the artery, either in the muscular layers or in the collagen structure, promotes development of an aneurysm. The degenerative hypothesis is supported by a belief that the arterial wall partially degenerates, producing a weakness through which the intimal layers gradually herniate. Contributing factors such as arterial hypertension act to aggravate and promote herniation

TABLE 44–1

Incidence of Intracranial Aneurysms by Arterial Distribution

Intracranial Artery	Incidence (%)
Cavernous segment internal carotid artery (ICA)	5
Supraclinoid ICA (includes supraclinoid segment of ICA, ophthalmic artery, posterior communicating artery, and anterior choroidal artery)	24–40
Anterior cerebral artery and anterior communicating artery	33
Middle cerebral artery	21–31
Vertebrobasilar system	5–12

From Wojner AW: Neurovascular disease. In: Kinney MR, Dunbar SB, Brooks-Brun JA, et al (eds): AACN Clinical Reference for Critical Care Nursing. St. Louis, Mosby–Year Book, 1998, pp 733–766.

further. The third hypothesis suggests that both congenital and degenerative processes contribute to the production of intracranial aneurysms and proposes that aneurysms are the result of an inherent vessel wall weakness that, over time, becomes subject to degenerative processes. Most neuroscientists accept that the latent onset of symptoms related to intracranial aneurysms, between 50 and 60 years of age, suggests that degenerative influences are most likely involved in the development of intracranial aneurysms.[20]

The brain's arterial vessels are different from arteries in the systemic circulation, in that they consist of thinner intimal and medial layers and a more conspicuous internal elastic lamina. At bifurcations, the tunica media of the brain's arteries is occasionally absent, a finding that appears to be related to the common development of aneurysms at these sites.[20]

Arteriovenous Malformations. Vascular malformations of the central nervous system (CNS) fall into one of five main categories: 1) AVMs; 2) telangiectases; 3) cavernous malformations; 4) venous malformations; and 5) varices.[30] The most commonly encountered vascular malformation of the brain is the AVM.[20, 30] Approximately 2000 new cases of AVM are diagnosed each year.[31] Because of the frequency of these lesions, further discussion of vascular malformations is limited to intracranial AVMs.

AVMs are the most clinically significant vascular malformation, composed of masses of arteries and arterialized veins that promote high vascular flow. These lesions are best described as a tangled array of dilated vessels that form an anomalous connection between the arterial and venous system that lacks the normally intervening capillary network.[8]

AVMs consist of developmentally immature vessels and are thought to be congenital lesions that occur during early fetal development. Neuroscientists believe that abnormalities in the development of CNS vasculature at a fetal age of approximately 3 to 12 weeks sets the stage for production of AVMs. AVMs often continue to develop over time, recruiting new blood vessels during childhood and early adulthood.[32] Familial and multiple AVMs are uncommon, a finding suggesting that the aberrant process responsible for their formation is not genetic, but instead is a developmental anomaly.

Usually, AVMs are found among middle cerebral artery (MCA) territory. AVMs are the second most common cause of spontaneous SAH after saccular aneurysms. AVMs occurring within the cerebral hemispheres are usually wedge-shaped lesions based at the cortical surface with an apex pointing toward the lateral ventricle. The feeding arteries of AVMs may also harbor saccular aneurysms.[30]

The size of an AVM varies from a few millimeters to a large mass of vessels that demand an increase in cardiac output. Varying luminal diameters and vessel thromboses are common within the lesion. The feeding arteries of an AVM lack normal CNS autoregulatory control, resulting in primarily passive blood flow within the structure. Veins within an AVM are often referred to as "arterialized veins" because of the lack of a discernible tunica elastica and because of the characteristically thick walls. The term "red veins" has also been used to describe an AVM's venous channels because of the admixture of arterial blood to the venous system.[8]

The nidus of an AVM represents the site of direct arteriovenous shunting. The nidus is usually located in the brain parenchyma, but choroid plexus and extra-parenchymal AVMs have also been observed.[8] Often, it is difficult to determine the site of bleeding within an AVM, but vessels with markedly thinned walls are believed to be the source.[30, 32]

Brain tissue located around an AVM often demonstrates reactive change related to persistent alterations in cellular perfusion. This tissue is abnormal and typically consists of gliotic or scarred brain parenchyma, signs of old hemorrhage and chronic inflammation, malformed or degenerative structures, signs of calcification, and varying degrees of necrosis.[30, 32] Examination of this abnormal brain tissue surrounding an AVM has contributed to the understanding of a "steal" phenomenon, a process by which AVMs produce focal neurologic findings. Low-pressure arterial feeders within an AVM divert blood away from surrounding brain tissue, thus "stealing" blood from normal perfusion pathways. The persistent "stealing" of blood from surrounding brain tissue promotes ischemia and permanent tissue changes producing focal neurologic deficit and seizures. Some AVMs may show enlargement and increased complexity of the nidus and vascular channels over time related to steal phenomena, whereas others remain stable in size.[30]

Assessment

The cardiovascular assessment of a stroke patient should include overall hemodynamic status. In the case of an intracranial aneurysm or AVM, the use of an oximetric pulmonary artery catheter and arterial line helps to determine the need for and the response to volume. Distal pulses and wound site in patients undergoing transfemoral canalization for angiographic or endovascular procedures should also be assessed.[8]

Respiratory status should be assessed as frequently as indicated by the overall clinical picture to ensure a patent airway, oxygenation, and ventilation. Mechanical ventilation may be required secondary to a decreased level of consciousness, an ineffective breathing pattern, and treatment methods used to manage increased intracranial pressure (ICP). Measurement of venous oxygen saturation (SvO_2) and pulse oximetry should be used to guide therapy in patients requiring mechanical ventilation. In a patient with an extremely moribund presentation, the use of mechanical ventilation may be deferred based on the patient's end-of-life wishes.[8]

Fluid and electrolyte balance and overall renal function should be assessed cautiously in the stroke patient. In hemorrhagic stroke, fluid and electrolyte imbalance may result secondary to aggressive preload augmentation to counteract vasospasm, hyponatremia, or diabetes insipidus. The nurse must cautiously assess the overall status of the patient and must carefully balance treatment goals against individual tolerance of requisite therapies.[8]

Ischemic Stroke

The clinical assessment findings of a patient with ischemic stroke vary according to the location of the brain infarction and its size. Table 44–2 provides an overview of neurologic deficit likely to occur based on the arterial distribution of the stroke process. A general understanding of gross neurologic anatomy and physiology supports the nurse's ability to localize a stroke lesion from clinical assessment data alone, before viewing the results of diagnostic testing.

Hemorrhagic Stroke

Although assessment of focal neurologic findings also plays a role in the diagnostic workup of hemorrhagic stroke, other clinical features specific to each of the hemorrhage subtypes are important.

Intraparenchymal Brain Hemorrhage

The clinical assessment findings occurring in IPBH vary by location of the hemorrhage within the brain. Seizures may be an early clinical finding when hemorrhage occurs within the cerebral cortex. Vomiting is a common finding in IPBH occurring in the posterior fossa, and it may be related to direct stimulation of the medulla's vomit center or the result of increased ICP. Headache as a clinical finding occurs in only one-third of patients with IPBH.[21]

Subarachnoid Hemorrhage

Ninety percent of intracranial aneurysms remain asymptomatic before rupture, but large aneurysms may produce symptoms without rupturing because of compression of an underlying neurologic structure. Unruptured aneurysms may reach a size of approximately 10 mm before producing symptoms.[20]

Although many studies have concluded that heavy physical exertion is not associated with aneurysmal rupture, many practitioners continue to believe in a relationship between aneurysm rupture and physical exertion.[27] Approximately 30 to 40% of patients experience aneurysm rupture at rest,[25] but most aneurysmal SAHs occur during ordinary, nonexertional activities of daily living (ADLs).[8] Processes that increase systemic arterial pressure, whether they be of physical or psychological onset, may increase the risk of

TABLE 44–2

Clinical Findings Associated With Stroke by Arterial Distribution*

Arterial Distribution	Possible Clinical Findings
Anterior Arterial Distribution	Contralateral hemiparesis
	Contralateral sensory deficits
	Aphasias (left-sided lesions in left cerebral dominance)
	Dysphagia
	Altered mental status
	Poststroke depression
	Unilateral neglect (visual and/or tactile; more common with right cerebral infarction)
	Gaze preference
	Apraxia
	Signs and symptoms of increased intracranial pressure when size of lesion produces mass effect
Posterior Arterial Distribution	Dysphagia
	Ataxia
	Visual field defects
	Gaze preference or disconjugate extraocular movements
	Nystagmus
	Motor and sensory deficits, including bilateral hemiparesis
	Altered level of consciousness
	Signs and symptoms of increased intracranial pressure when size of lesion produces mass effect

*Clinical signs and symptoms vary according to precise location of the stroke within the brain.

aneurysm rupture, but no conclusive evidence indicates that this is the case.

Spontaneous SAH may be a serious, although relatively rare, complication of pregnancy.[33] The dramatic cardiovascular changes occurring during pregnancy may predispose some women to hemorrhagic stroke. In pregnancy-related SAH, the source of hemorrhage has been equally attributed to aneurysm or AVM rupture. AVMs usually bleed earlier in pregnancy than do aneurysms, which are more likely to rupture toward the end of the gestational period. AVMs usually rupture during a woman's first pregnancy, whereas aneurysms may remain intact and rupture during subsequent pregnancies.[34]

The clinical signs associated with aneurysm rupture depend on the rate and amount of bleeding and on the location of the aneurysm. Clinical signs and symptoms may be relatively benign in patients with minimal SAH, or they may show evidence of acute intracranial hypertension and impending brain death in patients with massive hemorrhage.

Signs and symptoms of aneurysmal SAH include the abrupt onset of a severe, atypical headache, often described by patients as the "worst headache" of their life. Stimulation of pain fibers concentrated in the meninges and the basal and pial vessels is the likely origin of the SAH headache. The headache frequently radiates into the occiput and down the spine into the extremities.[20] Headache onset may or may not be associated with a brief loss of consciousness, nausea or vomiting, focal neurologic deficits, or meningismus. Older patients may not present with the "worst"

headache because of a reduced mass effect secondary to brain atrophy.[35] Subarachnoid hemorrhage also produces "sterile meningitis," often causing symptoms such as nuchal rigidity and Kernig's and Brudzinski's signs. Other signs associated with aneurysm rupture include report of a "popping" sensation and intermittent loss of hearing or vision.[20]

The warning leak phenomenon has become a well-identified sign associated with impending intracranial aneurysm rupture. Approximately 37 to 60% of patients who present with aneurysmal SAH give a history of having had unusual, atypical headaches for several weeks before the definitive event.[23, 35] Unfortunately, these patients are often misdiagnosed as having tension headache or neck pain referable to cervical spondylosis. An alarming 12% of persons with warning leak are denied medical attention secondary to misdiagnosis.[24] Once a warning leak has occurred, the interval between it and subsequent aneurysmal rupture is approximately 14 days.[23] History of significant headache should increase a diagnostician's index of suspicion, promoting positive identification of aneurysmal SAH.

The Hunt and Hess grading scale is often used to classify the severity of aneurysmal SAH.[36] Table 44–3 illustrates use of the scale in the identification of outcomes based on clinical assessment. Despite considerable advances in perioperative management, the overall prognosis for patients with aneurysmal SAH is poor. Only 65% of patients with aneurysmal SAH are selected to go on to interventional treatment, because of their moribund appearance at the time of hospital-

TABLE 44–3
Grade of Subarachnoid Hemorrhage and Associated Outcomes

Hunt and Hess Scale	
Grade	Neurologic Status
I	Asymptomatic, or minimal headache and slight nuchal rigidity
II	Moderate to severe headache, meningismus, no neurologic deficit other than cranial nerve palsy
III	Drowsiness, confusion, minimal focal neurologic deficit
IV	Stuporous, moderate to severe hemiparesis, possible early decerebrate rigidity and vegetative disturbances
V	Deep coma, decerebrate posturing, moribund appearance

Glasgow Outcome Scale	
Category	Outcome
1	Good recovery, independent lifestyle
2	Moderate disability, independent lifestyle
3	Severe disability, conscious but not independent
4	Vegetative
5	Dead

Data from Hunt WE, Hess RM: Surgical risk as related to time of intervention in the repair of intracranial aneurysms. J Neurosurg 28:14–20, 1968; Mendel RC, Carter LP: Evaluation and treatment of clinical vasospasm following subarachnoid hemorrhage. Contemp Neurosurg 16:1–6, 1994; Findley, JM: Perioperative management of subarachnoid hemorrhage. Contemp Neurosurg 17:1–5, 1995; National Stroke Association: Management of subarachnoid hemorrhage. Stroke Clin Updates 6:1–4, 1995. Reprinted from Wojner AW: Neurovascular disease. In: Kinney MR, Dunbar SB, Brooks-Brun JA, et al (eds): AACN Clinical Reference for Critical Care Nursing. St. Louis, Mosby–Year Book, 1998, pp 733–766.

ization.[27] Overall mortality related to aneurysmal rupture is between 5 and 60%, depending on severity of the SAH, and approximately 10 to 33% of patients with aneurysm die as a result of the initial major hemorrhage.[20, 22, 27] Unfortunately, among survivors of aneurysmal SAH, functionally significant morbidity has been documented to occur in 20 to 50% of patients.[20, 24]

In patients receiving nonsurgical, conservative treatment after acute aneurysm rupture, recurrent rupture carries a mortality rate of approximately 70%. The peak incidence for recurrent rupture is within 10 days of the initial hemorrhage. Most patients go on to receive surgical or endovascular obliteration of the aneurysm early in the course of treatment, given the grim statistics associated with conservative treatment.[24]

Aneurysm rupture and the potential for poor outcome could be avoided if asymptomatic, unruptured aneurysms could be detected early and treated before they ruptured. Current limitations for widespread screening include the need for angiography to define size, shape, and precise location in the asymptomatic patient. The risks and costs associated with routine screening by angiography make this an unrealistic option. Future improvement in magnetic resonance angiography (MRA) will, one hopes, provide a realistic mechanism for routine aneurysm screening in high-risk persons.[8]

Arteriovenous Malformation Hemorrhage

Theoretically present since birth, AVMs typically become symptomatic during the second, third, and fourth decades.[37] Although AVMs may come to medical attention in various ways, the most common clinical presentations include hemorrhage, headache, and seizure. Progressive neurologic deficit within surrounding brain tissue or signs related to mass effect with compression of normal neural and vascular tissue may also produce clinical findings suggestive of AVM.[38]

Hemorrhage is the most common presenting symptom associated with AVM. The effects of physical exertion on AVM rupture remain unclear, but no significant relationship has been found among preexisting or incidental hypertension, trauma, and AVM hemorrhage.[32] The peak incidence of AVM hemorrhage occurs in the late teens to early twenties and is believed to originate from the arterialized venous channels that form the nidus of the lesion.[39] The risk of rebleeding after an initial hemorrhage increases annually and carries a mortality rate as high as 65%.[38]

The size of the AVM is related to a presenting symptom of seizure or bleeding. Large AVMs have a lower risk of hemorrhage and a greater risk of seizure as the presenting symptom.[38] The average age of onset of a seizure disorder is 25 years.[37] Jacksonian seizures are common when the AVM is located within the

motor and sensory cortex, whereas AVMs of the temporal lobe commonly result in partial complex seizures.[32]

Headache may also be a presenting symptom of AVM. The mechanism responsible for headache is thought to be abnormal dilation of pain-sensitive structures, such as feeding arteries and draining veins or sinuses. A few patients may present with neurologic deficits that may originate from hemorrhage, mass effect, hydrocephalus, or steal phenomenon.[37]

Unlike the almost universal use of the Hunt and Hess scale for aneurysmal SAH, grading systems specific to AVM clinical presentation and outcome have not been used routinely by practitioners. The scale developed by Spetzler and Martin is displayed in Table 44–4. This scale shows promise as an easy-to-use grading system that incorporates elements known to relate to treatment outcomes.[30, 40]

Laboratory and Diagnostic Tests

All types of stroke follow a similar diagnostic course guided by the use of neurologic imaging systems. Computed tomography (CT) is always the first imaging technique used in the diagnostic workup for stroke; depending on CT findings, the workup may progress to the use of magnetic resonance imaging (MRI) to assist with diagnosis. MRI may be used to disclose occult ischemic changes, aneurysms, AVMs and surrounding brain ischemia, the distribution and

TABLE 44–4

Spetzler and Martin Arteriovenous Malformation (AVM) Grading System

Criteria	Corresponding Score*
Size of AVM Nidus	**AVM Score by Size**
Small: <3 cm	Small: 1
Medium: 3–6 cm	Medium: 2
Large: >6 cm	Large: 3
Eloquence of Adjacent Brain	**AVM Score by Eloquence**
Noneloquent	0
Eloquent	1
Deep Vascular Component	**AVM Score by Vascular Depth**
Limited to superficial	0
Deep component present	1

*Sum of AVM Scores = Total Score or AVM Grade

Data from Spetzler RF, Martin NA: A proposed grading system for arteriovenous malformations. J Neurosurg 65:476–483, 1986. Brain eloquence is defined as a region of the brain that harbors easily identifiable neurologic function that, if injured, would result in disabling neurologic deficit. The Spetzler and Martin system has demonstrated the highest overall correlation with operative difficulty and postoperative neurologic outcome. Reprinted from Wojner AW: Neurovascular disease. In: Kinney MR, Dunbar SB, Brooks-Brun JA, et al (eds): AACN Clinical Reference for Critical Care Nursing. St. Louis, Mosby–Year Book, 1998, pp 733–766.

site of hemorrhage, and the presence of a dilated ventricular system. Repeat CT or MRI may be helpful to confirm suspected brain infarction or hemorrhagic transformation of an ischemic lesion.[20]

The routine use of electroencephalogram (EEG) testing for suspected stroke has become rare. However, when seizure is suspected or is a known presenting symptom, EEG should be considered. Similarly, lumbar puncture (LP) may be eliminated from the clinical workup if CT or MRI has demonstrated the presence of SAH. When imaging findings prove negative and a high index of suspicion exists based on clinical presentation, diagnostic LP should be performed with care, so that minimal fluid is withdrawn to prevent a shift in pressure that may aggravate brain displacement within the skull. SAH is diagnosed by the presence of thousands of red blood cells and xanthochromic or fresh blood mixed with cerebrospinal fluid (CSF).[24]

Magnetic resonance angiography (MRA) has been shown to identify the presence of intracranial aneurysms and AVMs effectively. Unfortunately, MRA has not reached a level of resolution that permits the exact visualization of aneurysms or AVM geometry, including adjacent arterial branches in these lesions. Because of this limitation, exclusive use of this technology is not possible, but diagnosticians are hopeful that MRA may replace angiography in the future, as the systems undergo additional enhancements.[24, 41]

Angiography is still considered the current standard for diagnostic imaging and treatment planning for both aneurysms and AVMs. Angiography should be performed as soon as the diagnosis of SAH is made, except in the patient with devastating neurologic presentation, such as coma, in whom it may be withheld until a more favorable clinical presentation develops. Patients with IPBH may also go on to angiography, to distinguish primary IPBH from that associated with aneurysm or AVM rupture.[20]

Newer angiography methods record images electronically, through the use of digital subtraction angiogram (DSA). This type of angiography subtracts images of bone and soft tissue, leaving only the image of the intracranial vessels. Superselective angiography (SSA) is also performed by placing small, flexible, coaxial loaded catheters directly into the suspected arterial branch, thus enabling treatment planning for aneurysms and an examination of AVM hemodynamics, including transit time through the nidus and perfusion of surrounding normal vessels.[41]

Serial angiograms may be performed at several critical times throughout the perioperative course. Repeated studies assist in determining the success of surgical or endovascular obliteration therapy, in diagnosing the presence of vasospasm, and in identifying the source of hemorrhage, should rebleeding occur. In suspected aneurysmal SAH, approximately 5 to 25% of initial angiograms do not distinguish the source of bleeding. However, within 10 days of the initial angiogram, repeated studies disclose approximately 10% of aneurysms previously missed.[20, 24]

The use of transcranial Doppler (TCD) ultrasonography has become commonplace in the noninvasive diagnosis and repeated assessment of intracranial arterial vasospasm secondary to aneurysmal SAH. Most studies report good correlation with angiography, particularly in assessing blood flow along the MCA stem.[24]

TCD measures the velocity of intracranial arterial blood flow. As the lumen of an artery with vasospasm narrows, the velocity of blood flow increases similar to the effect achieved by placing a finger over a portion of a running water hose spout. Arterial velocities increase slightly on the first day after SAH. By days 4 to 6, velocity begins to accelerate. Mean intracranial velocity usually peaks by the ninth or tenth day and later returns to baseline in asymptomatic patients with vasospasm.[24] Velocity changes of 25% or greater from one examination to the next forewarn the onset of brain ischemia. This shift in velocity usually occurs between the seventh and eighth days and is followed by clinically symptomatic vasospasm in approximately 1 to 2 days.[20] Table 44–5 provides criteria that support the diagnosis of vasospasm by TCD.

Functional imaging of brain tissue can be conducted by single photon emission CT (SPECT) or xenon-enhanced CT. Images provided by these studies allow visualization of the vascular steal phenomenon and the identification of eloquent brain that may be at risk of ischemia after surgical excision or embolization.[30, 42] SPECT is a noninvasive study that provides direct anatomic correlation between brain tissue perfusion and neurologic function. SPECT is capable of documenting areas of decreased perfusion before the development of brain infarction.[43]

Xenon-enhanced CT produces useful clinical information for patients with hemorrhagic stroke. Xenon-enhanced CT and blood flow studies require the CT scanner to have integrated software and hardware for the measurement of vascular flow. This method provides information about blood flow and anatomic correlation and is important in the diagnosis of delayed ischemic deficit. Blood flow measures less than or equal to 20 mL/100 g of brain per minute correlate closely with neurologic deficit. Blood flow measures less than 15 mL/100 g of brain per minute correlate positively with brain infarction.[43] .

Diagnostic radiologic imaging procedures can be safely performed in pregnant women, but they require proper shielding of the fetus. Contrast agents used in angiography appear to pose no fetal threat. However, when operative procedures are planned on a pregnant woman with neurovascular disease, use of both a neurosurgical and an obstetric anesthesiologist is recom-

TABLE 44–5

Criteria for the Diagnosis of Vasospasm by Transcranial Doppler

Mean Middle Cerebral Artery Velocity (cm/sec)	Degree of Vasospasm
100–120	Borderline vasospasm
120–160	Mild vasospasm
160–200	Moderate vasospasm
>200	Severe vasospasm

From Wojner AW: Neurovascular disease. In: Kinney MR, Dunbar SB, Brooks-Brun JA, et al (eds): AACN Clinical Reference for Critical Care Nursing. St. Louis, Mosby–Year Book, 1998, pp 733–766.

mended, with cautious maternal and fetal monitoring provided throughout the case.[33,34]

Nursing Diagnoses

Patients with stroke require vigilant nursing care consisting of expert neurologic assessment, ongoing multiorgan system assessment, and delivery of nursing care in a nonstressful, healing environment. In patients with ischemic stroke or hemorrhagic stroke with an extremely moribund presentation, interdisciplinary providers must base decisions on providing aggressive care on the patient's expressed end-of-life wishes.

Table 44–6 contains a list of priority nursing diagnoses that may apply to patients with stroke. Interventions designed to provide holistic care must be delivered within a collaborative multidisciplinary en-

vironment and must be framed by goals aimed at preventing complications, ensuring early mobilization, and resuming self-care activities.[44]

Collaborative Management

Approximately 25 to 50% of stroke survivors suffer partial or total dependence in ADLs.[44] To enhance poststroke recovery, rehabilitative processes must begin during the acute phase of hospitalization to promote successful societal reintegration.[45]

In both ischemic stroke and nonsurgical hemorrhagic stroke, patients with minimal to severe deficits generally require few acute care interventions, yet they remain needy in the area of rehabilitative and convalescent custodial care. Recognizing this need, most hospitals in the United States now provide stroke care routinely beyond the traditional boundaries of the intensive care unit (ICU), in less costly, highly specialized stroke units.[7] The overall goals of care in these units include preventing complications, optimizing nutrition, and stabilizing physiologic status, so that the patient rapidly moves through the acute care phase, within approximately 5 days, toward placement in a suitable rehabilitative care facility. The use of structured care methodologies (SCM), such as critical pathways, protocols, order sets, and algorithms, helps to support this rapid movement, by providing a quality care framework for interdisciplinary practice.[8, 45] The interdisciplinary critical pathway for a patient with ischemic or nonoperative hemorrhagic stroke is an example of such a pathway (Figure 44–2).

TABLE 44–6

Nursing Diagnoses

Problem Statement	Etiologic Factors
Altered tissue perfusion, cerebral	Interruption in cerebral blood flow secondary to cerebral embolus, intracranial hemorrhage, cerebral edema, vasospasm, or steal phenomenon
Impaired verbal communication	Aphasia, dysarthria secondary to impaired cerebral circulation, neuromuscular impairment, or impaired level of consciousness
Sensory/perceptual alterations	Inability to receive, transmit, or integrate sensory data secondary to cerebral damage
Ineffective airway clearance	Ineffective cough secondary to dysphagia or impaired level of consciousness
Ineffective breathing pattern	Cerebral damage, brain stem dysfunction
Risk for aspiration	Ineffective cough, altered consciousness, absent gag reflex, neuromuscular dysfunction
Activity intolerance	Neuromuscular dysfunction secondary to cerebral damage, impaired level of consciousness
Self-care deficit	Limitations in neuromuscular functioning, sensory and perceptual alterations, impaired cognitive processes
Body image disturbance	Changes in neuromuscular functioning, sensory and perceptual alterations
Impaired swallowing	Neuromuscular/perceptual impairment
Altered nutrition, less than body requirements	Dysphagia, altered consciousness
Knowledge deficit	Condition, treatment strategies, self-care and discharge education and planning
Ineffective individual/family coping	Sudden change in health status of family member, uncertain prognosis, change in family roles

| HEALTH OUTCOMES INSTITUTE, INC.
Interdisciplinary Critical Pathway
DRG 014: Ischemic or Nonoperative Hemorrhagic Stroke | | | | Addressograph | |

DATE	DAY 1: _____	DAY 2: _____	DAY 3: _____	DAY 4: _____	DISCHARGE TARGET DAY 5: _____
CONSULTS	Neurology; social service; dietitian; physical and occupational therapists; consider speech and language pathologist	Physical medicine and rehabilitation (PM & R)			Consider consult for percutaneous gastrotomy tube
DIAGNOSTICS	Chest radiograph Brain CT scan 12-Lead ECG Chemistry 7 & 12 CBC and platelets PT/PTT Consider prealbumin	Consider carotid Doppler Anticoagulated: PT/PTT Consider transesophageal echocardiogram	Consider modified barium swallow study Anticoagulated: PT/PTT	Anticoagulated: PT/PTT Consider prealbumin	Anticoagulated: PT/PTT
ASSESSMENTS	Calculate National Institute of Health Stroke Scale score Calculate dysphagia risk score Neurologic assessment q2–4h Intake and output q8h	Complete PM&R therapy plan Neurologic assessment q2–4h Intake and output q8h	Neurologic assessment q4h Intake and output prn	Neurologic assessment q4–8h Intake and output prn	Neurologic assessment q8h and at discharge
TREATMENTS	Consider weight-based heparin protocol Consider rt-PA protocol Consider dysphagia protocol	Consider continency protocol	Consider warfarin therapy		Discontinue heparin
ACTIVITY	Begin stroke activity protocol; advance as directed by physical therapist	Stroke activity protocol Begin ADL retraining protocol; advance as directed by physical therapist	Stroke activity protocol ADL retraining protocol	Stroke activity protocol ADL retraining protocol	Stroke activity protocol ADL retraining protocol
NUTRITION	Nutrition risk screening Consider nutritional assessment Order diet to suit swallow competency and nutritional needs	Diet as ordered by registered dietitian	Diet as ordered by registered dietitian	Diet as ordered by registered dietitian	Diet as ordered by registered dietitian
PT/FAMILY EDUCATION	Introduction to stroke disease process	Individual care routine: ADLs	Nutritional management	Prevention of complications	Collaborate with patient/family to generate discharge care plan
DISCHARGE PLANNING	Complete patient assessment profile Assess for advance directive and durable power of attorney Notify payer	Patient and family counseling regarding discharge options Referral made to discharge site		Transfer/discharge plans finalized	Provide contact numbers for nursing, registered dietitian, speech and language pathologist, physical therapist, occupational therapist, physician, social worker Discharge

Figure 44–2

An example of a clinical pathway for ischemic or nonoperative hemorrhagic stroke. (Adapted from Health Outcomes Institute, Inc., The Woodlands, Texas.)

Common Ischemic and Hemorrhagic Stroke Problems and Interventions

Increased Intracranial Pressure

The three potential origins of increased ICP after stroke are ischemic brain edema, intracranial hemorrhage, and hydrocephalus. This section is primarily devoted to brain edema as the cause of increased ICP. Other causes of increased ICP are covered separately.

The development of brain edema after stroke insult is the direct result of failed cellular perfusion.[7] Edema results secondary to arterial occlusion in ischemic stroke. In hemorrhagic stroke, edema results from the hemorrhagic volume with its associated mass effect, producing an increase in ICP, and restriction of normal arterial perfusion to surrounding brain tissue.[20, 46]

In the case of increased ICP in stroke, drainage of CSF by ventriculostomy is usually considered a first-line treatment. Use of diuretic therapy for treatment of ICP associated with aneurysmal hemorrhage should be cautiously undertaken because loss of intravascular volume may exacerbate vasospasm.[8] Placing the patient in a pentobarbital coma is an aggressive measure that may be considered when ventriculostomy fails to reduce ICP.[47] Chart 44–3 presents a protocol for the use of pentobarbital in the treatment of increased ICP.

Hyperventilation therapy aimed at driving down arterial carbon dioxide levels should be cautiously undertaken in stroke patients with increased ICP, because of the potential for further reduction in cellular perfusion in the presence of a respiratory alkalosis.[8] When hyperventilation therapy is used, it should be guided by jugular venous oxygen saturation (JvO_2) monitoring to ensure that oxygen is released to brain tissues.[48] Use of adrenocorticosteroids is controversial in stroke patients with increased ICP, but some providers continue to advocate the use of these agents as a mechanism to control edema and to protect ischemic brain tissue. Nursing measures for the management of increased ICP are similar to those discussed in Chapter 41 on acute head trauma and consist of minimal stimulation, elevation of the head of the bed 15 to 30°, and careful positioning to maintain the head and neck in neutral alignment to facilitate jugular venous drainage. Nursing care may also extend to maintenance of ICP monitoring and ventriculostomy systems, based on the degree of neurologic compromise the patient exhibits and on the aggressiveness of the care regimen.

CHART 44–3

Pentobarbital Coma Protocol

1. Consult anesthesiologist for intubation, oximetric pulmonary artery catheter insertion, jugular bulb catheter insertion, and initiation of pentobarbital protocol.
2. Consult clinical pharmacist for ongoing medication and interaction monitoring.
3. Consult registered dietitian for comprehensive enteral nutritional support.
4. Move ventilator and intubation setup to bedside.
5. Place warming blanket on bed; make continuous temperature monitoring and automatic blanket temperature adjustments to maintain patient temperature between 97 and 100°F.
6. a. Administer loading dose of pentobarbital 10 mg/kg over 30 minutes IV.
   b. Follow with pentobarbital 5 mg/kg/hr for 3 hours to achieve a serum pentobarbital concentration greater than 2 mg/dL.
   c. Follow with a maintenance dose of 2.5 mg/kg/hr.
   d. If intracranial pressure (ICP) increases above 20 mm Hg, and the serum pentobarbital concentration is <3 mg/dL, administer an additional pentobarbital 5 mg/kg IV over 30 minutes to reduce ICP.
7. Administer morphine sulfate _____ mg IV every 2 hours for duration of pentobarbital therapy.
8. Administer _____ (paralytic agent) _____ mg IV _____ (frequency) for duration of pentobarbital therapy; assess depth of neuromuscular blockade every 15 minutes until 1–2 twitch response is achieved; follow with assessments of depth of neuromuscular blockade every 8 hours.
9. Obtain baseline arterial blood gases, hematocrit and hemoglobin, serum osmolality, and cardiac output with calculated hemodynamic profile within 1 hour of loading dose administration.
10. Draw serum pentobarbital levels at 4, 8, 12, and 24 hours after initial loading dose (therapeutic range, 2–4 mg/dL).
11. Monitor SvO_2, SpO_2, JvO_2, and temperature continuously.
12. Repeat cardiac output every 8 hours for first 24 hours, then once daily and as needed for duration of pentobarbital therapy.
13. Obtain serum pentobarbital levels once daily for duration of therapy; maintain level between 2 and 4 mg/dL.
14. Set ventricular drain at an overflow level of _____ mm Hg/cm H_2O; document ICP, cerebral perfusion pressure, and ventricular drainage hourly.

Adapted with permission from the Health Outcomes Institute, Inc., The Woodlands, TX.

Sensorimotor Disability

Early mobilization during the acute phase of stroke care is an important goal. However, in some patients mobilization may be limited to passive range of motion because of increased ICP, the effect of medications, or the presence of severe paralysis. The nurse should foster some degree of involvement in self-care activities, dictated by neurologic compromise, from the moment the patient enters the acute care system.[7]

Approximately 75% of stroke patients suffer hemiparesis as an outcome after stroke.[44] Skin integrity must be closely monitored in patients with hemiparesis. Provision of appropriate nutrition and hydration, routine cleansing, turning, positioning, and careful transfer technique contribute significantly to maintenance of skin integrity.[7]

Approximately 10% of stroke patients die annually from pulmonary embolus secondary to deep vein thrombosis (DVT). Low-molecular-weight or low-dose heparin may complement a sensorimotor rehabilitation program, thus reducing the risk of DVT by 45 to 47%.[44, 49]

Dysphagia and Nutritional Needs

Swallowing function is commonly insulted after stroke, yet many practitioners fail to assess swallow integrity completely. When neurologic impairment involves both voluntary and involuntary neurocontrol mechanisms in the motor and sensory cortex, subcortical regions, or brain stem, temporary or permanent dysphagia may result.[7] Interdisciplinary care of stroke patients with dysphagia should prevent aspiration, provide nutrition that meets individual protein and calorie needs, prevent dehydration, and when possible, aim to restore normal swallowing function.

Chart 44–4 lists important physical assessment findings associated with severe swallowing dysfunction requiring tube feeding after stroke. A speech and language pathologist should be consulted when preliminary bedside findings demonstrate potential dysphagia. Visualization of swallow integrity can be accomplished by modified barium swallow, when the patient's cognitive function and level of consciousness permit use of this diagnostic technique. An intact gag reflex alone does not indicate normal swallowing function. In fact, an intact gag reflex may be found in some patients with severe dysphagia who are at risk of aspiration.[7]

When the severity of dysphagia suggests the need for alternative feeding routes, the gut should be used unless contraindicated. A period as short as 3 days without adequate nutrition in stroke has been associated with untoward outcomes including fever of unknown origin requiring a septic workup, inability to wean from mechanical ventilation, activity intolerance reducing eligibility for rehabilitation, and an increased hospital length of stay.[50] The expertise of a nutrition support dietitian should be used to guide therapy and to measure the effectiveness of nutritional care. Nursing staff should carefully monitor all oral intake and should keep a suction apparatus on hand for use as needed.

Bowel and Bladder Dysfunction

Urinary incontinence is common after stroke because of neurologic deficit affecting the bladder, immobility, alteration in level of consciousness, inability to communicate needs, or cognitive inattention. The use of indwelling urinary catheters should be avoided to reduce the risk of infection. Use of a urinary continence protocol that includes defined toileting intervals, monitoring of fluid intake, or intermittent catheterization often leads to successful attainment of continence.[44]

Bowel incontinence, usually in the form of diarrhea, also occurs frequently after stroke and may be related to intolerance to a tube feeding formula, infection, or specific medications. Once infection has been ruled out, the dietitian and pharmacist should be consulted to assist with management of diarrhea. The presence of fecal impaction should also be ruled out.[7, 44]

Perceptual Deficit: Unilateral Neglect

Unilateral neglect is defined as a disturbance in spatial perception affecting the contralateral side.[7] Approximately 50% of patients with strokes affecting the right cerebral hemisphere and approximately 25% of those with left hemispheric strokes may develop neglect.[51]

Neglect challenges a stroke patient's ability to be functionally independent in ADLs because the patient disregards half of his or her world, including one-half of the body. Patients with neglect may wash and dress only half of their body, and yet they perceive their actions to be complete.[7] Similarly, activities involving independent mobility may result in collision with structures that are not recognized within the patient's

---

CHART 44–4

Clinical Findings Associated With Tube Feeding Dependency After Stroke

Wet voice after swallowing water
Cough, during or immediately after water swallow
Hypoglossal nerve dysfunction
Incomplete oral labial closure

Adapted from the work of Wojner AW, Walton MW, Dildy T, et al: Predictors of tube feeding dependency following acute stroke.

perceptual space. Unfortunately, research has yet to identify whether lasting benefit is achieved through the use of compensation therapies in the patient with this disorder.

Communication

Approximately 40% of stroke patients suffer from speech and language disorders.[44] Written and verbal assessments of language function should be performed early after admission for stroke. Consultation with a speech and language pathologist should occur when fluency of speech is altered by dysarthria, "word-finding" errors, or the presence of an expressive (ability to use written or spoken language to respond), receptive (ability to receive written or spoken language), or global aphasia (both an expressive and a receptive aphasia). Speech and language alterations reduce employability and quality of life and place the patient at risk of social isolation.[7] Family counseling should be provided to introduce special therapeutic techniques and to clarify both expectations and functional limitations. Alternative forms of communication should be considered by multidisciplinary providers.

Neuropsychological Outcomes

Approximately 68% of stroke survivors have been reported to suffer from poststroke depression (PSD).[44] In cases of aneurysmal SAH, over 50% of patients have been found to experience some degree of psychiatric dysfunction involving PSD or cognitive dysfunction.[22] Strokes involving the left anterior cerebral cortex, the basal ganglia, or the right posterior cerebrum may produce PSD. Paradoxical cheerfulness may result from strokes in the right anterior cortex.[7]

Warning signs signifying the presence of PSD include loss of appetite, tearfulness, reduced energy, disinterest in ADLs, and agitation.[7] Unfortunately, stroke patients suffering from depression carry increased mortality rates in the immediate 10 years after stroke; they have increased lengths of stay in rehabilitation and are more likely to suffer from failed social reintegration.[44, 52] Antidepressants and psychotherapy may successfully treat PSD, but they should be coupled with appropriate family support.[7]

Cognitive dysfunction is a common outcome after frontal lobe stroke. Patients with cognitive dysfunction have an alteration in orientation, memory, insight, judgment, or abstract reasoning skills.[7] The presence of cognitive dysfunction limits the successfulness of rehabilitation efforts, prolongs length of stay in both acute and rehabilitative care, and reduces both functional independence and socialization.[53] Cognitive retraining should begin during the acute care phase of recovery and should continue through rehabilitation, but the long-term effectiveness of these therapies has yet to be established in the literature.

Hemorrhagic Stroke Problems and Interventions

Hydrocephalus

Approximately 25% of patients with hemorrhagic stroke develop ventriculomegaly within 72 hours of the hemorrhagic event. Causes include intraventricular hemorrhage and CSF obstruction at the level of the subarachnoid cisterns or arachnoid villi. Hydrocephalus is classified as acute or chronic, depending on the time of its occurrence.[5, 37]

Patients with hydrocephalus require immediate treatment by lateral frontal ventriculostomy to reduce intracranial hypertension. More than half these patients demonstrate clinical improvement once the ventriculostomy is in place.[5, 22] Most commonly, patients requiring ventriculostomy management are easily weaned from the drain over a few days. Weaning consists of clamping the ventriculostomy drain for a designated period, during which the patient is closely assessed for clinical signs suggestive of increased ICP. When weaning is not tolerated, the system is unclamped and is returned to active monitoring and drainage, or a permanent shunt procedure is performed.[8]

Chronic ventriculomegaly develops between the tenth and thirtieth days after SAH.[5, 46] Fibrotic scarring of the ventricular system and the subarachnoid granulations produce long-term interference with CSF absorption. Most patients with chronic ventriculomegaly undergo placement of a permanent ventriculoperitoneal (VP) shunt.

Fluid and Electrolyte Imbalance

Fluid and electrolyte imbalance related to salt-wasting syndrome, syndrome of inappropriate antidiuretic hormone (SIADH), or diabetes insipidus (DI) may also occur in hemorrhagic stroke. Salt-wasting syndrome is thought to be caused by centrally elaborated atrial natriuretic factor,[22, 54] although the exact mechanism that triggers its onset is unknown. Most neuroscientists believe that hyponatremia in hemorrhagic stroke is due to this poorly understood syndrome, which produces a primary sodium loss typically associated with volume contraction.[55]

SIADH is still considered by some investigators to be the cause of hyponatremia in hemorrhagic stroke. The greatest risk of SIADH appears to occur in patients with hemorrhage in the area of the anterior communicating artery, which is thought to interfere with the supraoptic hypothalamic neurons that secrete antidiuretic hormone (ADH).[46] This process results in abnormal ADH production and release, unrelated to true serum osmolality or volume status. Water is retained by the kidneys in SIADH, resulting in hyponatremic expansion of extracellular fluid volume. Volume expansion suppresses aldosterone release, resulting in a secondary depletion of sodium from reduced tubular sodium reabsorption.[22]

In SIADH, fluid volume should be restricted, whereas salt-wasting syndrome may require rehydration guided by clinical assessment.[55] Both syndromes may include the administration of hypertonic (3%) saline to treat marked hyponatremia. Vigilant monitoring of hydration status is necessary in patients with aneurysmal SAH, because decreased hydration may trigger the onset of vasospasm.

DI may also occur in patients with hemorrhagic stroke through a similar mechanism as described for SIADH. In DI, urine outputs greater than or equal to 300 mL per hour are associated with a specific gravity less than 1.005 g/mL. Patients also present with polydipsia, elevated serum osmolality, and elevated serum sodium levels secondary to excessive fluid volume loss from failure to release ADH. Cautious intake and output records must be maintained. Volume must be replaced regularly, especially in patients at risk for the development of vasospasm. Aqueous ADH or desmopressin (1-deamine-8-D-arginine vasopressin [DDAVP]) may be ordered if replacement volumes become impractical.[22, 46]

Seizures

Seizures after hemorrhagic stroke have been reported in 10 to 30% of patients. Seizure development is thought to be related to direct cortical irritation by blood. Seizures usually occur only during the first few minutes after hemorrhage, but a few patients may go on to develop chronic epilepsy.[22, 46]

Anticonvulsants are used prophylactically during the acute phase of SAH management. The location of the hemorrhage within the brain may allow anticonvulsant use to be terminated, or it may mandate that it be continued for years after the stroke.[22] Phenytoin or phenobarbital should be considered for maintenance therapy. When these drugs are unsuccessful at controlling seizures, carbamazepine may be used with good results. Serum drug levels and hematologic and liver function tests should be followed in patients receiving anticonvulsant therapy.[47] Anticonvulsants should be avoided during pregnancy because of their known teratogenic effects.[34]

Hypertension

Hypertension after hemorrhagic stroke may be pronounced in patients with preexisting hypertension. In the face of increased ICP or vasospasm, abrupt reduction of arterial pressure may place patients at risk of an ischemic insult.[8] Preoperatively, when definitive obliteration of the bleeding source has not occurred, systolic blood pressures greater than 160 mm Hg, or a mean arterial pressure greater than 110 mm Hg, may place the patient at significant risk of rebleeding.[47, 56]

During any attempt to manipulate blood pressure, hemodynamics, neurologic status, cerebral perfusion pressure (CPP), and ICP should be closely monitored.

Blood pressure should be reduced modestly over time to optimize hemodynamics and to prevent reduction of intracranial blood flow resulting in neurologic deficit. Increased ICP should be treated by ventricular drainage and diuretic therapy, before manipulation of arterial pressure.[56]

Neurogenic Pulmonary Edema

Hemorrhagic stroke has also been associated with the development of neurogenic pulmonary edema (NPE).[46, 47] NPE is thought to be the result of hypothalamic irritation, secondary to an acute rise in ICP, which leads to a massive sympathetic, adrenergic discharge, systemic vasoconstriction, and systemic hypertension causing a shift of blood to the lower resistance pulmonary circuit. The acute shift in blood increases pulmonary capillary hydrostatic pressure, which triggers the development of noncardiogenic NPE.[57] Researchers believe that the homeostatic intention for the shift in blood volume is aimed at maintaining CPP after an acute rise in ICP.[46]

NPE occurs in patients lacking a history or clinical evidence of cardiac disease or volume overload. Its clinical signs include elevated pulmonary pressures, decreased lung compliance, alveolar fluid accumulation, and subsequent alveolar collapse associated with ventilation–perfusion mismatch and hypoxemia. Treatment of NPE includes ICP reduction and control, mechanical ventilation with positive end-expiratory pressure, and optimizing of cardiovascular function.[46]

Specific Management for Ischemic Stroke

Experimental Drug Therapy

The discovery of the metabolic cascade in brain ischemia has directed movement toward identification of drug agents that may arrest cellular destruction. Glutamate antagonists such as MK-801 are under study to determine whether inhibition of the cellular response to glutamate release can prevent irreversible cellular changes. Blockage of the N-methyl-D-aspartate (NMDA) receptor-mediated channels, which regulate calcium ion intake after glutamate release, is also under study, specifically identification of NMDA antagonists that will penetrate the blood–brain barrier.[12, 58]

Adenosine, which functions as a neuromodulator capable of preventing release of neurotransmitters including glutamate, is being investigated to determine whether this agent may play a role in inhibiting cellular destruction from stroke. Calpain inhibitors capable of countering the effects of this protease during intracellular acidosis are also under development.[12, 58]

The use of growth factors, specifically basic fibroblast growth factor (bFGF), a polypeptide with an ability to promote sprouting and survival of neurons, to stimulate glial cell division, and to foster angiogenesis, is also under investigation. The sprouting effects promoted by bFGF may provide a means to rewire injured neuronal networks because neuronal cells do not divide.[12, 58]

Antithrombotic Therapy

Use of antithrombotic therapy including heparin or heparinoids and warfarin is controversial in the patient with ischemic stroke. The rationale in support of antithrombotic therapy suggests that these agents may prevent stroke progression and recurrence through prevention of an additional occluding thrombus or thromboemboli at the site of occlusion. Practice varies widely among providers, but it is generally accepted that patients with cardioembolic stroke or those with progressing stroke or crescendo TIA are likely to benefit from antithrombotic therapy.[7] The risk of hemorrhagic transformation of an ischemic lesion must also be considered when undertaking antithrombotic therapy. The reported incidence of hemorrhagic transformation is between 1 and 7% and may be related to the use of antithrombotic agents, or it may occur spontaneously in patients who are not anticoagulated.[59]

Thrombolytic Therapy

Use of thrombolytic agents such as streptokinase, urokinase, and tissue plasminogen activator (tPA) in the acute treatment of ischemic stroke continues to be evaluated by neuroscientists. A randomized, double-blind trial of recombinant tPA (rtPA) in ischemic stroke found that the drug was beneficial when it was started within 3 hours of the onset of stroke symptoms (see Appendix, ACLS: Algorithm for Suspected Stroke Patients, Figure 12). Slightly more than 6% of patients who received rtPA developed intracranial hemorrhages within 36 hours of stroke occurrence.[60]

Thrombolytic agents for the treatment of acute ischemic stroke remain controversial. Neuroscience practitioners must weigh the risk of brain or systemic hemorrhage against possible therapeutic benefit. A checklist of patient inclusion and exclusion criteria for rtPA administration is presented in Chart 44–5, whereas Chart 44–6 represents an order set for administration of rtPA in ischemic stroke.

Specific Management for Intracranial Aneurysms

Aneurysm Occlusion

Approximately 20% of unoperated patients with ruptured intracranial aneurysm experience an episode of rebleeding that is frequently fatal.[46] Traditionally, neurosurgical teaching dictated a surgical delay of 10 to 14 days from the initial rupture of an aneurysm to

---

CHART 44–5

Recombinant Tissue Plasminogen Activator Ischemic Stroke Inclusion or Exclusion Criteria Checklist

Inclusion Criteria:

_____ Age ≥18 years and functionally independent before current presentation

_____ Clinical diagnosis of ischemic stroke with measurable neurologic deficit

_____ CT scan negative for intracranial hemorrhage

_____ Presentation within 180 minutes of symptom onset

Exclusion Criteria:

_____ Rapid improvement in neurologic function before treatment

_____ CT scan positive for intracranial hemorrhage

_____ Evolving infarction documented on CT scan with acute hypodensity or mass effect

_____ Presentation suggests subarachnoid hemorrhage in the face of a negative CT scan

_____ History of seizure before or during stroke event

_____ Extreme moribund presentation

_____ Inability to maintain systolic blood pressure <185 or diastolic blood pressure <110 mm Hg

_____ Aggressive hypertensive control requiring sodium nitroprusside

_____ Serum glucose <50 mg/dL or >400 mg/dL

_____ History of surgery or trauma within the past 14 days

_____ Arterial puncture at a noncompressible site

_____ Lumbar puncture within the past 7 days

_____ History positive for stroke within the last 3 months

_____ History of intracranial hemorrhage

_____ Possible postmyocardial pericarditis

_____ Lactating or pregnant woman

Reprinted with permission from the Health Outcomes Institute, Inc., The Woodlands, TX.

CHART 44–6

Recombinant Tissue Plasminogen Activator (rtPA) Ischemic Stroke Order Set

1. Complete inclusion and exclusion criteria checklist.
2. Call stroke response team stat.
3. Start two IV lines as follows:
   a. Dedicated rtPA infusion line
   b. Keep vein open (KVO) line for other fluid and medication administration
4. Insert Foley catheter if patient unable to void before start of rtPA infusion.
5. Calculate dosage of rtPA 0.9 mg/kg:
   Step A. Patient weight _____ kg × 0.9 mg = _____ **mg total rtPA dose.** (**Stop: Check dose;** if greater than 90 mg by calculation, give total of 90 mg only.)
   Step B. Administer 10% of total rtPA dose as an initial bolus: _____ mg total rtPA dose × 0.10 = _____ **mg bolus dose.**

Step C. Administer the balance of the rtPA over the next 60 minutes. _____ mg total rtPA − _____ mg bolus dose = _____ **mg infusion dose.**

6. Neurologic vital signs every 15 minutes for 1 hour; then begin once hourly for 5 hours, and then every 2 hours for 18 hours. Increase frequency of neurologic vital signs as indicated by the patient's clinical status. Notify MD stat of signs and symptoms of deterioration.
7. Cardiac monitoring for 24 hours.
8. After rtPA infusion, perform no nasoenteric or nasogastric tube insertions, Foley catheter insertions, or invasive lines or procedures for 24 hours unless clinically indicated.
9. Stat brain CT scan for signs and symptoms of clinical deterioration.
10. Stop anticoagulant or antiplatelet medications until further notice.

Adapted with permission from the Health Outcomes Institute, Inc., The Woodlands, TX.

beyond the peak period for vasospasm.[20] Current trends toward early operation have reduced the risk of rebleeding, although an overall effect on mortality and morbidity has not been achieved. Early surgical intervention with microsurgical clipping of the intracranial aneurysm suggests that patients undergo operation within the first 72 hours after SAH, or in an increasing number of institutions, immediately on presentation.[23, 61] Exceptions to early surgery are made for patients with morbid presentation. In these cases, practitioners must grapple with the possibility of prolonging a vegetative existence, instead of restoring meaningful neurologic function.[62]

Successful aneurysm clipping involves total obliteration of the aneurysm and preservation of all native vessels (Figure 44–3). Many types of clips are available for occluding saccular or fusiform aneurysms. Wrapping techniques may be used to reinforce the walls of an aneurysm that cannot be surgically clipped. Postoperatively, angiograms are performed to document complete obliteration.[8]

The emergence of Guglielmi detachable coils (GDCs) shows great promise as an endovascular treatment for aneurysms. The GDC method is particularly well suited for those aneurysms with narrow necks, from 5 mm to giant size, located within the ICA, MCA,

and basilar artery circulations.[63] The treatment is performed by an interventional neuroradiologist and is usually performed with the patient under local or general anesthesia.

The GDC coil is inserted through the aneurysm neck, into the dome, and an electrical current is passed through the coil to promote electrothrombosis within the aneurysm. At the same time, electrolysis of the system's wire occurs, detaching the platinum coil in the aneurysm without any traction. Coil therapy is now considered an alternative for inoperable aneurysms, but the long-term results are still not known.[63]

Vasospasm

Vasospasm is a delayed narrowing of the large arteries at the base of the brain after SAH. It is usually associated with evidence of reduced distal perfusion to brain tissue in affected arteries. Vasospasm typically has its onset at 3 to 5 days after the hemorrhagic event. Maximal narrowing of vasospastic arteries occurs between the fifth and fourteenth days after hemorrhage, followed by a gradual resolution over 2 to 4 weeks. Approximately 50% of patients suffering from vasospasm develop a neurologic ischemic deficit, which may resolve or may progress to permanent brain infarction.[5]

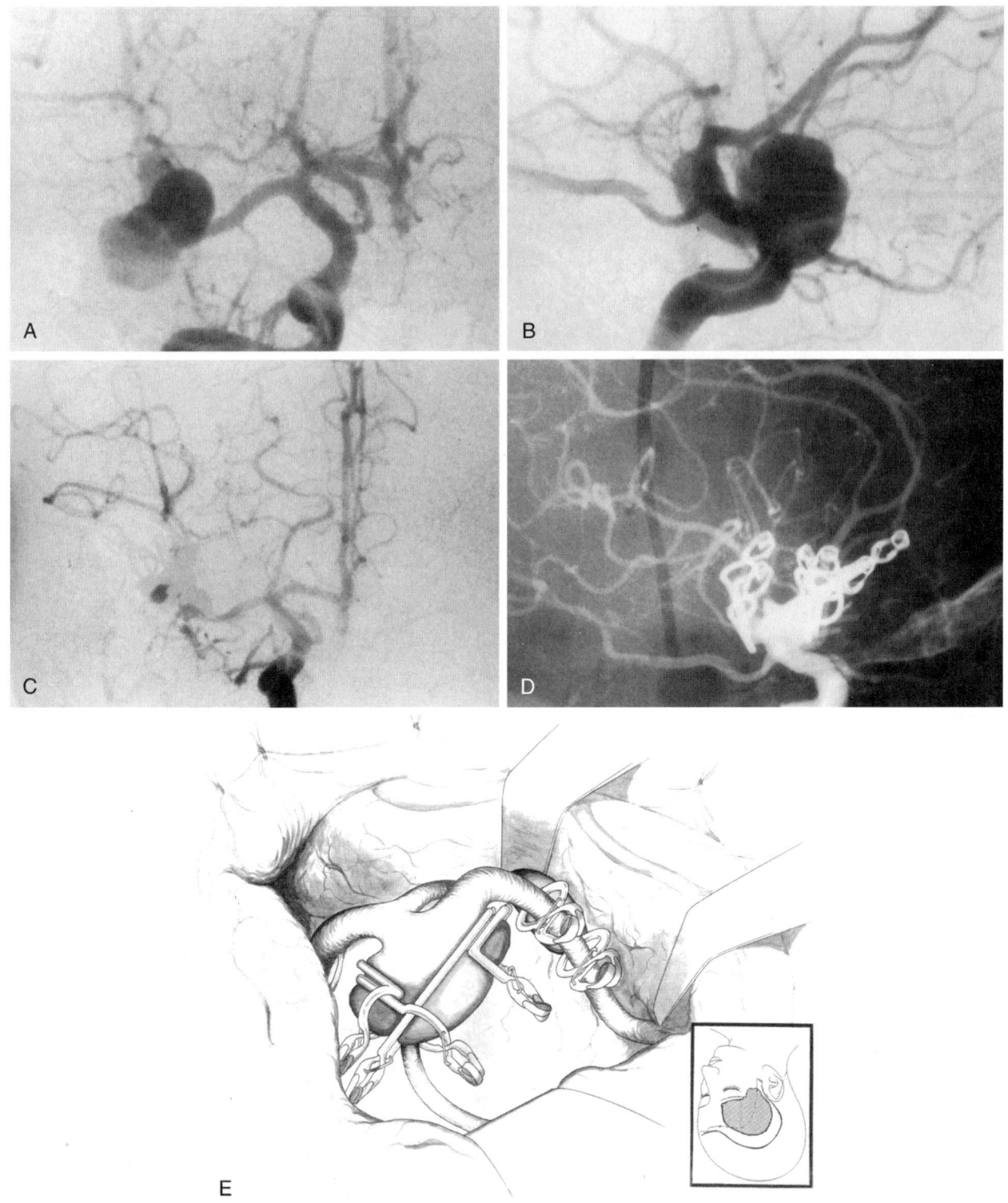

Figure 44–3

A giant middle cerebral artery aneurysm. *A* and *B*, Preoperative views of the right carotid artery. *C* and *D*, Right carotid angiograms 2 years after surgery show exclusion of the aneurysm. *E*, Illustration showing clipping. The body of the giant aneurysm was occluded with clips and then reinforced. Two angled-ring clips were used to occlude a fusiform dilatation of the distal portion of the aneurysm. The remaining portion of the neck of the aneurysm was wrapped with soft cellulose patty. (From Youmans JR: Neurological Surgery, 4th ed. vol. 2. Philadelphia, WB Saunders, 1996, p 1316.)

The pathogenesis of vasospasm has been studied for more than 20 years, yet today we remain uncertain of its origin. The most widely accepted theory explaining arterial vasospasm proposes that a substance within the blood itself acts on the smooth muscle in the walls of small arteries and arterioles to cause vasoconstriction. More than 30 vasoactive substances, including neurotransmitters, and blood constituents have been investigated.[8] Oxyhemoglobin is currently the focus of much study leading to an evaluation of the effect of antioxidants in the treatment of vasospasm.[64, 65]

Clinically apparent symptoms of brain ischemia secondary to vasospasm are found in only about one-third of patients with SAH, but up to 70% of patients with SAH demonstrate subclinical spasm documented on angiographic and TCD studies. Serial TCD examinations are helpful in detecting progressive increases in blood flow velocity resulting from vasospasm, but direct confirmation by angiogram remains the current standard for diagnosis.[22]

Triple "H" therapy remains at the center of vasospasm treatment. The combination of *hypertension*, *hypervolemia*, and *hemodilution* optimizes blood flow and oxygen delivery to brain tissues.[22, 23] When aggressive fluid administration is prescribed, use of a pulmonary artery catheter with calculation of cardiac performance indices should guide preload augmentation.

In "low-flow" states such as vasospasm, viscous resistance may become elevated to a point where blood flow stops completely. Hematocrit reduction with low-molecular-weight dextran or 5% albumin may enhance blood flow when hematocrit is reduced to approximately 30%. When hematocrit drops below 30%, the reduction in oxygen-carrying capacity overrides the benefit of reduced viscosity in the microcirculation.[66]

Vasopressors such as phenylephrine or dopamine may be administered to produce hypertension. Systolic blood pressure may be safely increased to 160 to 170 mm Hg in patients with unsecured aneurysms, whereas in those with secured aneurysms, systolic augmentation to a high of 200 mm Hg has been used successfully to block vasospasm.[22, 23] Pulmonary artery and arterial monitoring should be used in patients receiving aggressive hypertensive therapy to enhance assessment of cardiac system tolerance of significant afterload.

Balloon angioplasty dilation of vasospastic intracranial arteries has been shown to reestablish blood flow rapidly and to prevent ischemic insult to brain tissues. Vasospasm is thought to involve the reorganization and constriction of collagen fibers within arterial vessel walls by myofibroblast cells. Balloon angioplasty redistributes collagen, disrupting binding sites with myofibroblasts, and stretches the vessel wall's connective tissue matrix.[67, 68]

Balloon angioplasty catheters are floated into the carotid or vertebral artery system and are advanced to the point of constriction. Successive 8- to 10-second balloon inflations occur with each advancement along the constricted vessel until optimal anatomic vessel dilatation has been documented on angiography, and blood flow has been restored. The two primary complications associated with the procedure include vessel or aneurysm rupture and aggravated ischemia.[20]

Nimodipine is commonly used in patients with aneurysmal SAH. Initially, nimodipine was thought to reduce the incidence or severity of arterial vasospasm. Instead, the agent is now believed to exert a protective effect on brain tissues during vasospasm, thus reducing the incidence of brain infarction and improving functional outcomes.[69] Current dosage recommendations are oral nimodipine, 60 mg every 4 hours.

Specific Management for Intracranial Arteriovenous Malformations

AVMs pose a challenge to the neurosurgical team in terms of treatment decision making. Often, patients benefit from a combination of therapies that may not be available at smaller medical centers, thereby necessitating referral of therapy to an experienced neurosurgical colleague. This section discusses therapies that are available at most large medical centers to treat AVMs with the best current care.

Embolization and Combined Surgical Intervention

Preoperative embolization is used to reduce vascular shunting before surgical excision. This technique, combined with surgical resection, appears to reduce overall morbidity significantly. Embolization requires a team approach to care consisting of a neurosurgeon, a neurologist, an interventional neuroradiologist, a neuroanesthesiologist, and neuroscience nurses.[8]

Small intravascular catheters are used to embolize smaller nutrient arteries selectively in complex, deep AVMs. The microcatheter is fed inside the AVM to the point of the nidus. Embolization is then carried out using one of many different types of embolic substances including liquid glue, slurries, particulate matter, silk fibers, detachable balloons, or wire coils.[70–72]

CT or MRI scans are performed immediately after the procedure to document the effect of the embolization on surrounding brain tissue. Patients are observed clinically for signs and symptoms related to tissue ischemia that may occur secondary to the embolization itself or as a result of postprocedural edema. Embolization and definitive surgical intervention are typically separated by 7 days to allow for resolution of procedural edema before the surgical event.[73]

Surgical excision alone provides the most effective treatment for AVM. Without surgical removal, embolization may only result in subtotal occlusion and potential AVM revascularization. Microclips ranging in size from slightly larger than 1 mm to slightly larger than 4 mm are used to clip AVM vessels. After permanent vessel occlusion, the vessel is coagulated.[71]

Several complications may occur after surgical resection of an AVM, including postoperative edema secondary to surgical retraction, postoperative hemorrhage, normal perfusion pressure breakthrough, and vasospasm.[8] Vasospasm associated with AVM is uncommon, but when it complicates the postoperative course, it may be treated with the methods previously discussed for use in aneurysms. Postoperative hemorrhage is the most urgent postoperative complication, capable of producing rapid neurologic deterioration. Rebleeding has been reported to occur in approximately 1 to 6% of patients with AVM secondary to residual AVM or to insecure hemostasis. Patients experiencing rebleeding should be rapidly returned to the operating room for definitive management.[73]

Normal pressure perfusion breakthrough phenomenon may contribute to the development of postoperative hemorrhage or brain edema after AVM resection. This phenomenon occurs most commonly in patients with large, high-flow AVMs, demonstrating evidence of angiographic steal.[73] Normal perfusion pressure breakthrough is thought to occur as a result of failed autoregulatory processes within the AVM's vascular structure. The vessels outside an AVM are in a state of constant dilatation to ensure adequate tissue perfusion. After AVM resection, these vessels retain their dilated state and are bombarded with malignant pressures when normal pressure perfusion is reinstated.[8] Postoperative hemorrhage secondary to vessel rupture or brain edema from hyperperfusion results.

Stereotactic Radiosurgery

Stereotactic radiosurgery (SR) has been suggested as an alternative to surgical obliteration in patients with challenging, nonoperative AVMs.[71, 74, 75] The most common forms of SR are gamma knife SR, which uses cobalt-60 sources located within a shield that surrounds the head, and medical linear accelerator (LINAC) SR, which uses high-energy x-ray radiation. Similar outcomes are achieved with both SR systems.[75]

SR uses photon bombardment to produce physical changes in tissues through ionization. The goal of SR is delivery of high-dose radiation to a specified target while minimizing the dose to surrounding tissues. Multiple beams are fired from different directions to accomplish this goal.[75]

SR is typically an outpatient procedure. A stereotactic headframe is secured to the patient's head by four pins, which are twist drilled into the skull. After placement of the headframe, the patient undergoes diagnostic imaging by CT or MRI. After this phase, the patient is transferred to a holding area, where he or she remains with the headframe still attached for approximately 4 to 6 hours, while computer-driven, treatment planning is performed by the neurosurgical team. Activity and diet are generally ordered "as tolerated," with the patient free to move around the room independently or with assistance as needed.[75]

Once treatment plans have been completed, the patient is transported by wheelchair to the radiation suite and is placed onto the treatment couch. The headframe is locked in place to ensure pinpoint accuracy during irradiation. The total treatment varies between 30 and 60 minutes for this one-time therapy. After irradiation, the stereotactic headframe is removed, the pin insertion sites are cleansed and dressed with adhesive bandages, and the patient is returned to the outpatient unit for discharge.[75]

Time to development of radiation-induced tissue injury is directly related to the rate of cellular turnover, because cell loss after irradiation occurs in connection with cell division.[76] The tissues of the brain are slowly proliferating. Radiation injury to the CNS may take from months to years after irradiation, with a minimal latency period of 6 months. "Cure" in SR is defined as radiographically dead or inactive tissue. Patients are followed longitudinally to determine treatment effectiveness, because evidence of "cure" is not immediately available.[75]

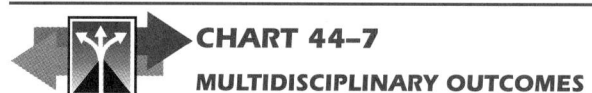

CHART 44–7
MULTIDISCIPLINARY OUTCOMES

Restoration of optimal intracranial hemodynamics

Restoration of neurologic function with minimal neurologic deficit

Promotion of adequate oxygenation and ventilation

Prevention of aspiration pneumonia

Restoration of effective cough and clear airway

Progressive participation in activities of daily living to optimal level of functioning

Successful societal reintegration

Resumption of optimal speech and language capacity

Restoration of adequate neuromotor swallow control

Achievement and maintenance of adequate nutrition and hydration

Prevention of complications related to limitations in mobility

Provision of adequate rest and sleep

Achievement of psychosocial balance

Effective individual and family coping

Staged radiosurgery is currently being studied as another form of treatment for AVMs. In staged procedures, endovascular AVM embolization is used before SR to reduce the size of the treatment area; SR then follows the embolization procedure.[70] Unfortunately, no outcomes data are currently available, but staged procedures may hold promise for AVMs deemed too large for SR treatment alone.

Multidisciplinary Outcomes

Some multidisciplinary outcomes of interest to providers caring for the stroke patient are listed in Chart 44–7. Individualized outcome statements are used both to guide the selection of multidisciplinary care and to measure the effectiveness of the care regimen.

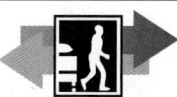 **CHART 44–8**

BEYOND THE ICU: CARE OF THE PATIENT WITH A STROKE

Care for the ischemic stroke patient has moved beyond the walls of the traditional ICU, to less costly, highly specialized stroke units. This philosophy is consistent with the needs of these patients, because beyond the administration of a thrombolytic agent, patients with ischemic stroke have few acute care needs. Acute care hospital days have declined as well in this population, with most programs moving patients to some form of rehabilitative or custodial care by the fifth to seventh day.

Hemorrhagic stroke remains more complex than ischemic stroke, in that the source of the hemorrhage must be determined, and certain untoward clinical sequelae may occur. Consequently, the patient with hemorrhagic stroke often begins a course of acute care in a traditional ICU environment. When intraparenchymal brain hemorrhage is diagnosed, the patient is generally transferred to the stroke unit and follows a similar course as the patient with ischemic stroke. However, in the case of aneurysmal subarachnoid hemorrhage or arteriovenous malformation, the patient may require long-term ICU management to combat the potential or actual untoward events associated with these disease processes.

A closer look at a typical stroke unit reveals a unit that provides care from admission to discharge. Multiple levels of care are typically provided in a stroke unit, thus enabling the patient to receive ventilator support if necessary, to traditional intermediate and general floor level care. Stroke units incorporate the rehabilitation philosophy of multidisciplinary collaborative practice, providing standardized care practices through the use of critical pathways, protocols, algorithms, and standard order sets. Patients and families are incorporated into all levels of planning, implementing, and evaluating care. Discharge planning begins on the day of admission and is a multidisciplinary team priority.

After discharge, certain care alternatives are available to the stroke patient and family. The National Institutes of Health Stroke Scale score has been used to predict discharge placement for stroke patients (see Figure 44–4). Patients with scores between 0 and 8 with minimal disability discharge to home with outpatient rehabilitative therapy. Scores of 9 to 17 define the classic inpatient rehabilitation candidate, and scores of 18 or higher represent a patient who must convalesce at a slower pace in a skilled nursing facility or subacute care center. Scores of 18 or higher also define those patients who may require prolonged custodial care.

Often, family members prefer to care for a chronically, critically ill stroke patient at home. Through preparation in the stroke unit, family members are able to assume the role of caregivers more efficiently and with less stress. Family members are involved in care delivery from the day of admission through to the day of discharge. Depending on the discharge plan, family members may assume total care of the patient for 2 to 3 days before discharge, under the supervision of the nurse. At discharge, the family is provided with contact numbers for key multidisciplinary staff members. A home health nurse assumes the role of care supervisor after discharge.

Advent of the subacute unit has greatly benefited stroke patients and families dealing with prolonged critical illness. These "chronically critically ill" patients lack acute care needs, but they require long-term support toward accomplishments such as ventilator weaning, improved level of consciousness, and enhanced functional status. Subacute units offer care to patients until they are eligible for transfer to an inpatient rehabilitation center and thus form a necessary bridge between acute and rehabilitative care for patients with long-term care needs.

Data from Wojner AW: Optimizing ischemic outcomes: an interdisciplinary approach to poststroke rehabilitation in acute care. Crit Care Nurs Q 19:1–15, 1997.

Continued rehabilitation and convalescence after discharge from an acute care setting also are important considerations after stroke. The severity of each patient's functional disability is used to drive the selection of an appropriate stroke program.[7] Figure 44–4, the National Institutes of Health Stroke Scale, is an example of a tool used to quantify a patient's disability after a stroke. Chart 44–8 provides a description of the continuum-based care sites where critical care nursing is provided to stroke patients.

Discharge to an inpatient rehabilitation center typically requires medical stability, the ability to tolerate 3 or more hours of continuous rehabilitation services, and the existence of more than one type of functional disability. Patients with complex medical problems requiring round-the-clock medical attention may be better suited for rehabilitative services at a slower pace, such as those provided at a skilled nursing facility or a subacute unit. Reassessment of the patient's appropriateness for transfer to a comprehensive rehabilitation center may then be conducted once convalescence is complete. In patients with minimal disability, rehabilitation may best be provided on an outpatient basis.[7, 44] Chart 44–9 provides an example of an ethical dilemma related to discharge planning for a stroke patient.

Optimal patient outcomes are best achieved when patients and their significant others are viewed as care partners in the recovery process. Hands-on participation enhances development of caregiver roles and improves translation of care delivery skills for continuation of therapeutic techniques after discharge.

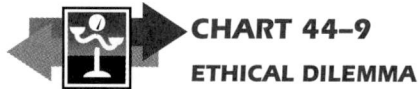

CHART 44–9

ETHICAL DILEMMA

A 43-year-old man is admitted to your unit from the emergency department with a diagnosis of acute ischemic stroke. The patient's past medical history is positive for primary hypertension, and he admits that he has not been taking his antihypertensive medications for over a year. He states that he has been unemployed and can no longer afford to fill his prescriptions or see his doctor. It has been more than 3 years since his last medical examination.

On neurologic examination, the patient is alert and oriented to time, place, and person. Visual fields are full, and extraocular movements are intact. Speech is fluent, with a mild dysarthric quality. Left hemiparesis is noted on gross motor examination, with the left arm measured at 2/5 and the left leg measured at 3/5. Partial left facial nerve palsy is noted, with flattened nasal labial folds. The patient tests positive for visual and tactile left spatial neglect. He is hemodynamically stable, and no other systems offer significant clinical findings.

The patient is an unemployed construction worker with a high school education. He has no medical insurance to cover his hospital or rehabilitative care. He is single, and he is without family to assist with medical expenses or to provide care during his recovery.

The physical medicine and rehabilitation service is consulted to determine a plan of care. The patient is found to be an excellent candidate for inpatient rehabilitation. Having no acute medical needs, he is deemed ready for transfer to a rehabilitation facility. A social worker and discharge planner make several referrals to rehabilitation centers within and surrounding the community, but none are willing to accept the patient because of his financial status. The only transfer option available is a Medicaid skilled nursing home. As the nurse caring for this patient, you are under intense pressure to expedite the discharge because the patient has no financial resources to pay for his hospital bill. Yet, you know that transfer to a nursing home may not be in the patient's best interests.

1. What is the nurse's role in identifying viable discharge options for this patient?
2. What is the patient's role in discharge planning and rehabilitation goal setting?
3. What additional information would be helpful to reconstruct a more suitable discharge plan?
4. What ethical principles support the nurse's position in this dilemma?

Indicator	Descriptor	Score
LOC	Alert, keenly responsive	0
	Drowsy, but arousable by minor stimulation to obey, answer, or respond	1
	Requires repeated stimulation to attend, or lethargic or obtunded, requiring strong or painful stimulation to make movements	2
	Responds only with reflex motor or autonomic effects, or totally unresponsive, flaccid, reflexless	3
LOC Questions The patient is asked the month and his/her age; only the initial answer is graded.		
	Answers both correctly	0
	Answers one correctly	1
	Answers both incorrectly	2
LOC Commands: The patient is instructed to open or close his or her hand or eyes. Only the initial response is graded; credit is given if an unequivocal attempt is made but not completed.		
	Obeys both correctly	0
	Obeys one correctly	1
	Answers both incorrectly	2
EOMS	Normal	0
	Partial gaze palsy. Score is given when gaze is abnormal in one or both eyes, but where forced deviation or total gaze paresis is not present	1
	Forced deviation or total gaze paresis is not overcome by the oculocephalic maneuver	2
Visual Fields: Test for hemianopia using moving fingers on confrontation with both patient's eyes open; double simultaneous stimulation is also performed. Use visual threat where LOC or comprehension limits testing. Score 1 only if clear-cut asymmetry is found; complete hemianopia (2) is recorded for dense loss extending to within 5 to 10 degrees of fixations.		
	No visual loss	0
	Partial hemianopia	1
	Complete hemianopia	2
Facial Palsy:	Normal	0
	Minor	1
	Partial	2
	Complete	3
Motor Arm: Patient is examined with arms outstretched at 90° if sitting, or at 45° if supine; request full effort for 10 seconds. If consciousness or comprehension is abnormal, cue the patient by actively lifting his or her arms into position as request for effort is orally given. Grade only the weaker limb.		
	Limb holds for 10 seconds	0
	Limb holds position but drifts before full 10 seconds	1
	Limb cannot hold position for full 10 seconds, but there is some effort against gravity	2
	Limb falls; no effort against gravity	3

Figure 44–4

The National Institutes of Health Stroke Scale. LOC, level of consciousness; EOMs, extraocular movements.

Illustration continued on following page

	Motor Leg:		
	While supine, patient is asked to maintain each leg at 30° for 5 seconds. If consciousness or comprehension is abnormal, cue the patient by actively lifting the leg into position as the request for effort is orally given. Grade only the weaker limb.		
	Leg holds 30° position for 5 seconds	0	
	Leg falls to intermediate position by the end of the 5 second period	1	
	Leg falls to bed by 5 seconds, but there is some effort against gravity	2	
	Limb falls to bed immediately with no effort against gravity	3	
Plantar reflex	Normal	0	
	Equivocal	1	
	Extensor	2	
	Bilateral extensor	3	

	Limb Ataxia:	
	Finger-to-nose and heel-to-shin tests are performed. Ataxia is scored only if clearly out of proportion to weakness. Limb ataxia is charted as "absent" in the hemiplegic; do not chart it as "untestable."	
	Absent	0
	Ataxia is present in one limb	1
	Ataxia is present in two limbs	2

	Sensory:	
	Test with pin; when consciousness or comprehension is abnormal, score sensory normal unless deficit is clearly recognized (i.e., grimacing, withdrawal). Only hemisensory losses are counted as abnormal.	
	Normal, no sensation loss	0
	Mild to moderate; patient feels pinprick is less sharp or is dull on affected side, or there is a loss of superficial pain with pinprick but patient is aware of being touched	1
	Severe to total sensation loss; the patient is not aware of being touched	2
Neglect	No neglect	0
	Visual, tactile, or auditory hemi-inattention	1
	Profound hemi-inattention to more than one modality	2
Dysarthria	Normal	0
	Mild to moderate; patient slurs at least some words; and, at worst, can be understood with some difficulty	1
	Patient's speech is so slurred as to be unintelligible (in the absence of, or out of proportion to any dysphasia)	2

	Language:	
	The patient is asked to name the items on the naming sheet and is then asked to read from the reading sheet. Comprehension is judged from responses to each of the commands in the preceding neurologic examination.	
	Normal	0
	Mild to moderate, as follows: Naming errors, word-finding errors, paraphasia, and/or impairment of comprehension or expressive disability	1
	Severe: Fully developed Broca's or Wernicke's aphasia (or variant)	2
	Mute or global aphasia	3
	TOTAL SCORE:	

Figure 44–4 *Continued*

Critical Thinking Exercise

Mr. X., a 52-year-old Asian man, is admitted with sudden onset, severe headache. Before an abrupt loss of consciousness, Mr. X. described the headache to his wife as the "worst" he had ever experienced. He now presents to you as lethargic, but responsive to verbal stimuli, disoriented to time and place, with a mild motor weakness of the right upper extremity (motor grade 4/5), and right facial nerve weakness. An emergency CT scan reveals the presence of SAH, so Mr. X. is sent for an immediate four-vessel intracranial angiogram. You are notified that the angiogram documented the presence of four intracranial aneurysms: right anterior cerebral artery (1); right MCA (1); left MCA (1); right posterior communicating artery (1). The left MCA aneurysm is the aneurysm suspected of rupturing. Mr. X. is taken for emergency operative clipping of the left MCA aneurysm and insertion of a ventriculostomy. He returns to you for postoperative admission to the neuroscience critical care unit, intubated and mechanically ventilated, with a pulmonary artery catheter, arterial line, and a peripheral intravenous line in place.

1. What is the rationale for insertion of a ventriculostomy in the patient with aneurysmal SAH?
2. Should Mr. X. develop vasospasm along the distribution of the left MCA, what additional clinical findings will he likely have on assessment?
3. Mr. X. is to be treated prophylactically for vasospasm with triple "H" therapy.
   A. Discuss the rationale that supports use of triple "H" therapy for treatment of vasospasm in aneurysmal SAH.
   B. What nursing care measures should be considered when providing triple "H" therapy to Mr. X.?

Key Concepts

⇒ Stroke results in minimal to catastrophic neurologic disability, threatening quality of life for both patients and family.

⇒ The two broad subtypes of stroke are ischemic and hemorrhagic.

⇒ Within the ischemic stroke category, thrombotic strokes are produced by a progressive narrowing of an arterial vessel wall due to atherosclerosis. Embolic strokes are caused by loss of blood flow due to an embolus lodging in an arterial vessel.

⇒ The hemorrhagic category of stroke is divided into strokes produced by an IPBH, aneurysmal SAH, and brain hemorrhages related to an AVM.

⇒ Although many new interventions exist, many more are needed to affect functional recovery adequately in stroke survivors.

⇒ The public's knowledge regarding stroke risk factors, symptoms, and the need for rapid entry into treatment must improve.

⇒ Nurses are challenged to play an important role in the future of stroke care, by enhancing consumer access to health services and by creating new interventions to optimize outcomes for future stroke survivors.

References

1. Sweeny PJ, Furlan AJ: "Stroke": origin of the term. Stroke 3:559, 1986.
2. Bronstein KS, Popovich JM, Stewart-Amidei C: Promoting Stroke Recovery. St. Louis, C.V. Mosby, 1991.
3. Ozer MN, Materson RS, Caplan LR: Management of Persons With Stroke. St. Louis, C.V. Mosby, 1994.
4. Wolf PA, Kannel WB, Verter J: Epidemiologic appraisal of hypertension and stroke risk. In: Guthrie GP, Kotchen TA (eds): Hypertension and the Brain. Mt. Kisco, NY, Futura, 1984, pp 221–246.
5. National Stroke Association: NSA Newslett 11:1, 3, 1994.
6. Ebrahim S: Clinical Epidemiology of Stroke. Oxford, Oxford University Press, 1990.
7. Wojner AW: Optimizing ischemic stroke outcomes: an interdisciplinary approach to poststroke rehabilitation in acute care. Crit Care Nurs Q 19:47–61, 1996.
8. Wojner AW: Outcomes management: from theory to practice. Crit Care Nurs Q 19:1–15, 1997.
9. Hacke W, Hennerici M, Gelmers HJ, et al: Cerebral Ischemia. Berlin, Springer, 1991.
10. O'Brien MD: The window of opportunity for the treatment of cerebral ischaemia. In: Hartmann A, Yatsu F, Kuschinsky W (eds): Cerebral Ischemia and Basic Mechanisms. Berlin, Springer, 1994, pp 1–5.
11. Heiss WD, Fink GR, Huber M, et al: Uncoupling flow and metabolism in early ischemic stroke. In: Hartmann A, Yatsu F, Kuschinsky W (eds): Cerebral Ischemia and Basic Mechanisms. Berlin, Springer, 1994, pp 9–17.
12. Allison M: Searching for moving targets: metabolic effects of brain injury. Headlines January/February: 3–8, 1993.
13. Symon L, Taylor DL, Obrenovitch TP: Aspects of acid–base homeostasis in ischemia. In: Hartmann A, Yatsu F, Kuschinsky W (eds): Cerebral Ischemia and Basic Mechanisms. Berlin, Springer, 1994, pp 52–57.
14. Hickey JV: The Clinical Practice of Neurological and Neurosurgical Nursing, 4th ed. Philadelphia, J.B. Lippincott, 1996.
15. Fox HM, Rizzo ND, Gifford S: Psychological observations of patients undergoing mitral surgery. Psychosom Med 16:186–208, 1954.
16. Brass L, Fayad PB: Intraoperative monitoring with Doppler ultrasonography during cardiac surgery and interventions. In: Babikian VL, Wechsler LR (eds): Transcranial Doppler Ultrasonography. St. Louis, C.V. Mosby, 1993, pp 222–231.
17. Wolf PA: Epidemiology of intracerebral hemorrhage. In: Kase CS, Caplan LR (eds): Intracerebral Hemorrhage. Boston, Butterworth–Heinemann, 1994, pp 21–30.
18. Broderick JP, Brott T, Tomsick T, et al: Intracerebral hemorrhage is more than twice as common as subarachnoid hemorrhage. J Neurosurg 78:188–191, 1993.
19. Kase CS: Aneurysms and vascular malformations. In: Kase CS, Caplan LR (eds): Intracerebral Hemorrhage. Boston, Butterworth–Heinemann, 1994, pp 153–178.
20. Smith RR, Zubkov YN, Tarassoli Y: Cerebral Aneurysms: Microvascular and Endovascular Management. New York, Springer, 1994.

21. Caplan LR: Clinical features of spontaneous intracerebral hemorrhage. In: Kaufman, HH (ed): Intracerebral Hematomas. New York, Raven Press, 1992, pp 31–47.

22. Crowell RM, Ogilvy CS, Gress DR, et al: General management of aneurysmal subarachnoid hemorrhage. In: Ojemann RG, Ogilvy CS, Crowell RM, et al (eds): Surgical Management of Neurovascular Disease, 3rd ed. Baltimore, Williams & Wilkins, 1995, pp 111–122.

23. Loftus CM: Perioperative management of spontaneous primary subarachnoid hemorrhage. Contemp Neurosurg 16:1–5, 1994.

24. National Stroke Association: Management of subarachnoid hemorrhage. Stroke Clin Updates 6:1–4, 1995.

25. de la Monte SM, Moore GW, Monk MA, et al: Risk factors for the development and rupture of intracranial berry aneurysms. JAMA 78:957–964, 1985.

26. Miller CA, Hill SA, Hunt WE: "De novo" aneurysms: a clinical review. Surg Neurol 24:173–180, 1985.

27. Lindley JG, Wirth FP: Epidemiology of cerebral aneurysms. In: Ratcheson RA, Wirth FP (eds): Ruptured Cerebral Aneurysms: Perioperative Management. Baltimore, Williams & Wilkins, 1994, pp 15–22.

28. Crowell RM, Ogilvy CS, Gress DR: Unruptured aneurysms. In: Ojemann RG, Ogilvy CS, Crowell RM, et al (eds): Surgical Management of Neurovascular Disease, 3rd ed. Baltimore, Williams & Wilkins, 1995, pp 305–322.

29. Lozano AM, Leblanc R: Familial intracranial aneurysms. J Neurosurg 66:522–528, 1987.

30. Marin N, Vinters H: Pathology and grading of intracranial vascular malformations. In: Barrow DL (ed): Intracranial Vascular Malformations. Park Ridge, IL, American Association of Neurological Surgeons, 1990, pp 1–30.

31. McNair N: Arteriovenous malformations. Crit Care Nurse 8:35–40, 1988.

32. Tatter SB, Ogilvy CS: Vascular malformations: general considerations. In: Ojemann RG, Ogilvy CS, Crowell RM, et al (eds): Surgical Management of Neurovascular Disease, 3rd ed. Baltimore, Williams & Wilkins, 1995, pp 387–403.

33. Diaz MS, Sekhar LN: Intracranial hemorrhage from aneurysms and arteriovenous malformations during pregnancy and the puerperium. Neurosurgery 27:855–866, 1990.

34. Carmel PW, Swift DM: Spontaneous intracranial hemorrhage occurring during pregnancy. In: Kaufman HH (ed): Intracerebral Hematomas. New York, Raven Press, 1992, pp 117–125.

35. Findley JM: Perioperative management of subarachnoid hemorrhage. Contemp Neurosurg 17:1–5, 1995.

36. Hunt WE, Hess RM: Surgical risk as related to time of intervention in the repair of intracranial aneurysms. J Neurosurg 28:14–20, 1968.

37. Woodard EJ, Barrow DL: Clinical presentation of intracranial vascular malformations. In: Barrow DL (ed): Intracranial Vascular Malformations. Park Ridge, IL, American Association of Neurological Surgeons, 1990, pp 53–61.

38. Wilkins RH: Natural history of arteriovenous malformations of the brain. In: Barrow DL (ed): Intracranial Vascular Malformations. Park Ridge, IL, American Association of Neurological Surgeons, 1990, pp 31–44.

39. Muraszko KM, Oldfield ED: Vascular malformations of the spinal cord and dura. Neurosurg Clin North Am 1:631–652, 1990.

40. Spetzler RF, Martin NA: A proposed grading system for arteriovenous malformations. J Neurosurg 65:476–483, 1986.

41. Choi IS: Endovascular treatment of aneurysms. In: Ojemann RG, Ogilvy CS, Crowell RM, et al (eds): Surgical Management of Neurovascular Disease, 3rd ed. Baltimore, Williams & Wilkins, 1995, pp 138–151.

42. Martin N, Dion JE: Imaging of intracranial vascular malformations. In: Barrow DL (ed): Intracranial Vascular Malformations.

Park Ridge, IL, American Association of Neurological Surgeons, 1990, pp 63–89.

43. Mendel RC, Carter LP: Evaluation and treatment of clinical vasospasm following subarachnoid hemorrhage. Contemp Neurosurg 16:1–6, 1994.

44. Agency for Health Care Policy and Research: Post-stroke Rehabilitation. Clinical practice guideline no. 16, AHCPR publication 95-0662. Rockville, MD, U.S. Department of Health and Human Services, Public Health Service, 1995.

45. Wojner AW: Outcomes management: the search for best practice. AACN Clin Issues 7:133–145, 1996.

46. Tresser SJ, Selman WR, Ratcheson RA: Pathophysiologic alterations following aneurysm rupture. In: Ratcheson RA, Wirth FP (eds): Ruptured Cerebral Aneurysms: Perioperative Management. Baltimore, Williams & Wilkins, 1994, pp 23–45.

47. Giannotta SL, Schneider JH: Perioperative management of intracranial arteriovenous malformations. In: Barrow DL (ed): Intracranial Vascular Malformations. Park Ridge, IL, American Association of Neurological Surgeons, 1990, pp 99–109.

48. Sikes PJ, Segal J: Jugular bulb oxygen saturation monitoring for evaluating cerebral ischemia. Crit Care Nurs Q 17:9–20, 1993.

49. Clagett GP, Anderson FA, Levine MN, et al: Prevention of venous thromboembolism. Chest 102(Suppl):391–407, 1992.

50. Hedberg A-M, Wojner AW: Incorporating Nutrition Care into Critical Pathways for Improved Outcomes. Columbus, OH, Ross Products Division, Abbott Laboratories, 1994.

51. Stone SP, Wilson B, Wroot A, et al: The assessment of visuospatial neglect after acute stroke. J Neurol Neurosurg Psychiatry 54:345–350, 1991.

52. Cushman LA: Secondary neuropsychiatric complications in stroke: implications for acute care. Arch Phys Med Rehabil 69:877–879, 1988.

53. Galski T, Bruno RL, Zorowitz R, et al: Predicting length of stay, functional outcome, and aftercare in the rehabilitation of stroke patients: the dominant role of higher-order cognition. Stroke 24:1794–1800, 1993.

54. Wijdicks EE, Ropper AH, Hunnicutt EF, et al: Atrial natriuretic factor and salt wasting after aneurysmal subarachnoid hemorrhage. Stroke 22:1519–1524, 1991.

55. Ritter AM, Robertson CS: Intensive care management of the neurosurgical patient. Contemp Neurosurg 16:1–7, 1994.

56. Kotchen TA, Halbritter KA, Boegehold MA: Hypertension and the brain. In: Kaufman HH (ed): Intracerebral Hematomas. New York, Raven Press, 1992, pp 23–29.

57. Knudsen F, Jensen HP, Perterson PL: Neurogenic pulmonary edema: treatment with dobutamine. Neurosurgery 29:269–270, 1991.

58. Candelise L: New treatments for acute ischemic stroke. In: Adams HP (ed): Handbook of Cerebrovascular Diseases. New York, Marcel Dekker, 1993, pp 415–432.

59. Marler JR: Antithrombotic and thrombolytic therapy for acute ischemic stroke. In: Adams HP (ed): Handbook of Cerebrovascular Diseases. New York, Marcel Dekker, 1993, pp 404–414.

60. National Institute of Neurological Disorders and Stroke rt-PA Study Group: Tissue plasminogen activator for acute ischemic stroke. N Engl J Med 353:1581–1587, 1995.

61. Kassel NF, Torner JC, Haley EC, et al: The International Cooperative Study on the Timing of Aneurysm Surgery. I. Overall management results: surgical results. J Neurosurg 73:18–47, 1990.

62. Schucart W, Wu J: Timing of operation for ruptured aneurysms: delayed surgery. In: Ratcheson RA, Wirth FP (eds): Ruptured Cerebral Aneurysms: Perioperative Management. Baltimore, Williams & Wilkins, 1994, pp 54–58.

63. Guglielmi G, Vinuela E, Dion J, et al: Electrothrombosis of saccular aneurysms via endovascular approach. 2. Preliminary clinical experience. J Neurosurg 75:8–14, 1991.

64. Macdonald RL, Weir BK: A review of hemoglobin and the pathogenesis of cerebral vasospasm. Stroke 22:971–982, 1991.

65. Steele JA, Stockbridge N, Malijkovic G, et al: Free radicals mediate actions of oxyhemoglobin on cerebrovascular smooth muscle cells. Circ Res 68:416–423, 1991.

66. Wood JH, Kee DB Jr: Hemorheology of the cerebral circulation in stroke. Stroke 16:765–772, 1985.

67. Higashida RT, Halbach VV, Cahan LD, et al: Transluminal angioplasty for treatment of intracranial arterial vasospasm. J Neurosurg 71:648–653, 1989.

68. Yamamoto Y, Smith RR, Bernanke DH: Mechanism of action of balloon angioplasty in cerebral vasospasm. Neurosurgery 30:1–6, 1992.

69. Pickard JD, Murray GD, Illingworth R, et al: Effect of oral nimodipine on cerebral infarction and outcome after subarachnoid haemorrhage: British Aneurysm Nimodipine Trial. BMJ 298:636–642, 1989.

70. Hacein-Bey L, Pile-Spellman J, Ogilvy CS: Embolization of brain arteriovenous malformations. In: Ojemann RG, Ogilvy CS, Crowell RM, et al (eds): Surgical Management of Neurovascular Disease, 3rd ed. Baltimore, Williams & Wilkins, 1995, pp 404–418.

71. Sundt TM: Operative techniques for arteriovenous malformations of the brain. In: Barrow DL (ed): Intracranial Vascular Malformations. Park Ridge, IL, American Association of Neurological Surgeons, 1990, pp 111–123.

72. Vinuela F, Dion JE, Fox AJ: Interventional neuroradiology for intracranial arteriovenous malformations. In: Barrow DL (ed): Intracranial Vascular Malformations. Park Ridge, IL, American Association of Neurological Surgeons, 1990, pp 169–178.

73. Korosue K, Heros RC: Complications of complete surgical resection of AVMs of the brain. In: Barrow DL (ed): Intracranial Vascular Malformations. Park Ridge, IL, American Association of Neurological Surgeons, 1990, pp 157–168.

74. Ogilvy CS: Radiation therapy for arteriovenous malformations: a review. Neurosurgery 26:725–735, 1990.

75. Wojner AW, Graves B: Stereotactic radiosurgery: new practice frontiers for the perioperative nurse. Semin Periop Nurs 4:177–183, 1995.

76. van der Kogel AJ: Radiation injury in the central nervous system. In: Alexander E, Loeffler JS, Lunsford LD (eds): Stereotactic Radiosurgery. New York, McGraw-Hill, 1993, pp 43–50.

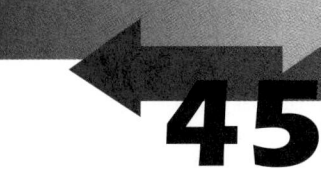

45

Seizure Disorders

Tess L. Sierzant

Objectives

After completing this chapter, the student will be able to:

1. Distinguish epilepsy from seizures.
2. Distinguish between causes of recurrent and nonrecurrent seizures.
3. Use components of seizure assessment accurately.
4. Plan patient care to include safety measures tailored to the patient's individual seizure type.
5. Manage a patient with status epilepticus effectively.
6. Relate causes of status epilepticus to associated collaborative management strategies.
7. Participate in planning collaborative care that extends across the patient's care continuum.
8. Incorporate psychosocial interventions into the patient's plan of care.
9. Relate pharmacokinetic properties of antiepileptic drugs with conditions that can alter these properties.
10. Differentiate among surgical interventions for epilepsy.

A seizure is a paroxysmal high-frequency or synchronous low-frequency discharge of neurons in the cerebral cortex. In other words, a group of neurons in the brain becomes abnormally and overly excited, the usual regulation by inhibitory substances fails to occur, and a seizure results. In fact, more than 20 different types of seizures are recognized, and one person's seizure activity can appear distinctively different from another's, depending on which neurons are misfiring and the rapidity with which they do so.

Seizures may be nonrecurrent, related to an acute medical, neurologic illness or neurosurgical procedure, such as head trauma, cerebrovascular accident, or cranial surgery for tumor excision. Nonrecurrent seizures are self-limited and do not recur after the illness has been treated. The term "epilepsy" refers to the chronic disorder characterized by a tendency toward recurrent, unprovoked seizures. Recurrent seizures (epilepsy) may be primary (idiopathic) or secondary (symptomatic). "Seizure disorder" may be perceived by some as a less threatening, less judgmental, and less stigmatizing term and is used to refer to situations in which nonrecurrent seizures are present, although the term is often used interchangeably with epilepsy.

In the United States, about 125,000 new cases of epilepsy are diagnosed each year.[1] The incidence (the number of new cases occurring in a defined population) is higher in children under 2 years of age and in adults over age 65. Males, African-Americans, and the socially disadvantaged also have a higher incidence.[1] The prevalence (the number of cases of a disease in a population at a specific point in time) of epilepsy in the United States is about 2 million, when defined as individuals with a history of epilepsy who have experienced a seizure or have taken antiepileptic drugs (AEDs) within the previous 5 years.[1] The nurse may encounter patients who have either recurrent or nonrecurrent seizures. Patients may be those with a preexisting diagnosis of epilepsy who have an unrelated illness, those who may be having epilepsy-related surgery, or those who develop seizures as a result of an illness or its treatment. Some of these causative factors may be direct insults to the central nervous system (CNS), such as craniocerebral trauma, and others may be related to toxic or metabolic conditions such as renal failure.

In patients with epilepsy, acute and chronic components to the disorder can challenge health care professionals in various ways. Patients with more severe types of epilepsy may endure repeated hospitalizations for management of status epilepticus. The chronic nature of the disorder may contribute to depression, lack of self-esteem, social isolation, and dependence on others. Awareness of the wide variation in expression of epileptic seizures, recognition of the clinical occurrence of seizures, the ability to describe and assess the effects on the patient accurately, and implementation of appropriate interventions to maintain patient safety and maximum functional level are essential skills of the nurse.

ETIOLOGY AND PATHOPHYSIOLOGY

An epileptic seizure can occur in anyone, given the right combination of circumstances. Numerous factors contribute to the development of this combination, including genetic and environmental factors as well as normal physiologic influences. Variations in our ability to adapt to changes in the external and internal environments account for the variability in seizure occurrence, such as why one person experiences seizures after stroke and another does not. Every person has a certain threshold for seizure activity determined by predisposing factors; when that threshold is passed, a seizure occurs. The cause is unknown for about two-thirds of people with epilepsy.[2] Lothman[3] states that although much is known about mechanisms of individual seizures, the pathophysiology underlying epilepsy is not well understood. In considering the underlying pathophysiology of epilepsy, many factors must be considered. Individual differences in genetic makeup interacting with environmental factors contribute to each person's susceptibility to seizures.[3] Stress, sleep deprivation, and diseases that are not direct insults to the CNS but have considerable effect on the brain's subsequent ability to manage disturbances in neuronal excitability and synchronization of electrical discharges play a role. Many factors have been clearly identified as contributors to the etiology of epilepsy (Chart 45–1).

Patients with systemic disease are often encountered in the critical care setting. Numerous medical illnesses and their subsequent treatments may result in seizures as a complicating factor. Patients with multiple organ dysfunction are particularly challenging to manage from a seizure perspective because of their delicate balance in physiologic status, multiple medications, and limitations in means of administering AEDs.[4] Factors lowering the seizure threshold in critically ill patients include electrolyte imbalance (particularly sodium, calcium, and magnesium), acid–base shifts, rapid fluid shifts, fever, cerebral hypoperfusion, hypoxemia, various medications, and the chronic sleep deprivation of the critical care setting.

Factors altering the effectiveness of AEDs relate to the administration, absorption, and metabolism of the drugs. Access to the gastrointestinal tract or its functioning may be altered, as in patients who are

---

CHART 45–1

Factors Associated With Increased Risk of Epilepsy

Family history of epilepsy or febrile seizures
Perinatal injuries such as toxemia during pregnancy, delivery problems, neonatal hypoxia or anoxia, low birth weight
Toxic and metabolic disturbances
Stroke
Anoxia
Craniocerebral trauma
Central nervous system infections such as viral encephalitis and bacterial and aseptic meningitis
Congenital cerebral malformations
Subarachnoid hemorrhage and vasospasm
Use of and withdrawal from alcohol and drugs
Alzheimer's disease
Multiple sclerosis
Tumors
Abrupt withdrawal of antiepileptic medications or sedatives used on a long-term basis

---

allowed nothing by mouth (are NPO), or who have ileus, bowel obstruction, fluid restriction, or emesis. Patients receiving enteral feedings can also present challenges in maintaining therapeutic drug levels, with a potential for increased transit time and decreased medication absorption. Alterations in hepatic and renal function can have significant effects on the metabolism of AEDs. Most AEDs are protein bound, and levels can fluctuate in the face of decreased protein levels. The critically ill patient usually receives multiple medications, a factor that increases the likelihood of drug interactions and the potential for side effects.[4] Some recently approved AEDs now provide options for patients with liver dysfunction because they are renally eliminated almost unchanged.

A broad range of systemic diseases, including cardiovascular, renal, respiratory, and hepatic conditions, can contribute to the development of seizure activity (Chart 45–2). Medications also can contribute to seizure activity. Most often, they play a role in lowering the seizure threshold, so careful consideration of the risk-to-benefit ratio must be undertaken. The nurse must be aware of pathophysiologic conditions in which seizures may occur and of medications that may lower the threshold for seizures (Table 45–1).

CHART 45–2

Conditions Contributing to the Development of Seizure Activity

Atrial fibrillation	Cerebral aneurysm rupture
Subacute bacterial endocarditis	Cardiac or respiratory arrest
Altered protein binding	Uremia
Dysequilibrium syndrome	Primary central nervous system infections
HIV infection	Neurocysticercosis
Intracranial structural lesions	Immunosuppression

From Boggs JG: Seizures in medically complex patients. Epilepsia 38(Suppl 4):S55–S59, 1997.

Classification of Epileptic Seizures

An understanding of the International Classification of Seizures[5] is essential in the diagnostic and treatment process for patients with seizures. The terminology within the classification more accurately reflects what occurs during a seizure; generalized tonic–clonic (GTC) provides a better description than grand mal, as does absence rather than petit mal. Accurate identification of a patient's seizure type provides the basis on which medication is prescribed, lifestyle changes are integrated, and coping strategies are developed. Important distinctions in seizure classification include the separation into partial and generalized seizures (Table 45–2) and whether or not consciousness is impaired. Partial seizures begin in one cerebral hemisphere; generalized seizures involve both.

The terms "ictal" or "ictus" are used to refer to the seizure activity itself. Technically, it means event or occurrence. Thus, preictal refers to the period of time and events before the seizure. The postictal period is that time during which the clinical seizure activity has ceased, the electroencephalogram (EEG) remains slowed, and the patient is returning to baseline, or pre-ictal, status.

Partial Seizures

Simple partial seizures are those in which consciousness is not impaired. These seizures are often referred to as auras or warnings. They may be experienced as altered sensory or motor activities. They may have an autonomic component, or they may be a psychic phenomenon, such as a feeling of fear. Simple partial

TABLE 45–1
Medications That May Lower the Seizure Threshold

Drug Classification	Examples
Antidepressants	Imipramine, amitriptyline, doxepin, nortriptyline, maprotiline, mianserin, nomifensine, bupropion
Antipsychotics	Chlorpromazine, thioridazine, perphenazine, trifluoperazine, prochlorperazine, haloperidol
Analgesics	Fentanyl, meperidine, pentazocine, propoxyphene, cocaine, mefenamic acid, tramadol
Local Anesthetics	Lidocaine, mepivacaine, procaine, bupivacaine, etidocaine
General Anesthetics	Ketamine, halothane, enflurane, propanidid, methohexital
Antimicrobials	Penicillin, synthetic penicillins (oxacillin, carbenicillin, ticarcillin), ampicillin, cephalosporins, metronidazole, nalidixic acid, isoniazid, cycloserine, pyrimethamine, imipenem
Antineoplastics	Chlorambucil, vincristine, methotrexate, cytarabine, misonidazole, BCNU, PALA, busulfan
Bronchodilators	Aminophylline, theophylline
Sympathomimetics	Ephedrine, terbutaline, phenylpropanolamine
Other	Insulin, antihistamines, anticholinergics, baclofen, cyclosporine, lithium, atenolol, disopyramide, phencyclidine, amphetamines, domperidone, doxapram, ergonovine, folic acid, camphor, methylxanthines, thyrotropin-releasing hormone, vitamin K oxide, aqueous iodinated contrast media, oxytocin, hyperosmolar parenteral solutions, hyperbaric oxygen, antiepileptic medications, methylphenidate, flumazenil

Adapted from Mastaglia FL: Iatrogenic (drug-induced) disorders of the nervous system. In: Aminoff MJ (ed): The Neurological Aspects of Medical Disorders. New York, Churchill Livingstone, 1989.

TABLE 45–2
International Classification of Seizures

Classification	Subclassification	Subtypes
Partial (Focal)	Simple partial (without impairment or loss of consciousness)	Motor signs Somatosensory or special sensory symptoms Autonomic symptoms or signs Psychic symptoms
	Complex partial (with impairment or loss of consciousness)	Simple partial onset, with progression to complex partial Onset with impairment of consciousness
	Partial seizures with secondary generalization	Simple partial with secondary generalization Complex partial with secondary generalization Simple partial to complex partial with secondary generalization
Generalized	Tonic–clonic Absence Myoclonic Atonic Tonic only Clonic only	—— —— —— —— —— ——
Unclassified	Seizures that do not meet any of the above criteria; often seen in neonates	

Adapted from Commission on Classification and Terminology of the International League Against Epilepsy: Proposal for revised clinical and electroencephalographic classification of epileptic seizures. Epilepsia 22:489–501, 1981.

seizures may go largely unnoticed to those around the patient, and it is important to determine whether the patient experiences any type of warning. These episodes may play a role in preventing injury if the seizure is prone to progression. Simple partial seizures range in expression widely, from varying tastes, smells, and sounds to focal motor activity, tachycardia, nausea, or a flushed feeling, depending on which area of the brain is involved. If the seizure is motor in expression, the patient may experience jerking of a single part of the body, such as the leg or face. Sometimes, it moves to other areas of the body. The important distinguishing characteristic is that consciousness is not impaired. Distinguishing consciousness from ability to respond may be significant with these types of seizures, because sometimes a patient may be completely aware of what is occurring, but the seizure prevents normal verbal expression. Simple partial seizures may be as brief as several seconds, or they can last for minutes or longer. The patient is usually able to resume previous activity immediately.

Complex partial seizures are those in which consciousness is impaired; the limbic system is involved. They have also been referred to as temporal lobe, psychomotor, or focal seizures. The patient may have a warning, or simple partial seizure, heralding the onset. Behaviors may range widely, including automatic activity, referred to as automatisms, such as walking, chewing, swallowing, activities in process at the time of the seizure, purposeless activity such as fumbling with

clothing or objects nearby, looking around or staring aimlessly, or those in which the patient continues with an action repetitively, such as rubbing the abdomen. The patient may mumble, speak in shortened phrases, or not speak at all. There may be evidence of fear, and the patient may try to run. In some situations, it is evident on the basis of visual observation that the patient has an alteration in consciousness; in others, this change may not be immediately evident without additional interaction. Duration may be from a minute to several minutes. Patients with complex partial seizures are often mistakenly believed to be intoxicated with alcohol or drugs or mentally ill. Postictally, the patient may be tired and confused and may have little or no recall of the events that occurred during the seizure.

Generalized Seizures

Generalized seizures manifest themselves in various ways. Certainly, the most commonly known seizure is the tonic–clonic, previously known as grand mal, seizure. Others, such as absence or myoclonic, may be more subtle and difficult to recognize.

Tonic–Clonic. Tonic–clonic seizures may begin with a simple or complex partial seizure that secondarily generalizes, or it may begin suddenly, typically with a sharp cry. The patient may fall and become rigid (tonic phase) in the face, trunk, arms, and legs. This phase is followed by jerking, or clonic, activity. The jerking is usually rhythmic, and muscles of the face, trunk, arms, and legs are involved. The clonic activity usually begins slowly, crescendos, then gradually subsides in frequency. The patient may demonstrate shallow or absent spontaneous breathing, increased secretions, biting of the tongue, deviation of the eyes, and changes in skin color. These changes include flushing, becoming pale or blue. A typical GTC seizure lasts approximately 90 seconds. Afterward, the patient may be sleepy and minimally responsive, sometimes for several hours.

Absence. Absence seizures are vastly different in expression than GTC seizures. They are much more subtle and may go unrecognized to the uneducated eye. Absence seizures are characterized by a blank stare, brief, rapid blinking of the eyes, and occasional chewing movements and are typified by those who experience them as "spacing out" for a few seconds. This type of seizure occurs primarily in children, although in rare situations, they persist into adulthood. Untreated children may have hundreds of these seizures per day, and the occurrence of these seizures has implications for the learning of new material.

Myoclonic. Myoclonic seizures, as the name implies, are characterized by brief, massive muscle jerks. They occur suddenly and, in severe cases, can result in falls and injury. They may involve the entire body or a single part of it. The experience is similar to nocturnal myoclonus, a common physiologic experience that occurs as we are falling asleep and abruptly awaken with a start from a dream in which we were in danger of injury or death. Myoclonic seizures last seconds, but they may occur serially.

Atonic. Atonic seizures are also known as drop attacks. The patient experiences a loss of muscle tone, an abrupt fall, and a loss of consciousness. This type of seizure is associated with an increased risk of injury. Recovery can take up to several minutes, after which the patient is able to walk again.

Unclassified Seizures

Some seizures, despite the best clinical description and video EEG documentation, do not lend themselves to classification in this schema. Many of these are seizures seen in neonates who have abnormal eye movements or swimming movements.

The International Classification of Epilepsies and Epileptic Syndromes[6] provides a framework for characterizing not only the patient's seizure type, but also the cause, precipitating factors, age of onset, severity, chronicity, diurnal and circadian cycling, family history, and prognosis.[7] This classification distinguishes between idiopathic and symptomatic epilepsies and can assist clinicians in providing effective management and in better education of patients and families about anticipated changes during the life span (Table 45–3).

Status Epilepticus

The Epilepsy Foundation of America's Working Group on Status Epilepticus[8] has defined status epilepticus as more than 30 minutes of continuous seizure activity or two or more sequential seizures without full recovery of consciousness between seizures. Any epileptic seizure can progress to status epilepticus. As with the International Classification of Seizures discussed earlier, status epilepticus is classified as generalized and partial. The condition is also divided into convulsive and nonconvulsive types. The term "status" is often used to refer to generalized convulsive status epilepticus (CSE), a life-threatening condition. Nonconvulsive status, which may take several forms, was once thought to be a benign condition, but now it is recognized that aggressive treatment may be important with some types.

Convulsive Type

CSE is a medical emergency. Because the patient is at risk of severe neuronal injury and death if seizures persist, prompt intervention to stop the seizures is imperative. Estimates of incidence of CSE range from 50,000 to 60,000 per year[2] to 250,000 per year.[9] Mortality related to CSE is estimated to be 3 to 35%.[2, 8] One of the most common causes of CSE in patients with epilepsy is withdrawal from AEDs.[10] Symptomatic causes include stroke, anoxia, tumor, craniocerebral trauma, fevers, infections, drugs, alcohol, and toxic or metabolic disorders. One-third of patients with CSE are susceptible as a result of an identifiable cause; and in another one-third of patients, CSE heralds epilepsy without an identifiable cause.[11]

Three factors contribute to mortality and morbidity secondary to status epilepticus: 1) direct damage to the brain caused by an acute insult that precipitates the condition; 2) systemic stress from repeated GTC seizures; and 3) injury from repetitive electrical discharges within the brain.[12] The neurons involved in the seizure activity fire more rapidly and thus produce increased amounts of potentially cerebrally toxic waste products; the injury results when cerebral circulation is unable to keep up with the clearance of these waste products. Numerous systemic complications can result from prolonged convulsive activity. These include hypoxia, lactic acidosis, carbon dioxide narcosis, hyperkalemia, hypoglycemia, early hypertension with late hypotension and circulatory failure, cardiac dysrhythmias, pulmonary edema, acute tubular necrosis, high-output failure, aspiration pneumonia, hyperpyrexia, rhabdomyolysis, leukocytosis and cerebrospinal fluid (CSF) pleocytosis, and other autonomic symptoms such as vomiting, electrolyte and fluid loss, detrusor muscle contraction leading to urinary incontinence, fecal incontinence, and increases in sweating,

TABLE 45–3
International Classification of Epilepsies and Epileptic Syndromes

Classification	Subclassification	Subtypes
Localization-Related (Focal, Partial)	Idiopathic with age-related onset	Benign childhood epilepsy with centrotemporal spike Childhood epilepsy with occipital paroxysms Primary reading epilepsy
	Symptomatic	Chronic progressive epilepsia partialis continua of childhood (Kojewnikow's syndrome) Syndromes characterized by seizures with specific modes of precipitation
	Cryptogenic	Cryptogenic epilepsies presumed to be symptomatic, origin unknown*
Generalized Epilepsies and Syndromes	Idiopathic (with age-related onset, listed in chronologic order)	Benign neonatal familial convulsions Benign neonatal convulsions Benign myoclonic epilepsy in infancy Childhood absence epilepsy (pyknolepsy) Juvenile absence epilepsy Juvenile myoclonic epilepsy (impulsive petit mal) Epilepsy with grand mal (GTCs) seizures on awakening Other generalized idiopathic epilepsies not defined above Epilepsies with seizures precipitated by specific modes of activation
	Cryptogenic or symptomatic (in order of age)	West syndrome (infantile spasms, Blitz–Nick–Salaam Krämpfe) Lennox–Gastaut syndrome Epilepsy with myoclonic–astatic seizures Epilepsy with myoclonic absences
	Symptomatic	Nonspecific origin: early myoclonic encephalopathy; early infantile epileptic encephalopathy with suppression burst; other symptomatic generalized epilepsies not defined above Specific syndromes: epileptic seizures may complicate many disease states; heading includes diseases in which seizures are a presenting or predominant feature
Epilepsies and Syndromes Undetermined Whether Focal or Generalized	Both generalized and focal seizures	Neonatal seizures Severe myoclonic epilepsy in infancy Epilepsy with continuous spike waves during slow-wave sleep Acquired epileptic aphasia (Landau–Kleffner syndrome) Other undetermined epilepsies not defined above
	Without unequivocal generalized or focal features	All cases with GTCs in which clinical and electroencephalographic findings do not permit classification as clearly generalized or localization related, such as in many cases of sleep grand mal (GTCs), which are considered not to have unequivocal generalized or focal features
Special Syndromes	Situation-related seizures	Febrile convulsions Isolated seizures or isolated status epilepticus Seizures occurring only in the presence of an acute metabolic or toxic event from factors such as alcohol, drugs, eclampsia, and nonketotic hyperglycemia

GTCs, generalized tonic–clonic seizures.
*This subtype differs from the previous one by lack of etiologic evidence.
Adapted from Commission on Classification and Terminology of the International League Against Epilepsy: Proposal for revised classification of epilepsies and epileptic syndromes. Epilepsia 30:389–399, 1989.

salivation, and tracheobronchial secretions.[13] Therefore, the condition must be recognized and treated immediately.

Nonconvulsive Type

Consciousness may be impaired or preserved in nonconvulsive status epilepticus. Situations in which consciousness is impaired include continuous absence seizures and complex partial status epilepticus. Absence status occurs primarily in children and is manifest by changes in level of consciousness (LOC) and behavior. Academic performance may decline if the condition occurs frequently. Complex partial status epilepticus is estimated to occur in approximately 20% of all patients with status epilepticus.[14] Presentation varies widely and may include cessation of speech or activity, automatisms, alteration of consciousness, and confusion, which may be attributed to other conditions in the critically ill patient.

Neuronal damage in patients experiencing complex partial status epilepticus is being studied. Serum neuron-specific enolase (s-NSE) is a marker of acute brain injury. Increased levels have been seen in patients with CSE and anoxic encephalopathy. DeGiorgio and colleagues[15] reported that elevations in s-NSE levels in patients with complex partial status epilepticus provide evidence that the condition causes brain injury, and these investigators advocate that complex partial status epilepticus should be considered a medical emergency.

In status with simple partial seizures, known as *epilepsia partialis continua* or focal status epilepticus, consciousness is preserved. Patients experience focal jerking of a body part, often the hand or foot, that may appear similar to myoclonic jerks. Its occurrence is uncommon and is often associated with certain CNS infections such as Rasmussen's encephalitis, atherosclerotic cerebrovascular disease, strokes, or tumors, although, like other seizures, it may be idiopathic.[16]

Assessment

Health History

Seizures may be mistaken for other conditions, including transient ischemic attacks, panic attacks, syncope, sleep disorder, cardiac dysrhythmias, hyperventilation, migraine syndromes, psychiatric disorders, toxic and metabolic disturbances, and nonepileptic seizures of psychogenic origin.[17, 18] A careful evaluation is essential to establishing the correct diagnosis. The context in which seizures occur is critical to developing the appropriate management plan. A detailed description of the event in question is essential. This may be obtained by interviewing the patient whenever possible and those with the patient when it happened.

Astute observations and documentation by health care professionals, particularly nurses, are essential. Nurses observe more seizures "live" than do most physicians and even neurologists. The registered nurse must be aware of the dynamic assessments that are required for accurate description of a seizure. The progress of a seizure is not linear; various aspects of the seizure may need to be assessed simultaneously and repeatedly while it is occurring. Data about the seizure must be gathered not only on the basis of sensory (e.g., visual, auditory) information, but also interactively, to determine the patient's LOC during the seizure, an important component in the correct classification of the event. Other aspects of the health history are listed in Table 45–4.

Signs and Symptoms of Seizure Disorders

Observation of seizure activity by the nurse contributes to the appropriate and successful management of the seizure. In the case of CSE, monitoring the length of time seizures last, the number of seizures, and the time between seizures is crucial. Assessment of a seizure includes data gathered during preictal, ictal, and postictal phases.[19]

The circumstances before the seizure itself actually begins should be documented. These include the presence of headache, sleep or wakefulness, observable behavior changes, sensory experiences of the patient, such as "a weird feeling," and changes in functional abilities, especially in patients who cannot express themselves. Information regarding precipitating factors should be gathered and may be psychological, social, emotional, metabolic, physical, and environmental.

The time of onset of the seizure should be noted. This time may be difficult to pinpoint, and it may be marked by the patient's report, the onset of observable altered physical activity, or behavior changes. Detailed knowledge of the patient's previous seizure activity contributes to early recognition and intervention.

LOC is an essential component of the assessment process. It is important to assess this parameter at intervals during the seizure, because LOC can vary during the course of a seizure, and failure to return to preictal LOC may indicate status epilepticus, necessitating more aggressive treatment. The degrees of responsiveness, awareness, and interaction with the environment and orientation are assessed. The ability to follow commands provides data about the patient's ability to hear, to process information, and to translate that into motor activity. Memory is often impaired during a seizure, and telling the patient with words or showing items to remember can be useful in determining the extent of the memory and speech impairment. Immediate and delayed memory should be assessed.

Motor activity can vary widely during seizure activity. The presence or absence of movement should be

TABLE 45-4
Components of a Health History After a Seizure

Category	Topics to Explore
Detailed Description of Events	Occurrences before seizure activity took place Initial onset of symptoms, including prodrome or aura Progression of seizure activity What happened during postictal period
Medical History	Past history of seizures, including febrile convulsions Predisposing factors such as head trauma, stroke, substance abuse, infections
Family History	Febrile seizures Seizure history in parents, siblings, immediate family Other neurologic disorders in the family
Psychosocial History	Coping patterns Discrimination Social exclusion Negative life events Stigma Support systems Occupation Recent travel

Data from Ellis C: Nursing assessment and intervention for the patient experiencing seizures: a structured approach. Clin Nurs Pract Epilepsy 1(2):4–7, 1993; and Leppik IE: Contemporary Diagnosis and Management of the Patient With Epilepsy, 3rd ed. Newtown, PA: Handbooks in Health Care, 1997.

noted. Motor activity may involve a specific part of the body for the duration of the seizure, it may spread, or it may be symmetric or rhythmic. The patient may wander about aimlessly or may become agitated. During complex partial seizures, motor activity may consist of purposeless movements such as picking at clothing or nearby objects. The progression and sequence of the movements should be noted. The arms and legs are often involved, but the nurse should note the motor activity of the head, jaw, face, eyes, tongue, and trunk as well. The eyes may twitch, deviate laterally or vertically, or blink repeatedly. Flexion or extension of the body may occur. Tone in the involved extremities and the Babinski response should be assessed.

Vocalization or verbalization may occur during a seizure. A GTC seizure is sometimes associated with a cry at its onset. Mumbling may occur. At times, during some complex partial seizures, the patient may seem coherent, based solely on an ability to speak, but further evaluation reveals a patient with an altered LOC.

Changes in autonomic regulation necessitate evaluation of pupillary size and reactivity. Heart rate, blood pressure, and respiratory character and rate should be closely monitored. The skin may become clammy and may appear ashen, cyanotic, pale, or flushed.

The exact time of the end of the seizure may be difficult to identify. The progression of the activity and associated times should be documented. Cessation of motor activity may occur gradually, or it may be abrupt. It may be the hallmark of the end of seizure ac-

tivity for some patients, but in those who exhibit minimal motor activity, this would be impossible to verify. In any case, the return of LOC to baseline should be monitored closely.

The description of the seizure and detailed documentation of these components are far more important than attempting to classify the type of seizure. Knowing the details about onset, progression, and cessation of seizure activity is essential for accurate diagnosis. This information is helpful in clarifying the areas of the brain involved, safety interventions needed, treatment options, and lifestyle implications.

Status Epilepticus

The importance of recognition and early intervention for CSE cannot be overemphasized. Of the assessment components discussed earlier, the most essential component to be monitored is the patient's LOC. Persistent seizure activity can lead to morbidity and mortality, as noted earlier. Therefore, the nurse must note the duration of the GTC activity, including any cessation and restarting between the seizures. Although motor activity may appear to be slowing down, the abnormal brain activity can persist. If GTCs are persistent, the muscles become tired, and the intense jerking evident at the onset probably will lessen considerably. It is important to observe the patient for even slight motor activity, such as subtle, low-amplitude twitching of the fingers, arms, or legs. This sign indicates continued seizure activity that could be detected only with an EEG.

The patient's ability to maintain air exchange must be monitored. During the clonic jerking, along with the associated autonomic stimulation, saliva production increases and can occlude or impair the airway. Turning the patient on the side is effective in clearing the airway, but it may not be possible during the clonic phase. Oral suctioning may be needed. A hard-tipped suction catheter is usually the most effective means of clearing the secretions.

Laboratory and Diagnostic Tests

A combination of tests is used in making the diagnosis of epilepsy. After a patient's first seizure, it is imperative to rule out the presence of a structural lesion. This can be done with a computed tomographic (CT) scan, although magnetic resonance imaging (MRI) is desirable. An EEG is another standard part of the diagnostic workup. An EEG can be done at the patient's bedside. Movement artifact is a common problem, especially in patients who may be restless or unable to remain still during the study. An EEG may not always provide evidence of abnormal electrical activity. In fact, it is common for patients to have normal EEGs after seizure activity. This finding is consistent with the episodic nature of the disorder, with abnormalities in brain activity occurring only during the abnormal clinical activity. Many patients have consistently normal EEGs despite periodic seizure activity. The term "epileptiform discharges" is used to refer to the abnormalities in brain activity. The common types are spikes, sharp waves, and spike-and-wave discharges. Each has a different duration and pattern on an EEG.

The current standard for diagnosis of seizure type, in addition to a detailed description of the event, is a video EEG recording of the seizure. Specialized epilepsy centers offer this technique for clarification of seizure diagnosis and determination of candidacy for surgical treatment. Patients are often recorded on video for several consecutive days in an effort to capture seizure activity on video simultaneously with the EEG recording.

Nursing Diagnoses

The care of patients experiencing seizures varies widely, depending on the cause and other coexisting conditions. Nurses practicing in any setting, from emergency department to intensive care, to group home or outpatient setting, must be able to recognize and document suspected seizure activity. Santilli[20] describes the spectrum of epilepsy and the interdependence between the physiologic and psychologic states. Patients with epilepsy can be described broadly as being in one of three categories: uncomplicated, compromised, and devastated[21] (Table 45–5). With this range of patient experience, associated nursing and collaborative diagnoses range from those related to maintenance of vital functions such as ineffective airway clearance to psychosocial aspects including altered coping and knowledge deficit (Table 45–6).

Nurses in critical care settings are more likely to encounter patients with physiologic diagnoses. The range of patient responses, however, must be assessed

TABLE 45–5
Spectrum of the Effects of Epilepsy

Category	Descriptions
Uncomplicated	Majority in this category Seizures controlled with medications Minimal side effects Well-established support system Rare academic, vocational, or psychological problems
Compromised	Seizures usually controlled Possible fluctuating difficulties in social, emotional, cognitive, functional domains, quality of life Possible altered health perceptions Without in-depth assessment, patients appear well adapted
Devastated	Multiple problems including impaired learning, motor, and emotional functioning Seizures often uncontrolled Possible associated cognitive dysfunction related to underlying brain disease (see Table 45–3) Support system stressed, with altered coping Epilepsy possibly the focus of a family's life Patients require continuous intervention and reassurance

Data from Santilli N: The spectrum of epilepsy. Clin Nurs Pract Epilepsy 1(1):4–7, 1993; and Marshall RH, Cupoli JM: Epilepsy and education: the pediatrician's expanding role. Adv Pediatr 33:159–180, 1986.

TABLE 45–6
Nursing Diagnoses

Problem Statement	Etiologic Factors
Acute Care	
Altered cerebral tissue perfusion	Prolonged generalized tonic–clonic seizure activity
Sensory or perceptual alteration	Seizure activity (partial, generalized)
Ineffective airway clearance	Generalized tonic–clonic seizure activity
Ineffective breathing pattern	Generalized tonic–clonic seizure activity
Risk for injury	Altered motor function during seizure activity
Impaired physical mobility	Altered functioning during postictal period
Impaired verbal communication	Altered functioning during postictal period
Knowledge deficit and learning need	Diagnosis, treatment strategies, self-care
Anxiety or fear	Sudden hospitalization, unknown prognosis
Personal identity disturbance	Perception of being out of control, stigma associated with seizures
Chronic Care*	
Knowledge deficit or learning need	Long-term management of disorder
Sensory or perceptual alteration	Medication side effects
Impaired physical mobility	Medication side effects
Altered thought processes	Medication side effects
Altered sexuality patterns	Physiologic effects of epilepsy, medication side effects
Anxiety or fear	Episodic generalized tonic–clonic seizures
Ineffective individual coping	Misconceptions, required lifestyle adaptations
Social isolation	Ineffective coping
Altered role performance	Activity restrictions (e.g., driving) imposed by disorder
Ineffective family coping	Concern for member with epilepsy, fear and inability of family system to successfully adapt to diagnosis

*In addition to items listed under acute care.
Data from Ozuna J: Nursing diagnoses in epilepsy: guidelines for reassessment. Clin Nurs Pract Epilepsy 1(1):11–13, 1993.

in any setting. The psychologic effects can play a significant role in patient healing.

Collaborative Management

A team approach to management of the patient with seizures is essential, whether in the critical care setting or elsewhere on the patient's continuum (Figure 45–1). In the most acute situation, CSE, early recognition and prompt intervention are essential for maintenance of optimal cerebral tissue perfusion. Most cases of CSE begin outside the hospital setting. Public health information recommends calling for emergency assistance if seizures persist for 5 minutes.[22] Nurses must be aware of the institution's protocol for management of CSE. Continuous, skilled nursing care of cardiac, respiratory, and metabolic status is essential to successful management of these patients.

Pharmacotherapy

The Epilepsy Foundation of America's Working Group on Status Epilepticus[8] suggests a timetable for treatment, beginning with the time of seizure onset. Immediate measures include basic life support, stabilization

of vital signs, and laboratory studies including complete blood count, serum chemistries including glucose, sodium, calcium, magnesium, blood urea nitrogen, and AED levels. Administration of 50 mL of 50% glucose and 100 mg intravenous thiamine is recommended, followed by initiation of intravenous AED therapy in the presence of continuing seizures. AED management can vary and usually involves administration of a short-acting drug, such as lorazepam or diazepam, followed by a longer-acting medication, such as fosphenytoin, the phenytoin prodrug, followed by phenobarbital (Table 45–7). In extreme situations, the patient may require intubation, usually related to the effects of the medications necessary to stop the seizures.

If the seizures persist, anesthetizing the patient with phenobarbital or pentobarbital may be required. The airway must be established and mechanical ventilation initiated. Electrocardiogram (ECG), arterial blood pressure, and EEG should be monitored continuously while the patient is receiving the infusion. With pentobarbital, the most commonly used agent, the loading dose is 5 to 20 mg/kg, titrated until the EEG shows a burst-suppression pattern. This pattern is characterized by brief bursts of mixed spikes, slow waves, and sharp waves, interrupted by longer periods of relative

ABBOTT NORTHWESTERN HOSPITAL
Minneapolis Neuroscience Institute
ALLINA HEALTH SYSTEM

CASE TYPE/DIAGNOSIS _____ **INTRACTABLE EPILEPSY / DIFFERENTIAL DIAGNOSIS** _____
OLD RECORDS: ☐ NONE ☐ MICROFILM ☐ ON UNIT
PLAN OF CARE INITIATED BY_____ CONFIRMED W/M.D. _____
IN-HOSPITAL TRANSPORT: ☐ Wheelchair ☐ Lifepack ☐ Cart ☐ O$_2$
☐ Other _____

Primary R.N./Team _____
Primary M.D. _____ # _____
Nursing Case Manager _____ # _____
Nursing Care Coordinator _____ # _____
Case Team Rounds _____

ALERT
Advance Directives? ☐ No ☐ Yes ☐ MD notified
Type _____ Location _____
DNR status: ☐ No ☐ Yes _____ ☐ ID band on
Next of kin/legal guardian _____
ER contact: Name/ph. #/relation _____

IV FLUIDS:
IV Team Draw ☐
Saline Lock _____ Last Site Change _____ △ q 72°
Central Line _____ Insertion _____ Last Drsg. _____
(Type) (Date) (Date)

VALUABLES

ITEM	NONE	DISPOSITION	DISPOSITION	DISPOSITION	DISPOSITION	DAY OF D/C PERSON RETURNED TO
Glasses/Contact Lenses						
Dentures ☐ Up ☐ Low						
Hear. Aid ☐ R ☐ L						
Prosthesis						
Jewelry						
Prescription Medications						
Other:						

TREATMENT / TEMPORARY ORDERS / PROTOCOLS / NOTIFICATIONS

SPECIMENS / CULTURES	C	U	RESULT

CONSULTANT	DATE SEEN	CODE #	SPECIALTY	OFFICE #
M.D.:				
M.D.:				
M.D.:				
M.D.:				
M.D.:				
M.D.:				
S.S.:				
Home Care:				
P.T.:				

CONSULTANT	DATE SEEN	CODE #	SPECIALTY	OFFICE #
O.T.:				
Speech:				
Chaplain:				
Dietitian:				
IV Therapy:				
R.C.:				
Other:				
Other:				
Other:				

DATE	PATIENT'S STORY / SIGNIFICANT EVENTS THIS ADMISSION

SEIZURE DESCRIPTION

ADMITTING PHYSICIAN SOC. SEC. # ADDRESS DOB PATIENT

MMC 475
AD 1274 (12/96)

MINNEAPOLIS NEUROSCIENCE INSTITUTE – INTRACTABLE EPILEPSY / DIFFERENTIAL DIAGNOSIS

PATIENT NAME: _____

DAY 1 DATE: DAY OF WEEK:	DAY 2 DATE: DAY OF WEEK:	DAY 3 DATE: DAY OF WEEK:	DAY 4 DATE: DAY OF WEEK:	DAY 5 DATE: DAY OF WEEK:	DISCHARGE OUTCOMES DAY 6 DATE: DAY OF WEEK:

OUTCOMES

LAB/DIAGNOSTIC/PROCEDURES:
☐ DAILY

MET NOT MET
☐ ☐ Verbalizes safety needs
☐ ☐ Verbalizes educational needs
☐ ☐ Follows safety guidelines
☐ ☐ Verbalizes rationale for reduction of AED's or med change
☐ ☐
☐ ☐
☐ OUTCOMES/DAILY PLAN OF CARE REVIEWED c̄ PT./FAMILY

MET NOT MET
☐ ☐ Follows safety guidelines
☐ ☐ Interacts with peers
☐ ☐
☐ ☐
☐ ☐
☐ ☐
☐ OUTCOMES/DAILY PLAN OF CARE REVIEWED c̄ PT./FAMILY

MET NOT MET
☐ ☐ Follows safety guidelines
☐ ☐
☐ ☐
☐ ☐
☐ ☐
☐ OUTCOMES/DAILY PLAN OF CARE REVIEWED c̄ PT./FAMILY

MET NOT MET
☐ ☐ Verbalizes understanding of basic education
☐ ☐ Follows safety guidelines
☐ ☐ Verbalizes home safety needs
☐ ☐
☐ ☐
☐ OUTCOMES/DAILY PLAN OF CARE REVIEWED c̄ PT./FAMILY

MET NOT MET
☐ ☐ Follows safety guidelines
☐ ☐ Verbalizes understanding of AED's
☐ ☐ Accurately sets up own med box
☐ ☐ Describes characteristics of own seizure type
☐ ☐
☐ OUTCOMES/DAILY PLAN OF CARE REVIEWED c̄ PT./FAMILY

MET NOT MET Verbalizes understanding of:
☐ ☐ Diagnosis
☐ ☐ Rationale for follow-up treatment
☐ ☐ Describes community resources available
☐ ☐ Demonstrates accurate self-medication
☐ ☐
☐ OUTCOMES/DAILY PLAN OF CARE REVIEWED c̄ PT./FAMILY

EVALUATION OF PLAN

☐ NO CHANGES ☐ PLAN MODIFIED ☐ SEE DAR NOTE (×6 columns)

SIGN N D E (×6 columns)

NURSING DIAGNOSES & PLAN
Knowledge deficit:
RT evaluation process, epilepsy & treatment
AEB

High risk for injury:
RT seizure activity

Ineffective coping individual/family:
RT
AEB

Figure 45–1

Sample care map for management of a patient during inpatient evaluation for clarification of seizure diagnosis or presurgical evaluation. (Courtesy of the Minneapolis Neuroscience Institute, Minneapolis, MN.)

COLLABORATIVE / MEDICAL PROBLEMS		

DISCHARGE PLAN
Evaluate home safety needs
Living situation:
  with whom _____
  ☐ House   ☐ Room   ☐ Apartment
  ☐ Health Care Facility   ☐ Home Health Care
  Name _____
  Ph. # _____
Prior use of home care services? ☐ Y ☐ N
Referral: ☐ Social Service ☐ Home Care
Can pt. return to current situation? ☐ Y ☐ N
Who can assist p̄ d/c?
  Name _____
  Relation _____

IF NO SEIZURES BY DAY 3 –
team to discuss need for:
☐ Sleep deprivation
☐ Further AED reduction
☐ Exercise
☐ _____

Discharge conference:
Date _____
Time _____

EDUCATION PLAN
Plan of Care developed:
  w/pt.? ☐ Yes ☐ No
  family? ☐ Yes ☐ No
See education flow sheet (on back)
☐ Review outpatient education checklist
   and incorporate into education plan

Assess needs for further outpatient teaching:
☐ Yes ☐ No ☐ NA   Compliance Clinic
☐ Yes ☐ No ☐ NA   Surgical Teaching
☐ Yes ☐ No ☐ NA   View own seizure video

COGNITIVE/PERCEPTUAL PLAN
Full scale IQ _____
Cognitive assessment: ☐ Yes ☐ No ☐ NA
If yes, plan _____
_____

SAFETY PLAN
Restraints _____

Safety devices/seizure precautions:
☐ Siderail padding x 2 _____ , x 4 _____
☐ Helmet
☐ Helmet with face mask
☐ Off-unit transportation: ○ W/C ○ litter
☐ Transfer belt: in chair
☐ Walk w/assist. only: ○ w/1 ○ w/2
☐ Padded sink & table edges
☐ Mouth guard
☐ Assess pt's. ability to do self-medication
☐ Assess need for med box

PSYCHOSOCIAL/COPING PLAN
For high-risk patients, plan interventions:
☐ Vulnerable adult
☐ Suicidal
☐ Post ictal psychosis
_____
_____
Encourage participation in group activities

ACTIVITY PLAN
VS: Routine
Off unit only with supervision
Up ad lib

NUTRITIONAL PLAN
Regular

PLACE BAR CODE HERE

PATIENT NAME:

Figure 45–1 *Continued*

EEG flattening. Reliance on EEG activity rather than the clinical evidence of seizures to determine whether the therapeutic goal has been met means that the nurse must have the skills to recognize this EEG pattern. Infusion ranges from 1 to 5 mg/kg per hour. For breakthrough seizure activity, additional boluses of up to 50 mg can be used. The infusion is usually continued for 12 to 24 hours after the last seizure. Recommendations for tapering range from discontinuation of the infusion to weaning 1 mg/kg per hour every 4 to 6 hours.

Medications are the cornerstone of treatment for epilepsy. Since phenobarbital was introduced in 1912, more than 20 additional medications have been introduced for treatment. Since 1993, several agents have been introduced, and more will be forthcoming (Chart 45–3). Characteristics of some of the more frequently used AEDs are summarized in Table 45–8. Most of the medications are metabolized by the liver. Some of the newer agents are eliminated by renal excretion and may be useful in patients with liver dysfunction. Collaboration among pharmacist, nurse, and physician in identifying the optimal medication regimen is essential in any setting.

Key principles of medication management include the following: 1) selection of the appropriate drug for the individual patient's seizure type; an accurate diagnosis of the seizure type is assumed; 2) balance between efficacy and side effects; 3) determination of therapeutic goals; in some patients, complete seizure control may not be realistic, but reduction in severity and frequency is; 4) gradual increase in dosage after introduction, to minimize CNS side effects; 5) identification of the patient's target therapeutic range, which can vary from patient to patient and may not be consistent with the laboratory "normal range," in which only 80% of individuals fall; the patient is assessed

TABLE 45-7
Major Drugs Used to Treat Status Epilepticus

	Diazepam	Lorazepam	Fosphenytoin	Phenobarbital
Adult IV dose (mg/kg)	0.15–0.25	0.1	15–20 phenytoin equiv	20
Maximal administration rate (mg/min)	5	2.0	150 phenytoin equiv	20
Minutes to cessation of convulsive status epilepticus	1–3	6–10	10–30	20–30
Duration of action (hr)	0.25–0.5	>12–24	24	>48
Elimination half-life (hr)	30	24	24	100
Volume of distribution (L/kg)	1–2	0.7–1.0	0.5–0.8	0.7
Potential side effects				
Depression of consciousness	10–30 min	Several hours	None	Several days
Respiratory depression	Occasional	Occasional	Infrequent	Occasional
Hypotension	Infrequent	Infrequent	Occasional	Infrequent
Cardiac dysrhythmias	—	—	In patients with heart disease	—

Data from Epilepsy Foundation of America's Working Group on Status Epilepticus: Treatment of convulsive status epilepticus. JAMA 270:845–859, 1993. Copyright 1993, American Medical Association; Treiman DM: General principles of treatment: responsive and intractable status epilepticus in adults. Adv Neurol 34:377–384, 1983; Treiman DM: Special treatment problems in adults. In: Smith DB (ed): Epilepsy: Current Approaches to Diagnosis and Treatment. New York, Raven Press, 1990, pp 155–172.

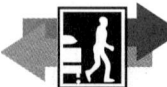 **CHART 45-3**

BEYOND THE ICU: CONVULSIVE STATUS EPILEPTICUS AND PROLONGED SEIZURE ACTIVITY

Episodes of convulsive status epilepticus and prolonged seizure activity have resulted in many trips for patients to the emergency department and admissions to critical care settings. Development of new formulations of medications that can be administered before the patient reaches an emergency department may improve patient outcomes and may result in fewer hospital admissions. First-response professionals, whether 911-dispatched emergency medical technicians or nurses caring for patients in a skilled nursing facility, group home, or home care setting, and parents or family members present during these potentially life-threatening conditions, will play an increasingly important role.

A patient can experience status epilepticus in any setting and at any time. Convulsive status epilepticus may present as the first seizure activity ever for a patient, or it may be recurrent in someone with severe brain disease or in the patient who is noncompliant with the prescribed medication program. The release of the phenytoin prodrug, fosphenytoin sodium, raises questions about initiation of treatment for status epilepticus outside of the acute care setting. This medication, unlike phenytoin, can be administered intramuscularly. It is rapidly absorbed after intramuscular injection (almost as fast as with intravenous administration) and raises possibilities that, in selected situations, patients could receive this early in an episode of status epilepticus and when intravenous access is not immediately possible.

Some children with recurrent episodes of prolonged seizures have endured repeated trips to the emergency department to stop the seizure activity. Use of rectal diazepam in selected situations has been successful in stopping seizures in the home setting. Release of a newer, more easily administered formulation may further expand the use of this agent in these situations. Clearly specifying the parameters within which care providers should use the medication, or transport the child to the emergency department, have been helpful in maintaining safety and in minimizing unnecessary trips to the hospital. This treatment plan cannot be used universally, however, and those who do participate must be knowledgeable of the child's seizure activity as well as competent to administer the medication and then monitor the child's response.

Prompt treatment of these two conditions outside the acute care setting may result in improved patient outcomes and fewer hospital admissions. Nurses employed in these settings need to be aware of the rapid changes occurring in the treatment of seizures. Self-education and education of care providers will be imperative, to provide optimal care to this patient population.

clinically in conjunction with the laboratory data; one must treat the patient, not the laboratory; 6) evaluation of AED levels at regular intervals, depending on the patient's response; and 7) knowledge of the pharmacokinetic profile of the drug, the extent of protein binding, the route of elimination, and drugs that induce hepatic enzymes.

Airway Support

Patients who have GTC seizures are at increased risk of airway compromise. The pharyngeal and ventilatory muscles are in a state of sustained contraction during the tonic phase. The clonic phase results in increased production of saliva and an inability to clear secretions independently. The simplest intervention is to turn the patient to the side when the clonic activity has begun to subside, thereby allowing gravity to drain the secretions from the side of the mouth. In situations of more prolonged seizure activity, oral suction may be necessary, as well as intubation. Patients may vomit during GTC seizures and are at increased risk of aspiration.

Safety Measures

Maintaining patient safety during seizure activity is essential. Removal of harmful objects from the environment, support of the patient's head, staying with the patient during seizures in which he or she may wander aimlessly, and gently guiding the patient to positions of safety, whether the patient is in bed or ambulatory, are key safety measures. The patient should not be restrained unless this is the only means of preventing further injury. Insertion of a tongue blade to prevent oral cavity injuries has been an area of controversy in seizure management. The Epilepsy Foundation of America recommends that no object be forced between the teeth during any seizure. Jaffe and Tosch[23] reported oral cavity injuries in 8 of 21 patients who experienced GTCs. Patients were managed in accordance with the foregoing recommendation. The study has merit, but the sample size in these preliminary data is too small from which to draw conclusions, and additional study is needed to determine the scientific basis for this practice.

Cardiovascular Support

During CSE, the patient becomes hypertensive and tachycardic because of the release of epinephrine and norepinephrine. Cardiac dysrhythmias may occur. Hypotension may follow the initial period of hypertension. Blood pressure and heart rate should be monitored closely. Support of blood pressure with vasopressors and ECG monitoring may become necessary.

Psychological Support

Patients and families require varying degrees of psychological and emotional support when they are living with seizures. In the critical care setting, the fear and stigma associated with seizures may need to be explored, especially with those who have not previously seen or experienced a seizure. The occurrence of seizures as a complication of another disease process introduces additional stressors (Chart 45–4). Families of those patients being treated with barbiturate coma often need repeated explanations for the use of this therapy and the therapeutic goal that is trying to be achieved.

Patients with epilepsy frequently need ongoing psychological support in dealing with the chronicity of the disorder, the associated lifestyle changes, self-esteem issues, and the concomitant medication side effects. Identification of current coping patterns, exploration of the current support system, and knowledge of and access to resources can be essential components in attaining the quality of life the patient seeks (Chart 45–5).

Surgical Interventions

Collaboration among team members is essential in working with patients who are candidates for surgical management of epilepsy. Not all patients who have epilepsy are candidates for surgery, and the evaluation process itself can be grueling for patients and families. A positive outcome is not guaranteed with any of the surgical interventions. An in-depth evaluation can provide sufficient information about the patient's potential for such an intervention. A surgical evaluation includes the following: 1) structural and functional brain imaging with MRI, positron emission tomography, or single photon emission CT; 2) clinical assessment; 3) neuropsychological evaluation to localize areas of altered cognitive function such as language and memory; 4) psychiatric evaluation to determine readiness for surgery and the ability to cope with the outcome (positive or negative); and 5) electrophysiologic studies with video EEG and sphenoidal electrodes. In addition to the extracranial studies noted earlier, intracranial studies, such as depth, subdural, and epidural electrodes, and the intracarotid amobarbital injection test,[24] may be used.[25]

The most common type of operation performed is the temporal lobe resection in patients whose seizures arise from the anterior temporal lobe. Functional mapping of the brain can maximize the amount of epileptic tissue removed and can minimize the removal of normal tissue. Success rates of 55 to 70% have been reported.[26] Extratemporal resections in the frontal, parietal, and occipital lobes are much less successful.

TABLE 45-8

Common Medications Used to Treat Epilepsy

Drug	Usual Maximal Adult Dosage	Time to Steady State	Half-Life	Elimination	Thera-peutic Range	Common Side Effects	Affected by AED*	Affect AED*
Carbamazepine (CBZ)	400–1200 mg/day BID–QID	4–6 wk; after induction 2–4 days	8–72 hr	1–3% unchanged in urine	4–14 µg/mL	Dizziness, diplopia, drowsiness, blurred and double vision, nausea, headache, leukopenia	Oral contraceptives, warfarin, theophylline, doxycycline	Fluoxetine, propoxyphene, erythromycin, cimetidine, FBM, phenobarbital, PHT
Felbamate (FBM)	3600 mg/day TID–QID	5–7 days	20–23 hr	50–60% metabolized; 40–60% unchanged in urine	Not defined	Anorexia, weight loss, vomiting, insomnia, nausea, headache, aplastic anemia,[†] hepatic failure[†]	PHT, VPA, CBZ and its epoxide	PHT, CBZ, VPA
Gabapentin (GBP)	900–1800 mg/day TID–QID	Renal function dependent; 1–2 days normal renal function	5–7 hr with normal function; up to 132 hr with anuria	Renal; not metabolized	Not defined	Fatigue, somnolence, weight gain, dizziness, ataxia	None	Aluminum hydroxide, magnesium hydroxide
Lamotrigine (LTG)	100–150 mg/day w/VPA; 300–500 mg/day without VPA BID–TID	3–15 days	Varies depending on monotherapy, presence of other enzyme inducers, VPA; range 11–113 hr	85% metabolized; 10% unchanged in urine	Not defined	Drowsiness, headache, tremor, diplopia, ataxia, abnormal thinking, nervousness, weight gain, nausea, vomiting	CBZ epoxide, VPA	PHT, CBZ, phenobarbital, primidone, VPA

Drug	Dose	Time to steady state	Half-life	Metabolism	Therapeutic level	Side effects	Drugs affecting level	Drugs affected
Phenytoin (PHT)	500–600 mg/day QD–TID	1–3 wk	7–42 hr	Over 90% to inactive metabolites	Total 10–25 µg/mL Unbound (free) 0.3–0.5 µg/mL	Nystagmus, ataxia, slurred speech, incoordination, gingival hyperplasia, folate deficiency, anemia	Oral contraceptives, bishydroxycoumarin, quinidine, vitamin D, folic acid	FBM, methsuximide, cimetidine, fluconazole, phenobarbital, alcohol, disulfram, isoniazid, warfarin, CBZ, antacids, VPA
Topiramate (TPM)	400–600 mg/day BID	4 days with normal renal function	21 hr	70% unchanged in urine; % metabolized increases with inducers	Not defined	Somnolence, fatigue, psychomotor slowing, decreased concentration, word-finding difficulties, kidney stones, nystagmus, paresthesias, weight loss	PHT, VPA, oral contraceptives, digoxin, CNS depressants, carbonic anhydrase inhibitors	PHT, CBZ, VPA
Valproate (VPA)	3000–5000 mg/day BID–QID	5–10 days	5–20 hr	Almost completely metabolized; some active metabolites	50–100 µg/mL	Nausea, vomiting, tremor, thrombocytopenia, increased appetite, alopecia, prolonged bleeding times, elevated liver enzymes	Phenobarbital FBM, LTG	Cimetidine, salicylates, phenobarbital, PHT, CBZ, LTG

*Partial listing of drug interactions.
†FBM should only be used when risk is fully weighed and is clearly understood by patient and family because of the high incidence of these side effects.

Data from Leppik IE, Wolff DL: Antiepileptic medication interaction. Neurol Clin 11:905–921, 1993; and Levy RH, Mattson RH, Meldrum BS (eds): Antiepileptic Drugs, 4th ed. New York, Raven Press, 1995.

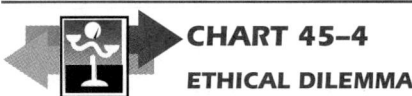

CHART 45–4
ETHICAL DILEMMA

Mr. J. is an 80-year-old man with a history of adenocarcinoma of the colon diagnosed 5 years ago. He was recently admitted from his home, where he has been living independently with his wife, because he was complaining of headaches, right-sided weakness, intermittent periods of disorientation, and confusion. An episode of combative behavior, unlike Mr. J.'s typical behavior, prompted his wife to call 911 for emergency assistance. On admission to the emergency department, he was oriented to his name, had +3 (0–5 scale) strength in all muscle groups of the right extremities, and insisted that he needed to get to the grocery store as soon as possible. Cognitive examination revealed one of three items recalled after 5 minutes, word-finding difficulty, and impaired judgment. A head computed tomography scan reveals presumed metastatic lesions to the brain. He is admitted to the neuroscience unit for further assessment and care.

Eight hours after admission, Mr. J. begins to have focal seizure activity of his right hand, which progresses to involve his arm, face, and leg and then generalizes. Lorazepam is administered, followed by a loading dose of fosphenytoin; however, generalized tonic–clonic seizure activity is persistent. Phenobarbital is ordered, and the seizure activity is finally controlled after 45 minutes. Intubation is required because of the respiratory depression, and his blood pressure is 86/72 mm Hg (admission, 118/82 mm Hg). He is transferred to the intensive care unit,

where you will be providing care to the patient. His blood pressure continues to drop, and dopamine is started.

Mr. J.'s medical record has his advance directive, in which he states that he does not wish extraordinary measures to be instituted should his cancer progress. He also states that he wishes to be kept comfortable with pain medications only. You discuss the advanced directive with the physician, who points out that if the seizures are controlled, Mr. J.'s cardiovascular and respiratory status should stabilize, and the dopamine and ventilator will no longer be needed. Mrs. J. is overwhelmed by the situation and expresses that her husband would never want all these "tubes and lines. He has had enough of this in the last 5 years." .

1. What is the nature of the conflict between the care being provided and Mr. J.'s advanced directive?
2. Which ethical principles play a role in this dilemma?
3. What additional information do you need from Mrs. J. and the physician to be able to take steps to resolve this conflict?
4. What is your role in working through this dilemma?
5. What other decisions about his care need to be made?

Corpus callosotomy, the sectioning or disconnecting of the anterior two-thirds of this band of white matter, is done to prevent the spread of seizures from one hemisphere to the other. Patients with seizures characterized by sudden, precipitous falls associated with recurrent injuries may be candidates for this operation. Hemispherectomy is most commonly performed in children who have seizures arising from one poorly functioning hemisphere and have weakness and loss of touch sensation and vision on the opposite side of the body. The affected cerebral hemisphere, including the amygdala and hippocampus, is removed.

Patients who arrive in the intensive care unit after a surgical procedure receive the same skilled level of neurologic assessment and intervention as any other patient who has experienced a craniotomy. They are at risk not only for seizures, but also for other complications of intracranial surgery, including hemorrhage, ischemic stroke, and infection.

Complications

The morbidity and mortality associated with status epilepticus are discussed earlier in this chapter. In addition to the potential for neuronal injury and death, the patient is also at risk for the psychological complications associated with seizures. In patients with nonrecurrent seizures, the stress of seizures in addition to the concurrent medical illness may be devastating. Whether the seizures are recurrent or nonrecurrent, the consequences to the patient may be the same.

Multidisciplinary Outcomes

Multidisciplinary outcomes in intensive care settings are focused on restoring balance to the physiologic patterns of the patient, such as activity and cognitive and metabolic functioning. In outpatient settings, focus

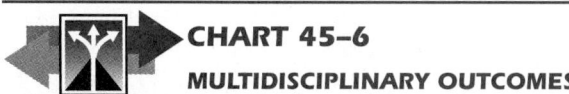

CHART 45-5

RESEARCH UTILIZATION: PREFERENCES CONCERNING EPILEPSY: OPINIONS OF NURSES, PHYSICIANS, AND PERSONS WITH EPILEPSY

Abstract: This descriptive study had two purposes: 1) to determine whether patients with epilepsy treated in outpatient settings would prefer to receive information about epilepsy and its treatment from physicians, nurses, or other health care professionals; and 2) to determine which health care professionals physicians and nurses believe are able to teach patients about epilepsy. Three samples of participants were used: 1) persons with epilepsy being treated in outpatient clinics; 2) neurologists and neurosurgeons in the investigators' state and resident neurologists and neurosurgeons in the study hospital; and 3) nurses working in outpatient settings and in neurology and neurosurgery units at metropolitan hospitals. A 41-item Health Educator Preference Questionnaire was used. It addressed five areas: 1) anatomy and physiology; 2) psychological factors; 3) medications; 4) seizure information; and 5) general lifestyle information. Results indicated that persons with epilepsy generally prefer to receive information about epilepsy and its treatment from physicians. Nurses received the most support for teaching general lifestyle information, although the number was still lower than that for physicians. Nurses and physicians agreed that nurses are preferred for providing information about psychological concerns and physicians are the preferred provider of information about the cause and treatment of epilepsy.

Critique: The responses of the nurse and physician participants may be representative only of those who have an interest in epilepsy, and results may be biased in favor of the role of the nurse as patient educator. Another limitation of the study is that the patients sampled obtained care in private physicians' offices and a hospital clinic for epilepsy patients. Patients who receive care at specialized epilepsy centers may have different opinions about receiving education from nurses. It is unclear whether nurses from these settings were included in the sample. Patients may have different perceptions of nurses who work in these settings.

Nursing Considerations: This study certainly challenges nursing's strong commitment to providing patient education. In all five categories, patients preferred to receive information about epilepsy from physicians. Further exploration of this perception is needed, and evidence of it in the critical care setting should be described. Nurses working in any setting should be aware of the potential for variation in patient preferences about education. They should continually challenge the assumption that they are the primary educators of patients, and they should ensure that they are working collaboratively with other health care professionals who are involved with the patient's care, both within the acute care setting and beyond.

Source: Dilorio C, Manteuffel B: Preferences concerning epilepsy education: opinions of nurses, physicians, and persons with epilepsy. J Neurosci Nurs 27:29–34, 1995.

CHART 45-6

MULTIDISCIPLINARY OUTCOMES

Acute Care: Restoration of adequate cerebral tissue perfusion by early recognition of and intervention for convulsive and nonconvulsive status epilepticus

Effective airway clearance by institution of proper positioning and suctioning during and after seizure activity

Effective respiratory patterns by prevention of aspiration and effective airway clearance during and after seizure activity

Prevention of injury during seizure activity by institution of measures appropriate to maintain safety during seizure activity

Restoration and maintenance of the sensorium by clarification of the patient's seizure experience, reorientation to the environment, and evaluation of medication and environmental effects on the patient

Chronic Care*: Self-management of therapeutic regimen by education, access to services, and social and psychological support

Restoration of psychosocial balance in patient

Restoration and maintenance of family dynamics

*In addition to items listed under acute care.

expands to other patterns including self-perception, roles, relationships, sexuality, coping, stress, and health management (Chart 45–6).

Critical Thinking Exercise

A 24-year-old woman with no significant previously known health problems is admitted to the emergency department and is responsive to deep pain only. Her roommate accompanies her and reports that she found the patient in bed early this morning, breathing heavily, but was unable to awaken her for work. The patient's hair, neck, and shirt are damp with saliva.

The neurologic assessment reveals a patient unresponsive to verbal stimuli, with withdrawal of all extremities to nail bed stimulation and slight twitching of her right hand. Pupils are equal and are briskly reactive to light. Her blood pressure is 100/60 mm Hg, heart rate is 100, and respiratory rate is 8. Her temperature is 37.0°C. Other aspects of her physical assessment are unremarkable. CT scan of the head is ordered. Complete blood count, glucose, and toxicology screen are ordered.

1. Identify signs and symptoms that lead you to suspect that the patient may be experiencing CSE.

Before the patient can be taken for the head CT, she begins to experience focal twitching of her right arm. The resident orders diazepam, 5 mg intravenously, which has no effect on the twitching. He orders a repeat dose of 5 mg, which likewise has no effect on the twitching.

2. Identify the focus of your nursing assessments and the rationale for these priorities.
3. What can you anticipate as the next interventions for this patient?

A loading dose of fosphenytoin sodium is ordered.

4. Identify the focus of your nursing assessments at this point and the rationale for these priorities.

The patient's vital signs remain stable during the infusion, and the twitching of the right arm stops. Her parents arrive and are anxious and fearful.

5. List your nursing diagnoses at this point and associated interventions and outcomes.

Key Concepts

⟹ Seizures can occur in any human being, given the right combination of circumstances in which abnormal cerebral activity exceeds the seizure threshold.

⟹ Many conditions seen in critical care settings can contribute to seizure occurrence.

⟹ Epilepsy is a chronic disorder, the hallmark of which is recurrent, unprovoked seizures.

⟹ Seizures may also be nonrecurrent when they are related to symptomatic, transient causes such as toxic or metabolic conditions. Self-limited seizures are not epilepsy.

⟹ The clinical expression of a seizure varies, depending on the area of the brain involved. Sensory, motor, autonomic, and cognitive components are highly variable, and the same patient may not have the identical, stereotypic seizure activity each time.

⟹ The two major classes of seizures are partial and generalized. Each class has several types of seizures that are uniquely expressed clinically and on EEG.

⟹ Accurate description and classification of seizures are essential in identifying appropriate treatment.

⟹ Knowledge of a patient's epileptic syndrome can assist in determining when to treat and for how long.

⟹ The hallmark of treatment for epilepsy is medication. Medications with newer mechanisms of action and newer formulations of standard medications are increasing the options for patients.

⟹ Some patients may be candidates for epilepsy surgery, but this group comprises the minority of patients. The type of surgical procedure used is based on the type of seizure and an extensive evaluation involving the multidisciplinary team.

⟹ The variability of seizure activity affects patients' lives in various ways.

⟹ Any seizure may progress to status epilepticus, or continuous seizure activity. Regardless of type, the seizures should be stopped. Some types are life-threatening.

⟹ CSE is a life-threatening condition that leads to neuronal injury and death. Seizures must be stopped as quickly as possible.

⟹ A team approach to the management of seizures and epilepsy is essential regardless of setting. The team brings knowledge of the clinical presentation of the seizure, the most effective treatment plan, and the patient's response to the plan.

⟹ A stigma about seizures and epilepsy continues to exist. Increased knowledge and understanding are essential in breaking down the barriers associated with the stigma.

⟹ Psychosocial support plays a key role in a patient's effectively coping with seizures. The continuum of uncomplicated, compromised, and devastated provides a framework for evaluating the effects of the disorder on the patient and family.

Acknowledgment

The author gratefully acknowledges the thorough review of this manuscript and thoughtful suggestions by Therese Bowman Cloyd, Nina Graves, Margaret Jacobs, and Elaine Hogan Miller.

References

1. Hauser WA: Epidemiology of seizure disorders and the epilepsies. In: Santilli N (ed): Managing Seizure Disorders: A Handbook for Health Care Professionals. Philadelphia, Lippincott–Raven, 1996.
2. Hauser WA: Status epilepticus: epidemiologic considerations. Neurology 40(Suppl 2):9–13, 1990.
3. Lothman EW: Functional anatomy: a challenge for the decade of the brain. Epilepsia 32 (Suppl 5):S3–S13, 1991.
4. Boggs JG: Seizures in medically complex patients. Epilepsia 38 (Suppl 4):S55–S59, 1997.
5. Commission on Classification and Terminology of the International League Against Epilepsy: Proposal for revised clinical and electroencephalographic classification of epileptic seizures. Epilepsia 22:489–501, 1981.
6. Commission on Classification and Terminology of the International League Against Epilepsy: Proposal for revised classification of epilepsies and epileptic syndromes. Epilepsia 30:389–399, 1989.
7. Dreifuss FE: Classification of the epilepsies: Influence on management. In: Santilli N (ed): Managing Seizure Disorders: A Handbook for Health Care Professionals. Philadelphia, Lippincott–Raven, 1996.
8. Epilepsy Foundation of America's Working Group on Status Epilepticus: Epilepsy Foundation of America: Treatment of convulsive status epilepticus. JAMA 270:854–859, 1993.
9. DeLorenzo RJ, Towne AR, Pellock JM, et al: Status epilepticus in children, adults, and the elderly. Epilepsia 33 (Suppl 4):S15–S25, 1992.
10. Browne TR, Mikati M: Status epilepticus. In: Ropper AH, Kennedy SF (eds): Neurological and Neurosurgical Intensive Care, 2nd ed. Rockville, MD, Aspen Publishers, 1988.
11. Hauser WA, Hesdorffer DC: Epilepsy Frequency, Causes and Consequences. New York, Demos Publications, 1990.
12. Leppik IE: Status epilepticus: the next decade. Neurology 40(Suppl 2):4–9, 1990.
13. Wasterlain CG, Fujikawa DG, Penix L, et al: Pathophysiological mechanisms of brain damage from status epilepticus. Epilepsia 34 (Suppl 1):S37–S53, 1993.
14. Krumholz A, Sung GY, Fisher RS, et al: Complex partial status epilepticus accompanied by serious morbidity and mortality. Neurology 45:1499–1504, 1995.
15. DeGiorgio CM, Gott PS, Rabinowicz AL, et al: Neuron-specific enolase, a marker of acute neuronal injury, is increased in complex partial status epilepticus. Epilepsia 37:606–609, 1996.
16. Schomer DL: Focal status epilepticus and epilepsia partialis continua in adults and children. Epilepsia 34 (Suppl 1):S29–S36, 1993.
17. Ellis C: Nursing assessment and intervention for the patient experiencing seizures: a structured approach. Clin Nurs Pract Epilepsy 1(2):4–7, 1993.
18. Leppik IE: Contemporary Diagnosis and Management of the Patient with Epilepsy, 3rd ed. Newtown, PA, Handbooks in Health Care, 1997.
19. American Association of Neuroscience Nursing: Seizure Assessment Guidelines. Chicago, American Association of Neuroscience Nursing, 1997.
20. Santilli N: The spectrum of epilepsy. Clin Nurs Pract Epilepsy 1(1):4–7, 14, 1993.
21. Marshall RH, Cupoli JM: Epilepsy and education: the pediatrician's expanding role. Adv Pediatr 33:159–180, 1986.
22. Santilli N: Anticipatory management of status epilepticus. Clin Nurs Pract Epilepsy 3(3):12–15, 1996.
23. Jaffe W, Tosch P: Myths and misconceptions: the tongue blade controversy. Clin Nurs Pract Epilepsy 1(2):9, 14, 1993.
24. Tackenberg JN, Ahern GL, Herring AM, et al: Nursing implications of the intracarotid amobarbital procedure. J Neurosci Nurs 26:309–318, 1994.
25. Sierzant T: Surgical options for individuals with epilepsy: opportunities for nursing interventions. Clin Nurs Pract Epilepsy 3(2):4–7, 1996.
26. National Institutes of Health Consensus Development Conference Statement: Surgery for epilepsy. Epilepsia 31:806–812, 1990.

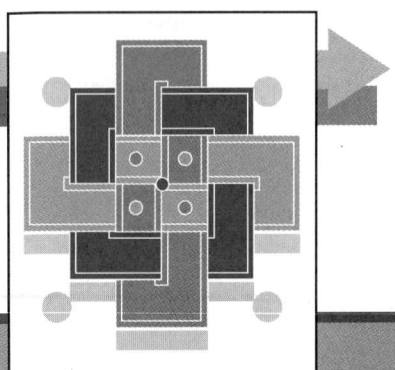

Multisystem Disorders

Challenge Met in Giving Burn Patient Back His Life

I was the admitting nurse for Lawrence, a 36-year-old man, transferred from another facility to our burn center. Before his arrival in our unit, we knew he had been involved in a motorcycle accident and had sustained full-thickness burns (third-degree) over 80% of his body. I was also told that the doctors at the referring facility believed that perhaps it would be best just to make him comfortable because the prognosis was so grim. From my 10-year experience as a burn nurse, I knew, before even seeing Lawrence, that his injury carried approximately a 75%+ mortality rate and that great disabilities often resulted from the injury. I also knew he would be facing at least a 3-month hospitalization and would have to undergo multiple surgical procedures, not to mention the pain, disfigurement, and emotional scars that are everlasting to the burn patient.

Lawrence arrived in our unit at 11:00 AM escorted by a transport team. Lawrence's eyes were swollen shut, and he appeared huge to me because of the total body edema. He was restless but seemed to hear me when I spoke. I kept reassuring him and explaining to him what we were doing. I remember feeling overwhelmed about his wounds, but I also remember feeling strangely consoled when I realized that most of the burns were too deep to hurt. The doctors and the other members of our burn team looked gloomy and shook their heads as we did a head-to-toe assessment while receiving report from the transport team. As I prepared the hydrotherapy tub for what would be the first of many "tubbings" for Lawrence, I was trying to focus on something positive and encouraging. Suddenly, it occurred to me that, although swollen, his face had been spared, as well as his hands and genitalia. I know from my experience that burns of the face, hands, and genitalia are difficult from a rehabilitation point of view. The attending physician who had accepted the patient looked particularly pensive, as if he were thinking out loud. I heard him whisper, "Perhaps they were right, the most merciful thing to do would be to just make him comfortable."

After making our initial assessment, our routine is to submerge the patient in our hydrotherapy tub. This is done to cleanse and decontaminate the wounds. Before placing him in the tub, I left the room to obtain some sedation and pain medication for Lawrence. While walking past the waiting room, I noticed a woman who was obviously praying. She met my eyes and said, "Please save my boy . . . He is a good boy." I realized that the badly burned 36-year-old man in our tub room was "her boy." I gave her a reassuring hug and told her the doctors would be out to speak to her in just a little while. She immediately returned to her praying. We tubbed Lawrence, and the doctors extended the escharotomies on his arms. I controlled the bleeding, and, with the help of our burn technician and physical therapist, I dressed his entire body in burn dressings and moved him to his room. In his room, I placed him on the cardiac monitor and oxygen saturation monitor, and the respiratory therapist placed him on a volume ventilator. I looked around and suddenly realized that the six-member transport team was gone, the burn resident and the attending doctor left to speak to the family, and the respiratory therapist was seeing to other patients. Lawrence was all mine. I realized that to an extent his survival depended on me and on all the nurses who would care for him. The nurse's knowledge and skills in assessing, reporting, alerting, intervening, and administering are instrumental in the patient's survival. The intravenous fluids must be titrated carefully to maintain urine output at a minimum of 30 mL per hour, to preserve kidney function. Burn patients survive if the burn care team can anticipate problems and can see that appropriate treatment is initiated in a timely fashion. Predictable infections must be treated before sepsis ensues, and subtle changes in the patient can alert the nurse to early signs of organ failure.

From the very first day, I began bonding with Lawrence. He was intubated and could not speak. His eyes were swollen shut so he could not see. In the initial hour he was with me, I became so busy treating his hypothermia and dealing with the coffee-ground returns from his Salem sump that I must have worked in silence. Suddenly, I felt him try to grab my arm in an almost desperate attempt to communicate. After that, I spoke to him constantly. The doctors returned to Lawrence's bedside after talking to his family and said, "The family wants everything possible done." The way the attending physician said those words was as if he were asking me my opinion. I remember blurting out with great conviction, "He can make it! We must give him a chance." I impressed on the doctors the positive aspects of our new patient, namely, his relatively young age, his previous good health, his loving and supportive family, and my observation that three major areas of the body were spared. I also felt I needed to put in a word for his mother, who was still praying in the waiting room. After our brief discussion, the attending physician said he would start scheduling multiple surgery times and instructed me to make the appropriate arrangements to begin culturing epithelium. Culturing skin is a technique of harvesting the patient's own skin in the laboratory from plugs taken from the patient's spared areas. The laboratory-grown skin is then used to autograft the patient, to cover areas where burn tissue is surgically débrided.

I was Lawrence's bedside nurse for 60 days of his 4-month hospitalization. I cared for Lawrence through dozens of hydrotherapy treatments, many Swan–Ganz catheter insertions, and multiple débridements. I assisted in many sessions in the operating room and helped apply the cultured epithelium when it finally arrived. I nursed him through dozens of blood transfusions and at least four septic episodes. The entire time I cared for him, his mother prayed at the bedside and other loving family members and his girlfriend visited. At times, people asked whether his mother was in my way because I rarely asked her to leave. Of course she was not in my way. She was an important member of the team, and I felt she was a driving force in his recovery. Most of the time I was too busy to hear what she was actually saying in her prayers, but on several occasions I heard her praying for me.

Lawrence was soon extubated and could speak; however, he was confused and often hallucinated. Decreased sensorium is often the first sign of sepsis. On more than one occasion, I reported my suspicions that he was septic, and lifesaving treatment was initiated without wasting precious time waiting for the cultures that eventually proved my suspicions. As if the septicemia were not enough, 4 weeks into his hospitalization he developed potentially lethal cardiac dysrhythmias, and several codes were called. After many episodes of bradydysrhythmias and ventricular standstills, an external pacemaker was added to the repertoire of equipment, procedures, and monitoring parameters I needed to watch closely. For several weeks, Lawrence had many setbacks, and several times the burn team doubted that his survival was a reasonable goal. After nearly a dozen surgical procedures, most of his body was covered with new skin, and his medical condition slowly improved. His mother appeared more and more confident as she prayed. She hugged me often, and I was thrilled when I could give her encouraging news. Lawrence's mind cleared, and he began venting his fears and concerns. He now needed a sounding board as he tried to put in perspective what had happened to him. I tried to sit and talk to him as much as time allowed, as did the other members of our burn team. I often included his family in our gab sessions because I recognized that support from his loved ones was now as critical to his long-term survival as the intensive monitoring was during the emergency phase of his injury.

Eventually, Lawrence was ready for transfer to a rehabilitation center so he could better prepare for his return to society. During his last days in our unit, he told me that he did not remember much of his early weeks here, but he said he remembered my reassuring voice. In hearing this I was so glad that I talked to him constantly even when I was overwhelmed with the tasks at hand. On one of his return visits, he told me he now remembers his short stay at the facility where he was originally admitted. He remembers being told in the emergency room there that they could make him comfortable but that he would most likely not survive. He is grateful to our team for having taken the enormous challenge of giving him back his life. He is complimentary to me for my involvement. He credits me with more than he should, but it certainly makes me feel good and makes me proud of our burn team.

Paula C. Fillari, RN, CCRN
Bothin Burn Center
Saint Francis Memorial Hospital
San Francisco, California

1997 AACN-3M Health Care Excellence in Clinical Practice Award Recipient

46

Human Immunodeficiency Virus Disease

Sharon Douglass and Frances B. Smith

Objectives

After completing this chapter, the student will be able to:

1. Relate the physiologic principles of the immune system to the pathophysiology of human immunodeficiency virus (HIV) disease.
2. Differentiate the major modes of transmission of HIV disease.
3. Select the primary components of assessment in screening patients for HIV disease.
4. Correlate the assessment findings and treatment strategies with the phase of development of HIV disease.
5. Select appropriate nursing interventions to address the major psychosocial problems confronted by patients with HIV.
6. Plan appropriate educational strategies for patients with HIV and their families.
7. Correlate management strategies with major physiologic symptoms found in patients with HIV.
8. Compare the major categories of drugs used in the treatment of HIV disease and the opportunistic infections associated with HIV disease.

Acquired immunodeficiency syndrome (AIDS) is currently referred to as HIV disease, although these two terms are often used interchangeably. As the pandemic known as HIV disease mounts, the costs from social, economic, and health perspectives continue to increase. Although the word "cure" is not yet associated with this illness, it is now viewed as a chronic disease with an increasingly hopeful prognosis. Hope for a cure depends on continued diligence and the search for the right combination of knowledge, attitudes, behavior changes, and pharmaceutical interventions. Even with remarkable drug therapies such as protease inhibitors, prevention efforts are vital to the control and elimination of the disease.

Patients with HIV disease may be admitted to a critical or intermediate care setting at any point in the course of their illness. These admissions may be due to an exacerbation of the HIV disease, or the patient with HIV may present with an unrelated illness such as trauma. For these reasons, the nurse needs a solid foundation in the pathophysiology, diagnostic workup, and treatment strategies related to the care of this population of patients.

ANATOMY OF THE IMMUNE SYSTEM

To appreciate, prevent, and manage the disease caused by HIV fully, the nurse needs to understand how the immune system functions in relation to this disease. The first lines of defense against disease-producing microorganisms and viruses are the body's chemical and physical barriers. Skin, when intact, is a perfect barrier against microbial invasion. Sweat, which is composed of lactic and fatty acids, also helps to repel bacteria. Mucosal membranes lining the inner surfaces of the body resist bacteria and remove them mechanically by the action of cilia, sneezing, or coughing. Body fluids (such as tears, saliva, and gastric juices) are bactericidal. In addition, tears, saliva, and urine also rid the body of unwanted bacteria. Body cavities contain "friendly" bacteria that suppress pathogens. Unfortunately, when these friendly bacteria are suppressed by antibiotics, unwanted flora usually proliferates. If the first line of defense is compromised, the second line of defense is activated and involves several organ systems.

The *thymus gland* is important in the maturation of a small to medium-size cell known as the *T cell*, which has a circulating life span of up to 5 years. This organ is also essential in the development of the immune response in newborns. When the thymus gland is removed early in life, the host becomes more susceptible to acute infectious diseases later in life. *Lymph nodes,* small pinhead to olive-size glands, filter foreign material such as bacteria to detain it from reaching the blood. Clustered in certain regions (neck, cervical; armpit, axillary; groin, inguinal), these nodes produce both lymphocytes and monocytes.

The *spleen* is important in embryonic development because it produces all types of blood cells. The adult spleen is responsible only for lymphocytes and monocytes, but it can produce various blood cells if bone marrow is damaged. The spleen filters blood and removes matter such as bacteria and dying red blood cells (RBCs) from circulation.

The *bone marrow* produces blood cells and determines hemoglobin. Lymphocytes comprise 20% to 50% of the total white blood cells. *B cells* originate from bone marrow and T-cells from the thymus. *Antibodies* develop in response to infection by an antigen or as the result of a vaccination. They may be transferred to the fetus from the mother in utero, or they may result from accidental, unknown exposure *(natural antibodies).* All antibodies belong to a group of serum proteins called immunoglobulins,

also referred to as IgA, IgG, IgM, IgE, and IgD (Table 46–1).

This antigen–antibody reaction forms the basis of immunity. *Complement,* an enzymatic protein manufactured in the liver, must be activated to phagocytize bacteria and other cells. Fourteen different components combine with the antigen–antibody complex to effect cell lysis. *Phagocytes* are the body's garbage disposal units, ingesting and destroying invading microorganisms, cells with their cellular debris, and dust particles. Phagocytes lack memory, so they are unable to distinguish among foreign invaders. When presented with the same microorganism, they will not speed up the phagocytic process. Phagocytic cells do, however, differentiate between self and non-self, as explained in the next section, on the physiology of the immune system.[1,2] Each component of the immune system is essential, if the body is to be protected; loss of one component affects the functioning of others and thus ultimately proves hazardous.

PHYSIOLOGY OF THE IMMUNE SYSTEM

Immunity, whether achieved passively or actively, is essential to a disease-free state. Under most circum-

TABLE 46–1
Types and Functions of the Immunoglobulins

Type	Function
IgM	Initial immunoglobulin produced by plasma cells in response to infection Lasts from several days to weeks Remaining IgM with greater affinity for antigen than the original Comprises only 7–10% of Igs in serum Largest of immunoglobulins Cannot cross placenta Found on B lymphocytes as sites for antigen binding
IgG	Produced after IgM Lasts for several weeks Responsible for protection of newborn during first 6 months of life Comprises 75–80% of Igs in serum Inactivates viruses and bacteria (extracelluarly) and toxins Coats antigens in preparation for phagocytosis Involved in hypersensitivity reactions
IgA	Found in external secretions like tears and saliva Found in mucosa in secretory IgA form to prevent attachment Chief defense of respiratory tract Provides local or topical immunity Comprises 10% of Igs in serum
IgE	Found in body secretions in response to allergies in large amounts Otherwise only found in trace amounts in serum
IgD	Found only in newborns Comprises less than 1% of Igs in serum Like IgM, can be found on B lymphocytes as sites for antigen binding

Data from Boyd RF: *Basic Medical Microbiology.* Boston, Little, Brown 1995; Galantino ML: *Clinical Assessment and Treatment of HIV Rehabilitation of a Chronic Illness.* Thorofare, NJ, Slack, 1992; and Flaskerud JH: *AIDS/HIV Infection: A Reference Guide for Nursing Professionals.* Philadelphia, W.B. Saunders, 1989.

stances, exposure to a disease-producing antigen elicits a protective response by the immune system, similar to the way in which a vaccine stimulates the immune system. In utero, an embryo conducts a "self" check, whereby all organs, tissues, and fluids are recognized as belonging to "self." This systems review is essential to identify an outside challenger as foreign later in life. Anything not documented in this initial review will elicit an antibody response. An example is sequestered fluid in the eyeball. If injury to the eye produces leakage, the immune system may target the fluid as foreign and may destroy the eye. In addition to this *innate* immunity, the body has two other mechanisms to protect itself: cell-mediated immunity and humoral immunity. These two responses to invading antigens, whether pollens, grafted tissues, microorganisms, or the individual's own cells, are also called *specific immunity,* or *adaptive,* because of antigen specificity and immunologic memory.[3]

Cell-mediated immune response refers to the production of T cells in response to antigens. These white blood cells migrate to the thymus, develop, and mature into T cells. Mature T cells travel to lymphoid tissue, wandering between blood and lymph. Three subtypes of T cells are known: 1) *T-helper cells,* which trigger the immune system and stimulate the production of antibody-forming cells from B lymphocytes; 2) *cytotoxic* or *killer T cells,* which are responsible for graft rejection and the death of infected or damaged cells; and 3) *suppressor T cells,* which suppress antibody-forming cells from B lymphocytes.[3]

Humoral immune response is the production of B cells (plasma lymphocytes) in response to antigen exposure, creating antibodies. Occasionally, this response produces not only immunity, but also hypersensitivity. In addition, there is a nonspecific immune response, which does not involve antibody production but includes complement activation, the inflammatory reaction, and phagocytosis of microorganisms (Table 46–2). The two types of immune response are primary and secondary. The primary response is the response first elicited when an organism makes its initial appearance. This situation causes an IgM response followed by an IgG response. Years later, when the organism again tries to enter the body, the secondary

response takes over. The time for production of IgM is shortened, as is the time for the appearance of IgG. The total antibody production exceeds the primary response, and more IgG is formed than IgM.

Primary Versus Secondary Immunodeficiency Disorder

Immune deficiencies are primary (genetic) or secondary (acquired). Primary deficiencies are rare and usually occur in young patients. Deficiencies can occur in B cells, hypogammaglobulin anemias (50% of cases), combined B and T cells (20–30%), isolated T cells (10–15%), and phagocytic cells (10%).[4]

A detailed history and physical examination usually point to secondary immunodeficiency. Many problems are associated with secondary immunodeficiency, including suppression by drugs, diseases of the lymph nodes, infectious diseases (HIV), age, systemic inflammatory diseases, problems with mucus production (cystic fibrosis), diabetes, and renal failure.[4]

Immunosuppression

At times, it is desirable to suppress the immune system. In organ transplantation, immune defenses must be suppressed to prevent antibodies from attacking the grafted tissue. The purpose of immunosuppression is to destroy the lymphocytes before they have a chance to recognize the antigen. Additionally, it is undesirable for the lymphocytes to multiply if inflammation is to be reduced. However, this manipulation allows microorganisms normally under control to reproduce. Powerful drugs that suppress lymphocytes also suppress other proliferating cells, including bone marrow. Anti-inflammatory agents are used to depress phagocyte chemotaxis. They also prevent the release of hydrolytic enzymes from the lysosomes that would otherwise destroy the graft. Specific drugs have been developed to target T cells directly, allowing other cells to remain intact. Radiation is used to destroy lymph tissue. Unfortunately, it must be done several days in

TABLE 46–2
Differences Between T and B Cells

T Lymphocytes (T Cells)	B Lymphocytes (B Cells)
Originate from Stem Cell Precursors of Lymphocytes in Bone Marrow	
Migrate to thymus cells	Migrate to bursa cells
60–70% of small lymphocytes in serum are T cells	30–40% of small lymphocytes in serum are B cells
Synthesize lymphokines after interaction with antigens	Synthesize antibodies after interaction with antigens
Control cell-mediated immunity	Control humoral immunity

advance of organ transplantation, and this approach is impossible for some candidates.[5]

Autoimmunity

Autoimmune diseases are caused when the body fails to recognize "self" molecules, so the body responds by making autoantibodies. Scientists do not yet know whether self-tolerance is the result of active suppression of self-antigen suppressor T cells (T8) or the absence of self-reactive T cells.[6] Occasionally, antigens produced in response to foreign microorganisms are similar to self-antigens. This situation causes the body to attack itself because of cross-reacting antigens. Viruses can sometimes cause an autoimmune response, if they change the surface antigen as they enter the host cell.[5] Examples of autoimmune diseases include rheumatoid arthritis (RA), insulin-dependent diabetes mellitus (IDDM), multiple sclerosis (MS), myasthenia gravis (MG), and systemic lupus erythematosus (SLE).[6]

Normal Structural and Functional Changes Associated With Aging

As the body ages, host susceptibility to infections increases. The following is a summary from the report of the Task Force on Immunology and Aging from the National Institute on Aging and the National Institute of Allergy and Infectious Diseases (NIAID).[7]

Immunity is the result of cells and chemicals working together to respond to invading organisms. The "memory" of B cells responsible for antibody production makes this system responsive to future invasions. As one ages, this function of T and B cells is lost or impaired. Memory to past encounters is retained, but memory to new encounters may be at risk. Cytokines, the mediators of the inflammatory and immune response, are produced by T cells. Loss of T cells, or altered balanced production of cytokines, can change immunity. Research is limited on other immune modulators, such as steroids, which affect immune system function. Antigen-presenting cells are important in the initial stages of immunity; however, it is not yet known whether aging affects their function. Much work is needed on the decline of the humoral and cellular responses during aging and the activation process of T and B cells, although some specific alterations in secondary signaling have been defined. The immune system is constantly removing and replenishing cells. This fine balance can be upset by the aging process, including the atrophy of the thymus, T-cell alterations and a decrease in B-cell precursors from the bone marrow. Aging also affects physical and chemical

first-line defenses. Whether because of changes in the host's cells or changes in the cellular environment, particular sites appear predisposed to infection in elderly persons. Few data exist on the effects of gender, race, and culture on immune defenses. Studies of the effects of aging on the mucosal membranes and the production of IgA are needed to develop more effective treatments against infectious diseases. Stem cells, the precursors of all other types, are being studied to determine whether aging influences their differentiation. As one ages, it is important to give the immune system a boost, either directly by enhancing immune response, or indirectly by vaccines. Studies are under way with a nonreplicating plasmid DNA that will trigger the appropriate pathways to produce antibodies and cytotoxic T cells to various viruses and bacteria. Further study of the aging immune system will allow scientists to target more specifically the component that is failing.

Murasko and colleagues[8] studied the thymus's inability to promote T-cell differentiation, leading to a decline in the proliferative capacity of T lymphocytes to mitogens and viruses. Delayed-type skin hypersensitivity (DTH) may be related to a decrease in lymphocytes. A defect in interleukin-2 (IL-2) adds to decreased lymphocyte responsiveness.[9] Peripheral lymphocytes were found to be significantly lower in elderly persons, whereas numbers of neutrophil phagocytes were increased.[10] In chronically ill elderly patients, nutritional deficits contribute to the impairment of immunoregulatory mechanisms.[11] Many elderly patients also show an inability to react to specific antigens (anergy) because of medications, acute and chronic diseases, stress, and depression. Anergy can sometimes be reversed by addressing the underlying problems.[12]

In summary, it is clear that the effectiveness of the immune system declines with age, and this decline places the elderly at high risk of overwhelming infectious diseases as well as nosocomial infections while hospitalized. Care should be planned such that invasive procedures (arterial lines and pulmonary artery catheters) are minimized whenever possible.

EPIDEMIOLOGY OF HIV DISEASE

In developed countries within the Western world, infectious diseases were thought to be under control by the 1980s. The incidence of childhood diseases and of epidemics such as smallpox and polio was greatly reduced. The causative agents for Legionnaires' disease and toxic shock syndrome were discovered so quickly that scientists began to believe that they could defeat anything. Basking in the new science of genetic engineering and microbial studies, the scientific community celebrated success, even as HIV was spreading through the world's populations. Silently, methodically, the virus passed from person to person undetected. In the June 5, 1981 issue of the *Morbidity and Mortality Weekly Report* (MMWR), the United States Centers for Disease Control and Prevention (CDC)[13] published a small paragraph on five homosexual men who had appeared at three different hospitals in Los Angeles suffering from *Pneumocystis carinii* pneumonia (PCP), two of whom had already died. "AIDS" had become an official disease, even though it had no name at that time. Doctors were urged to report similar cases to their local health department officials, who were responsible for reporting these cases to CDC. Twenty-six cases of PCP and Kaposi's sarcoma (KS) were subsequently reported in the July 3, 1981, issue of MMWR,[14] but no infectious agent had been identified. The gay community began to call the phenomenon the "gay plague," but by late 1981, it was apparent that intravenous (IV) drug users were also affected. The CDC knew by mid-1982 that the blood supply was at risk, as were heterosexual couples and patients with hemophilia. The label "AIDS" appeared in 1983, when maternal transmission was reported.[1,2]

The incidence of AIDS doubled during the first 3 years of the epidemic, as did rumors about its origins. These rumors included the possibility that amyl nitrate was a causative agent because of its use among homosexuals,[15] and they even included the theory of political germ warfare by the United States government to generate an AIDS epidemic among gay men[16] or blacks. The Soviet Union accused the United States of developing a "secret" weapon,[17] and others asserted that the United States deliberately contaminated a vaccine shipment to Africa.[18,19] Genetic engineering laboratories were scrutinized for possible viral escape.[11,15]

Although the epidemic is officially dated to 1981 in the United States, HIV antibodies were recovered in frozen serum as early as 1959 in Central Africa.[20] In 1980, a Canadian heterosexual man who had received a blood transfusion in Zaire in 1976 died of opportunistic infections (OIs). His stored blood was tested in 1983 and was found to be HIV positive, the first documented case of transfusion-related AIDS.[21] In Norway, HIV symptoms were documented in 1966, when a sailor who frequently visited Africa acquired the virus. His wife developed symptoms a year later and transmitted the disease to her 2-year-old child. This family was identified as having Europe's first three cases of AIDS, as well as the first known case of sexual transmission, maternal transmission, and pediatric AIDS.[22]

In the United States, the first case is thought to be a 15-year-old boy whose unusual death prompted physicians to freeze his tissue and serum in 1969.[23] An autopsy revealed he had died of complications of HIV infection. If one were to date the epidemic in the United States using clinical data rather than laboratory data, earlier cases could be dated back to 1952.[2,15] Scientists wonder whether this form of HIV was genetically different from the current one and whether it would have progressed had its carrier not died.

Myers and colleagues[24] proposed that the grandparent organism originated in West Central Africa. However, it split into HIV-1, HIV-2, and simian immunodeficiency virus (SIV) and was perhaps transmitted between humans and monkeys.[25] Eigen and Nieselt-Struwe[26] suggested that HIV-1 and HIV-2 diverged from a common ancestor more than 900 years ago. However, Myers, MacInnes, and Korber[24] asserted that HIV has been around for a century or two, perhaps as a less virulent strain than the current one. In his book, *Evolution of Infectious Disease*, Paul Ewald[25] suggested that sexual intercourse plays an important role in the increased virulence of HIV. Two reasons for the spread of HIV in Africa were identified by McCoy and Inciardi[27] as being demographic shifts from rural to urban living and increased heterosexual prostitution. Additionally, the sexual revolution in the United States increased the number of multiple partners among heterosexuals and homosexuals, thus increasing the opportunity for transmission of the virus. A low rate of condom use and a high incidence of lesion-producing venereal diseases also increased transmission.[28]

TRANSMISSION OF HIV DISEASE

The major modes of HIV transmission are 1) unprotected sexual activity, 2) blood-to-blood contact, and 3) transference from mother to infant. The CDC continues to investigate all reported cases of HIV infection to determine whether alternative routes of transmission exist.

Sexual Activity

The presence of sexually transmitted diseases (STDs), such as syphilis, herpes simplex virus 2 (HSV-2) infection, chancroid, and other ulcerative STDs, provides an opening to the blood or systemic system. In the United States, the epidemic initially spread fastest among homosexual men. New infections among older gay men may be stabilizing because of education and prevention initiatives. However, among young gay men, the incidence of new HIV infections continues to increase.

However, whether sexual behaviors occur between partners of the same sex or the opposite sex, it is not sexual orientation, but the sexual behavior itself that places a person at risk. Oral, anal (rectal), and vaginal sex carry respective risks of transmission. Transmission by oral sex is possible only if there are cuts, abrasions, or bleeding in the oral cavity. Anal intercourse carries the highest risk of sexual transmission, because the rectum is not designed as a depository. It is lined with paper-thin tissue over millions of CD4 cells, all subject to infection. The partner at greatest risk from anal sex is the passive receptive partner. This receptive rectum is torn and therefore is susceptible to infected semen. The active insertive partner is also at risk of HIV from the torn, bleeding tissue. Because some abrasions or lesions on the penis are microscopic, neither partner may realize the potential risk.

In vaginal intercourse, the second highest risk category, the male can contract the virus from infected CD4 cells, vaginal fluid, or menstrual blood. The female contracts the virus from infected semen and is generally at greater risk than the male because of the anatomy of the uterus, which provides more immediate access to the blood. Any lesions or abrasions in the vaginal cavity, such as those produced by STDs, cervical erosion, or vaginal dryness, will allow viral contact with the woman's systemic blood. This risk is increased in women with intrauterine devices (IUDs). Macrophages carrying HIV can penetrate the tissue of the cervix at the opening of the uterus. Moreover, sexual intercourse at the beginning of or during a woman's menstrual cycle increases access to HIV because of the tearing down and rebuilding of the uterine wall. Minority women who are of childbearing age are among the fastest growing AIDS populations.[29] Thirty-nine percent of the cases in women were attributed to sex with IV drug users, bisexual males, hemophiliacs, HIV-infected transfusion recipients, or an HIV-infected person whose risk has not been identified.[30] Drug use and sexual activity place one at dual risk. Use of drugs impairs judgment, thus reducing the likelihood of safer sex practices. Women who have little influence over their male counterparts are at increased risk because they are not always able to demand condom use.

Blood-to-Blood Contact

Among drug users, sharing drug paraphernalia used for IV use and skin popping contaminate the needle with blood. Blood often remains in the hub of the needle and becomes mixed with the drug. As several persons repeat this process, the potential for transmission of HIV, as well as other diseases such as hepatitis, increases. Statistically, 43% of cases of AIDS in women are attributed to IV drug use.[30] The risk of acquiring HIV through transfusion of blood or its components was greatly reduced in the United States when testing was made available in 1985. The incidence of HIV infection in patients with hemophilia has decreased because of intense heat processing of human donor clotting factors. Any blood-to-blood contact carries a degree of risk, such as needlesticks, tattoos, or any body piercing.

Mother-to-Infant Transmission

Transmission can occur transplacentally while the fetus is in the uterus, during vaginal delivery because the baby is exposed to maternal secretions and blood, or during breast-feeding through the milk or bleeding nipples. Babies who test positive at birth will either test negative about 18 to 24 months later, indicating that the initial positive test resulted from their mother's antibodies, or will continue to test positive, signifying they contracted the virus.

The NIAID and the National Institute of Child Health and Human Development[31] announced interim results of a randomized, multicentered, double-blind placebo-controlled clinical trial. In this study, HIV-positive women took oral zidovudine (ZDV, formerly known as azidothymidine or AZT) at 14 to 34 weeks of gestation, continuing with 500 mg daily throughout pregnancy. During labor, IV ZDV was administered in a loading dose of 200 mg/kg over 1 hour, followed by a continuous infusion (1 mg/kg/hr) until delivery. The newborn received ZDV syrup (2 mg/kg q6h) for the first 6 weeks of life, beginning 8 to 12 hours after birth. Results demonstrated a reduction in the transmission from mothers to their offspring in the treatment group from 34 to 8%. As a result of this study, pregnant women or those seeking pregnancy must be offered an HIV antibody test. Refusal must be documented in the patient's medical record. If the test is positive, the mother must be offered ZDV therapy. If she refuses drug therapy, it must be documented. It is anticipated that newer drugs and drug combinations will result in revisions of this protocol.

Global Transmission

As the HIV epidemic endures, three patterns have emerged. In Western Europe, Canada, and the United States, the epidemic began in the homosexual and IV drug communities. In Latin America and Central, Eastern and Southern Africa, heterosexual transmission occurred through infected persons. This was also true in Eastern Europe, the Middle East, North Africa, and Asia, in addition to transmission through medical equipment and imported blood. Developing countries are particularly vulnerable because persons with HIV are young or middle-aged workers representing the country's future. Failure to recognize, diagnose, and report HIV compounds the problem in developing countries. Testing in developing countries may cost as much as 100 times more than in the United States. In addition, these nations cannot afford to follow CDC recommendations to reduce transmission rates, nor can they afford the high cost of drugs to treat HIV or OIs, much less the cost of disposable syringes.[1]

The World Health Organization (WHO) predicts that 90% of all new cases will come from developing countries, and this prediction generates several ethical dilemmas. Do developed countries have a moral obligation to help developing nations in the fight against HIV? Who should subsidize the costs to fight this battle? Will assistance be contingent on cultural changes to reduce HIV transmission? The next century will likely reveal the answers to these questions.

ETIOLOGY AND PATHOPHYSIOLOGY

One pathophysiologic model for HIV suggests that although helper T cells are preferentially infected, HIV and suppressor T cells undergo a process of convergent selection, causing them to resemble each other over time and ultimately leading to autoimmunity.[32] When first introduced into the body, HIV elicits the same immune response as any other virus. What makes it so unique is that it targets the T-helper cell as its host cell to assist in viral replication, then turns on that host and destroys it. The initial response to HIV in 50% of cases mimics the common cold or flu, and therapy usually consists of self-treatment with over-the-counter (OTC) drugs. Once symptoms disappear, HIV infection has no observable manifestations. However, at the tissue level, cellular destruction begins with the lymph nodes. The follicular dendritic cells may transmit infection to other cells as they migrate through lymphoid follicles, producing a large reservoir of CD4 cells and macrophages that are latently infected.[33]

Phagocytes, having detected HIV-infected cells, digest these cells. As the macrophage destroys the cell, HIV antigens are displayed on the outer protein coat, next to its own identifying marker protein, major histocompatibility complex (MHC) protein, marking the macrophage as "self." After digestion, the macrophage migrates to the lymph node and presents its findings to the T-helper cell (T4 and CD4). The reaction of the antigen and MHC releases lymphokines, which stimulate either T or B cells. The antigen presented determines whether T or B cells are stimulated. The activated T cells stimulate the cytotoxic (killer) T cells to search for the MHC-foreign antigen combination on the surface of infected cells. Identified cells are rendered useless by a powerful protein that punches holes in the cell's membrane, causing death by leakage. Killer T cells also stimulate additional lymphokines at the initial site, and this process attracts additional macrophages to the site to sensitize them to the organism. Ordinarily, suppressor T cells turn the immune system off as the response to the original antigen stimulus lessens. However, HIV's infection of the CD4 cell ensures its continued production, forcing the immune system to keep up with viral production on a daily basis. As the sensitized macrophage wanders through the lymph node, it eventually locates a B cell containing the surface antibody molecule corresponding to the antigen. When the antibody–antigen combination is complete, the B cell is committed to producing antibodies specific to that antigen. Two thousand antibodies can be made each second. Set free, the antibodies search out the antigen that caused their production.

HIV's ability to target CD4 cells to produce thousands of copies makes it unique among antigens. Specific resistance is nullified over time, as viral replication depletes the cell's biochemicals and destroys its structure to supply the building blocks for viral parts. Unfortunately, replacement of CD4 cells requires 14 days, whereas HIV is replaced every 3 days. Thus, HIV simply outlasts the immune system.[34]

Considering the small number of CD4 cells originally infected, their death is not the complete explanation for the demise of the immune system, nor does natural or programmed death (apoptosis) of the CD4 cells totally explain the large numbers killed. One theory is that antibodies to gp120 and gp41 interfere with histocompatibility antigens on healthy cells because they are so similar. This interference impairs immune function of these cells. Another idea is that gp120 actually triggers an attack on healthy CD4 cells by killer T cells.[35] Anergy, the prevention of division of CD4 cells in response to a foreign antigen, may cause a drop in viable CD4 cells.[36] Uninfected CD4 cells also clump to infected CD4 cells. This large cell mass serves no purpose for immune system protection and is therefore targeted by killer T cells to destroy large numbers of CD4 cells effectively.

Phases of HIV Infection

In 1981, most health care practitioners working with HIV-infected individuals focused on diagnosis, treating the OIs, and dealing with accompanying psychosocial issues. The complexity of the disease was compounded by the number and type of OIs. Initially, drug treatment was limited to a single class of drugs, the antiretrovirals, and was therefore simple to manage. The number of new drugs and tests available today makes treatment more complex. Even before research is published, results are frequently applied in practice, requiring an enormous commitment to remain current.

Acute Retroviral Syndrome

When first exposed to HIV, most patients develop an acute retroviral syndrome that mimics the common cold or flu, a mild skin rash, or mononucleosis. Patients report fatigue, sore muscles, mild fevers, and swollen lymph nodes, indicating antibody production.

These symptoms can last up to 7 weeks.[37] When this syndrome passes, the patient has seroconverted. This is one of the most infectious periods, because of rapid viral replication.

The "window period" (the time from infection until antibodies appear) varies from 2 weeks to 6 months. Testing during this period yields a false-negative result because the virus is actually present, although the antibodies measured by the test have not yet developed (Table 46–3). Many persons demonstrate an antibody response after 3 months, others in 6 months, and rare persons may not test positive for up to 2 years (Figure 46–1). Unless they are tested, many persons do not suspect HIV infection and may treat the symptoms of the acute retroviral syndrome with OTC medications.

Asymptomatic Stage

After seroconversion, the patient enters the "clinical latency" or asymptomatic period when signs and symptoms of illness are barely detectable. Enlarged lymph nodes indicate the ongoing battle between CD4 cells and HIV, but test results are the only confirmation of infection. Routine laboratory tests help to stage the disease. Prophylactic immunizations should begin. Basically, this period is a time to observe the patient for acute infections and to focus on the patient's overall mental, emotional, and physical status. Management of the patient during this stage is likely to change in the future, as more is learned about the timing of the death of memory cells and the length of time that triple- or quadruple-drug therapy will delay symptoms. If the immune system is allowed to deteriorate to the point at which memory cells are depleted, any exposure to an opportunistic organism will be treated as a new infection. This is true no matter how many times the person is exposed. The asymptomatic period has lasted up to 15 years, with the average being 10 years.

Symptomatic Stage

The second stage of illness has been referred to as AIDS-related complex (ARC) or more recently as the "symptomatic stage." During this time, infected persons may suffer weight loss, diarrhea, fever, night sweats, fatigue, lymphadenopathy, and candidiasis (oral or esophageal thrush or, in women, recurrent vaginal yeast infections that are resistant to treatment). Their CD4 cell counts drop significantly (from a high of

TABLE 46–3
Comparison of Serologic Tests for HIV Infection

Test	Description
Enzyme-Linked Immunosorbent Assay (HIV-1 ELISA)	Usually the first test performed on a blood sample to identify whether a person is negative or positive for HIV antibodies
	A sensitive, although nonspecific test, ELISA to be confirmed by WB
	False-negative tests possible if the person is tested during the window period
	Most variants, except subtype O, detected by this test
	Combined HIV-1/HIV-2 test on the market used by the blood banks in the United States
	Average cost, $20
Immunofluorescent Assay (IFA)	A confirmatory test that uses a fluorescent dye to determine the presence of HIV antibodies
Western Blot (WB)	Used to verify ELISA findings
	An antibody test, uses the protein bands of the virus to test against
Polymerase Chain Reaction (PCR) p24 Antigen	Unlike antibody test, PCR searching for viral DNA attached to host DNA inside the nucleus of the cell
	A specific protein found in the core of the virus that signifies rapid replication of the virus
	Increased p24 antigen levels occurring twice during viral replication: shortly after the initial infection and again when the patient reaches the "AIDS" designation whereby the immune system is overpowered and unable to produce significant antibodies to fight the production of HIV
OraSure (Oral Transudate Test for HIV-1)	Has the same sensitivity as ELISA, but is easier to collect
	Must also be confirmed by WB
	Patient places collection pad (looks like a small toothbrush) between lower gum and cheek for 2–5 minutes
	Fluid (oral mucosal transudate) that may contain antibodies to HIV drawn through the cheek and gums onto pad
	Device then removed and placed into a small vial containing a preservative, then sent to laboratory for analysis

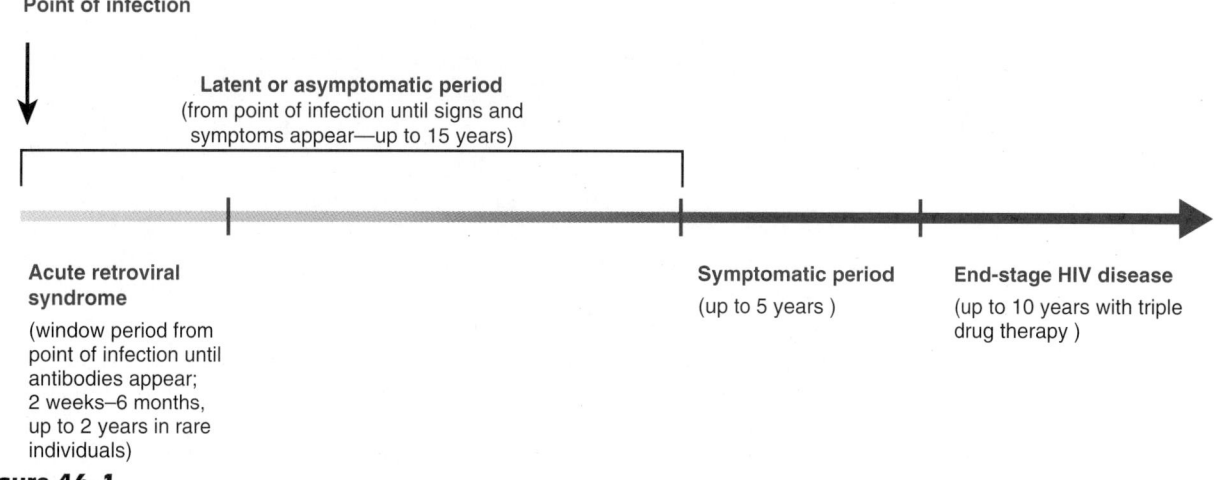

Figure 46–1

The human immunodeficiency virus (HIV) disease continuum.

around 800 to fewer than 400 cells/μL). Emotionally and physically, these patients are on a roller coaster and may exhibit labile emotions. One day, they feel healthy enough to work 8 hours; the next day, they may be bedridden. It is a time of vacillation between hope and despair. Prophylaxis against myriad OIs is essential. Antiretroviral therapy is initiated and, because of its many adverse effects (e.g., fatigue, diarrhea, anemia), many patients terminate therapy prematurely.

End-Stage Disease

End-stage HIV disease (the final stage) is the point at which the patient's CD4 count is less than 200, or one of the AIDS-defining conditions recognized by the CDC is present (Chart 46–1), or both. Once patients are classified as having end-stage HIV disease, the time to actual death can be 10 years or more. Current drug therapies have resulted in a shift of the labeling of HIV infection from a disease that produces a rapid death to a chronic disease.

The CDC classification system is used most frequently to categorize HIV infections and is based on the following criteria: 1) the presence of signs and symptoms; 2) clinical or laboratory findings; and 3) the chronology of their occurrence (Table 46–4). The Walter Reed Army Medical Center System offers an alternative classification system that consists of six stages based on signs and symptoms associated with immune dysfunction (Table 46–5).

Common Illnesses Associated with End-Stage HIV Disease

Numerous and often devastating illnesses develop in patients with end-stage HIV disease (see Chart 46–1).

Only the more common HIV-associated conditions are described here.

Tuberculosis

Before the appearance of HIV, tuberculosis (TB) was a controlled disease in most of the developed world. With the immunosuppression that results from HIV, TB has made a catastrophic comeback, recently in a multidrug resistant form (MDRTB). *Mycobacterium tuberculosis* (MTB), the causative agent of TB, is spread through inhaled airborne droplets containing the bacilli, and those patients with end-stage HIV disease are likely to succumb rapidly once exposed. Because MTB replicates slowly, treatment is long term. The emergence of MDRTB is due to several factors: 1) poor access to health care and preventive medicine; 2) poor assessment of the antimicrobials used to treat an individual patient; and 3) nonadherence, including discontinuing therapy prematurely. Mutations that occur during therapy require continuous reevaluation of drugs given. Within parts of Africa, the incidence of MDRTB has risen to over 3 million cases, and it is steadily increasing in the United States. Populations especially vulnerable include the homeless, IV drug users, alcoholics, the elderly, and prison inmates or others housed in close quarters.

Pneumocystis carinii Pneumonia

The first OI recognized in the HIV epidemic was *Pneumocystis carinii* pneumonia (PCP). Although the organism is usually benign in healthy persons, PCP is the second leading cause of death in patients with HIV infection (Table 46–6). The protozoan responsible multiplies rapidly in the alveoli, displacing oxygen and causing rapid labored breathing, a nonproductive cough, and anxiety. In 1989, the CDC recommended

CHART 46–1

AIDS Indicator Conditions

Bacterial infection, multiple or recurrent
Candidiasis of bronchi, trachea, or lungs
Candidiasis of esophagus
    Definitive diagnosis
    Presumptive diagnosis
Carcinoma, invasive, cervical
Coccidioidomycosis, disseminated or extra-
    pulmonary
Cryptococcosis, extrapulmonary
Cryptosporidiosis, chronic intestinal
Cytomegalovirus disease other than retinitis
Cytomegalovirus retinitis
    Definitive diagnosis
    Presumptive diagnosis
Herpes simplex, with esophagitis, pneumonitis, or
    chronic mucocutaneous ulcers
Histoplasmosis, disseminated or extrapulmonary
HIV encephalopathy (dementia)
HIV wasting syndrome
Immunosuppression, severe HIV-related*
Isosporiasis, chronic intestinal
Kaposi's sarcoma
    Definitive diagnosis
    Presumptive diagnosis
Lymphoid interstitial pneumonia or pulmonary lym-
    phoid hyperplasia†
    Definitive diagnosis
    Presumptive diagnosis

Lymphoma, Burkitt's (or equivalent term)
Lymphoma, primary in brain
Mycobacterium avium or *M. kansasii*, disseminated
    or extrapulmonary infection
    Definitive diagnosis
    Presumptive diagnosis
M. tuberculosis, disseminated or extrapulmonary in-
    fection
    Definitive diagnosis
    Presumptive diagnosis
M. tuberculosis, pulmonary infection‡
Mycobacterial disease, other, disseminated or extra-
    pulmonary
    Definitive diagnosis
    Presumptive diagnosis
Pneumocystis carinii pneumonia
    Definitive diagnosis
    Presumptive diagnosis
Pneumonia, recurrent
    Definitive diagnosis
    Presumptive diagnosis
Salmonella septicemia, recurrent
Toxoplasmosis of brain
    Definitive diagnosis
    Presumptive diagnosis

*Defined as CD4+ T-lymphocyte count or less than 200 cells/μL or a CD4+ percentage less than 14 in adults or adolescents who meet the AIDS surveillance case definition.
†Not applicable as an indicator of AIDS in adults or adolescents.
‡Not applicable as an indicator of AIDS in children.
Data from Centers for Disease Control and Prevention (CDC): HIV/AIDS Surveillance Report, vol. 7. Atlanta, GA, CDC, 1995, p 18.

that primary prophylaxis be instituted if 1) the CD4 count (T4 helper cells) is less than 200 cells/μL, 2) CD4 cells are less than 20% of total circulating lymphocytes, or 3) thrush or fever of unknown origin is present, regardless of the CD4 count. In primary prophylaxis, the goal is to prevent PCP, whereas secondary prophylaxis seeks to reduce recurrences once PCP has occurred.

The preferred drug combination for prevention is trimethoprim–sulfamethoxazole (TMP–SMX) (Bactrim or Septra), one double-strength tablet twice daily (800 mg of sulfamethoxazole and 160 mg of trimethoprim). A desensitization protocol for patients sensitive to TMP–SMX may help.[38] Other alternative drugs are dapsone,[39] dapsone in combination with pyrimethamine,[40] dapsone–pyrimethamine and pyrimethamine–sulfadoxine combinations,[41] and atovaquone.[42]

One treatment modality now used as an alternative when the more current drugs fail or when the patient is allergic to the drugs is pentamidine isethionate (Pentam-300). It is given in aerosolized form monthly, to kill the protozoan and to protect the lungs. However, it does little to protect other organs and is affected by the type of nebulizer used, the amount of drug, patient ventilation mechanics, pulmonary physiology, and body position. The aerosolized pentamidine may also affect the diagnostic accuracy of sputum induction or bronchoalveolar lavage, thereby making multiple lobe lavages and biopsies necessary. Aerosolized pentamidine may cause violent coughing, placing others at risk for TB, especially if the condition is undiagnosed in the patient. Ultraviolet lights used in the setting where pentamidine is administered

TABLE 46-4
CDC Classification of HIV Disease

Stage	Symptoms
Stage I	Acute HIV infection (resembling mononucleosis, aseptic meningitis)
Stage II	Asymptomatic
Stage III	Persistent generalized lymphadenopathy
Stage IV	Other disease
	A. Constitutional disease (fever, weight loss, diarrhea)
	B. Neurologic disease (dementia, myelopathy, peripheral neuropathy)
	C. Secondary infections
	1. CDC-defined AIDS-associated*
	2. Other specified infections†
	D. Secondary cancers (CDC-defined AIDS-associated)‡
	E. Other conditions attributed to HIV infection or immunosuppression

*Pneumocystis carinii pneumonia, toxoplasmosis, cryptococcosis, chronic cryptosporidiosis, extraintestinal strongyloidiasis, isoporiasis, candidiasis (esophageal, bronchial, or pulmonary), histoplasmosis, mycobacterial infection with Mycobacterium avium-intracellulare complex or M. kansasii, cytomegalovirus infection, chronic mucocutaneous or disseminated herpes simplex infection, and progressive multifocal leukoencephalopathy.
†Multidermatomal herpes zoster, oral hairy leukoplakia, nocardiosis, tuberculosis, recurrent Salmonella bacteremia, and oral candidiasis.
‡Kaposi's sarcoma, non–Hodgkin's high-grade lymphoma, primary central nervous system lymphoma.
From Centers for Disease Control and Prevention (CDC), Atlanta, GA.

reduces TB transmission, as does the use of a mask. Vigilant precautions may include testing for TB by tuberculin skin test, chest radiograph, sputum cultures, acid-fast bacilli (AFB) smears, and retesting every 6 months.[43]

Kaposi's Sarcoma

The second OI recognized in the HIV epidemic was KS, described by Moritz Kaposi as a cancer of the muscle and skin. Classic KS appears in Mediterranean men over 50 years of age as a slow-growing tumor, with a benign 10- to 15-year course. It is usually localized to the lower extremities, ankles, or soles of the feet.[44] In equatorial Africa, KS may resemble classic KS or a much more aggressive form often seen in younger patients. A third type with a poor prognosis appears in African prepubescent children with generalized lymphadenopathy.[45]

The KS secondary to HIV is not restricted to the lower extremities, but it may produce generalized pink, brown, blue, or purple plaque formations with edema or raised nodules protruding from the surface of the skin. The lungs, liver, spleen, digestive system, and other internal organs may be invaded. It is aggressive, but not fatal. Observed primarily in male homo-

TABLE 46-5
Walter Reed Army Medical Center Classification System for HIV Disease*

Stage	HIV Antibody or Virus	Chronic Lymph-adenopathy	Helper T Lymphocytes (per mm³)	Delayed Hyper-sensitivity	Thrush	Oppor-tunistic Diseases
WR0	Negative	Negative	>400	Normal	Negative	Negative
WR1	Positive	Negative	>400	Normal	Negative	Negative
WR2	Positive	Positive	>400	Normal	Negative	Negative
WR3	Positive	Positive or negative	<400	Normal	Negative	Negative
WR4	Positive	Positive or negative	<400	Partial	Negative	Negative
WR5	Positive	Positive or negative	<400	Partial or complete	Positive or negative	Negative
WR6	Positive	Positive or negative	<400	Partial or complete	Positive or negative	Positive

*Charts from exposure (WR0) through onset of infection (WR1) to destruction of immune system cells. WR5 is the stage at which the patient does not respond to any skin tests or thrush may appear. WR6 is equal to AIDS.
Data from Redfield RR, Wright DC, Tramont EC, et al: The Walter Reed Staging Classification for HTLV-III/LAV infection. N Engl J Med 314:131–139, 1986.

TABLE 46–6

AIDS Indicator Conditions in 73,380 Adults and Adolescents with AIDS

Most Frequently Reported Conditions*	Percentage of Cases (%)
Immunosuppression, severe HIV-related	85
Pneumocystis carinii pneumonia	18
HIV wasting syndrome	9
Candidiasis of esophagus	7
Kaposi's sarcoma	4
Herpes simplex disease	3
Mycobacterium avium complex	3
Pneumonia, recurrent	3

*Many persons with AIDS have more than one condition.
From Centers for Disease Control and Prevention (CDC): AIDS surveillance/epidemiology L178 slide series through 1995. Atlanta, GA, CDC, 1996.

sexuals, KS is rare in IV drug users, women, and children. It is evident that HIV does not directly cause KS, but rather contributes to its development through immunosuppression. Treatment of the lesions includes chemotherapy and radiation therapy. Two new drugs (SP-PG and AGM-1470) block the development of new blood vessels, which are necessary in the spread of KS.[1,2]

Mycobacterium avium Complex

This complex is one of the most common, disseminated bacterial infections in patients with HIV and is named for two organisms, *Mycobacterium avium* and *M. intracellulare* (MAC). The organisms that cause the complex are found in water, dust, soil, bird droppings, water mists, and vapors. MAC organisms enter the body by ingestion of contaminated food or water or, less commonly, through the lungs. Initially, these bacteria may grow in colonies in the intestines or lungs with few outward symptoms. When symptoms such as night sweats, fevers, loss of appetite, severe diarrhea, and weight loss occur, the organism is spreading and damaging tissue. Patients with CD4 counts less than 75 cells/μL are at greatest risk of acquiring MAC infection. Other symptoms may include cramping, abdominal pain, nausea, and vomiting. Once MAC spreads throughout the body, the patient may experience painful joints and bone, brain, and skin infections. The spleen, liver, and abdominal lymph nodes may be enlarged. MAC is difficult to diagnose in the early stages because the symptoms described could be the result of several other infections. Diagnosing MAC requires culturing blood, tissue, or bone mar-row over a period of several weeks. Obtaining these samples may require bone marrow aspiration, endoscopy, or bronchoscopy. Most physicians prescribe prophylaxis for patients while awaiting test

results, although prevention remains the best intervention.

Ways to minimize exposure to MAC include the following: 1) drinking boiled water; 2) avoiding raw food, especially salads, root vegetables, and unpasteurized milk and cheese; 3) rinsing and peeling fruits and vegetables; 4) minimizing animal contact, especially birds and their droppings; and 5) reducing or avoiding alcohol consumption because it can accelerate the development of MAC infection in people with HIV. Baking, boiling, or steaming foods kills MAC organisms.

Prophylactic treatment with rifabutin (Mycobutin), clarithromycin (Biaxin), or azithromycin (Zithromax) can prevent or delay the onset of MAC in persons with HIV. For patients whose CD4 count is less than 50, a regimen of clarithromycin (500 mg twice daily) or azithromycin (1200 mg once weekly) should be instituted. Rifabutin is used only when the other agents are not tolerated. Combination therapy, although effective, is not warranted because of the side effects and increased costs. Resistance to clarithromycin indicates the likelihood of resistance to azithromycin because the two drugs are closely related. Rifabutin, a different classification of drug, shows no evidence of cross-resistance with the other two drugs. Before the initiation of therapy, a chest radiograph and TB test should be done. If the patient tests positive, treating with a single drug could lead to cross-resistance with other TB drugs, such as rifampin (Rifadin) and should be avoided at all costs.

The United States Public Health Service Task Force recommended in 1993 that treatment include either clarithromycin or azithromycin plus ethambutol (Myambutol) as a second drug and one or more of the following as a third or fourth drug: rifabutin, rifampin, ciprofloxacin (Cipro), or amikacin (Amikin). Table 46–7 lists possible side effects of these drugs–drug interactions. Maintenance therapy should be strong enough to keep the organism under control while not risking the development of drug-resistant strains. Children and pregnant women should also receive MAC prophylaxis and treatment.

Many of the drugs used to treat HIV also have drug interactions with the drugs used to treat MAC. Patients taking protease inhibitors should most likely avoid rifabutin, unless it becomes the only combination available. Indinavir (Crixivan) plus rifabutin calls for a reduction of rifabutin by 50%. Clarithromycin may decrease levels of ZDV by as much as one-third. Another potential problem in treating MAC is the dysfunction of the immune system modulators or cytokines that are released by macrophages, lymphocytes, and other cells to fight infections. As a result of this dysfunction, two strategies have been suggested: 1) the use of granulocyte macrophage-colony stimulating factor (GM-CSF) in combination with azithro-

TABLE 46–7

Drugs Used to Treat *Mycobacterium avium* **Complex: Common Side Effects and Interactions**

Drug	Side Effects	Drug Interaction
Rifabutin	Rash, fever, gastrointestinal distress, hemolysis, decreased white blood count and platelets, uveitis, joint pain	Ketoconazole affects many drugs metabolized through liver; can reduce clarithromycin blood levels by 50%
Ethambutol	Liver toxicities, vision changes, vomiting, diarrhea	—
Clofazimine	Skin discoloration, itchy, dry skin, rash	—
Ciprofloxacin	Nausea, diarrhea, vomiting	Avoid antacids
Amikacin	Kidney, liver toxicity, hearing loss	Avoid amphotericin B, diuretics, penicillin
Clarithromycin	Nausea, reversible hearing loss	Can reduce zidovudine levels by one-third and increase rifabutin levels by 80%
Azithromycin	Nausea, loose stools, hearing loss	—
Sparfloxacin	Photosensitivity	—

mycin; and 2) encasing the drug in liposomes, which would be ingested by the macrophage, in which they would release their killing effect on the bacteria hidden inside.

Other Illnesses

Perhaps one of the hallmarks of the HIV epidemic is the number of different concurrent diseases (Table 46–8). From the protozoan family come PCP (discussed previously), toxoplasmosis, and cryptosporidiosis. Harden and Hair[46] found that toxoplasmosis was the first opportunistic protozoan infestation for 10 to 38% of AIDS patients. Toxoplasmosis (caused by *Toxoplasma gondii,* an obligate protozoan in humans, transmitted from domestic animals) produces a chronic, asymptomatic infection in 10 to 40% of adults in the United States[2] and in up to 90% of adults in some European countries.[47] The organism lies dormant in the reticuloendothelial system until it is reacti-

vated when the immune system is compromised. When the pathogen infects the brain, it causes cerebral edema, lesions, and encephalitis in more than 30% of HIV-infected patients. Laboratory tests and computed tomography (CT) scans may be needed to rule out neoplasms, mycobacterial encephalitis, and cryptococcal meningitis. TMP–SMX, used as prophylaxis against PCP, also helps to protect against toxoplasmosis. Other treatments include pyrimethamine alone (which may increase folic acid) or in combination with sulfadiazine or clindamycin (Cleocin). Because there is no cure, suppressive therapy with TMP–SMX or dapsone often continues.[48]

Cryptosporidium is another protozoan that can be found in persons whose immune systems are compromised. Cryptosporidiosis usually affects the small intestine, but in HIV-infected patients, it has been recovered throughout the entire gastrointestinal tract.[49] It causes unrelenting diarrhea, fluid and electrolyte imbalance, weight loss, malaise, cramping, abdominal

TABLE 46–8

Concurrent Diseases Seen in Patients With HIV

Respiratory System	Integumentary System	Eye	Gastrointestinal System	Neurologic System
Pneumocystis carinii pneumonia	HSV-1	Cytomegalovirus (CMV) retinitis	*Cryptosporidium muris*	*Toxoplasma gondii*
Cryptococcus species	Herpes simplex type 2 (HSV-2)	HSV-1	CMV	Papovavirus
Histoplasma capsulatum	Varicella-zoster virus (VZV)	VZV	HSV-1	Cryptococcal meningitis
Mycobacterium tuberculosis	KS		*Candida albicans*	CNS lymphomas
Coccidioides immitis	Bacillary angiomatosis		*Mycobacterium avium* complex	AIDS-dementia complex
Herpes simplex (type 1 HSV-1)			*Isospora belli*	
Kaposi's sarcoma (KS)			*Salmonella*	
			KS	
			Non–Hodgkin's lymphoma	

pain, anorexia, nausea, vomiting, malabsorption, malnutrition, and sometimes death. Up to 25 L of fluid can be lost from severe diarrhea.[2] Because current treatment is primarily palliative, prevention through good hygiene and hand washing is vital.[50] Experimental treatments (paromomycin, letrazuril, azithromycin) are being tested.[51]

Fungal infections include cryptococcosis, histoplasmosis, coccidioidomycosis, and candidiasis. *Cryptococcus* resides in the lungs of healthy persons, but in patients with HIV, it multiplies and spreads to the blood and brain, causing cryptococcal meningitis. Symptoms include piercing headaches, stiff neck, paralysis, mental dysfunction, and changes in behavior.[1] This fungus also appears in the lungs, myocardium, pericardium, mediastinum, peripheral lymph nodes, gastrointestinal tract, liver, spleen, prostate, bone marrow, joints, blood, eyes, and skin.[52] If untreated, cryptococcal meningitis is fatal.

Treatment includes IV amphotericin B (AMB) until laboratory data are negative. To prevent relapse, AMB is administered weekly. Side effects of the therapy often seem more severe than the disease and include fever, chills, stiffness, nausea, vomiting, hematuria, renal dysfunction, renal papillary necrosis, hypotension, and bowel ischemia. Liver function studies may be needed to monitor drug therapy. Ketoconazole (Nizoral), fluconazole (Diflucan), itraconazole (Sporanox), flucytosine (a pyrimidine derivative), and combinations of AMB and flucytosine offer new hope to these patients.[53] No matter which drug therapy is chosen, the patient must be monitored for side effects, allergic reactions, and drug interactions. Because most drugs are eliminated by the respiratory system, kidneys, and liver, each system should be monitored for changes from baseline.

Histoplasmosis often develops in HIV-infected patients who have a history of being in endemic areas such as the river valleys in the United States and results from reactivation of a latent infection. Clinical signs and symptoms can be severe and can include persistent fever, weight loss, abdominal pain, diarrhea, cough, fatigue, or a clinical syndrome resembling Gram-negative sepsis (hypotension, leukopenia, disseminated intravascular coagulation, acute respiratory distress syndrome, encephalopathy, hepatic insufficiency, and renal failure). Itraconazole or AMB is the treatment of choice. Rifampin, rifabutin, phenytoin (Dilantin), carbamazepine (Tegretol), and antacid therapy are contraindicated in patients receiving itraconazole.[51]

Coccidioidomycosis is a self-limiting fungal disease commonly found in California's San Joaquin Valley and in other southwestern states including Arizona, Nevada, New Mexico, Texas, and Utah.[52] In persons with impaired T-cell immunity, the fungus disseminates to the lungs, bone, skin, liver, or central nervous system (CNS), causing fever, weight loss, cough, and

fatigue. Diagnosis of such nonspecific symptoms depends on a history of being in endemic areas or a positive skin test. Treatment includes AMB, fluconazole, and itraconazole. Prophylaxis for systemic fungal infections is controversial, because these infections rarely appear until the CD4 is less than 100/μL. Prophylaxis should be considered for persons in endemic areas or with T-cell counts less than 50/μL.[52]

Candidiasis is one of the most frequent signals of HIV disease and is a recurring problem for both men and women (Figure 46–2). Risk of infections on the skin, gingivae, teeth, oropharynx, vagina, or large intestine increases with age or immunosuppression. Some antibiotics suppress normal flora and allow *Candida* to flourish. Dehydration or poor nutrition or hygiene increases vulnerability for infection through the skin. Oral candidiasis (thrush) is treated with "swish and swallow" liquid antifungal nystatin agents or a daily fluconazole tablet. Sometimes, clotrimazole troches (Mycelex) or ketoconazole tablets may be used, with some risk to the liver. The itching and pain of vaginal candidiasis (yeast infection) can cause severe discomfort in women; nystatin (Mycostatin) vaginal tablets, myconazole creams, or vaginal suppositories are given.[53]

In 1993, the CDC added cervical cancer to the list of AIDS-defining conditions and classified HIV-positive women with cervical cancer as having AIDS. Cervical cancer in these women occurs earlier (age 16–48 instead of 45–50 years), is more aggressive and less responsive to treatment, and has a poor prognosis.[51]

Other conditions affecting patients with HIV include cytomegalovirus (CMV), HIV-related encephalopathy, herpes simplex virus (HSV) disease, non–Hodgkin's lymphoma, recurrent pneumonia, progressive multifocal leukoencephalopathy, salmonellosis, and HIV wasting syndrome. Table 46–9 pro-

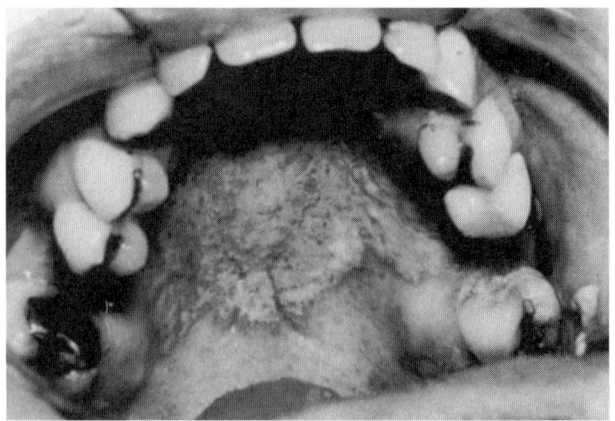

Figure 46–2

Pseudomembranous candidiasis. (From Greenspan JS, Greenspan D: Oral complications of HIV infection. In: Sande MA, Volberding PA (eds): The Medical Management of AIDS, 5th ed. Philadelphia, WB Saunders, 1995, p 170.)

TABLE 46–9
Opportunistic Diseases Found in Patients With HIV Infection

Organism or Disease	Clinical Presentation	Current Treatment Strategies
Cytomegalovirus (CMV)	CMV retinitis (loss of visual field, blurred vision) Pneumonitis (usually seen with other infection such as PCP or MAC, progressive shortness of breath, dyspnea on exertion, dry, nonproductive cough with or without fever) Encephalitis (personality changes, cognitive impairment, motor impairment) Colitis (weight loss, anorexia, fever) Esophagitis (ulcers) Adrenalitis (postural hypotension and sodium deficits)	Ganciclovir Foscarnet Colony-stimulating factor (investigational)
HIV Encephalopathy (AIDS-Dementia Complex)	Inability to concentrate, decreased memory, slowness in thinking, leg weakness, ataxia, clumsiness, apathy, reduced spontaneity, social withdrawal, irritability, hyperactivity, and anxiety without an identifiable cause to mania, delirium, euphoria, grandiose delusions	Zidovudine Didanosine Methylphenidate Dextroamphetamine
Herpes Simplex Virus (HSV) Disease	Oral lesions (ulcers on lips, tongue, pharynx or buccal mucosa, fever, pharyngitis cervical lymphadenopathy) Genital lesions (inguinal lymphadenopathy, dysuria) Perianal and anorectal lesions (localized pain, itching, pain on defecation, tenesmus, constipation, sacral radiculopathy, impotence, neurogenic bladder) HSV esophagitis (dysphagia, odynophagia, retrosternal pain) HSV encephalitis (headache, maningismus, personality change, fever, nausea, lethargy, confusion, cranial nerve deficits, seizures)	Acyclovir (intravenous, oral or topical) Foscarnet for acyclovir-resistant HSV-2 infection
Lymphoma, Non–Hodgkin's (NHL)	Nonspecific symptoms, unexplained fever, drenching night sweats, or weight loss >10% of total body weight HIV plus NHL, confusion, lethargy, memory loss, hemiparesis, aphasia, seizures, cranial nerve palsies, headache, numbness of the chin, and stiff neck.	Standard-dose chemotherapy for those with good immune function and no previous OIs Lower-dose chemotherapy for immunocompromised patients, history of OIs Regimens using chemotherapy, antiretrovirals, prophylaxis for PCP and colony-stimulating factors under investigation
Recurrent Pneumonia	Abrupt onset, with fever, cough with purulent sputum, and systemic toxic effects	Broad-spectrum antimicrobial therapy until organism identified, then appropriate antibiotic Additional treatment measures: fluids, antipyretic drugs, airway suction or postural drainage, bronchodilator for bronchospasm
Progressive Multifocal Leukoencephalopathy (PML)	Extremity weakness, cognitive dysfunction, visual loss, gait disturbances, limb incoordination, headache, speech or language disturbance, spastic hemiparesis, visual field loss, and altered mentation Cerebellar involvement: ataxia, limb dysmetria, dysarthria Cortical infection: aphasia, apraxia, Gerstmann's syndrome, prosopagnosia, left-sided neglect, and impaired spatial orientation	No effective therapy

Table continued on following page

TABLE 46-9
Opportunistic Diseases Found in Patients With HIV Infection *Continued*

Organism or Disease	Clinical Presentation	Current Treatment Strategies
Salmonellosis	Fever, chills, sweats, weight loss, diarrhea, and anorexia	Ampicillin and chloramphenicol most often used third-generation cephalosporin, amoxicillin, ciprofloxacin, and norfloxacin
HIV Wasting Syndrome	Anorexia, diarrhea, nausea or vomiting, oral lesions, dysphagia, taste or smell changes, physical limitations, neuropsychiatric symptoms including HIV encephalopathy, medication interactions and/or side effects, and allergies or intolerance Additional symptoms: odynophagia, steatorrhea, abdominal pain, polyuria, polydipsia, polyphagia, and neuropathy indicating presence of diabetes	Treatment for symptom control Oral supplements: Ensure, Sustacal and Resource Lipisorb, and Isosource Parenteral nutrition last resort
Mycobacterium Tuberculosis Infection (TB)	Fever, weight loss, night sweats and fatigue, lymphadenopathy, dyspnea, chills, hemoptysis, and chest pain Extrapulmonary sites or fluids with possible evidence of TB in HIV-positive patients: lymph nodes, bones, joints, bone marrow, liver, spleen, cerebrospinal fluid, skin, gastrointestinal mucosa, CNS, urine, blood, mass lesions, or tuberculosis bacteremia	Primary treatment protocol: isoniazid + rifampin + pyrazinamide and either streptomycin or ethambutol Second line of defense drugs: ciprofloxacin, ofloxacin, kanamycin, amikacin, capreomycin, ethionamide, cycloserine, para-aminosalicylic acid, and clofazimine.
Mycobacterium Avium Complex (MAC) Disease	Unexplained systemic symptoms of fever, with or without night sweats, weight loss and debilitation, chronic diarrhea, abdominal pain, anemia, malabsorption, extrahepatic biliary obstruction, intra-abdominal lymphadenopathy, pneumonia, arthritis, skin lesions, pericarditis, meningitis, endophthalmitis, osteomyelitis, and infection of lymph nodes and rectal mucosa in association with KS	Azithromycin, amikacin, clarithromycin, clofazimine, ethambutol, ciprofloxacin, rifampin, rifabutin, cycloserine, ethionamide, and streptomycin

OIs, opportunistic infections; PCP, *Pneumocystis carinii* pneumonia.
From Ungvarski PJ, Staats JA: Clinical manifestations of AIDS in adults. In: Flaskerud JH, Ungvarski PJ (eds): HIV/AIDS: A Guide to Nursing Care, 2nd ed. Philadelphia, W.B. Saunders, 1995, pp 81–133.

vides an overview of the clinical presentations and treatments for some of these organisms.

Assessment

Patients with HIV infection must be identified to facilitate early treatment and prevention of transmission of the disease to others. As the number of infected individuals from all socioeconomic levels grows, the responsibility of health care professionals to be well informed increases. Primary care providers (e.g., physicians and nurse practitioners) are usually able to manage patients during the asymptomatic period. As information expands, primary care providers should avail themselves of the knowledge and expertise of HIV specialists, the CDC, and agencies serving HIV-infected patients through consultation or referral.

Health History

When patients make a visit to their primary care provider or are admitted to an acute care setting, a thorough history should be obtained, starting with a description of their chief complaint, the reason they sought health care. The format that follows can be used as a guide by the nurse to collect pertinent subjective data related to the patient's health history.

The history of the present illness includes the patient's description of what has been happening usually over a finite period of time (days, weeks, perhaps months). The presenting illness often offers clues to the type of defect in the patient's immune response. Antibody defects may present as upper and lower respiratory infections. Viral, mycobacterial, fungal, and protozoal infections are the result of a T-cell defect. Recurrent mucosal infections, psoriasis, and eczema, especially when aggressive and difficult to treat, are possibly due to a default in phagocytosis.[4] One of the most important questions the nurse should ask is the person's HIV status. Because drug therapies can improve immune functions, delay infections, reduce complications, and postpone the onset of AIDS, it is a very important question. The nurse simply should ask patients whether they have been tested for HIV, because many undergo testing anonymously. In most states, an HIV test requires informed consent of the patient. If patients refuse to be tested, an assessment of high-risk behaviors should be completed (Chart 46–2). If patients have tested positive, ask how they have accepted the results and about their plans for coping. Ask which high-risk behaviors they have been engaging in since their diagnosis. Some patients think that suicide is their only alternative because they believe that HIV means a certain and imminent death. Establishing these baseline data is important for later comparisons.

The patient's past medical history should be obtained by exploring all childhood illnesses and interventions up to the present problem. In addition, the patient's past surgical history should also be explored. Questions about all surgical procedures and their outcomes should be reviewed. Finally, by securing a family history, the nurse may be alerted to clues to a specific diagnosis otherwise overlooked (e.g. a woman's baby has been in and out of the hospital with unexplained illnesses, suggestive of HIV, but as yet undiagnosed).

A medication history includes a review of all prescription and OTC drugs the patient is taking. This information provides important clues about the symptoms being treated. Many of the drugs used to treat HIV are highly toxic and interact with a host of other commonly prescribed drugs (Table 46–10). A patient's allergy history (drugs, food, environmental substances) should also be explored. When patients identify an allergy, specific descriptions of the allergic response should also be obtained.

When exploring the patient's social history, the nurse should assess for drug use, starting with simple questions about tobacco and alcohol use and moving into questions about the more potent drugs. If patients acknowledge using drugs, the nurse should ask what type, how often, whether they share drug paraphernalia, and when the drugs were last used.

A travel history provides information regarding possible exposure to areas of high HIV infection or areas with endemic OIs. Based on the patient's response, a skin test for TB, for example, may be indicated.

Obtaining a sexual history of all patients is important. In HIV screening, an assessment for high-risk behaviors should be conducted on all patients (see Chart 46–2). Questions asked should be open ended, straightforward, and nonjudgmental. First, the nurse should ask whether patients are sexually active or have been in the past. One should probably not ask whether a person is homosexual, heterosexual, or bisexual, but rather whether they have sex with men, with women, or both. Knowledge of specific sexual practices is necessary to determine risk. Patients engaging in anal intercourse are at greatest risk, followed by those engaging in vaginal intercourse and then oral sex. These questions should not be omitted because of embarrassment from discussing such private matters.[54] Many patients may not fully disclose all of their sexual activity initially, thus making this aspect of the history open to revision. The number of sexual partners is also important, because unprotected sex with multiple partners places patients at considerably higher risk for HIV. The nurse should phrase questions to encourage honesty. For example, one could ask, "Would you estimate that you have had over 10, 50, or more sexual partners?" as opposed to "How many people have you had sex with?" The use of condoms should be explored with men and women. Is use consistent, sporadic, or nonexistent? If a condom is used, the nurse should ask what types of condom and lubricant are used. Latex and polyurethane condoms prevent transmission of the virus; sheepskin (natural) condoms do not. With latex condoms, using a water-based rather than an oil-based lubricant helps to prevent deterioration. A history of other STDs is important because STDs increase susceptibility to HIV. If appropriate, immediate health education can begin, along with referrals (e.g., counseling for substance abuse).[55]

The patient's immunization history provides vital information necessary to protect the patient who may be immunosuppressed, especially if travel abroad is anticipated. Records should be up to date, and dis-

CHART 46–2

Recognized High-Risk Behaviors Related to HIV Disease

Unprotected anal, vaginal, or oral sex with a male or female partner

Multiple sex partners

Unprotected sexual intercourse with a partner who is known to be HIV positive or at high risk for HIV who or has an unknown risk

Sexual intercourse with an injecting drug user, especially someone who shares needles

The use of recreational drugs (marijuana) or the abuse of alcohol

History of a sexually transmitted disease

Blood transfusion before 1985

TABLE 46–10
Common Drug Interactions*

	Zidovudine (ZDV)†	Nevirapine	Rifabutin	Ritonavir
ZDV	XXX	↑ Antiviral activity in test tubes	↓ ZDV levels	↑ Antiviral activity in test tubes
Amphotericin B	↑ Risk of bone marrow toxicity	XXX	XXX	XXX
Acyclovir	↑ Antiviral activity in test tubes	XXX	XXX	XXX
Clarithromycin	May ↓ ZDV levels	May ↑ nevirapine levels; may ↑ risk of liver toxicity	May ↑ rifabutin levels by 80% and ↓ clarithromycin by up to 50%; ↑ risk of painful eye inflammation, arthritis, joint pain, tenderness or pain in muscles	↑ Clarithromycin levels by 80%
Dapsone	May ↑ risk of bone marrow toxicity	May ↑ dapsone levels	May ↓ dapsone levels	XXX
Stavudine (d4T)	May ↓ antiviral activity	XXX	XXX	XXX
Didanosine (ddI)	↑ Antiviral activity in test tubes	May ↑ antiviral activity in test tubes	XXX	XXX
Food in Stomach	May ↓ ZDV levels in blood	XXX	XXX	↑ Ritonavir levels
Ganciclovir	Hematologic toxicities; may require ↓ in AZT dose	XXX	XXX	XXX
Rifampin	Monitor for antiretroviral failure (↑ in viral loads or ↓ in CD4); may require ↑ in dose of ZDV	XXX	XXX	↓ Ritonavir level by 35%

*Drug interactions are either pharmacodynamic (synergistic or antagonistic) or pharmacokinetic (leading to changes in absorption, distribution, metabolism, or excretion). This table is just a small sample of the types of drug interactions facing HIV patients.
†Formerly known as azidothymidine (AZT).
XXX, No interaction.

eases common to the area of travel should be reviewed with the patient. Because transfusions of blood products always carry a risk for hepatitis and, in some countries, of HIV, it may be necessary to vaccinate the patient against hepatitis B.

Identifying the patient's psychosocial needs is paramount and should not be overlooked. The growing field of psychoneuroimmunology validates that emotions affect immunity. Particularly, stress and depression alter many biochemicals supporting immunity. If a detailed psychosocial history is not feasible because of time constraints, specific questions should focus on assessment of the patient's relationships, the availability of support systems, and a description of the patient's successful coping skills.

After the history is obtained, a review of systems should follow. This review involves asking the patient descriptive questions about current signs relative to each of the major body systems (neurologic; ears, eyes, nose, throat; pulmonary; cardiovascular; gastrointestinal; musculoskeletal; genitourinary; mental status; in-

tegumentary). For example, when exploring the pulmonary system, the nurse may ask whether the patient is experiencing a cough. If the answer is yes, the nurse should follow up with specific questions, such as the following:

- How often you do cough?
- When you cough, do you bring anything up?
- What color is it?
- At what time of the day do you find that you cough the most?
- Have you taken any medication for the cough?
- Have these medications been effective?

Once questions have been asked that cover each system, the nurse conducts the physical examination to verify the patient's complaints.

Physical Examination

Ideally, the review of systems should be validated by objective findings. The physical examination is the examination of each body system using auscultation, palpation, percussion, and inspection. For instance, if the patient reported a loss of appetite and diarrhea during the review of systems, then the patient should be weighed. A change in the patient's weight could objectively substantiate this subjective information. Together with a thorough history, the physical examination may determine the need for an HIV antibody test or, if the patient is HIV positive, may indicate the stage of the illness. Chart 46–3 is a list of the most common clinical signs and symptoms associated with HIV disease.

Diagnostic Tests

After the health history and physical examination, certain diagnostic data are usually collected and reviewed. Diagnostic data should not be reviewed in isolation. For example, absolute laboratory values are important, but out-of-range values versus slight fluc-

---

CHART 46–3

Most Common Signs and Symptoms Attributed to HIV Infection

Nonspecific Presentations

- Night sweats (profuse sweating during sleep; early sign of disease)
- Fever (low-grade)
- Weight loss (even in the presence of normal appetite)
- Diarrhea (nonresponsive to antidiarrheals)
- Cough (not related to smoking, cold, flu; may be productive or nonproductive)
- Hepatomegaly or splenomegaly (enlargement of the liver or spleen)
- Persistent generalized lymphadenopathy (disease of the lymph nodes throughout the body)
- Failure to thrive (generally seen in infants or preteens)

Skin Disorders

- Herpes zoster (shingles) and herpes simplex (genital organs)
- Kaposi's sarcoma (a cancer of the blood vessels under the surface of the skin, which manifests on the surface as a pinkish to brown to bluish lesion)
- Candida (a yeastlike fungus of the skin)
- Acne and pimples
- Cellulitis (inflammation of cellular or connective tissue that has spread through the tissue)
- Warts in the genital or perianal areas
- Impetigo (inflammatory skin disease marked with isolated pustules)
- Molluscum contagiosum (mildly infective skin disease characterized by tumor formations on the skin usually affecting children or young adults)
- Onychomycosis (disease of the nails due to a parasitic fungus)

- Itching around the anus caused by pinworms, hemorrhoids, fistula in the anus, or irritation
- Psoriasis (genetically determined dermatitis with dull-red itching lesions)
- Seborrheic dermatitis (inflammatory skin disease beginning on the scalp)
- Folliculitis (inflammation of a hair follicle caused most likely by staphylococci)
- Tinea corporis (a fungal skin disease of the body)
- Xerosis (abnormal dryness of skin, mucous membranes, or conjunctiva)

Mucous Membrane Problems

- Angular stomatitis (inflammation of the mouth, particularly the corners)
- Small ulcers
- Kaposi's sarcoma
- Oral hairy leukoplakia (white patches on the tongue)
- Oral thrush
- Periodontitis or gingivitis
- Vaginal candidiasis

Eye Problems

- Exudate
- Retinal hemorrhage
- Visual field defects

Other Problems

- Bacterial pneumonia
- Sinusitis
- Syphilis, gonorrhea, or other sexually transmitted diseases
- Tuberculosis

Adapted from Pottage JC, Samet JH, Soloway BH: The asymptomatic patient. Patient Care 30:35, 1996.

tuations from normal values are not always reliable indicators of the patient's state of illness. More often, changes in laboratory findings from the patient's baseline provide more significant information on the patient's well-being. A discussion of the common diagnostic tests used to assess the health status of patients with HIV disease follows.

Laboratory Tests

A complete blood count (CBC) with differential, with particular attention to leukocyte morphology, can demonstrate immunodeficiency associated with neutropenia, abnormal neutrophil forms, abnormal RBC forms, lymphopenia suggestive of T-cell deficiency, and thrombocytopenia. CBCs can identify the proportions of each white blood cell type. If normal, quantification of serum immunoglobulins (IgG, IgA, IgM) helps to determine primary and secondary immunodeficiencies or a low platelet count. It is possible for the total serum concentration to be normal and still have a deficient antibody-mediated immune response.

A white blood count (WBC) differentiates between granulocytes and agranulocytes. Granulocytes (neutrophils, eosinophils and basophils) are phagocytes responsible for the hypersensitivity reaction. Agranulocytes, monocytes (the largest phagocyte) and lymphocytes, are responsible for antibody production. The body produces specific white cells as necessary. Increases in the WBC indicate infection, whereas decreases indicate an increased risk of infection. In addition to the absolute count, a higher percentage of neutrophils indicates potential infection, especially in conjunction with signs and symptoms of infection such as fever, fatigue, weakness, or dehydration.

The CBC is also used to determine hematocrit, hemoglobin, RBC morphology, and CD4 and CD8 cell counts and ratios. CD4 counts are used to stage the immune system's response to infection and provide an indication for antiretroviral therapy (CD4 <500 cells/μL) or immune system failure.

Viral load indicates progression of disease. Extremely high viral loads (>10,000) may indicate a rapid progression to end-stage HIV disease, whereas those less than 10,000 usually signify a longer asymptomatic period. This test is used as a surrogate marker of viral progression. Viral load measures only free viral RNA floating in the blood, not that which is trapped inside tissue.

Serologic tests for Venereal Disease Research Laboratory (VDRL) or rapid plasma reagin (RPR) are often ordered to rule out untreated syphilis. These tests provide baseline data, as do *Toxoplasma* and CMV antibody titers.

Other tests frequently ordered include a blood chemistry panel (SMA 12, 14, or 20). This group of tests can indicate underlying hepatitis and can assess liver function, especially when new drugs are started. Spe-

cific liver function tests are done to detect hepatitis A, B, and C and to distinguish between acute and chronic hepatitis or other liver problems. Liver enzymes, serum oxaloacetic transaminase (SGOT) and serum glutamic pyruvic transaminase (SGPT), are released when the liver is damaged by acute or chronic hepatitis. Serum albumin levels reflect protein synthesis by the liver. Low levels may indicate poor nutrition or a chronic liver disorder.

Increased levels of serum alkaline phosphatase may signify cholestasis, kidney failure, or bone disease. Elevations in serum amylase may be due to inflammation of the pancreas and salivary glands. The patient should be observed for increases in amylase, especially once antiretroviral drug therapy is initiated. Increases in triglycerides, blood urea nitrogen (BUN), and creatinine are likely in patients with end-stage HIV disease.

A deficiency in glucose-6-phosphate dehydrogenase (G6PD) may lead to anemia resulting from destruction of RBCs. This test should be done in patients with an allergy to TMP–SMX who will be given dapsone. If G6PD is absent, dapsone will not be tolerated.

Frequently, a urinalysis is ordered. The presence of protein or liver enzymes may contribute further evidence of liver dysfunction. Finally, blood cultures for AFB may be ordered if CD4 counts are less than 75/μL.

Skin tests are ordered to rule out TB. Mantoux testing with purified protein derivative (PPD) is used for TB diagnosis. However, because HIV impairs the immune system, the patient's ability to respond is limited, often yielding a false-negative result or a reduced reaction (e.g., a 5-mm induration rather than the 10-mm induration normally seen in a positive response). Using two of these three antigens—*Candida albicans*, tetanus toxoid, or mumps—should elicit accurate results. However, it can be difficult to obtain and maintain these antigens.

Radiographic Tests

Investigators have reported that routine annual chest radiographs for patients with HIV disease are not necessary.[56] Baseline chest radiographs should be obtained and used for comparison when ruling out pulmonary illnesses, especially TB (Figure 46–3) and PCP (Figure 46–4).

Considering that HIV disease affects the brain, neuroimaging studies may help to identify the cause of symptoms. Headaches, seizures, changes in mental status, sensory deficits, and nerve palsies are all indications for radiographic studies (e.g., CT scan). Toxoplasmosis can cause both focal neurologic deficits and seizures as well as nonfocal symptoms such as confusion. Clinical features are not always consistent with the neurologic abnormality. The four distinct patterns in neuroradiologic findings are 1) cerebral atrophy

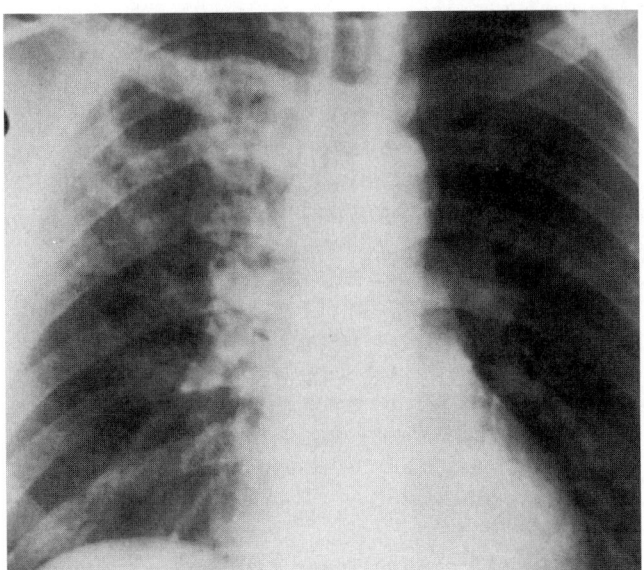

Figure 46–3

Tuberculosis. Note the opacities in the upper right lobe, where a large cavity is seen. Changes in the left upper lobe are minimal. This pattern is typical of reactivation tuberculosis in early stages of HIV infection. (From Saag MS: Cryptococcosis and other fungal infections (histoplasmosis, coccidioidomycosis). In: Sande MA, Volberding PA (eds): The Medical Management of AIDS, 5th ed. Philadelphia, WB Saunders, 1995, p 449.)

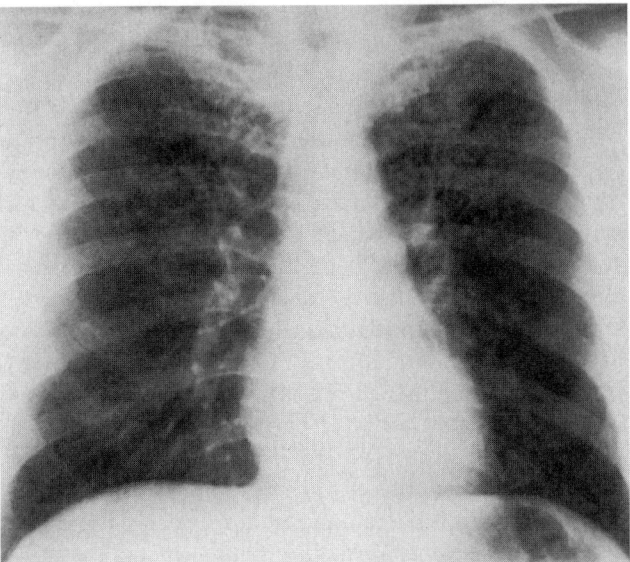

Figure 46–4

Pneumocystis carinii pneumonia. Note the upper lobe densities.

(HIV, CMV), 2) multiple mass lesions (toxoplasmosis, CNS lymphoma, *Candida* abscesses, cryptococcomas, herpes simplex encephalitis), 3) focal or diffuse white matter disease (CMV, papovavirus, varicella-zoster, herpes simplex), and 4) leptomeningeal or ependymal disease (HIV, CMV, fungi, syphilis, toxoplasmosis).[57]

Bone Marrow Aspiration

Hematologic problems are found in all stages of HIV infection and include bone marrow, blood, and coagulation abnormalities. Infection suppresses the young cells in the bone marrow and causes cytopenia, inhibiting the maturation of blood cells. The use of ZDV causes anemia, and other HIV drugs result in the myelosuppression of bone marrow, including ganciclovir (DHPG), foscarnet, TMP–SMX or other sulfa derivatives, and pentamidine.[58]

Indications for bone marrow examination may include cytopenia, persistent fever, diagnosis of lymphoma or MAC, and other OIs. Gluckman, Rosner, and Guarneri[59] reported that bone marrow examinations were useful in the diagnosis of disseminated opportunistic infection; however, in a retrospective review of bone marrow aspirates, Mazzulli and Salit[60] found little clinical utility in such examinations. Ciaudo and colleagues[61] also concluded that bone marrow examinations had little value in documenting the cause of cytopenia, but AFB bone marrow cultures were useful for lymphoma and fever of unknown origin, especially in CDC group II patients. Karcher

and Frost[62] found little correlation among bone marrow abnormalities, their origin, and the intervention used. However, these investigators recommended bone marrow examination in certain clinical situations. Martinez and associates[63] concluded that bone marrow studies were warranted for diagnosing OIs and lymphomas in patients with HIV disease. According to another study, conducted by Torda, Jones, and Beale,[64] bone marrow examinations proved most useful for lymphoma staging or MAC infection and also confirmed dysplasia and hypercellularity. Rodriguez and colleagues[65] found bone marrow examinations of little value in clarifying the origin of cytopenia and febrile syndromes. Although the value of bone marrow aspiration has not been consistently demonstrated, this test continues to be used frequently.

Specific Indicators of Immunosuppression

Many health care practitioners do not recognize the signs and symptoms of HIV infection (see Chart 46–3), a situation that leads to overreaction, in which one suspects that every illness indicates HIV, or underreaction, resulting in underreporting and delay of treatment. A history of previous infections, such as hepatitis, herpes, or syphilis, is important because these infections often recur in patients with HIV disease. Nurses should pay particular attention to the frequency and type of infections (thrush, oral hairy leukoplakia, canker sores) and should compare the incidence to that of persons of similar age and risk status. Other indications of immunosuppression include the need for prolonged or additional antibiotic therapy, the presence of unusual microorganisms (shingles in persons < 50 years of age), or the spread of infection to other anatomic sites. Perhaps the most important indicators of immunosuppression are fevers, night sweats, and weight loss. Like many of the other findings (diarrhea, fatigue, lymphadenopathy), these conditions are nonspecific indicators of generalized infection.

Sixty percent of patients with HIV disease present with PCP, usually with recurrent episodes. Mycobacterial TB, which occurs in approximately 10% of patients with HIV disease, has been found more frequently in IV drug users than in homosexual or bisexual men. CMV causes pneumonitis, which on radiography is difficult to distinguish from PCP. At present, there is no effective treatment for CMV pneumonia, and it is often found on autopsy of patients with HIV. Fungal pneumonias occur in less than 5% of patients with HIV and are usually endemic to certain parts of the United States. Although bacterial infections in patients with HIV are increasing, they can often be treated successfully with antibiotics if they are identified early.

Pulmonary involvement also occurs in 20% of patients with KS, usually homosexual or bisexual men. A form of HSV, KS is the manifestation of this virus in immunocompromised patients. Lymphocytic interstitial pneumonitis (LIP) is usually found in children under 13 years of age and occurs rarely in adults. AIDS-related lymphoma is a recognized AIDS-defining condition and a highly aggressive form of non–Hodgkin's lymphoma. Cardiac problems are often linked to pulmonary problems, and nuclear imaging scans help to differentiate diagnoses.

Six of the AIDS-defining conditions are gastrointestinal (see Chart 46–1). Because initial findings are subtle, double-contrast radiographic techniques are suggested for studies of the esophagus, stomach, and colon.[66] Abdominal and lower gastrointestinal films help to identify causative agents for enteritis, bowel obstructions, colitis, and neoplasms. Nuclear imaging or CT scans may also be needed.[63, 66]

Candida infections often occur in patients with HIV disease. Oral thrush occurs in the symptomatic stage, whereas esophageal candida is an AIDS-defining condition. Radiographs can help to differentiate between *Candida* and CMV and between neoplasms and infection; one must determine when endoscopic and culture techniques are necessary and aid in assessing the therapeutic response.[57, 66]

Nursing Diagnoses

Once patients have been diagnosed with HIV, the timeline varies as to when they will become symptomatic and require medical attention (see Figure 46–1). Because of complex nature of the disease and because patients present at different stages of illness, various diagnoses can be identified to direct interventions. Specific approaches to four of the most common emotionally related diagnoses for patients with HIV disease are discussed in detail. Additional diagnoses appropriate to these patients can be found in Table 46–11.

TABLE 46–11
Nursing Diagnoses

Problem Statement	Etiologic Factors
Anxiety	Changes in interpersonal relationships, decisions about sharing of information, concern about the future, fear of disapproval, fear of death
Altered family processes	Altered role functions; devastating illness of family member
Social isolation	Fear of rejection or actual rejection of others
Anticipatory grief	Multiple losses, lifestyle changes, threat to bodily functions and life
Confusion, chronic	HIV encephalopathy, medication side effects
High risk for infection	Immunosuppression, exposure to infectious agents by sexual behaviors, drug use, or nosocomial infections
Altered nutrition, less than body requirements	Oropharyngeal, esophageal, or other pain or discomfort due to OIs; lactose intolerance, HIV wasting syndrome, diarrhea, fever, and infection, side effects of medications
Risk for altered body temperature; hyperthermia	Infection, dehydration
Diarrhea	Pathogenic organisms, malabsorption syndrome, medication side effects
Fluid volume deficit	Fever, diarrhea, inadequate intake
Fatigue, activity intolerance	HIV wasting syndrome, OIs, inadequate nutrition, impaired respiratory function, fever, and infection
Ineffective breathing pattern, ineffective airway clearance, risk for aspiration, impaired gas exchange	OIs (e.g., *Pneumocystis carinii* pneumonia, cytomegalovirus pneumonia), fatigue
Sleep pattern disturbances	Night sweats, pain, medication regimen, urinary or bowel incontinence
Knowledge deficit	Complexity of HIV disease and medication regimen, need for coping strategies and self-care in chronic illness

OIs, opportunistic infections.

Ineffective Individual Coping

When patients are first informed that they are HIV positive, their emotional responses vary and may include the following: anger at the person who may have given them the virus;[67] guilt over their own role in exposing themselves to the virus;[68] despair over the prognosis, sometimes triggering suicidal acts; and fear of negative reactions from family, friends, and society. Many patients with HIV use the general guideline of sharing information on a "need to know" basis—only with those who have a legitimate reason to be informed. Others find it a relief and source of great support to be completely open from the beginning. Because each choice presents different problems and opportunities, the nurse can help patients to clarify their options and feelings by providing facts (e.g., current laws related to employment and insurance issues) and posing questions for consideration (e.g., what reactions does the patient anticipate from significant others?).

Although anger is frequently a normal response to the diagnosis of HIV and loss of health, it can also be harmful. Williams and Williams[69] cited research supporting their premise that "anger kills." Although the expression of anger has long been encouraged as a means of decreasing depression, Retzinger[70] cautioned that when persons express anger, the emotion can escalate and can lead to self-violence or violence against others. Nurses should provide a safe outlet for patients to express feelings of anger. The nurse should actively listen to patients' expressions of anger, should empathize, and should accept their feelings. Patients can be encouraged to write about their feelings (even if what is written is destroyed later) or to release their anger physically by punching or hitting something such as a pillow or by participating in an occupational therapy project that involves hammering. If patients like sports and are physically able, hitting balls or yelling while watching a game can also help to release anger.

If anger is expressed in destructive behaviors (e.g., biting, spitting, scratching, throwing feces, blood, or other body fluids), the nurse will need to intervene by setting limits. When informed patients continue actions that endanger others (e.g., unprotected sex without informing partners), a staff meeting may help to determine the best action as well as provide group support. State laws differ in relation to persons who knowingly infect a partner, and nurses need to keep current regarding these policies.

Anxiety and Fear

The patient with HIV faces many stressors (e.g., uncertain future, loss of health, isolation, financial responsibilities). These stressors can result in anxiety and fear and have shown to have a negative impact on the immune system.[71] In addition, anxiety and fear can affect the patient's physical well-being indirectly by influencing risk-taking behavior, adherence to treatment and health monitoring plans, and other health habits such as smoking, eating, or sleeping. Death anxiety, in particular, may influence health-seeking behavior.[72]

A positive, interpersonal support system is vital to the management of the patient's anxiety and fear. Patients who lack close relationships may need more support from the health care team. The nurse should also inform patients of local support groups and should encourage attendance. Research has shown that helper T cells and natural killer cells have been found to be higher and depression less frequent in patients with HIV who participated in a stress-management group compared with those who did not.[73] Group programs may also improve medication compliance and adherence.[74]

If the patient's customary recreational activities are safe and are not exhausting, the nurse should encourage continued participation. In particular, exercise discharges the epinephrine and stress chemicals stimulated in the "fight-or-flight" reaction. Less strenuous stress-reduction activities include music, warm baths, massage, yoga or meditation, humor, and relaxation techniques (e.g., deep breathing, progressive muscle relaxation, visual imagery, or autogenic body training, possibly in conjunction with biofeedback training). Bibliotherapy, such as readings in cognitive therapy, positive thinking, and inspirational or religious literature, may help patients to cultivate a reality-based, positive attitude and to control anxiety and fear.

Anticipatory Grieving

Grief is a normal response to the series of losses and anticipation of death experienced by the patient with HIV. The death of partners, close friends, or fellow support group members often precedes the patient's own diagnosis, increasing anticipatory fears of the disease. Resolution of grief requires the courage to mourn what is lost, to release it, and to embrace life's remaining joys. As the life span of patients with HIV increases, it is important that patients come to terms with *living* with HIV rather than anticipating imminent death.[75,76]

The nurse can assist with grief work and resolution by supporting the patient in dealing with unfinished business (e.g., making overtures to deal with significant interpersonal or family conflicts, making a will and advance directives, and planning one's memorial and bodily disposition). Grief work involves patients' expressions of feelings about their losses and what they mean.[77] These can include the disappearance of friends or partners, changes in sexual practices, changes in lifestyle, loss of health and body image culminating in the physical wasting that accompanies the disease, and impending death. For the patient who is experiencing an exceptional grief response, a psychiatric evaluation may be necessary. Suicide precautions, psychotherapy, or antidepressant medication can be initiated.

When death is imminent, the goal is to aid the patient in a peaceful death. The nurse's supportive presence can alleviate common fears of being alone and facing the unknown. If the patient lacks a supportive spiritual guide or belief system, the nurse should ask whether he or she desires contact with a sympathetic religious leader (e.g., hospital chaplain, a rabbi, priest, or clergy member of the patient's choice).

Survivors of patients dying of HIV disease have been identified as having particular problems in resolving grief.[78] The nurse should consider referring the survivors to Compassionate Friends, a self-help organization for parents who have lost a child at any age, local grief-support groups, or P-FLAGG (Parents and Friends of Lesbians and Gays Group), if applicable, for additional support.

Altered Thought Processes

As the HIV disease progresses, the patient's cognition is often affected by OIs or HIV encephalopathy (AIDS-dementia complex). Early manifestations include loss of focus and forgetfulness. Nursing interventions include patience and protection of the patient's self-esteem, limited and simple communication repeated as necessary, predictable routines, and use of audiovisual aids to promote orientation to person, place, and time (e.g., radios, clocks, calendars, signs, pictures, large name pins, and adequate lighting). Some patients with HIV exhibit a hyperactivity syndrome similar to the manic phase of bipolar disease, and AIDS-dementia complex later involves motor impairment. Restraints or antipsychotic medications may be necessary to ensure the safety of the patient or others. Recent use of antidepressants and anxiolytics indicates that these agents may be preferable to antipsychotics for some confused patients.[79] Staff education programs, directed at both staff attitudes and basic interventions (reducing stimuli, redirecting the patient's attention, and setting limits) have been evaluated as helpful in working with patients with similar alterations in thought processes.[80]

Collaborative Management

The care required by the patient with HIV in the acute care setting involves collaboration with numerous providers including physicians, nurses, case managers, clinical nurse specialists, respiratory therapists, dietitians, social workers, pharmacists, clergy, and the family. The nurse working in the intensive care unit (ICU) or the intermediate care unit needs to have a solid background in the treatment of the various HIV-related conditions (see Chart 46–1), because any of these conditions may be encountered by the HIV-infected patient over the course of the disease. It is impossible for nurses in general settings to know everything about HIV disease, because information on care and treatment changes rapidly. When available, HIV clinical nurse specialists should be consulted regarding management strategies.

One of the most crucial aspects of working with patients with HIV is the nurse's own attitude toward the disease and the patient (Chart 46–4). In a comprehensive review of research conducted during the 1990s, nursing knowledge and attitudes related to HIV were frequent topics.[81,82] Although acceptance of every patient is a standard of professional practice, it is critical for the patient with HIV for many unique reasons.

Fear of Acquiring the Virus

Even when gloves and other barrier protection are used properly, nurses may fear exposure to the virus. Unnecessary avoidance of contact further hinders the development of a therapeutic nurse–patient relationship. Although not all patients welcome touch, the appropriate use of touch can communicate caring and acceptance (e.g., backrub, hand-holding or a hug when sad). Being well informed generally helps nurses to differentiate irrational fear from appropriate precautions.[83] Some researchers found that nurses with more knowledge reported less fear of HIV-positive patients.[84–86] However, a 1-day workshop did not produce significant change,[87] and some nurses continued to feel vulnerable despite a good knowledge base.[88] Experience with HIV-positive patients has been associated with more positive attitudes and may be effective in changing some nurses' attitudes.[89]

Social Stigma Associated With HIV

Although improvements have been made in society's acceptance of patients with HIV, the general social stigma associated with the disease remains. HIV disease has been compared with leprosy, and fear of isolation was identified as a reason that HIV-positive patients keep their status secret.[90] A "matter-of-fact" attitude of acceptance of the disease is usually well received, as well as acceptance of the individual and his or her culture and attitudes.[91,92]

Judgments related to particular behaviors by which some patients acquire the virus have been reported. Many patients have experienced rejection or anticipate disapproval because IV drug use,[68] indiscriminate sexual activity, or anal sex, especially if between homosexuals. In studies of the attitudes of nurses and

CHART 46-4

RESEARCH UTILIZATION: NURSES' ATTITUDES TOWARD CARING FOR AIDS PATIENTS

Abstract: The purpose of this study was to identify nurses' attitudes toward caring for AIDS patients and to examine the relationship of these attitudes to the variables of nursing education and experience in caring for AIDS patients. An anonymous mail survey of 138 registered nurses was conducted using a modification of a Likert instrument from previous research by Scherer and associates.[1] This instrument was designed to measure five nursing attitudes: 1) fears and concerns about caring for AIDS patients; 2) attitudes toward the patients' use of health care services; 3) attitudes toward caring for terminally ill patients; 4) attitudes toward homosexuality; and 5) attitudes of significant others toward AIDS patients. Frequency distribution, independent t-tests, and analyses of variance were used to analyze data. Nurses with experience in caring for patients with AIDS demonstrated more positive attitudes toward patients' use of health care ($P < .05$) and more positive attitudes toward homosexuality ($P < .04$) than nurses without such experience. Educational background was not found to be a significant variable related to nurses' attitudes.

Critique: The review of literature cited several related studies and provided adequate rationale for both the need for the study and the selection of variables considered, although research literature on this subject is even more extensive.[2,3] Anonymity was assured, and participants were provided information about the study. Data were presented on the reliability and validity of the instrument. Researchers stated that the instrument was modified and piloted; more information or possibly more extensive testing of the instrument would assist the reader in evaluating the researchers' choice of an instrument. The researchers' use of the term "attitudes of significant others toward AIDS patients" is assumed to refer to the significant others of patients rather than the significant others of nurses; however, the latter is a factor in influencing those attitudes. Because this study focused on nurses' attitudes and their cultural and support systems, clarification would have been helpful.

The sample size of 138 from 250 surveys mailed was an acceptable return rate, but a larger and more representative sample would strengthen the study and would seem feasible with the mail-survey design described. The researchers acknowledged the limitation of all subjects being chosen from one Midwestern state, limiting generalization of findings.

The demographic data reported included age, sex, and education, but they did not include other categories such as race, which could be useful in analysis. The number of respondents in several categories was too small for meaningful analysis (males, nurses with higher degrees, and some age categories). For example, only 8.6% of respondents fell into the category of subjects less than 30 years old, and some categories were collapsed because of the small number of respondents in each cell. In the final analysis, the amount of experience respondents had with AIDS patients was collapsed into only two categories: nurses who had cared for at least one AIDS patient and nurses who had never cared for an AIDS patient. This difference in experience emerged as a major finding in the study. The reader must consider whether other factors may have influenced both the nurses' lack of experience with HIV-positive patients and the attitudes reported, such as the work setting. Preexisting attitudes may also have influenced nurses' experience with HIV-positive patients. For example, nurses with more positive attitudes may have elected to work with AIDS patients, whereas those with less positive attitudes may have avoided doing so. The researchers accurately reported only the association among the variables; a cause-and-effect relationship should not be inferred.

Implications for Nursing: Overall, this study heightens awareness of nurses' attitudes toward AIDS patients and provides valuable data with implications for future research and nursing practice. Assigning nursing students or registered nurses to care for AIDS patients in a supportive environment appears to be an important initial step to help overcome negativity. Such assignments should provide a basis for exploring nurses' attitudes in the clinical setting, as well as for studying whether attitudes change after this experience (e.g., replacing the independent t-test with a paired t-test; a pretest and a posttest with experience as the intervention and a multiple regression analysis with experience as an independent variable are possibilities). Other strategies that may be useful in alleviating fears and altering attitudes should also be pursued, such as group discussions or role play to explore nurses' feelings. Categories of subjects' educational background were based on formal educational degrees; the value of different approaches to continuing education should be explored as well as the AIDS curriculum of programs of nursing. Although attitudes

Chart continued on following page

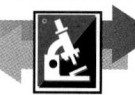

CHART 46–4 *Continued*

RESEARCH UTILIZATION: NURSES' ATTITUDES TOWARD CARING FOR AIDS PATIENTS

toward homosexuality were more positive among nurses with more experience with AIDS patients, nurses with fewer years of total nursing experience were found to have more positive attitudes toward homosexuality than nurses with more experience, a finding possibly indicating that more recent graduates are exposed to educational experiences that are more supportive of diversity.

The primary implications for both research and practice center around an increased awareness that nurses need support in dealing with their feelings to provide the supportive care needed by AIDS patients. Strategies should be integrated into the supervisory process to ensure that nurses become part of the solution, not part of the problem. After efforts are made to foster positive attitudes, nurses' self-

selection or volunteer assignment to work with HIV-positive patients may ultimately be preferable for the patients' welfare. Because of the chronic nature of the illness, the lack of support by some elements of society, and the suffering and death associated with HIV disease, patients need nurses who are accepting, supportive, and responsive to their needs and who are effective, committed patient advocates.

1. Scherer YK, Haughey BP, Wu YB: AIDS: What are nurses' concerns? Clin Nurse Specialist 3:48–54, 1989.
2. Bennett JA: Nurses' attitudes about acquired immunodeficiency syndrome care: what research tells us. J Prof Nurs 11:339–350, 1995.
3. Larson E, Ropka ME: An update on nursing research and HIV infection. Image: J Nurs Sch 23:4–11, 1991.

Source: Baylor RA, McDaniel AM: Nurses' attitudes toward caring for patients with acquired immunodeficiency syndrome. J Prof Nurs 12:99–105, 1996.

student nurses toward HIV-positive patients, homophobia was acknowledged as an issue,[84,93] but it was found to be decreasing in recent graduates, regardless of their age.[89]

Emotional Costs

The emotional costs of working with patients (many of whom are in the prime of their lives) with a poor prognosis are high. Although the prognosis for patients with HIV is improving, there is no cure; instead, these patients have repeated episodes of illness and, ultimately, they die. Nurses need to examine their feelings and abilities to reinvest continually in new patients while losing others to whom they have become attached. Many HIV experts caution nurses against burnout and emphasize that peer support, stress management, and a personal life that provides spiritual and emotional renewal are vital to personal well-being.[83] Some researchers conclude that empathic, involved relationships with patients actually prevent rather than contribute to burnout by increasing the rewards experienced by the nurse.[94,95] In summary, HIV-positive patients' suffering and impending death, combined with a lack of support by some elements of society, increase the need for nurses who are accepting, supportive, and responsive to these patients' needs.

The current management of patients with HIV is complex and involves physiologic and psychosocial dimensions. Interventions are categorized based on the phase of illness, with health promotion and main-

tenance and disease prevention the primary focus of care in the asymptomatic phase of HIV disease and symptom management the primary focus of care in the symptomatic and end-stage phases of HIV disease. In addition, patient education needs, strategies to control opportunistic infections, and pharmcotherapeutic interventions are discussed in detail. Finally, information related to occupational concerns facing health care providers (e.g., known or suspected exposure to HIV) is presented.

Health Promotion and Maintenance and Disease Prevention

Vigilant health monitoring (e.g., gynecologic exams, dental care, and routine screening by a provider knowledgeable about HIV disease) is essential during the early treatment of the asymptomatic patient with HIV. During this time, the prevention of other communicable diseases is critical. Each infection or illness depletes some of the patient's immune resources, thus increasing his or her vulnerability to the progression of HIV disease. In addition to adherence to prophylactic medication regimens, patients should increase attention to basic disease prevention measures such as hand washing.[96] Contact with communicable diseases and animal feces should be avoided, and patients are advised to use good hand washing technique if cleaning pet excrement[97] or bird droppings. Patients are also advised to maintain current immunizations and records.

Maintaining nutritional status and fluid and electrolyte balance in these patients is essential. Consultation with the dietitian early in the course of the disease is often beneficial. A healthy diet, including fresh foods and daily vitamin and mineral supplements, supports the immune system. Nutritionally complete drinks or electrolyte or glucose drinks should be added when patients are unable to meet nutritional requirements through a normal diet.

Patients are also advised to avoid caffeine, alcohol, tobacco, and mood-altering drugs or chemicals for several reasons. Such substances affect major organs and may hasten multisystem failure in end-stage HIV disease.[98] Substance use has been correlated with non-compliance with medication,[99] and some substances, including alcohol, interact with certain HIV drugs to increase the risk of pancreatitis.[100]

Inadequate sleep and rest reduce immunity. Many patients with HIV are young people whose lifestyle may fail to include adequate sleep and rest periods. Initially, some patients may deal with their prognosis by partying and overworking to "cram more life" into their shortened life span. The nurse's role in educating these patients can help to increase their acceptance of difficult lifestyle changes. As HIV disease progresses, fatigue becomes a major symptom, requiring patients to know how to set priorities and to conserve energy.

Sleep disturbances may also develop in patients with HIV. Remedies for insomnia include the following: warm milk, herbal tea, and a high-carbohydrate snack at bedtime; massage; exercise during the day with a quiet time before bedtime (e.g., quiet music, reading, stress-reduction techniques, or meditation); and a bedtime routine that includes retiring at the same time each night. Nurses should organize care to provide periods of undisturbed rest and to reduce noxious stimuli such as odors, or reduce the volume of beeping monitors, staff conversations, and telephones.

Early morning awakening occurs when one falls asleep at bedtime but awakens in the early hours of morning. This disturbance of deep sleep often occurs after drinking alcohol or is due to depression. Nightmares may result simply from eating rich food late at night, but they can be an early sign of habituation to an addicting drug. Any of these sleep disturbances may also arise from emotional conflict. If sleep disturbances persist, counseling and anxiolytic or antidepressant medications may be needed.

Maintaining an exercise program is important to the overall well-being of these patients. Even if they have some degree of fatigue, some exercise is needed to prevent the physiologic hazards of immobility. Regular exercise also promotes immune functions[101] and is associated with a lower incidence of some diseases. Exercise can reduce the physiologic and psychological consequences of stress, by using the excess energy to improve conditioning and to stimulate biochemicals that elevate mood.

In selecting exercise activities, patients should seek to avoid injury or overexertion. Short periods of walking, dancing, or swimming are usually good choices, provided the pool is chlorinated and is not used by children in diapers (fecal contimation).

Symptom Management

As the HIV disease progresses, patients are admitted to acute care settings for repeated episodes of illnesses. For example, patients may present to the ICU with PCP several times. Even with appropriate therapy, the damage done to the patient's lungs with each infection is additive and is complicated by a failing immune system. A multidisciplinary approach to care of these patients ensures that maximum patient outcomes are achieved. Nursing interventions are increasingly directed toward management of symptoms. In addition to treating specific aspects of OIs, interventions for the most frequent symptoms experienced by patients with symptomatic or end-stage HIV disease are discussed.

Pain

Patients with HIV may report with varying degrees of pain. Many of the stress-reduction techniques described previously are also useful in pain management. Other nonpharmacologic interventions include the use of acupuncture, biofeedback training for target symptoms, and the application of heat and cold. Patients may self-manage moderate pain such as headaches or joint pain with OTC analgesics or non-steroidal anti-inflammatory drugs (NSAIDs). If effective, these remedies are preferable to steroids, which further suppress immunity. Patients with bruising, bleeding, or gastrointestinal disturbances may need to avoid aspirin.

As both pain and the prognosis worsen, pain relief takes priority over concerns about addiction or the effect of the medication on major organs, and prescription-strength medications, including narcotics, are given. With severe pain, medication may be administered in successive increments until the patient obtains relief or falls asleep and then lowered slightly to provide relief while awake, yet still maintaining an effective blood level. Intravenous patient-controlled analgesia (PCA) is often preferable for patients whose mental status permits this degree of self-regulation, especially if injections must be limited because of bruising or bleeding.

When pain and discomfort are due to more specific symptoms, nursing interventions can be selected individually. For example, in some patients with neuropathy, numbness or burning of the feet is relieved several weeks after discontinuing antiretroviral medication.

Meanwhile, massage, exercise, relaxation, analgesics, or tricyclic antidepressant medication may provide relief.[73] Partial relief for a stiff neck, skin lesions, or bruises may be obtained through positioning and cushioning of affected areas.

Fever

For febrile patients, the nurse should diligently monitor the patient's temperature (avoiding rectal readings if the patient has diarrhea or bruises easily) and observe for sweating (diaphoresis, night sweats) and chills. In addition, patients may require an increase in fluid intake, the use of hypothermia blankets, special attention to skin care,[73] and the administration of antipyretic medications. Reducing room temperature slightly while providing extra cover for intermittent chills can increase patient comfort.

Respiratory Symptoms

Depending on the OI, patients with HIV experience various respiratory symptoms. The nurse, working with the respiratory therapist and physician, must monitor the patient's arterial blood gases (ABGs), respiratory rate and pattern, breath sounds, and secretions.[73] Nursing interventions may include the following: positioning the patient in Fowler's or semi-Fowler's position and encouraging range-of-motion exercises and ambulation as tolerated; humidification, such as a saline mist by nebulizer and increased fluid intake; promotion of coughing, deep breathing, use of assistive devices (e.g., incentive spirometry), or postural drainage; administration of antitussives or expectorants; maintenance of a patent airway by suctioning as needed; energy conservation techniques; and the teaching of relaxation exercises to decrease anxiety or to prevent hyperventilation by patients on a mechanical ventilator.[73]

Diarrhea

Some patients with HIV experience constipation, but as the disease progresses, as many as 60% of HIV patients experience serious diarrhea.[102] Diarrhea in these patients can be caused by the HIV disease, one of the OIs, sexually transmitted gastrointestinal pathogens, or 1 of at least 8 pathogens involving the small or large bowel, or it may be a side effect of HIV medications.[102] Patients may have more than 20 stools per day, with incomplete relief from traditional antidiarrheal medications. Such unrelenting diarrhea hastens progression of HIV disease by affecting nutritional status, fluid and electrolyte balance, skin integrity, socialization, and self-esteem.

Malabsorption syndrome can also develop, which is an inability of the gastrointestinal system to absorb fats and proteins. It is manifested by three to eight greasy, foul-smelling stools per day. Diagnosis of malabsorption syndrome can be confirmed with a D-xylose absorption test or Sudan stain, but it is usually assumed to be present if weight loss continues despite a caloric intake adequate to support body weight.[102]

Diagnosing the specific cause of diarrhea helps in targeting treatment when possible; however, this diagnosis requires time, and causes are often multiple. Nursing interventions involve four major areas: 1) administering medications prescribed to treat the cause of the diarrhea, if known; 2) administering antidiarrheal medications (e.g., kaolin, pectin, loperamide, atropine or diphenoxylate, opium, octreotide); 3) dietary changes; and 4) compensatory measures to decrease the negative effects of diarrhea.

A low-residue, high-protein, high-calorie diet may be ordered. Dietary recommendations include the following: 1) small, frequent feedings; 2) bland foods that are not mechanically irritating (e.g., raw vegetables), are not too spicy, or do not cause flatus; 3) elimination of caffeine, which stimulates peristalsis; 4) elimination of sorbitol (in some brands of liquid dietary supplements); 5) decreasing fat, especially greasy foods; 6) decreasing soluble fiber (e.g., breads or cereals with whole grain, especially bran, wheat germ, or granola; nuts, seeds, some vegetables with skins); 7) increasing protein and calories; 8) increasing insoluble fiber such as pectin (e.g., oatmeal, potatoes, bananas); and 9) correcting for lactose intolerance by use of *Lactobacillus acidophilus* capsules or special milk marketed with it as an additive or by substituting soy milk or a calorie-dense liquid such as Sustacal, Ensure, Resource, or Nutren.[103] Yogurt is a healthy food often tolerated well, especially if the diarrhea is partly due to destruction of intestinal flora by medications.

If these measures are inadequate, as in some cases of malabsorption syndrome, two types of liquid dietary supplements have been recommended: 1) medium-chain triglycerides (MCTs) (e.g., Lipisorb and Peptamen), or 2) complete elemental formulas, which, although unpalatable, demonstrate promise (e.g., Vivonex, total enteral nutrition).[102, 103]

It is also important to compensate for other negative effects of severe diarrhea. In addition to monitoring the frequency, quantity, and quality of stools and collecting specimens for culture, the nurse should monitor the patient's skin integrity and should teach the patient to do so. If diarrhea persists, rectal bags may be considered. An enterostomal therapist, when available, should be consulted for additional advice on skin care issues. It is particularly important to protect the patient's dignity and self-esteem as he or she experiences this loss of control over the body.

Wasting Syndrome

An unexpected loss of more than 10% of body weight is defined by the CDC as wasting, which differs from other types of weight loss in that it depletes muscles more than fat. An AIDS-defining diagnosis, wasting creates a vicious cycle of weakness and gastrointestinal impairment that makes it even more difficult to meet the patient's nutritional needs, thus hastening death. Nutritional supplements or total parenteral nutrition (TPN) may be necessary. The nurse should monitor the patient's daily weights and food intake. Decreased albumin and total protein levels suggest malnutrition.

Fluid and Electrolyte Imbalance

Diarrhea is the most frequent cause of fluid and electrolyte (potassium, magnesium) losses. Elevated serum levels of BUN and sodium with a normal creatinine indicate dehydration.[102] Fever and infection can also increase fluid requirements. Up to 3 L per day of electrolyte or glucose drinks are recommended. The nurse should monitor intake and output, IV fluid and electrolyte infusions, skin turgor, and serum albumin, hemoglobin, and hematocrit levels. As HIV progresses, many patients become incontinent. Males can often use external catheters. In considering indwelling catheters, advantages such as protection against skin breakdown and improving socialization must be weighed against the increased risk of infection. Bedclothes, linen, and skin should be kept clean and dry for the patient's comfort and to protect skin integrity.

Monitoring Effects of Medication

The nurse needs to know the therapeutic and adverse effects of all patients' medications—how they interact with each other, how they are affected by food and drink, how they are metabolized and excreted and affect body organs, and how they should be stored. For example, indinavir should not be taken with food, whereas ritonavir should be, and saquinavir should be taken within 2 hours either before or after meals.

Because of the large number of drugs used to treat HIV disease and OIs and the rapid changes in these prescriptions, nurses should consult with pharmacists as needed. For example, numerous drugs affect plasma levels of protease inhibitors, and a drug interaction screen should be conducted by the pharmacist for all patients taking these medications.[90]

The frequency of adverse effects associated with HIV drug treatment is high. These adverse effects can include fever and allergic reactions and may also affect other body systems (e.g., gastrointestinal effects such as nausea, vomiting, and diarrhea; CNS effects such as hypotension; hematologic effects such as leukopenia, thrombocytopenia, and azotemia; dermatologic effects such as severe skin rashes; and assaults on body organs such as pancreatitis, hepatitis, and nephritis).[73]

In administering medications and teaching patients about them, one must appreciate the risk of resistance or cross-resistance. All medications should be given on time, to maintain the appropriate blood level. If a dose is regurgitated or missed, the next dose should not be doubled. If adverse effects develop, the nurse (or patient) should not omit a dose, but should report the adverse effects immediately to the physician. Stopping a drug for several weeks (a drug holiday) before reintroducing it or changing medications has been recommended.[91] However, in triple-drug therapy, all three drugs must be discontinued, not just the one causing the problem.

Patient Education

The nurse's role in patient and family education is a key factor in the successful prevention, acute care, and long-term management of the patient with HIV disease. The use of an ongoing checklist to record the teaching provided to these patients is recommended (Figure 46–5). Patient educators are also encouraged to evaluate the reading level of all written material used for patients and to consider the general age, attention span, and interests of the audience when selecting or developing materials.[104, 105] Learning materials are more effective when targeted to the patient's cultural background. Examples of such efforts include guidelines developed by Walters, Canady, and Stein[106] for evaluating multicultural approaches in HIV and AIDS educational material research and by O'Donnell, SanDoral, and Vornfett[107] on developing videos for HIV prevention among Hispanics. For patients who do not speak English well, learning materials in their native language are imperative.[108]

Nurses teaching HIV-infected patients and their families regularly are encouraged to maintain a resource book and to catalog the teaching materials. For example, resources may be listed according to their appropriateness for the general public, patients with HIV, or health care professionals. Additional categories may be used to identify the source, cost, reading level, language, purpose, and medium (e.g., video, audiotape, pamphlet, novel) of the materials. Nurses should not limit their search of teaching materials to professional literature, but they should peruse what is available to the public, inviting patients to contribute to this effort as well (e.g., browse public libraries or bookstores, tape television programs, purchase movies, review plays or novels, and surf the Internet with the lay consumer in mind).

When teaching content that is emotionally laden, as is much of HIV education, the nurse should ask the patient to repeat the major points, to evaluate what has actually been learned. In addition, patients may not keep written materials, to protect their privacy. Overall, the long-term needs of these patients and the gravity of the diagnosis make teaching during all phases of the disease one of the nurse's most important functions.

TRANSMISSION ROUTES AND RISKS

Sexual behavior

Risk of major types of sexual activity

☐ Anal
☐ Vaginal
☐ Oral

Factors influencing risk

☐ Partners' status
☐ Partners' risk status
☐ Partners' contacts and their risk factors
☐ Window period

☐ Abrasions, open sores
☐ Other STDs
☐ Use of protection

Barrier protection (male or female condoms)

☐ Latex vs. polyurethane
☐ Sheepskin condoms
☐ Condition (storage, age, single use)
☐ Proper application technique

☐ Water-based lubricant
☐ Other tips
☐ Other barriers
☐ Dental dam

☐ Relative effectiveness
☐ Nonoxynol 9

Drug-related behavior

General risks

☐ Loss of inhibitions/control of self, partner
☐ Impact on general health and community
  ☐ Physiological effects of drugs used
  ☐ Indirect effects (diet, rest, safety)

Drug use involving needles

☐ Sharing needles
☐ Sharing drugs
☐ Sterile needles used once
☐ Ways to decrease risk
☐ Use of bleach
☐ Other

Maternal transmission

☐ Prenatal
☐ During birth process
☐ Sheepskin condoms
☐ Breast milk
☐ Prevention
  ☐ Protocol 076
  ☐ Contraceptives

Blood-to-blood or body fluid contact

☐ Standard precautions
☐ High-risk situations
  ☐ Needlesticks
  ☐ Invasive procedures
  ☐ Accidents, injuries, bites, etc.
  ☐ Children, diapers, feces

Other risks

☐ Food and fluids
  ☐ Raw eggs
  ☐ Swimming and drinking water
  ☐ Travel precautions

HIV Testing

☐ Referrals to testing sites
☐ Confidential vs. anonymous testing
☐ Types of tests (ELISA, IFA, Western blot)
  ☐ Limitations of the test
  ☐ Basic information (cost, waiting period, etc.)
  ☐ Support/motivation
  ☐ Overview of the pre-post test counseling sessions

General health promotion and maintenance

☐ Diet
☐ Vitamins
☐ Exercise
☐ Sleep and rest
☐ General stress reduction strategies
☐ Specific stress management techniques
☐ Use of caffeine, nicotine, alcohol, drugs

Referral to self-help support group

☐ Other support systems

Bibliotherapy

☐ Given educational materials
☐ Referred to educational materials

Immunizations

☐ Update of immunizations and records

Health Monitoring

☐ Dental examinations
☐ Gynecologic examinations
☐ Physical examinations
☐ Referral to HIV/professional for screening, monitoring
☐ Recognition of signs and symptoms of disease progression
☐ Significance of CD4 counts and viral loads

Medications

☐ Purpose/therapeutic effects
☐ Adverse effects
☐ Coping strategies
☐ What to report to primary care provider
☐ Schedule of administration
☐ Correct dosages
  ☐ Whether with food, drink
  ☐ What to do when dosage is missed

☐ Importance of "no drug holidays"
☐ Rationale for above
☐ Method(s) for keeping track of medications

Figure 46–5

Health education checklist.

Controlling Opportunistic Infections

Because of the recent changes in the health care industry, the treatment of patients with HIV in acute care settings has been minimized. As a result, local AIDS support groups, the home health care industry, and hospice organizations make important contributions to the management of these patients in the community (Chart 46–5). An overriding management goal is the prevention of or reduction in OIs in this patient population, and the use of prophylaxis is critical to this goal (Table 46–12).

The CDC offers guidelines for the prevention of OIs in patients with HIV as well as suggestions for manag-

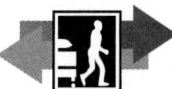

CHART 46–5

BEYOND THE ICU: MAINTAINING QUALITY OF LIFE FOR PATIENTS WITH HIV

One of the goals of caring for patients with HIV disease is to maintain them in their home environments as much as possible. To achieve this goal, it is desirable for the primary care provider to be experienced and knowledgeable in the care of HIV-infected patients and to have established an interdisciplinary network of other health care providers who are readily available to collaborate and contribute their expertise to the patients' care.

Such a network should include local AIDS support organizations (ASOs), grief support groups for patients and families, social services not already provided through ASOs such as Meals on Wheels, and at least one organization providing home health care. The ASO case managers, which include professional nurses, communicate with physicians, patients, and their significant others, third-party payers, and other personnel and agencies to assess the patients' needs; they also plan, organize, and coordinate services and evaluate outcomes and patient satisfaction. Ideally, one case manager should follow the patient from diagnosis through death, by monitoring changes in health status and facilitating the "best match" of appropriate services based on a growing awareness of the patient as a unique individual. However, because of large patient loads, case managers are divided into two groups. The general case manager often has responsibility for more than 100 patients in the asymptomatic and symptomatic stages. Once patients are diagnosed with AIDS, they are transferred to a Project AIDS Care (PAC) case manager. It is the responsibility of this case manager to see these patients through the social services maze and to continue to provide for them until their death. Given the severity of the situation, PAC case managers usually monitor up to 45 patients.

Home health care agencies usually have a combination of professional and auxiliary staff members, who provide services ranging from housekeeping, transportation, meal preparation, and hygienic care to high-technology, skilled nursing care with social workers, pharmacists, physical therapists, psychologists, psychiatric nurses, and nutritionists available as consultants.

The nutritionist working with HIV-infected patients can provide various services. Calculating the patient's caloric needs, based on body weight, activity, and the presence of fever or infection can provide a baseline for assessing weight loss, wasting, malabsorption syndrome, and other gastrointestinal problems. The nutritionist can provide education and help patients to plan high-protein, high-calorie meals that are nutritious and also reflect some of their food preferences. When diarrhea, thrush, or other gastrointestinal symptoms develop, the nutritionist can suggest changes to assist with these problems. If supplements or total parenteral nutrition regimens become necessary, the nutritionist can work with the patient and physician to arrive at the best formula and feeding schedule.

For patients to be maintained in their home environments, pain management must be provided. This may mean teaching family members how to give injections, providing a patient-controlled analgesia pump in the home, or referring patients to pain-management clinics. Such clinics usually offer various pain-reduction methods and work with patients to discover what combination works best. Adjuvant therapies such as acupuncture, natural herbs, biofeedback training, and various stress management techniques may be tried, as well as analgesics, nonsteroidal anti-inflammatory drugs, narcotics, sedatives, and various psychotropic medications, including antidepressants and anxiolytics.

By considering each patient's needs seriously and addressing these needs with whatever eclectic, interdisciplinary approaches can be applied, patients with HIV disease can spend more of their limited life span in their own environments, thus maintaining and even improving their quality of life.

---

ing recurrences. The overall goals are 1) to prevent exposure to the organism, 2) to provide a safe prophylactic regimen to prevent infection after exposure, and 3) to prevent recurrence of infections. The diseases for which prophylaxis is most likely implemented are PCP, toxoplasmosis, CMV, fungal infections, TB, and herpes simplex.[109] Before instituting medication prophylaxis, the health care team should consider the prevalence of the OI, the complications associated with the OI, the known benefits and risks of the prophylaxis, and the ability to treat acute infections successfully. Some diseases can be treated easily in the acute phase, such as candidiasis. By not providing prophylaxis with fluconazole, the development of resistance may be avoided or delayed. Medication use increases the potential for drug interactions. Many

TABLE 46–12

Prophylaxis for Opportunistic Diseases

Disease	Prevention of Exposure	Dosage	When to Start
Pneumocystis carinii pneumonia	TMP/SMX Dapsone Pentamidine Dapsone + pyrimeth-amine + leucovorin	1 DS tablet PO QD 50 mg PO BID or 100 mg PO QD 300 mg aerosol monthly 200 mg PO weekly + 75 mg PO weekly + 25 mg PO weekly	When CD4 cells drop below 200/μL; unexplained fever >100°F for ≥2 wks; history of oropharyngeal candidiasis
Toxoplasmic encephalitis	TMP/SMX Sulfadiazine + pyrimethamine + leucovorin	1 DS tablet PO QD 1.0–1.5 g PO q 6h + 25–75 mg PO QD + 10–25 mg PO QD	CD4 < 100/μL and IgG antibody to Toxoplasma
Tuberculosis Isoniazid sensitive	Isoniazid + pyridoxine	300 mg PO + 50 mg PO QD × 12 mo or isoniazid 900 mg PO + pyridoxine 50 mg PO BID × 12 mo	TST reaction of ≥ 5 mm
Isoniazid resistant Multidrug resistant	Rifampin Choice of drugs requires public health consultation	600 mg PO QD × 12 mo	Same as above
Disseminated infection with Mycobacterium avium complex	Rifabutin Azithromycin Clarithromycin	300 mg PO QD 1200 mg weekly 500 mg BID	CD4 < 50/μL
Candidiasis	Fluconazole	100–200 mg PO QD	CD4 < 50/μL
Cryptococcosis	Fluconazole	100–200 mg PO QD	CD4 < 50/μL
Histoplasmosis	Itraconazole	200 mg PO QD	CD4 < 50/μL or endemic regions
Coccidioidomycosis	Fluconazole	200 mg PO QD	CD4 < 50/μL or endemic regions
Cytomegalovirus (CMV) disease	Oral ganciclovir	1 g PO TID	CD4 < 50/μL or CMV antibody positive
Herpes simplex virus disease	Acyclovir	800 mg PO QID	CD4 < 200/μL

TMP/SMX, trimethoprim–sulfamethoxazole; DS, double strength; TST, tuberculosis skin test.

From Centers for Disease Control and Prevention: USPHS/IDSA Guidelines for the Prevention of Opportunistic Infections in Persons Infected with Human Immunodeficiency Virus: A Summary. MMWR Morb Mortal Wkly Rep 44:26, 1995.

medications are detoxified or eliminated by the kidneys or liver, adding strain on these organs that are already compromised by HIV disease. Cost can also be great, and adherence to the dosage schedule is extremely difficult, because times and dosages widely differ (Table 46–13).

The CDC has outlined specific methods to reduce exposure to OIs, because the desire for the patient to remain "normal" may translate into high-risk behaviors. Persons with HIV should use a condom during every sexual encounter. Avoiding sexual practices that bring one into contact with feces will reduce the possibility of acquiring intestinal infections (e.g., cryptosporidiosis, shigellosis, campylobacteriosis, amebiasis, giardiasis, and hepatitis A and B).

Workplaces also present a risk for exposure to several OIs. The risk of TB increases in health care facilities and crowded areas such as prisons and homeless shelters. Employees or volunteers in these settings may wish to be screened for TB on a more frequent basis. Persons infected with TB who also have children at day care centers, or who work at such facilities, are

at greater risk of CMV infection, cryptosporidiosis, hepatitis A, and giardiasis. Good hygiene reduces the risk (e.g., when changing diapers, wiping saliva, or cleaning up urine spills). Work with animals increases the risk of cryptosporidiosis, toxoplasmosis, salmonellosis, campylobacteriosis, and bartonellosis. The CDC does not recommend that patients give up such work, but that they be informed of the risk. In areas endemic for cryptosporidiosis and toxoplasmosis, gardening, cleaning chicken coops, and working on building excavation sites are high-risk activities.[110] Pets are also controversial; some primary care providers suggest that all pets be avoided, whereas others simply suggest extra precautions (Chart 46–6).

Patients with HIV should avoid raw or undercooked eggs or foods containing them (e.g., Hollandaise sauce, Caesar salad dressing, mayonnaise), raw or undercooked poultry, meat, or seafood, and unpasteurized dairy products. Uncooked meat should never come into contact with other foods. All uncooked fruits and vegetables should be scrubbed with a mild bleach and water solution, as should hands,

TABLE 46–13
Dosages and Conditions for Certain HIV Drug Regimens*

Drug	Dose	Conditions
Nevirapine	1 200-mg tablet	With breakfast
Zidovudine (ZDV)	2 100-mg capsules	
Lamivudine (3TC)	1 150-mg tablet	
Zalcitabine (ddC)	1 0.75-mg tablet	
Stavudine (d4T)	1 40-mg capsule	
Ritonavir	6 100-mg capsules	↓
Saquinavir	3 200-mg capsules	Within 2 hours of breakfast
Didanosine (ddI)	200-mg tablets	At least 2 hours after breakfast (and at least 1 hour before next meal)
Indinavir	2 400-mg capsules	↓
ZDV	2 100-mg capsules	With lunch
ddC	1 0.75-mg tablet	↓
Saquinavir	3 200-mg capsules	Within 2 hours of lunch
Indinavir	2 400-mg capsules	At least 2 hours after lunch (and at least 1 hour before next meal)
Nevirapine	1 200-mg tablet	With dinner
ZDV	2 100-mg capsules	
3TC	1 150-mg tablet	
ddC	1 0.75-mg tablet	
d4T	1 40-mg capsule	
Ritonavir	6 100-mg capsules	↓
Saquinavir	3 200-mg capsules	Within 2 hours of dinner
ddI	2 200-mg tablets	At least 2 hours after dinner (and at least 1 hour before next meal)
Indinavir	2 400-mg capsules	↓

*3TC should be given only if weight >50 kg; ddC (zalcitabine, Hivid) should not be taken concomitantly with ddI or taken simultaneously with antacids; d4T should be given only if weight >60 kg; ritonavir (Norvir) should be kept refrigerated and should be taken with meals; saquinavir (Invirase) should be taken within 2 hours of a full meal; when not taken with food, saquinavir may have little or no antiviral activity; ddI (didanosine, Videx) must be taken on an empty stomach, either 2 hours after or 1 hour before a meal; alcohol may exacerbate toxicity; indinavir (Crixivan) should be taken on an empty stomach, either 2 hours after or 1 hour before a meal; patients taking indinavir should drink at least 1.5 L of liquid daily or kidney stones may develop.

CHART 46–6

Pets

Pets are a controversial topic. Some physicians believe that all pets should be avoided, whereas others believe that taking extra precautions around a pet is all that is necessary. For instance, if the pet is experiencing diarrhea, the veterinarian should examine the pet for causes of the problem, and the owner should avoid the pet's fecal matter. If an HIV-positive person decides to acquire a new pet, he or she should avoid puppies and kittens under 6 months of age and obtain the pet from a reputable source. After playing with the pet, the person should wash the hands thoroughly. Special care needs to be taken with cats because of the risk of toxoplasmosis and *Bartonella* infections. Litter boxes pose a threat to those who are HIV infected, and good hand washing is required when changing litter. Cat scratches and bites should be avoided whenever possible. However, when accidents occur, thorough cleansing of the site and the application of antibiotic (Polysporin) ointment should hasten healing. A cat should never be permitted to lick human wounds. Flea control is also recommended.

Source: Centers for Disease Control and Prevention, Atlanta, GA.

cutting boards, counter surfaces, and knives and other utensils used in food preparation. Soft cheeses and ready-to-eat foods such as hot dogs and cold cuts can cause listeriosis and should be reheated before eating. Drinking water should always be tested or boiled if the purity is unknown. Similarly, patients with HIV should avoid swallowing water when swimming in a river, lake, or stream and should always use ear plugs when swimming.

When traveling in underdeveloped nations, patients with HIV have an increased risk of OIs from food and water sources. In addition, medical services may be substandard if an illness does develop. Precautions include eating only well-cooked foods and fruit that can be peeled and drinking only canned or bottled carbonated beverages or those made with boiling water (tea or coffee). Diarrhea should be treated immediately, and patients should be instructed to carry a good supply of antimicrobial agents. Prophylactic medication to prevent traveler's diarrhea is not recommended. All vaccinations are mandatory and should be of the inactivated form (e.g., chemoprophylaxis for malaria, protection against arthropod vectors, and treatment with immune globulin). Information about local diseases, modes of transmission, and areas affording the greatest protection against OIs have been identified by the CDC.[111]

Pharmacotherapeutics

In 1981, when a person was diagnosed with HIV disease, it was considered a "death sentence." Now, however, treatment can slow both the AIDS-defining conditions and viral replication. The first rule in designing effective therapy is that it must either kill the pathogen or prevent it from replicating. Because the virus is linked to DNA inside certain cells (e.g., CD4, macrophages, or brain cells), therapy directed at killing the pathogen destroys the host cell and ultimately the patient. Therefore, the goal of therapy becomes slowing viral replication. The second rule of therapy requires that the drug must not further damage or interfere with normal host functions. Many patients with HIV state that the toxic effects from drug therapies can seem worse than the disease.[1]

Drug manufacturers must consider the six steps in viral replication when designing drugs. The first step is the attachment of gp120 to the CD4 receptor site. One drug, AL721, which was made in many kitchens throughout the United States in the early days of HIV disease, competed with HIV for the active site on CD4. Another drug in this class was genetically engineered CD4. Problems arose when there was insufficient drug to keep all the active sites bound, thereby allowing HIV to attach as soon as a binding site became available. The second step is the release of the RNA–reverse transcriptase complex, in which nonnucleosides work. The third step is to interfere with

the provirus so that new HIV particles are not encoded. Drugs can also be targeted to stop the translation of genetic information into messenger RNA (mRNA)—the fourth step—as with antiretrovirals such as ZDV. The fifth step is the modification of viral proteins before they assemble with RNA to form new HIV particles. In the sixth step, the budding process releasing new HIV particles into the blood is halted, thus preventing replication (Figure 46–6).[1,2] Other pharmaceutical considerations include the side effects that may plague each type of cell, the ability of the drug to cross the blood–brain barrier without damaging brain cells, and the avoidance of drug interactions.[1]

Antiretrovirals

Antiretroviral therapy is recommended for anyone whose CD4 count is less than 500 cells/μL. Some primary care providers begin sooner if CD4 counts fall rapidly (velocity), and still others wait until counts are less than 200 cells/μL and symptoms are present. For counts of more than 500 cells/μL, monitoring should take place every 6 months. As the count nears 500 cells/μL, monitoring increases to every 3 months. The decision to start drug therapy is important because starting too soon can increase drug toxicity. An even bigger question facing patients today is which drugs to try first and in what combination. Monotherapy is recommended for patients with high CD4 counts, low viral load and no OIs, with dideoxyinosine (didanosine or ddI) being the preferred drug, followed by ZDV and stavudine (d4T).

The first of the nucleoside analogs, AZT (now known as ZDV), was developed to combat tumor growth in cancer in 1964 and was shelved because of its limited success. When HIV appeared, such "shelved" drugs were reexamined as potential warriors against HIV. Of the 300 tested, only 15 including AZT, showed any promise in interfering with HIV replication. Phase I clinical trials began in July 1985, placebo trials in 1986, and permission to market the drug came in 1987. By 1988, the name had been changed from AZT to ZDV and was sold under the trade name Retrovir. Reverse transcriptase uses deoxythymidine to link other nucleosides within the DNA chain. ZDV, which looks like deoxythymidine, fools reverse transcriptase into choosing it as the next link. This false link terminates the long-chain building of DNA and prevents the production of provirus by competitive inhibition. As ZDV competes for the active site on reverse transcriptase, other nucleosides cannot bind. Slowing viral replication, ZDV allows the immune system to regenerate, thus reducing fevers and OIs. The drug also reduces transmission from mother to fetus, the basis of protocol 076.

Two other drugs, ddI and dideoxycytidine (zalcitabine or ddC), provide similar interference with reverse transcriptase, but with fewer severe side

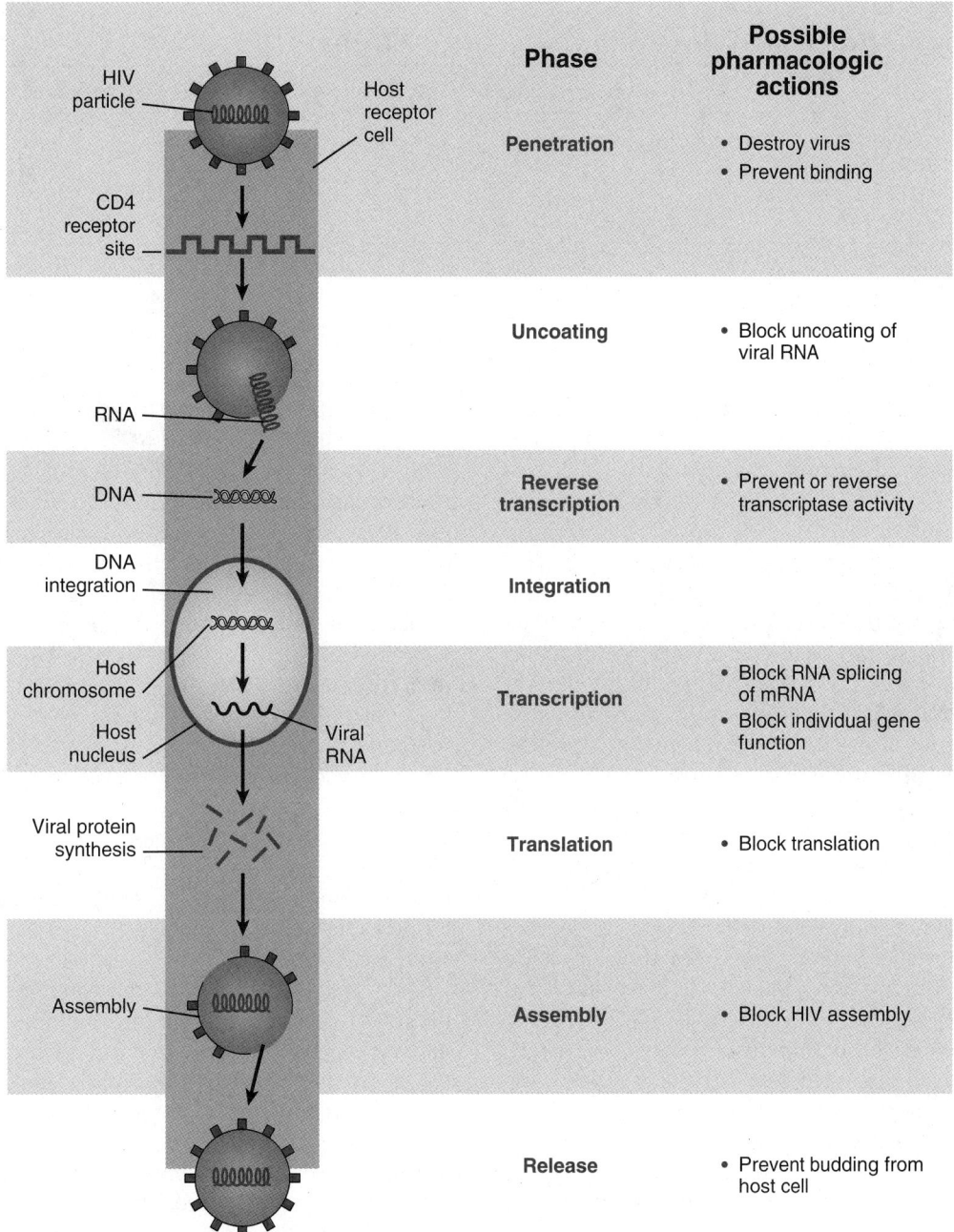

	Phase	Possible pharmacologic actions
HIV particle / Host receptor cell	**Penetration**	• Destroy virus • Prevent binding
CD4 receptor site		
RNA	**Uncoating**	• Block uncoating of viral RNA
DNA	**Reverse transcription**	• Prevent or reverse transcriptase activity
DNA integration	**Integration**	
Host chromosome / Host nucleus / Viral RNA	**Transcription**	• Block RNA splicing of mRNA • Block individual gene function
Viral protein synthesis	**Translation**	• Block translation
Assembly	**Assembly**	• Block HIV assembly
	Release	• Prevent budding from host cell

Figure 46–6

Schematic representation of the various pharmacologic sites for blocking human immunodeficiency virus (HIV) infection and viral replication.

effects. The United States Food and Drug Administration (FDA) granted early approval for ddI, because ZDV was so toxic. Side effects of ddI and ddC are similar and include headache, fevers, pain, pinprick or tingling in the extremities, and decreased touch and vibratory sensations.

A fourth nucleoside analog drug is d4T. Granted accelerated approval in 1994 by the FDA, d4T is used when other drugs have shown to be ineffective. Peripheral neuropathy and increase in liver enzymes are the most commonly reported side effects.

The last of the nucleoside analogs is lamivudine (3TC or Epivir). Like d4T, it was approved under the accelerated program for use with ZDV. In combination, ZDV–3TC has provided a much longer antiviral effect than either drug alone.[112]

Nonnucleoside analogs, nevirapine (Viramune), delavirdine (Rescriptor), loviride, DMP-266, and MKC-442, inhibit reverse transcriptase, but at a different site than nucleosides. A rapid resistance to HIV may develop if nevirapine is administered alone; however, in combination with nucleoside analogs, it decreases viral load profoundly. Metabolized by the liver, it may elevate transaminase. With a protease inhibitor, it may decrease plasma viral concentration. Delavirdine also causes a decline in viral load. Like

TABLE 46-14

Correlation of Viral Load With Progression of HIV Disease

Viral Load Level	Median Time to AIDS (Years)	Median Survival Time (Years)
<4,531 HIV RNA copies/mL	>10	>10
4,531–13,020 HIV RNA copies/mL	7.7	9.5
13,021–36,270 HIV RNA copies/mL	5.3	7.4
>36,270 HIV RNA copies/mL	3.5	5.1

Data from Mellors JW, Rinaldo CR, Gupta, et al: Prognosis in HIV-1 infection predicted by the quantity of virus in plasma. Science 272:1167–1170, 1996.

nevirapine, it is best used in combination with other nucleosides. Studies are being conducted comparing the results of monotherapy with the results from double-, triple-, or quadruple-drug therapy.

Protease Inhibitors

Protease inhibitors are the most recent class of drugs for the treatment of HIV. The goal of this class of medications is to fill the active site on protease and to inhibit its trimming action. In 1989, a three-dimensional structure of protease was developed, determining its role in viral replication. Protease trims the long protein chains to the smaller structures necessary to manufacture the protein coat. This can be thought of as a thread being pulled through the eye of a needle, and as it comes out the other side, small pieces are cut from the longer thread. If the eye of the needle is filled, it would be unable to make the smaller pieces. The smaller pieces are essential if the virus is to assemble into a mature form. Several generations of protease inhibitors had been developed by 1995, each reducing viral load and increasing CD4 counts. In 1996, the FDA approved three drugs; saquinavir (Invirase), indinavir (Crixivan), and ritonavir (Norvir). All three decrease viral load and reverse disease progression and death in up to 50% of cases.[1]

First-generation saquinavir had poor bioavailability and was not effective. More quickly metabolized by the liver than the others, it was given in triple-drug combinations. Second-generation saquinavir does not biodegrade as quickly.[113] Indinavir has demonstrated potent antiviral activity with modest side effects. In triple-drug therapy (ZDV, indinavir, and 3TC), viral loads were reduced significantly when compared with either the use of indinavir alone or the use of a nucleoside analog alone. Ritonavir, a third protease inhibitor, slowed progression of HIV disease in patients with CD4 counts less than 100/μL for up to 11 years.[114]

Nelfinavir (Viracept) is a fourth protease inhibitor with potent antiviral action that is enhanced when given in combination with d4T. It is currently used if other protocols fail, if other protease inhibitors cannot be tolerated, or if CD4 counts are less than 50/μL.

Four groups of initial viral load levels were correlated with progression of HIV disease and death (Table 46–14). The lower the viral load at initial testing, the longer the asymptomatic period and survival time.

Using these data, progression of HIV can be predicted as much as 10 years into the future. A major problem in the war against HIV is that the virus has developed resistance to all existing drugs. Nonnucleoside reverse transcriptase inhibitors (NNRTI) develop resistance quickly when given as monotherapy. The National Cancer Institute mapped the resistance patterns of 2500 NNRTI drugs and found that monotherapy creates a resistance to the initial drug used and a cross-resistance to all others in its class. However, at this time, for reasons yet to be understood, this resistance does not reduce clinical benefit. Some combinations also have a synergistic antiviral effect, allowing drugs to be paired to increase the time required for resistance to develop. Cross-reactivity with other drugs used to treat HIV-related diseases may also develop (e.g., ZDV crosses with ganciclovir to cause hematologic toxicities; therefore, if ganciclovir is needed to prevent CMV retinitis, another drug such as ddI or ddC must be substituted).[115–117]

The Office of AIDS Research convened a National Institutes of Health (NIH) panel to define principles of therapy for HIV infection, in part because of recent advances in the treatment and understanding of HIV disease. The aim was to identify therapies that would suppress the virus over long periods and would lessen damage to the immune system. In this rapidly changing environment, it would be unethical to establish "gold standards" for treatment. However, the panel developed 11 principles to help guide treatment decisions (Table 46–15).

Vaccines

Within the scientific community, the development of vaccines is a high priority. If the immune system could recognize specific antigens and could respond with antibodies, protecting against different strains of the organism, long-lasting immunity from free-floating virus and cells infected with the virus could be achieved. Two types of vaccines exist currently; inactivated virus, which is unable to multiply, and attenuated virus, which multiplies slowly. Whole-organism vaccines have the disadvantage of possible reproduction. Subunit vaccines are much safer because they are made up of viral particles that stimulate an immune response without infecting or reproducing inside cells.

TABLE 46–15
CDC Principles of Therapy

Principle	Statement	Explanation
Principle 1	"The goals of antiretroviral therapy of HIV infection should be to maintain immune function in as near a normal state as possible, protect from disease progression, prolong survival and preserve quality of life."	Antiretroviral therapy should be started before the immune system has suffered irreversible damage.
Principle 2	"CD4 + T cell count determinations permit assessment of an HIV individual's risk of developing specific opportunistic infections and when used in concert with viral load determinations, enhance the accuracy with which the risk of disease progression and death can be predicted."	CD4 counts indicate immune system health, whereas viral loads indicate progression toward disease.
Principle 3	"Decisions about when to initiate antiviral therapy for an HIV infected person should be based on their risk of disease progression and degree of immunodeficiency."	The greatest impact occurs when antiviral therapy begins before evidence of disease progression as measured by CD4 count and viral load, for instance, if CD4 cell counts are <500/μL or declining, if HIV RNA levels are increasing or are >3000 copies/mL, or if symptomatic illness or primary HIV infection occurs. Obviously, it would be beneficial to initiate therapy with >500 CD4 count and HIV RNA levels <3000 copies.
Principle 4	The "goal of antiviral therapy is to suppress HIV replication as much as possible for as long as possible."	Suppression to undetectable levels is the goal; although this does not affect a cure, any reduction will benefit. The biggest challenge in realizing this goal is patient adherence, an absolute requirement to decrease viral load and to minimize drug resistance.
Principle 5	"Drugs used in combination should show evidence of antiviral synergy, lack antagonistic pharmacokinetic or antiviral properties and possess non-overlapping toxicities. Ideally, the drugs chosen will display molecular interactions that increase the potency of antiviral therapy and/or delay the emergence of antiviral drug resistance."	To avoid cross-resistance, it is best to place patients on a drug regimen new to them or to look for combinations that enhance their current drug therapy. In combination therapy, all drugs should be introduced at the same time. Monotherapy is no longer recommended. Two nucleoside analog inhibitors combined with a potent protease inhibitor are recommended. For treatment-naive patients (i.e., those who have never received drug treatment), two nucleoside analogs and one non-nucleoside inhibitor may work well. If drugs fail or are toxic, one should change more than one component.
Principle 6	"As the number of effective non–cross-resistant antiviral drugs available is currently limited a decision to change antiviral therapy must be considered carefully."	Currently, there is no definition of treatment failure; one should consider a change if plasma HIV RNA is not suppressed to below detectable levels and HIV continues to replicate, previously undetectable levels of HIV RNA are increasing, or drug toxicity develops.
Principle 7	"The use of antiviral treatment in HIV-infected pregnant women presents important, unique concerns."	The United States government suggests and many states mandate counseling and testing of pregnant women. Protocol 076 decreased transmission from mother to child when zidovudine was taken from the second trimester until the end of pregnancy. For women who become pregnant while receiving combination therapy, all drugs should be stopped and reintroduced simultaneously in the second trimester. As with other patient populations, pregnant women should be followed with CD4 counts and viral load.

Table continued on following page

TABLE 46–15
CDC Principles of Therapy *(Continued)*

Principle	Statement	Explanation
Principle 8	"In HIV-infected children . . . the goal of antiviral therapy is to suppress HIV replication as much as possible for as long as possible."	The drugs chosen must be age appropriate. Viral loads tend to be higher in children than in adults who have been infected for a comparable period of time. The earlier treatment is started, the better.
Principle 9	"It has been suggested that antiviral therapy during primary infection may serve to favorably alter the subsequent clinical course of the infection; however, this has yet to be formally demonstrated."	It is recommended that combination therapy begin immediately and continue indefinitely and that research on treatment continue.
Principle 10	"Antiviral therapy following occupational exposure has been shown to decrease the risk of HIV infection."	The NIH panel agreed with recent CDC recommendations for treatment of occupational exposure to HIV.
Principle 11	"No data are available concerning the ability of HIV-infected persons with antiviral therapy–induced suppression of HIV replication to undetectable levels to transmit the infection to others."	Safer sex practices should continue.

Adapted from Centers for Disease Control and Prevention, Atlanta, GA.

A third recent vaccine is composed of synthetic microbial antigens (recombinant DNA).[1,2,19]

To design an "AIDS" vaccine, the pharmaceutical companies must consider a host of safety factors in their design. The use of a whole-organism vaccine could lead to the development of HIV disease in the recipient, whereas inactivated vaccines may not produce the necessary antibody response. In subunit vaccines, small viral particles enter chromosomes, causing tumors. A strong antibody response is elicited by HIV, as demonstrated by the long asymptomatic period. The goal is to find the HIV gene responsible for this reaction and to amplify it. A traditional vaccine provides immunity against future attacks through immune surveillance or sterilizing immunity. Therapeutic immunity refers to a vaccine that delays the onset of AIDS. Although this type of vaccine does not prevent future attacks, it prolongs life, slows progression, and could ultimately lead to the elimination of the virus. Viral load will be used by scientists to determine the vaccine's efficacy.[1,2,19]

To make the subunit vaccine more appealing to macrophages, adjuvant carriers are used. Reengineered to carry HIV genes within the viral genes, cowpox appears promising. When host animals are inoculated, they develop antibodies to the virus and HIV subunit. Salk proposed a whole-virus vaccine designed to provoke an antibody response to control free-floating virus while the immune system repairs itself. Others tested the theory that small amounts of SIV without the *nef* gene would protect the monkey when larger challenge doses of full-strength SIV were given. The animals maintained their CD4 levels with only small traces of SIV in tissue. In Africa, certain groups of women who have been repeatedly exposed to HIV are being studied because they appear to have natural protection. These women, who are infected with HIV-2 (the second identified strain of HIV), appear to be less likely to become infected with HIV-1. In subunit vaccines, each subunit requires a specific vaccine, a time-consuming factor in research. In whole-virus vaccine research, safety is always an issue, because of the possibility of infection instead of protection.[1,2,19]

Barriers to testing an HIV vaccine include 1) the lack of appropriate animal models, 2) the ongoing mutation of the virus requiring a vaccine for each mutation, and 3) the complexity of the virus responsible for HIV disease. For example, traditional vaccines may work against HIV if it did not make a provirus and hijack the cell's own material to replicate itself or if HIV were more extracellular or free floating. Antibodies seek viral proteins. When incorporated into the chromosomes, HIV in its proviral state is immune from such attack, because it is no longer a protein. One hopes that a vaccine against gp120 and gp41, the two parts of the virus that do not mutate, can be made and will delay the onset of symptoms.[1,2,19]

Occupational Concerns

In health care centers around the world, the occupational risk of HIV has been studied extensively.[118,119] Some investigators believe that transmission of HIV after exposure, such as a needlestick, depends on the quantity of the virus, the stage of the disease (highest at initial infection and during the advanced symptomatic period),[120] the volume of blood or body fluid transmitted,[121] the duration of contact, the condition of the surface contaminated (intact versus broken skin), the depth of penetration, the size of the needle, whether blood was injected directly,[122] and the status of the health care worker's immune system.[123] In reality, health care workers are probably better protected on the job than elsewhere (Table 46–16). However, some cases of occupational exposure are probably not tabulated by CDC because some states report only HIV disease and not HIV infection.

Determining exposure probability can be a challenge. Health care providers may not report the exposure because of denial or fear of criticism of their actions, or they may overestimate or underestimate the severity of the exposure (Chart 46–7). Exposure routes fall into four broad categories: 1) needlesticks (e.g., syringes, IV line needles, vacuum tube phlebotomy assemblies), of which an estimated 1,000,000 occur each year in the United States, 2) mucous membranes; 3) contamination of open wounds or lesions; and 4) contamination of broken skin. Each major category has subcategories. Needlesticks are divided into size and type of needle, depth of penetration, volume injected, and site. Contact with mucous membranes, wounds or lesions, and broken skin is divided into type, volume, and duration of contact. For wounds from sharps (needles), the site, wound appearance, amount of bleeding, and time the contaminating fluid was outside the body are reported. The HIV status of the source patient is not always known. Patients are not tested

without informed consent, and patient confidentiality must be protected.[2,124] However, if consent for testing is refused, clinical and epidemiologic data may help to estimate risk. Exposed health care providers should undergo a baseline test in case they seroconvert later. Follow-up testing should be performed at 6 weeks, 3 months, and 6 months. Some facilities may request 9- and 12-month tests. Counseling is important for the exposed health care provider, because many of the initial symptoms of the acute retroviral syndrome also mimic the signs of the common cold or flu. The CDC recommends that exposed persons either abstain from sex or practice safer sex and never share needles for 6 months to protect others. The same standards to protect health care providers should also apply to patients exposed to an employee who may be HIV positive.

Guidelines for treatment of health care providers exposed and possibly infected with HIV have been published.[122] In the June 7, 1996, issue of MMWR, the CDC issued provisional recommendations for exposed health care providers. Treatment is now recommended to begin within 1 to 2 hours after exposure to HIV. A triple-drug combination consisting of ZDV (200 mg three times daily or 300 mg twice a day), 3TC (150 mg two times daily), and indinavir (800 mg three times

TABLE 46–16

Health Care Workers With Documented and Possible Occupationally Acquired AIDS/HIV Infection, by Occupation Reported Through December 1997 in the United States*

Occupation	Documented Occupational Transmission† (No.)	Possible Occupational Transmission‡ (No.)
Dental worker, including dentist	—	7
Embalmer/morgue technician	1	2
Emergency medical technician/paramedic	—	12
Health aide/attendant	1	15
Housekeeper/maintenance worker	1	10
Laboratory technician, clinical	16	18
Laboratory technician, nonclinical	3	—
Nurse	22	32
Physician, nonsurgical	6	11
Physician, surgical	—	6
Respiratory therapist	1	2
Technician, dialysis	1	3
Technician, surgical	2	2
Technician/therapist, other than those listed above	—	9
Other health care occupations	—	3
Total	54	134

*Health care workers are defined as those persons, including students and trainees, who have worked in a health care, clinical, or HIV laboratory setting at any time since 1978. See MMWR 41:823–825, 1992.

†Health care workers who had documented HIV seroconversion after occupational exposure or had other laboratory evidence of occupational infection: 46 had percutaneous exposure, 5 had mucocutaneous exposure, 2 had both percutaneous and mucocutaneous exposures, and 1 had an unknown route of exposure. Forty-nine exposures were to blood from an HIV-infected person, 1 to visibly bloody fluid, 1 to an unspecified fluid, and 3 to concentrated virus in a laboratory. Twenty-five of these health care workers developed AIDS.

‡These health care workers have been investigated and are without identifiable behavioral or transfusion risks; each reported percutaneous or mucocutaneous occupational exposures to blood or body fluids, or laboratory solutions containing HIV, but HIV seroconversion specifically resulting from an occupational exposure was not documented.

From Centers for Disease Control and Prevention (CDC): HIV/AIDS Surveillance Report, vol 9, number 2. Atlanta, GA, CDC, 1997, p 21.

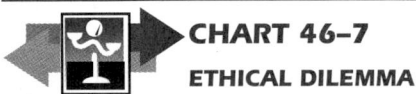

CHART 46–7

ETHICAL DILEMMA

June is a 20-year-old senior about to graduate from nursing school. She has been going to the university, taking full-time classes, and working part time as a nurse technician. Everyone said she was born to be a nurse, and she dreamed of the day when she would join the professional ranks. She recently received an employment offer from the medical center and will begin orientation shortly after graduation.

During her last clinical experience, just 2 weeks before graduation, she was asked to obtain a blood sample from her patient's central line. June was thinking about graduation as she prepared to draw the blood sample. She was not paying close attention to what she was doing, because this procedure was routine now. June experienced a needlestick during the procedure.

June knew that hospital policy required that the incident be reported to employee health, her supervisor, and her clinical instructor. The stick was just a glancing blow to her fingertip (through her glove) as she transferred the blood from the syringe to the test tube. The patient was unaware that anything had taken place. June washed her hands thoroughly with soap and water.

Immediately after, June went to the nurses' station and read through the patient's chart. Nothing in it led her to believe that the patient was HIV positive or at risk for the disease. As part of her course of study at the university, June had taken an HIV course and decided, based on the knowledge she obtained from that course and her review of the patient's chart, to ignore the incident.

June was experiencing many feelings, including the fear that she would lose her job offer at the medical center if she tested positive for HIV. Although her risk for transmission as a scrub nurse was small, she knew that the hospital had just come out with a policy that HIV-positive employees would be assigned to areas that presented little chance for transmission of the virus. In fact, if any employer knew of her status, June was afraid she would never get a job as a nurse. Given the stigma attached to this disease, she also believed that the fewer people who knew of the incident, the better

her life would be. She told no one of the incident, not even her closest friend.

June graduated on schedule and started in her new position. Her manner was always professional, and she was popular with coworkers, patients, and their families. Every once in a while, June would think of the needlestick. Five years passed, and she continued to enjoy good health. Then the unthinkable happened. June was cut with a scalpel during surgery. Before she knew it, a small amount of her blood had dropped onto the surgical wound. Because June had never been tested for HIV, she did not know her own status.

1. Even though June was afraid of losing her job offer, should she have reported the needlestick incident to the appropriate authorities? Defend your answer.
2. Should June be tested now? If she tests positive, what ethical obligation does June have to tell her employer about her previous needlestick injury?
3. Although no laws force health care providers to reveal their HIV status to patients, it is recommended that they remove themselves from certain positions, especially those that pose a greater threat of transmission than normal. Should June be transferred to a new position? Why or why not?
4. What ethical obligation does June have to tell the patient of his or her potential exposure, even if she subsequently tests negative? Should she tell the patient before she knows her own test results? If she tests negative, is it a moot point?
5. If June tests positive, can she claim worker's compensation?
6. Because June is also a sexually active person and has, on occasion, unprotected sex, how would she know which behavior, the needlestick incident or the unprotected sex, exposed her to HIV? Why or why not would this matter? Does she need to tell her sex partners now about their possible exposure? Defend your answers.

daily) for 4 weeks should be initiated. Most recently, a new ZDV formulation is being evaluated and will be a twice-daily dose. For persons exposed to a drug-resistant strain of HIV, expert consultation on alternate combinations is essential. All persons identified for postexposure prophylaxis (PEP) should receive expert medical care and appropriate counseling. Animal studies have shown that PEP is not effective in those whose initial therapy is begun after 24 to 36 hours, but the CDC recommends starting triple-drug therapy even if 2 weeks have elapsed in persons at the greatest risk of infection. If HIV is not eradicated, at least there may be some potential benefit. Some medical centers are even trying this triple-drug therapy for those exposed through sexual contact. Table 46–17 provides a summary of the initial care and continued management strategies for patients with HIV infection.

Multidisciplinary Outcomes

The patient with HIV disease presents numerous challenges to the health care team. Outcomes for these patients vary, based on the phase of the patient's illness. Many patients are not aware of their exposure to HIV until they reach the asymptomatic phase of the disease. Patient care, at this point, is best managed by physicians, nurse practitioners, and nurses. Dietitians may be involved at this stage if the patient has nutritional deficits. Counseling may also be appropriate. Multidisciplinary outcomes for this period are focused on supporting the patient's overall physical and emotional well-being. Currently, this phase may last as long as 15 years.

The patient in the symptomatic phase of HIV disease experiences wide variations in emotional and physical health. Multidisciplinary outcomes are directed at restoring or maintaining health because OIs and reduced CD4 counts place the patient at considerable risk of serious illness. During an acute illness, the physician and nurse work to coordinate the treatment plan. The involvement of respiratory therapists, pharmacists, dietitians, social workers, and clergy as needed ensures that the patient will benefit from the expertise of a variety of specialists. For example, the social worker may begin to work with the patient and others in the home environment while the patient is in the critical care unit. If the social worker is not involved at this point, he or she usually will join the team as the patient moves to an intermediate or general care unit. If patients are discharged back into the environment that contributed to their hospitalization, without appropriate changes, they are at risk of relapse and rehospitalization. Ensuring that patients are able to comply with discharge information is extremely important.

Depending on the extent of the patient's debilitation, the services of a physical therapist may be required. Range-of-motion exercises and assistance with ambulation may be necessary to prevent further loss of muscle tone and to maintain mobility. Often, the physical therapist continues to work with the patient throughout the recovery phase.

Patients with end-stage HIV disease have a greatly improved prognosis. Outcomes are focused on supporting these patients with aggressive drug therapies and other interventions as required by their presenting illnesses. Care is delivered in the acute care setting as

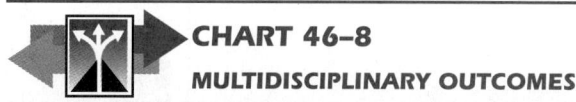

CHART 46–8
MULTIDISCIPLINARY OUTCOMES

Restoration and maintenance of previous level of health

Restoration and maintenance of optimal level of functioning

Prevention and elimination of opportunistic infections

Improvement and maintenance of nutritional status

Restoration and maintenance of adequate oxygenation

Stabilization and maintenance of CD4 counts > 250 cells/µL and viral loads below detectable levels

Self-management of therapeutic regimen

Restoration and maintenance of psychosocial balance

Preparation for peaceful death

well as in the home. When appropriate, hospice care is encouraged to facilitate a peaceful death. Chart 46–8 presents a list of the multidisciplinary outcomes related to the care of patients with HIV disease throughout the course of their illness.

Critical Thinking Exercise

Ms. J., a 26-year-old woman, presented at her doctor's office with cough, dyspnea, and a fever for 3 days. Bilateral interstitial infiltrates were seen on a radiograph. The patient was diagnosed with HIV 1 year ago. CD4 count at that time was 370, and her HIV RNA (viral load) was greater than 750,000 copies. Her pharmacotherapeutic history included ZDV monotherapy, followed by combination therapy with ddI and d4T. The patient is now taking 3TC and ZDV. Laboratory studies showed an increase in liver function tests, and a recent CT showed fatty diffuse infiltrates of the liver, but no masses. The hepatitis profile was negative for hepatitis B and C.

Ms. J. complains of peripheral neuropathy. There is some memory loss for which she is taking nevirapine (Viramune). She reports a history of molluscum contagiosum and thrush. She recently stopped smoking and does not drink alcohol. Her weight has been stable, although she has reported some intermittent nausea and vomiting over the past several days.

Other medications include dapsone, amitriptyline (Elavil), azithromycin (Zithromax), oxandrolone (Oxandrin), and multivitamins. She has no known allergies.

Physical examination findings include the following vital signs: blood pressure, 140/100; temperature, 103.0°F; pulse,

TABLE 46-17
Protocol for Initial Care and Continued Management of Patients With HIV Infection

Interventions	1st Office Visit	2nd Visit (1–2 Wk Later)	3rd Visit (1–2 Wk Later)	CD4 >500/μL	CD4 <500/μL	CD4 <200/μL	CD4 <100/μL	CD4 <50/μL
Physical examination	X	X	X	q3–6mo	q2–3mo	q1–2mo	PRN	PRN
Patient education	X	X	X	q3–6mo	q2–3mo	q1–2mo	PRN	PRN
Influenza virus vaccine	X	Once a year, every autumn						
Pneumococcal vaccine				Given at initial office visit if necessary				
Hepatitis B vaccine		No prior exposure, at risk, initiate immunization	Continue until series is complete					
Diphtheria-tetanus toxoids, absorbed	If needed							
Measles-mumps-rubella virus vaccine	If needed							
Complete blood count with differential	X	Review results	Follow-up if necessary	q3–6mo	q2–3mo	q1–2mo	PRN	PRN
Hepatitis B screen	X							
Chest film	X	Yearly after initial, unless symptoms warrant repeat			Only as symptoms warrant			
PPD and anergy panel	X			If negative without anergy at baseline, repeat until anergic twice q6mo in high prevalence areas				
Viral load assay	X			q3–6mo	q3–6mo or more frequently with drug changes or if viral load increases			

Procedure	Baseline	Follow-up	q3–6mo	q2–3mo	q1–2mo	PRN
T-cell profile	X		q3–6mo	q2–3mo	q1–2mo	PRN
Toxoplasma and cytomegalovirus	X					PRN; yearly until positive
Urinalysis	X					
VDRL or RPR test	X	Treat if necessary; Yearly screen	After initial screen, follow-up yearly as long as patient is sexually active	→	→	PRN
Serum chemistry panel	X	Review and follow-up; Yearly	q3–6mo	q2–3mo	q1–2mo	PRN
Pelvic examination with Pap smear	X		Yearly	q6mo	q6mo or PRN	q6mo or PRN
Referral to support groups	X					
Discuss advance directives (living will, DNR orders)	X	Initial discussion then review yearly	Review with patient on a yearly basis	→	→	
Mammogram	X	Yearly after initial	Annual screening mammograms for rest of life	→	→	
Dental examination	X		Oral examination by primary care provider, follow-up with routine dental visits q3–6mo	→	→	
Acid-fast bacillus, blood culture	X				X	X
Eye examination	X	Yearly		Encourage if symptomatic		PRN
Antiretrovirals		Initial discussion	Discuss risks and benefits if CD4 approaching 500 cells/μL	Encourage if symptomatic	q6mo; q4–6mo; Encourage use and monitor effectiveness, switch drug regimen if failure noted	PRN

PPD, purified protein derivative; RPR, rapid plasma reagin; VDRL, Venereal Disease Research Laboratory.
Data from Bradley-Springer L: HIV/AIDS Nursing Care Plans. El Paso, TX, Skidmore-Roth 1995; and Pottage JC, Samet JH, Soloway BH: The asymptomatic patient. Patient Care 30:27–30, 35–38, 43, 47–48, 49, 51, 1996.

102; respiratory rate, 24. Ms. J. looks acutely ill. Her mucous membranes are dry and her neck is supple. Diffuse crackles are heard on auscultation. Normal S_1, S_2, and postural changes in blood pressure indicate mild dehydration. Her abdomen is soft and nontender, and no masses are palpated. She has normal female genitalia, positive and strong peripheral pulses, no edema, and decreased sensation to cold at the level of both knees. The diagnosis is bilateral interstitial pneumonitis and HIV disease. Orders are to admit Ms. J. to general unit and to start IV fluids at 150 mL per hour, as well as IV TMP–SMX (Bactrim) and methylprednisolone (Solu-Medrol), and to obtain blood for PCP stain and culture and sensitivity, CD4 count with viral load, and ABGs on room air. Oxygen is given by nasal cannula at 4 L per minute after blood gases are drawn. Laboratory results are as follows: ABGs: pH, 7.56; $Paco_2$, 26; HCO_3^-, 21; Pao_2, 45. Identification is positive for Pneumocystis carinii. CD4 count is 15, and viral load is 750,000 copies.

During the hours that followed, Ms. J. proceeded to develop respiratory distress. The nasal cannula was replaced with a Venturi mask at 100%. The second set of ABGs were: pH, 7.29; $Paco_2$, 52; HCO_3^-, 22; Pao_2, 39. Finally, she was urgently intubated and moved to the ICU. She was now diagnosed with acute respiratory failure with severe hypoxemia. When admitted to ICU, the doctor ordered IV furosemide. An echocardiogram was ordered, and a pulmonary artery catheter was considered. The echocardiogram showed normal left ventricular function. Over the next several days, Ms. J. remained stable, and then, suddenly, she began to improve. By day 5, she was weaned from the ventilator. During the time she was intubated, she received quadruple-drug therapy through a nasogastric tube. She continued ZDV and 3TC; saquinavir and indinavir (protease inhibitors) were added. On day 6, Ms. J. was transferred to a general unit and was discharged several days later.

1. Why was Ms. J. ordered 150 mL per hour of IV fluids on arrival to the unit? What was the rationale for the TMP–SMX and methylprednisolone?
2. Why was the doctor considering the placement of a pulmonary artery catheter, in light of a normal echocardiogram?
3. If the admitting physician was concerned enough about Ms. J.'s state of hydration to order aggressive IV fluids, why did the physician in the ICU order furosemide?
4. The patient continued to receive the antiretrovirals and protease inhibitors, even though she was intubated. Why would the physician be so insistent that the medications be given by nasogastric tube and not withheld until she was extubated?

Key Concepts

➡ AIDS was identified in the 1980s and is currently referred to as HIV disease.

➡ HIV disease is an infectious, ultimately fatal disease with no vaccine and no cure. However, with recent pharmacologic advances, it is now viewed as a chronic illness with an increasingly hopeful prognosis.

➡ The major modes of transmitting HIV are through sexual contact, by blood-to-blood contact, or from mother-to-infant.

➡ HIV disease progresses from the point of infection through a "window period" in which the infected person tests negative to seroconversion, when antibodies appear and HIV tests become positive, to an asymptomatic latent period, to a symptomatic period with various infections, and to end-stage disease, with multisystem failure and death.

➡ The nurse must be knowledgeable of the pathophysiology of HIV in relation to immune system functioning, including changes associated with aging to care for patients with HIV disease competently.

➡ Methods of assessing the patient's health status in relation to HIV disease include initial HIV testing, comprehensive health history, complete physical examination, and specific diagnostic tests.

➡ Patients with HIV disease require careful screening and ongoing monitoring to evaluate the extent of their immunosuppression.

➡ Common opportunistic infections and AIDS-defining conditions include TB, PCP, KS, and MAC, as well as protozoan and fungal infections affecting various body systems.

➡ Medication regimens are prescribed both prophylactically, to slow progression, and aggressively, to treat acute episodes of OIs and end-stage illnesses.

➡ Drug research is evolving rapidly, with three categories of medications currently prescribed: antiretrovirals, nonnucleoside analogs, and protease inhibitors. Unfortunately, patients experience many side effects from these drugs, and the regimens are complicated.

➡ Adherence to the drug regimens is extremely important, because resistance develops among many HIV medications, and cross-resistance develops between HIV medications and medications used in treatment of diseases other than HIV infection.

➡ Methods of preventing HIV transmission and the development of opportunistic infections include adherence to standard precautions, preventive measures for different modes of transmission, and recommendations for special circumstances such as travel and pet care.

➡ Nursing interventions are derived from a holistic approach to patient care and address some of the major psychosocial problems (coping, anxiety, grief, altered thought processes) experienced by patients with HIV disease.

➡ Interventions for the goal of health promotion and maintenance and disease prevention in patients with HIV disease include vigilant health monitoring, prevention of other communicable diseases, maintenance of nutritional status and fluid and electrolyte balance, promotion of sleep and rest, and maintenance or initiation of exercise.

➠ As HIV disease progresses, nursing interventions are directed toward symptom management (pain, fever, respiratory symptoms, diarrhea, and wasting).

➠ Nurses play a major role in monitoring the effects of medications and in educating patients with HIV disease.

References

1. Alcamo IE: AIDS: The Biological Basis, 2nd ed. Chicago, William C. Brown, 1997.
2. Stine GJ: AIDS Update 1996: An Annual Overview of Acquired Immune Deficiency Syndrome. Upper Saddle River, NJ, Prentice-Hall, 1996.
3. Thomas CL (ed): Tabers Cyclopedic Medical Dictionary. Philadelphia, F.A. Davis, 1997.
4. Kavanaugh A: Evaluation of patients with suspected immunodeficiency. Am Fam Physician 49:1167–1172, 1994.
5. Boyd RF: Basic Medical Microbiology. Boston, Little, Brown, 1995.
6. Sinha A, Lopez T, McDevitt H: Autoimmune diseases: the failure of self tolerance. Science 248:1380–1387, 1990.
7. National Institute on Aging and National Institute of Allergy and Infectious Diseases: Report of the Task Force on Immunology and Aging. Bethesda, MD, National Institutes of Health, 1996, pp 1–7.
8. Murasko DM, Nelson BJ, Matour D, et al: Heterogeneity of changes in lymphoproliferative ability with increasing age. Exp Gerontol 26:269–279, 1991.
9. Jackola DR, Ruger JK, Miller RA: Age-associated changes in human T cell phenotype and function. Aging 6:25–34, 1994.
10. Wikby A, Johansson B, Ferguson F, et al: Age-related changes in immune parameters in a very old population of Swedish people: a longitudinal study. Exp Gerontol 29:531–541, 1994.
11. Delafuente JC, Meuleman JR: Immune aberrations in chronically ill aged subjects. J Clin Exp Gerontol 14:251–267, 1992.
12. Mulvihill M, Cohen C, Martemucci W, et al: Anergy in the frail elderly is associated with an increased rate of infection and mortality. Aging Immunol Infect Dis 6:1–13, 1995.
13. Centers for Disease Control: Pneumocystis pneumonia: Los Angeles. MMWR Morb Mortal Wkly Rep 30:250–252, 1981.
14. Centers for Disease Control: Kaposi's sarcoma and pneumocystis pneumonia among homosexual men: New York City and California. MMWR Morb Mortal Wkly Rep 30:305–308, 1981.
15. Shilts, R: And The Band Played On. New York, St. Martin's Press, 1987.
16. Altman D: AIDS in the Mind of America: The Social, Political, and Psychological Impact of the New Epidemic. Garden City, NY, Anchor Books, 1987.
17. New York Times, 5 November 1987, p A31.
18. Cantwell A: AIDS and the Doctors of Death: An Inquiry into the Origin of the AIDS Epidemic. Los Angeles, Aries Rising, 1988.
19. Schoub BD: AIDS and HIV in Perspective: A Guide to Understanding the Virus and Its Consequences. New York, Cambridge Press, 1994.
20. Rogan E, Jewell LD, Meilke BW, et al: A case of acquired immune deficiency syndrome before 1980. Can Med Assoc J 137:637–638, 1987.
21. Reichert C, Giliary T, Levens D, et al: Autopsy pathology in the acquired immune deficiency syndrome. Am J Pathol 112:357–382, 1983.
22. Froland SS, Jenum P, Lindboe CF, et al: HIV-1 infection in Norwegian family before 1970. Lancet 1;1344–1345, 1988.
23. Garry RF, Witte MH, Gottlieb A, et al: Documentation of an AIDS virus infection in the United States in 1968. JAMA 260:2085–2087, 1988.
24. Myers G, MacInnes K, Korber B: The emergence of simian/human immunodeficiency viruses. AIDS Res Hum Retroviruses 8:373–386, 1992.
25. Ewald PW: Evolution of Infectious Disease. New York, Oxford University Press, 1994.
26. Eigen M, Nieselt-Struwe K: How old is the immunodeficiency virus? AIDS 4(Suppl 1):S85–S93, 1990.
27. McCoy CB, Inciardi JA: Sex, Drugs, and the Continuing Spread of AIDS. Los Angeles, Roxbury, 1995.
28. Neequaye AR, Neequaye JE, Biggar RJ: Factors that could influence the spread of AIDS in Ghana, West Africa: knowledge of AIDS, sexual behavior, prostitution, and traditional medical practices. J Acquir Immune Defici Syndr 4:914–919, 1991.
29. Centers for Disease Control: HIV Testing among women aged 18–44 years: United States, 1991 and 1993. MMWR Morb Mortal Wkly Rep 45:733–737, 1996.
30. Centers for Disease Control and Prevention (CDC): Adult/adolescent female risk factors. In: HIV/AIDS Surveillance Report, vol. 9. Atlanta, GA, CDC, 1997, p 10.
31. Centers for Disease Control and Prevention: Zidovudine for the prevention of HIV transmission from mother to infant. MMWR Morb Mortal Wkly Rep 43:285–287, 1994.
32. Hoffmann GW: The T cell receptor and AIDS pathogenesis. Scand J Immunol 41:331–337, 1995.
33. Tsunetsugu-Yokota Y, Akagama K, Kimoto H, et al: Monocyte-derived cultured dendritic cells are susceptible to human immunodeficiency virus infection and transmit virus to resting T cells in the process of nominal antigen presentation. J Virol 69:4544–4547, 1995.
34. Hamann B: Disease: Identification, Prevention and Control. St. Louis, C.V. Mosby, 1994.
35. Greene W: AIDS and the immune system. Sci Am 269:99–105, 1993.
36. Schwartz RH: T cell anergy. Sci Am 269:62–63, 1993.
37. Radkowski M, Mian M, Laskus T, et al: Concomitant symptom syndrome of primary HIV infection. Pol Arch Med Wewn 90:226–229, 1993.
38. Fischl MA, Dickinson GM, La Voie L: Safety and efficacy of sulfamethoxazole and trimethoprim chemoprophylaxis for Pneumocystis carinii penumonia in AIDS. JAMA 259:1185–1189, 1988.
39. Hughes WT, Kennedy W, Dougdale M, et al: Prevention of Pneumosystis carinii pneumonia in AIDS patients with weekly dapsone. Lancet 336:1066, 1990.
40. Lavelle J, Falloon J, Morgan A, et al: Weekly dapsone and dapsone/pyrimethamine for PCP prophylaxis. Presented at Sixth International Conference on AIDS, San Francisco, June 20–23, 1990 [abstract WB-2207:233].
41. Grunewald T, Bergmann F, Eljaschewitsch J, et al: Antiprotozoal prophylaxis in AIDS patients: results from a prospective, randomized study comparing dapsone pyrimethamine and sulfadoxine pyrimethamine. Presented at Ninth International Conference on AIDS, Berlin June 7–11, 1993 [abstract WS-B13-3].
42. Falloon J, Boenning C, Pagano G, et al: The pharmacokinetics of atovaquone suspension on patients with HIV infection. Presented at First National Conference on Human Retroviruses and Related Infections, Washington, DC, December 12–16, 1993 [abstract 242].
43. Centers for Disease Control: Guidelines for prophylaxis against Pneumocystis carinii pneumonia for persons infected

with human immunodeficiency virus. MMWR Morb Mortal Wkly Rep 38(Suppl 5):1–9, 1989.

44. Safai B, Good RA: Kaposi's sarcoma: a review and recent developments. Clin Bull 10:62–69, 1980.

45. Templeton AC, Bhana D: Prognosis in Kaposi's sarcoma. J Natl Cancer Inst 55:1301–1304, 1975.

46. Harden CL, Hair LS: Diagnosis of central nervous system toxoplasmosis in AIDS patients confirmed by autopsy. AIDS 8:1188–1189, 1994.

47. Gellin B, Soave R: Coccidian infections in AIDS: Toxoplasmosis, cryptosporidiosis, and isosporiasis. Med Clin North Am 76:205–234, 1992.

48. Daar ES, Horowitz H: The spectrum of HIV infection. Patient Care, 27:99–128, 1993.

49. Bartlett JA: Cryptosporidiosis. PAACNOTES 5:110–112, 1993.

50. Church DL: Fatal diarrhea in an AIDS patient. Patient Care 26:280–283, 1992.

51. Ungvarski PJ, Staats JA: Clinical management of AIDS in adults. In: Flaskerud JH, Ungvarski PJ (eds): HIV/AIDS: A Guide to Nursing Care, 2nd ed. Philadelphia, W.B. Saunders, 1995, pp 81–133.

52. Saag MS: Cryptococcosis and other fungal infections (histoplasmosis, coccidioidomycosis). In: Sande MA, Volberding PA (eds): The Medical Management of AIDS. Philadelphia, W.B. Saunders, 1995, pp 437–459.

53. Greenspan JS, Greenspan D: Oral complications of HIV infection. In: Sande MA, Volberding PA (eds): The Medical Management of AIDS. Philadelphia, W.B. Saunders, 1996, pp 182–194.

54. Merrill JM, Laux LF, Thomby JL: Why doctors have difficulty with sex histories. South Med J 83:613–617, 1990.

55. Grimes DE, Grimes RM: AIDS and HIV Infection. Philadelphia, C.V. Mosby, 1994.

56. Schneider RF, Hansen NI, Rosen MJ, et al: Lack of usefulness of radiographic screening for pulmonary disease in asymptomatic HIV-infected adults: Pulmonary Complications of HIV Infection Study Group. Arch Intern Med 156:191–195, 1996.

57. Olsen WC, Cohen W: Neuroradiology of AIDS. In: Federle MP, Megibow AJ, Naidich DP: Radiology of AIDS. New York, Raven Press, 1988, pp 21–46.

58. Hambleton J, Abrams D: Hematologic Manifestations of HIV Infection. In: Sande MA, Volberding PA (eds): The Medical Management of AIDS. Philadelphia, W.B. Saunders, 1990, pp 182–194.

59. Gluckman RJ, Rosner F, Guarneri JJ: The diagnostic utility of bone marrow aspiration and biopsy in patients with acquired immunodeficiency syndrome. J Natl Med Assoc 81:119–125, 1989.

60. Mazzulli T, Salit IE: Clinical utility of bone marrow examinations in HIV-infected patients. International Conference on AIDS, Abstract n. F.B. 503 6(2), June 20–23, 1990, p 203.

61. Ciaudo M, Doco-Lecompte T, Guettier C, et al: Revisited indications for bone marrow examinations in HIV-infected patients. Eur J Haematol 53:168–174, 1994.

62. Karcher DS, Frost AR: The bone marrow in human immunodeficiency virus (HIV-related disease, morphology and clinical correlation). Am J Clin Pathol 95:63–71, 1991.

63. Martinez P, Ortega A, Sorlano V, et al: Usefulness of bone marrow aspirate examination in HIV-infected patients. National Conference on Human Retrovirus-Related Infection, 1993, p 142.

64. Torda A, Jones PD, Beale P: Evaluation of results and clinical utility of bone marrow examination in patients with HIV. Annual Conference of Australia's Society of HIV Medicine, 6:117, Nov. 3–6, 1994.

65. Rodriguez JN, Dieguez JC, Moreno MV, et al: Usefulness of bone marrow examination in patients with advanced HIV infection. Rev Clin Esp 196:213–216, 1996.

66. Magibow AJ, Wall SD, Balthazar EJ, et al: Gastrointestinal Radiology in AIDS patients. In: Federle MP, Magibow AJ, Naidich DP (eds): Radiology of AIDS. New York, Raven Press, 1988, pp 77–105.

67. Kübler-Ross E: On Death and Dying. New York, Macmillan, 1969.

68. Merritt P: Guilt and shame in recovering addicts. J Psychosoc Nurs Ment Health Serv 35:46–49, 1997.

69. Williams R, Williams V: Anger Kills: Seventeen Strategies for Controlling the Hostility That Can Harm Your Health. New York, Time Books, 1993.

70. Retzinger SM: Violent Emotions: Shame and Rage in Marital Quarrels. Newbury Park, CA, Sage, 1991.

71. McCain N: Stress and coping in the context of psychoneuroimmunology: a holistic framework for practice and research. Arch Psychiatr Nurs 4:221–227, 1994.

72. Knight KH: Relationship of death anxiety/fear to health-seeking beliefs and behaviors. Death Studies 20:23–31, 1996.

73. Lisanti P, Zwolski K: Understanding the devastation of AIDS. Am J Nurs 97:26–35, 1997.

74. Guinon J: The use of group programs to improve medication compliance in patients with chronic diseases. Patient Educ Counseling 26:189–193, 1995.

75. Lindsey E: Health within illness: experiences of chronically ill/disabled people. J Adv Nurs 24:465–472, 1996.

76. Davidhizar R: Disability does not have to be the grief that never ends: helping patients adjust. Rehabil Nurs 22:32–35, 1997.

77. Arnold J: Rethinking grief. Home Healthcare Nurse 14:777–783, 1996.

78. Houseman C, Pheifer WG: Potential for unresolved grief in survivors of persons with AIDS. Arch Psychiatr Nurs 2:296–301, 1988.

79. Lesseig DZ: Pharmacotherapy for long-term care residents with dementia-associated behavioral disturbance. J Psychosoc Nurs Ment Health Serv 36:27–31, 1998.

80. Montgomery P, Kitten M, Niemiec C: The agitated patient with brain injury and the rehabilitation staff: bridging the gap of misunderstanding. Rehabil Nurs 22:20–39, 1997.

81. Bennett JA: Nurses' attitudes about acquired immunodeficiency syndrome care: what research tells us. J Prof Nurs 11:339–350, 1995.

82. Larson E, Ropka ME: An update on nursing research and HIV infection. Image: J Nurs Sch 23:4–11, 1991.

83. Adinolfi A: The role of the nurse in the care of patients with HIV. In: Bartlett J (ed): Care and Management of Patients with HIV Infection. Durham, NC, Glaxo, 1993.

84. Byrne VA, Murphy JP: Research briefs: are we preparing future nurses to care for individuals with AIDS? J Nurs Educ 3:84–86, 1993.

85. Mueller CW, Cerny JE, Amundson MJ, et al: Nursing faculty and students' attitudes regarding HIV. J Nurs Educ 31:273–279, 1992.

86. Sherman DW: Taking the fear out of AIDS nursing: voices from the field. J NY State Nurses Assoc 27:4–8, 1996.

87. Williams RD, Benedict S, Pearson BC: Degree of comfort in providing care to PWA's: effect of a workshop for baccalaureate nursing students. J Nurs Educ 31:397–402, 1992.

88. Webb AA, Bower DA, Gill S: Satisfaction with nursing care: a comparison of patients with HIV/AIDS, non-HIV/AIDS infections, diseases, and medical diagnoses. J Assoc Nurses AIDS Care 8:39–46, 1997.

89. Baylor RA, McDaniel AM: Nurses' attitudes toward caring for patients with acquired immunodeficiency syndrome. J Prof Nurs 12:99–105, 1996.

90. Ungvarski PJ: Update on HIV infection. Am J Nurs 97:44–52, 1997.

91. Kagawa-Singer M: Cross-cultural views of disability. Rehabilitation 19:362–365, 1994.

92. Giger J, Davidhizar R: Transcultural Nursing: Assessment and Intervention, 2nd ed. St. Louis, C.V. Mosby, 1995.

93. Chitty KK: A national survey of AIDS education in schools of nursing. J Nurs Educ 28:150–155, 1989.

94. Benner P, Wrubel J: The Primacy of Caring: Stress and Coping in Health and Illness. Menlo Park, CA, Addison-Wesley, 1989.

95. Visintini R, Campanini E, Fossati A, et al: Psychological stress in nurses' relationships with HIV-infected patients: the risk of burnout syndrome. AIDS Care 8:183–194, 1996.

96. Valenti WM: Infection control, human immunodeficiency virus, and home health care: infection risk to the patient. Am J Infect Control 22:371–372, 1994.

97. Anastasi JB, Rivera J: Understanding prophylactic therapy for infections. Am J Nurs 94:36–42, 1994.

98. Caulker-Burnett I: Primary care screening for substance abuse. Nurse Pract 19:42–48, 1994.

99. Crispo-Fierro M: Compliance/adherence and care management in HIV disease. J Assoc Nurses AIDS Care 8:43–54, 1997.

100. LeMone P, Burke K: Medical-Surgical Nursing: Critical Thinking in Client Care. Reading, MA, Addison-Wesley, 1996.

101. Baigus-Smith J, Coombs V, Larson E: HIV infection, exercise, and immune function. Image J Nurs Sch 26:277–280, 1994.

102. Anastasi JB, Sun V: Controlling diarrhea in the HIV patient. Am J Nurs 96:35–42, 1996.

103. Anastasi JB, Lee VS: HIV wasting: how to stop the cycle. Am J Nurs 94:18–25, 1994.

104. Albright J: Readability of patient education materials: implications for clinical practice. Appl Nurs Res 77:139–143, 1996.

105. Wilson FL: Measuring patients' ability to read and comprehend: a first step in patient education. Nurs Connections 8:17–25, 1995.

106. Walters JL, Canady R, Stein T: Evaluating multicultural approaches in HIV/AIDS educational material. AIDS Educ Prev 6:446–453, 1994.

107. O'Donnell L, SanDoral A, Vornfett R: Reducing AIDS and other STDs among inner-city Hispanics: the use of qualitative research in the development of video-based patient education. AIDS Educ Prev 6:140–153, 1994.

108. Murphy J, Giger J, Davidhizar R: Strategies for teaching clients who do not speak English. J Healthcare Educ Teach 8:8–12, 1994.

109. Gallant JE, Masur H, Powderly WG: Prophylaxis: who, what, when, and why? Patient Care 30:77–97, 1996.

110. Centers for Disease Control: USPHS/IDSA guidelines for the prevention of opportunistic infections in persons infected with human immunodeficiency virus: a summary. MMWR Morb Mortal Wkly Rep 44:1–33, 1995.

111. Lange WR, Denny SC: Travel in Eastern Europe: guidelines for patients. Postgrad Med 89:143–147, 1991.

112. Davey RT, Goldschmidt RH, Sande MA: Anti-HIV therapy in 1996. Patient Care 30:55–72, 1996.

113. Saquinavir fact sheet. Project Inform, San Francisco, 1997.

114. Mellors JW, Rinaldo CR, Gupta P, et al: Prognosis in HIV-1 infection predicted by the quantity of virus in plasma. Science 272:1167–1170, 1996.

115. ddI fact sheet. Project Inform, San Francisco, 1997.

116. Whitfield L: 1998 Antiviral drug guide. J Test-Positive Aware Network, January/February, 1998, pp 28–42.

117. Protease inhibitors: choices and analysis. Project Inform, San Francisco, 1996.

118. Kuhls TL, Viker S, Parris NB, et al: Occupational risk of HIV, HBV and HSV-2 in health care personnel caring for AIDS patients. Am J Public Health 77:1306–1309, 1987.

119. Wormser GP, Joline C, Sivak S, et al: Human immunodeficiency virus infection: considerations for health care workers. Bull NY Acad Med 64:203–215, 1988.

120. Ho DD, Moudgil T, Alam M: Quantitation of human immunodeficiency virus type 1 in the blood of infected persons. N Engl J Med 321:1621–1625, 1989.

121. Mast S, Woolwine J, Gerberding JL: Efficacy of gloves to reducing blood volumes transferred during simulated needlestick injury. J Infect Dis 168:1589–1592, 1993.

122. Centers for Disease Control: Public Health Service Statement on Management of Occupational Exposure to Human Immunodeficiency Virus, Including Considerations Regarding Zidovudine Postexposure Use. MMWR (RR01): 1–14, 1990.

123. Clerici M, Levin JM, Kessler HA, et al: HIV-specific T-helper activity in seronegative health care workers exposed to contaminated blood. JAMA 271:42–46, 1994.

124. Gerberding JL: Management of occupational exposure to blood-borne viruses. N Engl J Med 332:444–451, 1995.

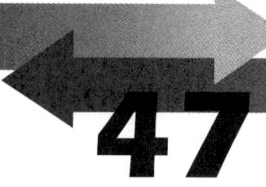

47

Shock

Kimmith M. Jones and Linda Bucher

Objectives

After completing this chapter, the student will be able to:

1. Differentiate the etiology and pathophysiologic pathways associated with hypovolemic, cardiogenic, and distributive shock.
2. Correlate the neural, hormonal, and other intrinsic compensatory mechanisms to maintain blood flow to the pathophysiology of shock states.
3. Assess the major body systems for clinical signs and symptoms related to shock states.
4. Identify appropriate nursing diagnoses for the patient experiencing shock.
5. Select appropriate definitive and supportive management strategies for patients experiencing hypovolemic, cardiogenic, or distributive shock.
6. Evaluate outcomes appropriate to patients experiencing shock.

Shock is an extremely common diagnosis in the critical care setting. Regardless of the cause, early recognition and prompt management of the patient with shock are vitally important to achieve positive patient outcomes. Skillful management requires knowledge of the most current technology, as well as an understanding of the devastating physiologic derangements that make shock so lethal. Mortality from most forms of shock is high despite advances in technology and pharmacology. Care of patients with shock remains a demanding and challenging task. This chapter discusses the mechanism of shock, the clinical presentation of shock, assessment of the patient with shock, and current management strategies.

ETIOLOGY

Shock is a condition that occurs when perfusion of the body's organs and tissues is inadequate to meet the oxygen and nutritional demands of the cells. Many different conditions can lead to shock states (e.g., traumatic blood loss, spinal cord injury, cardiac tamponade, infections, exposure to antigens). If shock is not interrupted, the end results include cellular dysfunction, organ failure, and death.[1,2]

Two criteria must be met before shock can be diagnosed. First, there must be a reduction in mean systemic blood pressure. Blood flow through the blood vessels remains constant through a mechanism termed "autoregulation." When a patient's mean arterial pressure (MAP) is between 60 and 130 mm Hg, the diameter of the blood vessels automatically adjusts to maintain a constant flow of blood to the tissues and cells of the body. When the MAP falls below 60 mm Hg, autoregulation fails and hypoperfusion results. The second criterion needed to diagnose shock is clinical evidence of hypoperfusion of vital organs.

Compensatory Mechanisms to Maintain Adequate Blood Flow

The body sets various compensatory mechanisms into motion in an attempt to return or maintain adequate blood flow to the tissues and cells of the body. These mechanisms are activated when the body recognizes that a low-perfusion state is occurring. The end result of these compensatory mechanisms is an improvement in tissue perfusion and prevention of tissue necrosis in the healthy person.

Unfortunately, the critically ill patient often reaches a point when the compensatory mechanisms can no longer support tissue perfusion. Decompensation occurs, and the patient's signs and symptoms worsen. If the shock state is not reversed at this time, the patient will die.

Neural Compensatory Mechanisms

Baroreceptor Reflex. Baroreceptors are located in the carotid body and aortic arch and function to monitor changes in arterial blood pressure. When there is a reduction in MAP, the amount of stretch of the arterial baroreceptors decreases. This stimulation of the baroreceptors is communicated within seconds to the vasomotor center, located in the medulla of the brain. A compensatory response is fully activated within 30 seconds of a drop in blood pressure. The outcome of this stimulation is the release of impulses to the sympathetic vasoconstrictor fibers located throughout the body in both arterial and venous systems (Figure 47–1). Consequently, blood is shunted away from nonpriority organs (lungs, skin, kidneys, gastrointestinal tract) and to the brain and heart (vital organs). The effects on the heart include increased contractility and heart rate (HR) in an effort to improve cardiac output (CO) and to increase blood pressure. In addition, the coronary arteries dilate, resulting in an increase in the delivery of oxygen to the myocardium.[1]

Central Nervous System Ischemic Response. When perfusion drops and the MAP falls below 50 mm Hg, the vasomotor center in the brain becomes ischemic, resulting in elevated carbon dioxide levels. Carbon dioxide is a potent sympathetic stimulator that leads to vasoconstriction. The central nervous system ischemic response begins within seconds of the drop in MAP and is completely activated within minutes.[3]

Reflex Venoconstriction. Sympathetic stimulation of the veins, resulting in venoconstriction, does not alter arterial blood pressure or total peripheral resistance significantly. The positive effect of sympathetic stimulation of veins is the decrease in the amount of blood they can hold. Benefits to the patient include increases in preload and, subsequently, CO.[3]

Stimulation of Chemoreceptors. Chemoreceptors are also located in the carotid bodies and aortic arch. Chemoreceptors are sensitive to changes in oxygen concentration and reductions in arterial blood pressure. When the chemoreceptors are stimulated, impulses travel to the vasomotor center of the brain, and a response, similar to the stimulation of the baroreceptors, is activated. The vasomotor center releases impulses to the sympathetic vasoconstrictor fibers, resulting in vasoconstriction of the arteries and veins. The chemoreceptor response is not a powerful mechanism in the control of blood flow to the tissues until systolic blood pressure falls below 80 mm Hg. However, this compensatory response plays a much greater role in the control of respiration than in the control of blood pressure.[3]

When perfusion to the lungs is reduced, alveoli are ventilated, but transport of oxygen is impaired. Consequently, physiologic dead space increases, and a ventilation–perfusion (V/Q) mismatch occurs. This impairment in gas exchange results in a decrease in arterial oxygen levels (hypoxemia). The compensatory response includes an increase in the rate and depth of ventilations.[1]

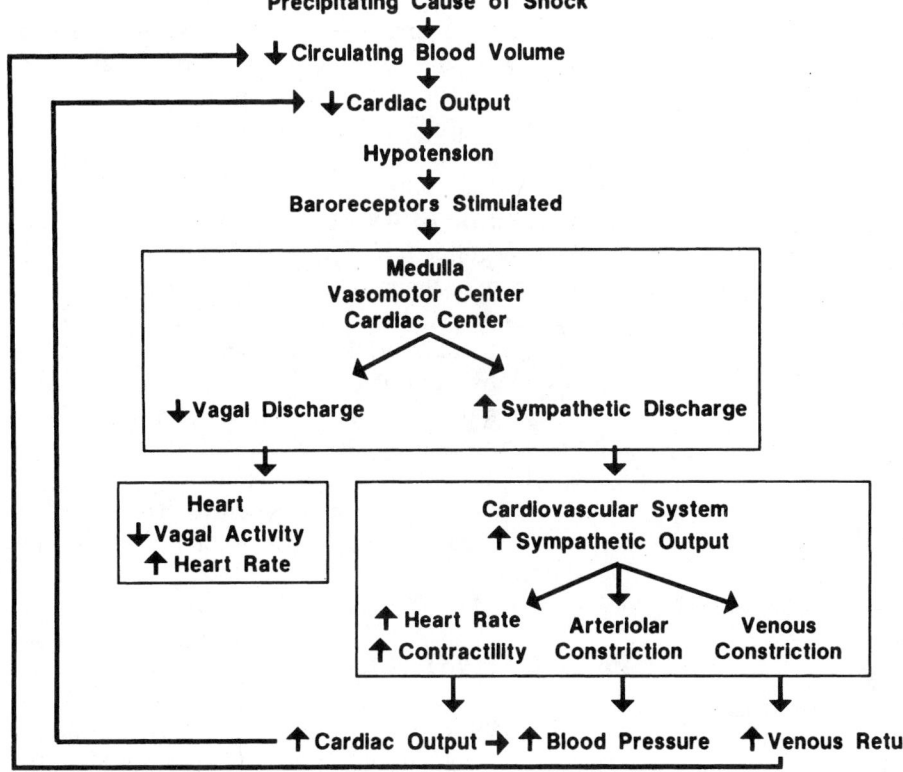

Figure 47–1

Compensatory mechanisms for the restoration of circulatory blood volume. (From Vary T, Kearny M: Pathophysiology of traumatic shock and multiple organ system failure. In: Cardona V, Hurn P, Bastinagel-Mason P, et al [eds]: Trauma Nursing From Resuscitation Through Rehabilitation, 2nd ed. Philadelphia, W.B. Saunders, 1994, p 116.)

Hormonal Compensatory Mechanisms

Norepinephrine–Epinephrine Vasoconstrictor Mechanism. Norepinephrine and epinephrine (catecholamines) are released from the adrenal medulla during stimulation of the vasomotor center and sympathetic nervous system. These "stress" hormones have several effects. Epinephrine acts as a vasoconstrictor to improve blood pressure, as a cardiac stimulant to increase HR and CO, and as a bronchodilator to relax the bronchioles. Norepinephrine functions primarily as a potent vasoconstrictor. These compensatory responses to physiologic stress can be sustained for hours or even days.[1,3]

Renin–Angiotensin System Activation. When blood flow to the kidneys is reduced, stimulation of the baroreceptors in the juxtaglomerular cells activates the renin–angiotensin system. The response of this system occurs within minutes of a drop in perfusion and becomes fully activated within 30 minutes. The renal hormone, renin, is released by the juxtaglomerular cells and converts renin substrate (angiotensinogen) to angiotensin I. Angiotensin I is then converted to angiotensin II by a substance called angiotensin-converting enzyme (ACE) (Figure 47–2). This conversion takes place primarily in the vascular epithelium of the lungs. Conversion of angiotensin I to angiotensin II also occurs in the heart, adrenal glands, kidneys, and brain. Angiotensin II is an extremely potent vasoconstrictor that causes widespread vasoconstriction in the arterioles and, to a lesser extent, in the venules.

The renin–angiotensin system also stimulates the release of aldosterone from the adrenal cortex. This hormone acts on the renal tubules by retaining sodium and, subsequently, water. This compensatory response is directed at increasing or maintaining intravascular volume.[1]

Antidiuretic Hormone. When blood pressure is reduced, the osmoreceptors in the hypothalamus are stimulated, causing the posterior pituitary gland to release antidiuretic hormone (ADH; vasopressin). The release of ADH has a vasopressor effect that functions to increase blood pressure. In addition, ADH acts on the renal tubules to retain water in an effort to restore or preserve intravascular volume.[1,3]

Release of Glucocorticoids. The anterior pituitary gland responds to the activation of the sympathetic nervous system by releasing adrenocorticotropic hormone (ACTH). This hormone stimulates the adrenal cortex to release glucocorticoids (e.g., cortisol). Glucocorticoids are involved in protein (glyconeogenesis) and carbohydrate (glycogenolysis) metabolism. The overall effect of these hormones is an increase in blood glucose levels. This glucose then becomes available to meet the increased metabolic needs of the cells.[1]

Additional Intrinsic Compensatory Mechanisms

Capillary Fluid Shifts. Arteriolar constriction during states of low blood flow leads to a reduction in venous pressure and a drop in capillary hydrostatic pressure. This change produces a shift of fluid from the interstitial and intracellular space to the intravascular space. Capillary fluid shifts start within minutes of a decrease in blood pressure and become completely activated within several hours.[3]

Constriction of Arterioles of the Kidneys. A decrease in systemic blood pressure results in a concurrent decrease in the renal artery blood pressure. In an attempt to maintain a constant blood flow to the kidney, the renal arterioles constrict. The effect of this constriction is a reduction in glomerular filtration and renal plasma flow. Ultimately, this condition results in the retention of sodium and water and the reduction of urine output. Like many of the compensatory mechanisms discussed, these consequences are aimed at restoring or maintaining intravascular volume and blood pressure.[3]

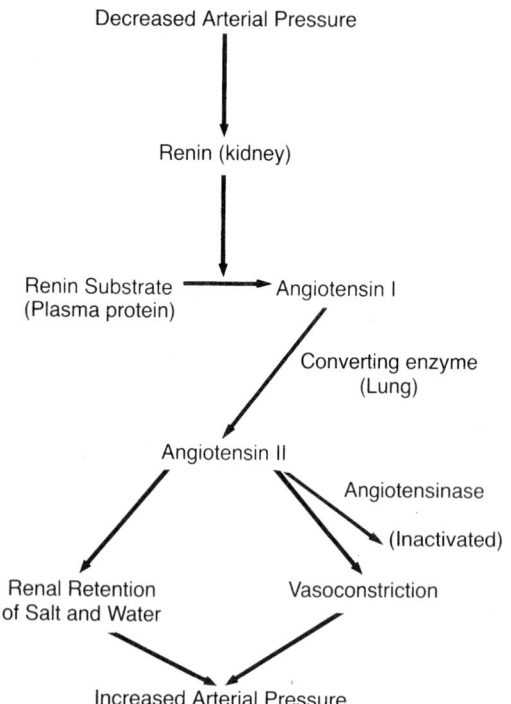

Figure 47–2

Renin–angiotensin vasoconstrictor mechanism for arterial pressure control. (From Guyton A, Hall J: Textbook of Medical Physiology, 9th ed. Philadelphia, W.B. Saunders, 1996.)

PATHOPHYSIOLOGY

In the normally functioning cell that is receiving an adequate oxygen supply, oxygen is used by the mitochondria to convert adenosine diphosphate (ADP) to adenosine triphosphate (ATP) through a process called oxidative phosphorylation in the Krebs cycle (Figure 47–3). The ATP that has been engineered is then used by the body to carry out its many functions. This process is also referred to as aerobic metabolism. When oxygen is not available, as in shock states, anaerobic metabolism occurs. ATP is still engineered; however, the process is less efficient. A smaller amount of ATP is produced, thus leading to a deficiency in the amount of energy available for bodily functions. In addition, anaerobic metabolism produces large amounts of pyruvic acid, which is converted to lactic acid. The accumulation of lactic acid produces metabolic acidosis (see Figure 47–3). As intracellular pH decreases, powerful enzymes are released that destroy the cell membrane and digest the cell contents. The consequences can range from cellular dysfunction to tissue destruction to organ system failure to death.

The end result of all shock states is the development of an imbalance between oxygen supply and oxygen demand in the body's cells and tissues. Oxygen supply becomes inadequate to meet the oxygen demand of the cells when the body's neuronal, hormonal, and intrinsic compensatory mechanisms fail. When the oxygen supply drops, the oxygen consumption (Vo_2) of the cells decreases and anaerobic metabolism occurs, along with an accumulation of an oxygen debt. The extent of the oxygen debt correlates with the seriousness and irreversibility of the shock state. The larger the oxygen debt, the more serious and irreversible the shock state becomes.

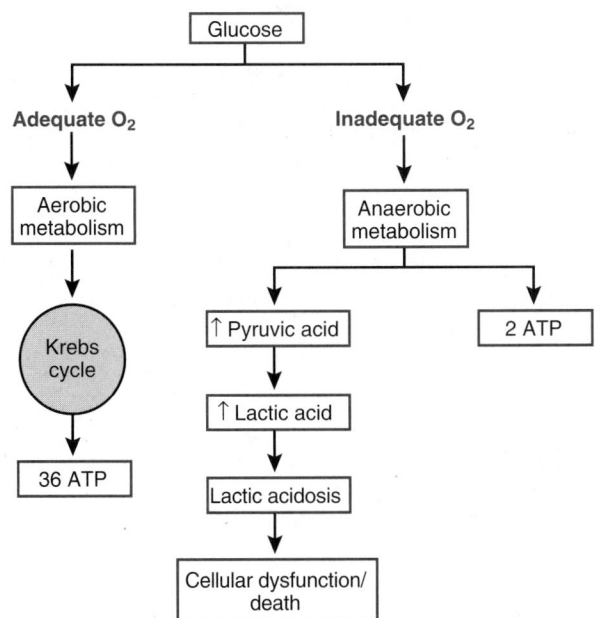

Figure 47–3

Aerobic and anaerobic metabolism.

Once the body's compensatory mechanisms begin to fail, cellular hypoxia develops and anaerobic metabolism begins. The anaerobic process is the same regardless of the cause of the low-perfusion or low-blood-flow state. This process can be reversed if interventions are promptly instituted. However, if a low-perfusion state persists for an extended period or if interventions are not successful, the process will become irreversible, and death will be imminent.[4]

Lactate levels are used as an indicator of decreased oxygen delivery to the cells. Elevated levels of lactate produce an acidic environment and can have dramatic effects on the arterial pH. Lactate levels of more than 5 mEq/L or more than 45 mg/dL have been associated with increased rates of mortality. The lactate blood level represents lactic acid production and correlates with the degree of hypoperfusion that has taken place. An elevated lactate level is a late indicator of hypoperfusion because it only occurs after maximal oxygen extraction by the cells. For lactate to be eliminated by the body, it must leave the cell and travel to the liver, where it is metabolized. Removal of lactate from the body during shock can take hours to correct. Progressive decreases in lactate levels are associated with restoration of blood flow to the body organs and tissues and improved patient outcomes. Early identification of hypoperfusion or shock states is crucial to avoiding the devastating consequences of anaerobic metabolism and lactic acid production.[2]

Systems Affected by Shock

Every body system is affected by hypoperfusion states.[5] Nurses caring for patients with shock need to conduct a thorough, baseline assessment of each body system when they first encounter the patient. Thereafter, nurses must frequently monitor these patients for changes in signs and symptoms in each body system (Table 47–1). The cardinal parameters of tissue perfusion include level of consciousness (LOC), skin, urine output, and vital signs (temperature, heart rate and peripheral pulses, respiratory rate, and blood pressure).[1] At times, some of these changes may be subtle. Trending of data provides critical information regarding the progression of the shock state as well as the effectiveness of the interventions.

Pulmonary System

During hypoperfusion states, alterations in the microcirculation of the lungs take place. Capillary permeability increases, and leaks develop, thus flooding the alveoli of the lung. Leukocytes, platelets, and fibrin accumulate in the alveoli as a result of the changes in the microcirculation. Further, damage to the endothelial lining of the capillary beds occurs, resulting in altered

TABLE 47–1
Clinical Manifestations of Shock

Body System	Early Findings	Late Findings
Cardiovascular*	Slightly increased blood pressure, slowly increasing heart rate → sinus tachycardia; bounding peripheral pulses	Steadily decreasing blood pressure (systolic blood pressure <90 mm Hg), MAP <60 mm Hg, steadily decreasing cardiac output, thready → nonpalpable pulses; delayed capillary refill, myocardial ischemia and infarction
Respiratory	Increased respiratory rate, respiratory alkalosis, hypoxemia	Respiratory acidosis, pulmonary edema, acute respiratory distress syndrome
Neurologic	Restlessness, apathy, anxiety, confusion, disorientation	Extreme lethargy, stupor, coma, cerebral edema, dysfunction of vital control centers
Renal	Decreased renal perfusion, decreased glomerular filtration rate, decreased urine output (<30 cc per hour	Oliguria, metabolic acidosis, uremia, renal failure
Integumentary†	Pallor (skin, lips, oral mucosa, conjunctiva); cool, moist skin or warm, flushed skin	Cyanosis, cold skin, edema, necrosis/ulceration
Gastrointestinal	Decreased gastrointestinal motility, gastrointestinal ulceration	Paralytic ileus, gastrointestinal hemorrhage, translocation of gut bacteria, gastrointestinal ischemia and infarction
Hepatic	Increased glucose production → decreased glucose production (hypoglycemia); decreased lactic acid conversion → lactic acidosis	Increased liver enzymes, decreased clotting factors → coagulopathies; jaundice, increased serum ammonia level, toxic levels of drugs due to hepatic failure
Musculoskeletal	Weakness, myalgias, increased lactate levels	Myoglobinemia, myoglobinuria

→, leading to; MAP, mean arterial pressure.
*Patients with neurogenic shock will demonstrate a persistent decreased blood pressure and heart rate due to the loss of sympathetic tone.
†Patients with early septic and neurogenic shock will demonstrate warm, flushed skin due to the global vasodilation. Patients with anaphylactic shock may demonstrate urticaria and angioedema.

functioning of type II pneumocytes. Consequences include a reduction in surfactant production, the collapse of the alveoli, and a decrease in lung compliance. If hypoxia persists, pulmonary shunting and V/Q mismatch occurs, predisposing the patient to the development of acute respiratory distress syndrome (ARDS).[4,5]

During the early stages of shock, the patient compensates for decreases in arterial oxygen levels with rapid and deep respirations, resulting in a decrease in carbon dioxide levels which leads to respiratory alkalosis. As the shock state progresses, the patient begins to hypoventilate because of exhaustion and depletion of energy reserves. Respirations often remain rapid but shallow, thereby precipitating high levels of carbon dioxide and, ultimately, respiratory acidosis and a poor prognosis.

Renal System

The kidneys are useful in monitoring shock and perfusion to end organs because they are susceptible to autoregulation during reduced blood flow. The kidney normally receives about 1.3 L per minute of blood; however, during shock, this amount can be reduced to 200 mL per minute. This drop in blood flow has a dramatic effect on the kidney. In addition to a reduction in glomerular filtration rate, blood flow within the kidney itself is also affected. Blood appears to be shunted from the outer cortex and medullary nephrons to the inner cortex. When the kidney senses a reduction in blood flow, the renin–angiotensin system is initiated (described earlier). If, however, the cells and nephrons of the kidney are damaged by hypoxia and the consequences of anaerobic metabolism, the compensatory mechanisms of the kidney can fail. The combination of the lack of oxygen and the resultant lack of ATP produces cellular sloughing and acute tubular necrosis. The patient with acute tubular necrosis is unable to generate and reabsorb bicarbonate or to excrete waste products such as acids, potassium, creatinine, and blood urea nitrogen (BUN). As renal failure progresses, urine output decreases, and uremia and metabolic acidosis develop.[1,4,5]

Cardiovascular System

During hypoperfusion states, the body responds by shunting blood to the central circulation and vital organs. The heart is one of the organs that receives increased blood flow during these times, even to the detriment of other organs. Through autoregulation, coronary perfusion pressure is maintained in an attempt to maintain myocardial function. Myocardial oxygen demands increase during shock, especially in the early phase, because of the tachycardia that occurs in response to the stimulation of the sympathetic nervous system. During times of low MAP, the oxygen extraction in the ventricles increases. This increase is generally not sufficient to overcome the negative effects of the alpha-adrenergic tone and extravascular tissue pressure that result from myocardial edema.[4,5]

If the shock state persists, compensatory mechanisms will begin to fail, and CO and blood pressure will decrease. This change results in a decrease in coronary perfusion pressure and an imbalance between myocardial oxygen supply and demand. Consequences of this imbalance include dysrhythmias and myocardial ischemia or infarction. These conditions further contribute to myocardial dysfunction and inadequate tissue and organ perfusion.

These sequelae are manifested in patients by changes in HR (tachycardia to bradycardia), pulse quality (<+2), systolic blood pressure (<90 mm Hg), MAP (<60 mm Hg), and capillary refill (>3 seconds).

Neurologic System

Early in the shock state, the brain also benefits from the shunting of blood to the central circulation. The cerebral blood flow may increase fivefold as a result of the autoregulation that accompanies the activation of the compensatory mechanisms. When the MAP drops below 60 mm Hg, the autoregulatory response begins to fail. As a result of sustained low blood flow, cerebral cells become ischemic, and lactate levels in the brain accumulate. Intracranial hypertension develops and cerebral perfusion pressure falls, contributing to further cerebral ischemia and infarction. Eventually, vital control centers fail to function, and death is inevitable.[1,4,5]

Changes in the neurologic system are primarily monitored by the patient's LOC. Early changes in the patient's LOC may be subtle and include anxiety, apathy, and restlessness. As the shock state progresses, the patient's LOC deteriorates. The patient may become confused and disoriented, and eventually he or she will not respond to verbal stimuli. If cerebral ischemia continues, the patient will eventually fail to respond to painful stimuli and will become comatose.[1]

Hepatic System

The hepatic system is extremely susceptible to the consequences of shock. The liver fails because of the cellular damage that occurs during anaerobic metabolism. The hepatocytes cannot generate the requisite ATP during anaerobic metabolism, thus leading to cellular membrane damage and a loss of liver function. As a result of

the inability of the liver to function properly, elevations in the liver enzymes (alanine aminotransferase [ALT], aspartate aminotransferase [AST], lactate dehydrogenase [LDH]) are observed. If the hypoperfusion state is limited or reversed, these values can return to normal.[4,5]

If the shock state persists, liver cell destruction will be inevitable and will be manifested clinically in several ways. The liver fails to conjugate bilirubin completely, and as it accumulates, patients develop jaundice. Waste products (e.g., ammonia, lactate) accumulate and may precipitate asterixis (flapping tremors) in patients. The failing liver cannot metabolize drugs, and toxic levels may develop. Finally, the patient with liver failure is at high risk of infection because the ability of the liver to neutralize invading microorganisms is lost.[1]

Gastrointestinal System

One of the initial responses of the body to hypoperfusion is the redirection of blood from nonessential areas, such as the gastrointestinal system, to the heart and brain. This change occurs through constriction of blood vessels in the splanchnic area. The gastrointestinal system is the first organ system to be affected in shock, and anatomic changes (e.g., mucosal ulceration) have been documented within hours after the onset of shock.[1] The reduction of blood flow to the splanchnic area (stomach, small intestine, large intestine, liver, gallbladder, and pancreas) results in damage to the epithelial lining of these organs and leakage of proteins and solutes into the intestinal lumen. Prolonged alterations in splanchnic blood flow result in a decrease in gastrointestinal motility and the development of paralytic ileus. In addition, patients are predisposed to the development of stress ulcers, which can interfere with the absorption of nutrients and may trigger acute gastrointestinal bleeding.[1] Finally, altered splanchnic blood flow damages the intestinal microvilli, which then allow bacteria to enter the systemic circulation. This translocation of gut bacteria (e.g., *Escherichia coli*) from the intestinal lumen places the critically ill patient at high risk of infection.[4,5]

Hematologic System

The hematologic system is also affected by hypoperfusion states. Sluggish blood flow through the blood vessels can lead to the development of microemboli, which can result in deep venous thrombosis or pulmonary embolism. Hypoperfusion of the liver and the resultant decrease in production of clotting factors can cause coagulopathies (e.g., disseminated intravascular coagulation). In the early stages of shock, leukopenia can occur, as a result of leukocytosis and the depletion of white blood cells (WBCs) in the blood and bone marrow.

Integumentary System

The skin responds differently, depending on the type of shock and the stage of shock (early versus late). Most often, peripheral vasoconstriction, in response to the efforts to maintain perfusion to vital organs, occurs, resulting in pale, cool, and moist (clammy) skin. When peripheral vasodilation occurs (e.g., neurogenic shock, early septic shock), the skin is warm, dry, and flushed. Patients with anaphylactic shock often present with flushed skin, urticaria, pruritus, and angioedema. When compensatory mechanisms fail in all types of shock, the patient's skin is extremely cool, cyanotic, and mottled. In extreme cases, areas of ulceration or necrosis may develop, especially on the distal extremities.[1]

CLASSIFICATION OF SHOCK

The three major classifications of shock are hypovolemic, cardiogenic, and distributive (or vasogenic). Each of these shock states results from physiologic changes that impair the delivery of oxygen to the tissues. Assessment findings and definitive management strategies vary, however, depending on the type of shock.

HYPOVOLEMIC SHOCK

Hypovolemic shock occurs as a result of a loss of intravascular blood volume. The amount of volume lost determines the severity of shock and, subsequently, the patient's clinical manifestations. The American College of Surgeons has developed the most widely recognized classification system of fluid and blood losses (Table 47–2).

Intravascular losses can result from either internal fluid shifts or external fluid losses. Internal fluid shifts refer to the loss of intravascular volume into the interstitial or intracellular spaces. If the shift is large enough, hypovolemia and shock can develop. For example, patients with internal bleeding (e.g., closed, long bone fractures; ruptured spleen; surgical procedures) and ascites (third spacing) are at high risk of developing hypovolemic shock.[1]

External fluid losses represent the majority of the causes of hypovolemic shock. Examples include patients with external hemorrhage (e.g., trauma), excessive gastrointestinal losses (e.g., vomiting, diarrhea), certain disease states (e.g., Addison's disease, diabetes insipidus), and excessive diuresis (e.g., hyperglycemic osmotic diuresis).

Assessment

It is difficult to identify a patient who has class I blood loss. In this class, the body's compensatory mechanisms can maintain a normal arterial blood pressure and CO. The only clinical evidence that may be seen with this degree of blood loss is a drop in hematocrit of 3 to 5% 24 hours after the initial event. In some cases, anxiety and restlessness are the first and earliest clues of a problem.

The compensatory mechanisms activated with class I fluid loss include sympathetic constriction of the blood vessels and the release of norepinephrine and epinephrine from the adrenal medulla, resulting in tachycardia. If the low blood-flow state continues, secretion of ADH, renin, and aldosterone occurs, along with a fluid shift from the interstitial space to the intravascular space. All these mechanisms are directed at maintaining intravascular volume. The patient who experiences class I blood loss is typically asymptomatic.[6–8]

TABLE 47–2
Classification of Fluid and Blood Losses*

	Class I	Class II	Class III	Class IV
Blood loss (mL)	≤750	750–1500	1500–2000	>2000
Blood loss (% blood volume)	≤15%	15–30%	30–40%	>40%
Pulse rate	<100	>100	>120	>140
Blood pressure	Normal	Normal	Decreased	Decreased
Capillary refill	Normal	Delayed	Delayed	Delayed
Respiratory rate	14–20	20–30	30–40	>35
Urine output (mL/hr)	>30	20–30	5–15	Negligible
Mental status	Slightly anxious	Mildly anxious	Anxious and confused	Confused, lethargic
Fluid replacement (3:1 rule)	Crystalloid	Crystalloid	Crystalloid and blood	Crystalloid and blood

*Amounts are based on the patient's initial presentation.
From American College of Surgeons Committee on Trauma. The Advanced Trauma Life Support Student Manual. Chicago, American College of Surgeons, 1993, p 86.

Class II blood loss is more easily recognizable, and the accompanying clinical signs and symptoms should lead the nurse to suspect hemorrhage. Class II blood loss occurs when the patient has an intravascular volume deficit of 15 to 30%. With this degree of volume loss, preload and, subsequently, CO and arterial blood pressure are reduced. In response to this altered perfusion state, compensatory mechanisms are activated, resulting in vasoconstriction and sympathetic adrenergic discharge. Blood pressure does not begin to drop until a 20% reduction in blood volume has occurred. However, orthostatic (postural) changes in blood pressure can be observed in patients with a 10 to 20% blood loss. Clinical manifestations resulting from these compensatory mechanisms can include an increase in HR and respiratory rate, pallor, diaphoresis, apprehension, restlessness, prolonged capillary filling, and decreased urine output (see Table 47–2).[6–8]

Patients with class III hemorrhage are immediately recognizable, and aggressive interventions are needed to prevent complications from developing. Class III hemorrhage occurs when blood volume loss reaches 30 to 40%. All compensatory mechanisms are in full action, and they may or may not be able to maintain adequate perfusion. Signs of hypoperfusion are readily identifiable. Any additional blood loss can result in rapid decompensation in CO, arterial blood pressure, and tissue perfusion. Patients with a blood volume loss of more than 30% are in a life-threatening situation and they have a high risk that shock may be irreversible. Irreversible shock occurs when the patient fails to respond to resuscitation measures and other therapeutic interventions.[6–8]

Class IV hemorrhage exists when the blood volume deficit is greater than 40%. At this point, compensatory mechanisms are exhausted and can no longer maintain tissue perfusion. Symptoms of impaired organ function are present and lead to multiple organ system failure. Irreversible shock is present in patients with class IV hemorrhage.[6–8]

Many hemodynamic changes can be observed in patients experiencing hypovolemic shock. These changes include decreases in stroke index (SI), left ventricular stroke work (LVSW), CO and cardiac index (CI), pulmonary artery pressure (PAP), and pulmonary artery occlusive pressure (PAOP). The reduced filling pressures and subsequent CO are a result of a decrease in preload secondary to the intravascular fluid loss. Systemic vascular resistance (SVR) is increased because of compensatory arterial vasoconstriction. Oxygen consumption (VO_2) is decreased secondary to a decreased CO and hypovolemia. Mixed venous oxygen saturation (SvO_2) is also decreased. A decreased SvO_2 is related to a de-

crease in CO and an increased oxygen extraction at the tissue level (Table 47–3).[1,2,9]

Nursing Diagnoses

The care of patients with hypovolemic shock is challenging, and the nurse needs to execute superior observational and assessment skills. Early and rapid interventions are essential to prevent the progression of the hypovolemic shock state. As members of a multidisciplinary team, nurses can be guided by nursing diagnoses that address the specific needs of these patients and their families. Table 47–4 presents actual and potential diagnoses for a patient with hypovolemic shock.

Collaborative Management

Definitive management strategies for the patient experiencing hypovolemic shock are directed toward correcting the cause of the volume depletion and restoring the intravascular volume.[1] For example, if the cause of the volume loss is external hemorrhage, it may be necessary to apply direct pressure to the bleeding site. For the postoperative patient who develops hypovolemic shock because of internal hemorrhage, a return to the operating room may be necessary to correct the cause of the bleeding. Patients who experience severe gastrointestinal losses secondary to vomiting or diarrhea need antiemetics or antidiarrheals to halt further fluid losses.

Rapid replacement of intravascular volume is the primary objective for the patient experiencing any degree of hemorrhage. Infusion of intravenous fluids is the fundamental treatment strategy. The most common intravenous fluids used for resuscitation are crystalloids (e.g., normal saline solution [NSS], Ringer's lactate solution). Volume replacement is continued until adequate MAP is achieved and tissue perfusion is reestablished.[10,11]

Controversy exists regarding the most appropriate intravenous fluid to infuse during the resuscitation of a patient with hemorrhage. It is thought that colloids (e.g., albumin) may help to decrease the risk of pulmonary edema by maintaining serum oncotic pressure. Because colloids remain in the intravascular space better than crystalloids, smaller volumes may be used to achieve successful resuscitation. However, colloids are much more expensive than crystalloids, and some of the synthetic colloids (e.g., hetastarch, dextran) have a tendency to alter normal coagulation, thus placing the patient at risk of bleeding complications.[1,4,12]

TABLE 47–3
Hemodynamic Patterns in Shock

	Cardiac Output	Pulmonary Artery Occlusive Pressure	Pulmonary Artery Pressure	Systemic Vascular Resistance	Svo₂	Vo₂	O₂Ext	Central Venous Pressure	Left Ventricular Stroke Work	Heart Rate	Stroke Index
Hypovolemic	↓	↓	↓	↑	↓	↓	↑	↓	↓	↑	↓
Cardiogenic	↓	↑	↑	↑	↓	↓	↑	↑	↓	↑	↓
Distributive*	↓	↓	↓	↓	↓	↓	↑	↓	↓	↑	↓

O₂Ext, oxygen extraction; Vo₂, oxygen consumption; Svo₂, venous oxygen saturation.
*A mixed picture may be present.
From Jones K: Shock. In: Clochesy J, Breu C, Cardin S, et al (eds): Critical Care Nursing, 2nd ed. Philadelphia, W.B. Saunders, 1996, p 1376.

TABLE 47–4
Nursing Diagnoses: Hypovolemic Shock

Problem Statement	Etiologic Factors
Fluid volume deficit	Blood and fluid losses from the intravascular fluid compartment
Altered tissue perfusion, peripheral	Blood and fluid losses from the intravascular compartment; impairment in delivery of oxygen and nutrients to cells
Decreased cardiac output	Decrease in preload secondary to intravascular fluid losses
Anxiety and fear	Impaired cerebral perfusion, sudden change in health, hospitalization, threat of death
Ineffective family coping	Changes in family roles, sudden critical illness of family member
Knowledge deficit	Limited experience with health care system, understanding of critical illness or events leading to critical illness, procedures, and treatment modalities
Altered nutrition, less than body requirements	Impairment in delivery of oxygen and nutrients to body cells

Crystalloids are distributed throughout the intravascular, interstitial, and intracellular spaces, depending on the concentration of the solution. To achieve successful resuscitation with crystalloids, three times the estimated volume loss is needed, to allow for the distribution of the fluids throughout the three spaces. The use of crystalloids may result in substantial hemodilution. A 1 to 3 g drop in hemoglobin can be observed during resuscitation of a patient with hypovolemic shock when only crystalloids are used. This hemodilution can result in decreased oxygen delivery to the tissues.[4, 12]

Specific blood products are often used to restore intravascular volume that has been depleted by blood loss. Autologous transfusions of fresh whole blood, using special collection devices, are considered whenever possible. Stored whole blood is rarely used because of the metabolic and biochemical changes that occur over time. Stored blood has increased levels of potassium and decreased amounts of platelets and clotting factors.[1] Packed red blood cells (PRBCs) contain an amount of hemoglobin equivalent to that in a unit of whole blood, but the volume has been reduced by removing the plasma portion of the blood. Using PRBCs in conjunction with crystalloids can improve the oxygen-carrying capacity of the blood while limiting the risk of fluid overload (see Table 47–2).[1]

There does not appear to be a difference in oxygen metabolism when the hematocrit is 30% versus 40%. Some researchers found little benefit in transfusing patients whose hemoglobin was greater than 10 mg/dL. However, patients with heart failure or decreased SvO_2 may require a higher hemoglobin level to achieve adequate oxygen delivery and may benefit from a blood transfusion.

In addition to these definitive management strategies, specific supportive strategies for managing patients with hypovolemic shock are also indicated. See the section later in this chapter on supportive strategies in the collaborative management of shock.

CARDIOGENIC SHOCK

Despite advances in the treatment of patients with cardiac disease, cardiogenic shock continues to be a leading cause of in-hospital mortality for this population.[1] Cardiogenic shock results from a reduction in oxygen delivery to the tissues secondary to pump (or heart) failure. Cardiogenic shock can be defined as a low CO and hypotension with clinical signs of inadequate blood flow to the tissues. These clinical manifestations can include low urine output, changes in mental status, decreased peripheral pulses, and cool and clammy skin.

The causes of cardiogenic shock can be classified as coronary or noncoronary (Chart 47–1).[1] Acute myocardial infarction (AMI) is the major event leading to coronary cardiogenic shock. The risk of cardiogenic shock increases as the area of myocardial necrosis increases. When more than 40% of the left ventricle is destroyed in the AMI process, cardiogenic shock is likely within 48 hours of the acute event. The risk of cardiogenic shock in patients with AMI accompanied by mechanical complications (e.g., papillary muscle dysfunction or rupture, interventricular septal defect) is compounded. Unfortunately, many of these patients may no longer be in the intensive care unit (ICU) when these complications occur. Overall mortality from cardiogenic shock is 75 to 90%, and occurs in 6 to 20% of all patients with AMI.[1, 13, 14]

Noncoronary cardiogenic shock develops in the absence of myocardial infarction. The failure of the heart to pump effectively may result from various conditions. Metabolic derangements, such as severe hypoxemia, acidosis, hypoglycemia, or hypocalcemia, can interfere with the pumping action of the heart. Pump failure may also result from obstructions to blood flow somewhere in the cardiovascular system. This type of noncoronary cardiogenic shock, called obstructive shock, can result from pulmonary embolism,

CHART 47-1

Etiology of Cardiogenic Shock

Coronary Cardiogenic Shock	Noncoronary Cardiogenic Shock
Acute myocardial infarction (AMI)	Metabolic derangements
Loss of critical left ventricular myocardium	Acidosis
Right ventricular failure	Hypoxemia
Mechanical complications of AMI	Hypocalcemia
Acute mitral regurgitation secondary to papillary	Hypoglycemia
muscle dysfunction or rupture	End-stage cardiomyopathy
Interventricular septal rupture	Myocardial contusion
Free wall rupture	Pulmonary embolus
Left ventricular aneurysm	Tension pneumothorax
Electrical complications of AMI	Pericarditis
Bradydysrhythmias	Left ventricular outflow tract obstruction
Tachydysrhythmias	Aortic stenosis
	Left ventricular inflow tract obstruction
	Mitral stenosis or regurgitation
	Left atrial myxoma
	Cardiac tamponade

Adapted from Califf R, Bengtson J: Cardiogenic shock. N Engl J Med 330:1724, 1994. Copyright © 1994 Massachusetts Medical Society. All rights reserved.

tension pneumothorax, cardiac tamponade, and atrial myxoma.[1,9,13,14]

A vicious cycle develops when patients present with cardiogenic shock (Figure 47–4). Cardiac output is reduced because of a drop in left ventricular systolic function. This change leads to hypotension, hypoperfusion, and hypoxemia. A decrease in coronary blood supply secondary to the drop in the arterial blood pressure further complicates the left ventricular dysfunction.[13]

In an attempt to correct the hypoperfusion state, compensatory mechanisms are initiated. These mechanisms work to increase blood volume and to maintain preload, the amount of stretch on the myocardium, at the end of diastole. These responses are not beneficial for the patient in cardiogenic shock because they further increase myocardial oxygen demand and the volume of blood in the heart. These consequences place an additional workload on an already impaired left ventricle.

Assessment

The patient with cardiogenic shock may experience many different classic symptoms including pulmonary edema, peripheral edema, and jugular vein distention. Left ventricular ejection fraction is usually less than 30%. Right-sided heart pressures (CVP, PAP) may be normal or elevated. Other signs and symptoms include hypotension and reduced CO secondary to a reduction in contractility of the heart. An increase in respiratory rate and the development of crackles may be observed secondary to pulmonary congestion that results from the passive transmission of blood volume from the left ventricle to the left atrium to the pulmonary circulation.[1] Urine output is decreased, and restlessness, agitation, or confusion can be seen as a result of reduced cerebral perfusion pressure. If the hypoperfusion state persists, renal failure and further reductions in LOC can develop.[15]

Patients experiencing cardiogenic shock develop some characteristic changes in hemodynamic parameters including decreases in CO and CI, despite an elevated pulmonary PAOP of more than 18 mm Hg. In addition, decreased SI and LVSW index result from left ventricular dysfunction. PAP and PAOP are increased as a result of an elevated left ventricular preload. Right atrial pressure is passively elevated secondary to an elevated left ventricular end-diastolic pressure (LVEDP) and the inability of the left ventricle to pump blood forward. During cardiogenic shock, an increase in preload results in an increased atrial stretch and the release of atrial natriuretic hormone from the atrial myocytes. This hormone produces renal artery vasodilation in an attempt to maintain renal blood flow.[1,2,9]

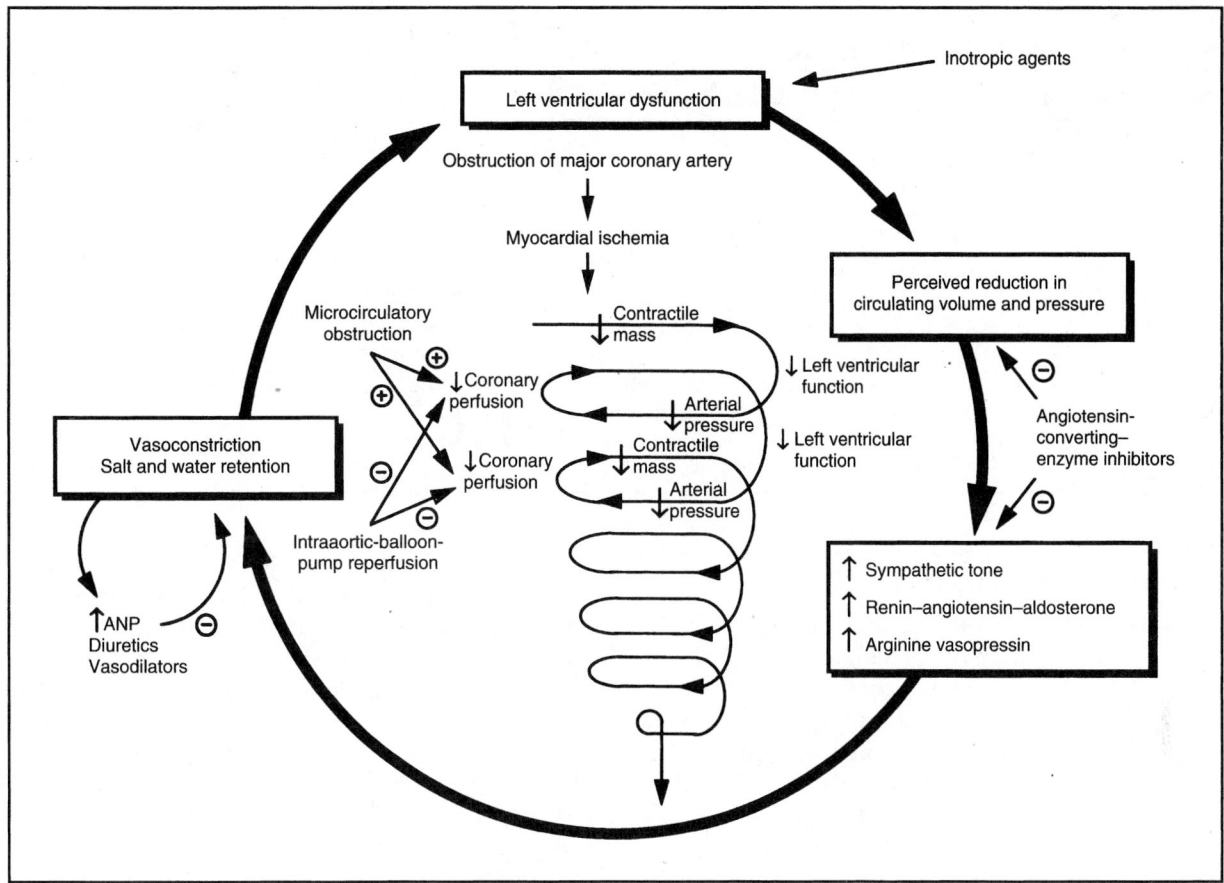

Figure 47–4

Mechanisms activated in cardiogenic shock. (From Califf R, Bengtson J: Cardiogenic shock. N Engl J Med 330:1725, 1994. Reprinted with permission from the New England Journal of Medicine.

In patients with cardiogenic shock, SVR is elevated secondary to compensatory vasoconstriction. Vo_2 is reduced because of the decline in the quantity of oxygen delivered to the tissues. Svo_2 is also reduced secondary to an increase in oxygen extraction at the cellular level (see Table 47–3).[1,2,9]

CI is an effective hemodynamic parameter to assess when determining the severity of cardiogenic shock. A CI of less than 1.8 L/m^2 per minute indicates cardiogenic shock. Clinical signs of hypoperfusion can be observed when the CI is between 1.8 and 2.2 L/m^2 per minute. These include diminished peripheral pulses, changes in LOC, and severe hypotension. Developing a bedside Starling curve to determine the most appropriate PAOP that will maximize CI can be extremely useful.[15]

The body's compensatory response to these changes, particularly the low blood pressure, is to stimulate the sympathetic nervous system. Sympathetic stimulation results in the release of the catecholamines epinephrine and norepinephrine. These hormones increase HR and contractility. Peripheral vasoconstriction also occurs and results in pale, cool,

and clammy skin. When these compensatory mechanisms fail, blood pressure drops, whereas HR continues to further increase.

Disturbances in HR can also add to inadequate pump function. CO is the product of HR and stroke volume (SV); therefore, bradydysrhythmias can reduce CO despite a normal or even increased SV. Tachydysrhythmias can reduce SV because of insufficient diastolic filling time, resulting in a reduction in CO despite the rapid HR.

Nursing Diagnoses

Patients experiencing cardiogenic shock may be acutely ill, as with an AMI, or chronically ill, as with end-stage cardiomyopathy. Regardless of the cause, these patients need intensive monitoring, ongoing assessment, and accurate interpretation of clinical signs and symptoms associated with a failing pump. Nursing diagnoses are formulated as one mechanism to guide and evaluate the effectiveness of interventions and to prevent or identify complications rapidly (Table 47–5).

TABLE 47–5
Nursing Diagnoses: Cardiogenic Shock

Problem Statement	Etiologic Factors
Decreased cardiac output	Ineffective myocardial contractility secondary to myocardial ischemia or necrosis, tamponade, electrolyte disturbances, dysrhythmias, valve dysfunction
Altered tissue perfusion, myocardial	Coronary artery disease, ischemia, occlusion
Altered tissue perfusion, peripheral	Impairment in delivery of oxygen and nutrients to cells secondary to decreased cardiac output
Impaired gas exchange	Impaired oxygen–carbon dioxide exchange secondary to pulmonary edema
Fluid volume excess	Impaired renal function secondary to hypoperfusion
Anxiety and fear	Sudden critical illness and hospitalization, inadequate cerebral perfusion, invasive procedures, threat of death
Altered nutrition, less than body requirements	Impairment in delivery of oxygen and nutrients to body cells
Ineffective family coping	Sudden critical illness of family member, change in family roles
Knowledge deficit	Disease process, treatments, procedures

Collaborative Management

Because the most common precursor to cardiogenic shock is AMI, definitive management strategies are directed at limiting or reducing myocardial damage during the AMI process. Additional definitive management strategies are aimed at improving the effectiveness of the pumping action of the heart and apply to all causes of cardiogenic shock.[1] Stabilization of the patient while attempting to establish an exact diagnosis is paramount for all patients with cardiogenic shock (Chart 47–2).[14]

Collaborative measures to reduce myocardial damage during an AMI event include the early identification of the AMI and rapid intervention with thrombolytics, angioplasty, or coronary revascularization. Additional measures entail the use of nitroglycerin and supplemental oxygen, the control of pain, and the provision of rest. Thrombolysis and primary angioplasty have had dramatic effects on the survival of patients experiencing an AMI and on the prevention of cardiogenic shock (see Chapter 10).

Improvement of heart function is critical to the treatment of a patient with cardiogenic shock. Intravenous fluids must be administered cautiously to obtain maximal stretch of the myocardial fibers and, ultimately, optimal contraction. In some instances, too much fluid in the intravascular space leads to the need for fluid removal (diuresis), even though the patient may be borderline hypotensive. Removing excess fluid allows the myocardial fibers to obtain maximal stretch. This change is reflected in an improvement in CO and blood pressure.[14]

Positive inotropic agents, such as dobutamine (Dobutrex), dopamine (Intropin), and amrinone (Inocor), are used to increase the force of myocardial contraction, HR, and systolic ejection of blood. Dobutamine is the preferred agent unless hypotension is present. Dobutamine is a beta-adrenergic agonist that leads to an improvement in CI, oxygen delivery (DO_2), and VO_2 and a reduction in PAP, PAOP, SVR, and pulmonary vascular resistance (PVR). Dobutamine does not affect these variables in patients who remain hypovolemic. Dobutamine has the advantages of augment-

CHART 47–2

Therapeutic Approaches to Cardiogenic Shock

General resuscitation
  Monitoring of rhythm and blood pressure
  Correction of hypoxia, electrolyte abnormalities, and acid–base imbalance
  Intravascular volume management
Improvement in systolic function
  Administration of catecholamines
  Intra-aortic balloon counterpulsation
  Restoration of coronary blood flow
    Thrombolysis
    Angioplasty
    Revascularization
Maximization of preload and afterload
  Administration of normal saline solution or diuresis
  Vasodilation
Diagnosis and management of mechanical dysfunction of intracardiac structure
  Mitral valve dysfunction
  Ventricular septal defect
  Ventricular free wall rupture

ing the diastolic coronary blood flow and the collateral blood flow to the ischemic areas of the heart while increasing the heart's contractility. Although dobutamine increases myocardial oxygen demand, the improvement in coronary blood flow and, therefore, the improvement in myocardial oxygen delivery are greater than the increased oxygen demand required for increased inotropy. Positive inotropic agents and vasopressors are typically started when the systolic blood pressure drops below 100 mm Hg.[14–16]

Dopamine is the preferred inotropic agent when hypotension is present. Dopamine produces vasoconstriction of the peripheral blood vessels, thereby increasing arterial blood pressure and perfusion to vital organs. Amrinone is a phosphodiesterase inhibitor that increases the contractility of the heart without stimulating the sympathetic nervous system. Use of amrinone leads to improved CO and PAP with less of an increase on myocardial work. All three of these agents improve myocardial contractility.[14, 15]

Vasoactive drugs, such as sodium nitroprusside (Nipride) and nitroglycerin (Tridil), are also used to improve the pumping action of the heart by reducing both preload and afterload. Nitroglycerin is not as potent as sodium nitroprusside as an arteriolar vasodilator; however, it does have the advantage of limiting coronary "steal," which is the preferential coronary blood flow to nonischemic vascular beds.

Intra-aortic balloon counterpulsation (IABC) is another treatment that can be used to stabilize the patient with cardiogenic shock. The primary objectives of IABC are to increase SV, to increase diastolic coronary artery perfusion, to decrease afterload, to decrease cardiac work, and to decrease myocardial V_{O_2}. Clinical outcomes that can be anticipated in patients with cardiogenic shock receiving IABC include increases in urine output and CO and decreases in HR and MAP. Seventy-five percent of patients who receive IABC as a management strategy demonstrate clinical improvements in their condition (Chart 47–3).[14–16]

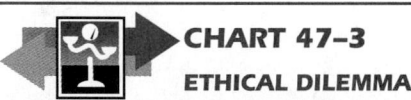

CHART 47–3

ETHICAL DILEMMA

Mr. F. is a 72-year-old man who sustained an AMI 2 days ago and developed cardiogenic shock. He is being mechanically ventilated and is receiving dopamine and dobutamine to maintain a blood pressure of 85/40 mm Hg. Mr. F. is not a candidate for coronary artery bypass surgery at this time because of his hemodynamic instability.

Mr. F. is married and has three children. His wife is 68 years old and is a retired chef. Mr. F. was an active man until this event; he played golf one to three times per week and rode a stationary bike 30 minutes three times per week. His children all live within a 30-mile radius of Mr. F. and his wife.

Mr. F. and his wife have talked about end-of-life issues. He told his wife that if anything were to happen to him, he did not want to have cardiopulmonary resuscitation performed on him or to be connected to a breathing machine. This is documented on his advance directive form and is attached to his chart.

The health care team believes that Mr. F. has a chance of surviving this event, although some evidence indicates that he sustained a stroke. A CT scan of his head revealed a right-sided density consistent with a stroke. Mr. F. is only minimally arousable, so a complete neurologic examination is not possible at this time. Mr. F.'s wife and children have spoken with the nurse and have expressed their interest in not

pursuing drastic measures concerning Mr. F.'s care because of the discussions they have had with him in the past regarding his quality of life. The cardiologist wants the family to give permission for the use of the intra-aortic balloon pump (IABP) to improve Mr. F.'s cardiac function. She explains to the family that this procedure will greatly improve Mr. F.'s chances of survival. The family members do not understand why the physician wants to be so aggressive.

1. Define the ethical dilemma in this situation.
2. What is the nurse's role as the patient's advocate in this dilemma? Is this role in conflict with the nurse's role as family advocate in this situation? Defend your response.
3. How would you respond to the family's confusion regarding the physician's interest in inserting the IABP?
4. Does Mr. F.'s advance directive help or hinder the resolution of this dilemma?
5. What institutional resources may be available to assist the family and health care team to resolve this dilemma?
6. Who has the legal authority to make the decisions for this patient? Could the enforcement of this legal authority possibly conflict with the ethical responsibility to adhere to the patient's expressed wishes and advance directive?

Cardiac transplantation is a more extreme strategy to manage the patient with cardiogenic shock. Because of the limited availability of donor organs, intermediate interventions may need to be instituted until a donor heart is available. In the critical care environment, artificial hearts and ventricular assist devices may be used to stabilize the patient who is waiting for a heart transplant.[14, 15]

In addition to these definitive management strategies, specific supportive strategies for managing patients with cardiogenic shock are also indicated. See the later section on supportive strategies in the collaborative management of shock.

DISTRIBUTIVE SHOCK

Distributive, or vasogenic, shock results in inadequate perfusion of the tissues through a maldistribution of blood flow. Intravascular volume and heart function are both normal in distributive shock; however, blood is not reaching the tissues. Distributive shock develops when acute vasodilation occurs without a simultaneous increase in intravascular volume. There are three types of distributive shock: septic shock, the most common, anaphylactic shock, and neurogenic shock.

Septic Shock

In the early 1990s, the American College of Chest Physicians and the Society of Critical Care Medicine convened a conference to clarify the terminology and definitions of systemic inflammatory response syndrome (SIRS), sepsis, and septic shock. The results of that conference are shown in Chart 47–4. SIRS is manifested by two or more of the following clinical manifestations: temperature higher than 38 or lower than 36° C; HR of more than 90 beats per minute; respiratory rate of more than 20 breaths per minute or $Paco_2$ less than 32 mm Hg; or a WBC count of more than 12,000 cells/mm^3, less than 4000 cells/mm^3, or more than 10% immature (bands) forms. SIRS can develop from various conditions (e.g., burns, pancreatitis, trauma, radiation). When SIRS develops in response to a confirmed infection, sepsis is said to be present.[17, 18]

Sepsis is the thirteenth leading cause of death in the United States and accounts for about 1 of 100 hospitalized patients, with an incidence of 500,000 to 800,000 cases a year. Sepsis accounts for 5 to 10 billion health care dollars spent annually and has a mortality rate of 40 to 60%.[1, 17] Under normal circumstances, the body has protective processes that help to keep infections under control. When these processes lose control, septic shock can result. Initially, an infection begins secondary to an alteration in the host defenses. Once the invading organism enters the body, a generalized inflammatory

CHART 47–4

Distinguishing Systemic Inflammatory Response Syndrome (SIRS), Sepsis, and Septic Shock

SIRS*

Temperature > 38.0 or < 36.0° C
Heart rate > 90 beats/min
Respiratory rate > 20 breaths/min or $Paco_2$ < 32 mm Hg
White blood cell count > 12,000 or < 4000 cells/mm^3 or > 10% immature bands

Sepsis

SIRS with a confirmed infection

Septic Shock

Sepsis with hypotension (systolic blood pressure < 90 mm Hg or a reduction of > 40 mm Hg from baseline) in the absence of other causes for hypotension that is unresponsive to adequate fluid resuscitation and occurs with perfusion abnormalities, as evidenced by, but not limited to, lactic acidosis, oliguria, or changes in mental status

*SIRS is manifested by two or more of the defining conditions.
Adapted from American College of Chest Physicians-Society of Critical Care Medicine. Consensus Conference: Definitions for sepsis and organ failure and guidelines for the use of innovative therapies in sepsis. Chest 101:1644–1655, 1992.

response is initiated. Immunogenic cells are directed to the site of infection (Figure 47–5). Initially, this response results in an elevation of blood flow and vascular permeability at the infectious site. This process facilitates the migration of specific immunogenic cells to the area. Once there, the cells begin to adhere to the foreign invaders, to identify and destroy foreign cells, and to engulf the foreign debris.[19]

The second aspect of the inflammatory response is the release of mediators from the immunogenic cells. More than 40 mediators have been implicated in the development of sepsis and septic shock. These chemical mediators cause several alterations in the vascular beds of the body. These responses are good when they are under control. When these processes do not remain under control, hypoperfusion, cellular derangements, and septic shock develop.[18, 20]

The complement cascade is activated when the body is invaded by bacteria. Activation of the comple-

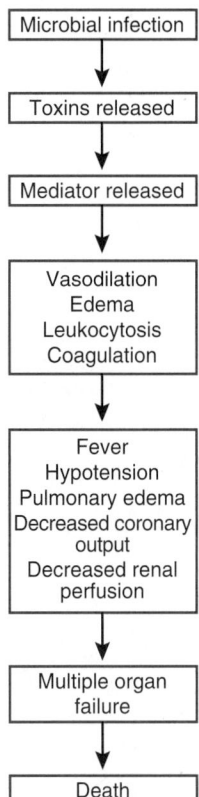

```
┌──────────────────┐
│ Microbial infection │
└──────────────────┘
         │
         ▼
┌──────────────────┐
│  Toxins released │
└──────────────────┘
         │
         ▼
┌──────────────────┐
│ Mediator released │
└──────────────────┘
         │
         ▼
┌──────────────────┐
│   Vasodilation    │
│      Edema        │
│   Leukocytosis    │
│   Coagulation     │
└──────────────────┘
         │
         ▼
┌──────────────────┐
│      Fever        │
│   Hypotension     │
│  Pulmonary edema  │
│ Decreased coronary│
│      output       │
│  Decreased renal  │
│    perfusion      │
└──────────────────┘
         │
         ▼
┌──────────────────┐
│  Multiple organ   │
│     failure       │
└──────────────────┘
         │
         ▼
┌──────────────────┐
│      Death        │
└──────────────────┘
```

Figure 47–5

Evolution of septic shock.

ment cascade initiates and enhances the inflammatory immune response. The result of complement cascade activation is the stimulation of WBC to the area of infection (chemotaxis), phagocytosis of the bacteria, WBC aggregation, vasodilation of the vascular beds, increased vascular permeability, release of leukotrienes, stimulation and the release of histamine, and stimulation of the clotting cascade. The release of large amounts of complement may promote organ dysfunction and activation of WBCs to release enzymes. These enzymes, called oxygen-derived free radicals, alter cell membrane integrity and contribute to cellular dysfunction and death.[19]

Sepsis is most commonly caused by Gram-negative bacteria (e.g., *E. coli, Pseudomonas, Klebsiella, Enterobacter, Serratia*) with Gram-positive bacteria representing the second most common causative organisms (e.g., *Staphylococcus, Streptococcus*). Gram-negative bacteria produce and release substances known as endotoxins. Endotoxins lead to the release of arachidonic acid from the membranes of cells. Once liberated, arachidonic acid is metabolized and results in the production of prostaglandin, thromboxane, leukotrienes, and prostacyclin (Figure 47–6). The end result of prostaglandin production is increased renal blood flow, bronchodilation, and venoconstriction. Thromboxane production produces platelet aggregation, vasoconstriction, and pulmonary hypertension. Leukotrienes lead to leuko-

cyte aggregation, leukocyte chemotaxis, increased vascular permeability, and venoconstriction. Prostacyclin production leads to the prevention of platelet aggregation, vasodilation, increased renal blood flow, and stimulation of renin release.[19]

The results of this inflammatory response include a maldistribution of circulating volume (distributive shock), an imbalance of oxygen supply and demand, and an alteration in cellular metabolism. The clinical manifestations of these pathophysiologic changes all relate to the compensatory mechanisms initiated to maintain blood flow to the tissues and the decompensation that results from low perfusion to the vital organs of the body.[17]

Assessment

Patients with septic shock can present in two states: an early (hyperdynamic) state or a late (hypodynamic) state. During early septic shock, the body's compensatory mechanisms respond to improve tissue perfusion. Signs of sympathetic stimulation can be observed and include an increase in HR, respiratory rate, myocardial contractility, and CO. Early septic shock is characterized by an increase in the amount of oxygen consumed by the tissues and cells. This increased Vo_2 must be balanced by an increase in the Do_2 to the tissues and cells. The body attempts to achieve this by increasing CO and minute ventilation (respiratory rate × tidal volume). To encourage tissue perfusion, CO increases and the blood vessels dilate, thus allowing more blood to flow forward. This change results in a fall in SVR. These responses are crucial to meet the oxygen demands of the cells. It is common to see young patients in early septic shock with a CO of more than 8 L per minute. Other signs and symptoms of a hyperdynamic state include warm, flushed skin, changes in LOC, fever and chills, hypoxemia, rapid, bounding peripheral pulses, and decreased urine output.[3,17,19]

The body cannot maintain this state indefinitely. If treatment is not initiated or if it is inadequate, a hypodynamic state will develop. A hypodynamic state develops when the body can no longer meet the oxygen demands of the tissues. The patient experiences a decreased CO with severe hypotension, weak, rapid, thready pulses, hypothermia, cold, clammy, mottled skin, and multiple organ failure. The key to managing this cascade of events is to recognize sepsis early and to initiate interventions quickly, to ensure adequate tissue perfusion and to avoid the sequelae of hypoperfusion.[3]

The nurse must realize that patients with septic shock can present with many different signs and symptoms. The classic signs and symptoms are fever,

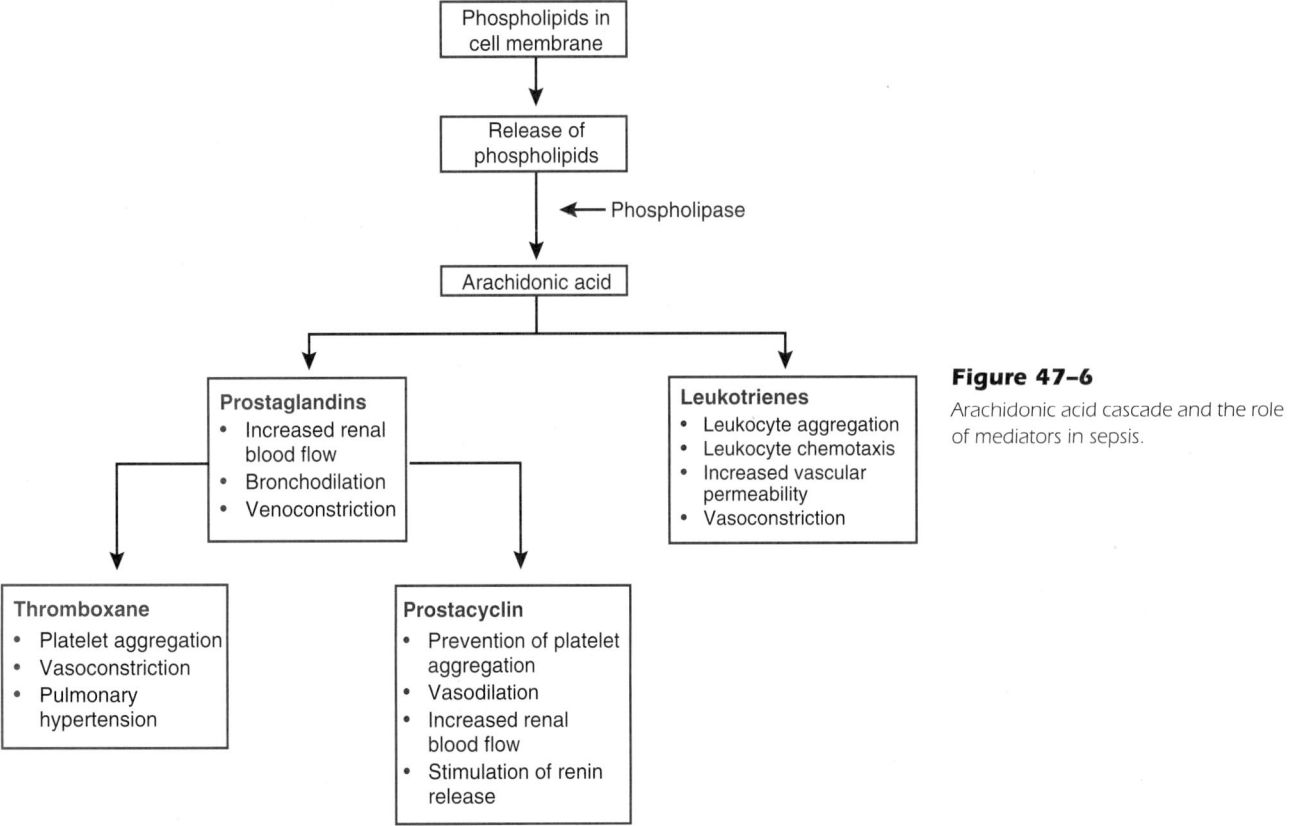

Figure 47–6
Arachidonic acid cascade and the role of mediators in sepsis.

increased HR, hypotension, and flushed skin. Additional manifestations are related to the progression of the shock state and may include tachycardia, myocardial depression from the release of myocardial depressant factor, decreased urine output, decreased LOC, metabolic acidosis related to the production of lactic acid from anaerobic metabolism, hyperventilation to compensate for the metabolic acidosis, hypoxemia, hyperglycemia or hypoglycemia, increased WBC count, decrease in platelets and clotting factors, and an elevation in fibrin split products. Ongoing assessment of the patient with septic shock is critical, to guide interventions and to evaluate the patient accurately for signs of improvement or deterioration (Chart 47–5).

Nursing Diagnoses

Patients suffering from distributive shock present unique challenges to the health care team. Although the final consequence of all distributive shock is hypoperfusion of the cells and tissues, the type of distributive shock the patient is experiencing must be considered. Nursing diagnoses appropriate for all classifications of distributive shock as well as those specific to septic shock are presented in Table 47–6.

Collaborative Management

Definitive management strategies for patients experiencing distributive shock depend on the specific type of distributive shock. Overall, management strategies for these patients are aimed at "filling the tank" and constricting the blood vessels. This is generally accomplished through the administration of intravenous fluids (e.g., normal saline, Ringer's lactate solution) and vasoconstrictors (e.g., dopamine).[17] These interventions are titrated to achieve an acceptable MAP and reestablish adequate perfusion to body organs. Additional management strategies are focused on correcting or reducing the cause of the specific shock state.

Definitive management strategies for patients experiencing septic shock include eliminating the source of infection and administering appropriate antibiotics. Eliminating the source of infection is a challenge for all members of the health care team. Specimens of blood, urine, sputum, wound drainage, peritoneal fluid, and spinal fluid may be ordered for culture and sensitivity in an attempt first to locate the source of infection. Once the source is identified, it may be appropriate to remove the nidus of infection. This may involve removing catheters or drains, débriding wounds, draining abscesses, and amputating gangrenous extremities.[1]

Antibiotic therapy should be initiated whenever sepsis is suspected. Often, a broad-spectrum antibiotic

CHART 47–5

RESEARCH UTILIZATION: ACCURACY OF FINGERSTICK GLUCOSE VALUES IN SHOCK PATIENTS

Abstract: Bedside glucose monitoring has become standard in many critical care settings. A combination of cost effectiveness and the need for rapid treatment has driven the acceptance of this practice. The purpose of this replication study was to determine the accuracy of fingerstick blood glucose measurements in patients with shock. The researchers hypothesized that there would be no differences in the mean glucose values obtained by fingerstick method, venous specimens analyzed on the bedside glucometer, and venous samples analyzed by the laboratory. In addition, they hypothesized that there would be no differences in the diagnoses and treatments subjects received as a result of the three glucose measurements. Thirty-eight critically ill patients with signs of inadequate tissue perfusion were conveniently selected, and one set of data was collected on each patient. Results indicated that mean fingerstick blood glucose values were significantly lower than the mean laboratory glucose values (P = .004), and no differences were seen in the venous specimens analyzed in the bedside glucometer versus the laboratory; thus, the first hypothesis was not supported. Further, 12 patients would have received an incorrect insulin dose (less than ordered) based on the fingerstick glucose measurements; thus, the second hypothesis was not supported. The results of this study did support previous research findings.[1]

Critique: The importance of replication research cannot be overstated. Although the researchers used a convenient sample, they did clearly define a patient with inadequate tissue perfusion. Internal validity may have been threatened by the use of multiple data collectors, although the researchers attempted to control for this by having the principal investigator train each data collector. Because of the small number of subjects, data could not be analyzed based on use of vasopressors among the sample.

Nursing Considerations: Many critically ill patients require accurate glucose monitoring as a part of their management. Patients with impaired tissue perfusion, such as those with shock, may be at risk for errors in insulin administration (specifically, undermedication) based on fingerstick glucose measurements. Although the use of vasopressors may have accounted for the observed differences in glucose measurements in this study, these agents are ordered frequently in patients with impaired tissue perfusion.

Nurses are often in position to make the decisions regarding the method of blood collection for bedside glucose analysis. The results of this and prior research have demonstrated that patients with shock are inappropriate candidates for fingerstick blood glucose analysis. This blood collection method should not be used in patients with clinical evidence of impaired tissue perfusion. Instead, nurses should use venous bedside glucose measurements or laboratory glucose results to guide clinical decisions regarding glucose monitoring and insulin administration.

1. Atkin SH, Dasmahapatra A, Jakar MA, et al: Finger stick glucose determination in shock. Ann Intern Med 114: 1020–1024, 1991.

Source: Sylvain HF, Pokorny ME, English SM, et al: Accuracy of fingerstick glucose values in shock patients. Am J Crit Care 4:44–48, 1995.

is ordered before the results of the cultures and sensitivities are known. Specific pharmacotherapy includes an aminoglycoside (e.g., gentamicin [Garamycin]) for Gram-negative bacteria, a third-generation cephalosporin (e.g., cefotaxime [Claforan]) for both Gram-negative and Gram-positive bacteria, a penicillin agent (e.g., nafcillin [Nafcil]) for Gram-positive bacteria, chloramphenicol (Chloromycetin) for anaerobic bacteria, and fluconazole (Diflucan) for fungi.[1] When administering antibiotics, the nurse needs to monitor patients for signs of effectiveness and any side effects of the drug. Many antibiotics are nephrotoxic or hepatotoxic, and monitoring kidney and liver function is important, especially if these organs are already suffering from hypoperfusion. Nurses are encouraged to consult with pharmacists to evaluate drug side effects as well as any possible drug interactions.

Currently, much pharmacologic research has been directed at halting the cascade of events that occur with sepsis and septic shock. One area of attention has

TABLE 47–6
Nursing Diagnoses: Distributive Shock

Problem Statement	Etiologic Factors
For All Classifications of Distributive Shock	
Altered tissue perfusion, peripheral	Maldistribution of intravascular blood volume; impairment in delivery of oxygen and nutrients to cells
Fluid volume deficit	Relative intravascular blood loss secondary to massive vasodilation and maldistribution of intravascular blood volume
Altered nutrition, less than body requirements	Impairment in delivery of oxygen and nutrients to cells
Anxiety and fear	Sudden critical illness and hospitalization, inadequate cerebral perfusion, invasive procedures, unknown prognosis, threat of death
Altered nutrition, less than body requirements	Impairment in delivery of oxygen and nutrients to cells
Knowledge deficit	Critical illness, prognosis, treatments, procedures
Ineffective family coping	Sudden critical illness of family member, changes in family roles
For Septic Shock	
Decreased cardiac output	Impaired myocardial contractility secondary to toxins and chemical mediators; decrease in preload secondary to vasodilation and increased capillary permeability
Ineffective thermoregulation	Invading microorganisms, inflammatory response
Impaired gas exchange	Pulmonary interstitial edema secondary to increased capillary permeability
For Anaphylactic Shock	
Decreased cardiac output	Massive vasodilation secondary to the release of vasoactive mediators in response to antigen–antibody reaction
Ineffective breathing pattern	Stridor, wheezing, bronchoconstriction secondary to chemical mediators, limited chest wall expansion
Impaired gas exchange	Pulmonary interstitial edema secondary to increased capillary permeability
Risk for impaired skin integrity	Pruritus, urticaria
For Neurogenic Shock	
Decreased cardiac output	Loss of sympathetic vasomotor tone
Hypothermia	Exposure to environmental temperatures less than body temperature

been on the inactivation of endotoxins. Endotoxin has been shown to activate the complex events associated with the immune response. The development of monoclonal antibodies against specific antigens, such as endotoxins, holds promise. These antibodies are specific for one antigen and work by binding to the antigen and signaling the body to destroy it. The destruction of the antigen or endotoxin, as in the case of sepsis, is thought to block the interaction of endotoxin with neutrophils and macrophages, thus interrupting the sepsis cascade.[21]

Additional research has studied the effects of cyclooxygenase inhibitors, such as ibuprofen (Motrin), on patients with septic shock. Cyclooxygenase inhibitors reduce the production of arachidonic acid metabolites involved in the inflammatory response activated in sepsis and septic shock (see Figure 47–6). The use of nonsteroidal anti-inflammatory agents, such as ibuprofen, also shows promise, although more research is needed.[21]

Finally, the use of naloxone (Narcan) in patients with septic shock has been studied. Endorphins, endogenous opiates, are released during septic shock and contribute to the generalized vasodilation and cardiovascular instability. Naloxone, a narcotic antagonist, is given as a continuous infusion and works by competing for the opiate receptor sites. This competition ultimately inhibits the binding of the endorphins to receptor sites. Some studies have demonstrated an increase in systolic blood pressure and MAP when naloxone is given early in the shock state.[19,21]

In addition to these definitive management strategies, specific supportive strategies for managing patients with septic shock are also indicated. See the later section on supportive strategies in the collaborative management of shock.

Anaphylactic Shock

Anaphylactic shock, the second example of distributive shock, is the most severe manifestation of allergy and can occur after exposure of sensitized persons to drugs, foods, insect venoms, or other allergens. The

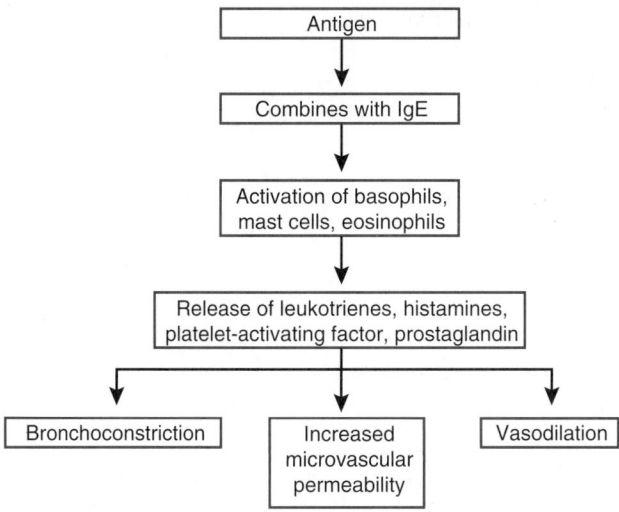

Figure 47-7

Evolution of anaphylactic shock.

mechanism of shock is distributive because the accompanying release of histamine and vasoactive compounds from mast cells leads to massive vasodilation and increased capillary permeability.[1]

During anaphylactic shock, an antigen attaches to immunoglobulin E (IgE) and activates basophils, mast cells, and eosinophils. These cells are responsible for producing and releasing leukotrienes, histamine, platelet-activating factor, prostaglandins, and other mediators that increase microvascular permeability, vasodilation, and bronchoconstriction (Figure 47-7).[9]

Assessment

Signs and symptoms of anaphylactic shock can begin within 20 minutes of exposure to the allergen. The severity of the reaction is greater if the signs and symptoms occur soon after the exposure to the allergen. The clinical manifestations of anaphylactic shock can progress from the earliest sign of the patient feeling "warm" to the later signs of urticaria, pruritus, and angioedema. Some patients report a sense of "impending doom." Laryngeal edema may develop and can result in hoarseness and stridor. Severe bronchoconstriction may also occur and results in wheezing, cyanosis, and severe respiratory distress.

Peripheral vasodilation and increased capillary permeability produce pooling of blood in the periphery and a decrease in right ventricular preload. This decrease can be severe enough to reduce left ventricular preload, with a resultant increase in HR and decrease in CO and blood pressure. Hemodynamic monitoring of patients with anaphylactic shock may show a decreased SVR secondary to dilation of the peripheral

vessels, decreased CO and CI, and decreases in CVP, PAP, and PAOP. SvO_2 is also decreased because of the reduction in CO and increased extraction of oxygen from the blood that is reaching the tissues (see Table 47-3).[1,9]

Anaphylactic shock can progress to death quickly. It is vital that the nurse rapidly assess the patient to provide the necessary emergency interventions and to monitor the effectiveness of these interventions.

Nursing Diagnoses

Nursing diagnoses for all classifications of distributive shock, as well as those specific to anaphylactic shock, are presented in Table 47-6.

Collaborative Management

Definitive management strategies for patients experiencing anaphylactic shock include the identification and removal of the causative antigen and the reversal of the effects of the chemical mediators. For example, if the anaphylactic response is a result of a blood transfusion or an antibiotic reaction, the nurse should stop the infusion immediately. Other measures may include removing a bee stinger or performing gastric lavage to remove the causative agent from the stomach. In some instances, removal of the antigen may not be possible (e.g., anaphylactic reactions to contrast dye), or the antigen may not be known.[1]

Management strategies directed at reversing the effects of the mediator substances include the administration of epinephrine to restore arterial blood pressure, the use of antihistamines (e.g., diphenhydramine [Benadryl]) to reverse the effects of histamine, and the use of aminophylline (theophylline) or other bronchodilators (e.g., Albuterol [Proventil]) to reduce bronchoconstriction. The use of corticosteroids may also be considered to reverse the adverse effects of the immune response.[1] Prostaglandin, leukotriene, and platelet-activator inhibitors are currently under investigation for use in patients with anaphylactic shock.[17] Patients with anaphylactic shock present with a life-threatening and dramatic clinical situation. Nurses, physicians, and respiratory therapists are called on to intervene quickly, to halt the cascade of events that occur in this type of shock.

In addition to these definitive management strategies, specific supportive strategies for managing patients with anaphylactic shock are also indicated. See the later section on supportive strategies in the collaborative management of shock.

Neurogenic Shock

A third type of distributive shock is neurogenic shock. Neurogenic shock primarily occurs in patients with spinal cord injuries or diseases above the midthoracic region. It may also occur in patients who sustain direct injury to the medullary vasomotor center in the brain, who receive high spinal anesthesia, or who experience severe pain or emotional distress. These conditions result in the loss of sympathetic vasoconstrictor tone and cause the patient to experience global vasodilation. This maldistribution of the blood results in decreased preload, SV, CO, and blood pressure. Bradycardia develops as a result of the inhibition of the baroreceptor response. The loss of reflex tachycardia further compromises CO and tissue perfusion (see Table 47–3). Finally, patients with neurogenic shock develop impaired thermoregulation because of the loss of vasomotor tone in the cutaneous blood vessels. Consequently, patients become poikilothermic; that is, they assume the temperature of the environment. Although neurogenic shock is rare and usually transitory, the effects are serious. As with other forms of shock, tissue perfusion and cellular metabolism are impaired and, if not corrected, can result in organ failure and death.[1,22]

Assessment

Patients can develop neurogenic shock within 60 minutes after a spinal cord injury, and the shock state can continue for several weeks. The presenting signs and symptoms usually include hypotension, HR less than 60, warm, dry skin, and hypothermia.[1,22] Additional signs of hypoperfusion can include a decrease in urine output, changes in LOC, decrease in peripheral pulses, and a capillary refill of more than or equal to 3 seconds. Patients who have neurogenic shock related to a spinal cord injury should also be assessed for changes in respiratory patterns (rate, rhythm, depth).

Nursing Diagnoses

Nursing diagnoses for all classifications of distributive shock, as well as those specific to neurogenic shock, are presented in Table 47–6.

Collaborative Management

Definitive management strategies for patients experiencing neurogenic shock vary according to the cause. For patients with spinal cord injuries, early and proper stabilization of the spinal cord is critical to preventing or limiting neurogenic shock. If neurogenic shock is a result of severe pain, appropriate analgesia is imperative. Postoperatively, nurses must properly position patients who receive spinal anesthesia, to prevent blockage of sympathetic outflow.[1]

In addition to these definitive management strategies, specific supportive strategies for managing patients with neurogenic shock are also indicated. See the next section of this chapter.

Collaborative Management of Shock: Supportive Strategies

In addition to the definitive management strategies for the various types of shock, supportive management strategies are initiated to increase Do_2, to establish and maintain tissue perfusion, and to preserve normal cell function.[1] Measures to improve Do_2 include establishing and maintaining the patient's airway. Establishing an effective airway may involve simple positioning, the placement of an oropharyngeal or nasopharyngeal airway, or the insertion of an endotracheal or tracheostomy tube. Once the airway is established, maintenance of the airway becomes critical. Nurses, together with respiratory therapists, should provide chest physical therapy and suctioning as needed.

Measures to improve ventilation early in the shock state may include deep breathing and coughing, incentive spirometry, and supplemental oxygen (e.g., oxygen by nasal cannula). As shock progresses, however, patients begin to hypoventilate because of respiratory muscle fatigue. Mechanical ventilation with high concentrations of inspired oxygen is usually required to provide adequate ventilation and to correct hypoxemia. If the shock state and hypoxemia are not corrected quickly, positive end-expiratory pressure (PEEP) may need to be added to improve the patient's blood oxygen level. The nurse, in collaboration with the physician and respiratory therapist, needs to monitor the patient's clinical response to mechanical ventilation (e.g., arterial blood gases, pulse oximetry, and respiratory rate and rhythm).[1,17]

Establishing and maintaining adequate tissue perfusion depend on several variables. Optimal intravascular volume is critical to the delivery of oxygen to the cells. Fluids are ordered as needed, and nurses must evaluate the patient's clinical response to the fluid therapy. Evaluation parameters are usually determined by the physician and vary among individual patients. For example, an adequate intravascular volume may be determined by systolic pressure of more than 90 mm Hg, CO more than 4 L per minute, normal filling pressures, MAP more than 75 mm Hg, +2 peripheral pulses, capillary refill less than 3 seconds, urine output more than 30 mL per hour, and an appropriate LOC.[1]

Often, adequate CO cannot be achieved in spite of an adequate intravascular volume, and pharmacologic interventions are required. Drugs that influence myocardial contractility, filling pressures, and SVR are frequently given in combination. For example, a positive inotropic agent, such as dobutamine, may be given to increase myocardial contractility, SV, and CO. Concurrently, nitroprusside may be administered to reduce preload, afterload, and myocardial oxygen demand and to improve CO. The nurse monitoring patients who receive multiple drug therapies to improve CO must realize that the effects of these drugs are optimized when hypoxemia, acidosis, and electrolyte imbalances are corrected.[1] Careful monitoring of these patients for signs of improved perfusion is critical when titrating these drugs. Target parameters are determined in consultation with the physician, and the minimum dose needed to achieve the desired effect is administered.

A minimal MAP is essential to tissue perfusion and organ preservation during shock. If parenteral fluid administration and cardioselective drug therapies do not improve blood pressure, it may be necessary to consider vasopressors (e.g., norepinephrine [Levophed], dopamine). These drugs work by increasing peripheral resistance (SVR) and must be titrated cautiously to achieve minimal perfusion pressures. Because these drugs constrict blood vessels in nonvital organs, tissue perfusion and DO_2 to these areas are impaired. The nurse must carefully monitor the patient's periphery for signs of cyanosis and diminished or absent pulses. In addition, nonvital organs (e.g., liver, gastrointestinal tract) should be assessed frequently for signs of dysfunction or failure. These devastating effects result from the prolonged administration of vasoconstrictors and are usually poor prognostic indicators.[1]

Other variables that promote adequate tissue perfusion include adequate red blood cell volume and SaO_2. Blood transfusions are ordered as needed to achieve and maintain a hemoglobin of more than 7 g/dL. Continuous pulse oximetry is initiated, and a saturation of more than 93% is targeted. In addition to ensuring adequate hemoglobin and SaO_2, the nurse must determine whether or not the oxygen is being released at the cellular level. The nurse should monitor variables that influence the release of oxygen from hemoglobin (e.g., normal pH and serum phosphate level, normothermia) to facilitate optimal use of oxygen at the cellular level.[1]

Finally, it may be necessary to initiate supportive strategies aimed at restoring metabolic balance in patients with shock. As previously discussed, metabolic acidosis results from anaerobic metabolism and from impaired renal function, both secondary to hypoperfusion states. Hyperventilation may be used to facilitate the removal of excess carbon dioxide, and, in severely acidotic states, sodium bicarbonate may be added to parenteral fluids. Ventilatory changes and adjustments in drug dosages are guided by arterial blood gases and the patient's response to the interventions. Attention to the patient's electrolyte balance and temperature status is also necessary when providing metabolic support. The nurse must monitor the patient for signs and symptoms of electrolyte disturbances and must administer replacement electrolytes as needed. The patient should be normothermic, and antipyretics and cooling or warming blankets are used accordingly. Adequate nutrition and gut protection also play an important role in supporting the patient's metabolic needs. The nurse consults with the physician and dietitian to determine the optimal route for providing nutrition to the patient with shock.[1]

In summary, the management of the patient in shock is a collaborative effort that relies on the health care team to apply the definitive and supportive strategies necessary to improve perfusion to the cells and to maintain cellular function.

Multidisciplinary Outcomes

The multidisciplinary outcomes for the patient with shock relate primarily to the stabilization of the patient, identification and treatment of the underlying cause of the hypoperfusion state, and return of the patient to an optimal level of functioning. The health care team is responsible for working collaboratively to develop an appropriate plan of care directed toward achieving the best possible patient outcomes (Chart 47–6). Patients who survive shock have experienced a life-threatening situation that may have lasted less than an hour (e.g., anaphylactic shock) or several weeks (e.g., septic shock). The patient and family must be included in the development and implementation of the plan, to ensure realistic expectations (Chart 47–7).

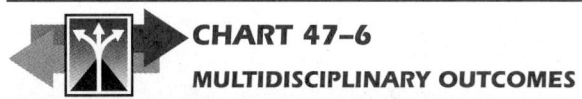

CHART 47–6
MULTIDISCIPLINARY OUTCOMES

Restoration and maintenance of adequate fluid volume
Restoration of adequate tissue perfusion
Stabilization of hemodynamic parameters
Normalization of ventilation and gas exchange
Stabilization of temperature
Prevention of complications related to acute illness
Stabilization of psychosocial well-being
Normalization of nutritional status
Self-management of therapeutic regimen
Achievement of optimal level of functioning

CHART 47-7

BEYOND THE ICU: STRATEGIES TO PREVENT SHOCK AND TO FACILITATE RECOVERY AFTER SHOCK

Patients at risk for developing shock are often not located in critical care units. Nurses in noncritical care settings must be able to identify these patients and to prevent shock whenever possible. Vigilant nursing care that includes thorough nursing histories, astute observation skills, and ongoing assessments is paramount to identifying these patients. For example, all postoperative patients are at risk of developing hypovolemic shock. Prevention strategies should include ongoing assessment of vital signs, including the cardinal parameters of tissue perfusion. Should overt bleeding occur, the nurse can minimize blood loss by quickly applying direct pressure to the bleeding site and notifying the surgeon.

Similarly, anaphylactic shock can be prevented by first obtaining a detailed history of a patient's allergies. For patients with impaired communication, the family should be consulted. Extreme caution should be taken when administering the initial dose of any intravenous medication. When transfusing blood or blood products, the nurse must follow institutional policies regarding patient identification and match. Patients should be monitored closely for signs of an allergic reaction, especially during the first 15 minutes of the transfusion. If a reaction is suspected (e.g., flushing, dyspnea, pruritus), the nurse must immediately discontinue the transfusion, maintain a patent intravenous line with normal saline solution, and notify the physician.

The prevention and early detection of sepsis and septic shock in hospitalized patients are critical. Nurses must first identify patients at risk for sepsis (e.g., age > 65 years, presence of chronic illnesses, use of invasive catheters) and must strive to protect them from infections. Strict attention to aseptic technique and hand washing in addition to careful monitoring of the patient for signs of local (e.g., redness, drainage) and systemic (e.g., temperature, elevated WBC count) infections are important nursing roles.

In spite of the best nursing efforts, some patients develop shock. Although the prognosis is often poor, many patients survive. Unfortunately, the cost of survival may be emotionally or physically high. Once these patients leave the critical care unit, nursing care is focused on recovery. Recovery varies, based on the type and extent of shock the patient experienced. For example, patients surviving cardio-

genic shock from an acute myocardial infarction are faced with severe myocardial dysfunction that may limit their ability to resume previous lifestyles. Cardiac rehabilitation is often recommended, and nurses in this setting work with patients and families to maximize their level of functioning. Other patients may be severely debilitated and may be placed on a waiting list for heart transplantation.

Patients recovering from neurogenic shock secondary to spinal cord injury are often transferred to a rehabilitation facility. There, nurses work closely with the patient and his or her support group to facilitate physical and emotional adjustment to the devastating life role changes.

Anaphylactic shock from foreign antigens, such as insect bites, often occurs in previously healthy persons. Surviving a potentially life-threatening event may leave patients frightened and in need of education regarding prevention and treatment of further reactions. Nurses should encourage all patients to obtain and wear medic alert identification regarding their allergies. In addition, it is often recommended that patients carry emergency drugs (e.g., epinephrine) with them. Patients and their families need to be taught the proper method of injecting the drugs as well as the importance of obtaining emergency help should an anaphylactic reaction occur outside the hospital.

Shock states predispose patients to organ dysfunction or failure. Acute tubular necrosis secondary to renal ischemia is a common complication of shock. Many times, patients require dialysis while the kidney heals. This need may continue even after the patient is discharged. Pulmonary complications (e.g., acute respiratory distress syndrome) are also frequently seen in patients with prolonged periods of shock. Most patients require intubation and mechanical ventilation. Weaning from mechanical ventilation may be prolonged in the presence of coexisting illnesses (e.g., chronic obstructive pulmonary disease). Patients may need to be transferred to transitional care units to facilitate the weaning process.

The physical and emotional consequences of shock can be far-reaching, affecting the patient and the patient's family long after the acute event. Nurses in various settings need to provide technical as well as psychological interventions to maximize the recovery of a patient who survives shock.

Data from Rice V: Shock: A Clinical Syndrome, 2nd ed. Aliso Viejo, CA, American Association of Critical Care Nurses, 1997.

Critical Thinking Exercise

Mr. K. is a 34-year-old man who was thrown from his trail bike. He was wearing a helmet at the time of his accident. Mr. K. was found by a neighbor, who called for an ambulance, which arrived about 15 minutes later. At the scene, Mr. K.'s vital signs were as follows: blood pressure, 168/92; HR, 98; and respiratory rate, 24. An intravenous infusion of Ringer's lactate solution was started. Mr. K. did not lose consciousness during the event and was able to remember what happened. He complained of left upper quadrant pain and of multiple bruises and lacerations to his arms and legs. He was placed on a backboard with a cervical collar and was transported to the emergency department (ED).

Mr. K.'s vital signs upon arrival in the ED were as follows: blood pressure, 180/92; HR, 118; and respiratory rate, 28. A second intravenous line was started, and additional fluids were infused. A CT scan of the abdomen was performed and revealed a splenic laceration with active bleeding. Cervical and lumbar spine radiographs were negative. Initial laboratory studies revealed the following: WBC count, 29.1; hemoglobin, 13; hematocrit, 39; platelet count, 283; prothrombin time/partial thromboplastin time, 12.8/21.3 seconds; and lactate level, 7.4 (normal lactate level, 0.5–2.8 mEq/L). In the ED, Mr. K. received 4 L of NSS, 1 U of dextran, and 2 U of PRBCs. Mr. K.'s urine output was 250 mL on insertion of a Foley catheter, but it has been minimal since then. During this time, Mr. K. became anxious and confused. He was transported to the operating room and underwent a splenectomy. Estimated blood loss was 10 L preoperatively and 4 L postoperatively. He was in the operating room for 3 hours.

Mr. K. arrived in the ICU with a blood pressure of 106/54, a HR of 95, a respiratory rate of 14 on mechanical ventilation, and Sao$_2$ of 100%. Two hours later, his blood pressure dropped to 80/30, and his HR increased to 145. His intravenous fluids were increased to wide open. He was returned to the operating room, where surgeons found that rebleeding had occurred. Two hours later, Mr. K. returned to the ICU.

On return to the ICU, Mr. K.'s vital signs were as follows: blood pressure, 114/60; HR, 104; and respiratory rate, 16 on mechanical ventilation. Laboratory results revealed the following: WBC count, 18; hematocrit, 9.3; hemoglobin, 3.2; platelets, 23; and lactate, 11.5. Mr. K. received 4 U of PRBCs along with his intravenous fluids, which were being infused at a rate of 250 mL per hour. Urine output was 15 mL per hour.

Over the next 6 hours, Mr. K.'s intravascular volume was replaced. Throughout the day, he received 5 additional U of PRBCs. By the next morning, his laboratory results were as follows: hematocrit, 28; hemoglobin, 9.6; platelets, 70; and lactate, 1.4. Mr. K. was breathing on his own and was successfully weaned and extubated. On postoperative day 2, Mr. K. spiked a temperature of 39.2°C and complained of difficulty in breathing (respiratory rate, 26).

1. Why were PRBCs selected to restore Mr. K.'s hemodynamic status?
2. Provide rationales for the administration of crystalloids and a plasma expander (in addition to the PRBCs) in the initial treatment of Mr. K. in the ED.
3. If Mr. K.'s spleen was ruptured and he was bleeding into his abdomen, why was his blood pressure in the ED 180/92 mm Hg?
4. What class of blood loss did Mr. K. experience? Identify the clinical evidence that supports your selection.
5. What is the significance in the changes in Mr. K.'s lactate levels?
6. Provide possible explanations for the clinical changes in Mr. K. on postoperative day 2. What orders would you expect based on these changes and why?

Key Concepts

➡ Two criteria are necessary for the diagnosis of shock: reduction in MAP to less than 60 mm Hg and clinical evidence of hypoperfusion of vital organs.

➡ When a low-perfusion state occurs, compensatory mechanisms are activated to improve tissue perfusion and to preserve tissue function.

➡ Neural compensatory mechanisms include the baroreceptor reflex, central nervous system ischemic response, reflex venoconstriction, and chemoreceptor stimulation. In general, these mechanisms respond by causing vasoconstriction and an increase in the rate and depth of respirations.

➡ Hormonal compensatory mechanisms include the norepinephrine–epinephrine vasoconstrictor mechanism, renin–angiotensin system activation, and the release of ADH and glucocorticoids. These complex responses result in increases in blood pressure (vasoconstriction) and heart rate (cardiac stimulation), decreases in urine output (fluid preservation), and release of glucose (energy substrates).

➡ During periods of hypoperfusion (shock), oxygen supply to the cells is inadequate, resulting in a change from aerobic to anaerobic metabolism.

➡ Metabolic acidosis develops when the by-product of anaerobic metabolism, lactic acid, accumulates. As cellular pH drops, the integrity of the cell is lost and the cell dies.

➡ Lactic acid levels are used as a prognostic indicator of hypoperfusion states.

➡ The consequences of hypoperfusion are manifested in every body system. Careful and frequent assessment of patients is necessary to monitor the progression of shock as well as the effectiveness of interventions.

➡ The cardinal parameters of tissue perfusion include LOC, skin, urine output, and vital signs (temperature, HR, respiratory rate, peripheral pulses, blood pressure).

➡ Changes in the pulmonary microcirculation during shock can precipitate acute respiratory distress syndrome.

➡ When compensatory mechanisms fail, patients in shock are at risk of acute tubular necrosis, further acidosis, and death.

➡ If the shock state is prolonged, hepatic failure can occur, and the patient can develop jaundice, asterixis, coagulopathies, and drug toxicities.

➡ The three major classifications of shock are hypovolemic, cardiogenic, and distributive. Distributive shock includes septic shock, anaphylactic shock, and neurogenic shock.

➡ External fluid losses represent the majority of causes of hypovolemic shock. Definitive management strategies include correcting the cause of the volume depletion and restoring intravascular volume.

➡ Often, a combination of crystalloids and blood products is used to restore intravascular volume.

➡ Cardiogenic shock from an AMI results in the loss of the body's ability to pump blood forward. Definitive management strategies are directed toward preserving left ventricular function and improving the effectiveness of the pumping action of the heart.

➡ Treatment of cardiogenic shock can include the administration of positive inotropic agents, vasopressors, and vasodilators. In addition, IABC, left ventricular assist devices, and heart transplantation may be considered.

➡ Septic shock develops as a consequence of overactivity of the patient's immune system in response to an infection. Patients with septic shock may present in either a hyperdynamic (early) state or a hypodynamic (late) state.

➡ Definitive management strategies for patients with septic shock include eliminating the source of the infection and initiating antibiotic therapy.

➡ Anaphylactic shock, the most severe form of allergy, is treated with epinephrine to restore arterial blood pressure, with antihistamines (e.g., diphenhydramine) to reverse the effects of histamine, with aminophylline (theophylline) or other bronchodilators to reduce bronchoconstriction, and with corticosteroids to reverse the adverse effects of the immune response.

➡ Patients with neurogenic shock suffer massive vasodilation because of the loss of sympathetic tone,

and management strategies are related to the cause. For example, if the patient has suffered a spinal cord injury, stabilization of the spine is critical.

➡ Supportive management strategies for patients with shock are directed toward increasing oxygen delivery (DO_2), establishing and maintaining tissue perfusion, and preserving cell function.

➡ Although the prognosis for patients with shock varies according to the type of shock, the length of the shock state, and preexisting patient factors, patients do survive. Recovery from this life-threatening event can be complex and extensive.

References

1. Rice V: Shock: A Clinical Syndrome, 2nd ed. Aliso Viejo, CA, American Association of Critical Care Nurses, 1997.
2. Cornwell E, Kennedy F, Rodrigues J: The critical care of the severely injured patient. Surg Clin North Am 76:959–969, 1996.
3. Vary T, Kearney M: Pathophysiology of traumatic shock and multiple organ system failure. In: Cardona V, Hurn P, Bastinagel-Mason P, et al (eds): Trauma Nursing from Resuscitation Through Rehabilitation, 2nd ed. Philadelphia, W.B. Saunders, 1994, pp 114–150.
4. Leier C: Approach to the patient with hypotension and shock. In: Kelley W (ed): Textbook of Internal Medicine, 3rd ed. Philadelphia, Lippincott–Raven, 1997, pp 361–370.
5. Britt L, Weireter L, Riblet J, et al: Priorities in the management of profound shock. Surg Clin North Am 76:645–660, 1996.
6. American College of Surgeons: The Advanced Trauma Life Support Student Manual. Chicago, American College of Surgeons, 1993.
7. Baron B, Scalea T: Acute blood loss. Emerg Med Clin North Am 14:35–55, 1996.
8. McQuillan K: Initial management of traumatic shock. In: Cardona V, Hurn P, Bastinagel-Mason P, et al (eds): Trauma Nursing from Resuscitation Through Rehabilitation, 2nd ed. Philadelphia, W.B. Saunders, 1994, pp 152–178.
9. Jones K: Shock. In: Clochesy J, Breu C, Cardin S, et al (eds): Critical Care Nursing, 2nd ed. Philadelphia, W.B. Saunders, 1996, pp 1371–1380.
10. Daleiden A: Physiology and treatment of hemorrhagic shock during the early postoperative period. Crit Care Q 16:45–59, 1993.
11. Phlederer T: Emergency fluid management for hypovolemia. Postgrad Med 100:243–254, 1996.
12. Rodgers K: Cardiovascular shock. Emerg Med Clin North Am 13:793–810, 1996.
13. Astiz ME, Rackow EC, Weil MH: Pathophysiology and treatment of circulatory shock. Crit Care Clin 9:183–203, 1993.
14. Califf R, Bengtson J: Cardiogenic shock. N Engl J Med 330:1724–1728, 1994.
15. Astiz ME, Rachow EC: Assessing perfusion failure during circulatory shock. Crit Care Clin 9:299–312, 1993.
16. Howell J: Acute myocardial infarction and congestive heart failure. Emerg Med Clin North Am 14:83–91, 1996.
17. Ferguson K, Brown L: Bacteremia and sepsis. Emerg Med Clin North Am 14:185–195, 1996.
18. American College of Chest Physicians–Society of Critical Care Medicine Consensus Conference: Definitions of sepsis and organ failure and guidelines for the use of innovative therapies in sepsis. Crit Care Med 20:862–875, 1992.

19. Clochesy J: Patients with systemic inflammatory response syndrome. In: Clochesy J, Breu C, Cardin S, et al (eds): Critical Care Nursing, 2nd ed. Philadelphia, W.B. Saunders, 1996, pp 1359–1370.

20. Crowley S: The pathogenesis of septic shock. Heart Lung 25:124–134, 1996.

21. Wiessner WH, Casey LC, Zbilut JP: Treatment of sepsis and septic shock: a review. Heart Lung 24:380–392, 1995.

22. Nolan S: Current trends in the management of acute spinal cord injury. Crit Care Nurs Q 17:64–78, 1994.

48

Burns

Elisabeth Greenfield

Objectives

After completing this chapter, the student will be able to:

1. Relate the pathophysiology of thermal injury to the plan of care for the patient who has suffered burn injury.
2. Implement appropriate patient assessment strategies for the resuscitation and acute phases of burn management.
3. Relate the pathophysiology of thermal injury to the major systemic effects of burn injury.
4. Evaluate the adequacy of fluid resuscitation for a patient who has suffered burn injury.
5. Select appropriate measures for burn wound management.
6. Implement appropriate psychosocial interventions in the plan of care for the patient after burn injury.
7. Formulate a collaborative plan of care that extends across the three phases of burn injury.
8. Select appropriate interventions for patients with different types of thermal injuries and exfoliative skin conditions through the three phases of recovery.
9. Evaluate effects of collaborative care on anticipated outcomes for the patient with burn injury.

Over the past several decades, the improvement in survival after thermal injury and exfoliative skin diseases that pose problems similar to burns has been dramatic. Advances in fluid resuscitation, ventilatory support, nutritional support, infection-control policies, and wound care have contributed significantly to improved patient outcomes. Of all the challenges a nurse faces, caring for the critically ill burn patient is one of the greatest. Because of the multiorgan physiologic response elicited by this catastrophe, this group of patients has often been referred to as the universal trauma model.[1]

ANATOMY AND PHYSIOLOGY OF THE SKIN

As the body's largest organ, the skin has distinct and vital functions (Table 48–1). The skin is composed of two distinctive layers, the dermis and the epidermis. The epidermis, or outer layer, is thinner, ranging from 0.5 to 1.0 mm. It is avascular and is composed primarily of epithelial cells, but it also contains melanocytes that produce pigmentation, Langerhans' cells that provide immunologic protection, Merkel cells that serve as mechanoreceptors, and keratinocytes that produce keratin. Sebaceous glands, hair follicles, and sweat glands are epidermal appendages that extend into the dermis. The dermis is approximately 10 times thicker than the epidermis and contains sensory fibers for pain, pressure, temperature, and touch. The superficial papillary layer, or the first layer of the dermis, contains a rich lymphatic and vascular supply that plays a major role in skin metabolism and nourishment. The next layer is the reticular layer, which contains primarily fibroblasts. Fibroblasts are active in both collagen and elastin production and provide mechanical strength and elasticity to the skin. In addition, the reticular layer contains macrophages that produce an immunologic response and histamine-and-heparin producing mast cells that play an important role in the inflammatory response to local injury.

Below the dermis is the hypodermis or subcutaneous tissue. This tissue is composed of fat and supports the blood vessels and nerves that pass from the tissue below to the dermis above. It also contains the panniculus adiposus, the connective tissue responsible for fat formation. Fat provides heat insulation, acts as a

TABLE 48–1
Functions of the Skin

Function	Description
Thermoregulation	Prevents heat loss
	Allows for rapid cooling through evaporation of sweat and dermal vasodilatation
Neurosensory role	Provides sensory contact with the environment
	Is organ of sensation for pain, heat, cold, and touch
Fluid and electrolyte balance	Prevents excessive losses of fluids, proteins, and electrolytes
	Helps to control fluid and electrolyte excretion
Protective barrier	Protects from harmful environmental elements such as heat, cold, and radiation
Immunologic role	Protects against infection by interfering with the entrance of microorganisms
	Uses the process of desquamation to dispose of bacteria
	Possesses antibacterial properties
Metabolism	Produces vitamin D
Cosmesis	Provides personal identity
	Plays a role in physical attraction and body image

mechanical shock absorber, and serves as a calorie reservoir. Figure 48–1 depicts a diagram of normal skin and associated burn depth injury.

ETIOLOGY AND PATHOPHYSIOLOGY

Etiology

Thermal injury results from exposure to open flames or radiation or contact with hot liquids, caustic chemicals, or electric current. Frostbite, another form of

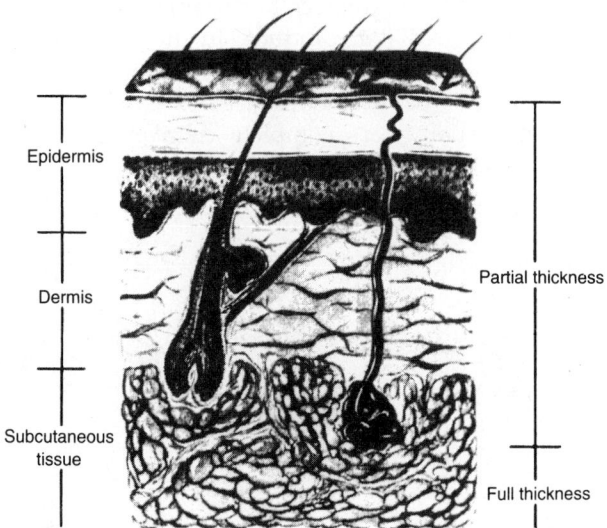

Figure 48–1

Schematic illustration of skin and subcutaneous tissue, demonstrating the relationship between the depth of burn and the corresponding anatomic structures. Partial-thickness burns heal because dermal elements necessary to generate new skin remain. In full-thickness burns, these elements are destroyed; the wound does not heal and must be closed by skin grafting. (From Pruitt BA et al: Burns including cold, chemical, and electrical injuries. In: Sabiston DC (ed): Textbook of Surgery: The Biological Basis of Modern Surgical Practice. Philadelphia, W.B. Saunders, 1996, p. 222.)

thermal injury, results from prolonged exposure to extreme cold. Some of the influential factors in the causes and risks of burn injury and death include age, occupation, economic status, season of the year, and geographic location. Persons of low economic status, children, and the elderly are at greater risk for injury from burns. Exposure to flames, usually from house fires or ignition of clothing, is the predominant cause of adult admissions to burn centers, whereas the most common cause in children under the age of 5 years is scalding from hot liquids.[2] Sources estimate that approximately 1.4 million people in the United States are burned each year, and of these, 270 people per million require hospitalization for burn injury annually. Approximately 82 people per million are considered to have a major burn injury. The American Burn Association (ABA) has classified burn injuries according to severity and has made recommendations for patients requiring transfer to a recognized burn center based on the of the extent of injury, associated injuries, pre-existing disease, and the presence or absence of involvement of critical areas.[3] Chart 48–1 summarizes burn injury classification by the severity of burn injury.

Pathophysiology

Mechanism of Injury

Thermal injury causes coagulation necrosis from denaturation of cellular proteins that may involve both the skin and the underlying tissue. With prolonged exposure to temperatures of 44°C (111°F) or greater, cellular dysfunction becomes evident. Impairment of the sodium membrane pump, which results in a high intracellular sodium content and swelling, is a primary example of loss of cellular homeostasis. The depth and severity of tissue injury are determined by the tem-

CHART 48-1

American Burn Association Criteria for Burn Center Referral

Burns with TBSA >10%, <10 years, partial-thickness burns

Burns with TBSA >10%, >50 years, partial-thickness burns

Burns with TBSA >20%, other ages

Burns with TBSA >5%, full-thickness burns

Any burns that involve the hands, feet, face, perineum, or major joints

Circumferential burns of the chest or extremities

Electrical injury

Extensive chemical injury

Significant associated injuries that could complicate recovery

Suspicion of inhalation injury

Major preexisting disease

TBSA, total body surface area.

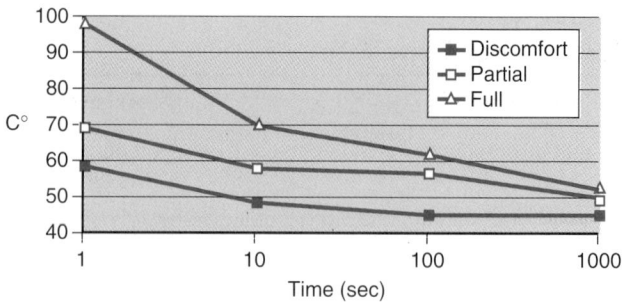

Figure 48-2

This graph depicts the time–surface temperature thresholds at which cutaneous burning occurs.

perature of the heat source, the duration of contact time with the injuring agent, the amount of tissue exposed to the source, and the body's ability to dissipate the thermal energy. As depicted in Figure 48–2, the extent of tissue damage increases in direct proportion to temperature and exposure time. Tissue destruction can occur in 3 to 5 seconds with exposure to temperatures of 140°F or 60°C. Because of their thinner skin, children and the elderly are at greater risk of injury from lower temperatures and shorter durations of contact.

Local Response

Figure 48–3 shows the most common method of depicting the relation of tissue effects to severity of injury and ultimate tissue viability in the three zones of injury described by Jackson.[4] The innermost zone, or zone of coagulation, represents the area of cellular death. The penetration or extension of the zone of coagulation into the dermis determines the depth of injury. The adjacent zone is the zone of stasis. Because damage in this area is less severe and most cells are initially viable, tissue injury is potentially reversible. Restoration of blood flow and attenuation of the inflammatory response are key to maintaining tissue viability. This area may rapidly progress to ischemia and necrosis in the absence of adequate fluid resuscitation. The outermost zone is the zone of hyperemia and is characterized by minimal cellular damage. As a result of vasoactive mediators produced by the initial inflammatory response, blood flow and vasodilatation increase in this area. In the absence of trauma or infection, one usually sees complete cellular and tissue recovery in this area.

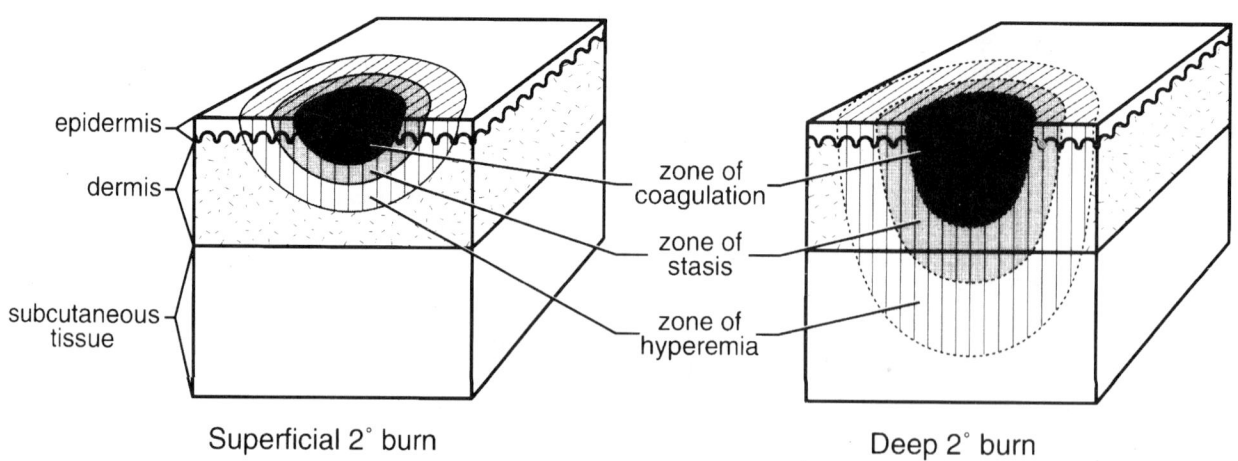

Figure 48-3

A diagrammatic rendition of Jackson's three zones of burn injury. If the zone of stasis progresses to necrosis, the potential for conversion of partial-thickness injury to full-thickness injury exists. (From Williams G, Phillips L: Pathophysiology of the burn wound. In: Herndon DN (ed): Total Burn Care. London, W.B. Saunders, 1996.)

Stages of Wound Healing

Three phases of wound healing are recognized. The first phase, the inflammatory response, begins within minutes of injury and may continue for several days after cellular injury has occurred. It is characterized by erythema, edema, heat, and tenderness resulting from increased cellular permeability and blood flow to the area. An increase in microvascular permeability is attributed to the release of multiple mediators such as products of platelet aggregation and the complement cascade, prostaglandins, and leukotrienes, which increase vascular permeability. Vasoactive substances such as histamine are released from mast cells, and this release causes an increase in fluid and protein leakage from microvessels.[5,6] The second phase of wound healing is the fibroblastic phase and occurs 4 to 20 days after injury. During this phase, cells for wound healing proliferate, fibroblasts synthesize collagen, and myofibroblasts pull wound edges together. Exaggerated wound contractures may result from excessive collagen production and may lead to severe functional and cosmetic compromise. The final phase, the maturation phase, starts about 20 days after injury and may continue for several years. During this phase, tissue develops strength as scars form from collagen deposits.

Systemic Response

Virtually every organ system is affected by thermal injury. The extent of dysfunction is proportional to the total body surface area (TBSA) involved. Maximum edema occurs between 8 and 48 hours after burn injury, depending on burn size. The systemic response to injury is biphasic, with early hypofunction followed rapidly by hyperfunction. Organ function gradually returns to normal as the wounds heal or are surgically excised and grafted.

Burn Shock

Burn shock has historically been the leading cause of burn mortality and results from inadequate fluid resuscitation that leads to hypotension, tissue hypoxia, and renal failure. Burn shock is characterized by decreased cardiac output, increased peripheral vascular resistance, and increased capillary permeability with fluid shifts from the intracellular to the extracellular space. It results from both hypovolemic and cellular shock. The vascular shifts that result from burn injury far exceed those encountered after other types of trauma. Changes in systemic microcirculation that increase capillary permeability both systemically and locally are attributed to the release of multiple mediators such as products of platelet aggregation and the

complement cascade, prostaglandins, and leukotrienes. In addition, the release of histamines causes an increase in both fluid and protein leakage from microvessels.

Although the rate of fluid and protein losses diminishes after the first 2 postburn days, increased protein permeability of tissue capillaries may persist for several weeks, producing significant evaporative losses and hypernatremia. Consideration of these losses must be accounted for early during the resuscitation period and must continue until all wounds are closed. Chart 48–2 provides a formula used to guide estimation of fluid losses and corresponding requirements for fluid replacement. Replacement of insensible fluid losses must be carefully balanced against intravascular fluid gains from edema resorption.[7]

CHART 48–2

Calculation of Evaporative Water Loss and Required Fluid

Formula for Estimating Evaporative Losses:

Insensible water loss (mL/hr)
$$= (25 + \% \text{ TBSA burned}) \times \text{TBSA in m}^2$$

Example for a 70-kg Patient:

Weight:	70 kg
TBSA burn:	50%
TBSA:	1.7 m^2
Urine output for past 24 hours:	2000 mL
Nasogastric tube losses past 24 hours:	500 mL

Calculations for This Patient:

$$(25 + 50) \times 1.7 = 125 \text{ mL/hr}$$

or

$$125 \text{ mL/hr} \times \text{hr/day} = 3000 \text{ mL/day}$$

Fluid required = evaporative loss
+ other losses

Fluids Required for This Patient:

Evaporative loss	3000 mL/day
Urine	2000 mL/day
Nasogastric tube	500 mL/day
Total Fluid Required	5500 mL/day

TBSA, total body surface area.

Hemodynamic Response

The immediate neurohormonal response after injury is characterized by a marked decrease in cardiac output, as much as 50%, and a significant increase in peripheral vascular resistance that is proportional to burn size. Systemic vascular resistance and afterload are also increased from the release of vasoconstrictors and increased blood viscosity secondary to hemoconcentration, to provide adequate perfusion to essential viscera in the early postburn period and to redistribute blood flow to vital organs.[7]

After the first 24 hours of a burn injury, cardiac output gradually rises to supranormal levels as the hyperdynamic state evolves, and systemic vascular resistance gradually falls to subnormal levels. Mild to modest tachycardia (100–120 beats/min) from persistently elevated catecholamines is commonly present and is accentuated by hypothermia, hypoxemia, and pain. Patients unable to generate or maintain this tachycardia are less likely to survive. Likewise, arterial blood pressure may initially be low, but it should respond to fluid resuscitation. Further evaluation of arterial blood pressure is discussed in the section of this chapter on assessing fluid resuscitation. These early manifestations of postburn hypermetabolism continue until the wounds are closed and healing is complete.[8]

During the early hypermetabolic state associated with the early postresuscitation period, a significant increase in oxygen consumption also occurs. Other clinical manifestations related to hypermetabolism include an increase in body temperature by 1 to 2°F, an increase in gluconeogenesis, a decrease in glucose tolerance, an increase in catabolism, and an increase in oxygen consumption of 50 to 100%. If lactic acidosis is present, as manifested by hyperventilation, low arterial pH, and possibly dysrhythmias, it usually indicates inadequate tissue perfusion and can usually be corrected by improving oxygen delivery and blood flow.

Pulmonary Response

As with systemic vascular resistance, pulmonary vascular resistance also increases in response to burn injury. It is usually associated with a modest decrease in lung compliance and arterial oxygen tension. Unlike the rise in systemic vascular resistance, the rise in pulmonary vascular resistance is more dramatic and lasts longer, and this phenomenon may provide a protective mechanism against pulmonary edema during the early postburn resuscitative phase. In patients who develop hypovolemia, minute ventilation is initially depressed, but then it may increase after resuscitation in excess of twice the normal minute ventilation. Hyperventilation may be associated with mild hypoxemia and respiratory alkalosis during edema resorp-

tion. As the burn wounds heal or are closed by grafting, this hypermetabolic response usually decreases.

Host Defense Mechanisms

Although the mechanisms for many of the immune deficiencies evoked by burn injury are unclear, investigators have proposed complex interactions of major metabolic, hormonal, and immunologic changes. In the period immediately after injury, the arachidonic acid cascade and the inflammatory cytokine cascade are activated and are accompanied by early translocation of bacteria and endotoxins. After 3 to 4 days, another endotoxemic peak appears to occur and to cause functional changes in leukocytes, neutrophils, and macrophages. These changes interfere with the host's ability to fight invading pathogens and produce cell damage and death, probably as a result of toxic intracellular metabolite formation.[9]

Renal Response

During the initial hypometabolic period, the renal response is usually manifested by oliguria related to a decrease in both plasma flow and glomerular filtration rate. As cardiac output increases, oliguria is followed by modest diuresis. Diuresis may be masked by evaporative water losses and slow mobilization of edema fluid.

Metabolic Response

Hypermetabolism is one of the most significant alterations after burn injuries of more than 30% of the TBSA. As stated earlier, increased catecholamine production has a profound effect on hemodynamic status. Peak metabolic rates are usually reached between the sixth and tenth days after burn injury, as a result of an increase in catecholamine production required to support wound healing. Besides TBSA, age, sex, preburn nutritional status, preexisting medical conditions, and nutrient intake affect the amount of protein wasting and weight loss. Requirements for nutritional support to compensate for these changes are covered later in this chapter.

Gastrointestinal Response

Patients with burns over more than 25% of TBSA are subject to myriad gastrointestinal complications secondary to hypovolemia and the neurologic and endocrine responses to injury. The two most commonly seen complications are stress ulceration and paralytic ileus.

Superficial stomach and duodenal erosions that can progress to frank ulceration, from which life-threatening gastrointestinal hemorrhage can occur, are not uncommon in patients with burns of more than 25% TBSA. To prevent hemorrhagic complications, these patients must be protected with antacids or histamine (H_2) receptor antagonists.

In the early phase, when blood flow is redistributed to vital organs, blood is shunted away from the gastrointestinal tract and this may cause paralytic ileus. Patients require a nasogastric tube for gastric decompression to prevent aspiration until gastrointestinal motility is restored in the postresuscitation phase. Bowel sounds should be assessed every 4 hours. Hourly gastric pH monitoring is essential. Antacids or H_2 blockers are administered to maintain a gastric pH greater than 5, to prevent ulcer formation.

Neuroendocrine Response

Neurologic manifestations of burn injury are numerous. They are usually late sequelae, although in the presence of early hypovolemia and hypoxemia, agitation and restlessness are not uncommon. Many confounding factors make central nervous system assessment in the early postinjury period difficult. The neurologic effects of inhaled toxic materials or circulating drugs and alcohol at the time of injury cannot be excluded. Other factors that obscure an adequate assessment include sepsis, pain medication and anxiolytics, and sensory deprivation associated with the intensive care unit (ICU) environment.

An endocrine response related to burn size develops early in the postburn period, as manifested by an elevation in glucagon, cortisol, and catecholamine levels. Additionally, triiodothyronine (T_3), thyroxine (T_4), and insulin levels are decreased.

Classification of Burn Injuries

Assessing Depth of Burn Injury

Depth of injury is an important determinant of morbidity and mortality, as well as of healing, surgical management, wound management, and ultimate function and cosmesis. Depth of injury is most commonly described as superficial (first-degree burns), partial thickness (second-degree burns), and full thickness (third-degree burns) (see Figure 48–1). Some sources describe fourth-degree burns that involve injuries to muscle, bone, and subcutaneous fat, whereas others refer to these injuries as full-thickness burns.

Patients with first-degree burns, most commonly seen in the form of sunburn, are not admitted for inpatient treatment except in rare instances. Partial-thickness injuries can be either superficial, in which only the epidermis is involved, or deep, in which portions of the dermis are also involved. Superficial partial-thickness wounds are typically characterized by blister formation, a bright red color, and exquisite pain. If protected from infection or other trauma, these wounds generally heal without surgical intervention in 10 to 21 days. Although deep partial-thickness wounds may involve a significant portion of the dermis, dermal appendages such as hair follicles and sweat glands that contain germinal epithelium are usually spared. Although these wounds may heal spontaneously in 3 to 5 weeks, they frequently heal by contracture and hypertrophic scarring and require later grafting for optimum functional and cosmetic results. Causes and clinical characteristics of partial-thickness and full-thickness burn injuries are detailed in Table 48–2.

Determining Burn Size

Burn injury severity is directly proportional to both the extent of TBSA burned and the depth of injury. The extent of injury is the greater determinant of pathophysiologic changes. Assessment of the extent and depth of burn injury is crucial to the successful management of burn patients. The extent of injury is calculated and expressed as a percentage of TBSA burned. Three methods for calculating TBSA burned are commonly used. The most common method in the emergency room and prehospital setting is the rule of nines (Figure 48–4). It is a means of rapidly estimating TBSA by dividing the body into various anatomic regions, each of which represents 9% of the TBSA or a multiple thereof, whereas the genitalia represent 1%.[10] A more reliable method of assessing extent of burn injury is the use of a burn diagram such as that of Lund and Browder.[11] Figure 48–5 is a burn diagram that takes into consideration the changes in TBSA accompanying aging. A third method of calculating the extent of burn injury is the "rule of the palm," a method that is particularly useful when estimating small or widely dispersed burns.[12] The patient's palm represents approximately 1% of the patient's TBSA. By adding up the number of hands it would take to cover the burns, one can estimate burn size.

Laser Doppler flowmetry is used to assess and classify wound depth.[13] It is currently not in widespread use because of its cost and limitations.

Types of Thermal Injuries

Several types of injury result from thermal trauma and include thermal (heat or cold), chemical, electrical, and radiation. In addition, certain exfoliative skin conditions, such as toxic epidermal necrolysis syndrome (TENS), Stevens–Johnson syndrome (SJS), and staphylococcal scalded skin syndrome (SSSS), require specialized wound care in a burn center because of the extensive skin loss associated with these syndromes. Direct thermal injuries

TABLE 48-2
Burn Depth Characteristics

Burn Depth	Usual Causes	Morphologic Localization of Injury	Physical Characteristics	Healing Time
Partial-Thickness (Superficial Second-Degree)	Brief exposure to flash flame and dilute chemicals; brief contact with steam or hot objects	Epidermis; more dermal damage than in superficial burn	Mottled, moist, bright pink or red color; blister formation; blanches with pressure; tactile and pain sensation	Within 21 days
Deep Dermal Partial-Thickness (Deep Second-Degree)	Longer contact with hot liquids or solids; flash flame, direct flame; intense radiant energy	Entire epidermis and more dermal involvement than in superficial partial-thickness burns; intact hair follicles and sweat glands	Pale waxy appearance; no blanching with pressure; dry appearance; decreased pinprick sensation but pressure sensation intact; very painful	Prolonged healing period > 21 days; contracture formation; possible conversion to full-thickness injury; frequently requires grafting
Full-Thickness (Third-Degree)	Prolonged contact with flames, hot liquids, steam; chemicals; high voltage electric current	Epidermis, dermis, epidermal appendages; portion of subcutaneous fat; possible connective tissue involvement	Dry, leathery, insensate, avascular; white to brown or black; possibly charred; thrombosed vessels	Incapable of self-regeneration; requires grafting

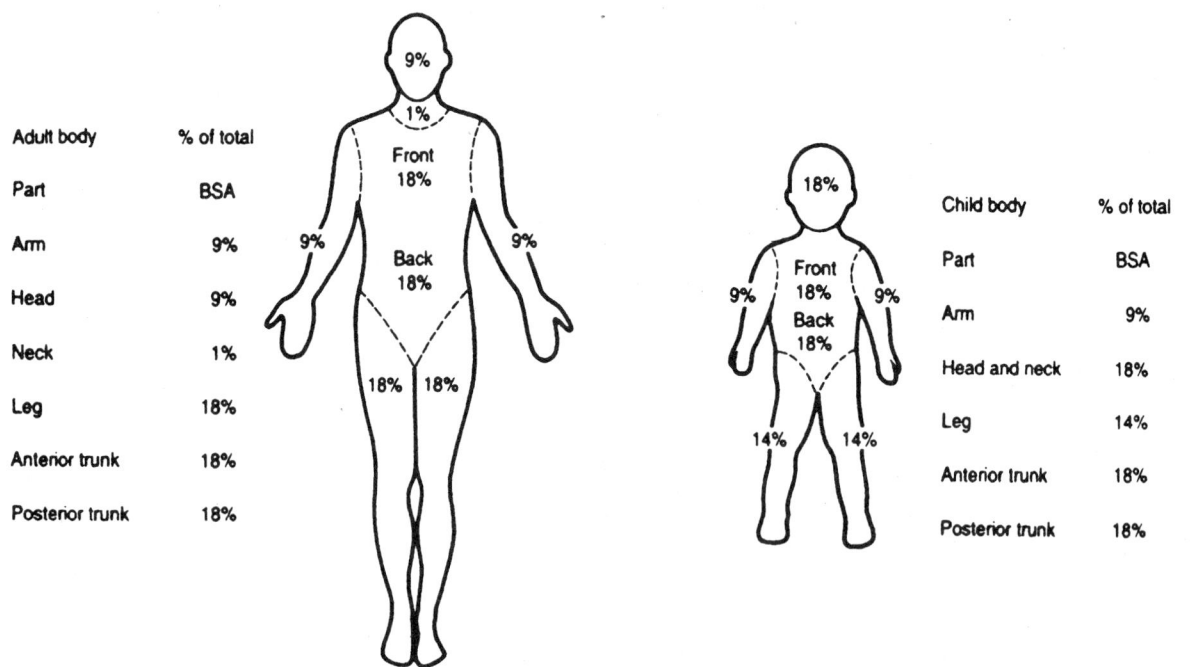

Figure 48-4

The "rule of nines" is useful in estimating the extent of burn injury. Note the differences between adults and children. BSA, body surface area. (From Micak RP, et al: Prehospital management, transportation, and emergency care. In: Herndon DN (ed): Total Burn Care. London, W.B. Saunders, 1996.)

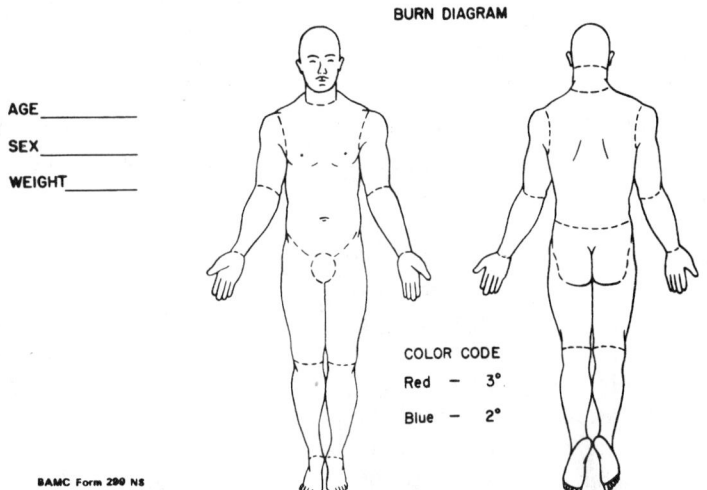

AGE vs AREA

Area	Birth 1 yr	1 – 4 yr	5 – 9 yr	10 – 14 yr	15 yr	Adult	2°	3°	Total	Donor Areas
Head	19	17	13	11	9	7				
Neck	2	2	2	2	2	2				
Ant Trunk	13	13	13	13	13	13				
Post Trunk	13	13	13	13	13	13				
R Buttock	2½	2½	2½	2½	2½	2½				
L. Buttock	2½	2½	2½	2½	2½	2½				
Genitalia	1	1	1	1	1	1				
R U Arm	4	4	4	4	4	4				
L.U. Arm	4	4	4	4	4	4				
R L Arm	3	3	3	3	3	3				
L L Arm	3	3	3	3	3	3				
R Hand	2½	2½	2½	2½	2½	2½				
L Hand	2½	2½	2½	2½	2½	2½				
R Thigh	5½	6½	8	8½	9	9½				
L. Thigh	5½	6½	8	8½	9	9½				
R Leg	5	5	5½	6	6½	7				
L Leg	5	5	5½	6	6½	7				
R. Foot	3½	3½	3½	3½	3½	3½				
L Foot	3½	3½	3½	3½	3½	3½				
						TOTAL				

BURN DIAGRAM

AGE _____

SEX _____

WEIGHT _____

COLOR CODE
Red — 3°.
Blue — 2°

BAMC Form 290 NS
1 May 74

Figure 48–5

This is the burn diagram used by the United States Army Institute of Surgical Research. It is based on the Lund and Browder chart using the Berkow formula to take into account the anatomic and age differences in body size. This diagram is also used to map the patient's extent of injury and color code depth of injury for partial-thickness and full-thickness burns.

result from contact with flame, hot liquids, or another direct heat source such as space heaters and barbeque grills. The mechanism of injury in these types of burns is described previously in this chapter.

Chemical Injuries

Cutaneous chemical injuries differ from thermal injuries in that they may cause both local tissue damage and systemic toxicity. Although wounds from chemical injuries are deceptively similar to thermal injuries in appearance, protein destruction and cellular damage continue until all traces of the chemical disappear. The severity of injury is determined by the chemical nature of the substance, the concentration of the chemical, the duration of contact with the skin, and the agent's mechanism of action. The mechanism of action on the skin and the chemical class of the agent are used to classify chemical injury.

Mechanisms of Action. The first classification of a chemical injury is based on the agent's activity. Table 48–3 lists examples of chemical agents by mechanism of action. Damage from heat rarely plays a major role in chemical injury, except in the case of concentrated acids or alkalis that react with water exothermically.

Chemical Classes. Classification of chemical injury is also based on the agent's chemical activity or the secondary activities it initiates. The chemical's ability to alter pH (acidity or basicity) is one of the most important characteristics of a chemical and is a major consideration in clinical management of cutaneous chemical injuries. The concentration of the chemical is also significant because as concentration increases, so do viscosity, reactivity, and hygroscopicity. Moreover, as the concentration of the chemical agent increases, so does heat production during neutralization or lavage.[14]

Strong acids are common industrial chemicals, but they are also found in household agents such as metal

TABLE 48–3

Examples of Chemical Agents and Their Mechanism of Injury

Mechanism of Action	Chemical Agents
Corrosives cause tissue denaturation	Phenol Lye White phosphorus
Desiccants cause cellular dehydration	Sulfuric acid Muriatic acid
Oxidizers oxidize on contact with skin	Chromic acid Sodium hypochlorite Potassium permanganate
Protoplasmic Poisons impair cellular function by coagulation	Acetic acid Hydrofluoric acid Hydrochloric acid Formic acid
Vesicants cause blister formation	Warfare chemicals Cantharides Poisonous gases

polishes, rust removers, glass and tile cleaners, and acidic substances used in home swimming pools. Inactivation of common acids that cause burns is by dilution with water. Continuous lavage for 30 to 60 minutes normally stops tissue damage.

Alkalis can cause denaturation and can dissolve cellular and structural molecules. Because they bind infinitely more tenaciously with tissue than acids, they are more difficult to remove and cause more severe damage than acids. Water lavage is measured in hours for alkali burns. If the agents are in powder form, they must be brushed away from the skin before water irrigation. Alkalis are found in many cleaning products and include ammonia, sodium and potassium hydroxide, and lime.

Organic compounds are capable of producing severe local and systemic effects by direct chemical reaction. If phenols are absorbed systemically, they can cause central nervous system depression, hypotension, hypothermia, intravascular hemolysis, pulmonary edema, and even death. Petroleum-based compounds such as gasoline cause cell membrane injury and dissolution of lipids that results in tissue necrosis. The release of hydrocarbons from the lungs may lead to chemical pneumonitis and bronchitis.

Hydrofluoric acid is a strong inorganic acid that is widely used both at home and in industry for glass etching and certain chemical manufacturing processes. Hydrofluoric acid produces dehydration and corrosion of tissue by freeing hydrogen ions, which produce skin necrosis. Unless treated, hydrofluoric acid burns cause full-thickness injury and even underlying bone decalcification. Systemic hydrofluoric acid exposure is manifested by hypocalcemia and hypomagnesemia. The initial treatment for these burns is the application of a topical calcium gluconate–based gel. Local injection of 10% calcium carbonate directly into the tissues is also effective. Intra-arterial calcium solution may be required to stop the pain. Patients who have suffered significant exposure require cardiac monitoring and serial serum calcium and magnesium evaluations.

Electrical Injuries

Although electrical injuries account for fewer than 5% of all admissions to burn centers, they are associated with higher morbidity and mortality than thermal injuries.[15] Tissue damage results from the conversion of electrical energy into heat, which is affected by voltage, type of current, pathway of the current, and duration of contact or by the flash caused by electrical arcing. Alternating current is considered more dangerous than direct current because it has a greater likelihood of producing life-threatening complications such as cardiopulmonary arrest and a tetanic effect. Electrical injuries are usually categorized as high-voltage, low-voltage, or lightning injuries.

High-Voltage Injuries. Because the intense heat produced by high-voltage current (>1000 volts) frequently results in a flash flame that causes clothes to catch fire and produces deep skin burns, the concomitant injury from the passing electric current may be overlooked. Tissue injury is greatest at contact points, where the density of the current is highest, and at the sites where the current arcs. Superficial tissues cool more rapidly than deep tissues, which are less likely to sustain deep tissue necrosis.

As high-voltage electric current passes under the skin, not only does it have direct heat effects, but also it causes devascularization from destroyed blood vessels and tissue necrosis. Damage to nerves and muscles may also occur from increased compartment pressures. Figure 48–6 illustrates characteristic changes on an upper limb with high-voltage electrical injury and the extent of débridement required to remove nonviable tissue. Vascular thrombosis and thermal necrosis of tissue may cause severe dysfunction and may necessitate amputation.[15]

The nurse must monitor and evaluate both systemic and local changes in patients with high-voltage electrical injury. A summary of complications associated with electrical injuries is presented at Table 48–4, and monitoring and evaluation criteria are summarized at Table 48–5. In addition to cardiopulmonary monitoring and support for potential early postinjury cardiac dysrhythmias, pulmonary dysfunction, and cardiopulmonary arrest, peripheral perfusion and muscle com-

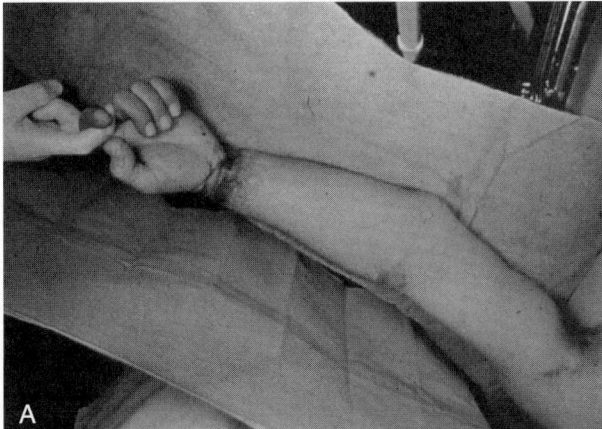

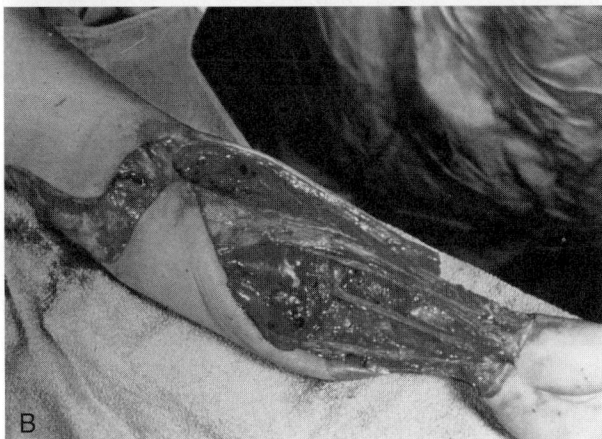

Figure 48–6

A, Note the cyanosis and flexion deformity of the digits, characteristic of severe high-voltage electrical injury. Burns of the flexor surface of the wrist and antecubital space represent the effects of arcing. B, Stony hardness of the forearm muscle compartments necessitated exploration of the forearm and débridement of nonviable tissue.

TABLE 48–4
Complications of Electrical Injury

Cause	Complication
Direct or delayed effect of electric current	Deep tissue necrosis
	Cardiopulmonary arrest and early death
	Cataract formation
	Neurologic deficits
Underestimation of fluid resuscitation requirements based on size of surface injury	Oliguria
	Acute renal failure
Muscle destruction	Hyperkalemia
	Myoglobinuria

Other systemic effects associated with high-voltage electrical injury include pulmonary dysfunction from central nervous system–related hypoventilation and chest wall compliance impairment, acute central nervous system dysfunction, long bone fractures and joint dislocations, and cataract formation.

Low-Voltage Injuries. Low-voltage injuries are more common in children than in adults. Sucking on the end of a live extension cord and biting on electrical wires are the leading causes of burns in children 1 to 2 years of age.[15] The oral wounds that result from these injuries may become extremely edematous. Edema usually subsides in approximately 5 to 10 days, and sloughing of local necrotic tissue begins; bleeding from the labial artery may occur.

Because low-voltage injuries may result in cardiac dysrhythmias and ventricular fibrillation, electrocardiographic (ECG) monitoring is advisable for 24 hours. Tetany and muscle spasm from alternating current may cause fractures.

Lightning Injuries. Mortality associated with lightning injuries is high. A direct lightning strike occurs when a person acts as a grounding site. When lightning changes direction after hitting another object, it is called a flash discharge and is less severe than a direct strike. As with other electrical injuries,

partment pressures must also be carefully monitored. Because fluid resuscitation is often underestimated in patients with electrical injury and large quantities of myoglobin may be released from injured muscle, patients are also at relatively high risk of renal failure. Appropriate fluid resuscitation and treatment for this group of patients are discussed later in this chapter.

TABLE 48–5

Monitoring and Evaluation of Local and Systemic Changes in Patients With Electrical Injuries

Systemic Changes	Local Changes
Vital signs and neurologic checks, particularly level of consciousness	Frequent Doppler ultrasound determinations of extremity blood flow
Hourly urine output, pH, and urine pigmentation (presence of myoglobin)	Frequent assessment for possible nerve compression
Serial hematocrits	Measurement of compartment pressures
Serum electrolytes (especially potassium) and clotting factors	
Cardiac monitoring and serial electrocardiograms for possible dysrhythmias	

lightning causes cardiovascular (myocardial depolarization), central nervous system (transient loss of consciousness), and musculoskeletal and skin injuries similar to those incurred with high-voltage electricity. Treatment for systemic involvement is supportive. Treatment for skin and musculoskeletal injuries is as described for other injuries.

Inhalation Injury

Inhalation injury may occur with or without cutaneous injury. It is usually a consequence of respiratory tract exposure to direct heat, toxic chemical damage, or carbon monoxide poisoning and is usually classified according to the proximity of the injury to the glottis. Upper respiratory tract injuries affect the nasal cavity, pharynx, larynx, glottis, trachea, and larger bronchi. Lower respiratory tract injuries involve the smaller bronchi, bronchioles, and alveoli. Injuries sustained in an enclosed space, where the concentration of carbon monoxide and potentially irritating and toxic gases is likely to be high, are more likely to result in inhalation injury. People with decreased levels of consciousness related to drug overdose, alcohol intoxication, or head injury are more prone to inhalation injury because of an inability to detect and avoid prolonged exposure to smoke and products of incomplete combustion. Pulmonary injury from direct heat is rare and usually affects only the upper airways. The pulmonary consequences of inhalation injury include a progressive decrease in functional residual capacity, which may lead to atelectasis, ventilation–perfusion mismatch, respiratory failure, and eventual death.

A patient presenting with facial burns, singed nasal hairs, and carbonaceous sputum is highly suspect for an underlying inhalation injury. Specific clinical manifestations of inhalation injury include dyspnea, brassy cough, stridor, wheezing, hoarseness, bronchorrhea, unexplained hypoxemia, disorientation, obtundation, and coma. Approximately 56% of patients with inhalation injury present with three or more of the aforementioned signs and symptoms.[16] A summary of clinical indicators of respiratory injury after thermal injury is presented at Chart 48–3. Although highly indicative of inhalation injury, these clinical findings are often inconclusive. Chest radiographs are often normal in the early postburn period, even in the presence of inhalation injury, and are therefore unreliable as a diagnostic measure. Fiberoptic bronchoscopy and xenon-133 ventilation scanning are required for definitive diagnosis.

Carbon Monoxide Toxicity. Carbon monoxide poisoning is one of the leading causes of death associated with fire. Carbon monoxide is released as a colorless, odorless, and tasteless gas as a result of incomplete combustion. Inhaled carbon monoxide preferentially binds with hemoglobin to form carboxyhemoglobin, which reduces the oxygen-carrying capac-

---

CHART 48–3

Clinical Indicators of Respiratory Injury

Facial burns

Presence of carbonaceous sputum or soot around mouth and nares

Signs of hypoxia, including tachycardia, dysrhythmias, or anxiety

Evidence of respiratory difficulty manifested by use of accessory muscles, intercostal or sternal retractions, stridor, or hoarseness

Abnormal breath sounds

Arterial blood gases outside normal limits

---

ity of blood and leads to tissue hypoxia. Because carbon monoxide causes a shift to the left of the oxyhemoglobin dissociation curve, oxygen unloading may be impaired at the tissue level. Severe myocardial depression characterized by low cardiac output that is unresponsive to fluid challenges or inotropic support may result from prolonged exposure to carbon monoxide.

A definitive diagnosis of carbon monoxide toxicity can only be made by direct determination of serum carboxyhemoglobin levels. Depending on geographic location, carboxyhemoglobin levels of 10% or greater are diagnostic of carbon monoxide poisoning. Arterial oxygen tension (PaO_2) is an unreliable indicator because the chemical alteration of hemoglobin by carbon monoxide does not affect the amount of oxygen dissolved in the plasma. Clinical signs of toxicity may include headache, confusion, fatigue, visual disturbances, and combativeness.

Fiberoptic Bronchoscopy. Fiberoptic bronchoscopy permits detailed examination of the major airways and identification of the early inflammatory changes such as tracheal hyperemia, mucosal sloughing, and ulceration indicative of inhalation injury. In addition, it facilitates immediate therapy such as intubation and pulmonary hygiene when severe inhalation injury is present or airway obstruction is imminent. The diagnostic accuracy of fiberoptic bronchoscopy approaches 100% in normotensive and euvolemic patients.

Xenon-133 Ventilation–Perfusion Scan. Intravenous xenon-133 ventilation–perfusion scanning is useful in identifying regions of incomplete or complete small airway obstruction. However, it may produce false-positive results in patients with a history of chronic obstructive pulmonary disease, tracheobronchitis or pneumonia from aspiration, or preexisting pulmonary infection.

TABLE 48–6

Treatment of the Physiologic Consequences of Inhalation Injury

Severity	Problem	Treatments
Mild	Hypoxemia Copious secretions Bronchorrhea	Supplemental oxygen Incentive spirometry Chest physiotherapy Nasotracheal suction
Moderate	Wheezing Mucus plugging Bronchospasm	Humidification Bronchoscopy (therapeutic) Aerosolized heparin Aminophylline
Severe	Respiratory failure	Endotracheal intubation Mechanical ventilation Tracheostomy

The treatment of inhalation injury is primarily supportive and is guided by the patient's pulmonary dysfunction. Table 48–6 summarizes common treatments for the physiologic consequences of inhalation injury. The pulmonary dysfunction induced by inhalation injury may require intubation, mechanical ventilation, and positive end-expiratory pressure (PEEP).

High-frequency interrupted-flow positive-pressure ventilation has been associated with less parenchymal injury and barotrauma and an improvement in survival after inhalation injury.[16] Advantages of the use of high-frequency ventilation include ventilation at lower peak and mean airway pressures, adequate oxygenation at a lower fraction of inspired oxygen (FIO_2), an increase in secretion clearance, and recruitment of collapsed alveoli from the oscillatory nature of high-frequency ventilation.

Hyperbaric Oxygen. Although hyperbaric oxygen therapy unquestionably accelerates the elimination of carbon monoxide, clinical trials have not conclusively demonstrated its superiority to 100% humidified oxygen in improving long-term neurologic sequelae and in increasing survival.[8] It is difficult to monitor and care for patients adequately in a small chamber, and large chambers expose nurses and physicians to the risks of "diving" with the patient. One study reported that hyperbaric treatment was related to cardiac arrests, seizures, and cardiac dysrhythmias in 7 of 10 patients, a finding that leaves reasonable doubt about whether the potential benefits of hyperbaric treatment outweigh the risks.[17]

Exfoliative Skin Disorders

Because of the extensive skin losses that are tantamount to partial-thickness injury, severe exfoliative disorders of the skin pose significant problems similar to those seen in patients with major burns. Two major varieties of exfoliative skin disorders are seen in burn centers today. As depicted by their clinical presentation, summarized in Table 48–7, the clinical characteristics of these disorders often overlap, and final diagnosis relies on histopathologic examination.[18–20]

Toxic Epidermal Necrolysis Syndrome and Stevens–Johnson Syndrome

Approximately 77 to 94% of cases of TENS and SJS have a drug-induced origin. The most commonly implicated drugs are sulfonamides, anticonvulsants, nonsteroidal anti-inflammatory drugs (NSAIDs), and analgesics.

Patients with either TENS or SJS experience a prodrome 2 to 4 days before cutaneous slough manifestations. These symptoms are similar to those found with respiratory tract infections and include malaise, sore throat, fevers, rhinitis, anorexia, and coughing. Lesions initially present as a diffuse, tender erythema or pruritus with substantial mucosal membrane involvement. After 24 to 96 hours, the involved areas begin to form blisters and large bullae. The epidermis separates from the dermis with only mild pressure, known as a positive Nikolsky's sign. As the bullae rupture, the patient

TABLE 48–7

Characteristics of Toxic Epidermal Necrolysis and Stevens–Johnson Syndrome

Characteristics	Stevens–Johnson Syndrome	Toxic Epidermal Necrolysis
Onset	4–8 days with skin tenderness and burning sensation	1–2 day onset with skin sensations same as Stevens–Johnson syndrome
Lesions	Pattern of distribution varies; erythema and vesicles; Nikolsky's sign positive	Generalized and diffuse; no target lesions; positive Nikolsky's sign
Involvement of mucosa	Severe involvement of two or more surfaces	Same as Stevens–Johnson syndrome
Diagnostic histopathology	Intense dermal infiltrate, areas of epidermal detachment	Minimal dermal infiltrate, larger area of epidermal detachment
Mortality	0–38%	25–80%

becomes covered with large areas of denuded skin, leaving a bright red superficial partial-thickness wound. Skin loss can be 100% of TBSA.

Severe oral, conjunctival, and pharyngeal mucosal involvement is characteristic of these diseases as manifested by hemorrhagic erosion of the lips, palate, and buccal mucosa that may extend into the larynx, trachea, bronchi, and esophagus. Urethral, perianal, and vaginal skin is frequently inflamed and can develop erosions. These manifestations are not related to the percentage of total skin loss.

Both disorders are frequently associated with serious systemic complications, including esophagitis and gastrointestinal ulcerations, desquamation of alveolar lining cells, bronchopneumonia, and hepatic dysfunction.[21] These patients are also at significant risk of pulmonary complications that include hyperventilation and hypoxemia, as well as pulmonary edema during fluid resuscitation.[22] The long-term ocular sequelae can lead to blindness. These patients require fluid resuscitation, wound care, and nutritional support and are best treated in a burn ICU setting.

Transient hematologic abnormalities such as leukopenia, neutropenia, lymphopenia, and thrombocytopenia are common findings in patients with TENS. Of these findings, the most significant is leukopenia, which places the patient at greater risk of infection and neutropenia, which is associated with a higher mortality.[22–24]

Corticosteroids are useful if they are initiated before skin sloughing. They can decrease tissue sloughing by attenuating the sloughing process. However, once epidermal–dermal separation has commenced, corticosteroids retard the healing process. Other treatment modalities currently in use with varying degrees of success include plasmapheresis,[25] anticoagulants,[26] and cyclosporine.[27]

The goal of therapy is to protect the exposed dermis from desiccation, mechanical trauma, and infection. In addition to meticulous wound and oral care, these patients require intense nutritional support. Oral nutrition is difficult if not impossible because of oral lesions. Enteral feeding is preferred unless tube placement is difficult because of severe esophagitis. Nutritional requirements and wound care for these patients are comparable to those prescribed for patients with comparable burn injury.

Patients describe the pain associated with the acute phase of exfoliative skin diseases as excruciating and unrelenting. Elimination of pain may have a positive impact on the patient, both physiologically and psychologically.[28] Pain-management strategies for all types of burns are addressed later in this chapter.

Staphylococcal Scalded Skin Syndrome

SSSS, or Ritter's disease, is a dermatologic condition seen primarily in infants and children.[29] In adults, the disease is usually associated with chronic renal insufficiency, immunocompromise, and malignancy, and it carries a significantly higher mortality rate than in children.[30–32] The most common causative toxin is exfoliatin A.[33] The exfoliatins are usually produced at an initial distal site of staphylococcal infection and are transported to the skin by the blood. The early stages of the disease are manifested by fever, general malaise, and tenderness and usually precede skin lesions, which commonly begin on the face as reddened areas that spread within 24 to 48 hours to form large, soft, fragile vesicles that may involve the entire body surface. Unlike in TENS and SJS, oral mucosal lesions are uncommon. The lesions typically resemble blisters similar to those of scald injury, and the vesicles eventually rupture, leading to the skin peeling in leaflike sheets. As with TENS and SJS, Nikolsky's sign is positive, and a definitive diagnosis requires a wound biopsy.

Initial treatment of SSSS requires aggressive parenteral administration of antistaphylococcal antibiotics. Methicillin is the usual drug of choice for community-acquired SSSS because most staphylococci have demonstrated resistance to penicillin, whereas methicillin-resistant strains should be considered for nosocomial infections.[21] Steroids are contraindicated in the treatment of SSSS. Wound care is directed at preventing secondary infection until healing has occurred. SSSS usually responds rapidly to appropriate antibiotic therapy, and skin lesions most frequently heal in 7 to 10 days.

Assessment

Initial Assessment and Primary Survey

The Nebraska Burn Institute has established guidelines for advanced burn life support for patients with moderate and major burns.[34] These guidelines are like those for any trauma patient and begin with a primary survey that includes a rapid assessment of airway, breathing, circulation, and, when indicated, cervical spine immobilization. Figure 48–7 summarizes priorities for the primary survey.

Secondary Survey

Except for chemical injuries, the burn wound is often the most obvious injury. However, other associated life-threatening injuries may be present. To ensure that these injuries are appropriately recognized and managed, a thorough assessment is required. Initial management and definitive care are based on priorities of care, the mechanism of action, the severity of injury, and the patient's response to injury. Circumstances surrounding the accident provide valuable information for

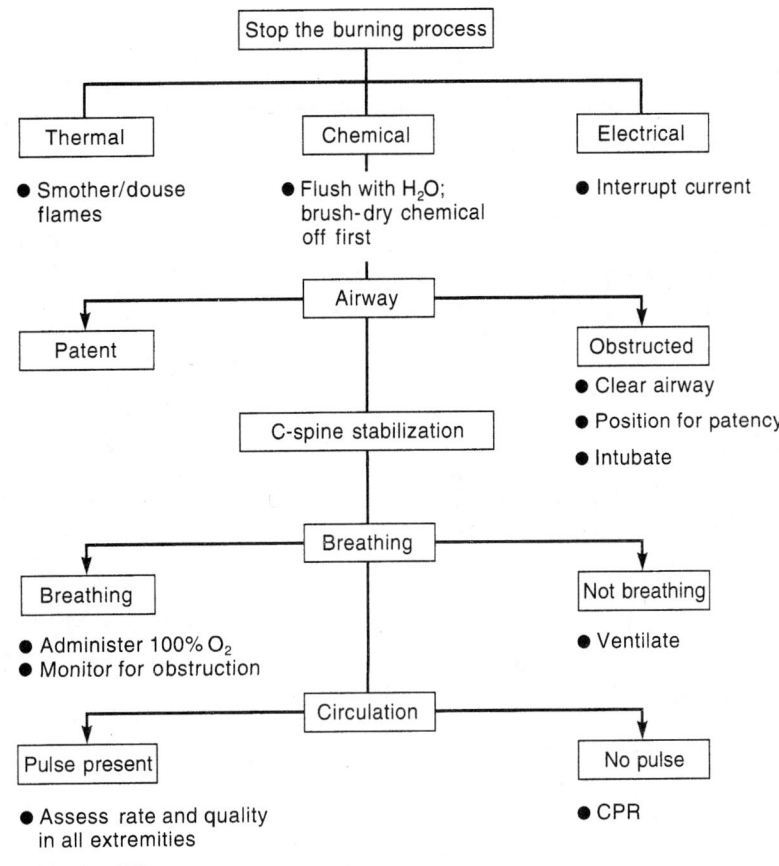

Figure 48–7

An example of a critical path for major burns during the resuscitation phase. BP, blood pressure; CPR, cardiopulmonary resuscitation. (From Hartshorn JC, et al: Introduction to Critical Care, 2nd ed. Philadelphia, W.B. Saunders, 1997, p 533.)

assessing the patient for associated trauma. Details of the accident, such as the time and cause of the burn, events leading to the accident, location of the accident (closed or open space), the presence or absence of hazardous chemicals, a history of loss of consciousness or difficulty in breathing, are examined. A current and past medical history that includes any preexisting disease such as diabetes or cardiac or renal disease, food or drug allergies, current medications, tetanus immunization status, and any history of alcohol or drug use and smoking is important. Figure 48–8 is a summary of guidelines for a secondary assessment.

Diagnostics

Initial laboratory studies are, to a degree, based on the cause of injury. However, because burn injury can lead to major organ dysfunction, baseline studies include hematocrit, serum electrolytes, blood urea nitrogen (BUN), urinalysis, and chest roentgenogram. Arterial blood gases (ABG) are indicated if there is any question of inhalation injury or facial burns. ECG is obtained in all patients with electrical injuries or in the presence of preexisting cardiac disease. Carboxyhemoglobin is analyzed when the history indicates a closed-space fire or the presence of hazardous chemicals, and blood glucose levels are determined in children.

Nursing Diagnoses

In both the resuscitative and acute phases of injury, assessment by the nurse must focus on early detection or prevention of complications associated with moderate and severe burns. Frequent monitoring is required to assess indices of essential organ function. A comprehensive list of actual or potential nursing diagnoses for patients with thermal injuries in the resuscitative, acute, and rehabilitative phases of care is presented in Table 48–8.

Collaborative Management

It is well documented that care of burn patients is best provided by a multidisciplinary approach that includes a team of physicians, nurses, occupational and physical therapists, respiratory therapists, dietitians, social workers, and chaplains. Many teams also include a burn clinical nurse specialist and a psychiatric clinical nurse specialist. Critical pathways or care maps are often useful in providing guidelines for a consistent approach to assessment, intervention and for evaluation and facilitation of a collaborative practice.[35] One example is included in this chapter, and several others have been developed and published by

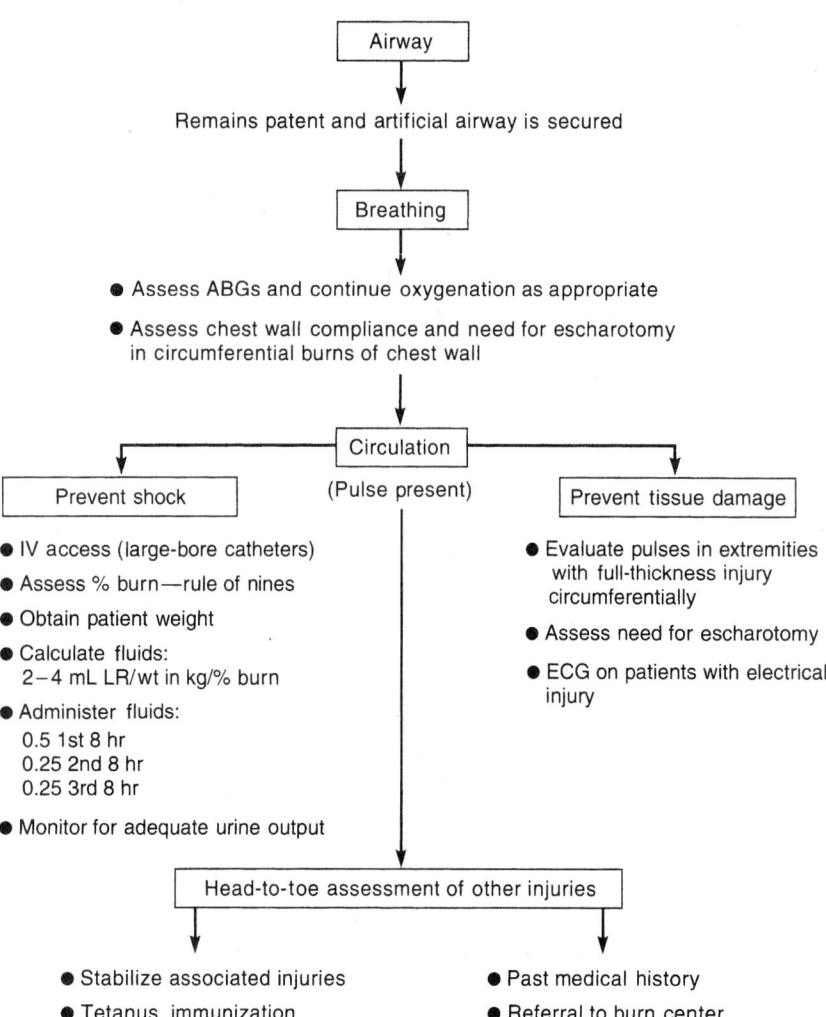

Figure 48–8

Summary of guidelines for secondary assessment of burn injuries. ABG, arterial blood gas; ECG, electrocardiogram; IV, intravenous; LR, lactated Ringer's solution. (From Hartshorn JC, et al: Introduction to Critical Care, 2nd ed. Philadelphia, W.B. Saunders, 1997, p 534.)

major burn centers across the United States (Figure 48–9).[36]

Prehospital Management

The most important priority of care at the scene of the accident is to stop the burning process. It is important not only to prevent further injury to the patient but also to prevent injury to oneself.[34] Flames may be extinguished by rolling the patient on the ground or by smothering flames with blankets or dousing with water. Thermal injuries not involving flames, such as scald burns from hot liquids, should be cooled with water. Ice is not used for cooling because it promotes vasoconstriction and leads to further tissue injury. All clothing should be removed from the involved area unless it is burned into the skin. Rings, watches, and jewelry can compromise distal circulation and should also be removed.

Chemicals continue the burning process for as long as the chemical is in contact with the skin and should therefore be removed immediately by continuous water lavage. All clothing should be removed, and powdered chemicals should be brushed off from clothing and skin before instituting water lavage. If the

burn involves the eye, the eye should be irrigated with water or physiologic saline until evaluated by an ophthalmologist. Neutralizing agents are never used because they increase heat production when they come in contact with the chemical agent and increase tissue injury.

In the case of electrical injury, the patient should be immediately removed from the electrical source. The rescuer should also be protected from injury and should recognize that thermal injury can also occur if clothing is ignited.

All patients with major burn injury, as well as those suspected of inhalation injury, should receive 100% humidified oxygen delivered by face mask. Ventilatory support in the form of endotracheal intubation may be required early in patients with facial edema and inhalation injury. Hypoxia may also occur in patients who have sustained electrical injury as a result of tetanic contractions of the respiratory muscles.

Although hypovolemic shock is rare in the early postburn period, the patient may have evidence of shock in the presence of internal or external injuries. A common complication of electrical injury is cardiac dysrhythmias or cardiac arrest caused by heat damage

TABLE 48–8
Nursing Diagnoses

Problem Statement	Etiologic Factors
Resuscitative Phase	
Ineffective airway clearance	Tracheal edema secondary to inhalation injury
Impaired gas exchange	Interstitial pulmonary edema
Fluid volume deficit	Fluid shifts out of the vascular compartment into the interstitium, diuresis, or evaporative water loss secondary to thermal injury
Altered peripheral tissue perfusion	Impaired vascular perfusion in extremities with circumferential burns
Risk for infection	Loss of integument and invasive therapy
Colonic constipation	Ileus secondary to hypovolemia
Hypothermia	Decreased heat production and increased external heat loss secondary to thermal injury
Pain	Thermal injury
Ineffective individual/family coping	Acute stress of injury and potential life-threatening crisis
Impaired skin integrity	Thermal injury
Altered nutrition, less than body requirements	Increased metabolic demands secondary to physiologic stress and wound healing
Impaired physical mobility	Therapeutic splinting or contractures
Self-care deficit	Therapeutic splinting or contractures
Altered family processes	Acute illness of family member and potential lifestyle and family role changes
Knowledge deficit, learning need	Treatment plan
Acute Care Phase	
Risk for infection	Loss of integument and invasive therapy
Hypothermia	Decreased heat production and increased external heat loss secondary to thermal injury
Pain	Thermal injury
Risk for injury	Gastrointestinal hemorrhage secondary to stress response
Ineffective individual/family coping	Acute stress of injury and potential life-threatening crisis
Fluid volume deficit	Diuresis or evaporative water loss
Altered nutrition, less than body requirements	Increased metabolic demands secondary to physiologic stress and wound healing
Impaired physical mobility	Therapeutic splinting or contractures
Self-care deficit	Therapeutic splinting or contractures
Altered family processes	Acute illness and potential lifestyle and family role changes
Constipation	Immobility and side effects of narcotic analgesics
Knowledge deficit, learning need	Treatment plan and prognosis
Rehabilitative Phase	
Impaired physical mobility	Therapeutic splinting or contractures
Self-care deficit	Therapeutic splinting or contractures
Risk for impaired skin integrity	Itching secondary to healing
Pain	Mobilization of injured body parts
Altered family processes	Long-term consequences of illness and potential lifestyle and family role changes
Knowledge deficit, learning need	Rehabilitation plan and long-term management of thermal injuries
Altered role performance	Disfigurement or dysfunction secondary to thermal injury
Body image disturbance	Disfigurement or dysfunction secondary to thermal injury
Self-esteem disturbance	Disfigurement or dysfunction secondary to thermal injury

to the cardiac muscle or electrical interference with normal cardiac electrical activity.

Peripheral pulses are monitored frequently to assess adequate circulation to extremities. Both burned and unburned extremities are assessed because vascular compromise may occur early in the postburn period from a compartment syndrome that results from direct heat damage to compartment contents, multiple attempts at arterial or venous access, or previous vascular problems. The subsequent swelling may contribute to a decrease in quality or loss of a pulse. Palpable peripheral pulses are frequently obscured by swelling from full-thickness circumferential burns and require hourly assessments by Doppler ultrasound. Burned extremities should be elevated above the level of the patient's heart to facilitate circulation.

CLINICAL PATHWAY: MAJOR BURNS: RESUSCITATION PHASE

Attending MD _____   % Partial-thickness injury _____

Primary nurse _____   % Full-thickness injury _____

This pathway is a guideline only.

Standard of Care	Day 1	Day 2	Day 3
Location:	→ICU	ICU	ICU
Consultations	• Burn specialist • Ophthalmologist • Social services • Other clinical specialists as required	→	→
Assessments	• ED→Primary/secondary surveys • ICU: assess % burned using Lund and Browder chart • Vital signs q1h to monitor for adequate fluid resuscitation • Urine output q1h = 30–50 mL/h • Assess peripheral pulses q1h in extremities with circumferential burns • Pulmonary q1h to assess airway patency and adequate O_2 saturation • Assess metabolic function • Assess GI function q2h (gastric pH) • Assess pain status q1h	→ Continue assessment per requirements of patient condition	→
Laboratory and Diagnostic Tests	• CBC, ECG, ABG, chemistry panel, chest radiograph (daily if intubated) • ABG as required • Electrolytes, BUN, creatinine qPM as needed • Bronchoscopy and xenon scan for possible inhalation injury	• Reduce unnecessary laboratory tests to conserve blood volume	→ Review need for PM laboratory results
Interventions	• Bed rest • Range of motion to all extremities BID • Elevate extremities • Vital signs q1h • Assess peripheral pulses q1h • I&O q1h (urinary catheter required) • Functional positioning devices initiated • Wound care per unit protocol: all wounds cleansed and hair shaved from wound areas • Weights BID • Nasogastric tube to low continuous suction; assess for occult blood q2h • Heat lamps and room temperature control to maintain body temperature	→ • Cardiac output measurements low for first 12 h then return to normal or supranormal after this time • Consider discontinuing peripheral pulse monitoring in extremities with circumferential burns • Reassess need for daily weights • Maximum weight gain from fluid resuscitation occurs within 24 hours	→ Weight loss begins with diuresis; should lose no more than 10% of weight gain per day until preburn weight is achieved

Figure 48–9

An example of a critical pathway for the resuscitation phase of a major burn.

CLINICAL PATHWAY: MAJOR BURNS: RESUSCITATION PHASE *Continued*

Standard of Care	Day 1	Day 2	Day 3
	• Safety measures in place: ensure all jewelry is removed, no constriction of extremities with monitoring devices, tubes secured with cloth ties, ears protected from pressure with foam donuts, no pillows used if neck burns present, facial tube ties do not put pressure on ears or nares		
Medications	• Short-acting narcotics (morphine sulfate is drug of choice) IV bolus q1–2h until hemodynamic stability is achieved • Histamine (H_2) blockers and antacids to maintain gastric pH >7 • Anxiolytics as needed • No IM medications until hemodynamic stability achieved • Topical antimicrobial wound agents per MD orders BID	→ • Consider continuous narcotic medication through IV therapy or patient-controlled analgesia	→
Nutrition	• NPO until gastric ileus is resolved	• Consider inserting feeding tube for enteral nutrition	→
Wound Care	• Photos after initial wound cleansing • Cleanse wounds daily in bed • Eye lubricants q1h to prevent complications from drying	• Consider for surgical excision and grafting when hemodynamic stability achieved	→
Emotional Support and Teaching	• Explain all procedures to patient/family • Offer support services to family • Provide information to patient/family as needed • Involve family in care planning and allow frequent access to patient • Place picture of patient near room to assist staff in relating to preburn state		→ Reassess family state of coping mechanisms and provide resources as needed Initiate multidisciplinary discharge planning

Figure 48–9 *Continued*

It is important to evaluate patients for neurologic deficits early in the postburn period. Patients are typically awake, alert, and oriented after the injury. If a problem is noted with the patient's mental status, other causes such as preexisting diseases, associated trauma, hypoxia, or substance abuse must be investigated.

Once stabilized, the patient should be prepared for transfer to the emergency department or burn center. The patient is covered with a clean, dry sheet and blanket to prevent further wound contamination and to maintain body temperature. The use of space blankets should be considered if a lengthy transport time is expected. Keeping the patient warm not only provides comfort but also protects the wound from further tissue damage caused by circulatory compromise.

Intravenous fluids should be started if transport is expected to take longer than 30 minutes or if indicated for other associated injuries. Narcotic administration should also be avoided until arrival at the emergency department, to avoid the risk of hypotension, respiratory depression, and inaccurate neurologic assessment. To prevent vomiting and aspiration, the patient should take nothing by mouth. Because they are at higher risk for paralytic ileus, patients with more than 20% TBSA burn should have a nasogastric tube inserted before transport.

Emergency Department Management

On arrival at the emergency department, the patient should be reassessed for patency of airway and ventilatory and circulatory status. Special attention should be given to full-thickness circumferential burns of the extremities and the thorax.

Assessing Peripheral Perfusion

Blood flow to underlying or distal tissue may be impaired by mechanical compression, vasospasm, or destruction of vessels underlying full-thickness circumferential burns of the extremities. As edema forms beneath an encircling eschar of the burned extremity, tissue pressure increases, and blood flow to underlying muscle compartments and unburned tissue is compromised. The usual clinical signs of impaired blood flow, such as cyanosis, impaired capillary refill, and neurologic signs such as deep tissue pain and parathesia, are relatively unreliable in burned tissue. The loss of a Doppler ultrasound signal of the palmer arch vessel in the upper extremities and the posterior tibial artery pulse in the lower extremities is the most reliable indicator of the need for an escharotomy.

Escharotomies are usually performed without the use of either general or local anesthesia because the incisions are made through full-thickness insensate eschar. Escharotomy incisions should extend through the eschar and the superficial fascia to a level deep enough to allow the cut eschar edges to separate but not deep enough to incise unburned tissue. If distal blood flow is not restored after the first incision, a second incision should be made on the contralateral midline of the extremity.[8]

Assessing Impaired Ventilation

Ventilation may also be impaired by edema that develops after full-thickness burns of the anterior and lateral chest wall from inelastic eschar that restricts chest wall movement. A chest wall escharotomy may be required to restore ventilatory exchange. Chest wall escharotomy incisions are made along both anterior axillary lines and extend from the clavicle to the intercostal margin. It is sometimes necessary to connect anterior axillary escharotomies with a transverse subcostal incision.

Edema that results from high-voltage electrical injuries, injuries involving muscle and associated soft tissue, long bone, or vascular injury, occurs beneath the investing fascia. Therefore, escharotomies may not

restore blood flow, and fasciotomies are required. Fasciotomies are performed in the operating room, with the patient under general anesthesia, to release the investing fascia of all involved compartments where potential injuries to deeper tissues can also be directly assessed.

Intravenous Access

Intravenous access is established using at least one and preferably two large-bore catheters. The preferred site for catheter insertion is unburned skin. When an unburned skin site is not available, the catheter should be inserted through burned skin. The third preference is a venous cutdown. The use of central lines is discouraged until arrival at a burn center because of potential complications encountered during insertion and infection-control considerations. If a central line is the only option, the femoral vein is the preferred site. Fluid resuscitation is initiated in the emergency department using Ringer's lactate solution.

Fluid Resuscitation

At a 1978 National Institutes of Health consensus conference, participants agreed that, regardless of formula implemented, the goal of fluid resuscitation was to provide the smallest amount of fluid necessary for adequate vital organ perfusion without creating further cardiovascular and pulmonary complications from either excessive or inadequate fluid administration, and the optimum fluid should replace sodium lost from the intravascular fluid compartment.[37, 38] Several formulas have been introduced as guidelines for optimal fluid replacement, and two are summarized in Chart 48–4.

Even since that conference, controversy still exists over which fluids to use during resuscitation. A study by Baxter[39] demonstrated that, during the first 24 hours, Ringer's lactate solution was as effective in maintaining normal plasma volume as the administration of plasma. Pruitt and Mason[40] found that, during the first 24 hours after burn injury, the addition of colloid-containing fluids to crystalloids did not increase intravascular volume to any greater extent than an equal volume of crystalloid fluids, and only after the first 24 hours after burn injury did colloid-containing fluids expand intravascular volume more than did crystalloid fluids.

Ringer's lactate continues to be the preferred and most widely used resuscitation fluid during the first 24 hours after burn injury. All resuscitation requirements are based on the time of burn and not the time of arrival to the emergency department or burn center. When estimating requirements for the first 24 hours after injury, the period between occurrence of injury and initiation of fluid resuscitation must be considered. For example, a patient whose injury was sustained 3 hours before initiation of fluid resuscitation should have the first 8 hours of calculated fluid requirements infused over a 5-hour period.

CHART 48–4

Fluid Resuscitation Formulas

Baxter (Parkland) Formula:

During the first 24 hours after injury, administer
  4 mL lactated Ringer's solution/% TBSA burn/kg body weight
  Half the volume in first 8 postburn hours and the second half evenly distributed over the next 16 hours
During the second 24 hours, administer
  Plasma or albumin to replace plasma volume and maintain hemodynamic stability
In addition to the above, administer 5% dextrose in water to maintain desired urinary output

Modified Brooke Formula

During the first 24 hours, administer
  2–4 mL lactated Ringer's solution/% TBSA burn/kg body weight

TBSA, total body surface area.

Start with smallest amount required to maintain urinary output >30 mL/hr
Administer half the volume in the first 8 postburn hours;
  One-quarter of the volume over the next 8 hours, and the remaining quarter in the last 8 hours
During the second 24 hours,
  Administer albumin diluted to plasma equivalent in normal saline using the following as a guideline:
  0.3 mL/% burn/kg body weight for 30–40% TBSA burns
  0.4 mL/% burn/kg body weight for 50–69% TBSA burns
  0.5 mL/% burn/kg body weight for 70+% TBSA burns

In patients with larger burns, usually greater than 30% TBSA, colloid replacement is initiated at the beginning of the second 24 hours after injury. The crystalloid fluid is changed to a hypotonic solution in the form of 5% glucose solution.

Assessing Adequacy of Resuscitation. Fluid resuscitation formulas are only guidelines based on TBSA burned and weight in kilograms. Age is also a consideration for the very young and the elderly. The adequacy of fluid resuscitation is continuously assessed and is guided by several clinical indices. The increased sympathetic tone caused by the early release of catecholamines in the early postburn period may produce blood pressure readings that are misleading. Cuff pressures in an edematous burned limb may also be misleading because of the difficulty encountered with auscultation or palpation. Additionally, invasive arterial line pressures may also be inaccurate in patients with massive burn injury because of vasospasm produced by catecholamines and other vasoactive substances. The mean arterial pressure required to maintain adequate perfusion and tissue oxygenation must be individualized for each patient and should be determined by observing the patient's response to the administration of fluids. Heart rate is often a more valuable monitoring parameter in the early postburn period. If fluid resuscitation is adequate, the heart rate should be less than 120 beats per minute or in the upper limits of normal for age. A higher heart rate may indicate a need for additional fluid, or it may reflect inadequate pain control. Heart rate is less useful in elderly patients or in patients with preexisting cardiac disease because they commonly are less able to increase their heart rate in response to hypovolemia.

As a result of the hyperdynamic response to burn injury, invasive cardiac monitoring through a pulmonary artery catheter is indicated in only a few patients. Pulmonary artery occlusive pressure (PAOP) is usually normal to low in the early postburn period, even when perfusion is adequate, and left ventricular filling pressures are normally low during the first 24 hours after burn injury. The natural tendency to improve these filling pressures to normal range often leads to overresuscitation. As a result, the associated risks of catheter insertion may exceed the benefits of monitoring adequate perfusion. Swan–Ganz catheter placement should be considered only for patients whose fluid requirements far exceed those predicted, for elderly patients who have suffered significant smoke inhalation injury, or for patients with preexisting cardiac disease. Likewise, cardiac index may not indicate adequate delivery of oxygen to injured tissues because of the hyperdynamic response related to burn wound size. Oxygen delivery may be better monitored using mixed venous oxygen tension as an index of success. In the absence of heart disease or smoke inhalation, however, mixed venous oxygen tension measurement is not usually required.

Hourly urine output is often considered the most useful indicator of adequate renal perfusion and effectiveness of fluid resuscitation because it is generally reliable, provided glycosuria is not present and no hyperosmolar solutions, such as mannitol or dextran, have been administered. A urine output of 30 to 50 mL per hour for an adult is considered adequate. Greater urine outputs usually require increased fluid administration that may lead to iatrogenic edema. Ruling out intrinsic renal disease increases the reliability of urine output as an index of tissue perfusion.

Special Considerations. Patients with large amounts of hemochromagens in their urine from high-voltage electrical injury, those with extensive mechanical soft tissue injury, or those with deep full-thickness burns that involve muscle are more prone to acute renal failure. Greater fluid volumes to increase urine output to 75 to 100 mL per hour may be required to clear the urine and to decrease the risk of renal failure. Diuretics may be required if urine output does not respond to increased fluid volume. Mannitol is commonly used as the diuretic of choice; 12.5 g of mannitol are added to each liter of intravenous fluid until the pigmentation clears and the desired hourly urine output is achieved. Occasionally, a 25-g mannitol bolus is administered before instituting the mannitol infusion. If diuretics have been administered, urine output is no longer a reliable index of adequate fluid resuscitation, and other indices such as invasive cardiac monitoring may be needed to assess resuscitation.

Inotropic Support. In the presence of persistent oliguria or other signs of inadequate perfusion despite aggressive fluid resuscitation, inotropic support may be required during the first 24 hours after burn injury. In such cases, adequacy of fluid resuscitation should be confirmed by placement of a pulmonary artery catheter before initiating inotropic support. If the primary goal is to improve renal perfusion and urine output, low-dose or renal-dose dopamine (1–4 μg/kg/min) is administered. Dopamine doses of 5 to 10 μg/kg per minute improve cardiac output to a normal to high-normal range and increase myocardial contractility. Dobutamine yields the same results with less tachycardia. Digoxin should be avoided during the early periods, to prevent digitalis toxicity associated with rapid fluid shifts.

Other objective parameters that require close monitoring during fluid resuscitation include chest radiography, arterial blood gases, serum electrolytes, serum bicarbonate, BUN, and blood glucose. Patients with electrical injuries also require ECGs for at least 24 hours after injury. Preburn or baseline body weight should be obtained as soon as possible after admission and should be used to calculate fluid requirements, drug dosages, and nutritional requirements. Daily weights thereafter assist in monitoring fluid balance and nutritional adequacy.

Nutritional Support

The resting energy expenditure (REE) after severe burn injury can increase by as much as 100% above normal predicted levels, as determined by use of standard tables for age, size, sex, and weight. Increased heat loss from the burn wound and an increase in beta-adrenergic activity are thought to be largely responsible for this phenomenon.

Nitrogen balance must be restored by supplying substantial calories and large quantities of dietary nitrogen to compensate for the effects of elevated energy expenditure and to maintain a lean body mass. Studies have shown that even if parenteral feedings are started immediately, they are less effective than enteral feedings in the thermally injured patient. Patients with smaller burns can usually be adequately supported with an oral diet. Patients with larger burns generally cannot meet their nutritional requirements with an oral diet and usually require nasogastric or nasoenteric feedings. Patients with gastric ileus may require transpyloric feedings by means of a feeding tube that is passed beyond the pylorus and into the duodenum or jejunum.

Enteral feedings are started as soon as possible after burn injury to avoid a nutrient deficiency. Many sources believe that early nutrition reduces morbidity associated with septic complications by preserving host defenses and gut barriers.[43] When nutrient needs decrease and oral intake increases, tube feedings can be weaned. Tube feedings are usually discontinued when 80 to 90% of the patient's diet can be consumed orally.[44]

Many formulas are available to estimate caloric requirements based on predicted basal energy expenditure for a given age, sex, and body size. The bedside metabolic cart has provided another method of estimating nutritional requirements. Using indirect calorimetry, nutritional estimates are based on measurements of oxygen consumption and carbon dioxide production. Metabolic cart measurements should be made frequently over several days to obtain data to formulate nutritional therapy.

Nutritional status should be monitored using daily weights, calorie counts, and nitrogen balance. Although comparisons of intake and output records and changes in weight provide an estimate of alterations in lean body mass, they are not always a sensitive measure because retained fluid can be mistaken for lean body mass. Serum electrolytes, BUN, serum and urine creatinine, serum albumin, and urea levels are also useful in assessing nutritional status.

Pain Management

Pain and anxiety are intimately related in the burn patient, particularly in the acute period. Pain management not only presents a challenge to the care provider, but also it is of paramount importance to the patient. Elimination of most burn pain has been shown to have a positive impact on patient outcomes.[45] Pharmacologic therapy is often required for the management of both pain and anxiety. Pain is best managed with the use of narcotics, whereas anxiety is usually managed with benzodiazepines.

Pain control is best achieved using small, incremental, intravenous doses of narcotics. Morphine is most commonly used, although meperidine is also given. A consistent level of analgesia can be obtained by using a continuous intravenous infusion, but it should be limited to patients who are mechanically ventilated. If patients are awake and alert, narcotics may also be delivered by means of a patient-controlled analgesia (PCA) pump. This method gives the patient some control over pain relief and accommodates the wide interpatient variations in analgesic requirements. Subcutaneous and intramuscular injections are not used during the resuscitative phase because of impaired soft tissue circulation. Once hemodynamic stability is achieved, pain medication may be administered intravenously, intramuscularly, or orally. Table 48–9 provides a summary of pain and anxiety strategies currently in use.

Pain assessment is an even greater challenge for the nurse. Assessing pain based on the patient's perception of pain is key to effective, individualized pain management. Various pain-assessment tools are currently in use, but their efficacy is often questioned. Chart 48–5 provides more detail regarding the use of pain-assessment tools and patient preferences for these tools. The ultimate goal of pain management is for the patient to be satisfied with the implementation of the pain-management plan, whereas the expected outcome is for patients to achieve a delicate balance between active participation in activities of daily living and comfort levels that promote required rest and sleep.

Management of the Burn Wound

Initial Management

After the patient has reached the burn center and is hemodynamically stable, attention is turned to the burn wound. Total exposure of the wound is necessary to allow for complete assessment of burn depth and size. To reduce the risk of hypothermia and to increase patient comfort, initial wound care is provided in a warm environment. Cleansing is achieved using a

TABLE 48–9

Current Interventions for the Management of Pain and Anxiety in the Thermally Injured Patient

Interventions	Resuscitation Phase	Acute Phase	Rehabilitation Phase
Analgesics	Morphine Continuous infusion PCA IV push Meperidine (Demerol) Fentanyl IV push Continuous infusion Transcutaneous Ketamine Nitrous oxide Methadone	Morphine Continuous infusion PCA IV push Meperidine (Demerol) Fentanyl IV push Transcutaneous Oxycodone (Percocet) Sustained-release morphine (MS Contin)	Oxycodone (Percocet) NSAIDs (Ibuprofen) Acetaminophen Diphenhydramine (Benadryl) (itching) Hydroxyzine (Atarax) (itching)
Anxiolytics	Diazepam Lorazepam Midazolam	Diazepam Lorazepam Alprazolam	Administer as needed
Nonpharmacologic interventions	Hypnosis Transcutaneous nerve stimulation Distraction	Hypnosis Relaxation therapy Behavior modification Stress reduction Transcutaneous nerve stimulation Acupuncture	Relaxation therapy Behavior modification Stress reduction

IV, intravenous; NSAIDs, nonsteroidal anti-inflammatory drugs; PCA, patient-controlled analgesia.

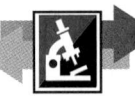

CHART 48–5

RESEARCH UTILIZATION: SELECTING APPROPRIATE PAIN-ASSESSMENT TOOLS

Abstract: The most commonly used pain-assessment tools were identified in a 1994 survey of national burn centers. Of those that responded, 67% used the visual analog scale (VAS), and 33% used an adjective scale.

Forty patients were enrolled in this ongoing prospective multicenter study. Visual analog and color scales were used during a 3-day cycle, and adjective scales and faces were used during another 3-day cycle. Pain levels were assessed twice each day, once during a quiet time and once immediately after a painful activity. At the end of each 3-day cycle, the patient was asked which tool he or she preferred. At the completion of the study period, the patient was asked to select the overall preferred tool of pain assessment.

After the cycle during which adjectives and faces were used, patients showed a significant preference for the faces tools (72.5% versus 27.5%, $P = .006$). After the cycle during which colors and VAS were used, patients noted a significant preference for the colors tool (82.5% versus 17.5%, $P = .006$). Considering all four scales after both cycles, there were also significant preferences ($P = .007$): adjectives, 12.5%; faces, 40%; VAS 10%; and colors 37.5%. The faces tool was preferred significantly over VAS and adjectives, and the colors tool was preferred over VAS.

This study indicated that patients preferred the faces and color scales over the most commonly used VAS and adjective scales. Further research is needed to determine the potential impact of preferred tools on pain management. The results may also lead burn centers to reevaluate current pain-assessment tool selection.

Critique: Although this is a multicenter study, the sample size is small, and the centers are located within one geographic location. Further studies using a broader geographic base and larger sample sizes are recommended.

Nursing Considerations: Assessment and management of pain for the critically ill or injured patient are challenges for nurses. Without appropriate pain assessment, it is difficult to achieve adequate pain management. It has been reported that physiologic and psychological outcomes have been significantly improved by eliminating or reducing pain related to injury or treatment.

Consequently, the management of pain in the critically ill or injured patient is not only a challenge, but a necessity. Management of pain is critical to survival and social recovery.

The unique challenges of the critically ill or injured patient make objective, physiologic assessment measurements of pain both complex and difficult. Multiple studies have shown that nurses' assessments of patients' pain are inadequate, primarily because they do not correlate well with patients' subjective assessments. Accurate assessment and adequate pain management are crucial to positive outcomes for these patients.

Because nurses are the only health care providers who are at the patient's bedside continuously, they have the responsibility for taking the initiative for pain assessment and for evaluating adequate pain management. Improved pain management and therefore patient comfort during hospitalization not only will reduce the average length of stay, but also will significantly improve ultimate patient recovery and quality of life by allowing for earlier mobilization and exercise that can reduce functional deformities and the development of chronic pain.

Source: Gordon M, Greenfield E, Marvin J: Use of pain assessment tools: is there a preference? J Burn Care Rehabil 19:451–454, 1998.

mild soap, such as 4% chlorhexidine, and is followed by copious irrigation with water.[46] Intact blisters and loose, nonviable tissue are débrided, and hair on the burn wound, to include a 3- to 4-inch margin surrounding the wound, is shaved to reduce the risk of infection and to improve visualization of TBSA burned. During the procedure, pain is controlled by administering small incremental doses of intravenous narcotics. Once the wounds are cleaned and débrided and

the extent of injury is assessed, the patient should be weighed.

Daily Wound Care
Patient outcomes largely depend on the prevention and treatment of infection through daily topical burn wound care, burn wound monitoring, and early wound excision and closure. The goals of wound care procedures and protocols are to remove nonviable

tissue, to control microbial colonization, to promote reepithelialization, and to achieve wound coverage as early as possible.

Daily cleansing with a surgical scrub solution containing an antibacterial agent that is then rinsed with warm saline or tap water is essential. Daily hygiene can be accomplished by transporting the patient to the shower or by giving a bed bath to hemodynamically unstable patients who cannot be taken to the shower. Immersion in water is contraindicated because of the potential to increase contamination of uncolonized wounds with organisms from other contaminated sites. All necrotic tissue, exudates, and loose debris should be removed from the wound bed to promote healing and to control bacterial proliferation. The cleansed, exposed burn wounds should then be covered with topical antimicrobial agents.

Some institutions employ chemical débridement through the use of commercially prepared topical agents such as sutilains, collagenase (Santyl), or fibrinolysin–desoxyribonuclease (Elase). These agents facilitate eschar removal by selectively digesting necrotic tissue.

Topical antimicrobial agents, which provide a broad-spectrum means of controlling organisms that may have colonized the wound during or after injury, have been the mainstay of local wound care for more than 30 years. Predisposition to microbial opportunistic colonization depends on burn size, in that the larger the burn size, the more the burn wound is predisposed to microbial opportunistic colonization. Such colonization may be the first step in a progression of microbial proliferation leading to invasion of viable tissue. Topical antimicrobials do not necessarily prevent burn wound colonization. They are, however, the most effective means of delaying colonization, preventing bacterial proliferation in the burn wound eschar, and maintaining low microbial density in the wound.

Their ideal characteristics include their ability to penetrate eschar, broad antimicrobial activity, lack of interference with wound healing, and minimal systemic absorption and toxicity.

Three major topical antimicrobial agents are commonly used in burn centers for the treatment of extensive burns. Specific indications, advantages, limitations, and nursing considerations for use of these agents must be reviewed before their use are summarized in Table 48–10.

Mafenide acetate (Sulfamylon) 11.1% cream is especially active against Gram-negative organisms such as *Pseudomonas aeruginosa* and also has anticlostridial activity. Because it is highly soluble, it readily penetrates burn eschar, a property that makes it invaluable in the treatment of extensive, deep wounds into which bacteria have penetrated and proliferated. Sulfamylon can cause carbonic anhydrase inhibition and hyperventilation, which predispose the patient to metabolic acidosis from renal bicarbonate wasting and depletion of the total body buffer base. These toxicities are rare and are readily manageable, and they do not indicate a need to discontinue use of the agent. The severe pain that can last for up to 30 minutes after application of Sulfamylon cream is effectively controlled by administering analgesics before application.

Silver sulfadiazine (Silvadene) is available as a 1% cream. Like Sulfamylon, it has a broad spectrum of antimicrobial coverage, but it penetrates the wound poorly. It is painless on application and is not associated with acid–base imbalances. In about 5% of the patient population, Silvadene causes transient leukopenia manifested by decreased neutrophil counts. A return to previous values can be expected when use of the cream is stopped.

Both Sulfamylon and Silvadene creams are applied directly to the burn wound in a thickness of approximately 1/16th of an inch using a sterile glove or

TABLE 48–10
Characteristics of Topical Antimicrobial Agents

Agent	Activity	Advantages	Disadvantages
Mafenide acetate cream 11.2% (Sulfamylon)	Broad-spectrum activity against Gram-positive and Gram-negative organisms. Persistent activity against *Pseudomonas*	Good eschar penetration because of high solubility	Pain for 20–30 min after application. Possible metabolic acidosis from hyperventilation. Occasional hypersensitivity
Silver sulfadiazine cream 1% (Silvadene)	Activity against Gram-negative and Gram-positive organisms	Painless application. Effectiveness against yeasts	Rare hypersensitivity. Poor eschar penetration. Transient leukopenia (rare)
Silver nitrate 0.5% soaks	Effectiveness against a wide spectrum of pathogens, including fungal infections	No contribution to ongoing allergic reactions in toxic epidermal necrolysis. Decreased evaporative heat loss from dressings	Limited joint motion. Equipment and environment staining. Poor eschar penetration

spatula, and they are reapplied if these agents are inadvertently removed by patient activity. In patients with TBSA burns larger than 20%, the agents are applied alternately. Because of the pain associated with its application, Sulfamylon burn cream is applied in the morning after wound hygiene, and Silvadene burn cream is applied in the evening. In patients with less than 20% TBSA, Silvadene is usually the sole agent.

Silver nitrate is a 0.5% solution that also provides a broad spectrum of antimicrobial coverage. It is applied by saturating multilayered dressings and placing them over the wound. Pain may be experienced on removal of the dressings. When applied over joints, these dressings may impede motion. Silver nitrate does not penetrate eschar and precipitates immediately on contact. This precipitation leads to a brownish discoloration of unburned skin and virtually everything else with which it comes in contact. The use of silver nitrate 0.5% solution may be associated with alkalosis, electrolyte abnormalities, and water loading. Loss of sodium, potassium, chloride, and calcium, which are leeched from the wound, may incur a requirement for sodium supplements to prevent hyponatremia, and fluids must be adjusted to prevent or correct overhydration. Silver nitrate soaks are used as topical antimicrobial therapy for patients with allergies to sulfonamides and are commonly used in the treatment of wounds incurred from exfoliative skin disorders.

Both an open method and a closed method of treatment are used in burn wound care. Because both methods have advantages and disadvantages, protocols and procedures differ among burn centers. Sulfamylon and Silvadene creams may be used with either the open method (exposure) of wound care or the closed method, which employs dry, bulky dressings. Silver nitrate 0.5% solution must always be applied with wet dressings.

The stated advantages of the exposure method are that it allows for continuous wound observation and early detection of wound changes while enhancing patient mobility. Although closed wound care inhibits patient activity, requires painful dressing changes, and may facilitate microbial proliferation by maintaining a warm, moist environment at the wound surface, the dressings reduce evaporative water loss, especially for patients in air-fluidized beds and lessen radiative heat losses. Dressings also minimize air currents, to which superficial dermal burns are initially sensitive.

Care of Special Areas
Burns of the ears are prone to infection and inflammation and require special treatment. Sulfamylon 11.1% cream is always used for antimicrobial topical therapy. Special positioning devices such as foam donuts with a hole for the ear to rest in while the patient is in a lateral position are required to alleviate pressure and to prevent breakdown.

Burns of the eyes require consultation with an ophthalmologist. Frequent application of an ophthalmic ointment or artificial tears helps to prevent corneal and conjunctival drying and adherence.

Burns of the hands and feet may lead to permanent disability. Their care is directed at preservation of function. The position of comfort is the position of dysfunction. Therefore, active or passive range of motion is initiated as soon as possible after injury to prevent muscle atrophy, to reduce ligament shortening, and to reduce edema. Edema can be further reduced by keeping the hands and feet elevated. Splinting devices are used to maintain function and to prevent deformities. During ambulation, the lower extremities should be wrapped with an elastic bandage to prevent pooling of blood, and the bandage should be removed when the lower extremities are elevated.

Monitoring the Burn Wound
Burn wounds require frequent observation and an evaluation of general wound appearance (particularly changes in wound appearance), wound characteristics, exudates, and odor. To ensure early detection and identification of colonizing organisms and to facilitate early recognition of cross-contamination between patients, burn wound monitoring includes routine surface cultures. Unexpected changes in burn wound appearance or clinical signs indicative of burn wound infection mandate a burn wound biopsy to determine the presence of burn wound invasion. Burn wound invasion may be diagnosed and staged by the histologic examination of a wound biopsy sample.

The usual signs of systemic infection are often unreliable in burn patients because they resemble the hypermetabolism present even in uninfected patients. Burn wound biopsies are a critical tool in differentiating colonized but not infected burn wounds from microbial invasion of viable tissue. Early identification of microbial burn wound invasion permits early surgical wound excision and decreases mortality from wound invasion.

Burn Wound Excision
Early surgical excision of the burn wound has contributed significantly to the survival of patients with massive burns. Advantages of early excision and grafting include a decrease in the duration and magnitude of injury-related physiologic stress, a decrease in the duration of risk for wound infection, early ambulation, and a reduction in length of hospital stay.[47] Conversely, early excision is associated with greater anesthetic and operative risks, large blood losses, and transfusion-related immunosuppression and disease transmission.

Wound Closure
The amount of uninfected burn wound that is surgically excised at any one time is usually limited by

blood loss or by length of operating time. Generally, 20% or less of the TBSA is excised in a single procedure. However, in the presence of microbial invasion, the entire burn wound must be excised if the patient is to survive.

Autologous skin is the replacement material of choice for wound closure. Autologous skin, or the patient's own skin, may be applied either as a sheet or a meshed graft. In smaller injuries (<20% TBSA), expansion by meshing is usually not required. Meshed grafts are often cosmetically undesirable because of the mesh-patterned scar that forms after healing. However, because available donor sites may be limited in patients with large injuries, meshed autografts are required. In massive burn injuries, burns greater than 50%, autologous donor skin is limited, and alternative methods to achieve initial temporary wound coverage must be employed. Sheet grafts or meshed grafts without expansion are generally used over flexion points and hands. The unexpanded mesh graft prevents fluid collections under the graft site and allows better motion while reducing the interstitial healing required for expanded mesh grafts.

Fresh human cadaver allograft, allogenic skin, is the most common alternative method to autologous skin grafting. It reduces water, electrolyte, and protein losses, reduces the risk of wound infection, and minimizes pain. However, allograft carries a small risk of bloodborne pathogen transmission and is of limited supply.

Wounds that cannot be permanently closed by autografting require temporary wound coverage. The goal of synthetic wound coverage is to mimic physiologic epidermis and dermis. The importance of a dermal component to provide permanent wound adherence and to reduce wound contracture after skin grafting is now more clearly understood, and several investigators are seeking to develop dermal substitutes and bilaminate skin replacements.[48] Many of these products are under investigation, but several have demonstrated promise in early clinical trials.

As stated earlier, donor sites are limited in massive burn injuries, thus making permanent wound closure in these patients both difficult and time consuming. A period of 7 to 10 days is required for first-harvest split-thickness skin graft donor sites to heal. Each time the same donor site is reharvested, healing takes longer and the new grafts are of inferior quality. Additionally, while waiting for repeated harvestings, patients remain at risk of infection.

Cultured autologous keratinocytes or cultured epithelial autografts have been offered as one alternative to split-thickness autografts for permanent burn wound coverage.[49–51] Although cultured keratinocytes were initially perceived as an ideal permanent wound cover for massive burn injury, successful grafts have been limited. Allogenic cultured keratinocytes are now

being explored as alternate approach to wound closure. They offer the immediate advantage of being readily available, a feature that eliminates the 3- to 4-week waiting time required to culture autografts. Although studies have not supported their use as a permanent wound cover, investigators have suggested that even with brief contact, epithelial allografts appear to stimulate reepithelialization of partial-thickness burns and promote the formation of granulation tissue in full-thickness injury.[51, 52]

Temporary Wound Coverage

Wound coverage materials that are temporary must be replaced by reepithelialization or autologous skin grafts. Temporary wound covers are not used on heavily colonized wounds and should be used only on superficial partial-thickness wounds. Wound covers serve as substitute barriers for lost epidermal function until definitive wound closure can occur. They provide a microbial barrier for the wound bed to prevent infection and to minimize pain by protecting the wound surface from ambient air currents. Biobrane (Dow Hickam Pharmaceuticals, Inc.) and calcium alginate dressings such as Curasorb (Kendall Co.) and Kalginate (DeRoyal Wound Care) are commonly used biosynthetic dressings and have been effective in the treatment of scald injuries[53, 54] and TENS.[55] Examples of temporary wound covers and their properties are provided in Table 48–11.

Donor Site Care

Management of donor sites, which are surgically created partial-thickness wounds, is essential in burn wound management. If these sites become infected, they may convert to full-thickness wounds and require grafting. Several products are commercially available for donor site care, and the product choice is usually made by the physician or burn center. Table 48–12 provides a summary of the description for each of these products.[56, 57]

Infection

Mortality from burn wound infection has decreased significantly in the past two decades, largely because of the use of topical antimicrobials and early excision and grafting. Pneumonia, presenting primarily as bronchopneumonia, has emerged as the most frequent septic complication of burn injury. Other common site-specific infections in burn centers include blood infections, urinary tract infections, chondritis, and suppurative thrombophlebitis.

Patients with severe thermal injury are at high risk of infection because they are frequently immunosuppressed, they are subjected to long-term intubation and mechanical ventilation, they have reduced gut permeability, they are transfused with multiple units of blood products, and they lack the natural barriers to

TABLE 48–11
Temporary Biologic Wound Covers

Type	Characteristics
Cutaneous Allograft	Composed of skin transplanted from another human and can be used to cover extensive wounds, widely meshed grafts, or partial-thickness wounds
	Decreases bacterial proliferation, wound desiccation, and evaporative water loss
	Fresh allograft preferred to cryopreserved allograft because it is better vascularized
	Tissue can transmit viral disease and undergo rejection
Cutaneous Xenograft (Porcine)	Usually harvested from pigs
	Can be used on clean partial-thickness wounds and patients with toxic epidermal necrolysis
	Promotes epithelialization of partial-thickness burns
	Has limited shelf life and can cause bacterial contamination
Biobrane	Bilaminate wound dressing composed of nylon mesh enclosed in collagen with a Silastic epidermal analog outer membrane
	May be used on superficial partial-thickness burns and freshly excised full-thickness burns
Integra (Artificial Dermis)	Bilaminate dressing composed of thin Silastic epidermal analog and collagen-based dermal analog
	Inhibits inflammation and wound contraction
	Biologically compatible

microbial invasion afforded by intact skin. Other major sources of opportunistic infection are invasive devices such as indwelling urinary catheters and intravascular lines.

Prevention and Control Strategies. The goal of an infection-control program in a burn center is to reduce the transmission of both endogenous and exogenous organisms while supporting the existing defense mechanisms in an immunocompromised patient.[58]

McManus and colleagues[59] demonstrated that the use of single-bed isolation significantly delayed the onset of colonization with *Pseudomonas aeruginosa,* as well as the incidence of bacteremia, pneumonia, and burn wound invasion by this pathogen.

The primary sources of exogenous or hospital-acquired infections are other patients. Therefore, to reduce cross-contamination between patients, nursing care of burn patients requires adherence to barrier precautions and reverse isolation techniques appropriate

TABLE 48–12
Donor Site Dressings

Dressing	Description
Fine Mesh Gauze	Cotton gauze placed directly on a donor site
	Crust forms as gauze dries, and wound epithelialization occurs under the dressing
Synthetic Films	
Opsite	Thin, occlusive, elastic films that are waterproof but permeable to moisture, vapor, and air
Tegaderm	Fluids may pool and require dressing removal and replacement
Biocclusive	
Synthetic gels	
Omniderm	Absorptive gel-like dressing containing a moist environment for wound healing
Duoderm	
Synthetic Laminates	
Epigard	Designed to replicate skin and contain two or more layers of synthetic or biologic material
Biobrane	Outer layer permeable to water vapor
	Inner layer allows for migration of fibroblasts
Vigilon	Colloidal suspension on a polyethylene mesh support that provides a moist environment and is permeable to gases and water vapor
Calcium alginate	
Kaltostat	Hydrophilic, nonwoven fiber that converts to firm gel when activated by wound exudate
	Nonadherent to the wound

for immunosuppressed patients. The importance of hand washing before and after each patient contact cannot be overemphasized. In addition to standard precautions, gowns, head covers, masks, and gloves are required of all personnel entering a patient's room to perform activities involving contact with the patient. Medical supplies and equipment should be designated for individual patient use to prevent cross-contamination between patients.

Microbial surveillance is an important aspect of an infection-control program. Routine wound, sputum, and urine cultures provide early identification of colonizing organisms and cross-contamination between patients, assist in monitoring the effectiveness of topical antimicrobial treatment, and eliminate the need for empiric choice of antibiotic use if infection occurs at a monitored site. Most burn centers obtain routine admission cultures, and many routinely obtain surveillance cultures two or three times per week.

Psychosocial Considerations

Burn injury is often described as one of the most physically and psychologically devastating injuries. The threat of survival and the uncertainty of the long-term effects of the injury on future lifestyle evoke major stress and can precipitate a major crisis for both patient and family. Chart 48–6 presents some of the major ethical decisions faced by both patient and family and the nurse's role is assisting with the decision-making process.

Many psychosocial issues require consideration during recovery from major burn injury (Chart 48–7). The stages of psychological adaptation after burn injury are presented in Chart 48–8. Although not all patients experience the manifestations of all these stages, both patient and family require support to reduce psychosocial morbidity.[28]

Discharge Planning

As with most patients, discharge planning for the critically ill burn patient begins with admission. Short-term and long-term disabilities that result from burn injury should be assessed early, with consideration for available financial resources and other support systems. Multidisciplinary discharge planning and patient and family education should provide information and guidance with regard to physical, psychological, and social needs.

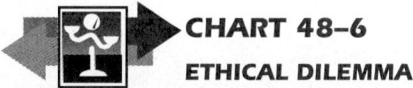

CHART 48–6

ETHICAL DILEMMA

Mr. S. is a 72-year-old man who has just been admitted to the burn center following massive burn injury. He was trapped in a house fire and sustained full-thickness burns to 85% of his body. Although a definitive diagnosis has not been made, there is a strong suspicion that he also has an inhalation injury. He has no advance directive. A team of nurses and physicians is at his bedside performing escharotomies to both lower extremities and his chest wall to relieve constricting circumferential burns, inserting a pulmonary artery catheter and intra-arterial line, and obtaining laboratory results and cultures. His wife suddenly arrives and wishes to see him. At the moment he is awake and able to communicate verbally, although his condition is rapidly deteriorating. Endotracheal intubation and mechanical ventilation are imminent.

You have taken a few minutes to explain to his wife what has happened and that his prognosis is poor. She states that she wishes to see him now while he is still capable of recognizing her. She only wants to stay 1 or 2 minutes to let him know that

she is here and that she loves him. You go to the anteroom door and tell his primary physician, Dr. J., that the patient's wife is here and would like to see her husband while he is still capable of recognizing her.

Dr. J. realizes the importance of letting the wife see her husband and is willing to "hold in place" for a few minutes to allow her to visit. Dr. S., the resident, is less willing, and they proceed to argue vehemently at the patient's bedside. Meanwhile, Mr. S.'s wife is becoming frantic at the thought of losing her husband before she has a chance to see him.

1. What is your position regarding the wife's visit?
2. What is your first reaction to the physicians' arguing?
3. How will you approach them to assist in the decision-making process?
4. What is your role in the decision-making process?
5. What do you tell the wife about this obvious dilemma?

CHART 48–7

Psychosocial Recovery After Burn Injury

Learning new skills for reentry into the school or workplace

Fear of being perceived as handicapped

Fear of social interaction and initiating new relationships

Fear of rejection

Loss of self-esteem

Dealing with feelings of fear, guilt, and anger

Loss of sexual identity and fear of resuming sexual intimacy

Coping with sadness and depression

Fear of never fully recovering

Rehabilitation

Functional rehabilitation and therapeutic exercise should begin on the day of admission. Reduction of the immobilizing effects of edema and maintenance of muscle strength and joint movement are key to every exercise program. To be effective in contracture prevention, positioning and splinting programs require continuous attention. The limiting effects of scarring and contracture formation caused by immature connective tissue shortening can be minimized with gentle stretching of healing skin. A progressive program that includes muscle-strengthening exercises, cardiovascular exercises to improve endurance, and functional exercises designed to improve the performance of the daily activities of living is developed by the multidisciplinary team. The program combines both active and passive motion, although active motion is preferred because it preserves strength and flexibility. Occupational and physical therapy personnel often manufacture antideformity positioning and splinting devices to prevent contractures and breakdown, to provide strength training, and to assist in the development of self-sufficiency in preparation for return to home, school, or work.

Rehabilitation can be a long process and often involves several years of multiple reconstructive surgical procedures. Comprehensive, multidisciplinary discharge planning must prioritize its approach to achieve maximum function and optimal cosmetic appearance. The rehabilitation staff can assist in preparing for discharge needs based on size and location of

CHART 48–8

Stages of Postburn Psychological Adaptation

Survival Anxiety

This stage is manifested by lack of concentration, easy startle response, tearfulness, social withdrawal, and inappropriate behavior. The nurse should allow patient time to verbalize concerns and fears. Increased reports of pain are frequently associated with high levels of anxiety.

Search for Meaning

During this stage, the patient repeatedly recounts the events leading to the injury, in an effort to determine a logical, emotionally acceptable explanation. The nurse should not judge the patient's reasoning, but should listen and actively participate in the discussions with the patient.

Investment in Recuperation

This is a period of increased cooperation with the treatment regimen. The patient is motivated to be independent and takes pride in small accomplishments. The nurse should educate the patient concerning discharge goals and should involve the patient and family in planning for a program of increased self-care. The patient requires much praise and verbal encouragement in this phase.

Investment in Rehabilitation

The patient is focused on regaining maximum preburn function. Depression may occur as new losses in function are realized. This phase usually occurs after the patient is discharged from the hospital and is undergoing outpatient rehabilitation. Praise, support, and continued information are beneficial strategies.

Reintegration of Identity

The patient accepts losses and recognizes that changes have occurred. Adaptation is completed, and staff involvement is terminated.

Adapted from Watkins P, Cook E, May S, et al: Psychological stages in adaptation following burn injury: a method for facilitating psychological recovery of burn victims. J Burn Care Rehabil 9:376–384, 1988.

the injury, the patient's prior functional status, the patient's living environment, and community resources.

Multidisciplinary Outcomes

Patients suffering from thermal injury or similar exfoliative skin disorders are best cared for by a multidisciplinary team approach. The role of the nurse extends from prevention through rehabilitation (Chart 48–9). The ABA published burn care outcomes and critical indicators to assist care providers in assessing the quality of care delivery and to identify quality improvement activities.[60] Chart 48–10 summarizes the multidisciplinary outcomes that can be expected for this patient population, as well as the appropriate clinical parameters that support the achievement of these outcomes.

A 28-year-old male electrician was working in his yard cutting the upper branches of his trees. His family found him on the ground after an undetermined period of time. He was awake, but he did not remember the events surrounding his accident. His clothing was charred. His family noticed a break in the high-voltage wires that ran above the trees where he was working. When EMS arrived on the scene, his respiratory rate was 26 breaths per minute, and he had an irregular heart rate of 98 beats per minute.

On arrival at the emergency department, the patient was found to have a contact wound in his right hand and an exit wound in his right shoulder. Once his charred clothing was removed, burns to his chest and abdomen, right arm, and the anterior portions of both thighs were revealed. His weight was 75 kg.

1. What management priorities should be initiated before transporting the patient to the local medical

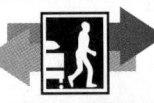

CHART 48–9
BEYOND THE ICU: MANAGING BURN CARE IN THE HOME SETTING

The primary role of the nurse as a care provider is to make a difference in patient outcomes. In the past, the nurse has always made this difference in the hospital setting, and more specifically at the patient's bedside. Today, that role is expanding in many directions, and burn care is no exception.

Burn nurses are actively involved as case managers, educators, researchers, clinical nurse specialists, rehabilitation nurses, outpatient and home health care providers, and directors of community outreach programs. In addition, many institutions utilize burn nurses as hospital-wide wound and skin care consultants.

Recently, a burn center in California collaborated with a home health agency to provide specialized education in burn wound management and functional rehabilitation. These home health nurses spend several weeks in the burn center being educated by nurse experts. Their educational process is both clinical and didactic. In fact, some of the burn nurses are now a part of this home health program. The net result is shorter length of stay for many patients who, for various reasons, would not otherwise be able to go home and return for daily outpatient treatments. Many of these patients are also able to reenter the workforce or school earlier, a factor that contributes to their psychological well-being. Follow-up evaluation has indicated no differences in the critical indicators of outcome between this group of patients and those who were hospital-

ized because they do not meet the criteria for this program. No difference was noted in graft loss, contracture formation, or infection rate.

In many burn centers, the outpatient clinic serves three populations: 1) acute burn outpatients; 2) patients requiring rehabilitative care; and 3) patients who may need surgical reconstruction. The nurse is an integral multidisciplinary team member in each of these areas.

In a study consisting of 642 children with a range in burn size from 0.5 to 19% (mean, 2.9%) who were treated for minor and moderate burns in an outpatient setting from 1988 to 1992, 88% of them healed without inpatient admission. The study supported outpatient management of minor to moderate injuries in a pediatric population. Attention to patient and family education contributed to the achievement of optimal outcomes.

In addition to outpatient management, the nurse plays a major role in burn prevention education. Evidence of a burn center's participation in burn prevention programs is one of the requirements for American Burn Association (ABA) Burn Center Verification. Burn nurses are involved in community outreach programs, schools, and fire departments. To reinforce the role in burn prevention education, the ABA presents a Burn Prevention Award at its annual meeting to persons who have made major contributions to this aspect of burn care.

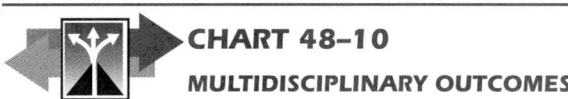

CHART 48–10
MULTIDISCIPLINARY OUTCOMES

Maintenance of Optimal Cardiac and Circulatory Status as Manifested by

Vital signs appropriate for age

Urine output 30–50 mL/hr until diuretic phase begins in 48–72 hr after burn

Absence of tissue loss secondary to hypovolemia or restrictive circumferential eschar

Absence of cardiac dysrhythmia resulting in hemodynamic compromise

Blood pressure adequate in relation to pulse and urinary output

Cardiac output and pulmonary artery occlusive pressure (PAOP) that are low the first 6–12 hours, followed by a normal or supranormal cardiac output with normal PAOP until wound closure

Strong, palpable pulses in all extremities with good capillary refill

Maintenance of Optimal Pulmonary and Airway Status (Assuming No Acute Respiratory Insult) as Manifested by

Patent airway, with clear breath sounds after pulmonary hygiene

Absence of respiratory infection

O_2 saturation >90%

Normal pulmonary examination

Preinjury arterial blood gas values

Decreased dyspnea and work of breathing with appropriate positioning

Ability to cough effectively and to produce clear secretions.

Achievement of an Acceptable Level of Pain and Anxiety Control or Clinical Indicators That Pain is Reduced as Manifested by

Patient communicating need for pain intervention

Patient communicating reduction in pain based on measurable scale after pain intervention

Noncommunicative patient exhibiting signs of comfort during periods of rest and after intervention for pain

Adequate respirations and hemodynamic stability after administration of narcotic analgesia

Decrease in perceived pain level based on a subjective scale or change in physiologic parameters

Identification of factors that contribute to pain

Achievement and Maintenance of a Balanced Metabolic State as Manifested by

Absent or controlled shivering

Body temperature <101.3°F

Electrolytes within established parameters

pH within normal parameters

Glucose between 60 and 200 mg/dL

Improvement in serum protein levels

Achievement and Maintenance of Optimal Fluid and Electrolyte Balance as Manifested by

Appropriate weight gain in first 48 hours with diuresis occurring over next 8–10 days at a weight loss rate of no more than 10% of weight gain/day

Urine output in first 48 hours of 30–50 mL/hr (75–100 mL/hr with electrical injuries)

Urine specific gravity that normalizes to 1.010–1.020 after diuresis

Normal urinary sugar and acetone levels

Electrolytes within normal limits after adequate replacement therapy

Absence of Local or Systemic Infection as Manifested by

Body temperature between 99 and 101°F

Negative sputum, blood, and urine cultures

Absence of wound infection as evidenced by normal wound biopsy

Acceptable white blood cell and platelet counts, coagulation times, and serum glucose

Absence of purulence, erythema, or pain around invasive catheter sites

Adherence of allograft or autograft skin to granulation tissue

Skin Integrity of Unburned Skin Remaining Intact and Graft Take >90% as Manifested by

Intact skin in nonburned areas

Wound closure within an appropriate time frame after burn injury or donor skin harvesting

Grafts vascularized, adherent, and intact

Evidence of progressive epithelialization of interstices of meshed grafts

No evidence of graft breakdown secondary to pressure or shearing

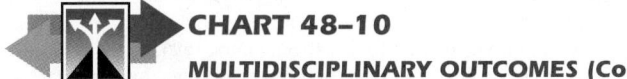

CHART 48–10

MULTIDISCIPLINARY OUTCOMES (Continued)

Restoration of Preinjury Gastrointestinal Functioning as Manifested by

Absence of aspiration
Gastric pH greater than 5
Heme-negative stools and gastric contents
Presence of formed stools

Maintenance of Optimum Nutritional Status as Manifested by

Positive nitrogen balance
≥85% consumption of prescribed caloric intake, based on appropriate formulas for caloric needs
Weight remaining within 10% of preburn weight
Verbalization by patient and family of understanding of nutritional requirements

Demonstration of Optimum Physical Mobility and Function as Manifested by

Range of motion of all joints equal to the preburn level unless presence of new dysfunction secondary to associated trauma at the time of injury
Maximum participation in activities of daily living
Joint strength in noninjured areas remaining equal to preburn strength

Evidence of Effective Patient and Family Coping as Manifested by

Verbalization of goals of the treatment regimen
Initiation of steps to access appropriate support systems
Expression of concerns or fears
Demonstration of adaptive behavior by seeking relevant information and setting appropriate goals

---

center, which is about 20 minutes away by ambulance?

2. How would you estimate this patient's TBSA burn?
3. How would you calculate this patient's fluid requirements?
4. How would you administer these fluids?

A secondary survey is initiated, and associated injuries are excluded. The patient's history is negative for cardiac, pulmonary, or other diseases. He has had a tetanus immunization within the past 3 years. His airway is patent, and he is experiencing no difficulty breathing.

5. What laboratory or other diagnostic tests would you anticipate at this point and why?
6. What wound care should be initiated at this time?
7. Should this patient be transferred to a burn center?

The emergency department decides to transfer this patient to a nearby burn center. Once the patient arrives at the burn center, he is reevaluated for hemodynamic stability. He is taken to the shower to be cleaned and to reevaluate the extent and depth of his injuries. The patient is complaining of exquisite pain during this procedure.

8. What interventions could you offer him?

It has now been 6 hours since the accident. The patient's initial wound care has been completed. You are preparing his plan of care.

9. How would you evaluate the adequacy of his fluid resuscitation?
10. What other nursing considerations would you include in his plan of care for the next 24 to 72 hours?

Key Concepts

⟹ Thermal injury results from exposure to open flames, radiation, contact with hot liquids, or electric current. Caustic chemical agents and certain exfoliative skin diseases also create injuries that resemble thermal injury.

⟹ The extent of tissue damage is directly proportional to the temperature of and duration of exposure to the heat source.

⟹ Assessment of burn depth is an important determinant of morbidity and mortality.

⟹ Burn injury severity is directly proportional to both the extent of TBSA burned and the depth of injury. The extent of injury is the greater determinant of pathophysiologic changes.

⟹ Cutaneous chemical injuries may cause both local tissue damage and systemic toxicity. Alkalis bind more tenaciously with tissue than acids and cause more severe damage.

⟹ Electrical injuries associated with a higher morbidity and mortality are usually categorized as high-voltage, low-voltage, or lightning injuries.

⟹ Inhalation injury may occur with or without cutaneous injury and is usually a consequence of respiratory tract exposure to toxic chemical damage or carbon monoxide poisoning. High-frequency interrupted-flow positive-pressure ventilation has improved survival after inhalation injury.

⟹ TENS and SJS are often associated with serious systemic complications such as esophagitis, gastrointestinal ulcerations, desquamation of alveolar lining cells, bronchopneumonia, and hepatic dysfunction.

➡ The most important priority of care at the scene of the accident is to stop the burning process.

➡ Peripheral perfusion requires constant monitoring by Doppler ultrasound because blood flow to underlying or distal tissue may be impaired by mechanical compression, vasospasm, or destruction of vessels underlying full-thickness circumferential burns of the extremities.

➡ The goal of fluid resuscitation is to provide the smallest amount of fluid necessary for adequate vital organ perfusion without creating further cardiovascular and pulmonary complications from either excessive or inadequate fluid administration.

➡ Resuscitation formulas generally recommend 2 to 4 mL of Ringer's lactate solution per kilogram body weight per percentage of TBSA burned. Half the calculated volume is given during the first 8 hours *after injury*, and the remaining half is given over the subsequent 16 hours. Adequacy of fluid resuscitation is continuously assessed and is guided by several clinical indices. One of the most reliable indices is urine output.

➡ Patients with large amounts of hemochromagens in their urine from high-voltage electrical injury, patients with extensive mechanical soft tissue injury, or those with deep full-thickness burns that involve muscle are more prone to acute renal failure and require greater fluid volumes to decrease the risk of renal failure.

➡ The ultimate goal of pain management is for the patient to be satisfied with the implementation of the pain-management plan, whereas the expected outcome is for patients to achieve a delicate balance between active participation and comfort levels that promote required rest and sleep.

➡ Patient outcomes largely depend on the prevention and treatment of infection through daily topical burn wound care, burn wound monitoring, and early wound excision and closure.

➡ Patients with severe thermal injury are at high risk of infection because they are frequently immunosuppressed, they are subjected to long-term intubation and mechanical ventilation, they have reduced gut permeability, they are transfused with multiple units of blood products, and they lack the natural barriers to microbial invasion afforded by intact skin.

➡ Reduction of the immobilizing effects of edema and maintenance of muscle strength and joint movement are key to every exercise program.

References

1. Pruitt BA Jr: The universal trauma model. Bull Am Coll Surg 70:2, 1985.
2. Pruitt BA Jr, Mason AD Jr: Epidemiological demographic and outcome characteristics of burn injury. In: Herndon DN (ed): Total Burn Care. London, W.B. Saunders, 1996.
3. American Burn Association: Hospital and pre-hospital resources for optimal care of patients with burn injury: guidelines for operation and development of burn centers. J Burn Care Rehabil 11:2, 1990.
4. Jackson DM: The diagnosis of the depth of burning. Br J Surg 40:588, 1953.
5. Ferrara JJ, Dyess DL, Collins JN, et al: Effects of Pentafraction administration on microvascular permeability alterations induced by graded thermal injury. Surgery 115:182–189, 1994.
6. Lund T, Onaheim H, Reed RK: Pathogenesis of edema formation in burn injuries. World J Surg 16:2–9, 1992.
7. Demling RH: Burn care in the immediate resuscitation period. In: Wilmore DW, Cheung LY, Harken AH, et al (eds): Scientific American Surgery. New York, Scientific American, 1995.
8. Pruitt BA Jr, Goodwin CW, Cioffi WG: Thermal injuries. In: Davis JH, Sheldon GF (eds): Surgery: A Problem Solving Approach. St. Louis, C.V. Mosby, 1995.
9. Munster AM: The immunological response and strategies for intervention. In: Herndon DN (ed): Total Burn Care. London, W.B. Saunders, 1996.
10. Berkow SG: A method for estimating the extensiveness of lesions (burns and scalds) based on surface area proportions. Arch Surg 8:138, 1924.
11. Lund CC, Browder NC: Estimation of areas of burns. Surgery, Gynecology and Obstetrics 79:352, 1944.
12. Sheridan R, Petras L, Basha G, et al: Planimetry study of the percent of body surface represented by the hand and palm: sizing irregular burns is more accurately done with the palm. J Burn Care Rehabil 16:605–606, 1995.
13. Atiles L, Mileski W, Purdue G, et al: Laser Doppler flowmetry in burn wounds. J Burn Care Rehabil 16:388–393, 1995.
14. Milner SM, Rylah LT, Nguyen TT, et al: Chemical injury. In: Herndon DN (ed): Total Burn Care. London, W.B. Saunders, 1996.
15. Demling RH: Electrical injury. In: Wilmore DW, Cheung LY, Harken AH, et al (eds): Scientific American Surgery. New York, Scientific American, 1995.
16. Fitzpatrick JC, Cioffi WG: Diagnosis and treatment of inhalation injury. In: Herndon DN (ed): Total Burn Care. London, W.B. Saunders, 1996.
17. Grube BJ, Marvin JA, Heimbach DM: Therapeutic hyperbaric oxygen: help or hindrance in burn patients with carbon monoxide poisoning. J Burn Care Rehabil 9:249–252, 1988.
18. Patterson R, Dyewicz MS, Gonzales A, et al: Erythema multiforme and Stevens–Johnson syndrome: descriptive and therapeutic controversy. Chest 98:331–336, 1990.
19. Rasmussen JE: Erythema multiforme, Steven–Johnson syndrome, and toxic epidermal necrolysis. Dermatol Nurs 7:37–43, 1995.
20. Roujeau JC, Guillaume JC, Fabre JP, et al: Toxic epidermal necrolysis (Lyell syndrome): incidence and drug etiology in France, 1981–1985. Arch Dermatol 126:37–42, 1990.
21. Hollyoak M, Muller MJ, Desai MN: Exfoliative and necrotizing conditions of the integument. In: Herndon DN (ed): Total Burn Care. London, W.B. Saunders, 1996.
22. Roujeau JC, Chosidow O, Saiag P: Toxic epidermal necrolysis (Lyell syndrome). J Am Acad Dermatol 23:1039–1062, 1990.
23. Avakian R, Flowers F, Araujo O, et al: Toxic epidermal necrolysis: a review. J Am Acad Dermatol 25:69–79, 1991.
24. Bradley T, Brown R, Kucan J, et al: Toxic epidermal necrolysis: a review and report of the successful use of Biobrane for early wound coverage. Ann Plast Surg 35:124–132, 1995.
25. Kamanabroo D, Schmitz-Landgraf W, Czarnetski B: Plasmapheresis in severe drug-induced toxic epidermal necrolysis. Arch Dermatol 121:1548–1549, 1985.

26. Roujeau JC: Drug induced toxic epidermal necrolysis. II. Current aspects. Clin Dermatol 11:493–500, 1993.

27. Heng M, Allen S: Efficacy of cyclophosphamide in toxic epidermal necrolysis. J Am Acad Dermatol 25:778–786, 1991.

28. Molter NC: When is the burn injury healed?: Psychosocial implications of care. AACN Clin Issues Crit Care 4:424–432, 1993.

29. Resnick S: Staphylococcal toxin mediated syndromes in childhood. Semin Dermatol 11:11–18, 1992.

30. Khuong MA, Chosidow O, El Solh N, et al: Staphylococcal scalded skin syndrome in an adult: possible influence of nonsteroidal anti-inflammatory drugs. Dermatology 186:153–154, 1993.

31. Ginsburg CM: Staphylococcal toxin syndromes. Pediatr Infect Dis J 199:319–321, 1991.

32. Cribier B, Piemont Y, Grosshans E: Staphylococcal scalded skin syndrome in adults. J Am Acad Dermatol 30:319–324, 1994.

33. Gemmell CG: Staphylococcal scalded skin syndrome. J Med Microbiol 43:318–327, 1995.

34. Nebraska Burn Institute: Advanced burn life support course. Lincoln, Nebraska Burn Institute, 1994.

35. Greenfield E: Critical pathways: what they are and what they are not. J Burn Care Rehabil 16(Suppl 2):196–197, 1995.

36. Gordon M, Greenfield E, Marvin J: The truth about critical pathways. J Burn Care Rehabil 17(Suppl 6):1–36, 1996.

37. Schwartz SL: Consensus summary on fluid resuscitation. J Trauma 19(11 Suppl):876, 1979.

38. Shires GT: Proceedings of the Second NIH Workshop on Burn Management. J Trauma 19(11 Suppl):862, 1979.

39. Baxter CR: Early surgical excision and immediate grafting. In: Artz CP, Moncrief JA, Pruitt BA Jr (eds): Burns: A Team Approach. Philadelphia, W.B. Saunders, 1979.

40. Pruitt BA Jr, Mason AD Jr: Hemodynamic studies of burned patients during resuscitation. In: Matter P, Barclay TL, Konickova Z (eds): Research in Burns. Berne, Hans Huber, 1971.

41. Warden GD: Burn shock resuscitation. World J Surg 16:16–23, 1992.

42. Merrell SW, Saffle JR, Sullivan JJ, et al: Fluid resuscitation in thermally injured children. Am J Surg 152:664, 1986.

43. Alexander J, Gottschlich M: Nutritional immunomodulation in burn patients. Crit Care Med 18(2 Suppl):S149–S153, 1990.

44. Hildreth M, Gottschlich M: Nutritional support of the burned patient. In: Herndon DN (ed): Total Burn Care. London, W.B. Saunders, 1996.

45. Erleben C, Still J: Psychosocial morbidity and pain. Proc Am Burn Assoc Meet 17:abstract 104, 1985.

46. McManus WF, Pruitt BA: Thermal injury. In: Feliciano D, Moore E, Mattox K (eds): Trauma. Stamford, CT, Appleton & Lange, 1996.

47. Heimbach DM: Early burn wound excision and grafting. In: Boswick JA (ed): The Art and Science of Burn Care. Rockville, MD, Aspen, 1987.

48. Hansbrough JF: Wound Coverage With Biologic Coverings and Cultured Skin Substitutes. Austin, TX, Landes, 1992.

49. Cooper ML, Spielvogel RL: Artificial skin for wound healing. Clin Dermatol 12:183, 1994.

50. Phillips TJ: Keratinocyte grafts for wound healing. Clin Dermatol 12:171, 1994.

51. Phillips TJ: Biologic skin substitutes. J Dermatol Surg Oncol 19:794, 1993.

52. Phillips TJ, Bhawan J, Leigh IM, et al: Cultured epidermal autografts and allografts: a study of differentiation and allograft survival. J Am Acad Dermatol 23:189, 1990.

53. Bishop J: Pediatric considerations in the use of Biobrane in burn wound management. J Burn Care Rehabil 16:331–334, 1995.

54. Demling RH: Use of Biobrane in the management of scalds. J Burn Care Rehabil 16:329–330, 1995.

55. Kucan JO: Use of Biobrane in the treatment of toxic epidermal necrolysis. J Burn Care Rehabil 16:324–328, 1995.

56. Hansbrough JF: Use of Biobrane for extensive posterior donor site wounds. J Burn Care Rehabil 16:329–330, 1995.

57. Bettinger D, Gore C, Humphries Y: Evaluation of calcium alginate skin graft donor sites. J Burn Care Rehabil 16:59–61, 1995.

58. Weber JM, Tompkins DM: Improving survival: infection control and burns. AACN Clin Issues Crit Care Nurs 4:414–423, 1993.

59. McManus AT, Mason AD, McManus WF, et al: A decade of reduced Gram-negative infections and mortality associated with improved isolation of burn patients. Arch Surg 129:1306–1309, 1994.

60. American Burn Association Committee on Organization and Delivery of Burn Care: Burn care outcomes and clinical indicators. J Burn Care Rehabil 17:17A–40A, 1996.

49

Multiple Organ Dysfunction Syndrome

Karen K. Carlson

Objectives

After completing this chapter, the student will be able to:

1. Describe the evolution of multiple organ failure (MOF), the systemic inflammatory response syndrome (SIRS), and the multiple organ dysfunction syndrome (MODS).
2. Differentiate the pathophysiology of SIRS, sepsis, MODS, and disseminated intravascular coagulation (DIC).
3. Describe the systemic manifestations of the cellular pathophysiology of MODS.
4. Relate the assessment findings associated with each system's dysfunction to the pathophysiology.
5. Select appropriate nursing interventions for a patient experiencing MODS.
6. Outline the key interventional goals in the patient with MODS or DIC.
7. Evaluate the current therapies employed in caring for the patient with MODS or DIC.

ETIOLOGY AND PATHOPHYSIOLOGY

Health care professionals in the 1980s and 1990s have witnessed the manifestation of a new problem, the progressive deterioration of organ function in critically ill patients, initially termed "multiple organ failure." MOF, defined as the failure of two or more organ systems as a result of malignant intravascular inflammation,[1] was often described interchangeably with sepsis. Malignant intravascular inflammation describes an abnormal host response to a generalized, persistent activation of the immune system. In early MOF research, investigators believed that infection was an important and mandatory part of the syndrome. Studies in the late 1980s showed that not only can this organ system dysfunction occur in the absence of infection, but also it can be produced experimentally by infusing the spectrum of mediators of inflammation.[2]

In an effort to describe this malignant intravascular inflammation better, independent of its cause, the term "systemic inflammatory response syndrome" was developed in 1991.[3] SIRS is seen in patients with many different insults, and its presence is demonstrated by one or more of the clinical manifestations described in

Table 49-1.[3] To be considered significant, these manifestations should appear in the absence of known causes of the changes, such as in a patient receiving chemotherapy. In addition to infectious causes, in which the inflammatory response would be called sepsis, certain noninfectious causes are known, including such disorders as shock, tissue injury, ischemic conditions, and pancreatitis.

As knowledge about MOF grew, it became apparent that there were no universally accepted definitions of any given organ failure, a finding that led researchers to modify the name and to use MODS rather than MOF. The term "dysfunction" implies a continuum of physiologic derangements rather than the presence or absence of organ failure.[3]

Developing as a complication of SIRS, MODS has been defined as the presence of altered organ function in the acutely ill patient such that homeostasis cannot be maintained without intervention.[3] Dysfunction can include complete organ failure or chemical failure of an organ that may or may not result in a significant clinical findings.[4]

MODS can be viewed as either primary or secondary. Primary MODS is the direct result of a well-

TABLE 49-1
Clinical Manifestations of Systemic Inflammatory Response Syndrome

Clinical Manifestation	Description
Altered body temperature	Hypothermia (<36°C) or Hyperthermia (>38°C)
Tachycardia	Heart rate >90 beats/min
Tachypnea	Respiratory rate >20 breaths/min or Hyperventilation demonstrated by $Paco_2$ <32 mm Hg
Altered white blood cell count	>12,000 or <4,000, or >10% band cells (immature cells)

defined insult; organ dysfunction occurs early and is directly related to the insult.[3] The abnormal and excessive inflammatory response is less evident than in secondary MODS. Conversely, secondary MODS results from the effects of the persistent presence and actions of the inflammatory response mediators on the body, rather than the injury itself.

Patients who develop MODS are survivors of major surgery or a traumatic event to the body. MODS is associated with many different triggers. Secor[5] grouped the triggers into the following six broad categories, in an effort to organize the most common triggers:

1. Mechanical tissue damage such as seen in burns, crush injuries, and surgical procedures.
2. Any type of abscess.
3. Ischemic or necrotic tissue, which stimulates the immune system and can include disorders from myocardial infarction to pancreatitis to DIC.
4. Any type of microbial invasion, often related to sepsis-induced MODS. Patients most at risk in this category are those who are immunosuppressed, undergoing surgery or having experienced trauma, or any type of nosocomial or community exposure to infection.
5. Any bacterial source responsible for the release of endotoxin such as Gram-negative organisms. Failure of the gastrointestinal (GI) tract and the associated translocation of bacteria also fit into this group.
6. Any clinical state that creates a perfusion deficit that could be a trigger for MODS. This group includes any global perfusion deficits, such as seen in shock states or cardiopulmonary arrest.

Regional perfusion deficits such as vascular injury, any vascular repair procedure, or thrombolic event can also lead to MODS.

MODS is deemed by many clinicians to be a final common pathway for many critically ill patients; it accounts for most deaths, with mortality greater than 50%, in noncoronary critical care units. The absolute prevalence of MODS is difficult to determine. As our health care and insurance environments are changing, more consumers without health care access may delay seeking care. The incidence of MODS is pre-

dicted to increase, thus providing a future of critical care units entirely filled with patients with MODS (Chart 49–1).

Mortality related to MODS is linked to the patient's prior state of health, the patient's age, the duration of a system's dysfunction, and the number of systems that are dysfunctional. In patients with systems that had been dysfunctional for more than 3 days, the mortality rate was 40% when one system was involved, 60% when two systems were involved, approaching 100% when three systems were involved, and 100% when four or more systems were involved.[1] A more recent study, utilizing a simple scoring system based on dysfunctional systems on the first day of a critical care stay, found that mortality could be accurately predicted approximately 75% of the time.[6] The average length of stay for the patient with MODS is estimated at 21 days.[4]

Activation of Interrelated Systems

When the body is injured or insulted, it responds by activating a series of interrelated systems with the intent of protecting the host, limiting the extent of injury, and promoting rapid healing. All these systems are designed to be beneficial. When these protective mechanisms are initiated but host defense fails, the body is overwhelmed by the impact of the inflammatory responses, and MODS develops. Bone proposed that, as a result of this inflammatory response, the body mounts a compensatory anti-inflammatory response syndrome (CARS).[7] If the response is sufficient, it will cause clinical anergy, increased susceptibility to infection, or both. Although we have much to learn about the relationship between the inflammatory response and proposed CARS, Bone viewed it as a battle of opposing, and often unequal, forces. If these countermediators balance and the initiating cause is eliminated, homeostasis occurs. If not, SIRS and CARS result in the coexistence of inflammatory and anti-inflammatory mediators. These theories provide new avenues for research and may assist in explaining the relative lack of progress currently seen in treating MODS.

CHART 49-1

RESEARCH UTILIZATION: INFLUENCE OF MULTIPLE ORGAN DYSFUNCTION SYNDROME ON PATIENT OUTCOMES

Abstract: Critically ill surgical patients are major consumers of health care resources. Infectious complications are not uncommon in this patient population and may lead to the development of multiple organ dysfunction syndrome (MODS). Critical care health care professionals hypothesized that the development of MODS could be used as a predictor of patient outcomes. This study evaluated the relationship between the degree of MODS patients developed and their associated length of stay. Data in this study were collected from a surgical intensive care unit (SICU) of a university medical center. Utilizing a prospective review of a large population (N = 2646), the data revealed that even modest degrees of MODS were related to a critical care stay of nearly 3 weeks (115 patients stayed in the SICU for >21 days). Retrospectively, the study data were used to analyze whether the magnitude of MODS could differentiate between survivors and nonsurvivors in those patients with the prolonged SICU stay. APACHE II and APACHE III scores were calculated. Additionally, the Marshall MODS score was calculated daily. Not surprisingly, the data suggest that survival is enhanced if the patient's condition can be improved early in the critical care stay.

Critique: Many health care professionals agree that increasing our ability to predict patient outcomes in certain situations would be valuable as we continue our movements toward high-quality, yet cost-contained care. This study certainly suggests that the earlier the interventions, the more likely we are to be able to make a difference in patient outcomes. Whereas this study examined data from a large sample, the data were collected only from patients in one SICU. Therefore, it is difficult to ascertain whether the findings would be applicable to other critically ill patient populations.

Nursing Considerations: Caring for the patient in MODS is a collaborative effort. These patients demand that critical care nurses utilize their best assessment and monitoring skills and report findings in a timely fashion. This study reinforces the notion that early detection is key to managing outcomes. Nursing assessment is the one of the keys that will allow the health care team to make progress in treating these complex patients.

One data collection tool that may be used more frequently in the future is the Marshall MODS score. This score can be calculated rapidly, objectively, and easily from available data, and it grades the severity of dysfunction of 6 organ systems: cardiac, central nervous, hematologic, hepatic, pulmonary, and renal. Each system can receive 4 points, for a maximum of 24 points. The potential exists for this tool to be incorporated into other nursing assessments and completed by nursing staff.

Source: Barie PS, Hydo LJ: Influence of multiple organ dysfunction syndrome on duration of critical illness and hospitalization. Arch Surg 131:1318-1324, 1996.

Normal Inflammatory Response

The normal response to any stimulant of the immune system includes steps to eliminate infectious organisms and to clear cellular debris and foreign materials. With any damage to the endothelium, generalized activation of the inflammation systems occurs.[8] If the response becomes "malignant" or uncontrolled, the result is further damage to the endothelium and direct cytotoxicity, which impairs organ function. This malignant intravascular inflammation can occur either because the body is overrun by bacteria and bacterial by-products or because the inflammatory responses are unregulated by the body. Widely diverse processes, as described with SIRS, initiate the inflammatory response.

When the body sustains an injury, several interrelated systems of inflammation are activated simultaneously. These systems are summarized in Table 49-2.[9] The first system to be activated is the complement system, resulting in neutrophil aggregation and movement of white blood cells (WBCs) to the area of injury. Leukotaxis and leukoagglutination are promoted; foreign cells are lysed and opsonized. Cellular components are also activated, playing a major role in host defense, because these cellular components are the source of many different mediators.

The dominant neutrophils in the body, polymorphonuclear neutrophils (PMNs) have as their primary function to phagocytize foreign particles. During phagocytosis, PMNs undergo increased metabolic activity, and as PMNs become sequestered in organs, such as the liver and lungs, mediators are released. The primary mediators released include leukotrienes, thromboxane, oxygen-free radicals, and interleukin-1.

TABLE 49-2
Systems Activated in Response to Inflammation

System	Actions
Complement System	Stimulation of cellular components (white blood cells, platelets, mast cells): neutrophil aggregation, leukotaxis and leukoagglutination, opsonization, phagocytosis resulting in release of the mediator, histamine Polymorphonuclear cells: phagocytosis of foreign particles resulting in release of the mediators: leukotrienes, thromboxane, oxygen-free radicals, and interleukin Monocytes and macrophages: elimination of foreign materials and cellular debris resulting in release of the mediators: tumor necrosis factor, interleukin-1, thromboxane, and coagulation factors Lymphocytes: T cells responsible for direct cytotoxicity and enhanced B-cell activity; B cells responsible for antibody production Platelets: coagulation and inflammation
Kinin System	Release of the mediator bradykinin
Renin–Angiotensin–Aldosterone System	Renin splitting from angiotensin from angiotensinogen, which is converted from angiotensin II, resulting in vasoconstriction and increased sodium and water reabsorption
Clotting System	Clotting cascade stimulation leading to hypercoagulability and microemboli formation
Sympathetic Nervous System	Epinephrine and norepinephrine release Renin–angiotensin–aldosterone system stimulation
Other	Endogenous opiate release Myocardial depressant factor

Adapted from Carlson KK: Multiple organ dysfunction syndrome. In: Urban NA, Greenlee KK, Krumberger JM, et al (eds): Guidelines for Critical Care Nursing. St Louis, C.V. Mosby, 1995, p 619.

Mast cells are stimulated, and histamine is released. Histamine, also released by platelets and basophils after complement stimulation or direct cell trauma, causes vasodilation, increased capillary permeability, myocardial depression, and smooth muscle contraction.

Monocytes and macrophages are the body's primary defense against foreign invasion of the tissue and an additional source of mediator release. These cells attempt to remove all foreign materials and cell debris. The primary mediators released by these cells include tumor necrosis factor (TNF), interleukin-1, thromboxane, and coagulation factors. Lymphocytes, a major cellular component of lymph nodes and the spleen, regulate, stimulate, or suppress, as needed in an injury situation. There are two types of lymphocytes, T cells and B cells, each with different functions. Direct cytotoxicity, enhancement of B cell activity, regulation of the immune response through activation and suppressor activity, and the release of mediators are all T cell functions, whereas B cells are responsible for antibody production and the cloning of memory cells.

Platelet release is also stimulated. Platelets have an important role in both coagulation and inflammation processes, and they also release mediators, thromboxane, and complement activator.

A second system activated by injury is the kinin system. When stimulated, the kinin system releases a peptide or mediator called bradykinin. Bradykinin works in a fashion similar to that of histamine, by causing vasodilation and increased capillary permeability. Augmented by the adhesion of the activated leukocytes to blood vessel walls, which potentiates local inflammation, bradykinin facilitates fluid exudate and increases vascular compliance.

The renin–angiotensin–aldosterone system is stimulated in response to states of low volume or low renal perfusion. Renin, released from the juxtaglomerular apparatus on the afferent arteriole of the kidney, circulates and splits angiotensin I from angiotensinogen. Angiotensin I travels to various tissues, where angiotensin-converting enzyme converts it to angiotensin II, a powerful vasoconstrictor. Angiotensin II also stimulates the release of aldosterone, resulting in increased sodium reabsorption from the renal tubules. The overall result is an increased blood pressure and increased vascular volume, secondary to the increase in sodium (Na^+) and water reabsorption.

The clotting cascades are also activated, resulting in hypercoagulability and the formation of microemboli. Decreased blood flow and tissue perfusion, secondary to the thrombosis, result in further microemboli, leading to tissue ischemia and hemolysis. Consumption of platelets and clotting factors is not uncommon and may ultimately lead to DIC.

In addition to the systems activation already described, the sympathetic nervous system is also stimulated. Epinephrine and norepinephrine are released and cause vasoconstriction. Antidiuretic hormone (ADH) is released, causing increased water reabsorption in the renal tubule. The renin–angiotensin–aldosterone system, as already described, is also activated by the sympathetic nervous system.

Endogenous opiates called endorphins are released. Endorphins, found in the brain, are morphine-like substances, with receptor sites in both central and peripheral nervous systems. When these receptors are stimulated, vasodilatation results.

Myocardial depressant factor (MDF) is released from the pancreas after any period of hypotension-induced pancreatic ischemia. Circulating to the heart, it has a negative inotropic effect.

Mediators

Certain mediators facilitate the cell-to-cell communication responsible for malignant inflammation. Some are meant to be beneficial, whereas other have a detrimental effect. Over time, the impact of all these mediators is detrimental to the body as their impact is unchecked.

Bradykinin, released by the kinin system, causes vasodilatation, increased capillary permeability, and bronchoconstriction. Histamine, coming from mast cells, has similar effects and also depresses the myocardium and causes smooth muscle contraction.

Released by PMN cells, macrophages, and B cells when activated by endotoxin, interleukin-1 is another mediator that stimulates leukocytosis and enhances both B-cell and T-cell activity. Like TNF, it causes fever and decreased responsiveness to catecholamines.

Leukotrienes, released as part of the arachidonic acid cascade, cause bronchoconstriction, pulmonary vasoconstriction, neutrophil activation, increased capillary permeability, and activation of phagocytosis, and they potentiate the inflammatory response. Prostacyclin, another arachidonic acid cascade by-product, causes vasodilatation and antiaggregation (see Figure 47–6).

Oxygen-free radicals, an active form of oxygen, act to oxidize fatty acids, which are an important component of the membranes of many cells. When the cell membrane oxidizes, cellular metabolic systems are damaged. Nervous system tissue is most susceptible because of the high lipid content of cell membrane. Additionally, oxygen-free radicals stimulate the clotting cascades.

When bacterial cells are destroyed, their cell walls release a substance called endotoxin. Produced primarily by the macrophages after activation by this endotoxin, TNF is believed to mediate the toxic effects of endotoxin and to produce many of the signs and symptoms seen in the patient in shock. TNF produces

hypotension, tachycardia, tachypnea, hyperglycemia, metabolic acidosis, third spacing, and gastrointestinal ischemia.[10] It also produces alveolar thickening, acute tubular necrosis, and profound changes in temperature. Therefore, TNF is believed to be the major mediator of septic shock and MODS. There has been extensive animal research into TNF synthesis, metabolism, activity, and treatment potential. Specific actions in the body believed to be mediated by TNF include enhanced PMN function, fever induction, decreased vascular responsiveness to catecholamines, and the production of anorexia and wasting, probably secondary to the effect on the hypothalamus and gastric emptying. The actions of many of the mediators seen in the patient with MODS are described in Table 49–3.[9]

All these systems are interrelated and communicate in a cell-to-cell fashion, a characteristic that adds to the "malignant" intravascular inflammation origin of MODS. All the pathophysiologic mechanisms activated by injury manifest in systemic consequences. These include the maldistribution of blood flow, oxygen supply and demand imbalance, and various metabolic abnormalities.

Systemic Consequences

The maldistribution of blood flow results from the mix of vasodilatation, vasoconstriction, and vascular occlusion found secondary to system and mediator activation. Vasodilatation, from histamine and bradykinin, is the primary abnormality. With many vascular beds dilating, others are vasoconstricting from the circulating epinephrine, norepinephrine, and angiotensin II, as well as from compensatory mechanisms activated in response to the insult. Vascular occlusion adds to the maldistribution of blood flow. When the clotting cascades are activated, microemboli result, adding to the vascular occlusion. Complement activation and its resultant damage to the endothelial wall enhance emboli formation. With the increased capillary permeability that results from histamine and bradykinin release, fluid leaks into the interstitial space, thereby decreasing circulating volume, increasing blood viscosity, and enhancing emboli formation. Neutrophil and platelet aggregation also slow blood flow and add to the possibility of vascular occlusion.

Changes in blood flow occur as the many mediators attempt to match circulation and oxygen need. Initially, mediators may be successful, but with continued inflammation, compensatory mechanisms become exhausted, resulting in an imbalance in oxygen supply and demand. After any injury, the body raises its demand for oxygen and becomes hypermetabolic as the body attempts to defend itself. Depending on the injury, the body's demand for oxygen may be further increased by fever, pain, and increased work of breath-

TABLE 49–3
Mediators of Inflammation

Mediators	Actions
Bradykinin	Vasodilation
	Increased capillary permeability
	Bronchoconstriction
Histamine	Vasodilation
	Increased capillary permeability
	Myocardial depression
	Smooth muscle contraction
Interleukin-1	Stimulation of leukocytosis
	Enhanced B- and T-cell activity
	Fever induction
	Decreased vascular responsiveness to catecholamines
Leukotrienes	Bronchoconstriction
	Pulmonary vasoconstriction
	Neutrophil activation
	Increased capillary permeability
	Activation of phagocytosis
	Potentiation of inflammatory response
Oxygen-free radicals	Destruction of cell membranes leading to abnormal intracellular enzyme system functioning
Prostacyclin	Vasodilation
	Antiaggregation
Tumor necrosis factor	Enhanced polymorphonuclear cell function
	Fever induction
	Decreased vascular responsiveness to catecholamines
	Production of anorexia
Thromboxane A$_2$	Myocardial depression
	Vasoconstriction
	Enhanced platelet aggregation

Adapted from Carlson KK: Multiple organ dysfunction syndrome. In: Urban NA, Greenlee KK, Krumberger JM, et al (eds): Guidelines for Critical Care Nursing. St. Louis, C.V. Mosby, 1995, p 620.

ing. Additionally, oxygen supply is diminished. Pulmonary edema, ventilation–perfusion mismatch or shunt, and decreased cardiac output, common to these patients, decrease available oxygen. Many patients experience subnormal hemoglobin levels, thus decreasing oxygen carrying sites. Strong evidence indicates that cellular deficits occur, resulting in an oxygen extraction deficit at the tissue level and decreased cellular utilization of oxygen.

Metabolism of carbohydrates, fats, and proteins is altered as intracellular enzyme systems fail. In response to the body's hypermetabolic state, the liver initially increases the amount of glucose released from glycogenolysis. As the cells become depleted and glucose stores are decreased, synthesis of new sugar is inhibited, and patients becomes hypoglycemic. Also common is resistance to the exogenous administration of substrate. As a result of these metabolic abnormalities, catabolism occurs, and protein stores are used for fuel.

The interrelationships among the mediators of the inflammatory response are extremely sophisticated and are difficult to interrupt when host defense fails. Little agreement exists in the literature on exact defini-

tions to explain the individual system effects of this host defense. Bone and colleagues[3] suggested that a comprehensive and continuously updated database is necessary to validate criteria clinically for identifying MODS in each system.

Multiple Organ Dysfunction Syndrome, Sepsis, and Disseminated Intravascular Coagulation

MODS, sepsis, and DIC are all multidimensional processes that represent dysfunctional cellular interactions among organ systems, rather than isolated processes of a single organ dysfunction. Many of the mediators discussed are common to all three and are affected by complicated feedback loops, autoactivation, and impaired regular mechanisms. Having discussed sepsis (SIRS driven by an infectious focus) and MODS, DIC is defined as the inappropriate, accelerated, systemic activation of the coagulation cascades.

DIC always develops as a secondary process. The initiators of DIC are classified as intrinsic or extrinsic, defined by the initiator's location relative to the body. Examples of intrinsic triggers of DIC include anything that damages or results in damage to the endothelium, such as endotoxin release and sepsis, shock, red blood cell damage, and vasculitis. Examples of extrinsic triggers include crush injuries, burns, and brain injury. Although these lists are not comprehensive, any factor on these lists, along with many others, may trigger the clotting cascades causing the formation of fibrin in the vascular space and the deposit of fibrin in the microcirculation. This excessive and inappropriate formation of fibrin initiates the depletion of necessary clotting factors. As clotting continues to be stimulated, clots impair circulation and consume platelets and other clotting factors. Fibrinolysis is activated and, coupled with abnormal clotting, results in ischemic tissue damage and bleeding. When inappropriate clots are formed, a normal, stable clot cannot be formed, if needed, at the site of an insult. The extent to which a patient may bleed depends on the balance between the rate of fibrin formation and the rate at which the body is able to clear the products of fibrin breakdown (fibrin split products [FSP]). DIC can be perpetuated by the circulating FSP because they are themselves anticoagulants. DIC is considered to be the most profound example of hematologic dysfunction, because it can be life-threatening and can profoundly alter the function of many other organ systems.[11] The pathophysiology of DIC is summarized in Figure 49–1.[11]

Assessment

MODS is a complex disorder. To assist with understanding of the impact of the foregoing pathophysiologic effects of MODS on individual organ systems, Table 49–4 summarizes effects as they create dysfunction in each system. Likewise, Table 49–5 summarizes the clinical assessment findings that result from each system's dysfunction.

Respiratory System

As a result of the complement system and attraction of neutrophils to the area, the endothelium of the lungs becomes damaged. Mediators such as leukotrienes cause bronchoconstriction and pulmonary vasoconstriction. As a result, the lungs develop a massive capillary leak, which alters hydrostatic and oncotic pressures. This change leads to interstitial edema and a potentially increased ventilation–perfusion mismatch.

When these patients are assessed, clinical manifestations of the foregoing physiologic features are manifest. Patients can either be bradypneic (respirations <10 breaths per minute) or tachypneic (respirations >20 breaths per minute) as a reflection of their fluid overload, possible hypoxia, and attempt to compensate for developing acid–base disorders, primarily metabolic acidosis. Patients are often dyspneic and have increased work of breathing for similar reasons. On auscultation, crackles and/or wheezes are heard, and the chest radiograph shows diffuse infiltrates, reflecting consolidation and possible infection.

The patient's arterial blood gases (ABG) demonstrate hypoxia, usually with a partial arterial pressure of oxygen (PaO_2) less than 60 mm Hg on a fraction of inspired oxygen (FIO_2) greater than 50% because of hypermetabolism, decreased oxygen-carrying sites, consolidation, ventilation–perfusion mismatching or shunt, and pulmonary interstitial edema. The partial pressure of carbon dioxide ($PaCO_2$) is often greater than 45 mm Hg because of inadequate air exchange. From an acid–base standpoint, ABGs may initially be normal and may then show either metabolic acidosis or respiratory alkalosis or a combination of the two. FIO_2 may need frequent manipulation to maintain adequate oxygenation, often with positive end-expiratory pressure (PEEP) greater than 5 cm H_2O to maintain an adequate functional residual capacity. Pulmonary compliance is generally decreased. These patients often demonstrate refractory cyanosis, the result of a combination of hypoxia, hypercarbia, poor gas exchange, and cellular oxygen utilization deficits.

Renal System

Not a protected organ, the kidney sustains prolonged vasoconstriction from circulating epinephrine and angiotensin II. The renal system appears to attract circulating microemboli, which lead to renal ischemia. The

Figure 49–1

Schematic illustration of the pathophysiology of disseminated intravascular coagulation. (From Dressler DK: Patients with coagulopathies. In: Clochesy JM, et al (eds): Critical Care Nursing. Philadelphia, W.B. Saunders, 1996, p 1148.)

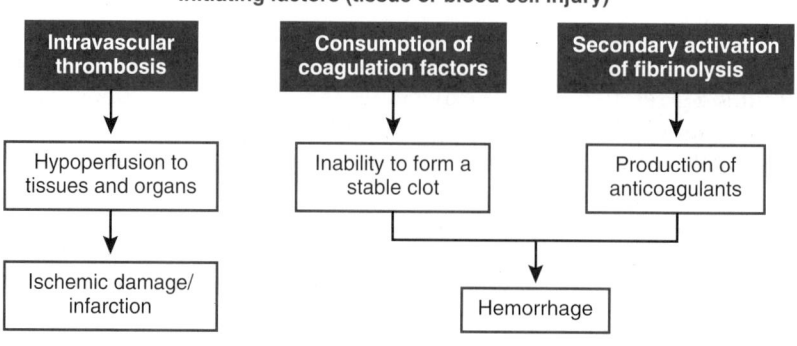

TABLE 49–4
Pathophysiology of Multiple Organ Dysfunction Syndrome by System

System	Pathophysiologic Effects
Respiratory System	Endothelial lung damage Bronchoconstriction and pulmonary vasoconstriction Massive capillary leak Altered hydrostatic and oncotic pressure Interstitial edema Potential ventilation–perfusion mismatch
Renal System	Endothelial damage Renal vasoconstriction Microemboli resulting in renal ischemia Renal interstitial edema
Cardiovascular System	Myocardial ischemia Decreased contractility
Gastrointestinal System	Gastrointestinal ischemia Gastric ulceration Splanchnic blood flow impairment Increased bacterial load resulting in systemic bacterial translocation
Central Nervous System	Cerebral ischemia Cerebral hemorrhage Cerebral vasodilation Decreased cerebral perfusion pressure
Hematologic System	Consumption of hematologic and clotting factors Absolute numbers of individual blood components (white blood cells, red blood cells, platelets) increased: predominantly immature and nonfunctional cells

circulating mediators damage the endothelial membranes, and capillaries become leaky, leading to renal interstitial edema. All these conditions create a situation placing the patient at high risk of development of renal failure.

Patients are often oliguric (<400 mL of urine in 24 hours) and may become anuric because of renal dysfunction from hypoxia and decreased perfusion. Serum osmolality is usually greater than 295 mOsm/kg as a result of fluid shifts into the interstitial space because of the leaky capillaries. In evaluating laboratory tests, creatinine clearance is often less than 30 mL per minute, the result of the hypoxia and decreased perfusion.

Urine Na^+ varies with the type of renal failure. In prerenal failure, urine Na^+ is low, less than 20 mEq/L, because reabsorption of Na^+ is increased in the attempt to increase renal perfusion. In intrarenal failure, urine Na^+ is generally greater than 30 mEq/L because of the loss of Na^+ reabsorptive ability. Specific gravity is variable, depending on fluid and renal status. In prerenal failure, specific gravity is often greater than 1.020 because of the kidney's inability to eliminate fluid, whereas in intrarenal failure, it is more likely to be less than 1.010 because of the loss of concentrating ability. Another laboratory test is serum creatinine, which is greater than 2.0 mg/dL or double the patient's admission creatinine. Blood urea nitrogen (BUN) is greater than 20 mg/dL. Both these changes result from decreased renal filtering and excretion, secondary to poor perfusion, actual renal damage, or both.

Various electrolyte abnormalities may be seen. Potassium (K^+) and phosphate (PO_4) are generally higher than normal as excretion is decreased. K^+ is often greater than 5 mEq/L, whereas PO_4 is greater than 4.5 mg/dL. Na^+, calcium (Ca^{++}), and magnesium (Mg^{++}) are all lower than normal because excretion is increased. Na^+ is less than 130 mEq/L, Ca^{++} is less than 8.5 mg/dL, and Mg^{++} is low, less than 1.5 mEq/L.

Cardiovascular System

The cardiovascular system is affected by all other system dysfunction. The myocardium does sustain direct damage, primarily from the ischemia propagated by the decreased blood flow and mediators. Contractility is diminished as the result of the usually present acidosis and circulating MDF.

Patients are generally tachycardic, reflecting sympathetic nervous system intervention, as well as the body's attempt to compensate for the fluid overload and hypoxia. The character of pulses may change as a

TABLE 49–5

Assessment Findings in Multiple Organ Dysfunction Syndrome

System	Findings
Respiratory System	Bradypnea or tachypnea Dyspnea with increased work of breathing Crackles or wheezes Chest radiograph showing diffuse infiltrates Arterial blood gases: Pao_2 <60 mm Hg; $Paco_2$ >45 mm Hg; metabolic acidosis, respiratory alkalosis, or both Pulmonary compliance decreased Refractory cyanosis

Renal System	Oliguria or anuria
	Serum osmolality >295 mOsm/kg
	Creatinine clearance <30 mL/min
	Urine sodium and specific gravity vary with the type of renal failure:
	    Prerenal failure: urine sodium <20 mEq/L; specific gravity >1.020
	    Intrarenal failure: urine sodium >30 mEq/L; specific gravity <1.010
	Laboratory tests:
	    Serum creatinine >2.0 mg/dL or double the patient's admission creatinine
	    Blood urea nitrogen >20 mg/dL
	    Potassium >5 mEq/L
	    Phosphate >4.5 mg/dL
	    Sodium <130 mEq/L
	    Calcium <8.5 mg/dL
	    Magnesium <1.5 mEq/L

Cardiovascular System	Tachycardia Bounding or diminished pulses Mean arterial pressure <70 mm Hg Intractable dysrhythmias Pulmonary artery pressures variable Pulmonary artery occlusive pressures <12 mm Hg Central venous pressures <8 mm Hg Cardiac output initially >8 L/min; later <4 L/min Cardiac index initially >4 L/min; later <2.5 L/min Skin initially warm, later cool and clammy Skin pale Peripheral edema S_3 heart sound

Gastrointestinal System	Anorexia, nausea, vomiting, stress ulcers
	Ileus with nasogastric tube output >600 mL/24 hr
	Constipation, diarrhea
	Hematemesis
	Melena
	Guaiac-positive nasogastric tube output and stool
	Jaundice
	Bleeding tendencies
	Laboratory tests:
	    Bilirubin >2.0 mg/dL
	    Lactate dehydrogenase and serum glutamic-oxaloacetic transaminase (aspartate transaminase) >50% above normal
	    Albumin <2.8 g/dL
	    Hyperglycemia initially, hypoglycemia later

Central Nervous System	Altered level of consciousness Headache Glasgow Coma Scale <6 Intracranial pressure >15 mm Hg Respiratory depression Hypothermia or hyperthermia

TABLE 49–5
Assessment Findings in Multiple Organ Dysfunction Syndrome (Continued)

System	Findings
Hematologic System	Bleeding tendencies
	Increased susceptibility to infection
	Petechiae or purpura
	Evidence of bleeding in other systems, including unexplained nausea, headache, diarrhea or consti-
	pation, changes in urine output
	Laboratory tests:
	Prothrombin time >25% above normal
	Activated partial thromboplastin time >25% above normal
	Thrombin time prolonged
	Fibrin split products >10 μg/mL
	Fibrinogen decreased
	Hemoglobin and hematocrit decreased
	Platelets <100,000/mL
	White blood cells initially: >10,000/mm^3, later <5,000/mm^3
	D-Dimer positive
	Plasminogen low
	Antithrombin III assay low

reflection of fluid status and may be either bounding or diminished. Patients with MODS with cardiac involvement commonly have a mean arterial pressure (MAP) less than 70 mm Hg from the acid–base imbalances, TNF, fluid shifts, MDF, and vasodilation from mediators. The patient may have intractable dysrhythmias, which are refractory to the usual antidysrhythmic therapy, because of electrolyte imbalances, acidosis, and hypoxia. If pulmonary artery monitoring is done, pulmonary artery pressures (PAP) are often lower than normal, although they may be high initially while compensatory mechanisms are still functional. Pulmonary artery occlusive pressures (PAOP) are often less than 12 mm Hg, and central venous pressures (CVP) are less than 8 mm Hg as a result of fluid shifts to interstitium and mediator-driven vasodilation. Cardiac output (CO) is initially high, greater than 8 L per minute, because of inflammatory mediators and systemic vasodilation; later, CO is less than 4 L per minute as sympathetic stimulation decreases and as myocardial ischemia and hypoxia increase. Cardiac index follows CO, initially being greater than 4 L per minute and later becoming less than 2.5 L per minute for the same reasons as CO changes. Systemic vascular resistance (SVR) reflects the predominant problem, caused by the inflammatory mediators, vasodilation. This results in an SVR of less than 800 dynes/cm^{-5} per second. To touch, the patient's skin is often initially warm, then it turns cool and clammy as perfusion decreases. The skin is generally pale. A patient's weight is elevated as a reflection of the fluid overload and interstitial shifts. Peripheral edema is common, again, because of the movement of fluid into the interstitial space. It is common for patients with MODS to have an S$_3$ heart sound from the fluid overload.

Gastrointestinal System

Because it has such a high metabolic rate, the gut is extremely sensitive to ischemic injury. In a normally functioning gut, bacteria are removed before they have an opportunity to infiltrate and infect the body. As perfusion falls, the GI tract is at risk of becoming dysfunctional as it loses its usual defense mechanisms with splanchnic blood flow impairment. The liver is also affected in a similar fashion. The liver is stressed by the lack of perfusion, and it may be unable to filter an increased bacterial load coming from the GI tract. If bacteria are not removed in the GI tract or liver, they will be transported to the rest of the body, resulting in seeding of bacteria. Both the pathophysiologic mechanisms at play in MODS and the interventions used to treat the manifestations of such mechanisms put patients at risk of GI dysfunction and potential infection from the translocation of bacteria that may occur.[12] Additionally, with the body in a stressed state, the patient often has increased stomach acid production that may lead to ulceration.

Assessment of the GI tract is linked to other systems. Patients may experience anorexia, nausea, vomiting, stress ulcers, ileus accompanied by nasogastric tube output of greater than 600 mL in 24 hours, constipation or diarrhea, hematemesis, melena, guaiac-positive nasogastric tube output or stool, jaundice, and bleeding tendencies. All are related to GI tract hypoxia, decreased motility, and decreased use. Bilirubin is greater than 2.0 mg/dL because of the loss of bilirubin conjugation with liver dysfunction. Liver enzymes such as lactate dehydrogenase (LDH) and serum glutamic-oxaloacetic transaminase (SGOT) (aspartate transaminase [AST]) are more than 50% above normal. Albumin synthesis is compromised, so serum albumin is less than 2.8 g/dL. Glucose homeostasis is altered, generally resulting in a patient who is initially hyperglycemic but who becomes hypoglycemic as MODS progresses.

Neurologic System

There is little evidence that the patient with MODS suffers from primary neural dysfunctional, but rather, the central nervous system is affected by other system dysfunction. For example, the high ammonia levels that result from hepatic insufficiency alter neurologic function. The bleeding that may occur from thrombocytopenia can lead to bleeding in the brain. The uremia seen in renal dysfunction can change the level of consciousness (LOC), and the hypoxia and hypercarbia associated with acute respiratory distress syndrome (ARDS) all affect neural function. When the MAP falls, cerebral perfusion pressure falls, causing cerebral vessels to vasodilate in an attempt to increase cerebral perfusion. As decreased perfusion continues, ischemic damage to the brain may occur.

A change in LOC is usually the first clinical assessment seen and can range from disorientation to unconsciousness to coma. A patient's Glasgow Coma Scale is often less than 6, and if intracranial pressure (ICP) monitoring is being done, ICP will be greater than 15 mm Hg. Depending on how the brain is affected, additional signs may include respiratory depression, hypothermia or hyperthermia, and headache. All result from hypoxia, acid–base imbalances, hypoperfusion, and uremic toxins.

Hematologic System

The hematologic system becomes dysfunctional as it is exhausted by the SIRS and as consumption of hematologic and clotting factors occurs. Investigators also believe that the system is directly affected by the action of the mediators on the spleen, bone marrow, and individual blood components. Often, absolute numbers of blood factors increase, but these cells are predominantly immature and nonfunctional.

The primary clinical manifestations of hematologic dysfunction are bleeding tendencies and increased susceptibility to infection. Bleeding may occur from multiple sites and may range from oozing to frank bleeding. Rebleeding (new bleeding from a site when hemostasis was formerly achieved) is common. Patients may have no overt bleeding, but they may develop petechiae or purpura. Evidence of bleeding in other systems may be hidden, so consideration should be given to unexplained nausea, headache, diarrhea or constipation, and changes in urine output. All sources of output should be checked for occult blood.

Laboratory tests, including coagulation studies, are abnormal as follows. Both the prothrombin time (PT) and the activated partial thromboplastin time (aPTT) are greater than 25% above normal. Thrombin time is also prolonged. FSPs are elevated, generally greater than 10 µg/mL, whereas fibrinogen is decreased. Hemoglobin and hematocrit are decreased; hematocrit is below 33% without evidence of blood loss. Platelets are decreased below 100,000/mL, and WBCs are elevated, greater than 10,000/mm^3, usually with a high percentage of band (immature) cells because of inflammatory mediators, infection, and circulating catecholamines, and later falling to less than 5000/mm^3 because of bone marrow exhaustion. The D-dimer is positive, plasminogen is low, and the antithrombin III assay is low.

Nursing Diagnoses

As with any critically ill patient, caring for the patient with MODS demands the best assessment skills the health care team has to offer. Care is multifaceted, balancing the needs of one system against the demands of another, and trying to maximize overall homeostasis. Nursing diagnoses appropriate for the patient with MODS are determined by the systems involved and the manifestations of the overall pathophysiologic sequelae. Table 49–6 outlines the nursing diagnoses with associated etiologic factors.

Collaborative Management

No single treatment plan exists for MODS. Rather, therapies must focus on each dysfunctional system. Three commonly identified overall goals are treatment of the underlying cause, removal, if possible, of the initial insult, and aggressive support of dysfunctional systems. Some evidence suggests that MODS can be reversed if infection is prevented or controlled and if tissue oxygenation remains adequate.[13] Treatment for patients with MODS must be tailored to fit the whole patient because therapy designed to support one system may damage another. Treatment must also be individually tailored because different patients have different systems affected.

Nursing care of the patient with MODS is equally challenging. Interventions that benefit one system may harm another. The five primary goals of care are to prevent or control infection, to ensure appropriate circulating volume, to ensure adequate oxygenation, to maximize the effectiveness of the heart as a pump, and to provide support for the patient and family.

In general, patients with MODS often have acid–base disturbances. These disorders should be treated aggressively with sodium bicarbonate and dialysis or continuous renal replacement therapy

TABLE 49–6
Nursing Diagnoses

Problem Statement	Etiologic Factors
Airway clearance, ineffective	Mechanical ventilation
	Increased work of breathing
	Intubation
	Secretions
Gas exchange, impaired	Pulmonary edema
	Shunting
	Collapsed alveoli
	Ventilation–perfusion mismatching
Ineffective breathing pattern	Increased work of breathing
	Fluid volume excess
	Hypoxia
	Muscle weakness
Tissue perfusion, altered	Fluid volume deficit
	Stimulation of clotting cascade
	Altered capillary dynamics
	Mixed vasodilation and vasoconstriction
Decreased cardiac output	Myocardial depressant factor
	Endotoxin
	Hypoxemia
	Electrolyte imbalances
	Dysrhythmias
Fluid volume excess	Impaired renal function
	Volume administration
	Leaky capillaries
	Third spacing
Infection, risk for	Uremic toxins
	Use of invasive lines or catheters
	Compromised skin integrity
	Compromised nutritional status
Nutrition, less than body requirements	Hypermetabolic state
	Gastrointestinal distress
	Fatigue
	Cellular abnormalities
Anxiety	Disease processes
	Knowledge deficit about procedures, therapies
Thermoregulation, ineffective	Altered cerebral perfusion
	Disease processes
Impaired verbal communication	Intubation
	Confusion
Family coping: compromised, ineffective	Disease process, change in family roles

(CRRT), as needed. Encephalopathy, with or without increased ICP, is an ominous sign. Efforts to decrease ICP may include hyperventilation and the use of mannitol or furosemide. Coagulation disturbances are also grave indicators because DIC further complicates treatment. Management of DIC is discussed later in this chapter.

Changes in LOC should be monitored every hour. The nurse should reorient the patient to person, place, and time as needed. The bed should be kept in a low position with side rails up, for safety reasons. The nurse should institute seizure precautions as needed. Cerebral perfusion pressure is calculated during every shift, if an ICP catheter is in place.

Prevention and Control of Infection

A high priority must be given to the prevention of infection. If required, patients should be taken to the operating room and wounds débrided. Fractures should be stabilized, to minimize tissue trauma. Depending on the injury or insult, consideration should be given to use of prophylactic antibiotics. Panculturing (sputum, urine, blood, and catheter tips) is often done before instituting antibiotics to ensure that correct antibiotics are used. If fever occurs, antipyretics and use of a hypothermia blanket may be indicated.

Strict attention must be given to aseptic technique in all procedures to minimize patient's risk of infection. Other measures to prevent infection include maintaining skin integrity, excellent skin and mouth care to minimize breakdown, overall hygiene measures, and protection from visitors or other patients who are infected. Close monitoring of temperature, noting trends, is imperative as well as monitoring for early signs of infection such as malaise, abnormal WBC, and positive cultures.

There has been controversy about the appropriateness of selective decontamination of the GI tract to avoid bacterial translocation from the gut. Such therapy generally utilizes broad-spectrum antibiotics and therefore may contribute to colonization, so it has not been universally recommended.[14] Current studies have shown that selective decontamination has no impact on reducing mortality or cost.[14,15]

Early stabilization of the GI tract is essential. Early institution of nutritional support may minimize catabolism. Some centers are using slow-drip (for example, 5–10 mL/hr) enteral feedings to maintain gastrointestinal integrity while using total parenteral nutrition to meet the balance of nutritional needs. These patients must have a prescribed diet, including high caloric intake and frequent feedings. A nasogastric tube is inserted and is attached to low intermittent suction, as needed. The nurse monitors gastric output (color, amount) and guaiac testing of all stools, emesis, and nasogastric tube drainage to assess for occult bleeding. Gastric alkalization (antacids, H_2 blockers) is provided according to gastric pH. The nurse provides frequent oral hygiene, using a soft toothbrush and ice chips, as indicated, to maintain intact oral membranes.

Establishing Adequate Oxygenation

Maintaining adequate tissue oxygenation in patients with MODS is often difficult. Maintenance of adequate cardiac function, adequate hemoglobin levels, and adequate oxygen saturation are necessities. Treatment objectives for the patient in respiratory failure are focused on achieving acceptable gas exchange while minimizing damage to the lung. Early, aggressive ventilation, often with PEEP, is aimed at keeping the PaO_2 greater than 80 mm Hg. Some centers are utilizing inverse ratio ventilation (IRV) in the severely hypoxic, PEEP-resistant patient with MODS. IRV reverses the inspiratory and expiratory phases of the respiratory cycle, thus making the inspiratory time long and the expiratory time short. Concurrently, these patients are ventilated, utilizing pressure-control ventilation to maintain the mean airway pressures as low as possible. Use of IRV may be uncomfortable, so sedation and paralysis should be considered.

Collaboratively, nursing and respiratory therapy staff members work to maintain a patent airway to maximize air exchange. Pulmonary hygiene such as suctioning, chest physical therapy, incentive spirometry, and turn, cough, and deep breathing maneuvers should be implemented to assist in mobilizing secretions and promoting ventilation. These patients generally benefit from early intubation. Early, aggressive mechanical ventilation, including PEEP, helps to increase the patient's functional residual capacity before alveoli collapses and promotes oxygen delivery. The patient's ventilatory compliance and minute ventilation should be monitored. Oxygenation should be closely monitored using ABGs, oximetry, or oximetric catheter (when evaluating ABGs, the $PaO_2/PaCO_2$ ratio and the FIO_2/PaO_2 relationship are assessed). Patients requiring intubation should be evaluated for the need for restraints to maintain an intact endotracheal tube. The nurse monitors the patient's respiratory status hourly. This assessment should include respiratory rate, effort and pattern, and breath sounds. Bronchodilators may be utilized to enhance ventilation. The nurse should attempt to maximize blood flow to the lungs by changing the patient's position. Any change in body position requires an evaluation of its impact on the patient's hemodynamic status and oxygenation. This method assists in identifying positions of maximal ventilation without hemodynamic compromise. Suction (using in-line suction catheters if the patient is PEEP dependent) is performed as needed to maintain a patent airway and to maximize oxygen and carbon dioxide exchange. Use of paralytic agents should be considered when an acceptable PaO_2 cannot be reached. The use of paralytic agents decreases oxygen consumption by respiratory muscles and decreases chest wall pressure, thereby decreasing the pressures required to ventilate. If paralytic agents are used, the nurse should ensure that the patient is adequately sedated, to minimize anxiety. Pulmonary artery monitoring is instituted early in care, to follow fluid status carefully and to avoid fluid overload and pulmonary edema.

Establishing Adequate Circulating Volume

Fluid balance is a challenge in the patient with MODS and requires meticulous attention to both cardiovascular and renal systems. Attempts are made to avoid fluid overload. Use of diuretics and low-dose dopamine may be instituted to minimize pulmonary edema. At the same time, consideration must be given to adequate fluid balance to support renal function. Hemodialysis or CRRT may be initiated to allow additional fluid or parenteral nutrition administration.[16] Pulmonary artery monitoring is essential to evaluate fluid balance and the success of interventions. Continued debate exists around the use of crystalloids or colloids in management of these patients. Although hypoalbuminemia is common in the patient with MODS, albumin and other colloids must be administered with extreme caution. In the presence of increased capillary permeability, colloid administration may exacerbate vascular fluid movement into the interstitium. Fluid therapy must be individualized to each patient and fluid challenges may be necessary.

Attempting to maintain normal renal function is a challenge. Antibiotics should be administered carefully because dose alterations may be necessary if renal function is diminished. The nurse should monitor the patient's BUN and creatinine values when administering renal toxic antibiotics. Laboratory values (electrolytes, BUN, creatinine, hemoglobin, hematocrit, platelet count, PT, PTT, WBC with differential, ABGs) should be monitored, with abnormal laboratory values corrected as needed. The nurse should monitor for signs and symptoms of fluid and electrolyte imbalances as well as signs and symptoms of acid–base and electrolyte interactions. Skin turgor and mucous membranes should be noted during every shift. The nurse should monitor the patient's daily weights and should note trends. Careful intake and output should be performed every hour. One should maintain fluid restriction or provide for careful fluid administration and consider the use of low-dose dopamine (1–3 μg/kg/min) to enhance renal blood flow. The nurse should prepare the patient for dialysis or CRRT, if indicated. A Foley catheter is maintained to enable more accurate measurement of urine output. However, the Foley catheter should be removed if the patient becomes anuric or has a minimal urine output because it is a source of potential infection. If hypervolemia occurs, diuretics and antihypertensive agents should be administered as ordered. Specific gravity is monitored during every shift, to assess the concentrating ability of the kidney and the patient's fluid status.

The treatment of DIC is considered when attempting to establish adequate circulating volume. If a patient bleeds excessively, maintenance of an adequate circulating volume will be difficult. Therapy is often complicated because all three abnormalities—clotting, bleeding, and fibrinolysis—are occurring simultaneously. Initial therapy should be addressed at the precipitating event, with aggressive support given to systems affected by the coagulation abnormalities. Vigorous fluid administration, ventilation and oxygenation, inotropic and vasopressor support, and hemodialysis or renal replacement therapy should be instituted to support tissue perfusion and oxygenation and to treat circulatory shock. Pharmacologic interventions may include heparin, antiplatelet agents, and antifibrinolytic agents.

The use of all of these agents is considered controversial by many investigators, partially because of the lack of randomized, clinical trials providing evidence of success. Heparin acts to prevent further fibrin deposits in the microvasculature by activating the antithrombin III system, thus interrupting the intravascular formation of thrombin. Although it does nothing to eliminate established clots, it slows the coagulation processes enough that coagulation factor regeneration is possible. Platelet inhibitors, such as aspirin and nonsteroidal anti-inflammatory agents, have also been used in some patients. Antifibrinolytic agents have been given in conjunction with heparin.

The use of blood products in DIC is also considered controversial. The decision to administer blood products is made, balancing the positive impact of replacement of lost products with the addition of more clotting factors to an already dysfunctional system. The choice of product, be it whole blood, packed cells, platelets, fresh frozen plasma (FFP), or cryoprecipitate, is based on the patient's clinical situation. All components or any combination of components may be used.

Plasmapheresis is undergoing research for use in the treatment of DIC, the thought being that it will remove the circulating FSP, and through use of exchange transfusions, fresh clotting factors are administered. It is useful to understand that even with the most aggressive treatment, DIC is a difficult clinical entity to treat. Mortality related to DIC is extremely high.

Cardiovascular Support

Therapies directed at cardiac failure are focused on the patient's symptoms because these vary, depending on whether the patient is also septic. Continuous cardiac monitoring is instituted, and dysrhythmias are treated as indicated with appropriate antidysrhythmic agents. Frequently, however, patients in MODS continue to have dysrhythmias despite what appears to be adequate antidysrhythmic therapy. The nurse monitors CO, cardiac index, and SVR every 4 hours and as needed to evaluate the effect of PEEP and to maximize the patient's fluid status. The nurse monitors the patient's vital signs, PAP, PAOP, and CVP at least hourly. Inotropic or vasopressor medications are given as ordered to maximize cardiac function. Vasopressor agents, such as dopamine, phenylephrine, and norepinephrine, are commonly used when patients are hypotensive despite fluid interventions. Dobutamine, isoproterenol, or amrinone may be indicated, and the choice is determined by the patient's individual situation. Generally, patients who maintain high CO and low SVR do not require vasodilator therapy. However, in MODS and sepsis, patients may progress to low-CO states with a high SVR. In this situation, agents such as nitroprusside may be helpful.

Crystalloids rather than colloids are used in fluid replacement to minimize movement of fluid into interstitial space. Diuretics are administered as needed to avoid fluid overload and to manage heart failure. The nurse monitors distal pulses, as well as temperature, color, and capillary refill in extremities to assess peripheral perfusion. Mechanical assist devices (pacemaker, intra-aortic balloon pump) are used as necessary to enhance cardiac function.

To maximize fluid balance, the nurse monitors the patient for bleeding from all sites. Blood collection is grouped to minimize blood waste and to maximize tissue perfusion. Blood and blood products are given as needed to maximize tissue perfusion.

Patient and Family Support

Patients with MODS are extremely ill. Both patients and their families need frequent, clear information. Unit routines, equipment, and test results are just a few examples of information that needs to be communicated to patients and families. Regularly scheduled team meetings that include the family may help the family to feel well informed and may decrease their stress and the number of interruptions team members receive. These patients that could benefit from having both a primary nurse and a primary physician, along with a well-defined health care team. Attempts should be made to control the chaotic environment of the critical care unit by being attentive to both sensory overload and sensory deprivation of meaningful stimuli.

Future Trends

Our knowledge of appropriate interventions for patients with MODS will continue to change as research and technology advance. Along with our progress in treating MODS, the number of ethical dilemmas may increase as our ability to treat individual dysfunctional systems improves (Chart 49–2). The use of monoclonal

CHART 49–2

ETHICAL DILEMMA

Mrs. J., a 53-year-old widow, was admitted through the emergency department after a neighbor found her unresponsive, on the floor, at home. It was estimated that she had been unresponsive for more than 24 hours. A complete workup was done, including a CT scan to the head, as a result of which it was identified that she had suffered a large stroke, possibly related to a tumor that was visualized. During the CT scan, Mrs. J. became severely hypotensive and experienced cardiac arrest. Initially resuscitated, she was transferred to the critical care unit; she was on the ventilator, with a dopamine drip to keep her blood pressure greater than 90 mm Hg systolic and a lidocaine drip as follow-up to her ventricular tachycardic arrest. Efforts to contact her family were futile.

After 3 days of aggressive therapy, Mrs. J. remained on the ventilator, was dopamine dependent, and had suffered two additional episodes of ventricular tachycardia. Her morning laboratory tests and vital signs showed the following results: temperature, 99.9°F; heart rate, 129 beats per minute; blood pressure, 92/64 mm Hg; respirations, 22 per minute; blood urea nitrogen, 60 mg/dL; cre-atinine, 3.2; potassium, 5.9 mEq/L; and sodium, 128 mEq/L.

Her health care team believes that dialysis or continuous renal replacement therapy should be initiated immediately. Mrs. J. is intermittently conscious and, when lucid, wants no further therapy. Her family members (two daughters) were found and have flown in from out of state. They want every possible therapy available to their mother initiated. The older daughter has the health care power of attorney for her mother.

1. At this point in care, who has the final authority for making decisions about treatment?
2. What should the nurse's response be if asked by the family whether or not to proceed with additional interventions?
3. Suppose the medical staff members choose to listen to the family over the patient. What should your response as the nurse be?
4. Identify additional information and resources that you could make available to the patient and family that may assist with their decision making.

antibodies offered promise, but it has been shown to be ineffective in patients with MODS and sepsis. Another study suggests that the use of human recombinant interleukin-1 receptor antagonist may prove favorable. Investigation of the use of anti-TNF antibodies is being suggested.

The time spent by a patient with MODS in the critical care unit is a small percentage of the overall time this patient needs to recover. Rehabilitation can be extensive and long, requiring care in different settings. Chart 49–3 addresses the focus of care after discharge from the critical care unit for these patients.

Multidisciplinary Outcomes

The outcomes for the patient with MODS are related to the systems that have been dysfunctional, so they vary from patient to patient. They include all or some combination of the following:

1. Identification of the initiating injury, insult, or infectious source.
2. Restoration of dysfunctional organ systems.
3. Restoration of hemodynamic values.
4. Restoration of fluid, electrolyte, and acid–base imbalances.
5. Control of infection, if present.
6. Suppression of the body's inflammatory response.
7. Rehabilitation of the patient.

Multidisciplinary outcomes for the patient with MODS progress as the patient moves through the health care system. Table 49–7 summarizes outcomes as the patient's progress is seen through critical care, intermediate care, and rehabilitation.

Critical Thinking Exercise

Ms. J., a 35-year-old woman, was admitted to the hospital with a diagnosis of lower abdominal pain. Her past medical history was significant for hysterectomy, oophorectomy, vaginectomy, and partial colectomy for vaginal cancer a year before admission. The day after her admission, Ms. J.'s pain continued, and a rectal tube was placed with some symptomatic relief. By the evening of the second day, her blood pressure and urine output fell. A Foley catheter was placed to monitor her urine output. Over the next 8 hours,

CHART 49–3

BEYOND THE ICU: CARE OF THE PATIENT IN REHABILITATION AFTER MULTIPLE ORGAN DYSFUNCTION SYNDROME

Early identification and intervention are essential to the patient with multiple organ dysfunction syndrome (MODS). If a patient survives the intensive care phase, recovery will depend on the patient's age and preinjury health status. Rehabilitation time may be prolonged. The patient's focus during rehabilitation is regaining muscle mass and neuromuscular function. The focus of collaborative management is to assist the patient to adjust to an environment other than the ICU and to increase independence in his or her activities. As recovery continues and it becomes apparent that a patient will survive MODS, plans for discharge should begin. The intensive care phase of MODS is often prolonged, and a gradual transition is needed to assist the patient and family from this environment to a progressive care unit and then to home. The patient may be faced with a lengthy rehabilitation in a transitional care or rehabilitation facility once he or she leaves the hospital. The goals and expected outcomes of this rehabilitation phase should be openly discussed with the patient and family so that they may begin the necessary psychological adjustments.

The nursing diagnosis that is a priority in the rehabilitation phase is activity intolerance, with an associated outcome of the patient being able to perform his or her own activities of daily living. The patient may continue to have an ineffective breathing pattern from overall muscle weakness and prolonged intubation. The expected outcome is a normal breathing effort and pattern and an ability to maintain normal arterial blood gases. The health care team needs to continue to collaborate, including physical and occupational therapy, to design and implement a plan for progressive activity. The team should provide for adequate rest and nutrition for the patient to promote strength and healing. The overall goal during rehabilitation is to return the patient to his or her optimal level of functioning.

---

she was given 3 L of lactated Ringer's solution (LR) to try to increase her urine output and to maintain her systolic blood pressure above 90 mm Hg. Her heart rate increased to 120, her respiratory rate to 40, and her LOC became depressed.

Ms. J. was taken to surgery at 3 AM. She was found to have 5 feet of necrotic bowel with gross peritonitis and hemorrhagic ascites totaling 4600 mL. On admission to critical care, her blood pressure was labile (80–120/50–60 mm Hg). She was volume dependent, requiring more than 1 L of LR every 30 minutes to maintain her blood pressure above 90 mm Hg. She received a total of 10 L of fluid in the first 4 hours. A pulmonary artery catheter was placed, and the following values were obtained: PAP, 25/15 mm Hg; PAOP, 20 mm Hg; CVP, 18 mm Hg; CO, 5.28 L per minute; cardiac index, 3.57; SVR, 1151; and temperature, 96.6°F.

Ms. J. was intubated during surgery and remains on the ventilator. Her settings included the following: tidal volume, 650; rate, 10(A/C); FiO_2, 40%; and ABGs: pH, 7.02; $PaCO_2$, 52; PaO_2, 63; and HCO_3^-, 12. After these ABGs, her rate was increased to 18, FiO_2 to 60%, and 4 ampules of HCO_3^- were given. Her pulmonary status continued to deteriorate. Later the same day, her FiO_2 was up to 80%, and PEEP of 5 was added, with the following ABGs: pH, 7.36; $PaCO_2$, 32; PaO_2, 74; HCO_3^-, 18.

Ms. J.'s evening shift nurse noted some oozing on the abdominal dressing as well as around her Swan and catheter intravenous insertion sites. Her urine was heme positive. A coagulation screen was drawn: PT, 37; PTT, more than 100; platelets, 47,000; and fibrinogen, 74. Then 2 U FFP, an eight-pack of platelets, and 15 U of cryoprecipitate were given with the following results: PT, 21.2; PTT, more than 100; platelets, 120,000; and fibrinogen 230.

After an additional 2 U of FFP, her PT and PTT dropped further, to 14.9 and 56.1. Later in the day, her blood pressure was falling again, despite large amounts of blood and LR (70/55 mm Hg; heart rate, 145). Dopamine was started and titrated to keep the blood pressure above 90 mm Hg. Fluids were to be titrated to keep her PAOP in the range of 15 to 18 mm Hg.

Her urine output continued to drop over the next 36 hours, despite large amounts of fluid and furosemide. By her third ICU day, her weight had increased to 68 kg (admission weight, 48 kg). Laboratory results were as follows: creatinine, 2.8; BUN, 33; K^+, 6.2; and Ca^{++}, 7.7. ABGs were as follows: pH, 7.28; $PaCO_2$, 39; PaO_2, 94; HCO_3^-, 19 (80%, PEEP 5).

An ampule of 50% dextrose and 10 U of regular insulin intravenously along with an ampule of HCO_3^- were given: Her K^+ dropped to 4.5. It was thought that her hypocalcemia was due to binding with the citrate in the banked blood. An ampule of calcium chloride was given. Renal replacement was instituted early because of her extreme weight gain and rapid development of renal failure. Her blood pressure was labile during dialysis, requiring dopamine support. She went into atrial fibrillation while receiving renal replacement and required diltiazem to convert her rhythm to sinus tachycardia. Her course continued to be

TABLE 49–7
Multidisciplinary Outcomes

Phase of Recovery	Outcomes
Critical care	Stabilization and maintenance of airway and breathing pattern
	Normalization and stabilization of normal cardiac output and tissue perfusion
	Identification and stabilization of initial injury, insult, or infection
	Restoration of fluid, electrolyte, and acid–base imbalances
Intermediate care	Maintenance of tissue perfusion
	Maintenance of adequate cardiac output
	Maintenance of adequate oxygenation
	Restoration of patient and family psychological well-being
Rehabilitation	Normalization and stabilization of mobility and muscle strength
	Normalization and stabilization of activities of daily living
	Maintenance of psychological well-being
	Restoration of previous roles

rocky for another 6 days with CRRT, blood pressure support, abnormal coagulation tests, development of a small GI hemorrhage, climbing bilirubin to 8 mg/dL, and temperature spikes. She returned to surgery 8 days after her first operation and was found to have necrotizing fasciitis. The skin, muscle, and fascia over a large area of her abdominal wall were surgically removed. She is now improving daily. Coagulation studies are back to normal, her blood pressure is stable, and she is being weaned from the ventilator. She has required multiple surgical procedures.

1. Within the first several days of her hospitalization, what signs and symptoms does Ms. J. have of the development of MODS?
2. After her initial surgery, what should the focus of your care have been?
3. After her abnormal coagulation studies, what do you believe that she is developing and what is your plan of care?
4. What interventions would you consider for her blood pressure drop after improvement of her coagulation studies?
5. Discuss the developments that contributed to each system's becoming dysfunctional.

Key Concepts

⟹ MODS can be viewed as either primary or secondary.

⟹ Patients who develop MODS are survivors of major surgery or of a traumatic event to the body.

⟹ MODS is viewed by many as the final pathway for many critically ill patients, accounting for most deaths, with a mortality rate of greater than 50%, in noncoronary critical care units.

⟹ MODS, sepsis, and DIC are all multidimensional processes that represent dysfunctional cellular interactions among organ systems rather than isolated processes of a single organ dysfunction.

⟹ DIC development is always a secondary process with intrinsic and extrinsic initiators.

⟹ Mediators cause vasoconstriction and bronchoconstriction of the pulmonary vasculature that lead to the development of a massive capillary leak.

⟹ Chest radiographs reveal diffuse infiltrates reflecting consolidation and possibly infection.

⟹ The kidneys sustain prolonged vasoconstriction from the circulating epinephrine and angiotensin II, which increase the risk of development of renal failure.

⟹ The cardiovascular system is affected by MODS because of the dysfunction of the other systems.

⟹ As perfusion rates decrease, the GI tract and the liver also become at risk of dysfunction.

⟹ If bacteria are not removed from the GI tract or the liver, they will be transported to the rest of the body, resulting in seeding of bacteria.

⟹ A change in LOC is usually the first assessment seen, but it can range from disorientation to unconsciousness to coma.

⟹ The hematologic system becomes affected as it is exhausted by the SIRS and consumption of hematologic and clotting factors occurs.

⟹ No single treatment plan for MODS exists.

References

1. Knaus WA, Wagner DP: Multiple systems organ failure: epidemiology and prognosis. Crit Care Clin 5:221–232, 1989.
2. Sculier JP, Brom D, Verboven N, et al: Multiple organ failure during interleukin-2 and LAK cell infusion. Intensive Care Med 14:666–667, 1988.
3. Bone RC, Balk RA, Cerra FB, et al: Definitions for sepsis and organ failure and guidelines for the use of innovative therapies in sepsis. Chest 101:1644–1655, 1992.
4. Beal AL, Cerra FB: Multiple organ failure syndrome in the 1990's: systemic inflammatory response and organ dysfunction. JAMA 271:226–233, 1994.
5. Secor VH: Multiple Organ Dysfunction: Pathophysiology and Clinical Implications. St. Louis, Mosby–Year Book, 1996.

6. Herbert PC, Drummond RN, Singer J, et al: A simple multiple system organ failure scoring system predicts mortality of patients who have sepsis syndrome. Chest 104:230–235, 1993.

7. Bone RC: Sir Isaac Newton, sepsis, SIRS, and CARS. Crit Care Med 24:1125–1127, 1996.

8. Pinsky MR, Matuschak GM: Multiple systems organ failure: failure of host defense homeostasis. Crit Care Clin 5:199–220, 1989.

9. Carlson KK: Multiple organ dysfunction syndrome. In: Urban NA, Greenlee KK, Krumberger JM, et al (eds): Guidelines for Critical Care Nursing. St. Louis, C.V. Mosby, 1995, pp 618–628.

10. Tracey KJ, Cerami A: Tumor necrosis factor: an updated review of its biology. Crit Care Med 21:S415–S422, 1993.

11. Dressler DK: Patients with coagulopathies. In: Clochesy JM, Breu C, Cardin S, et al (eds): Critical Care Nursing. Philadelphia, W.B. Saunders, 1996, pp 1147–1161.

12. Stechmiller JK, Treloar D, Allen N: Gut dysfunction in critically ill patients: a review of the literature. Am J Crit Care 6:204–209, 1997.

13. Macho JR, Luce JM: Rational approach to the management of multiple systems organ failure. Crit Care Clin 5:379–392, 1989.

14. Hammond JMJ, Potgieter PD, Saunders L: Selective decontamination of the digestive tract in multiple trauma patients—is there a role? Results of a prospective, double-blind, randomized trial. Crit Care Med 22:33–39, 1994.

15. Vandenbroucke-Grauls CM, Vandenbroucke J: Effect of selective decontamination of the digestive tract on respiratory tract infections and mortality in intensive care. Lancet 338:859–862, 1991.

16. Van Bomel EF: Should continuous renal replacement therapy be used for "non-renal" indications in critically ill patients in shock? Resuscitation 33:257–270, 1997.

50

Trauma

Linda Laskowski-Jones

Objectives

After completing this chapter, the student will be able to:

1. Analyze the epidemiology of trauma as a public health problem.
2. Define the components of a trauma care system.
3. Describe the etiology and pathophysiology of injury for the major body regions.
4. Define the approach to the initial assessment of the adult trauma patient.
5. Differentiate the initial management priorities for the acutely injured adult trauma patient.
6. Describe the elements of the diagnostic phase of care for trauma patients.
7. Select appropriate nursing and collaborative trauma care interventions.
8. List specific considerations for care of the elderly trauma patient.
9. Evaluate the effectiveness of trauma care as related to anticipated outcomes.
10. Define the roles of the nurse in promoting trauma prevention.

EPIDEMIOLOGY

The term "trauma" is derived from the Greek word for wound. Although the general public tends to associate the word "trauma" with any crisis, such as a heart attack or severe psychological stress, the term actually refers to bodily injury. Traumatic injury is the number 1 cause of death for persons under the age of 45 years and is the fourth leading cause of death in the United States overall.[1] Each year, approximately 150,000 people die as a result of both intentional and unintentional injury, the foremost public health problem in America today.[1]

Although trauma affects persons across the life span, those in the highest risk group statistically are males between the ages of 15 and 24 years.[2] Because trauma is a disease of young people, more years of life are lost annually than for all other causes of death. However, death is only one measure of trauma's impact; permanent disability and varying degrees of physical impairment are other potential outcomes. Each year, approximately 2.1 million people hospitalized for traumatic injury survive to be discharged.[3] The cost to society is great, considering medical care, nursing home care, rehabilitation, lost wages, and property damage. The real cost to patients and families in terms of human suffering and lifestyle disruption cannot be calculated in dollar amounts, but it must be recognized as the most significant sequela of traumatic injury. Because nurses witness firsthand the devastation brought about by traumatic events that are often preventable, they are ideally prepared to share their insights with patients and the general public. Chart 50–1 describes the way in which nurses can incorporate injury reduction and prevention strategies into health teaching opportunities.

SYSTEMS OF TRAUMA CARE DELIVERY

A trauma center is a specialty care facility that has been formally evaluated according to state, regional, or national standards and has been found to meet criteria established to ensure competent and expedient provision of care to injured patients. Perceptions differ about what constitutes a trauma center, even among some hospitals that self-report their status incorrectly.[4] It is important to understand that not all hospitals that offer 24-hour emergency services are considered trauma centers. The real trauma center designation is a hard-earned status based on stringent requirements that reflect institutional commitment to optimal trauma care given the available resources.

Today's civilian trauma centers are direct descendants of wartime mobile army surgical hospital

CHART 50-1

BEYOND THE ICU: TRAUMA PREVENTION

Like cancer and heart disease prevention efforts, effective strategies exist to reduce the incidence and severity of traumatic injury. The first challenge is to overcome the pervasive view that trauma is simply an "act of God" for which victims have no control, similar to the occurrence of a natural disaster. Measures to prevent trauma not only can reduce the likelihood of an injury-producing event, but also they can lessen the impact if one should occur. For example, seat belts are 42% effective in preventing fatalities in motor vehicle collisions; the addition of an airbag increases the effectiveness by 12%.[1] Child safety seats offer significant protection to children if secured and positioned properly in the vehicle. A reduction in the accessibility of firearms may limit the homicide rate in the United States, now the tenth leading cause of death in all age groups and ranked in the top five causes for people 1 to 44 years of age.[2] Dedicated efforts to increase public awareness about the risks of drinking and driving may reduce the overall incidence of alcohol-related crashes. A wealth of resource information exists on trauma and injury prevention in the health care literature and through multiple agencies and safety organizations.

Nurses in all settings who care for trauma patients are in an ideal role to promote trauma prevention. Nurses comprehend the magnitude of the pain, suffering, disability, and overall crisis incurred by victims and their significant others, and they can offer realistic prevention messages in their health teaching. The two major fronts for trauma-prevention intervention are the individual trauma patient and the general public.

Individual trauma patients require an assessment of the factors that brought them into the trauma care system. Questions to consider may include the following points: Were seat belts or other recommended safety devices used properly? Did alcohol or drugs play a role in the event? Is the home environment safe? Were firearms and ammunition readily accessible? Was the incident gang-related? Is the patient a victim of interpersonal or domestic violence, abuse, or neglect? The answers to these questions may come from several sources: patterns of injury, laboratory results from drug and alcohol screenings, prehospital or police information, and statements made during conversation with the patient, family, or significant others.

Among adolescents and young adults, high-risk behaviors such as drug and alcohol use, delinquency, and reckless driving are commonly associated with traumatic injury and trauma recidivism; being a trauma victim is a recognized risk factor for subsequent trauma.[3] In both the pediatric and geriatric trauma population, a careful assessment of home safety may be indicated. In addition, the question whether a debilitated elderly person should continue to drive a car or live alone may require consideration. Based on an exploration of the circumstances surrounding the traumatic injury, the nurse can incorporate pertinent trauma-prevention information into the health teaching plan. In addition, initiating patient referrals to drug or alcohol rehabilitation programs, child protective services, social services, psychiatric services, or community programs that address high-risk behaviors may be necessary.

The community is another target for trauma-prevention interventions. The nurse may take on multiple roles—health care educator, political activist, and safety advocate. Experience in caring for trauma patients and knowledge of prevention strategies make the nurse an effective educator for schools, businesses, and community groups. Trauma-prevention education should be directed to address frequent causes of traumatic injury in the particular community as well as in high-risk groups; statistics from hospital or state trauma registries can help to define the areas of need for prevention efforts. Ideally, an evaluation of the presentation's effectiveness also should be planned when possible. Political activity is another nursing function related to trauma prevention. In this role, the nurse may need to educate and seek the support of legislators and community members to enable passage of bills to promote trauma prevention. Typical legislative initiatives related to trauma prevention include enactment of seat belt and helmet laws, strict drinking-and-driving statutes, weapon-control measures, and mandatory protection features in automobiles and homes and on roadways. Finally, the nurse can serve as a safety advocate by encouraging the use of appropriate safety devices in occupational settings, sports activities, and recreational pursuits.

References

1. Viano DC: Restraint effectiveness, availability and use in fatal crashes: implications to injury control. J Trauma 38:538–546, 1995.
2. The Violence Prevention Task Force of the Eastern Association for the Surgery of Trauma: Violence in America: a public health crisis—the role of firearms. J Trauma 38:163–168, 1995.
3. Smeltzer SC, Redeker NS: A framework of trauma and trauma recidivism in adolescents and young adults. J Trauma Nurs 2:93–99, 1995.

(MASH) units from the era of the Vietnam and Korean conflicts. Rapid transport from the battlefield to a facility staffed with qualified surgeons and other medical and nursing personnel who were immediately available to initiate lifesaving interventions dramatically reduced mortality rates of injured soldiers. The concepts of organized care and resources prioritized to the needs of the trauma patient eventually, but slowly, spread to civilian hospitals beginning in the 1960s and 1970s.

In 1976, the American College of Surgeons (ACS) published the first guidelines for classification of trauma centers in the United States.[5] However, not until the 1980s did the widespread growth of trauma centers across the United States become a reality. Research began to validate the assumption that trauma centers save more lives: a 1979 landmark study in California clearly demonstrated a significant reduction in injury-related mortality when trauma victims were treated at a trauma center, as opposed to being treated at the closest community hospital.[6] The focus of the 1990s became the development of trauma systems, with the recognition that a trauma center is only as good as the mechanisms in place to transport the patient to the facility and to provide for community reintegration through appropriate rehabilitation services. To facilitate trauma system development across America, the Trauma Care Systems Planning and Development Act of 1990 (P.L. 101-590) made funding available to states that were willing to submit an application and commit resources to form a state trauma system. In 1992, the United States Public Health Service, Health Resources and Services Administration, offered the Model Trauma Care System Plan to states as a general framework for creating their own individualized system.[7] The plan identified the following mandatory trauma care system components, with the objective of including all health care providers or facilities that could render trauma care resources: leadership; system development; legislation; finance; public information or education and prevention; human resources; prehospital care including communications, medical direction, triage, and transport; definitive care encompassing trauma care facilities, interfacility transfer, and rehabilitation; and evaluation.[8]

The ACS guidelines have evolved to include not only the standards for the various levels of trauma centers, but also the entire system of trauma care delivery as outlined in the Model Trauma Care System Plan.[9] Four levels of trauma centers are currently defined and characterized by the ACS: level I (highest capability), level II, level III, and level IV.[9] Nurses, as consumers of health care as well as providers, need to have a clear understanding of the resources for trauma care available in their own communities. When such resources are critically reviewed, significant gaps in services are often encountered, particularly in areas of the United States that do not have an organized trauma system. Nurses are in an ideal position as health care advocates to pursue community and legislative action to help establish a coordinated system inclusive of the essential components that will provide optimal care to injured patients. Although not every community requires or could even support a level I or level II trauma center, at minimum a plan should be in place to transfer trauma patients to facilities best prepared to meet their needs, even if that means transferring persons out of their own community. A summary of the major distinguishing features of each level of trauma center follows, based on ACS standards.[9]

Level I Trauma Center

The ACS defines a level I trauma facility as a "regional resource trauma center" with the ". . . capability of providing leadership and total care for every aspect of injury, from prevention through rehabilitation."[9] Clinical capabilities that differentiate level I centers from other levels of trauma center include cardiac surgery, hand surgery, microvascular surgery for replantation of severed limbs, an in-house general surgeon, nuclear scanning, neuroradiology, cardiopulmonary bypass, and acute hemodialysis capabilities, to name a few. Usually a university-based or major teaching hospital, the level I trauma center assumes responsibilities that extend beyond the clinical aspects to encompass trauma education for all levels of staff, research, community injury prevention and outreach programs, and trauma systems planning. Most level I trauma centers are located in urban areas.[4]

Level II Trauma Center

The level II trauma center is generally a community hospital with the same requirements for "initial definitive trauma care," trauma education, and trauma prevention as a level I center.[9] However, it is recognized that some patients may require transfer to a level I center to receive care for complex injuries. Conducting research is desired, but it is not considered essential for level II status.

Level III Trauma Center

A level III trauma center provides a critical link to communities that do not have level I or level II facilities. At this center, the goal is rapid initial resuscitation and stabilization of the patient and then transfer to a higher-capability trauma center with resources to meet the patient's needs.[9] In some cases, surgery may be necessary to stabilize the patient before transfer. Level

III centers must have transfer agreements with level I or level II centers and must use standard treatment protocols for trauma management. A general surgeon must be readily available.

Level IV Trauma Center

In rural or remote areas that do not have access to a level I, level II, or level III trauma center, or perhaps even a physician, a clinic or similar facility may serve as the initial point of entry into the trauma system. Requirements for level IV status include having personnel who are trained in advanced trauma life support, standard treatment protocols, and transfer agreements with higher-capability trauma centers.[9] As is the case for all levels of trauma centers, participation in quality audits to evaluate the trauma care provided is essential.

MECHANISM OF INJURY

"Mechanism of injury" (MOI) is the term used to describe the manner in which the patient sustained injury, including the forces involved. It is vital to learn the MOI when obtaining a history from the prehospital care providers and, when possible, from the patient. MOI serves as a triage marker for trauma team activation and can help to predict injury patterns, injury severity, and, sometimes, eventual outcomes (Figure 50–1). The terms *blunt trauma* and *penetrating trauma* are discussed because they denote two of the most common injury-producing mechanisms. Other significant traumatic mechanisms may result from chemical, thermal, electrical, or radiation energy forces.

Blunt Trauma

Blunt trauma occurs from impact forces such as motor vehicle crashes, falls, sports injuries, and assault with fists, kicks, or a blunt object such as a baseball bat. The force or speed of impact is a significant factor. Acceleration–deceleration forces in a high-speed motor vehicle collision or a fall from a height play a major role in causing compression, tearing, and shearing of bone, soft tissues, and blood vessels. In a motor vehicle crash, for example, three collisions actually occur: the vehicle itself, the occupant within the vehicle, and the occupant's internal organs and structures; whether or not the occupant is restrained with a seat belt determines the pattern of injury. In any significant MOI, focusing only on the obvious external injuries is a critical error in judgment. One must always maintain a high index of suspicion that the patient is at great risk of occult internal injury.

Penetrating Trauma

Penetrating trauma is a result of injury from a knife, bullet, shotgun blast, sharp object, or projectile. Patterns of injury vary, based on the nature of the penetrating object and the body cavities violated. As a case in point, knife wounds often look small, nonbleeding, and innocuous by external appearance. However, the knife may have perforated multiple internal organs, blood vessels, and structures, depending on its length, the angle in which it was inserted, and, perhaps, the way it was moved about in the body.

With a firearm, injuries are determined by the type of weapon (e.g., handgun, rifle, shotgun), the muzzle velocity, the characteristics of the bullet or projectile (e.g., size or caliber, presence of a jacket), the distance between the victim and the weapon, and the body regions penetrated (Figure 50–2). Bullets can enter and exit the victim, lodge in soft tissue or organs, or strike bone and ricochet inside the body, thus producing multiple injuries. Bullets do not always take a straight path. Some types of bullets (soft-point and hollow-point bullets) are manufactured to deform or mushroom readily when they enter the body, to increase wounding potential. High-velocity projectiles such as those fired from an automatic weapon can produce a large zone of injury because they create a temporary cavity from tissue stretch as the bullet passes through the body; this tissue may become devitalized later, thereby increasing wound severity. Wounds from shotguns vary according to the distance between the gun and the victim and the type of shot loaded in the gun. A characteristic spray of pellets is the typical wounding pattern observed in shotgun wounds. However, a close-range shotgun blast may cause enormous tissue destruction. Conversely, pellet wounds can be superficial if the distance between the gun and the victim is sufficient. In explosions from bombs or volatile chemicals, injuries are related to the blast force itself, as well as to shrapnel liberated from the explosion or the surrounding area. In this case, the patient must also be evaluated for blunt force injuries from blast effect.

ETIOLOGY AND PATHOPHYSIOLOGY

The etiology and pathophysiology of traumatic injury are determined by numerous variables: MOI; gender, age, and previous health status of the victim; body region injured; severity of injury; use of protective devices; and history of substance use or abuse. Special populations such as the elderly have unique risks related to their physiologic status. For example, age-related changes and preexisting diseases in the elderly trauma patient often complicate diagnosis and man-

TRIAGE CRITERIA FOR TRAUMA CODE

Step I — **Vital Signs & Level of Consciousness**
1. Witnessed arrest
2. BP < 90 despite ALS
3. Obvious ventilatory compromise**
4. GCS < 8

YES → Initiate trauma code

NO ↓

**(e.g. RR >35 or <10 with retractive breathing and diminished breath sounds)

Step II — **Assess Anatomy of Injury**
1. Obvious major vascular injury with external hemorrhage
2. Severe maxillofacial injury with potential airway compromise
3. Large open wounds (e.g. degloving)
4. Multiple open fractures
5. Major amputation proximal to elbow and knee
6. Suspected head injury (GCS < 12) with major torso or extremity injury suspected or present

YES → Initiate trauma code

NO ↓

Step III — **Assess Mechanism of Injury**
1. Gunshot wounds to neck, trunk or groin
2. Shotgun or buckshot wounds
3. Major impaling injury to neck, torso, or proximal extremity

YES → Initiate trauma code

NO ↓

Step IV — **Logistical**
1. Hemodynamic deterioration of previously stable patient
2. Simultaneous arrival of three or more multitrauma patients

YES → Initiate trauma code

Also consider Trauma Alert or Trauma Code for:
- Severe Animal Bites
- Envenomations
- Drowning
- Hypothermia
- Major Surgical Crises
- Hangings

IF IN DOUBT, INITIATE TRAUMA CODE

CHRISTIANA CARE
Trauma Program

TRIAGE CRITERIA FOR TRAUMA ALERT

Step I — **Vital Signs & Level of Consciousness**
1. Systolic BP < 90
2. Respiratory rate < 10 or > 30
3. Unresponsive to voice (GCS ≤ 12)

YES → Initiate trauma alert

NO ↓

Step II — **Assess Anatomy of Injury**
1. All penetrating injuries to head, neck, torso and extremities proximal to elbow and knee
2. Flail chest
3. Combination trauma with burns of 10% or inhalation injuries
4. Two or more proximal long-bone fractures
5. Pelvic fractures
6. Limb paralysis
7. Amputation proximal to wrist and ankle

YES → Initiate trauma alert

NO ↓

Step III — **Assess Mechanism of Injury**
1. Ejection from automobile
2. Death in same passenger compartment
3. Extrication time >20 minutes
4. Falls >20 feet
5. Roll-over
6. High-speed auto crash – Initial speed >40 mph
   Velocity change >20 mph
   Major auto deformity >20"
   Intrusion into passenger compartment >12"
7. Auto-pedestrian injury with significant (>5 mph) impact
8. Pedestrian thrown or run over
9. Motorcycle crash >20 mph or with separation of rider and bike

YES → Consider trauma alert*

NO ↓

Step IV — **Assess for Co-Morbid Factors**
1. Extremes of age <12 years or >60 years of age
2. Hostile environment (such as extremes of heat or cold)
3. Medical illnesses (such as COPD, CHF, renal failure, etc.)
4. Presence of intoxicants
5. Pregnancy

YES → Consider trauma alert*

*Initiate trauma alert if significant injury is present or suspected (i.e., extremity deformity, rigid abdomen, abdominal pain, decreased breath sounds, etc.)

Also consider Trauma Alert or Trauma Code for:
- Severe Animal Bites
- Envenomations
- Drowning
- Hypothermia
- Major Surgical Crises
- Hangings

IF IN DOUBT, INITIATE TRAUMA CODE

CHRISTIANA CARE
Trauma Program

Figure 50–1

Triage criteria for trauma team activation. ALS, advanced life support; BP, blood pressure; CHF, congestive heart failure; COPD, chronic obstructive pulmonary disease; GCS, Glasgow Coma Score; RR, respiratory rate. (Courtesy of Christiana Care Health Services, Newark, DE.)

agement and lead to higher morbidity and mortality rates from less severe injuries.[10]

Alcohol deserves special attention because of its well-established link with traumatic injury and its popularity and widespread consumption, especially among young people. It is estimated that almost half of all trauma patients admitted to hospitals in the United States were injured while under alcohol's influence.[11] Alcohol and other drugs confound management of a trauma patient by masking the effects of injury, by altering action and metabolism of drugs, and by producing withdrawal symptoms during hospitalization.[12] In addition, chronic alcoholism leads to organ dysfunction that can complicate resuscitation

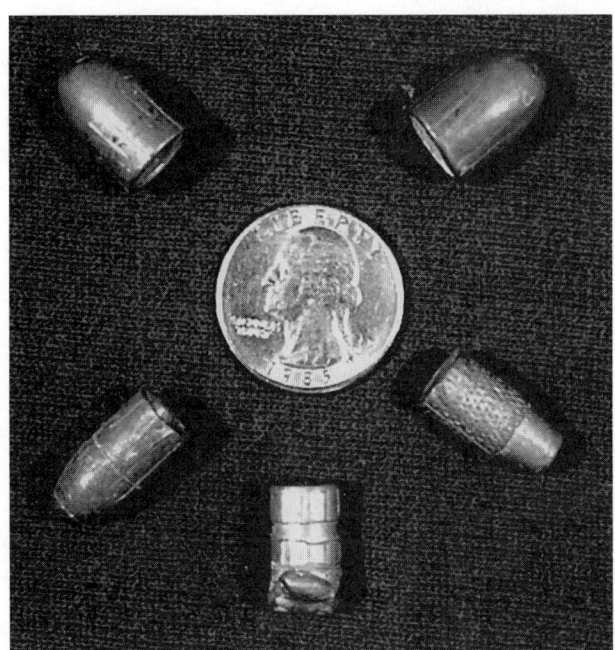

Figure 50–2

Comparison of various-caliber bullets with the size of a quarter. (Courtesy of Charles Fort, RN.)

and recovery, including liver impairment with resultant blood clotting abnormalities, poor nutritional status, and increased infection risk.[12]

With the multiple variables that may contribute to the etiology and pathophysiology of traumatic injury, it is no wonder that each individual trauma patient poses a unique set of challenges to the trauma team. The overall plan of trauma care must be individualized to address specific patient needs after generic resuscitation priorities are accomplished. A discussion reviewing the basic etiology and pathophysiology of trauma for all major body regions follows.

Head

The head is the most frequently injured body part in victims of multisystem trauma; alcohol is a major contributing factor.[13] After hemorrhage, head injury is the leading cause of death in trauma patients. It is also responsible for varying degrees of permanent disability, with significant physical, social and economic consequences. Common etiologic factors associated with head trauma include motor vehicle collisions, falls, pedestrian injury, interpersonal violence, occupational injury, and sports injury.[14] Failure to wear appropriate protective head gear (e.g., hard hats or motorcycle, bicycle, and football helmets) places persons at much higher risk of serious head injury.

Although the brain is encased by a rigid skull for protection, significant impact can fracture bone and

compress or otherwise harm neural tissue. Shear forces related to acceleration–deceleration mechanisms also produce brain injury by causing the brain to slide within the cranial vault and sustain damage from contact with bony protuberances, particularly at the base of the skull. *Coup–contrecoup* injuries are one example of this phenomenon. The brain is especially susceptible to damage from lateral impacts.[15] Cerebral hemorrhage or hematoma (subdural, epidural, subarachnoid, and intraparenchymal) and cerebral edema are common, but potentially deadly, sequelae of head trauma.

Intracranial pressure (ICP) can rise because of the mass effect from a hematoma, cerebral edema from the brain injury itself, and impaired absorption of cerebrospinal fluid (CSF), as may occur in subarachnoid hemorrhage (communicating hydrocephalus). Intracranial hypertension (usually defined as an ICP >15 mm Hg) can lead to cerebral ischemia, infarct, and, ultimately, brain herniation if uncorrected. Equally important to consider in the trauma patient is cerebral perfusion pressure (CPP), defined as the difference between mean arterial pressure (MAP) and ICP.

The brain requires a CPP of at least 70 mm Hg to maintain delivery of oxygen and glucose to cerebral cells. Hypotension from shock states or cardiovascular dysfunction reduces CPP, resulting in secondary brain injury from inadequate perfusion. Even relatively minor brain injuries can be significantly worsened by uncorrected or prolonged hypotension. Thus, the trauma team must consider the *whole* patient, not just the brain injury, when planning management. The main points to remember are that elevations in intracranial pressure *and* decreases in cerebral perfusion pressure must be managed promptly to preserve the brain from further insult. For this reason, hematomas that produce a mass effect and lead to deterioration in neurologic status generally require surgical evacuation. Cerebral edema is usually managed medically with diuretics and other measures to reduce brain swelling (see Chapter 41).

Neck

Injury to the neck occurs from blunt and penetrating trauma mechanisms. The most frequent causes of neck trauma are the acceleration–deceleration forces associated with motor vehicle collisions.[16] Penetrating trauma to the neck from sharp implements and missiles, as well as the compressive and shearing forces of blunt trauma mechanisms, can produce cervical spine injury with or without spinal cord involvement, vascular injury, and injury to the pharynx, larynx, trachea, and esophagus. In penetrating trauma, the path of a bullet or knife can expose multiple structures in the neck to harm; the energy dissipated in the blast effect alone can produce significant injury.[16] Blunt force, hyperextension, and rotation of the neck can cause blunt carotid artery trauma that may lead to arterial disruption, carotid–cavernous fistula formation, pseudoaneurysm, arterial dissection, or thrombosis, with significant risk of neurologic impairment.[16, 17] Because major blood vessels course through the neck in proximity to the airway, vascular injury with the formation of a hematoma can potentially block the airway. Similarly, soft tissue injury with resultant edema in proximity to the airway, or involving airway structures, also threatens airway integrity and patency.

Mechanisms associated with cervical spinal injury include hyperextension, hyperflexion, rotation, axial loading (also known as vertical compression), distraction, and penetrating trauma. The risk to the spinal cord is great: these mechanisms can produce spinal cord edema, contusion, compression, rupture, or transection. If an area within the spinal cord is deprived of blood supply by edema or injury, it will become ischemic and will ultimately infarct, resulting in permanent neurologic deficits below the spinal cord lesion.

Hyperextension is typically associated with rear-end collisions and falls striking the chin; the victim's head is thrust backward beyond the limits of range of motion, with potential damage to the cervical spinal cord. Conversely, hyperflexion is most often due to front-end collisions in which the victim's head is thrust downward toward the chest when it hits the steering wheel, windshield, or roof. This mechanism can produce ligamentous injury in the cervical spine and may lead to vertebral column instability with subsequent risk to the spinal cord. Rotational forces also may be involved in hyperextension and hyperflexion mechanisms; such forces are associated not only with spinal injury, but also with vascular injury.[16] Axial loading or vertical compression occurs from falls on the head. The impact force of the landing is transmitted to the cervical vertebrae and classically produces a *vertebral burst fracture* with a high probability of spinal cord injury. Distraction (such as occurs with a hanging) causes a stretch injury of the vertebral column with potential rupture of the spinal cord. Finally, penetrating trauma can result in transection of the spinal cord with or without bony injury, thus producing a permanent neurologic deficit (see Chapter 42).

Thorax

Thoracic trauma accounts for approximately one-quarter of deaths related to trauma in the United States. Both blunt and penetrating mechanisms are re-

sponsible. Motor vehicle crashes, falls, and blows to the chest are the typical blunt injury mechanisms. Stab wounds and gunshot wounds represent common penetrating injuries; trauma to any structure within the chest is possible. For both mechanisms, life-threatening hemorrhage and tension pneumothorax are the most immediate concerns.

Blunt chest trauma can range in severity from simple chest wall contusion or rib fracture to multiple rib fractures, contusive injury to the heart and lung tissue, tracheobronchial disruption, and cardiac rupture. Of particular concern is the presence of rib fractures involving the first through third ribs. Because these ribs are relatively well protected by the clavicle, significant force is required to produce fractures in this area. A high probability of concurrent vascular, neurologic, or tracheobronchial injuries exists with this injury pattern.

Even with simple rib fractures, pain can be significant during movement or breathing; hypoventilation from splinting and atelectasis can impair ventilation and may lead to respiratory failure in an otherwise healthy patient. Patients who are elderly or obese or who have preexisting pulmonary disease are at particularly high risk of compromise.[18] Blunt cardiac injury (also known as a "cardiac contusion") can disrupt the heart's normal conduction system, cause dysrhythmias, and impair ventricular function. Cardiac tamponade, caused by trauma to myocardial tissue or coronary vessels, occurs when the pericardial sac fills with blood and compresses the heart, subsequently impairing cardiac output. Pulmonary contusion, frequently associated with rib fractures and flail chest (defined as three or more adjacent ribs broken in two or more places), produces extravasation of blood into the lung parenchyma; hemoptysis is expected. Large areas of pulmonary contusion appear as a white-out on a chest radiograph, similar to acute respiratory distress syndrome (ARDS), and can pose a critical threat to the patient's oxygenation status. Tracheobronchial disruption can jeopardize the patient's airway and also produce profound ventilatory impairment. Cardiac rupture is an uncommon, but usually fatal, outcome of severe blunt chest trauma.

Acceleration–deceleration forces in high-speed motor vehicle collisions or falls from a significant height are also responsible for shearing or tearing of thoracic structures such as the aorta, vena cava, and lymphatic vessels. Of particular concern is thoracic aortic disruption. The aorta is fixed at three points in the chest: at the aortic root, at the ligamentum arteriosum just distal to the left subclavian artery, and at the diaphragm. Shear forces from motor vehicle crashes most commonly tear the aorta at the ligamentum arteriosum; falls, or vertical deceleration injuries, usually produce disruption at the aortic root. The mortality rate is extremely high. Those patients who survive to hospital admission have a pseudoaneurysm or a contained rupture of the thoracic aorta; urgent to emergency surgical intervention is the general standard of care.

Both blunt and penetrating chest trauma can produce a pneumothorax, or air in the pleural space that causes collapse of the affected lung. In blunt trauma, rib fractures or a sudden compressive force to the chest can produce a rent in the lung parenchyma. The latter mechanism is best likened to the bursting of an inflated paper bag from impact. A stab wound or gunshot wound allows the normally negative intrapleural pressure to become positive as atmospheric air enters the pleural space through the violation in the chest wall. Consequently, in both blunt and penetrating mechanisms, the air mass that accumulates in the pleural space has the potential to expand and to shift the mediastinal structures toward the unaffected lung; elevated intrathoracic pressure and compression of the vena cava impair cardiac filling and produce profound respiratory distress and hypotension. Breath sounds are typically absent on the *affected* side. The trachea may deviate toward the *unaffected* side, although tracheal deviation is a late sign. This condition is referred to as a *tension pneumothorax*. Bilateral tension pneumothoraces can occur as well. Positive-pressure ventilation, despite its necessity in resuscitation of the critically injured patient, rapidly exacerbates this condition. Ultimately, cardiovascular collapse ensues without effective chest decompression (discussed later in this chapter).

Abdomen

The abdomen is composed of solid organs such as the spleen, pancreas, and liver and air-filled hollow visceral structures such as the stomach, small bowel, and colon. Blunt or penetrating abdominal trauma places these structures at significant risk of injury. As expected, the immediate threat after abdominal trauma is hemorrhage; the later threat is peritonitis.

Direct impact to the abdomen can cause lacerations or compressive injuries to the solid organs as well as burst injuries to the air-filled structures. Trauma to the lower rib cage also may be associated with concurrent abdominal injury. Acceleration–deceleration forces can tear not only blood vessels themselves, but also organs such as the liver and spleen away from their points of attachment to major vasculature, producing life-threatening hemorrhage. Damage to the mesenteric vessels that provide blood supply to the bowel can cause bowel ischemia and, ultimately, infarct. Stomach, pancreas, and small bowel injury may permit leakage of digestive enzymes into the abdominal cavity; rupture of the large bowel results in spillage of feces, the end result of which is the development of

peritonitis that, if not properly treated, causes intra-abdominal sepsis and eventual death.

Blunt or penetrating trauma can also violate the integrity of the diaphragm, the primary muscle of respiration that divides the abdominal cavity from the thoracic cavity. Penetrating trauma is actually the more common cause of diaphragmatic rupture.[19] Because the liver occupies the space under the diaphragm on the right side of the body, injuries to the diaphragm are more often diagnosed on the left side. The risk here is that abdominal contents, which are under positive pressure relative to the negative intrathoracic pressure, will herniate into the thorax and produce ventilatory compromise as well as harm to the abdominal structures. Bowel sounds can sometimes be heard in the chest cavity. Respiratory distress is frequently encountered because the abdominal contents compete for the space normally occupied by the lung. A chest radiograph that reveals herniation of the stomach or bowel into the thorax confirms diaphragmatic rupture. Prompt surgical intervention is necessary.

Pelvis

Pelvic fractures are a major source of morbidity and mortality in trauma patients (Figure 50–3). Injuries to the pelvis can produce a range of consequences from pain and impaired mobility to life-threatening hemorrhage and death. Violation of the structural integrity of the pelvis "serves a marker of substantial energy transfer to the patient as a whole, resulting in potentially severe injuries to all organ systems."[20] Compression and vertical shear forces give rise to pelvic fractures. The most common mechanisms, in descending order of frequency, are motor vehicle crashes, pedestrian injury, falls, motorcycle collisions, and crush injuries.[20]

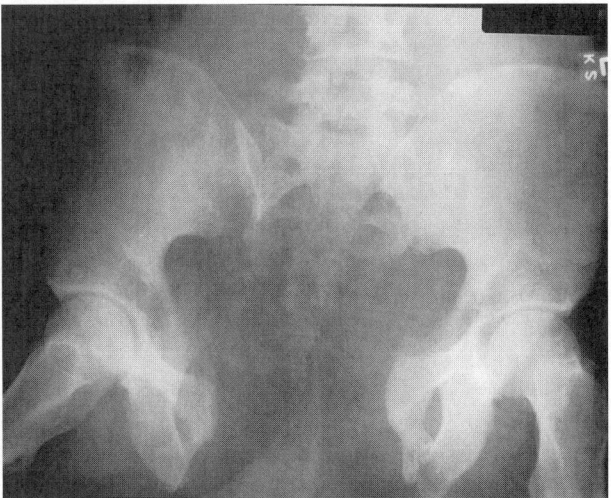

Figure 50–3

Open-book pelvic fracture sustained by the driver of a motorcycle thrown over the handlebars in the collision.

With respect to motor vehicle crashes, severe front-impact collisions are commonly associated with pelvic fractures. Of interest, however, is a study that found pelvic fractures to be most prevalent in side-impact collisions at lower speeds involving compact and subcompact cars; seat belts did not appear to prevent pelvic fractures in side-impact collisions in this study.[21]

The pathophysiology of pelvic fractures depends on the location and severity of the injury, as well as on the presence of concurrent injuries to blood vessels and other pelvic organs and structures. Genital and urinary tract injuries are common associated injuries that must be suspected and fully evaluated.[20] Pelvic fractures may be stable and may need no further intervention besides pain management and physical therapy to enhance patient comfort and mobility. Unstable pelvic fractures, however, produce significant pain and require some means of internal or external fixation before the patient can be mobilized; as with any fracture, bleeding is expected and can contribute to anemia that may necessitate intervention in the hospitalized trauma patient. At the far extreme, pelvic bone fragments or the injury-producing force itself can damage arteries and veins, producing severe life-threatening hemorrhage into the retroperitoneal space. These patients have a high mortality risk and demand intensive resuscitation efforts with fluid and multiple units of blood products. Measures typically employed to control hemorrhage in this situation include the pneumatic antishock garment (PASG) (also known as military antishock trousers or MAST suit), external pelvic fixation, internal pelvic fixation, and pelvic vessel embolization.[20]

Extremity

Various types and patterns of extremity injuries are commonly found in trauma patients. Extremity injuries are not considered a priority in the *initial* management of the trauma patient unless they are the source of significant hemorrhage or pose an immediate threat to limb viability. However, extremity injuries can lead to infection and disability if they are not managed appropriately and in a timely manner. MOIs include blunt trauma from direct blows, compression, twisting, and shearing forces, as well as penetrating trauma and burns. As in other body regions, extremity trauma occurs as a result of motor vehicle collisions, pedestrian injury, falls, violence, sports, and occupational activities. Typical injuries consist of soft tissue trauma, fractures, dislocations, vascular trauma, nerve impairment, and amputations.

Because the pathophysiologic consequences of extremity trauma vary depending on the nature of the injuries, only general concepts are presented here. Penetrating wounds, lacerations, contusions, hematomas, muscle injury, and burns constitute the general range of soft tissue injury. When the inevitable inflammatory response ensues, soft tissue swelling and pain can limit range of motion and may impair the patient's physical mobility. Any time skin integrity is disrupted, the patient is at high risk of infection; tetanus prophylaxis is necessary, as discussed later. Fractures may present in various ways: they may be stable or unstable, closed or open, displaced or nondisplaced, simple or comminuted. A joint dislocation may or may not be complicated by the presence of a fracture. Fractures, dislocations, and soft tissue trauma are often associated with vascular and nerve injury that can threaten the viability of the limb and may result in significant functional impairment for the patient. Management of extremity injuries may be complicated by the development of compartment syndrome, vascular occlusion from thrombus or embolism, pulmonary embolism or fat embolism syndrome, and infection.

Assessment and Management

Priorities in Trauma Care

Providing initial care to a trauma victim can be an overwhelming experience because of the critical nature of the patient's injuries as well as the influence of other factors inherent in emergency situations: remaining ever cognizant of the patient's potential for rapid physiologic deterioration; intervening without prior knowledge of the patient's medical history or allergies; being confronted with the need to manage multiple clinical problems and issues at once; and dealing with the intense psychosocial demands of the patient and family members, who are experiencing a crisis. To remain focused on priorities and to keep the situation under control, the nurse must use an organized approach that is applicable to *every* trauma patient and that simultaneously allows rapid evaluation and treatment of the most immediate threats to life.

The ACS provides the nationally accepted framework for initial trauma assessment and management through the Advanced Trauma Life Support (ATLS) course for physicians.[22] The ATLS methodology is the basis for trauma education and the development of trauma care standards for all levels of health care providers. Evidence exists that the ATLS course has reduced morbidity and mortality in trauma patients.[23] To address the education and certification needs of registered nurses, the Emergency Nurses Association offers the Trauma Nursing Core Course (TNCC) "to present core-level knowledge and psychomotor skills associated with implementing the trauma nursing process."[24]

The ability to set priorities accurately is a prerequisite to the provision of competent trauma care. All members of the trauma team must be "on the same wavelength" to expedite care delivery. Even the resuscitation room itself should be designed and stocked to allow ready access to the patient, trauma supplies, and equipment, including emergency drugs.

Trauma management begins with finding and treating immediate life threats and proceeds through a series of assessments and interventions aimed at addressing problems in a decreasing order of priority from most significant to least significant. The steps in the process include performing a rapid primary survey with simultaneous resuscitative interventions as indicated, completing additional resuscitative phase activities, conducting a comprehensive secondary survey to assess for other injuries and to elicit pertinent history information, and initiating laboratory and diagnostic studies. Documentation of all trauma assessment findings and resuscitation activities is a nursing responsibility; a well-organized trauma flow sheet that follows the typical pace and flow of initial trauma care is instrumental in facilitating accurate record keeping (Figure 50–4).[25]

In any discussion of resuscitation priorities, consideration must also be given to the protection of trauma team members from the risk of acquiring infectious disease from pathogens spread by contact with blood, body fluids, or inhalation. Pathogens of particular concern are human immunodeficiency virus (HIV), hepatitis B virus (HBV), and *Mycobacterium tuberculosis*.[26] Because the typical trauma patient population consists of many persons who engage in risk-taking behavior such as unprotected sex, violence, and substance abuse, the potential for infection is higher than average. In one study of the seroprevalence of HIV and HBV in an urban trauma center, the researchers found critically injured young urban trauma patients to have a 12 to 21% infection rate, or an infection rate two to three times higher than the general trauma patient population.[27] *Standard precautions attire must be worn* by all personnel involved in direct patient contact, even by those in close proximity to the patient, because splash contamination is likely in cases of free-flowing blood or during performance of invasive procedures. Standard precautions attire for trauma resuscitation include the use of impermeable cover gowns, gloves, a face mask, and eye protection or a face shield. Shoe covers and surgical caps are also advisable. Any garb that becomes obviously contaminated should be changed as soon as possible.[26]

Primary Survey and Resuscitation

The primary survey is an assessment technique to evaluate and treat *immediate threats to life* rapidly. These threats are best thought of as alterations that will result in imminent death if not immediately and effectively addressed. This is not the time for performance of an in-depth assessment; the opportunity for a more comprehensive examination follows in the secondary survey. The primary survey consists of the "ABC's" of trauma care: airway and cervical spine (A), breathing (B), circulation (C), disability (D), and exposure (E). Resuscitation efforts are *simultaneous* with each component of the primary survey. With a trauma team, many procedures can be performed at once. Although multiple problems or injuries may exist, it is important to remain mindful of the initial priorities and to direct all team efforts at managing needs identified in the primary survey *before* proceeding to activities of lower priority that can be accomplished later (i.e., splinting limbs and cleansing or closing wounds).

A: Airway and Cervical Spine

Ensuring an adequate airway is the highest-priority component of the primary survey as well as in overall trauma care. Human beings cannot live without an airway. The brain requires a constant supply of oxygen to be viable. After just minutes without oxygen, permanent changes occur in cerebral tissue that cause varying degrees of neurologic deficit; if the situation is unresolved, anoxic brain death will certainly ensue.

A basic tenet of trauma care is that *all trauma patients require supplemental oxygen administration*.[22] The rate of oxygen and type of device used depends on the method of airway management employed. As a general rule, a non-rebreather mask is used for spontaneously breathing patients who do not require ventilatory assistance to deliver maximum oxygen concentrations. A bag–valve–mask (BVM) device attached to a source of 100% oxygen and a mechanical ventilator are other modalities for oxygen delivery to the intubated patient. The goal is to start high in terms of fraction of inspired oxygen (FIO_2) and then reduce oxygen concentrations after initial assessment and resuscitation when the patient's condition permits.

Initial airway assessment should focus on the presence of any debris that can be cleared from the airway, either manually or with suction devices. If the patient can speak clearly, the airway is patent. However, stridor, a crowing noise with air movement, or a gurgling sound indicates airway obstruction. Potential causes include obstruction by the victim's tongue, blood, vomitus, secretions, teeth, or edema and structural disruption from injury to the face or neck. Hoarseness in the voice, changes in voice quality, or subcutaneous emphysema in the neck region can indicate laryngeal injury. Victims of smoke inhalation who present with carbonaceous sputum or singed nasal hair are at high risk of airway burns, which can result in laryngeal edema. Head trauma and the presence of intoxicants such as drugs or alcohol can produce an alteration in level of consciousness and an impaired gag

Date_____   Patient Name_____   Medical Record #_____   ☐ Male ☐ Female   Last Tetanus_____

Time Injured (military): _____   **Mode of Arrival:**   Ambulance   BLS   ALS   Helicopter   Self   Other   Transferred from _____

Time Arrived (military): _____   Medical History_____

Allergies _____   ☐ Unknown   Meds_____   ☐ Hx not available

CIRCLE ALL APPROPRIATE

MECHANISM

AUTOMOBILE: Driver   Passenger   Pedestrian / Front Seat   Back Seat / Seatbelt: Yes   No   Restraint Unk

Lap Belt   Shoulder Belt   Air Bag / Child Restraint: Yes   No / Auto vs_____   Describe:_____

BICYCLE / MOTORCYCLE: Driver   Passenger / Helmet   No Helmet / vs _____

ASSAULT: Gunshot   Shotgun   Stab Wound / Other   Describe: _____

OTHER: Fall _____ ft. / Fire / Home / Industrial / Other   Describe: _____

PRIMARY SURVEY / FINDINGS

Airway - On Arrival	Breathing	Cardiovascular	MAST Trousers

Airway - On Arrival

Patent   Obstructed   CRIC

NET tube # _____   OET tube # _____

Airway: Nasal   Oral

AMBU: Mask   Tube

O₂: Mask   Cannula   O₂ _____ L / min

Trachea: Midline   Deviated   R   L

C-Spine

Cervical collar:	Yes	No
CID:	Yes	No
Backboard:	Yes	No
Taped to board:	Yes	No

Breathing

Spontaneous / Unlabored
Shallow   Labored
Slow   Rapid
Assisted

Breath Sounds

Clear	R	L
Wheezing	R	L
Decreased	R	L
Rales / rhonchi	R	L
Absent	R	L
Crepitus	R	L

Cardiovascular

Radial Pulses:	Yes	No
Femoral Pulses:	Yes	No
Carotid Pulses:	Yes	No
Neck Vein Status:	Flat	Distended
Heart Sounds:	Clear	Muffled
	Absent	

Cardiac Rhythm _____

Skin

Dry	Warm	Pale
Moist	Cool	Cyanotic

MAST Trousers

	Inflate Time	Deflate Time
Abdomen	_____	_____
Right Leg	_____	_____
Left Leg	_____	_____

Neurological Status

Loss of Conciousness

Yes   Duration _____

No   Unk   Amnesia

Pupils

Size / Reaction

R _____ mm	L _____ mm
Brisk	Brisk
Sluggish	Sluggish
Non-Reactive	Non-Reactive

SECONDARY SURVEY

Abdomen: nontender   soft   tender   distended   firm   **Rectal Exam Heme:**   +   -

Narrative: _____

Extremity Assessment Key   ☐ No Obvious Injury

/ Laceration
X Fracture
► Penetration
※ Burn
Abrasion
● Hematoma

FRONT   BACK   R   L   FRONT   BACK

PROCEDURES AT HOSPITAL

TIME

_____ O₂ Nasal / Mask_____ L/min
_____ Ambu bag
_____ NET#_____ OET#_____
_____ Airway: Nasal / Oral
_____ Cervical collar applied
_____ NG tube   OG tube   size_____
_____ Foley _____ Fr
_____ Chest tube   R   Size _____
_____ Chest tube   L   Size _____
_____ Diagnostic Peritoneal Lavage
        ☐ Closed ☐ Open
        ☐ Neg ☐ Pos ☐ Equivocal
_____ Central Line   Site _____ L R
_____ Level 1 Infuser   Site _____

TIME

_____ Arterial Line   Site _____ L R
_____ Cricothyroidotomy
_____ Thoracotomy
        L   R
_____ # sponges opened _____
_____ # sponges counted_____
_____ Pericardiocentesis
_____ 12-Lead ECG
_____ Suturing site_____
_____ Suturing site_____
_____ Splint Application Site_____
_____ Other_____
_____ Other_____

X-RAYS

TIME COMPLETED

_____ C-spine lateral
_____ Chest Supine
_____ Pelvis
_____ Chest Erect
_____ Other_____
_____ Other_____

TIME COMPLETED

_____ Other_____
_____ CT Scan_____ Contrast_____
_____ CT Scan_____ Contrast_____
_____ Arteriogram_____
Time to X-Ray_____
Time to CT Scan_____

GLASGOW COMA SCALE

ADULT		PEDIATRIC
Eye Opening		**Eye Opening**
Spontaneous	4	Spontaneous
To Voice	3	To Speech
To Pain	2	To Pain
None	1	None
Verbal Response		**Verbal Response**
Oriented	5	Coos, Babbles
Confused	4	Irritable Crying
Inappropriate Words	3	Cries to Pain
Incomprehensible	2	Moans to Pain
None	1	None
Motor Response		**Motor Response**
Obeys Commands	6	Normal, Spontaneous Movements
Localizes Pain	5	Withdraws to Touch
Withdraw (Pain)	4	Withdraw Pain
Flexion (Pain)	3	Abnormal Flexion
Extension (pain)	2	Abnormal Extension
None	1	None

TOTAL 3 - 15   ☐

Figure 50–4

An example of a trauma flow sheet used to document care during the initial phase of trauma assessment and management. (Reprinted with permission from Christiana Care Health Services, Newark, DE.)

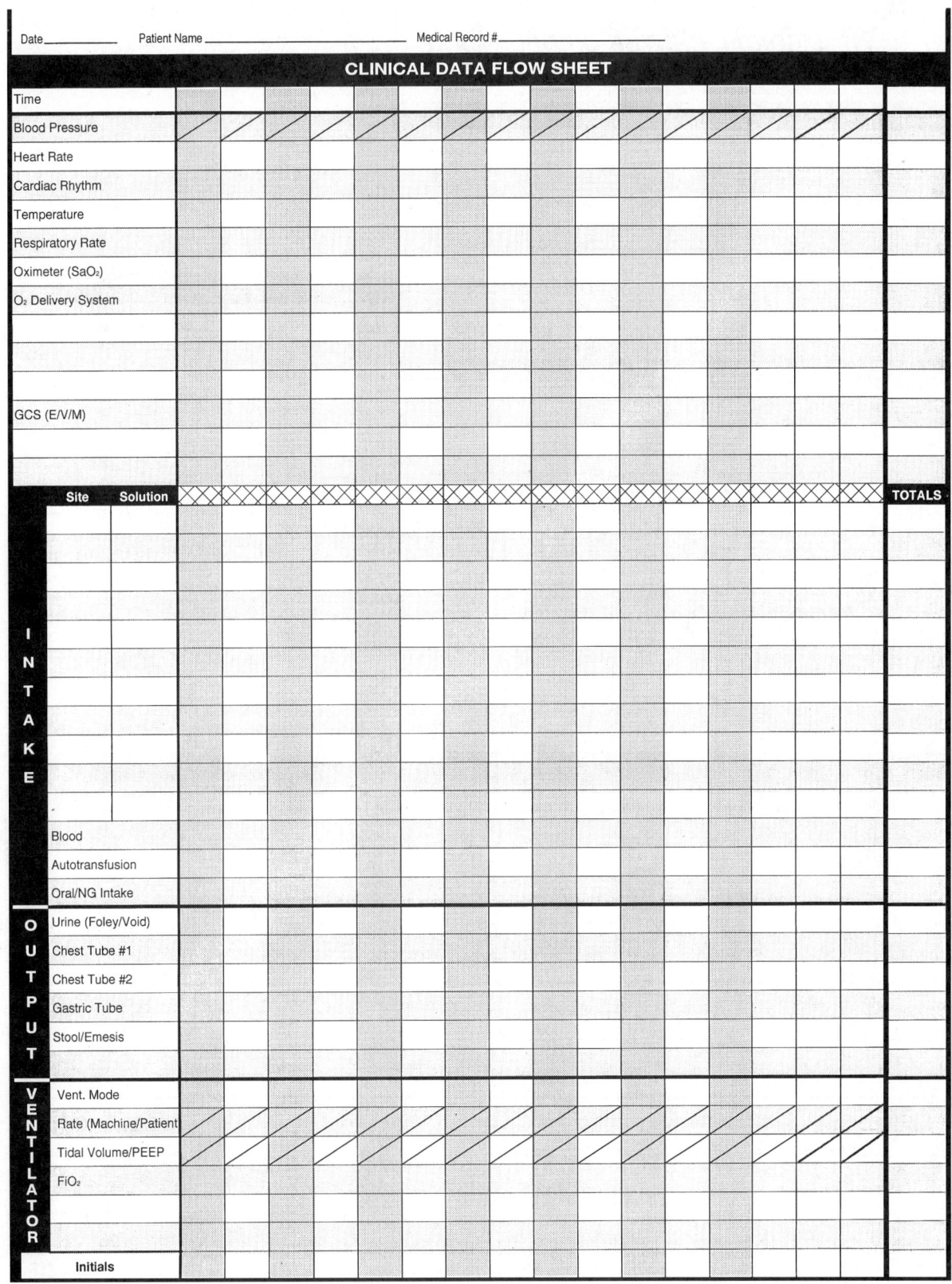

Figure 50–4 Continued

Illustration continued on following page

MEDICAL CENTER OF DELAWARE
TRAUMA FLOW SHEET

LABORATORY STUDIES

Time Completed

_____ TRA (CBC with differential, SMA-6, Glucose, ETOH, Amylase, CK, PT, PTT)

_____ TRP (CBC with differential)

_____ Type and Screen

_____ T & C _____ units _____

_____ UA

_____ TRAU (UA, benzodiazapines, Cocaine, Opiates)

_____ Pregnancy Test

_____ Dipstick Heme: Neg   Sm   Med   Lg

Time Completed

_____ Critical Care Profile

_____ ABGs

_____ Tox Screen   Urine   Blood

_____ Peritoneal Fluid

_____ Cell count / Spun Hct (purple)

_____ Amylase / Bile (red)

_____ Gram Stain (yellow)

_____ Other _____

_____ Other _____

_____ Other _____

MEDICATIONS

Time	Medication	Dose	Route	Given By	Ordered By:
	DT (Lot #)	0.5 cc	IM		

TRAUMA TEAM MEMBERS

☐ Consult   Time_____   ☐ Code   Time_____

☐ Alert   Time_____

Nurse Recorder Signature _____

✻ **Trauma Team Members**	Name	Time Present
ED Attending		
ED Resident		
Surgical Resident		
Surgical Resident		
Trauma Attending		
Nurse		
Nurse		
Respiratory		
X-Ray		
Anesthesia		
Neurosurgeon		
Orthopedics		
Consultant		

✻ Notification is Code or Alert time unless otherwise noted.   **PTA** - Prior to Patient Arrival   **OA** - On Patient Arrival

Time | Nursing Notes

Disposition

OR _____   Rm# _____   Morgue/ME _____

Home _____   AMA _____   Expired _____   Transfer _____ to _____

Signatures	Print Name / Date	Signatures	Print Name / Date	Doctors Signature
				_____ M.D.
				Print Name / Date

18743S (36840) (0495)C   CHART COPY   **I-20**

Figure 50–4 *Continued*

reflex. These factors can threaten the airway by placing the patient at increased risk of obstruction and aspiration.

Jaw Thrust Maneuver. Protection of the cervical spine during any maneuver to procure a patent airway is critical in the trauma patient with the potential for spine injury. The neck must not be hyperextended as in the head tilt, chin lift method of opening an airway, nor should it be flexed. The standard of trauma care is to maintain the cervical spine manually in a neutral, in-line position when establishing an airway. A jaw thrust maneuver is the initial approach to open the airway; this maneuver, performed by grasping the angle of the patient's jaw and moving the jaw forward, prevents the tongue from occluding the airway. If the trauma patient should suddenly vomit, a rapid but controlled log roll to the side with preservation of spinal alignment to clear the airway and to prevent aspiration of gastric contents is required.

Oropharyngeal and Nasopharyngeal Airways, Endotrachial Intubation. If jaw thrust maneuver and suctioning are insufficient to establish an adequate airway, other measures are necessary. Oropharyngeal and nasopharyngeal airways are adjuncts to the jaw thrust that help to maintain an open air passageway. For patients whose airway cannot be maintained because of a high risk of obstruction, aspiration, or structural trauma, emergency endotracheal intubation is required to provide definitive airway control. As a general rule, patients with a Glasgow Coma Scale score of less than or equal to 8 require a definitive airway.[22] The nasotracheal route may be selected only for patients who are spontaneously breathing. Nasotracheal intubation is contraindicated in patients who are apneic, because the usual technique is "blind" (i.e., no laryngoscope is used; air movement through the tube confirms placement), and in those with facial fractures or basilar skull fractures, because these patients are also at risk of cranial intubation and infection. Thus, the orotracheal route has advantages over nasotracheal intubation: it is safe to perform in patients with facial trauma and basilar skull fractures, and it is not associated with the incidence of sinus infection linked to nasotracheal intubation.

Cricothyroidotomy. For patients with severe maxillofacial trauma in whom anatomic landmarks are obscured through tissue disruption or hemorrhage, or for those who cannot be intubated on an emergency basis, a cricothyroidotomy is indicated as the emergency airway technique of choice.[22] A cricothyroidotomy is a procedure in which a puncture is made in the cricothyroid membrane of the trachea in a location higher than that selected for a formal tracheostomy. It can be performed with a large-bore needle (12 to 14 gauge in adults) as a short-term interim measure to ventilate the patient. A transtracheal jet ventilator or another device that delivers oxygen under high pressure ($\geq$50 psi) is required to provide adequate ventilation. This type of ventilation can be likened to breathing through a narrow straw; hypoxia, hypercarbia, and barotrauma are potential complications. Therefore, a more definitive airway should be established within 45 minutes of needle cricothyrotomy.[22]

The other method of performing a cricothyroidotomy is through a surgical incision with subsequent placement of a cuffed tracheostomy tube; the distal end of an endotracheal tube can also be used on a temporary basis. Because the adult larynx is at risk of injury if the device placed into it is too large (>9 mm outer diameter), care must be taken to ensure that the tube inserted is equal to or less than 9 mm in outer diameter (i.e., a no. 4 or no. 6 Shiley tracheostomy tube or a no. 7 endotracheal tube or smaller is appropriate).[28] A cricothyroidotomy is not considered a long-term means of airway maintenance; it should be converted to a formal tracheostomy if prolonged airway placement is anticipated, to avoid the associated complication of subglottic stenosis. Contrary to a commonly held belief, a *tracheostomy* is not recommended as an emergency surgical airway technique because it is difficult, requires more time to complete, and is associated with more bleeding as compared with a cricothyroidotomy.[22]

Maintaining Cervical Spine Alignment. Throughout the resuscitation, the patient's neck and spine must remain immobilized either manually or with adjuncts such as a cervical collar, spine board, head blocks, or other appropriate devices. To move the patient, a properly performed log roll or coordinated lift is necessary. The person maintaining cervical spine alignment is in charge of directing personnel; this person gives all the commands during the logroll or lift. A cervical collar alone is only a *stabilization* device; when spinal *immobilization* is required because of the nature of the patient's injuries, additional immobilization techniques are needed.

B: Breathing

After the patient's airway is assessed and initially managed, the next priority of the primary survey is breathing. Not only should the assessment include the determination of whether or not the patient is breathing, but just as important, the *effectiveness* of ventilatory efforts. At this point, breath sounds must be auscultated bilaterally; chest expansion, respiratory effort, and any evidence of chest wall trauma also must be noted.

Causes of significant ventilatory impairment that can be readily identified in the primary survey include multiple rib fractures, flail chest, and tension pneumothorax. Head trauma, intoxicants, and spinal cord injury are other potential causes. These disorders produce a range of respiratory compromise from apnea to ineffective or inadequate respiratory efforts. Two key interventions that may be required in this phase of the primary survey are ventilatory support and chest decompression.

Ventilatory Support. Patients who are apneic as well as those with ineffective breathing efforts (i.e., very slow, shallow, or too rapid) require ventilatory support. A BVM device is used to provide manual ventilation until definitive airway control is established and a mechanical ventilator is available. If cardiopulmonary resuscitation (CPR) becomes necessary, the patient must be disconnected from the mechanical ventilator and must be manually ventilated to sequence breaths with compressions and to gain a sense of lung compliance by the perceived difficulty of squeezing the bag.

Chest Decompression. A critical threat to breathing and circulation is the development of a tension pneumothorax, defined as a large collection of air in the pleural space that shifts the mediastinal structures toward the uninjured side and significantly impedes cardiac filling and, subsequently, cardiac output (see Chapter 19). If unrelieved, a tension pneumothorax will rapidly cause death. A tension pneumothorax can develop as a result of barotrauma from BVM or other positive-pressure ventilation, blunt or penetrating chest trauma, and expansion of a simple pneumothorax. Tension pneumothorax is a clinical diagnosis, not one that is confirmed by radiograph—the patient may not survive any delay in intervention. Clinical indicators of a tension pneumothorax include the absence of breath sounds on the affected side, profound respiratory distress, hypotension, and increased resistance to ventilation (decreased lung compliance) that can be appreciated when manually ventilating the patient with a BVM or when peak airway pressure dramatically increases on the ventilator. The patient is truly in a state of extremis. Tracheal deviation to the unaffected side and cyanosis also occur, but they are usually late findings. Once identified, the immediate intervention is chest decompression to vent the trapped air.

Chest decompression can be accomplished in two ways: needle thoracostomy and tube thoracostomy. Needle thoracostomy may be performed rapidly, but it is only a temporary emergency maneuver until a chest tube (i.e., tube thoracostomy) can be inserted. The procedure is straightforward: a large-bore needle (14- or 16-gauge intravenous catheter, 3–6 cm in length) is inserted into the second intercostal space in the midclavicular line; a rush of air is expected as the trapped air is expelled from the pleural space under pressure.[22] The nurse should document the occurrence of the rush

of air in the medical record to substantiate the presence of a tension pneumothorax.

After needle thoracostomy, tube thoracostomy is required, even if no air is released from the chest. The very act of inserting a needle into the chest can produce a pneumothorax by itself. Because other types of traumatic injury can mimic a tension pneumothorax, it is certainly not unheard of to perform needle chest decompression and to find no trapped air. A chest tube is inserted in the fifth intercostal space, just anterior to the midaxillary line. Chest tube placement in this location facilitates both air and fluid drainage. The nurse should prepare a chest tube drainage system, preferably one that has the capability for autotransfusion (i.e., a device that allows collection and subsequent reinfusion of shed blood) in anticipation of a hemothorax, to connect to the chest tube once inserted. Any sudden release of air, the presence of an air leak in the water seal chamber, and the character and amount of drainage should be noted in the medical record.

C: Circulation

Once effective ventilation is ensured, threats to the patient's circulation must be assessed. The main threat to circulation in trauma is *hemorrhage* leading to hypovolemic shock (see Chapter 47). Circulatory assessment and interventions in the primary survey serve to identify and to control life-threatening hemorrhage, as well as to establish vascular access. *External bleeding* is best controlled with firm, direct pressure over the site with a dry, absorbent dressing. Although external hemorrhage is usually obvious, *internal hemorrhage* represents a hidden danger that must be considered in any trauma patient who has sustained significant penetrating or blunt force injuries. Ongoing blood loss produces the clinical manifestations of shock, with resultant impairment of circulatory function and organ perfusion. After an initial compensatory period when blood pressure may be "normal," the patient exhibits pale skin that is cool and moist to the touch and has diminished peripheral pulses, decreasing blood pressure, and delayed capillary refill. Blood pressure can be quickly estimated based on the presence of peripheral and central pulses:

Presence of a radial pulse: blood pressure at least 80 mm Hg systolic
Presence of a femoral pulse: blood pressure at least 70 mm Hg systolic
Presence of a carotid pulse: blood pressure at least 60 mm Hg systolic

By the time hypotension ensues, the compensatory mechanisms that produced vasoconstriction have been exhausted, and significant blood loss has occurred.

Assessment of pulse rate deserves mention in any discussion of shock. Although tachycardia is classically associated with hypovolemic shock, failure to mount a tachycardic response should not lessen the suspicion that a shock state exists.[29] Many cardiac medications, particularly beta blockers, as well as increased vagal tone can inhibit the effects of the sympathetic nervous system and may produce a relative bradycardia (heart rate <100) in shock states.[29] Furthermore, elderly patients often lack the reserve to increase heart rate when under extreme physiologic stress. Thus, pulse rate should be evaluated for trends, but it should not be used to rule out hypovolemia by itself.

Vascular Access. Initial vascular access is best achieved by insertion of two large-bore peripheral intravenous catheters, 14 or 16 gauge in size, in the antecubital fossae. If peripheral access cannot be established or is inadequate to meet the resuscitation needs, femoral, external jugular, and subclavian venous access sites are other options for the trauma team. Large-bore (≥8.5-Fr) vascular access devices for central venous catheterization are commercially available in kits for the trauma resuscitation setting. The intravenous tubing also should have a large internal diameter to allow for rapid infusion of crystalloid solutions. Rapid infusion devices that both deliver a high flow rate and warm fluids and blood products should be utilized when significant fluid volume replacement or blood transfusion is anticipated; a large-bore Y-type blood administration set may work well if rapid infusion units are not immediately available. Standard resuscitation solutions are lactated Ringer's and 0.9% normal saline solution (NSS). If blood products are ordered, 0.9% NSS is the only appropriate solution to infuse in the same line; lactated Ringer's solution and dextrose-containing preparations cause hemolysis of red blood cells if these agents are administered through the same intravenous line as blood. Intravenous fluids and blood products should be warmed using appropriate warming devices to prevent hypothermia from rapid infusion of cold solutions and banked blood. As a general rule, when significant hypotension persists despite infusion of 2 L of crystalloid solution, transfusion of blood products is usually necessary. In addition, if more than 2 U of banked blood are to be administered to a trauma patient, or if the trauma patient is already hypothermic, blood products should be warmed to body temperature.[30] Hypothermia is a primary cause of coagulopathy in the trauma patient.

Application of a Pneumatic Antishock Garment. A temporary strategy to address hemorrhagic shock in the circulatory assessment and intervention phase of the primary survey is application of the PASG. The PASG is a three-chambered suit resembling trousers that is applied to the patient's legs and abdomen and is inflated with a foot pump connected to valves in proper sequence (i.e., the two leg chambers first, the abdominal chamber last) until the Velcro straps start to "pop." Physiologically, inflation has two main effects: it increases peripheral resistance in the patient's lower extremities and produces an elevation in blood pressure, and it controls hemorrhage by compressing bleeding vessels within the confines of the garment. Once the PASG is inflated, the garment is removed only after the patient has been adequately resuscitated with fluid or blood products; deflation must proceed slowly, with continual monitoring of blood pressure. With every 5-mm Hg fall in blood pressure, deflation is halted, and the blood pressure is allowed to stabilize with further resuscitation if necessary. Too rapid deflation can produce profound hypotension and can result in death. The main indication for use of PASG is stabilization of a fractured pelvis and control of the associated life-threatening hemorrhage; the PASG acts to tamponade bleeding pelvic vessels. However, the use of PASG is considered controversial when it is used solely as an adjunct to elevate blood pressure in patients in hemorrhagic shock. If the bleeding site lies above the confines of the PASG (e.g., in the chest), the PASG is contraindicated because bleeding can potentially increase. Other contraindications include pulmonary edema and known diaphragmatic rupture. Compartment syndrome is a potential complication.

Pericardial Tamponade. Auscultation of heart sounds and observation of jugular veins are other components of the circulatory assessment. Pericardial tamponade is caused by a rapid accumulation of blood or fluid in the pericardial sac that profoundly impedes cardiac filling and, subsequently, cardiac output (Figure 50–5). Clinical manifestations include muffled heart sounds, jugular vein distention, narrowed pulse pressure, and hypotension. In a critical situation, pericardial tamponade is treated with pericardiocentesis or emergency thoracotomy. In pericardiocentesis, the physician inserts a spinal needle attached to a large syringe into the pericardium using a subxiphoid approach. The objective is to aspirate blood or fluid, to decompress the pericardial sac, and to improve cardiac output until a more definitive procedure can be performed in the operating room.

Another approach to managing pericardial tamponade as well as other types of life-threatening thoracic hemorrhage (most commonly from penetrating trauma involving the heart or great vessels) is emergency thoracotomy. Emergency thoracotomy is performed by a physician at the patient's bedside, usually in the emergency department. Once the chest is opened, the goals are to release pericardial tamponade, to control major vascular or cardiac hemorrhage temporarily, and to perform internal cardiac massage; the aorta may also be cross-clamped to limit hemor-

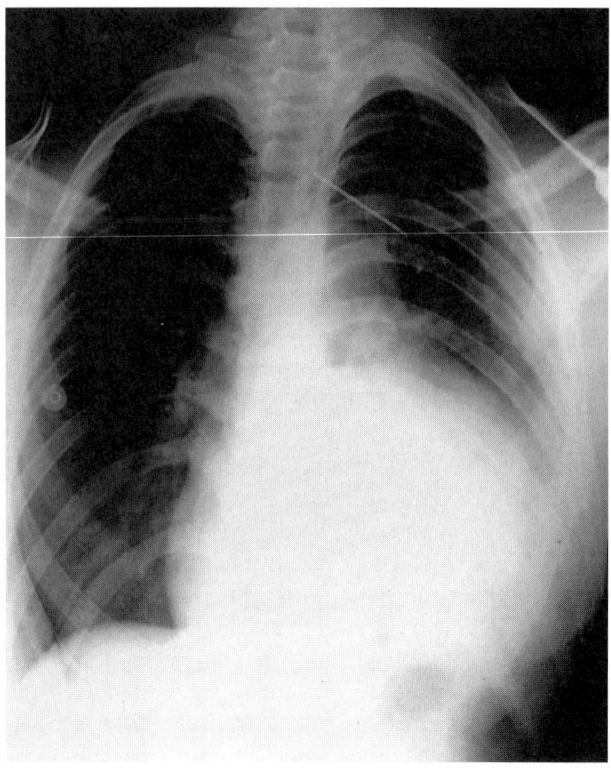

Figure 50–5

Chest radiograph revealing pericardial tamponade in a patient who sustained a precordial stab wound. Notice the rounded appearance of the heart resulting from distention of the pericardial sac with blood.

rhage occurring below the diaphragm.[31] Internal defibrillator paddles should be available because ventricular fibrillation may occur while the patient's chest is open. The patient is then taken to the operation room on an emergency basis for definitive repair of injuries.

D: Disability

The purpose of this component of the primary survey is to obtain a baseline evaluation of the patient's neurologic status, to gauge subsequent improvement or deterioration. A commonly used, simple mnemonic to facilitate rapid assessment of level of consciousness is "AVPU":

A: Alert
V: Responsive to voice
P: Responsive to pain
U: Unresponsive

Considering the interventions performed to this point, the observations for the AVPU assessment have already been made. Another excellent measure of level of consciousness that is internationally accepted and provides more information regarding neurologic function is the Glasgow Coma Scale (see Figure 50–4). Factors that can impair level of consciousness include hypoxia, head trauma, and intoxicants such as drugs and alcohol. Frequent reassessment is necessary to

detect any changes quickly that could represent either recovery or further compromise.

E: Exposure

The last step of the primary survey is exposure, by removing all the patient's clothing, to allow the entire body to be examined for evidence of trauma. Clothing should be cut when necessary to provide rapid access and to prevent exacerbation of injury that may occur while one attempts to undress the patient in the normal manner. Every attempt should be made to preserve any forensic evidence on the patient's body or clothing, including bullets, impaled objects, weapons, and drugs. All clothing and other miscellaneous items should be handled according to the institutional policy for preservation of evidence and maintenance of chain of custody. Police departments typically investigate traumatic injury cases; although the patient's physical needs are always the highest priority, cooperation with the investigation is an important aspect of overall care. The nurse may be even called to testify in court regarding observations made during resuscitation and injury management.

Once the patient's clothing is removed, hypothermia ($\leq 36°C$) is a significant risk that can depress the patient's body systems and may impede resuscitation.[32] The effects of hypothermia in the trauma patient complicate management by causing vasoconstriction, difficulty with venous access and arterial assessment, impaired oxygenation and ventilation, coagulopathy, increased bleeding, and slowed drug metabolism in the liver.[32] Measures to prevent hypothermia include monitoring body temperature, removing any wet sheets or clothing, immediately covering the patient with blankets, warming solutions and blood products before or during infusion, maintaining the room temperature at 75 to 80°F, and utilizing external warming devices such as heat lamps and warming blankets. Severe hypothermia requires core rewarming methods such as warmed gastric or bladder lavage or cardiopulmonary bypass.

Resuscitation Phase Activities

After the activities performed to address immediate threats to life in the primary survey, other interventions that may be necessary in the resuscitation phase include attachment of monitoring devices, insertion of additional intravenous access lines, placement of urinary and gastric catheters, and stabilization of impaled objects. If not already in place, a cardiac monitor should be connected for a continuous electrocardiographic (ECG) display with a digital readout of heart rate. A noninvasive blood pressure monitor (initially set to take the patient's blood pressure at least every 5 minutes) and a continuous pulse oximeter are also essential monitoring devices. A respiratory rate monitor is a useful adjunct. If the patient is intubated, a continuous end-tidal carbon dioxide monitor is also recommended.

Insertion of a urinary catheter attached to a urimeter is necessary for all critically injured patients, especially those who receive large volumes of resuscitation fluids, for accurate measurement of urinary output and as an indicator of end-organ perfusion. A real concern is urethral injury, which is far more common in males because of the length of the urethra. Therefore, before catheter insertion, a rectal examination must be performed to check the rectum for blood, which is evidence of an open pelvic fracture or colon injury, and a high-riding prostate, which could indicate urethral transection. Female patients should also have a vaginal examination. In addition, the urethral meatus must be inspected for blood or other signs of trauma. If urethral injury is suspected, a retrograde urethrogram (a dye study of the urethra) is performed before insertion of the catheter. In the presence of urethral injury, placement of a suprapubic cystostomy catheter may be necessary. Urethral injury is frequently associated with pelvic fractures. Blood in the urine (hematuria) may indicate renal or genitourinary trauma and requires further evaluation.

Insertion of a gastric tube (Salem sump) to decompress the stomach is another resuscitation phase intervention necessary for any trauma patient at significant risk of aspiration of gastric contents. It may also yield important diagnostic information regarding the presence or absence of blood in the stomach. Gastric tubes can be inserted nasally or orally. Nasogastric tubes are generally contraindicated in patients with head trauma or midface fractures; the tube may enter the cranial vault on passage through the nose if the cribriform plate (the bony structure that divides the sinuses from the brain) is disrupted. Therefore, inserting an orogastric tube is a safer alternative for these patients. After tube placement is confirmed, stomach contents should be evacuated using gastric suction.

If the patient has an impalement injury, the protruding object should be carefully stabilized with bulky dressings and *left in place* at this time; the surgical team will remove the object only after they have fully evaluated the structures penetrated and are in a position to provide adequate hemorrhage control, usually in the operating room (Figure 50–6).

Secondary Survey

The secondary survey follows the primary survey and resuscitation only after immediate threats to life have been identified and managed. The secondary survey encompasses a thorough hands-on, head-to-toe physical examination that seeks to locate evidence of all other significant injuries sustained by the patient. If the patient shows any signs of deterioration in this

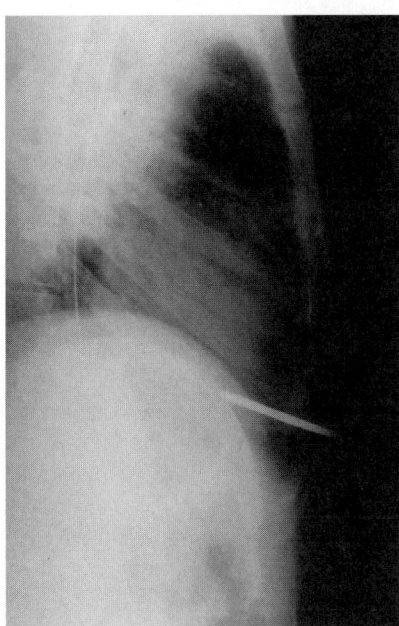

Figure 50–6
Anterior chest radiographic views showing a nail impaled in the heart. The patient, who had sustained the injury from a nail gun at a construction site, developed pericardial tamponade and survived the injury after thoracotomy and right ventricular repair.

phase of care, an immediate return to the primary survey with reassessment of the ABCs is warranted.

Vital Signs
At this stage, monitoring devices should already be attached to the patient. A full set of vital signs, including heart rate and rhythm, respiratory rate, pulse oximetry readings, blood pressure, and temperature, should be recorded. The frequency of these assessments is best determined by the patient's condition. In the highly unstable patient, documentation of vital signs is often required every 3 to 5 minutes. Otherwise, every 5 to 15 minutes is usually adequate during the first 30 to 60 minutes of resuscitation.

The nurse should not overlook temperature measurement as a vital sign parameter. Hypothermia is insidious and is best prevented or addressed before physiologic consequences occur. Trends in heart rate can be useful in evaluating effects of therapy. For example, if the heart rate trends downward toward a "normal" range (60–100) from an initial tachycardia, it may be evidence that fluid volume deficits have been corrected or that pain or anxiety is better controlled. Conversely, an increasing heart rate could signal deterioration. In the presence of head trauma, a falling heart rate could also indicate increased ICP: bradycardia, hypertension, and alterations in respiration are components of Cushing's triad, a sign of impending brain herniation. Cardiac dysrhythmias may indicate myocardial ischemia from a poor perfusion state or from direct trauma to the heart, as in blunt cardiac injury. Tachypnea or bradypnea may forewarn of the need for mechanical ventilation if the patient's breathing becomes ineffective. Pulse oximetry is a useful adjunct to assess oxygenation. Finally, to ensure accuracy and correlation of noninvasive blood pressure measurements with those of manual cuff pressures, manual cuff blood pressure should be taken and recorded for *each* arm.

Head-to-Toe Physical Examination

The head-to-toe examination portion of the secondary survey is a systematic method of inspection, palpation, percussion, and auscultation performed to discover signs of traumatic injury and other significant medical information about the patient that can be gleaned from examination. The survey begins at the patient's head, scalp, and face and then carefully proceeds through the neck, thorax, abdomen, pelvis, and extremities. To complete a full survey, the patient is properly log rolled onto the side, so that the posterior neck, back, buttocks, and legs can be visualized and assessed. Each area of the body is evaluated for any disruption in skin integrity, bleeding, contusions or discoloration, hematoma, edema, deformity, tenderness or pain, crepitus, drainage, neurovascular compromise, old or healing scars, and a medical identification bracelet or tag.

Other pertinent assessment considerations should be kept in mind as the survey progresses from head to toe. Pupil size, symmetry, and reactivity should be documented for all patients and reassessed frequently for any patient sustaining possible brain injury. If ocular trauma is suspected, a more thorough ophthalmologic examination is necessary. A quick check of visual acuity may be performed by simply asking the patient to read words on forms or whatever reading material is available in the room. The ears are observed for otorrhea and the nares for rhinorrhea, indicators of basilar skull fracture. An otoscope is used to detect hemotympanum, or blood behind the tympanic membrane, another sign of basilar skull fracture. The mouth is examined for loose or avulsed teeth and other intraoral trauma. The neck is evaluated for tracheal deviation, indicative of a possible pneumothorax or hematoma in the acute trauma setting, and subcutaneous emphysema from tracheobronchial tree or lung injury. Heart and breath sounds are auscultated again to reassess for changes or abnormalities. Chest expansion and respiratory effort are observed for any evidence of compromise. The abdomen is assessed for contusion, distention, guarding, rigidity, and pain, all indications of intra-abdominal trauma that may require operative intervention. The presence or absence of bowel sounds in an acutely injured patient may not have real clinical significance at this early stage. Finally, the extremities are also evaluated for any signs of neurovascular compromise and gross

sensory/motor deficits. A thorough sensory/motor examination is usually deferred until later in the diagnostic phase of care or after the patient's initial acute needs have been met.

The reality is that injuries may be missed in the secondary survey because of the presence of multiple or serious injuries that can distract attention from less obvious problems or because of the patient's inability to cooperate with the physical assessment secondary to impaired level of consciousness or cognitive function. Trauma can be thought of as "evolutionary"—injuries can evolve over time and may manifest later in the course of hospitalization. In addition to remaining attentive to the evolutionary nature of trauma, a *tertiary survey* should be performed within the first 24 hours of admission to evaluate the patient more fully for occult injuries.

"AMPLE" History

An accurate history is essential in planning care to meet the overall needs of the injured patient during acute hospitalization as well as during rehabilitation or community reentry. "AMPLE" is a common, simple mnemonic that can aid in collecting a relevant patient history:

A: Allergies
M: Medication history
P: Past medical history
L: Last meal
E: Events or environment preceding the injury

If the patient's level of consciousness and cognitive function are impaired, history information should be obtained from any available source: family or significant others, prehospital care personnel, medical identification bracelets or tags, and documents in the patient's wallet or handbag if available.

Allergies. Often, significant gaps in history can pose potential hazards for the patient. For example, lack of knowledge regarding drug or food allergies creates an increased risk of anaphylactic reactions. Extreme caution is necessary when medications are administered, particularly analgesic agents and antibiotics, because these agents are commonly given in the early phase of hospital trauma care. The nurse must remain vigilant to detect any sign of impending anaphylaxis and must immediately discontinue the drug and institute appropriate treatment as prescribed.

Medication History. Knowing the patient's prior medication history is also critical. Anticoagulant medication such as warfarin (Coumadin), for example, exacerbates bleeding in the traumatized patient. Because correction of the resulting coagulopathy with vitamin K may take more than 6 hours from the time of administration, fresh frozen plasma and clotting factor replacement also may be necessary to control hemorrhage. Aspirin and nonsteroidal anti-inflammatory drugs (NSAIDs) are other agents that can potentiate bleeding by impairing coagulation.

If the patient is a steroid user for a medical condition such as chronic obstructive pulmonary disease (COPD) or rheumatoid arthritis, adrenal insufficiency may occur in the physiologic stress state produced by traumatic injury; the patient may not be able to mount the necessary physiologic response to compensate.[29] Unless this problem is discovered and addressed, the patient becomes hypotensive, deteriorates clinically, and ultimately dies. Resuscitation efforts may not be effective unless exogenous or "stress doses" of steroids are administered. The recommended drug is hydrocortisone sodium succinate in a 100-mg dose given intravenously every 6 to 8 hours for an adult.[29]

Another class of commonly prescribed drugs that deserve mention in this regard are beta blockers (e.g., propranolol [Inderal] and atenolol [Tenormin]). These agents block the effects of the sympathetic nervous system and may prevent the patient from mounting a compensatory response to the shock state. The patient may show a poor response to resuscitation especially in the case of beta blocker overdose. Glucagon, administered by bolus and continuous intravenous infusion, has been found to be an effective reversal agent for beta blocker overdose.[33]

Also important is the patient's tetanus immunization status. *Clostridium tetani* is the anaerobic organism that enters tissue through a disruption in skin integrity and causes "lockjaw" or human tetanus. In the trauma setting, all wounds are typically considered tetanus-prone.[34] If 5 or more years have elapsed since the patient's last tetanus immunization was given, adult tetanus/diphtheria toxoid, adsorbed (Td), 0.5 mL intramuscularly, is indicated as a booster to confer *active* immunity against *C. tetani*. For patients who have not completed a full course of tetanus immunization (three doses), or for those whose immunization status is unknown, administration of tetanus immune globulin (TIG) (Hypertet), 250 to 500 U intramuscularly, is *also* necessary to provide *passive* immunity. The nurse gives this injection in a site different from that of the Td. Pain, induration, erythema, swelling, and muscle stiffness are common side effects of tetanus immunizations; as with any drug, anaphylactic reactions can occur.

Past Medical History. Past medical history can certainly affect the outcome of the patient with traumatic injury. Comorbid disease has been found to increase trauma-related mortality significantly.[35] Disorders of particular significance include congenital coagulopathy, cirrhosis of the liver, diabetes, COPD, and ischemic heart disease.[35] The presence of these health problems may seriously complicate management, may prolong recovery, and may increase the risk of dying in the trauma patient.

Last Meal. It is necessary to determine whether the patient has a full stomach, which increases the risk of vomiting and aspiration, especially if surgical procedures with anesthetic agents are anticipated. Anesthetic agents cause loss of the protective airway reflexes and thus place the patient at risk of airway compromise. As previously mentioned, a gastric tube is placed during the resuscitation phase to decompress the stomach when necessary. A word of caution is needed, however: the size of the usual gastric tube is 18 French; the tube diameter may not be large enough to evacuate more than fluid and air from the stomach. If the patient has recently ingested a meal, aspiration of large chunks of partially or undigested food still remains a risk despite gastric decompression. Again, because trauma is generally unplanned, the nurse must remain vigilant in the care of the injured patient who enters the health care system "unprepared" for medical or surgical interventions that typically require nothing by mouth (NPO) status as a routine.

Events or the Environment Preceding Injury. The final component of an adequate history for the trauma patient is the events or the environment related to the injury. This section focuses on information related to the MOI and relevant environmental factors such as weather conditions, temperature, contact with hazardous materials, and inhalation of toxic gases. Prehospital care providers can often provide the most accurate portrayal of the factors involved in the injury-producing incident because they are usually present at the scene. Knowing the MOI is helpful in predicting injury patterns and, sometimes, prognosis for recovery. Environmental factors must also be addressed when they pose a continued threat to the patient. For example, if skin or clothing is contaminated with hazardous chemicals, appropriate decontamination measures are required to protect the patient and hospital personnel from toxins.

Laboratory and Diagnostic Studies

Laboratory Studies

Initial laboratory studies are usually obtained at the time intravenous access is established for trauma patients in the resuscitation setting. Routine laboratory studies include a complete blood count (CBC), glucose, electrolytes, amylase, prothrombin time (PT), and partial thromboplastin time (PTT). In addition, arterial blood gases (ABGs), serum lactate, creatinine kinase (CK), and an ethanol level or a toxicology screen may be requested. A type and crossmatch or a type and screen for blood products should be performed for any trauma patient with actual or potential hemorrhage. A pregnancy test must be done on all female trauma patients of childbearing years as well. A specimen for urinalysis should be collected when the urinary catheter is inserted; if no catheter is inserted, the patient should be asked to give a voided specimen. Failure to produce a specimen may necessitate passing a straight catheter to collect the urine.

Because transport from the scene of the injury is generally quick in urban settings unless the patient was entrapped or treatment was delayed, initial laboratory values do not usually reflect changes that indicate acute hemorrhage. For example, the initial hemoglobin and hematocrit in the CBC may be within normal limits for patients experiencing rapid, acute blood loss. With fluid and blood replacement, dilution and equilibration occur; subsequent blood counts more accurately demonstrate the actual clinical values.

Blood glucose determination is essential in any patient with an alteration in level of consciousness or a history of diabetes. Hypoglycemia can impair consciousness and may be the proximate cause of the traumatic injury (i.e., car crash, fall). If the condition is uncorrected, death can ensue. Hyperglycemia can also produce stupor or coma, but it is less likely to be the cause of traumatic injury because it occurs over a much longer period than hypoglycemia.

Initial serum electrolytes should also be reviewed as baseline values. Many patients take pharmacologic agents at home such as blood pressure medications and diuretics, which can produce alterations in fluid and electrolyte balance that may require correction. Certainly, as resuscitation continues, dilutional electrolyte abnormalities may occur with fluid infusion. In addition, serum potassium levels can rise (hyperkalemia) with administration of banked blood from red cell hemolysis; serum calcium levels can drop (hypocalcemia) from binding with the citrate preservative in banked or autologous blood.

A serum amylase test may be ordered to detect signs of pancreatic injury. Because amylase is also found in the salivary glands, a high serum amylase level in the presence of facial trauma cannot be reliably interpreted to indicate an abdominal disorder. The amylase must be fractionated in the laboratory to analyze the origin of the enzyme; this study may take several days, depending on the capability of the laboratory.

A PT/PTT or a coagulation profile is ordered to detect any preexisting clotting disorders from anticoagulant use or disease (i.e., cirrhosis, hemophilia). If massive blood transfusion is required to resuscitate the patient, coagulopathies are anticipated. In this case, subsequent coagulation profiles are sent to guide the correction of clotting abnormalities with fresh frozen plasma, platelets, cryoprecipitate, or specific factor replacement therapy as indicated.

ABGs provide a measure of the adequacy of oxygenation and ventilation. In the initial resuscitation setting, hypoxia and hypercarbia must be rapidly corrected by airway interventions and provision of effective ventilatory support. To gauge the adequacy of resuscitation efforts, ABG results and serum lactate levels also provide indicators of tissue oxygenation and perfusion status. Uncorrected metabolic acidosis (pH < 7.35), a base deficit (≤6 mmol/L), and an elevated serum lactate level (>2 mmol/L) indicate anaerobic metabolism from inadequate tissue perfusion and oxygen debt, clinical manifestations of hypovolemia in the trauma patient.[36] In the critically injured trauma patient, this generally means that resuscitation has been inadequate to meet the physiologic needs of the patient.

Elevation in CK is an indicator of skeletal muscle injury. Myoglobin, derived from skeletal muscle breakdown, is a pigment that can potentially block renal tubules.[37] Myoglobin in the urine produces a classic tea color and is called myoglobinuria. The risk associated with myoglobinuria is acute renal failure. When CK levels are high (common in crush injuries, electrical injuries, or burns), the goal of therapy is to prevent renal failure by maintaining a urine output of at least 100 mL per hour with fluids and mannitol if necessary and by alkalinizing the urine with administration of intravenous sodium bicarbonate.[37]

An ethanol level is a common component of laboratory studies ordered for trauma patients; many trauma victims enter the health care system intoxicated to the point that their level of consciousness is depressed. A general serum toxicology screen may also be ordered to detect any substances that may be responsible for alteration in level of consciousness, that may have toxic metabolic or cardiovascular consequences, or that may have a potential interaction with anesthetic agents or other drugs.

Blood type and crossmatch should be drawn for the patient experiencing hemorrhage. The number of units of blood ordered is determined by the severity of the acute blood loss or the potential for further loss with surgical intervention. After massive transfusion, often defined as a transfusion of 10 U or more of blood within 24 hours or the amount necessary to replace the patient's own blood volume totally, another type and crossmatch may be necessary because the character of the patient's blood will have changed since the original study. If the need for blood transfusion is uncertain, a type and screen may be ordered. In a type and screen, no units of blood are requested, but the blood bank has the blood type and antibody information necessary to proceed with a type and crossmatch on request. In any event, because typed and crossmatched blood may require 30 to 40 minutes for preparation, patients who require immediate transfusion in life-threatening hemorrhage should be given *uncross-matched*, type O, Rh-negative blood until type-specific blood is available. In an emergency, women beyond childbearing age and men may also be given type O, Rh-positive blood if the supply of type O, Rh-negative blood is low.

Blood or urine must be sent for a pregnancy test for all female trauma patients of childbearing age. Although the basic standards of trauma management should not change for the pregnant patient, certain precautions such as lead shielding of the pelvis during radiologic studies can be undertaken. In addition, obstetric consultation is indicated to assist in patient management.

A urinalysis is a routine laboratory study ordered for the trauma patient. Of particular significance is the presence of blood in the urine. Hematuria can be gross or microscopic, seen only as red blood cells under the microscope in the urinalysis. Gross hematuria requires prompt diagnostic evaluation to rule out injury to the kidneys or genitourinary structures. Microscopic hematuria is a common finding in the trauma patient that requires follow-up to ensure resolution without renal or genitourinary sequelae; repeat urinalysis is necessary until the urine is negative for red blood cells.

Diagnostic Studies

Radiography. The three standard radiographs taken during initial resuscitation of the trauma patient are the lateral cervical spine, the supine chest, and the pelvis. If an overhead x-ray unit is not available in the trauma bay, a portable x-ray machine is needed because the patient should not be moved outside the resuscitation setting at this point. Additional films will be ordered as injuries are better defined in the secondary survey. Once the patient has been evaluated to be clinically stable, traveling to the radiology department for better-quality films is acceptable as long as appropriate personnel and monitoring equipment are available to accompany the patient.

The lateral cervical spine radiograph is only a screening film to find any gross evidence of cervical fracture or subluxation. To be adequate, all seven cervical vertebrae must be visualized, including the top of T1. Pulling the patient's arms downward better enables visualization of C7 on T1, the cervicothoracic junction. A negative lateral cervical spine film alone cannot reliably rule out injury to the cervical spine.[38] In the presence of neck pain, intoxicants, pain medication, or other significant injury that produces distracting pain, further diagnostic studies are required to ensure that the spine is not injured. These studies may include a three- to five-view cervical spine series of radiographs, flexion–extension films of the neck, a computed tomography (CT) scan to further define any questionable areas on the plain films, and perhaps

magnetic resonance imaging (MRI) if neck pain persists or is accompanied by neurologic deficit.

The chest radiograph is arguably the most important film during initial trauma resuscitation. It may reveal many findings that can affect the survival of the patient, such as pneumothorax or hemothorax, rib fractures, pulmonary contusion, diaphragmatic rupture, and evidence of tracheobronchial tree injury. A widened mediastinum on the chest radiograph is also an indicator of traumatic aortic disruption (Figure 50–7). Supine chest radiographs commonly demonstrate a widened mediastinum because of the patient's position; however, if the widened mediastinum persists on an upright chest film, or if the upright position is contraindicated, other diagnostic studies such as a thoracic arteriogram or a transesophageal echocardiogram are indicated to rule out aortic injury.

A pelvic radiograph is necessary if the patient has pain or tenderness over the pelvic bones, or if there was significant MOI to produce a pelvic fracture. It is especially important in the presence of a femur fracture because hip dislocations and acetabular fractures are common concurrent injuries. Severe pelvic fractures can produce exsanguinating blood loss; the nurse should anticipate fluid and blood product administration.

Diagnostic Peritoneal Lavage. The cause of hypotension in a trauma patient must be discovered without delay. Diagnostic peritoneal lavage (DPL) is a surgical technique performed at the patient's bedside to determine rapidly the presence of blood in the peritoneal space, an indication of intra-abdominal hemorrhage. Also known as a peritoneal tap, this procedure

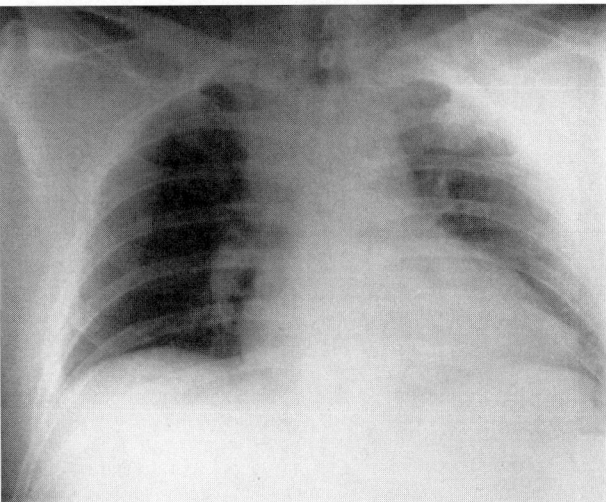

Figure 50–7

Chest radiograph demonstrating a widened mediastinum, a significant finding in the trauma patient, signifying possible thoracic aortic disruption.

is considered for the patient who is hypotensive despite initial fluid resuscitation and is unable to safely travel to CT scan because of hemodynamic instability. Before DPL, a gastric tube and urinary catheter *must* be inserted to decompress the patient's stomach and bladder to avoid risk of perforation. After properly preparing the skin and anesthetizing the area, the physician makes a small incision in the abdomen, inserts a catheter into the peritoneum, and attempts to aspirate blood from the catheter with a syringe. If more than or equal to 10 mL of gross blood is aspirated, the study is considered positive, and the patient is taken to the operating room for an emergency exploratory laparotomy (celiotomy)[39] (Figure 50–8).

If no gross blood is aspirated, then the peritoneum is lavaged by instilling up to 1 L of warmed lactated Ringer's solution or 0.9% NSS through peritoneal dial-

ysis tubing connected to the peritoneal catheter. Macrodrip intravenous tubing also can be used instead of peritoneal dialysis tubing as long as the intravenous tubing does not contain one-way valves. Once the solution has been instilled and the patient's abdomen has been gently agitated to enhance mixing with any peritoneal fluid, the intravenous bag and tubing are positioned below the abdomen on the floor to allow drainage of the peritoneal fluid back into the intravenous bag. As a helpful hint, the nurse should not let all the solution flow from the intravenous bag into the abdomen during instillation; the small amount of fluid that remains in the bag and tubing serves to create a siphon effect and facilitates drainage.

Once drainage is complete, the peritoneal catheter is removed, the incision site is sutured closed, and a small dressing is applied. The lavage fluid is observed for blood and particulate matter (food particles and stool). If the fluid appears so bloody that printed words cannot be read through the solution, the tap is again considered grossly positive. For indeterminate taps, lavage fluid also may be drawn from the intravenous bag and sent for laboratory analysis. The usual studies ordered are a cell count, Gram stain, bile, and amylase. Positive findings that indicate a need for surgery include a red blood cell count of more than $100,000/mm^3$ or a white blood cell count of $500/mm^3$ or greater, or the presence of bile or particulate fibers.[39]

Pertinent nursing activities include assisting with the procedure, monitoring the patient, and observing the incision site for drainage or signs of infection after the DPL. The only absolute contraindication to DPL is the presence of any injury that poses an obvious need for laparotomy.[22] Although the DPL is 98% sensitive for bleeding within the peritoneum, a limitation is that it does not reveal retroperitoneal bleeding or injuries to organs such as the duodenum, pancreas, and kidneys[22]; therefore, one must maintain a high index of suspicion for any patient at risk of intra-abdominal injury who has a negative DPL.

Ultrasonography. Ultrasonography performed in the resuscitation setting as a rapid screening test for free fluid in the abdomen is gaining support as a diagnostic tool in the evaluation of blunt abdominal trauma.[40] Unlike typical abdominal ultrasound studies commonly performed to diagnose organ disorders, emergency abdominal ultrasound is done in the acutely injured patient only as an attempt to visualize free fluid in the abdomen.

Free fluid indicates hemoperitoneum or bleeding into the peritoneal space. Once this condition is discovered, the physician has to make the decision whether to take the patient to the operating room for surgical intervention or to order further diagnostic studies to better define the injury. Ultrasound offers

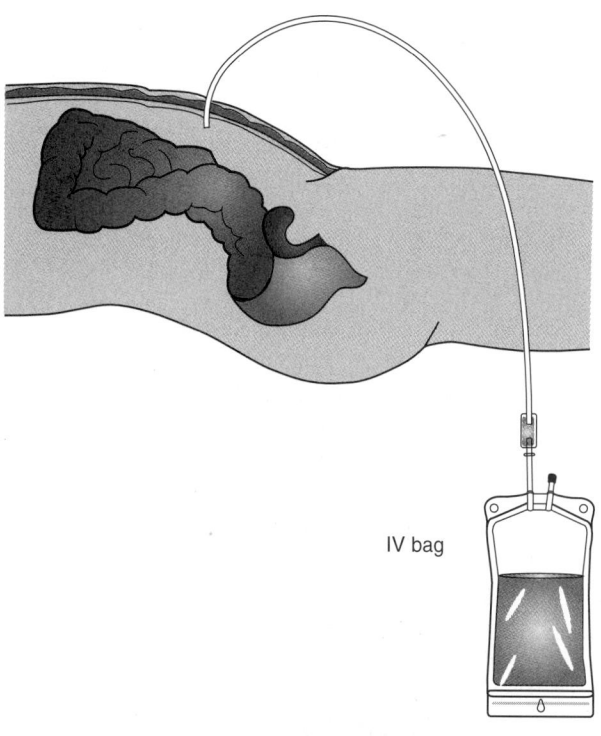

IV bag

INTERPRETATION OF RESULTS

Positive result	Aspiration of gastrointestinal contents, particulate fibers, bile
	Free-flowing blood on aspiration ($\geq$ 10 mL of gross blood)
	Grossly bloody lavage return
	>100,000 RBC/mm³
	>500 WBC/mm³
	Exit of lavage fluid from urinary or thoracic catheters
Negative result	<50,000 RBC/mm³
	<100 WBC/mm³

Figure 50–8

Diagnostic peritoneal lavage.

the advantages of being portable, noninvasive, and quick to perform. In research reviewing the results of 800 ultrasound studies performed to detect free fluid in patients with blunt abdominal trauma, the average study time was 10.6 minutes, with a range of 2 to 26 minutes.[41] In addition, the reported overall accuracy rate was 97.1%.[41] Surgeons and emergency department physicians can be taught to accomplish and interpret the study, to avoid the need for a radiologist.[40] Results are immediately available to the person making the management decisions. The patient benefits from the noninvasive nature of the test. Nursing care and patient monitoring can continue uninterrupted while the study is under way.

Computed Tomography. CT scanning is now a fundamental study in the diagnostic phase of care for most seriously injured patients at trauma centers. From the resuscitation setting, the trauma patient moves to the CT suite unless an emergency trip to the operating room is warranted because of the patient's instability. With newer CT technology, studies can be performed rapidly that can yield essential information for planning patient management. If the patient has suffered a loss of consciousness or has impaired consciousness, a CT scan of the head is in order. For the patient with evidence of abdominal trauma, a CT scan of the abdomen is indicated to determine the potential sites of bleeding or injury. CT scans of the chest, pelvis, and specific areas of the spine may also be obtained to locate or to define injuries further. CT scans demonstrate solid organ injury, define fractures, and reveal brain injury, hematoma, and edema. CT scans may be performed with or without administration of contrast media; whenever intravenous contrast is given, the nurse must monitor the patient for a potential allergic or anaphylactic reaction. In addition, intravenous contrast media can cause renal impairment and, in some cases, may precipitate acute renal failure. The nurse should closely monitor the patient's blood urea nitrogen, creatinine, and urinary output as indicators of renal function.

One significant limitation of CT scanning in the trauma patient is that subtle bowel, pancreatic, and diaphragmatic injury may go undiscovered.[39] Therefore, a "negative" CT scan of the abdomen should not be presumed to indicate no abdominal injuries are present. Ongoing clinical assessment is always necessary in this patient population to remain vigilant for evolving injuries. Another notable issue is that the patient needs to remain still for the duration of the study. The nurse attending the patient during the CT scan must be prepared to administer sedative medications as prescribed. For patients who fail to cooperate because of the effects of head injury or intoxication, the physician may choose to intubate and pharmacologi-

cally paralyze the patient if the perceived benefits of the diagnostic study prevail over the risks of intubation.

Arteriography. An arteriogram is a dye study performed to evaluate the patency and integrity of arteries. A radiologist injects contrast material into the vessel of interest and obtains films. Indications for arteriography in the trauma patient include evaluation for arterial disruption when evidence suggests vascular compromise after blunt or penetrating injury mechanisms and exclusion of a diagnosis of tears of the aorta. Cerebral arteriography may be ordered to establish a diagnosis of cerebral aneurysm, sometimes the proximate cause of traumatic injury. Nursing considerations include the patient's potential for an allergic reaction to the intravenous contrast material, renal impairment from the contrast load, and vessel injury with hematoma formation from needle puncture or catheter placement.

Magnetic Resonance Imaging. MRI is not routinely ordered as a diagnostic test in the initial phase of trauma management unless the patient's need for the study outweighs the potential risks inherent in the MRI environment. Aside from the well-known claustrophobic effects that often require the administration of sedative agents, the patient must be able to tolerate a supine position in the MRI tube for 40 minutes to 1 hour. The trauma team has extremely limited access to the patient during this time. Because no ferrous metal can be brought into the MRI suite, monitoring equipment and a mechanical ventilator may not be available options unless the facility owns such MRI-compatible equipment. Therefore, the MRI suite is an unsuitable place for trauma patients who lack physiologic stability.

With that said, MRI offers a real diagnostic advantage in the trauma evaluation of spinal cord injury. MRI is an excellent tool to define spinal cord compression from bony injury, ligamentous disruption, or hematoma formation. Because expedient surgery to decompress the spinal cord may be indicated in an attempt to reduce a neurologic deficit, the benefits of an MRI in this case justify the risks. Later in the course of hospitalization or in the outpatient setting, MRI is an excellent study to determine the extent of traumatic injury to the brain, soft tissues, intervertebral discs, tendons, and ligaments.

Definitive Care

The definitive care phase begins when wounds are closed, fractures are splinted and stabilized, and any injuries requiring surgical intervention are addressed in the operating room. Definitive care also encompasses general management of the trauma patient in the critical care unit, the step-down unit, and the surgical unit. For the patient suffering severe or multisystem injuries, resuscitation may actually continue from the emergency department through the operative phase and into the early critical care phase. The basic resuscitation principles previously presented apply. At this point, however, more sophisticated laboratory and diagnostic information is generally available to guide or refine resuscitation efforts to meet specific patient needs (e.g., electrolyte replacement, correction of clotting abnormalities, optimizing hemodynamic values).

Airway and ventilatory maintenance remains a top nursing priority in the definitive care phase. Thoracic and abdominal injury, surgery, neurotrauma, prolonged bed rest, and intubation and mechanical ventilation are some of the major factors that place trauma patients at significant risk of pulmonary compromise. ARDS is a potential sequela of shock, sepsis, multiple organ dysfunction syndrome, and aggressive fluid resuscitation; it carries significant morbidity and mortality for the trauma patient. Nursing interventions to promote pulmonary integrity include measures to prevent or correct physiologic compromise, coughing and deep breathing maneuvers, incentive spirometry, suctioning, turning, positioning, and early ambulation when possible. Monitoring the results of chest radiographs, ABG analyses, and sputum cultures is also a necessary nursing function, to detect early evidence of respiratory complications.

Prevention of shock states and maintenance of normal hemodynamic and laboratory values in the trauma patient require collaboration with the interdisciplinary health team. Hemodynamic monitoring lines such as arterial catheters and pulmonary artery catheters offer essential information when a clear knowledge of fluid volume and oxygenation status is required to optimize critical care management, particularly tissue perfusion. This approach is especially important in the elderly trauma victim, for example, who may have preexisting cardiovascular dysfunction. Hypotension from hypovolemia in the elderly should be managed in the same aggressive manner as in younger trauma patients, but with keen attention to "precise cardiopulmonary assessment measurements" to guide therapy.[10]

For the trauma patient who has undergone aggressive resuscitation with blood products and large volumes of crystalloid fluids, the nurse should be vigilant for hypocalcemia and clotting abnormalities. Citrate, a preservative found in banked blood products and autologous blood, binds serum calcium and produces hypocalcemia in patients who receive multiple blood transfusions. Ionized calcium levels should be carefully monitored in these patients, and calcium supplementation (i.e., calcium chloride) should be pro-

vided as clinically indicated. Furthermore, the nurse should be aware that continued bleeding, infusion of large volumes of fluids, and multiple transfusions of packed red blood cells (which are devoid of platelets and other clotting factors) eventually lead to coagulopathies from depletion and dilution of the normal clotting elements in blood. The potential need for platelets, fresh frozen plasma, and cryoprecipitate should be anticipated.

The pharmacology of trauma management most commonly consists of pain medication and antibiotic therapy. Pain control is a high priority in overall trauma care. Adequate pain management is often directly linked to the patient's ability to assist with pulmonary hygiene measures and early mobilization or rehabilitation efforts. Strategies must be individualized for each patient and typically include the use of opiate narcotics delivered by intermittent intravenous injection, patient-controlled analgesia pumps, or epidural catheters. Eventually, oral pain medication is substituted for intravenous formulations as the patient recovers. Achieving optimal pain control can be complicated in trauma patients who have preexisting substance abuse with physical dependence and tolerance to opiate drugs. A pain-management team, psychiatrist, or addiction specialist can be consulted for assistance in these challenging cases.

Interventions to treat and to prevent infection are other essential nursing responsibilities. Antibiotic therapy is typically instituted for pneumonia and sepsis, as well as for infections associated with contaminated wounds, open fractures, and bowel injuries. Wounds, pin sites, and surgical incisions must be carefully assessed for evidence of infection and treated with strict aseptic technique as indicated. Intravenous access lines placed in the field or in the resuscitation phase of care under suboptimal conditions should be replaced as soon as possible (generally in <24 hours) to reduce the risk of line sepsis and infections at the insertion site. Even invasive lines placed in an ideal hospital setting must be suspect if they are accessed frequently or left in place for a prolonged period. A descriptive research study investigating intravascular site care by nurses in two metropolitan hospitals documented wide variation in technique as well as inappropriate deviations from accepted standards, including low compliance with preprocedural hand washing.[42] Unfortunately, these findings are probably representative of the practices in many health care facilities. Institutions should have research-based protocols that dictate how often invasive lines should be changed and the type of site care required. The nurse should adhere to these protocols and act as a patient advocate, so that the patient receives optimal care.

During all aspects of the definitive care phase, the nurse must assess for any threats to the trauma

TABLE 50–1
Nursing Diagnoses

Problem Statement	Etiologic Factors
Gas exchange, impaired	Airway obstruction
	Pulmonary contusion and laceration
	Pneumothorax
	Hemothorax
Breathing pattern, ineffective	Rib fractures
	Flail chest
	Neurologic injury
Tissue perfusion, altered	Hemorrhagic shock
	Neurogenic shock
	Vascular injury
Fluid volume deficit	Blood loss
	Body fluid loss (burns, wound drainage)
Decreased cardiac output	Tension pneumothorax
	Hemorrhage
	Cardiac tamponade
	Blunt cardiac injury
Pain	Contusions
	Wounds
	Sprains and strains
	Fractures and dislocations
Tissue integrity, impaired	Lacerations
	Abrasions
	Avulsions
	Penetrating wounds
Physical mobility, impaired	Brain injury
	Spinal cord injury
	Extremity fractures and other injuries
Nutrition less than body requirements, altered	Abdominal or gastrointestinal trauma
	Facial fractures or wired jaws
	Neurologic injury
Infection, risk for	Disruption in tissue or skin integrity
	Iatrogenic (invasive procedures, vascular access or monitoring lines, intubation or mechanical ventilation)
	Shock states (bacterial translocation)
	Aspiration
Body image disturbance	Disfiguring injuries
	Physical impairment or limitations

patient's physiologic integrity such as fluid and electrolyte imbalances, infection, pulmonary embolism, and hematologic, cardiovascular, or pulmonary compromise. Thorough patient evaluation, accurate recording of intake and output measurements, and routine review of laboratory and diagnostic data are basic expectations of the trauma nursing role. Abnormalities should be promptly communicated to the responsible health team member. Volume replacement therapy, nutritional support, prevention of deep vein thrombosis, maintenance of skin integrity, and other interventions to address the patient's physiologic needs must be integrated into the management scheme.

The demands of providing physical care to the critically injured patient seem to leave little time for addressing the psychosocial issues. Meeting the psychosocial needs of the trauma patient and family can be challenging for the nurse. However, it is important to keep in mind that trauma is an unplanned catastrophic event that has the potential to alter functional abilities and life patterns permanently. Trauma does not simply affect one person; it affects significant others in ways that the health team may not fully appreciate. Roles change. Financial status is jeopardized. Even if the patient survives the trauma, he or she may become a different person with mental and physical limitations who no longer fits into the same place once occupied in society. Grief over real and potential losses is expected and can be overwhelming. The way in

> ### CHART 50–2
> #### ETHICAL DILEMMA
>
> Mrs. H. is a 77-year-old woman who sustained a spinal cord injury from a fall down basement stairs while visiting her son's home. A diagnostic evaluation revealed that Mrs. H. has a C5–C6 subluxation with quadriplegia. In the critical care unit, Mrs. H. is alert and fully oriented, with a Glasgow Coma score of 15. She exhibits diaphragmatic respiration and complains of difficulty in breathing. Her motor and sensory function are markedly impaired, with neurologic deficits characteristic of a spinal cord lesion at the C5 level. She was placed in Gardner–Wells tongs cervical traction by the neurosurgeon to reduce her subluxation.
>
> Despite the severity of her injury, Mrs. H. tells the nurse that she wants everything possible done to save her life, even if the paralysis is permanent. She says that life is precious to her; she wants to see her first grandchild born. Over the next 8 hours, Mrs. H. requires endotracheal intubation and mechanical ventilation to treat her worsening pulmonary status. She communicates by mouthing words and blinking her eyes.
>
> On day 4 of her hospitalization, Mrs. H. becomes progressively less responsive to verbal stimulation; assessment of her cognitive status is difficult. She has evidence of pneumonia and urosepsis. Because of her impaired state, she can no longer give consent for her own treatment. Her only immediate relative is her son. During his visit, he adamantly tells the nurse that he wants no further treatment initiated for his mother. He wants the endotracheal tube removed so that his mother can die a "peaceful death" instead of being "kept alive by machines." He firmly believes that his mother really would not want to live anymore in her condition.
>
> 1. How should the nurse respond to the son's statements?
> 2. Should aggressive trauma care continue based on the statements made by Mrs. H. while she was alert, or should her son's requests be honored at this time?
> 3. How should the issue of consent be handled if the son is the only legally recognized next-of-kin?
> 4. How would the nurse's beliefs regarding quality of life affect his or her course of action in this case?
> 5. What resources would assist the health care team in determining their action plan?

which patients and families cope with the traumatic event can be positively influenced by nursing interventions. When possible, the nurse should encourage the patient to verbalize feelings during routine care. If the patient is intubated, the nurse should obtain assistance from a speech therapist to facilitate alternative forms of communication. If the patient has an altered state of consciousness, the nurse should explain all procedures and talk to the patient, with the expectation that the communication is understood. Providing hope to the patient and family is essential. "Hope provides life-sustaining energy that can assist the family to cope with a multitrauma crisis."[43] If the nurse cannot spend the necessary time with family members, collaboration with social workers, pastoral care staff, psychiatric liaison nurses, or psychosocial support teams can provide the family with resources they need. If a family support group is available, it can also offer opportunities for family members to share their stories, to obtain information from group facilitators, and to gain coping skills by interacting with other group members.[44]

Nursing Diagnoses

Research has shown that total injury care, including early fracture stabilization, is associated with a significant reduction in morbidity and mortality in trauma patients.[45] Providing optimal trauma care requires an interdisciplinary team effort. Potential nursing diagnoses pertinent to the management of the acutely injured trauma patient should be considered when planning and delivering individualized care based on the nature and extent of the patient's injuries (Table 50–1).

Multidisciplinary Outcomes

The definitive care phase marks the start of convalescence for the trauma patient that culminates in recovery, rehabilitation, placement in a long-term care facility, or death. Ethical dilemmas are part of the reality of trauma care and must be addressed in this phase (Chart 50–2). Although optimal resuscitation care is

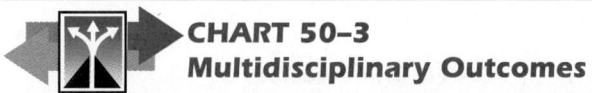

CHART 50-3
Multidisciplinary Outcomes

Maintenance of a patent airway and effective ventilation
Provision of adequate tissue perfusion
Maintenance of adequate fluid and electrolyte balance
Maintenance of adequate cardiac output
Relief of pain
Maintenance of skin and tissue integrity
Prevention of infection
Maintenance of nutritional support
Prevention of immobility complications
Provision of emotional and psychosocial support
Realistic patient expectations of instituted therapies
Timely initiation of rehabilitation services to facilitate community reentry

critical to the initial survival of the patient, the day-to-day medical, nursing, and allied health team management in this phase frequently determines the level of recovery possible and the ultimate outcome for the patient. Because health care quality management programs focus on outcome measures to evaluate the effectiveness of care delivery systems and interventions, it is necessary to consider the desired outcomes when planning overall care of the trauma patient (Chart 50–3). The trauma field is ripe for nursing research to investigate best practices and most cost-effective methods to achieve desired patient outcomes (Chart 50–4).

Critical Thinking Exercise

Ms. J. is a 27-year-old female unrestrained driver brought to the emergency department by paramedics after a motor vehicle crash with rollover during a rain storm; she was ejected from the car. On arrival, Ms. J. is awake, alert, and able to follow commands, but she is oriented only to name and place. She repeatedly asks the whereabouts of her family and states she is going to die. Ms. J. complains of severe left-sided abdominal pain with radiation into her back. She has a non-rebreather mask in place, with an oxygen flow rate of 15 L. Breath sounds are equal and clear bilaterally; chest expansion is normal. Peripheral pulses are palpable. The only obvious external bleeding source is a su-

perficial scalp laceration. Her skin is pale and cool. She has one peripheral intravenous access site started by paramedics in the field with 0.9% NSS infusing at a wide-open rate through macrodrip tubing. The rest of her clothing is cut away to facilitate evaluation. Her initial vital signs reveal a heart rate of 94 beats per minute, blood pressure of 108/60 mm Hg, a respiratory rate of 24, and a temperature of 36°C. Remarkable physical assessment findings include the superficial scalp wound and left upper quadrant pain on palpation. A second peripheral intravenous line is inserted, and another bag of warmed 0.9% NSS is hung at a wide-open rate through high-volume blood and fluid administration tubing.

Over the next 20 minutes during her trauma evaluation in the emergency department, Ms. J.'s blood pressure drops to 80 mm Hg systolic despite 2 L of intravenous crystalloid infusion. Her heart rate remains in the 90s. Her anxiety escalates; she is adamant that she is going to die and asks to see her 6-year-old son. Radial pulses become nonpalpable. A DPL is performed and reveals more than 10 mL of gross blood on initial aspiration. Two units of uncrossmatched type O negative blood are ordered and are transfused through a rapid infuser and warming device. She is transported immediately to the operating room.

1. List *initial* assessment findings provided in the case study organized according to the primary and secondary survey framework.
2. Is Ms. J. showing signs and symptoms of shock? If so, define the probable nature of the shock state and list pertinent clinical manifestations from the case study. Name at least three laboratory indicators of hypovolemic shock.
3. What sizes of peripheral intravenous catheters are indicated for an adult trauma patient in the resuscitation setting? What are appropriate insertion sites for these catheters?
4. Name two crystalloid solutions that are appropriate for trauma resuscitation. Which solution(s) can be administered in the same line with blood?
5. Is Ms. J. at risk of hypothermia? Why? List at least three interventions to prevent hypothermia in the trauma patient.
6. Why was DPL performed in the emergency department? How should Ms. J. be prepared before the DPL?

CHART 50-4

RESEARCH UTILIZATION: RESEARCH PRIORITIES FOR TRAUMA NURSING

Abstract: There is an identified lack of trauma nursing research in the current literature. To gain insight into trauma nursing research problems and priorities, this study was conducted using a 3-round Delphi technique to solicit and analyze expert opinions regarding research needs from experienced trauma nurses at each of the 25 accredited trauma centers in Pennsylvania. The first round included a request for 3 or more trauma nursing research questions from each participant. Data were categorized, and three major research themes emerged: interventions and treatments (N = 123); complications and sequelae (N = 71); and nursing issues (N = 61). Round 2 sought information regarding how the nurse respondents would rank each research problem in terms of its impact on patient welfare and its value for nursing practice. Round 3 asked participants to rate each question on whether it should be primary nursing research or a collaborative effort with other health team members. Final results were tabulated from the responses of the 137 nurses who completed all 3 rounds of the study. A list of the top 20 research priorities for trauma nursing was established and revealed a wide range of clinical and professional issues that deserve exploration through nursing and interdisciplinary research.

Critique: A limitation of the study is that it included only nurses from trauma centers in Pennsylvania. The extent to which the results can be generalized to other areas of the United States is uncertain. The researchers urge replication of the study on a national scale, better to capture diversity in nursing practice and patient populations; research questions and priorities may change.

Nursing Considerations: Research provides the scientific basis for nursing practice. To validate existing beliefs or to generate new knowledge, research is an essential component of nursing practice. This study sets forth trauma nursing research needs and priorities derived from expert practitioners at the bedside, in education, and administration who have a real sense of what research questions could yield the greatest potential improvement in patient outcomes and quality of nursing care. Interestingly, the top two research questions were the same in separate study categories regarding "impact on patient welfare" and "value for practicing nurses": 1) "What are the most effective nursing interventions in the prevention of pulmonary and circulatory complications in trauma patients?" 2) "What are the most effective methods for preventing aspiration in the trauma patient during the postoperative phase?" Other questions covered a broad subject range including pain control, coping and adaptation, oxygenation techniques, infection control, prevention of complications, behavior modification, family dynamics, documentation, and nursing stress. Of concern is the study authors' observation that only 2 of the 111 research questions generated dealt with trauma prevention; they infer that tertiary care nurses may have a limited awareness of prevention activities or lack support for personal involvement. This observation has implications for promoting active involvement of bedside nurses in trauma-prevention initiatives.

The study authors state that "the priorities identified by this study can guide the development of a theoretical and scientific foundation for trauma nursing." Nurses pursuing trauma-related research topics can use the study results to determine their own research agenda and to prioritize selected areas for investigation. Certainly, the results of this study will serve to validate that a particular research topic listed among the top 20 research questions has been objectively identified as a research priority. Such validation may be extremely important when applying for funding through the research grant application process.

Source: Bayley EW, Richmond T, Noroian EL, et al: A Delphi study on research priorities for trauma nursing. Am J Crit Care 3:208–216, 1994.

Key Concepts

⇒ The term "trauma" refers to bodily injury.

⇒ Trauma is the leading cause of death for people under age 45 years and the fourth leading cause of death overall; males between the ages of 15 to 24 years are at highest risk.

⇒ A trauma center is a specialty care facility that has been evaluated and meets criteria established to ensure competent and expedient provision of care to injured patients.

⇒ A trauma system represents organized local, state, or regional resources prioritized to meet the needs of the injured patient.

➥ The term "mechanism of injury" describes the manner in which the patient sustained injury, including the forces involved. Blunt and penetrating trauma are typical examples.

➥ Alcohol consumption is a major contributing factor in injury occurrence.

➥ In head trauma, measures to decrease intracranial pressure and to ensure adequate cerebral perfusion pressure are essential in preserving the brain from further insult.

➥ Penetrating trauma to the neck as well as blunt trauma can produce cervical spine injury, vascular injury, and injury to the pharynx, larynx, trachea, and esophagus.

➥ Pain from rib fractures can produce hypoventilation atelectasis; respiratory failure can ensue. Effective pain management and pulmonary hygiene methods are indicated to prevent pulmonary compromise.

➥ A widened mediastinum on the chest radiograph is an indication of thoracic aortic disruption.

➥ Blunt and penetrating chest trauma both can produce a pneumothorax or air in the pleural space that causes collapse of the affected lung; a tension pneumothorax is life-threatening and can result in cardiovascular collapse.

➥ The primary threats in abdominal trauma are hemorrhage and peritonitis.

➥ Pelvic fractures can produce a range of consequences from pain and impaired mobility to life-threatening hemorrhage and death; genital and urinary tract injuries are common concurrent injuries.

➥ Fractures, dislocations, and soft tissue trauma are often associated with vascular and nerve injury that can threaten limb viability and may result in functional impairment.

➥ The priorities in trauma care include a rapid primary survey with simultaneous resuscitation to address immediate threats to life, a comprehensive secondary survey, an AMPLE history, a diagnostic phase, and definitive care.

➥ Standard precaution attire must be worn when the potential for contamination with blood or body fluids exists (may include gloves, impervious gown, cap, mask, eye protection, and shoe covers).

➥ The primary survey addresses immediate threats to life; the components include the following: A, airway; B, breathing; C, circulation; D, disability; and E, exposure.

➥ Ensuring an adequate airway is the highest-priority component of the primary survey.

➥ All trauma patients require supplemental oxygen.

➥ The cervical spine must be immobilized in a neutral, in-line position when there is potential for cervical spine injury; a jaw thrust maneuver is the initial approach to open the airway. A co-

ordinated logroll is necessary when moving the patient.

➥ For patients in whom nasotracheal or orotracheal intubation is not possible, a cricothyroidotomy is the emergency airway technique of choice.

➥ Barotrauma from positive-pressure ventilation can produce a pneumothorax.

➥ Clinical indicators of a tension pneumothorax include the absence of breath sounds on the affected side, profound respiratory distress, hypotension, and increased resistance to ventilation (decreased lung compliance); tracheal deviation to the unaffected side and cyanosis are late findings.

➥ Chest decompression can be accomplished through needle or tube thoracostomy.

➥ The main threat to circulation in trauma is hemorrhage producing hypovolemic shock.

➥ External hemorrhage should be controlled with firm, direct pressure.

➥ Shock states may not always be associated with tachycardia.

➥ Large-bore intravenous catheters (14 or 16 gauge) and warmed crystalloid solutions (0.9% NSS and lactated Ringer's) are indicated in initial resuscitation for hypovolemic shock.

➥ 0.9% NSS is the only solution compatible in the same line as blood.

➥ Clinical manifestations of pericardial tamponade (caused by accumulation of blood or fluid in the pericardial sac) include muffled heart sounds, jugular vein distention, narrowed pulse pressure, and hypotension.

➥ In the disability assessment component of the primary survey, the AVPU scale or the Glasgow Coma Scale may be used to evaluate neurologic function.

➥ All clothing must be removed from the trauma patient to facilitate thorough assessment; hypothermia is a significant risk to the critically injured patient.

➥ Impaled objects must be stabilized in place; the surgical team will remove the object only after they can provide adequate hemorrhage control.

➥ If the patient's condition should deteriorate in the secondary survey, an immediate return to the primary survey and reassessment are warranted.

➥ The mnemonic AMPLE is defined as follows: A, allergies; M, medications; P, past medical history; L, last meal; and E, events or environment related to the injury.

➥ Initial laboratory values may not reflect hemorrhage if blood loss has been acute and rapid.

➥ Serum lactate level and base deficit are indicators of adequacy of resuscitation.

➥ A normal lateral cervical spine radiograph alone cannot reliably rule out injury to the cervical spine.

➡ DPL is a surgical technique used primarily to determine the presence of blood in the peritoneal space rapidly; a gastric tube and urinary catheter must be inserted before the procedure.

➡ Whenever intravenous contrast medium is given for diagnostic studies, the patient must be monitored for potential allergic and anaphylactic reactions and renal impairment.

➡ No ferrous metal can be brought into an MRI suit; monitoring capability is limited.

➡ The definitive care phase begins when wounds are closed, fractures are splinted and stabilized, and any injuries requiring surgical intervention are addressed in the operating room; this phase also includes patient management in critical care units and surgical units.

➡ Trauma care requires an interdisciplinary team effort.

References

1. U.S. Bureau of the Census: Statistical Abstract of the United States, 116th ed. Washington, DC, U.S. Government Printing Office, 1996.
2. National Safety Council: Accident Facts, 1996 ed. Itasca, IL, National Safety Council, 1996.
3. Morris JA, Limbird TJ, MacKenzie E: Rehabilitation in the trauma patient. In: Feliciano DV, Moore EE, Mattox KL (eds): Trauma, 3rd ed. Stamford, CT, Appleton & Lange, 1996, pp 1013–1022.
4. Bazzoli GJ, MacKenzie EJ: Trauma centers in the United States: identification and examination of key characteristics. J Trauma 38:103–110, 1995.
5. American College of Surgeons, Committee on Trauma: Optimal hospital resources for the care of the seriously injured. Bull Am Coll Surgeons 61:15–22, 1976.
6. West JG, Trunkey DD, Lim RC: Systems of trauma care: a tale of two counties. Arch Surg 114:455–460, 1979.
7. U.S. Department of Health and Human Services, Public Health Service, Health Resources and Services Administration: Model Trauma Care System Plan. Rockville, MD, U.S. Public Health Service, 1992.
8. Braslow JB, Snyder JA: Trauma system development and future directions. Prehosp Disaster Med 8:111, 114, 1993.
9. American College of Surgeons, Committee on Trauma: Resources for Optimal Care of the Injured Patient. Chicago, American College of Surgeons, 1993.
10. Stamatos CA: Geriatric trauma patients: initial assessment and management of shock. J Trauma Nurs 1:45–54, 1994.
11. Gentilello L, Donovan D, Dunn C, et al: Alcohol interventions in trauma centers: current practice and future directions. JAMA 274:1043–1048, 1995.
12. Sommers MS: Alcohol and trauma: the critical link. Crit Care Nurse 14:82–93, 1994.
13. Valadka AB, Narayan RK: Injury to the cranium. In: Feliciano DV, Moore EE, Mattox KL (eds): Trauma, 3rd ed. Stamford, CT, Appleton & Lange, 1996, pp 267–278.
14. Hussain K, Wijetunge DB, Grubnic S, et al: A comprehensive analysis of craniofacial trauma. J Trauma 36:34–47, 1994.
15. Ryan GA, McLean AJ, Vilenius ATS, et al: Brain injury patterns in fatally injured pedestrians. J Trauma 36:469–476, 1994.
16. Thal ER: Injury to the neck. In: Feliciano DV, Moore EE, Mattox KL (eds): Trauma, 3rd ed. Stamford, CT, Appleton & Lange, 1996, pp 329–343.
17. Cogbill TH, Moore EE, Meissner M, et al: The spectrum of blunt injury to the carotid artery: a multicenter perspective. J Trauma 37:473–479, 1994.
18. Laskowski-Jones L: Meeting the challenge of chest trauma. Am J Nurs 95:23–29, 1995.
19. Asensio JA, Demetriades D, Rodriguez A: Injury to the diaphragm. In: Feliciano DV, Moore EE, Mattox KL (eds): Trauma, 3rd ed. Stamford, CT, Appleton & Lange, 1996, pp 461–485.
20. Cryer HG, Johnson E: Pelvic fractures. In: Feliciano DV, Moore EE, & Mattox KL (eds): Trauma, 3rd ed. Stamford, CT, Appleton & Lange, 1996, pp 635–660.
21. Gokcen EC, Burgess AR, Siegel JH, et al: Pelvic fracture mechanism of injury in vehicular trauma patients. J Trauma 36:789–796, 1994.
22. American College of Surgeons, Committee on Trauma: Advanced Trauma Life Support for Doctors, Student Course Manual, 6th ed. Chicago, American College of Surgeons, 1997.
23. Jabbour M, Osmond MH, Klassen TP: Life support courses: are they effective? Ann Emerg Med 28:690–698, 1996.
24. Emergency Nurses Association: Trauma Nursing Core Course Instructor Manual, 4th ed. Park Ridge, IL, Emergency Nurses Association, 1995.
25. Bartley MK, Laskowski-Jones L: The Medical Center of Delaware's trauma flow sheet. J Emerg Nurs 22:586–590, 1996.
26. Martin RW, Rhodes RS: Protective surgical wear. Adv Trauma Crit Care 9:81–88, 1994.
27. Sloan EP, McGill BA, Zalenski R, et al: Human immunodeficiency virus and hepatitis B virus seroprevalence in an urban trauma population. J Trauma 38:736–741, 1995.
28. Salvino CK, Dries D, Gamelli R, et al: Emergency cricothyroidotomy in trauma victims. J Trauma 34:503–505, 1993.
29. Mullins RJ: Management of shock. In: Feliciano DV, Moore EE, Mattox KL (eds): Trauma, 3rd ed. Stamford, CT, Appleton & Lange, pp 159–180.
30. Judkins D, Neff J: Innovations in care: The cutting edge: fluid and blood warming systems. J Trauma Nurs 2:105–109, 1995.
31. Reed RA, Moore EE, Moore JB: Emergency department thoracotomy. In: Feliciano DV, Moore EE, Mattox KL (eds): Trauma, 3rd ed. Stamford, CT, Appleton & Lange, 1996, pp 193–206.
32. Sedlak SK: Hypothermia in trauma: the nurse's role in recognition, prevention, and management. Int J Trauma Nurs 1:19–26, 1995.
33. Duffy N: A 33-year-old woman with a propranolol and chlorpromazine overdose, with applied nursing diagnoses. J Emerg Nurs 19:13–16, 1993.
34. Scaletta TA, Schaider JJ: Emergent Management of Trauma. New York, McGraw-Hill, 1996.
35. Morris JA, MacKenzie EJ, Edelstein SL: The effect of preexisting conditions on mortality in trauma patients. JAMA 263:1942–1946, 1990.
36. Cassidy C, Marcher J: Base deficit: an indicator of tissue hypoperfusion. Int J Trauma Nurs 1:108–112, 1995.
37. Hoyt DB, Mackersie RC, Mehta RL: Renal failure. In: Feliciano DV, Moore EE, Mattox KL (eds): Trauma, 3rd ed. Stamford, CT, Appleton & Lange, 1996, pp 1133–1154.
38. Davis JW, Phreaner DL, Hoyt DB, et al: The etiology of missed cervical spine injuries. J Trauma 34:342–346, 1993.
39. Fabian TC, Croce MA: Abdominal trauma, including indications for celiotomy. In: Feliciano DV, Moore EE, Mattox KL (eds): Trauma, 3rd ed. Stamford, CT, Appleton & Lange, 1996, pp 441–459.
40. Boulanger BR, McLellan BA, Brenneman FD, et al: Emergent abdominal sonography as a screening test in a new diagnostic algorithm for blunt trauma. J Trauma 40:867–874, 1996.
41. Healey M, Simmons MB, Winchell RJ, et al: A prospective evaluation of abdominal ultrasound in blunt trauma: is it useful? J Trauma 40:875–885, 1996.

42. Roach H, Larson E, Bartlett DB: Intravascular site care: are critical care nurses practicing according to written protocols? Heart Lung 25:401–408, 1996.

43. Johnson LH, Roberts SL, Cheffer ND: A hope and hopelessness model applied to the family of the multitrauma patient. J Trauma Nurs 3:72–83, 1996.

44. Harvey C, Dixon M, Padberg N: Support group for families of trauma patients: a unique approach. Crit Care Nurse 15:59–63, 1995.

45. Bone LB, McNamara K, Shine B, et al: Mortality in multiple trauma patients with fractures. J Trauma 37:262–265, 1994.

Appendix
Algorithms for Advanced Cardiac Life Support*

*From the American Heart Association. *Advanced Cardiac Life Support.* © American Heart Association, 1997.

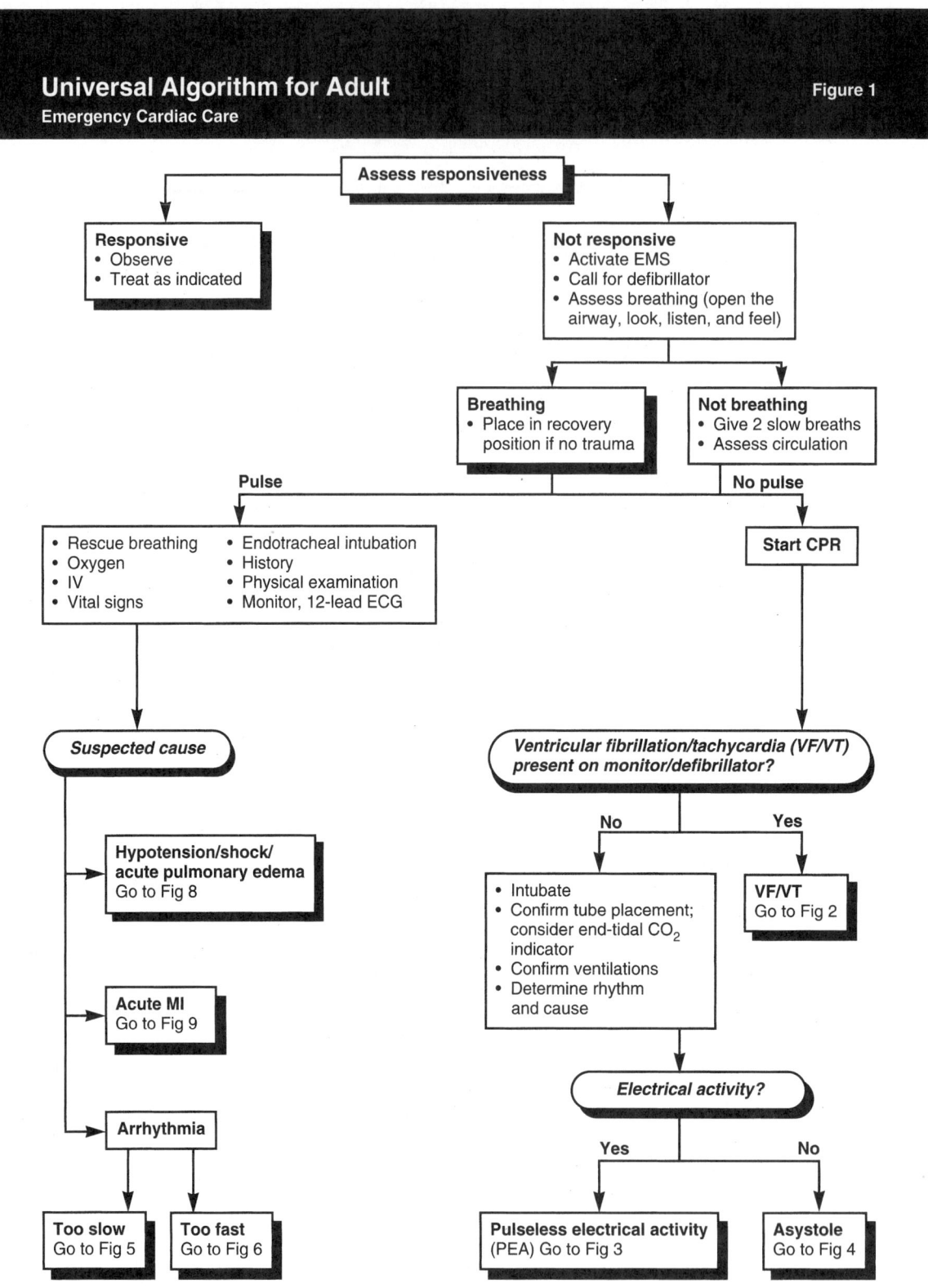

Universal Algorithm for Adult
Emergency Cardiac Care

Figure 1

Assess responsiveness

Responsive
• Observe
• Treat as indicated

Not responsive
• Activate EMS
• Call for defibrillator
• Assess breathing (open the airway, look, listen, and feel)

Breathing
• Place in recovery position if no trauma

Not breathing
• Give 2 slow breaths
• Assess circulation

Pulse

No pulse

• Rescue breathing
• Oxygen
• IV
• Vital signs
• Endotracheal intubation
• History
• Physical examination
• Monitor, 12-lead ECG

Start CPR

Suspected cause

Ventricular fibrillation/tachycardia (VF/VT) present on monitor/defibrillator?

No

Yes

Hypotension/shock/ acute pulmonary edema
Go to Fig 8

• Intubate
• Confirm tube placement; consider end-tidal CO_2 indicator
• Confirm ventilations
• Determine rhythm and cause

VF/VT
Go to Fig 2

Acute MI
Go to Fig 9

Arrhythmia

Electrical activity?

Yes

No

Too slow
Go to Fig 5

Too fast
Go to Fig 6

Pulseless electrical activity
(PEA) Go to Fig 3

Asystole
Go to Fig 4

Ventricular Fibrillation/Pulseless Ventricular Tachycardia (VF/VT) Algorithm

Figure 2

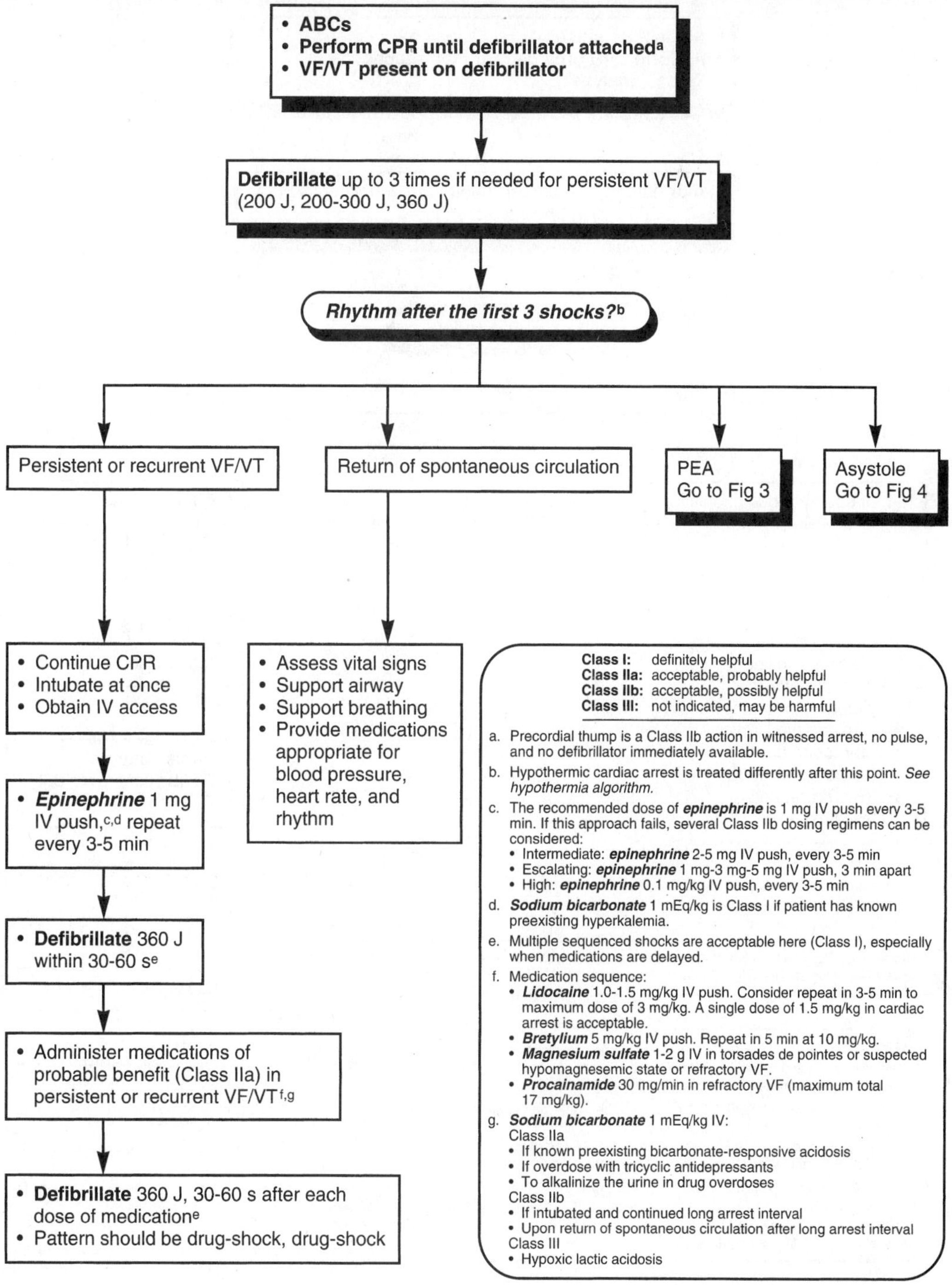

- **ABCs**
- **Perform CPR until defibrillator attached**[a]
- **VF/VT present on defibrillator**

↓

Defibrillate up to 3 times if needed for persistent VF/VT (200 J, 200-300 J, 360 J)

↓

Rhythm after the first 3 shocks?[b]

Persistent or recurrent VF/VT | Return of spontaneous circulation | PEA Go to Fig 3 | Asystole Go to Fig 4

Persistent or recurrent VF/VT:
- Continue CPR
- Intubate at once
- Obtain IV access

↓

- **Epinephrine** 1 mg IV push,[c,d] repeat every 3-5 min

↓

- **Defibrillate** 360 J within 30-60 s[e]

↓

- Administer medications of probable benefit (Class IIa) in persistent or recurrent VF/VT[f,g]

↓

- **Defibrillate** 360 J, 30-60 s after each dose of medication[e]
- Pattern should be drug-shock, drug-shock

Return of spontaneous circulation:
- Assess vital signs
- Support airway
- Support breathing
- Provide medications appropriate for blood pressure, heart rate, and rhythm

Class I: definitely helpful
Class IIa: acceptable, probably helpful
Class IIb: acceptable, possibly helpful
Class III: not indicated, may be harmful

a. Precordial thump is a Class IIb action in witnessed arrest, no pulse, and no defibrillator immediately available.

b. Hypothermic cardiac arrest is treated differently after this point. *See hypothermia algorithm.*

c. The recommended dose of **epinephrine** is 1 mg IV push every 3-5 min. If this approach fails, several Class IIb dosing regimens can be considered:
   - Intermediate: **epinephrine** 2-5 mg IV push, every 3-5 min
   - Escalating: **epinephrine** 1 mg-3 mg-5 mg IV push, 3 min apart
   - High: **epinephrine** 0.1 mg/kg IV push, every 3-5 min

d. **Sodium bicarbonate** 1 mEq/kg is Class I if patient has known preexisting hyperkalemia.

e. Multiple sequenced shocks are acceptable here (Class I), especially when medications are delayed.

f. Medication sequence:
   - **Lidocaine** 1.0-1.5 mg/kg IV push. Consider repeat in 3-5 min to maximum dose of 3 mg/kg. A single dose of 1.5 mg/kg in cardiac arrest is acceptable.
   - **Bretylium** 5 mg/kg IV push. Repeat in 5 min at 10 mg/kg.
   - **Magnesium sulfate** 1-2 g IV in torsades de pointes or suspected hypomagnesemic state or refractory VF.
   - **Procainamide** 30 mg/min in refractory VF (maximum total 17 mg/kg).

g. **Sodium bicarbonate** 1 mEq/kg IV:
   Class IIa
   - If known preexisting bicarbonate-responsive acidosis
   - If overdose with tricyclic antidepressants
   - To alkalinize the urine in drug overdoses
   Class IIb
   - If intubated and continued long arrest interval
   - Upon return of spontaneous circulation after long arrest interval
   Class III
   - Hypoxic lactic acidosis

Automated External Defibrillation (AED) Treatment Algorithm Figure 2A

Emergency cardiac care pending arrival of ACLS personnel

- **ABCs if no pulse**[a]
- **Perform CPR until defibrillator attached***
- **Press "analyze"**

↓

Defibrillate up to 3 times if needed for persistent VF/VT (200 J, 200-300 J, 360 J)[b,c]

↓

Check pulse[d]

Pulse present — **No pulse**

Pulse present:

Return of spontaneous circulation

↓

- Assess vital signs
- Support airway
- Support breathing
- Provide medications appropriate for blood pressure, heart rate, and rhythm

No pulse:

CPR for 1 min

↓

Check pulse, if absent

↓

- Press "analyze"
- **Defibrillate** up to 360 J
- Repeat 3 times

↓

CPR for 1 min

↓

Check pulse, if absent

↓

Repeat sets of three stacked shocks with up to 360 J[e]

*Health professionals with a duty to respond to a person in cardiac arrest should have a defibrillator available immediately or within 1-2 min.

a. The single rescuer with an AED should verify unresponsiveness, open the airway (**A**), give two respirations (**B**), and check the pulse (**C**). If a full cardiac arrest is confirmed, the rescuer should attach the AED and proceed with the algorithm.

b. Pulse checks not required after shocks 1, 2, 4, and 5 unless "no shock indicated" message is displayed.

c. If no shock is indicated, check pulse, repeat 1 min of CPR, check pulse again, and then reanalyze. After three "no shock indicated" messages, repeat "analyze" period every 1-2 min.

d. For hypothermic patients limit shocks to 3. See hypothermia algorithm.

e. If VF persists after 9 shocks, repeat sets of three stacked shocks with 1 min of CPR between each set until no "shock indicated" message is received. Shock until VF is no longer present or the patient converts to a perfusing rhythm.

Pulseless Electrical Activity (PEA) Algorithm
(Electromechanical Dissociation [EMD])

Figure 3

Includes
- Electromechanical dissociation (EMD)
- Pseudo-EMD
- Idioventricular rhythms
- Ventricular escape rhythms
- Bradyasystolic rhythms
- Postdefibrillation idioventricular rhythms

- Continue CPR
- Intubate at once
- Obtain IV access

- Assess blood flow using Doppler ultrasound, end-tidal CO_2, echocardiography, or arterial line

---

Consider possible causes
(Parentheses = possible therapies and treatments)

- Hypovolemia (volume infusion)
- Hypoxia (ventilation)
- Cardiac tamponade (pericardiocentesis)
- Tension pneumothorax (needle decompression)
- Hypothermia (see hypothermia algorithm)
- Massive pulmonary embolism (surgery, ***thrombolytics***)

- Drug overdoses such as tricyclics, digitalis, β-blockers, calcium channel blockers
- Hyperkalemia[a]
- Acidosis[b]
- Massive acute myocardial infarction (go to Fig 9)

- ***Epinephrine*** 1 mg IV push,[a,c] repeat every 3-5 min

- If absolute bradycardia (<60 BPM) or relative bradycardia, give ***atropine*** 1 mg IV
- Repeat every 3-5 min to a total of 0.03-0.04 mg/kg[d]

Class I: definitely helpful
Class IIa: acceptable, probably helpful
Class IIb: acceptable, possibly helpful
Class III: not indicated, may be harmful

a. ***Sodium bicarbonate*** 1 mEq/kg is Class I if patient has known preexisting hyperkalemia.

b. ***Sodium bicarbonate*** 1 mEq/kg:
Class IIa
- If known preexisting bicarbonate-responsive acidosis
- If overdose with tricyclic antidepressants
- To alkalinize the urine in drug overdoses
Class IIb
- If intubated and continued long arrest interval
- Upon return of spontaneous circulation after long arrest interval
Class III
- Hypoxic lactic acidosis

c. The recommended dose of ***epinephrine*** is 1 mg IV push every 3-5 min. If this approach fails, several Class IIb dosing regimens can be considered:
- Intermediate: ***epinephrine*** 2-5 mg IV push, every 3-5 min
- Escalating: ***epinephrine*** 1 mg-3 mg-5 mg IV push, 3 min apart
- High: ***epinephrine*** 0.1 mg/kg IV push, every 3-5 min

d. The shorter ***atropine*** dosing interval (3 min) is possibly helpful in cardiac arrest (Class IIb).

Asystole Treatment Algorithm   Figure 4

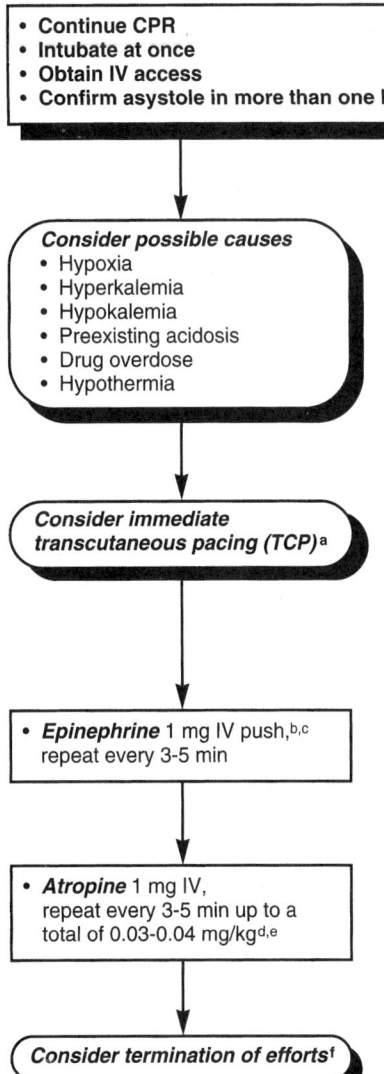

- **Continue CPR**
- **Intubate at once**
- **Obtain IV access**
- **Confirm asystole in more than one lead**

Consider possible causes
- Hypoxia
- Hyperkalemia
- Hypokalemia
- Preexisting acidosis
- Drug overdose
- Hypothermia

Consider immediate transcutaneous pacing (TCP)[a]

- **Epinephrine** 1 mg IV push,[b,c] repeat every 3-5 min

- **Atropine** 1 mg IV, repeat every 3-5 min up to a total of 0.03-0.04 mg/kg[d,e]

Consider termination of efforts[f]

Class I: definitely helpful
Class IIa: acceptable, probably helpful
Class IIb: acceptable, possibly helpful
Class III: not indicated, may be harmful

a. TCP is a Class IIb intervention. Lack of success may be due to delays in pacing. To be effective TCP must be performed early, simultaneously with drugs. Evidence does not support routine use of TCP for asystole.

b. The recommended dose of **epinephrine** is 1 mg IV push every 3-5 min. If this approach fails, several Class IIb dosing regimens can be considered:
- Intermediate: **epinephrine** 2-5 mg IV push, every 3-5 min
- Escalating: **epinephrine** 1 mg-3 mg-5 mg IV push, 3 min apart
- High: **epinephrine** 0.1 mg/kg IV push, every 3-5 min

c. **Sodium bicarbonate** 1 mEq/kg is Class I if patient has known preexisting hyperkalemia.

d. The shorter **atropine** dosing interval (3 min) is Class IIb in asystolic arrest.

e. **Sodium bicarbonate** 1 mEq/kg:
Class IIa
- If known preexisting bicarbonate-responsive acidosis
- If overdose with tricyclic antidepressants
- To alkalinize the urine in drug overdoses
Class IIb
- If intubated and continued long arrest interval
- Upon return of spontaneous circulation after long arrest interval
Class III
- Hypoxic lactic acidosis

f. If patient remains in asystole or other agonal rhythm after successful intubation and initial medications and no reversible causes are identified, consider termination of resuscitative efforts by a physician. Consider interval since arrest.

Bradycardia Algorithm
(Patient is not in cardiac arrest)

Figure 5

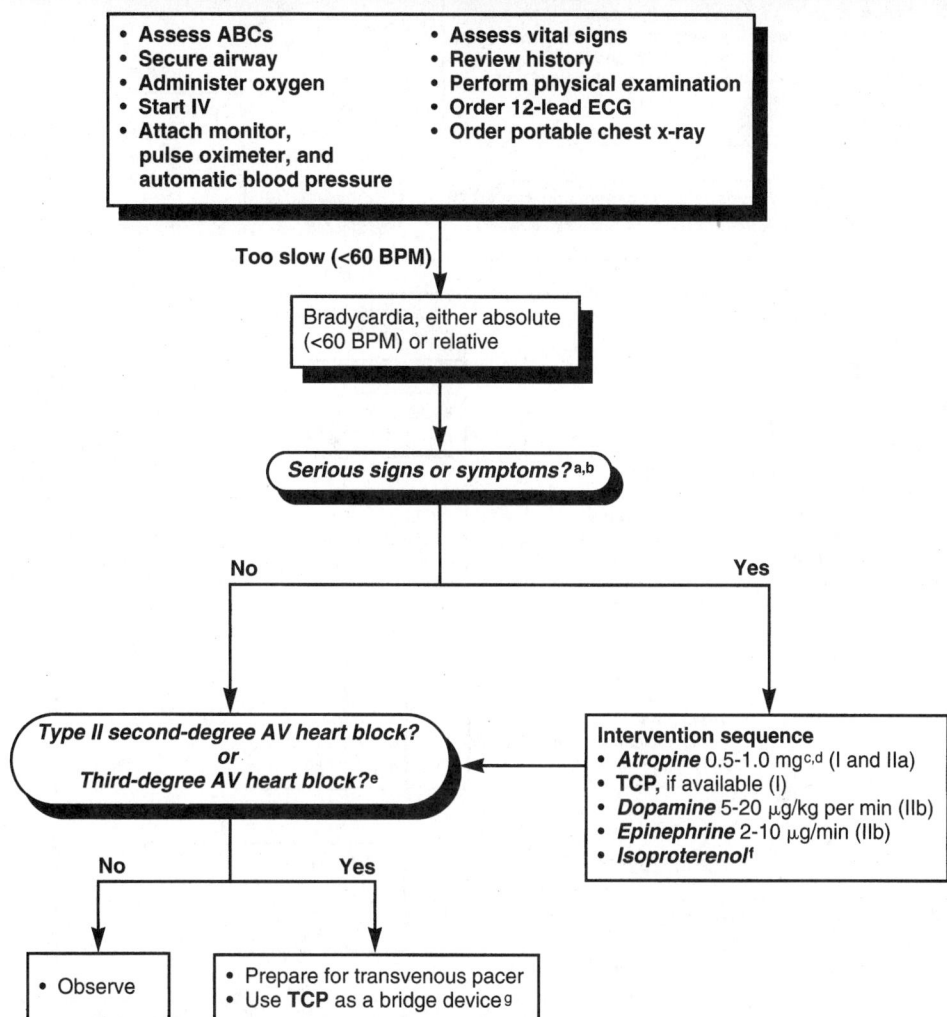

- Assess ABCs
- Secure airway
- Administer oxygen
- Start IV
- Attach monitor, pulse oximeter, and automatic blood pressure
- Assess vital signs
- Review history
- Perform physical examination
- Order 12-lead ECG
- Order portable chest x-ray

Too slow (<60 BPM)

Bradycardia, either absolute (<60 BPM) or relative

Serious signs or symptoms?[a,b]

No — Yes

Type II second-degree AV heart block?
or
Third-degree AV heart block?[e]

Intervention sequence
- *Atropine* 0.5-1.0 mg[c,d] (I and IIa)
- *TCP,* if available (I)
- *Dopamine* 5-20 μg/kg per min (IIb)
- *Epinephrine* 2-10 μg/min (IIb)
- *Isoproterenol*[f]

No — Yes

- Observe

- Prepare for transvenous pacer
- Use **TCP** as a bridge device[g]

a. Serious signs or symptoms must be related to the slow rate. Clinical manifestations include
  - Symptoms (chest pain, shortness of breath, decreased level of consciousness)
  - Signs (low BP, shock, pulmonary congestion, CHF, acute MI)

b. Do not delay TCP while awaiting IV access or for *atropine* to take effect if patient is symptomatic.

c. Denervated transplanted hearts will not respond to *atropine.* Go at once to pacing, *catecholamine* infusion, or both.

d. *Atropine* should be given in repeat doses every 3-5 min up to total of 0.03-0.04 mg/kg. Use the shorter dosing interval (3 min) in severe clinical conditions. It has been suggested that *atropine* should be used with caution in atrioventricular (AV) block at the His-Purkinje level (type II AV block and new third-degree block with wide QRS complexes) (Class IIb).

e. Never treat third-degree heart block plus ventricular escape beats with *lidocaine.*

f. *Isoproterenol* should be used, if at all, with extreme caution. At low doses it is Class IIb (possibly helpful); at higher doses it is Class III (harmful).

g. Verify patient tolerance and mechanical capture. Use analgesia and sedation as needed.

Tachycardia Algorithm   Figure 6

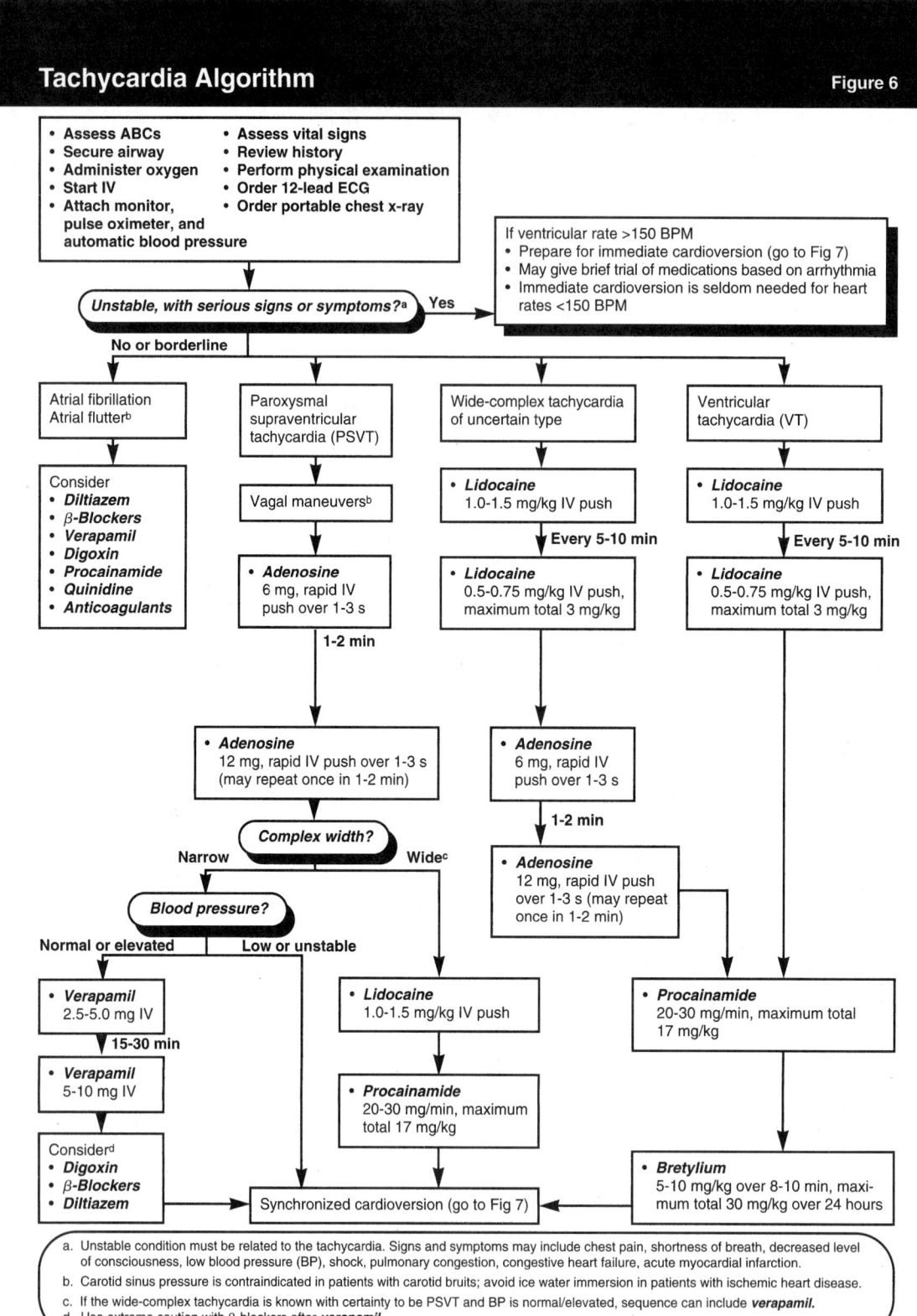

a. Unstable condition must be related to the tachycardia. Signs and symptoms may include chest pain, shortness of breath, decreased level of consciousness, low blood pressure (BP), shock, pulmonary congestion, congestive heart failure, acute myocardial infarction.

b. Carotid sinus pressure is contraindicated in patients with carotid bruits; avoid ice water immersion in patients with ischemic heart disease.

c. If the wide-complex tachycardia is known with certainty to be PSVT and BP is normal/elevated, sequence can include *verapamil.*

d. Use extreme caution with β-blockers after *verapamil.*

Electrical Cardioversion Algorithm

Figure 7

(Patient is not in cardiac arrest)

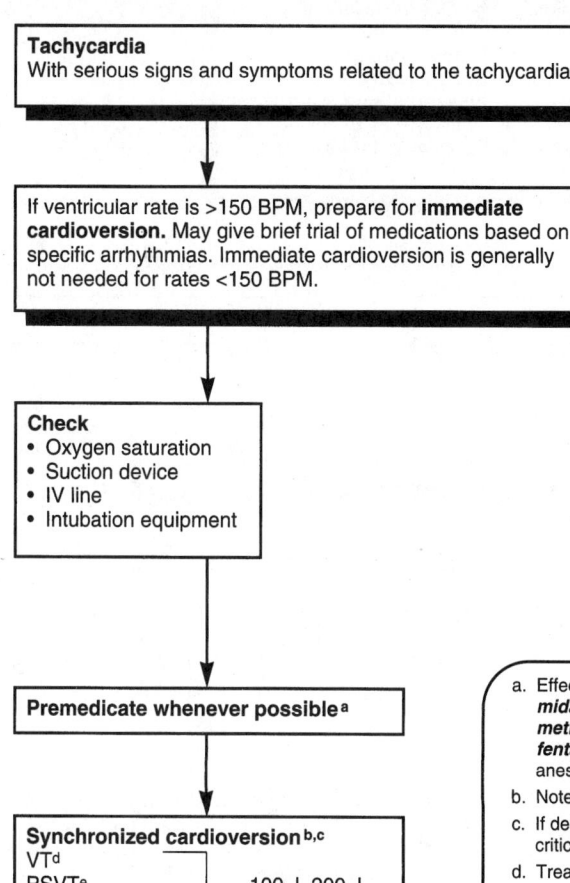

Tachycardia
With serious signs and symptoms related to the tachycardia

If ventricular rate is >150 BPM, prepare for **immediate cardioversion.** May give brief trial of medications based on specific arrhythmias. Immediate cardioversion is generally not needed for rates <150 BPM.

Check
• Oxygen saturation
• Suction device
• IV line
• Intubation equipment

Premedicate whenever possible [a]

Synchronized cardioversion [b,c]
VT [d]
PSVT [e] — 100 J, 200 J
Atrial fibrillation — 300 J, 360 J
Atrial flutter [e]

a. Effective regimens have included a sedative (eg, *diazepam, midazolam, barbiturates, etomidate, ketamine, methohexital)* with or without an analgesic agent (eg, *fentanyl, morphine, meperidine).* Many experts recommend anesthesia if service is readily available.

b. Note possible need to resynchronize after each cardioversion.

c. If delays in synchronization occur and clinical conditions are critical, go to immediate unsynchronized shocks.

d. Treat polymorphic VT (irregular form and rate) like VF: 200 J, 200-300 J, 360 J.

e. PSVT and atrial flutter often respond to lower energy levels (start with 50 J).

Acute Pulmonary Edema/Hypotension/Shock Algorithm

Figure 8

Clinical signs of hypoperfusion, congestive heart failure, acute pulmonary edema
- Assess ABCs
- Secure airway
- Administer oxygen
- Start IV
- Attach monitor, pulse oximeter, and automatic blood pressure
- Assess vital signs
- Review history
- Perform physical examination
- Order 12-lead ECG
- Order portable chest x-ray

What is the nature of the problem?

Volume problem
Includes vascular resistance problems

Pump problem

Rate problem

Administer
- Fluids
- Blood transfusions
- Cause-specific interventions
- Consider vasopressors, if indicated

What is the blood pressure (BP)?[a]

Too slow
Go to Fig 5

Too fast
Go to Fig 6

Systolic BP
<70 mm Hg[b]
Signs and symptoms of shock

Systolic BP
70-100 mm Hg[b]
Signs and symptoms of shock

Systolic BP
70-100 mm Hg[b]
No signs and symptoms of shock

Systolic BP[e]
>100 mm Hg
Patients in acute pulmonary edema

Consider
- *Norepinephrine*
  0.5-30 µg/min IV or
- *Dopamine*
  5-20 µg/kg per min

- *Dopamine*[c]
  2.5-20 µg/kg per min IV
  (Add *norepinephrine* if *dopamine* is >20 µg/kg per min)

- *Dobutamine*[d]
  2-20 µg/kg per min IV

- *Nitroglycerin* start 10-20 µg/min IV (use if ischemia persists and BP remains elevated. Titrate to effect)
  and/or
- *Nitroprusside* 0.1-5.0 µg/kg per min IV

Consider
further actions, especially if the patient is in acute pulmonary edema

First-line actions
- *Furosemide* IV 0.5-1.0 mg/kg
- *Morphine* IV 1-3 mg
- *Nitroglycerin* SL
- *Oxygen*/intubate PRN

Second-line actions
- *Nitroglycerin* IV if BP >100 mm Hg
- *Nitroprusside* IV if BP >100 mm Hg
- *Dopamine* if BP <100 mm Hg
- *Dobutamine* if BP >100 mm Hg
- Positive end-expiratory pressure (PEEP)
- Continuous positive airway pressure (CPAP)

Third-line actions
- *Amrinone* 0.75 mg/kg then 5-15 µg/kg per min (if other drugs fail)
- *Aminophylline* 5 mg/kg (if wheezing)
- *Thrombolytic* therapy (if not in shock)
- *Digoxin* (if atrial fibrillation, supraventricular tachycardias)
- Angioplasty (if drugs fail)
- Intra-aortic balloon pump (bridge to surgery)
- Surgical interventions (valves, coronary artery bypass grafts, heart transplant)

a. Base management after this point on invasive hemodynamic monitoring if possible. Guidelines presume clinical signs of hypoperfusion.
b. Fluid bolus of 250-500 mL normal saline should be tried. If no response, consider sympathomimetics.
c. Move to *dopamine* and stop *norepinephrine* when BP improves. Avoid *dopamine* (consider *dobutamine*) if no signs of hypoperfusion.
d. Add *dopamine* (and avoid *dobutamine*) if systolic BP drops below 90 mm Hg.
e. Consider *nitroglycerin* if initial blood pressures are in this range; reduces preload in patients with acute pulmonary edema.

Acute Myocardial Infarction Algorithm

Recommendations for early management of patients with chest pain and possible AMI

Figure 9

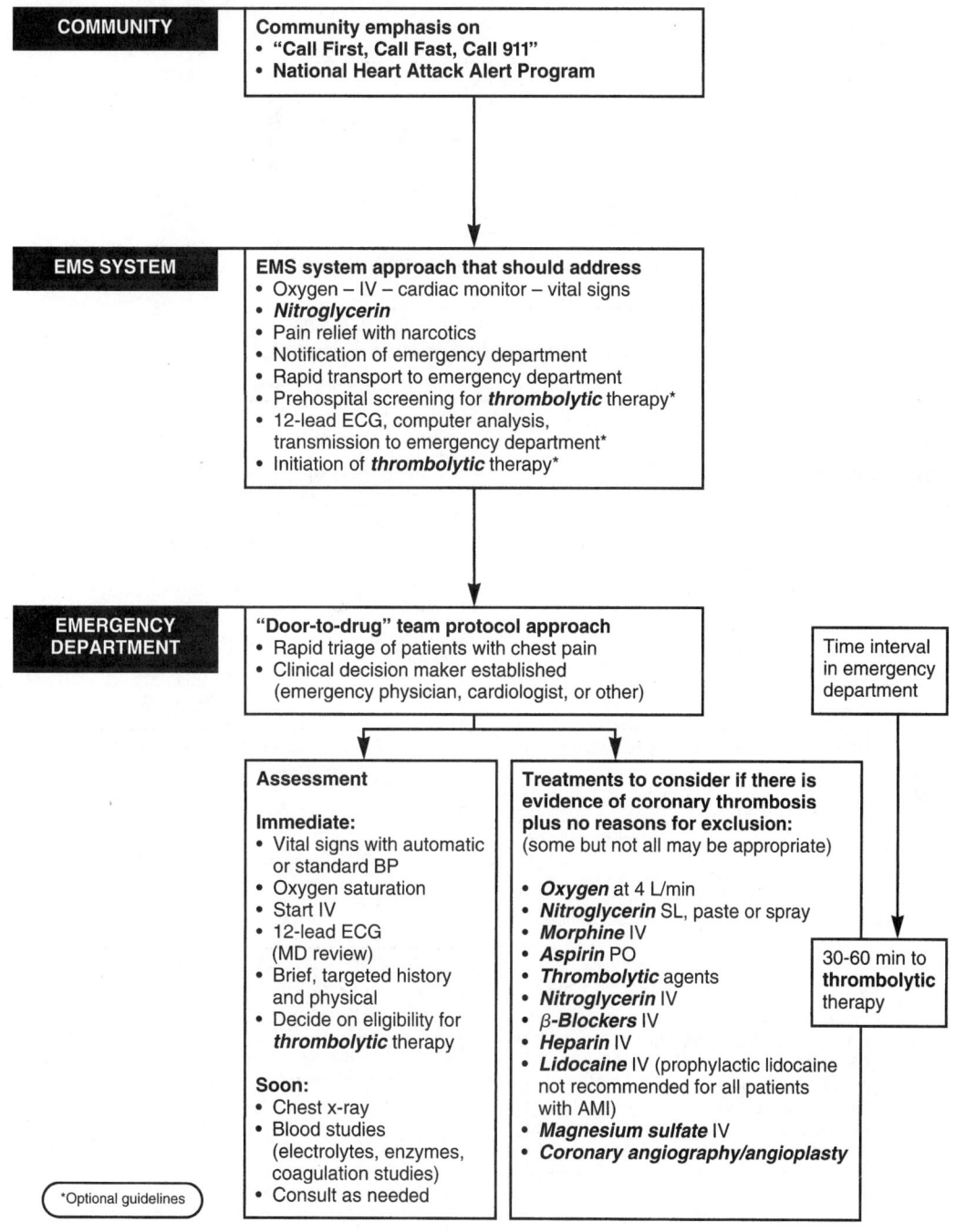

COMMUNITY

Community emphasis on
- "Call First, Call Fast, Call 911"
- National Heart Attack Alert Program

EMS SYSTEM

EMS system approach that should address
- Oxygen – IV – cardiac monitor – vital signs
- *Nitroglycerin*
- Pain relief with narcotics
- Notification of emergency department
- Rapid transport to emergency department
- Prehospital screening for *thrombolytic* therapy*
- 12-lead ECG, computer analysis, transmission to emergency department*
- Initiation of *thrombolytic* therapy*

EMERGENCY DEPARTMENT

"Door-to-drug" team protocol approach
- Rapid triage of patients with chest pain
- Clinical decision maker established (emergency physician, cardiologist, or other)

Time interval in emergency department

30-60 min to **thrombolytic** therapy

Assessment

Immediate:
- Vital signs with automatic or standard BP
- Oxygen saturation
- Start IV
- 12-lead ECG (MD review)
- Brief, targeted history and physical
- Decide on eligibility for *thrombolytic* therapy

Soon:
- Chest x-ray
- Blood studies (electrolytes, enzymes, coagulation studies)
- Consult as needed

Treatments to consider if there is evidence of coronary thrombosis plus no reasons for exclusion:
(some but not all may be appropriate)

- *Oxygen* at 4 L/min
- *Nitroglycerin* SL, paste or spray
- *Morphine* IV
- *Aspirin* PO
- *Thrombolytic* agents
- *Nitroglycerin* IV
- *β-Blockers* IV
- *Heparin* IV
- *Lidocaine* IV (prophylactic lidocaine not recommended for all patients with AMI)
- *Magnesium sulfate* IV
- *Coronary angiography/angioplasty*

*Optional guidelines

Hypothermia Algorithm   Figure 10

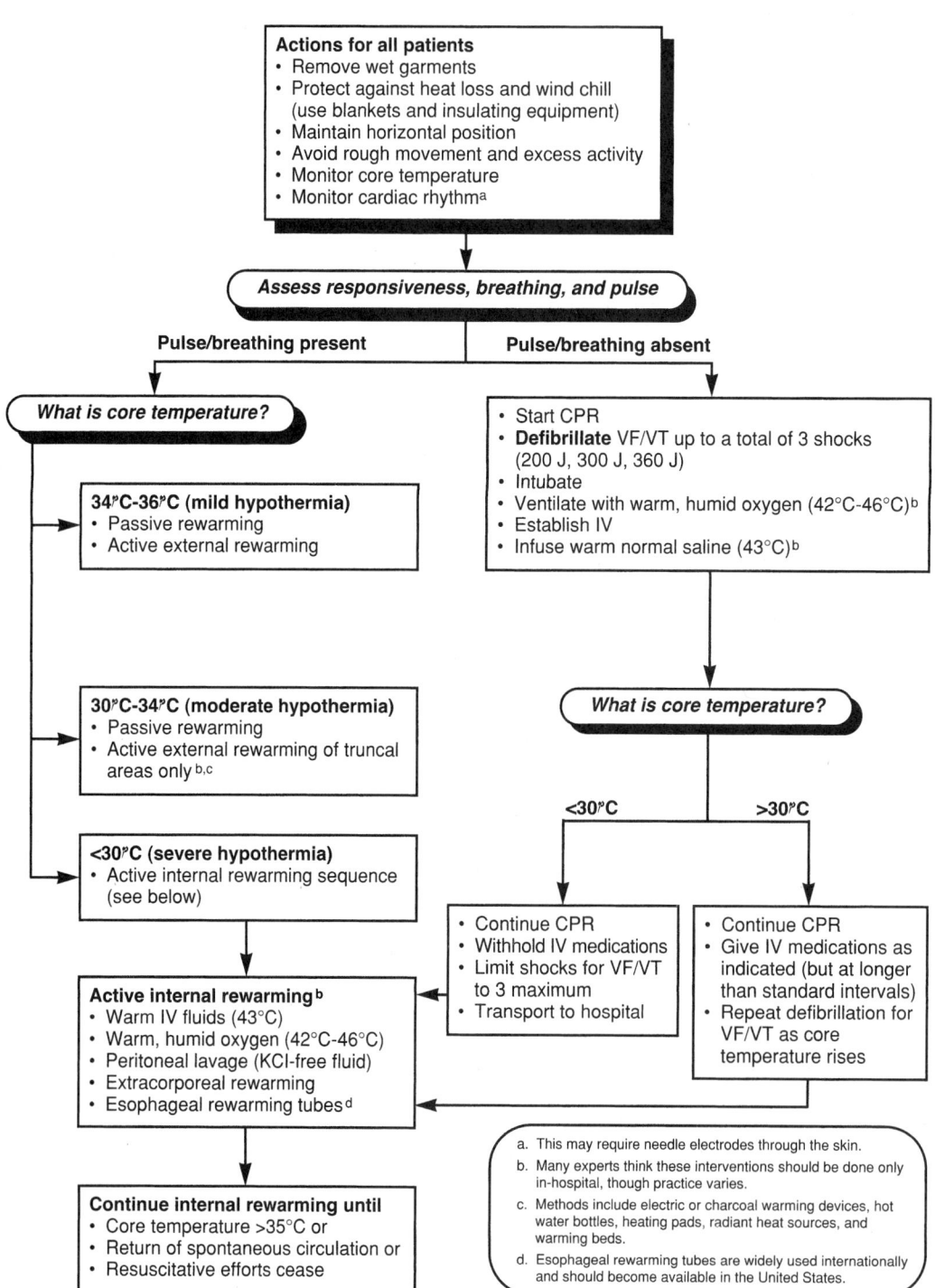

Actions for all patients
- Remove wet garments
- Protect against heat loss and wind chill
  (use blankets and insulating equipment)
- Maintain horizontal position
- Avoid rough movement and excess activity
- Monitor core temperature
- Monitor cardiac rhythm[a]

Assess responsiveness, breathing, and pulse

Pulse/breathing present

Pulse/breathing absent

What is core temperature?

- Start CPR
- **Defibrillate** VF/VT up to a total of 3 shocks
  (200 J, 300 J, 360 J)
- Intubate
- Ventilate with warm, humid oxygen (42°C-46°C)[b]
- Establish IV
- Infuse warm normal saline (43°C)[b]

34°C-36°C (mild hypothermia)
- Passive rewarming
- Active external rewarming

30°C-34°C (moderate hypothermia)
- Passive rewarming
- Active external rewarming of truncal
  areas only [b,c]

What is core temperature?

<30°C   **>30°C**

<30°C (severe hypothermia)
- Active internal rewarming sequence
  (see below)

- Continue CPR
- Withhold IV medications
- Limit shocks for VF/VT
  to 3 maximum
- Transport to hospital

- Continue CPR
- Give IV medications as
  indicated (but at longer
  than standard intervals)
- Repeat defibrillation for
  VF/VT as core
  temperature rises

Active internal rewarming[b]
- Warm IV fluids (43°C)
- Warm, humid oxygen (42°C-46°C)
- Peritoneal lavage (KCl-free fluid)
- Extracorporeal rewarming
- Esophageal rewarming tubes[d]

Continue internal rewarming until
- Core temperature >35°C or
- Return of spontaneous circulation or
- Resuscitative efforts cease

a. This may require needle electrodes through the skin.

b. Many experts think these interventions should be done only
   in-hospital, though practice varies.

c. Methods include electric or charcoal warming devices, hot
   water bottles, heating pads, radiant heat sources, and
   warming beds.

d. Esophageal rewarming tubes are widely used internationally
   and should become available in the United States.

Ischemic Chest Pain Algorithm

Figure 11

1
Chest Pain:
Pain Suggestive of Ischemia

2
Immediate assessment (<10 min)
- Vital signs with automatic or standard BP cuff
- Oxygen saturation
- Obtain IV access
- Obtain 12-lead ECG (physician reviews)
- Brief, targeted history and physical exam; focus on eligibility for thrombolytic therapy
- Initial serum cardiac marker levels
- Initial electrolyte and coagulation studies
- Portable chest x-ray (<30 min)

3
Immediate general treatment
- Oxygen at 4 L/min
- Aspirin 160-325 mg
- Nitroglycerin SL or spray
- Morphine IV (if pain not relieved with nitroglycerin)

Memory: "MONA" greets all patients

4
Much of the immediate assessment and treatment ("MONA") is appropriately performed by the EMS system, including the initial 12-lead ECG and review for thrombolytic therapy indications.

5 *Assess initial 12-lead ECG*

6
ST elevation or new or presumably new BBB: strongly suspicious for injury

13
ST depression or T-wave inversion: ECG strongly suspicious for ischemia

21
Nondiagnostic ECG: absence of changes in ST segment or T waves

7
Consider adjunctive treatments
(as indicated; no reperfusion delay)
- β-Blockers IV
- Nitroglycerin IV
- Heparin IV (especially with TPA)
- ACE inhibitors

14
Consider adjunctive treatments
(as indicated; no contraindications)
- Heparin IV
- Nitroglycerin IV
- β-Blockers IV

22 *Meets criteria for unstable or new-onset angina?*

Yes

No

8 *Time from onset of symptoms?*   >12 hours

15 *Assess clinical status*

9   <12 hours
Select a reperfusion strategy

16
High-risk patient
- Persistent symptoms
- Recurrent ischemia
- Depressed LV function
- Widespread ECG changes
- Prior AMI, PTCA, CABG

19
Clinically Stable

23
Consider
- Admission to ED chest pain unit
In ED follow
- Serial serum markers
- Serial/continuous ECGs
- Consider imaging study (2D echocardiography or radionuclide)

10
Thrombolytic therapy selected
(no contraindications)
- Front-loaded alteplase, or
- Streptokinase, or
- Reteplase
Goal: door-to-drug <30 min

Or equivalent alternative

11
Patients selected for primary PTCA or with contra-indications to thrombolytic therapy

17 *Perform cardiac catheterization: anatomy suitable for revascularization?*

No   Yes

24 *Evidence of ischemia/infarction over 8-12 hours?*

12
Primary PTCA selected. Goal:
- Door-to-dilatation interval, or
- Arrival-in-cath lab interval <60 min

18   **Yes**
Revascularization
- PTCA
- CABG

20
Admit to CCU/monitored bed
- Continue or start adjunctive treatments, as indicated
- Serial serum markers
- Serial/continuous ECGs
- Consider imaging study (2D echocardiography or radionuclide)

25   **No**
Discharge acceptable
- Arrange follow-up

This algorithm provides general guidelines that may not apply to all patients. For all treatments, carefully consider the presence of proper indications and the absence of contraindications.

Based on Figures 1, 3, 4, and Table 4 in ACC/AHA "Guidelines for the management of patients with AMI." *J Am Coll Cardiol.* 1996;28:1328-1428.

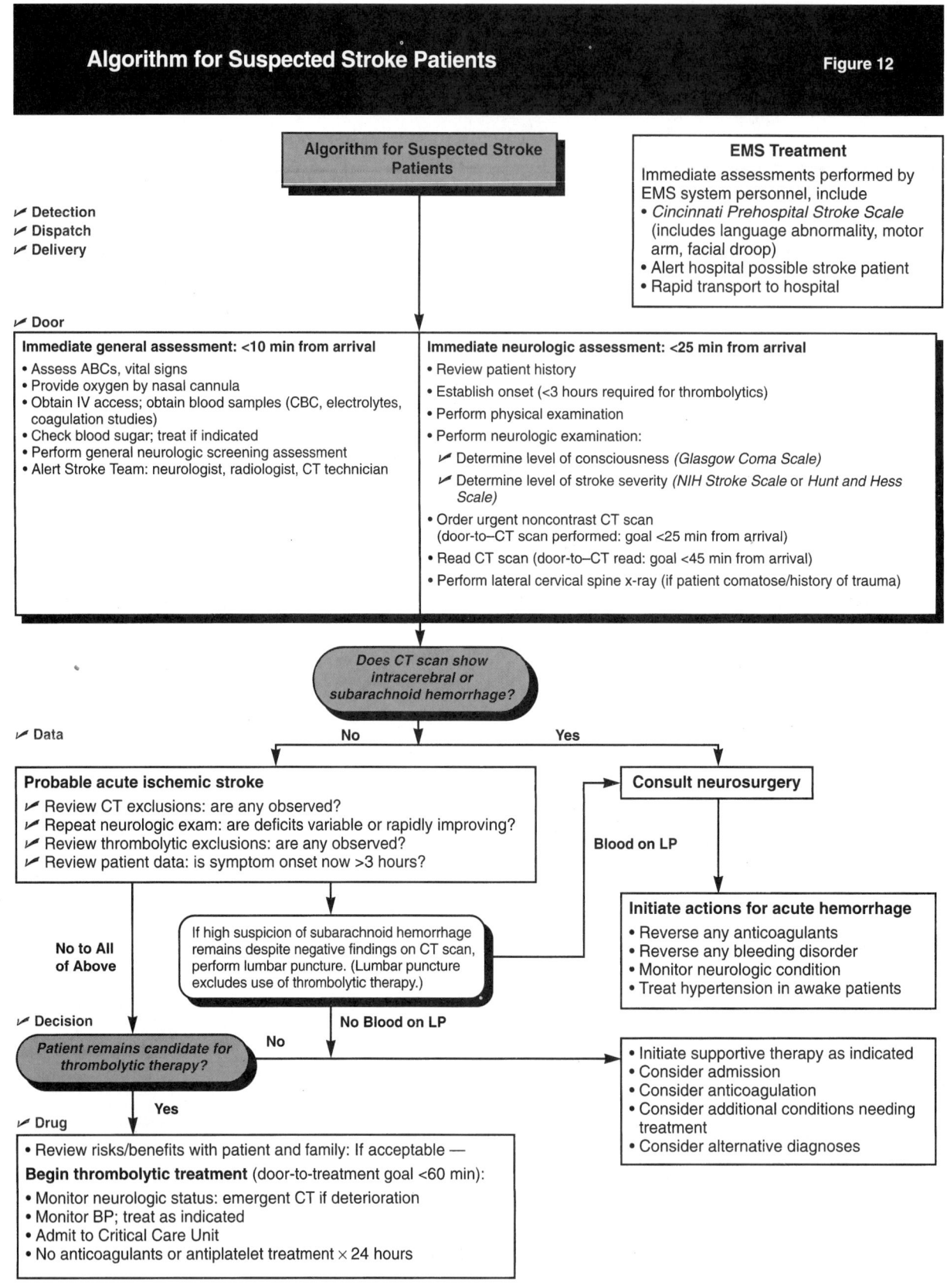

Algorithm for Suspected Stroke Patients

Figure 12

Algorithm for Suspected Stroke Patients

EMS Treatment

Immediate assessments performed by EMS system personnel, include
- *Cincinnati Prehospital Stroke Scale* (includes language abnormality, motor arm, facial droop)
- Alert hospital possible stroke patient
- Rapid transport to hospital

✔ Detection
✔ Dispatch
✔ Delivery

✔ Door

Immediate general assessment: <10 min from arrival
- Assess ABCs, vital signs
- Provide oxygen by nasal cannula
- Obtain IV access; obtain blood samples (CBC, electrolytes, coagulation studies)
- Check blood sugar; treat if indicated
- Perform general neurologic screening assessment
- Alert Stroke Team: neurologist, radiologist, CT technician

Immediate neurologic assessment: <25 min from arrival
- Review patient history
- Establish onset (<3 hours required for thrombolytics)
- Perform physical examination
- Perform neurologic examination:
  ✔ Determine level of consciousness *(Glasgow Coma Scale)*
  ✔ Determine level of stroke severity *(NIH Stroke Scale or Hunt and Hess Scale)*
- Order urgent noncontrast CT scan (door-to–CT scan performed: goal <25 min from arrival)
- Read CT scan (door-to–CT read: goal <45 min from arrival)
- Perform lateral cervical spine x-ray (if patient comatose/history of trauma)

Does CT scan show intracerebral or subarachnoid hemorrhage?

✔ Data

No   Yes

Probable acute ischemic stroke
✔ Review CT exclusions: are any observed?
✔ Repeat neurologic exam: are deficits variable or rapidly improving?
✔ Review thrombolytic exclusions: are any observed?
✔ Review patient data: is symptom onset now >3 hours?

Consult neurosurgery

Blood on LP

No to All of Above

If high suspicion of subarachnoid hemorrhage remains despite negative findings on CT scan, perform lumbar puncture. (Lumbar puncture excludes use of thrombolytic therapy.)

Initiate actions for acute hemorrhage
- Reverse any anticoagulants
- Reverse any bleeding disorder
- Monitor neurologic condition
- Treat hypertension in awake patients

✔ Decision

Patient remains candidate for thrombolytic therapy?

No

No Blood on LP

- Initiate supportive therapy as indicated
- Consider admission
- Consider anticoagulation
- Consider additional conditions needing treatment
- Consider alternative diagnoses

✔ Drug

Yes

- Review risks/benefits with patient and family: If acceptable —
Begin thrombolytic treatment (door-to-treatment goal <60 min):
- Monitor neurologic status: emergent CT if deterioration
- Monitor BP; treat as indicated
- Admit to Critical Care Unit
- No anticoagulants or antiplatelet treatment × 24 hours

Glossary

AACN. *See* American Association of Critical Care Nurses.

ABG. *See* arterial blood gas.

Ablation. An intracardiac catheter used to deliver energy to destroy localized areas of the dysrhythmia origin.

Absence Seizure. A blank stare associated with brief, rapid blinking of the eyes and loss of consciousness of a few seconds' duration; occurs most frequently in children.

Acculturation. An adaptation process in which one gradually acquires the dominant group's culture.

Acid. A substance that releases or liberates hydrogen (H^+) ions.

Acidemia. Arterial blood (plasma) with a pH < 7.35.

Acidosis. Respiratory or metabolic process causing an acidemia (pH < 7.35).

Acquired Immunodeficiency Syndrome (AIDS). A disabling or life-threatening illness caused by the human immunodeficiency virus (HIV).

ACTH. *See* adrenocorticotropic hormone.

Action Potential. The positive electrical potential recorded when a cell is activated by an electrical impulse or current.

Activated Clotting Time (ACT). Test done on venous whole blood to determine the time it takes to clot; may be used to monitor and regulate heparin therapy in patients requiring anticoagulation.

Activated Partial Thromboplastin Time (aPTT). Test using venous blood to detect deficiencies in all clotting factors, except VII and XIII, and platelet abnormalities; commonly used to monitor and regulate heparin therapy in patients requiring anticoagulation.

Active Immunity. Immunity resulting from the development within the body of substances that render a person immune; produced either as a result of antigen stimulation or by means of a vaccination.

Acute Care Nurse Practitioner. Advanced practice nurse encompassing the roles of researcher and practitioner to facilitate high-quality comprehensive care for the acutely ill patient.

Acute (Cellular) Rejection. The formation of T cells by the immune system that directly attack and destroy foreign tissue.

Acute Head Injury. Injury to the head and its structures; also called traumatic brain injury or brain injury.

Acute Myocardial Infarction (AMI, MI). The necrosis of some segment of myocardium usually due to a sudden occlusion of a coronary artery.

Acute Renal Failure. An abrupt and marked decrease in renal function that results in serious compromise to the patient.

Acute Respiratory Distress Syndrome (ARDS). A group of clinical manifestations associated with serious insult to lung tissue. Also referred to as adult respiratory distress syndrome.

Acute Respiratory Failure (ARF). The sudden and severe impairment in the lung's ability to maintain adequate oxygenation and ventilation.

Acute Retroviral Syndrome. Acute or primary HIV infection; may present as a mononucleosis-like syndrome within 3 months of the infection.

Addiction. Psychological dependence and compulsive drug use, characterized as a continuous craving for the narcotic and the need to use it for effects other than pain relief.

Addison's Disease. Disease characterized by an adrenal insufficiency.

Adenosine (Adenocard). A naturally occurring nucleotide that has vasodilating properties; used in nuclear studies to induce coronary artery dilation in patients who cannot exercise.

Adenosine Diphosphate (ADP). Precursor to adenosine triphosphate.

Adenosine Triphosphate (ATP). Substance that is used by cells as energy to carry out all the metabolic functions.

ADH. *See* antidiuretic hormone.

ADP. *See* adenosine diphosphate.

Adrenal Crisis. Condition in which there is an acute adrenal insufficiency characterized by severe hypotension, weakness, dehydration, progressing to shock and coma.

Adrenal Insufficiency. State of inadequate adrenal cortex release of cortisol.

Adrenocorticotropic Hormone. Hormone secreted by the anterior pituitary gland that stimulates secretion of other hormones by the adrenal cortex.

Advance Directives. Legal documents that allow individuals to give instructions about their future health care if they should become incapable of decision-making. Two types of advance directives are instruction directives (living wills) and proxy directives (durable health care powers of attorney).

Aerobic Metabolism. The method by which adenosine triphosphate is produced, using oxygen as the energy source.

Afterload. The force of resistance against which the heart has to pump to eject blood during systole.

AIDS Dementia Complex. Neurologic complications of HIV infection; may include inflammation of the brain (or of the membrane surrounding the brain), infections of the brain, brain or spinal cord tumors, nerve damage, difficulties in thinking, behavioral changes, and stroke.

AIDS-Related Complex (ARC). A term not officially defined or recognized by the Centers for Disease Control and Prevention that has been used to describe a variety of symptoms and signs found in some persons with HIV infection.

Aldosterone. A mineralocorticoid steroid hormone produced by the adrenal cortex that acts to regulate sodium and potassium balance in the blood.

Alkalemia. Arterial blood (plasma) with a pH > 7.45.

Alkalosis. Respiratory or metabolic process causing an alkalemia (pH > 7.45).

Allograft. Composed of skin transplanted from another human, usually a cadaver; can be either fresh or cryopreserved.

Alveolar. Pertaining to the alveoli sac, the site of gas exchange in the lungs.

Alveolar Ventilation. Gas exchange at the alveolar level.

Amebiasis. Inflammation of the intestines caused by infestation with an ameba and characterized by frequent, loose stools flecked with blood and mucus.

American Association of Critical Care Nurses (AACN). A professional specialty organization for nurses practicing or interested in critical care nursing; provides and supports education and research related to critical care nursing.

AMI. *See* acute myocardial infarction.

Amylase. A class of enzymes that split or hydrolyze starch.

Amylin. A 37–amino acid peptide hormone produced by the pancreatic beta cells and co-secreted with insulin in response to nutrient intake.

Anabolic. The constructive phase of metabolism concerned with the body's ability to synthesize protoplasm for growth and repair.

Anaerobic Metabolism. The pathway used by the cell to produce adenosine triphosphate when oxygen is not available.

Androgens. Steroidal hormones responsible for the development of secondary sexual characteristics.

Anemia. A lower than normal number of red blood cells.

Anergy. The loss or weakening of the body's immunity to an irritating agent or antigen.

Aneurysmal Subarachnoid Hemorrhage. The accumulation of blood in the subarachnoid space, most often at the base of the brain; usually caused by a ruptured intracranial aneurysm.

Angina. Substernal or precordial pain associated with a decrease in oxygen delivered to a portion of the myocardium; may be intermittent or prolonged and may radiate to the shoulders, neck, back, jaw, ears, or arms.

Angiography. X-ray visualization of the blood vessels after the intravascular introduction of radiopaque contrast medium.

Angiotensin I. The precursor to angiotensin II; angiotensin I is primarily converted to angiotensin II in the lung.

Angiotensin II. A potent vasoconstrictor; the end result of the renin–angiotensin pathway.

Angular Cheilitis. Inflammation of the corners of the mouth.

Anion Gap. A test that measures the difference between sodium (Na^+) and potassium (K^+) ion concentrations and the sum of chloride (Cl^-) and bicarbonate (HCO_3^-).

Anorexia. Loss of appetite.

Anterior Cord Syndrome. An incomplete, or partial, spinal cord injury usually caused by the compression of the anterior spinal artery; the most common of spinal cord injuries.

Anterior Horn. The anterior gray matter of the spinal cord containing the motor cells that send messages to the muscles for movement.

Antibiotic. An antimicrobial agent produced semisynthetically or derived from cultures of microorganisms; used to treat infections.

Antibodies. A protein substance produced by the body in response to, and interacting specifically with, an antigen.

Antidiuretic Hormone (ADH). Pituitary hormone that regulates fluid balance by increasing the permeability of the distal collecting tubules in an effort to retain water; also known as vasopressin.

Antigen. A substance that induces the formation of antibodies that react specifically with it.

Antiretroviral Agents. Substances used against retroviruses such as HIV.

Antithrombin. A substance that prevents blood coagulation or clotting by counteracting the effects of thrombin.

Antiviral. A substance or process that destroys a virus or suppresses its replication.

Anuria. No urine output.

Anxiety. A disorder characterized by excessive worry, difficulty controlling the worry, restlessness, irritability, decreased ability to concentrate, and disturbed sleep.

Apical Impulse. Point of maximal impulse (PMI); a visible pulsation seen in the left fifth intercostal space/midclavicular line that occurs with each contraction or thrust of the left ventricle.

Apoptosis. Cellular suicide, also known as programmed death of older cells.

ARC. *See* AIDS-related complex.

ARDS. *See* acute respiratory distress syndrome.

Areflexia. The absence of reflexes.

ARF. *See* acute respiratory failure.

Arterial Blood Gas (ABG). Measurement of gases and pH in arterial blood.

Arterial Oxygen Content (CaO$_2$). The amount of oxygen in the arterial blood.

Arterial Puncture. Percutaneous puncture of an artery for arterial blood gas sampling.

Arteriogram. A contrast study performed to radiographically evaluate arterial blood vessels.

Arteriovenous Fistula. Surgical anastomosis of an artery and vein resulting in increased blood flow and pressure in the venous system beyond the anastomosis; allows for placement of large-gauge needles to establish adequate extracorporeal blood flow.

Arteriovenous Graft. Surgical placement of a conduit between an artery and vein for easy needle placement to obtain adequate extracorporeal blood flow.

Arteriovenous Malformation. A mass of arteries and arterialized veins that forms an anomalous connection between the arterial and venous system, without a normally intervening capillary network.

Arthralgia. Pain in a joint.

Artifact. An electrocardiographic waveform that arises from sources other than the myocardium.

Ascites. Accumulation of free serous fluid in the abdominal cavity as a result of severe right-sided congestive heart failure, kidney or liver disease, or abdominal cancer.

Aspergillosis. A fungal infection (resulting from the fungus *Aspergillus*) of the lungs that can spread through the blood to other organs.

Assist/Control (A/C). A ventilator mode characterized by mandatory breaths and assisted spontaneous breaths.

Asymptomatic. Without symptoms.

Ataxia. An uneven, distorted gait; a common neuromuscular symptom.

Atelectasis. Alveolar collapse resulting from failure of alveolar expansion or reabsorption of alveolar air; incomplete expansion of the lungs.

Atheroma. An area of atherosclerotic plaque or lesion.

Atherosclerosis. Narrowing of the interlumen of an artery caused by the proliferation of cells and the accumulation of cholesterol, calcium, and other minerals.

Atonic Seizure. Seizures characterized by loss of muscle tone, abrupt fall, and loss of consciousness; also known as drop attacks.

ATP. *See* adenosine triphosphate.

Atrial Natriuretic Peptide. A substance secreted from atrial myocytes in the heart muscle; thought to counteract fluid conservation effort by the kidneys, resulting in increased filtration and decreased reabsorption of sodium.

Autoantibody. An antibody that is active against some of the tissues of the organism that produced it.

Autoimmune. A response of the immune system against one's own body in which antibodies are produced and attack healthy tissue.

Autologous Skin Graft. A patient's own skin is used to permanently cover an excised burn wound; can be a sheet or meshed graft. Also known as an autograft.

Autonomic Dysreflexia (Hyperflexia). A potentially life-threatening complication of a spinal column injury that occurs with injury at thoracic level 6 (T6) or above; a variety of stimuli can cause the syndrome, including a distended bladder, a full bowel, infection, skin breakdown, pain, or sudden changes in the ambient environmental temperature.

Autonomy. An ethical principle of independence and self-determination.

Autoregulation. The ability of vasculature to change the diameter of the blood vessels in an attempt to maintain a constant flow of blood to an area of the body.

Autotransfusion. The collection and reinfusion of the patient's shed blood from an appropriate device, such as a chest tube drainage system.

Axial Loading. Vertical compression forces applied to the head and transmitted to the spine.

Axis. Direction of an ECG waveform in the frontal plane, measured in degrees.

Axon. The message-carrying fibers of the nervous system.

Azidothymidine (AZT). A nucleoside analog that suppresses replication of HIV; now known as zidovudine.

Azotemia. Accumulation of uremic toxins, as seen in acute and chronic renal failure.

AZT. *See* azidothymidine.

B Lymphocytes. Essential cell for antibody-mediated immunity; when activated by lymphokines will become antibody-producing plasma cells. Also called humoral immunity.

Baroreceptors. Sensory nerve terminals sensitive to blood pressure changes.

Barotrauma. Injury to the alveoli caused by internal pressure.

Base. A substance that combines with hydrogen.

Base Excess. Total amount of buffering or base in a solution.

Baseline. A known value or quantity with which an unknown is compared when measured or assessed.

Basophil. A type of white blood cell, also called a granular leukocyte, filled with granules of toxic chemicals that can digest microorganisms.

Beneficence. The ethical principle of doing good.

Bilirubin. A bile pigment whose measurement can be used as an indication of the health of the liver; small amounts of bilirubin normally enter the bloodstream and circulate until they reach the liver and are excreted. Normal value is 0.1 to 1.5 mg per liter of blood.

Binding Antibody. An antibody that attaches to some part of the HIV virus; binding antibodies may or may not adversely affect the virus.

Biologic Age. Age of an individual's tissues and organ systems as determined by damage from environmental factors, lifestyle patterns, and diseases.

Bipolar. On an ECG, refers to those leads that have positive points of reference (i.e., standard limb leads I, II, and III). In pacemaker leads, refers to a pacing wire that has the positive and negative poles located at the tip of the pacing wire.

Biventricular Heart Failure. Inadequacy of both left and right ventricles of the heart to maintain their pumping action; results in physiologic decline.

Bleb. A blister formation.

Blinded Study. A clinical trial in which participants are unaware as to whether they are in the experimental or the control arm of the study.

Blood–Brain Barrier. The barrier between brain blood vessels and brain tissues whose effect is to restrict what may pass from the blood into the brain.

Blood Urea Nitrogen (BUN). A waste product resulting from the metabolic breakdown of protein, normally excreted by the kidney.

Blunt Trauma. Injury from impact forces or acceleration/deceleration mechanisms.

Bonadaptation. Positive outcome after a crisis-provoking event; successful and effective adaptation.

Bradypenic. Respirations less than 10 breaths per minute.

Brain Death. Cessation of cerebral blood flow and all vital brain stem functions, including pupillary reflexes, extraocular reflexes, corneal reflex, cough, gag, and breathing.

Brain Injury. An injury to the brain itself; also called traumatic brain injury or acute head injury.

Breakthrough Infection. An infection, caused by the infectious agent the vaccine is designed to protect against, that occurs during the course of a vaccine trial. These infections may be caused by exposure to the infectious agent before the vaccine has taken effect, or before all doses of the vaccine have been given.

Bronchoscopy. Method of assessing the airways using a flexible scope; can be used to assess, biopsy, or obtain specimens.

Bronchospasm. Spasmodic constriction of the bronchial tubes.

Brown-Séquard Syndrome. A partial injury of the spinal cord resulting from a hemisection of the spinal cord; frequently seen in penetrating injury to the spinal cord.

Bullae. Vesicular bubble-type formation larger than 1 cm.

Burkitt's Lymphoma. A lymphatic cancer that involves not only the lymphatic and the associated reticuloendothelial systems but also other body tissues.

Burst Fracture. *See* comminuted fracture.

Cachexia. General ill health and malnutrition, marked by weakness and emaciation, usually associated with serious disease. *See also* wasting syndrome.

Calyces. Hollow fingerlike projections extending from the center indented area of the kidney to the apex of the renal pyramids to collect urine.

Candidiasis. A fungal infection with a species of *Candida*; most commonly involves the skin, oral mucosa, respiratory tract, and vagina. Candidiasis of the esophagus, trachea, bronchi, or lungs is an indicator disease for AIDS.

CAPD. *See* continuous ambulatory peritoneal dialysis.

Capitation. Prepayment, per patient per month, by an organization to a health care provider.

Capnography. A wave tracing of exhaled carbon dioxide; usually measured with end-tidal CO_2 sensors.

Carbonic Anhydrase III. A protein found in skeletal muscle, released into the bloodstream when skeletal tissue is injured.

Cardiac Cycle. A single episode of electrical and mechanical activation and recovery of a myocardial cell or of the entire heart.

Cardiac Index. Amount of blood ejected by the heart per minute divided by body surface area; normal at rest > 3.0 L/min.

Cardiac Output. Amount of blood ejected by the heart per minute; normal at rest ≥ 5.0 L/min.

Cardiogenic Shock. Shock caused from the inability of the heart to pump effectively.

Cardiopulmonary Exercise Testing (CPX). Determines an individual's exercise capacity, peak heart rate, maximal oxygen consumption, respiratory gas exchange ratio, and ventilatory equivalent for oxygen.

Catabolism. The degradation or destructive phase of metabolism concerned with the breakdown by the body of complex compounds usually with liberation of energy.

Catecholamines. Adrenal medulla hormones that produce a fight or flight response by stimulation of the sympathetic nervous system; epinephrine and norepinepherine are the primary catecholamines.

Cation. A positively charged ion.

CBC. Complete blood cell count.

CD4 (T4) or CD4 Cells. Cells that orchestrate the immune response, signaling other cells in the immune system to perform their special functions; alternative term for T4 or T-helper cell.

CD8 (T8) Cells. A protein embedded in the cell surface of suppressor T lymphocytes; also called cytotoxic T cells.

Cell Lysis. Rupture and destruction of a cell.

Cell-Mediated Immunity. The branch of the immune system in which the reaction to foreign material is performed by specific defense cells (such as killer cells, macrophages, and other white blood cells) rather than antibodies.

Central Cord Syndrome. An incomplete, or partial, spinal cord injury associated with a hyperextension–flexion injury in a patient with cervical spondylosis (spurring of the cervical vertebrae from osteoarthritis) or cervical stenosis.

Cerebral Autoregulation. Mechanisms that control cerebral blood flow, including metabolic, myogenic, and chemical mechanisms.

Cerebral Edema. Swelling of the brain.

Cerebral Perfusion Pressure. The difference between mean arterial pressure and intracranial pressure.

Chemoreceptor. End organ sensitive to certain chemical stimuli.

Cholesterol. Steroid synthesized by the liver or ingested by humans.

Chronic (Humoral) Rejection. The formation of B cells by the immune system that stimulate the formation of memory cells that continue to recognize and attempt to destroy foreign tissue.

Chronic Renal Insufficiency. A gradual and progressive reduction in renal function.

Chronologic Age. Age of a person in years.

Chvostek's Sign. Spasm of the facial muscles after stimulation on one side of the face over the area of the facial nerve; secondary effect of hypocalcemia.

Chylothorax. Accumulation of milky lymphatic drainage in the pleural space.

Clinical Latency. The state or period of an infectious agent, such as a virus or bacterium, living or developing in a host without producing clinical symptoms.

Clinical Nurse Specialist. Advanced practice nurse encompassing the roles of educator, consultant, researcher and manager.

Clonic Seizure. Repetitive contraction and relaxation of muscle jerking, as seen in tonic-clonic seizures. The tonic phase of the seizure may not occur, hence it is referred to as a clonic seizure.

Closed-Head Injury. A blunt injury to the brain that does not result in an open-skull fracture.

CMV. *See* continuous mandatory ventilation.

CMV. *See* cytomegalovirus.

Collaboration. Working together in multidisciplinary problem-solving and decision-making to provide comprehensive care for critically ill patients.

Collateral Coronary Circulation. Minute anastomoses that exist between the smaller coronary arteries that dilate during times of acute coronary occlusion; the amount of collateral circulation varies among individuals.

Colloid. Intravenous fluids used to replace fluids that are lost; colloids contain proteins that help to keep the fluid in the vascular space.

Comminuted Fracture. The result of an axial loading injury, the vertebral body is shattered and bone may actually penetrate the spinal cord; also known as a burst fracture.

Complete Spinal Cord Injury. Injury that results in an irreversible total loss of motor and sensory function below the level of the injury; also known as complete transection of the cord.

Complex Partial Seizure. A partial seizure associated with impaired consciousness and a variety of clinical expressions ranging from no movement to wandering and automatisms; may start as a simple partial seizure and then progress.

Compliance. Pulmonary volume change produced by a pressure change.

Compression Injury. An injury in which the vertebral body is dislocated and moves posteriorly to compress the anterior spinal artery and the anterior spinal cord.

Computed Tomography (CT). A radiologic test in which the x-ray source rotates around the patient and produces images of specific planes in the body.

Continuous Ambulatory Peritoneal Dialysis (CAPD). A type of peritoneal dialysis in which approximately four fluid exchanges are administered throughout the day.

Continuous Cycle Peritoneal Dialysis/Automated Peritoneal Dialysis. Peritoneal dialysis using automated equipment (usually during night/sleep period) to perform multiple fluid exchanges.

Continuous Mandatory Ventilation (CMV). A mode of ventilation featuring totally controlled ventilation.

Continuous Renal Replacement Therapy (CRRT). Extracorporeal system that removes water, excess electrolytes, and end-products of metabolism; similar to hemodialysis but requires slower blood flows and results in minimal hemodynamic changes.

Contractility. The ability of muscle to develop tension and thereby shorten and contract.

Contraindication. A specific circumstance when the use of certain treatments could be harmful.

Contrast Medium. In radiography, a material opaque to x-rays administered intravenously to enhance x-ray imaging.

Contusion. Injury that results in small hemorrhages and bruising of the spinal cord.

Coping. Constantly changing cognitive and behavioral efforts to manage specific external and internal demands considered taxing or that exceed the resources of the person.

Cor Pulmonale. Right ventricular enlargement and/ or failure as a result of lung tissue or vessel disease causing higher than normal pulmonary pressures.

Coronary Angiography. Catheter-based procedure; dye is injected into the coronary arteries and radiographic images are recorded to determine the extent of occlusion present.

Corrosive Agents. Chemical agents that cause massive protein denaturation through corrosion.

Cortex. The tissue layer of the kidney immediately beneath the renal capsule; the glomeruli of the nephrons reside within this layer.

Corticotropin-Releasing Hormone (CRH). Secreted by the hypothalamus to stimulate release of ACTH by the anterior pituitary.

Cortisol. A steroid hormone produced naturally by the adrenal cortex and synthetically for pharmacologic use.

Coup-Contrecoup. A brain injury at both the impact site and the site opposite the impact, caused by movement of the brain within the cranial vault.

Creatinine. A waste product resulting from creatine metabolism, normally produced in predictable amounts and excreted by the kidney; an increase in serum creatinine may indicate renal dysfunction.

Creatinine Clearance. The measurement of glomerular filtration rate by determining the amount of creatinine filtered through the glomerulus and excreted in the urine; usually measured over a 24-hour period.

Crescendo Murmur. A murmur that increases from quiet to louder.

Crescendo-Decrescendo Murmur. A murmur that progresses from quiet to loud, to quiet.

CRH. *See* corticotropin-releasing hormone.

Cricothyroidotomy. A percutaneous or surgical procedure to access the trachea at the cricothyroid membrane to establish an emergency airway.

Critical Care Nursing. Nursing that involves caring for patients and families undergoing life-threatening illness or injury or potentially life-threatening illness or injury.

Critical Thinking. An attitude and an approach to ideas or decisions; willingness to give fair and equal consideration to all possible ideas or decisions, and accepting an idea or a decision after careful reflection.

CRRT. *See* continuous renal replacement therapy.

Cryptococcal Meningitis. A life-threatening infection of the membranes (meninges) that line the brain and the spinal cord, found in soil contaminated by bird droppings.

Crystalloid. Intravenous fluids used to replace fluids that are lost; crystalloids contain electrolytes and are pH balanced.

CT. *See* computed tomography.

Cyanosis. Bluish discoloration of the skin, mucous membranes, nailbeds, lips, and extremities.

Cytokines. Immune system proteins involved in the normal regulation of the immune response.

Cytomegalovirus (CMV). A herpes virus that is a common cause of opportunistic diseases in people with immune suppression.

Cytomegalovirus Retinitis. An eye disease common among patients infected with HIV.

Cytopenia. Deficiency in the cellular elements of the blood.

Cytotoxic. An agent or process that is toxic to cells; causes suppression of function or cell death.

Cytotoxic T Lymphocyte. Cell that attacks antigen-infected cells; also a host cell for HIV; activated by lymphokines of T-helper cells. Also called killer T cell.

Dead Space to Tidal Volume Ratio (V_D/V_T). The portion of V_T that does not participate in gas exchange (25%–35%).

Dead Space (V_D) Ventilation. Wasted ventilation occurring when alveoli are ventilated but the capillaries interfacing the alveoli are poorly perfused, or not perfused at all.

Decrescendo Murmur. A murmur that decreases from loud to quieter.

Decubitus X-Ray. Chest radiograph taken with the patient in a side-lying position on the affected side; used to assess fluid in the pleural space.

Delirium. Acute confusional state characterized by an abrupt onset that can develop over hours.

Dementia. Chronic intellectual impairment that affects a person's ability to function in a social or occupational setting.

Demyelination. The degeneration and removal of myelin from the axon of peripheral nerves.

Deoxyribonucleic Acid (DNA). The molecular chain found in genes within the nucleus of each cell that carries the genetic information enabling cells to reproduce.

Depolarization. A condition that alters the permeability of the cell membrane, thus allowing positively charged ions to cross into the cell.

Dermatitis. Inflammation of skin evidenced by itching, redness, and skin lesions.

Desiccants. Chemical agents that cause cellular damage by extracting water from the cells leading to cellular dehydration.

Diabetes Insipidus (DI). Disease resulting from the lack of antidiuretic hormone (ADH) or inability of the kidney to respond to ADH.

Diabetic Ketoacidosis (DKA). Severe insulin deficiency resulting in the inability of muscle and adipose tissue to use glucose, resulting in severe dehydration, electrolyte imbalance, metabolic acidosis, coma, or death.

Diagnosis. The determination of the presence of a specific disease or infection, usually accomplished by evaluating clinical symptoms and laboratory tests.

Diagnostic Peritoneal Lavage (DPL). A surgical technique primarily employed to rapidly determine the presence of blood in the peritoneal space.

Dialysate. A solution of water and ions (electrolytes and trace metals) compatible with human serum used in the vascular compartment of an artificial kidney.

Dialysis. Any system that uses a semi-permeable membrane to move substances by means of filtration, diffusion, or ultrafiltration from one compartment to another; used to treat the imbalances associated with renal failure, edematous states, and drug overdose.

Dialyzer. A disposable unit that includes a biocompatible, semi-permeable membrane (blood compartment) and a surrounding space for dialysate in which filtration, diffusion, and ultrafiltration occur to achieve hemodialysis.

Diaphoresis. Perceptible perspiration.

Diarrhea. Uncontrolled, loose, and frequent bowel movements; severe or prolonged diarrhea can lead to weight loss and malnutrition.

Diastole. Period when either the ventricles or the atria of the heart are relaxing.

DIC. *See* disseminated intravascular coagulation.

Diffuse Injury. Microscopic or neuronal injury.

Diminished Renal Reserve. Earliest stage of renal disease that can be clinically identified, usually by elevated serum creatinine, blood urea nitrogen, and decreased creatinine clearance; a patient may exhibit no symptoms, and electrolyte balance and fluid volume remain normal.

Dipyridamole (Persantine). A vasodilator medication used in nuclear stress testing to dilate coronary arteries in patients who are unable to exercise.

Direct Angioplasty. Repair of the occluded coronary artery using a percutaneous transluminal approach.

Dislocation. Occurs when one vertebra overrides another with unilateral or bilateral dislocation of the facets; usually results from torn or stretched ligaments.

Disseminated Intravascular Coagulation (DIC). The inappropriate, accelerated, systemic activation of the coagulation cascade.

Distributive Shock. Shock caused from the maldistribution of fluid in the intravascular space secondary to massive vasodilation.

Diuretic. A pharmacologic agent or method promoting the excretion of urine.

DKA. *See* diabetic ketoacidosis.

DNA. *See* deoxyribonucleic acid.

Dobutamine. Inotropic intravenous medication that enhances cardiac contractility by direct stimulation of the β receptors found in myocardial tissue; may cause an increase in myocardial oxygen demand by increasing myocardial contractility, heart rate, and blood pressure.

Dormancy. *See* latency.

Dressler's Syndrome. A collection of signs and symptoms that occur from 1 week to several months after an acute myocardial infarction and are indicative of pericarditis; includes chest pain, especially on deep inspiration, pericardial friction rub, diffuse ST-segment changes, fever, arthralgias, and pericardial effusion.

Durable Power of Attorney. A proxy advance directive in which another individual (agent) is designated to make health care and treatment decisions for a person if he or she becomes unable to do so.

Dysarthria. A dysarticulation or slurring of speech.

Dysmenorrhea. Painful menstruation.

Dysphagia. Loss of integrity of the swallowing mechanism that may occur after stroke when neurologic impairment involves both voluntary and involuntary neurocontrol mechanisms in the motor and sensory cortex, subcortical regions, or brain stem.

Dysplasia. Any abnormal development of tissue or organs.

Dyspnea. Difficult or labored breathing.

EBV. *See* Epstein-Barr virus.

Echocardiogram. Cardiac test that takes pictures of the heart with sound waves, revealing structural and functional problems.

Ectopic. An impulse arising from a focus other than the heart's sinus node.

Eczema. Acute or chronic cutaneous inflammatory condition with erythema, papules, vesicles, pustules, scales, crusts, or scabs alone or in combination.

Einthoven's triangle. An equilateral triangle composed of three limb leads, I, II, and III, providing an orientation for electrical information on the frontal plane.

Ejection Fraction. Percentage of blood that fills the ventricle and is subsequently pumped out during each systole; used as an indicator of ventricle contractility. Normal ejection fraction is 60% to 65%.

Electrocardiogram. A graphic recording of electrical activity generated by the heart.

Electrode. An electrical contact placed on the skin and connected to the ECG recorder.

Electrolytes. Chemical substances, such as salts, acids, and bases, that ionize and dissociate in water and are capable of conducting an electrical current.

Electrophysiologic Study (EPS). An invasive procedure to evaluate the electrical conduction system of the heart.

ELISA. *See* enzyme-linked immunosorbent assay.

Embolectomy. Removal of an obstructing blood clot in a blood vessel.

Emic. The cultural view of the insider or inhabitant of a culture.

Empyema. Purulent drainage in the pleural space or other body cavity.

Enculturation. The socialization of an individual into the ways of a culture or subculture.

Endocardium. Endothelial membrane lining the interior of the heart.

Endotoxin. A substance released from gram-negative bacteria that initiates a series of cascades resulting in vasodilation, bronchoconstriction, and increased microvascular permeability.

Endotracheal Tube (ETT). A large catheter passed through the glottis into the trachea to maintain a patent airway to facilitate controlled positive-pressure ventilation.

End-Stage Disease. Final period or phase in the course of a disease leading to a person's death.

End-Stage Renal Disease (ESRD). Occurs when renal function is reduced acutely or over time until kidneys can no longer support the body and chronic dialysis intervention or transplantation is required.

End-Tidal Carbon Dioxide (PETCO$_2$). Partial pressure of CO_2 in the end-expiratory air; a close estimate of alveolar partial pressure of CO_2.

Enteritis. Inflammation of the intestine.

Enzyme. Protein that accelerates a specific chemical reaction without altering itself.

Enzyme-Linked Immunosorbent Assay (ELISA). A laboratory test to determine the presence of antibodies to HIV in the blood. A positive ELISA generally is confirmed by the western blot test.

Eosinophil. A type of white blood cell that can digest microorganisms.

Epicardium. Outer aspect of the myocardial wall adjacent to the pericardial lining.

Epidemic. A disease that spreads rapidly through a demographic segment of the human population, such as everyone in a given geographic area or everyone of a certain age or sex within a region. Spreads from person to person or from a contaminated source such as food or water.

Epidemiology. A branch of medical science that deals with the incidence, distribution, and control of a disease in a population.

Epidural Hematoma. Hemorrhage found between the dura mater and the skull.

Epilepsy. A chronic disorder characterized by recurrent, unprovoked seizures.

Epogen/Epoetin Alfa. Synthetic erythropoietin created with recombinant gene technology, administered intravenously or subcutaneously to patients with end-stage renal disease to correct anemia caused by erythropoietin insufficiency.

EPS. *See* electrophysiologic study.

Epstein-Barr Virus (EBV). A contagious herpeslike virus that causes mononucleosis; associated with Burkitt's lymphoma and hairy leukoplakia.

Erythrocytes. Red blood cells whose major function is to carry oxygen to cells.

Erythropoietin. A hormone-type substance secreted by the endothelial cells of the peritubular capillaries in the renal cortex that stimulates production of red blood cells in the bone marrow.

Eschar. Nonviable tissue resulting from burn injury; it contracts rapidly, causing restriction of vessels, soft tissue, and underlying organs.

Escharotomy. A linear incision of constricting eschar, performed for circumferential burns of the extremities or chest wall permitting the cut edges to separate and restore blood flow to unburned tissue distal to the eschar.

ESRD. *See* end-stage renal disease.

Estrogen. Produced by the ovaries and conversion of adrenal androgens to estrogen; responsible for the development of secondary sex characteristics.

Ethnocentrism. The belief that the values, beliefs, and practices of one's own culture are the right ones, the best, or the only ones.

Ethnonursing. Leininger's approach to culturally congruent nursing care based on her theoretical model of Culture Care Diversity and Universality.

Etic. The view of the culture from an outsider's perspective.

ETT. *See* endotracheal tube.

Express Consent. Consent that is directly given, either verbally or in writing.

Expressive Aphasia. Altered ability to respond using written or spoken language.

Extracorporeal Membrane Oxygenation. Invasive technique used to supplement mechanical ventilation with direct oxygenation of the blood.

Factor V:Q506. A gene mutation responsible for resistance to activated protein C, thus allowing the development of blood clots and recurrent thrombophlebitis.

Febrile. Feverish; pertaining to a fever.

FEV$_{1.0}$. *See* forced expiratory volume in 1 second.

Fiberoptic Bronchoscopy. A tubular instrument used to visualize the major airways.

Fibrin. An insoluble protein derived through the activity of thrombin on fibrinogen.

Fibrinogen. A dissolved blood plasma protein that is converted into fibrin by the enzymatic action of thrombin.

Fibrinolysis. Blood clot dissolution.

Fidelity. The ethical principle of faithfulness to commitments made to self and others.

FIo$_2$. Fraction of inspired oxygen.

First Pass. During nuclear scans, a technetium tracer is injected and tagged to red blood cells. Images of the tracer on its initial pass through the left ventricle are obtained, allowing the heart to be assessed within a few seconds.

Flaccid Paralysis. Absence of voluntary muscle movement and loss of transmission of reflex arcs between sensory and motor neurons.

Flail Chest. Three or more contiguous ribs broken in two or more places producing an unstable segment of chest wall.

Focal Injury. Produces a macroscopic lesion.

Follicle-Stimulating Hormone (FSH). Stimulates ovarian follicle growth and maturation in the female; stimulates and maintains spermatogenesis in the male.

Follicular Dendritic Cells. Cells found in the germinal centers of lymphoid organs forming a weblike network to trap invaders.

Fomite. An inanimate object that can harbor pathogenic microorganisms and thus serve as an agent of transmission of an infection.

Forced Expiratory Volume in 1 Second (FEV$_{1.0}$). After taking as deep a breath as possible, the amount of air exhaled during the first second during a forced expiration.

Forced Vital Capacity (FVC). Maximal forceful exhaled volume after a maximal inspiration.

Frontal Plane. A vertical plane of the body lying perpendicular to both the horizontal and sagittal planes.

FSH. *See* follicle-stimulating hormone.

Full-Thickness Burn. Caused by prolonged exposure to a heat source, chemicals, or high-voltage electric current, involving the entire epidermis, dermis, and epidermal appendages; may involve a portion of the subcutaneous fat and connective tissue; also known as third degree burn.

Functional Antibody. An antibody that binds to an antigen and has an effect.

Functional Status. An individual's mobility and ability to perform activities of daily living.

FVC. *See* forced vital capacity.

Gallop. A cadence of heart sounds heard during auscultation that may be an indication of heart failure.

Gamma Interferon. A T cell–derived stimulating substance that suppresses virus reproduction; stimulates other T cells and activates macrophage cells.

Generalized Seizures. Those seizures indicative of involvement of both cerebral hemispheres; tonic, clonic, tonic-clonic, atonic, absence, and myoclonic are types of generalized seizures.

Genitourinary Tract. The system of organs concerned with the production and excretion of urine and with reproduction.

GFR. *See* glomerular filtration rate.

Giardiasis. A common protozoal infection of the small intestine spread through contaminated food and water and direct person-to-person contact.

Glasgow Coma Scale. A scale used to objectively assess level of consciousness; composed of eye opening, verbal, and motor score components.

Global Aphasia. Presence of both an expressive and receptive aphasia, compromising the individual's ability to use or receive written or spoken language.

Glomerular Filtration Rate (GFR). The rate (usually calculated per minute) at which a volume of blood is cleared of a substance in glomerulus; normal GFR is approximately 125 mL/min.

Glomerulonephritis. Inflammation of the kidney's glomeruli, resulting in an inability of the kidney to work properly.

Glomerulus. The filtering capillary bed of the nephron; blood enters this capillary bed and is filtered, removing metabolic waste products, water, electrolytes, and trace minerals.

Glucagon. A polypeptide secreted by the pancreas that causes glycogenolysis and hyperglycemia; can be administered in an emergency for severe hypoglycemia.

Gluconeogenesis. The formation of glucose by the liver from noncarbohydrate sources.

Glycolysis. The process of conversion of carbohydrate in tissue to pyruvic acid or lactic acid with release of energy.

Glycoprotein. A conjugated protein in which the nonprotein group is a carbohydrate; also called glucoprotein.

Glycosylated Hemoglobin. This concentration represents the average blood glucose level over the previous 3 to 4 months.

GnRH. *See* gonadotropin-releasing hormone.

Gonadotropin-Releasing Hormone (GnRH). Hypothalamic hormone that stimulates the anterior pituitary to secrete growth hormone.

Granulocyte. A cell type of the immune system filled with granules of toxic chemicals that enable them to digest microorganisms.

Growth Hormone. Anterior pituitary hormone that acts directly on the tissues to promote protein synthesis and tissue growth.

Gynecomastia. Abnormal enlargement of breast tissue in males secondary to follicle-stimulating hormone/luteinizing hormone stimulation.

Hairy Leukoplakia. A whitish, slightly raised lesion that appears on the side of the tongue.

Hampton's Hump. A wedge-shaped consolidation or a semicircular opacity at the peripheral pleural space observed on chest radiograph; a late sign of pulmonary infarction.

Hangman's Fracture. Fracture through the arch of the C2 vertebra.

Healthy People 2000. A document that outlines plans for significant improvement of the health of U.S. citizens by the year 2000.

Heart Rate. The number of times the heart beats per minute.

Helper T Cell. A T lymphocyte that releases lymphokines after being activated by an antigen-bearing macrophage; the host cell of HIV; also called T4 or CD4 cell.

Hematocrit. A laboratory measurement that determines the percentage of packed red blood cells in a given volume of blood.

Hematoma. A blood clot or collection of blood from a hemorrhage.

Hematuria. Blood in the urine.

Hemodialysis. An extracorporeal system that allows for the filtration of end products of metabolism, excess water, and diffusion of electrolytes and other trace elements when a patient's kidney no longer functions.

Hemoglobin. The component of red blood cells that carries oxygen.

Hemolysis. The rupture of red blood cells.

Hemophilia. An inherited disease that prevents the normal clotting of blood.

Hemoptysis. Presence of blood in expectorated secretions from the larynx, trachea, or lower respiratory tract.

Hemothorax. Accumulation of blood in the pleural space.

Hemotympanum. Blood behind the tympanic membrane.

Hepatitis. An inflammation of the liver caused by certain viruses and other factors such as alcohol abuse, some medications, and trauma; can sometimes lead to liver failure and death.

Hepatojugular Reflex (HJR). Assessment technique done by compressing upper right abdomen for 30 to 45 seconds while patient is sitting at a 45-degree angle. A positive HJR is present if the level of neck vein filling rises and the jugular pulses become more prominant; usually a sign of right ventricular failure.

Hepatomegaly. Enlargement of the liver.

Herniation. Displacement of brain tissue from compressing and displacing adjacent structures; types of herniation include cingulate, transtentorial, central or rostral caudal, and infratentorial.

Herpes Varicella Zoster Virus. The varicella virus causes chickenpox in children and may reappear in adults as herpes zoster, consisting of painful blisters on the skin that follow nerve pathways; also called shingles.

Heterotopic Ossification. A pathologic condition in which bone arises in tissues not in the osseous system, such as in connective tissues.

Hierarchy of Resort. The stages of seeking relief of symptoms of sickness or illness, from popular, to folk, to professional systems.

Histoplasmosis. A fungal infection, commonly of the lungs.

HIV Infection. The condition wherein HIV exists as a provirus in the nucleus of its host cells and the infected person has mild nonspecific symptoms such as fatigue, mild fever, and swollen lymph nodes.

HLA. *See* human leukocyte antigens.

Holter Monitoring. Continuous long-term ECG monitoring of one or more leads to detect rhythm abnormalities.

Homan's Sign. Pain behind the knee or in the calf with dorsiflexion of the foot that may indicate deep calf vein thrombosis.

Human Immunodeficiency Virus Type I (HIV-1). The retrovirus isolated and recognized as the etiologic agent of AIDS.

Human Immunodeficiency Virus Type II (HIV-2). A virus closely related to HIV-1 that has been found to cause immune suppression; most common in Africa.

Human Leukocyte Antigens (HLA). Histocompatibility antigens that identify genetic identity and relationships; degree compatibility or sharing is predictive of transplant graft survival.

Humoral Immunity. The production of B cells in response to antigen exposure.

Hyperacute Rejection. The destruction of transplanted tissue or organ by circulating antibodies that immediately recognize the transplanted material as foreign.

Hypercapnia. Abnormally high blood concentrations of carbon dioxide.

Hypercapnic Respiratory Failure. Acute respiratory failure due to ventilatory issues, characterized by abnormally high carbon dioxide levels.

Hypercoagulability. Increased ability to develop coagulation or clots in the blood.

Hyperemia. An increase in cerebral blood flow in relationship to demand; often a result of an increase in cerebral blood volume.

Hyperextension Injury. Injury caused by the backward and downward movement of the head, causing the spinal cord to stretch and suffer contusion and ischemia.

Hyperflexion Injury. Injury usually the result of sudden deceleration of the head.

Hyperglycemic Hyperosmolar Nonketotic Coma (HHNK). Extreme hyperglycemia resulting from a decrease in urine output causing severe dehydration and decrease in glomerular filtration rate.

Hyperinsulinemia. Insufficient insulin secretion as required by dietary intake; diabetes.

Hyperlipidemia. Excessive amounts of lipids (fatty acids) in the serum.

Hypernatremia. Serum sodium value more than 145 mEq/L.

Hyperpnea. Increase in depth and rate of respiration.

Hypertension. Persistently high arterial blood pressure.

Hyperthyroidism. A condition resulting from an excessive production and secretion of thyroid hormone causing an increased metabolic rate.

Hyperventilation. Greater than normal exchange of air between the alveoli and the atmosphere, characterized by low $PaCO_2$ values.

Hypervolemia. Excess extracellular fluid volume, especially in the intravascular space.

Hypocapnia. Less than normal levels of carbon dioxide in the blood.

Hyponatremia. Serum sodium value less than 135 mEq/L.

Hypotension. Decrease of systolic and diastolic blood pressure below normal.

Hypothalamic–Pituitary–Adrenal Axis. Activation of the hypothalamic–pituitary–adrenal axis can initiate the host defense response, releasing catecholamines that interact with glucocorticoids to assist in the maintenance of vascular tone; the inhibitory response is responsible for the termination of host defense response.

Hypothermia. Body temperature less than or equal to 35°C.

Hypothyroidism. Inadequate production and secretion of thyroid hormone resulting in a decreased metabolic rate.

Hypotonia. Less than normal muscle tone.

Hypoventilation. Less than normal exchange of air between the alveoli and the atmosphere; characterized by elevated $PaCO_2$.

Hypovolemia. Low blood volume from blood loss or dehydration.

Hypovolemic Shock. Shock caused from a loss of fluid from the intravascular space.

Hypoxemia. Insufficient oxygenation of the blood.

Hypoxemic Respiratory Failure. Acute respiratory failure due to abnormalities of oxygenation; characterized by low PaO_2.

Hypoxia. The lack of oxygen at the cellular level.

Ictal. The time during which a seizure is actually occurring.

I : E Ratio. The ratio of duration of inspiration to duration of expiration.

Immune Complex. Clusters formed when antigens and antibodies bind together.

Immune Deficiency. A breakdown or inability of certain parts of the immune system to function, thus making a person susceptible to certain diseases that they would not ordinarily develop.

Immune Response. The complex functions of the body that recognize foreign agents or substances, neutralize them, and recall the response later when confronted with the same challenge.

Immunity. A natural or acquired resistance to a specific disease; may be partial or complete, long-lasting or temporary.

Immunocompetent. Capable of developing an immune response; possessing a normal immune system.

Immunodeficiency. A deficiency of immune response or a disorder characterized by deficient immune response; classified as antibody, cellular, combined deficiency, or phagocytic dysfunction disorders.

Immunogen. A substance also called an antigen, capable of provoking an immune response.

Immunosuppression. State due to an immune system that is damaged and does not perform its normal functions; may be induced by drugs or result from certain disease processes.

Impedance Plethysmography. Noninvasive diagnostic examination to determine venous obstruction and volume changes in an extremity by measuring electrical resistance and impedance during inspiration and expiration.

Implied Consent. Consent that is given by a person's actions or inactions, rather than verbally or in writing.

Incomplete Spinal Cord Injury. An incomplete or partial injury resulting in a mixed loss of motor and sensory function because of the sparing of some of the spinal cord tracts; degree of loss depends on the level of injury and the specific nerve tracts damaged.

Incubation Period. The time interval between the initial exposure to infection and appearance of the first symptom or sign of disease.

Infarct. An area of necrosis in an organ resulting from obstruction in its blood supply.

Informed Consent. Consent based on the patient's knowledge and understanding. Requires the physician to provide the patient with information concerning diagnosis, treatment, benefits and risks of treatment, alternatives, and prognosis.

Insulin. Hormone secreted by the beta cells of the pancreas in response to increased levels of glucose in the blood.

Interleukin-2 (IL-2). One of a family of molecules that control the growth and function of many types of lymphocytes; an immune system protein produced in the body by T cells with potent effects on the proliferation, differentiation, and activity of a number of immune system cells.

Intermediate Care Unit. Units in an acute care facility that are equipped to provide advanced monitoring but not at the level of intensive care units; also known as telemetry or step-down units.

International Classification of Seizures. Developed by the International League Against Epilepsy to provide a framework for characterization of seizures and determination of medications and to provide a common language for clinicians and scientists.

Intraaortic Balloon Counterpulsation. Insertion of a balloon into the aorta to assist the heart; deflates when the heart is contracting and creates a potential space in the aorta for the blood; inflates when the heart relaxes, pushing blood back toward the heart to perfuse the coronary arteries.

Intracranial Pressure. Pressure within the cranium determined by the influence of blood, brain, and cerebrospinal fluid volumes.

Intraparenchymal Brain Hemorrhage. Direct release of blood into the brain tissues resulting from high arteriolar pressure.

Intrarenal Failure. Chronic or acute renal failure that is the result of functional impairment or organic structural abnormalities within the kidneys.

Intrinsicoid Deflection. Occurring in the initial portion of the QRS complex, represents a change from maximal positivity to maximal negativity, or vice versa.

Inverse Ratio Ventilation (IRV). Reversal of the inspiratory and expiratory phases of the respiratory cycle, making the inspiratory time long and the expiratory time short.

Ischemia. Transient and reversible insufficiency of blood flow to an organ that is so severe that it disrupts the function of the organ; in the heart it is often accompanied by precordial chest pain and diminished contraction.

Ischemic Fingerprint. A unique 12-lead ECG pattern related to the anatomical location of the infarcted coronary artery; often monitored as a means to assess reperfusion and/or acute reocclusion.

Ischemic Penumbra. A zone of ischemia that develops after loss of arterial blood flow; the penumbra is made up of severely ischemic core tissue surrounded by tissue that may be potentially viable.

Isoelectric Line. A horizontal line on an ECG recording that forms a baseline, representing neither a positive nor a negative electrical potential.

J Point. Junction of the QRS complex and the ST segment.

Kaposi's Sarcoma. A form of cancer that attacks the connective tissue, bones, cartilage and muscles of the body, characterized by abnormal growths of blood vessels that develop into purplish or brown lesions.

Ketogenesis. The formation of ketone bodies from the breakdown of free fatty acids.

Ketone Body. Any of the compounds that simultaneously increase blood and urine in ketoacidosis, starvation, pregnancy, after some anesthesia agents, and other conditions.

Ketosis. A condition is which ketones are present in blood and urine in excessive amounts.

Killer T Cells. Cytotoxic T lymphocytes.

Kussmaul's Respiration. The deep, gasping respiration associated with diabetic ketoacidosis; a compensatory response to metabolic acidosis.

LAS. *See* lymphadenopathy syndrome.

Latency. The period when an organism is in the body and not producing any ill effects.

Left Ventricular Dysfunction. Inability of the left ventricle to contract with the same force consistently and/or inability of the left ventricular wall to contract completely.

Left Ventricular End-Diastolic Pressure. Pressure exerted against the fibers of the left ventricle by the amount of blood in the ventricle just before systole.

Left Ventricular End-Diastolic Volume. The amount of blood (fluid) in the left ventricle, just before systole; also known as preload.

Lentivirus. Slow virus characterized by a long interval between infection and the onset of symptoms; HIV is a lentivirus.

Leukocytes. All white blood cells.

Leukocytosis. An increase in white blood cells.

Leukopenia. A decrease in the number of white blood cells; the threshold value for leukopenia is usually taken as less than 5000 white blood cells per cubic millimeter of blood.

LH. *See* luteinizing hormone.

LH-RH. *See* luteinizing hormone–releasing factor.

LIP. *See* lymphoid interstitial pneumonia.

Lipoprotein. Conjugated proteins consisting of simple proteins combined with lipid components (e.g., cholesterol, phospholipid, and tryglycerides).

Liquid Ventilation. The administration of liquid fluorocarbon into the endotracheal tube of a patient to transport dissolved oxygen to the alveolar unit and remove carbon dioxide.

Living Will. An instruction advance directive containing a written instruction of a person's treatment wishes, most often concerning use or withdrawal of life support in end-of-life situations.

Lobectomy. Surgical removal of an entire lobe of an organ.

Loculated. Containing several small cavities or divided into several small spaces.

Long-Term Care. Transitional care that focuses on support and provides services to patients requiring assistance with chronic illnesses; also known as extended care.

Lung Compliance. Calculated value indicating volume change per unit of pressure change, measuring lung distensibility.

Lung Fields. Areas of the lung seen on chest radiograph that appear dark or black.

Lung Injury Scoring System. Classifies the extent of pulmonary damage sustained by septic patients.

Lung Scan. Radiologic examination of the lungs to determine pulmonary function.

Luteinizing Hormone (LH). Stimulates production of testosterone in males; triggers ovulation and maintenance of the corpus luteum in females.

Luteinizing Hormone–Releasing Factor (LH-RH). Hypothalamic hormone that stimulates the anterior pituitary to secrete luteinizing hormone and follicle-stimulating hormone.

Lymph Nodes. Lymphatic tissue found in the neck, armpit, or groin that produces lymphocytes and monocytes and that acts as a filter for the bloodstream.

Lymphadenopathy Syndrome (LAS). Swelling of the lymph nodes, adenoids, and other tissues of the immune system.

Lymphocyte. A white blood cell present in the blood, lymph, and lymphoid tissue.

Lymphoid Interstitial Pneumonia (LIP). A form of pneumonia involving the lower lung lobes, with extensive alveolar infiltration by mature lymphocytes, plasma cells, and histiocytes.

Lymphokines. Products of the lymphatic cells that stimulate the production of disease-fighting agents and the activities of other lymphatic cells; include interferon gamma and interleukin-2.

Lymphoma. Cancer of the lymphoid tissues.

Lysis. Rupture and destruction of a cell.

Macrophage. A large immune cell that devours invading pathogens and other intruders; stimulates other immune cells by presenting them with small pieces of the invader.

Macule. Flat discolored spot or patch on the skin.

Magnetic Resonance Imaging (MRI). Radiofrequency used in a magnetic field to produce detailed medical imaging.

Major Histocompatibility Antigen (MHC). Antigens present on the surface of body cells unique for that particular individual; act as recognition sites during the immune process.

Malnutrition. Impaired nutritional function due to intake of nutrients less than the body requires.

Mantoux Reaction. Reaction to intracutaneous injection of old tuberculin; if active or inactive tuberculous infection is present, the area becomes hard (indurated) and red within 24 to 72 hours.

Mast Cell. A granulocyte found in tissue, responsible for the symptoms of allergy.

Maximal Inspiratory Pressure. Measure of respiratory muscle strength during inspiration.

Mediators. Substances released by the inflammatory response systems that potentiate inflammation and can become detrimental over time.

Melanocyte-Stimulating Hormone (MSH). Stimulates the production of melanocytes, which contain a dark tanning pigment.

Memory Cells. A subset of T lymphocytes that have been exposed to specific antigens and can then proliferate on subsequent immune system encounters with the same antigen.

Mental Status. The cognitive status of an individual consisting of arousal, attention, affect, orientation, perceptual ability, thought processes, and judgment.

Mesh Graft. A split-thickness skin graft that is removed with a dermatome and then meshed with a special instrument called a mesher; used when there are insufficient donor sites available because it can cover a larger surface area than an unmeshed graft or sheet grafts.

Messenger RNA. Also referred to as mRNA. An RNA (ribonucleic acid) that carries the genetic code for a particular protein from the nuclear DNA to a ribosome in the cytoplasm and acts as a template, or pattern, for the formation of that protein.

MI. *See* acute myocardial infarction.

Microvascular Permeability. An increase in the distance between the cells of the endothelium of the capillaries, allowing fluid and particles to travel between the intravascular and interstitium spaces.

Military Antishock Trousers (MAST). *See* pneumatic antishock garment.

Minute Ventilation. Total air flow per minute; measured as tidal volume times frequency per minute.

Mitosis. Type of cell division of somatic cells in which each daughter cell contains the same number of chromosomes as the parent cell; the process by which the body grows, and by which somatic cells are replaced.

Mixed Venous Oxygen Saturation (SvO_2). Venous oxygen saturation that reflects the adequacy of oxygen supply in meeting the demands of the tissues. Normal range is 60% to 80%.

Mixed Venous Partial Pressure of Oxygen (PvO_2). Measure of venous partial pressure of oxygen; usually sampled from a pulmonary artery catheter.

MODS. *See* multiple organ dysfunction syndrome.

MOF. *See* multiple organ failure.

Molluscum Contagiosum. A disease of the skin and mucous membranes caused by a poxvirus, characterized by scattered flesh-toned white papules; most frequently occurs in children and young adults with impaired immune response.

Monoclonal Antibodies. Antibodies produced by a hybridoma or antibody-producing cell source for a specific antigen; useful as a tool for identifying specific protein molecules.

Monocyte. A large white blood cell that ingests microorganisms or other cells and foreign particles. When a monocyte enters tissues, it develops into a macrophage.

Morbidity. The disability, complications, and costs of an illness or disease.

MSH. *See* melanocyte-stimulating hormone.

Multigated Acquisition Scan (MUGA). Nuclear scan in which a technetium tracer is tagged to red blood cells throughout the blood in the body. As the blood circulates through the heart, a certain number of frames or "gates" are taken of each heart beat; the R wave on the ECG signal is used to initiate when images are to be taken. Images are then combined to calculate ejection fraction.

Multiple Organ Dysfunction Syndrome (MODS). A complication of systemic inflammatory response syndrome; the presence of altered organ function in the acutely ill patient such that homeostasis cannot be maintained with intervention.

Multiple Organ Failure (MOF). The failure of two or more organ systems as a result of malignant intravascular inflammation.

Myalgia. Tenderness or pain in the muscles.

Myelin. The protective insulation covering the axon of nerve fibers that promotes rapid impulse conduction.

Myoclonic Seizure. Seizure characterized by sudden, massive muscle jerks involving either a part of the body or the entire body; injury can result.

Myoglobin (Mgb). An oxygen-binding protein found in skeletal and cardiac muscle tissue and released into circulation within 2 to 6 hours of injury.

Myoglobinuria. Myoglobin in the urine; indicative of skeletal muscle injury with subsequent release of myoglobin, a pigment that can potentially block renal tubules.

Myxedema Coma. A severe, life-threatening form of decompensated hypothyroidism usually precipitated by a physiologic or emotional stressor; symptoms include hypothermia, respiratory distress, lethargy.

Natural Antibodies. An antibody present in a person without known exposure to the specific antigen; may be the result of unknown, accidental exposure.

Natural Killer Cells (NK). A type of lymphocyte that attacks and kills tumor cells and protects against a wide variety of infectious microbes.

Near-Death Experience. A phenomena reported by patients who are successfully resuscitated after sudden death; common core experiences include a feeling of calm and peace.

Necrosis. Death of areas of tissue.

Negligence. An area of tort law and professional nursing liability, including the elements of duty, breach of duty, causation, and damages.

Neoplasm. An abnormal and uncontrolled growth of tissue; a tumor.

Nephron. Structural and functional unit of the kidney with both vascular and tubular components.

Nephronenic DI. Disease developing because of a decreased ability of the kidney to save water despite ADH presence; causes include hypercalcemia, hypokalemia, and the drug lithium.

Nephrotoxic Agents. Substances that cause toxic reactions within the functioning units of the kidney, decreasing the kidney's ability to filter waste products or regulate hormone production.

Neurogenic Bladder. Dysfunctional bladder resulting from a lesion in the nervous system.

Neurogenic Pulmonary Edema. The development of a noncardiogenic pulmonary edema in the patient with an acute rise in intracranial pressure.

Neurogenic Shock. The loss of sympathetic outflow that occurs shortly after injury at the T6 level or above; a form of distributive shock that manifests itself by hypotension.

Neuronenic DI (Central DI). DI developing due to lack of antidiuretic hormone from the hypothalmus and/or pituitary in spite of a high plasma osmolality; causes include brain injury, brain surgery, and an idiopathic variety.

Neuropathy. A group of disorders involving nerves; symptoms range from a tingling sensation or numbness in the toes and fingers to paralysis.

Neuroprotectant. Investigational drugs aimed at treating or altering some of the pathologic pathways that occur in ischemia.

Neutralizing Antibody. An antibody that keeps a virus from infecting a cell, usually by blocking receptors on the cell or the virus.

Neutropenia. An abnormal decrease in the number of neutrophils (the most common type of white blood cells) in the blood; associated with acute leukemia, infection, rheumatoid arthritis, and other conditions.

Neutrophil. A white blood cell that engulfs and kills foreign microorganisms; also called a polymorphonuclear neutrophil (PMN).

Nitric Oxide. A gas that can be administered to promote relaxation; vasodilatation effect is short and is selective to the pulmonary vasculature when inhaled.

Nonmaleficence. The ethical principle to do no harm.

Nonrecurrent Seizures. Seizures related to an acute medical or neurologic illness, or neurosurgical procedure; seizures are self-limited and do not recur after effective treatment of the illness.

Normal Aging. The changes that occur in the individual that can be ascribed only to aging rather than to environmental factors or disease.

Nuclear Scan. A diagnostic technique that uses an injected or ingested radioactive material and a scanning device for determining the size, shape, location, and function of organs and tissue.

Nucleoside Analog. Synthetic compounds similar to one of the components of DNA or RNA; a general type of antiretroviral drug.

Oligemic Cerebral Hypoxia. Low cerebral blood flow that may result in ischemia.

Oliguria. A urine output less than 400 mL/24 hours or 30 mL or less per hour.

Opportunistic Infection. An illness caused by an organism that usually does not cause disease in a person with a normal immune system.

Orthopnea. Shortness of breath when reclining or in the supine position.

Osmolarity. Concentration of osmotically active particles in solution.

Outcomes of Critical Illness. The consequences of critical illness, such as morbidity, mortality, functional status, pain, quality of life.

Oxidants. Chemical agents that cause damage by inserting oxygen, halogen, or sulfur into viable body proteins leading to cellular dysfunction.

Oxygen Consumption (Vo_2). Amount of oxygen used at the tissue level; normal = 250 mL/min.

Oxygen Debt. The negative balance that is present when oxygen supply does not match oxygen demand.

Oxygen Delivery. Amount of oxygen transported to the tissues of the body; expressed as arterial oxygen content times cardiac output.

Oxygen Demand. The amount of oxygen required by the body's cells to meet metabolic needs.

Oxygen Saturation of Arterial Blood (Sao_2). Percentage of available oxygen combined with hemoglobin.

Oxygen Supply. The amount of oxygen that is being carried to the tissues in the blood.

Oxygenation. Exchange of oxygen between the alveoli and the mixed venous blood entering the lungs.

Oxyhemoglobin Dissociation. Relationship between partial pressure of oxygen and oxygen saturation of hemoglobin.

Oxytocin. Stimulates uterine contractions during labor and is responsible for the letdown response that allows breast feeding to occur.

$Paco_2$. Partial pressure of carbon dioxide in arterial blood; normal = 35 to 45 mm Hg.

PAD. *See* pulmonary artery diastolic pressure.

Palliative. Serving to relieve or alleviate without curing.

Palpitations. Awareness of the heart beating, often noticing irregular beats.

PAM. *See* pulmonary artery mean pressure.

Pandemic. A disease prevalent throughout an entire country, continent, or the world.

Panhypopituitarism. Loss of pituitary function resulting in deficiency of all pituitary releasing hormones.

Pansystolic Murmur. A murmur that lasts throughout systole.

Pao_2. Partial pressure of oxygen in arterial blood; normal = 80 to 100 mm Hg.

Papillary Muscle Rupture. A structural complication of a myocardial infarction; tissue supporting the muscle of the mitral valve becomes necrotic secondary to coronary artery occlusion and breaks off, requiring emergency mitral valve replacement surgery.

Papule. Red elevated area on the skin that is solid and circumscribed.

Paradoxical Embolus. Embolus originating in a vein that passes into an artery via an atrial or ventricular septal defect in the heart.

Paralysis. A total loss of motor functioning below the level of a lesion; starts as a flaccid paralysis, but after spinal shock is over, a spastic paralysis occurs.

Parasite. A plant or animal that lives and feeds on or within another living organism; does not necessarily cause disease.

Parathyroid Hormone. Hormone secreted by the parathyroid glands that acts to maintain a constant concentration of calcium in the extracellular fluid.

Parenteral. Not in or through the digestive system.

Paresthesia. Sensation of numbness, prickling, or tingling; heightened sensitivity.

Partial-Thickness Burn. Caused by brief exposure to flash flame and dilute chemicals or brief contact with steam or hot objects; tissue involvement is primarily at the epidermal level but may involve portions of the dermis. Also known as a second-degree burn.

PAS. *See* pulmonary artery systolic pressure.

Passive Immunity. Immunity acquired in utero from antibodies that pass from the mother to the fetus through the placenta or are acquired by breast feeding.

Pathogen. Any disease-producing microorganism or material.

PAWP. *See* pulmonary artery wedge pressure.

PCIRV. *See* pressure-controlled inverse-ratio ventilation.

Peak Inspiratory Pressure (PIP). Maximal airway pressure during inspiration.

PEEP. *See* positive end-expiratory pressure.

Penetrating Trauma. Injury as a result of a knife, bullet, shotgun blast, sharp object, or projectile.

Perfusion ($\dot{Q}$). Blood flow.

Pericardial Tamponade. Accumulation of blood or fluid in the pericardial sac of a sufficient quantity to impede cardiac output.

Pericardiocentesis. Aspiration of the pericardium with a needle and syringe in the presence of an actual or suspected pericardial tamponade.

Pericarditis. Inflammatory condition of the lining of the heart characterized by chest pain on deep inspiration, a pericardial friction rub, and persistent ST-segment elevation.

Peritoneal Dialysis (PD). Instillation and drainage of a solution in the peritoneal cavity to achieve removal of end-products of metabolism, excess water, and diffusion of electrolytes and other trace elements.

Peritonitis. Inflammation of peritoneal structures due to infection.

Persistent Generalized Lymphadenopathy (PGL). Chronic, diffuse, noncancerous lymph node enlargement; typically found in patients with immune system disturbances who develop frequent and persistent bacterial, viral, and fungal infections.

PETco₂. Pressure of end-tidal carbon dioxide; usually measures 1 to 5 mm Hg less than $PaCO_2$.

PGL. *See* persistent generalized lymphadenopathy.

Phagocyte. A cell that is able to ingest and destroy foreign matter, including bacteria.

Phagocytosis. The process of ingesting and destroying a virus or other foreign matter by a phagocyte.

Pharyngitis. Inflammation of the pharynx.

Pheochromocytoma. Adrenal medulla tumor-induced hypertensive crisis.

Physiologic Reserve. The amount of used functional capacity the individual or an organ system can recruit under stressful conditions.

PIP. *See* peak inspiratory pressure.

Placebo. An inactive substance against which investigational treatments are compared for efficacy.

Plasma Cells. Large antibody-producing cells that develop from B cells.

Plasmapheresis. The process of removing plasma in exchange for either albumin or fresh frozen plasma usually for the process of diluting circulating antibodies in an autoimmune disease state.

Plasmin. A proteolytic enzyme from plasminogen present in the body.

Plasminogen. A globulin that is the inactive precursor of plasmin and is present throughout the body, including in clots.

Plateau Murmur. A murmur with the same intensity, or loudness, throughout.

Platelets. Active agents of inflammation when damage occurs to a blood vessel; fragments released by megakaryocyte cells.

Pleural Effusion. Presence of fluid in the pleural space.

Pleurodesis. Creation of adhesions between the visceral and parietal pleural layers by introduction of a mechanical or chemical irritant into the pleural space to promote inflammation and seal off pleural leaks to maintain lung reexpansion.

P-Mitrale. Double-humped P waves in lead II of the ECG; possibly indicative of left atrial strain, abnormality, or hypertrophy.

PMN. *See* neutrophil.

Pneumatic Antishock Garment (PASG). Three-chamber, inflatable trousers applied to a patient's lower extremities and abdomen to raise blood pressure in shock states; also known as military antishock trousers (MAST).

***Pneumocystis carinii* Pneumonia (PCP).** A life-threatening lung infection that can affect people with weakened immune systems.

Pneumomediastinum. Presence of free air in the mediastinal space of the thoracic cavity.

Pneumonectomy. Surgical removal of an entire lung.

Pneumothorax. Partial or complete collapse of the lung due to accumulation of air in the pleural space.

Point-of-Care Testing. Laboratory testing that is operated by clinicians in nonlaboratory settings, specifically testing done at the patient's side.

Polydipsia. Increased water intake.

Polymerase. Enzymes that catalyze the formation of DNA or RNA from precursor substances in the presence of preexisting DNA or RNA acting as templates.

Polymorphonuclear Neutrophil. *See* neutrophil.

Polyneuropathy. Disease affecting the peripheral nervous system; symptoms vary based on the sites of degeneration.

Polypharmacy. The situation in which an individual is taking multiple medications, including prescribed and over-the-counter medications.

Polyuria. Urine output of greater than 3 L per day.

Positive End-Expiratory Pressure (PEEP). An adjunct to mechanical ventilation in which some amount of positive pressure is continuously applied at the end of expiration to assist in maintaining open alveoli.

Postictal. The period immediately after a seizure; recovery after a seizure may be immediate or may last up to several hours, depending on the type and duration of seizure activity.

Postrenal Failure. Chronic or acute renal failure as a consequence of a structural or functional impairment of the lower urinary tract.

Postthrombotic Syndrome. Chronic condition after deep vein thrombosis resulting in leg swelling, calf pain, lower leg pigmentation and induration, and ulceration, as a result of shunting of blood from the deep leg veins to the superficial leg veins.

P-Pulmonale. Peaked P waves in lead II of the ECG; possibly indicative of right atrial strain, abnormality, or hypertrophy.

Precordial. Situated on the thorax, directly overlying the heart.

Precordium. The anterior chest wall overlying the heart and the great vessels.

Precursor Cells. Cells from which other cells are formed by natural processes.

Preictal. The time just preceding a seizure; patients may experience a prodrome or warning that a seizure is going to occur.

Preload. Volume or pressure generated at the end of diastole when the ventricle filled with blood; left ventricular preload is measured by the pulmonary capillary wedge pressure.

Prerenal Failure. Chronic or acute renal failure due to conditions that occur before the kidney structures themselves.

Pressure Control. A ventilator mode characterized by preset inspiratory pressures and fluctuating tidal volumes, depending on lung compliance.

Pressure-Controlled Inverse-Ratio Ventilation (PCIRV). A mode of ventilation designed to reverse the normal inspiratory time and expiratory ratios (I:E ratios) to prolong inspiratory time and deliver gas at a preset inspiratory pressure.

Pressure Support. A ventilator mode characterized by positive-pressure augmentation of spontaneous breaths.

Primary Adrenal Insufficiency. Disease caused by an inadequately functioning or malfunctioning adrenal gland. Inadequate levels of mineralocorticoids, glucocorticoids, and sex hormones are produced by the adrenal medulla and cortex.

Primary Injury. Occurring at the time of injury or impact.

Primary Pneumothorax. Lung collapse due to an undetectable underlying cause.

Primary Survey. An initial assessment method to rapidly assess and intervene to address immediate threats to life, including airway, breathing, circulation, disability, and exposure.

Prinzmetal's Angina. Angina caused by vasospasm; may or may not be associated with atherosclerosis and the presence of transient ST-segment elevation.

Process Standards. Working standards, such as protocols or procedure manuals.

Progesterone. Hormone that prepares the uterus for pregnancy and stimulates breast for lactation.

Programmed Electrical Stimulation. The use of electrical stimulation to produce an arrhythmia.

Prolactin. Anterior pituitary hormone that stimulates milk production in the mammary glands of the breast.

Prophylaxis. Treatment that helps to prevent a disease or condition before it occurs or recurs.

Protease. An enzyme that hydrolyzes proteins to their component peptides.

Protein C. A blood plasma protein constituent that prevents blood clotting.

Protein S. Vitamin K–dependent blood plasma protein constituent required as a cofactor for the antithrombotic functions of protein C.

Proteins. Any of the group of highly complex organic compounds found in all living cells.

Prothrombin. A plasma protein also known as thrombinogen or factor II; an inactive precursor of thrombin.

Protoplasmic Poisons. Chemical agents that interfere with normal cellular function by binding or inhibiting inorganic ions.

Pruritus. Severe itching.

Psoriasis. A common, genetically determined dermatitis consisting of discrete pink or dull-red lesions surmounted by characteristic silvery scaling; usually chronic.

PT/PTT. Prothrombin time/partial thromboplastin time.

Pulmonary Artery Diastolic Pressure (PAD). Taken during ventricular diastole; normal PAD pressure is 10 to 20 mm Hg.

Pulmonary Artery Mean Pressure (PAM). Mean pulmonary artery pressure; normal PAM pressure is 10 to 15 mm Hg.

Pulmonary Artery Pressures. Measurements by means of a flow-directed balloon-tipped catheter of pressure in the pulmonary artery during various stages of ventricular activity.

Pulmonary Artery Systolic Pressure (PAS). Taken during ventricular systole; normal PAS pressure is 20 to 30 mm Hg.

Pulmonary Artery Occlusive Pressure (PAOP). Also known as pulmonary artery wedge pressure (PAWP). Taken when pulmonary artery catheter balloon is inflated, thereby blocking off right ventricular influence and indirectly measuring left ventricular filling or left atrial pressure; normal PAOP is 4 to 12 mm Hg.

Pulmonary Contusion. Bruising of the lung parenchyma.

Pulmonary Embolus. Occlusion of a pulmonary blood vessel by fragments of a thrombus or other foreign material.

Pulmonary Infarction. Necrotic area in the lung caused by an obstruction of blood flow, usually by a clot.

Pulmonary Vascular Resistance (PVR). Measurement of blood flow resistance in the lung against which the right ventricle must pump; calculated by subtracting the mean left atrial or pulmonary wedge pressure from the mean pulmonary arterial pressure and then dividing by the cardiac output.

Pulse Oximetry. Noninvasive method of estimating arterial oxygen saturation level.

PVC. Premature ventricular contraction.

PVR. *See* pulmonary vascular resistance.

Q̇. *See* perfusion.

Quad-Assist Cough. A maneuver done by the care provider to assist the tetraplegic patient to mobilize and expel secretions.

Quadriplegia. The complete loss of motor power to all four extremities; may or may not exhibit complete loss of sensation. Now known as tetraplegia.

Quality of Life. Measure of a person's satisfaction with life; usually composed of activity level, ability to care for self, amount of resources, symptoms, mood, social support, and perceived health.

Racism. The belief that members of one race (usually one's own) are superior to all other races.

Radiolucent. Penetrable by x-ray.

Radionuclide Ventriculography. Nuclear scan that uses a radioactive tracer to mark red blood cells; allows the outlining of the ventricles and their function to be assessed.

Radiopaque. Impenetrable by x-ray; observed as white on the radiograph.

Rales. An abnormal sound heard on auscultation of the chest, produced by passage of air through bronchi that contain secretion or exudate or that are constricted by spasm or a thickening of their walls; may be heard on inspiration or expiration.

Rebleeding. New bleeding from a site when hemostasis was formerly achieved.

Receptive Aphasia. Alteration in the ability to receive written or spoken language.

Receptor. A molecule on the surface of a cell that serves as a recognition or binding site for antigens, antibodies, or other cellular or immunologic components.

Rehabilitative Care. A level of transitional care that provides an intensive program for patients usually recovering from traumatic, neurologic, and/or orthopedic injuries.

Renal Capsule. Collagenous covering of the kidney.

Renal Insufficiency. A stage of renal disease in which the presence of end-products of metabolism and electrolyte imbalance in the blood indicates inadequate renal excretion, usually resulting from the loss of 75% or less of renal function.

Renal Osteodystrophy/Osteoporosis. Bone disease caused by alterations in calcium–phosphorus–parathormone levels and balance secondary to renal failure.

Renal Threshold. The plasma concentration at which maximum reabsorption of a substance in the nephron is exceeded and excretion of that substance begins; usually describes the excretion of glucose in hyperglycemia.

Renin–Angiotensin. A potent vasoconstrictive system that begins with the secretion of renin in the juxtaglomerular apparatus of the nephron; the end-product of angiotensin II has multiple effects on mechanisms to control or correct hemodynamic status.

Reocclusion. The abrupt closure of a coronary artery previously opened either spontaneously or by one of the currently available reperfusion techniques.

Reperfusion. The reestablishment of blood flow through a previously occluded coronary artery.

Reperfusion Rhythm. The development of transient dysrhythmias associated with the establishment of blood flow through a previously occluded coronary artery; usually self-limiting and include accelerated idioventricular rhythms, ventricular tachycardia, and atrioventricular blocks.

Repolarization. Condition in which the inside of the cell is markedly positive in relation to the outside of the cell. This condition is maintained by a pump in the cell membrane, and it is distributed by the arrival of an electrical current.

Rescue Angioplasty. A second-line approach to reperfusion when thrombolytic therapy has failed; involves repair of the occluded coronary artery using a percutaneous transluminal approach.

Respiration. The physical and chemical processes by which tissues exchange gases.

Restless Legs Syndrome. Physiologic need to move legs to relieve sensations caused by accumulation of end-products of metabolism in the renal failure patient.

Restraint. Chemical or physical means of inhibiting free movement.

Reticuloendothelial Cells. A system of interstitial cells that includes all the phagocytic cells; protects against invading organisms in the connective tissue of the body.

Retrograde Urethrography. A contrast study of the urethra performed to detect urethral injury.

Retroperitoneal. The area behind the peritoneum within the abdomen.

Retrovirus. Viruses that carry their genetic material in the form of RNA and that have the enzyme reverse transcriptase to convert its RNA into DNA, which is then integrated into the host cell DNA.

Reverse Transcriptase. The enzyme of the HIV virus that converts the single-stranded viral RNA into DNA, the form in which the cell carries its genes.

Ribonucleic Acid (RNA). A nucleic acid, found mostly in the cytoplasm of cells, that is important in the synthesis of proteins.

S1. The first heart sound, produced when the mitral and tricuspid valves close. S1 marks the end of diastole and the start of ventricular systole.

S2. The second heart sound, produced when the aortic and pulmonic valves close. S2 marks the end of ventricular systole and the start of diastole.

S3. The third heart sound, produced during rapid ventricular filling early in diastole. A pathologic S3 often indicates left-ventricular failure. May be a normal finding in children and young adults.

S4. The fourth heart sound, produced during atrial contraction at the end of ventricular diastole, caused by decreased ventricular compliance.

Saddle Embolus. Blood clot that straddles a bifurcation of an artery so that both branches of the vessel are occluded.

Sao$_2$. *See* oxygen saturation of arterial blood.

Seborrhea. Functional disease of the sebaceous glands marked by increase in the amount and often alteration of the quality of the sebaceous secretion.

Secondary Adrenal Insufficiency. Disease caused by inadequate stimulation of the adrenal gland by the pituitary gland and other feedback mechanisms; inadequate levels of mineralocorticoids, glucocorticoids, and sex hormones are produced by the adrenal medulla and cortex.

Secondary Injury. Results from events that follow a primary injury, affecting oxygenation and perfusion of the brain tissue.

Secondary Pneumothorax. Lung collapse as a result of underlying pulmonary disease.

Secondary Survey. The phase of initial trauma care directed at taking a complete set of vital signs and performing a complete physical examination.

Second-Degree Burn. *See* partial-thickness burn.

Segmental Resection. Surgical removal of a segment of an organ.

Seizure. A symptom of brain dysfunction resulting from abnormal neuronal discharges, occurring suddenly in the gray matter; each of the many types of seizures has its own characteristic clinical and electroencephalographic profile.

Seizure Threshold. An individual's threshold for seizure activity, determined by a combination of genetic and environmental factors; when abnormal cerebral activity cannot be regulated sufficiently and passes this threshold, seizure activity occurs.

Sepsis. Intravascular inflammation that occurs as the result of a bacterial invasion.

Seroconversion. The development of antibodies to a particular antigen.

Severity of Illness. The amount of physiologic alteration that happens as a result of injury or illness.

Shigellosis. The disease produced by infection with *Shigella,* a non–lactose-fermenting, nonmotile, gram-negative rod that causes digestive disturbances ranging from mild diarrhea to a severe and often fatal dysentery.

Shingles. *See* herpes varicella zoster virus.

Shock. A clinical syndrome resulting from the lack of adequate perfusion to the tissues.

Shunt. Blood that bypasses the normal gas exchange mechanism.

SIADH. *See* syndrome of inappropriate antidiuretic hormone.

Simple Partial Seizure. Motor, sensory, autonomic, or psychic phenomena during which consciousness is not impaired; involves a limited area of the cerebral hemisphere. Also known as an aura.

SIMV. *See* synchronized intermittent mandatory ventilation.

SIRS. *See* systemic inflammatory response syndrome.

Skilled Care. A level of transitional care that addresses the needs of recently hospitalized patients with multiple, complex needs such as complex wound care or total parenteral nutrition.

Somatic. Pertaining to nonreproductive cells or tissues.

Somatosensory Evoked Potential Studies. A prognostic tool in spinal cord injuries in which an electrical stimulus is applied to a peripheral nerve in the arm or leg and the path of that message through the spinal cord to the brain is recorded.

Specific Immunity. *See* humoral immunity.

Spinal Shock. A complication of spinal cord injury that occurs after injury and lasts 7 to 10 days; symptoms include complete flaccid paralysis of all muscle groups below the level of injury, complete loss of sensation below the level of the injury, loss of bowel and bladder functioning, and loss of temperature regulation.

Spleen. Organ responsible for the production and storage of blood cells; also acts as a filter for blood.

Splenomegaly. Enlargement of the spleen.

Split-Thickness Skin Graft. Graft that includes the upper layer of the skin and part of the under layer; do not prevent regeneration of the skin at the site from which they are taken.

SpO_2. Saturation of hemiglobin with oxygen as measured by exterior pulse oximetry.

Spontaneous Pneumothorax. Lung collapse not resulting from physical injury.

Standards. Serve as guides for the provision of care and as criteria to evaluate care.

Status Epilepticus. More than 30 minutes of continuous seizure activity or two or more sequential seizures without full recovery of consciousness between seizures; classified as convulsive or nonconvulsive. Generalized convulsive status epilepticus is life threatening.

Stem Cells. Cells from which all blood cells derive; bone marrow is rich in stem cells.

Stenosis. Narrowing of an opening (e.g., valve).

Stereotactic Radiosurgery. The administration of high-dose radiation to a specified intracranial target, while minimizing the dose given off to surrounding tissues; usually administered through a linear accelerator or gamma knife system.

Stereotype. The belief or attitude that all members of a specific group are the same without individualizing characteristics.

Sterilizing Immunity. An immune response that completely eliminates an infection.

Stridor. A harsh, vibrating sound produced during respiration, usually due to acute narrowing of the upper airways.

Stroke Volume. The amount of blood ejected with each systole; stroke volume (SV) = cardiac output (CO)/heart rate (HR). Normal stroke volume is 60 to 100 mL per beat.

Subacute Care. A level of transitional care that includes patients who are severely impaired but medically stable, such as ventilator-dependent patients, who require continuous monitoring and therapy.

Subarachnoid Hemorrhage. Bleeding between the arachnoid membrane and pia mater.

Subcutaneous Emphysema. Air under the skin.

Subdural Hematoma. Hemorrhage found between the dura mater and the arachnoid membrane of the meninges.

Subendocardial Infarction. Necrosis of the innermost layer of the heart muscle resulting from an occlusion of a coronary artery.

Super PEEP. PEEP levels greater than 15 cm H_2O (conventional levels are usually between 5 and 15 cm H_2O). The use of high PEEP has the goal of a PaO_2 of 60 or greater and a pulse oximetry reading of greater than 90%.

Suppressor T Lymphocyte. Also called suppressor T cell; dampens the activity of the immune system by turning off cytotoxic T lymphocytes.

Surfactant. A mixture of phospholipids secreted by alveolar cells that reduces the surface tension and contributes to the elasticity of pulmonary tissue; synthetic versions may be administered to decrease atelectasis and improve oxygenation.

Surrogate Decision-Making Statutes. State laws that identify individuals (such as spouse or parent) authorized to make decisions on behalf of incompetent patients with no advance directives.

SvO₂. Saturation of venous hemiglobin with oxygen as measured in venous blood.

SVR. *See* systemic vascular resistance.

Synchronized Intermittent Mandatory Ventilation (SIMV). A ventilator mode characterized by mandatory breaths synchronized with the patient's spontaneous breaths; most spontaneous breaths are not augmented by the ventilator.

Syncope. Temporary loss of consciousness due to lack of blood flow; may be secondary to dysrhythmias.

Syncytia. Giant cells that are dysfunctional multicellular clumps formed by cell-to-cell fusion.

Syndrome of Inappropriate Antidiuretic Hormone (SIADH). Disease resulting from excess ADH in the presence of a dilute serum and hyponatremia.

Systemic Inflammatory Response System (SIRS). A host defense response mechanism initiated by severe insults to the body.

Systemic Vascular Resistance (SVR). Measurement of blood flow resistance in the body.

Systole. Period when either the ventricles or the atria are contracting.

Tachycardia. Abnormally high heart rate.

Tachypnea. Abnormally high respiratory rate.

Tachypneic. Respirations faster than 20 breaths per minute.

TB. *See* tuberculosis.

Tenckhoff Catheter. Implanted catheter surgically placed in the peritoneal cavity to provide the conduit for inflow and outflow of peritoneal dialysis solution.

Tension Pneumothorax. Lung collapse in which air is trapped in the intrapleural space, resulting in excessive pressures and compression of surrounding areas; cardiovascular collapse will ensue if untreated.

Terminal Weaning. Weaning from the ventilator with expectation of resultant death.

Tertiary Survey. A complete reassessment of the patient within 24 hours after traumatic injury to discover evolving or occult injuries.

Tetraplegia. The complete loss of motor power to all four extremities; may or may not exhibit complete loss of sensation. Formerly known as quadriplegia.

Thallium-201. A radioactive tracer used to detect myocardial perfusion and viability.

T-Helper Cell. Alternative term for T4 cell.

Therapeutic Communication. Interactive verbal and nonverbal strategies that focus on the needs of the patient and facilitate a goal-directed communication process.

Thermoregulation. The regulation of body temperature.

Third-Degree Burn. *See* full-thickness burn.

Thoracentesis. Removal of pleural fluid.

Thoracostomy. A hole or opening in the chest; may be performed with a needle or surgical instrument (with insertion of a chest tube) to decompress the chest in the presence of a pneumothorax.

Thrill. A palpable vibration associated with turbulent blood flow.

Thrombin. A blood enzyme derived from prothrombin that assists in forming a blood clot by converting fibrinogen into fibrin.

Thrombinogen. A plasma protein also known as prothrombin or factor II that is the inactive precursor of thrombin.

Thrombocytopenia. A decreased number of blood platelets (cells important for clotting).

Thromboendarterectomy. Surgical removal of a blood clot along with the intimal lining of the obstructed blood vessel.

Thrombolysis. Destruction of a blood clot that obstructs flow through a blood vessel.

Thrombolytic. Substance able to dissolve a blood clot.

Thrombolytic Agents. Drugs that dissolve or lyse thrombi in blood vessels.

Thrombomodulin. A substance that decreases the blood-clotting activity of thrombin, thereby acting as protection against thrombosis.

Thrush. Sore patches in the mouth caused by the fungus *Candida albicans;* one of the most frequent early symptoms of an immune disorder.

Thymus. An organ located in the mediastinal cavity anterior to and above the heart; produces T lymphocytes.

Thyroid Crisis. A severe, life-threatening form of decompensated hyperthyroidism usually precipitated by a physiologic or emotional stressor; symptoms include hyperthermia, tachycardia, and restlessness.

Thyroid-Releasing Hormone (TRH). Hypothalamic hormone that stimulates the anterior pituitary to secrete thyroid-stimulating hormone (TSH).

Thyroid-Stimulating Hormone (TSH). Anterior pituitary hormone, also known as thyrotropin, produced in response to thyroid-releasing hormone. TSH stimulates the thyroid gland to release T_4 (thyroxine) and T_3 (triiodothyronine).

Thyroxine (T₄). A hormone produced by the thyroid gland that is physiologically inactive.

Tidal Volume (V_T). Amount of air inhaled or exhaled with each breath during normal breathing at rest.

Tolerance. Physiologic response to a narcotic after repeated administration when it takes more drug for the same analgesic effect.

Tonic Seizure. State of muscle contraction; characterized by abrupt stiffening of arms and legs and may be associated with falls.

Tonic-Clonic Seizure. Formerly referred to as grand mal, during which the patient may cry out suddenly, become rigid, fall, and experience muscle jerking; may be associated with altered breathing patterns, including temporary suspension of breathing, changes in skin color, and incontinence.

Toxic Epidermal Necrolysis. An exfoliative dermatitis usually associated with mucosal involvement of conjunctival, oral, and/or urogenital areas.

Toxoplasmosis. An infection caused by a protozoan parasite; the most common site of toxoplasmosis is the brain.

Tracheostomy. The formation of an opening into the trachea.

Tracheostomy Tube. A large specially constructed catheter placed into the trachea through a surgically created opening.

Transcription. Process of constructing a messenger RNA molecule using a DNA molecule as a template with the resulting transfer of genetic information to the messenger RNA.

Transducer Probe. A device that transmits ultrasound waves to body structures and receives echoes that are reflected back as electrical signals displayed on an oscilloscope.

Transitional Care. Refers to a variety of health care settings, including subacute, skilled, rehabilitative, and long-term care.

Transmural Infarction. Necrosis in an area of the heart muscle extends through all layers (endocardium, myocardium, and epicardium) and results from an occlusion of a coronary artery.

Transverse Plane. Horizontal plane of the body that lies perpendicular to both the frontal and sagittal planes.

Traumatic Brain Injury. Brain injury that results from a traumatic event; also called acute head or brain injury.

Traumatic Pneumothorax. Lung collapse as a result of physical injury.

TRH. *See* thyroid-releasing hormone.

Triage. Sorting or selecting patients based on needs and priority of treatment.

Triiodothyronine (T₃). Hormone that helps control metabolism and body temperature; also acts to inhibit the secretion of thyrotropin by the pituitary by a negative feedback system.

Trousseau's Sign. A muscular contraction resulting from pressure applied to nerves and vessels of the upper arm; indicative of hypocalcemia and latent tetany; also occurs in osteomalacia.

TSH. *See* thyroid-stimulating hormone.

Tuberculosis (TB). A bacterial infection spread by airborne droplets expelled from the lungs causing infection in the air sacs of the lungs.

Type 1 Diabetes. An autoimmune disease with a possible viral trigger, precipitating absolute insulin deficiency.

Type 2 Diabetes. Non–insulin-dependent diabetes mellitus; obesity is a classic hallmark.

Ultrafast CT. Similar to conventional computed tomography; an electron beam is magnetically directed to create x-ray images of a patient at a much faster rate (50 to 100 msec per slice).

Ultrafiltrate. The solution filtered in the glomerulus of the kidney including both water and all of the solutes in blood except for plasma proteins, red blood cells, and white blood cells.

Ultrasonography. Technique of imaging deep structures of the body by measuring and recording the reflection of pulsed or continuous high-frequency sound waves.

Unilateral neglect. A disturbance in spatial perception affecting the contralateral side of the body; may involve the visual and/or tactile spatial domains.

Unlicensed Assistive Personnel (UAP). Employees who assist in the delivery of patient care, usually trained by an employing agency and not required to be licensed in the state in which they work.

Unstable Angina. Angina marked by increasing frequency, duration, and intensity; associated with atherosclerosis.

Uremia. Accumulation of end products of metabolism in the blood due to the failure of the kidneys to properly excrete these products.

Uremic Toxins. Waste products of metabolic processes; when allowed to accumulate systemically in the presence of acute or chronic renal failure, these substances have a toxic effect.

V̇. *See* ventilation.

Vaccination. Inoculation of a substance (vaccine) into the body for the purpose of producing active immunity against a disease; usually a weakened culture of the agent causing the disease.

Valsalva Maneuver. An activity that stimulates the vagus nerve by increasing intraabdominal and intrathoracic pressure during bearing down, breath holding, and so on; can result in sudden changes in heart rate and blood pressure.

Vascular Access. A surgically created conduit allowing for the removal of blood from the body to perform hemodialysis.

Vasoconstriction. Narrowing of the blood vessels.

Vasopressin. *See* antidiuretic hormone.

Vasospasm. A delayed narrowing of the large arteries at the base of the brain after subarachnoid hemorrhage; usually associated with evidence of reduced distal perfusion to brain tissue in affected arteries.

VATS. *See* video-assisted thoracic surgery.

V_D. *See* dead space ventilation.

V_D/V_T. *See* dead space to tidal volume ratio.

Vector. A nonpathogenic bacterium or virus used to transport an antigen into the body to stimulate protective immunity.

Venogram. X-ray of a vein after injection of an intravenous radioisotope or a radiopaque dye.

Venous Duplex Doppler Study. Noninvasive diagnostic examination to determine the patency of various veins throughout the body.

Venous Oxygen Content. Total amount of oxygen in venous blood.

Venous Oxygen Return (VR). Amount of oxygen returned in venous blood to the right ventricle after tissue oxygen consumption.

Venous Sinuses. Slightly dilated areas in the veins in which blood flow may be sluggish.

Venous Thrombus. A blood clot occurring in a vein.

Ventilation ($\dot{V}$). Movement of air between the external environment and the alveoli.

Ventilation–Perfusion ($\dot{V}/\dot{Q}$) Mismatch. A state in which abnormal amounts of ventilation and/or perfusion of the alveoli occurs when ventilation is decreased while perfusion is maintained. High $\dot{V}/\dot{Q}$ ratio mismatching occurs when perfusion is decreased while ventilation is maintained; demonstrated during pulmonary embolism and cardiogenic shock.

Ventricular Aneurysm. A structural complication of an acute myocardial infarction that results in a thin-walled, noncontractile outpouching of the (usually left) pumping chamber of the heart.

Ventricular Septal Rupture. A section of the tissue dividing the right and left sides of the heart becomes necrotic secondary to coronary artery occlusion and breaks open; may require emergency repair of the defect, depending on the size of the opening.

Vesicants. Potent chemical warfare agents that are characterized by their ability to produce cutaneous blisters.

Viable Myocardium. Myocardial cells that are "alive" yet ischemic and receiving blood flow. Cell function may improve after revascularization or reperfusion.

Vicarious Liability. Imputed liability, referring to the responsibility one has for the actions of other individuals due to a special relationship between them.

Video-Assisted Thoracic Surgery (VATS). Surgery utilizing an endoscopic approach, thus avoiding thoracotomy.

Viral Load (Burden). The amount of virus in the circulating blood.

Virchow's Triad. Three variances identified as the etiology of venous thrombosis including alterations in vein wall, blood flow, and blood coagulability.

Viremia. The presence of virus in the bloodstream.

Virus. Organism composed mainly of nucleic acid within a protein coat; can be either DNA or RNA nucleic acids but need the host cell's chemical energy and protein to replicate.

Vital Capacity (VC). Maximal exhaled volume after a maximal inspiration (60 to 80 ml/kg).

Volutrauma. Summarizes all elements of ventilator-induced lung injury. Techniques associated with volutrauma are high peak inspiratory pressures, high mean airway pressures, high PEEP, large tidal volumes, and rapid ventilator rates.

V_{O_2}. *See* oxygen consumption.

$\dot{V}/\dot{Q}$. Ratio of ventilation to perfusion in the lungs.

VR. *See* venous oxygen return.

V_T. *See* tidal volume.

Wasting Syndrome. Involuntary weight loss of 10% of baseline body weight plus either chronic diarrhea or chronic weakness and documented fever in the absence of a concurrent illness or condition other than HIV infection.

Wedge Resection. Surgical removal of a small peripheral part of an organ.

Westermark's Sign. Radiographic findings on chest radiography of dilation of pulmonary vessels proximal to a pulmonary embolus with drastic reduction of blood content and vascular markings in the pulmonary vessels distal to a pulmonary embolus.

Western Blot. A laboratory test for the presence of specific antibodies to the protein bands of HIV; more accurate than the ELISA.

Whole-Brain Death. The permanent, irreversible cessation of the functioning of all areas of the brain; the most frequently used criterion for determining death.

Xenograft. Skin that is harvested from another species, most commonly from a pig; used to promote granulation tissue for autografting.

Xenon-133 Scan. Intravenous injection of a radionuclide used for ventilation–perfusion scanning; useful in identifying regions of complete or incomplete small airway obstruction and therefore facilitates a definitive diagnosis of inhalation injury.

ZEEP. Zero end-expiratory pressure.

Zone of Infarction. Area of the myocardium that contains necrotic tissue; frequently identified electrocardiographically by the presence of a pathologic Q wave.

Index

Note: Page numbers in *italics* refer to illustrations; page numbers followed by t refer to tables.

Ethical Dilemmas